AACN
PROCEDURE
MANUAL *for*
PEDIATRIC ACUTE
and CRITICAL CARE

AACN

AMERICAN ASSOCIATION of CRITICAL-CARE NURSES

PROCEDURE MANUAL *for* PEDIATRIC ACUTE *and* CRITICAL CARE

Edited by

Judy Trivits Verger,
PhD, CRNP, CCRN
Pediatric Nurse Practitioner
The Children's Hospital of Philadelphia
Program Director, Pediatric Critical Care Nurse Practitioner
and Neonatal Nurse Practitioner Programs
School of Nursing
University of Pennsylvania
Philadelphia, Pennsylvania

Ruth M. Lebet,
MSN, CCNS, CCRN
Clinical Nurse Specialist
Nemours/Alfred I. duPont Hospital for Children
Wilmington, Delaware

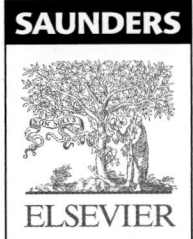

SAUNDERS

ELSEVIER

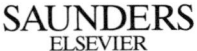

SAUNDERS
ELSEVIER

11830 Westline Industrial Drive
St. Louis, Missouri 63146

AACN Procedure Manual for Pediatric Acute and Critical Care   ISBN: 978-0-7216-0640-8

Copyright © 2008 by Saunders, an imprint of Elsevier Inc.

Notice

Knowledge and best practice in this field are constantly changing. As new research and experience broaden our knowledge, changes in practice, treatment and drug therapy may become necessary or appropriate. Readers are advised to check the most current information provided (i) on procedures featured or (ii) by the manufacturer of each product to be administered, to verify the recommended dose or formula, the method and duration of administration, and contraindications. It is the responsibility of the practitioner, relying on their own experience and knowledge of the patient, to make diagnoses, to determine dosages and the best treatment for each individual patient, and to take all appropriate safety precautions. To the fullest extent of the law, neither the Publisher nor the Editors assumes any liability for any injury and/or damage to persons or property arising out or related to any use of the material contained in this book.

The Publisher

ISBN: 978-0-7216-0640-8

Executive Publisher: Barbara Nelson Cullen
Associate Developmental Editor: Mayoor Jaiswal
Senior Developmental Editor: Jennifer Ehlers
Publishing Services Manager: Jeff Patterson
Design Direction: Paula Ruckenbrod

Printed in United States of America

Last digit is the print number: 9 8 7 6 5 4 3 2 1

Working together to grow
libraries in developing countries

www.elsevier.com | www.bookaid.org | www.sabre.org

ELSEVIER   BOOK AID International   Sabre Foundation

Dedication

We are fortunate to have worked with many extraordinary nurses whose dedication to caring for infants and children is beyond measure. These nurses represent only a small fraction of the pediatric nurses around the world who each day provide care to one of the most vulnerable patient populations, often in extremely challenging situations. This book is dedicated to each and every one of these caring, compassionate, bright, and talented individuals.

Contributors

Paula M. Agosto, RN, BSN, MHA
Director of Critical Care and Transport Nursing
The Children's Hospital of Philadelphia
Philadelphia, Pennsylvania
Protective/Restraint Devices: Application and Monitoring

Chris Angeletti, RN, BSN, CCRN
Patient Service Manager
Cardiac Intensive Care Unit
Children's Hospital of Pittsburgh
Pittsburgh, Pennsylvania
Continuous Renal Replacement Therapy

Dean Barone, MPAS, PAC, AT-C
Instructor, Department of Surgery
Division of Neurosurgery
Robert Wood Johnson Medical School
University of Medicine and Dentistry of New Jersey
Clinical Assistant Professor
School of Health Related Professions
Robert Wood Johnson University Hospital
New Brunswick, New Jersey
Halo Traction: Application and Care
Cervical Collar: Placement and Management

Cheryl N. Bartke, RN, MSN, APRN-BC, CPNP-AC
Instructor of Pediatrics
Penn State University, College of Medicine
Department of Pediatrics
Hershey, Pennsylvania
Pediatric Critical Care Nurse Practitioner
Penn State Children's Hospital
Hershey, Pennsylvania
*Balloon Gastrostomy and Low-Profile Balloon
    Gastrostomy: Reinsertion*

Dorothy M. Beke, RN, MS, CPNP
Clinical Nurse Specialist
Cardiac Intensive Care Unit
Children's Hospital
Boston, Massachusetts
Left Atrial Intracardiac Line: Care and Management
Left Atrial Intracardiac Line Removal: Perform

Kathryn A. Beauchamp, RN, MSN, CCRN
Clinical Nurse Specialist
Critical Care Medicine
MassGeneral Hospital for Children
Boston, Massachusetts
*Unit XVI Editor: Safety and Transitioning of Pediatric
    Patients*
Discharge

Amy C. Binck, RN, MSN, CPNP
Lecturer
School of Nursing
University of Pennsylvania
Philadelphia, Pennsylvania
Extubation: Assist
Intubation: Assist
Extubation: Perform
Intubation: Perform, Including Laryngeal Mask Airway

Beth Bolick, RN, MS, APRN-BC, CPNP-AC, CCRN
Assistant Professor
College of Nursing
Rush University Medical Center
Chicago, Illinios
Unit VII Editor: Musculoskeletal System

Kimberly R. Bookout, MSN, RN, CPNP, CWOCN
Associate Professor
Texas Women's University School of Nursing
Wound Ostomy Continence Nurse Practitioner
Children's Medical Center
Dallas, Texas
Closed Surgical Drain: Care and Management
Ostomy Appliance: Change

Michele J. Borisuk, RN, MSN, CPNP
Nurse Practitioner, Cardiac Center
The Children's Hospital of Philadelphia
Philadelphia, Pennsylvania
Pericardial Catheter: Management
Staple Removal

Karen C. Bowe, RN, MSN
Nurse Manager
Pediatric Intensive Care Unit
Nemours/Alfred I. duPont Hospital for Children
Wilmington, Delaware
Peripheral Nerve Stimulator

Eric A. Bowles, MSN, FNP-BC
Pediatric Intensive Care Nurse Practitioner
Primary Children's Medical Center
Pediatric Intensive Care Unit
Salt Lake City, Utah
Cricothyroidotomy: Assist
Postural Drainage with Percussion and Vibration
Cricothyroidectomy: Perform

Janet A. Koehler Boyce, RN, MSN, CCRN
Clinical Nurse III
Pediatric Intensive Care Unit
The Children's Hospital of Philadelphia
Philadelphia, Pennsylvania
Indices of Oxygenation and Ventilation
Mixed Venous Oxygen Saturation: Continuous Monitoring
Auto-PEEP Calculation

Lori Boyle, RN, BSN, CCRN
Clinical Level IV
Pediatric Intensive Care Unit
Children's Hospital of Philadelphia
Philadelphia, Pennsylvania
Noninvasive Oxygen Delivery Devices

Lee Brady, RN, BSN
Coordinator Patient/Family Education—International
    Center for Limb Lengthening
Sinai Hospital of Baltimore
Baltimore, Maryland
External Fixator Lengthening Device: Adjustments

Catherine Brailer, MSN, CPNP-AC
Pediatric Critical Care Nurse Practitioner
Children's Hospital of Eastern North Carolina
Pitt County Memorial Hospital
Greenville, North Carolina
Sedation for Procedures

Chris Breen, BSN, CNN
Home Program Coordinator—Dialysis Unit
The Children's Hospital of Philadelphia
Philadelphia, Pennsylvania
Hemodialysis: Assist

Eileen Briening, MSN, CRNP, CCRN
Pediatric Critical Care Nurse Practitioner
Nemours/Alfred I. duPont Hospital for Children
Wilmington, Delaware
End Tidal Carbon Dioxide Measurement
Noninvasive Positive Pressure Ventilation
Pronation Therapy
Arterial Catheter Insertion: Perform

Debbie Brinker, RN, MSN, CCRN, CCNS
Clinical Instructor, Child Health Faculty
Intercollegiate College of Nursing
Washington State University
Spokane, Washington
Unit XII Editor: Pain Management and Sedation
Pain Assessment Scales

Beth Broering, MSN, CEN, CCRN
Trauma Coordinator
Vanderbilt University Medical Center
Nashville, Tennessee
Vacuum-Assisted Closure (VAC) System: Management of
    Negative Pressure Therapy
Arterial Catheter: Blood Sampling

Joel M. Brown II, BS, RRT
Respiratory Staff Development Specialist
Cristiana Care Hospital
Newark, Delaware
Aerosolized Medication: Metered Dose Inhaler

Louise Callow, RN, MSN
Pediatric Cardiology
Clinical Nurse Practitioner
Congenital Heart Center
University of Michigan
Ann Arbor, Michigan
Pulmonary Artery Intracardiac Line: Care and
    Management
Pulmonary Artery Intracardiac Line Removal: Perform

Susan M. Campisciano, RN, MSN, APRN-BC
Lecturer, Clinical Instructor
University of Pennsylvania
Philadelphia, Pennsylvania
Tracheostomy Tube: Stoma Care and Tie Change
Tracheostomy Tube: Change
Tracheostomy Tube: Suctioning
Tracheostomy Tube: Decannulation

Amy Carnall-Grogan, RN, RNFA, MSN, CPNP
Pediatric Nurse Practitioner
Pediatric Intensive Care Unit
St. Christopher's Hospital for Children
Philadelphia, Pennsylvania
Externalized Ventricular Shunts and Drains: Catheter Management
Ventriculoperitoneal Shunt Tap: Assist
Ventriculoperitoneal Shunt Tap: Perform

Constance E. Cephus, MSN, RN, CNNP, CPNP
Nurse Practitioner, Cardiology
Texas Children's Heart Center
Texas Children's Hospital
Houston, Texas
Transvenous Pacemaker Insertion: Perform

Orlando R. Chapa, RN, BSN, MS, CCRN
Pediatric Intensive Care Educator
Cook Children's Medical Center
Fort Worth, Texas
Percutaneous Peritoneal Lavage: Assist

Catherine A. Cochran, RN, BSN
Director, Pediatrics, PICU
Moses Cone Health System
Greensboro, North Carolina
pH Monitoring Study: Care and Management

Bridget Connolly, RN
Mahopac, New York
Cerebrospinal Fluid Drainage: Assessment

Dyana Burns Conway, RN, MSN, CRNP
Pediatric Critical Care Nurse Practitioner
University of Maryland Medical System
Baltimore, Maryland
Enteral Nutrition: Administration
Orogastric/Nasogastric Tubes: Insertion, Care, and Management
Enteral Nutrition: Initiation and Advancement

Julie Creaden, RN, MSN, CPNP
Complemental Faculty
Rush University
Chicago, Illinois
Pediatric Nurse Practitioner
Division of Pediatric Cardiovascular and Thoracic Surgery
Children's Memorial Hospital
Chicago, Illinois
Emergency Medication Preparation and Administration

James A. Cullen, RN, BSN
Clinical and Financial Systems Manager
The Children's Hospital of Philadelphia
Philadelphia, Pennsylvania
Extracorporeal Membrane Oxygenation

Dawn Marie Daniels, DNS, RN
Clinical Faculty
Indiana University School of Nursing
Indianapolis, Indiana
Pediatric Trauma Research Program Coordinator—Injury Free Coalition for Kids of Indianapolis
Riley Hospital for Children
Indianapolis, Indiana
Intracompartment Pressure Monitoring

Gretchen Delametter, RN, MSN
Clinical Nurse Specialist
Moses Cone Health System
Greensboro, North Carolina
Gastric Lavage
pH Monitoring Study: Care and Management

Antoinette DeSalis, RN, CCRN, BSN
Certified Child Passenger Safety Technician
Clinical Level IV
The Children's Hospital of Philadelphia
Philadelphia, Pennsylvania
Intracranial/Intraparenchymal Catheter: Insertion Assist, Set-up, and Care

Holly DeWald, RN
Registered Nurse, Staff Nurse, Preceptor
Nemours/Alfred I. duPont Hospital for Children
Wilmington, Delaware
Decompression Tube: Insertion and Care

Kathryn M. Dodds, RN, MSN, CRNP
Nurse Practitioner
Cardiac Center
The Children's Hospital of Philadelphia
Philadelphia, Pennsylvania
Unit II Editor: Cardiovascular System

Marcella L. Donkin, MSN, RN, CPNP, CCRN
Nurse Practitioner
St. Louis Children's Hospital at Washington University Medical Center
St. Louis, Missouri
Central Venous Non-tunneled Catheter Insertion: Perform

Peggy Dorr, MS, CRNP
Pediatric Nurse Practitioner
Division of Pediatric Cardiology
University of Maryland Hospital
Baltimore, Maryland
Pressure Transducer Systems
Arterial and Venous Sheath Removal

Jacqueline Simpson Dunne, RN, MS, CPNP, CPON
Adjunct Professor
Columbia University School of Nursing
Hunter College
Pediatric Nurse Practitioner
Memorial Sloan-Kettering Cancer Center
New York, New York
Greenwich Hospital/Pediatrics
Greenwich, Connecticut
Skin Assessment Techniques

E. Marsha Elixson, RNC, MS, CCRN, FAHA
Adjunct Clinical Instructor
Maternal Child Nursing
University of Illinois
Chicago, Illinois
Associate Professor Child Health Division
Courtesy Faculty
Yale School of Nursing
Hartford, Connecticut
Education/Conference Coordinator
Sibley Heart Center Cardiology
Educational Consultant
Pediatric Critical Concepts, Inc.
Atlanta, Georgia
Intrahospital Transport

Dana Etzel-Hardman, RN, BSN, CPN
Training and Education Specialist
Children's Hospital of Pittsburgh
Pittsburgh, Pennsylvania
Totally Implantable Central Venous Port: Accessing, Management, and De-accessing

Laurie S. Finger, MN, APRN, CCRN, CCNS
Adjunct Faculty
Our Lady of the Lake College School of Nursing, New Orleans Campus
Baton Rouge, Louisiana
Clinical Nurse Specialist
Tulane Hospital for Children at Tulane University Hospital and Clinic
New Orleans, Louisiana
Arterial Blood Gas Analysis
Pulse Oximetry
Manual Ventilation Devices

Kelly S. Finkbeiner, MSN, CPNP
Pediatric Nurse Practitioner
Pediatric Surgery (General)
Children's Memorial Hospital
Chicago, Illinois
Intradermal Injection
Intramuscular Injection
Subcutaneous Injection

Maggie Fischer, RN, MSN
Testamur NASPExAM, 2005
Field Clinical Representative
Guidant Corporation
St. Paul, Minnesota
Permanent Pacemaker: Assessing Function
Transvenous and Epicardial Pacing: Monitoring

Annette M. Fleck, RN, BSN, CCRN
Staff Nurse
Children's Hospital of Pittsburgh
Pittsburgh, Pennsylvania
Obtaining an Accurate Temperature Measurement
Warming Devices: Radiant

Desiree Fleck, MSN, CRNP, CCRN
Nurse Practitioner for the Philadelphia Adult Congenital Heart Center
The Children's Hospital of Philadelphia and the
Hospital of the University of Pennsylvania
Philadelphia, Pennsylvania
Intraaortic Balloon Pump: Management

Pamela Meadors Fox, RN, MSN, CPNP-AC
Pediatric Critical Care Nurse Practitioner
Pitt County Memorial Hospital
Greenville, North Carolina
Sedation for Procedures

Anne Marie Frey, RN, CRNI, BSN
Clinical Level IV
The Children's Hospital of Philadelphia
Philadelphia, Pennsylvania
Central Venous Tunneled Catheter: Permanent Catheter Repair (Broviac or Other Brand)
Unit X Editor: Vascular Access

Laurene Fry, RN
Clinical Nurse II
Children's Hospital/Los Angeles
Rancho Palos Verdes, California
Implanted Cardioverter/Defibrillator

Robyn Neely Funk, BSN, RN, EMT-P, CMTE
Team Leader
MedCenter Air (Carolinas Healthcare System/Levine Children's Hospital)
Charlotte, North Carolina
Outside Facility Transport

Dana Garver, RN, MSN
Staff RN, Pediatric Intensive Care Unit
The Johns Hopkins Children's Center
Baltimore, Maryland
Peripheral Nerve Stimulator

Rhonda Gengler, RN, BSN, CCRN
Staff Nurse/CRRT Coordinator CICU/PICU
Children's Hospital of Pittsburgh
Pittsburgh, Pennsylvania
Continuous Renal Replacement Therapy

Mary Astor Gomez, RN, MSN, CPNP
Transport Team
Children's Memorial Hospital
Chicago, Illinois
Blood Glucose Monitoring

Cynthia Gould, RN, MS, CRNP
Pediatric Nurse Practitioner
Penn State Children's Hospital
Hershey, Pennsylvania
Intra-abdominal Pressure Monitoring

Mary Jo Grant, PhD, PNP
Pediatric Nurse Practitioner
Pediatric Critical Care
Primary Children's Medical Center
Salt Lake City, Utah
Unit I Editor: Respiratory System

Dan Graves, RN, MSN CRNP
Pediatric Critical Nurse Practitioner
Speciality Health Education, Inc.
Blue Bell, Pennsylvania
*Flow Directed Pulmonary Artery Catheter: Cardiac
    Output Measurement*
Flow Directed Pulmonary Artery Catheter: Insertion Assist

Margaret Grover, RN
Staff Nurse
The Children's Hospital of Philadelphia
Philadelphia, Pennsylvania
*Skin Puncture for Collection of Blood Samples: Fingerstick
    and Heelstick*
Venipuncture for Blood Sampling

Roberta L. Hales, BS, RRT-NPS, RN
Clinical Educator
Center for Simulation, Innovation and Education
Respiratory Therapist
Respiratory Care Department
The Children's Hospital of Philadelphia
Philadelphia, Pennsylvania
High Frequency Oscillatory Ventilation
Negative Pressure Ventilation
Noninvasive Positive Pressure Ventilation

Debra Hanisch, RN, MSN, CPNP
Assistant Clinical Professor
Family Health Care Nursing
University of California–San Francisco
San Francisco, California
Nurse Practitioner, Pediatric Cardiology
Lucile Packard Children's Hospital at Stanford
Palo Alto, California
Atrial Electrogram
Transesophageal Pacing: Assist

Elsie M. Hartigan, MSN, CRNP
Nurse Practitioner
Philadelphia, Pennsylvania
Tracheostomy Tube: Stoma Care and Tie Change
Tracheostomy Tube: Change
Tracheostomy Tube: Suctioning
Tracheostomy Tube: Decannulation

Cathy Haut, MS, CPNP, CCRN
PNP, Department of Critical Care Medicine
The Children's Hospital at Sinai
Baltimore, Maryland
Deputy Director
Pediatric Nursing Certification Board
Gaithersburg, Maryland
*Central Venous Catheters for Hemodialysis or
    Hemofiltration: Blood Sampling*

Harriet S. Hawkins, RN, CCRN, FAEN
Resuscitation Education Coordinator
Children's Memorial Hospital
Chicago, Illinois
Intraosseous Needle: Care and Management
Intraosseous Needle Placement: Perform

Elizabeth M. Henry, RN, CCRN
Clinical Level III
Peri-Anesthesia Care Unit
The Children's Hospital of Philadelphia
Philadelphia, Pennsylvania
Cervical Traction Maintenance

Kathleen Hinoki, RN, MSN, CNS
Nursing Instructor
California State University, Los Angeles
Los Angeles, California
Implanted Cardioverter/Defibrillator

Patricia A. Hubbs, RN, MBA, CCRN
Nurse Manager
Pediatric Intensive Care Unit
The Children's Hospital of Philadelphia
Philadelphia, Pennsylvania
Protective/Restraint Devices: Application and Monitoring

Diane Hudson-Barr, PhD, RN
Adjunct Assistant Professor
University of North Carolina at Chapel Hill
Clinical Nurse Specialist, Neonatology
North Carolina Children's Hospital
University of North Carolina Hospitals
Chapel Hill, North Carolina
Skin to Skin Contact/Kangaroo Care

Rémi Hueckel, RN, MSN, APRN
Pediatric Critical Nurse Practitioner
Duke University School of Medicine
Durham, North Carolina
pH Monitoring Study: Care and Management

Joy Hultman, RN, MSN
Head Nurse, PICU
Bristol-Myers Squibb Children's Hospital at
Robert Wood Johnson University Hospital
New Brunswick, New Jersey
Dressing Wounds with Drains

Larissa Hutchins, RN, MSN, CCRN
Clinical Nurse Specialist
Progressive Care Unit
Pediatric Intensive Care Unit
The Children's Hospital of Philadelphia
Philadelphia, Pennsylvania
Bispectral Index Monitoring

Sharon Y. Irving, RN, MSN, CRNP
Project Manager
Feeding and Energy Balance: Infants with CHD
University of Pennsylvania, School of Nursing
Nurse Practitioner
Division of Critical Care
The Children's Hospital of Philadelphia
Philadelphia, Pennsylvania
Parenteral Nutrition: Administration
Parenteral Nutrition: Initiation and Advancement

Laurie DeMondo Jaffe, RN
Freehold, New Jersey
Burn Wound Care
Donor Site Care
Skin Graft Care

Dena L. Jarog, MSN, CCNS
Clinical Nurse Specialist
Pediatric Critical Care
Saint Joseph's Children's Hospital
Marshfield, Wisconsin
Endotracheal Tube: Suctioning and Care
Endotracheal Tube: Taping
Nasopharyngeal Suctioning
Drain Removal

Tammara L. Jenkins, RN, MSN
Program Analyst, Research Coordinator
National Center for Rehabilitation Research
National Institutes of Health
Bethesda, Maryland
Unit VI Editor: Hematology/Oncology System

Aimee Jennings, RN, MSN
Pediatric Nurse Practitioner
Riley Hospital for Children
Clarian Health Partners
Indianapolis, Indiana
Right Atrial Intracardiac Line: Care and Management
Right Atrial Intracardiac Line Removal: Perform

Amanda Johnson, RN, APN
Nursing Staff, Neurosurgery
Department of Surgery
The University of Chicago
Chicago, Illinois
External Fixation Device: Pin Care

Cynthia Keel, RN, MSN, CPNP-AC
Pediatric Critical Care Nurse Practitioner
Pitt County Memorial Hospital
Pediatric Intensive Care Unit
Greenville, North Carolina
Sedation for Procedures

Mildred Kenney-Lau, CRNP, MSN
Lecturer
School of Nursing
University of Pennsylvania
Philadelphia, Pennsylvania
Unit XV Editor: Neonatal Issues
Umbilical Vessel Cannulation and Removal: Perform

Gail Keyser, RN, CNOR, RNFA
Clinical Coordinator for the Cardiac OR
The Children's Hospital of Philadelphia
Philadelphia, Pennsylvania
Open Sternotomy: Assist

Karen Kilian, RN, MS, CPNP, CCRN
Clinical Faculty
University of Washington School of Nursing
Pediatric Nurse Practitioner
Emergency Department
Children's Hospital & Regional Medical Center
Seattle, Washington
Atrial Overdrive Pacing
Transcutaneous Pacing: Initiation and Monitoring

Andrea M. Kline, RN, MS, PCCNP, CCRN
Nurse Practitioner
Pediatric Intensive Care Unit
Children's Memorial Hospital
Chicago, Illinois
Unit X Editor: Vascular Access
Vacuum-Assisted Closure (V.A.C) System: Management of
Negative Pressure Therapy
Arterial Puncture: Perform

Lisa M. Kohr, RN, MSN, CPNP, MPH
Pediatric Nurse Practitioner
Cardiac Center
The Children's Hospital of Philadelphia
Philadelphia, Pennsylvania
Unit II Editor: Cardiovascular System

Kathryn Carnighan Kuhn, MSN, CPNP
Pediatric Nurse Practitioner
Pediatric Oncology Branch
Center for Cancer Research
National Cancer Institute
National Institutes of Health
Bethesda, Maryland
Bone Marrow Aspiration and Biopsy: Assist
Bone Marrow Aspiration and Biopsy: Perform

Cecilia Lang, MSN, CCRN, CPRN, BC
Unit-Based Advanced Practice Nurse Intermediate
Intensive Care
Children's Hospital of Wisconsin
Milwaukee, Wisconsin
Hydration and Rehydration: Fluid Calculations
Aerosolized Medication: Nebulized Medication
Intranasal Medication

Kelly A. Lankin, RN, BSN, CCRN
Staff Nurse/Clinical Expert
Children's Memorial Hospital
Chicago, Illinois
Central Venous Non-tunneled Catheter: Insertion Assist
Central Venous Non-tunneled Catheter: Central Venous
Pressure Monitoring

Ruth M. Lebet, MSN, CCNS, CCRN
Clinical Nurse Specialist
Pediatric Intensive Care Unit
Nemours/Alfred I. duPont Hospital for Children
Wilmington, Delaware
Pericardiocentesis: Assist
Continuous Bladder Irrigation
Indwelling Urinary Catheter: Insertion and Removal
Suturing Wounds
Transpyloric Feeding Tube: Insertion

Charlene Leonard, MSN, CPNP, CPNP-AC
Pediatric Critical Care Nurse Practitioner
Wolfson Children's Hospital
Jacksonville, Florida
Continuous Bladder Irrigation

Sarah S. LeRoy, RN, MSN, CPNP, HRS, NAPSE
Testamur
Pediatric Nurse Practitioner
Pediatric Cardiology
University of Michigan Hospitals
Ann Arbor, Michigan
Electrocardiogram: Obtaining and Monitoring a 12-Lead
Electrocardiogram

Patricia Lincoln, RN, MS
Clinical Nurse Specialist
Cardiac Intensive Care Unit
Children's Hospital
Boston, Massachusetts
Left Atrial Intracardiac Line: Care and Management
Left Atrial Intracardiac Line Removal: Perform

Grace Macek, RN, MSN, APRN-BC, CCRN
Pediatric Cardiac Surgical Nurse Practitioner
University of Chicago Hospital
Chicago, Illinois
Blood and Blood Component: Administration and Blood
Pump Use

Maureen A. Madden, CPNP-AC, CCRN, FCCM
Bristol-Myers Squibb Children's Hospital at
Robert Wood Johnson University Hospital
New Brunswick, New Jersey
Unit VIII Editor: Skin
Drain Removal

Susan Ingrid Maeder-Chieffo, MSN-FNP, CCRN, PHRN
Clinical Leader
Emergency Transport Services
The Children's Hospital of Philadelphia
Philadelphia, Pennsylvania
Outside Facility Transport

Rosita Y. Maley, MSN, CCRN
Cardiac Clinical Specialist
Children's Hospital of Orange County
Heart Institute
Orange County, California
Ventricular Assist Device: Management

Kelly Keefe Marcoux, MSN, PCCNP
Bristol-Myers Squibb Children's Hospital at
    Robert Wood Johnson University Hospital
New Brunswick, New Jersey
Unit III Editor: Neurologic System
Intracranial/Intraparenchymal Catheter: Insertion Assist,
    Set-up, and Care
Intraventricular Catheter: Insertion Assist, Monitoring,
    and Care
Externalized Ventricular Shunts and Drains: Catheter
    Management
Intracranial Pressure Monitoring

Heidi Martin, RN
Clinical Level IV
Pediatric Intensive Care Unit
The Children's Hospital of Philadelphia
Philadelphia, Pennsylvania
Intraventricular Catheter: Insertion Assist, Monitoring,
    and Care

Sarah A. Martin, RN, MS, PCCNP, CPNP
Pediatric Nurse Practitioner
Pediatric Surgery (General)
Children's Memorial Hospital
Chicago, Illinois
Unit XI Editor: Medication Administration
Oral Medication

Rizalina Mauricio, RN, MSN, CCRN, CPNP-AC
Texas Children's Hospital
Houston, Texas
Bowel Irrigation

Shannon Stone McCord, MS, RN, CPNP, CNS, CCRN
Pediatric Nurse Practitioner
Wound, Ostomy and Continence
Texas Children's Hospital
Houston, Texas
Gastrostomy and Jejunostomy Tubes: Care and
    Management

Barbara McFadden, RNC, MSN, NNP
NNP Track Director
The University of Texas Health Science Center School of
    Nursing
NNP/NICU Educator
The Woman's Hospital of Texas
Houston, Texas
Neonatal Positioning

Jacqueline M. McGrath, PhD, RN, NNP, FNAP
Associate Professor
Virginia Commonwealth University
School of Nursing
Richmond, Virginia
Neonatal Thermoregulation

Kathleen M. McLane, MSN, RN, CPNP, CWON, WOC,
    PNP
Texas Children's Hospital
Houston, Texas
Closed Surgical Drain: Care and Management
Ostomy Appliance: Change

Susan Mills, RN, MSN
Nursing Lecturer and Clinical Instructor, Pediatrics
Widener University
Chester, Pennsylvania
Urine Culture: Indwelling Catheter or Suprapubic Tube

Lisa Milonovich, RN, MSN, PCCNP
Nurse Practitioner
Pediatric Critical Care Services
Children's Medical Center
Dallas, Texas
Unit V Editor: Renal System

Marisa Mize, RN, MSN, CCRN, CPNP
Pediatric Nurse Practitioner
Washington, DC
Suturing Wounds
Arterial Catheter: Insertion Assist and Management

Nancy L. Moureau, BSN, CRNI
President
PICC Excellence, Inc.
Orange Park, Florida
Peripherally Inserted Central Venous Catheter: Care,
    Management, and Removal
Peripherally Inserted Central Catheter (PICC) Insertion:
    Perform

Melissa Mullen, RN
Staff Nurse
The Children's Hospital of Philadelphia
Philadelphia, Pennsylvania
Open Sternotomy: Assist

Judith A. Mulloney, BS, RN
Clinical Leader, Pediatric ICU
The Children's Hospital at Sinai
Baltimore, Maryland
Pleural Catheter: Care

Kelly Murawski, MSN, RN, PNP
Pediatric Critical Care Nurse Practitioner
Cardinal Glennon Children's Medical Center
St. Louis, Missouri
Abdominal Paracentesis: Assist
Abdominal Paracentesis: Perform

Eileen Nelson, RN, BSN
Clinical Level IV Nurse
The Children's Hospital of Philadelphia
Philadelphia, Pennsylvania
Nasopharyngeal and Oropharyngeal Airway:
   Insertion and Care
Noninvasive Oxygen Delivery Devices

Delia R. Nickolaus, MSN, RN, CPNP
Pediatric Neurosurgery Nurse Practitioner
Phoenix Children's Hospital
Phoenix, Arizona
Cerebrospinal Fluid Sampling from Ventriculostomy/
   External Ventricular Drain

Lorri Nielsen, RN, MSN, CPNP
Nurse Practitioner
Children's Memorial Hospital
Chicago, Illinois
Continuous Intravenous Medication Infusion
Intravenous Medication: Heparin Lock Method

Jo Ann Nieves, MSN, CPN, ARNP-BC
Nurse Practitioner, Pediatric Cardiology
Miami Children's Hospital
Miami, Florida
Pulmonary Hypertension: Management

Linda L. Oakes, MSN, CCNS
Pain Clinical Nurse Specialist
St. Jude Children's Research Hospital
Memphis, Tennessee
Epidural Catheter: Care and Management
Locally Administered Anesthetic Infusions
Patient Controlled Analgesia

Kerri Oates, RN, MSN, CRNP, MJ
Pediatric Nurse Practitioner in the Cardiac Center
The Children's Hospital of Philadelphia
Philadelphia, Pennsylvania
Pericardiocentesis: Assist

Patricia O'Brien, RNC, MSN, PNP
Nurse Practitioner
Cardiac Surgery Service
Cardiovascular Program
Children's Hospital
Boston, Massachusetts
Epicardial Pacing Wire Removal: Perform

Patricia O'Connor, RN, MSN, CPNP
PICU Clinical Nurse Specialist
Bristol-Myers Squibb Children's Hospital at
Robert Wood Johnson University Hospital
New Brunswick, New Jersey
Peritoneal Dialysis Catheter Exit Site Care
Peritoneal Dialysis: Pass Management
Cleansing, Irrigating, Culturing, and Dressing Wounds

Lucy R. Paskus, RN, MSN, CPNP
Staff RN, Pediatric ICU
St. Vincent's Children's Hospital
Indianapolis, Indiana
Esophagogastric Tamponade Tube: Care and Management
Admission

Mary Frances D. Pate, DSN, RN
Oregon Health & Science University
Portland, Oregon
Sedation Assessment Scales

Terie Pearl, RN
Staff Nurse
The Children's Hospital of Philadelphia
Philadelphia, Pennsylvania
Open Sternotomy: Assist

Vittoria Pontieri-Lewis, MN, WOCN
Advanced Practice Nurse
Wound Ostomy Continence
Robert Wood Johnson University Hospital
New Brunswick, New Jersey
Fistulas/Wounds: Care and Management

Suzanne Porfyris, MSN, PCCNP
Anesthesia Pain Service Nurse Practitioner
Children's Memorial Hospital
Chicago, Illinois
Indwelling Urinary Catheter: Irrigation
Indwelling Urinary Catheter: Urinalysis Collection

Elizabeth M. Preze, RN, MSN, CPNP-AC
Pediatric Nurse Practitioner Cardiovascular and Thoracic
Children's Memorial Hospital
Chicago, Illinois
Intravenous Medication: Drip Method
Intravenous Medication: Syringe Pump Method

Kristin M. Print, RN, MSN, CCRN, APRN-BC
Pediatric Critical Care Nurse Practitioner
Primary Children's Medical Center
Salt Lake City, Utah
Negative Inspiratory Force Measurement
Respiratory Rate: Obtaining an Accurate Measurement

Kelly Pruden, MSN, CPNP, CCRN
Staff Nurse
Nemours/Alfred I. duPont Hospital for Children
Wilmington, Delaware
Urine Culture: Intermittent Catheterization

Karen Helton Rapoport, RNC, MSN, NNP
Neonatal Nurse Practitioner
Children's Hospital Los Angeles
Los Angeles, California
Umbilical Vessel Catheter: Care and Management

Elizabeth Ristuccia-Semegran, RN, CCRN
Staff Nurse: Leader
Children's Intensive Care Unit
Children's Healthcare of Atlanta at Egleston
Atlanta, Georgia
Intrahospital Transport

Kathryn E. Roberts, RN, MSN, CRNP, CCRN, CCNS
Clinical Nurse Specialist, PICU
The Children's Hospital of Philadelphia
Philadelphia, Pennsylvania
Unit I Editor: Respiratory System

Denise Ruffalo, RN, BSN, CCRN
Staff Nurse
Pediatric Intensive Care Unit
Children's Hospital of Pittsburgh
Pittsburgh, Pennsylvania
Hypo/hyperthermia Blanket and Use of BAIR Hugger®
  Warming Unit and Warming Cover

Mary Rummell, BSN, MN, CPNP, CNS
Clinical Nurse Specialist, Pediatrics
Providence St. Vincent Medical Center
Portland, Oregon
Cardioversion
Defibrillation: External

Ann Schwoebel, RN, MSN, NNP
Clinical Nurse Specialist
Pennsylvania Hospital
Philadelphia, Pennsylvania
Phototherapy

Kerry Shields, RN, MSN, PCCNP, MBE
Adjunct Lecturer at Rush University
Chicago, Illinois
Pediatric Critical Care Nurse Practitioner
Neurotrauma Intensive Care Unit
Children's Medical Center
Dallas, Texas
Chest Tube Placement: Assist
Chest Tube Removal: Assist
Closed Chest Drainage System: Set Up and Management

Marvin Siegel, RN, CRNI
Director of Nursing
Town Total Health
New York, New York
Central Venous Tunneled Catheter: Care and Management
Peripheral Intravenous Line: Insertion

Shari L. Simone, RN, MS, CRNP, CCRN, FCCM
Pediatric Critical Care Nurse Practitioner
University of Maryland Medical Center
Baltimore, Maryland
Unit XIII Editor: Nutrition

Margaret C. Slota, RN, MN
Director, Critical Care Services
Children's Hospital of Pittsburgh
Pittsburgh, Pennsylvania
Unit XIV Editor: Thermoregulation

Phyllis Slutsky, RN, BSN, MEd
Education Nurse Specialist
The Children's Hospital of Philadelphia
Department of Nursing Education
Philadelphia, Pennsylvania
Aerosolized Medication: Metered Dose Inhaler

Lara G. Smith, MSN, CPNP
Pediatric Nurse Practitioner
St. Louis Children's Hospital
St. Louis, Missouri
Central Venous Non-tunneled Catheter: Care and
  Management

Cynthia L. Smitka, RN, BSN
Department of Apheresis
University of Michigan Health System
Ann Arbor, Michigan
Apheresis: Assist

Lauren Sorce, RN, MSN, CCRN, CPNP
Nurse Practitioner
Pediatric Intensive Care Unit
Children's Memorial Hospital
Chicago, Illinois
Unit IX Editor: Fluid and Electrolyte Management
Hydration and Rehydration: Fluid Calculations

Michelle A. Sorscher, MSN, CPNP
Instructor of Pediatrics
University of Medicine and Dentistry
Robert Wood Johnson Medical School
Clinical Coordinator of Inpatient Pediatrics
Bristol-Myers Squibb Children's Hospital at
  Robert Wood Johnson University Hospital
New Brunswick, New Jersey
Lumbar Puncture: Assist
Lumbar Puncture: Perform

Erika Lynne Speier, RN, MSN, RNFA, PCCNP
Nurse Practitioner
Arizona State University
Pediatric Critical Care Nurse Practitioner
Cardiothoracic Surgery
Phoenix Children's Hospital
Phoenix, Arizona
Pleural Pigtail Catheter: Insertion

Carrie C. Steele, MSN
Neonatal Nurse Practitioner
The Children's Hospital of Philadelphia
Philadelphia, Pennsylvania
Lecturer
School of Nursing
The University of Pennsylvania
Philadelphia, Pennsylvania
Umbilical Vessel Cannulation and Removal: Perform

Rebecca A. Steinmann, RN, CEN, CCRN, CCNS
Complemental Faculty
Department of Women's and Children's Health Nursing
Rush University College of Nursing
Clinical Educator
Emergency Department
Children's Memorial Hospital
Chicago, Illinois
Fluid Administration: Rapid Infusion

Deb Templin, MSN, CCRN
Pediatric Critical Care Nurse Practitioner
Primary Children's Medical Center
Salt Lake City, Utah
Thoracentesis: Assist
Chest Tube Placement: Perform
Chest Tube Removal: Perform
Needle Thoracostomy: Perform
Thoracentesis: Perform

Bridget A. Thomas, RN, MSN, APRN-BC
Instructor
Rush University College of Nursing
Nurse Practitioner–Faculty Practice
Rush University Medical Center
Chicago, Illinois
Brace and Splint Application

Lisa Thompson, RN, CPNP
Children's Medical Center
Dallas, Texas
Providing a Safe Environment

Lucy Thompson, RN, MN, CCRN
APRN, Cardiac Intensive Care Unit
Children's Hospital of Pittsburgh
Pittsburgh, Pennsylvania
Red Cell Exchange Transfusion: Manual and Automated
Whole Blood Exchange Transfusion

Andrea Torzone, RN, MSN, PCCNP
Nurse Practitioner
Division of Cardiothoracic Surgery
St. Christopher's Hospital for Children
Philadelphia, Pennsylvania
Heart Rate and Blood Pressure: Obtaining an Accurate Measurement

Jamie A. Tumulty, RN, MS, CRNP
Pediatric Critical Care Nurse Practitioner
University of Maryland Medical System
Baltimore, Maryland
Breast Milk: Administration, Collection, and Storage
Enteral Nutrition: Selection of Formulas and Fortification
Growth Assessment: Obtaining Anthropometric Measurements

Helen Turner, MSN, APRN-C, RN-C,
Instructor
Oregon Health & Science University
Clinical Nurse Specialist, Pediatric Pain Management
Doernbecher Children's Hospital/OHSU
Portland, Oregon
Pain Assessment Scales

Andrea J. Velasco, RN, BSN
Department of Veterans Affairs Outpatient Clinic
Oakland Park, Florida
Jugular Venous Saturation Monitor: Insertion Assist, Monitoring and Care

Judy Trivits Verger, PhD, CRNP, CCRN
Program Director, Pediatric Critical Care Nurse Practitioner Program
Neonatal Nurse Practitioner Program
School of Nursing
University of Pennsylvania
Pediatric Nurse Practitioner, Progressive Care Unit
The Children's Hospital of Philadelphia
Philadelphia, Pennsylvania
Transpyloric Feeding Tube: Insertion

Wallis Halperin Wallis, RN, MSN, PCCNP
Clinical Nurse Specialist
CHOC at Mission
Mission Viejo, California
Cerebral Tissue Oxygenation Monitoring: Insertion Assist, Monitoring, and Care
Intracranial Pressure Monitoring

Holly F. Webster, MS, PNP
University of Utah College of Nursing
Pediatric Critical Care Nurse Practitioner
Primary Children's Medical Center
Pediatric Intensive Care Unit
Salt Lake City, Utah
Mixed Venous Oxygen Saturation: Continuous Monitoring
Mechanical Ventilation: Conventional Modes
Weaning from Mechanical Ventilation

Barbara A. Weintraub, RN, MSN, MPH, CPNP-AC, CEN
Manager, Pediatric Emergency Services
Northwest Community Hospital
Arlington Heights, Illinois
Ophthalmic Medication
Otic Medication

Joyce Weishaar, BSN, MSN, CCNS, MBA
Clinical Nurse Specialist/APN
Children's Memorial Hospital
Chicago, Illinois
Transfusion Reaction: Management

Kimberly Windt, RN, BSN, CNN
Staff Nurse
The Children's Hospital of Philadelphia
Philadelphia, Pennsylvania
Hemodialysis: Assist

Sheryl A. Woloskie, BSN, HP (ASCP)
Educational Nurse Coordinator
University of Michigan Health System
Ann Arbor, Michigan
Apheresis: Assist

Colleen Salazar Young, RNC, MSN, NNP
Clinical Nurse Specialist
Neonatal Nurse Practitioner
Presbyterian Intercommunity Hospital
Whittier, California
Umbilical Vessel Catheter: Care and Management

Maria Teresa Zapata, RN, BSN
Staff RN
Pediatric Sedation Services
Oregon Health & Science University
Doernbecher Children's Hospital
Portland, Oregon
Sedation Assessment Scales

Roni L. Zarge, RN, MSN, PNP, WOCN
Gastroenterology, Nutrition, and Hepatology Clinic
Mary L. Johnson Pediatric Ambulatory Care Center
Lucile Packard Children's Hospital at Stanford
Palo Alto, California
Rectal Medication

Tresa E. Zielinski, RN, MS
Pediatric Nurse Practitioner
Kidney Disease/Kidney Transplantation
Children's Memorial Hospital
Chicago, Illinois
Urine Culture: Suprapubic Aspirate

Reviewers

Judith A. Ascenzi, MSN, RN
Johns Hopkins Hospital
Baltimore, Maryland

Nancy Blake, MN, RN, CCRN, CNAA
Children's Hospital of Los Angeles
Los Angeles, California

Ann-Marie Brown, MSN, CPNP, CCRN
Akron Children's Hospital
Akron, Ohio

Mary Bolhuis, RN
Children's Hospital of Wisconsin
Milwaukee, Wisconsin

Margaret-Ann Carno, PhD, MBA, RNC, CCRN
School of Nursing
University of Rochester
Center for High Risk Children and Youth
Golisano Children's Hospital
Rochester, New York

Lorna Cisler-Cahill, MS, RN
Children's Hospital of Wisconsin
Milwaukee, Wisconsin

Suzanne E. Courtwright-Andersen, MS, CPNP
Children's Hospital of New York Presbyterian
Columbia Presbyterian Medical Center
New York, New York

Lauren Daly, MD
Nemours/Alfred I. dufont Hospital for Children
Wilmington, Delaware

Amy Flannigan Dittmer, MSN, ARNP(c)
St. Joseph's Children's Hospital
Tampa, Florida

Sharron L. Docherty, PhD, RN, CPNP
School of Nursing
Duke University Medical Center
Durham, North Carolina

Kasey Kochinski, MSN, APRN-BC
St. Louis Children's Hospital
St. Louis, Missouri

Jessica Strohm Farber, MSN, RN, CCRN
Children's National Medical Center
Washington, District of Columbia

Heidi L. Hillman, RN, BSN
Children's Hospital of Wisconsin
Milwaukee, Wisconsin

Kathleen M. Leack, RN, BSN
Children's Hospital of Wisconsin
Milwaukee, Wisconsin

Patricia A. Moloney-Harmon, MS, RN,
  CCNS, CCRN, FAAN
Sinai Hospital
Baltimore, Maryland

Mark Brenton Moore, MSN, RN, CPNP
Cardiac Surgical Associates
Tampa Children's Hospital at St. Josephs
Tampa, Florida

Lorri M. Phipps, MSN, RN, CPNP
Milton S. Hershey Medical Center
Penn State Children's Hospital
Hershey, Pennsylvania

Devon Draffen Plumer, MSN, RN, CPNP, CCRN
New Hanover Regional Medical Center
Wilmington, North Carolina

Karin Reuter-Rice, PhD, CFNP, CPNP, CCRN
Children's Hospital and Health Center
San Diego, California

Bonnie Anne Rice, MSN, ARNP, CCNS
All Children's Hospital
St. Petersburg, Florida

Lisa Marie Ring, MSN, CPNP
Children's National Medical Center
Washington, District of Columbia

Melanie Beth Jacobsen Schuster, MSN,
PCCNP, CCRN, CNOR
Cook Children's Medical Center
Ft. Worth, Texas

Andrea M. Cardis Sorbello, MSN, APRN-BC
Arnold Palmer Hospital
Orlando, Florida

Danica Fulbright Sumpter, MSN, CRNP
University of Pennsylvania
Philadelphia, Pennsylvania

Belen Terrazas-Ponce, RN, BSN, CPNP
Providence Memorial Hospital
El Paso, Texas

Beth Helen Wieczorek, MS, CACP, CASBM
Kennedy Krieger Institute
Baltimore Maryland

Michele A. Wilson, MS, RN, PCCNP, CNS
Loma Linda University Children's Hospital
Loma Linda, California

Martha Yee, PCCNP
NPs on Demand!
El Paso, Texas

Preface

The *AACN Procedure Manual for Pediatric Acute and Critical Care* was created to fill an existing void for a comprehensive manual of procedures that addresses the specific care needs of infants and children in the acute and critical care setting. The template for this manual originated from the fifth edition of the *AACN Procedure Manual for Critical Care*. Like any younger sibling, we have imitated our older sister, and the user-friendly format of the adult manual has been retained. We have, however, put our own individual stamp on this manual, ensuring that each procedure highlights the unique information needed to safely and competently care for infants and children and their families. After much discussion and quite a long gestation period, the first edition of the *AACN Procedure Manual for Pediatric Acute and Critical Care* is a reality, thanks to the many acute and critical care nurses across the country who have provided their time and expertise.

Patient safety has always been a priority for practitioners caring for infants and children. In this manual we have made every effort to incorporate all appropriate patient safety–related recommendations from The Joint Commission (formerly the JCAHO) into each procedure. We make the assumption that each organization has procedures in place to ensure that all electrical and mechanical equipment is maintained appropriately and is safe to use in a pediatric setting. We also assume that as professionals, practitioners remain current with regard to their state practice act. This is especially important with regard to the advanced practice procedures.

Within the manual, the procedures are organized so they are quickly and easily retrievable. The manual contains 16 units and begins with procedures that support the respiratory system. Each unit is further divided into sections. In each section, procedures addressing general practice are followed by those requiring advanced practice skills. To support the clinical practice of advanced practice nurses, advanced procedures have been grouped together so they are easy to locate.

Each procedure follows a focused format and is built around the nursing process. A short statement defining the procedure and its purpose is below the title and is the starting point for each procedure. *Prerequisite Knowledge*, in bullet-point format, provides information that is essential for the practitioner to understand before performing the procedure. The *Child and Family Assessment* section lists key assessments of the child and the family that are done in preparation for the procedure. The next section describes *Child and Family Education*. This section stresses the importance of preparing the child and family in a developmentally appropriate manner to minimize any negative impact related to performing the procedure. The *Equipment* required to complete the procedure is identified immediately prior to the steps of the procedure. The *Procedure* steps are then listed, along with rationale and considerations. The information included in the *Rationale* and *Consideration* columns is important to understanding the special issues related to growth, development, and other concerns associated with caring for infants and children. *Expected and Unexpected Outcomes* contrast the desired outcomes of the procedure with potential complications. The section on *Monitoring and Care of the Child* describes the assessment and monitoring required after the procedure is completed. Rationale and reportable conditions are included within this table. The *Documentation* section lists the required documentation. At the end of each procedure, the references cited within the procedure and some additional readings, including useful websites, are provided.

The use of evidence to identify best practice is an essential element of the *AACN Procedure Manual for Pediatric Acute and Critical Care*. Pediatric-specific research studies are referenced whenever they were obtainable to support the steps of each procedure. Levels of evidence are added when available to identify the strength of the recommended step within the procedure. The leveling system is borrowed from our older siblings, *AACN Procedure Manual for Critical Care* and *AACN Protocols for Practice,* and will be familiar to many readers. The levels are defined here and are included at the bottom of each procedure page where evidence exists to support practice.

Level I: Manufacturer's recommendations only

Level II: Theory based, no research data to support recommendations; recommendations from expert consensus group may exist

Level III: Laboratory data only; no clinical data to support recommendations

Level IV: Limited clinical studies to support recommendations

Level V: Clinical studies in more than one or two different patient populations and situations to support recommendations

Level VI: Clinical studies in a variety of patient populations and situations to support recommendations

Our goal throughout this project has been to develop a manual that is a useful resource based on the best available evidence for acute and critical care practitioners caring for infants and children. As practitioners use the procedure manual and examine the available evidence, it will become clear that there are many opportunities for research to clarify best practice!

We are fortunate to have authors with expertise in a variety of pediatric specialties from across the country. The depth and breadth of their knowledge are evident throughout the manual. We have made every effort to include the most current information, but even as you read this, information is being discovered. It is our hope that when we start work on the second edition, our colleagues will have provided us with an even richer research base from which to draw!

Judy Trivits Verger
Ruth M. Lebet

Acknowledgments

No undertaking this size is ever possible without the hard work of many individuals. First, we are especially thankful to the leadership at the American Association of Critical-Care Nurses, particularly Ellen French for understanding the importance of a pediatric procedure manual for acute and critically ill infants and children. Ellen's ongoing support and patience were felt throughout this process. In addition, many people at Elsevier played important roles in making this project a reality and deserve our thanks. Barbara Cullen, our editor at Elsevier, is the patient individual who provided direction, feedback, and sometimes a strong dose of motivation. Despite our growth pains as first-time editors, Barbara held the course until completion, and we are very grateful. Adrienne Simon is the developmental editor who started us out on our long journey. Her enthusiasm for the project was key in getting us organized and under way. We had the opportunity to work with three additional developmental editors, each of whom contributed significantly to keeping us on track: Laura Sieh Chu, Mayoor Jaiswal, and Jennifer Ehlers. Jeanne Genz, the project manager, did wonderful work in copyediting and in helping us to make up time. Her sense of humor was vital in getting us through the last stages of the project.

Our neonatal and pediatric colleagues who contributed their knowledge and expertise as well as their time to this project are the group who made the vision a reality. Section editors, procedure authors, and reviewers from across the country contributed countless hours to ensure that each procedure contained the most current and most valid information available. Their high standards and high-quality work will ensure this manual serves its intended purpose.

Our families and colleagues are also owed a huge thank you. Judy would like to thank her family and colleagues: To Carey, my lifelong partner, who allows me to pursue my dreams and only with his support would they become a reality. To my children, Jennie, Emily, and George, who have given up countless mommy hours and yet saw the importance of my work. To my colleagues, especially those in the critical care division and progressive care unit at The Children's Hospital of Philadelphia, who make me proud to be a nurse and keep me inspired. My gratitude also goes to the nurses and physicians that I worked with in the PICU at Johns Hopkins Children's Center. Those early years showed me the importance of a true culture of teamwork and the high value of nursing in the care of sick children. The greatest of my thanks, however, must go to Ruth Lebet. She is tenacious and insightful, sees the good in all, and is a true friend. Thanks, Ruth! Ruth would like to thank her colleagues in the PICU at the Nemours/Alfred I. duPont Hospital for Children, who remind me every day through the care they provide to critically ill infants and children why this project is important. I would also like to thank the many pediatric nurses I have had the opportunity to work with at The Johns Hopkins Children's Center and the Children's Hospital of Philadelphia, who taught me what it really means to be a pediatric nurse. I would also like to thank my parents, who introduced me early to pediatric nursing (I was the oldest daughter in a family of six children!) and my entire family, who have shown incredible patience and support throughout this process. Finally, I would like to thank Judy for her vision in moving this project from a concept to a reality. We are truly blessed.

Contents

UNIT I: RESPIRATORY SYSTEM

Unit Editors: Kathryn E. Roberts and Mary Jo Grant

SECTION ONE: Airway Management

UNIT II: CARDIOVASCULAR SYSTEM

Unit Editors: Kathryn M. Dodds and Lisa M. Kohr

SECTION NINE: Special Cardiac Procedures

UNIT III: NEUROLOGIC SYSTEM

Unit Editor: Kelly Keefe Marcoux

SECTION TEN: Neurologic Monitoring

SECTION ELEVEN: Special Neurologic Procedures

UNIT VI: ONCOLOGY/HEMATOLOGY SYSTEM

Unit Editor: Tammara L. Jenkins

SECTION SIXTEEN: Oncology/Hematology Procedures

UNIT VII: MUSCULOSKELETAL SYSTEM

Unit Editor: Beth Bolick

SECTION SEVENTEEN: Musculoskeletal Procedures

UNIT VIII: SKIN

Unit Editor: Maureen A. Madden

SECTION EIGHTEEN: Burn Wound Management

UNIT IX: FLUID AND ELECTROLYTE MANAGEMENT

Unit Editor: Lauren Sorce

UNIT X: VASCULAR ACCESS

Unit Editors: Anne Marie Frey and Andrea M. Kline

UNIT XI: MEDICATION ADMINISTRATION

Unit Editor: Sarah A. Martin

UNIT XII: PAIN MANAGEMENT AND SEDATION

Unit Editor: Debbie Brinker

UNIT XIII: NUTRITION

Unit Editor: Shari L. Simone

UNIT XIV: THERMOREGULATION

Unit Editor: Margaret C. Slota

UNIT XV: NEONATAL ISSUES

Unit Editor: Mildred Kenney-Lau

UNIT XVI: SAFETY AND TRANSITIONING OF PEDIATRIC PATIENTS

Unit Editor: Kathryn A. Beauchamp

AACN
Procedure Manual *for* Pediatric Acute *and* Critical Care

PROCEDURE **1**

Cricothyroidotomy: Assist

P U R P O S E : To establish a temporary airway in the child whose airway cannot be secured with usual methods

Eric A. Bowles

PREREQUISITE KNOWLEDGE

- Child development as it relates to clinical assessment and procedure
- Airway anatomy and physiology, including structural characteristics specific to the infant and child[1-3] (Figure 1-1)
    - ❖ A child's airway is both absolutely and relatively smaller in diameter and shorter than an adult's airway.
    - ❖ The tongue is large in relation to the mandible and the oropharynx.

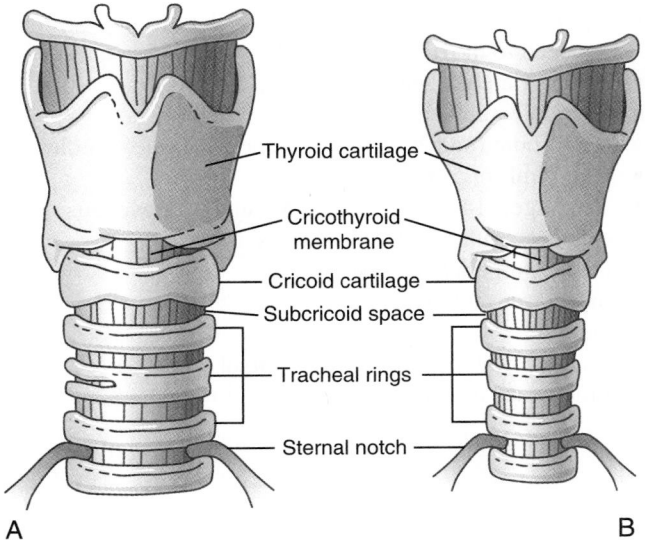

A   B

FIGURE 1-1 Anatomy of the Larynx. **A,** Older child/adult. **B,** Infant.

- ❖ The child's funnel-shaped larynx is higher and more cephalad.
- ❖ Vocal cords are 50% cartilage and attached lower and more anteriorly.
- ❖ The infant's epiglottis is floppy, long, and narrow and projects more posteriorly than that of the older child.
- ❖ The subglottic airway is smaller and more compliant, with the cartilage less developed than in the adult.
- ❖ Because the thyroid does not assume its adult configuration until puberty, the cricoid cartilage is the easiest landmark for identification in children.
- ❖ The cricoid cartilage is the narrowest portion of the upper airway in children less than 10 years of age. It lies at the level of the third cervical vertebrae in the infant and descends to the sixth cervical vertebrae at puberty.
- ❖ In teenagers and adults, the larynx is a cylinder, with its narrowest portion at the glottic inlet at the level of the vocal cords.
- ❖ The cricothyroid membrane is a dense fibroelastic membrane between the two largest cartilages in the larynx: the thyroid cartilage (located above the membrane) and the circumferential ring of the cricoid cartilage (located below the membrane).
- Mastery of pediatric advanced life support competencies, including principles of artificial airway establishment (e.g., bag-mask ventilation, oropharyngeal suctioning, proper positioning) and oxygen delivery systems[1]
- Principles of gas exchange
- Signs and symptoms of inadequate oxygenation and ventilation

❖ Cricothyroidotomy, also called cricothyrotomy, is a rare procedure accomplished with direct placement of a needle or angiocatheter percutaneously into the trachea through the cricothyroid membrane and is only attempted after oral tracheal and nasal tracheal intubation has failed[1] (see Figure 13-1).

❖ Success of percutaneous cricothyroidotomy is related to skill and training and is considered when complete airway obstruction cannot be resolved with standard treatment measures.[1,6] Percutaneous cricothyroidotomy has been effectively used for ventilation and oxygenation during administration of anesthesia with jet ventilation.[1,7]

❖ Surgical cricothyroidotomy requires surgical training and carries a significant risk, especially for infants and toddlers.[1,8,9] A short transverse incision is made across the cricothyroid membrane, and a large catheter is then threaded downward into the trachea.[2,8,9] If a surgical cricothyroidotomy is necessary, additional equipment is needed, such as scalpels with #11 and #15 blades, trachea hooks, a trousseau dilator (trachea dilator), curved Mayo scissors, curved hemostats, a small vascular clamp, a needle holder, sutures, a syringe with a 25-gauge needle for lidocaine with epinephrine, an appropriately sized tracheostomy tube, and appropriately sized endotracheal tubes.[8]

• A cricothyroidotomy is useful in foreign body obstruction if the obstruction is above or at the glottis. For an obstruction below the level of the cricoid cartilage, a cricothyroidotomy is not likely to be effective.[1]

• A cricothyroidotomy can produce adequate oxygenation but has limited capacity in the provision of adequate ventilation.[10,11] This adequate oxygenation may be sufficient to support survival in children who are seriously ill because hypercarbia, caused by suboptimal ventilation, may be tolerated.[12]

• Although reports do exist of percutaneous transtracheal ventilation in adults, few reports exist for children[7,13,14]

CHILD AND FAMILY ASSESSMENT

• Child's developmental level and ability to interact ➤➤**Rationale:** Influences preparation and interaction.

• Child's and family's understanding of the reasons for and risks and benefits of cricothyroidotomy ➤➤**Rationale:** Evaluates child's and family's understanding of the procedure and provides a gauge for ongoing education.

• Respiratory status, including chest wall movement and lung sounds ➤➤**Rationale:** Carbon dioxide (CO_2) retention may occur because of the small size of the catheter necessary for cricothyroidotomy.

• Signs and symptoms of inadequate oxygenation and ventilation ➤➤**Rationale:** Indication of effective pulmonary function.

• Presence of hemodynamic instability ➤➤**Rationale:** Hemodynamic instability may accompany respiratory failure.

• Last enteral intake of food or liquids ➤➤**Rationale:** Children with a full stomach are at risk for aspiration of gastric contents during airway manipulation.

CHILD AND FAMILY EDUCATION

Individualized, developmentally appropriate education is provided to the family and to the child based on desire for knowledge, readiness to learn, and overall neurologic and psychosocial state.

• Explain the cricothyroidotomy procedure, including steps and rationale ➤➤**Rationale:** Providing information decreases fear and anxiety.

• Inform the parents that a cricothyroidotomy is an emergency procedure used to attain a temporary airway and that a more stable and long-term airway will be placed ➤➤**Rationale:** Anticipatory guidance is provided, and the family is prepared for further intervention. The parents must understand that this life-saving measure is temporary and that surgery is needed to secure a stable airway.

• Explain that the child's pain will be managed ➤➤**Rationale:** Parents may be comforted to know the child's pain will be addressed.

• Encourage and answer questions as they arise ➤➤**Rationale:** Reinforcement of information is needed during periods of stress and is especially important given the emergent nature of the procedure.

EQUIPMENT

• Personal protective equipment, including gloves
• Appropriately sized manual ventilation bag (MVB) attached to the oxygen source
• Appropriately sized mask
• Suction equipment
• Small-bore (one 20-gauge and one 22-gauge) needles
• One 3-mL or 5-mL syringe
• 12-gauge, 14-gauge, and 16-gauge intravenous (IV) catheters with needle introducers
• One 3-mm tracheal tube adaptor
• Sterile gauze pads
• Tape
• Aseptic swab (or other antimicrobial solution)
• Emergency and procedural medications

Procedure for Cricothyroidotomy: Assist

Steps	Rationale	Considerations
1. Ensure child and family understand procedure and questions are answered.	Evaluates and reinforces understanding of previously taught information.	Developmental, cognitive, and anxiety levels determine approach and effectiveness of teaching. Given emergent nature of a cricothyroidotomy, procedure explanation may be delayed.
2. Gather needed equipment and supplies.	Facilitates completion of the task in a timely manner.	This step may occur as child is positioned.
3. Monitor child's vital signs and indications of inadequate oxygenation and ventilation before, during, and after procedure.	A child in respiratory failure has vital sign changes and may need additional intervention.	Pulse oximetry and a cardiorespiratory monitor are used when possible. At a minimum, periodic vital signs are taken. Use arterial or venous blood gasses when indicated.
4. Wash hands and put on gloves and other protective equipment.	Reduces transmission of infection. Protects personnel health.	
5. Position child supine with the head midline.	Positioning assists in the correct placement of the catheter.	Use caution when a cervical spine injury is a possibility.
6. Place a small shoulder/neck roll under the child.	Brings trachea anterior and simplifies landmark identification. May assist with stabilization of trachea. Controls any movement of trachea during instrumentation.	With cervical spine injuries, placement must be done with extreme caution.
7. Once airway is in place, attach a 3-mm endotracheal tube adapter connected to an oxygen source.	The small tube used for cricothyroidotomy limits air movement.	Oxygen flow rates should be relatively low (average, 110 mL/kg/min; maximum, 1 to 5 mL/min).[1] Child needs longer expiratory times or pauses between insufflations to promote loss of CO_2, especially in complete airway obstruction.[1] A high-pressure oxygen source has been suggested as an alternative.[15]
8. Secure airway to the child after catheter is in place.	Prevents dislodgement.	
9. Remove protective items and wash hands.	Reduces transmission of infection. Protects personnel health.	

Expected Outcomes
- Successful placement of a temporary airway
- Adequate oxygenation and ventilation
- A bridge is provided until a more stable airway is obtained
- Child shows acceptable level of comfort

Unexpected Outcomes
- Failure of catheter placement inside the trachea
- Inadequate oxygenation and ventilation
- Neurologic impairment from hypoxemia
- Death
- Unmanaged pain and irritability

Monitoring and Care of the Child

Activities and Interventions	Rationale	Reportable Conditions
1. Continuously monitor oxygenation and ventilation.	Because of small diameters, IV catheters produce high resistance and may cause air trapping or CO_2 retention from impaired passive exhalation.	• Physical examination that indicates inadequate oxygenation or ventilation; change in color, skin temperature, or level of consciousness • Decreasing or inadequate chest rise and fall • Abnormal blood gases: rising $PaCO_2$ and falling pH levels • A decreased oxygen saturation level (SaO_2)
2. Monitor vital signs.	Trending the vital signs helps to guide treatment.	• Abnormal vital signs
3. Continuously evaluate airway security.	Loss of airway could be fatal.	• Loss of airway
4. Assess effectiveness of pain management strategies and provide appropriate interventions.	Early identification of the child's comfort allows for immediate attention.	• Unresolved pain and discomfort • Continued irritability or changes in physiologic condition

Documentation

- Airway establishment, including date, time, and circumstances that necessitated the procedure
- Preprocedural and postprocedural physical assessment, including vital signs
- Comfort assessment, including interventions provided
- Additional interventions necessary
- Child's response to procedure
- Child and family education
- Unexpected outcomes and related treatments

References

1. Hazinski MF, et al: *Pediatric advanced life support provider manual,* Dallas, American Heart Association, 2002.
2. Curley MAQ, Thompson J: Oxygenation and ventilation. In Curley MAQ, Moloney-Harmon P, editors: *Critical care nursing of infants and children,* ed 2, Philadelphia, Saunders, 2001.
3. Thompson A: Pediatric airway management. In Fuhrman B, Zimmerman J, editors: *Pediatric critical care,* ed 3, Philadelphia, 2005, Elsevier.
4. McCance K, Huether S: *Pathophysiology: the biologic bases for disease in adults and children,* Philadelphia, Mosby, 2002.
5. Thibodeau G, Patton K, editors: *Anatomy and physiology,* ed 5, Philadelphia, Mosby, 2003.
6. Wong D, et al: What is the minimum training required for successful cricothyroidotomy: a study of mannequins, *Anesthesiology* 98(2): 349-353, 2003.
7. Depierraz B, et al: Percutaneous transtracheal jet ventilation for paediatric endoscopic laser treatment of laryngeal and subglottic lesions, *Can J Anesth* 41: 1200-1207, 1994.
8. Strange GR, Niederman LG: Surgical cricothyroidotomy. In Henretig FM, King BR, Loiselle J, et al, editors: *Textbook of pediatric emergency procedures,* Philadelphia, Williams & Wilkins, 1997.
9. Mathers L, Frankel L: Stabilization of the critically ill child. In Behrman R, et al, editors: *Nelson's textbook of pediatrics,* ed 17, Philadelphia, Saunders, 2004.
10. Brofelt BT, et al: An easy cricothyrotomy approach: the rapid four step technique, *Acad Emerg Med* 3(11): 1060-1063, 1996.
11. Cote CJ, et al: Cricothyroidotomy membrane puncture: oxygenation and ventilation in a dog model using an intravenous catheter, *Crit Care Med* 16: 615-619, 1988.
12. Golstein B, et al: Supercarbia in children: a clinical course and outcome, *Crit Care Med* 18: 166-168, 1990.
13. Smith RB, et al: Percutaneous transtracheal ventilation for anaesthesia and resuscitation: a review and report of complications, *Can Anesth Soc J* 22: 607-612, 1975.
14. Barrachina R, et al: Percutaneous dilational cricothyroidotomy: outcome with 44 consecutive patients, *Intensive Care Med* 22: 937-940, 1996.
15. Peak DA, Roy S: Needle cricothyroidotomy revisited, *Pediatr Emerg Care* 15: 224-226, 1999.

Additional Reading
Cummins R, editor: ACLS: *principles and practice,* Dallas, American Heart Association, 2003.

Endotracheal Tube: Suctioning and Care

PURPOSE: To maintain a patent airway, promote oxygenation and ventilation, prevent facial skin and mucosal breakdown, and provide oral hygiene

Dena L. Jarog

PREREQUISITE KNOWLEDGE

- Child development as it relates to clinical assessment and procedure
  - ❖ Anatomy and physiology of the pediatric pulmonary system, including structural characteristics specific to the infant and child[1-4]
  - ❖ A child's airway is both absolutely and relatively smaller in diameter and shorter than an adult's (see Figure 1-1).
  - ❖ Because the thyroid does not assume its adult configuration until puberty, the cricoid cartilage is the easiest landmark for identification in children. The cricoid cartilage is the narrowest portion of the upper airway in children less than 10 years of age.
  - ❖ In teenagers and adults, the larynx is a cylinder with its narrowest portion at the glottic inlet at the level of the vocal cords.
  - ❖ The quantity of alveoli increases until 8 years of age and thereafter increases in size and complexity. Peripheral airway resistance is disproportionately higher in the child.[1]
  - ❖ During inspiration, the infant's intercostal muscles stiffen and a downward movement of the diaphragm occurs, which results in negative intrathoracic pressure and air movement into the lungs. Because the infant's chest wall is compliant and flexible, it characteristically collapses inward (see Figure 23-1).

- Signs and symptoms of inadequate oxygenation and ventilation
  - ❖ Mastery of pediatric advanced life support competencies, including indications for an artificial airway, use of a manual resuscitation/ventilation system, and other adjuncts used to support ventilation.[1]
  - ❖ Endotracheal (ET) tubes help to maintain a patent airway and facilitate mechanical ventilation. Because the ET tube impairs coughing and secretion removal, periodic suctioning is necessary for removal of secretions and promotion of ventilation and oxygenation.
  - ❖ For reduction of the likelihood of airway contamination and prevention of nosocomial infection, suctioning is performed with sterile technique.[5-9]
  - ❖ Indications for suctioning include secretions in the ET tube, auscultation of adventitious lung sounds, increased peak airway pressures during volume-controlled mechanical ventilation or decreased tidal volume during pressure-controlled ventilation, changes in flow and pressure graphics during mechanical ventilation, increased work of breathing, sustained coughing and a decrease in blood oxygen saturations either arterial (SaO_2) or via pulse oximetry (SpO_2), and inability to generate an effective spontaneous cough.[10]
  - ❖ To decrease the likelihood of mucosal trauma, the frequency of suctioning is based on individual need rather than "unit routine."[1,5,10-13]

5

- ❖ Instillation of normal saline solution as a routine procedure for facilitation of suctioning of secretions is not evidence based.[9,11,14-17]
  - ❖ Stimulation of the vagus nerve during catheter insertion may lead to alterations in heart rate and rhythm.[1]
- Negative side effects of ET suctioning, including hypoxia, pulmonary artery hypertension, dysrhythmia, trauma to the trachea and bronchi, bronchospasm, infection, and hypertension or hypotension [5,6,14,17-20]
- For a reduction in the risk of hypoxemia, a frequency of no more than 10 to 15 seconds per suction pass is recommended.[21]
  - ❖ Proper humidity, hydration, and temperature levels assist in the maintenance of thinner secretions and facilitation of suctioning[9,14-17]
  - ❖ The size of the suction catheter can be estimated by doubling the ET tube size and using the next French (F) size (i.e., 4.5-cm ET tube = 8F suction catheter). A size no larger than half the diameter of the ET tube is typically needed.[9,20,22]
  - ❖ The two common methods of suctioning are:
    - ○ Open suction technique: The ventilation device is disconnected, and a suction catheter is introduced into the open end of the ET tube.

- ○ Closed suction technique: A specially designed multiple-use catheter that is enclosed in a sterile plastic sleeve for prevention of contamination is used. The catheter is attached in-line with the ventilation device, which allows for maintenance of oxygenation and ventilation. This method is particularly useful in children who need high levels of inspired oxygen or positive end-expiratory pressure (PEEP) (Figure 2-1).[4,23,24]
- ❖ Skin breakdown can occur from the tape used to secure the ET tube and from the pressure of the tube itself on the nares or lips
- ❖ Ventilator-associated pneumonia increases ventilator days and morbidity and mortality and appears to be related to aspiration of secretions from the stomach and mouth and colonization of the mouth that occurs in association with dental plaque.[8,25,26]
- Principles of oral hygiene and skin care

CHILD AND FAMILY ASSESSMENT

- Child's developmental level and ability to interact
  ➤**Rationale:** Influences preparation and interaction.

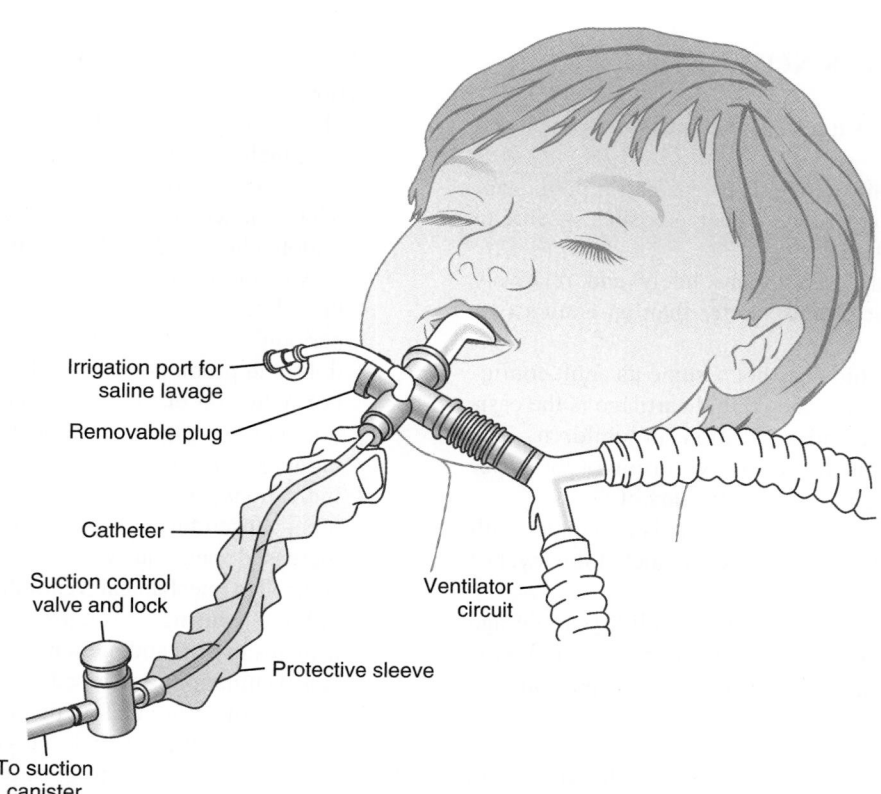

Irrigation port for
saline lavage

Removable plug

Catheter

Suction control
valve and lock

Protective sleeve

Ventilator
circuit

To suction
canister

FIGURE 2-1   Closed-Suctioning Technique.

- Child's and family's understanding of the reasons for and risks and benefits of ETT suctioning ➤➤*Rationale:* Evaluates child's and family's understanding of procedure and provides a gauge for ongoing education.
- Desire of family members to be present during the procedure ➤➤*Rationale:* The presence of family may provide comfort and support; although family members should have the choice not to remain with the child.
- Signs and symptoms of airway secretions and inadequate oxygenation and ventilation, including visible secretions in the airway, inspiratory wheezes, expiratory crackles, restlessness, ineffective coughing, decreased level of consciousness, diminished breath sounds, tachypnea, tachycardia or bradycardia, cyanosis, hypertension or hypotension, and shallow respirations,[22] ➤➤*Rationale:* The physical presence of secretions in the airway can result in obstruction of the airway and poor gas exchange.
- Increased peak pressures on the ventilator ➤➤*Rationale:* Secretions can increase resistance to airflow.
- Maintenance of cardiac and respiratory stability during manual ventilation ➤➤*Rationale:* Determines the need for a second person to perform hyperoxygenation or hyperventilation, the necessity of premedication, and the urgency of procedure completion.
- Endotracheal tube security, including tape integrity and tube movement ➤➤*Rationale:* ET tube security is ensured, and the ET tube is assessed for whether it needs to be secured again.
- Pressure areas and skin around and under tape and ET tube ➤➤*Rationale:* Reduction of skin breakdown and elimination of a potential source for infection.
- Oral cavity, including plaque buildup ➤➤*Rationale:* An association between ventilator-associated pneumonia and dental plaque has been suggested.[8,25,26]

CHILD AND FAMILY EDUCATION

Individualized, developmentally appropriate education is provided to the family and to the child based on desire for knowledge, readiness to learn, and overall neurologic and psychosocial state.

- Explain the suctioning procedure, including the purpose, steps, and rationale ➤➤*Rationale:* Providing information decreases fear and anxiety.[9,22]
- Discuss with the child and family that suctioning may be uncomfortable and may cause coughing and shortness of breath for a brief period of time ➤➤*Rationale:* Reduces anxiety and fear for the child and family and prepares the child for the experience.[9]
- Explain the importance of the having the child assist with secretion removal by coughing during the procedure ➤➤*Rationale:* The explanation elicits cooperation and improves the effectiveness of the procedure by facilitating removal of secretions from the tracheobronchial tree.

- Encourage questions and answer questions as they arise ➤➤*Rationale:* Reinforcement of information is needed during periods of stress.

EQUIPMENT (OPEN–SUCTIONING SYSTEM)

- Personal protective equipment, including eye protection, mask, and gown
- Appropriately sized disposable suction catheter
- Suction source (wall regulator or portable machine)
- Collection container
- Connecting tube (large-bore non-collapsible)
- Sterile water and cup for catheter clearance
- Sterile gloves
- Manual ventilation bag (MVB; self-inflating or flow-inflating) connected to an oxygen-flow meter
- Appropriately sized mask
- Positive end-expiratory pressure valve, depending on child's need for PEEP (>5 cm H_2O)
- Stethoscope
- Premedications as indicated

EQUIPMENT (CLOSED–SUCTIONING SYSTEM)

- Personal protective equipment
- Closed-suction setup with an appropriately sized catheter
- Suction source (wall regulator or portable machine)
- Collection container
- Connecting tube (large-bore non-collapsible)
- Manual ventilation bag (self-inflating or flow-inflating) connected to an oxygen-flow meter
- Appropriately sized mask
- Sterile saline solution lavage containers (as necessary)
- Individual catheters for oral and nasal suctioning (wide-bore pliable plastic suction catheter and rigid pharyngeal tonsil tip catheter)
- Clean gloves
- Stethoscope
- Premedications as indicated

EQUIPMENT (SKIN AND ORAL CARE)

- Personal protective equipment, including eye protection and mask
- Gauze pad or wash cloth
- Saline solution or water
- Soft toothbrush with suction if available or Toothette swab
- Hydrogen peroxide (1.5%) mouth rinse, as indicated
- Water-based moisturizer
- Other skin care items as needed

Procedure for Endotracheal Tube: Suctioning and Care

Steps	Rationale	Considerations

Open-Suction Technique

1. Ensure child and family understand procedure and questions are answered.

Evaluates and reinforces understanding of previously taught information.[22]

Developmental, cognitive, and anxiety levels determine approach and effectiveness of teaching.

2. Gather needed equipment and supplies including selection of appropriately sized suction catheter (Table 2-1).

Facilitates completion of task in a timely manner.
Suction catheter varies according to size of ET tube.
Include premedication as indicated.

Suction catheter should be no larger then half the diameter of the ET tube.[9,17,20,22]

Some children who are especially vulnerable to physiologic change during suctioning need premedication.

TABLE 2-1	Suction Catheter Size		

Age	ET Tube Size (mm)	Suction Catheter Size (F)
Newborn	3.0-3.5 uncuffed	6-8
6 mo	3.5-4 uncuffed	8
1-2 y	4-4.5 uncuffed 4.0 cuffed	8
4-6 y	5.0-5.5 uncuffed 4.5-5.0 cuffed	10
>8 y	6.0-8.0 cuffed	12

Curley MAQ, Thompson JE: Oxygenation and ventilation. In Curley MAQ, Moloney-Harmon PA, editors: *Critical care nursing of infants and children,* Philadelphia, 2001, Saunders.
Hazinski MF et al, editors: *Pediatric advanced life support provider manual,* Dallas, 2002, American Heart Association.

3. Ensure an appropriately sized MVB and mask are at the bedside.

Provides intervention if the ET tube becomes dislodged or completely removed.

MVB can be used for the duration of the child's stay but should be changed if any secretions are inside the opening of the oxygen delivery portion.

4. Monitor child's vital signs and indications of inadequate oxygenation and ventilation before, during, and after suctioning. (*Level II**)

Identifies signs and symptoms of complications from suctioning, such as decreased oxygen saturation (SpO_2), cardiac dysrhythmia (specifically bradycardia from stimulation of the vagus nerve), bronchospasm, respiratory distress, increased blood pressure, increased intracranial pressure (ICP), and anxiety.

Termination of suctioning is needed with cardiac dysrhythmia, hemodynamic instability, or significant changes in oxygenation or ventilation indices.

5. Wash hands and put on personal protective equipment, including eye protection; mask, and gown (as indicated).

Reduces transmission of infection.
Protects personnel health.

Use a gown in cases of copious secretions and strong cough reflex or in infectious situations (e.g., respiratory syncytial virus).

6. Assess lung sounds before suctioning.

Verifies patency and tube placement.
A comparison is necessary for post-suctioning auscultation.[7,27]

* Level II: Theory-based; no research data to support recommendations; recommendations from expert consensus group may exist

Procedure for Endotracheal Tube: Suctioning and Care—*Continued*		
Steps	**Rationale**	**Considerations**
7. Turn on the suction device and set the vacuum regulator between 80 and 150 mm Hg. *(Level VI*)*	Sufficient pressure should be applied for effective removal of secretions. Limiting the amount of negative pressure helps decrease damage to the tracheal epithelium.[9,13,20,23]	Appropriate suggested negative pressures: Infants (<1 yr), 60 to 80 mm Hg; children (1 to 8 yr), 80 to 120 mm Hg; children (>8 yr), 120 to 150 mm Hg.[9,13,20,23] Suction pressure is checked with occlusion of the end of the suction tubing.
8. Verify the appropriate insertion length of catheter with standard centimeter markings on the suction catheter with the ET tube. *(Level III*)*	Advancement of the suction catheter to the point of resistance causes tissue damage.[20]	
9. Open the packaging of the catheter with the inside of the package as a sterile field.	Provides a sterile field to prevent transmission of bacteria.	
10. Pour a small amount of sterile water in the sterile container.	Prepares flush solution for the catheter.	Sterile water can be used for up to 24 hours after opening. The date and time of opening should be written in a prominent spot on the container.
11. Put on gloves with sterile technique.	Reduces transmission of infection. Protects personnel health.	Although sterile suctioning technique is recommended for reduction of the likelihood of airway contamination, some institutions use clean technique for the suctioning procedure. See institution-specific protocol for variation.
12. Pick up the suction catheter with the dominant hand.		
13. With the non-dominant hand, pick up the connecting tube and secure it to the suction catheter.		
14. Suction a small amount of fluid from the container with sterile solution.	Assures properly functioning equipment.	
15. Hyperoxygenate and hyperinflate for at least 30 seconds.[9,11,13,21,22] Disconnect the ventilator tubing from the ET tube, attach the MVB to the ET tube with the nondominant hand, and give five to six breaths for 30 seconds. *(Level VI*)* For the child to remain on ventilation, press the hyperoxygenation button on the ventilator *or* increase the baseline fraction of inspired oxygen (FiO$_2$) level on the ventilator.	Hyperoxygenation increases arterial oxygen levels in preparation for suctioning, and hyperinflation assists in mobilization of secretions.[9-11,13,17,24,28] Minimizes risks of suctioning.[9,13,24,28] A ventilator equipped with this function may provide hyperventilation by delivering a "sigh" breath.	Ensure adequate PEEP levels (especially with >5 cm H$_2$O). For the child who is especially vulnerable to changes in oxygenation or ventilation, consider the use of a second person to deliver hyperoxygenation. The flow meter is typically set at 15 L/min. On blender, set at 100%. Hyperoxygenation with 100% FiO$_2$ is not recommended in certain medical conditions, including certain congenital heart defects and hypoxic respiratory drive.

Procedure continues on following page

* Level III: Laboratory data; no clinical data to support recommendations
Level VI: Clinical studies in a variety of patient populations and situations to support recommendations

Procedure for Endotracheal Tube: Suctioning and Care—*Continued*

Steps	Rationale	Considerations
		Without appropriate exhalation time or with too large a tidal volume, hyperinflation may cause pneumothorax.
16. With the suction off, gently insert the catheter with the dominant hand and advance the catheter 1 to 2 cm past the end of the ET tube.	Suctioning removes oxygen. Only apply as needed to remove secretions. Advancement of the suction catheter to the point of resistance causes tissue damage.[20]	If resistance is felt, pull the catheter back 0.5 to 1 cm and then apply suction. *(Level III*)* If difficulty arises in insertion of the suction catheter, assess for a kink in the ET tube or a kink in the suction catheter.
17. Place the non-dominant thumb over the control vent and apply continuous suction while withdrawing the catheter from the ET tube. As you withdraw, rotate the catheter with a twisting motion with the thumb and forefinger.[1] *(Level II*)*	Provides adequate removal of secretions.	Use brief suction periods of 10 seconds or less to minimize decreases in arterial oxygenation and to decrease airway trauma.[1,9,11,13,14,23] If bradycardia or significant changes in vital signs or clinical appearance occur, withdraw the catheter and provide oxygen until the levels return to baseline.[1]
18. Provide 30 seconds of hyperoxygenation before and after each pass of the suction catheter. *(Level VI*)*	Reduces risk of a decrease in arterial oxygen and allows for recovery of arterial oxygen saturations.	If secretions remain in the airway after two or three passes, place the child on ventilation and allow a rest period before additional passes are made.[9,17,22] Hyperoxygenation with 100% FiO_2 is contraindicated in certain medical conditions, including certain congenital heart defects and hypoxic respiratory drive.
19. As needed, flush and rinse the catheter with sterile solution.	Assists in maintenance of catheter patency. Rinsing decreases the chances of deposits of upper airway secretions in the lower respiratory tract.	
20. Once the ET tube is cleared of secretions, suction the oral and nasal pharynx.	Prevents contamination of the lower airways with upper airway organisms.	Care is taken to avoid trauma to the nasal and oral passages and gagging during suctioning.
21. For catheter disposal, wrap the catheter around the dominant hand and pull the glove off inside out. The catheter remains in the glove. Remove the other glove and discard in a waste container.	Reduces risk of microorganism transmission.	
22. Turn off the suction device.		
23. Discard the remaining saline solution and the solution container.		

* Level II: Theory-based; no research data to support recommendations; recommendations from expert consensus group may exist
  Level III: Laboratory data; no clinical data to support recommendations
  Level VI: Clinical studies in a variety of patient populations and situations to support recommendations

Procedure	for Endotracheal Tube: Suctioning and Care—*Continued*	
Steps	**Rationale**	**Considerations**
24. Assess breath sounds to determine whether any pertinent changes have occurred after suctioning.	Evaluates the effectiveness of suctioning.[9,22]	
25. Remove protective items and wash hands.	Reduces transmission of infection. Protects personnel health.	
26. Change the tubing and collection container at least every 72 hours or whenever the canister is full.[9,22] *(Level I*)*	Reduces transmission of infection.	

Closed-Suction Technique

1. Follow steps 1 to 6 as previously described.		
7. Put on clean gloves.	The catheter is enclosed in a sterile covering; therefore, sterile gloves are not necessary for this technique.	
8. Secure the connecting tube to the closed system suction port following the manufacturer's directions.		
9. Determine the proper catheter level for suctioning: Ensure the tip of the Y adaptor touches a marked whole centimeter number on the ET tube (e.g., 18 cm on the ET tube). Add 5.5 cm to the whole number in the previous step for the correct catheter length (e.g., 18 cm + 5.5 cm = 23.5 cm).	For alignment of the catheter under the lavage port before application of suction. *(Level I*)*	
10. Set the suction regulator at the appropriate suction level while the thumb port of the catheter is depressed. *(Level I*)*	Prepares for suctioning. Limits the amount of negative pressure to decrease damage to the tracheal epithelium.[9,13,21,23]	Adequate pressure should be applied to effectively remove secretions. Follow the manufacturer's directions for suction pressure levels with closed suction systems. *(Level I*)*
11. Hyperoxygenate by: Pressing the hyperoxygenation button on the ventilator. Alternatively increasing the baseline FiO$_2$ level on the ventilator.	Hyperoxygenation increases arterial oxygen levels in preparation for suctioning.[1,9,10,13,17,19,22,24]	Hyperoxygenation with 100% FiO$_2$ is contraindicated in certain medical conditions, including certain heart defects and hypoxic congenital respiratory drive.
12. If child is ventilated with an oscillator, pause oscillations before suctioning.		Resume oscillations between suctioning passes. Suctioning on high frequency oscillation ventilation (HFOV) can result in significant lung de-recruitment. Minimization of ET suctioning during the first 24 to 48 hours after initiation of HFOV is recommended.[29]

Procedure continues on following page

* Level I: Manufacturer's recommendations only

Procedure for Endotracheal Tube: Suctioning and Care—*Continued*

Steps	Rationale	Considerations
13. Advance the catheter until the measured number is aligned with the lavage port (Figure 2-2, *A*).		The most efficient catheter advancement occurs when the bag that covers the catheter bunches up behind the fingers.
14. When the catheter is at the correct depth, depress suction and hold while slowly withdrawing the catheter (Figure 2-2, *B*).		Support the catheter at the ET tube with one hand while withdrawing the catheter with the other hand to prevent extubation. Use brief suction periods of 10 seconds or less to minimize decreases in arterial oxygen saturations.[13,23]
15. Provide 30 seconds of hyper-ventilation between suctioning passes.[9,11,13,22]	Allows for recovery of arterial oxygen saturations.	

16. To clean the catheter:
    Withdraw the black tip of the catheter into the middle of the cleaning chamber.
    Depress suction first, and then gently squeeze saline solution into the chamber.
		Flush the catheter between each pass of the catheter while watching the catheter window.

17. Lock the suction catheter when finished suctioning and cleaning the catheter.	Prevents movement.	
18. Once the ET tube is cleared of secretions, use another suction device to suction the oral and nasal pharynx.	Prevents contamination of the lower airways with upper airway organisms.	This catheter should be changed with each suctioning event.
19. Assess breath sounds to deter-mine whether any pertinent changes have occurred after suctioning.[9,17]	Evaluates effectiveness of suctioning.	
20. Remove protective items and wash hands.	Reduces transmission of infection. Protects personnel health.	
21. Change closed suction set-up every 24 hours. Change tubing and collection container at least every 72 hours or whenever the canister is full.[9,17] *(Level I*)*	Reduces transmission of infection.	
Skin and Oral Care		
1. Ensure child and family understand procedure and questions are answered.	Evaluates and reinforces understanding of previously taught information.	Developmental, cognitive, and anxiety levels determine approach and effectiveness of teaching.
2. Wash hands and put on gloves.	Reduces transmission of infection. Protects personnel health.	
3. Gather needed equipment and supplies.	Facilitates completion of the task in a timely manner.	

Procedure continues on p. 14

* Level I: Manufacturer's recommendations only

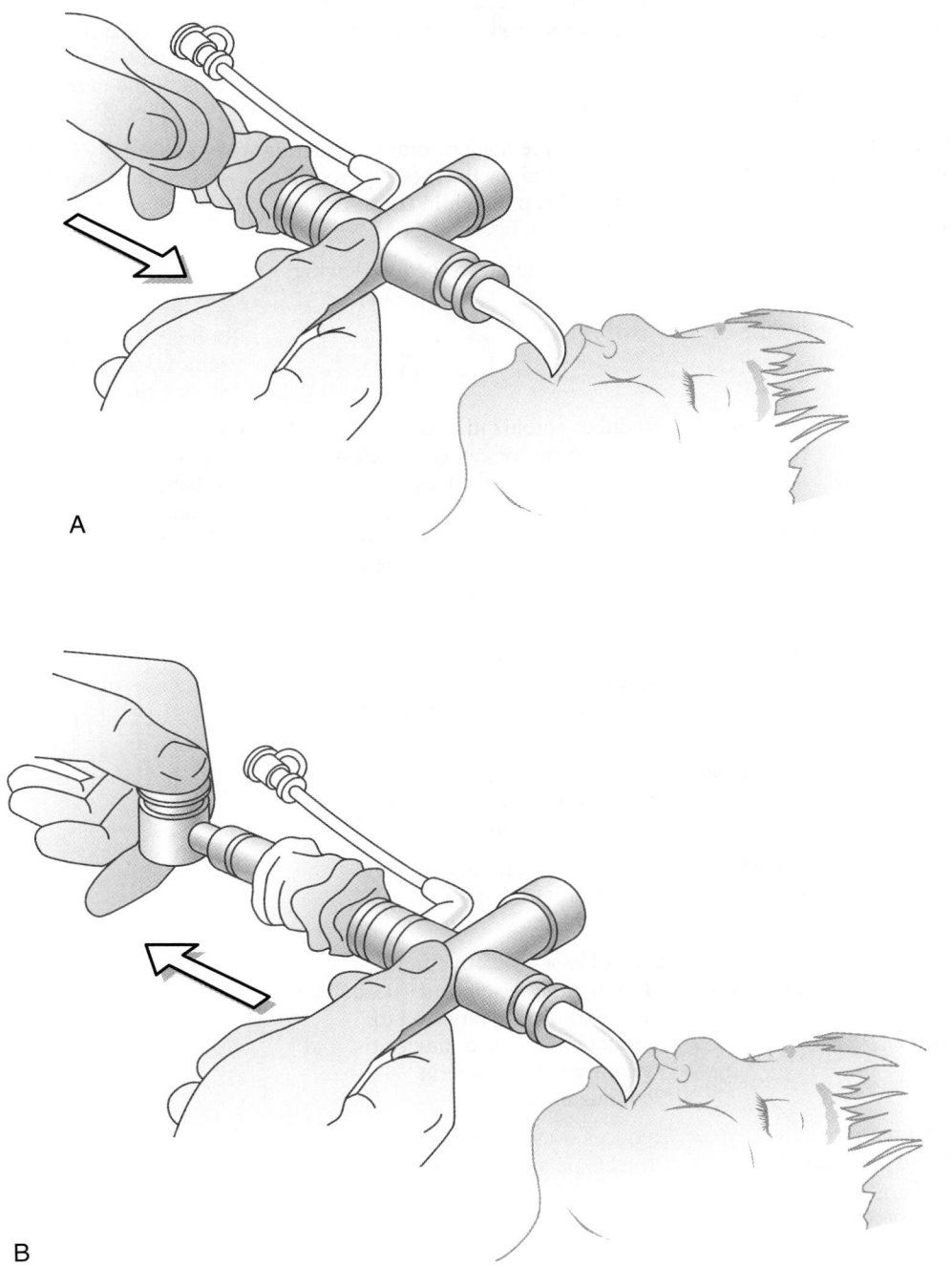

FIGURE 2-2 Closed-Suction Technique. **A,** Advance the catheter with the thumb and forefinger with small strokes. **B,** Withdraw the catheter with continuous or intermittent suction.

Procedure for Endotracheal Tube: Suctioning and Care—*Continued*

Steps	Rationale	Considerations
4. Assess the skin under and around the tape and ET tube.	Reduces skin breakdown and eliminates a potential source for infection.	Consider repositioning or retaping the ET tube if skin is reddened or if the tube has remained in the same area of the nares or mouth (see Procedure 3).
5. Assess the child's oral cavity and lips for oral dysfunction and for contraindications to oral care (oral trauma).[7,27]	Evaluates the level of oral dysfunction and determines the most appropriate care to keep the child comfortable and prevent complications.[7,27]	At least a daily inspection of the mouth is needed.
6. Suction oral secretions.	Clears the mouth for better viewing and cleaning.	
7. Connect a suction toothbrush or Toothette to the tubing.		Toothettes are less effective in plaque removal and mucosal tissue stimulation.[30]
8. Brush teeth and remove plaque with 1.5% hydrogen peroxide mouth rinse for 1 to 2 minutes. *(Level IV*)* Apply suction at completion and as needed during brushing.	Reduces colonization of the oropharyngeal cavity, which is related to ventilator-associated pneumonia.[8,25,26] Safety and efficacy are supported for 1% to 3% hydrogen peroxide as a cleaner for plaque and overall gingival health.[12,15,27]	Oral care is recommended every 2 to 4 hours.[7,27] For babies, use a gauze pad wrapped around the finger and moistened with sterile water to gently rub the gum.
9. Brush the tongue surface gently.	Reduces colonization of the oropharyngeal cavity, which is related to ventilator-associated pneumonia. *(Level IV*)*	
10. Suction any remaining fluid from the oral cavity. *(Level IV*)*	Removes accumulated secretions. Reduces the risk of ventilator-associated pneumonia.[8]	
11. Clean around the ET tube with gauze or cotton swabs and saline solution.	Removes secretions that could cause pressure and skin breakdown.	
12. Apply mouth moisturizer or lip balm to lips and areas exposed to the air to maintain mucosal integrity. *(Level IV*)*	Saliva has a protective function. Drying may occur with mechanical ventilation and may lead to reduction in saliva, mucositis, and gram-negative bacteria colonization.[28]	
13. Remove personal protective equipment and wash hands.	Reduces transmission of infection. Protects personnel health.	

* Level IV: Limited clinical studies to support recommendations

Expected Outcomes

- Removal of airway secretions
- Alleviation of clinical signs or symptoms of need for suctioning
- Support of oxygenation and ventilation
- Maintenance of recruited lung and PEEP
- Maintenance of skin integrity and oral mucosa
- Reduction of dental plaque
- Hemodynamic stability
- Maintenance of ICP within acceptable limits
- Acceptable level of comfort for the child

Unexpected Outcomes

- Inability to clear secretions
- Respiratory Instability
- Inadequate oxygenation and ventilation, including hypoxemia
- Bronchospasm
- Ventilator-associated pneumonia
- Mucosal breakdown or bleeding
- Skin breakdown
- Cardiac dysrhythmia and hemodynamic instability
- Increase in ICP
- Unmanaged pain and irritability

Monitoring and Care of the Child

Activities and Interventions	Rationale	Reportable Conditions
1. Monitor physiologic stability, including vital signs, ICP, and clinical appearance.	Signs and symptoms of complications from suctioning should be observed.	• Persistent dysrhythmia • Significant changes in oxygen saturation and arterial or venous blood gases • Bronchospasm • Unresolved increase in work of breathing • Changes in peripheral perfusion • Cyanosis • Increase in ICP • Anxiety, agitation, or changes in mental status
2. Assess signs and symptoms of airway secretion and changes in oxygenation or ventilation indices. *(Level II*)*	Pre-assessment determines the need for suctioning, and post-assessment shows whether any improvement has occurred after the suctioning procedure.[9,22]	• Diminished breath sounds • Significant changes in oxygenation saturation and arterial or venous blood gases • Increased peak airway pressures • Persistent coughing • Increased work of breathing • Inability to pass suction catheter • Change in quantity and characteristics of secretions
3. Suction the ET tube as needed.	Maintains patency of airway.	
4. Reconfirm security and position of the ET tube.	Ensure the tube is secure, which allows for immediate attention if needed.	• A change in position of the ET tube
5. Assess skin and oral integrity at least q 8 hours and provide interventions to maintain skin and oral integrity q 2 to 4 hours.	Early recognition promotes quick intervention. Maintain skin and oral integrity.	• Skin redness and breakdown • Mucosal bleeding • Excessive plaque buildup • Necrosis • Ulcerations • Trauma to lungs, tongue, or roof of mouth
6. Assess comfort and provide appropriate interventions. Allow the family to assist with non-pharmacologic comforts and to support the child.	Early identification of the child's comfort allows for immediate attention.	• Unresolved pain and discomfort • Continued irritability or changes in physiologic condition

* Level II: Theory-based; no research data to support recommendations; recommendations from expert consensus group may exist

Documentation

- Presuctioning and postrespiratory assessment findings, including vital signs, breath sounds, coughing, secretions in the tube, etc.
- ET tube size and position
- Date, time, and frequency of the procedure
- Color, amount, consistency, and odor of secretions
- Comfort assessment and any specific interventions provided
- Findings of skin and oral assessment
- Interventions performed in oral care and for promotion of skin integrity
- Additional interventions necessary before, during, and after suctioning
- Child's response to suctioning and care
- Child and family education
- Unexpected outcomes and related treatment

References

1. Hazinski MF, et al, editors: *Pediatric advanced life support provider manual,* Dallas, 2002, American Heart Association.
2. Thompson A: Pediatric airway management. In Fuhrman B, Zimmerman J, editors: *Pediatric critical care,* ed 3, Philadelphia, 2005, Elsevier.
3. McCance K, Huether S: *Pathophysiology: the biologic bases for disease in adults and children,* Philadelphia, 2002, Mosby.
4. Thibodeau G, Patton K, editors: *Anatomy and physiology,* ed 5, Philadelphia, 2003, Mosby.
5. Ridling DA, et al: Endotracheal suctioning with or without instillation of isotonic sodium chloride solution in critically ill children, *Am J Crit Care* 12(3): 212-217, 2003.
6. Spence K, et al: Deep versus shallow suction of endotracheal tubes in ventilated neonates and young infants, *Cochrane Database Syst Rev* 3: 2003.
7. Simmons-Trau D: Reducing VAP with 6 Sigma, *Nurs Manage* 35(6):41-45, 2004.
8. Centers for Disease Control and Prevention: Guidelines for preventing health-care associated pneumonia, 2003: recommendations of the CDC and the Healthcare Infection Control Practices Advisory Committee, *MMWR Morbid Mortal Wkly Rep* 53(RR-3): 1-40, 2004.
9. Day T, et al: An evaluation of a teaching intervention to improve the practice of endotracheal suctioning in intensive care units, *J Clin Nurs* 10(5):682-696, 2001.
10. Wrightson DD: Suctioning smarter: answers to eight common questions about endotracheal suctioning in neonates, *Neonatal Network* 18(1):51-55, 1997.
11. Blackwood B: Normal saline instillation with endotracheal suctioning: primum non nocere (first do no harm), *J Adv Nurs* 27(4):728-734, 1997.
12. Marshall M, et al: Hydrogen peroxide: a review of its use in dentistry, *J Periodontol* 66:789-796, 1995.
13. Swartz K, et al: A national survey of endotracheal suctioning techniques in the pediatric population, *Heart Lung* 25(1):52-60, 1996.
14. Turner BS, Loan LA: Tracheobronchial trauma associated with airway management in neonates, *AACN Clin Issues: Adv Pract Acute Crit Care* 11(2):283-277, 2000.
15. Shibly O, et al: Clinical evaluation of a hydrogen peroxide mouth rinse, sodium chlorhexidine, for prophylaxis against oral infections and associated bicarbonate dentifrice and mouth moisturizer on oral health, *J Clin Dent* 8:145-149, 1997.
16. Akgül S, Akyolcu N: Effects of normal saline on endotracheal suctioning, *J Clin Nurs* 11(6):826-830, 2002.
17. Gemma M, et al: Intracranial effects of endotracheal suctioning in the acute phase of head injury, *J Neurosurg Anesthesiol* 14(1):50-54, 2002.
18. Baun MM, et al: Endotracheal suctioning: open versus closed with and without positive end-expiratory pressure, *Crit Care Nurs Q* 25(2):13-26, 2002.
19. Kerr ME, et al: Effect of endotracheal suctioning on cerebral oxygenation in traumatic brain-injured patients, *Crit Care Med* 27(12):2776-2781, 1999.
20. Curley MAQ, Thompson JE: Respiratory support. In Curley MAQ, Moloney-Harmon PA, editors: *Critical care nursing of infants and children,* Philadelphia, 2001, Saunders.
21. AARC Clinical Practice Guideline: Endotracheal suctioning of mechanically ventilated adults and children with artificial airways, *Respir Care* 38(5):500-504, 1993.
22. Day T, et al: Tracheal suctioning: an exploration of nurses' knowledge and competence in acute and high dependency ward areas, *J Adv Nurs* 39(1):35-45, 2002.
23. Choong K, et al: Comparison of loss in lung volume with open versus in-line catheter endotracheal suctioning, *Pediatr Crit Care Med* 4(1):69-73, 2003.
24. Paul-Allen J, Ostrow CL: Survey of nursing practices with closed-system suctioning, *Am J Crit Care* 9(1):9-19, 2000.
25. Fourrier F, et al: Colonization of dental plaque, a source of nosocomial infections in intensive care patients, *Crit Care Med* 26:432-437, 1998.
26. Garrouste-Orgeas M: Oropharyngeal or gastric colonization and nosocomial pneumonia in adult intensive care unit patients: a prospective study based on genomic DNA analysis, *Am J Respir Crit Care Med* 156:1647-1655, 1997.
27. Schleder B, et al: The effect of a comprehensive oral care protocol on patients at risk for ventilatory-associated pneumonia, *J Advocate Healthcare* 4(1):27-30, 2002.
28. Pritchard MA, et al: Systematic review of the role of pre-oxygenation for tracheal suctioning in ventilated newborn infants, *J Paediatr Child Health* 39(3):163-165, 2003.
29. Arnold JH: High-frequency ventilation in the pediatric intensive care unit, *Pediatr Crit Care Med* 1(2):93-99, 2000.
30. Pearson LS, Hutton JL: A controlled trial to compare the ability of foam swabs and toothbrushes to remove dental plaque, *J Adv Nurs* 37:480-487, 2002.

Additional Readings

Czarnik CE, et al: Differential effects of continuous versus intermittent suction on tracheal tissue, *Heart Lung* 20(2): 144-151, 1991.

Hazinski MF: Pulmonary disorders. In Hazinski MF, editor: *Manual of pediatric critical care,* St Louis, 1997, Mosby.

Schwenker D, et al: A survey of endotracheal suctioning with instillation of normal saline, *Am J Crit Care* 7(4):255-260, 1998.

Endotracheal Tube: Taping

PURPOSE: To ensure that the endotracheal (ET) tube remains secure

Dena L. Jarog

PREREQUISITE KNOWLEDGE

- Child development as it relates to clinical assessment and procedure
- Anatomy and physiology of the pediatric pulmonary system, including structural characteristics specific to the infant and child[1-4]
  - ❖ A child's airway is both absolutely and relatively smaller in diameter and shorter than an adult's (see Figure 1-1).
  - ❖ Because the thyroid does not assume its adult configuration until puberty, the cricoid cartilage is the easiest landmark for identification in children. The cricoid cartilage is the narrowest portion of the upper airway in children less than 10 years of age.
  - ❖ In teenagers and adults, the larynx is a cylinder with its narrowest portion at the glottic inlet at the level of the vocal cords.
  - ❖ The quantity of alveoli increases until 8 years of age and thereafter increases in size and complexity. Peripheral airway resistance is disproportionately higher in the child.
  - ❖ During inspiration, the infant's intercostal muscles stiffen and a downward movement of the diaphragm occurs, which results in negative intrathoracic pressure and air movement into the lungs. Because the infant's chest wall is compliant and flexible, it characteristically collapses inward (see Figure 23-1).
- Signs and symptoms of inadequate oxygenation and ventilation

- Mastery of pediatric advanced life support competencies, including indications for artificial airways and adjuncts used to support ventilation[5]

CHILD AND FAMILY ASSESSMENT

- Child's developmental level and ability to interact ➤*Rationale:* Influences preparation and interaction.
- Child's and family's understanding of the reasons for and risks and benefits of endotracheal tube taping ➤*Rationale:* Evaluates child's and family's understanding of the procedure and provides a gauge for ongoing education.
- Desire of family members to be present during the procedure ➤*Rationale:* The presence of family may provide comfort and support, although family members should have the choice not to remain with the child.
- Child's level of consciousness, anxiety, and activity ➤*Rationale:* Determines the need for a sedative or muscle relaxant before retaping.
- Inadequate oxygenation and ventilation ➤*Rationale:* Changes may indicate that the ET has migrated or been dislodged.
- Endotracheal tube security, including integrity of the tape and tube movement ➤*Rationale:* Indicates a need for resecuring or retaping the ET tube.
- Pressure areas and the skin around and under the tape and ET tube ➤*Rationale:* Identifies any skin breakdown or other possible areas of tissue compromise.

CHILD AND FAMILY EDUCATION

Individualized, developmentally appropriate education is provided to the family and to the child based on desire for knowledge, readiness to learn, and overall neurologic and psychosocial state.

- Explain the taping procedure, including the purpose, steps, and rationale ➤➤*Rationale:* Providing information decreases fear and anxiety.
- Encourage questions and answer questions as they arise ➤➤*Rationale:* Reinforcement of information is needed during periods of stress.

EQUIPMENT

- Personal protective equipment, including gloves and eye protection
- Adhesive skin preparation (e.g., tincture of benzoin)
- Skin barrier (e.g., Duoderm [Convatec, Bristol-Myers Squibb, Princeton, NJ])
- Cloth tape, 1-inch wide
- Gauze and water for cleaning of skin
- Manual ventilation bag (MVB; self-inflating or flow-inflating)
- Appropriately sized mask
- Stethoscope
- Tape measure
- Luer lock syringe (for cuffed tubes), 5 to 10 mL
- Premedications as indicated

Procedure for Endotracheal Tube: Taping

Steps	Rationale	Considerations
1. Ensure child and family understand procedure and questions are answered.	Evaluates and reinforces understanding of previously taught information.	Developmental, cognitive, and anxiety levels determine approach and effectiveness of teaching.
2. Gather needed equipment and supplies.	Facilitates completion of task in a timely manner.	
3. Monitor indications of inadequate oxygenation and ventilation during and after the procedure.	ET tube may migrate from correct position.	
4. Provide sedation, analgesia, and muscle relaxant as indicated.	Ensure that child is comfortable and does not move during the procedure. Flexion of head and neck moves the tube farther into airway, and extension of head displaces tube farther out of the airway.[5]	The medications used are child specific and depends on physiologic condition.
5. Wash hands.	Reduces transmission of infection. Protects personnel health.	
6. Cut the skin barrier to fit from the corner of the child's mouth to 2 cm from the angle of the jaw.[6] *(Level II*;* Figure 3-1)	If the skin barrier is loose, the tube may dislodge and cause airway trauma.	Several companies offer skin barrier materials (e.g., Duoderm [Convatec, Bristol-Myers Squibb, Princeton, NJ]).
7. Tear two pieces of white cloth adhesive tape to the appropriate length for the size of the child.	Cloth tape is used over other types because of its adhesive quality.[1,6] *(Level II*)*	
8. Tear each piece of tape in half lengthwise, with at least 1 to 1.5 inches left whole at the end.		The length of the skin barrier can be covered to allow for optimal adhesion of the tape. The piece of tape resembles a Y shape.
9. Assess lung sounds before securing or resecuring the ET tube.	Affirms placement of tube in the proper place.	
10. Put on gloves and other personal protective equipment as indicated.	Reduces transmission of infection. Protects personnel health.	

* Level II: Theory-based; no research data to support recommendations; recommendations from expert consesus group may exist

Procedure	**for Endotracheal Tube: Taping**—*Continued*	
Steps	**Rationale**	**Considerations**

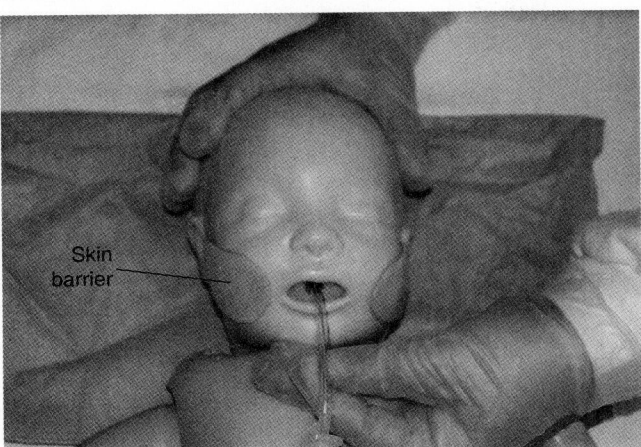 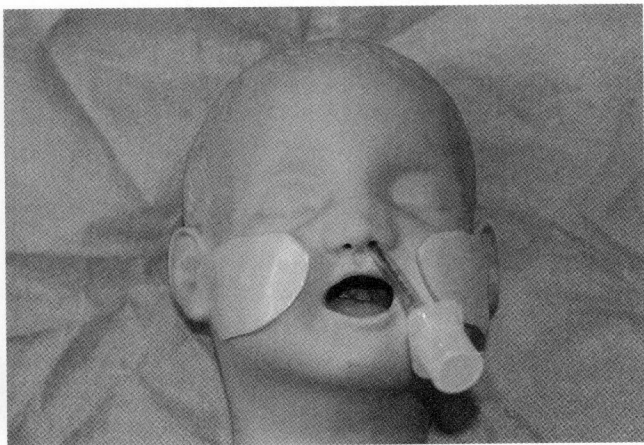

Skin barrier

A   B

FIGURE 3-1   **A,** Skin barrier for an oral ET tube. Tape is cut to fit from the corner of the mouth to 2 cm from the angle of the jaw. **B,** Skin barrier applied for a nasal ET tube.

11. If tube has been previously secured:
    Measure length of protruding tube from lip or nares to the cut end of tube.
    Remove old tape with care to avoid dislodging the tube.
	Provides ongoing monitoring of security of the ET tube.
	Confirms tube's location.
		Tape should be resecured as soon as it loosens. Fresh tape and fresh skin preparations are used with each change of tape.
		Distance marker from the lip or nares should be documented in medical record.

12. Assess skin of face, nares, and mouth for any breakdown or reddened areas.	Reduces skin breakdown and eliminates a potential source for infection.	ET tube can be moved from one side of mouth to the other to reduce chance of breakdown. *(Level II*)* Before a cuffed tube is moved, the cuff is deflated with a 5-mL to 10-mL syringe to prevent trauma.[1]
13. Clean and dry skin.	Reduces risk of skin breakdown. Improves tape adherence to the face.	
14. Paint upper lip, cheeks, and tube with adhesive skin preparations.	Protects the skin. Provides an optimal area for the tape adherence. *(Level II*)*	
15. After adhesive skin preparation dries to a sticky consistency, place precut skin barrier patches on the cheeks (Figure 3-1).		Allows for multiple applications and removal of tape without skin irritation.[6]
16. Paint patches with skin preparations and let them dry to a sticky consistency (Figure 3-2).		A thicker skin barrier (e.g., Duoderm) may stay in place longer than a liquid skin preparation.

17. Apply tape.
    Starting on one side of face, apply the whole end of tape to cover the prepared skin (Figure 3-3).
    Spiral top half of the split tape (Y portion) securely around the tube away from child, starting over the top of tube (Figure 3-4).
		With each spiral up the tube, tape must adhere to the tube rather than wrap over applied tape.

Procedure continues on following page

* Level II: Theory-based; no research data to support recommendations; recommendations from expert consesus group may exist

Procedure **for Endotracheal Tube: Taping**—*Continued*

Steps	Rationale	Considerations

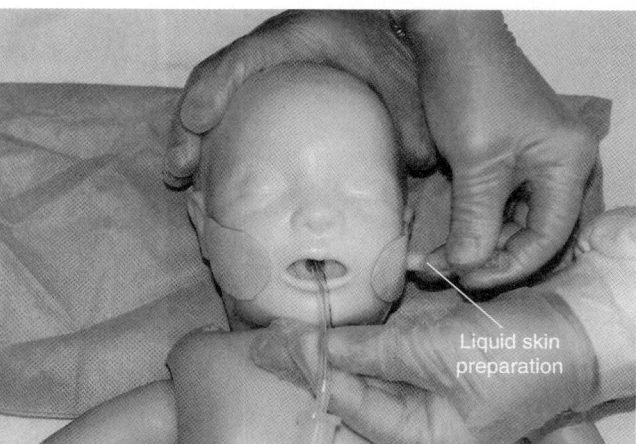

FIGURE 3-2   Painting of the liquid skin barrier for the securing of the oral ET tube.

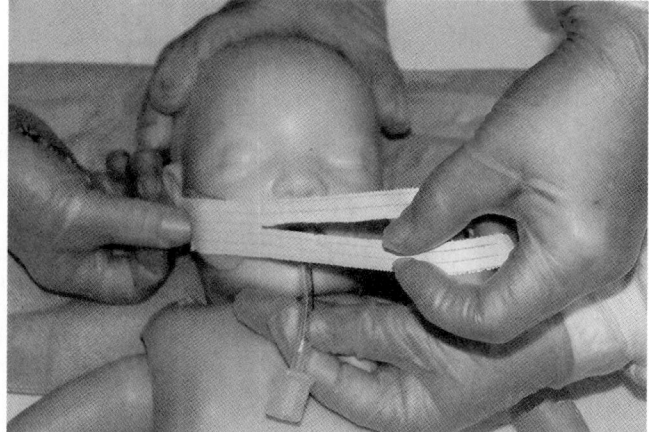

FIGURE 3-3   Application of the tape to the face for the securing of the oral ET tube.

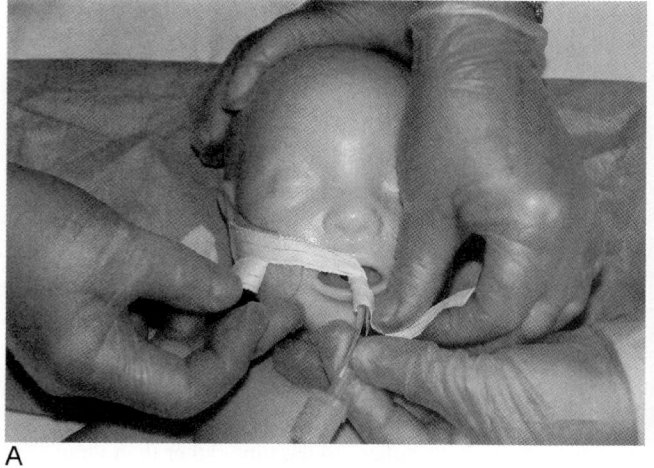
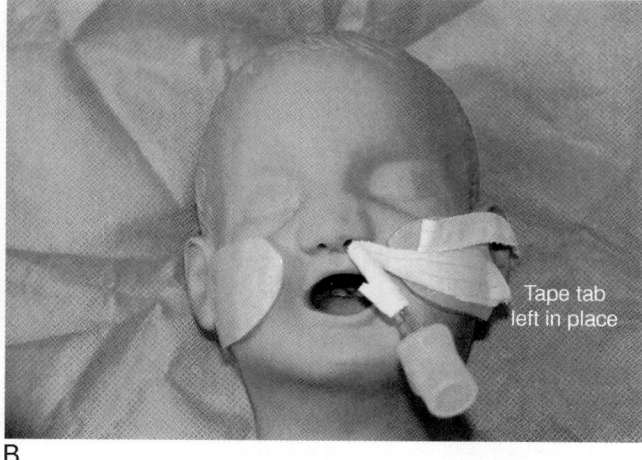

FIGURE 3-4   **A,** Spiraling of the tape on the tube for the securing of the oral ET tube. **B,** Spiraling of the tape on the tube for the nasal ET tube.

Procedure	for Endotracheal Tube: Taping—*Continued*	
Steps	**Rationale**	**Considerations**

Leave a piece of tape turned over at the end to aid removal.		
18. Secure bottom half of the split tape across the top lip of child, with extension to opposite cheek and on to prepared skin (Figure 3-5).	Bringing the bottom half of tape up and over the top half secures first piece to lip, keeping tube tight. *(Level II*)*	
19. With measuring tape, measure length of tube from the edge of lip to the cut end of tube.		Distance from the lip or nares should be documented in medical record.
20. Repeat steps 7 to 9 for opposite side of the face (Figure 3-6).		
21. Assess lung sounds.	Assures ET tube is in place and was not dislodged during procedure.	
22. Remove protective items and wash hands.	Reduces transmission of infection. Protects personnel health.	

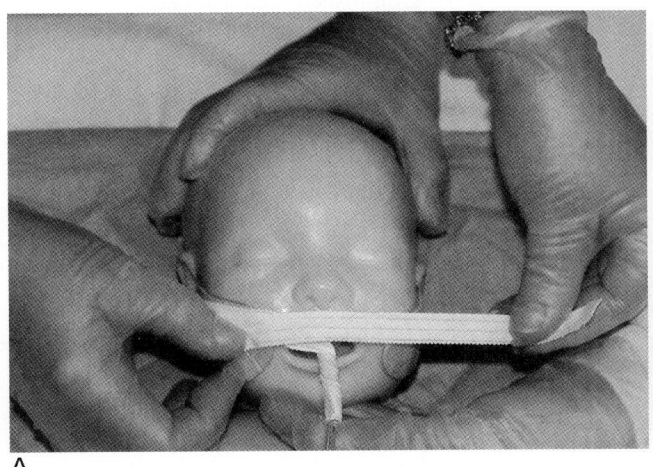
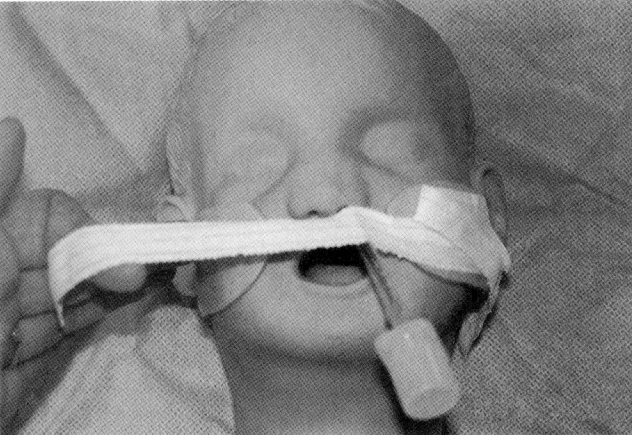

A   B

FIGURE 3-5   **A,** Securing of the tape on the cheek for the oral ET tube. **B,** Securing of the first piece of tape on the face.

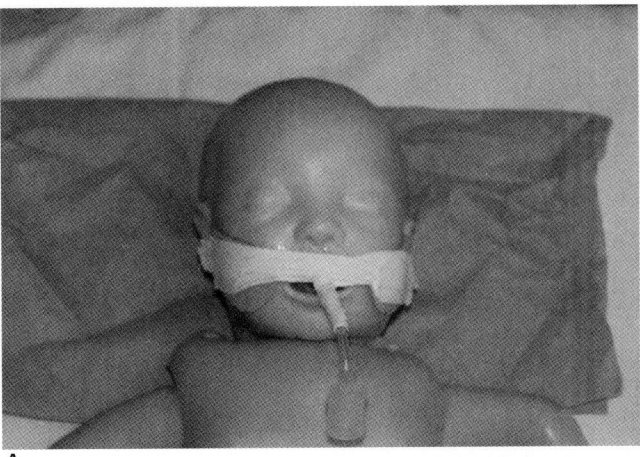
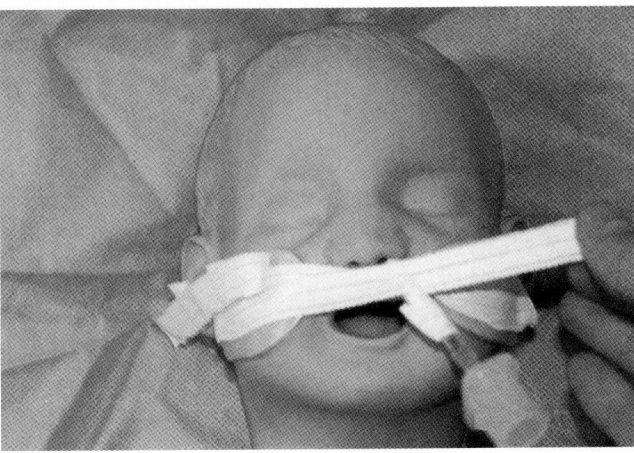

A   B

FIGURE 3-6   **A,** The ET tube is secured with tape. **B,** Securing of the second piece of tape on the opposite side of the face.

* Level II: Theory-based; no research data to support recommendations; recommendations from expert consesus group may exist

Expected Outcomes

- ET tube remains securely in place, and airway is maintained
- Adequate ventilation and oxygenation
- Skin integrity is intact
- Hemodynamic stability
- Acceptable level of comfort

Unexpected Outcomes

- Artificial airway migrates from correct position
- Inadequate oxygenation and ventilation
- Skin breakdown
- Hemodynamic instability
- Unmanaged pain and discomfort

Monitoring and Care of the Child

Activities and Interventions	Rationale	Reportable Conditions
1. Assess and care for skin, nares, and mouth.	Prevents breakdown and ulcerations of oral mucosal.	• Redness, open lesions • Necrosis, ulcerations • Trauma to lips, tongue, or mouth
2. Monitor security of the ET tube.	Assures that child is not inadvertently extubated.	• ET tube migration or dislodgement
3. Monitor oxygenation and ventilation.	ET tube may migrate during retaping.	• Significant changes in vital signs • Changes in skin color or skin temperature • Changes in level of consciousness • Diminished breath sounds • Increased work of breathing • A decrease in oxygen saturations or abnormal arterial or venous blood gases
4. Assess comfort and provide appropriate interventions. Allow the family to assist with nonpharmacologic comfort and to support the child.	Early identification of the child's comfort allows for immediate attention.	• Unresolved pain and discomfort • Continued irritability or changes in physiologic condition

Documentation

- Postprocedure physical assessment, including vital signs
- Size of ET tube and whether it is cuffed or uncuffed
- Position of ET tube: Left or right, mouth or nare, centimeter marking at gum line, lip or edge of nare
- Length of tube from lip or nare or gum line to cut of tube
- Findings of skin and oral assessment
- Comfort assessment and intervention if provided
- Child's response to procedure
- Additional interventions necessary
- Unexpected outcomes and related treatment
- Child and family education

References

1. Curley MAQ, Thompson JE: Oxygenation and ventilation. In Curley MAQ, Moloney-Harmon PA, editors: *Critical care nursing of infants and children,* Philadelphia, 2001, Saunders.
2. Thompson A: Pediatric airway management. In Fuhrman B, Zimmerman J, editors: *Pediatric critical care,* ed 3, Philadelphia, 2005, Elsevier.
3. McCance K, Huether S: *Pathophysiology: the biologic bases for disease in adults and children,* Philadelphia, 2002, Mosby.
4. Thibodeau G, Patton K, editors: *Anatomy and physiology,* ed 5, Philadelphia, 2003, Mosby.
5. Hazinski MF, et al, editors: *Pediatric advanced life support provider manual,* Dallas, 2002, American Heart Association.
6. Page NE, et al: Intubation complications in the critically ill child, *AACN Clin Issues Adv Pract Acute Crit Care* 9(1): 25-35, 1998.

Extubation: Assist

PURPOSE: Removal of the endotracheal tube (ET)

Amy C. Binck

PREREQUISITE KNOWLEDGE

- Child development as it relates to clinical assessment and extubation procedure
- Anatomy and physiology of the pediatric pulmonary system, including structural characteristics specific to the infant and child[1-4]
  - ❖ A child's airway is both absolutely and relatively smaller in diameter and shorter than an adult's (see Figure 1-1).
  - ❖ Because the thyroid does not assume its adult configuration until puberty, the cricoid cartilage is the easiest landmark for identification in children. The cricoid cartilage is the narrowest portion of the upper airway in children less than 10 years of age.
  - ❖ In teenagers and adults, the larynx is a cylinder with its narrowest portion at the glottic inlet at the level of the vocal cords.
  - ❖ The quantity of alveoli increases until 8 years of age and thereafter increases in size and complexity. Peripheral airway resistance is disproportionately higher in the child.
  - ❖ During inspiration, the infant's intercostal muscles stiffen and a downward movement of the diaphragm occurs, which results in negative intrathoracic pressure and air movement into the lungs. Because the infant's chest wall is compliant and flexible, it characteristically collapses inward (see Figure 23-1).
- Mastery of pediatric advanced life support competencies, including use of artificial airways, oxygen delivery systems, and principles of airway management[4]

- Signs and symptoms of inadequate oxygenation and ventilation
- Criteria for extubation include mechanical ventilation is no longer needed to maintain adequate oxygenation and ventilation, and resolution of the underlying condition that led to the need for an artificial airway. A specific ventilator weaning protocol and predictors of extubation success have not been developed for the heterogeneous pediatric population, therefore individualized assessment measures are necessary.[5,6]
- Complications of extubation, including hypoxemia and hypercapnia
- Complications of prolonged intubation, including sinusitis, vocal cord injury, laryngeal injury and stenosis, tracheal injury, and pulmonary infection[7]
- Medical interventions for immediate complications of extubation, including laryngospasm, bronchospasm, postextubation stridor, and hypoxia

CHILD AND FAMILY ASSESSMENT

- Child's developmental level and ability to interact ➜*Rationale:* Influences preparation and interaction.
- Child's and family's understanding of the reasons for and risks and benefits of extubation ➜*Rationale:* Evaluates child's and family's understanding of procedure and provides a gauge for ongoing education.
- Desire of family members to be present during the procedure ➜*Rationale:* The presence of family may provide

comfort and support, although family members should have the choice not to remain with the child.

- Duration and indication of intubation ➛➛*Rationale:* Assists determining whether the child is ready for extubation. Extubation failure rates may be disease specific.[5] Extubation should be considered at the earliest appropriate time when conditions for intubation have resolved.[7]
- Past history of preexisting respiratory conditions ➛➛*Rationale:* Preexisting respiratory conditions may predispose the child to extubation failure.[5]
- Neurologic status and level of consciousness ➛➛*Rationale:* Ensures that the desired level of consciousness is achieved before extubation.[7]
- Ability to maintain an airway, including the presence of cough and gag reflexes ➛➛*Rationale:* Assists in determining the child's ability to protect the airway and clear secretions.[1]
- Secretions, including amount, viscosity, and suctioning requirements ➛➛*Rationale:* Large amounts of secretions may make extubation more difficult and predispose the child to reintubation.
- Current level of ventilator support ➛➛*Rationale:* Assists in determining whether the child is ready for extubation.
- Work of breathing during minimal ventilator support ➛➛*Rationale:* Minimal ventilator assistance closely resembles independent breathing, and signs and symptoms of respiratory distress should be assessed.[8]
- Adequate oxygenation, hemodynamic stability, and the ability to initiate an inspiratory effort during a spontaneous breathing trial ➛➛*Rationale:* A spontaneous breathing trial in children who are undergoing mechanical ventilation for respiratory failure can help to determine the ability of the child to remain extubated.[9]
- Air leak around the endotracheal (ET) tube ➛➛*Rationale:* The incidence of postextubation stridor is highest in patients less than 7 years of age and those with an air leak around ET tube of more than 20 mm Hg.[10]
- Indications for administration of prophylactic corticosteroid ➛➛*Rationale:* Prophylactic administration of dexamethasone before elective extubation reduces the incidence rate of postextubation stridor in individual neonates and children.[11]
- Child's feeding status ➛➛*Rationale:* A child with a full stomach is predisposed to aspiration, and a regimen of nothing by mouth (NPO) for a minimum of 4 hours before extubation is recommended.

CHILD AND FAMILY EDUCATION

Individualized, developmentally appropriate education is provided to the family and to the child based on desire for knowledge, readiness to learn, and overall neurologic and psychosocial state.

- Explain the extubation procedure, including indications, criteria, steps, and rationale ➛➛*Rationale:* Providing information decreases fear and anxiety.
- Provide the rationale for the timing of NPO status before and following extubation ➛➛*Rationale:* The explanation alleviates fear and anxiety regarding holding nutrition and gives anticipatory guidance regarding the expected time of NPO status.
- Explain the expected outcomes after extubation, including possible stridor and continued need for supplemental oxygen ➛➛*Rationale:* Postextubation stridor may occur and may be frightening to the child and family.
- Discuss the possibility of reintubation ➛➛*Rationale:* Provides anticipatory guidance in the event of reintubation.
- Discuss the importance of suctioning, coughing, and deep breathing exercises after extubation ➛➛*Rationale:* Encourages cooperation and augments the care necessary to maintain airway and clear secretions.
- Explain that the child's voice may be hoarse after extubation ➛➛*Rationale:* Provides anticipatory guidance and minimizes child and family fear and anxiety in the event of sore throat and difficulty with vocalization.
- Encourage questions and answer questions as they arise ➛➛*Rationale:* Reinforcement of information is needed during periods of stress and is especially important given the emergent nature of the procedure.

EQUIPMENT

- Personal protective equipment, including gloves
- Oxygen source
- High-volume suction source
- Appropriately sized wide-bore rigid pharyngeal suction tip catheter
- Appropriately sized pliable tracheal suction catheters of a size to fit the ET tube
- Appropriately sized manual ventilation system (self-inflating or flow-inflating)
- Appropriately sized mask
- Appropriately sized oral and pharyngeal airways
- Translaryngeal intubation equipment (laryngoscope blades, handles, batteries, and stylettes)
- ET tubes of various sizes
- Pulse oximeter
- Supplies for arterial puncture and blood gas analysis (as indicated)
- Oxygen delivery equipment, including nasal cannula, oxygen mask, or hood
- Scissors
- 10-mL syringe
- Stethoscope
- Emergency cart available

Procedure for Extubation: Assist

Steps	Rationale	Considerations
1. Ensure child and family understand procedure and questions are answered.	Evaluates and reinforces understanding of previously taught information	Developmental, cognitive, and anxiety levels determine the approach and effectiveness of teaching.
2. Assess environment.	Extubation should occur in an environment in which child can be appropriately monitored and in which emergency medical equipment is available.[7]	
3. Gather needed equipment and supplies.	Facilitates completion of task in a timely manner.	
4. Monitor child's vital signs and indications of inadequate oxygenation and ventilation.	Identifies signs and symptoms of respiratory insufficiency.	Pulse oximetry is often used to continuously monitor oxygen saturations (SpO_2) to provide an indication of gas exchange. Consider arterial or venous blood gases when indicated.
5. Raise head of bed at least 45 degrees unless contraindicated by the child's condition. A small padding may be placed under the shoulders of child.	Respiratory muscles are more effective in an upright position. This position facilitates clearing of secretions and reduces risk of aspiration if vomiting occurs. Padding under shoulders maintains the head in the "sniffing" position to keep airway open.	Infants and small children may be supported with pillows to achieve the appropriate position.
6. Wash hands and put on personal protective equipment.	Reduces transmission of infection. Protects personnel health.	
7. Hyperoxygenate and suction ET tube and pharynx.	Hyperoxygenation increases arterial oxygen levels in preparation for extubation. Hyperinflation assists in mobilization and removal of secretions. Removes secretions.	Hyperinflation volumes of 100% to 150% have been recommended. Hyperoxygenation with 100% FiO_2 is not recommended for children with certain congenital heart defects and with hypoxic respiratory drive.
8. Assist with removal of tape used to secure the ET tube.	Frees tracheal tube from child's face for easier removal.	
9. Support and encourage child during extubation.	Provides reassurance and comfort for child during extubation.	
10. Assess lung sounds and work of breathing after extubation.	The child is especially vulnerable to respiratory insufficiency in the immediate period after extubation.	
11. Encourage child to cough and deep breath as developmentally appropriate.	Promotes hyperinflation and helps remove secretions	Nasopharyngeal and oropharyngeal suctioning may be used to help stimulate cough in younger child or in children who cannot follow commands.

Procedure continues on following page

Procedure for Extubation: Assist—*Continued*

Steps	Rationale	Considerations
12. Administer supplemental oxygen and aerosolized respiratory treatments as indicated.	Helps to prevent hypoxemia.	Cool humidification may be used to help minimize upper airway swelling. Racemic epinephrine treats upper airway edema and stridor.[12]
13. Remove protective items and wash hands.	Reduces transmission of infection. Protects personnel health.	

Expected Outcomes

- Atraumatic extubation
- Adequate oxygenation and ventilation without artificial airway
- Maintenance of energy and ability to breath spontaneously
- Acceptable level of comfort for child

Unexpected Outcomes

- Trauma to airway
- Inadequate oxygenation and ventilation that necessitate reintubation
- Laryngospasm
- Fatigue from increased work of breathing that necessitates reintubation
- Unmanaged pain

Monitoring and Care of the Child

Activities and Interventions	Rationale	Reportable Conditions
1. Assess vital signs, oxygenation and ventilation indices, and oxygen requirements.	Changes in vital signs after extubation may indicate respiratory deterioration and necessitate reintubation. The child's ability to effectively breathe may change without an artificial airway.	• Tachycardia • Tachypnea • Blood pressure of more than 110% of baseline • Oxygen saturation of less than 92% • Increased work of breathing, including grunting, nasal flaring, and retractions • Cyanosis • Irritability
2. Assess lung sounds before and after extubation.	For assessment of air movement, symmetric breath sounds, and adventitious sounds.	• Asymmetric air entry • Stridor • Wheezing
3. Continually assess comfort and level of consciousness.	Irritability and fatigue are signs of respiratory compromise. Early identification of the child's comfort allows for immediate attention.	• Significant irritability • Decreased level of consciousness • Reduced response to pain • Unresolved pain and discomfort • Changes in physiologic condition
4. Provide supplemental oxygen and aerosolized medications as needed.	Decreases incidence rate of oxygen desaturation immediately after extubation.	• Hypoxemia despite supplemental oxygen
5. Encourage coughing, deep breathing, and early mobilization as developmentally and medically appropriate.	Prevents atelectasis and secretion accumulation.	• Ineffective cough
6. Suction the oropharynx after extubation as needed.	Assists in clearing of secretions and prevents secretion accumulation.	• Inability to handle secretions

Documentation

- Preextubation and postextubation assessment findings including vital signs, breath sounds, coughing, and additional signs of adequate oxygenation and ventilation
- Date and time of extubation
- Comfort assessment, including specific interventions provided
- Child's response to extubation
- Unexpected outcomes after extubation with related treatments
- Additional interventions necessary before, during, and after extubation
- Child and family education

References

1. Curley MQ, Thompson JE: Oxygenation and ventilation. In Curley MQ, Moloney-Harmon PA, editors: *Critical care nursing of infants and children,* Philadelphia, 2001, Saunders.
2. Thompson A: Pediatric airway management. In Fuhrman B, Zimmerman J, editors: *Pediatric critical care,* ed 3, Philadelphia, 2005, Elsevier.
3. McCance K, Huether S: *Pathophysiology: the biologic bases for disease in adults and children,* Philadelphia, 2002, Mosby.
4. Hazinski MF, et al, editors: *Pediatric advanced life support provider manual,* Dallas, 2002, American Heart Association.
5. Kurachek SC, et al: Extubation failure in pediatric intensive care: a multiple-center study of risk factors and outcomes, *Pediatr Crit Care Med* 31(11):2657-2664, 2003.
6. Randolph AG, et al: Effect of mechanical ventilator weaning protocols on respiratory outcomes in infants and children: a randomized controlled trial, *JAMA* 288(20):2561-2568, 2002.
7. AARC Clinical Practice Guideline: Removal of the endotracheal tube, *Respir Care* 44 (1):85-90, 1999.
8. Manczur TI, et al: Comparison of predictors of extubation from mechanical ventilation in children, *Pediatr Crit Care Med* 1(1):28-32, 2000.
9. Evidence-based guidelines for weaning and discontinuing ventilatory support; a collective task force facilitated by the American College of Chest Physicians, the American Association for Respiratory Care, and the American College of Critical Care Medicine, *Respir Care* 47(1):69-90, 2002.
10. Mhanna MJ, et al: The "air leak" test around the endotracheal tube, as a predictor of postextubation stridor, is age dependent in children, *Crit Care Med* 30(12):2639-2643, 2002.
11. Markovitz BP, Randolph AG: Corticosteroids for the prevention of reintubation and postextubation stridor in pediatric patients: a meta-analysis, *Pediatr Crit Care Med* 3(30):223-226, 2002.
12. Davies MW, Davis PG: Nebulized racemic epinephrine for extubation of newborn infants, *Cochrane Database System Rev* (2):CD000506, 2000.

Additional Reading

Popernack ML, et al: Decreasing unplanned extubations: utilization of the Penn State Children's Hospital Sedation Algorithm, *Pediatr Crit Care Med* 5(1):58-62, 2004.

Intubation: Assist

PURPOSE: An endotracheal tube (ET) is placed into the trachea via the oral or nasal route to maintain airway patency, facilitate clearance of secretions, enable positive pressure ventilation, and provide a route for emergency medication delivery

Amy C. Binck

PREREQUISITE KNOWLEDGE

- Child development as it relates to clinical assessment and intubation procedure
- Anatomy and physiology of the pediatric pulmonary system, including structural characteristics specific to the infant and child[1-4]
  - ❖ A child's airway is both absolutely and relatively smaller in diameter and shorter than an adult's (see Figure 1-1).
  - ❖ The child's funnel-shaped larynx is higher and more cephalad and lies below the vocal cords. The vocal cords are 50% cartilage and are attached lower and more anteriorly.
  - ❖ The infant's epiglottis is floppy, long, and narrow and projects more posteriorly than that of the older child. The subglottic airway is smaller and more compliant, with the cartilage less developed than in the adult.
  - ❖ The cricoid cartilage is the easiest and the only landmark for identification in children because the thyroid does not assume its adult configuration until puberty. The cricoid cartilage is the narrowest portion of the upper airway in children less than 10 years of age.
  - ❖ In teenagers and adults, the larynx is a cylinder with its narrowest portion at the glottic inlet at the level of the vocal cords.
  - ❖ The quantity of alveoli increases until 8 years of age and thereafter increases in size and complexity. Peripheral airway resistance is disproportionately higher in the child.
  - ❖ During inspiration, the infant's intercostal muscles stiffen and a downward movement of the diaphragm occurs, which results in negative intrathoracic pressure and air movement into the lungs. Because the infant's chest wall is compliant and flexible, it characteristically collapses inward (see Figure 23-1).
- Mastery of pediatric advanced life support competencies, including principles of an artificial airway establishment (such as bag-mask ventilation, oropharyngeal suctioning, and proper positioning) and oxygen delivery systems[1]
- Principles of gas exchange
- Signs and symptoms of inadequate oxygenation and ventilation
- Indications for intubation, including upper airway obstruction, apnea, ineffective clearance of secretions, and high risk of aspiration and respiratory distress
- Indications and contraindications of each route of intubation: oral and nasal

  Two types of resuscitation bags are commonly used for manual ventilation: a self-inflating manual resuscitator and a flow-inflating manual resuscitator. Although both resuscitators serve the same purpose, differences are seen in technique (see Procedure 27).[1,5-8]
- Physiologic effects of laryngoscopy and intubation
- Predictors of difficult intubations
- Principles of airway and ventilator management
- Blood gas analysis
- Pharmacologic approach and indications for intubation techniques, including awake, sedated without paralyzing agents, and anesthetized intubations

❖ In the in-hospital setting a cuffed endotracheal (ET) tube is as safe as an uncuffed tube for infants beyond the newborn period and in children.[9] Cuffed tubes are typically used for children older than 8 to 10 years of age and for smaller children who need high inspiratory pressures.[1,10] The narrowest segment of the small child's airway is the cricoid ring. Cuffed tubes in young children may contribute to subglottic damage if the pressure exerted by the tube or cuff exceeds mucosal capillary pressure. Keep cuff inflation pressure < 20 cm H_2O.[9] As long as the cuff is closely monitored, cuffed tubes have not been shown to have greater complication rates than uncuffed tubes.[11-13]

❖ An appropriately sized mask provides a tight seal and fits to extend from the bridge of the nose to the cleft of the chin, encompassing the mouth and nose but keeping away from the eyes[1] (see Figure 8-1).

❖ Orotracheal intubation is preferred, especially in an emergency situation, because this approach is usually accomplished more quickly than the nasal approach.[1]

❖ Several methods are used in determination of ET tube size (internal diameter)[1,3]:

❖ For children less than 1 year of age, the following sizes are recommended: premature infant, 2.5 to 3.0; newborn, 3.0; newborn to 6 months, 3.5; 6 to 12 months, 3.5 to 4.0 ET tube size is more reliably based on a child's body length. Length-based resuscitation tapes are helpful for children up to approximately 35 kg.[9]

❖ For children older than 2 years of age, the following formulas can be used:
  ○ For uncuffed tubes: 16 + age(yr)/4
  ○ For cuffed tubes: age(yr)/1.1+3/4

• Complications of intubation, including sinusitis, vocal cord injury, laryngeal injury and stenosis, tracheal injury, and pulmonary infection[14]

❖ Head position affects ET tube position. Neck flexion results in the tip of the tube moving closer to the carina, whereas extension of the neck withdraws the tube toward the glottis.

❖ If an intubated patient's condition deteriorates, consider the following possibilities (DOPE)
  ○ Displacement of the tube from the trachea
  ○ Obstruction of the tube
  ○ Pneumothorax
  ○ Equipment failure

CHILD AND FAMILY ASSESSMENT

• Child's developmental level and ability to interact ➤➤*Rationale:* Influences preparation and interaction.

• Child's and family's understanding of the reasons for and risks and benefits of intubation[1] ➤➤*Rationale:* Evaluates child's and family's understanding of the procedure and provides a gauge for ongoing education.

• Desire of family members to be present during the procedure ➤➤*Rationale:* The presence of family may provide comfort and support, although family members should have the choice not to remain with the child.

• Level of anxiety, consciousness, and respiratory compromise ➤➤*Rationale:* Determines the need for sedation or paralytic agents and the child's ability to lie supine for intubation.

• Last enteral intake of food or liquids ➤➤*Rationale:* Children with a full stomach are at risk for aspiration of gastric contents during airway manipulation.

• Presence of head injury and history of trauma ➤➤*Rationale:* Laryngoscopy causes increased intracranial pressure (ICP) and may change the pharmacologic approach to intubation.

• Presence of cervical spine injury ➤➤*Rationale:* In-line cervical stabilization is used during intubation to prevent further neurologic injury during laryngoscopy.

• Presence of hypovolemia ➤➤*Rationale:* Fluid resuscitation may be necessary to prevent cardiovascular collapse.

• Presence of respiratory failure and hemodynamic instability ➤➤*Rationale:* Hemodynamic instability may accompany respiratory failure. Existing hemodynamic instability may become worse with sedation from loss of sympathetic tone. The pharmacologic approach should be individualized.

• Presence of intravenous (IV) access ➤➤*Rationale:* IV access is important in the delivery of medications and IV fluids if needed for intubation.

CHILD AND FAMILY EDUCATION

Individualized, developmentally appropriate education is provided to the family and to the child based on desire for knowledge, readiness to learn, and overall neurologic and psychosocial state.

• Explain the intubation procedure, including rationale and risks ➤➤*Rationale:* Information decreases fear and anxiety.

• Provide anticipatory guidance related to expected duration of intubation ➤➤*Rationale:* Guidance allows the parents to gauge the child's progress in recovery to independent respiratory functioning.

• Discuss appropriate expected outcomes of intubation ➤➤*Rationale:* Allows the family and medical team to formulate similar goals and expectations.

• Explain that the child will be unable to speak while the ET tube is in place ➤➤*Rationale:* Providing information decreases anxiety and fear.

• Explain that pharmacologic sedation and immobilization interventions may be necessary for the safety of the child and for prevention of accidental tube dislodgment and that such interventions are used only as necessary ➤➤*Rationale:* Pharmacologic agents and immobilization interventions may be necessary to ensure safety and secure position of the ET tube.

• Review the adjunct monitoring and support that ensues after intubation, such as blood gas sampling, ventilator assistance, and chest radiographs ➤➤*Rationale:* Provides assistance and guidance to the family in understanding a new plan of care and medical interventions.

- Explain the sensory implications of an airway in the nose or mouth ➤➤**Rationale:** Anticipatory guidance helps decrease anxiety and fear.
- Encourage questions and answer questions as they arise ➤➤**Rationale:** Reinforcement of information is needed during periods of stress and is especially important given the emergent nature of the procedure.

EQUIPMENT

- Personal protective equipment
- Suction equipment, including wall suction
- Wide-bore rigid pharyngeal tonsil tip suction catheter
- Pliable suction catheter of appropriate size
- Appropriately sized manual ventilation bag (self-inflating or flow-inflating)
- Oxygen source
- Appropriately sized mask
- Oropharyngeal airway or bite block
- Laryngoscope blade (Miller-straight or Macintosh-curved) with working light source (see Figure 15-1, A-B)
- Appropriate ET tubes: one tube the estimated necessary size, one tube 0.5 mm smaller, and one tube 0.5 mm larger (see Figure 15-2, A-B)
- Appropriately sized stylet
- Laryngoscope handle with batteries
- Magill forceps for nasal intubation or for removal of foreign body

- Luer-tip syringe for cuff inflation with a cuffed ET tube
- Tape
- Stethoscope
- Appropriate monitoring equipment, including continuous pulse oximetry, continuous cardiac monitor, appropriately sized blood pressure cuff, and end tidal carbon dioxide monitor (ETCO$_2$) or ETCO$_2$ detector cap
- Appropriate intubation and emergency medications
- Adhesive solution
- Anesthetic spray or local anesthetic jelly (nasal ET tube placement)

Pharmacologic Approach

The pharmacologic approach to intubation depends on numerous factors and may range from no pharmacologic intervention to induction of anesthesia. A flaccid child in cardiopulmonary arrest who needs intubation does not need pharmacologic interventions to achieve appropriate conditions for intubation. Alternatively, children with severe head trauma or those at risk of aspiration need an individualized pharmacologic approach. Although numerous medication combinations exist for intubation, they all fall into the categories of providing amnesia, sedation, or muscle paralysis or drugs that modulate the physiologic response to intubation. Consult a drug formulary before administration of any medications to review the appropriate dosage, route, and side effects. The timing of administration in relation to intubation is also highly individualized and depends on the child's hemodynamic status, risk of aspiration, and indication for intubation (see Table 15-2).

Procedure | for Intubation: Assist

Steps	Rationale	Considerations
1. Ensure child and family understand procedure and questions are answered. Obtain a signed consent if procedure is not emergent.	Evaluates and reinforces understanding of previously taught information. Ensures medical-legal compliance, as suggested by the Joint Commision on Accreditation Healthcare Organization (JCAHO).	Developmental, cognitive, and anxiety levels determine approach and effectiveness of teaching. Given the often emergent nature of intubation, the procedure explanation may be delayed.
2. Gather needed equipment and supplies.	Facilitates completion of task in a timely manner.	This step may occur as child is positioned.
3. Wash hands.	Reduces transmission of infection. Protects personnel health.	
4. Throughout the procedure, monitor child's vital signs, and check for indications of inadequate oxygenation and ventilation before, during, and after the procedure.	Hypoxia and bradycardia are possible complications of direct laryngoscopy, and hypotension may result from underlying hemodynamic instability or medication administration.	This step is especially important after medications are administered and as tube is placed before the airway is secured. Alert others to signs of deterioration. Pulse oximetry is often used to

Procedure for Intubation: Assist—*Continued*		
Steps	**Rationale**	**Considerations**
		continuously monitor oxygen saturations to provide an indication of gas exchange. Consider arterial or venous blood gases as indicated.
5. Calculate and prepare dosages of selected medications (see Table 15-2).	Modulates physiologic response to intubation.	The pharmacologic approach to intubation depends on numerous factors and may range from no pharmacologic intervention to induction of anesthesia. Intubation drugs often include those that provide amnesia, sedation, or muscle paralysis.
6. Put on gloves and personal protective equipment.	Reduces transmission of infection. Protects personnel health.	Protective eyewear is worn to prevent exposure to secretions.
7. Ensure suction apparatus is functional. Connect suction tubing to rigid suction-tip catheter. Have pliable suction catheters available.	Prepares for oropharyngeal suctioning as needed.	
8. Assist in positioning the child's head[10]: Position child supine so that oropharyngolaryngeal axes are aligned (see Figure 15-4, *A*). *Infant:* Head in neutral position. *Older child:* Elevate occiput to sniffing position and extend head at atlantooccipital joint (see Figure 15-4, *B*). *Suspected or confirmed spinal cord injury:* Maintain head in a neutral position with in-line cervical spine immobilization (see Figure 15-4, *C*).	Aligns axes for visualization of vocal cords. The infant's proportionately large occiput raises the head to align axes. Extension of the head without elevation of occiput anteriorly rotates the larynx. Prevents secondary injury.	Given the urgency that often occurs with intubation, this step may be done simultaneously with other steps. For infant, padding under torso may provide proper alignment of mouth, trachea, and pharynx.[1] Hyperextension is not typically necessary. A pillow under child's head may help with positioning. Neck flexion and extension should only be performed if neck trauma is not suspected.
9. Administer intubation medications as indicated.	Modulates physiologic response to intubation.	Sequencing and timing of drug administration is situational and child dependent.
10. Assist in preoxygenation with a bag-valve-mask device attached to oxygen source for 3 to 5 minutes (see Procedure 27).	Helps prevent hypoxemia.	For successful preoxygenation, airway must first be opened and a sufficient volume administered to ensure chest rise.[1] Hyperoxygenation with 100% FiO_2 is not recommended for children with certain congenital heart defects and with hypoxic respiratory drive.
11. Apply cricoid pressure (Sellick maneuver) as directed by the person performing the intubation (Figure 5-1).	Occludes esophagus by compressing the cricoid cartilage posterior against the vertebral body. May decrease incidence rate of passive regurgitation of stomach contents into the trachea and gastric distention during intubation.[15,16]	Cricoid pressure is initiated when the child is paralyzed and continued until the tube is placed in the trachea, with pressure maintained throughout intubation. Reflux regurgitation can occur when cricoid pressure is released.

Procedure continues on following page

Procedure | **for Intubation: Assist**—*Continued*

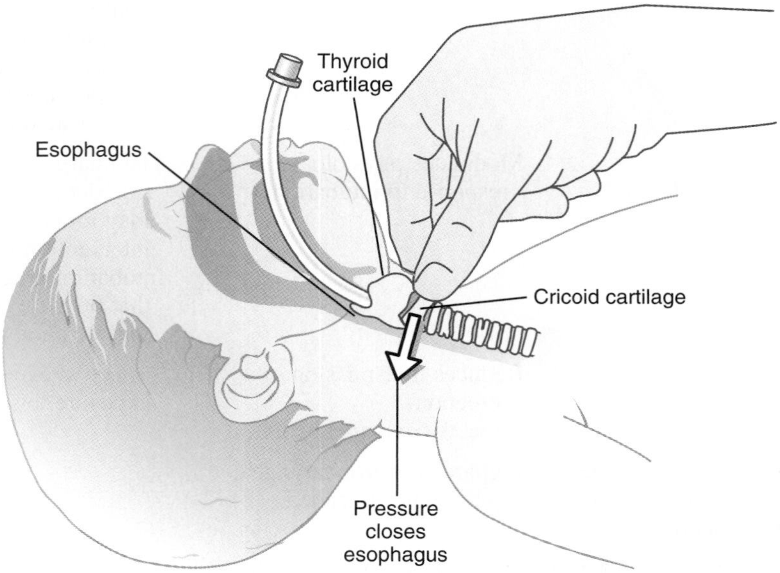

Steps	Rationale	Considerations

FIGURE 5-1   Sellick maneuver for cricoid pressure during endotracheal intubation.

Steps	Rationale	Considerations
12. Once tube is placed, assess lung fields.	Assesses for air movement, symmetric breath sounds, and adventitious sounds.	
13. Assess for air leak around ET tube.[13] Place stethoscope on the anterior neck overlying trachea with child's head in neutral position. With an aneroid manometer connected to ventilation bag, give positive pressure ventilation while auscultating for an air leak.	Assists in determination of whether tracheal tube size is correct. Inspiratory pressure at which air leaks around tube is the air leak, measured in centimeters of water (H_2O).	Maintenance of an air leak of 20 to 25 cm H_2O is desired and may reduce postextubation stridor in older children.[13] Absence of an air leak may indicate that tracheal tube is too large, that tube cuff is excessively inflated, or that laryngospasm is occurring.[1]
14. Assist with securing ET tube once it is in the correct position (see Procedure 3).	Securing artificial airway is a priority once airway is established.	
15. Remove protective items and wash hands.	Reduces transmission of infection. Protects personnel health.	
16. Confirm correct tube placement through primary and secondary means. (*Level II**)	Confirmation of placement is a critical step in establishment of an artificial airway.	ETCO$_2$ monitoring also has been used for verification of ET tube placement.[1,17-19] Chest radiograph is the definitive confirmation of correct ET tube placement.[1]

* Level II: Theory-based; no research data to support recommendations; recommendations from expert consensus group may exist

Expected Outcomes	Unexpected Outcomes
• Placement of a patent, correctly positioned and sized ET tube	• Intubation of esophagus or main stem bronchus
	• Large air leak around ET tube that indicates the tube size is too small
• Properly secured ET tube	• Migration of ET tube
• Improved oxygenation and ventilation	• Inadequate oxygenation and ventilation
• Decreased work of breathing	• Hypoxemia from inappropriate bag or mask ventilation technique or poor intubation skills
• Improved secretion clearance	• Aspiration
• Hemodynamic stability	• Hemodynamic instability from medications or vagal stimulation
• No traumatic injury	• Vocal cord or tracheal trauma
	• Broken teeth
• Acceptable level of comfort	• Unmanaged pain and discomfort

Monitoring and Care of the Child

Activities and Interventions	Rationale	Reportable Conditions
1. Assess lung sounds immediately after intubation, every 2 to 4 hours, and with changes in status.	Allows for detection of tube migration or dislodgment.	• Absent, decreased, or unequal breath sounds
2. Record position of tube at lip or nose with centimeter markings on tube as a reference.	Allows identification of tube migration or dislodgement.	• Tube movement from original position
3. Continually assess ET stability and integrity of the tape.	Prevents movement and dislodgement of the tube.	• Unplanned extubation • Poor tape integrity necessitating retaping
4. If present, assess ET tube cuff pressure every 4 hours and maintain the cuff pressure at less than 20 mm Hg.	Inflate the cuff to the minimal pressure necessary to seal an air leak and allow effective ventilation. High cuff pressures may precipitate tracheal damage	• Cuff pressure >20 mm Hg
5. Hyperoxygenate and suction the ET tube as needed (see Procedure 2).	Prevents obstruction of ET tube	• Inability to pass a suction catheter through the ET tube • Significant changes in the amount or character of secretions
6. After intubation, assess comfort and provide appropriate interventions; allow family to assist with non-pharmacologic means to comfort and support child.	Early identification of the child's comfort allows for immediate attention	• Unresolved pain and discomfort • Continued irritability or changes in physiologic condition

Documentation

- Preintubation and postintubation respiratory assessment findings, including vital signs, breath sounds, coughing, and tracheal secretions in tube
- Route of intubation: oral or nasal
- Size of ET tube and presence of cuff
- Medications given for intubation
- Confirmation of tube placement with indication of how placement was confirmed and depth of ET tube insertion (centimeters at lipline or nose)
- Presence of a leak
- Comfort assessment and any specific interventions provided
- Child's response to procedure
- Additional interventions necessary before, during, and after intubation
- Child and family education
- Unexpected outcomes and related interventions

References

1. Hazinski MF, et al, editors: *Pediatric advanced life support provider manual,* Dallas, 2002, American Heart Association.
2. Curley MAQ, Thompson J: Oxygenation and ventilation, In Curley MAQ, Moloney-Harmon P, editors: *Nursing care of critically ill infants and children,* ed 2, Philadelphia, 2001, Saunders.
3. Thompson A: Pediatric airway management. In Fuhrman B, Zimmerman J, editors: *Pediatric critical care,* ed 3, Philadelphia, 2005, Elsevier.
4. McCance K, Huether S: *Pathophysiology: the biologic bases for disease in adults and children,* Philadelphia, 2002, Mosby.
5. Trimble T: Using anesthesia bags, *Emerg Nursing World,* no date, accessed August 3, 2005, from http://www.enw.org/A-Bags.htm
6. American Academy of Pediatrics: Parts of a flow inflating bag, video 2, no date, accessed August 3, 2005, from http://www.aap.org/nrp/educational/educational_cdvideos_02.html
7. American Academy of Pediatrics: Parts of a self inflating bag, video 3, no date, accessed Aug 3, 2005, from http://www.aap.org/nrp/educational/educational_cdvideos_03.html
8. Hussey S., et al: Comparison of three manual ventilation devices using an intubated mannequin, *Arch Dis Child Fetal Neonatal Edition* 89(6):F490-493, 2004.
9. 2005 American Heart Association Guidelines for Cardiopulmonary Resuscitation and Emergency Cardiovascular Care, Supplement to *Circulation.* 2005; 112(24).
10. Deakers TW, et al: Cuffed tracheal tubes in pediatric intensive care, *J Pediatr* 125:57-62, 1994.
11. Westhorpe RN: The position of the larynx in children and its relationship to the ease of intubation, *Anaesth Intensive Care* 15:384-388, 1987.
12. Khine HH, et al: Comparison of cuffed and uncuffed endotracheal tubes in young children during general anesthesia, *Anesthesiology* 86(3):627-631, 1997.
13. Mhanna MJ, et al: The "air leak" test around the endotracheal tube, as a predictor of post extubation stridor, is age dependent in children, *Crit Care Med* 30(12):2639-2643, 2002.
14. AARC Clinical Practice Guideline: Removal of the endotracheal tube, *Respir Care* 44(1):85-90, 1999.
15. Moynihan RJ, et al: The effect of cricoid pressure on preventing gastric insufflation in infants and children, *Anesthesiology* 78:652-656, 1993.
16. Sellick BA: Cricoid pressure to control regurgitation of stomach contents during induction of anesthesia, *Lancet* 2:404-406, 1961.
17. Bhende MS, et al: Utility of an end-tidal carbon dioxide detector during stabilization and transport of critically ill children, *Pediatrics* 89:1042-1044, 1992.
18. Bhende MS, Alledn WD: Evaluation of a Capno-Flo resuscitator during transport of critically ill children, *Pediatr Emerg Care* 18(6):414-416, 2002.
19. Ward K, Yealy D: End-tidal carbon dioxide monitoring in emergency medicine, part 1: basic principles *Acad Emerg Med* 5:628-638, 1998.

Additional Readings

Guidelines 2000 for Cardiopulmonary Resuscitation and Emergency Cardiovascular Care: International Consensus on Science: Adjuncts to oxygenation, ventilation and airway control, *Circulation* 102(Suppl):95-104, 2000.

Newth CJ, et al: The use of cuffed versus uncuffed endotracheal tubes in pediatric intensive care, *J Pediatr* 144(3):333-337, 2004.

Sanders KC, et al: End tidal CO_2 detection in emergency intubation of four groups of patients, *J Emerg Med* 12:771-777, 1994.

Schaller R: Comparison of a colorimetric end-tidal CO_2 detector and an esophageal aspiration device for verifying endotracheal tube placement in the prehospital setting: a six-month experience, *Prehospital Disaster Med* 12:57-63, 1997.

Nasopharyngeal and Oropharyngeal Airways: Insertion and Care

P U R P O S E : Nasopharyngeal (NP) and oropharyngeal (OP) airways are used in the maintenance of upper airway patency and facilitation of removal of secretions from the posterior pharynx

Eileen Nelson

PREREQUISITE KNOWLEDGE

- Child development as it relates to clinical assessment and procedure
- Anatomy and physiology of the pediatric pulmonary system, including structural characteristics specific to the infant and child[1-4]
  - ❖ A child's airway is both absolutely and relatively smaller in diameter and shorter than an adult's (see Figure 1-1).
  - ❖ The tongue is large in relation to the mandible and oropharynx.
  - ❖ The child's funnel-shaped larynx is higher and more cephalad.
  - ❖ Vocal cords are 50% cartilage and are attached lower and more anteriorly.
  - ❖ The infant's epiglottis is floppy, long, and narrow and projects more posteriorly than the older child's.
  - ❖ The subglottic airway is smaller and more compliant with the cartilage less developed then in the adult.
  - ❖ Because the thyroid does not assume its adult configuration until puberty, the cricoid cartilage is the easiest landmark for identification in children.
  - ❖ The cricoid cartilage is the narrowest portion of the upper airway in children less than 10 years of age. It lies at the level of the third cervical vertebrae in the infant and descends to the sixth cervical vertebrae at puberty.
  - ❖ In teenagers and adults, the larynx is a cylinder with its narrowest portion at the glottic inlet at the level of the vocal cords.
  - ❖ The cricothyroid membrane is a dense fibroelastic membrane between the two largest cartilages in the larynx: the thyroid cartilage (above) and the circumferential ring of the cricoid cartilage (below).
  - ❖ The quantity of alveoli increases until 8 years of age and thereafter increases in size and complexity. Peripheral airway resistance is disproportionately higher in the child.
  - ❖ During inspiration, the infant's intercostal muscles stiffen and a downward movement of the diaphragm occurs, which results in negative intrathoracic pressure and air movement into the lungs. Because the infant's chest wall is compliant and flexible, it characteristically collapses inward (see Figure 23-1).
- Mastery of pediatric advanced life support competencies, including principles of artificial airway establishment (such as bag-mask ventilation, suctioning, proper positioning) and oxygen delivery systems[1]
- Principles of gas exchange
- Signs and symptoms of inadequate oxygenation and ventilation
- Indications for intubation, including upper airway obstruction, apnea, ineffective clearance of secretions, high risk of aspiration, and respiratory distress despite nasopharyngeal (NP) or oropharyngeal (OP) airway
- Knowledge of characteristics, indications, advantages, and disadvantages of NP and OP airways
  - ❖ NP airways
    - ○ NP airways are soft rubber or plastic tubes with a hollow shaft that are inserted into the nose and positioned posteriorly at the base of the tongue to provide a conduit from the nares to the pharynx (Figure 6-1).

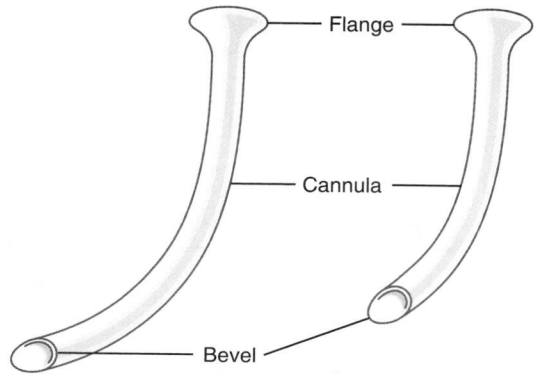

FIGURE 6-1   Nasopharyngeal Airway Characteristics.

○ NP airways are used in conscious children (with cough and gag), unconscious chil dren, and unco operative children.[1,2]
○ Advantages of an NP airway
  ○ NP airways are better tolerated than oral airways and are more comfortable, with less gagging and vomiting, which decreases the risk of aspiration.
  ○ A suction catheter can pass into the posterior pharynx and allow removal of secretions.[2,5]
○ Contraindications to use of the NP airway
  Facial fractures that cause nasal obstruction
  Basilar skull fractures: placement of NP airways in children with cerebrospinal fluid (CSF) leaks can lead to meningitis by impeding drainage and providing a tract for bacteria to enter the brain.[1]
  Ongoing anticoagulation therapy; children undergoing anticoagulation therapy are at risk of epistaxis as are children with hemorrhage disorders.[1,5]
❖ OP airways
  ○ OP airways are plastic, hard, and disposable (Figure 6-2).
  ○ The OP airway resembles the curvature of the tongue and soft palate and is designed to go over the tongue to secure it (and the soft hypopharyngeal structure) out from the posterior pharynx wall.[1,2,5]
  ○ The tip of the OP airway should end cephalad to the mandibular angle so that it lines up with the glottic opening.[1]

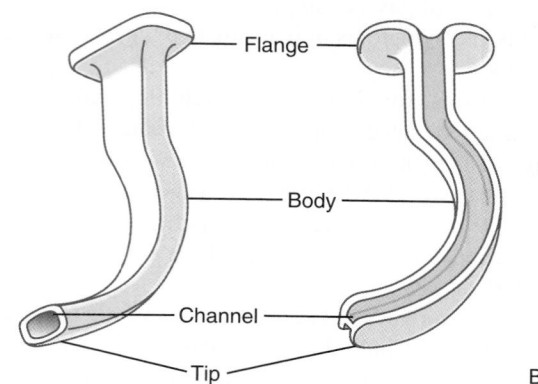

FIGURE 6-2   Oropharyngeal Airway Characteristics. **A,** Guerdel. **B,** Berman.

○ Advantages of an OP airway
  An OP airway positions the tongue away from the posterior pharyngeal wall to maintain patency of the hypopharynx. Although NP airways are preferred, OP airways may be used in an unconscious child if repositioning maneuvers do not open the airway.[1]
  The OP airway can also be used to prevent biting on the oral endotracheal (ET) tube.[1,6]
○ Disadvantages of an OP airway:
  The airway can stimulate gagging and vomiting and increase the risk for aspiration and should preferentially not be used in a child with an intact gag reflex.[1]
  This airway has the potential for trauma to the lips, mouth, and teeth.[1,2]

CHILD AND FAMILY ASSESSMENT

- Child's developmental level and ability to interact ➻**Rationale:** Influences preparation and interaction.
- Child's and family's understanding of the reasons for and risks and benefits of NP/OP airway placement ➻**Rationale:** Evaluates child's and family's understanding of procedure and provides a gauge for ongoing education.
- Desire of family members to be present during the procedure ➻**Rationale:** The presence of family may provide comfort and support, although family members should have the choice not to remain with the child.
- History of nasal or oral deformity or airway obstruction disorder ➻**Rationale:** Assists in decision making regarding appropriateness of airway choice.
- History of anticoagulant therapy ➻**Rationale:** Children who receive anticoagulants can have increased bleeding times.
- History of obstruction disorders ➻**Rationale:** Placement of a NP or OP airway in children with a history of stenosis, adhesions, or webbing may exacerbate these conditions.
- Child's level of consciousness and presence of gag and cough reflex ➻**Rationale:** Status influences airway choice.
- Last enteral intake of food or liquids ➻**Rationale:** Children with a full stomach are at risk for aspiration of gastric contents during airway manipulation.

CHILD AND FAMILY EDUCATION

Individualized, developmentally appropriate education is provided to the family and to the child based on desire for knowledge, readiness to learn, and overall neurologic and psychosocial state.

- Explain the procedure, including the purpose, steps, and rationale ➻**Rationale:** Information decreases fear and anxiety.
- Explain the sensory implications of an airway in the nose or mouth ➻**Rationale:** Anticipatory guidance is helpful in decreasing anxiety and fear.
- Explain that during tube insertion the child may gag or vomit ➻**Rationale:** Open communication with this information decreases anxiety and fear.

- Encourage questions and answer questions as they arise
  ➥*Rationale:* Reinforcement of information is needed during periods of stress.

EQUIPMENT

- Personal protective equipment
- Clean gloves
- Water-soluble lubricant
- Appropriate size of NP or OP airway
- Tape
- Suction equipment
- Gauze
- Flashlight for visualization if needed
- Topical anesthetic as indicated

TABLE 6-1	Oropharyngeal Airway Sizing Guidelines
Age	**Airway Size**
Premature infant	000
Newborn	00
Infant	0
1 to 3 y	1
3 to 6 y	2
6 to 18 y	3
≥ 18 y	4

Perry AG, Potter P: *Clinical nursing skills and techniques*, ed 5, Philadelphia, 2004, Elsevier.

Procedure for Nasopharyngeal and Oropharyngeal Airways: Insertion and Care

Steps	Rationale	Considerations
1. Ensure child and family understand procedure and questions are answered.	Evaluates and reinforces understanding of previously taught information.	Developmental, cognitive, and anxiety levels determine approach and effectiveness of teaching.
2. Gather needed equipment and supplies.	Facilitates completion of the task in a timely manner.	
3. Wash hands and put on personal protective equipment.	Reduces transmission of infection. Protects personnel health.	
4. Select appropriate size of airway.	Sizing of OP and NP airways depends on age and size of child.	Oral airways range in length from 4 to 10 cm (Guedel airway sizes, 000 to 4). (see Table 6-1). Sizes of NP airways range from 12F to 36F. A 12F size is typically used for a full-term infant.[1,2]
Oropharyngeal Put airway against the side of face. Length of airway should equal the distance between mouth flange at the corner of with mouth and the mandible (angle of jaw) (Figure 6-3, *A*).[1,2]	External diameter of the NP airway should be slightly smaller than the opening of the nares.[5]	When OP airway is too large, the tube hits the epiglottis (obstructing the larynx). If airway is too short, it may push tongue posteriorly and obstruct the airway.[1,2,5]
Nasopharyngeal Measure the distance from tip of the nose to tragus of the ear (Figure 6-4, *A*). *(Level II*[1,2,5]		A shortened ET tube may be used for an NP airway. If NP airway is too long, it can cause bradycardia from vagus stimulation or injury to the epiglottis or vocal cords.[1] Laryngospasm may also occur if airway is too long.[2]
5. Consider positioning of child in a supine semi-Fowler's position.	May promote comfort and ease insertion. Promotes good visualization of oral and nasal passages and decreases the risk of trauma.	Hyperextension of the neck can also be used, if indicated (and not contraindicated), with the head-tilt, chin-left technique.

Procedure continues on following page

* Level II: Theory-based; no research data to support recommendations; recommendations from expert consensus group may exist

Procedure	**for Nasopharyngeal and Oropharyngeal Airways: Insertion and Care**—*Continued*	
Steps	**Rationale**	**Considerations**

Steps	Rationale	Considerations
6. Remove excessive secretions from nares and mouth with suctioning as necessary.	Allows for visualization.	
7. Insert airway.		

Oropharyngeal

Steps	Rationale	Considerations
a. Pull tongue forward with a piece of gauze around the tongue or use a tongue depressor to compress tongue.	With tongue held away from posterior pharyngeal wall, obstruction of airway is prevented.	Some techniques suggest insertion of oral airway upside down and advancement in the oral cavity when airway reaches oral pharynx, with rotation of 180 degrees (Figure 6-3, *B*).[7,8]
b. Place airway into mouth, following curve of the tongue. The crossed-finger technique to open the mouth may be helpful.		Otherwise, rotate airway slightly if resistance is met or remove it and try again.[5,6,9]
c. Hold airway with curved end and advance over the base of tongue until flange is parallel to the face.		To decrease trauma, do not force either airway into position. When the airway is positioned properly, it extends below base of the tongue.[1,2]

Nasopharyngeal

Steps	Rationale	Considerations
a. Lubricate tip and sides of tube with a water-soluble lubricant or anesthetic gel.[6] *(Level II*)*	Helps facilitate passage through nares to decrease trauma during insertion.	Check with prescribing practitioner, or institution-specific protocol in regard to use of anesthetics and indications.

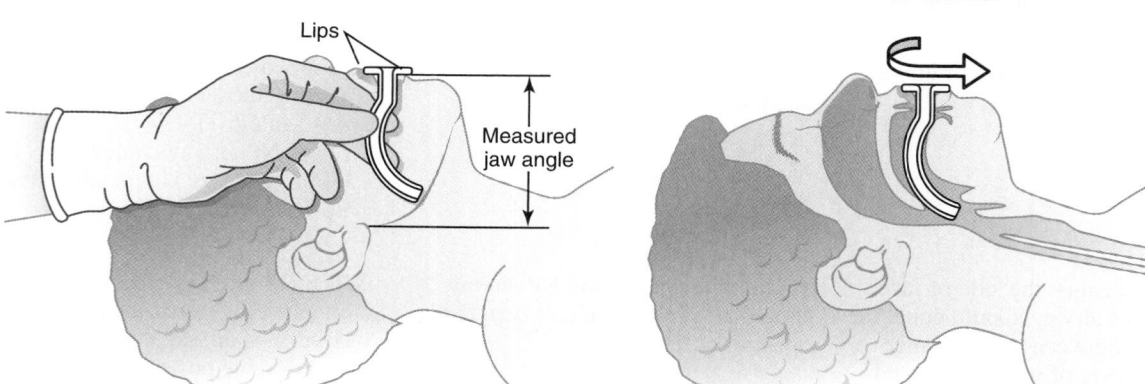

FIGURE 6-3   Sizing and Placement of Oropharyngeal Airway **A,** Correct measurement. **B,** Insertion location.

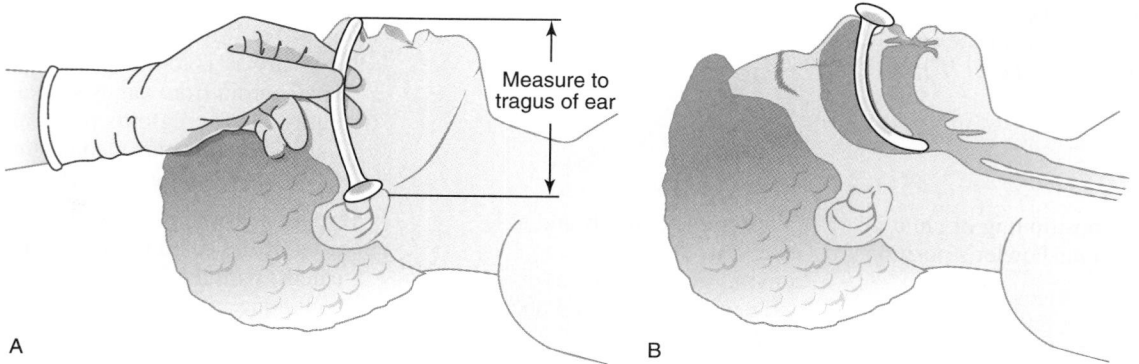

FIGURE 6-4   Sizing and Placement of Nasopharyngeal Airway. **A,** Correct measurement. **B,** Insertion location.

* Level II: Theory-based; no research data to support recommendations; recommendations from expert consensus group may exist

Procedure	for Nasopharyngeal and Oropharyngeal Airways: Insertion and Care—*Continued*	

Steps	Rationale	Considerations
b. Insert tube posteriorly through the nose with the bevel facing down. Gently advance the tube. (Figure 6-4, *B*)		
9. Assess lung sounds bilaterally for verification of airway patency.	Validates the effectiveness of the airway.	
10. Secure airway at the external end with taping around flange to the surrounding skin (Figure 6-5).	A flange is frequently incorporated into airway at the opening to prevent airway from migrating posteriorly.	
11. Suction airway as needed.	Maintains patency.	Small or extremely soft airways can become obstructed by mucus, vomitus, and soft tissue.
12. Reassess lung sounds and indices of oxygenation and ventilation.	Indicates effectiveness of airway.	If aeration is decreased, recheck the position of airway.
13. Remove protective items and wash hands.	Reduces transmission of infection. Protects personnel health.	

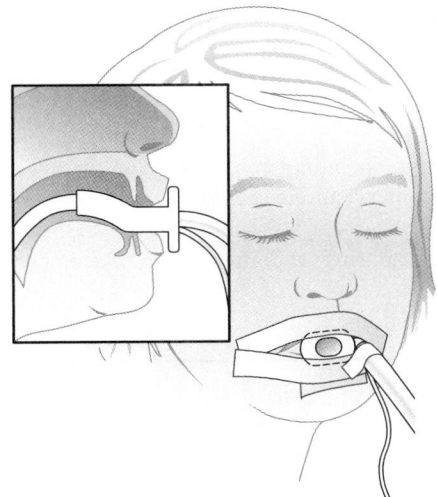

FIGURE 6-5 Securing of oral airway used as a biteblock for an oral endotracheal tube. *Modified from Mims, et al: Critical care skills, ed 2, Philadelphia, 2004, Saunders.*

Expected Outcomes

- Patency of airway is maintained
- Improved secretion clearance

- Improved oxygenation and ventilation
- Atraumatic insertion of airway

Unexpected Outcomes

- Obstructed airway
- Airway obstruction from mucous, emesis, or soft tissues
- Inadequate oxygenation and ventilation
- Trauma to nose, oral cavity, or pharynx

Monitoring and Care of the Child

Activities and Interventions	Rationale	Reportable Conditions
1. Assess vital signs and respiratory status every 1 to 2 hours. Check work of breathing, respiratory effort, and quality and presence of lung sounds.	Presence of tachycardia and bradycardia is an indicator of respiratory failure.	• Worsening respiratory status • Tachypnea • Decreased oxygen saturation (SaO_2) • Stridor • Retractions
2. Assess stability and patency of NP or OP airway.	Small airways can become occluded easily in the presence of secretions.	• Airway obstruction • Misplaced airway
3. Suction airway as needed.	Maintains patency of the airway.	• Airway obstruction
4. Inspect skin and mouth. Provide skin and oral care every 2 to 4 hours. Use lip balm to moisturize lips.	The pressure from the airway may cause cuts, ulcers, and necrosis. Early recognition promotes quick intervention. Lips may become cracked. Decreases chance of oral infections.	• Swelling • Mucosal bleeding • Skin redness • Necrosis • Ulcerations • Trauma to lips, tongue, and roof of mouth
5. Assess comfort and provide appropriate interventions. Allow family to assist with nonpharmacologic means to comfort and support the child.	Early identification of child's comfort allows for immediate attention.	• Unresolved pain and discomfort • Continued irritability or changes in physiologic condition

Documentation

- Assessment before and after airway placement
- Date, time, type, and size of airway inserted
- Appearance of tracheal and oral secretions, including consistency, color, and amount
- Assessment of comfort and any specific interventions provided
- Child's response to the procedure
- Additional interventions necessary before, during, and after airway placement
- Child and family education
- Unexpected outcomes and related interventions

References

1. Hazinski MF, et al, editors: *Pediatric advanced life support provider manual,* Dallas, 2002, American Heart Association.
2. Curley MAQ, Thompson JE: Oxygenation and ventilation. In Curley MAQ, Moloney-Harmon PA, editors: *Critical care nursing of infants and children,* ed 2, Philadelphia, 2000, Saunders.
3. Thompson A: Pediatric airway management. In Fuhrman B, Zimmerman J, editors: *Pediatric critical care,* ed 2, Philadelphia, 1998, Mosby.
4. McCance K, Huether S: *Pathophysiology: the biologic bases for disease in adults and children,* Philadelphia, 2002, Mosby
5. Barnhart SL, Czervinske MP: *Clinical handbook of perinatal and pediatric respiratory care,* Philadelphia, 1995, Saunders.
6. Hazinski MF: *Manual of pediatric critical care,* St. Louis, 1999, Mosby.
7. Lynn-McHale Wiegand DJ, Carlson K, editors: *AACN procedure manual for critical care,* ed 5, Philadelphia, 2005, Saunders.
8. Mims, et al: *Critical care skills,* ed 2, Philadelphia, 2004, Saunders.
9. Kelly KJ: Respiratory care of the neurologically injured child. In Koff PB, et al, editors: *Neonatal and pediatric respiratory care,* ed 2, St. Louis, 1993, Mosby.

Nasopharyngeal Suctioning

PURPOSE: To maintain a patent nasopharyngeal (NP) airway and promote oxygenation and ventilation

Dena L. Jarog

PREREQUISITE KNOWLEDGE

- Child development as it relates to clinical assessment and procedure
- Airway anatomy and physiology, including structural characteristics specific to the infant and child[1-4]
  - ❖ A child's airway is both absolutely and relatively smaller in diameter and shorter than an adult's (see Figure 1-1).
  - ❖ The child's funnel-shaped larynx is higher and more cephalad and lies below the vocal cords. The vocal cords are 50% cartilage and attached lower and more anteriorly.
  - ❖ The infant's epiglottis is floppy, long, and narrow and projects more posteriorly than the older child's. The subglottic airway is smaller and more compliant, with the cartilage less developed than in the adult.
  - ❖ The cricoid cartilage is the easiest and the only landmark for identification in children because the thyroid does not assume its adult configuration until puberty. The cricoid cartilage is the narrowest portion of the upper airway in children less than 10 years of age.
  - ❖ In teenagers and adults, the larynx is a cylinder with its narrowest portion at the glottic inlet at the level of the vocal cords.
- Mastery of pediatric advanced life support competencies, including principles of artificial airway establishment (e.g., bag-mask ventilation, suctioning, proper positioning) and oxygen delivery systems[1]
- Principles of gas exchange

- Signs and symptoms of inadequate oxygenation and ventilation
- Nasopharyngeal (NP) suctioning clears the airway of a child who is unable to do so independently.
- Contraindications to NP suctioning include facial fractures that cause nasal obstruction and basilar skull fractures; children who are undergoing anticoagulation therapy are at risk of epistaxis, as are children with hemorrhage disorders[1,5]

CHILD AND FAMILY ASSESSMENT

- Child's developmental level and ability to interact ➤*Rationale:* Influences preparation and interaction.
- Desire of family members to be present during the procedure ➤*Rationale:* The presence of family may provide comfort and support, although family members should have the choice not to remain with the child.
- Monitoring of the child's vital signs before, during, and after suctioning *(Level II*)* ➤*Rationale:* Identifies signs and symptoms of complications from suctioning, such as laryngospasm, bronchospasm, hemodynamic changes, gagging, and coughing.
- Presence of airway secretions ➤*Rationale:* The physical presence of secretions in the airway can result in obstruction of the airway and poor gas exchange.

---

* Level II: Theory-based; no research data to support recommendations; recommendations from expert consensus group may exist

- Last enteral intake of food or liquids ➻*Rationale:* Children with a full stomach are at risk for aspiration of gastric contents during airway manipulation.

CHILD AND FAMILY EDUCATION

Individualized, developmentally appropriate education is provided to the family and to the child based on desire for knowledge, readiness to learn, and overall neurologic and psychosocial state.

- Explain the suctioning procedure, including the purpose, steps, and rationale ➻*Rationale:* Providing information decreases fear and anxiety.
- Discuss with the child and family that suctioning may be uncomfortable and may cause coughing and shortness of breath for a brief period of time ➻*Rationale:* This discussion reduces anxiety and fear for the childand family and prepares the child for the experience.
- Encourage questions and answer questions as they arise ➻*Rationale:* Reinforcement of information is needed during periods of stress.

EQUIPMENT

- Personal protective equipment, including sterile gloves, mask, and eye protection
- Appropriately sized disposable suction catheter
- Suction source (wall regulator or portable machine)
- Collection container
- Connecting tube (large-bore noncollapsible)
- Normal saline solution or sterile water
- Disposable sterile container
- Water-soluble lubricant
- Wide-bore rigid pharyngeal tonsil tip suction catheter

Procedure for Nasopharyngeal Suctioning

Steps	Rationale	Considerations
1. Ensure child and family understand procedure and questions are answered.	Evaluates and reinforces understanding of previously taught information.	Developmental, cognitive, and anxiety levels determine the approach and effectiveness of teaching.
2. Gather needed equipment and supplies.	Facilitates completion of the task in a timely manner.	
3. Wash hands and put on personal protective equipment.	Reduces transmission of infection. Protects personnel health.	
4. Place child in semi-Fowler's position if tolerated.	Promotes lung expansion and effective coughing.[6]	Use pillows to splint any surgical sites or if child has paralysis to promote a stronger cough.
5. Turn on suction device and set vacuum regulator between 80 and 150 mm Hg. *(Level VI*)*	Readies device for suctioning. Use of higher pressures can cause trauma of the mucosa without increased secretion removal.[6]	Appropriate negative pressures: Infants (<1 yr), 60 to 80 mm Hg; children (1 to 8 yrs), 80 to 120 mm Hg; children (>8 yr), 120 to 150 mm Hg.[7-10] Suction pressure is checked with occlusion of the end of the suction tubing.
6. Determine appropriate insertion length of catheter from the tip of nose to the tragus of ear. *(Level III*)*	Advancement of suction catheter to the point of resistance causes tissue damage.[2]	
7. Open packaging of catheter with inside of package as a sterile field.	Provides a sterile field to prevent transmission of bacteria.	
8. Pour a small amount of sterile water in sterile basin.	Prepares flush solution for the catheter.	
9. Put on gloves with sterile technique.	Maintains a sterile technique. Reduces transmission of infection. Protects personnel health.[11]	Although sterile suctioning technique is recommended for reduction of the likelihood of airway contamination, some institutions use clean technique for the suctioning procedure (see institutional procedure for variation).

* Level III: Laboratory data; no clinical data to support recommendations
Level VI: Clinical studies in a variety of patient populations and situations to support recommendations

Procedure for Nasopharyngeal Suctioning—*Continued*

Steps	Rationale	Considerations
10. With maintenance of sterility, pick up the suction catheter with the dominant hand.	Reduces transmission of infection.	
11. With nondominant hand, pick up connecting tube and secure it to suction catheter.		
12. Suction a small amount of fluid from sterile solution in container.	Assures properly functioning equipment.	
13. Dip end of catheter in a water-soluble lubricant to aid with insertion.	Assists with insertion of the catheter into nasal passage and decreases incidence rate of trauma.	Catheter should be small enough to fit comfortably into nares with use of a water-soluble lubricant. Consider neosynephrine or phenylephrine nasal drops to prevent or decrease bleeding.
14. Without application of suction, insert catheter into the nose next to septum and advance it caudally to predetermined catheter length. Roll catheter between fingers to assist with advancement through the turbinates until child begins to cough.	Decreases chances of trauma to the mucosa of nasal passage.	If no history of nasal problems exists, alternate suctioning between the nostrils to minimize traumatic injury.
15. Place nondominant thumb over the control vent of suction catheter and apply continuous suction while withdrawing the catheter from nare. Rotate catheter between the thumb and forefinger during withdrawal.[6]		
16. Allow at least 20 to 30 seconds between passes of catheter.	Allows child to recover between passes.	Between passes, wrap the catheter around the dominant hand for prevention of contamination.
17. Flush catheter with sterile solution from the basin and rinse off any secretions on exterior of the catheter.	Flushing ensures patency if catheter is needed for a subsequent suctioning pass. Rinsing decreases chances of upper airway secretions being deposited in the lower respiratory tract.	
18. Repeat procedure until airway is clear.		
19. Wrap catheter around the dominant hand and pull off glove inside out. The catheter remains in the glove. Remove other glove.	Reduces risk of microorganism transmission.	
20. Flush connecting tubing with normal saline solution.	Cleans the tubing.	
21. Discard any remaining normal saline solution and solution container.		

Procedure continues on following page

Procedure for Nasopharyngeal Suctioning—*Continued*

Steps	Rationale	Considerations
22. Remove protective items and wash hands.	Reduces transmission of infection. Protects personnel health.[9,12]	
23. Assess breath sounds for determination of any pertinent changes after suctioning.	Evaluates effectiveness of suctioning[9,12]	

Expected Outcomes

- Removal of airway secretions
- Improved oxygenation and ventilation
- Alleviation of clinical signs or symptoms of need for suctioning
- Atraumatic procedure
- Child has acceptable level of comfort

Unexpected Outcomes

- Inability to clear secretions
- Inadequate oxygenation and ventilation, including hypoxemia
- Bronchospasm or laryngospasm
- Bloody nose or other mucosal trauma
- Unmanaged pain

Monitoring and Care of the Child

Activities and Interventions	Rationale	Reportable Conditions
1. Monitor child's vital signs and assess for changes in oxygenation and ventilation indices.	Preassessment determines need for suctioning; post-assessment determines improvement after suctioning. Identifies signs and symptoms of complications from suctioning.	• Laryngospasm, bronchospasm, or hemodynamic changes • Epistaxis • Unresolved increased work of breathing • Signs of changes in oxygen saturation
2. Monitor for gagging or prolonged coughing spells.	Gagging and coughing can cause child to vomit, and aspiration can occur.	• Unresolved gagging or coughing
3. Suction as needed.	Maintains patency of airway.	• Inability to pass suction catheter • Changes in quantity and characteristics of secretions
4. Assess comfort and provide appropriate interventions. Allow family to assist with nonpharmacologic comfort and support for child.	Early identification of child's comfort allows for immediate attention.	• Unresolved pain and discomfort • Continued irritability or changes in physiologic condition

Documentation

- Date, time, and reason for suctioning and the technique used
- Amount, color, consistency, and odor of secretions
- Pre-suctioning and post-respiratory assessment findings, including vital signs, breath sounds, work of breathing, and coughing
- Comfort assessment and any specific interventions provided
- Additional interventions needed before, during, and after suctioning
- Child's response to suctioning and care
- Child and family education
- Unexpected outcomes of suctioning and related treatment

References

1. Hazinski MF, et al, editors: *Pediatric advanced life support provider manual,* Dallas, 2002, American Heart Association.
2. Curley MAQ, Thompson JE: Oxygenation and ventilation. In Curley MAQ, Moloney-Harmon PA: *Critical care nursing of infants and children,* ed 2, Philadelphia, 2000, Saunders.
3. Thompson A: Pediatric airway management. In Fuhrman B, Zimmerman J, editors: *Pediatric critical care,* ed 3, Philadelphia, 2005, Elsevier.
4. McCance K, Huether S: *Pathophysiology: the biologic bases for disease in adults and children,* Philadelphia, 2002, Mosby.
5. Barnhart SL, Czervinske MP: *Clinical handbook of perinatal and pediatric respiratory care,* Philadelphia, 1995, Saunders.
6. Buchfa VL, Fries CM: Respiratory care. In Weinstock D, Bedard RA, Johnson PH, Cohen-Kligerman B, editors: *Nursing procedures,* Springhouse, PA, 2000.
7. AARC Clinical Practice Guideline: Endotracheal suctioning of mechanically ventilated adults and children with artificial airways, *Respir Care* 38(5):500-504, 1993.
8. Choong K, et al: Comparison of loss in lung volume with open versus in-line catheter endotracheal suctioning, *Pediatr Crit Care Med* 4(1):69-73, 2003.
9. Day T, et al: An evaluation of a teaching intervention to improve the practice of endotracheal suctioning in intensive care units, *J Clin Nurs* 10(5):682-696, 2001.
10. Swartz K, et al: A national survey of endotracheal suctioning techniques in the pediatric population, *Heart Lung* 25(1):52-60, 1996.
11. Blackwood B: Normal saline instillation with endotracheal suctioning: primum non nocere (first do no harm), *J Adv Nurs* 29(4):928-934, 1999.
12. Day T, et al: Tracheal suctioning: an exploration of nurses' knowledge and competence in acute and high dependency ward areas, *J Adv Nurs* 39(1):35-45, 2002.

Noninvasive Oxygen Delivery Devices

P U R P O S E : Noninvasive oxygen delivery devices supply supplemental oxygen to children as a first-line treatment for hypoxia and respiratory distress

Lori Boyle and Eileen Nelson

PREREQUISITE KNOWLEDGE

- Child development as it relates to clinical assessment and implications for oxygen delivery devices
- Anatomy and physiology of the pediatric pulmonary system, including structural characteristics specific to the infant and child[1-4]
  - ❖ A child's airway is both absolutely and relatively smaller in diameter and shorter than an adult's (see Figure 1-1).
  - ❖ Because the thyroid does not assume its adult configuration until puberty, the cricoid cartilage is the easiest landmark for identification in children. The cricoid cartilage is the narrowest portion of the upper airway in children less than 10 years of age.
  - ❖ In teenagers and adults, the larynx is a cylinder with its narrowest portion at the glottic inlet at the level of the vocal cords.
  - ❖ The quantity of alveoli increases until 8 years of age and thereafter increases in size and complexity. Peripheral airway resistance is disproportionately higher in the child.
  - ❖ During inspiration, the infant's intercostal muscles stiffen and a downward movement of the diaphragm occurs, which results in negative intrathoracic pressure and air movement into the lungs. Because the infant's chest wall is compliant and flexible, it characteristically collapses inward (see Figure 23-1).
- Mastery of pediatric advanced life support competencies, including oxygen delivery devices[1]

- Principles of oxygen delivery and gas exchange[1]
- Signs and symptoms of inadequate oxygenation and ventilation
- Knowledge of physiologic signs of respiratory distress[5]
- Oxygen is a drug and is administered in the lowest concentration possible for support of oxygenation and work of breathing.[2]
- Blood gas analysis
- Oxygen delivery systems can be divided into low-flow and high-flow systems. In low-flow systems, 100% oxygen mixes with room air during inspiration. The delivered concentration of oxygen is dependent on the child's minute ventilation. In high-flow systems, the flow rate meets the total inspired flow requirements of the child and entrapment of room air does not occur. This method delivers a more reliable concentration of oxygen and is used in emergency situations.[1]
- Masks are often poorly tolerated in infants and toddlers. Nasal prongs may be a preferable alternative. Because of an infant's smaller tidal volume, high concentrations of oxygen can be delivered with nasal prongs.

CHILD AND FAMILY ASSESSMENT

- Child's developmental level and ability to interact
  ➡️*Rationale:* Influences preparation and interaction.
- Child's and family's understanding of the reasons for and risks and benefits of supplemental oxygen
  ➡️*Rationale:* Evaluates child's and family's understanding

the procedure and provides a gauge for ongoing education.

- Signs and symptoms of inadequate oxygenation and ventilation ➥**Rationale:** Indicates effective pulmonary function.
- Level of anxiety, consciousness, and respiratory compromise ➥**Rationale:** Determines the need for additional support.
- Any pertinent medical history or condition that predisposes the child to a chronically lower than normal oxygen saturation ➥**Rationale:** Despite low oxygen saturation, certain medical conditions do not necessitate supplemental oxygen to support physiologic stability.

CHILD AND FAMILY EDUCATION

Individualized, developmentally appropriate education is provided to the family and to the child based on desire for knowledge, readiness to learn, and overall neurologic and psychosocial state.

- Explain the chosen oxygen delivery device, including rationale and risks ➥**Rationale:** Providing information decreases fear and anxiety and improves compliance.[6]
- Provide anticipatory guidance related to the expected duration of supplemental oxygen delivery ➥**Rationale:** Parents can gauge the child's progress to independent respiratory functioning in recovery.

- Discuss appropriate expected outcomes of oxygen delivery ➥**Rationale:** The family and medical team can formulate similar goals and expectations.
- Explain hypoxemia ➥**Rationale:** With knowledge of the meaning of hypoxemia, the child and family can better understand the need for the noninvasive oxygen delivery.
- Explain the necessary assessments during supplemental oxygen delivery ➥**Rationale:** Knowledge of continuous monitoring of the child decreases anxiety and fear.
- Encourage and answer questions as they arise ➥**Rationale:** Reinforcement of information is needed during periods of stress.

EQUIPMENT

- Oxygen source (wall supply or portable oxygen cylinder)
- Appropriate prescribed delivery device (i.e., nasal cannula, simple mask, partial rebreather mask, nonrebreather mask, venturi mask/fixed performance mask, oxygen tent, oxygen hood)
- Oxygen analyzer
- Flow meter
- Humidifier
- Appropriate tubing
- Pulse oximeter
- Supplies to secure the tubing to the child's face as needed (i.e., tape, tegaderm, etc)

Procedure | for Noninvasive Oxygen Delivery Devices

Steps	Rationale	Considerations
1. Ensure child and family understand procedure and questions are answered.	Evaluates and reinforces understanding of previously taught information.	Developmental, cognitive, and anxiety levels determine approach and effectiveness of teaching.
2. Review prescribing practitioner's order.	Oxygen is considered a drug, and inappropriate use can be dangerous.[7]	
3. Select appropriate noninvasive oxygen delivery device (Table 8-1).[5,8]	A variety of noninvasive devices are available for safe administration of oxygen therapy.	In addition to desired oxygen concentration, age, development, and clinical condition are considered in the right delivery system choice.[1] If one method of oxygen delivery is upsetting to the child, a change in delivery devices may be helpful.
4. Gather additional needed equipment and supplies.	Facilitates completion of task in a timely manner.	
5. Wash hands and put on personal protective equipment as indicated.	Reduces transmission of infection. Protects personnel health.	
6. Monitor vital signs and assess respiratory status, including signs of inadequate oxygenation and ventilation.	Supplemental oxygen can help in the maintenance of adequate oxygenation and respiratory and hemodynamic stability.	Pulse oximetry is often used for continuous monitoring of oxygen saturations to provide an indication of gas exchange. Consider arterial/venous blood gases as indicated.

Procedure continues on following page

Procedure for Noninvasive Oxygen Delivery Devices—*Continued*

Steps	Rationale	Considerations
7. Adjust flow meter to deliver correct amount of oxygen.		
8. Apply and secure noninvasive oxygen delivery device and ensure it is correctly sized.	Ensures optimal oxygen delivery and reduces risk of skin breakdown. Helps to ensure that child receives prescribed amount of oxygen.	Masks should cover mouth and nose but not the eyes (Figure 8-1). Too small a mask may decrease fraction of inspired oxygen (FiO_2), and too large a mask adds to dead space.[2] Use adhesives for nasal cannula or elastic strap for face mask.
9. Assess child's respiratory status and need for increased or decreased oxygen therapy.	Directs intervention for reduction of the effects of hypoxemia.	For avoidance of oxygen-related complications, changes in oxygen delivery are based on child's condition and availability of alternative methods to support oxygenation.[7]
10. Remove personal protective equipment and wash hands.	Reduces transmission of infection. Protects personnel health.	

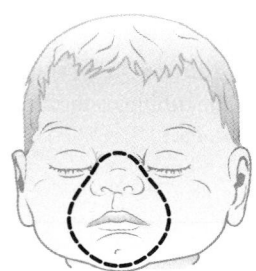
Correct
Covers mouth and nose but not eyes
A

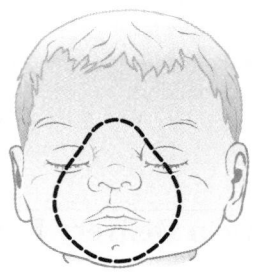
Too Large: Covers eyes
B

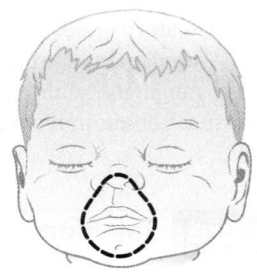
Incorrect
Too Small: Does not cover mouth and nose
C

FIGURE 8-1   Positioning of Facial Mask. **A,** Proper size and positioning, with covering of mouth and nose only. **B,** Improper size and positioning, with mask covering eyes. **C,** Improper size and positioning, with mask not covering mouth and nose.

TABLE 8-1   Noninvasive Oxygen Delivery Devices

Device	Description	Indications	Considerations
Nasal cannula	Nasal cannula are light weight and have two soft prongs that fit in each nare and attach on each side to tubing.[2] Different sizes are available.[8]	Children who need less than 0.50 FiO_2.[8] Allows child to eat, talk, and cough.	FiO_2 inconsistent. Most commonly used O_2 delivery device.[2,6] Child's size and tidal volume alter the oxygen concentration child receives despite same flow rate.[1] Blenders may be used to wean O_2 in the neonate to allow for more precise titration of flow rates.[2,8] May cause drying of nasal mucous membranes, especially at high flow rates (>4 to 5 L/min).[1,6,8] Nasal cannula is more comfortable than mask.[6]

TABLE 8-1	Noninvasive Oxygen Delivery Devices—Cont'd

Device	Description	Indications	Considerations
Simple mask 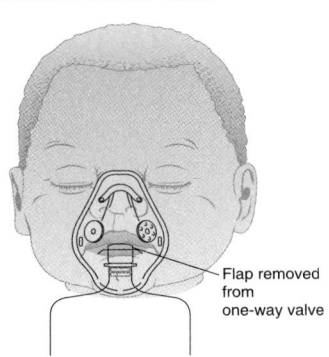	Mask sits on face and over mouth and nose, with elastic strap to secure. Available in variety of sizes.[2]	Low-flow device for children who need FiO_2 of approximately 0.30 to 0.60 oxygen.[8]	Inconsistent FiO_2 delivery. Monitor for signs of hypercarbia.[9] Delivers 5 to 10 L/min.[7] Elastic strap may cause irritation. Minimum of 6 L/min must be maintained to ensure enough oxygen is delivered and to prevent rebreathing of carbon dioxide.[1,2]
Partial rebreather mask	Mask sits on face and over mouth and nose and has elastic strap. Similar to simple mask but with reservoir bag attached that fills with 100% oxygen and child's exhaled gas.[8]	Children who need 0.40 to 0.70 FiO_2.[7] Good for short-term therapy in children who need larger concentrations of oxygen.[7]	Inconsistent FiO_2 delivery. Monitor for signs of hypercarbia.[9] Exhaled gas in reservoir bag is oxygen rich because it comes from upper airway.[1] Rebreathing of carbon dioxide is prevented if flow is maintained at higher than child's minute ventilation.[1] Oxygen flow rate of 10 to 12 L/min is typically necessary.[1] May be uncomfortable for some children.[7] Elastic strap may cause irritation. Adjust flow to prevent reservoir from collapsing on inhalation. Because of mixing of gases (exhaled and supplemental O_2), less flow is needed than for some other devices.[10]
Nonrebreather mask 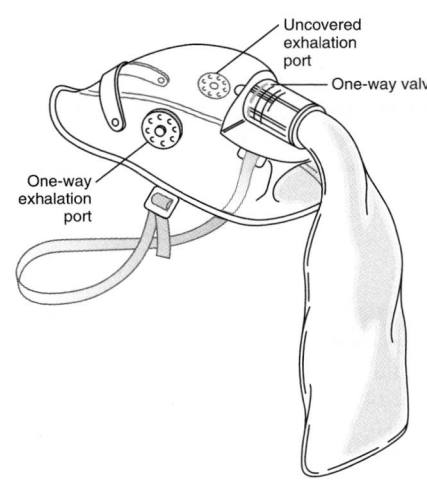	Mask sits on face and over mouth and nose and has elastic strap. Attached reservoir bag has one-way valve to prevent mixing of exhaled gases with oxygen supply.	High-flow system for children who need highest amount of oxygen (usually for short periods) without intubation.[7]	Inconsistent FiO_2 delivery. Monitor for signs of hypercarbia.[9] Elastic strap may cause irritation. Adjust flow to prevent reservoir from collapsing on inhalation.[7] One-way valve provides higher inhaled oxygen concentrations.[10]

Flap removed from one-way valve

Uncovered exhalation port

One-way valve

One-way exhalation port

Continued

TABLE 8-1	Noninvasive Oxygen Delivery Devices—Cont'd

Device	Description	Indications	Considerations
Venturi mask/fixed performance mask	Mask sits on face and over mouth and nose and has air entrainment port, with elastic strap.	Children who need 0.24 to 0.50 FiO_2.[7] Children who need low consistent oxygen concentration not affected by child flow.[6]	Inconsistent FiO_2 delivery. Monitor for signs of hypercarbia.[9] Air-entrapment mask allows constant flow at low to moderate FiO_2 level. Most commonly used mask device.[7] Elastic strap may cause irritation. Humidification can alter oxygen concentration with this device.
Oxygen tent	Clear plastic tent encloses child's body[2,8]	Children who need cool humidity and less than 0.50 FiO_2 (although oxygen tents cannot practically deliver more than 0.30 FiO_2)[8].	Inconsistent FiO_2 delivery. Tent can be cumbersome.[2] Creates cool and wet environment.[5] Tents may become foggy and make assessment of child difficult without breaking seal of tent.[8] Electric toys, percussors, or vibrators should not be allowed in tent.[8] Need analyzer in tent to monitor FiO_2 level.[8]
Oxygen hood	Clear plastic box covers child's head.[2] Oxygen can be delivered either via blender or nebulizer.[8]	For neonates or infants who need oxygen.[5] Inspired oxygen concentration of 80% to 90% can reliably be delivered.[1]	Monitor for signs of hypercarbia.[9] Prolonged therapy can limit mobility.[9] High flow is needed to achieve appropriate oxygen concentrations and decrease hypercarbia.[9] Nasal cannula may be needed when infant is feeding and other nursing care is performed.[10] Temperature needs to be monitored in tent.[10] Creates moist environment.

Labels: Opening exhaled air, Venturi barrel, Oxygen supply, Nose clip, Room air

Expected Outcomes

- Signs of improved oxygenation
- A decrease in hypoxemia-related side effects, including anxiety
- Respiratory, cardiovascular, and neurologic stability

- Maintenance of skin integrity
- Child has an acceptable level of comfort

Unexpected Outcomes

- Signs of inadequate oxygenation
- Increased work of breathing
- Complications of supplemental oxygen
- Increasing cardiovascular, respiratory, or neurologic compromise[7]
- Skin breakdown
- Unmanaged pain and anxiety

Monitoring and Care of the Child

Activities and Interventions	Rationale	Reportable Conditions
1. Assess signs and symptoms of changes in oxygenation/ventilation indices, including oxygen saturation monitoring.	Indicative of changes in effectiveness of supplemental oxygen. Pulse oximetry can be used to monitor effectiveness of oxygen therapy.	• Diminished breath sounds • Significant changes in oxygenation saturation and arterial/venous blood gases • Increased work of breathing • Dysrhythmias, including tachycardia to bradycardia
2. Monitor physiologic stability, including vital signs and clinical appearance.	With hypoxemia, changes in respiratory, cardiovascular, and neurologic status occur.	• Hypertension to hypotension • Changes in level of consciousness[7] • Changes in peripheral perfusion
3. Check and maintain the proper fit of the child's noninvasive oxygen delivery device.	Ensures that the child receives desired oxygen content. Optimizes comfort.	
4. Assess skin every 4 hours and as necessary.	Reduces skin breakdown and eliminates potential source for infection. The bridge of the nose and the cheeks are prone to skin breakdown.[6]	• Any noted breakdown of skin integrity associated with the device
5. Assess for signs of hypercarbia in child with oxygen hood and face masks.	Danger of hypercarbia exists if the flow of gas is too low.[9,10]	• Increasing agitation • Rapid and deep respiration • Dyspnea • Progressive lethargy
6. Assess for signs of dry mucous membranes and dehydration.	Dry and sore mucous membranes can occur with the delivery of oxygen.[6]	• Signs of dehydration and dry or cracked mucous membranes
7. Consider humidification with delivery of higher oxygen concentrations and when supplemental oxygen delivery is necessary for a prolonged period of time.[6]	Thick secretions are more difficult to mobilize.[6]	

Documentation

- Delivery device and amount of oxygen delivered
- Respiratory status, including work of breathing, lung sounds, and pulse oximeter reading
- Vital signs
- Pulse oximeter reading
- Child's response to supplemental oxygen
- Comfort assessment and any specific interventions provided
- Additional interventions necessary
- Child and family education
- Unexpected outcomes and related treatment

References

1. Hazinski MF, et al, editors: *Pediatric advanced life support provider manual,* Dallas, 2002, American Heart Association.
2. Curley MAQ, Thompson JE: Oxygenation and ventilation. In Curley MAQ, Moloney-Harmon P, editors: *Critical care nursing of infants and children,* ed 2, Philadelphia, 2001, Saunders.
3. Thompson A: Pediatric airway management. In Fuhrman B, Zimmerman J, editors: *Pediatric critical care,* ed 3, Philadelphia, 2005, Elsevier.
4. McCance K, Huether S: *Pathophysiology: the biologic bases for disease in adults and children,* Philadelphia, 2002, Mosby.
5. Wong DL, Hockenberry MJ: *Nursing care of infants and children,* Philadelphia, 2003, Mosby.
6. Porter-Jones G: Short-term oxygen therapy, *Nurs Times* 98(40):53-56, 2002.
7. Pruitt WC, Jacobs M: Breathing lessons: basics of oxygen therapy, *Nursing* 33(10):43-45, 2003.
8. Barnhart SL, Czervinske MP: *Clinical handbook of perinatal and pediatric respiratory care,* Philadelphia, 1995, Saunders.
9. Frey B, Shann F: Oxygen administration in infants, *Arch Dis Childhood* 88(2):84-88, 2003.
10. Myers TR: Selection of an oxygen delivery device for neonatal and pediatric patients-2002 revision and update, *Respir Care* 47(6):707-714, 2002.

Postural Drainage with Percussion and Vibration

PURPOSE: Postural drainage with percussion and vibration mobilizes secretions and increases alveolar ventilation

Eric A. Bowles

PREREQUISITE KNOWLEDGE

- Child development as it relates to clinical assessment and procedure
- Anatomy and physiology of the pediatric pulmonary system, including structural characteristics specific to the infant and child[1-4]
  - A child's airway is both absolutely and relatively smaller in diameter and shorter than an adult's (see Figure 1-1).
  - Because the thyroid does not assume its adult configuration until puberty, the cricoid cartilage is the easiest landmark for identification in children. The cricoid cartilage is the narrowest portion of the upper airway in children less than 10 years of age.
  - In teenagers and adults, the larynx is a cylinder with its narrowest portion at the glottic inlet at the level of the vocal cords.
  - The quantity of alveoli increases until 8 years of age and thereafter increases in size and complexity. Peripheral airway resistance is disproportionately higher in the child.
  - During inspiration, the infant's intercostal muscles stiffen and a downward movement of the diaphragm occurs, which results in negative intrathoracic pressure and air movement into the lungs. Because the infant's chest wall is compliant and flexible, it characteristically collapses inward (see Figure 23-1).

- Signs and symptoms of inadequate oxygenation and ventilation
- Mastery of pediatric advanced life support competencies, including use of artificial airways, oxygen delivery systems, and tracheal suctioning[4]
- Knowledge of physiologic symptoms of respiratory distress
- Postural drainage, percussion, and vibration involve manipulation of the child and the application of hand techniques for promotion of drainage of secretions to the bronchial tree[5,6] (Figure 9-1).
- Postural draining includes positioning of the child for use of gravity to facilitate mobilization of secretions.
- Percussion involves painless rhythmic clapping of the chest wall with cupped hands, with fingers and thumbs tightly together. The entire outer portion of the hand makes contact with the chest wall and creates an air pocket that acts as a cushion. A percussion cup is also available and is especially useful for infants. Manual vibration is sustained downward vibrating pressure with the flat part of the palm of the hand and is effective during exhalation. Hand-held vibrators are also used to provide chest vibration.[1,7]
- Conditions that may benefit from postural drainage, percussion, and vibration include bronchitis, cystic fibrosis, pneumonia, atelectasis, and ineffective cough.[8,9]
- Some contraindications to consider before postural drainage with percussion and vibration include large

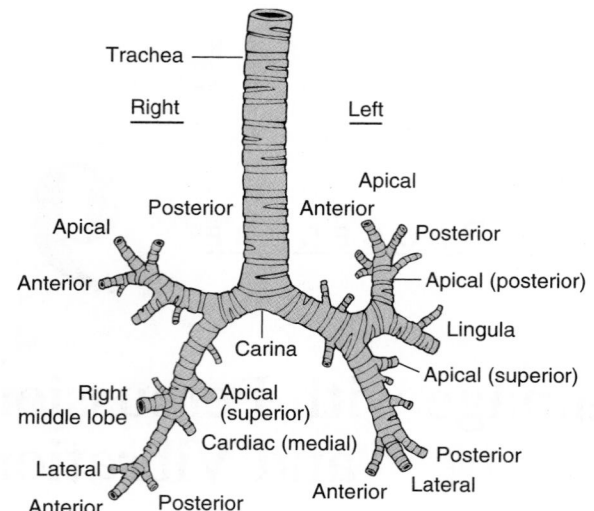

FIGURE 9-1   Bronchial Tree. *Modified from Frownfelter DL, Dean E:* Principles and practice of cardiopulmonary therapy, *ed 3, St. Louis, 1996, Mosby.*

pleural effusions, active hemoptysis, rib fracture, untreated pneumothorax, pulmonary embolism, spinal injury or recent spinal surgery, foreign body aspirations, head and neck injury until stabilization, abnormal coagulation profile, and increased intracranial pressure.[7,10]

- For children undergoing aerosolized antibiotic therapy, administration of the medication after postural drainage, percussion, and vibration may be preferable because the greatest surface area of the airway is exposed after the procedure.

CHILD AND FAMILY ASSESSMENT

- Child's developmental level and ability to interact ➻*Rationale:* Child's developmental level influences preparation and interaction.
- Child's and family's understanding of the reasons for and risks and benefits of postural drainage, percussion, and vibration ➻*Rationale:* Evaluates child's and family's understanding of the procedure and provides a gauge for ongoing education.
- Desire of family members to be present during the procedure ➻*Rationale:* The presence of family may provide comfort and support; although family members should have the choice not to remain with the child.
- Observation of the trend of oxygen requirement and improvement in the chest x-ray ➻*Rationale:* Indicates the effectiveness of the therapy.
- Signs and symptoms of airway secretions and inadequate oxygenation and ventilation, including visible secretions in the airway, inspiratory wheezes, expiratory crackles,

restlessness, ineffective coughing, decreased level of consciousness, diminished breath sounds, tachypnea, tachycardia or bradycardia, cyanosis, hypertension/hypotension, and shallow respirations ➻*Rationale:* Secretions in the airway can result in obstruction of the airway and poor gas exchange.

- For children undergoing mechanical ventilation, increased peak pressures on the ventilator should be noted ➻*Rationale:* Secretions can increase resistance to airflow.

CHILD AND FAMILY EDUCATION

Individualized, developmentally appropriate education is provided to the family and to the child based on desire for knowledge, readiness to learn, and overall neurologic and psychosocial state.

- Explain the procedure, including the purpose, steps, and rationale ➻*Rationale:* Providing information decreases fear and anxiety.
- Discuss appropriate expected outcomes of the procedure ➻*Rationale:* The family and medical team can formulate similar goals and expectations.
- If appropriate, explain the importance of the child assisting with secretion removal with coughing during the procedure ➻*Rationale:* This explanation elicits cooperation and improves the effectiveness of the procedure with facilitation of removal of secretions from the tracheobronchial tree.
- Instruct the family to encourage the child to play games that promote the clearance of mucus (i.e., blowing a cotton ball across a table, blowing a pinwheel, or blowing bubbles) ➻*Rationale:* Active deep inhalation with long forced exhalation forces the air behind the secretions and aids in their mobilization and improved alveolar ventilation.
- Encourage questions and answer questions as they arise ➻*Rationale:* Reinforcement of information is needed during periods of stress.

EQUIPMENT

- Appropriately sized disposable suction catheters
- Suction source (wall regulator or portable machine)
- Collection container
- Connecting tube (large-bore noncollapsible)
- Sterile water and cup for clearing the catheter
- Manual ventilation bag (MVB) connected to an oxygen flow meter (if child has an artificial airway)
- Personal protective equipment, including eye protection, mask, and gown as indicated)
- Stethoscope

Procedure for Postural Drainage with Percussion and Vibration

Steps	Rationale	Considerations
1. Ensure child and family understand procedure and questions are answered.	Evaluates and reinforces understanding of previously taught information.	Developmental, cognitive, and anxiety levels determine approach and effectiveness of teaching.
2. Gather needed equipment and supplies.	Facilitates completion of the task in a timely manner.	
3. Wash hands and put on personal protective equipment as indicated.	Reduces transmission of infection. Protects personnel health.	Use a gown in cases of copious secretions and strong cough reflex or infectious situations (e.g., respiratory syncytial virus [RSV]).
4. Administer bronchodilators as directed.	Opens airways to facilitate the mobilization of secretions.	Ideally administered 20 minutes before the procedure begins. Monitor child's response to the bronchodilators for bronchospasm.
5. Position child and provide percussion/vibration at specifically identified location.[7]	Optimization of child's position facilitates movement of secretions from each area of the lungs.	Child should undergo percussion for 5 to 7 minutes in each area.

Upper lobes

Anterior apical bronchi: Child sits upright at a 30-degree to 45-degree angle. Percussion at shoulders and fingers at clavicles in front (Figure 9-2, *A*).

Posterior apical bronchi: Child sits Percussion upright and leans over a pillow. on either side of upper spine (Figure 9-2, *B*).

Anterior bronchi: Child is supine in neutral alignment. Hand is just below the clavicles (Figure 9-2, *C*).

Percussion and vibration assist in mobilizing secretions.

Ability to position and use percussion and vibration to specific areas of the lung depends on child's clinical condition; positioning is modified.

The use of pillows under knees in Trendelburg's position and at the back with side lying is recommended.[7]

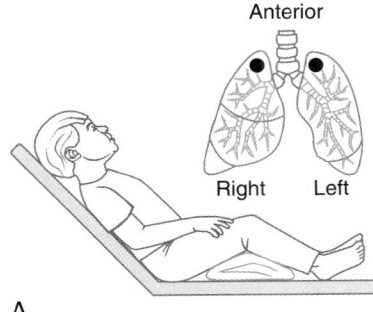

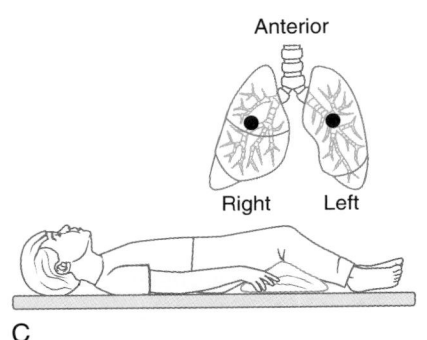

FIGURE 9-2   Positions for Postural Drainage—Upper Lobes.
From Thompson JM, et al, editors: Mosby's clinical nursing, ed 4, St. Louis, 1997, Mosby.

Procedure continues on following page

Procedure   for Postural Drainage with Percussion and Vibration—*Continued*

Steps	Rationale	Considerations

Upper lobes, cont'd

Posterior segment: Child is prone with a roll under the hips to expose desired flank (Figure 9-2, *D* and *E*).

Right middle lobe bronchus: Child is in left side lying position with the foot of bed elevated approximately 30 to 45 degrees. Percussion is to the right of the nipple below the axilla (Figure 9-2, *F*).

Lingular bronchus: Child is in right side lying position with the foot of the bed elevated approximately 30 to 45 degrees. Percussion is lateral to the left nipple below the axilla (Figure 9-2, *G*).

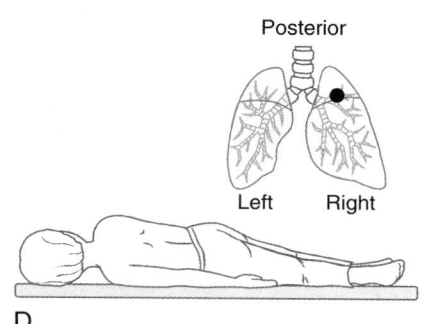

D

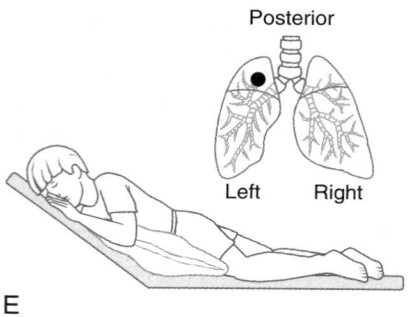

E

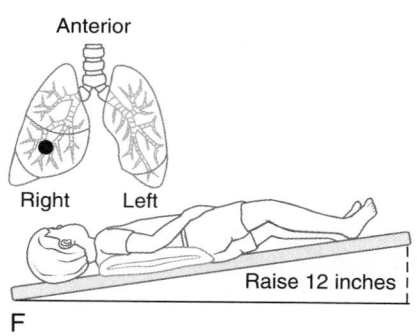

F

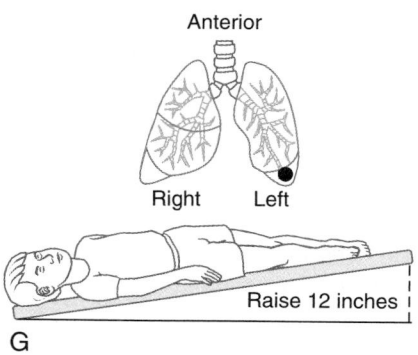

G

FIGURE 9-2, CONT'D   Positions for Postural Drainage—Upper Lobes.

Procedure	for Postural Drainage with Percussion and Vibration—*Continued*	
Steps	**Rationale**	**Considerations**

Lower lobes

Anterior bronchi: Child is prone, and the foot of the bed is elevated approximately 30 to 45 degrees. Percussion is over the lower anterior ribs on both sides (Figure 9-2, *H*).

Lateral bronchus: Child is positioned on each side one at a time with desired flank exposed, and the foot of bed is elevated at least 30 to 45 degrees. Percussion is over the right side of the chest below scapulas posterior to midaxillary line (Figure 9-2, *I* and *J*).

Basal bronchi: Child is prone, and the foot of bed is elevated approximately 30 to 45 degrees. Percussion is over the lower posterior ribs on either side of the spine (Figure 9-2, *K*).

Superior bronchi: Child is prone, and a pillow is under the abdomen. Percussion is below the scapulas on either side of the spine (Figure 9-2, *L*).

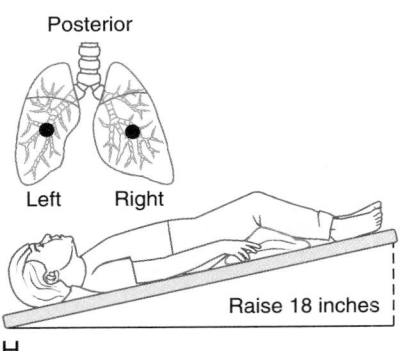

H

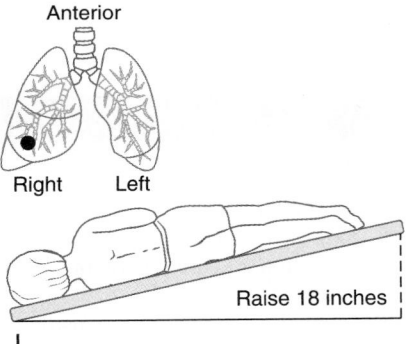

I

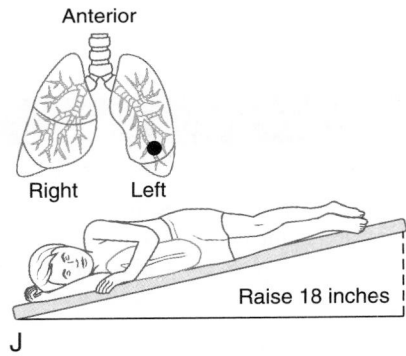

J

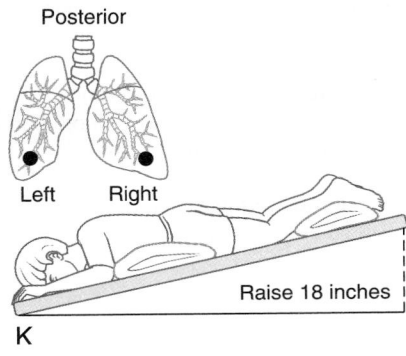

K

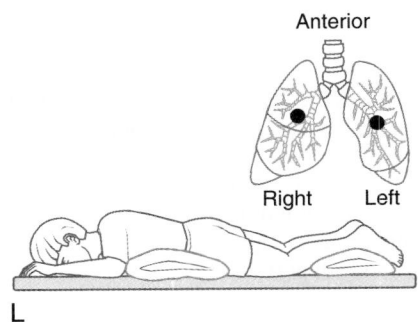

L

FIGURE 9-2, CONT'D   Positions for Postural Drainage—Lower Lobes.

Procedure continues on following page

Procedure for Postural Drainage with Percussion and Vibration—*Continued*

Steps	Rationale	Considerations
6. Encourage cough and suction the airway as indicated. See Procedure 2 and Procedure 7.	Further mobilizes and clears secretions from airway.	Therapy may be less effective if child is unable to cough. In this case, aggressive suctioning to clear the upper airway should be done.
7. Remove personal protective equipment and wash hands.	Reduces transmission of infection. Protects personnel health.	
8. Assess postprocedural respiratory status, including lung sounds and signs of inadequate oxygenation and ventilation.	Provides an assessment of the effectiveness of the procedure.	

Expected Outcomes

- Signs of improved oxygenation and alveolar ventilation
- Improved clearance of secretions from the airway
- Child has an acceptable level of comfort
- Procedure performed without complications

Unexpected Outcomes

- Signs of inadequate oxygenation and ventilation
- Inability to mobilize secretions
- Unmanaged pain and anxiety
- Traumatic injury, including rib fractures

Monitoring and Care of the Child

Activities and Interventions	Rationale	Reportable Conditions
1. Monitor physiologic stability, including vital signs and clinical appearance.	Stimulation may cause an increase in oxygen consumption. Child may have dysrhythmias associated with suctioning.	• Dysrhythmias • Significant changes in oxygen saturation and arterial/venous blood gases • Changes in peripheral perfusion
2. Assess signs and symptoms of airway secretion and changes in oxygenation and ventilation indices.	Child's respiratory rate and work of breathing should return to baseline after the treatment has ended. Percussion therapy can cause desaturation episodes.	• Tachypnea • Diminished breath sounds • Significant changes in oxygenation saturation and arterial/venous blood gases • Increased peak airway pressures (with mechanical ventilation) • Persistent coughing • Increased work of breathing
3. Interpret chest radiograph.	Identify the lung area that benefits from postural drainage, percussion, and vibration.	• Worsening lung changes noted on chest radiograph results
4. Assess comfort and provide appropriate interventions. Allow family to assist with nonpharmacologic means to comfort and support the child.	Identification of child's comfort allows for immediate attention.	• Unresolved pain and discomfort

Documentation

- Date, time, frequency, and length of procedure
- Pre-procedure and postrespiratory assessment, including lung sounds and work or breathing
- Vital signs
- Color, amount, consistency and odor of secretions
- Comfort assesment and any specific interventions provided
- Additional interventions required pre-, post-percussion, vibration, and postural drainage
- Child's response to percussion, vibration, and postural drainage
- Unexpected outcomes and related treatment

References

1. Thompson A: Pediatric airway management. In Fuhrman B, Zimmerman J, editors: *Pediatric critical care,* ed 3, Philadelphia, 2005, Elsevier.
2. McCance K, Huether S: *Pathophysiology: the biologic bases for disease in adults and children,* Philadelphia, 2002, Mosby.
3. Curley MAQ, Thompson JE: Oxygenation and ventilation. In Curley MAQ, Moloney-Harmon PA, editors: *Critical care nursing of infants and children,* ed 2, Philadelphia, 2000, Saunders.
4. Hazinski MF, et al, editors: *Pediatric advanced life support provider manual,* Dallas, 2002, American Heart Association.
5. Oberwaldner B: Physiotherapy for airway clearance in pediatrics, *Eur Respir J* 15:196-204, 2000.
6. Houtmeyers E, et al: Regulation of mucociliary clearance in health and disease, *Eur Respir J* 13:1177-1188, 1999.
7. Perry AG, Potter PA: *Clinical nursing skills and techniques,* ed 5, St. Louis, 2004, Mosby.
8. Wallis C, Prasad A: Who needs chest physiotherapy? *Arch Dis Child* 80:393-397, 1999.
9. Kirlloff L, Owens G, Roger R, et al: Does chest physical therapy work? *Chest* 88:436-444, 1985.
10. AARC Clinical Practice Guideline: Postural drainage therapy, *Respir Care* 36:1418-1426, 1991.

Additional Reading

Pryor J: Physiotherapy for airway clearance in adults, *Eur Respir J* 14:1418-1424, 1999.

Tracheostomy Tube: Stoma Care and Tie Change

P U R P O S E : Tracheostomy stoma care and tie change are performed for preservation of skin integrity, decrease in the risk of infection, and maintenance of airway security

Elsie M. Hartigan and Susan M. Campisciano

PREREQUISITE KNOWLEDGE

- Child development as it relates to clinical assessment and procedure
- Anatomy and physiology of the pediatric pulmonary system, including structural characteristics specific to the infant and child[1-6]
  - ❖ A child's airway is both absolutely and relatively smaller in diameter and shorter than an adult's (see Figure 1-1).
  - ❖ Because the thyroid does not assume its adult configuration until puberty, the cricoid cartilage is the easiest landmark for identification in children. The cricoid cartilage is the narrowest portion of the upper airway in children less than 10 years of age and lies at the level of the third cervical vertebrae in the infant and descends to the sixth cervical vertebrae at puberty.
  - ❖ In teenagers and adults, the larynx is a cylinder with its narrowest portion at the glottic inlet at the level of the vocal cords.
  - ❖ The quantity of alveoli increases until 8 years of age and thereafter increases in size and complexity. Peripheral airway resistance is disproportionately higher in the child.
  - ❖ During inspiration, the infant's intercostal muscles stiffen and a downward movement of the diaphragm occurs, which results in negative intrathoracic pressure and air movement into the lungs. Because the infant's chest wall is compliant and flexible, it characteristically collapses inward (see Figure 23-1).
- Signs and symptoms of inadequate oxygenation and ventilation[2]

- Mastery of pediatric advanced life support competencies, including indications for an artificial airway, use of a manual resuscitation/ventilation system, and other adjuncts used for ventilation support[5]
- Tracheotomy is a surgical procedure that involves the construction of a channel between the trachea and the skin surface of the neck in the midline (see Figure 11-1). An incision is made through the second, third, and fourth tracheal rings. Placement too close to the first ring risks cricoid cartilage damage with subsequent subglottic stenosis.[1,5] A tracheostomy is the opening or stoma made with the tracheotomy incision.
- Clinical indications for the child's tracheotomy and date of original tube placement
  - ❖ Some possible indications from tracheotomy include upper airway obstruction, craniofacial abnormalities that interfere with natural airway patency, prolonged ventilatory support, prevention of aspiration, and removal of secretions.[2,3,5,7-9] Some common abnormalities that lead to tracheostomy tube placement for infants and children include chronic lung disease, subglottic stenosis, tracheal stenosis, laryngotracheomalacia, and neuromuscular weakness and neurologic impairment.[2,3,5,7-9]
- Tracheostomy tubes are available (or can be custom made) with different characteristics, including the size of the internal diameter and outer diameter, tube length, presence or absence of a cuff, presence or absence of an internal cannula, and presence or absence of fenestration.[2,5,10,11] Pediatric tubes are generally made of plastic and are single cannula (Figure 10-1).

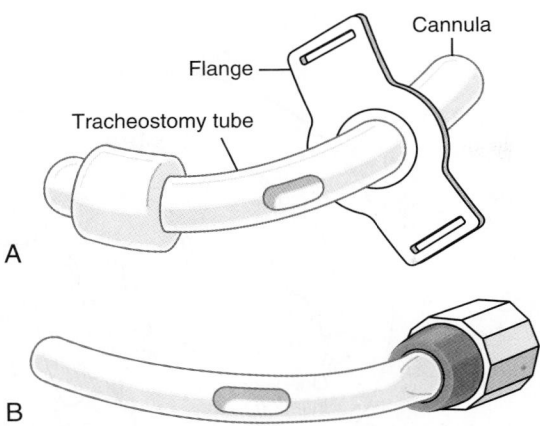

FIGURE 10-1   Pediatric Tracheostomy Tube. **A,** Pediatric tracheostomy tube. **B,** Pediatric tracheostomy tube with obturator.

- The difference between neonatal, pediatric, and adult tracheostomy tubes of the same diameter is the length of the tube. As with adult tracheostomy tubes, some pediatric tubes for older children and adolescents have cuffs to minimize leak and an inner cannula to ease cleaning and to reduce the frequency of tracheostomy tube change (Figure 10-2).
- Tracheostomy tubes also come fenestrated (with openings) to let air into the upper airway so the child can speak (Figure 10-3).
- Advantages of a tracheostomy tube, over an endotracheal tube, include improved comfort and security, ability to provide a mechanism for speech, increased mobility,

easier removal of secretions, and prevention of further airway injury from the endotracheal tube.[3,10]
- Children with tracheostomy tubes do not have the upper airway to humidify the air that is breathed, so a humidification device (humidifier or heat-moisture exchanger) is needed to prevent tracheal secretions from becoming viscous and potentially occluding the airway.[1,11-14]
- A second caregiver is essential with a tie change.[13] Extra hands can reduce the risk of accidental decannulation. Assessment of developmental, cognitive, and anxiety levels determines the need for a third person to prevent the child's accidental decannulation.
- Many children are discharged home with a tracheostomy tube and later return to the hospital for decannulation.[15]

CHILD AND FAMILY ASSESSMENT

- Child's developmental level and ability to interact →→**Rationale:** Influences preparation and interaction.
- Child's and family's understanding of the reasons for and risks and benefits of the procedure →→**Rationale:** Evaluates child's and family's understanding of the procedure and provides a gauge for ongoing education.
- Desire of family members to be present during the procedure →→**Rationale:** The presence of family may provide comfort and support, although the family should have the choice to not remain with the child.
- Characteristics and production of tracheal secretions →→**Rationale:** Assists in identifying underlying pathology and direction of intervention. Irritation of mucosa results in increased production of secretions.
- Cardiopulmonary assessment, including vital signs, visual inspection of breathing patterns and chest wall movement, auscultation of lung fields, and signs of inadequate oxygenation and ventilation, such as decreased arterial oxygen saturation, cardiac arrhythmias, increased work of breathing, cyanosis, increased blood pressure, elevated intracranial pressure, anxiety, agitation, and changes in

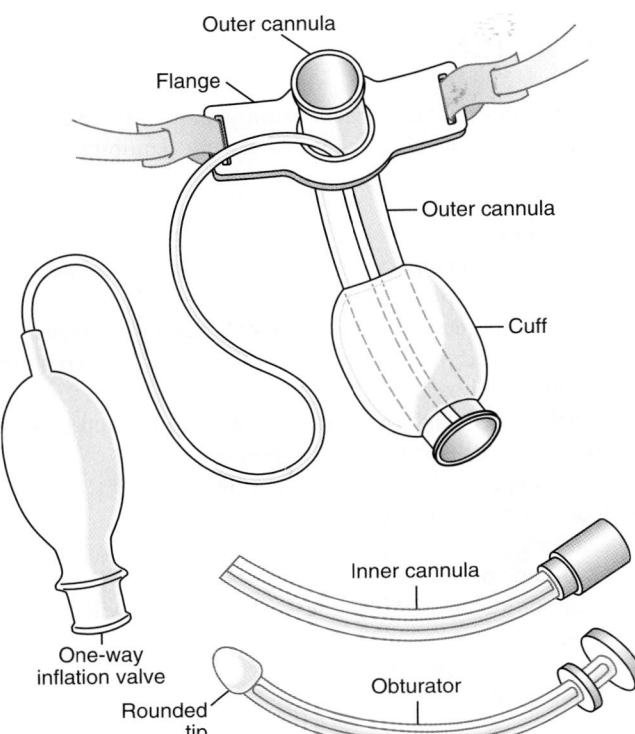

FIGURE 10-2   Tracheostomy tube with inner cannula and inflatable cuff.

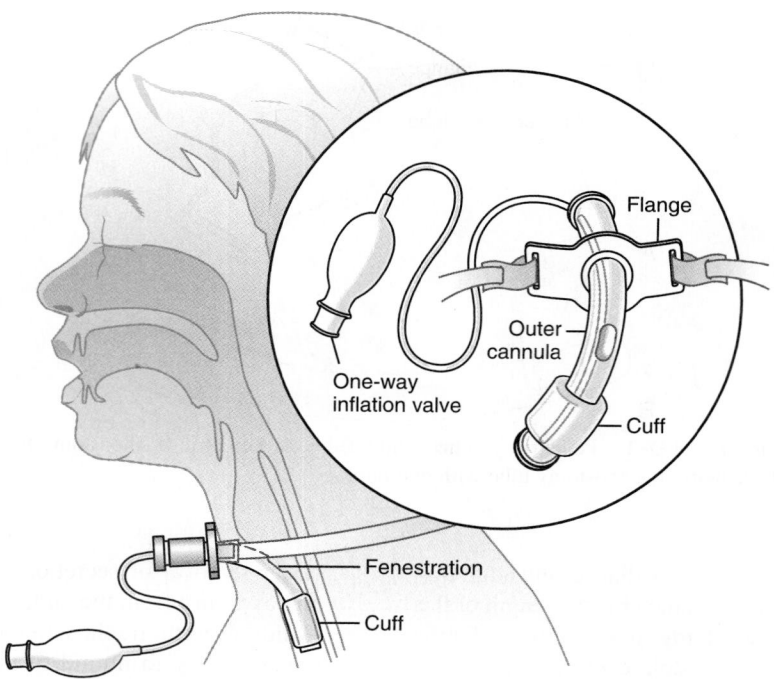

FIGURE 10-3   Fenestrated Tracheostomy Tubes.

level of consciousness ➻*Rationale:* Evaluates the child's cardiopulmonary status provides valuable information in determination of clinical condition and the child's ability to tolerate tracheostomy stoma care.

- Skin around and under ties and tracheostomy tube ➻*Rationale:* Reduces skin breakdown and eliminates a potential source for infection.
- Presence and characteristics of peristomal secretions and condition of tracheostomy ties and dressing ➻*Rationale:* Reduces skin breakdown and eliminates a potential source for infection.

CHILD AND FAMILY EDUCATION

Individualized, developmentally appropriate education is provided to the family and to the child based on desire for knowledge, readiness to learn, and overall neurologic and psychosocial state.

- Explain the procedure for tracheostomy tie change and stoma care, including the purpose, steps, and rationale ➻*Rationale:* Providing information decreases fear and anxiety and provides a basis for a home teaching plan.[7]
- If developmentally appropriate, explain to children how they can assist in the stoma care ➻*Rationale:* Stoma care is completed in a more timely manner if children are cooperative.

- Encourage questions and answer questions as they arise ➻*Rationale:* Reinforcement of information is needed during periods of stress.

EQUIPMENT

Some institutions use tracheostomy care kits that may contain some or all of the following equipment and supplies.

- Clean gloves
- Additional personal protective equipment as indicated, including eye protection, mask, and gown
- Applicators (cotton swabs) and 4×4 dressing sponges
- Fenestrated drainage sponges (4×4 or 2×2) or moisture absorptive dressing
- Sterile water (tap water that has been boiled and cooled may be used)/normal saline solution
- 1/2-strength hydrogen peroxide as desired
- Container to hold water or hydrogen peroxide
- Scissors
- Twill tape or Velcro ties
- Foam or moleskin with adhesive backing (if twill ties are used)
- Hemostat or tweezers
- Blanket roll

Procedure for Tracheostomy Tube: Stoma Care and Tie Change

Steps	Rationale	Considerations
1. Ensure child and family understand procedure and questions are answered.	Evaluates and reinforces understanding of previously taught information.	Developmental, cognitive, and anxiety levels determine approach and effectiveness of teaching.
2. Gather necessary equipment and supplies.	Facilitates completion of procedure in a timely manner.	

3. When changing ties:
    Cut the correct length of foam (or moleskin), first measuring the distance around the neck between the tracheostomy tube flanges with enough room to allow one finger to easily pass under the foam.
    Cut the correct length of twill tape by measuring at least twice the length of foam and then cut on a diagonal to a point.
	Ties and foam (or other securing device) need to fit snugly to prevent accidental decannulation.
	Allowing one finger to pass under the foam minimizes skin breakdown and maintains airway security. *(Level IV*)*
	Cutting ties on a diagonal helps insertion of ties through the tracheostomy islet.
		Developmental and cognitive levels influence the selection of securing device.
		As an alternative to twill tape, Velcro ties and trim can be used appropriately. With Velcro ties, bring the ends together and straighten ties. Although Velcro fasteners are softer and preferred because of ease of use, they may not be appropriate for children at increased risk for decannulation (e.g., a small infant, an active toddler, or a child who is agitated).[13] *(Level IV*)*

4. Wash hands and put on clean gloves.[16]	Reduces transmission of infection. Protects personnel health.	This step may occur earlier in the procedure. Put on additional personal protective equipment as indicated, including eye protection, mask, and gown.
5. Fill container with water, normal saline solution, or equal parts water and hydrogen peroxide, as per institutional guidelines. *(Level IV*)*	Choice of cleaning agent depends on cleaning need and skin sensitivity.	The use of hydrogen peroxide may be unnecessary for adequate cleaning and may be too harsh for the skin of some children.
6. Monitor vital signs and indications of inadequate oxygenation and ventilation.	Decompensation may occur during the procedure.	Consider child's status in selection of appropriate monitoring.
7. Position child so the head is slightly extended and stoma site is visible and easily accessible. Place a blanket roll under shoulders to hyperextend the neck.	Assists in visualization of the neck, which allows for a thorough assessment of skin that surrounds stoma site and for thorough cleansing.	Attention to ensured adequate visibility of stoma site is especially important in infant or obese child with a small neck that limits visualization.
8. Older adolescents may have a tracheostomy tube with an inner cannula (Figure 10-4, *A*). In this case, remove the inner cannula. Place inner cannula in hydrogen peroxide solution (saline solution or water alone can also be used), clean it with a small brush, and rinse it with saline solution. Reinsert internal cannula and lock it in place[10] (Figure 10-4, *B* and *C*).	Cleans secretions from inner cannula to promote airway patency.	The outer cannula remains in place to maintain the airway. This step may occur later in the procedure.
9. One caregiver holds the tracheostomy tube while a second caregiver cuts or loosens the securing device.	Maintaining the airway is critical throughout the procedure.	The caregiver holding the tracheostomy tube is responsible for ensuring that the tube stays in place until the new tracheostomy ties are secure.[12,13,16]
10. Remove soiled pads if present.	Microorganisms grow in a warm moist environment.[13]	Routine cleaning of stoma site should also occur independent of tie changes.
11. Moisten sponges and cotton swabs and clean surrounding skin and stoma site. Allow skin to completely dry. Pat dry if necessary.	Provides friction to remove debris. A dry surface reduces the likelihood of microorganism growth and skin breakdown.	Cotton swabs are helpful in removal of debris at the juncture of the stoma and tracheostomy tube. Never use a cut 4×4 gauze pad

Procedure Continues on following page

* Level IV: Limited clinical studies to support recommendations

Procedure | for Tracheostomy Tube: Stoma Care and Tie Change—*Continued*

Steps	Rationale	Considerations

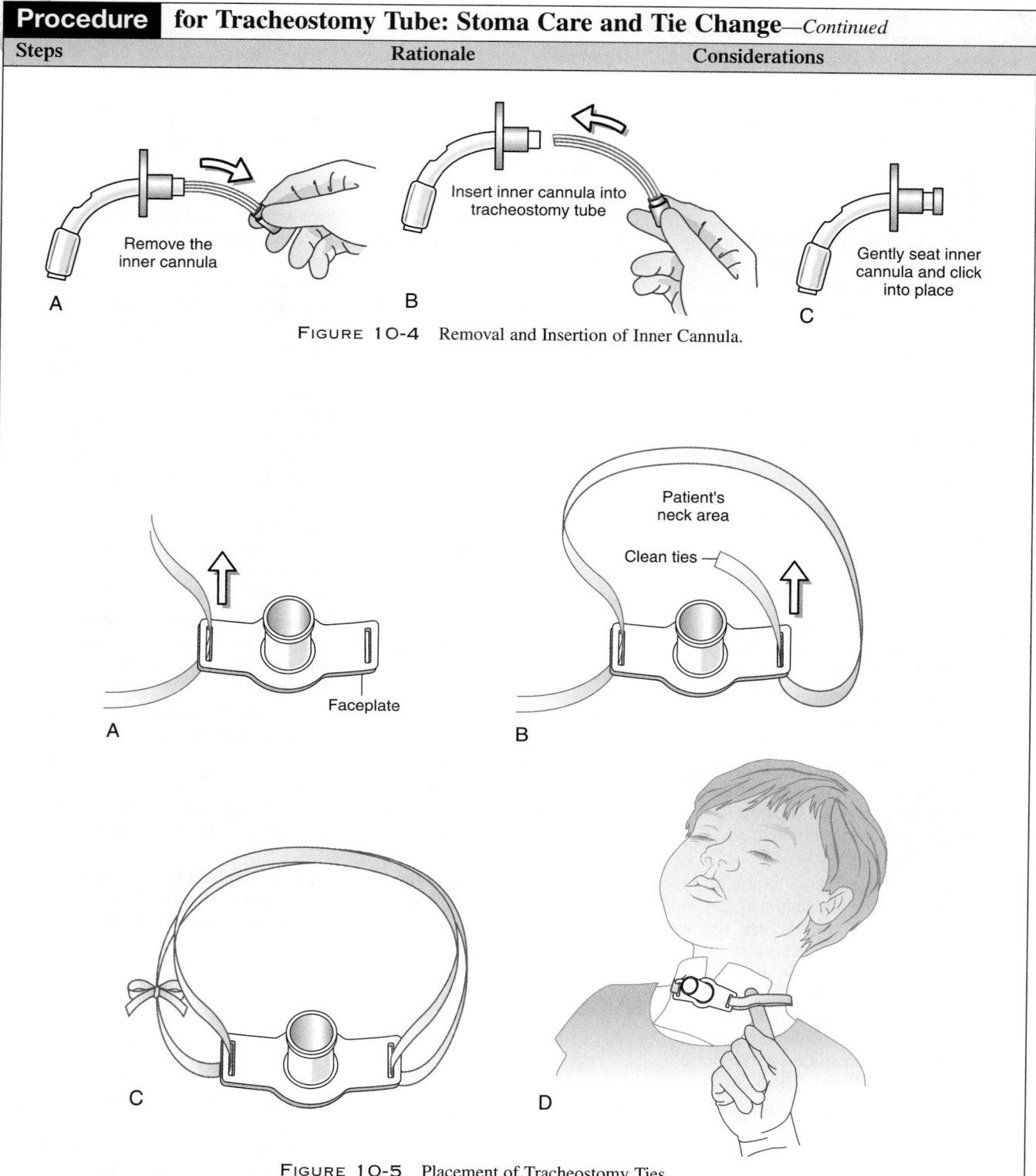

Remove the inner cannula

A

Insert inner cannula into tracheostomy tube

B

Gently seat inner cannula and click into place

C

FIGURE 10-4   Removal and Insertion of Inner Cannula.

Faceplate

A

Patient's neck area

Clean ties

B

C

D

FIGURE 10-5   Placement of Tracheostomy Ties.

Procedure for **Tracheostomy Tube: Stoma Care and Tie Change**—*Continued*

Steps	Rationale	Considerations
		because edges fray and provide a potential source for infection or aspiration.[16]
12. Thread new ties through neck plate or tracheostomy tube flange (Figure 10-5, *A*). Use hemostat or tweezers if necessary. With twill tape use, attach foam (or moleskin) to ties. Do not allow foam to cover tracheostomy tube flange.	Secures tracheostomy tube. Foam or moleskin provides a cushion to reduce risk of skin breakdown.	With each tie change, use opposite side to begin threading so that knot alternates between left and right sides of the tracheostomy tube. With use of Velcro ties, bring ends together and straighten ties.
13. Bring ties, encased in foam (or Velcro ties), around the neck and thread the bottom tie through the opposite hole in the neck plate (Figure 10-5, *B*).	Promotes security of the tracheostomy tube.	
14. Knot tracheostomy ties. Initially use a single slip knot (Figure 10-5, *C*). Place one finger between ties and neck[5] (Figure 10-5, *D*). Readjust ties if necessary to an acceptable tension. Secure with a triple knot. *The assistant may now release the tracheostomy tube.*	Maintains security of tracheostomy tube.[13,16] Ties that are excessively tight can lead to skin breakdown and cause jugular venous distention.[5] *(Level IV*)*	The tightness of the ties varies depending on the child's comfort and cognitive and developmental levels.
15. If indicated, replace tracheostomy pads. *(Level IV*)*	Promotes absorption of drainage under tracheostomy tube flange.[13]	Placing tracheostomy pads between the skin and tube flanges may not be necessary if child's tracheostomy stoma does not have significant drainage.[1] In addition, use of tracheostomy pads varies on the basis of individual child's needs and institutional policies.
16. Discard gloves and soiled equipment and supplies appropriately and wash hands.	Prevents spread of infection and maintains standard precautions.	
17. Perform postprocedural clinical assessment.	Decompensation may occur during procedure.	

* Level IV: Limited clinical studies to support recommendations

Expected Outcomes	**Unexpected Outcomes**
• Ties are tight yet comfortable • Maintenance of airway position and patency • Dry and intact stoma site • Cardiopulmonary stability • Acceptable level of comfort	• Excessively loose or tight ties • Decannulation • Skin ulceration • Stoma infection • Cardiac or respiratory decompensation • Unmanaged pain and irritability

Monitoring and Care of the Child

Activities and Interventions	Rationale	Reportable Conditions
1. Assess the skin integrity around the entire circumference of the neck, with particular attention to skin folds.[2]	Moisture promotes maceration and skin breakdown at the stomal opening.	• Skin redness and breakdown • Necrosis • Ulcerations
2. Monitor secretions (color, amount, and consistency).	Changes in secretions may indicate infection.	• Copious drainage, purulent drainage, excessively thick secretions
3. Assess respiratory status and physiologic stability, including vital signs, clinical appearance, and signs and symptoms of inadequate oxygenation and ventilation.	May indicate a change in position of the tracheostomy tube.	• Diminished breath sounds • Significant changes in oxygenation saturation and arterial/venous blood gases • Increased peak airway pressures • Persistent coughing • Increased work of breathing • Changes in peripheral perfusion • Changes in color • Anxiety, agitation, and change in mental status
4. Ensure that scissors and an extra tracheostomy tube are visible at the child's bedside.	Obstruction of the trachea necessitates immediate intervention.	
5. Assess comfort and provide appropriate interventions. Allow the family to assist with nonpharmacologic means to comfort and support the child.	Early identification of the child's comfort allows for immediate attention.	• Unresolved pain and discomfort • Continued irritability

Documentation

- Pre-respiratory and postrespiratory assessment findings, including vital signs, breath sounds, and work of breathing
- Assessment of tracheal stoma site, including skin condition (note presence/extent of granulation tissue or breakdown) and presence of any drainage at stoma site, including the amount, color, odor and consistency
- Child's response to stoma care
- Comfort assessment and any specific interventions provided
- Additional interventions necessary before, during, and after the procedure
- Child and family education
- Unexpected outcomes and related treatment

References

1. Gera T, Matthew JL: *Tracheostomy/long term care,* 2000, retrieved March 5, 2005, from http://pedsccm.wustl.edu/All-Net/english/pulmpage/trache/trachlong.html.
2. Curley MAQ, Thompson JE: Oxygenation and ventilation. In Curley MAQ, Moloney-Harmon P, editors: *Critical care nursing of infants and children,* ed 2, Philadelphia, 2001, Saunders.
3. Jardine D, Martin L: Specific disease of the respiratory system and upper airway. In Furham B, Zimmerman J, editors: *Pediatric critical care,* ed 3, Philadelphia, 2005, Elsevier.
4. Katz R: Function and physiology of the respiratory system. In Furham B, Zimmerman J, editors: *Pediatric critical care,* ed 2, Philadelphia, 1998, Mosby.
5. Hazinski MF, et al, editors: *Pediatric advanced life support provider manual,* Dallas, 2002, American Heart Association.
6. Froh D: Alterations of pulmonary function in children. In McCance K, Huether S, editors: *Pathophysiology: the biologic basis for disease in adults and children,* ed 4, Philadelphia, 2002, Mosby.
7. Panitch HB, et al: Guidelines for homecare of children with chronic respiratory insufficiency, *Pediatr Pulmonol* 21(1):52-56, 1996.
8. Lee W, et al: Indications for tracheotomy in pediatric intensive care unit population, *Arch Otol Head Neck Surg* 128:1249-1252, 2002.
9. Lewis C, et al: Tracheostomy in pediatric patients: a national perspective, *Arch Otol Head Neck Surg* 129(5):523-529, 2003.

10. Skillings K, Curtis B: Procedure 12 tracheostomy tube care. In Lynn-McHale Wiegand DJ, Carlson K, editors: *AACN procedure manual for critical care,* ed 5, Philadelphia, 2004, Saunders.
11. American Thoracic Society: Care of the child with a chronic tracheostomy, *Am J Respir Crit Care Med* 161:297-308, 2000.
12. Hooper M: Nursing care of the patient with a tracheostomy, *Nurs Stand* 10(34):40-43, 1996.
13. Woodrow P: Managing patients with a tracheostomy in acute care, *Nurs Stand* 16(44):39-48, 2002.
14. Griggs A: Tracheostomy: suctioning and humidification, *Nurs Stand* 13(2):49-53,55-56, 1998.
15. Edwards EA, et al: Sending children home on tracheostomy dependent ventilation: pitfalls and outcomes, *Arch Disabled Child* 89:251-255, 2004.
16. Serra A: Tracheostomy care, *Nurs Stand* 14(42):45-55, 2000.

Additional Reading
Carr M, Poje C, Kingston L, et al: Complications in pediatric tracheotomies, *Laryngoscope* 111:1925-1928, 2001.

Tracheostomy Tube: Change

PURPOSE: Tracheostomy tube change is performed for maintenance of artificial airway patency, assurance of adequate gas exchange, and reduction of the risk of infection

Susan M. Campisciano and Elsie M. Hartigan

PREREQUISITE KNOWLEDGE

- Child development as it relates to clinical assessment and the procedure
- Anatomy and physiology of the pediatric pulmonary system, including structural characteristics of the upper and lower respiratory tract that are specific to the infant and child[1-5]
  - ❖ A child's airway is both absolutely and relatively smaller in diameter and shorter than an adult's (see Figure 1-1).
  - ❖ The child's funnel-shaped larynx is higher and more cephalad and lies below the vocal cords. The vocal cords are 50% cartilage and are attached lower and more anteriorly.
  - ❖ The infant's epiglottis is floppy, long, and narrow and projects more posteriorly than in the older child. The subglottic airway is smaller and more compliant, with the cartilage less developed than in the adult.
  - ❖ Because the thyroid does not assume its adult configuration until puberty, the cricoid cartilage is the easiest landmark for identification in children. The cricoid cartilage is the narrowest portion of the upper airway in children less than 10 years of age. It lies at the level of the third cervical vertebrae in the infant and descends to the sixth cervical vertebrae at puberty.
  - ❖ In teenagers and adults, the larynx is a cylinder with its narrowest portion at the glottic inlet or at the level of the vocal cords.

- ❖ The quantity of alveoli increases until 8 years of age and thereafter increases in size and complexity. Peripheral airway resistance is disproportionately higher in the child.
- ❖ During inspiration, the infant's intercostal muscles stiffen and a downward movement of the diaphragm occurs, which results in negative intrathoracic pressure and air movement into the lungs. Because the infant's chest wall is compliant and flexible, it characteristically collapses inward (see Figure 23-1).
- Signs and symptoms of inadequate oxygenation and ventilation[6]
- Mastery of pediatric advanced life support competencies, including indications for an artificial airway, use of a manual resuscitation/ventilation system, and other adjuncts used for ventilation support[5]
- Tracheotomy is a surgical procedure that involves the construction of a channel between the trachea and the skin surface of the neck in the midline.[5] An incision is made through the second, third, and fourth tracheal rings (Figure 11-1).
- Placement too close to the first ring risks cricoid cartilage damage with subsequent subglottic stenosis.
- A tracheostomy is the opening or stoma made with the tracheotomy incision.
- Clinical indications for the child's tracheotomy and date of original tube placement
  - ❖ Some possible indications for tracheotomy include upper airway obstruction, craniofacial abnormalities

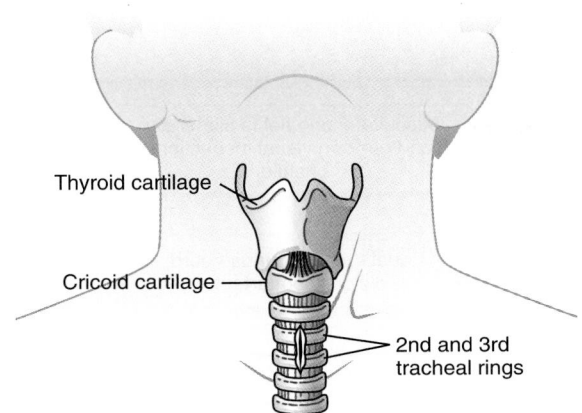

Thyroid cartilage

Cricoid cartilage

2nd and 3rd
tracheal rings

FIGURE 11-1   Tracheotomy Incision.

that interfere with natural airway patency, prolonged ventilatory support, prevention of aspiration, and removal of secretions.[3,5-9] Some common abnormalities that lead to tracheostomy for infants and children include chronic lung disease, subglottic stenosis, tracheal stenosis, laryngotracheomalacia, neuromuscular weakness, and neurologic impairment.[3,6-9]

- Advantages of a tracheostomy tube, over an endotracheal tube, include improved comfort and security, ability to provide a mechanism for speech, increased mobility, easier removal of secretions, and prevention of further airway injury from an endotracheal tube[3,6]
- Tracheostomy tubes are available (or can be custom made) with different characteristics, including the size of the internal diameter and outer diameter, tube length, presence or absence of a cuff, presence or absence of an internal cannula, and presence or absence of a fenestration.[5,6,10,11] Pediatric tubes are generally made of plastic and are single cannula (see Figure 10-1). The difference between neonatal, pediatric, and adult tracheostomy tubes of the same diameter is the length of the tube. As with adult tracheostomy tubes, some pediatric tubes for older children and adolescents have cuffs to minimize leak and an inner cannula to ease cleaning and reduce the frequency of tracheostomy tube change[10] (see Figure 10-2). Tracheostomy tubes also come fenestrated (with openings) to let air into the upper airway so the child can speak (see Figure 10-3).
- The first tracheostomy change is generally performed by the physician service that initially placed the tracheostomy tube.[12] Subsequent tube changes are performed by trained staff, including nurses, respiratory therapists, physicians, or trained family members on a routine basis and whenever an obstruction is suspected.[6]
- Routine tracheostomy tube changes occur weekly to monthly. Two caregivers are needed during the tube change, and children should have nothing by mouth for at least 1 hour before the procedure.[13,14]
- Emergency tracheostomy tube change for airway obstruction or accidental tube dislodgement is performed on the basis of acute clinical deterioration and respiratory compromise as indicated by nasal flaring, use of accessory muscles, increased respiratory rate, increased heart rate, bradycardia or respiratory arrest, cyanosis, or decrease in oxygen saturation. For children who are dependent on a ventilator, an increase in peak inspiratory pressure or loss of inspiratory pressure may indicate a need for a tracheostomy tube change.[1,13,14]
- Troubleshooting protocol for tracheostomy tube change[11,13-16] (Figure 11-2).

CHILD AND FAMILY ASSESSMENT

- Child's developmental level and ability to interact ➥*Rationale:* Influences preparation and interaction.
- Child's and family's understanding of the reasons for and risks and benefits of the procedure ➥*Rationale:* Evaluates child's and family's understanding of the procedure and provides a gauge for ongoing education.
- Desire of family members to be present during the procedure ➥*Rationale:* The presence of family may provide comfort and support, although family members should have the choice not to remain with the child.
- History of upper airway anomalies, presence of a critical airway, and neurologic status ➥*Rationale:* Evaluates the child's ability to maintain a patent airway provides valuable information in determination of the child's ability to tolerate tracheostomy tube change.
- Presence of cardiac or pulmonary disease, degree of ventilator dependence (ventilator settings, including oxygen requirement), and tolerance of brief periods without mechanical ventilation ➥*Rationale:* Children with underlying respiratory or cardiac disease may decompensate during tracheostomy tube change because of an increase in oxygen consumption and a decrease in oxygen reserves.
- Timing of most recent feeding ➥*Rationale:* A full stomach may lead to vomiting or aspiration during the procedure. For avoidance or minimization of this risk, nothing by mouth should be maintained.[14]
- Characteristics and production of tracheal secretions ➥*Rationale:* Assists in identifying underlying pathology and direction of intervention. Irritation of mucosa results in increased production of secretions.
- Cardiopulmonary assessment, including vital signs, visual inspection of breathing patterns and chest wall movement, auscultation of lung fields, and signs of inadequate oxygenation and ventilation, such as decreased arterial oxygen saturation, cardiac arrhythmias, increased work of breathing, cyanosis, increased blood pressure, elevated intracranial pressure, anxiety, agitation, and changes in level of consciousness ➥*Rationale:* Evaluating cardiopulmonary status provides valuable information in determination of the child's need for and ability to tolerate the procedure. Routine tracheostomy tube change is performed when the child is clinically stable and shows signs of optimal gas exchange.

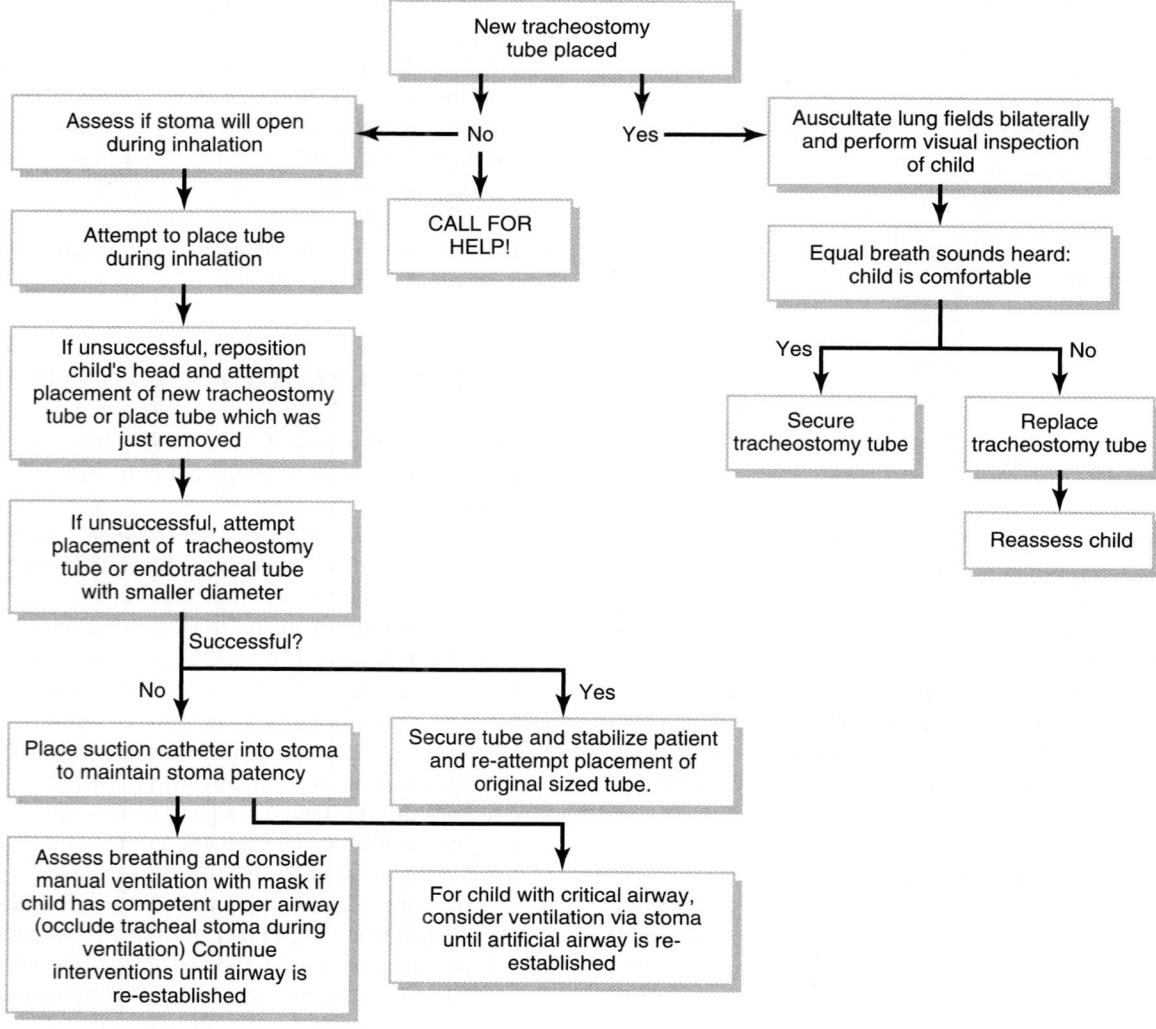

FIGURE 11-2   Troubleshooting.

CHILD AND FAMILY EDUCATION

Individualized, developmentally appropriate education is provided to the family and to the child based on desire for knowledge, readiness to learn, and overall neurologic and psychosocial state.

- Explain the procedure for tracheostomy tube change, including the purpose, steps, and rationale ➥*Rationale:* Providing information decreases fear and anxiety and helps build a plan for tracheostomy teaching.
- If appropriate for the child's current cognitive and developmental level, explain the procedure to the child and consider use of a child life specialist in assisting with the child's preparation for the procedure ➥*Rationale:* Involving the child with the preparation for tracheostomy change can increase the feeling of control and increase tolerance to the procedure.
- Explain that child may experience anxiety and discomfort during the procedure ➥*Rationale:* Involving the child

and family with the preparation for tracheostomy change can increase the feeling of control and increase tolerance to the procedure.

- Encourage questions and answer questions as they arise ➥*Rationale:* Reinforcement of information is needed during periods of stress.

EQUIPMENT

- Clean gloves
- Additional personal protective equipment as indicated, including eye protection, mask, and gown
- Sterile tracheostomy tube of appropriate size with obturator as indicated
- Spare emergency tracheostomy tube of appropriate size
- Tracheostomy tube or endotracheal tube with an internal diameter one half size smaller than the child's current tube size[14,16]
- Syringe to deflate cuff, if tube is cuffed

- Twill tape or Velcro ties
- Foam or moleskin with adhesive backing (with twill tie use)
- Scissors
- Hemostat or tweezers
- Manual ventilation bag (MVB) with oxygen source as needed

- Suction equipment
- Stethoscope
- Blanket roll
- Water-soluble lubricant

Procedure for Tracheostomy Tube: Change

Steps	Rationale	Considerations
1. Ensure child and family understand procedure and questions are answered.	Evaluates and reinforces understanding of previously taught information.	Developmental, cognitive, and anxiety levels determine approach and effectiveness of teaching.
2. Gather equipment and supplies at the bedside.	Facilitates completion of procedure in a timely manner.	Application of tracheostomy tube ties (Velcro or twill tape and foam) to new tracheostomy tube, in advance, may minimize time that tube is not secure.
3. Verify new tracheostomy tube is correct size, including internal diameter, external diameter, and length. Inspect tube to ensure it has no manufacturer or acquired defects. *(Level II*)*	The pediatric trachea has a smaller diameter than the adult trachea. Individual variations of tracheal length and carina position are found in children. Some children need a tracheostomy tube with a custom length.[14]	The internal and outer diameter measurements of many tracheostomy tubes are found on tube flange. For length measurement, refer to manufacturer packaging. *(Level I*)*
4. Prepare the new tube with the tracheal tube tip kept sterile. If child has a cuffed tracheostomy tube, inflate cuff with air or water to ensure it works properly. Be sure cuff is deflated before insertion of a new tube. If tracheostomy tube needs an obturator for insertion, put obturator into the tracheostomy tube before placement. If tracheostomy tube has an inner cannula, remove inner cannula and insert obturator into the new tracheostomy tube.	Avoidance of contamination of the tube tip reduces risk of contamination with microorganisms. A child may need a cuffed tracheostomy tube for maintenance of an adequate seal for optimal delivery of ventilation or for minimization of the risk of aspiration.[15-17] Many tracheostomy tubes have obturators for assistance with insertion of tubes into tracheal stomas. Adolescents with adult tracheostomy tubes have an inner cannula.[16]	Whether the cuff is inflated with water or air is determined by the manufacturer of the tracheostomy tube. *(Level I*)*
5. Wash hands and put on gloves and appropriate personal protection equipment.	Reduces transmission of infection and protects personnel health. The trachea has colonization with bacteria; therefore, clean technique may be acceptable as an approach to tracheostomy tube change.[16]	Use of sterile or aseptic technique may be indicated on the basis of the child's clinical status or institutional policies. For home caregiver training, use of clean technique is recommended.[14]
6. Monitor child's vital signs and indications of inadequate oxygenation and ventilation before, during, and after procedure.	Routine tube change is performed when child's condition is clinically stable and optimal gas exchange is seen.	Consider the child's status and experience with tracheostomy tube change in selection of monitoring.

Procedure continues on following page

* Level I: Manufacturer's recommendations only
Level II: Theory-based; no research data to support recommendations; recommendations from expert consensus group may exist

Procedure for **Tracheostomy Tube: Change**—*Continued*

Steps	Rationale	Considerations
7. Suction tracheostomy tube as indicated.	Secretions that are present in trachea before tube change may be pushed further into the airway if not removed before a new tracheostomy tube is inserted.[6]	See Procedure 12.
8. Position child so head is slightly extended and stoma site is visible and easily accessible.	Allows visualization of neck and stoma for tracheal tube change.[13]	Placement of a blanket roll under the shoulders for hyperextension of the neck is helpful.
9. Provide increased ventilatory support, hyperoxygenation before procedure, and pharmacologic sedation as indicated.	Children with significant cardiac or pulmonary disease or those who are critically ill may need hyper-oxygenation, increased ventilatory support or oxygen flow, or sedation for prevention of significant decompensation.	
10. The first caregiver holds current tracheostomy tube securely, and the second caregiver cuts and removes ties. *(Level II*)*	When tracheostomy tube is not secured, a caregiver must hold tube in place in the stoma for prevention of dislodgement.[14]	
11. The second caregiver removes new tracheostomy tube from package and prepares to insert the tracheostomy tube.	The second caregiver must be ready before tracheostomy tube is removed.	The second caregiver determines the initiation of the tracheostomy tube change once the new tracheostomy tube is ready for insertion.
12. If child has a cuffed tube, deflate the cuff before removal with withdrawal of air or water from cuff with a syringe.	Prevents trauma to tracheal tissue.	
13. Once second caregiver is ready, first caregiver removes current tracheostomy tube from the stoma followed immediately by second caregiver inserting new tube with the curve pointing downward and following curve of the tracheal stoma (Figure 11-3, *A* and *B*).	Tracheostomy tube removal occurs just before reinsertion.	Placement of a small amount of water-soluble lubricant on the tracheostomy tube tip may assist with placement of the tube in the stoma. If resistance occurs in replacement of the tracheostomy tube, remove and

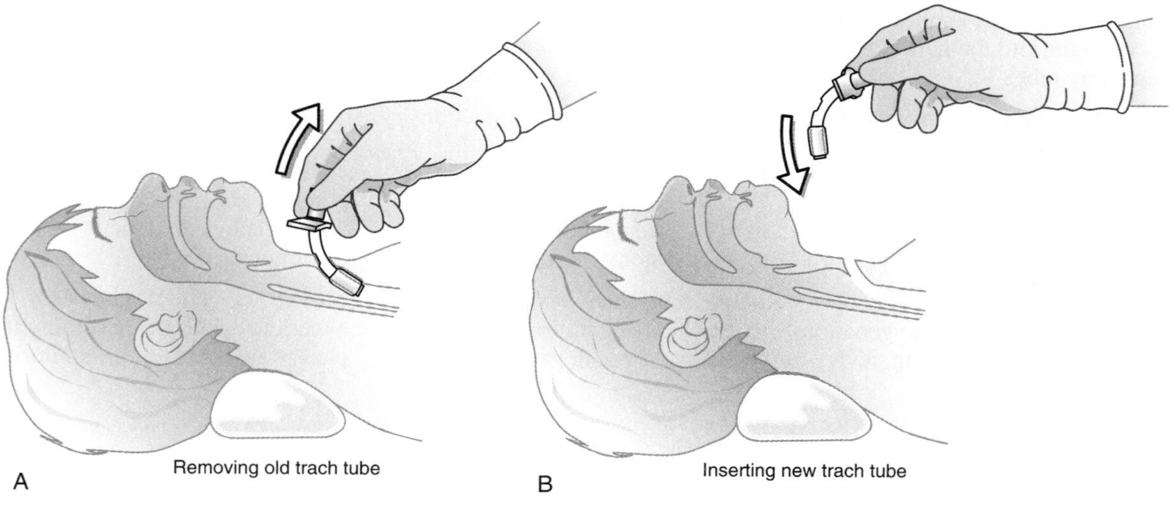

A   Removing old trach tube   B   Inserting new trach tube

FIGURE 11-3   Tracheostomy Tube Change.

* Level II: Theory-based; no research data to support recommendations; recommendations from expert consensus group may exist.

Procedure for Tracheostomy Tube: Change—*Continued*

Steps	Rationale	Considerations
With obturator use, the second caregiver maintains pressure on the obturator and removes the obturator after insertion. If tracheostomy tube has an inner cannula, it should be inserted and locked into place after obturator is removed.	Pressure prevents obturator from becoming displaced during insertion.	try again. *Do not force.* With new tracheotomies, the tracheostomy tube may be easily inserted into the paratracheal tissue.[13] (See troubleshooting flow chart in Figure 11-2.)
14. The first caregiver attaches ventilator tubing or oxygen delivery device to new tracheostomy while the second caregiver holds new tube securely.	Minimizes duration of disconnect from ventilatory support or oxygen delivery.	
15. The first caregiver auscultates child's breath sounds bilaterally and performs a clinical respiratory assessment.	Auscultation of equal breath sounds bilateral with equal expansion of the chest confirms that tracheostomy tube has been placed correctly in trachea.[13,14]	Monitor the child for unequal breath sounds or signs of respiratory distress. (See trouble-shooting flow chart in Figure 11-2.) An end tidal carbon dioxide monitor can also be used in an intensive care unit for confirmation of tube placement.
16. Continue careful clinical assessment of the child's cardiopulmonary status with visual examination and appropriate monitoring devices.	The child's condition may not return to baseline respiratory status for several minutes.	
17. Secure tracheostomy tube with twill tape or Velcro ties.		See Procedure 10.
18. Remove and discard protective items and wash hands.	Reduces transmission of infection. Protects personnel health.	

Expected Outcomes / Unexpected Outcomes

Expected Outcomes	Unexpected Outcomes
• New tracheostomy tube is patent and correctly placed in the child's airway • Atraumatic insertion of tracheostomy tube • Adequate oxygenation and ventilation with baseline clinical examination, ventilatory support, and oxygen requirement • Acceptable level of comfort	• Decannulation • Inadvertent placement of tracheostomy tube in right bronchus or tracheal blind pouch • Trauma to trachea or stoma site • Inadequate oxygenation and ventilation • Cardiopulmonary arrest • Unmanaged pain and agitation

Monitoring and Care of the Child

Activities and Interventions	Rationale	Reportable Conditions
1. Assess respiratory status and physiologic stability, including vital signs, clinical appearance, and signs and symptoms of inadequate oxygenation and ventilation.	May indicate a need for additional assessment and intervention. Temporary removal of the artificial airway may alter the child's physiologic stability. Confirms correct tube placement.	• Diminished breath sounds • Significant changes in oxygenation saturation and arterial/venous blood gases • Increased peak airway pressures • Persistent coughing • Increased work of breathing • Persistent dysrhythmias, including bradycardia and tachycardia • Changes in peripheral perfusion

Continued

Monitoring and Care of the Child—Cont'd

Activities and Intervention	Rationale	Reportable Conditions
		• Cyanosis • Anxiety, agitation, or changes in mental status
2. Assess the stoma for bleeding, ulceration, or granulation tissue and provide stoma care (see Procedure 10).	Assessment provides direction for intervention. Ensures that the stoma site is clean and dry.	• Redness, ulceration, granulation tissue, or traumatic injury to the site
3. Suction the tracheostomy tube as indicated (see Procedure 12).	Secretions may be pushed down into the trachea with tube change. Removal of secretions may be necessary for maintenance of airway patency.	• Change in quantity and characteristics of secretions
4. Assess comfort and provide appropriate interventions. Allow the family to assist with nonpharmacologic means to comfort and support the child.	Early identification of the child's comfort allows for immediate attention.	• Unresolved pain and discomfort • Continued irritability

Documentation

- Prerespiratory and postrespiratory assessment findings, including vital signs, breath sounds, and work of breathing
- Note ease or difficulty in placement of new tracheostomy tube
- Assessment of tracheal stoma site, including skin condition (note the presence and extent of granulation tissue or breakdown) and the presence of any drainage at the stoma site, including amount, color, odor, and consistency
- Child's involvement and response to tracheal tube change
- Comfort assessment and any specific interventions provided
- Additional interventions necessary before, during, and after tracheostomy tube change
- Child and family education
- Unexpected outcomes and related treatment

References

1. Gera T, Matthew JL: *Pediatric tracheostomy,* 2000, retrieved February 5, 2005, from http://pedsccm.wustl.edu/All-Net/english/pulmpage/trache/trachetitle.html.
2. Froh D: Alterations of pulmonary function in children. In McCance K, Huether S, editors: *Pathophysiology: the biologic basis for disease in adults and children,* ed 4, Philadelphia, 2002, Mosby.
3. Jardine D, Martin L: Specific disease of the respiratory system and upper airway. In Furham B, Zimmerman J, editors: *Pediatric critical care,* ed 3, Philadelphia, 2005, Elsevier.
4. Katz R: Function and physiology of the respiratory system. In Fuhrman B, Zimmerman J, editors: *Pediatric critical care,* ed 3, Philadelphia, 2005, Elsevier.
5. Hazinski MF, et al, editors: *Pediatric advanced life support provider manual,* Dallas, 2002, American Heart Association.
6. Curley MAQ, Thompson JE: Oxygenation and ventilation. In Curley MAQ, Moloney-Harmon P, editors: *Critical care nursing of infants and children,* ed 2, Philadelphia, 2001, Saunders.
7. Panitch HB, Downes JJ, Kennedy JS, et al: Guidelines for homecare of children with chronic respiratory insufficiency, *Pediatr Pulmonol* 21(1):52-56, 1996.
8. Lee W, et al: Indications for tracheotomy in pediatric intensive care unit population, *Arch Otol Head Neck Surg* 128:1249-1252, 2002.
9. Lewis C, et al: Tracheostomy in pediatric patients: a national perspective, *Arch Otol Head Neck Surg* 129(5):523-529, 2003.
10. Skillings K, Curtis B: Procedure 12 tracheostomy tube care. In Lynn-McHale Wiegand DJ, Carlson K, editors: *AACN procedure manual for critical care,* ed 5, Philadelphia, 2004, Saunders.
11. American Thoracic Society: Care of the child with a chronic tracheostomy, *Am J Respir Crit Care Med* 161:297-308, 2000.
12. Deutsch ES: Early tracheostomy tube change in children, *Arch Otolaryngol Head Neck Surg* (124):1237-1238, 1998.
13. Buzz-Kelly L, Gordin P: Teaching CPR to parents of children with tracheostomies, *MCN* (18):158-163, 1993.
14. Dougherty JM, Kandrak G, Kinney Z, et al. Pediatric tracheostomy and ventilator care, *Nurs Spec Career Fitness Online* CE:131, 2003.
15. Hooper M: Nursing care of the patient with a tracheostomy, *Nurs Stand* 10(34):40-43, 1996.
16. Serra A: Tracheostomy care, *Nurs Stand* 14(42):45-55, 2000.
17. Woodrow P: Managing patients with a tracheostomy in acute care, *Nurs Stand* 16(44):39-48, 2002.
18. Edwards EA, et al: Sending children home on tracheostomy dependent ventilation: pitfalls and outcomes, *Arch Disabled Child* 89:251-255, 2004.

Additional Reading

Carr M, Poje C, Kingston L, et al: Complications in pediatric tracheotomies. *Laryngoscope* 111:1925-1928, 2001.

Tracheostomy Tube: Suctioning

P U R P O S E : Tracheostomy tube suctioning removes tracheal secretions, maintains airway patency, and provides a method for acquiring tracheal aspirates for laboratory analysis

Susan M. Campisciano and Elsie M. Hartigan

PREREQUISITE KNOWLEDGE

- Child development as it relates to clinical assessment and the procedure
- Anatomy and physiology of the pediatric pulmonary system, including structural characteristics of the upper and lower respiratory tract that are specific to the infant and child[1-6]
  - ❖ A child's airway is both absolutely and relatively smaller in diameter and shorter than an adult's (see Figure 1-1)
  - ❖ Because the thyroid does not assume its adult configuration until puberty, the cricoid cartilage is the easiest landmark for identification in children.
  - ❖ The cricoid cartilage is the narrowest portion of the upper airway in children less than 10 years of age. It lies at the level of the third cervical vertebrae in the infant and descends to the sixth cervical vertebrae at puberty.
  - ❖ In teenagers and adults, the larynx is a cylinder with its narrowest portion at the glottic inlet at the level of the vocal cords.
  - ❖ The quantity of alveoli increases until 8 years of age and thereafter increases in size and complexity. Peripheral airway resistance is disproportionately higher in the child.
  - ❖ During inspiration, the infant's intercostal muscles stiffen and a downward movement of the diaphragm occurs, which results in negative intrathoracic pressure and air movement into the lungs. Because the infant's chest wall is compliant and flexible, it characteristically collapses inward (see Figure 23-1).
- Signs and symptoms of inadequate oxygenation and ventilation[5]
- Mastery of pediatric advanced life support competencies, including indications for an artificial airway, use of a manual resuscitation/ventilation system, and other adjuncts used to support ventilation[4]
- Tracheotomy is a surgical procedure that involves the construction of a channel between the trachea and the skin surface of the neck in the midline. An incision is made through the second, third, and fourth tracheal rings[4] (see Figure 11-1). Placement too close to the first ring risks cricoid cartilage damage with subsequent subglottic stenosis.
- A tracheostomy is the opening or stoma made by the tracheotomy incision.
- Clinical indications for the child's tracheotomy and date of original tube placement
  - ❖ Some possible indications for tracheotomy include upper airway obstruction, craniofacial abnormalities that interfere with natural airway patency, prolonged ventilatory support, prevention of aspiration, and removal of secretions.[2,5-10]
  - ❖ Some common abnormalities that lead to tracheostomy tube placement for infants and children include chronic lung disease, subglottic stenosis, tracheal stenosis, laryngotracheomalacia, neuromuscular weakness, and neurologic impairment.[2,5-10]

- Tracheostomy tubes are available (or can be custom made) with different characteristics, including the size of the internal diameter and outer diameter, tube length, presence or absence of a cuff, presence or absence of an internal cannula, and presence or absence of a fenestration.[4,5,10,11] Pediatric tubes are generally made of plastic and are single cannula (see Figure 10-1).
- The difference between neonatal, pediatric, and adult tracheostomy tubes of the same diameter is the length of the tube. As with adult tracheostomy tubes, some pediatric tubes for older children and adolescents have cuffs to minimize leakage and an inner cannula to ease cleaning and to reduce the frequency of tracheostomy tube changes[11] (see Figure 10-2).
- Tracheostomy tubes also come fenestrated (with openings) to let air into the upper airway so the child can speak (see Figure 10-3).
- Children with tracheostomy tubes do not have the upper airway to humidify the air that is breathed, so a humidification device (humidifier or heat-moisture exchanger) is needed to prevent tracheal secretions from becoming viscous and potentially occluding the airway.[1,10,12,13]
- Tracheostomy tube suctioning is often most effective after chest physiotherapy, percussion, vibration, the use of a mechanical device such as an in-exsufflator or intrapulmonary percussive ventilation, and other respiratory therapies. The use of adjunct therapy to maintain airway patency is especially important for the child with an ineffective cough from neuromuscular weakness.[10]
- Pharmacologic therapy, such as inhaled or nebulized mucolytic agents or bronchodilators, can enhance the effectiveness of removal of tracheal and lower airway secretions during suctioning.
- Suctioning can be performed with either open suction technique, which involves a disconnecton from the ventilator circuit or oxygen source, or closed (inline) suctioning technique. Closed suctioning technique is particularly useful in children who need maintenance of high levels of inspired oxygen or positive end expiratory pressure (Table 12-1).[14,15]
- Indications for suctioning include audible tracheal secretions, auscultation of adventitious lung sounds, and signs of respiratory compromise, including increased work of breathing, increased respiratory rate and heart rate, sustained coughing, decreased blood oxygen saturations either arterial (SaO_2) or via pulse oximetry (SpO_2), and inability to generate an effective spontaneous cough. Suctioning may also be indicated with ventilator dependence with increased peak airway pressures during volume-controlled mechanical ventilation or decreased tidal volume during pressure-controlled ventilation, changes in flow, and pressure graphics during mechanical ventilation.[12,14]
- Selection of catheter size is based on the internal diameter of the tracheostomy tube (Table 12-2).
  - ❖ As a general rule, the outer diameter of the suction catheter should be no greater than one half the inner diameter of the artificial airway.[1,7,10,14,16,17]
- Instillation of normal saline solution into the tracheostomy tube is not recommended. Many authors have suggested that this practice is ineffective in enhancing removal of tracheal secretions.[12,17,18]

CHILD AND FAMILY ASSESSMENT

- Child's developmental level and inability to interact ➥*Rationale:* Influences preparation and interaction.
- Child's and family's understanding of the reasons for and risks and benefits of the procedure ➥*Rationale:* Evaluates child's and family's understanding of the procedure and provides a gauge for ongoing education.
- Desire of family members to be present during the procedure ➥*Rationale:* The presence of family may provide comfort and support, although remaining with the child should always be a choice.
- History of upper airway anomalies, presence of a critical airway, and neurologic status ➥*Rationale:* Evaluates the child's ability to maintain a patent airway provides valuable information in determination of the child's ability to tolerate suctioning.
- Presence of cardiac or pulmonary disease, degree of ventilator dependence (ventilator settings, including oxygen requirement), and tolerance of brief periods without ventilatory support ➥*Rationale:* Children with underlying

TABLE 12-1	Recommended Wall Suction Pressure
Infant	50 to 100 mm Hg
Child	80 to 120 mm Hg
Adult	100 to 120 mm Hg*

* Maximum pressure, 150 mm Hg.
For portable suction units, refer to portable suction unit procedural manual.
Carroll P: Improve your suctioning technique, *RN* 66:30ac2-30ac6,30ac8, 2003.
Griggs A: Tracheostomy: suctioning and humidification, *Nurs Stand* 13(2):49-53,55-56, 1998.

TABLE 12-2	Suction Catheter Size
Tracheostomy Size	**Recommended Catheter Size**
2.5 to 3.5 mm	6F
3.5 to 4.5 mm	8F
5.0 to 5.5 mm	10F
6.0 to 6.5 mm	12F
7.0 to 8.0 mm	14F

General rule to guide selection: outer diameter of suction catheter should be no greater than one half internal diameter of artificial airway.[10]
Carroll P: Improve your suctioning technique, *RN* 66:30ac2-30ac6,30ac8, 2003.
Gera T, Matthew JL: *Pediatric tracheostomy,*.2000, retrieved August 15, 2005, from http://pedsccm.wustl.edu/All-Net/english/pulmpage/trache/trachetitle.html.
Griggs A: Tracheostomy: suctioning and humidification, *Nurs Stand* 13(2):49-53,55-56, 1998.
Joanna Briggs Institute for Evidence Based Nursing and Midwifery: Tracheal suctioning of adults with an artificial airway, *Best Practice: Evidence based practice information sheets for health professionals* 4(4):1-6, 2000. Text available at http://www.joannabriggs.edu.au/pdf/bpsuc.pdf.
Panitch HB, Downes JJ, Kennedy JS, et al: Guidelines for homecare of children with chronic respiratory insufficiency, *Pediatr Pulmonol* 21(1):52-56, 1996.

respiratory or cardiac disease may experience decompensation during the suctioning procedure because of an increase in oxygen consumption and decreased oxygen reserves.[14,17] These children may benefit from hyperoxygenation before the procedure or use of closed (inline) suctioning technique.

- Characteristics and production of tracheal secretions ➧➧*Rationale:* Assists in identifying underlying pathology (i.e., bacteria infection) and direction of interventions.
- Cardiopulmonary assessment, including vital signs, visual inspection of breathing patterns and chest wall movement, auscultation of lung fields, and signs of inadequate oxygenation and ventilation, such as decreased arterial oxygen saturation, cardiac arrhythmias, increased work of breathing, cyanosis, increased blood pressure, elevated intracranial pressure, anxiety, agitation, and changes in level of consciousness ➧➧*Rationale:* Evaluates the child's cardiopulmonary status furnishes valuable information in determination of the child's need for and ability to tolerate suctioning.
- Timing of most recent feeding and presence of gastroesophageal reflux disease ➧➧*Rationale:* Infants have an incompetent lower esophageal sphincter and an increased incidence rate of gastroesophageal reflux, which can cause vomiting or aspiration during the procedure. To avoid or minimize this risk, tracheal suctioning should be performed before feedings whenever possible.

CHILD AND FAMILY EDUCATION

Individualized, developmentally appropriate education is provided to the family and to the child based on desire for knowledge, readiness to learn, and overall neurologic and psychosocial state.

- Explain the procedure for tracheostomy tube suctioning, including the purpose, steps, and rationale ➧➧*Rationale:* Providing information decreases fear and anxiety and helps build a plan for tracheostomy teaching.[11]
- If appropriate for the child's current cognitive and developmental level, explain the procedure to the child and consider the use of a child life specialist in assisting with the child's preparation for the procedure ➧➧*Rationale:* Involving the child in understanding the procedure can increase the feeling of control and increase tolerance to the procedure.
- Explain to the child and family that the child may feel the need to cough or gag and may experience discomfort during the procedure ➧➧*Rationale:* Involving the child with preparation for suctioning can increase the feeling of control and increase tolerance to the procedure.
- Encourage questions and answer questions as they arise ➧➧*Rationale:* Reinforcement of information is needed during periods of stress.

EQUIPMENT

Open Suctioning System
- Appropriately sized disposable suction catheters clearly marked with numbers
- Personal protective equipment, including eye protection, mask, and gown as indicated
- Suction source (wall regulator or portable machine) with connector tubing and container
- Gloves
- Measuring tape to obtain premeasured suctioning depth (if not already obtained)
- Manual ventilation bag (MVB; self-inflating or flow-inflating) connected to an oxygen flow meter (if clinically indicated)
- Stethoscope
- Normal saline solution in disposable vial or sterile water/normal saline solution and cup

Closed (Inline) Suctioning System
- Gloves and personal protective equipment as indicated
- Closed tracheal suction system (i.e., elbow adaptor or Y adaptor)
- Suction source (wall regulator or portable machine) with connector tubing and container
- Manual ventilation bag (self-inflating or flow-inflating) connected to an oxygen flow meter (if clinically indicated)
- Normal saline solution in disposable vial or sterile water/normal saline solution and cup

Procedure	for Tracheostomy Tube: Suctioning	
Steps	Rationale	Considerations
1. Determine appropriate suctioning technique (open or closed). *(Level IV*)*	Closed suctioning technique is particularly useful in children who need maintenance of high levels of inspired oxygen, inspiratory pressures, and positive end-expiratory pressure.[14,15]	Additional presence of respiratory therapy staff or other experienced personnel may be indicated in the child in whom tracheal suctioning is not tolerated.

Procedure continues on following page

---

* Level IV: Limited clinical studies to support recommendation

Procedure	**for Tracheostomy Tube: Suctioning**—*Continued*	
Steps	**Rationale**	**Considerations**

Open Suctioning System

Steps	Rationale	Considerations
2. Ensure child and family understand procedure and questions are answered.	Evaluates and reinforces understanding of previously taught information.[19]	Developmental, cognitive, and anxiety levels determine approach and effectiveness of teaching.
3. Assess child's respiratory status, including clinical signs of need for tracheal suctioning.	Provides a comparison for postsuctioning auscultation. Tracheal suctioning is performed when clinically indicated, not on a routine schedule.[7,12,14]	
4. Gather needed equipment and supplies.	Facilitates completion of task in a timely manner.	Ensure that an appropriately sized MVB is at the bedside.
5. Monitor child's vital signs and indications of inadequate oxygenation and ventilation before, during, and after suctioning. (*Level II**)	Because of temporary occlusion of the airway, decompensation may occur during the procedure.	Termination of suctioning is needed with cardiac dysrhythmia, hemodynamic instability, or a significant change in oxygenation/ventilation indices.
6. Ensure suction is turned on and pressure is within recommended range (see Table 12-1). (*Level IV**)	Adequate negative pressure is necessary for effective removal of tracheal secretions. Suctioning with pressures higher than recommended can cause mucosal damage to the trachea.[12,14,16]	Follow manufacturer's directions for suction pressure levels with closed suction systems.
7. Wash hands.	Reduces transmission of infection. Protects personnel health.	
8. Select appropriate size of suction catheter on the basis of internal diameter of the artificial airway[10] (see Table 12-2). Use of multi-eyed catheters is preferred over use of single-eyed catheters.	Suction catheter size varies according to the size of the tracheostomy tube. Use of a catheter with too large an external diameter can cause hypoxia or atelectasis.[1,12,14,16,17] Multi-eyed catheters cause less trauma to tracheal tissue.[14] (*Level IV**)	The external diameter of the suction catheter should be less than half the internal diameter of the tracheostomy tube. If the catheter is too small for effective removal of tracheal secretions, the child may benefit from a tracheostomy tube with a larger internal diameter.
9. Verify measured length for catheter insertion before tracheal suctioning.[10] Measure length of child's tracheostomy tube (with numbers marked on suction catheter). Add on length of any adaptors or connections. Add 0.5 to 1.0 cm to ensure suction catheter will clear end of tracheostomy tube.	Because of the smaller length of pediatric trachea and individual variations of tracheal length and carina position, use of premeasured catheter technique is essential in children. Advancement of suction catheter to the point of resistance causes damage of tracheal mucosa and formation of granulation tissue, which can lead to tracheal obstruction.[7,12,14]	The length of catheter insertion measurement is recorded in the child's record and at the bedside. Be sure to use the correct tracheostomy tube in obtaining measurement. Some children may have tracheostomy tubes cut to a custom length.
10. Put on gloves with sterile technique or according to institutional policy. Put on personal protective equipment, including eye protection, mask, and a gown (as indicated).	Reduces transmission of infection. Protects personnel health.	Although sterile suctioning technique is recommended to reduce the likelihood of airway contamination, some institutions use clean technique for suctioning procedure (see institutional procedure for variation).[7,14,19]

* Level II: Theory-based, no research data to support recommendations; recommendations from expert consensus group may exist
   Level IV: Limited clinical studies to support recommendations

Procedure	for Tracheostomy Tube: Suctioning—*Continued*	
Steps	**Rationale**	**Considerations**
		A gown is indicated in cases of copious secretions and strong cough reflex or infectious situations (e.g., respiratory syncytial virus [RSV]).
11. With nondominant hand, pick up and manipulate suction connecting tubing while using the dominant hand to hold suction catheter.	Avoids contamination of catheter before insertion in to trachea.	
12. Disconnect child from ventilator circuit or oxygen source with non-dominant hand (or with a second person if clinically indicated) and administer hyperventilation and hyperoxgenation to the child with MVB.	Hyperoxygenation increases arterial oxygen levels in preparation for suctioning.[4,5,20] Hyperinflation assists in mobilization of secretions. Providing oxygen or manual ventilation can increase child's ability to tolerate the procedure. On the basis of the child's clinical condition, a second trained person may be needed during tracheal suctioning.	If child is undergoing mechanical ventilation, increased oxygen flow via the ventilator circuit or use of manual breath option on the ventilator is an appropriate alternative to a MRB.[17] Hyperoxygenation with 100% fraction of inspired oxygen (FiO_2) is not recommended in certain medical conditions, including certain congenital heart defects and hypoxic respiratory drive.
13. Insert suction catheter into the tracheostomy tube to premeasured length without application of suction (Figure 12-1, *A*). *(Level V*)*	Suctioning is not performed on insertion to minimize trauma to tracheal tissue.[1,12,14,16,17]	
14. Put thumb over the suction port and apply suction while withdrawing the catheter. As catheter is withdrawn, use a twisting motion (Figure 12-1, *B*).	Effective removal of tracheal secretions occurs during removal of the catheter. The rotating motion allows tracheal secretions that have adhered to sides of the tube to be dislodged.	Rotation of the suction catheter is not essential with a multieyed suction catheter.[14] Use brief periods (maximum, 10 to 15 seconds) to minimize decreases in arterial oxygenation and airway trauma.[7,14] *(Level IV*)*

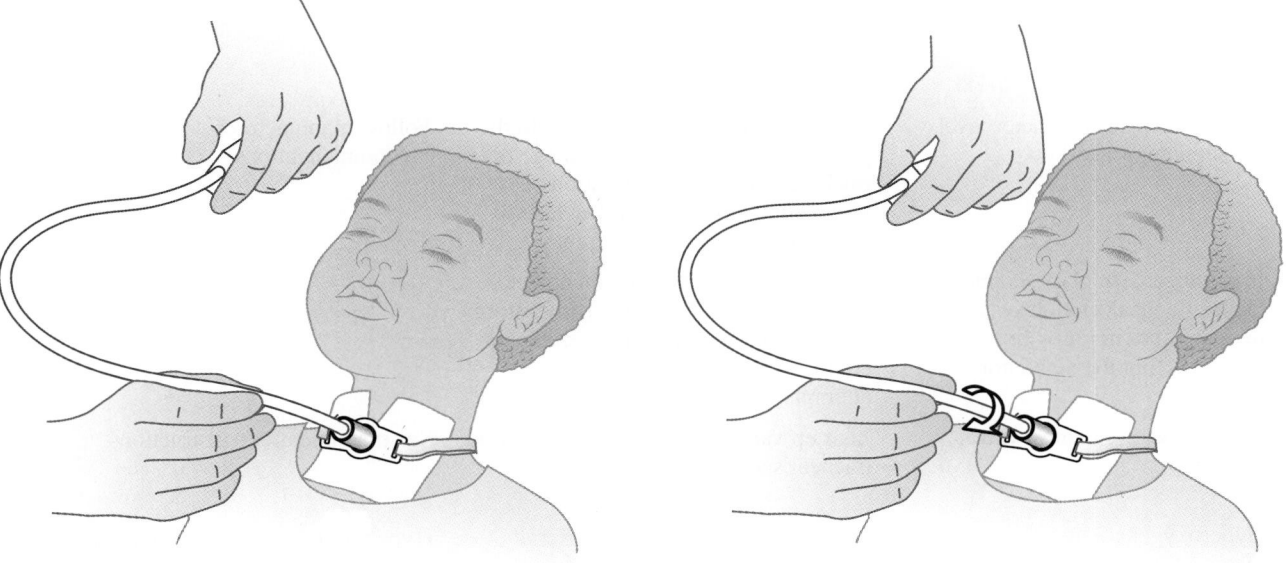

A   B

FIGURE 12-1 Suctioning of Tracheostomy Tube. **A,** Insert suction catheter with suction port open (without application of suction) to premeasured length. **B,** Withdraw catheter and apply suction by occluding suction port with thumb. Use rotating or circular motion.

Procedure continues on following page

* Level IV: Limited clinical studies to support recommendations.
Level V: Clinical studies in more than one or two patient populations and situations to support recommendations.

Procedure for Tracheostomy Tube: Suctioning—*Continued*

Steps	Rationale	Considerations
15. Return child to ventilator circuit or oxygen source. Administer hyperoxygenation or hyperventilation with MVB as clinically indicated.	The level of support is determined by child's clinical condition and child's tolerance of procedure.[7,14,16]	
16. Reassess need for further passes of the suction catheter and repeat steps 11 to 15.	Several passes of suction catheter may be indicated to effectively clear the pediatric tracheostomy tube because of its small internal diameter.[1,12]	Allow child sufficient recovery time between passes of the suction catheter. If tracheal secretions do not clear after repeated passes of suction catheter, the tracheostomy tube may need to be changed (see Procedure 11).
17. To dispose of catheter, wrap it around the dominant hand and pull the glove off inside out. Remove other glove and discard it in a waste container.	Reduces risk of microorganism transmission.	
18. Remove personal protective equipment and discard.	Reduces transmission of infection. Protects personnel health.	
19. Flush connecting tubing with saline solution or sterile water.	Clears tubing of debris.	
20. Turn off suctioning device and secure suction at bedside in clear view for future suctioning needs.	Unsecured suction equipment left in proximity of child can cause contamination of suction equipment or suction burns if the suction catheter inadvertently has contact with patient skin.	
21. Perform postassessment of breath sounds to determine any pertinent changes after suctioning.	Evaluates effectiveness of suctioning.	
22. Wash hands.		
Closed Suctioning Technique See previous Steps 1-7, pp. 77-78.		
8. Determine proper catheter level for suctioning.	Advancement of suction catheter to the point of resistance causes damage of tracheal mucosa and formation of granulation tissue, which can lead to tracheal obstruction.[7,12,14]	Follow manufacturer's recommendations.
9. If not already in place, connect closed tracheal suction system in ventilator circuit by briefly disconnecting the ventilator circuit.	This technique allows suction catheter to be inserted through the tracheostomy tube without disconnecting ventilator circuit with future suctioning attempts.[14,15]	
10. Unlock locking control valve. (*Level I**)	This step varies depending on the closed tracheal suction system used.	See manufacturer's instructions.
11. Hyperoxygenate by pressing the hyperoxygenation button on the ventilator or increase the baseline FiO_2 on ventilator.	Hyperoxygenation increases arterial oxygen levels in preparation for suctioning.[4,5,20]	Hyperoxygenation with 100% FiO_2 is not recommended in certain medical conditions, including certain congenital heart defects and hypoxic respiratory drive.

* Level I: Manufacturer's recommendations only

Procedure	for Tracheostomy Tube: Suctioning—*Continued*	
Steps	**Rationale**	**Considerations**
12. Advance inline suction catheter with dominant hand (while holding tracheostomy tube with nondominant hand) to the premeasured distance (measured number is aligned with the lavage port; see Figure 2-2). No suction is applied during catheter insertion.	Suctioning or use of negative pressure is not applied during insertion of catheter because this can cause tracheal trauma.[1,12,14,16,17]	
13. When catheter is at the correct depth, apply suction while slowly withdrawing the catheter (see Figure 2-2). Continue to secure tracheostomy tube by holding with nondominant hand.	Limiting time of catheter insertion minimizes the duration of airway occlusion in a child who is critically ill.[14,15]	Use brief periods (maximum, 10 to 15 seconds) to minimize decreases in arterial oxygenation and airway trauma.[7,14] *(Level IV*)*
14. Allow child to recover with several ventilator breaths between insertions of the catheter.	Continual assessment of child during procedure, including visual inspection and use of monitoring devices, alerts the caregiver to indicators of respiratory compromise.[7,14]	Increase oxygen flow as needed to maintain oxygen saturation.
15. Reassess need for further passes of the suction catheter and repeat Steps 12 to 14.	Several passes of suction catheter may be indicated to effectively clear pediatric tracheostomy tube because of its small internal diameter.[1,12]	Assess for presence of clinical indicators of need for suctioning as mentioned previously. Allow child sufficient recovery time between passes of suction catheter. If tracheal secretions are not cleared after repeated passes of suction catheter, tracheostomy tube may need to be changed (see Procedure 11).
16. To clean catheter, withdraw black tip of catheter into middle of the cleaning chamber, depress suction, and then gently squeeze saline solution into chamber. *(Level I*)*	Ensures that tubing remains free of debris.	Check recommendations of each manufacturer for specific information for each catheter.
17. Lock suction catheter when finished and turn off suctioning device.	Prevents movement.	
18. Flush the connecting tubing with saline solution or sterile water.	Clears the tubing of debris.	
19. Perform postassessment of breath sounds to determine any pertinent changes after suctioning.	Evaluates effectiveness of suctioning.	
20. Remove and discard personal protective items and wash hands.	Reduces transmission of infection. Protects personnel health.	

* Level I: Manufacturer's recommendations only
  Level IV: Limited clinical studies to support recommendations

Expected Outcomes	Unexpected Outcomes
• Removal of airway secretions and alleviation of clinical signs and symptoms of need for suctioning	• Inability to clear secretions
	• Airway occlusion
• Artificial airway patency	
• Cardiopulmonary stability with adequate oxygenation and ventilation	• Inadequate oxygenation and ventilation
	• Cardiopulmonary arrest
	• Atelectasis
	• Infection
	• Cardiac dysrhythmias (i.e:, bradycardia)
	• Hemodynamic instability
• No traumatic injury as a result of the suctioning procedure	• Tracheal tissue damage or granuloma formation
	• Hemorrhage
• Acceptable level of comfort	• Unmanaged pain, irritability, or agitation

Monitoring and Care of the Child

Activities and Intervention	Rationale	Reportable Conditions
1. Assess respiratory status and physiologic stability, including vital signs, clinical appearance, and signs and symptoms of inadequate oxygenation and ventilation. *(Level II*)*	Preassessment determines the need for suctioning, and post-assessment shows changes after the suctioning procedure. With temporary occlusion of the airway, oxygen saturation may decrease. Heart rate may be increased related to agitation or decreased related to vagus nerve stimulation.	• Bronchospasm • Changes in peripheral perfusion • Cyanosis • Anxiety, agitation, or changes in mental status • Altered respiratory patterns that fail to return to baseline within 5 to 10 minutes after suctioning • Diminished breath sounds • Significant changes in oxygenation saturation and arterial/venous blood gases • Increased peak airway pressures • Persistent coughing • Unresolved increased work of breathing
2. Assessment of color, consistency, and amount of tracheal secretions suctioned from the tracheostomy tube.	Changes in tracheal secretions can indicate infection or airway trauma.	• Purulent or blood-tinged tracheal secretions or any change in baseline tracheal secretions
3. Assess comfort and provide appropriate intervention. Allow the family to assist with nonpharmacologic means to comfort and support the child.	Early identification of the child's comfort allows for immediate attention.	• Unresolved pain and discomfort • Continued irritability

* Level II: Theory-based, no research data to support recommendations; recommendations from expert consensus group may exist

Documentation

• Presuctioning and postsuctioning respiratory assessment findings, including vital signs, breath sounds, and increased work of breathing
• Date, time, and frequency of procedure
• Color, amount, consistency, and odor of secretions
• Child's response to suctioning
• Comfort assessment and any specific interventions provided
• Additional interventions necessary before, during, and after suctioning
• Child and family education
• Unexpected outcomes and related treatment

References

1. Gera T, Matthew JL: *Pediatric tracheostomy,* 2000, retrieved February 5, 2005, from http://pedsccm. wustl.edu/All-Net/english/pulmpage/trache/ trachetitle.html.
2. Jardine D, Martin L: Specific disease of the respiratory system and upper airway. In Furham B, Zimmerman J, editors: *Pediatric critical care,* ed 3, Philadelphia, 2005, Elsevier.
3. Froh D: Alterations of pulmonary function in children. In McCance K, Huether S, editors: *Pathophysiology: the biologic basis for disease in adults and children,* ed 4, Philadelphia, 2002, Mosby.
4. Hazinski MF, editors: *Pediatric advanced life support provider manual,* Dallas, 2002, American Heart Association.
5. Curley MAQ, Thompson JE: Oxygenation and ventilation. In Curley MAQ, Moloney-Harmon P, editors: *Critical care nursing of infants and children,* ed 2, Philadelphia, 2001, Saunders.
6. Katz R: Function and physiology of the respiratory system. In Fuhrman B, Zimmerman J, editors: *Pediatric critical care,* ed 3, Philadelphia, 2005, Elsevier.
7. Panitch HB, et al: Guidelines for homecare of children with chronic respiratory insufficiency, *Pediatr Pulmonol* 21(1):52-56, 1996.
8. Lee W, et al: Indications for tracheotomy in pediatric intensive care unit population, *Arch Otolaryngol Head Neck Surg* 128:1249-1252, 2002.
9. Lewis C, Jeffrey C, Perkins J, et al: Tracheostomy in pediatric patients: a national perspective, *Arch Otolaryngol Head Neck Surg* 129(5):523-529, 2003.
10. American Thoracic Society: Care of the child with a chronic tracheostomy, *Am J Respir Crit Care Med* 161:297-308, 2000.
11. Skillings K, Curtis B: Procedure 12 tracheostomy tube care. In Wiegand DJ, Carlson K, editors: *AACN procedure manual for critical care,* ed 5, Philadelphia, 2004, Saunders.
12. Hooper M: Nursing care of the patient with a tracheostomy, *Nurs Stand* 10(34):40-43, 1996.
13. Woodrow P: Managing patients with a tracheostomy in acute care, *Nurs Stand* 16(44):39-48, 2002.
14. Griggs A: Tracheostomy: suctioning and humidification, *Nurs Stand* 13(2):49-53, 55-56, 1998.
15. Oschreither JM: Closed tracheal suctioning: advantages, drawbacks, and research recommendations, *Online J Knowledge Synthesis Nurs* 2(doc2):Online14,1-8, 1995.
16. Carroll P: Improve your suctioning technique, *RN* 66:30ac2-30ac6,30ac8, 2003.
17. Joanna Briggs Institute for Evidence Based Nursing and Midwifery: Tracheal suctioning of adults with an artificial airway, *Best Practice: Evidence based practice information sheets for health professionals* 4(4):1-6, 2000. Text available at http://www.joannabriggs.edu.au/pdf/bpsuc.pdf.
18. Raymond SJ: Normal saline instillation before suctioning: helpful or harmful? a review of the literature, *Am J Crit Care* 4(4):267, 1995.
19. Centers for Disease Control and Prevention: Guidelines for preventing health-care associated pneumonia, 2003: recommendations of the CDC and the Healthcare Infection Control Practices Advisory Committee, *MMWR Morbidity Mortality Weekly Report* 53(No. RR-3):1-40, 2004.
20. Pritchard MA, et al: Systematic review of the role of preoxygenation for tracheal suctioning in ventilated newborn infants, *J Paediatr Child Health* 39(3):163-165, 2003.

Additional Readings

Buglass E: Tracheostomy care: tracheal suctioning and humidification, *Br J Nurs* 8(8):500-504, 1999.

Carr M, et al: Complications in pediatric tracheostomies, *Laryngoscope* 111:1925-1928, 2001.

Edwards EA, et al: Sending children home on tracheostomy dependent ventilation: pitfalls and outcomes, *Arch Disabled Child* 89:251-255, 2004.

AP
Cricothyroidotomy: Perform

P U R P O S E : To establish a temporary airway in the child whose airway cannot be secured with usual methods

Eric A. Bowles

PREREQUISITE KNOWLEDGE

- Child development as it relates to clinical assessment and procedure
- Airway anatomy and physiology, including structural characteristics specific to the infant and child[1-4] (see Figure 1-1)
  - ❖ A child's airway is both absolutely and relatively smaller in diameter and shorter than an adult's airway.
  - ❖ The tongue is large in relation to the mandible and oropharynx.
  - ❖ The child's funnel-shaped larynx is higher and more cephalad.
  - ❖ Vocal cords are 50% cartilage and are attached lower and more anteriorly.
  - ❖ The infant's epiglottis is floppy, long, and narrow and projects more posteriorly than in the older child.
  - ❖ The subglottic airway is smaller and more compliant with the cartilage less developed than in the adult.
  - ❖ The cricoid cartilage is the easiest and the only landmark for identification in children because the thyroid does not assume its adult configuration until puberty.
  - ❖ The cricoid cartilage is the narrowest portion of the upper airway in children less than 10 years of age. It

lies at the level of the third cervical vertebrae in the infant and descends to the sixth cervical vertebrae at puberty.
  - ❖ In teenagers and adults, the larynx is a cylinder with its narrowest portion at the glottic inlet at the level of the vocal cords.
  - ❖ The cricothyroid membrane is a dense fibroelastic membrane between the two largest cartilages in the larynx: the thyroid cartilage (above) and the circumferential ring of the cricoid cartilage (below; see Figure 1-2).
- Mastery of pediatric advanced life support competencies, including principles of artificial airway establishment (such as bag-mask ventilation, orophayngeal suctioning, proper positioning) and oxygen delivery systems[1]
- Principles of gas exchange
- Signs and symptoms of inadequate oxygenation and ventilation
- Cricothyroidotomy (cricothyrotomy) is a rare procedure accomplished with direct placement of a needle or angio-catheter percutaneously into the trachea through the cricothyroid membrane and is only attempted after oral tracheal and nasal tracheal intubation has failed[1] (Figure 13-1).
- Success of percutaneous cricothyroidotomy is related to skill and training and is considered when complete airway obstruction cannot be resolved with standard treatment measures.[1,5] Percutaneous cricothyroidotomy has been effectively used for ventilation and oxygenation during anesthesia with jet ventilation.[1,6]
- Surgical cricothyroidotomy requires surgical training and carries significant risk, especially for infants and

---

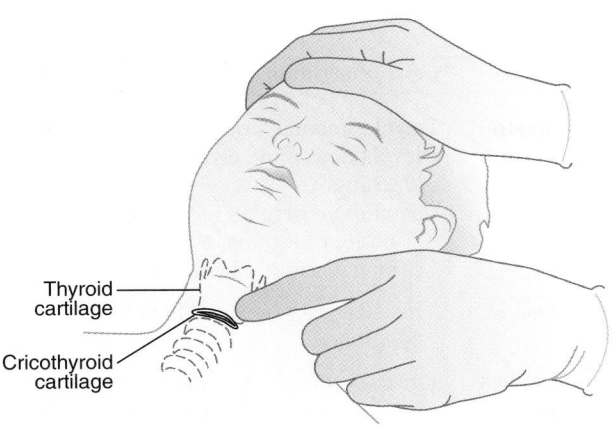

Thyroid cartilage

Cricothyroid cartilage

FIGURE 13-1   Location of Cricothyroidotomy.

toddlers.[1,7] A short transverse incision is made across the cricothyroid membrane, and a large catheter is then threaded downward into the trachea.[2,7,8] If a surgical cricothyroidotomy is necessary, additional equipment is needed, such as scalpels with #11 and #15 blades, trachea hooks, trousseau dilator (trachea dilator), curved mayo scissors, curved hemostats, small vascular clamp, needle holder, suture, syringe with 25-gauge needle for lidocaine with epinephrine, appropriately sized tracheostomy tube, and appropriately sized endotracheal (ET) tubes.[8]

- A cricothyroidotomy is useful in foreign body obstruction if the obstruction is above or at the glottis. For an obstruction below the level of the cricoid cartilage, a cricothyroidotomy is likely not effective.[1]
- A cricothyroidotomy can produce adequate oxygenation but has limited capacity to provide adequate ventilation.[9,10] This ventilation may be sufficient to support survival in seriously ill children because hypercarbia, caused by ventilation that is suboptimal, may be tolerated.[11]
- Although reports exist of percutaneous transtracheal ventilation in adults, few reports exist for children.[6,12,13]

CHILD AND FAMILY ASSESSMENT

- Child's developmental level and ability to interact ➡*Rationale:* Influences preparation and interaction.
- Child's and family's understanding of the reasons for and risks and benefits of cricothyroidotomy ➡*Rationale:* Evaluates child's and family's understanding of the procedure and provides a gauge for ongoing education.
- Respiratory status, including chest wall movement and lung sounds ➡*Rationale:* Carbon dioxide (CO_2) retention may occur because of the small size of the catheter needed for cricothyroidotomy.

- Signs and symptoms of inadequate oxygenation and ventilation ➡*Rationale:* Indication of effective pulmonary function.
- Presence of hemodynamic instability ➡*Rationale:* Hemodynamic instability may accompany respiratory failure.
- Last enteral intake of food or liquids ➡*Rationale:* Children with a full stomach are at risk for aspiration of gastric contents during airway manipulation.

CHILD AND FAMILY EDUCATION

Individualized developmentally appropriate education is provided to the family and to the child based on desire for knowledge, readiness to learn, and overall neurologic and psychosocial state.

- Explain the cricothyroidotomy procedure, including steps and rationale ➡*Rationale:* Providing information decreases fear and anxiety.
- Inform the parents that a cricothyroidotomy is an emergency procedure to attain a temporary airway and a more stable and long-term airway will be placed ➡*Rationale:* This information provides anticipatory guidance and prepares the family for further intervention. The parents must understand that this life-saving measure is temporary and that surgery is needed to secure a stable airway.
- Explain that the child's pain will be managed ➡*Rationale:* Parents may be comforted to know the child's pain will be addressed.
- Encourage questions and answer questions as they arise ➡*Rationale:* Reinforcement of information is needed during periods of stress and is especially important given the emergent nature of the procedure.

EQUIPMENT

- Personal protective equipment, including gloves
- Appropriately sized manual ventilation bag (MVB) attached to oxygen source
- Appropriately sized mask
- Suction equipment
- Small-bore (one 20-gauge and one 22-gauge) needles
- One 3-mL or 5-mL syringe
- 12-gauge, 14-gauge, and 16-gauge intravenous (IV) catheters with needle introducers
- One 3-mm tracheal tube adaptor
- Sterile gauze pads
- Tape
- Aseptic swab (or other antimicrobial solution)
- Emergency and procedural medications

Procedure   for Cricothyroidotomy: Perform

Steps	Rationale	Considerations
1. Ensure child and family understand procedure and questions are answered.	Evaluates and reinforces understanding of previously taught information.	Developmental, cognitive, and anxiety levels determine effectiveness of teaching. Given the emergent nature of a cricothyroidotomy, the procedure explanation may be delayed.
2. Gather needed equipment and supplies.	Facilitates completion of task in a timely manner.	This step may occur as the child is positioned.
3. Monitor child's vital signs and indications of inadequate oxygenation and ventilation before, during, and after the procedure.	A child in respiratory failure has vital sign changes and may need additional intervention.	Pulse oximetry and a cardiorespiratory monitor are used when available. At a minimum, periodic vital signs are taken. Use arterial or venous blood gasses when indicated.
4. Wash hands and put on personal protective equipment and gloves.	Reduces transmission of infection. Protects personnel health.	Timing may vary.
5. Place a neck role behind child's shoulders.[1]	Hyperextension of neck brings the trachea more anterior and makes identification of landmarks easier.	Placement can be performed by an assistant. With cervical spine injuries, placement must be performed with extreme caution.
6. Prepare site.	Reduces transmission of infection.	
7. Stabilize trachea with left hand.[1]	Immobilizes trachea during the procedure.	Be careful that the blood flow is not occluded through the carotid arteries.
8. Locate cricothyroid membrane with index finger of left hand with finding the anterior and transverse indentation or dip between thyroid and cricoid cartilage[1] (Figure 13-1).	With tip of finger, the space between thyroid and cricoid cartilages can be identified.[1]	This space is narrow in infants and may only be identifiable with the fingernail.[1]
9. Insert a small-bore (20-gauge or 22-gauge) needle attached to a syringe through cricothyroid membrane and aspirate air as the needle is advanced (aimed directly downwards)[1,7] (see Figure 13-2).	Only air should be aspirated through the needle with correct location in trachea.	The cricoid membrane is relatively avascular.[1] Care must be taken not to advance needle through the posterior wall of trachea.[7] An alternative is use of a modified Sellinger's technique with insertion of a small-bore needle, a wire threaded through needle, and then a dilator put over needle.[1]

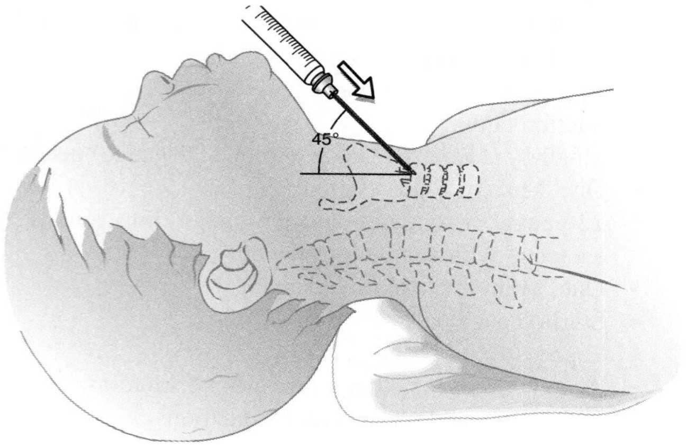

FIGURE 13-2   Needle Positioning for Percutaneous Cricothyroidotomy.

Procedure for Cricothyroidotomy: Perform—*Continued*

Steps	Rationale	Considerations
10. If air is aspirated, remove the needle and insert a large IV catheter (12-gauge to 16-gauge) through the previous needle track. Aspirate air from the syringe.	The aspiration of air signifies entry into the trachea lumen.	The needle mark is the landmark for catheter placement.
11. Advance catheter through the cricothyroid membrane into trachea with the needle directed at a 45-degree angle through midline caudally and posterior.[1,2]	Positions catheter in airway.	Redefine all landmarks before the insertion of the catheter.
12. Recheck placement with aspiration of air through catheter.	Aspiration of air confirms entry into trachea and correct placement.	
13. Attach a 3.0-mm adapter from an ET tube on the end of the IV cannula.[1]	Facilitates ventilation.	
14. Connect to oxygen source or MVB.	The small tube used for cricothyroidotomy limits air movement.	Oxygen flow rates should be relatively low (average, 100 mL/kg/min; maximum, 1 to 5 L/min).[1] The child needs longer expiratory times or pauses between insufflations to promote loss of CO_2, especially in complete airway obstruction.[1] A high-pressure oxygen source has been suggested as an alternative.[14]
15. Check lung sounds and ensure airway is secured after catheter is in place.	Prevents dislodgement.	
16. Remove protective items and wash hands.	Reduces transmission of infection. Protects personnel health.	

Expected Outcomes

- Successful placement of temporary airway
- Adequate oxygenation and ventilation
- A bridge is provided until a more stable airway is obtained
- Child has acceptable level of comfort

Unexpected Outcomes

- Failure to place the catheter inside the trachea
- Inadequate oxygenation and ventilation
- Neurologic impairment from hypoxemia
- Death
- Unmanaged pain and irritability

Monitoring and Care of the Child

Activities and Interventions	Rationale	Reportable Conditions
1. Continuous monitoring of oxygenation and ventilation.	Because of the small diameter, IV catheters produce high resistance and may cause air trapping. CO_2 retention from impaired passive exhalation.	• Physical examination results that indicate inadequate oxygenation/ventilation: change in color, skin temperature, or level of consciousness • Decreasing or inadequate chest rise and fall • Abnormal blood gases: a rising $PaCO_2$ and a falling pH • Decreased oxygen saturation (SaO_2)

Monitoring and Care of the Child—Cont'd

Activities and Interventions	Rationale	Reportable Conditions
2. Monitor vital signs.	Trending the vital signs helps to guide treatment.	• Abnormal vital signs
3. Continuously evaluate airway security.	Loss of airway could be fatal.	• Loss of airway
4. Assess effectiveness of pain management strategies and provide appropriate interventions.	Early identification of the child's comfort allows for immediate attention.	• Unresolved pain and discomfort • Continued irritability or changes in physiologic condition

Documentation

- Preprocedural and postprocedural physical examination results, including vital signs
- Stepwise explanation of airway insertion, including date, time, site preparation, and circumstances necessitating the procedure
- Comfort assessment, including interventions provided
- Additional interventions necessary
- Child's response to procedure
- Child and family education
- Unexpected outcomes and related treatments

References

1. Hazinski MF, et al, editors: *Pediatric advanced life support provider manual,* Dallas, 2002, American Heart Association.
2. Curley MAQ, Thompson JE: Oxygenation and ventilation. In Curley MAQ, Moloney-Harmon P, editors: *Critical care nursing of infants and children,* ed 2, Philadelphia, 2001, Saunders.
3. Thompson A: Pediatric airway management. In Fuhrman B, Zimmerman J, editors: *Pediatric critical care,* ed 3, Philadelphia, 2005, Elsevier.
4. McCance K, Huether S: *Pathophysiology: the biologic bases for disease in adults and children,* Philadelphia, 2002, Mosby.
5. Wong D, et al: What is the minimum training required for successful cricothyroidotomy? A study of mannequins, *Anesthesiol* 98(2)349-353, 2003.
6. Depierraz B, et al: Percutaneous transtracheal jet ventilation for paediatric endoscopic laser treatment of laryngeal and subglottic lesions, *Can J Anesth* 41:1200-1207, 1994.
7. Mathers L, Frankel L: Stabilization of the critically ill child. In Behrman R, et al, editors: *Textbook of pediatrics,* ed 17, Philadelphia, 2004, Saunders.
8. Strange GR, Niederman LG: Surgical cricothyroidotomy. In Henreting FM, et al, editors: *Textbook of pediatric emergency procedures,* 1997, Williams & Wilkins.
9. Brofelt BT, et al: An easy cricothyrotomy approach: the rapid four step technique, *Acad Emerg Med* 3(11):1060-1063, 1996.
10. Cote CJ, et al: Cricothyroidotomy membrane puncture: oxygenation and ventilation in a dog model using an intravenous catheter, *Crit Care Med* 16:615-619, 1988.
11. Golstein B, et al: Supercarbia in children: a clinical course and outcome, *Crit Care Med* 18:166-168, 1990.
12. Smith RB, et al H: Percutaneous transtracheal ventilation for anaesthesia and resuscitation: a review and report of complications, *Can Anesth Soc J* 22:607-612, 1975.
13. Barrachina R, et al: Percutaneous dilational cricothyroidotomy: outcome with 44 consecutive patients, *Intensive Care Med* 22:937-940, 1996.
14. Peak DA, Roy S: Needle cricothyroidotomy revisited, *Pediatr Emerg Care* 15:224-226, 1999.

Additional Readings

Cummins R, editor: *ACLS: principles and practice,* Dallas, 2003, American Heart Association.
Thibodeau G, Patton K, editors: *Anatomy and physiology,* ed 5, Philadelphia, 2003, Mosby.

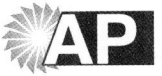

Extubation: Perform

P U R P O S E : Removal of the endotracheal tube (ET)

Amy C. Binck

PREREQUISITE KNOWLEDGE

- Child development as it relates to clinical assessment and extubation procedure
- Anatomy and physiology of the pediatric pulmonary system, including structural characteristics specific to the infant and child[1-4]
  - ❖ A child's airway is both absolutely and relatively smaller in diameter and shorter than an adult's (see Figure 1-1)
  - ❖ Because the thyroid does not assume its adult configuration until puberty, the cricoid cartilage is the easiest landmark for identification in children. The cricoid cartilage is the narrowest portion of the upper airway in children less than 10 years of age.
  - ❖ In teenagers and adults, the larynx is a cylinder with its narrowest portion at the glottic inlet at the level of the vocal cords.
  - ❖ The quantity of alveoli increases until 8 years of age and thereafter increases in size and complexity. Peripheral airway resistance is disproportionately higher in the child.
  - ❖ During inspiration, the infant's intercostal muscles stiffen and a downward movement of the diaphragm occurs, which results in negative intrathoracic pressure

and air movement into the lungs. Because the infant's chest wall is compliant and flexible, it characteristically collapses inward (see Figure 23-1).
- Mastery of pediatric advanced life support competencies, including use of artificial airways, oxygen delivery systems, and principles of airway management[4]
- Signs and symptoms of inadequate oxygenation and ventilation
- Criteria for extubation include mechanical ventilation is no longer needed to maintain adequate oxygenation and ventilation, and resolution of the underlying condition that led to the need for an artificial airway. A specific ventilator weaning protocol and predictors of extubation success have not been developed for the heterogeneous pediatric population, therefore individualized assessment measures are necessary.[5,6]
- Complications of extubation, including hypoxemia and hypercapnia
- Complications of prolonged intubation, including sinusitis, vocal cord injury, laryngeal injury and stenosis, tracheal injury, and pulmonary infection[7]
- Medical interventions for immediate complications of extubation, including laryngospasm, bronchospasm, postextubation stridor, and hypoxia

CHILD AND FAMILY ASSESSMENT

- Child's developmental level and ability to interact ➥*Rationale:* Influences preparation and interaction.
- Child's and family's understanding of the reasons for and risks and benefits of intubation ➥*Rationale:* Evaluates

child's and family's understanding of the procedure and provides a gauge for ongoing education.

- Desire of family members to be present during the procedure ➤➤*Rationale:* The presence of family may provide comfort and support, although family members should have the choice not to remain with the child.
- Duration and indication of intubation ➤➤*Rationale:* Assists in determining whether the child is ready for extubation. Extubation failure rates may be disease specific.[5] Consider extubation at the earliest appropriate time when conditions for intubation have resolved.[7]
- History of preexisting respiratory conditions ➤➤*Rationale:* Preexisting respiratory conditions may predispose the child to extubation failure.[5]
- Neurologic status and level of consciousness ➤➤*Rationale:* The desired level of consciousness is ensured before extubation.[7]
- Ability to maintain an airway, including the presence of cough and gag reflexes ➤➤*Rationale:* Assists in determining the child's ability to protect the airway and clear secretions.[1]
- Secretions, including amount, viscosity, and suctioning requirements ➤➤*Rationale:* Large amounts of secretions may make extubation more difficult and predispose the child to reintubation.
- Current level of ventilator support ➤➤*Rationale:* Assists in determining whether the child is ready for extubation.
- Work of breathing during minimal ventilator support ➤➤*Rationale:* Minimal ventilator assistance closely resembles independent breathing, and signs and symptoms of respiratory distress should be assessed.[8]
- Adequate oxygenation, hemodynamic stability, and the ability to initiate an inspiratory effort during a spontaneous breathing trial ➤➤*Rationale:* A spontaneous breathing trial in children undergoing mechanical ventilation for respiratory failure can help to determine ability to remain extubated.[9]
- Air leak around the endotracheal (ET) tube ➤➤*Rationale:* The incidence rate of postextubation stridor is greater in older children (≥7 yr) with an air leak at more than 20 mm Hg.[10]
- Indications for administration of prophylactic corticosteroid ➤➤*Rationale:* Prophylactic administration of dexamethasone before elective extubation reduces the incidence rate of postextubation stridor in individual neonates and children.[11]
- Child's feeding status ➤➤*Rationale:* A child with a full stomach is predisposed to aspiration, and nothing by mouth (NPO) status for a minimum of 4 hours before extubation is recommended.

CHILD AND FAMILY EDUCATION

Individualized, developmentally appropriate education is provided to the family and to the child based on desire for knowledge, readiness to learn, and overall neurologic and psychosocial state.

- Explain the extubation procedure, including indications, criteria, steps, and rationale ➤➤*Rationale:* Providing information decreases fear and anxiety.
- Provide the rationale for the timing of NPO status before and following extubation ➤➤*Rationale:* Alleviation of fear and anxiety regarding holding nutrition and anticipatory guidance regarding the expected time of NPO status.
- Explain expected outcomes after extubation, including possible stridor and continued need for supplemental oxygen ➤➤*Rationale:* Postextubation stridor may occur and may be frightening to the child and family.
- Discuss the possibility of reintubation ➤➤*Rationale:* Anticipatory guidance in the event of reintubation.
- Discuss the importance of suctioning, coughing, and deep breathing exercises after extubation ➤➤*Rationale:* Encourages cooperation and augments the care necessary to maintain airway and clear secretions.
- Explain that the child's voice may be hoarse after extubation ➤➤*Rationale:* The explanation provides anticipatory guidance and minimizes the child's and family's fear and anxiety in the event of sore throat and difficulty with vocalization.
- Encourage questions and answer questions as they arise ➤➤*Rationale:* Reinforcement of information is needed during periods of stress and is especially important given the emergent nature of the procedure.

EQUIPMENT

- Personal protective equipment, including gloves
- Oxygen source
- High-volume suction source
- Appropriately sized wide-bore rigid pharyngeal suction tip catheter
- Appropriately sized pliable tracheal suction catheters of a size to fit the ET tube
- Appropriately sized manual ventilation system (MVB; self-inflating or flow-inflating)
- Appropriately sized mask
- Appropriately sized oral and pharyngeal airways
- Translaryngeal intubation equipment (laryngoscope blades, handles, batteries, stylettes)
- ET tubes of various sizes
- Pulse oximeter
- Supplies for arterial puncture and blood gas analysis (as indicated)
- Oxygen delivery equipment, including nasal cannula, oxygen mask, or hood
- Scissors
- 10-mL syringe
- Stethoscope
- Emergency cart available

Procedure for Extubation: Perform

Steps	Rationale	Considerations
1. Ensure child and family understand procedure and questions are answered.	Evaluates and reinforces understanding of previously taught information.	Developmental, cognitive, and anxiety levels determine approach and effectiveness of teaching.
2. Assess environment.	Extubation should occur in an environment in which the child can be appropriately monitored and in which emergency medical equipment is available.[7]	
3. Ensure all equipment and supplies have been collected and are working properly.	Facilitates completion of task in a timely manner.	
4. Ensure child's vital signs and indications of inadequate oxygenation and ventilation are monitored.	Identifies signs and symptoms of respiratory insufficiency.	Pulse oximetry is often used to continuously monitor oxygen saturations (SpO_2) to provide an indication of gas exchange. Consider arterial/venous blood gases as indicated.
5. Wash hands and put on personal protective equipment.	Reduces transmission of infection. Protects personnel health.	
6. Ensure that child is optimally positioned.	Respiratory muscles are more effective in an upright position. This position also facilitates clearing of secretions and reduces risk of aspiration if vomiting occurs. Padding under shoulders maintains the head in the "sniffing" position to keep airway open.	Unless contraindicated, head is elevated at least 45 degrees. Infants and small children may be supported with pillows to achieve appropriate position. A small padding placed under the shoulders of child may be helpful.
7. Hyperoxygenate and suction ET tube and pharynx.	Hyperoxygenation increases arterial oxygen levels in preparation for extubation. Hyperinflation assists in mobilization and removal of secretions.	Hyperinflation volumes of 100% to 150% have been recommended. Hyperoxygenation with 100% FiO_2 is not recommended for children with certain congenital heart defects and hypoxic respiratory drive.
8. Attach syringe to the one-way valve in pilot balloon if a cuffed tracheal tube is in place.	Prepares for cuff deflation. Cuff must be deflated before extubation to prevent trauma to airway.	
9. Assist in removal of tape from face to free the tube.	Frees tracheal tube from child's face for easier removal.	
10. Apply positive pressure with MVB, deflate cuff (if present), and remove tube during peak inspiration.	Positive pressure promotes hyperinflation, clears tracheal tube of foreign material, and assists in clearing secretions. Vocal cords are maximally abducted at peak inspiration.	For a child with a cuffed tube, the cuff must be deflated before extubation.
11. Assess lung sounds and work of breathing after extubation.	The child is especially vulnerable to respiratory insufficiency in the immediate period after extubation.	
12. Encourage child to cough and deep breathe as developmentally appropriate.	Promotes hyperinflation and helps remove secretions.	Nasopharyngeal and oropharyngeal suctioning may be used to help stimulate cough in a younger child who cannot follow commands.

Procedure continues on following page

Procedure for Extubation: Perform—*Continued*

Steps	Rationale	Considerations
13. Administer supplemental oxygen and aerosolized respiratory treatments as appropriate.	Helps prevent hypoxemia.	Cool humidification may be used to help minimize upper airway swelling. Racemic epinephrine treatments may be used if upper airway edema or stridor is present.[12]
14. Remove protective items and wash hands.	Reduces transmission of infection. Protects personnel health.	

Expected Outcomes

- Atraumatic extubation
- Adequate oxygenation and ventilation without artificial airway

- Maintenance of energy and ability to breath spontaneously
- Child has acceptable level of comfort

Unexpected Outcomes

- Trauma to airway
- Inadequate oxygenation and ventilation that necessitates reintubation
- Laryngospasm
- Fatigue from increased work of breathing that necessitates reintubation
- Unmanaged pain

Monitoring and Care of the Child

Activities and Interventions	Rationale	Reportable Conditions
1. Assess vital signs, oxygenation and ventilation indices, and oxygen requirements.	Changes in vital signs after extubation may indicate respiratory deterioration and necessitate reintubation The child's ability to effectively breath may change without an artificial airway.	• Tachypnea • Blood pressure of more than 110% of baseline • Oxygen saturation of less than 92% • Increased work of breathing, including grunting, nasal flaring, and retractions • Cyanosis • Irritability
2. Assess lung sounds before and after extubation.	Assessment for air movement, symmetric breath sounds, and adventitious sounds.	• Asymmetric air entry • Stridor • Wheezing
3. Continually assess comfort and level of consciousness.	Irritability and fatigue are signs of respiratory compromise. Early identification of the child's comfort allows for immediate attention.	• Significant irritability • Decreased level of consciousness • Reduced response to pain • Unresolved pain and discomfort • Changes in physiologic condition
4. Provide supplemental oxygen and aerosolized medications as needed.	Decreases incidence rate of oxygen desaturation immediately after extubation.	• Hypoxemia despite supplemental oxygen • Ineffective cough
5. Encourage coughing, deep breathing, and early mobilization as developmentally and medically appropriate.	Prevents atelectasis and secretion accumulation.	
6. Suction oropharynx after extubation as needed.	Assists in clearing secretions and prevents secretion accumulation.	• Inability to handle secretions

Documentation

- Preextubation and postextubation assessment findings, including breath sounds, coughing, and additional signs of adequate oxygenation and ventilation
- Date and time of extubation
- Comfort assessment, including specific interventions provided
- Child's response to extubation
- Additional interventions necessary before, during, and after extubation
- Child and family education
- Unexpected outcomes and related treatments

References

1. Curley MAQ, Thompson JE: Oxygenation and ventilation. In Curley MAQ, Moloney-Harmon P, editors: *Critical care nursing of infants and children,* ed 2, Philadelphia, 2001, Saunders.
2. Thompson A: Pediatric airway management. In Fuhrman B, Zimmerman J, editors: *Pediatric critical care,* ed 3, Philadelphia, 2005, Elsevier.
3. McCance K, Huether S: *Pathophysiology: the biologic bases for disease in adults and children,* Philadelphia, 2002, Mosby.
4. Hazinski MF, et al, editors: *Pediatric advanced life support provider manual,* Dallas, 2002, American Heart Association.
5. Kurachek SC, et al: Extubation failure in pediatric intensive care: a multiple-center study of risk factors and outcomes, *Pediatr Crit Care Med* 31(11):2657-2664, 2003.
6. Randolph AG, et al. Effect of mechanical ventilator weaning protocols on respiratory outcomes in infants and children: a randomized controlled trial, *JAMA* 288(20):2561-2568, 2002.
7. AARC Clinical Practice Guideline: Removal of the endotracheal tube, *Respir Care* 44(1):85-90, 1999.
8. Manczur TI, et al: Comparison of predictors of extubation from mechanical ventilation in children, *Pediatr Crit Care Med* 1(1):28-32, 2000.
9. Evidence-based guidelines for weaning and discontinuing ventilatory support: a collective task force facilitated by the American College of Chest Physicians, the American Association for Respiratory Care, and the American College of Critical Care Medicine, *Respir Care* 47(1): 69-90, 2002.
10. Mhanna MJ, et al: The "air leak" test around the endotracheal tube, as a predictor of postextubation stridor, is age dependent in children, *Crit Care Med* 30(12):2639-2643, 2000.
11. Markovitz BP, Randolph AG. Corticosteroids for the prevention of reintubation and postextubation stridor in pediatric patients: a meta-analysis, *Pediatr Crit Care Med* 3(30):223-226, 2002.
12. Davies MW, Davis PG: Nebulized racemic epinephrine for extubation of newborn infants, *Cochrane Database System Review* (2):CD000506, 2000.

Additional Reading

Popernack ML, Thomas NJ, Lucking SE: Decreasing unplanned extubations: utilization of the Penn State Children's Hospital Sedation Algorithm, *Pediatr Crit Care Med* 5(1):58-62, 2004.

AP

Intubation: Perform, Including Laryngeal Mask Airway

P U R P O S E :   An endotracheal tube (ET) is placed into the trachea via the oral or nasal route to maintain airway patency, facilitate clearance of secretions, provide positive pressure ventilation, and supply a route for emergency medication delivery. A laryngeal mask airway (LMA) provides an emergency airway during resuscitation of a child who is profoundly unconscious.

Amy C. Binck

PREREQUISITE KNOWLEDGE

- Child development as it relates to clinical assessment and securing an artificial airway
- Anatomy and physiology of the pediatric pulmonary system, including structural characteristics specific to the infant and child[1-4]
  - ❖ A child's airway is both absolutely and relatively smaller in diameter and shorter than an adult's (see Figure 1-1).
  - ❖ The tongue is large in relation to the mandible and oropharynx.
  - ❖ The child's funnel-shaped larynx is higher and more cephalad.
  - ❖ Vocal cords are 50% cartilage and attached lower and more anteriorly.
  - ❖ The infant's epiglottis is floppy, long, and narrow and projects more posteriorly than the older child's.
  - ❖ The subglottic airway is smaller and more compliant with the cartilage less developed than in the adult.
  - ❖ Because the thyroid does not assume its adult configuration until puberty, the cricoid cartilage is the easiest landmark for identification in children.

- ❖ The cricoid cartilage is the narrowest portion of the upper airway in children less than 10 years of age. It lies at the level of the third cervical vertebrae in the infant and descends to the sixth cervical vertebrae at puberty.
- ❖ In teenagers and adults, the larynx is a cylinder with its narrowest portion at the glottic inlet or at the level of the vocal cords.
- ❖ The cricothyroid membrane is a dense fibroelastic membrane between the two largest cartilages in the larynx: the thyroid cartilage (above) and the circumferential ring of the cricoid cartilage (below).
- ❖ The quantity of alveoli increases until 8 years of age and thereafter increases in size and complexity. Peripheral airway resistance is disproportionately higher in the child.
- ❖ During inspiration, the infant's intercostal muscles stiffen and a downward movement of the diaphragm occurs, which results in negative intrathoracic pressure and air movement into the lungs. Because the infant's chest wall is compliant and flexible, it characteristically collapses inward (see Figure 23-1).
- Mastery of pediatric advanced life support competencies, including principles of artificial airway establishment (such as bag-mask ventilation, oropharyngeal suctioning, and proper positioning) and oxygen (O_2) delivery systems[1]
- Principles of gas exchange
- An appropriately sized mask provides a tight seal and fits so that it extends from the bridge of the nose to the cleft

of the chin, encompassing the mouth and nose but keeping away from the eyes[1] (see Figure 8-1).

- Proficiency in using self inflating manual resuscitator and flow inflating manual resucitator equipment (see Procedure 27).[1,5-7]
- Signs and symptoms of inadequate oxygenation and ventilation
- Indications for placement of an artificial airway, including upper airway obstruction, apnea, ineffective clearance of secretions, high risk of aspiration, and respiratory distress
- Indications and contraindications of each route of intubation: oral and nasal
- Orotracheal intubation is preferred, especially in an emergency situation, because this approach is usually accomplished more quickly than the nasal approach.[1]
- Complications of intubation, including sinusitis, vocal cord injury, laryngeal injury and stenosis, tracheal injury, and pulmonary infection[8]
- Physiologic effects of laryngoscopy and airway intubation
- Predictors of difficult airway intubations
- Principles of airway and ventilator management
- Chest radiograph interpretation
- Blood gas analysis
- Endotracheal (ET) tube size varies with age and size (Table 15-1)
- Several methods are used in determining ET tube size (internal diameter)[1,2,9]
  - ❖ For children less than 1 year of age, the following sizes are recommended: premature infant, 2.5 to 3.0; newborn, 3.0; newborn to 6 months, 3.5; 6 to 12 months, 3.5 to 4.0
  - ❖ For children older than 2 years of age, the following formula can be used:
    For uncuffed tubes: 16 + age (yr)/4
    For cuffed tubes: age (yr)/1.1 + 3/4
- Cuffed tubes are typically used for children older than 8 to 10 years of age and for smaller children who need high inspiratory pressures.[1] Cuffed tubes in young children may contribute to subglottic damage if the pressure exerted by the tube or cuff exceeds mucosal capillary pressure. As long as the cuff is closely monitored, cuffed tubes have not been shown to have greater complication rates than uncuffed tubes.[10,11]
- Pharmacologic approach to artificial airway placement, including awake, sedated without paralyzing agents, and anesthetized intubations (Table 15-2).
- Head position effects ET tube position; neck flexion results in the tip of the tube moving closer to the carina, and neck extension results in the tube withdrawing toward the glottis.
- A laryngeal mask airway (LMA) is a supraglottic airway management device used to secure the airway of a child who is unconscious.[1,4,12]
- Indications for LMA use include.[1,4,12]
  - ❖ Need for an airway during resuscitation of children who are unconscious with absent glossopharyngeal and laryngeal reflexes when ET intubation is not possible

TABLE 15-1	Age, Endotracheal Tube, and Laryngoscope Blade Size for Intubation	
Age	**Endotracheal Tube (mm)**	**Laryngoscope Blade**
Premature infant	2.5 uncuffed	Miller 0
	3.0 uncuffed	
Newborn	3.0 uncuffed	Miller 0-1
		Wis-Hipple 1
Newborn to 6 months	3.5 uncuffed	Miller 0-1
		Wis-Hipple 1
6 to 12 months	3.5 uncuffed	Miller 1
	4.0 uncuffed	Wis-Hipple 1 1/2
	4.5 uncuffed	
1 to 2 years	4.0 uncuffed	Miller 2
	4.0 cuffed	Macintosh 2
		Flagg 2
4 to 5 years	5.0 uncuffed	Miller 2
	5.5 uncuffed	Macintosh 2
	4.5 cuffed	Flagg 2
6 to 7 years	5.5 uncuffed	Miller 2
	6.0 uncuffed	Macintosh 2
	5.0 cuffed	Flagg 2
8 to 10 years	6.0 cuffed	Miller 2
	6.5 cuffed	Macintosh 2
12 years to adolescent	7.0 cuffed	Macintosh 3
	8.0 cuffed	Miller 3

For children older than 2 years, the following formula can be used:
  For uncuffed tubes: 16 + age(yr)/4
  For cuffed tubes: age (yr)/1.1 + 3/4

Curley MAQ, Thompson J: Oxygenation and ventilation. In Curley MAQ, Moloney-Harmon P, editors: *Nursing care of critically ill infants and children*, ed 2, Philadelphia, 2001, Saunders.

Thompson A: Pediatric airway management. In Fuhrman B, Zimmerman J, editors: *Pediatric critical care*, ed 2, Philadelphia, 1998, Mosby.

Hazinski MF, et al, editors: *Pediatric advanced life support provider manual*, Dallas, 2002, American Heart Association.

Wiegand DLM, Carlson K, editors: *AACNs procedure manual for critical care*, ed 5, Philadelphia, 2004, Elsevier.

  - ❖ Achievement and control of the airway during routine and emergency anesthetic procedures
  - ❖ Known or unexpected difficult airway situations
  - ❖ Children with oropharyngeal trauma may benefit from an LMA when all other means of airway establishment fail and when the risks of insertion are weighed against the need to establish an airway.
- Contraindications and limitations of LMA use[1,12]
  - ❖ Children who are conscious with intact gag reflex
  - ❖ Children with delayed gastric emptying, fullstomachs, or undetermined last enteral intake. The LMA does not protect the airway from aspiration of stomach contents.
  - ❖ Children with decreased pulmonary compliance that necessitates high ventilator pressures. The LMA provides a low-pressure seal.
  - ❖ Use may be problematic during transport, compared with an ET tube, because maintenance of the LMA's proper position during movement may be more difficult.

TABLE 15-2	Pediatric Intubation Drugs	
Drug	**Dose Duration**	**Comments**
Anesthetic Agents		
Thiopental	2-4 mg/kg 5-10 min	Myocardial depression, apnea, ↓PVR, ↓CBF, ↓ICP
Etomidate	0.3 mg/kg 3-5 min	Minimal cardiovascular effects, apnea, ↓ICP, ↓CBF
Ketamine	0.5-2 mg/kg 10-15 min	Catecholamine release (↑HR, ↑BP), ↑ICP, bron- chodilation, laryngospasm
Propofol	2-3 mg/kg 4-8 min	Dose-dependant cardiovascular depression
Sedatives and Narcotics		
Midazolam	0.05-0.1 mg/kg 1-2 h	Occasional respiratory depression, amnesia
Fentanyl	1-5 mcg/kg 0.5-1.5 h	Respiratory depression, occasional chest wall rigidity and bradycardia if given rapidly
Morphine	0.1-0.2 mg/kg 2-4 h	Respiratory depression, histamine release, ↓BP, ↓arterial and venous tone, bronchospasm
Neuromuscular Blocking Agents		
Succinylcholine	1-2 mg/kg 5-10 min	Depolarizing, ↓HR, ↑ICP, ↑IOP, ↑serum potassium, triggers malignant hyperthermia
Cisatracurium besylate	0.1-0.2 mg 15-20 min	Mild histamine release, ↓BP, neither renal nor hepatic function necessary for excretion
Vecuronium bromide	0.1-0.15 mg/kg 35-70 min	Minimal cardiovascular effect, prolonged effect in hepatic failure
Pancuronium bromide	0.1-0.15 mg/kg 30-90 min	↑HR, prolonged effect in renal failure
Rocuronium	0.6-1.2 mg/kg 45-60 min	Minimal cardiovascular effect, prolonged effect in hepatic failure, rapid onset with larger doses
Adjunctive Medications		
Atropine	0.02-0.03 mg/kg	Used to prevent bradycardia, salivation, bron- chospasm
Glycopyrrolate	0.01 mg/kg	Used to prevent bradycardia, salivation, bronchospasm
Lidocaine	1-2 mg/kg	IV dose before intubation or suctioning may prevent ↑ICP

PVR, Peripheral vascular resistance; *CBF,* cerebral blood flow; *ICP,* intracranial pressure; *HR,* heart rate; *BP,* blood pressure; *IOP,* intraocular pressure.
Data from Hazinski MF, et al, editors: *Pediatric advanced life support provider manual,* Dallas, 2002, American Heart Association.
Curley MAQ, Moloney-Harmon P, editors: *Nursing care of critically ill infants and children,* ed 2, Philadelphia, 2001, Saunders.
Fuhrman B, Zimmerman J, editors: *Pediatric critical care,* ed 2, Philadelphia, 1998, Mosby.

- Components of an LMA[12] (Figure 15-1)
- When inflated via the pilot balloon, the mask's cuff con- forms to the contours of the hypopharynx, positioning the opening of the air tube directly over the laryngeal opening.
- Several types of LMA devices and a variety of methods of insertion are seen (Table 15-3).
- A range of sizes are available. The sizes based on weight are an approximation and should be used as a guide (Table 15-4).
- Informed consent is required unless procedure is emergent.

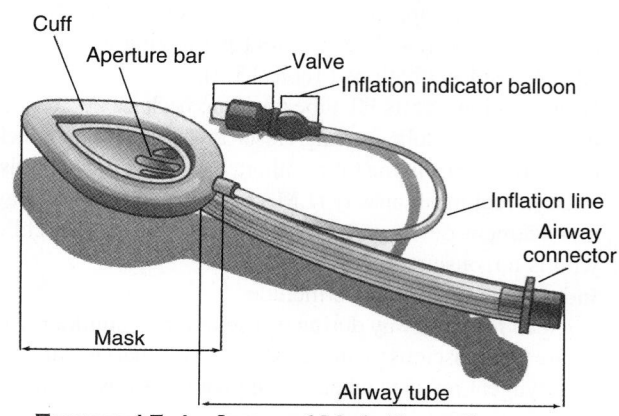

FIGURE 15-1   Laryngeal Mask Airway Components.

TABLE 15-3	Laryngeal Mask Airway Device Summary	
LMA Device (Year of Introduction)	**Use**	**PPV**
LMA Classic (1992)	Reusable General anesthetic cases	Up to 20 cm water
LMA ProSeal (2000)	Reusable Cases that need higher seal pressures to deliver higher PPV and those that need access to gastrointestinal tract thorough drain port	Up to 30 cm water
LMA Unique (1997)	Disposable General anesthetic cases and stocking crash carts for rescue airway	Up to 20 cm water

PPV, Positive pressure ventilation.

The Laryngeal Airway Mask Airway Limited: *LMA airway instruction manual,* San Diego, 2004, LMA North America. Text available at http://www.lmana.com/prod/content/education/LMA_Airways_Manual.pdf.

TABLE 15-4	Laryngeal Mask Airway Selection Guidelines	
LMA Airway Size	**Child Size**	**Maximum Cuff Inflation Volume (Air)**	**Test Cuff Overinflation Volumes (Air)**
---	---	---	---
1	Neonates/infants, up to 5 kg	4 mL	6 mL
1 ½	Infants, 5-10 kg	7 mL	10 mL
2	Infants/children, 10-20 kg	10 mL	15 mL
2 ½	Children, 20-30 kg	14 mL	21 mL
3	Children, 30-50 kg	20 mL	30 mL
4	Adults, 50-70 kg	30 mL	45 mL
5	Adults, 70-100 kg	40 mL	60 mL
6	Adults, >100 kg	50 mL	75 mL

Information from The Laryngeal Airway Mask Airway Limited: *LMA airway instruction manual,* San Diego, 2004, LMA North America. Text available at http://www.lmana.com/prod/content/education/LMA_Airways_Manual.pdf.

CHILD AND FAMILY ASSESSMENT

- Child's developmental level and ability to interact ➥*Rationale:* Influences preparation and interaction.
- Child's and family's understanding of the reasons for and risks and benefits of artificial airway ➥*Rationale:* Evaluates child's and family's understanding of the procedure and provides a gauge for ongoing education.
- Desire of family members to be present during the procedure ➥*Rationale:* The presence of family may provide comfort and support, although family members should have the choice not to remain with the child.
- History of difficult artificial airway placement ➥*Rationale:* Previous difficult intubations suggest structural abnormalities that may not be evident on physical examination.
- Assessment of the child's head, face, mouth, and neck ➥*Rationale:* Malformations such as micrognathia, facial clefts, facial hypoplasia, facial asymmetry, masses, small mouth, and a short neck may impede effective bag and mask ventilation and visualization of the larynx. The number of teeth and presence of loose teeth are noted in case of dislodgement with the laryngoscope blade.
- Assesses the child's temporomandibular joint or cervical spine mobility ➥*Rationale:* Limited mobility can make laryngoscopy and tracheal tube placement difficult.
- Presence of head injury and history of trauma ➥*Rationale:* Laryngoscopy causes undesirable physiologic responses that increase intracranial pressure and change the pharmacologic approach to intubation.
- Presence of cervical spine injury ➥*Rationale:* Inline cervical stabilization should be used during artificial airway placement to prevent further neurologic injury during laryngoscopy.
- Level of anxiety, consciousness, and respiratory compromise ➥*Rationale:* Determines need for sedation, paralytic agents, and the child's ability to lie supine for artificial airway placement.
- Degree and indications of respiratory failure ➥*Rationale:* Indicates need for artificial airway placement.
- Last enteral intake of food or liquids ➥*Rationale:* Children with a full stomach are at risk for aspiration of gastric contents during airway manipulation.
- Presence of hypovolemia ➥*Rationale:* Fluid resuscitation may be necessary to prevent cardiovascular collapse.
- Presence of hemodynamic instability ➥*Rationale:* Hemodynamic instability may accompany respiratory failure. Existing hemodynamic instability may become worse with sedation because of loss of sympathetic tone. Pharmacologic approach should be individualized.
- Presence of intravenous (IV) access ➥*Rationale:* IV access is important in the delivery of medications and IV fluids if needed during artificial airway placement.

CHILD AND FAMILY EDUCATION

Individualized, developmentally appropriate education is provided to the family and to the child based on desire for knowledge, readiness to learn, and overall neurologic and psychosocial state.

- Discuss the indication for artificial airway placement specific for the child ➥*Rationale:* Providing information decreases anxiety and fear.

- Discuss the risks associated with placement of an artificial airway ➤➤*Rationale:* The family must be provided with this information to understand the possibility of adverse events.
- Provide anticipatory guidance related to expected duration of artificial airway placement ➤➤*Rationale:* Parents can gauge the child's progress in recovery to independent respiratory functioning.
- Discuss appropriate expected outcomes of artificial airway placement ➤➤*Rationale:* The family and health care team can formulate similar goals and expectations.
- Explain that the child will be unable to speak while the artificial airway is in place ➤➤*Rationale:* Providing information decreases anxiety and fear.
- Explain that pharmacologic sedation and immobilization interventions may be necessary for the safety of the child and prevention of accidental tube dislodgment and that such interventions are used only as necessary ➤➤*Rationale:* Pharmacologic agents and immobilization interventions may be necessary to ensure safety and secure position of the artificial airway.
- Review adjunct monitoring and support that will ensue after artificial airway placement, such as blood gas sampling, ventilator assistance, endotracheal suctioning, and chest roentgenograms ➤➤*Rationale:* The family receives assistance and guidance in understanding the new plan of care and medical interventions.
- Explain the sensory implications of an airway in the nose or mouth ➤➤*Rationale:* Anticipatory guidance is helpful in decreasing anxiety and fear.
- Encourage questions and answer questions as they arise ➤➤*Rationale:* Reinforcement of information is needed during periods of stress and is especially important given the emergent nature of the procedure.

EQUIPMENT

- Personal protective equipment
- Suction equipment, including wall suction
- Wide-bore rigid pharyngeal tonsil tip suction catheter
- Pliable suction catheter of appropriate size
- Appropriately sized manual ventilation (MVB; self-inflating or flow-inflating; minimal size, 450 to 500 mL)[1]
- Oxygen source
- Appropriately sized mask
- Oropharyngeal airway/bite block
- Laryngoscope blade (Miller [straight] or Macintosh [curved]) with working light source
- Appropriately sized ET tubes: one tube the estimated required size, one tube 0.5 mm smaller, and one tube 0.5 mm larger
- Appropriately sized stylet
- Laryngoscope handle with batteries
- Magill forceps for nasal intubation or removal of foreign body
- Luer-tip syringe for cuff inflation with use of a cuffed ET tube and an LMA
- Tape
- Stethoscope
- Appropriate monitoring equipment, including continuous pulse oximetry, continuous cardiac monitor, appropriately sized blood pressure cuff, and end tidal carbon dioxide monitor ($ETCO_2$) or $ETCO_2$ detector cap
- Appropriate intubation and emergency medications
- Adhesive solution
- Anesthetic spray or local anesthetic jelly (nasal ET tube placement)
- LMAs(2), as needed

Procedure for Intubation: Perform, Including LMA		
Steps	**Rationale**	**Considerations**
Endotracheal Intubation 1. Ensure child and family understand procedure and questions are answered. Acquire informed consent unless procedure is emergent.	Evaluates and reinforces understanding of previously taught information. Ensures medical-legal compliance as suggested by Joint Commission of Accreditation of Health Care Organization.	Developmental, cognitive, and anxiety levels determine approach and effectiveness of teaching. Given the often emergent nature of intubation, the procedure explanation may be delayed. For emergencies, refer to institution-specific policy for assumption of consent.
2. Wash hands.	Reduces transmission of infection. Protects personnel health.	
3. Select appropriate laryngoscope blade (see Table 15-1): • *Infants and young children*: straight blade (Miller; Figure 15-2, *A*).	Allows for easier visualization of the vocal cords. Lifts base of the tongue to expose vocal cords. A straight blade is typically preferred in infants and toddlers because it affords better visuali-	The most important characteristic of the blade is the length.

Procedure	for Intubation: Perform, Including LMA—*Continued*	
Steps	**Rationale**	**Considerations**

| | zation of relatively cephalad and anterior glottis. | |
| • *Children older than 2 to 3 years*: curved blade (Macintosh; Figure 15-2, *B*). | A curved blade is broader and provides better control of child's larger tongue and exerts less leverage on child's upper teeth. | The base of curved blades may obstruct the practitioner's line of vision because of the infant's small mouth. |

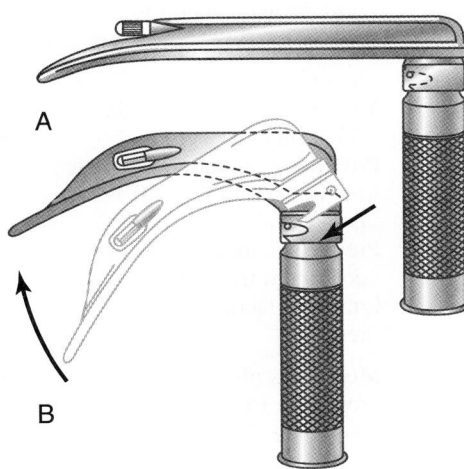

FIGURE 15-2   Laryngoscope Blades. **A,** Straight blade. **B,** Curved blade.

| 4. Select appropriate size of ET tubes[1] (see Table 15-1).   Choose a cuffed or uncuffed tube (Figure 15-3). | ET tubes that are too small result in increased resistance to air flow and may produce a large air leak around tube. ET tubes that are too large produce increased pressure to airway and may result in ischemia or stenosis. Cuffed tubes are typically used in children older than 8 to 10 years of age and in younger children who need high inspiratory pressures. | Three ET tubes should be immediately available during intubation: one tube the estimated required size, one tube 0.5 mm smaller, and one tube 0.5 mm larger.[1] If a cuffed tube is chosen, calculate size based on age and reduce tracheal tube size by 0.5 to 1mm. Using a cuffed ET tube may reduce the risk of aspiration; allow for more accurate measurement of $ETCO_2$ monitoring and inhalation gas concentration, reduce the number of intubations necessary |

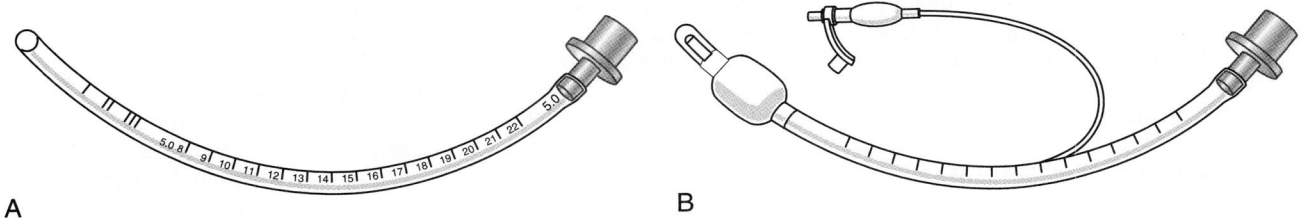

FIGURE 15-3   Endotracheal Tubes. **A,** Uncuffed tube. **B,** Cuffed tube.

Procedure continues on following page

Procedure	**for Intubation: Perform, Including LMA**—*Contintued*	
Steps	**Rationale**	**Considerations**
		to achieve an appropriately sized tube, and prevent ventilator management difficulties in the case of poor lung compliance or high airway resistance.[10,11,13]
5. Select appropriately sized stylet: 6F, 10F, or 14F.	The stylet is used to change shape of ET tube for a child with airway anatomy.	Intubation may be performed without a stylet.
6. Check to ensure preparation of all other equipment and supplies. • Check laryngoscope batteries. • Use a syringe to inflate and completely deflate cuff on the tube. • With use of a stylet, insert it into ET tube. Ensure that tip of stylet does not extend past the end of tracheal tube.	Facilitates completion of task in a timely manner. Verifies that equipment is functional. Provides adequate light source. Identifies that tube cuff is patent and without leaks. Prevents damage to vocal cords and trachea. Lubricant facilitates stylet removal	A stylet provides rigidity to the ET tube and helps guide it through the vocal cords. Minimal resistance should be present in removal of the stylet. The stylet should be recessed by at least 0.5 inch from the distal end of the tracheal tube. A water-soluble lubricant may be applied to end of stylet.
7. Ensure intubation medications are drawn and ready to administer (see Table 15-2).	Modulates physiologic response to intubation.	The pharmacologic approach to intubation depends on numerous factors and may range from no pharmacologic intervention to induction of anesthesia. Intubation drugs often include those that provide amnesia, sedation, muscle paralysis, or drugs.
8. Ensure child's vital signs and indications of inadequate oxygenation and ventilation are monitored.	Hypoxia and bradycardia are possible complications of direct laryngoscopy, and hypotension may result from underlying hemodynamic instability or medication administration.	Pulse oximetry is often used to continuously monitor O_2 saturations to provide an indication of gas exchange. If child is in cardiac arrest, intubate without stopping for physiologic monitors.[1] Consider arterial/venous blood gases as indicated.
9. Put on gloves and personal protective equipment.	Reduces transmission of infection. Protects personnel health.	Protective eyewear is worn to prevent exposure to secretions.
10. Position child supine so that oropharyngolaryngeal axes are aligned.[14] *Infant:* Place head in a neutral position on a flat surface with chin in sniffing position (Figure 15-4, *A*). *Older child:* Elevate occiput to the sniffing position and extend the head at the atlantooccipital joint (Figure 15-4, *B*). *Suspected or confirmed spinal cord injury:* Maintain head in a neutral position with inline cervical spine immobilization (Figure 15-4, *C*).	Alignment allows for visualization of the vocal cords. The infant's proportionately large occiput raises head to align the axes. Extension of head without elevation of the occiput anteriorly rotates the larynx. Prevents secondary injury.	Given the urgency that often occurs with intubation, this step may be done simultaneously with other steps. For the infant, padding under the torso may provide proper alignment of the mouth, trachea, and pharynx.[1] Because of a relatively large occiput with placement on a flat surface, anterior displacement occurs naturally and aligns the mouth, pharynx, and trachea.[1] Hyperextention is not typically necessary. A pillow under the child's head may help with positioning. Neck flexion and extension should only be performed if neck or head trauma is not suspected. If cervical spine injury is present or suspected, the cervical spine should be immobilized.

Procedure	for Intubation: Perform, Including LMA—*Continued*	
Steps	**Rationale**	**Considerations**

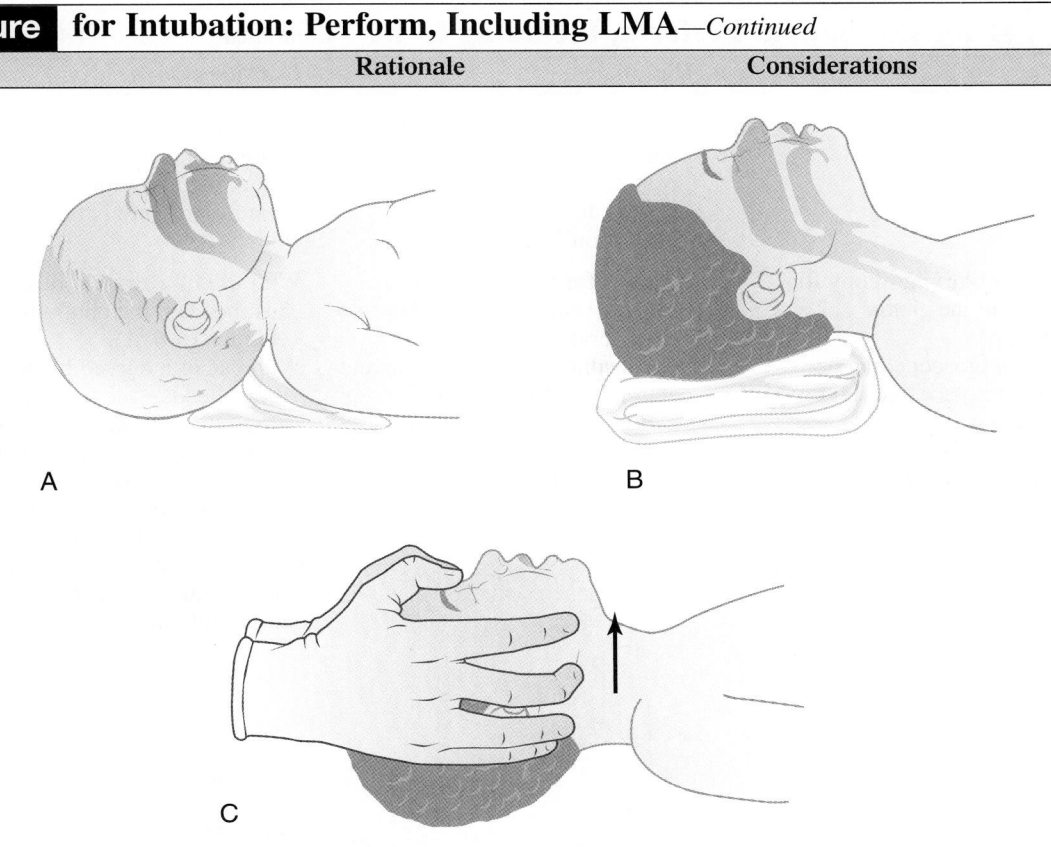

A

B

C

FIGURE 15-4 Head and Neck Position. **A,** Infant with head in neutral position and neck slightly extended with chin in sniffing position. **B,** Older child with occiput elevated into sniffing position and head extended at atlantooccipital joint, aligning oral, pharyngeal, and tracheal axes. **C,** Child with suspected or confirmed neck injury: maintain head in neutral position.

11. Ensure intubation medications are administered.	Modulates physiologic response to intubation.	
12. When child has a perfusing rhythm, ensure that child undergoes preoxygenation with a self-inflating MVB with mask attached to O$_2$ source for 3 to 5 minutes (unless rapid sequence intubation)[1] (see Procedure 21).	Helps prevent hypoxemia.	For successful preoxygenation, airway must first be opened and a sufficient volume administered to ensure chest rise.[1] Preoxygenation with a mask is most effective when provider stands at child's head and ensures a firm seal while airway is kept open by a head tilt and a mandibular jaw thrust.[15] Hyperoxygenation with 100% fraction of inspired oxygen (FiO$_2$) is not recommended for certain congenital heart defects and hypoxic respiratory drive. If rapid sequence intubation is necessary, avoid bag mask ventilation because of the increased risk of vomiting.[1]
13. Consider having assistant apply gentle cricoid pressure (Sellick's maneuver) in the unconscious child without a cough and gag[16] (see Figure 5-1).	Occludes esophagus by compressing cricoid cartilage posterior against the vertebral body.	Cricoid pressure should be continued until the tube is correctly placed into the trachea.

Procedure continues on following page

Procedure | for Intubation: Perform, Including LMA—*Continued*

Steps	Rationale	Considerations
	May decrease incidence rate of passive regurgitation of stomach contents into the trachea and gastric distention during intubation.[16,17]	Pressure is maintained throughout intubation. Reflux regurgitation can occur when cricoid pressure is released.[1]
14. Perform direct laryngoscopy for visualization of the glottis (Figure 15-5). Grasp laryngoscope handle (with blade in place and light on) in the left hand. Open child's mouth with right hand with a scissor-like motion. Insert blade into the right side of the child's mouth, advancing it to the base of the tongue and pushing tongue to the left.	Prepares for blade placement. Provides visualization and access to the oral cavity. With displacement of tongue and epiglottis anteriorly, the glottic opening is exposed. Allows for correct placement of the tube into trachea.[1]	With use of a straight blade, extend it just beneath the epiglottis (Figure 15-6, *A*). With use of a curved blade, insert it in the vallecula (the space between the epiglottis and the base of the tongue) to displace the tongue anteriorly (Figure 15-6, *B).*[1] Do not use child's teeth as a fulcrum when lifting the blade. Keeping left wrist stiff and lifting from the shoulder and arm prevents pressure on the teeth and gums.

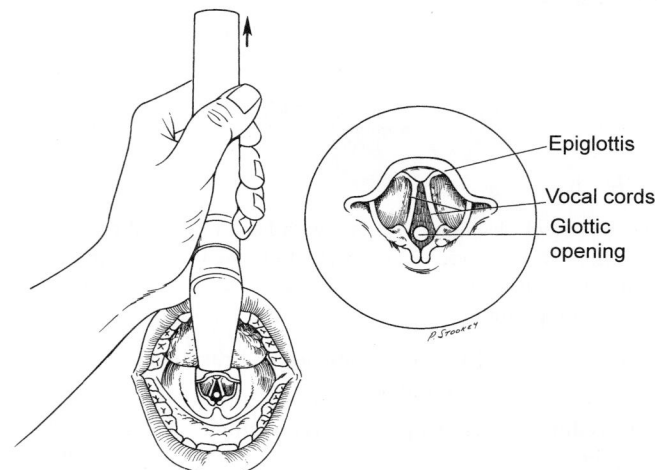

Epiglottis

Vocal cords

Glottic opening

FIGURE 15-5   Perform direct laryngoscopy to visualize glottis.

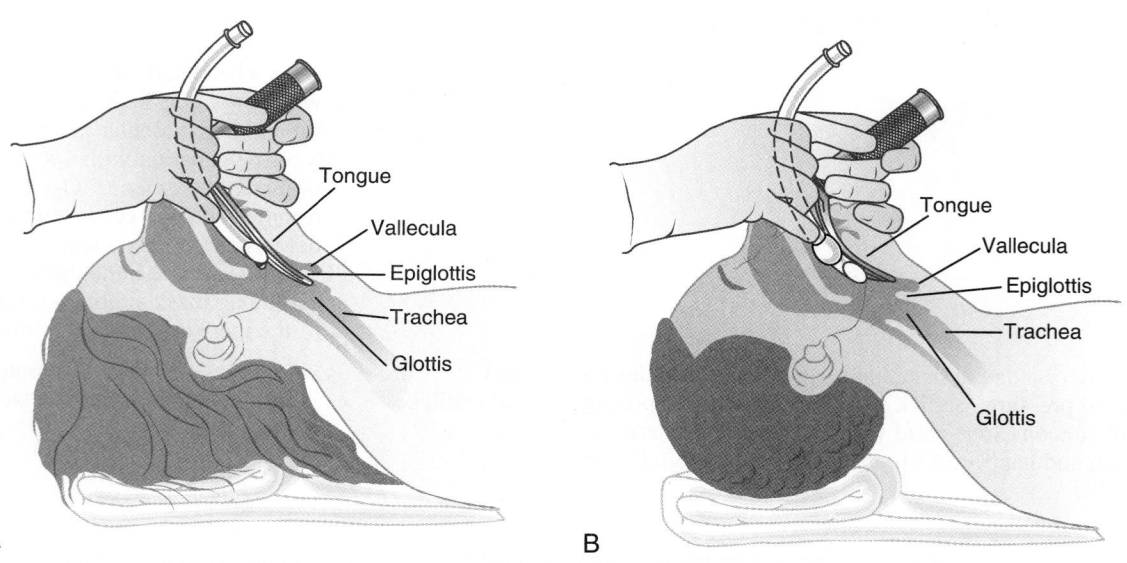

Tongue

Vallecula

Epiglottis

Trachea

Glottis

Tongue

Vallecula

Epiglottis

Trachea

Glottis

A

B

FIGURE 15-6   Position of Laryngoscope Blade. **A,** Use of straight laryngoscope blade, extending beneath epiglottis. **B,** Use of curved laryngoscope blade, with blade placed in vallecula.

Procedure	for Intubation: Perform, Including LMA—*Continued*	
Steps	**Rationale**	**Considerations**

With blade in correct placement, lift the handle outward and upward at a 45-degree angle to the bed.

Continue to lift laryngoscope handle until vocal cords are visualized.

Oral Intubation

15. Once vocal cords are visualized, ET tube is held in right hand and inserted at the right corner of child's mouth in a plane that intersects with laryngoscope blade at level of the glottis. Advance ET tube through the vocal cords to the appropriate depth with one of the following methods: a. Vocal cord mark inscribed on the tube. b. Depth of insertion for children more than 2 years of age[1] (cm): $[\text{Age (yr)}/2] + 12$	Visualization of ET tube passing through the vocal cords ensures proper placement. Ensures correct placement.	If intubation is unsuccessful within 30 seconds or if the child shows signs of hemodynamic instability, remove the tube and resume bag/mask ventilation with O_2 before another attempt is made (unless the provider's judgment indicates that intubation is of higher priority than transient decreases in oxygenation and heart rate).[1] Infants are especially vulnerable because of increased O_2 requirements and small lung volume.[1] When mark is placed at the vocal cords, tube should be in correct placement when head is in neutral position. Cuffed tubes are placed so that cuff is just below vocal cords.[1]

Nasotracheal Intubation

16. Instill appropriate dose of anesthetic or nasal vasoconstrictor to the nares. Lubricate tip of ET tube with water-soluble lubricant. Insert tip of the ET tube into the nare and advance until the tip of the tube is visible in the oropharynx. Use direct laryngoscopy to visualize the glottis as described previously. Advance ET tube at nasal end. Use forceps to direct tip through vocal cord.	Decreases incidence rate of epistaxis. Allows ease in insertion and prevents nasal trauma. Visualization of tip allows the use of forceps to direct the tube tip. Direct laryngoscopy assists with proper placement. Ensures proper placement.	May be contraindicated in children with hypertension, hyperthyroidism, or heart disease. Forceps may damage vocal cords and should not be used to push tip through the vocal cords.
17. Confirm ET tube placement with primary and secondary confirmation while providing positive pressure ventilation.[1]	Use of a combination of primary and secondary confirmation techniques reduces risk of undetected tube misplacement.	Outside of chest radiograph, no single confirmation technique is completely reliable under all circumstances.[1] The child's underlying disease process may make this assessment less reliable.

Primary confirmation[1]:

Assess for chest rise. *(Level II*)* Assess lung sounds for symmetry over peripheral lung fields, with assessment *(Level II*)* Auscultate for breath sounds over the upper abdomen.	Symmetric bilateral chest rise, equal breath sounds over peripheral lung fields, and absent breath sounds over abdomen are indicative of correct tracheal tube placement.	Children in cardiac arrest or with severe airway obstruction may not have detectable CO_2 levels.[1,21] Esophageal detector devices have been effective in verification of tube placement and can be used in older children.[1,21,22]

Procedure continues on following page

* Level II: Theory-based; no research data to support recommendations; recommendations from expert consensus group may exist

Procedure for Intubation: Perform, Including LMA—*Continued*

Steps	Rationale	Considerations
Secondary confirmation: Monitor exhaled ETCO$_2$ content.[1,18-20] Assess for improvement in or sustained O$_2$ saturation. Chest radiograph. *(Level II*)*	Exhaled CO$_2$ should be detected within six manual breaths if the tube is in trachea of a child who weighs more than 2 kg and has a perfusing cardiac rhythm.[1] O$_2$ saturations usually increase or remain excellent with successful intubation and administration of 100% O$_2$. This is most reliable method to visualize correct tube placement; however, it is not usually feasible for immediate assessment.	If doubt exists about correct ET tube position, revisualization of the airway may be necessary.
18. Assess for air leak around ET tube. Place a stethoscope on anterior neck overlying trachea with child's head in neutral position. With an aneroid manometer connected to ventilation bag, give positive pressure ventilation while auscultating for an air leak.	Assists in determination of whether tracheal tube size is correct. The inspiratory pressure at which air leaks around the tube is the air leak, measured in cm H$_2$O.	Maintenance of an air leak of 20 to 25 cm H$_2$O is desired and may reduce postextubation stridor in older children.[23] The absence of an air leak may indicate the tracheal tube is too large, the tube cuff is excessively inflated, or laryngospasm is occurring.[1]
19. Clean face and secure ET tube while child's head is in neutral position (see Procedure 3).	Prevents migration of the ET tube.	
20. Remove protective items and wash hands.	Reduces transmission of infection. Protects personnel health.	
Laryngeal Mask Airway (LMA-Unique) Insertion		
1. Ensure child and family understand procedure and questions are answered.	Evaluates and reinforces understanding of previously taught information.	Developmental, cognitive, and anxiety levels determine approach and effectiveness of teaching. Given the often emergent nature of LMA placement, procedure explanation may be delayed.
2. Gather equipment and supplies.		
3. Ensure child's vital signs and indications of inadequate oxygenation and ventilation are monitored.	Hypoxia and bradycardia are possible with airway placement. Hypotension may result from underlying hemodynamic instability.	Pulse oximetry is often used to continuously monitor O$_2$ saturations to provide an indication of gas exchange. Consider arterial/venous blood gases as indicated.
4. Wash hands.	Reduces transmission of infection. Protects personnel health.	
5. Put on gloves and personal protective equipment.	Reduces transmission of infection. Protects personnel health.	Protective eyewear is worn to prevent exposure to secretions.
6. Ensure a spare LMA of the same size is immediately available. *(Level I*)*	Provides back-up if initial device should fail.	

* Level I: Manufacturer's recommendations only

Level II: Theory-based; no research data to support recommendations; recommendations from expert consensus group may exist

Procedure for Intubation: Perform, Including LMA—*Continued*

Steps	Rationale	Considerations
7. Remove LMA from package and inspect the exterior for obvious damage and the interior of the tube for particles. *(Level I*)*	Ensures that LMA is not defective.	
8. Perform inflation and deflation tests (Figure 15-7).[12] *(Level I*)*	Ensures that LMA is not defective and works as indicated.	Discard LMA if structural defects are visible during inspection and inflation/deflation test.

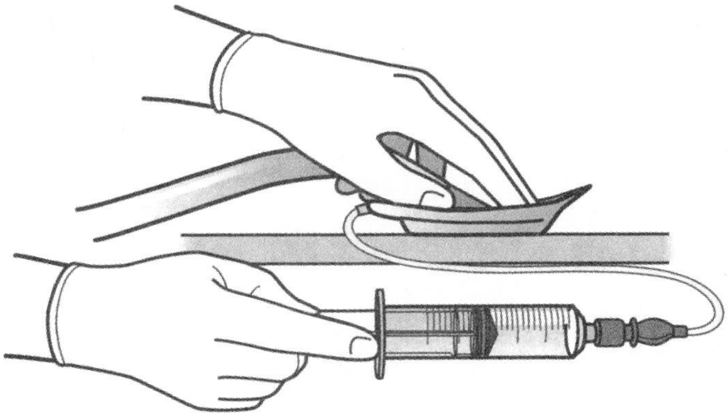

FIGURE 15-7   Inflation and Deflation Tests for LMA.

9. Attach appropriate size Luer-tip syringe to the pilot balloon valve.		
10. Pull back the syringe plunger to completely deflate cuff and examine cuff to ensure that it remains fully deflated.		
11. Remove syringe from the balloon valve and fill syringe with appropriate volume of air for LMA size (see Table 15-4).		
12. Reattach balloon to valve and inflate cuff.		
13. Ensure cuff inflates symmetrically without bulges and that pilot balloon is elliptical.		Instill 50% more air than the maximum clinical inflation volume. Any tendency of the cuff to deflate becomes evident within 2 minutes.
14. Deflate cuff by placing it aperture side down on a hard flat surface and smooth out any wrinkles as air is withdrawn from cuff (Figure 15-8).	Facilitates smooth insertion and avoids deflection of the epiglottis or entry of the tip into the glottis.	The cuff should appear smooth and without wrinkles before insertion.

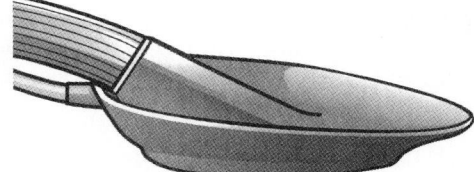

FIGURE 15-8   Deflating Cuff for LMA.

Procedure continues on following page

* Level I: Manufacturer's recommendations only

AP   This procedure should be performed only by physicians, advanced practice nurses, and other health care professionals (including critical care nurses) with additional knowledge, skills, and demonstrated competence per professional licensure or institutional standard.

Procedure | for Intubation: Perform, Including LMA—*Continued*

Steps	Rationale	Considerations
15. Lubricate posterior tip of cuff with water-soluble lubricant.	Facilitates smooth insertion.	Lubricant should not spread to anterior portion of cuff because it may be aspirated.
16. Assume a position at child's head and position child's head in a sniffing position.		Child's head may be left midline if contraindicated by child's condition, such as cervical spine injury.
17. Hold LMA so that dominant hand's index finger and thumb grasp airway tube just behind the cuff as if holding a pen (Figure 15-9, *A*).		The mask aperture should face toward the child's feet, and the black line on the airway tube should face toward the child's nose.
18. During direct visualization, insert LMA into child's mouth and direct it upward toward hard palate (Figure 15-9, *B*).		If the LMA does not flatten against the hard palate, begin again.

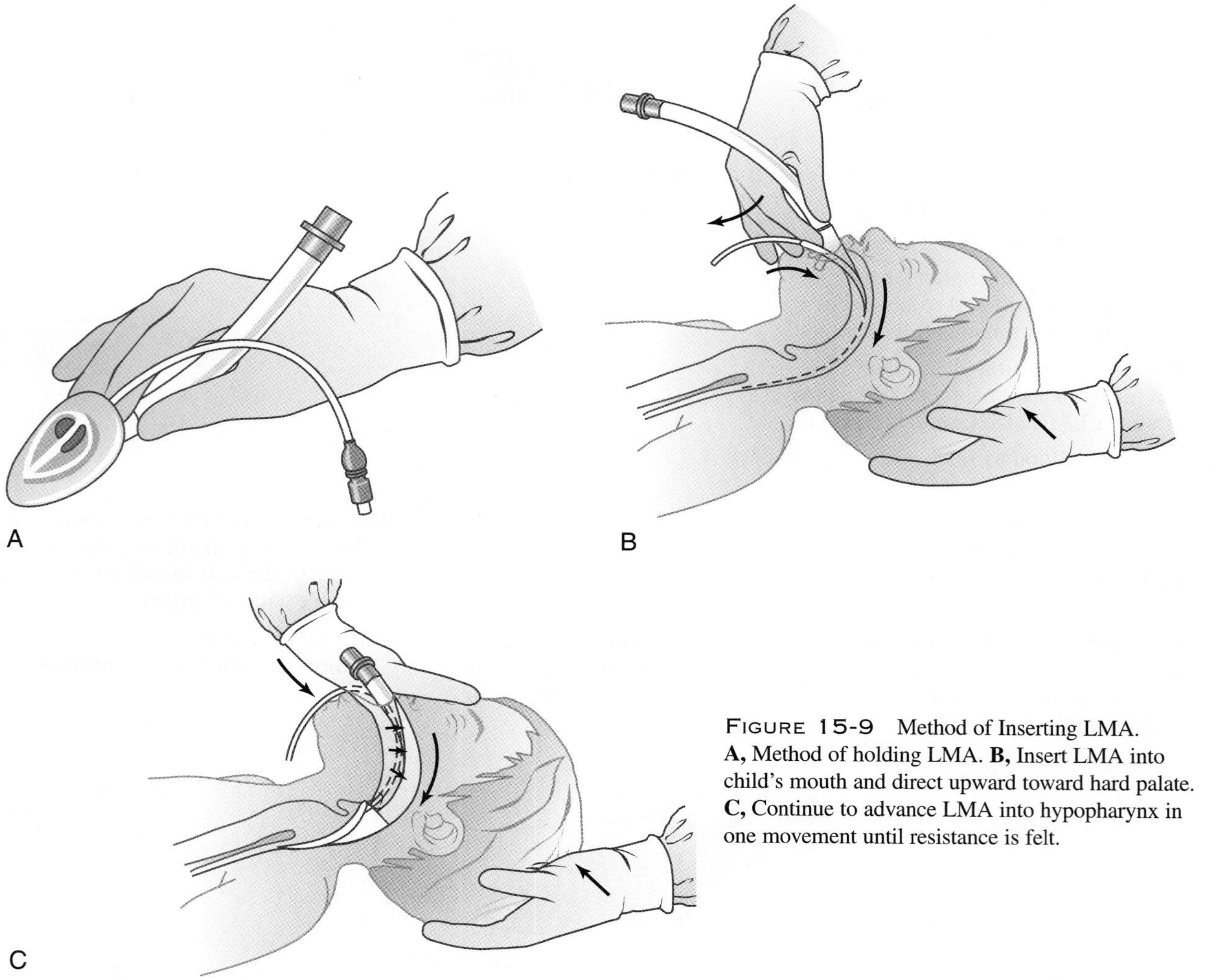

FIGURE 15-9   Method of Inserting LMA. **A,** Method of holding LMA. **B,** Insert LMA into child's mouth and direct upward toward hard palate. **C,** Continue to advance LMA into hypopharynx in one movement until resistance is felt.

Procedure for Intubation: Perform, Including LMA—*Continued*

Steps	Rationale	Considerations
19. With index finger, continue to advance LMA into the hypopharynx in one movement until resistance is felt (Figure 15-9, *C*).	Moves LMA into proper position.	Excessive force should be avoided.[12] Do not continue to hold the jaw open while advancing the LMA because this causes the epiglottis and tongue to drop downwards, preventing the mask from passing.
20. Release the airway tube and inflate the cuff with appropriate amount of air (see Table 15-4).	Inflating cuff creates a seal.	
21. Observe for one or more signs of correct placement and inflation, including slight outward movement of the airway, slight bulging of neck around the cricothyroid area, or no cuff visible in the mouth.	Ensures correct position.	After correct insertion, tip of the LMA is positioned in esophagus. The LMA opening is positioned at the glottis so that air passes into trachea through the tube.[1] If none of these signs of placement are observed, consider deflating cuff and removing the LMA.
22. Connect male adapter to the bag-valve device and gently give positive pressure ventilation with peak pressures of less than 20 cm water.	Maintenance of low ventilatory pressures prevents overriding the pressure in the cuff, which creates a leak and forces air into stomach.	The cuff may leak air with first few breaths as it settles into correct position. If leaking continues, ensure that positive pressures are less than 20 cm water.
23. Remove protective gear and wash hands.	Reduces transmission of infection.	

Expected Outcomes

- Placement of a patent and correctly positioned and sized ET tube or LMA

- Properly secured ET tube or LMA
- Improved oxygenation and ventilation
- Decreased work of breathing

- Improved secretion clearance
- Hemodynamic stability

- No traumatic injury

- Child maintains an acceptable level of comfort

Unexpected Outcomes

- Intubation of esophagus or main stem bronchus
- Large air leak around the tube indicates that the tube size is too small
- Migration of ET tube/LMA
- Inadequate oxygenation and ventilation
- Hypoxemia from inappropriate bag/mask ventilation technique or poor intubation skills
- Aspiration
- Hemodynamic instability from medications or vagal stimulation
- Vocal cord or tracheal trauma
- Broken teeth
- Unmanaged pain and discomfort

Monitoring and Care of the Child

Activities and Interventions	Rationale	Reportable Conditions
1. Assess lung sounds immediately after airway placement, every 2 to 4 hours, and with changes in status.	Allows for detection of tube migration or dislodgment.	• Absent, decreased, or unequal breath sounds
2. Record the position of the tube at the lip or nose with centimeter markings on the tube as reference.	Allows for identification of tube migration/dislodgement.	• Tube movement from the original position

Continued

Monitoring and Care of the Child—Cont'd

Activities and Interventions	Rationale	Reportable Conditions
3. Continually assess tube stability and integrity of the tape.	Prevents movement and dislodgement of the tube	• Unplanned extubation • Poor tape integrity that necessitates retaping • Cuff pressure of more than 20 mm Hg
4. If a cuff is present, assess the tube cuff pressure every 4 hours and maintain cuff pressure at less than 20 mm Hg.	Inflate cuff to minimal pressure necessary to seal an air leak and allow effective ventilation. High cuff pressures may precipitate tracheal damage.	
5. Hyperoxygenate and suction the tube as needed (see Procedure 2).	Prevents obstruction of the tube.	• Inability to pass a suction catheter through the tube • Significant change in amount or character of secretions
6. After airway placement, assess comfort and provide appropriate interventions. Allow family to assist with nonpharmacologic means to comfort and support the child.	Early identification of the child's comfort allows for immediate attention.	• Unresolved pain and discomfort • Continued irritability or changes in physiologic condition

Documentation

- Respiratory assessment findings before and after airway placement, including vital signs, breath sounds, coughing, and tracheal secretions in tube
- Route of artificial airway placement
- Size of airway and presence of cuff
- Medications administered
- Confirmation of airway placement with indication of how placement was confirmed and depth of insertion (centimeters at lip line or nose)
- Presence of a leak
- Comfort assessment and any specific interventions provided
- Child's response to the procedure
- Additional interventions necessary before, during, and after artificial airway placement
- Child and family education
- Unexpected outcomes and related interventions

References

1. Hazinski MF, et al, editors: *Pediatric advanced life support provider manual,* Dallas, 2002, American Heart Association.
2. Thompson A: Pediatric airway management. In Fuhrman B, Zimmerman J, editors: *Pediatric critical care,* ed 3, Philadelphia, 2005, Elsevier.
3. McCance K, Huether S: *Pathophysiolog: the biologic bases for disease in adults and children,* Philadelphia, 2002, Mosby.
4. The Laryngeal Airway Mask Airway Limited: *LMA airway instruction manual,* San Diego, 2004, LMA North America. Text available at http://www.lmana.com/prod/content/education/LMA_Airways_Manual.pdf.
5. Trimble T: (2005) Using anesthesia bags, Emergency Nursing World, retrieved August 3, 2005, from http://www.enw.org/A-Bags.htm.
6. American Academy of Pediatrics: *Parts of a flow inflating bag, video 2,* retrieved August 3, 2005, from http://www.aap. org/nrp/educational/educational_cdvideos_02.html.
7. American Academy of Pediatrics: *Parts of a self inflating bag, video 3,* retrieved August 3, 2005, from http://www.aap.org/nrp/educational/educational_cdvideos_03.html.
8. American Association of Respiratory Therapy Clinical Practice Guideline: Removal of the endotracheal tube, *Respir Care* 44 (1):85-90, 1999.
9. Curley MAQ, Thompson J: Oxygenation and ventilation. In Curley MAQ, Moloney-Harmon P, editors: *Nursing care of critically ill infants and children,* ed 2, Philadelphia, 2001, Saunders Inc.
10. Deakers TW, et al: Cuffed tracheal tubes in pediatric intensive care, *J Pediatr* 125:57-62, 1994.
11. Khine HH, et al: Comparison of cuffed and uncuffed endotracheal tubes in young children during general anesthesia, *Anesthesiology* 86(3):627-31, 1997.
12. Day M: Procedure 7 laryngeal mask airway. In Wiegand DJ, Carlson K, editors: *AACN procedure manual for critical care,* ed 5, Philadelphia, 2004, Saunders.
13. Newth CJ, et al: The use of cuffed versus uncuffed endotracheal tubes in pediatric intensive care, *J Pediatr* 144(3): 333-337, 2004.

14. Westhorpe RN: The position of the larynx in children and its relationship to the ease of intubation, *Anaesthesia Intens Care* 15:384-388, 1987.

15. Beers M, Berkow R, editors: Cardiac and respiratory arrest and cardiopulmonary resuscitation, *The Merck manual of diagnosis and therapy,* ed 17, 2005, Merck Company Inc.

16. Sellick BA: Cricoid pressure to control regurgitation of stomach contents during induction of anesthesia, *Lancet* 2:404-406, 1961.

17. Moynihan RJ, et al: The effect of cricoid pressure on preventing gastric insufflation in infants and children, *Anesthesiology* 78:652-656, 1993.

18. Bhende MS, et al: Utility of an end-tidal carbon dioxide detector during stabilization and transport of critically ill children, *Pediatrics* 89:1042-1044, 1992.

19. Bhende MS, Alledn WD: Evaluation of a Capno-Flo resuscitator during transport of critically ill children, *Pediatr Emerg Care* 18(6):414-416, 2002.

20. Ward K, Yealy D: End-tidal carbon dioxide monitoring in emergency medicine, part 1: basic principles, *Acad Emerg Med* 5:628-638, 1998.

21. Schaller R: Comparison of a colorimetric end-tidal CO2 detector and an esophageal aspiration device for verifying endotracheal tube placement in the prehospital setting: a six-month experience, *Prehospital Disaster Med* 12:57-63, 1997.

22. International Consensus on Science: Guidelines 2000 for cardiopulmonary resuscitation and emergency cardiovascular care: adjuncts to oxygenation, ventilation and airway control, *Circulation* 102(Suppl):95-104, 2000.

23. Mhanna MJ, et al: The "air leak" test around the endotracheal tube, as a predictor of post extubation stridor, is age dependent in children, *Crit Care Med* 30(12):2639-2643, 2002.

Additional Readings

American Society of Anesthesiologists Task Force on Difficult Airway Management: Practice guidelines for management of the difficult airway, *Anesthesiology* 98:1269-1277, 2003.

Hussey S, et al: Comparison of three manual ventilation devices using an intubated mannequin, *Arch Dis Childhood Fetal Neonatal Ed* 89(6):F490-493, 2004.

Sanders KC, et al: End tidal CO_2 detection in emergency intubation of four groups of patients, *J Em Med* 12: 771-777, 1994.

16

AP

Tracheostomy Tube: Decannulation

P U R P O S E : Tracheostomy tube decannulation is the removal of a tracheostomy tube to allow the child to breathe through the natural airway independent of the artificial airway

Elsie M. Hartigan and Susan M. Campisciano

PREREQUISITE KNOWLEDGE

- Child development as it relates to clinical assessment and the procedure
- Anatomy and physiology of the pediatric pulmonary system, including structural characteristics of upper and lower respiratory tract that are specific to the infant and child[1-5]
  - ❖ A child's airway is both absolutely and relatively smaller in diameter and shorter than an adult's (see Figure 1-1)
  - ❖ The child's funnel-shaped larynx is higher and more cephalad and lies below the vocal cords. The vocal cords are 50% cartilage and are attached lower and more anteriorly.
  - ❖ The infant's epiglottis is floppy, long, and narrow and projects more posteriorly than the older child's. The subglottic airway is smaller and more compliant with the cartilage less developed than in the adult.
  - ❖ Because the thyroid does not assume its adult configuration until puberty, the cricoid cartilage is the easiest landmark for identification in children
  - ❖ The cricoid cartilage is the narrowest portion of the upper airway in children less than 10 years of age. It lies at the level of the third cervical vertebrae in the infant and descends to the sixth cervical vertebrae at puberty.

  - ❖ In teenagers and adults, the larynx is a cylinder with its narrowest portion at the glottic inlet at the level of the vocal cords.
  - ❖ The quantity of alveoli increases until 8 years of age and thereafter increases in size and complexity. Peripheral airway resistance is disproportionately higher in the child.
  - ❖ During inspiration, the infant's intercostal muscles stiffen and a downward movement of the diaphragm occurs, which results in negative intrathoracic pressure and air movement into the lungs. Because the infant's chest wall is compliant and flexible, it characteristically collapses inward (see Figure 23-1).
- Signs and symptoms of inadequate oxygenation and ventilation[1]
- Mastery of pediatric advanced life support competencies, including indications for an artificial airway, use of a manual resuscitation/ventilation system, and other adjuncts used to support ventilation[4]
- Tracheotomy is a surgical procedure that involves the construction of a channel between the trachea and the skin surface of the neck in the midline. An incision is made through the second, third, and fourth tracheal rings[4] (see Figure 11-1). Placement too close to the first ring risks cricoid cartilage damage with subsequent subglottic stenosis.
- A tracheostomy is the opening or stoma made by the tracheotomy incision.
- Clinical indication for the child's tracheotomy and date of original tube placement

- Some possible indications for tracheotomy include upper airway obstruction, craniofacial abnormalities that interfere with natural airway patency, prolonged ventilatory support, prevention of aspiration, and removal of secretions.[1,2,4,6-10]
  - Some common abnormalities that lead to tracheostomy tube placement for infants and children include chronic lung disease, subglottic stenosis, tracheal stenosis, laryngotracheomalacia, neuromuscular weakness, and neurologic impairment.[1,2,4,6-10]
- Decannulation refers to the removal of the tracheostomy tube
- Indications for decannulation include reversal or improvement of the underlying condition that led to the need for an artificial airway, including airway obstruction and lung disease; capacity to independently clear the airway; minimal risk of aspiration; and no need for invasive mechanical ventilation[3,10]
- Many children are discharged home with a tracheostomy tube and, after a lengthy stabilization and weaning period, return to the hospital for decannulation[11] (Figure 16-1).
- At best, tracheal decannulation is a planned procedure, and the child must be closely monitored (typically in an intensive care unit or stepdown unit). The length of hospital stay varies on the basis of the child's to decannulation and clinical condition. Typically, a minimum of 24 to 48 hours is necessary.
- Before planned decannulation, the tracheostomy tube is gradually downsized with successively smaller tubes to progressively narrow and restrict the tube lumen until the smallest tube is in place and the child is breathing without difficulties.[6]

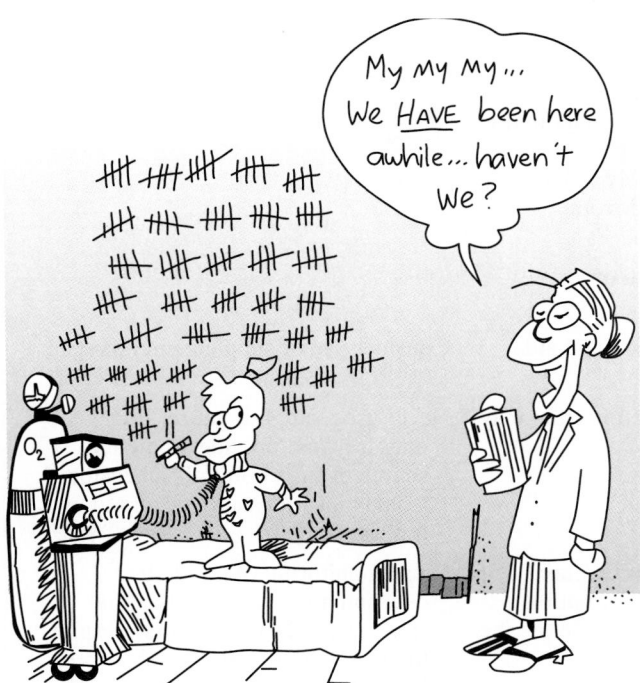

FIGURE 16-1 Image as it appears in Edwards EA, et al: Sending children home on tracheostomy dependent ventilation: pitfalls and outcomes, *Arch Disabled Child* 89:255, 2004.

- Before planned decannulation, diagnostic laryngotracheobronchoscopy allows for direct visualization of the airway and helps in identification of issues that are likely to impede effective breathing.[2]
- Complications after decannulation include tracheomalacia, tracheocutaneous fistula, airway obstruction from granular tissue on the tracheal wall, significant laryngeotracheal stenosis, and reduced movement of the vocal cords.[8,12]
- Children with chronic lung disease and upper airway obstruction appear to have a greater chance for success after decannulation.[12] Older children appear to have worse decannulation results.[8]

CHILD AND FAMILY ASSESSMENT

- Child's developmental level and ability to interact ➤➤*Rationale:* Influences preparation and interaction.
- Child's and family's understanding of the reasons for and risks and benefits of the procedure ➤➤*Rationale:* Evaluates child's and family's understanding of the procedure and provides a gauge for ongoing education.
- Desire of family members to be present during the procedure ➤➤*Rationale:* The presence of family may provide comfort and support; although remaining with the child should always be a choice.
- History of upper airway anomalies, presence of a critical airway, and neurologic status ➤➤*Rationale:* Evaluates child's ability to maintain a patent airway and provides valuable information in determining the child's ability to tolerate decannulation.
- Timing of most recent feeding ➤➤*Rationale:* A full stomach may lead to vomiting or aspiration during the procedure. To avoid or minimize this risk, maintain nothing by mouth.[6]
- Cardiopulmonary assessment, including vital signs, visual inspection of breathing patterns and chest wall movement, auscultation of lung fields, and signs of inadequate oxygenation and ventilation, such as decreased arterial oxygen saturation, cardiac arrhythmia, increased work of breathing, cyanosis, increased blood pressure, elevated intracranial pressure, anxiety, agitation, and changes in level of consciousness ➤➤*Rationale:* Evaluating the child's cardiopulmonary status provides valuable information as to the ability and preparedness of the child to tolerate decannulation.

CHILD AND FAMILY EDUCATION

Individualized, developmentally appropriate education is provided to the family and to the child based on desire for knowledge, readiness to learn, and overall neurologic and psychosocial state.

- Explain the procedure for decannulation, including the purpose, steps, and rationale ➤➤*Rationale:* Providing information decreases fear and anxiety.
- If appropriate for the child's current cognitive and developmental level, explain the procedure to the child and consider use of a child life specialist in assisting with the child's preparation for the procedure ➤➤*Rationale:*

Involving the child with the preparation for decannulation can increase the feeling of control and increase tolerance to procedure.

- Encourage questions and answer questions as they arise ➤*Rationale:* Reinforcement of information is needed during periods of stress.

EQUIPMENT

- Gloves
- Additional personal protective equipment as indicated, including eye protection, mask, and gown
- Sterile tracheostomy tube of appropriate size (with obturator as indicated)
- A tracheostomy tube with an internal diameter a half size smaller than the child's current tube size[4,6]
- Syringe to deflate cuff (if tube is cuffed)
- Scissors
- Manual ventilation bag (MVB) and appropriately sized face mask
- Oxygen source as
- Stethoscope
- Suction equipment
- Endotracheal intubation supplies
- Emergency cart readily available

Procedure | for Performing Decannulation

Steps	Rationale	Considerations
1. Ensure child and family understand procedure and questions are answered.	Evaluates and reinforces understanding of previously taught information.	Developmental, cognitive, and anxiety levels determine approach and effectiveness of teaching.
2. Gather equipment and supplies at bedside.	Preparation facilitates completion of the procedure in a timely manner.	
3. Monitor child's vital signs and indications of inadequate oxygenation and ventilation.	Removal of artificial airway may cause significant respiratory compromise.	Ensure that a pulse oximeter is reading accurately and that the cardiac monitor is on.
4. Wash hands and put on gloves and appropriate personal protection equipment.	Reduces transmission of infection. Protects personnel health.	
5. For those children with a cuffed tube, ensure that cuff is deflated.	Prevents trauma to tracheal tissue.	
6. Cut and remove twill tape.	Readies tube for removal.	
7. Instruct child to deep breathe.	Promotes hyperinflation.	
8. At peak of a deep inspiration, remove the tracheostomy tube in one motion.	During peak of inspiration, the child's vocal cords are maximally abducted. Cough response after decannulation is likely to have more force if started from maximal inspiration.[1,2,6]	
9. Suction pharynx as indicated.	Assists in maintenance of airway patency.	
10. After decannulation, encourage child to cough and deep breathe.	Promotes hyperinflation and aids airway clearance.	Consider use of supplemental oxygen.
11. Place a dry sterile 4×4 dressing over stoma after decannulation.	Helps to contain secretions that may seep out of stoma.	Never use a cut 4×4 gauze. Edges may fray and provide a potential source of infection.[13] Tracheostomy stoma closure usually occurs in a few days.[1,2,6,14]
12. Continue careful clinical assessment of child's cardiopulmonary status with visual examination and appropriate monitoring devices.	Ongoing assessment is essential and provides valuable information about child's ability to tolerate the decannulation.	Close monitoring of child after decannulation remains essential (for at least 24 to 48 hours) despite the length and vigilance of process leading up to decannulation.[1,2,6,14]

AP This procedure should be performed only by physicians, advanced practice nurses, and other health care professionals (including critical care nurses) with additional knowledge, skills, and demonstrated competence per professional licensure or institutional standard.

Expected Outcomes	Unexpected Outcomes
• Natural airway supports oxygenation and ventilation	• Fatigue and respiratory failure leading to recannulation
• Nontraumatic decannulation without subsequent complications	• Laryngospasm
• Closure of tracheal stoma	• Cardiorespiratory arrest
	• Trauma to trachea or soft tissue
	• Persistent hoarseness
• Cough is effective in clearing secretions	• Ineffective cough and swallowing
• Effective swallowing	• Aspiration
• Acceptable level of comfort	• Unmanaged pain and agitation

Monitoring and Care of the Child

Activities and Interventions	Rationale	Reportable Conditions
1. Assess respiratory status and physiologic stability, including vital signs, clinical appearance, and signs and symptoms of inadequate oxygenation and ventilation.	May indicate a need for additional assessment and intervention. Removal of the artificial airway may alter the child's physiologic stability.	• Diminished breath sounds • Significant changes in oxygenation saturation and arterial/venous blood gases • Increased peak airway pressures • Persistent coughing • Increased work of breathing • Persistent dysrhythmias, including bradycardia and tachycardia • Changes in peripheral perfusion • Cyanosis • Anxiety, agitation, or changes in mental status
2. Promote optimal oxygenation with supplemental oxygen and humidification as needed.	Decreases incidence rate of oxygen desaturation immediately after decannulation.	• Oxyhemoglobin saturation of less than 90%
3. Assess swallowing and effectiveness of cough.	Long-term tube placement may result in harm to swallowing.	• Inability to swallow
4. Monitor for aspiration related to pooled secretions.	Child may have pooled secretions and be unable to clear airway.	• Inability to manage secretions
5. Assess comfort and provide appropriate interventions. Allow the family to assist with nonpharmacologic means to comfort and support the child.	Early identification of the child's comfort allows for immediate attention.	• Unresolved pain and discomfort • Continued irritability

Documentation

- Predecannulation and postdecannulation respiratory assessment findings, including vital signs, breath sounds, and work of breathing
- Assessment of the tracheal stoma site, including skin condition (note the presence or extent of granulation tissue or breakdown) and the presence of any drainage at the stoma site including of amount, color, odor, and consistency
- Comfort assessment and any specific interventions provided
- Additional interventions necessary before, during, and after decannulation
- Child and family education
- Unexpected outcomes and related treatment

References

1. Curley MAQ, Thompson JE: Oxygenation and ventilation. In Curley MAQ, Moloney-Harmon P, editors: *Critical care nursing of infants and children,* ed 2, Philadelphia, 2001, Saunders.

2. Thompson A: Pediatric airway management. In Fuhrman B, Zimmerman J, editors: *Pediatric critical care,* ed 3, Philadelphia, 2005, Elsevier.

3. Froh D: Alterations of pulmonary function in children. In McCance K, Huether S, editors: *Pathophysiology: the biologic basis for disease in adults and children,* ed 4, Philadelphia, 2002, Mosby.

4. Hazinski MF, et al, editors: *Pediatric advanced life support provider manual,* Dallas, 2002, American Heart Association.

5. Katz R: Function and physiology of the respiratory system. In Fuhrman B, Zimmerman J, editors: *Pediatric critical care,* ed 3, Philadelphia, 2005, Elsevier.

6. Gera T, Matthew JL: *Pediatric tracheostomy,* 2000, retrieved February 5, 2005, from http://pedsccm.wustl.edu/All-Net/english/pulmpage/trache/trachetitle.html.

7. Panitch HB, et al: Guidelines for homecare of children with chronic respiratory insufficiency, *Pediatr Pulmonol* 21(1):52-56, 1996.

8. Lee W, et al: Indications for tracheotomy in pediatric intensive care unit population, *Arch Otolaryngol Head Neck Surg* 128:1249-1252, 2002.

9. Lewis C, et al: Tracheostomy in pediatric patients: a national perspective, *Arch Otolaryngol Head Neck Surg* 129(5):523-529, 2003.

10. American Thoracic Society: Care of the child with a chronic tracheostomy, *Am J Respir Crit Care Med* 161:297-308, 2000.

11. Carr M, et al: Complications in pediatric tracheostomies, *Laryngoscope* 111:1925-1928, 2001.

12. Edwards EA, et al: Sending children home on tracheostomy dependent ventilation: pitfalls and outcomes, *Arch Disabled Child* 89:251-255, 2004.

13. Serra A: Tracheostomy care, *Nurs Stand* 10(34):40-43, 2000.

14. Gray RF: Tracheostomy decannulation in children: approaches and techniques, *Laryngoscope* 108:8-12, 1998.

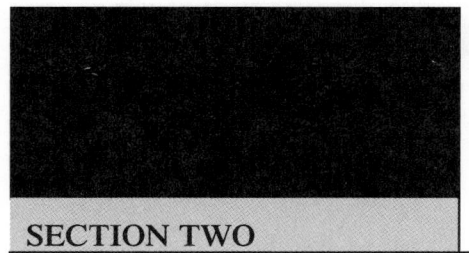

P R O C E D U R E **17**

Arterial Blood Gas Analysis

P U R P O S E : Arterial blood gases (ABGs) are analyzed to determine the child's acid base balance, oxygenation, and ventilatory status

Laurie S. Finger

PREREQUISITE KNOWLEDGE

- Child development as it relates to clinical assessment and interpretation of arterial blood gases (ABG)
- Anatomy and physiology of the pediatric pulmonary system
- Signs and symptoms of inadequate oxygenation and ventilation
- Principles of oxygen delivery and gas exchange (Table 17-1)
  - ❖ Transfer of oxygen across the alveolar-capillary membrane
  - ❖ Transfer of oxygen is dependent on the ventilation/perfusion (V/Q) match
    - ○ Oxygen-carrying capacity
    - ○ Capacity is determined by hemoglobin level
    - ○ Oxygen delivery
    - ○ Delivery is determined by cardiac index and arterial oxygen content
  - ❖ Oxygen release from the hemoglobin molecule
    - ○ Release is determined by the oxyhemoglobin dissociation curve
  - ❖ Cell utilization of oxygen
    - ○ Utilization is determined by oxygen extraction and oxygen consumption
- Dynamics of the oxyhemoglobin dissociation curve (Figure 17-1)
- Blood gas analysis is a systematic process of evaluation of oxygenation, ventilation, and acid/base balance providing information about pH, $paCO_2$, SaO_2, HCO_3^-, and base deficit/excess (Figure 17-2).
- Indications for arterial blood gas analysis are child specific and include monitoring status of respiratory distress/failure,

acid-base balance, shock, cardiopulmonary resuscitation, and therapies, such as ventilator management.
- Normal arterial blood gas values (Table 17-2)
- Capillary and mixed venous blood gases may augment monitoring of oxygenation and ventilation (Table 17-3).
- Chronic conditions, such as bronchopulmonary dysplasia, cystic fibrosis, and congenital heart disease, may alter the acceptable normal arterial blood gas values.

CHILD AND FAMILY ASSESSMENT

- Child's developmental level and ability to interact ➤➤*Rationale:* Influences preparation and interaction.
- Child's and family's understanding of the underlying condition, the reasons for ABG analysis, the results, and their significance ➤➤*Rationale:* Evaluates child's and family's understanding of the procedure and provides a gauge for ongoing education.
- Any pertinent medical history or current condition that predisposes the child to alterations in oxygenation, ventilation, and acid/base balance ➤➤*Rationale:* Some medical conditions and therapies predispose the child to changes in arterial blood gas values (e.g., hypoplastic left heart syndrome, diabetic ketoacidosis, and supplemental oxygen therapy).
- Assessment of the child's respiratory status, including respiratory rate, work of breathing, and breath sounds ➤➤*Rationale:* ABGs are only a part of an assessment of the child.
- Signs and symptoms of inadequate oxygenation and ventilation ➤➤*Rationale:* Indicates effective pulmonary function and need for blood gas analysis.

TABLE 17-1	Indicators of Oxygenation		
Indices of Oxygenation	**Definition**	**Equation**	**Normal Values***
Ventilation/perfusion (V/Q) match	Transfer of oxygen across alveolar-capillary membrane		4/5 (0.8) L/min
Oxygen carrying capacity (Hgb level)	1 g Hgb carries 1.34 mL of oxygen		10 to 16 g/dL* In neonates, normal level is 14 to 22 g/dL
Oxygen delivery (DO_2)	Amount of oxygen delivered to tissues each minute	$DO_2 = CI \times CaO_2 \times 10$	18 to 20 mL/dL
Cardiac index (CI)	Amount of blood ejected by heart each minute divided by body surface area	$CI = CO/BSA\ (M^2)$	3.5 to 5.5 L/min/M^2
Arterial oxygen content (CaO_2)	Amount of oxygen carried by arterial Hgb plus oxygen carried by plasma ($PaO_2 \times 0.003$)	$CaO_2 = (Hgb \times 1.34 \times SaO_2) + (PaO_2 \times 0.003)$	18 to 20 mL/dL
Oxygen utilization (VO_2)	Amount of oxygen consumed by tissues	$VO_2 = CI \times C(a{-}v)O_2 \times 10$	15 mL/dL
Oxygen extraction ratio (O_2ER)	Ratio of amount of VO_2 and DO_2	$O_2ER = \dfrac{C(a{-}v)O_2}{CaO_2} \times 100$	25%

*This number may vary by laboratory and age.

BSA = Body Surface Area (a and v are defined as a part of their respective equations; thus, CaO_2 is arterial oxygen content and Vo_2 is oxygen utilization. See above).

CHILD AND FAMILY EDUCATION

Individualized, developmentally appropriate education is provided to the family and to the child based on desire for knowledge, readiness to learn, and overall neurologic and psychosocial state.

- Explain the underlying condition, the reasons for ABG analysis, the results, and their significance ➧➧*Rationale:* Providing information decreases fear and anxiety and improves compliance.
- Encourage questions and answer questions as they arise ➧➧*Rationale:* Reinforcement of information is needed during periods of stress.

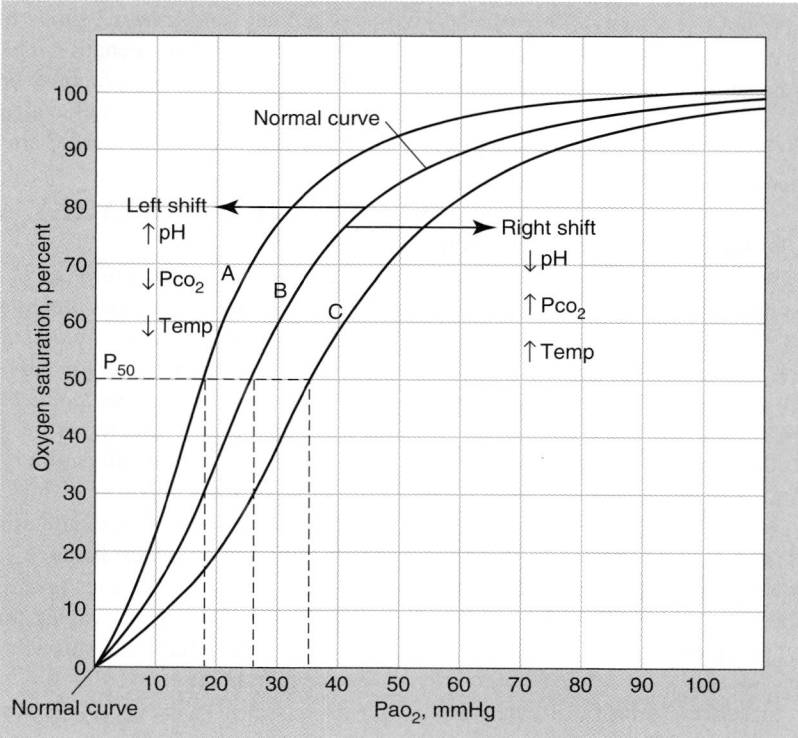

FIGURE 17-1   Oxyhemoglobin Dissociation Curve. *Powers A: Acid-base balance. In Curley MAQ, Moloney-Harmon P, editors:* Critical care nursing of infants and children, *ed 2, Philadelphia, 2001, Saunders. Curley MAQ, Thompson JE: Oxygenation and ventilation. In Curley MAQ, Moloney-Harmon P, editors:* Critical care nursing of infants and children, *ed 2, Philadelphia, 2001, Saunders.*

TABLE 17-2	Normal Arterial Blood Gases	
Indicator	**Definition**	**Normal Values**
pH	Concentration of free hydrogen ions (H^+) in blood produced by acid/base reactions; thus, pH refers to acid-base balance of blood	7.35 to 7.45
Pa_{CO_2}	Partial pressure of dissolved carbon dioxide in blood and is controlled in lungs through ventilation	35 to 45 mm Hg
Pa_{O_2}	Partial pressure of dissolved oxygen in blood	80 to 100 mm Hg Normal 60 to 80 mm Hg
Sa_{O_2}	Percent of hemoglobin saturated with oxygen	95% to 100%
HCO_3^-	Concentration of bicarbonate ions (HCO_3^-) in blood that is excreted or retained by kidneys to regulate pH	22 to 26 mEq/L
Base excess/deficit	Milliequivalents of bicarbonate in excess or deficient per liter of extracellular water	+2 to −2

Data from Curley MAQ, Thompson JE: Oxygenation and ventilation. In Curley MAQ, Moloney-Harmon P, editors: *Critical care nursing of infants and children*, ed 2, Philadelphia, 2001, Saunders.

Doerschug K, et al: *Arterial blood gas analysis, systematic analysis of blood gases*, 1999, retrieved March 5, 2005, from www.vh.org/adult/provider/internalmedicine/abg/ABGHome.html.

Hornick D: *An approach to the analysis of arterial blood gases and acid-base disorders*, 2003, retrieved March 5, 2005, from http://www.vh.org/adult/provider/ internalmedicine/bloodgases/.

Powers A: Acid-base balance. In Curley MAQ, Moloney-Harmon P, editors: *Critical care nursing of infants and children*, ed 2, Philadelphia, 2001, Saunders.

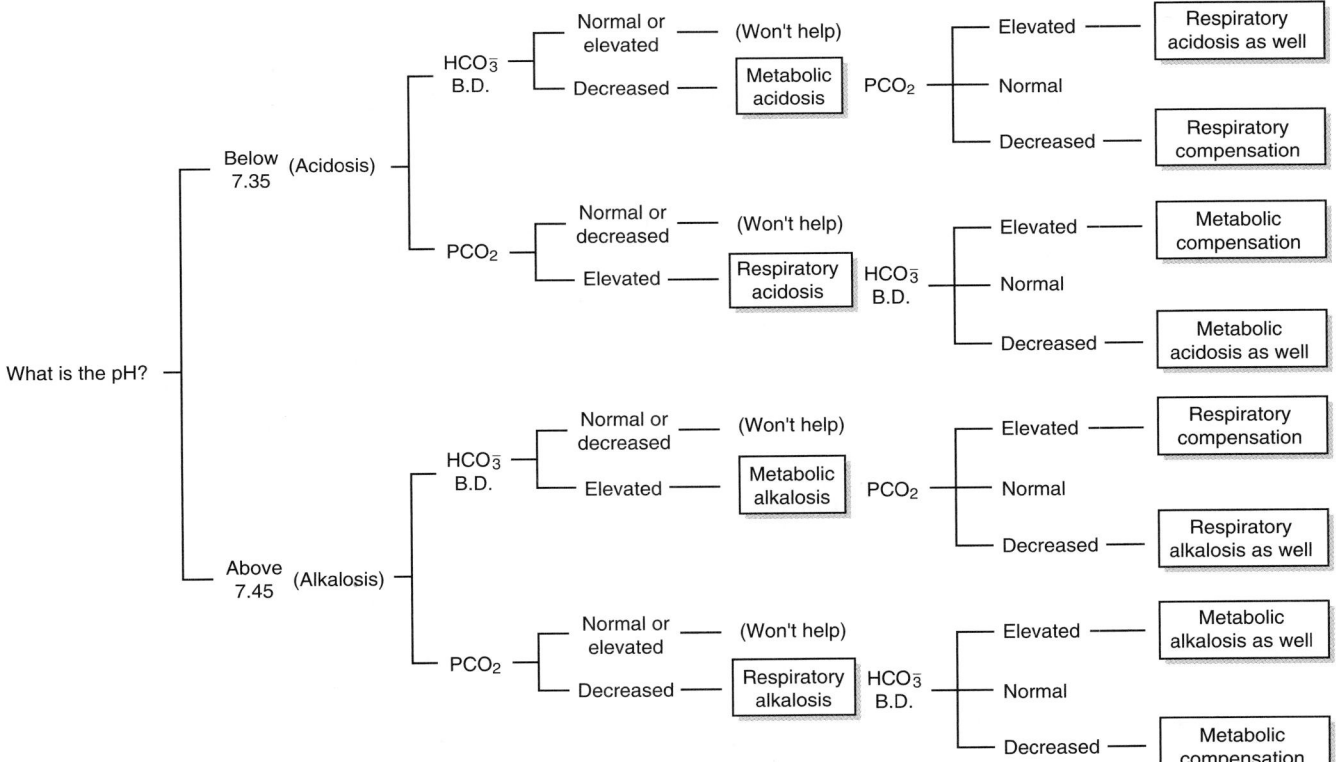

B.D. = Base deficit

FIGURE 17-2   Arterial Blood Gas Analysis. *Powers A: Acid-base balance. In Curley MAQ, Moloney-Harmon P, editors:* Critical care nursing of infants and children, *ed 2, Philadelphia, 2001, Saunders.*

TABLE 17-3	Capillary and Venous Blood Gas Vaues	
Parameter	Capillary	Mixed Venous
pH	7.35 to 7.45	7.31 to 7.41
PaO_2	<Arterial	35 to 40 mm Hg
O_2 saturation	<Arterial	70% to 75%
$PaCO_2$	35 to 45 mm Hg	40 to 50 mm Hg
HCO_3^-	22 to 26 mEq/L	22 to 26 mEq/L
Total CO_2 content	20 to 27 mEq/L	20 to 27 mEq/L
Base excess	+2 to −2	+2 to −2

Powers A: Acid-base balance. In Curley MAQ, Moloney-Harmon P, editors: *Critical care nursing of infants and children,* ed 2, Philadelphia, 2001, Saunders.

Procedure for Arterial Blood Gas Analysis

Steps	Rationale	Considerations
1. Ensure child and family understand procedure and questions are answered.	Evaluates and reinforces understanding of previously taught information.	Developmental, cognitive, and anxiety levels determine approach and effectiveness of teaching.
2. Examine pH level.	Determine whether acidosis, alkalosis, or normal acid base balance is present.	If the pH level is normal, then the blood gas level may be normal or the child may have a chronic condition for which the body has had time to compensate. If the pH level is abnormal, then the condition is acute and the body has not yet had time to compensate.
3. Examine $PaCO_2$ level.	If $PaCO_2$ level is abnormal, the derangement is of a respiratory origin.	A change in $PaCO_2$ level of 10 mm Hg results in a pH shift of 0.08 units in the opposite direction.[1-3] If the $PaCO_2$ level is abnormal and the actual pH level is different from the calculated pH level, check the HCO_3^-) level for a mixed component. For example, a $PaCO_2$ level of 50 mm Hg should result in a pH level of 7.32 in a pure respiratory acidosis. If, however, the pH level is 7.13 with the same $PaCO_2$ level of 50 mm Hg, a metabolic component must exist; check the HCO_3^-.
4. Examine HCO_3^- level.	If HCO_3^- level is abnormal, derangement is metabolic in origin.	A change in HCO_3^- level of 10 mEq/L results in a pH shift of 0.15 units in the same direction.[1-3] If the HCO_3^- level is abnormal and the actual pH level is different from the calculated pH level, check the $PaCO_2$ level for a mixed component. For example, a HCO_3^- level of 15 mEq/L should result in a pH level of 7.25 in a pure metabolic acidosis. If, however, the actual pH level is 7.13, a respiratory component must exist; check the $PaCO_2$ level.

Procedure for Arterial Blood Gas Analysis—*Continued*

Steps	Rationale	Considerations
5. Check HCO_3^- level for compensation if pH level is normal, or almost normal, and $PaCO_2$ level is abnormal.	When pH level is abnormal, the body attempts to compensate through lungs or kidneys. Respiratory compensation occurs immediately to conserve or remove CO_2 via hypoventilation or hyperventilation. Metabolic compensation occurs over several hours to several days to retain or excrete acids or bases in child with healthy kidneys.	In chronic respiratory failure, the child's $PaCO_2$ level is "normally" high and the HCO_3^- level is also "normally" high to compensate and maintain the pH level within the normal range. For example, a typical ABG in a child with chronic respiratory failure may show a pH of 7.40, a $PaCO_2$ of 56 mm Hg, a HCO_3^- of 34 mEq/L, and a base excess of +7.
6. Determine whether a base excess or base deficit is present.	A base excess indicates that more base is present than acid; a base deficit indicates that more acid is present than base.	
7. Evaluate oxygenation: PaO_2 and SaO_2.	A PaO_2 level of less than 60 mm Hg (<50 mm Hg in neonates) is considered clinically significant hypoxemia. SaO_2 level is most important single reflection of arterial oxygen content because almost all oxygen in blood exists as oxyhemoglobin.[1,2,4]	Hemoglobin (Hgb) level must also be evaluated. Because most oxygen is carried by Hgb, the Hgb level must be (at least) normal for maximum oxygen carrying capacity.[1,2,4]
8. Interpret arterial blood gas results (Table 17-4).		

TABLE 17-4   Acid Base Disturbances

Active Base Disturbance	Values	Causes
Respiratory Acidosis Uncompensated/acute respiratory acidosis	↓ pH, ↑↑± $PaCO_2$, and base deficit	*CNS depression:* narcotic overdose, increased ICP, neuromuscular disorders, central hypoventilation syndrome
Compensated/chronic respiratory acidosis	Normal (or close to normal) pH, ↓ $PaCO_2$, ↑ HCO_3^-, and less of base deficit	*Decrease in ventilation:* obstructed airways, obstructed ETT, external compression of airway, atelectasis, pneumonia *Decreased lung compliance:* BPD, ARDS, cystic fibrosis *Traumatic injuries:* broken ribs, pneumothorax, hemothorax, pulmonary contusion, phrenic nerve paralysis
Metabolic Acidosis Uncompensated/acute metabolic acidosis sepsis, CHF	↓ pH, ↓ HCO_3^-, and base deficit	*Decreased tissue perfusion (resulting in lactic acidosis):* dehydration, hypovolemia
Compensated/chronic metabolic acidosis	Normal (or close to normal) pH, ↓ HCO_3^-, ↓ $PaCO_2$, and less of base deficit	*Renal abnormalities (resulting in increase in organic acids):* renal failure, acute tubular necrosis *Loss of base:* renal tubular acidosis, diarrhea

Continued

TABLE 17-4	Acid Base Disturbances—Cont'd	

Active Base Disturbance	Values	Causes
Respiratory Alkalosis		
Uncompensated/acute respiratory alkalosis	↑ pH, ↓ $PaCO_2$, and base excess	Alveolar hyperventilation from hypoxemia CNS irritation Pain
Compensated/chronic respiratory alkalosis	Normal (or close to normal) pH, ↓ $PaCO_2$, ↑ HCO_3^-, and less of base excess	Iatrogenic causes Mechanical ventilation
Metabolic Alkalosis		
Uncompensated/acute metabolic alkalosis	↑ pH, ↑ HCO_3^-, and base excess	Loss of acid gastric suctioning, vomiting *Loss of H^+ via kidneys:* chronic diuretic therapy
Compensated/chronic metabolic alkalosis	Normal (or close to normal) pH, ↑ HCO_3^-, ↑ $PaCO_2$, and less of base excess	Adding base infusion of too much Na HCO_3^- Multiple blood transfusions or exchange transfusion with blood preserved with citrate

CNS = Central nervous system, ICP = intracranial pressure, ETT = endotracheal tube, BPD = bronchopulmonary dysplasia, ARDS = acute respiratory distress syndrome, CHF = congestive heart failure.

Monitoring and Care of the Child

Activities and Interventions	Rationale	Reportable Conditions
1. Assess child's respiratory status at least every 2 hours and as necessary.	Arterial blood gas levels are only a part of the respiratory assessment. Subtle changes in level of consciousness, rate and depth of respirations, breath sounds, and work of breathing may indicate worsening respiratory status before blood gas levels become abnormal. These subtle changes may occur rapidly.	• Worsening respiratory status • Changes in respiratory rate in a child who is in respiratory distress
2. Monitor ABGs as needed in children at high risk for respiratory or metabolic derangements.	Arterial blood gas levels provide information regarding the child's ventilation, oxygenation, and metabolic processes.	• Abnormal arterial blood gas levels • Arterial blood gas results as appropriate after interventions or changes in status

Documentation

- Respiratory assessment
- Arterial blood gas analysis results
- Interventions in response to ABG results
- Ventilator settings and supplemental oxygen use
- Child's response to interventions
- Child and family education

References

1. Doerschug K, et al: *Arterial blood gas analysis, systematic analysis of blood gases,* 1999, retrieved March 5, 2005, from www.vh.org/adult/provider/internalmedicine/abg/ABGHome.html.
2. Hornick D: *An approach to the analysis of arterial blood gases and acid-base disorders,* 2003, retrieved March 5, 2005, from http://www.vh.org/adult/provider/internalmedicine/bloodgases/.
3. Powers A: Acid-base balance. In Curley MAQ, Moloney-Harmon P, editors: *Critical care nursing of infants and children,* ed 2, Philadelphia, 2001, Saunders.
4. Curley MAQ, Thompson JE: Oxygenation and ventilation. In Curley MAQ, Moloney-Harmon P, editors: *Critical care nursing of infants and children,* ed 2, Philadelphia, 2001, Saunders.

Additional Reading

Shapiro B, et al: *Clinical application of blood gases,* ed 5, St. Louis, 1994, Mosby.

End-Tidal Carbon Dioxide Measurement

P U R P O S E : An end-tidal carbon dioxide (CO_2) monitor (capnograph) noninvasively measures expired CO_2. Capnography is a useful tool in detection of life-threatening conditions, such as displacement of endotracheal tubes, impending ventilatory failure, and circulatory failure[1-3]

Eileen Briening

PREREQUISITE KNOWLEDGE

- Child development as it relates to clinical assessment
- Anatomy and physiology of the pediatric pulmonary system
- Principles of ventilation
  - CO_2 is a byproduct of the oxygen (O_2) used by the cells after aerobic metabolism
  - CO_2 diffuses into the alveoli from the capillary bed for elimination
- Knowledge of mechanical ventilation
  - Positive pressure ventilation can be delivered invasively through an endotracheal (ET) tube or a tracheostomy tube or noninvasively through a face or nasal mask or prongs.[4]
  - Modes of mechanical ventilation include pressure ventilation, volume ventilation, continuous positive airway pressure (CPAP), and bi-level positive airway pressure (BiPAP).[4]
  - In positive pressure ventilation, a preset gas mixture is cyclically delivered to the upper airway and a pressure gradient between the upper airway and the lungs drives the gases into the lungs.[4]
- Indications for end-tidal CO_2 (ETCO$_2$) monitoring include determination of a CO_2 waveform and the partial pressure of ETCO$_2$, airway patency and breathing, pulmonary blood flow during cardiopulmonary resuscitation, and improper feeding tube placement.[5]
- Principles of ETCO$_2$ monitoring

- ETCO$_2$ represents partial pressure of CO_2 (PaCO$_2$) of all the ventilated alveoli whether or not they are perfused.
- ETCO$_2$ concentration is 1 to 5 mm Hg lower than the PaCO$_2$ value.[6] Any condition that reduces pulmonary perfusion increases the difference between the ETCO$_2$ measurement and the PaCO$_2$ value.[7]
- A capnograph determines the amount of CO_2 in an expired gas sample on the basis of the absorption properties of CO_2. The exhaled gas is exposed to a range of wave lengths of infrared light.[7]
- ETCO$_2$ monitors use two different sampling techniques: mainstream and sidestream.[2]
- Mainstream capnometers (patient-ventilator interface) have an airway adaptor cuvette attached in line and close to the endotracheal tube. The cuvette incorporates an infrared light source and sensor that detects carbon dioxide absorption with measurement of exhaled ETCO$_2$.[2,7]
- Sidestream capnometers (diverted to a monitor) use a sampling line that attaches to a T-piece adaptor at the ET/tracheostomy tube opening that allows continuous aspiration of tidal airway gas for analysis of CO_2[2,7]
- Capnography can be used noninvasively in children with spontaneous breathing to monitor adequacy of ventilation.[2]
- The normal ETCO$_2$ waveform has the following characteristics:
  - Exhalation begins at zero (baseline) as the dead space gas exits the large airways. Next is a rapid rise as the

gas exits the intermediate airways and a flat plateau as the gas exits the alveoli. Finally, a rapid decline is seen as the next breath is inhaled[8] (Figure 18-1).

CHILD AND FAMILY ASSESSMENT

- Child's developmental level and ability to interact ➤➤*Rationale:* Influences preparation and interaction.
- Child's and family's understanding of the underlying condition, the reasons for $ETCO_2$ monitoring, the results, and their significance ➤➤*Rationale:* Evaluates child's and family's understanding of procedure and provides a gauge for ongoing education.
- History of respiratory disease, including bronchospasm, chronic pulmonary disease and upper airway disease, and apnea ➤➤*Rationale:* These conditions may affect $ETCO_2$ waveforms.

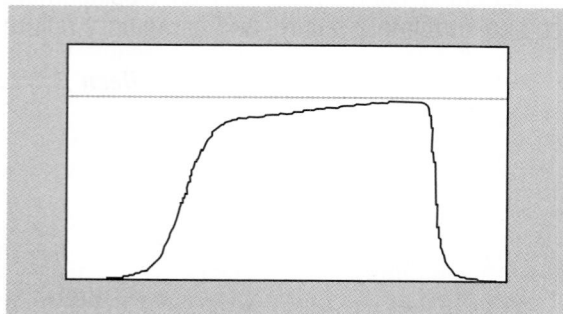

FIGURE 18-1   Normal Capnogram.

- Assessment of the child's respiratory status, including respiratory rate, work of breathing, and breath sounds ➤➤*Rationale:* $ETCO_2$ monitoring is only a part of an assessment of the child.
- Signs and symptoms of inadequate oxygenation and ventilation ➤➤*Rationale:* Indicates effective pulmonary function and need for blood gas analysis.

CHILD AND FAMILY EDUCATION

Individualized, developmentally appropriate education is provided to the family and to the child based on desire for knowledge, readiness to learn, and overall neurologic and psychosocial state.

- Provide information about the $ETCO_2$ monitor, including use and attachments ➤➤*Rationale:* Providing information decreases fear and anxiety and improves compliance.
- Encourage and answer questions as they arise ➤➤*Rationale:* Reinforcement of information is needed during periods of stress.
- Review with the parents and child the capnograph alarm ➤➤*Rationale:* Providing information about the $ETCO_2$ monitor alarm reduces anxiety and fear.

EQUIPMENT

- End-tidal CO_2 monitor
- Cable and airway adaptor

Procedure for ETCO₂ Measurement

Steps	Rationale	Considerations
1. Assemble all equipment and assess proper functioning of equipment.	Ensures reliability of $ETCO_2$ values and waveforms.	
2. Wash hands and put on proper protective equipment.	Reduces transmission of micro-organisms; standard precautions.	
3. Connect capnograph into grounded wall outlet and cable into display monitor.	Decreases incidence rate of electrical interference.	If applicable, check capnograph battery capacity and charging time (see operator's manual).
4. Perform calibration. *(Level I*)*	Failure to calibrate properly may result in erroneous $ETCO_2$ values.	See the operator's manual for calibration instructions.
5. Assemble airway adaptor and sensor. Attach to the child's ET/tracheostomy tube per manufacturer's instructions.	Appropriate placement of sensor decreases incidence rate of improper gas sampling.	See the operator's manual for instructions.
6. With use of a sidestream sampling port for a child who is or is not intubated, be sure sampling port is placed at a right angle to ET tube, nasal cannula, or ventilator circuit.[3]	Decreases secretion accumulation on CO_2 port where gas is drawn for sampling.[2]	

* Level I: Manufacturer's recommendations only

Procedure for ETCO$_2$ Measurement—*Continued*

Steps	Rationale	Considerations
7. Set age-appropriate alarms for respiratory rate, apnea default, and high and low ETCO$_2$ readings.	Alerts staff to potentially life-threatening problems.	See the operator's manual for details.
8. Wash hands. *(Level VI*)*	Reduces transmission of infection. Protects personnel health.	

* Level VI: Clinical studies in a variety of patient populations and situations to support recommendations

Expected Outcomes	Unexpected Outcomes
• Normal capnogram results that confirm placement of the ET tube (see Figure 18-1) • Detection of significant changes in ventilation • Confirmation of adequate pulmonary blood flow during closed cardiac chest compressions	• Display of inaccurate measurements of ETCO$_2$ that result from calibration drift or contamination of the sensor with moisture or secretions • Equipment malfunction

Monitoring and Care of the Child

Activities and Interventions	Rationale	Reportable Conditions
1. Ensure child and family understand procedure and questions are answered.	Evaluates and reinforces understanding of previously taught information.	• Developmental, cognitive, and anxiety levels determine approach and effectiveness of teaching
2. Wash hands. *(Level VI*)*	Reduces transmission of infection. Protects personnel health.	
3. Gather equipment and supplies.	Improves efficiency.	
4. Observe waveform for confirmation of airway patency.	Poor waveform may be indicative of improper placement of the ET tube.[8]	• Endotracheal or tracheal tube dislodgement[8]
5. Observe waveform for poor plateau.	May be indicative of inadequate expiration[8] (Figure 18-2)	• Bronchospasm or any obstruction that limits expiration[8]

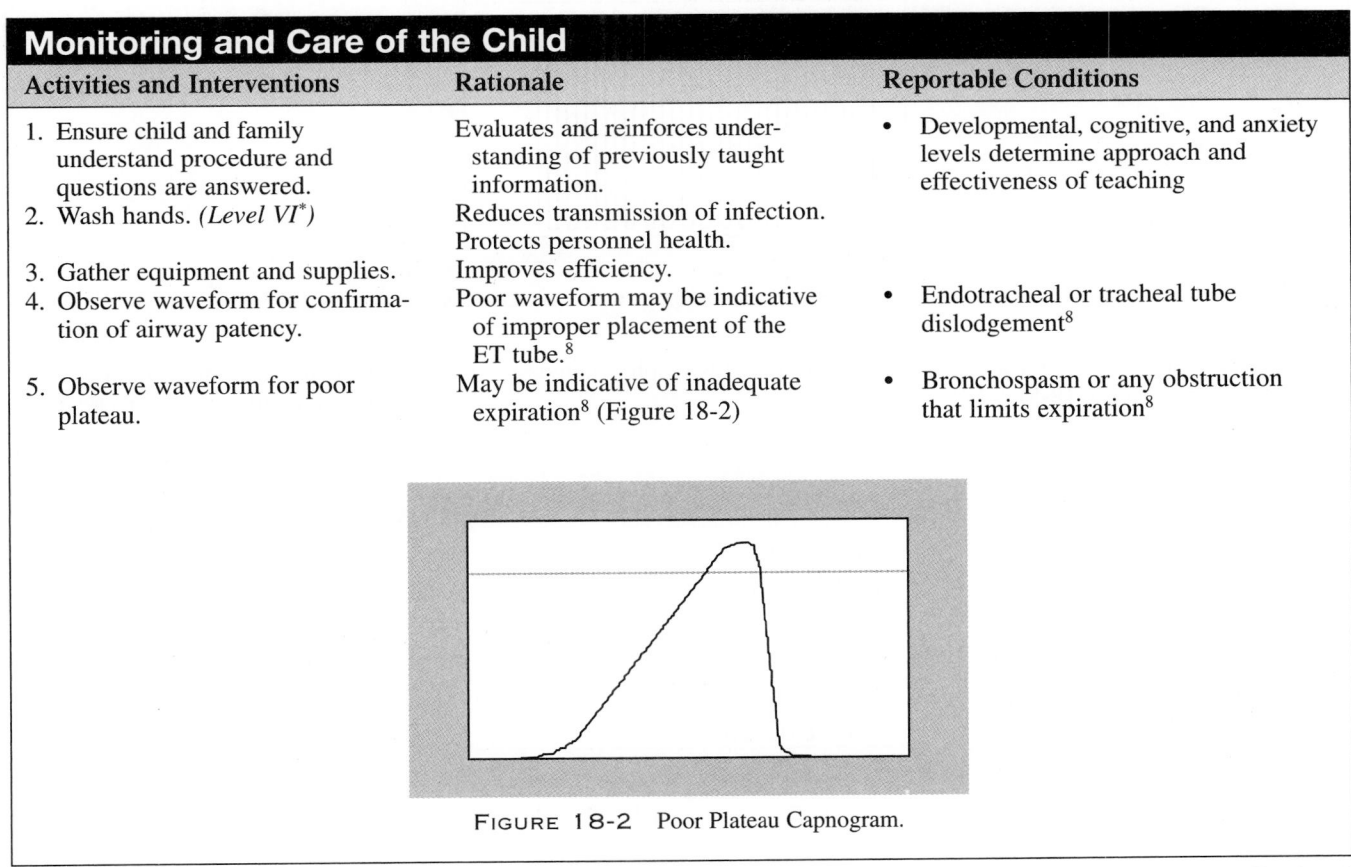

FIGURE 18-2 Poor Plateau Capnogram.

* Level VI: Clinical studies in a variety of patient populations and situations to support recommendations.

Continued

Monitoring and Care of the Child—Cont'd

Activities and Interventions	Rationale	Reportable Conditions
6. Observe waveform for a humped or "camel" configuration (Figure 18-3).	May be indicative of changes in endotracheal tube position or expiration.[8]	• Lateral position or tube touching the carina[8]

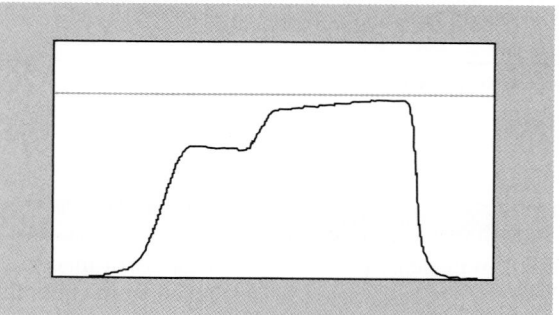

FIGURE 18-3   Humped or "Camel" Capnogram.

7. Observe ETCO$_2$ trends for a slow decrease on the graph (Figure 18-4).	Trending of ETCO$_2$ is useful to observe adequate ventilation.[8]	• May indicate hyperventilation, decrease in body temperature, or poor lung or peripheral perfusion[8]

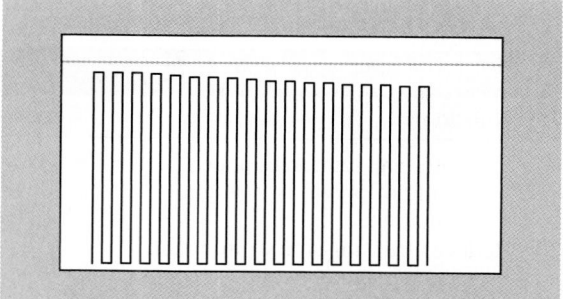

FIGURE 18-4   Trends Graph with Slow Decrease.

8. Observe ETCO$_2$ trends for a sudden drop (Figure 18-5).	A decline in trends graph is noted.[8]	• May indicate a leak in the circuit (i.e., deflated cuff, bronchospasm, or leak in sampling tube)[8]

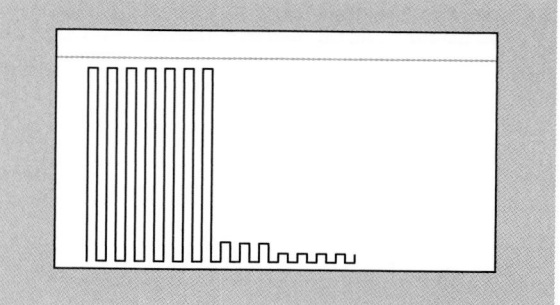

FIGURE 18-5   Trends Graph with Sudden Drop.

Monitoring and Care of the Child—Cont'd

Activities and Interventions	Rationale	Reportable Conditions
9. Observe ETCO$_2$ trends for an exponential decline (Figure 18-6).	An exponential decline in trends graph is noted.[8]	• May be indicative of circulatory arrest, embolism, or sudden severe hyperventilation[8]

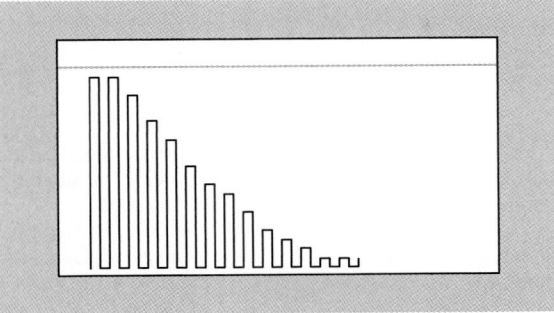

FIGURE 18-6   Trends Graph with Exponential Decline.

10. Observe ETCO$_2$ trends for a gradual increase (Figure 18-7).	A rise in trends graph is noted.[8]	• May indicate hypoventilation or a rapidly rising body temperature[4]

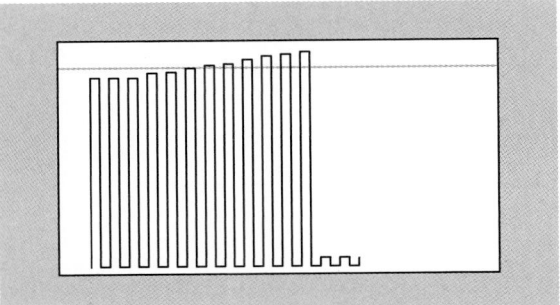

FIGURE 18-7   Trends Graph with Gradual Increase.

11. Observe ETCO$_2$ trends for a sudden increase (Figure 18-8).	A sudden rise in trends graph is noted.[8]	• May be observed with injection of sodium bicarbonate[8]

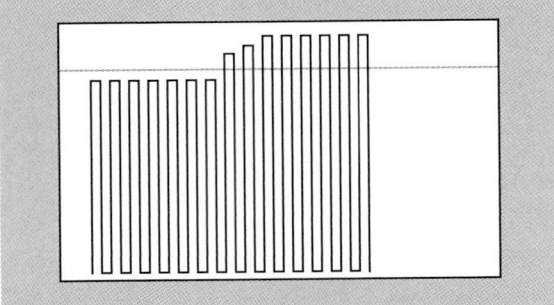

FIGURE 18-8   Trends Graph with Sudden Rise.

Documentation

- $ETCO_2$ numeric readings
- Baseline $ETCO_2$ waveform and any change in waveform
- Respiratory assessment, including work of breathing, breath sounds, and respiratory rate
- Child's response to interventions if necessary
- Child and family education
- Unexpected outcomes and related treatment

References

1. Bhende MS: End-tidal carbon dioxide monitoring in paediatrics: concepts and technology, *J Postgraduate Med* 47(2):153-156, 2001.
2. Good VS: Continuous end-tidal carbon dioxide monitoring. In Lynn-McHale DJ, Carlson K, editors: *AACN procedure manual for critical care,* ed 5, Philadelphia, 2005, Elsevier.
3. Kodali BS: *Capnography in pediatrics,* 2004, retrieved February 12, 2005, from http://www.capnography.com/Homepage/HomepageM.htm.
4. Pollack C: Mechanical ventilation and noninvasive ventilatory support. In Rosen, editor: *Emergency medicine: concepts and clinical practice,* St. Louis, 2002, Mosby, Inc.
5. Bhende MS: End-tidal carbon dioxide monitoring in paediatrics: clinical applications, *J Postgraduate Med* 47(3):215-218, 2001.
6. St. John R: End tidal CO_2 monitoring. In Bursn S, editor: *American Association of Critical Care Nurses technology series,* Aliso Viejo, CA, 1996, American Association of Critical Care Nurses.
7. Dobyns E: Assessment and monitoring of respiratory function. In Fuhrman B, Zimmerman J, editors: *Pediatric critical care,* ed 3, Philadelphia, 2006, Mosby.
8. Sainsbury D: *CO_2 monitoring,* retrieved February 12, 2005, from http://www.health.adelaide.edu.au/paedanaes/talks/CO2/capnography.html

Indices of Oxygenation and Ventilation

P U R P O S E : The calculation and trending of the indices of oxygenation is a tool in the management of pediatric respiratory failure. The calculation of the oxygenation indices assists in the early identification of trends in oxygen delivery and consumption, shunting as a mechanism of hypoxemia, and the impact of ventilation therapies.

Janet A. Koehler Boyce

PREREQUISITE KNOWLEDGE

- Oxygen is transported to the body dissolved in plasma or bound to hemoglobin (oxyhemoglobin). The total oxygen content is the amount of oxygen carried by the hemoglobin (approximately 97%) and the amount dissolved in the plasma (approximately 3%). The oxygen saturation is the percentage of oxygen bound to hemoglobin (Hgb), which can be of arterial (SaO_2) or mixed venous (SvO_2) origin.
- The oxygen content of arterial blood (CaO_2) and mixed venous blood (CvO_2) can be calculated with the individual saturations and hemoglobin concentration.
- Normal oxygen consumption (VO_2) is higher in children when compared with adults, which reflects the higher metabolic demands of growth and development and limited oxygen reserves.[1] Small variations in VO_2 can reflect major changes in the child's cardiorespiratory status from a decreased preload, depressed myocardial function, sepsis, anemia, low oxygen saturations from hypoxemia from worsening lung disease or from cyanotic heart disease, or complications of positive pressure ventilation (PPV) or positive end-expiratory pressure (PEEP).
- Cardiac output (CO) directly affects oxygen utilization. If the CO falls, oxygen delivery (DO_2) falls with higher oxygen extraction by the tissues from arterial blood, reflected in lowered CvO_2 values. If the body's compensatory mechanisms do not maintain adequate blood flow, anaerobic metabolism results with lactic acidosis as a consequence. Lactate levels may be drawn as an assessment tool in low output states.
- CO and cardiac indexes (CI) per kilogram are higher for children than for adults. A normal CI for children is 3.0 to 4.5 $L/min/M^2$ BSA (body surface area).[2] Children need higher CO and DO_2 because of the higher metabolic rates from growth and development. A child's stroke volume (SV) is relatively small, and low output states are compensated by an increase in heart rate. Small changes in heart rate may significantly influence cardiac output[2] and thus, DO_2. Children have higher resting heart rates than do adults, and bradycardia is an ominous sign of potential deterioration. Normal vital signs are not always appropriate in the critically ill child and must be evaluated in terms of the overall hemodynamic status.
- The PaO_2 (arterial oxygen tension) is determined by the fraction of inspired oxygen concentration (FiO_2), barometric pressure (P_{bar}), alveolar ventilation, diffusion of oxygen across the alveolar-capillary membrane, CO_2 levels in the alveoli, and matching of ventilation and perfusion in the lung.
- The PAO_2 (alveolar partial pressure of oxygen) is representative of all the oxygen pressures within the alveoli of the lungs. The PAO_2 is dependent on the same variables as the PaO_2. In the normally functioning lung, the PAO_2 should approximate the PaO_2.
- The estimation of intrapulmonary shunting (perfusion but lacking ventilation of the lung units) can be determined by

127

calculating the a:A ratio (partial pressure of arterial oxygen to alveolar oxygen ratio, or as the PaO_2:PaO_2 ratio), the PaO_2:FiO_2 ratio (partial pressure of arterial oxygenation to fraction of inspired oxygen ratio, or as the P/F ratio), and the oxygenation index (OI). These indices take into account the current FiO_2 during mechanical ventilation and can be useful in trending the degree of shunting in the lung. If a significant shunt exists, changes in the FiO_2 do not have an impact on the PaO_2. If the shunt is insignificant, changes in the PaO_2 and FiO_2 are in direct proportion.

- Procedures for arterial blood and mixed venous blood sampling
- Blood gas analysis by cooximetry of both arterial and mixed venous blood
- Current Hgb level
- Mean airway pressure and (FiO_2) from the ventilator values
- Refer to Table 19-1 for a synopsis of the indices of oxygenation

CHILD AND FAMILY ASSESSMENT

- Child's developmental level and ability to interact ➸***Rationale:*** Influences preparation and interaction.
- Child's and family's understanding of the underlying condition and current therapies ➸***Rationale:*** Evaluates child's and family's understanding of the procedure and provides a gauge for ongoing education.

Table 19-1 Summary of Oxygenation Indices

Oxygenation Index	Description	Considerations	Norms
A-vDO_2	Arterial-venous oxygen difference	Reflects oxygen utilization by the body by the difference between arterial and venous oxygen contents Requires the determination of both the arterial oxygen content (C_aO_2) and the venous oxygen content (C_vO_2) by cooximetry Inversely proportional to oxygen delivery by cardiac output Widening difference may be due to inadequate oxygen delivery or increased oxygen extraction by the tissues Low difference may be due to high oxygen delivery or decreased extraction by the tissues Affected by low cardiac output, hypoxemia, presence of dyshemoglobins (carboxyhemoglobin, methemoglobin) Requires the use of a pulmonary artery catheter to obtain mixed venous blood gases	A-vDO_2 = 3 – 5.5 ml/dl C_aO_2 = 18-20 mlO_2/dl blood[4] C_vO_2 = 15 ml/dl blood[3]
A-aDO_2	Alveolar-arterial oxygen difference	Reflects the relationship between alveolar to arterial uptake of oxygen in the lungs Increased if an intrapulmonary shunt exists even with a normal PaO_2 secondary to an increased FiO_2 Requires the calculation of the alveolar oxygen tension	50-70 mmHg on an FiO_2 1.0[2] <20-25 mmHg in room air[4]
a-A ratio	Partial pressure of arterial oxygen to alveolar oxygen ratio	Estimation of intrapulmonary shunting High ratios reflect adequate lung function Small ratios reflect a larger degree of shunting Requires the calculation of the alveolar oxygen tension	0.8-1.0[1] <0.6 reflects inadequate oxygenation requiring supplemental oxygen[6] <0.15 indicates refractory hypoxemia due to significant shunting[6]
PaO_2/FiO_2	Partial pressure of arterial oxygenation to fraction of inspired oxygen ratio	Also known as the P/F ratio Estimation of intrapulmonary shunting The smaller the ratio, the greater degree of intrapulmonary shunting	>300 200-300 is reflective of acute lung injury ≤200 is associated with ARDS (acute respiratory distress syndrome)[2]
OI	Oxygenation index	Estimation of intrapulmonary shunting Used to assess oxygenation in relation to respiratory therapy Accounts for the mean airway pressures during mechanical ventilation Accounts for changing FiO_2	Less than 10 >10 significant for respiratory compromise >25–35 significant for respiratory failure[4]

- Family barriers to learning, such as stress, anxiety, or language ➤➤*Rationale:* Effective communication of therapeutic goals.
- Signs and symptoms of oxygenation and ventilation and related impact on organ systems
  - ❖ Respiratory parameters: rise or fall in arterial oxygen tension measurements, changes in the mean airway pressures, total respiratory rate (spontaneous and ventilated breaths), adventitious breath sounds, presence or absence of retractions, and trends in pulse oximetry
  - ❖ Hemodynamic parameters: tachycardia, bradycardia, dysrhythmias, peripheral perfusion, and blood pressure trends
  - ❖ Renal parameters: urine output and presence or absence of metabolic acidosis
  - ❖ Neurologic parameters: changes in behavior, such as anxiety, restlessness, agitation, confusion, lethargy, and ability to follow commands
  - ❖ Hematologic parameters: Hgb level and presence or absence of cyanosis ➤➤*Rationale:* Inadequate oxygenation and ventilation is reflected in the function of the major organ systems.
- Determine PaO_2 with arterial blood gas analysis and arterial saturation ➤➤*Rationale:* Hypoxemia and inadequate oxygenation are indicated by falling PaO_2 values and arterial desaturation.
- Determine the trends of the oxygenation indices ➤➤*Rationale:* Trends in the oxygenation indices show stasis, improvement or deterioration in the child's oxygenation status, and the response to changes in mechanical ventilation management.
- Conditions that may result in increased oxygen consumption: fever, shivering, anxiety, increased work of breathing, procedures such as repositioning, endotracheal suctioning, and portable chest x-ray ➤➤*Rationale:* Increased oxygen consumption may lead to tissue hypoxia.
- Conditions that may decrease oxygen consumption: hypothermia, sleep or rest, neuromuscular blockade, and sedation ➤➤*Rationale:* Decreased metabolic demands.

CHILD AND FAMILY EDUCATION

Individualized, developmentally appropriate education is provided to the family and to the child based on desire for knowledge, readiness to learn, and overall neurologic and psychosocial state.

- Explain the child's underlying condition, the overall oxygenation status, and the means by which this status is evaluated ➤➤*Rationale:* Providing information decreases fear and anxiety and improves compliance.
- Discuss the overall relationship between oxygenation and hypoxemia ➤➤*Rationale:* Explanations are based on the level of understanding and how testing relates to the therapeutic goals for the child.
- Encourage questions and answer questions as they arise ➤➤*Rationale:* Reinforcement of information is needed during periods of stress.

EQUIPMENT

- Calculator
- Equations for the calculation of the indices of oxygenation
- Pulmonary artery catheter

Procedure	**for Indices of Oxygenation and Ventilation**	
Steps	**Rationale**	**Considerations**
1. **Calculate arterial-venous oxygen difference (a-vDO$_2$).** a. Obtain arterial and mixed venous blood gases with cooximetry. *(Level VI*)* b. Determine and record the value to be used throughout all calculations for oxygen-carrying capacity (either 1.39 or 1.34).[4] *(Level II*)*	Data collection for the SaO$_2$ and SvO$_2$. Data collection for the current hemoglobin. Consistency in data collection.	Mixed venous blood drawn from the distal port of the pulmonary artery catheter reflects the true mixing of superior vena cava (SVC), inferior vena cava (IVC), and coronary artery circulations.[3] Institutional preferences on the value utilized for oxygen carrying capacity.
c. Calculate arterial oxygen content (CaO$_2$) with the modified Fick's equation[1,4]: **CaO$_2$ = [1.39 (or 1.34)] × Hgb × % SaO$_2$** (use decimal point). *(Level V*)*	Data collection.	In some institutions, the dissolved oxygen content is used in the calculation of the a-vDO$_2$. With use of this parameter, the equation is[1,4]: CaO$_2$ = 1.39 (or 1.34) × Hgb × % SaO$_2$ + (0.003 × PaO$_2$).

Procedure continues on following page

* Level II: Theory-based; no research data to support recommendations; recommendations from expert consensus group may exist
Level V: Clinical studies in more than one or two patient populations and situations to support recommendations
Level VI: Clinical studies in a variety of patient populations and situations to support recommendations

Procedure for Indices of Oxygenation and Ventilation—*Continued*		
Steps	**Rationale**	**Considerations**
d. Calculate the CvO_2 with the modified Fick's equation[1,4]: $CvO_2 = 1.39$ **(or 1.34)** $\times$ **Hgb** $\times$ **% SvO_2** (use decimal point). *(Level V*)*	Data collection.	With use of the dissolved oxygen content, the equation is[1,4]: $CvO_2 = 1.39$ (or 1.34) $\times$ Hgb $\times$ % SvO_2) + (0.003 $\times$ PaO_2).
e. Subtract CvO_2 from CaO_2[1,4]: **a-vDO_2 = CaO_2 – CvO_2**	Results in the a-vDO_2 value.	The a-vDO_2 is only an approximation and not a direct measurement of oxygenation.
f. Compare the current a-vDO_2 with previous measurements and report results.	Trending changes in the a-vDO_2 may indicate the need for altering care strategies in relation to tissue oxygenation.	Changes may be needed in ventilation parameters and hemodynamic support.
2. Calculate the alveolar-arterial oxygen difference (A-aDO_2).[5] *(Level VI*)*	The A-aDO_2 measurement reflects the relationship between alveolar and arterial uptake of oxygen in the lungs.	The blood gas must be obtained on 100% FiO_2 for the A-aDO_2 calculation. For all other calculations, the FiO_2 recorded is the current FiO_2 on the ventilator.
a. Obtain an arterial blood gas value.	Data collection.	
b. Calculate the PaO_2.[5] $PAO_2 = FiO_2 (Pbar – PH_2O) – (PaCO_2/RQ)$ $PAO_2 = FiO_2 (750 – 47) – (PaCO_2/0.8)$ FiO_2 = fraction of inspired oxygen P_{bar} = barometric pressure or 750 mmHg PH_2O = pressure of water vapor or 47 mmHg $PaCO_2$ = partial pressure of arterial carbon dioxide tension RQ = respiratory quotient or 0.8	Data collection.	
c. Obtain the PaO_2 value from the arterial blood gas.	Data collection.	
d. Subtract PaO_2 from PAO_2: **A-aDO_2 = PAO_2 – PaO_2**	Results in the A-aDO_2 gradient.	
3. Calculate the a:A ratio.[5] *(Level V*)* **(PaO_2/PAO_2)** PAO_2 = partial pressure of alveolar oxygen obtained from the A-aDO_2 equation	The estimation of the a-A ratio reflects the degree of intrapulmonary shunting.	Partial pressure of arterial oxygen to alveolar oxygen ratio.
4. Calculate (P/F) ratio (partial pressure of arterial oxygenation to fraction of inspired oxygen ratio ($PaO_2:FiO_2$)[3,5]: **(PaO_2/FiO_2)** Partial pressure of arterial oxygen (PaO_2) obtained from the arterial blood gas. Fraction of inspired oxygen (FiO_2) obtained from the oxygen analyzer on mechanical ventilator. *(Level V*)*	The P/F ratio reflects the degree of intrapulmonary shunting.	

* Level V: Clinical studies in more than one or two patient populations and situations to support recommendations
  Level VI: Clinical studies in a variety of patient populations and situations to support recommendations

Procedure	for Indices of Oxygenation and Ventilation—*Continued*	
Steps	**Rationale**	**Considerations**
5. Calculate the oxygenation index (OI)[3,5]: $\dfrac{(FiO_2)\ MAP}{PaO_2}$ Fraction of inspired oxygen (FiO_2) obtained from the oxygen analyzer on mechanical ventilator. Mean airway pressure (MAP) in cm H_2O obtained from ventilator measurements. Partial pressure of arterial oxygen (PaO_2) obtained from the arterial blood gas. *(Level V*)*	The calculation of the OI assists in trending the degree of respiratory failure.	

* Level V: Clinical studies in more than one or two patient populations and situations to support recommendations

Expected Outcomes

- Adequate oxygenation as reflected in the profile calculations

- Decrease in the FIO_2 necessary as oxygenation improves
- Titration of the ventilation settings, particularly the positive end-expiratory pressures (PEEP)
- Hemodynamic support as necessary to maintain adequate perfusion
- Adequate sedation or neuromuscular blockade to decrease oxygen consumption

Unexpected Outcomes

- Signs of oxygen toxicity from prolonged exposure to high levels of oxygen (>0.5 FIO_2) that may be exhibited by increased shunting, decreased lung compliance, or increasing A-aDO_2

- Complications of positive pressure ventilation (barotrauma or pneumothorax)
- Hemodynamic instability that may result in oxygenation disturbances
- Inadequate sedation or neuromuscular blockade

Monitoring and Care of the Child

Activities and Interventions	Rationale	Reportable Conditions
1. Observe for trends in the a-vDO_2 values.	The trend of a-vDO_2 values is often used as a sign of hypoxia. Causes of hypoxia are related to hypoventilation, impaired transport of oxygen across the alveolar-capillary membrane, ventilation or perfusion mismatches, or decreased hemoglobin concentrations.[6,7] Trending a-vDO_2 values can give insight into the child's hemodynamic status related to increased intrathoracic pressures from PPV (positive pressure ventilation) and hyperdynamic or hypodynamic perfusion states and can assist in management of the child's cardiorespiratory care. Adequate sedation decreases oxygen consumption.	• Any acute change in the a-vDO_2 values, either high or low

Continued

Monitoring and Care of the Child—Cont'd

Activities and Interventions	Rationale	Reportable Conditions
2. Monitor trends in the oxygenation indices from baseline to subsequent ventilation interventions. 3. Monitor for increasing PaO_2 and SaO_2 values.	Shunting, as the mechanism of hypoxemia, is reflected in oxygenation indices. Trending indices may show worsening respiratory failure or improvement and the effects of ventilation therapy. An adequate PaO_2 and SaO_2 with an FiO_2 of 0.4 or less is not reflective of shunting as the mechanism of hypoxemia. High oxygen concentrations are necessary to maintain oxygenation in the presence of a significant shunt.	• Significant differences from previous oxygenation profiles

Documentation

- Child and family education, including the content and level of understanding
- Arterial blood gas and the mixed venous blood gas values if obtained
- Time, ventilator settings, FiO_2, hemoglobin, child's position, and sedation used at the time the blood gases were drawn
- Changes in the child's hemodynamic status or changes in hemodynamic support
- Nursing interventions, such as positioning or sedation, that may improve oxygenation
- Changes in the ventilation management and the child's response to those changes
- Unexpected outcomes and related treatment

References

1. Curley MAQ, Thompson JE: Oxygenation and ventilation. In Curley MAQ Moloney-Harmon PA, editors: *Critical care nursing of infants and children,* ed 2, Philadelphia, 2001, Saunders.
2. Hazinski MF: Pediatric evaluation and monitoring considerations. In Darovic GO, editor: *Hemodynamic monitoring: invasive and noninvasive clinical applications,* ed 3, Philadelphia, 2002, Saunders.
3. Hazinski MF: *Manual of pediatric critical care,* St. Louis, 1999, Mosby.
4. Burns S: Arterial-venous oxygen difference calculation. In Lynn-McHale DJ, Carlson K, editors: *AACN procedure manual for critical care,* ed 5, Philadelphia, 2005, Elsevier.
5. Burns S: Indices of oxygenation: alveolar-arterial oxygen difference, partial pressure of arterial oxygenation to fraction of inspired oxygen ration, partial pressure of arterial oxygen to alveolar oxygen ration. In Lynn-McHale DJ, Carlson KK, editors: *AACN procedure manual for critical care,* ed 5, Philadelphia, 2005, Elsevier.
6. Matthews PJ, Gregg BL: Monitoring and management of the patient in the ICU. In Scanlan CL, et al, editors: *Egan's fundamentals of respiratory care,* ed 7, St. Louis, 1999, Mosby.
7. Misasi RS, Keyes JL: Pathophysiology of hypoxia, *Crit Care Nurs* 14(4):55-64, 1994.

Additional Readings

AARC Clinical Practice Guideline: Blood gas analysis and hemoximetry: 2001 revision & update, *Respir Care* 46:498-505, 2001.
Ahrens T: Changing perspectives in the assessment of oxygenation, *Crit Care Nurs* 13(4):78-83, 1993.

Ahrens TS: Concepts in the assessment of oxygenation, *Focus Crit Care* 14(1):36-44, 1987.
Ahrens TS., Powers CC: Pulmonary clinical physiology. In Kinney MR, Dunbar SB, et al, editors: *AACN clinical reference for critical care nursing,* ed 4, St. Louis, 1998, Mosby.
Berry BE, Pinard AE: Assessing tissue oxygenation, *Crit Care Nurs* 22(3):22-42, 2002.
Darovic GO: Monitoring oxygenation. In Darovic GO, editor: *Hemodynamic monitoring: invasive and noninvasive clinical application,* ed 3, Philadelphia, 2002, Saunders.
Darovic GO, Zbilut JP: Pulmonary anatomy and physiology. In Darovic GO, editor: *Hemodynamic monitoring: invasive and noninvasive clinical application,* ed 3, Philadelphia, 2002, Saunders.
Des Jardins T: *Cardiopulmonary anatomy and physiology. essentials for respiratory care,* ed 3, Albany, NY, 1998, Delmar Publishers.
Downs JB: Has oxygen administration delayed appropriate respiratory care? Fallacies regarding oxygen therapy, *Resp Care* 48(6):611-620, 2003.
Leach RM, Treacher DF: ABC of oxygen: oxygen transport – 2. tissue hypoxia, *BMJ* 17:1370-1373, 1998.
Misasi RS, Keyes JL: Matching and mismatching ventilation and perfusion in the lung, *Crit Care Nurs* 16(3):23-40, 1996.
Scanlan CL, Wilkins RL, Stoller JK, editors: *Egan's fundamentals of respiratory care,* ed 7, St. Louis, 1999, Mosby.
Shoemaker WC: Monitoring and management of acute circulatory problems: the expanded role of the physiologically oriented critical care nurse, *Am J Crit Care* 1(1):38-53, 1992.
Treacher DF, Leach RM: ABC of oxygen: oxygen transport – 1. basic principles, *BMJ* 17:1302-1306, 1998.

Mixed Venous Oxygen Saturation: Continuous Monitoring

P U R P O S E : Continuous mixed venous oxygen saturation monitoring (SvO_2) is performed to assist in the assessment of the balance between oxygen delivery (DO_2) and oxygen consumption (VO_2). Mixed venous oxygen saturation values are obtained through the use of a fiber optic pulmonary artery (PA) catheter connected to a computer and display monitor for measurement of the oxygen saturation of the mixed venous blood from the PA.

Janet A. Koehler Boyce and Holly F. Webster

PREQUISITE KNOWLEDGE

- The basic principles of invasive hemodynamic monitoring, including an understanding of the anatomy and physiology of the cardiopulmonary system and the physiologic and technical aspects of invasive monitoring[1]
- An ability to identify transduced waveforms of the right atrium (RA), right ventricle (RV), PA, and pulmonary capillary wedge (PCWP) (Figure 20-1)
- Knowledge of normal pressure values for RA, PA, and PCWP
- The identification of basic arrhythmias
- An understanding of the basic physiologic principles of oxygenation (delivery and consumption), blood gas interpretation and cooximetry
- Superior vena cava (SVC) saturations are typically higher than inferior vena cava (IVC) saturations. A mixing of these two blood volumes begins in the RA and is complete in the PA; therefore, the blood in the PA is an *admixture* (or an average) of all systemic venous blood that has returned to the right side of the heart.
- Trending of arterial oxygen saturation (SaO_2) with SvO_2 provides an indicator of adequacy of cellular oxygenation. A decreasing SaO_2 with an increasing SvO_2 may be observed with progressive cellular death. Conversely, an increasing SaO_2 with a decreasing SvO_2 can indicate adequacy of cellular oxygenation or failure of cellular oxygen uptake (as seen in sepsis).[2]
- Indications for use of SvO_2 monitoring include: low cardiac output (CO) state unresponsive to fluid resuscitation or necessitating pharmacologic support, pulmonary hypertension, and severe respiratory disease.
- The SvO_2 monitoring system consists of the *fiber optic PA catheter* that encases the fiber optic filaments, the *optic module* that houses the light-emitting diodes (LEDs), and the *oximeter computer* that contains a microprocessor that converts light information into an electronic display (continuous graphic trends, numerics, or both; Figure 20-2).
- The principle of SvO_2 monitoring is based on the reflective spectrophotometry. The LEDs in the optic module transmit various light wavelengths. The photodetector receives the light reflected back. Oxygenated blood easily reflects light back, whereas deoxygenated blood absorbs the light, thus decreasing light reflection. The optic module determines the percent of hemoglobin (Hgb) that is oxygenated.
- Due to the physiologic demands for growth and development, children have a higher delivery and consumption of

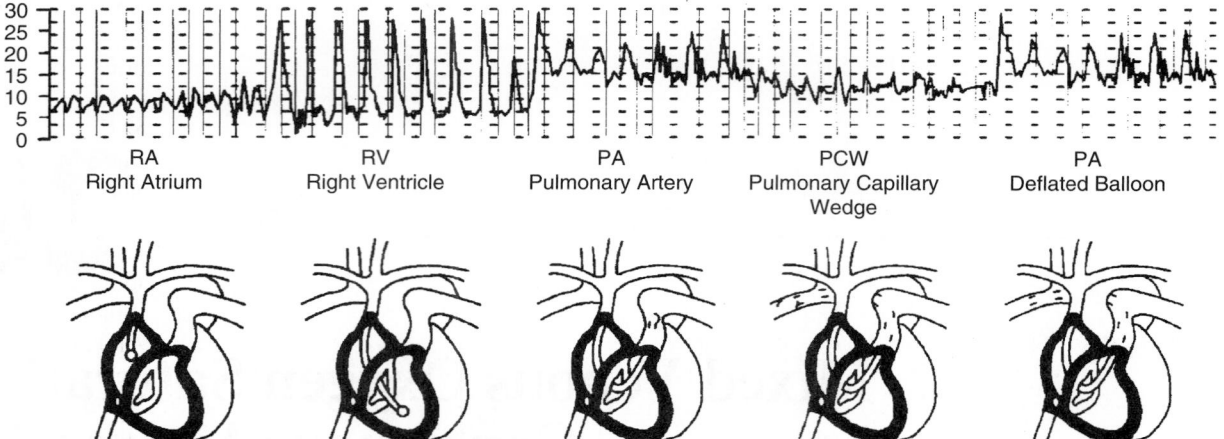

FIGURE 20-1   Pulmonary artery catheter progression through the heart with waveforms. *From Abbott Critical Care Systems, Mountain Views, CA.*

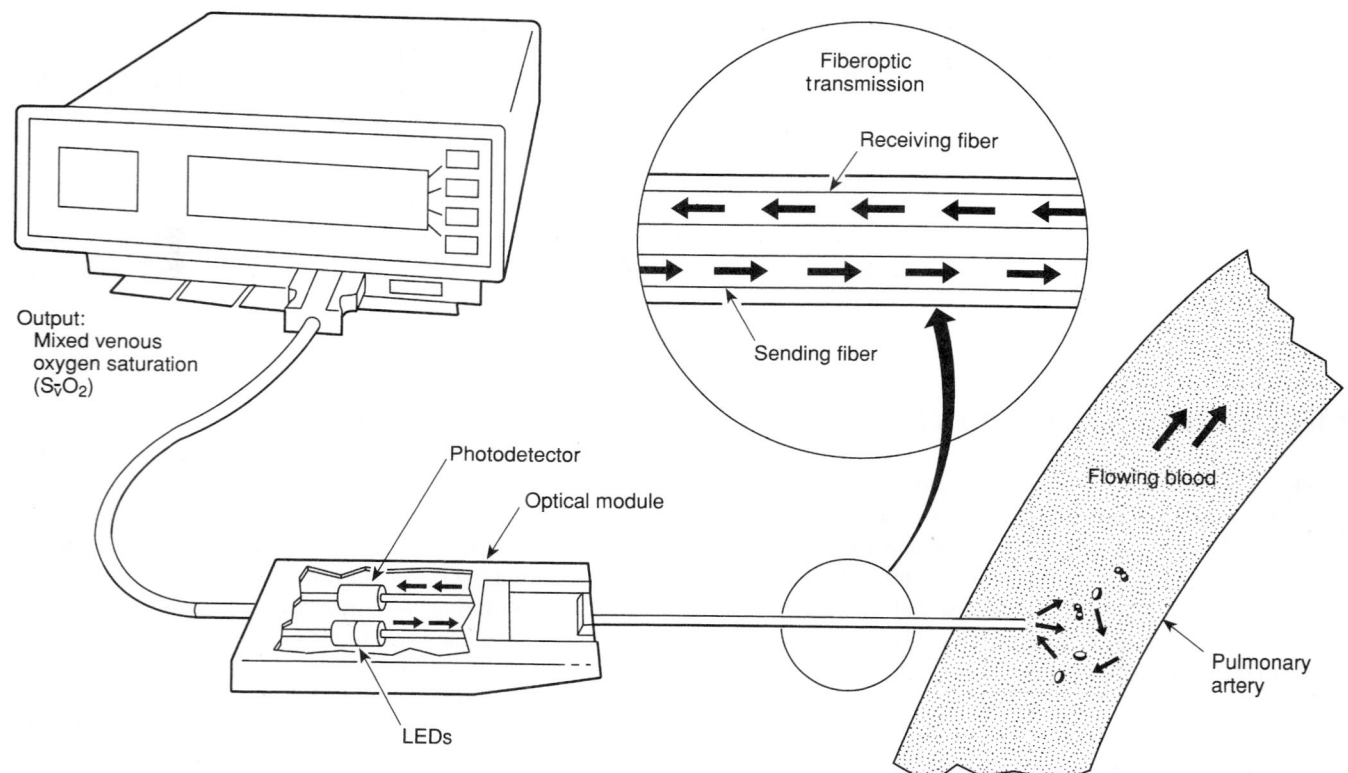

FIGURE 20-2   The SvO_2 system with reflection spectrophotometry. *From American Edwards Laboratories: Understanding continuous mixed venous oxygen saturation monitoring with the Swan-Ganz oximetry TD system, Irvine, CA, 1987.*

oxygen than adults. With any situation that decreases or impairs DO_2 or causes an increase in O_2, the pediatric patient is at risk for development of rapid progressive tissue hypoxia.[3]

• Typical blood gas analyzers *calculate* SvO_2 (or SaO_2) rather than directly *measuring* the SvO_2. A cooximeter *measures* the SvO_2; therefore, the value more closely represents the true SvO_2 of the child.[4]

• The SvO_2 reflects the interrelationship among all the variables that impact oxygen delivery and consumption: arterial partial pressure of oxygen (PaO_2), arterial blood saturation of oxygen (SaO_2), Hgb, and CO. With any threat to oxygen balance, the body responds with compensatory mechanisms by increasing CO or increasing oxygen extraction in an effort to preserve oxygen venous reserves. If the compensatory mechanisms become ineffective, a fall in the SvO_2 occurs, which indicates that the child is drawing on the venous reserve. A normal SvO_2 is 60% to 80%. Changes in the SvO_2 of 5% to 10% for greater than 5 minutes are significant. The interpretation of the SvO_2 values should be viewed in the context of the dynamic state of the child with variable oxygen demands.[2,5,6]

- Various conditions may alter Do_2 and Vo_2 at any given moment (Table 20-1). Low SvO_2 values (less than 60%) represent decreased DO_2 or increased oxygen demand. Elevated SvO_2 values (greater than 80%) represent an increase in arterial oxygen content from an increased DO_2 or a decreased oxygen demand. Tissue oxygen extraction may vary with the child's condition (such as sepsis). An alteration in SvO_2 is used as a prompt to further evaluate the determinants of Do_2 and Vo_2.
- Knowledge of the impact of the diagnosis, nursing care activities, procedures, and conditions such as fever, pain, agitation, or anxiety can affect the SvO_2
- Knowledge of the function, correct set-up, maintenance, and calibration of the bedside monitoring equipment

CHILD AND FAMILY ASSESSMENT

- Child's developmental level and ability to interact ➤➤*Rationale:* Influences preparation and interaction.
- Child's and family's understanding of the underlying condition, the reasons for SvO_2 monitoring, and the results and their significance ➤➤*Rationale:* Evaluates child's and family's understanding of the procedure and provides a gauge for ongoing education.
- A complete assessment of child, including sampling of relevant laboratory tests such as arterial blood gas, complete blood count (CBC), weight, and height ➤➤*Rationale:* Ensuring the physiologic stability of the child's condition minimizes or prevents adverse events during the procedure. Hgb and hematocrit (Hct) impact the interpretation of SvO_2. while height and weight are used for other derived calculations using the PA catheter.
- Assess intracardiac waveforms before SvO_2 measurement ➤➤*Rationale:* Confirms correct placement of PA catheter tip.
- Assess level of sedation and pain ➤➤*Rationale:* Unrelieved pain and anxiety may result in an increased oxygen demand and cause a decrease in the SvO_2 from increased oxygen extraction.

TABLE 20-1	SvO_2 Values Related to Oxygen Supply and Demand
Low SvO_2: Decrease Oxygen Delivery	**Low SvO_2: Increase Oxygen Consumption**
<ul><li>Anemia</li><li>Hypoxemia from presence of dysfunctional hemoglobin (carboxyhemoglobin, methemoglobin)</li><li>Hypoventilation</li><li>Pulmonary conditions, such as atelectasis, pulmonary edema, pneumothorax</li><li>Airway obstruction from mucus plugging, kinked or dislodged endotracheal tubes</li><li>Low cardiac output from hypovolemia, bradyarrythmias/tachyarrythmias, increased afterload, cardiac dysfunction</li><li>Sepsis</li><li>Hypotension</li></ul>	<ul><li>Increased metabolic demands from fever/shivering, pain/anxiety, cold stress</li><li>Increased work of breathing</li><li>Seizure activity</li><li>Procedural stress from repositioning, endotracheal tube suctioning, chest x-rays, bathing, weights</li><li>Sepsis</li></ul>
Elevated SvO_2: Increased Oxygen Delivery	**Elevated SvO_2: Decreased Oxygen Consumption**
<ul><li>Blood transfusions</li><li>Improved cardiac function as result of inotrope infusions, afterload reduction, volume repletion, correction of arrhythmias</li><li>Effective ventilation strategies improving oxygenation</li><li>Hyperoxia from increased FiO_2</li></ul>	<ul><li>Reversal of high metabolic states</li><li>Normothermia (antipyretic usage, maintenance of neutral thermal environment)</li><li>Neuromuscular blockade</li><li>Effective control of pain and anxiety</li><li>Control of seizure activity</li><li>Cellular dysfunction in uptake of oxygen</li><li>Effective ventilatory support with patient-ventilator synchrony</li></ul>

FIo_2, Fractional concentration of oxygen in inspired gas.
Data from Davidson LJ, Brown S: Continuous SvO_2 monitoring: a tool for analyzing hemodynamic status, *Heart Lung* 15(3):287-292, 1986.
Des Jardins T: *Cardiopulmonary anatomy and physiology: essentials for respiratory care,* ed 3, Albany, 1998, Delmar Publishers.
Enger EL, Holm K: Perspectives of the interpretation of continuous mixed venous oxygen saturation, *Heart Lung* 19(5):578-580, 1990.
Gawlinski A, Henneman EA: Evaluating oxygen delivery and oxygen utilization with mixed venous oxygen saturation monitoring: a case study approach, *Heart Lung* 19(5):566-570, 1990.
Headley JM: New trends in oxygen delivery, consumption and debt assessment: global and regional indices, *AACN News* 19(7):16,19, 2002.
Headley JM: Invasive hemodynamic monitoring: applying advanced technologies, *Crit Care Nurs Q* 21(3):73-84, 1998.

CHILD AND FAMILY EDUCATION

Individualized, developmentally appropriate education is provided to the family and to the child based on desire for knowledge, readiness to learn, and overall neurologic and psychosocial state.

- Provide information about the Svo_2 monitoring, including indications for use, equipment, procedure for catheter placement and risks involved ➤➤*Rationale:* Providing information decreases fear and anxiety and improves compliance.
- Relate the significance of Svo_2 monitoring and the body's use of oxygen ➤➤*Rationale:* A fall in the Svo_2 values may be caused by overstimulation of the child, which may require the caregivers and family to cluster or refrain from bedside activities to allow for adequate rest.

- Encourage and answer questions as they arise ➤➤*Rationale:* Reinforcement of information is needed during periods of stress.

EQUIPMENT

- Fiber optic PA catheter of the appropriate size for the child (sizes are approximate)[3,7]
  $\leq$4 kg, 3.5F to 5.0F
  <15 to 18 kg, 5F to 5.5F/6.0F
  >18 to 20 kg, 7.0F to 7.5F
- Monitoring equipment per institution-specific protocol optic module, bedside monitor or oximeter computer, printer
- Equipment for PA line placement (see Procedure 66)

Procedure | for Continuous Svo_2 Monitoring

Steps	Rationale	Considerations
1. Ensure child and family understand procedure and questions are answered.	Evaluates and reinforces understanding of previously taught information.	Developmental, cognitive, and anxiety levels determine approach to and effectiveness of teaching.
2. Obtain weight and height if other values are to be derived using the PA catheter measurements.	Weight and height are needed for the calculation of other parameters including CO and oxygen indices.	
3. Assemble equipment for PA catheter insertion, pressure monitoring, and continuous Svo_2 monitoring per institution-specific protocol (see Procedure 60).	Equipment must be ready and functional before insertion procedure.	
4. Select the optimal lead for an artifact-free electrocardiograpm (ECG) on monitor.	Simultaneous ECG tracing can assist in proper PA waveform identification.[9] Dysrhythmias may occur during insertion and with migration.	Use a lead that provides a clear p, QRS and t wave to facilitate recognition of deviation from a normal sinus rhythm.
5. Identify the chld with appropriate patient and procedure verification process (e.g., "Time out").	Confirms correct patient, procedure, and site as recommended by the Joint Commission on Accreditation of Healthcare Organizations (JCAHO); prevents unnecessary medical procedures.	
6. Turn on the computer after connection to power source to allow for adequate warm-up time and internal system checks by the computer.[3,5,6,8] *(Level II*)*	The optics monitor must be turned on and warmed up before use.	For bedside monitor, access Svo_2 module and verify functionality. Warm-up times vary per manufacturer.[3,5,6,8]
7. Wash hands and use standard precautions.	Reduces transmission of micro-organisms.	Insertion procedure is done under sterile conditions.

* Level II: Theory-based; no research data to support recommendations; recommendations from expert consensus group may exist

Procedure for Continuous SvO₂ Monitoring—*Continued*

Steps	Rationale	Considerations
8. Connect the optics module to the computer/module.	Allows transfer of data.	Maintain sterility of catheter package.
9. Preinsertion catheter light source calibration: in vitro calibration.[3,5,6,8] a. Access inner package with optic connector and catheter. b. Connect the optics computer to the optics connector of the PA catheter. c. Enter the required data, Hgb, and Hct, into the computer. d. Assess the light intensity of the catheter for brightness. e. Perform the calibration per manufacturer's requirements. *(Level I*)*	An in vitro calibration must be performed to ensure that the catheter is functional and provides accurate readings. The preinsertion calibration assures fiber optic integrity and adequate light intensity at the tip of the catheter.	Catheter tip must remain isolated in the tray. Some catheter lumens should remain dry until after in vitro calibration. Check manufacturer's instructions. Incorrectly entered data values result in inaccurate SvO₂ values for two wavelength modules. Three wavelength modules automatically recalibrate the optics module as the child's Hgb and Hct values change. The light intensity should be clearly visible and within the size specifications for the manufacturer.
10. Join ports to transducer system; flush and zero (see Procedure 63). If balloon catheter is used, balloon inflation is tested before insertion, and the volume of air necessary to inflate the balloon is noted.	Ensures the equipment is operable and system is ready for monitoring. The balloon is never inflated with greater than the recommended volume of air.	The balloon configuration should be round and inflate evenly in all directions.
11. Insert the PA catheter per hospital guidelines and manufacturer instructions. Observe the waveforms and light emission intensity as the catheter is advanced into the distal PA (see Procedure 60).[5,6,8] *(Level V*)*	Observation of the waveforms correlates with the advancement of the catheter into the distal PA. Adequate light intensity verifies that catheter fiber optics are intact. Kinks or breaks may occur during catheter insertion and interrupt the emission of light and result in a low light intensity and erroneous readings. The light intensity displayed during a wedge procedure should remain within the manufacturer's guidelines.[3,5,8]	During insertion, the balloon may be partially inflated in children with tricuspid regurgitation, pulmonary valve (PV) abnormalities, pulmonary hypertension and low CO to facilitate insertion through the PV. In younger children, the passage of the balloon through the PV may cause momentary occlusion of flow, dysrhythmias and a decrease in SaO₂. If the catheter tip is placed too close to the vessel wall during a wedge procedure, the light reflects off the vessel wall, increases the intensity of light reflection, and gives falsely high SvO₂ values.
12. Verify PA catheter tip location by observing a normal PA pressure tracing (see Figure 20-1).	Correct PA placement is necessary for optimal position for SvO₂ monitoring. Ideally the tip is located in zone 3 of the lung, or as far distally that allows a normal PA waveform, and a PAWP with less than maximum balloon volume.	An accurate SvO₂ is measured from the distal PA catheter tip. The RA or SVC measurements are not accurate or predictable of a true PA sample.[10] Marking the insertion point on the catheter and daily chest x-rays are useful for monitoring of catheter tip position.

Procedure continues on following page

* Level I: Manufacturer's recommendations only
Level V: Clinical studies in more than one or two patient populations and situations to support recommendations

Procedure for Continuous Svo_2 Monitoring—*Continued*

Steps	Rationale	Considerations
13. Apply site dressing per institution-specific protocol.	Reduces contamination by environmental organisms.	Line-related sepsis is a significant cause of morbidity.[11]
14. Secure optic module near child.	Avoid tension on the catheter or module, which may damage the optic filaments.	
15. Set high and low alarms.[3,5,6] *(Level V*)*	Alarm parameters, set according to the child's condition, alert the clinician to changes in the child's status.	Svo_2 alarms are typically set 10% above and 10% below the child's baseline.[3,5,6]
16. After catheter calibration and insertion, obtain a baseline set of oxygenation values.	Postinsertion data provide a baseline for ongoing comparisons after interventions to support oxygen supply and demand. Fiberoptic technology detects only oxyhemoglobin and reduced Hgb.[10]	Cooximetry is performed to detect the presence of dyshemoglobins (carboxyhemoglobin or methemoglobin).[5,12]

17. Perform an in vivo calibration of the Svo_2 monitor according to manufacturer's guidelines.[3,5,6]
  a. Obtain a mixed venous blood gas and send for cooximetry analysis (see Procedure 64).
  b. Place the Svo_2 computer to the in vivo calibration mode.
  c. Compare the monitored Svo_2 value with the mixed venous Svo_2.
  d. Adjust the Svo_2 monitor according to manufacturer guidelines if the values differ by more than 5%.[5] *(Level I*)*
	An in vivo calibration verifies the accuracy of the Svo_2 values after catheter insertion by comparing the monitored Svo_2 value with the obtained Svo_2 value from the mixed venous blood sample analyzed with cooximetry.[3,5,6]	In vivo calibrations are often performed every 12 to 48 hours but may vary per institution or manufacturer guidelines.
		In vivo calibrations are also done if catheter integrity or Svo_2 values are in doubt.[3,5,6]
		When drawing sample, do not aspirate with excessive negative pressure because this may cause sampling of arterialized (capillary) blood, giving an erroneously high Svo_2 measurement.

18. Continuously monitor the Svo_2 values, light signal strength, and PA waveform.	Ongoing assessments of the PA waveform detect catheter migration or spontaneous wedging. The light signal strength on the Svo_2 monitor detects position changes of the catheter or the formation of a clot at the catheter tip.	Immediate intervention can be accomplished if catheter malfunction is suspected or an acute change in the child's status occurs.
19. If the child needs to be transported while Svo_2 monitoring is conducted, disconnect only the cable, not the catheter, from the computer.[5]	The memory chips inside the optical cable and computer save all the prior information from the initial calibration if only the cable is disconnected.[5]	If the catheter is disconnected, an in vivo calibration needs to be performed. If only the cable is disconnected, monitoring may continue without the need for an in vivo calibration.[5]

* Level I: Manufacturer's recommendations only
  Level V: Clinical studies in more than one or two patient populations and situations to support recommendations

Expected Outcomes	**Unexpected Outcomes**
• Svo_2 values do not fluctuate beyond 5% to 10% from the baseline for greater than 5 minutes	• Svo_2 values trend greater than 5% to 10% from baseline (or <60% or >75% to 80%) for greater than 5 minutes after appropriate intervention
• Child's condition remains hemodynamically stable	• Child's condition is hemodynamically unstable
	• Arrhythmias
• The PA catheter tip is positioned in the distal PA	• Pulmonary ischemia or infarction
• Transducer waveforms are accurately visible and monitored	• Inaccurate waveforms and pressure monitoring
• Child remains infection free	• Line sepsis from the presence of the PA catheter
• All equipment functions properly without deleterious mechanical complications	• Balloon rupture, thromboemboli from the formation of clots at the catheter tip, rupture from spontaneous or persistent wedging, or catheter breakage[3]

Monitoring and Care of the Child

Activities and Interventions	Rationale	Reportable Conditions
1. Observe and trend Svo_2 continuously, especially with changes in child's clinical condition and during interventions that may affect Svo_2 values.	Changes in Svo_2 values may indicate a significant clinical change. A variation of more than 5% indicates a need for further assessment and trouble shooting of system. Abrupt changes in the Svo_2 values may indicate inaccuracy of the monitoring system.	• Svo_2 values less than 60% or greater than 75 % for more than 5 minutes
2. Assess the integrity of the PA catheter for kinks or bends hourly or per hospital protocol.	Fiberoptics are prone to damage with any twisting, bending, or stretching. Overtightening of the connector can pinch fibers, impairing transmission of light wave lengths.	• Changes in PA waveform or Svo_2 more than 5% to 10% from baseline.
3. Monitor the PA waveform continuously for changes in the amplitude (dampening), configuration, rising baseline, or widening of the PA pulse pressure (see Figure 64-3 in Procedure 64).	The PA catheter may migrate and cause an erroneous elevation of the Svo_2 into the postcapillary arterialized blood or from the catheter lodging against the vessel wall. Clot formation at the distal tip of the PA catheter may cause erroneously high or low values. A widening PA pulse pressure may be indicative of catheter slippage into the right ventricle. A migrating PA catheter poses the risk of PA infarction or rupture.	• Any changes in the PA waveform configuration, spontaneous wedging, or widening PA pulse pressures may indicate catheter complications or erroneous readings
4. Check pressure lumens for bubbles or clots every 4 hours or per institution protocol.	A continuous column of fluid from the child to the module is necessary for accurate transmission of pressure measurements.	
5. Consider clustering or refraining from nursing interventions.	A fall in the Svo_2 values may be caused by overstimulation of the child, which may require the caregivers and family to cluster or refrain from bedside activities to allow for adequate rest.	
6. Monitor arterial blood pressure (ABP).	A precipitous change in ABP may be an indication of PA infarction, pulmonary embolus, or PA rupture.	• Significant changes in ABP

Continued

Monitoring and Care of the Child—Cont'd

Activities and Interventions	Rationale	Reportable Conditions
7. Continuous ECG monitoring.	Retrograde migration of catheter tip toward PV or RV may cause dysrhythmias.	• Dysrhythmias
8. Assess insertion site for signs of infection and bleeding.	Assures early recognition of treatable complications.	• Excessive bleeding, redness, or swelling around insertion site

Documentation

- Child's tolerance of procedure
- Volume of air needed to obtain a PAWP waveform
- Insertion distance
- Changes in Svo_2 that occur with changes in medications, nursing interventions, or child-induced changes, such as movement or shivering
- Print and evaluate PA and PAWP waveform every 12 hours or per institution protocol
- Record of Svo_2 with hemodynamic measurements per institution-specific protocol
- Child's response to additional interventions
- Unexpected outcomes
- Child and family education

References

1. Edwards JD, Mayall RM: Importance of the sampling site for measurement of mixed venous oxygen saturation in shock, *Crit Care Med* 26(8):1356-1360, 1998.
2. Curley MAQ, Thompson JE: Oxygenation and ventilation. In Curley MAQ, Moloney-Harmon PA, editors: *Critical care nursing of infants and children,* ed 2, Philadelphia, 2001, Saunders.
3. Hazinski MF: Pediatric evaluation and monitoring considerations. In Darovic GO, editor: *Hemodynamic monitoring: invasive and noninvasive clinical application,* ed 3, Philadelphia, 2002, Saunders.
4. Polderman K, Girbes A: Central venous catheter use: part 2: infectious complications, *Intens Care Med* 28(10):18-28, 2002.
5. Darovic GO: Monitoring oxygenation. In Darovic GO, editor: *Hemodynamic monitoring: invasive and noninvasive clinical application,* ed 3, Philadelphia, 2002, Saunders.
6. Headley JM: Continuous mixed venous oxygen saturation monitoring. In Lynn-McHale Wiegand DJ, Carlson K, editors: *AACN procedure manual for critical care,* ed 5, Philadelphia, 2005, Saunders.
7. Robotham JL, et al:Cardiorespiratory interactions. In Rogers MC, editor: *Textbook of pediatric intensive care,* ed 2, Baltimore, 1996, Williams and Wilkins.
8. Sanders CL: Making clinical decisions using Svo_2 in PICU patients, *Dim Crit Care Nurs* 16(5):257-264, 1997.
9. American Association of Critical Care Nurses (5/04) Practice Alert: Pulmonary Artery Measurement http://www.aacn.org//AACN/practice Alert.nsf/Files/PAPMonitoring4-7-04/$file/PAPMonitoring.pdf accessed July 26, 2006
10. White KM: Using continuous Svo_2 to assess oxygen supply/demand balance in the critically ill patient, *AACN Clin Issues* 4(1):134-147, 1993.
11. Abbott Critical Care Systems: Flow-directed thermo-dilution fiberoptic pulmonary artery catheter model P575, 1998.
12. AARC Clinical Practice Guideline: Blood gas analysis and hemoximetry: 2001 revision and update, *Resp Care* 46: 498-505, 2001.

Additional Readings

Bridges EJ: Monitoring pulmonary artery pressures: just the facts, *Crit Care Nurs* 20(6):59-78, 2000.
Cathelyn JL, Samples DA: Svo_2 monitoring: tool for evaluating patient outcomes, *Dim Crit Care Nurs* 17(2):58-66, 1998.
Copel LC, Stolarik A: Continuous Svo_2 monitoring. a research review, *Dim Crit Care Nurs* 10(4):202-209, 1991.
Darovic GO: Pulmonary artery pressure monitoring. In Darovic GO, editor: *Hemodynamic monitoring: invasive and noninvasive clinical application,* ed 3, Philadelphia, 2002, Saunders.
Davidson LJ, Brown S: Continuous Svo_2 monitoring: a tool for analyzing hemodynamic status, *Heart Lung* 15(3):287-292, 1986.
Des Jardins T: *Cardiopulmonary anatomy and physiology: essentials for respiratory care,* ed 3, Albany, 1998, Delmar Publishers.
Enger EL, Holm K: Perspectives of the interpretation of continuous mixed venous oxygen saturation, *Heart Lung* 19(5):578-580, 1990.
Gawlinski A, Henneman EA: Evaluating oxygen delivery and oxygen utilization with mixed venous oxygen saturation monitoring: a case study approach, *Heart Lung* 19(5):566-570, 1990.
Hazinski MF: *Manual of pediatric critical care,* St. Louis, 1999, Mosby.
Headley JM: New trends in oxygen delivery, consumption and debt assessment: global and regional indices, *AACN News* 19(7):16-19, 2002.
Headley JM: Invasive hemodynamic monitoring: applying advanced technologies, *Crit Care Nurs Q* 21(3):73-84, 1998.
Mims BC: Physiologic rationale of Svo_2 monitoring, *Crit Care Nurs Clin North Am* 1(3):619-628, 1989.
Shoemaker WC: Monitoring and management of acute circulatory problems: the expanded role of the physiologically oriented critical care nurse, *Am J Crit Care* 1(1):38-53, 1992.
Whalen DA, Kelleher RM: Cardiovascular patient assessment. In Kinney MR, Dunbar SB, et al, editors: *AACN clinical reference for critical care,* ed 4, St. Louis, 1998, Mosby.
White KM, Winslow EH, Clark AP, et al: Physiologic basis for continuous mixed venous oxygen saturation monitoring, *Heart Lung* 19(5):548-551, 1990.
Yu DT, et al: Relationship of pulmonary artery catheter use to mortality and resource utilization in patients with severe sepsis. *Crit Care Med* 31(12):2734-2741, 2003.

Negative Inspiratory Force Measurement

PURPOSE: Negative inspiratory force (NIF) quantifies respiratory muscle strength. Measurement assists in determination of respiratory insufficiency

Kristin M. Print

PREREQUISITE KNOWLEDGE

• Child development as it relates to procedure
• Anatomy and physiology of the pediatric pulmonary system, including structural characteristics specific to the infant and child
• Negative inspiratory force measurement is also referred to as negative inspiratory pressure (NIP) or maximal inspiratory pressure (MIP).
• Negative inspiratory force is a measure of inspiratory respiratory muscle strength and is a strong negative predictor (but poor positive predictor) of extubation success.
• The most common threshold cited for NIF is −20 cm H_2O or less; however, a NIF of −30 cm H_2O or less indicates adequate muscle strength for normal respiratory effort.[1,2] NIF of more than −20 cm H_2O indicates potential for inadequate muscle strength for sustained effective respirations.[1,2]
• If applicable, understanding of the reason for mechanical ventilation: procedural (i.e., operative procedure) versus physiologic (i.e., acute respiratory distress syndrome, infant botulism)
• Measurements of NIF are used in children with neuromuscular disease as a sign of possible deterioration of muscle strength and respiratory insufficiency that may necessitate mechanical ventilation.
• Adequate NIF measurements are not a direct marker of successful extubation. Other indicators must be considered, such as resolution of underlying disease process, normal inspiratory drive, and ability to sustain spontaneous respirations without excessive effort.

• Inadequate NIF measurements alone are not a contraindication for extubation or intubation.
• Measurements of NIF are negatively affected by use of sedation and neuromuscular blockade and by other disease processes, such as Duchenne's muscular dystrophy, infant botulism, and spinal muscle atrophy.

CHILD AND FAMILY ASSESSMENT

• Child's developmental level and ability to interact ➤*Rationale:* Influences preparation and interaction.
• Child's and family's understanding of the reasons for NIF measurement ➤*Rationale:* Evaluates child's and family's understanding of the procedure and provides a gauge for ongoing education.
• Desire of family members to be present during the procedure ➤*Rationale:* The presence of family may provide comfort and support, although family members should have the choice not to remain with the child.
• Signs and symptoms of inadequate ventilation, such as shallow or irregular respirations, tachypnea or bradypnea, dyspnea, restlessness, confusion, lethargy, tachycardia, and rising arterial carbon dioxide level ➤*Rationale:* Signs of inadequate ventilation, along with a poor NIF measurement, may predict a need for mechanical ventilation.
• Level of consciousness and cognitive ability ➤*Rationale:* Determines whether the child is ready to take breaths for measurements.
• History of neuromuscular disease, abnormal anatomy such as scoliosis that causes restrictive lung disease, or

pathophysiologic process that affects current lung function ➤➤*Rationale:* These conditions may negatively affect the NIF measurement.
- Patency of endotracheal tube (ETT) and status of respiratory tract ➤➤*Rationale:* Excessive secretions cause increased resistance and may interfere with accurate NIF measurement.

CHILD AND FAMILY EDUCATION

Individualized, developmentally appropriate education is provided to the family and to the child based on desire for knowledge, readiness to learn, and overall neurologic and psychosocial state.

- Explain the procedure for NIF measurements, including purpose of the measurement, steps in obtaining a quantifiable number, and the meaning of the value in relation to the child ➤➤*Rationale:* Providing information decreases anxiety and fear.
- If developmentally appropriate, explain how the child can assist with obtaining the measurement, such as deep breathing when indicated by the practitioner ➤➤*Rationale:* Accurate measurements are obtained more easily with a cooperative child.
- Explain that the child may need suctioning before the procedure ➤➤*Rationale:* Suctioning before the procedure reduces airway resistance and enhances a more accurate NIF measurement.
- Explain that the child may cough during the procedure ➤➤*Rationale:* Manipulation of the ETT to attach the manual ventilation bag can result in stimulation of the trachea and result in coughing.
- Encourage questions and answer questions as they arise ➤➤*Rationale:* Reinforcement of information is needed during periods of stress.

EQUIPMENT

- Mask
- One-way exhalation valve attached to manometer
- Nonsterile gloves

Procedure   for Negative Inspiratory Force Measurement

Steps	Rationale	Considerations
1. Ensure child and family understand procedure and questions are answered.	Evaluates and reinforces understanding of previously taught information.	Developmental level, cognitive ability, and anxiety level determine approach to and effectiveness of teaching.
2. Collect all necessary equipment and supplies.	Preparing all materials before procedure facilitates completion in a timely manner.	
3. Ensure appropriate cardiopulmonary monitoring.	Child may decompensate during the procedure.	Children are susceptible to agitation, bradycardia, and desaturations.
4. Wash hands and put on clean gloves.	Reduces transmission of infection. Protects personnel health.	
5. Consider suctioning child if indicated.	Secretions in the airway may cause resistance and prevent accurate NIF measurements.	
6. Disconnect ETT from ventilator and attach tube to one-way valve or place mask with one-way valve attachment over child's face with a secure seal (Figures 21-1 and 21-2).	Pressure manometer is used to measure NIF.	Be sure that one-way exhalation valve is connected to a manometer. The NIF measurement may be uncomfortable because the child cannot take an effective ventilation breath during the procedure. Stop measurement if child does not tolerate procedure.
7. Instruct child to take deep breath (if developmentally appropriate) and measure the NIF of at least three spontaneous breaths.	The goal is to obtain the child's best effort over a 20-second time lapse per each measurement.[3]	The valve is capped for the measurement (see Figures 21-1 and 21-2).

Procedure for Negative Inspiratory Force Measurement—*Continued*

Steps	Rationale	Considerations

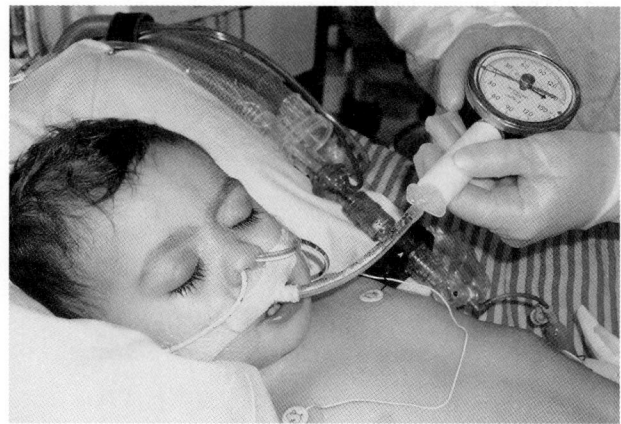

FIGURE 21-1   Disconnect endotracheal tube from ventilator and attach tube to one-way valve.

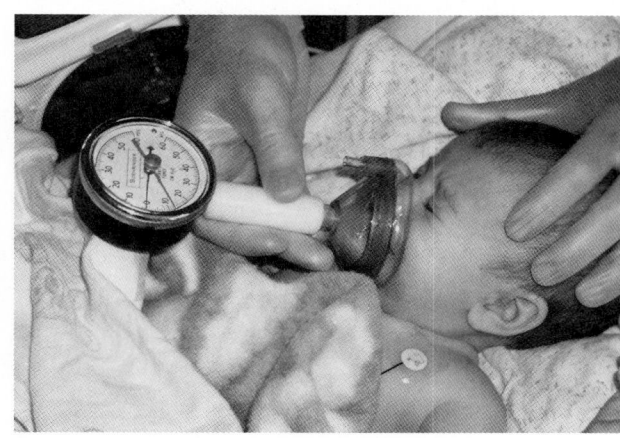

FIGURE 21-2   Place mask with one-way valve attachment over child's face with secure seal.

Steps	Rationale	Considerations
8. Record the most negative breath in centimeters H$_2$O.	Establishes trends in NIF measurements.	Discard invalid or unreliable measurements.
9. Reconnect child to ventilator or remove mask from child's face.	Allows child time to readjust to either positive-pressure ventilation or normal respiration.	

Expected Outcomes

- Accurate NIF measurement without complications

Unexpected Outcomes

- Unintentional extubation
- Increased ventilatory support as result of continued coughing, decreased oxygen saturations, or cyanosis
- Need for intubation indicated by sustained decreased saturations, cyanosis, or hemodynamic instability refractory to increased oxygen therapy

Monitoring and Care of the Child

Activities and Interventions	Rationale	Reportable Conditions
1. Monitor child's tolerance to NIF measurement.	Changes in child's condition may indicate complications from NIF measurement.	- Unintentional extubation - Continued coughing, decreased oxygen saturations, or cyanosis - Need for escalation in respiratory support measures

Documentation

- Best NIF measurements
- Additional interventions necessary before, during, and after measurement
- Child's response to measurement
- Unexpected outcomes and related treatment
- Child and family education

References

1. Durbin CG, et al: AARC clinical practice guideline: removal of the endotracheal tube, *Respir Care* 44:85-90, 1999. Text available at http://www.rcjournal.com/online_resources/cpgs/rotecpg/html.
2. Khan N, et al: Predictors of extubation success and failure in mechanically ventilated infants and children, *Crit Care Med* 24:1568-1579, 1996.
3. Lynn-McHale Wiegand DJ, Carlson KK: *AACN procedure manual for critical care,* ed 5, Philadelphia, 2005, Elsevier.

Additional Readings

Baum GL, et al: *Textbook of pulmonary diseases,* ed 6, Philadelphia, 1998, Lippincott.

Burton GG, et al: *Respiratory care: a guide to clinical practice,* ed 4, Philadelphia, 1997, Lippincott.

El-Khatib MF, et al: Inspiratory pressure/maximal inspiratory pressure: does it predict successful extubation in critically ill infants and children? *Intensive Care Med* 22:264-268, 1996.

Kacmarek RM, et al: *The essentials of respiratory care,* ed 3, St. Louis, 1990, Mosby.

Kacmarek RM, et al: *Monitoring in respiratory care,* ed 1, St Louis, 1993, Mosby.

Shapiro BA, et al: *Clinical application of respiratory care,* ed 4, St Louis, 1991, Mosby.

Venkataraman ST, et al: Validation of predictors of extubation success and failure in mechanically ventilated infants and children, *Crit Care Med* 28:2991-2996, 2000.

Pulse Oximetry

P U R P O S E : Pulse oximetry provides a continuous non-invasive estimate of arterial oxyhemoglobin saturation

Laurie S. Finger

PREREQUISITE KNOWLEDGE

- Child development as it relates to clinical assessment
- Anatomy and physiology of the pediatric pulmonary system[1]
- Pulse oximetry measures the absorption of two wavelengths of light by oxygenated and deoxygenated hemoglobin in pulsatile tissue (Figure 22-1). Hemoglobin (Hgb) that is saturated with oxygen absorbs light differently from unsaturated Hgb. Thus, the pulse oximeter measures the amount of absorption present and uses this in the calculation of the ratio of saturated Hgb to total Hgb. The monitor then displays the ratio as a percentage.[1-3]
- The oxygenation status of the child is dependent on the amount of Hgb present, how well the Hgb moves throughout the body, and how easily the oxygen leaves the Hgb and enters the cells.[1,2,4]
- Normal pulse oximetry values vary by age and condition, but a generally accepted range is 92% to 100%.[2,5-7] Children with sickle cell disease may have lower pulse oximetry readings than the actual partial pressure of oxygen (PaO_2) value.[8,9]
- Children with decreased Hgb concentrations (from anemia or hemorrhage) can have a saturation level of 100% and yet still be hypoxemic and cyanotic. The Hgb present may be fully saturated, but the child does not have adequate Hgb to carry enough oxygen to meet the needs of the body.
- Children with decreased perfusion (from shock, bradycardia, or vascular disease) may initially have 100% of

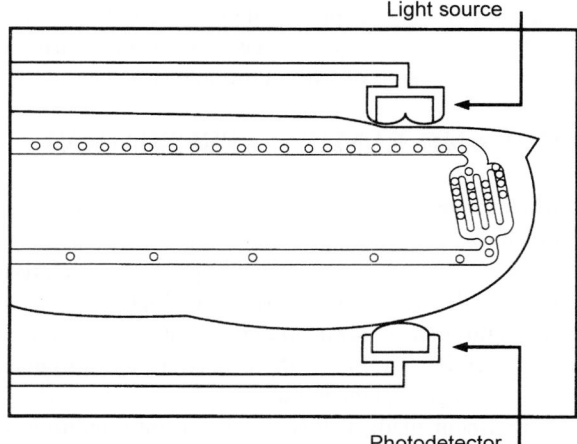

Light source

Photodetector

FIGURE 22-1 Pulse oximeter probe uses light source that emits red and infrared light and photodetector placed opposite it that measures amount of each wavelength of light absorbed by Hgb in blood as it moves past probe site. *Reprinted with permission of Nellcor Puritan Bennett Incorporated, Pleasanton, Calif.*

Hgb saturated with oxygen. Because of decreased blood flow, the Hgb is in prolonged contact with cells. The demand for oxygen by the cell is increased; the Hgb is stripped of its oxygen and takes longer to return to the lungs for reoxygenation.
- Dynamics of the oxyhemoglobin dissociation curve (ODC; see Figure 17-1)

- ❖ A shift to the right in the ODC represents a decrease in the Hgb's affinity for oxygen at the alveolar level. Oxygen is readily released from Hgb at the cellular level.
  - ❖ A shift in the ODC to the left represents an increase in the hemoglobin's affinity for oxygen at the alveolar level. Oxygen is bound more tightly to the Hgb and is released less readily at the cellular level.
- Pulse oximetry readings are altered by motion artifact, presence of intravascular dyes, ambient light, low perfusion states, dark skin pigmentation, and nail polish and artificial nails.[1-3]
- Pulse oximetry does not differentiate between carboxyhemoglobin, methemoglobin, and normal Hgb. Therefore, saturation levels in the presence of carbon monoxide (CO) poisoning or with nitric oxide (NO) administration may be misleading. In these cases, arterial Po_2 levels should be monitored directly, as should carboxyhemoglobin and methemoglobin levels.[1-3,10]
- A high rate of false alarms (primarily from movement artifact) and inaccuracies in quantification of saturations of less than 70% has been reported.[1,3,8,11-15] The standard pulse oximeter is also inconsistent in its ability to quantify the degree of hyperoxemia.
- Newer pulse oximeters are more reliable at quantification of hyperoxemia and show an improvement in measurement of saturations during movement and in low perfusion states.[1,3,11,12,13,14,16,17]
- Pulse oximetry is not appropriate for all children. Arterial blood gas analysis may be necessary for monitoring pH and partial pressure of carbon dioxide ($Paco_2$).

CHILD AND FAMILY ASSESSMENT

- Child's developmental level and ability to interact ➥*Rationale:* Influences preparation and interaction.
- Child's and family's understanding of the underlying condition, the reasons for pulse oximetry, the results, and their significance ➥*Rationale:* Evaluates child's and family's understanding of the procedure and provides a gauge for ongoing education.
- Any pertinent medical history or current condition that predisposes the child to alterations in oxygenation, ventilation, and acid/base balance ➥*Rationale:* Some medical conditions and therapies predispose the child to changes in oxygen saturation (e.g., hypoplastic left heart syndrome, supplemental oxygen therapy).
- Assess the child's respiratory status, including respiratory rate, work of breathing, and breath sounds ➥*Rationale:* Pulse oximetry is only a part of an assessment of the child.

- Signs and symptoms of inadequate oxygenation and ventilation ➥*Rationale:* Indicates effective pulmonary function and need for blood gas analysis.
- Note the child's serum Hgb level ➥*Rationale:* Children with decreased Hgb concentrations (from anemia or hemorrhage) can have a saturation level of 100% and yet still be hypoxemic and cyanotic.
- Assess for conditions (presence of CO poisoning, NO administration) that prevent accurate monitoring of oxygen saturation with pulse oximeter ➥*Rationale:* Pulse oximetry does not differentiate between carboxyhemoglobin, methemoglobin, and normal Hgb.
- Assess the intended site of probe placement for adequacy of perfusion, presence of nail polish, or altered skin integrity ➥*Rationale:* If the perfusion to the intended site is poor, or nail polish is over the intended site, the probe does not function properly. If a break in skin integrity is found at the intended site, the presence of the probe may worsen the break.[1-3,18-21]

CHILD AND FAMILY EDUCATION

Individualized, developmentally appropriate education is provided to the family and to the child based on desire for knowledge, readiness to learn, and overall neurologic and psychosocial state.

- Explain the child's underlying condition, the reasons for pulse oximetry monitoring, and the meaning of the oxygen saturation reading ➥*Rationale:* Providing information decreases fear and anxiety and improves compliance.
- Review with the parents and child the pulse oximeter alarm and explain the possibility of false alarms, including causes of false alarms, such as movement and ambient light interference ➥*Rationale:* Decreases child's and family's anxiety in response to alarms and increases knowledge of trouble-shooting techniques to prevent false alarms.
- Encourage questions and answer questions as they arise ➥*Rationale:* Reinforcement of information is needed during periods of stress.

EQUIPMENT

- Appropriately sized pulse oximeter probes (adult, pediatric, or infant; see Figure 22-2)
- Pulse oximetry monitor or module
- Pulse oximetry cable
- Fingernail polish remover (if needed)

Procedure | for Pulse Oximetry

Steps	Rationale	Considerations
1. Ensure child and family understand the procedure and questions are answered.	Evaluates and reinforces understanding of previously taught information.	Developmental level, cognitive ability, and anxiety level determine approach to and effectiveness of teaching.
2. Wash hands. *(Level VI*)*	Reduces transmission of infection. Protects personnel health.	
3. Gather equipment and supplies.	Improves efficiency.	Probes come in adult, pediatric, and infant sizes. Clip-on probes are primarily used for spot checks, and circumferential tape probes are primarily used for continuous monitoring (Figure 22-2).
4. Select an appropriate oximeter site (see Figure 22-2).	Site selection can affect the accuracy of the pulse oximeter readings.	Avoid sites distal to arterial lines or noninvasive blood pressure (BP) cuffs or on the same side as a Blalock-Taussig shunt.[1,2,19] *(Level V*)* In children with cyanotic heart disease, a preductal saturation can be obtained in the right arm and a postductal saturation may be obtained in the left arm or in either foot.[1] *(Level V*)*
5. Apply the probe to the child, ensuring that the light source is directly opposite the photodetector and that the probe fits snugly without any gaps between the probe and the skin. *(Level VI*)*	For accurate measurement of the saturation, the light source and the photodetector must be directly opposite each other.[1,2,19] Ensure that the pulse oximeter light source passes through tissue to the photodetector.	Do not apply the probe too tightly so that the probe interrupts blood flow to or from the site. Tissue perfusion can be impaired by circumferential restriction of arterial flow, or venous return and venous congestion may lead to venous pulsations and false readings.[1,2,19]
6. Protect the probe from excessive ambient light. *(Level VI*)*	Excessive ambient light interferes with the photodetector's ability to measure saturation accurately.[1-3] Measurement inaccuracies occur when the photodetector erroneously uses an alternative light source, called "optical shunting."[1,2,19]	If the child uses bilirubin lights or is under a bright examination light, a blanket or some other light-blocking material may be necessary to cover the probe.
7. Plug the oximeter into a grounded outlet, plug the cable into the oximeter or oximetry box, and plug the probe into the cable.	Grounded outlets reduce the chance of electrical interference; connection of all the components is necessary for monitoring of saturations.	Portable pulse oximeters must be plugged into an electrical outlet to keep the battery charged.
8. Turn the oximeter on, with allowance for a 15-second initialization period.	An initializing period is necessary for detection and averaging of pulse rate and saturations.	For "spot-checking" of saturations, allow the oximeter several minutes to average and obtain a reliable saturation reading. *(Level II*)*
9. Set the appropriate alarm parameters.	Setting the appropriate alarm parameters decreases the incidence rate of false alarms. *(Level V*)*	Pulse oximeter alarms should be set 3% less than the child's baseline saturation and ±20 bpm from the child's baseline heart rate. *(Level II*)*

Procedure continues on p. 149

---

* Level II: Theory-based; no research data to support recommendations; recommendations from expert consensus group may exist
Level V: Clinical studies in more than one or two patient populations and situations to support recommendations
Level VI: Clinical studies in a variety of patient populations and situations to support recommendations

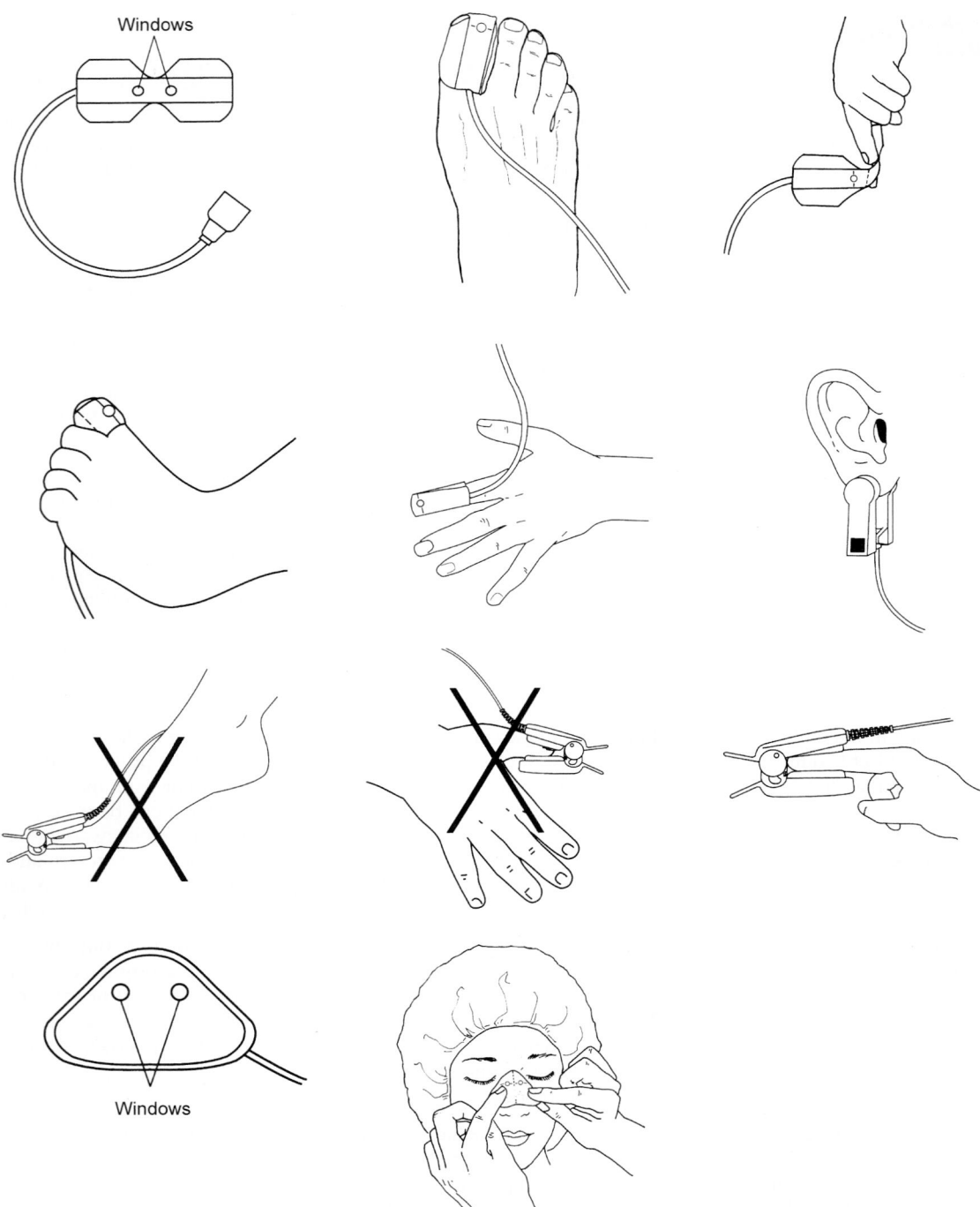

FIGURE 22-2   Sensor Types and Appropriate Sites for Placement Sensor types and sensor sites for pulse oximetry monitoring. Use "wrap"-style sensors on fingers and toes. Clip-style sensors are appropriate for fingers and earlobe. For all sensor types and sensor sites, windows for light source and photodector must be placed directly opposite each other on each side of arteriolar bed to ensure accuracy of pulse oximetry (SpO_2) measurements. *Reprinted with permission of Nellcor Puritan Bennett Incorporated, Pleasanton, California.*

Procedure for Pulse Oximetry—*Continued*

Steps	Rationale	Considerations
10. Verify the accuracy of the pulse oximeter reading by correlating the child's heart rate to the reading from the pulse oximeter. Analyze the size and shape of waveform and height and fluctuation of graphical display bar. At selected intervals, compare the monitored saturation level with the child's measured oxygen saturation from an arterial blood gas. *(Level VI*)*	Assures accuracy of the pulse oximeter value. The child's measured electrocardiogram or palpated heart rate should match the heart rate displayed by the pulse oximeter.	Some oximeters display the pulse wave graphically, in which case the pulse waveform should resemble an arterial waveform without a dicrotic notch. If the pulsatile flow past the probe is sluggish, the waveform may be dampened and the reading may be in error. The heart rate is also displayed as a pulsatile bar in a rectangle. As long as the pulsation of the bar correlates with the heart rate and the height of the bar fills at least 75% of the rectangle, the pulse oximeter reading is accurate.[2,3,15]
11. Wash hands. *(Level VI*)*	Reduces transmission of infection. Protects personnel health.	

* Level VI: Clinical studies in a variety of patient populations and situations to support recommendations

Expected Outcomes

- Oxyhemoglobin saturation levels are continuously monitored
- The need for invasive monitoring of oxygenation status is reduced
- All periods of desaturation are identified and appropriate action is taken
- Reduced number of false alarms

- Skin integrity is maintained

Unexpected Outcomes

- Pulse oximetry saturation readings do not correlate with measured saturation from arterial blood gases
- Equipment failure

- Child decompensates without identifying changes in pulse oximetry
- Excessive motion or decreased tissue perfusion interferes with proper functioning of the pulse oximeter
- The pulse oximeter probe causes breakdown in tissue integrity

Monitoring and Care of the Child

Activities and Interventions	Rationale	Reportable Conditions
1. Physiologic stability, including vital signs, respiratory status, and clinical appearance.	Pulse oximetry only provides one piece of data. The child's physiologic status must be considered to gain a complete assessment of the child's condition.	- Signs of hypoxia: decreased level of consciousness, tachypnea and tachycardia, increased work of breathing, cyanosis, and a decreased oxygen saturation level
2. Assess the probe site for breakdown every 2 hours and rotate the site at least every day or as per institution-specific policy.[19,21,22]	Skin probes have the potential to cause skin injury.[19,21,22] Certain conditions, such as low perfusion states, use of norepinephrine and other vasoconstrictive infusions, hypoxia, hypotension, prolonged probe contact, prolonged arterial catheterization in the same extremity as the pulse oximeter probe, and hypothermia, seem to increase the likelihood of injury.[20,22]	- Skin discoloration, decreased capillary refill, cooler temperatures, or skin breakdown at or distal to the probe site

---

Documentation

- Pulse oximetry readings
- Condition of probe site
- Child's physical assessment
- Amount and delivery method of supplemental oxygen (if used)
- Episodes of desaturation
- Child's response to interventions if necessary
- Child and family education
- Unexpected outcomes and related treatment

References

1. Curley MAQ, Thompson JE: Oxygenation and ventilation. In Curley MAQ, Moloney-Harmon P, editors: *Critical care nursing of infants and children,* ed 2, Philadelphia, 2001, Saunders.
2. Schultz S: Oxygen saturation monitoring by pulse oximetry. In Lynn-McHale Wiegand DJ, Carlson K, editors: *AACN procedure manual for critical care,* ed 5, Philadelphia, 2005, Elsevier.
3. Sayler JW: Neonatal and pediatric pulse oximetry, *Resp Care* 48(4):386-398, 2003.
4. Casey G: Oxygen transport and the use of pulse oximetry, *Nurs Stand* 15(47):46-55, 2001.
5. Hunt CE, et al: Longitudinal assessment of hemoglobin oxygen saturation in healthy infants during the first 6 months of age, *J Pediatr* 135(5):580-586, 1999.
6. Richmond S, et al: Routine pulse oximetry in the asymptomatic newborn, *Arch Dis Child Fetal Neonatal Ed* 87:F83-F88, 2002.
7. Urschitz MS, et al: Reference values for nocturnal home pulse oximetry during sleep in primary school children, *Chest* 123(1):96-101, 2003.
8. Blaisdell C, et al: Pulse oximetry is a poor predictor of hypoxemia in stable children with sickle cell disease, *Arch Pediatr Adolesc Med* 154(9):900-903, 2000.
9. Fitzgerald R, Johnson A: Pulse oximetry in sickle cell anemia, *Crit Care Med* 29(9):1803-1806, 2001.
10. Wong ALW, et al: Normal pulse oximeter reading in a cyanotic infant, *J Pediatr Child Health* 37:94-95.
11. Bohnhurst B, et al: Pulse oximeters' reliability in detecting hypoxemia and bradycardia: comparison between a conventional and two new generation oximeters, *Crit Care Med* 28(5):1565-1568, 2000.
12. Bonhurst B, et al: Detection of hyperoxaemia in neonates: data from three new pulse oximeters, *Arch Dis Child Fetal Neonatal Ed* 87:F217-F219, 2002.
13. Miyasaka K: Pulse oximetry in the management of children in the PICU, *Anesth Analg* 94(1):S44-S46, 2002.
14. Poets C, et al: Pulse oximetry in the neonatal intensive care unit: detection of hyperoxemia and false alarm rates, *Anesth Analg* 94(1):S41-S43, 2002.
15. Wouters PF, et al: Accuracy of pulse oximeters: the European multi-center trial, *Anesth Analg* 94(1):S13-S18, 2002.
16. Malviya S, et al: False alarms and sensitivity of conventional pulse oximetry versus the Masimo SET™ technology in the pediatric postanesthesia unit, *Anesth Analg* 90(6):1336-1340, 2000.
17. Rheineck-Leyssius AT, Kalkman CJ: Advanced pulse oximeter signal processing technology compared to simple averaging: effect on frequency of alarms in the operating room, *J Clin Anesth* 11:192-195, 1999.
18. Hamber EA, et al: Delays in the detection of hypoxemia due to site of pulse oximetry probe placement, *J Clin Anesth* 11:113-118, 1999.
19. McConnell EA: Performing pulse oximetry, *Nursing* 99:1999.
20. Villanueva R, et al: Effect of peripheral perfusion on accuracy of pulse oximetry in children, *J Clin Anesth* 11:317-322, 1999.
21. Lindo D, et al: Toe deformity from prolonged pulse oximetry, *Arch Dis Child* 87(6):533, 2002.
22. Wille J, et al: Pulse oximeter-induced digital injury: frequency rate and possible causative factors, *Crit Care Med* 28(10):3555-3557, 2000.

Additional Readings

AARC Clinical Practice Guideline: *Pulse oximetry,* 1991, from http://www.rcjournal.com/online_resources/cpgs/pulsecpg.html.

Bell C, et al: Effect of probe design on accuracy and reliability of pulse oximetry in pediatric patients, *J Clin Anesth* 11:323-327, 1999.

DeNicola L, et al: Noninvasive monitoring in the pediatric intensive care unit, *Pediatr Clin North Am* 48(3):573-588, 2001.

Iyer P, et al: Accuracy of pulse oximetry in hypothermic neonates and infants undergoing cardiac surgery, 1996. Cited in: Hamber EA, et al: Delays in the detection of hypoxemia due to site of pulse oximetry probe placement, *J Clin Anesth* 11:113-118, 1999.

Jones N, Gupta R: Postoperative monitoring of pediatric toe-to-hand transfers with differential pulse oximetry, *J Hand Surg* 26A(3):525-529, 2001.

Respiratory Rate: Obtaining an Accurate Measurement

P U R P O S E : Respiratory rate is an external assessment of ventilation. Accurate measurements are essential in monitoring for clinical signs of changes in work of breathing.

Kristin M. Print

PREREQUISITE KNOWLEDGE

- Child development as it relates to clinical assessment and procedure
- Anatomy and physiology of the pediatric pulmonary system, including structural characteristics specific to the infant and child[1-3]
  - ❖ Infants and young children inhale a small amount of air relative to exhalation volumes.
  - ❖ Infants and young children have fewer alveoli and consequently less alveolar surface area for gas exchange.
  - ❖ Normal respirations of infants and young children can be irregular.[4,5]
  - ❖ Ratio of inspiratory time to expiratory time is typically 1:2.
  - ❖ Respiratory rates are approximately inversely proportional to the child's age (Table 23-1).
  - ❖ A higher metabolic rate contributes to increasing respiratory rates.
  - ❖ Medications, such as narcotics, may decrease respiratory rates.
  - ❖ The position of the child may impede ventilatory movements.
  - ❖ Pain can increase or decrease rate of respirations.
  - ❖ Increased activity, anxiety, fear, and fever can all increase rate and depth of respirations.
  - ❖ Pathologic states, such as head injury, hemorrhage, infection, anemia, lung disease, meningitis, and

TABLE 23-1	Variations in Respiratory Rate by Age	
Age	**Rate (breaths/min)**	**Average**
1 yr	20-40	30
3 yr	20-30	25
6 yr	16-22	19
10 yr	16-20	18
Adult	12-20	16

Note that respiratory rate values are inversely proportional to age. From Engel J: *Mosby's pocket guide for pediatric assessment,* ed 5, St. Louis, 2006, Mosby.

tetanus, can all impact respiratory rate, rhythm, and depth (Table 23-2).
- Cardiopulmonary monitors detect respiratory rate through chest rise and fall; movement of the child may interfere with the accuracy of the respiratory rate measurement displayed on the screen.
- A child with previous tachypnea who had increased work of breathing and now has a decreased respiratory rate may be having eminent respiratory failure.
- The most accurate respiratory rate measurements are taken on a calm infant or child, often before more intrusive procedures are begun.

CHILD AND FAMILY ASSESSMENT

- Child's developmental level and ability to interact
  ➥*Rationale:* Influences preparation and interaction.

151

TABLE 23-2	Illustrations and Descriptions of Various Altered Respiratory Patterns

Pattern	Description
Dyspnea	Difficult or labored breathing; indicated by presence of retractions.
Bradypnea	Abnormally slow rate of breathing; rhythm regular.
Tachypnea	Abnormally fast rate of breathing.
Hyperpnea	Rapid, deep respirations.
Apnea	Absence of respirations.
Cheyne-Stokes respiration (periodic breathing)	Periods of deep, rapid breathing alternating with periods of apnea. Commonly seen in infants, and can be seen normally in children during deep sleep. Abnormal causes include drug-induced depression and brain damage.
Kussmaul's respiration	Abnormally deep breathing. Can be rapid, normal, or slow. Commonly associated with metabolic acidosis.
Biot's respiration (ataxic breathing)	Unpredictable, irregular breathing. Seen with lower brain damage and respiratory depression.

From Engel J: *Mosby's pocket guide for pediatric assessment,* ed 5, St. Louis, 2006, Mosby.

- History of cardiac or respiratory disorders, including apnea and asthma ➛*Rationale:* These conditions often influence respiratory rate.
- Medications ➛*Rationale:* Certain medications may increase or decrease respiratory rate.
- Presence of respiratory infections ➛*Rationale:* Infection of the respiratory tract affects respiratory rate.
- Level of consciousness and cognitive ability ➛*Rationale:* Self-consciousness may alter the respiratory rate once the child understands that someone is measuring respirations. A decreased respiratory rate may be an indication of decreased perfusion or hypoxia.
- Artificial airway or ventilatory support ➛*Rationale:* Artificial ventilatory support alters the child's ventilation.

CHILD AND FAMILY EDUCATION

Individualized, developmentally appropriate education is provided to the family and to the child based on desire for knowledge, readiness to learn, and overall neurologic and psychosocial state.

- Provide information about respiratory rate, including purpose of the measurement, steps in obtaining a quantifiable number, and the meaning of the value in relation to the child ➛*Rationale:* Providing information decreases anxiety and fear.
- Explain that the respiratory rate value displayed on the cardiopulmonary monitor may reflect lead displacement or body movement instead of the child's true respiratory rate ➛*Rationale:* Cardiopulmonary monitors measure respiratory rate with detection of chest rise and fall; the child's movement may interfere with this measurement and lead to an inaccurate respiratory rate value displayed on the screen.
- Encourage questions and answer questions as they arise ➛*Rationale:* Reinforcement of information is needed during periods of stress.

EQUIPMENT

- Stethoscope, if needed
- Watch or clock with a second hand

Procedure | for Obtaining an Accurate Respiratory Rate

Steps	Rationale	Considerations
1. Ensure child and family understand steps and rationale for obtaining a respiratory rate.	Evaluates and reinforces understanding of previously taught information.	Developmental level, cognitive ability, and anxiety level determine approach to and effectiveness of teaching.
2. Collect stethoscope and watch.	Preparation facilitates completion of the procedure in a timely manner.	
3. Wash hands.	Reduces transmission of organisms.	
4. Approach child on the basis of development level and degree of anxiety.	A fearful or crying child has an altered respiratory rate.	A pacifier may help calm a crying infant or young child. Restlessness and anxiety can be related to hypoxia.
5. Position child so that chest can be easily auscultated.	Chest should be easily accessible and visualized for an accurate measurement.	Infants and small children often tolerate assessments better if they are held in a parent's arms or in a comfortable position.
6. Count respiratory rate with one of the following methods: • Auscultate breath sounds for 1 full minute via stethoscope. • Directly visualize abdominal movements in infants or chest movements in children.[1,4-8]	The strategy chosen is based on child's condition. Respirations are diaphragmatic in infants.[4,5]	Warm the bell of the stethoscope before placing it on the skin. Measurement of the respiratory rate when counting the pulse may be helpful to decrease the child's self-awareness.[5] Respiratory rates of children may be counted for 30 seconds if the pattern is regular.[4]
7. Note depth and pattern of respirations, the presence of anxiety, restlessness, irritability, retractions, and color.	Restlessness or irritability can be signs of respiratory distress and hypoxia.	
8. Record results as breaths per minute and compare results with normal for individual child and age range.	Documentation allows for trending the respiratory rate and communicates findings to the health care team.	

Expected Outcomes

- Accurate respiratory rate measurement
- Normal respiratory rate for child's age

Unexpected Outcomes

- Inaccurate respiratory rate measurement
- Altered respiratory pattern
- Altered respiratory rate and pattern
- Increased work of breathing

Monitoring and Care of the Child

Activities and Interventions	Rationale	Reportable Conditions
1. Monitor child's respiratory rate during normal routine assessment and as indicated by condition.	A change in respiratory rate or pattern may indicate a change in child's condition.	• Apnea • Abnormal respiratory rate and pattern • Increased work of breathing, use of accessory muscles, tachypnea, grunting, and nasal flaring

Documentation

- Respiratory rate
- Work of breathing
- Child and family education
- Unexpected outcomes and related treatment (e.g., O_2, repositioning)

References

1. Curley MAQ, Moloney-Harmon PA: *Critical care nursing of infants and children,* ed 2, Philadelphia, 2001, Saunders.
2. Thompson A: Pediatric airway management. In Fuhrman B, Zimmerman J, editors: *Pediatric critical care,* ed 3, Philadelphia, 2006, Elsevier.
3. McCance K, Huether S: *Pathophysiology the biologic bases for disease in adults and children,* Philadelphia, 2002, Mosby.
4. Bowden VR, Greenberg CS: *Pediatric nursing procedures,* ed 1, Philadelphia, 2003, Lippincott.
5. Skale N: *Manual of pediatric nursing procedures,* ed 1, Philadelphia, 1992, Lippincott.
6. Engel J: *Pocket guide to pediatric assessment,* ed 4, St. Louis, 2002, Mosby.
7. Hazinski MF: *Manual of pediatric critical care,* ed 1, St. Louis, 1999, Mosby.
8. Wong DL, Hockenberry MJ: *Wong's clinical manual of pediatric nursing,* ed 6, St. Louis, 2004, Mosby.

Additional Readings

Edmonds ZV, Mower WR, Lovato LM, et al: The reliability of vital sign measurements, *Ann Emerg Med* 39:233-237, 2002.
Hazinski MF: *Nursing care of the critically ill child,* ed 2, St. Louis, 1992, Mosby.
Henretig FM, King C: *Textbook of pediatric emergency procedures,* 1997, Williams and Wilkins.
Wong D, Hockenberry MJ: *Nursing care of infants and children,* ed 7, St. Louis, 2003, Mosby.

PROCEDURE **24**

Auto Positive End-Expiratory Pressure Calculation

P U R P O S E : Dynamic gas trapping at the alveolar level can occur during mechanical ventilation and result in auto positive end-expiratory pressure (auto-PEEP). This calculation is performed to quantify the level of auto-PEEP and assess the need for changes in ventilation therapy.

Janet A. Koehler Boyce

PREREQUISITE KNOWLEDGE

- Child development as it relates to clinical assessment
- Anatomy and physiology of the pediatric pulmonary system
- Basic principles of positive end-expiratory pressure (PEEP)
- Auto-PEEP is also known as occult PEEP, intrinsic PEEP, or inadvertent PEEP.
- Auto-PEEP occurs at end exhalation as the result of dynamic air trapping in the alveoli. Auto-PEEP is PEEP generated above the set PEEP during mechanical ventilation. When inspiratory flow begins, before the conclusion of expiratory flow, inadequate exhalation and the stacking of breaths result. The level of auto-PEEP is dynamic and can change quickly (Figure 24-1).[1,2]
- The presence of auto-PEEP could lead to alveolar overdistention and result in volutrauma, barotrauma, and impaired gas exchange.
- Auto-PEEP is associated with obstructive lung disease, bronchospasm, obstructive airway disease (in particular status asthmaticus), and nonhomogeneous lung disease.
- Assessment of auto-PEEP becomes important when mechanical ventilation includes a high minute ventilation, long inspiratory time, insufficient expiratory time, high respiratory rate, or small endotracheal tube (ET).[1-4]

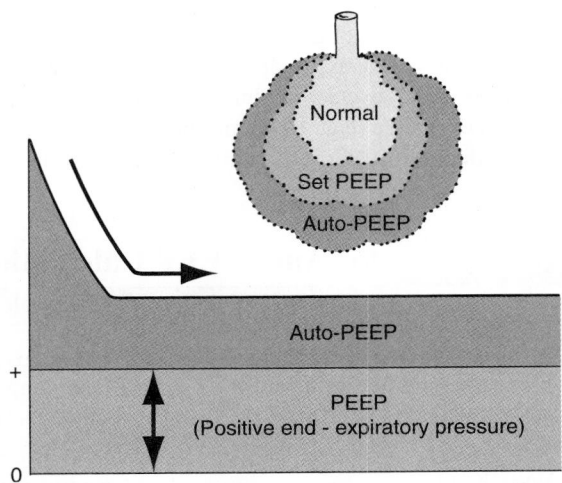

FIGURE 24-1 Auto-PEEP. *From Kinney M, et al:* AACN clinical reference for critical care nursing, *ed 4, St Louis, 1998, Mosby.*

- Auto-PEEP may cause an increased work of breathing as the child's diaphragm becomes flattened from lung distention. An asynchrony between the child's breaths and the ventilator's breaths may occur with increased inspiratory work of breathing. A ventilator breath may be triggered in an effort to overcome the presence of auto-PEEP. The set sensitivity on the ventilator may be inadequate to overcome the auto-PEEP. Auto-PEEP elevates the plateau pressure, and if undetected, the static compliance calculation is altered.[1,5-7]

- Adverse effects of auto-PEEP include increased work of breathing with associated development of fatigue, barotrauma with air leak syndrome, and hemodynamic compromise as a result of decreased venous return from the elevated intrapleural pressures.[2,6]
- Auto-PEEP is a desired consequence of pressure-controlled inverse ratio ventilation from nonhomogeneous lung disease. Auto-PEEP facilitates alveolar recruitment by increasing functional residual capacity and reducing intrapulmonary shunt.[1]
- Minimization of auto-PEEP can be achieved by decreasing the airflow obstruction (through the use of bronchodilators, ET suctioning), by adjusting the ventilatory settings (decreasing inspiratory time, increasing expiratory time, decreasing the set rate, changing the mode of ventilation, adjusting the level of set PEEP), or by replacing a faulty expiratory valve that impedes expiratory flow from malfunction or moisture accumulation.[1,5,6,8-10]

CHILD AND FAMILY ASSESSMENT

- Child's developmental level and ability to interact ➡*Rationale:* Affects preparation and interaction with the child.
- Child's and family's understanding of the reasons for and risks and benefits of assessing auto-PEEP ➡*Rationale:* Evaluates child's and family's understanding of the procedure and provides a gauge for ongoing education.
- Assess for presence of auto-PEEP with notation of child-ventilator asynchrony, increased work of breathing, decreased chest excursion during exhalation, signs of poor gas exchange (e.g., rising partial pressure of arterial carbon dioxide [$PaCO_2$]), hemodynamic compromise,

signs of air leak syndromes from barotrauma, increase in frequency of bronchospasm, progressive fatigue, and changing values on the ventilator display (if available), such as decreased expiratory volume, increasing mean airway pressure, or changes in the graphic waveform displays[1,2,4,10-12] ➡*Rationale:* Auto-PEEP increases the work of breathing. With auto-PEEP, the child is at risk for barotrauma and hemodynamic compromise. Clinical conditions with elevated airway resistance, such as status asthmaticus, may contribute to the presence of auto-PEEP.[3]

CHILD AND FAMILY EDUCATION

Individualized, developmentally appropriate education is provided to the family and to the child based on desire for knowledge, readiness to learn, and overall neurologic and psychosocial state.

- Discuss with the family and the child the overall respiratory status of the child in terms of therapies and progress ➡*Rationale:* Reinforced learning contributes to the general understanding of the child's respiratory status and progress.
- Discuss the concept of auto-PEEP in relationship to the child's status ➡*Rationale:* Fear and anxiety may be diminished if the concepts and reasons for interventions are understood in relation to the child's progress.
- Encourage questions and answer questions as they arise ➡*Rationale:* Reinforcement of information is needed during periods of stress.

EQUIPMENT

- Manual airway manometer (if the ventilator in use does not provide an end-expiratory hold button)

Procedure for Auto-PEEP Calculation		
Steps	**Rationale**	**Considerations**
1. Ensure child and family understand procedure and questions are answered.	Evaluates and reinforces understanding of previously taught information.	Developmental level, cognitive ability, and anxiety level determine approach to and effectiveness of teaching.
2. Wash hands.	Reduces transmission of microorganisms.	
3. Locate the end-expiratory hold button on the ventilator. (*Level I**)	During exhalation, the ventilator circuit is exposed to atmospheric pressure through the exhalation valve. The expiratory hold button closes the ventilator to the atmosphere at end exhalation, which allows for the equalization of pressure within the circuit.[1]	Not all ventilators have an end-expiratory hold button. If the ventilator does not have an end-expiratory hold button, a pressure manometer may be necessary at the exhalation port of the ventilator. Consult with the respiratory therapist for specific ventilator functions related to performing an end-expiratory hold maneuver.[1,13,14]

* Level I: Manufacturer's recommendations only

Procedure for Auto-PEEP Calculation—*Continued*

Steps	Rationale	Considerations
4. Depress the end-expiratory hold button at end exhalation. *(Level I*)*		
5. Assess for baseline changes on the airway manometer, digital readout, or graphic waveform display. *(Level V*)*	Auto-PEEP is present if the end-expiratory pressure reading remains elevated above the set PEEP level. The expiratory portion of a graphic waveform does not return to the baseline PEEP set but remains elevated.[5,8-10,14]	To accurately assess the presence of auto-PEEP, the child must be compliant and breathing in synchrony with the ventilator. The child may need sedation to reduce agitation or need neuromuscular blockade.
6. Record the total PEEP and the set PEEP. Auto PEEP (cm H_2O) = Total PEEP (cm H_2O) – Set PEEP (cm H_2O).	If no difference is found between the total PEEP and the set PEEP, auto-PEEP is not present.	To accurately estimate respiratory compliance, auto-PEEP is subtracted from the total PEEP.[15]
7. Record the level of auto-PEEP on the appropriate document.	Data communication.	

* Level I: Manufacturer's recommendations only
  Level V: Clinical studies in more than one or two patient populations and situations to support recommendations

Expected Outcomes

- Detection and degree of auto-PEEP
- Child's condition remains stable throughout measurement
- Auto-PEEP is monitored when desired in pressure-controlled inverse ratio ventilation

Unexpected Outcomes

- Barotrauma
- Hemodynamic compromise
- Inadequate mechanical ventilation

Monitoring and Care of the Child

Activities and Interventions	Rationale	Reportable Conditions
1. Ongoing evaluations for the presence of auto-PEEP.	Prevention of complications associated with auto-PEEP. Permissive hypercarbia may be desirable as a lung protection strategy for prevention of barotrauma. Sedation or neuromuscular blockade or both may be needed to allow for child-ventilator synchrony.[1,2]	• Presence of auto-PEEP at a level of 1 to 3 cm H_2O may not produce clinical symptoms, but auto-PEEP is dynamic and may change rapidly[2]
2. Assess for signs of barotrauma.	Barotrauma that results from the overdistention of the alveoli could result in air leak syndromes.	• Abrupt changes in heart rate, blood pressure, central venous pressure, pulse oximetry • Decreased or absent breath sounds unilaterally • Abrupt increase in work of breathing
3. Assess for signs of hemodynamic compromise.	Increased alveolar pressure compresses the pulmonary capillary bed, which could lead to a decrease in cardiac output and hypotension.	• Signs of altered perfusion or oxygenation related to a decreased cardiac output

---

Documentation

- Presence or absence of auto-PEEP
- Changes in ventilation management and response to changes in therapy
- Child's response to additional interventions, if necessary
- Child and family education
- Unexpected outcomes and related treatment

References

1. Burns SM: Auto-PEEP calculation. In Lynn-McHale Wiegand DJ, Carlson KK, editors: *AACN procedure manual for critical care,* ed 4, Philadelphia, 2005, Elsevier.
2. Curley MAQ, Thompson JE: Oxygenation and ventilation. In Curley MAQ, Moloney-Harmon PA, editors: *Critical care nursing of infants and children,* ed 2, Philadelphia, 2001, Saunders.
3. Briening EP: Management of children in status asthmaticus, *Crit Care Nurs* 18(1):74-82, 1998.
4. Hicks GH, Scanlan CL: Initiating and adjusting ventilatory support. In Scanlan DL, Wilkins RL, Stoller JK, editors: *Egan's fundamentals of respiratory care,* ed 7, St Louis, 1999, Mosby.
5. Holt TO: Physics and physiology of ventilatory support. In Scanlan CL, Wilkins RL, Stoller JK, editors: *Egan's fundamentals of respiratory care,* ed 7, St Louis, 1999, Mosby.
6. Kastens VM: Nursing management of "Auto-PEEP," *Focus Crit Care-AACN* 18(5):419-412, 1991.
7. Pruitt WC: Ventilator graphics made easy, *RT* 15(1): 23-24,50, 2002.
8. Aloi A, Burns SM: Continuous airway pressure monitoring in the critical care setting, *Crit Care Nurs* 15(2):66-74, 1995.
9. Burns SM: Continuous airway pressure monitoring, *Crit Care Nurs* 21(3):66-71, 2001.
10. Burns SM: Working with respiratory waveforms: how to use bedside graphics, *AACN Clin Iss* 14(2):133-144, 2003.
11. Hazinski MF: *Nursing care of the critically ill child,* ed 2, St Louis, 1992, Mosby.
12. Hazinski MF: *Manual of pediatric critical care,* St Louis, 1999, Mosby.
13. AARC Clinical Practice Guideline: Patient-ventilator system checks, *Respir Care* 37:882-886, 1992.
14. Matthews PJ, Gregg BL: Monitoring and management of the patient in the ICU. In Scanlan CL, Wilkins RL, Stoller JK, editors: *Egan's fundamentals of respiratory care,* ed 7, St Louis, 1999, Mosby.
15. Ruggles L: Auto-PEEP: measurement issues and nursing interventions, *Crit Care Nurs* 15(2):30-38, 1995.

Additional Readings

American Thoracic Society: International consensus conference in intensive care medicine: ventilator-associated lung injury in ARDS, *Am J Respir Crit Care Med* 166:2118-2124, 1999.

Burns SM: Measurement of compliance and resistance. In Lynn-McHale Wiegand DJ, Carlson KK, editors: *AACN procedure manual for critical care,* ed 5, Philadelphia, 2005, Elsevier.

Carlo WA, Ambalavanan N: Conventional mechanical ventilation: traditional and new strategies, *NeoRev,* 117-126, 1999.

Cheifetz IM: Invasive and noninvasive pediatric mechanical ventilation, *Respir Care* 48(4):442-453, 2003.

Connors CA, Rosenthal-Dichter C: Components of breathing: pediatric ventilatory challenges, *Crit Care Nurs* 17(1):60-70, 1997.

Heulitt MJ, et al: Effects of continuous positive airway pressure/positive end-expiratory pressure and pressure-support ventilation on work of breathing: using an animal model, *Respir Care* 48(7):689-696, 2003.

Jubran A: Advances in respiratory monitoring during mechanical ventilation, *Chest* 116(5):1416-1425, 1999.

Kercsmar CM: Current trends in neonatal and pediatric respiratory care: conference summary, *Respir Care* 48(4):459-464, 2003.

Kress JP, et al: Clinical examination reliably detects intrinsic positive end-expiratory pressure in critically ill, mechanically ventilated patients, *Am J Respir Crit Care Med* 159:290-294, 1999.

Lu Q, Rouby JJ: Measurement of pressure-volume curves in patients on mechanical ventilation: methods and significance, *Crit Care* 4(2):91-100, 2000.

Malinowski C, Wilson B: Neonatal and pediatric respiratory care. In Scanlan DL, Wilkins RL, Stoller JK, editors: *Egan's fundamentals of respiratory care,* ed 7, St Louis, 1999, Mosby.

Marraro GA: Innovative practices of ventilatory support with pediatric patients, *Pediatr Crit Care Med* 4(1):8-20, 2003.

Tobin MJ, et al: Patient-ventilator interaction, *Am J Respir Crit Care Med* 163(5):1059-1063, 2001.

Tobin MJ: Critical care medicine in AJRCCM 200: year in review, *Am J Respir Crit Care Med* 165:565-583, 2002.

Werner H: Status asthmaticus in children: a review, *Chest* 119(6):1913-129, 2001.

Wright J, Gong H: Auto-PEEP: incidence, magnitude, and contributing factors, *Heart Lung* 19(4):352-357, 1990.

Extracorporeal Membrane Oxygenation

P U R P O S E : Extracorporeal membrane oxygenation (ECMO) is used to provide cardiopulmonary support for children with reversible life-threatening heart or lung disease that is unresponsive to maximal conventional treatment

James A. Cullen

PREREQUISITE KNOWLEDGE

- Child development as it relates to clinical assessment and implications for extracorporeal membrane oxygenation (ECMO)
- Anatomy and physiology of the pediatric pulmonary system, including structural characteristics specific to the infant and child[1-4]
- Signs and symptoms of inadequate oxygenation and ventilation[1-2]
- Mastery of pediatric advanced life support competencies, including indications for an artificial airway and other adjuncts used to support ventilation[1]
- Extracorporeal membrane oxygenation is used to facilitate heart and lung rest and recovery.[5] The amount of time a child may need ECMO support varies according to the primary disease being treated and complications that may arise during therapy. The overall survival rate has been reported as more than 50%.[6]
- Children who undergo ECMO therapy have a variety of underlying conditions.[6-10] Indications for ECMO include cardiac or respiratory failure that is not responsive to maximal conventional therapy, cardiac arrest, lack of improvement on maximal conventional therapy, weaning failure from cardiopulmonary bypass, postoperative cardiac failure, and bridge to transplantation.[6,9]
- The selection criteria for ECMO for a child includes a gestational age of greater than 34 weeks, no significant coagulopathy or active bleeding complications, no signif-icant intracranial bleeding, less than 10 to 14 days of mechanical ventilation, and no lethal congenital anomalies.
- Understanding of the role of the bedside nurse and ECMO specialist
  - ❖ During ECMO, the bedside nurse is responsible for all of the routine care that the critically ill child needs. In collaboration with the ECMO specialist, the nurse is accountable for clinical assessment and the nursing care necessary to ensure safety. The bedside nurse must also be prepared to provide increased ventilatory support and resuscitation in the event of an acute ECMO circuit failure.
  - ❖ The ECMO specialist is a specially trained nurse, respiratory therapist, or perfusionist who monitors and maintains the ECMO circuit. All procedures related to the ECMO circuit are performed by the ECMO specialist. Responsibility for clinical assessment is shared between the ECMO specialist and the bedside nurse.
- Methods of treatment
  - ❖ Veno-arterial (V-A) ECMO: V-A ECMO provides support for the heart and lungs. Blood is drained by gravity from the right atrium into the ECMO circuit, pumped through the membrane oxygenator for gas exchange, and returned to the aorta (Figure 25-1).
  - ❖ Veno-venous (V-V) ECMO: V-V ECMO is used for pulmonary support only. Blood is drained from the right atrium into the circuit and returned to the right atrium after gas exchange (Figure 25-2).

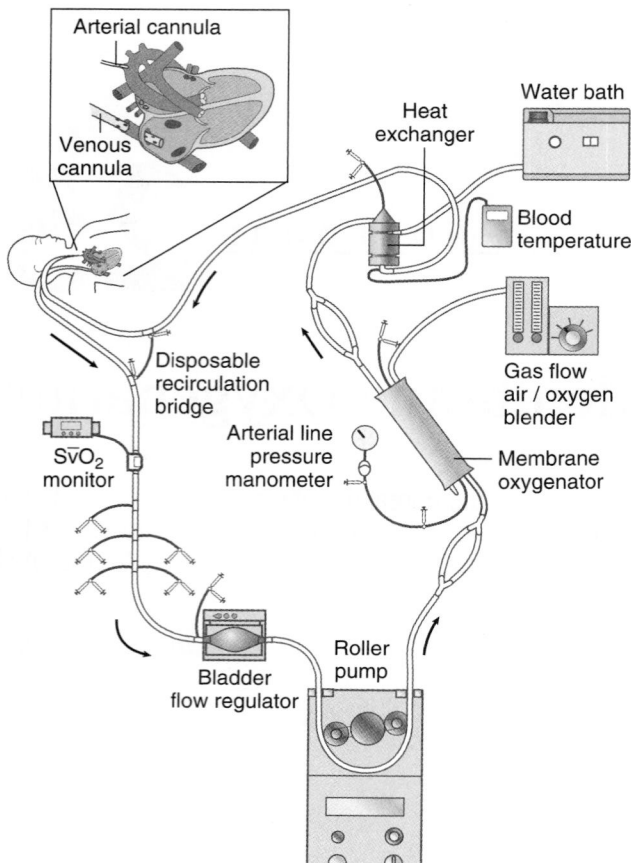

FIGURE 25-1 Veno-arterial ECMO support. Veno-arterial ECMO with cervical cannulation. *From Dalton H: Extracorporeal life support. In Fuhrman B, Zimmerman J, editors:* Pediatric critical care, *ed 2, Philadelphia, 2005, Elsevier.*

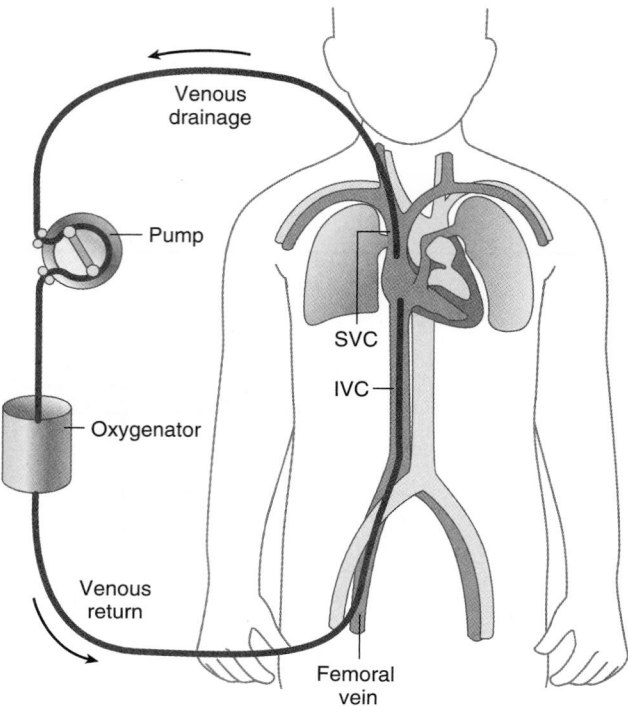

FIGURE 25-2 Veno-venous ECMO support. Veno-venous ECMO with superior vena cava to right atrium as venous outflow tract and femoral vein to inferior vena cava as inflow tract. *From Dalton H: Extracorporeal life support. In Fuhrman B, Zimmerman J, editors:* Pediatric critical care, *ed 2, Philadelphia, 2005, Elsevier.*

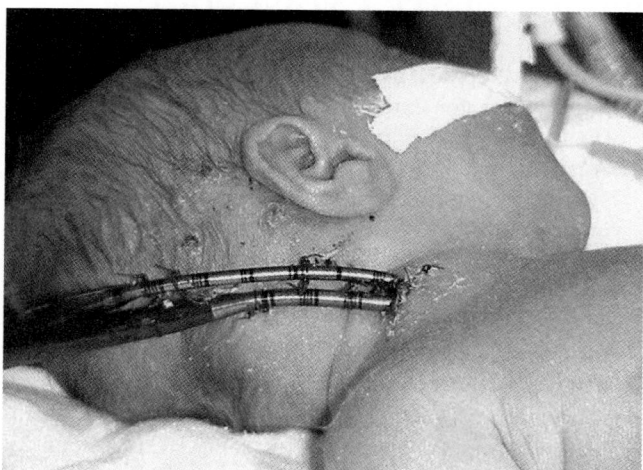

FIGURE 25-3 Veno-arterial cannulation.

- Vascular access: The ECMO cannulas can be placed with open procedure under direct vision or by percutaneous cannulation.[6,11]
  - Veno-arterial ECMO: The right internal jugular vein and right common carotid artery are the primary sites used for cannulation (Figure 25-3). Transthoracic cannulation of the right atrium and aorta is used for some children with cardiac disease. When additional venous drainage is needed, the femoral veins can also be cannulated.
  - Veno-venous ECMO: In neonates, V-V ECMO can be performed with a double-lumen cannula that is placed in the right atrium via the right internal jugular vein (Figure 25-4).[12] For older patients, the femoral veins are used for venous drainage and the jugular vein is cannulated for returning the oxygenated blood to the heart.
- Anticoagulation therapy during ECMO: Exposure of the child's blood to the artificial surfaces of the ECMO circuit activates coagulation via the intrinsic clotting cascade.[13] Platelets and other clotting factors are consumed over time and need replacement. Heparin is used to prevent excessive clotting in the cannulas and ECMO circuit during treatment. Anticoagulation therapy begins during

cannulation with a loading dose of 50 to 100 units/kg intravenously (IV). A continuous infusion is started after cannulation and is titrated to maintain the activated clotting time (ACT) between 180 and 200 seconds. The ACT is measured hourly by the ECMO specialist. The heparin infusion is typically administered via infusion ports on the ECMO circuit.[14]
- Extracorporeal membrane oxygenation flow mechanics: Drainage to the ECMO circuit is gravity dependent. Factors that affect venous drainage include the size and position of the venous cannulas, the size of the blood

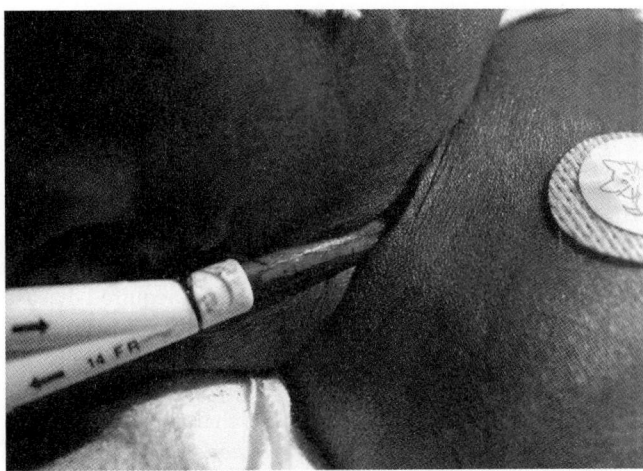

FIGURE 25-4 Veno-venous cannulation with double-lumen cannula.

tubing on the venous side of the circuit, the position of the child, the intravascular volume, and the height of the bed. Blood return to the child is limited by the size and position of the arterial cannula.

❖ Gas exchange on ECMO is the result of the combined contributions of the membrane oxygenator and the child's lungs. For children with primary pulmonary disease, little or no contribution may be made by the native lungs to gas exchange. Control of gas exchange in the membrane oxygenator is achieved by adjusting the gas flow rate (sweep gas) and fraction of inspired oxygen (FiO$_2$).[6]

❖ Systemic perfusion on ECMO is related to the method used and the amount of pump flow. For children undergoing V-V ECMO, systemic perfusion is a function of cardiac output. V-V ECMO provides no cardiac support. With V-A ECMO, the adequacy of perfusion reflects the combined contributions of ECMO pump flow and native cardiac function. For children with primary cardiac disease, the systemic perfusion may be supplied entirely by the ECMO circuit.

• The potential complications of ECMO include:

❖ Third spacing and edema: When ECMO is initiated, contact between the child's blood and the ECMO circuit surfaces initiates an inflammatory response, in which cytokines and other mediators of increased capillary permeability are released.[13,14] As a result, intravascular volume is lost and must be replaced to maintain adequate ECMO flow. This process is self limiting but can result in significant edema formation.

❖ Inadequate venous drainage ("cutting out"): Whenever venous drainage to the circuit is less than the pump flow rate, the ECMO pump controller reduces flow or shuts down the system temporarily. Impaired venous drainage can result from low intravascular volume, cannula placement problems, impaired venous return to the heart, the position of the child, or pneumothorax or hemothorax that, if severe, can cause mediastinal shift, compressing the heart and reducing blood flow.[6,15]

❖ Thrombocytopenia: Platelet activation and consumption is routinely seen during ECMO as a result of contact with the artificial surfaces of the circuit. Replacement transfusions are necessary when the platelet count falls below the threshold determined by the prescribing practitioner.[14]

❖ Coagulopathy: Clot formation in the ECMO circuit may trigger coagulopathy. Prolonged clotting times, bleeding, and failure of the membrane oxygenator may result. Platelets and fibrinogen need to be replaced when levels fall below the threshold set by the ordering practitioner. If repeated replacement transfusions do not correct the deficiency, the ECMO circuit may need to be replaced.

❖ Hemolysis: Red blood cells can be hemolyzed from shear stresses created by flow through the blood pump and arterial cannula. Excessive hemolysis can impair renal function and cause coagulopathy.[16]

❖ Hemorrhage: Anticoagulation therapy and clotting factor consumption increase the risk of bleeding during ECMO

❖ Infection: ECMO necessitates a surgical procedure to place the cannulas, which remain in place for several days to weeks[6]

• Lung function is decreased in the early phase of treatment because of the effects of reduced ventilatory support and pulmonary edema caused by capillary leak. Breath sounds are diminished or absent, and chest movement is equally reduced. For children with primary lung disease, gas exchange is largely accomplished by the membrane lung, so blood gases and oxygen saturation (SaO$_2$) should be normal. Reduced flow causes decreases in arterial and mixed venous oxygen saturations. As healing progresses and lung volumes increase, with improvement in breath sounds and chest movement, SaO$_2$ also increase, permitting a reduction in ECMO support.

• For children undergoing V-A ECMO, systemic perfusion is driven primarily by nonpulsatile flow from the ECMO circuit. Mean arterial pressure should be within normal limits, but the arterial tracing is dampened in proportion to the ECMO flow rate. Some children with primary cardiac disease may have limited left ventricular function. Peripheral pulses are diminished, and pulse oximeters may not function. Mixed venous saturation (SvO$_2$) should also be normal if the ECMO flow rate is adequate. Severe left ventricular dysfunction may cause severe pulmonary edema and may necessitate intervention in the form of a balloon septostomy.[9] Rising SaO$_2$ with a falling mixed venous saturation can indicate cardiac dysfunction. With V-V ECMO, cardiac assessment is not altered and deterioration in cardiac function is a potential emergency that could necessitate resuscitation and conversion to V-A ECMO. In contrast to children undergoing V-A ECMO, these patients have lower SaO$_2$ with higher mixed venous saturations from the recirculation of oxygenated blood back to the circuit that was not ejected by the right heart.

- Third-space fluid loss can be profound in the first days of treatment and is reflected by increased body weight and edema. Blood product transfusions needed to replace depleted clotting factor levels and decreased hemoglobin can add to the problem if renal function is impaired. Heparin is excreted in urine, and changes in urine output alter the amount of circulating heparin and affect activated clotting times.

CHILD AND FAMILY ASSESSMENT

- Child's developmental level and ability to interact ➼*Rationale:* Influences preparation and interaction.
- Child's and family's understanding of the reasons for and risks and benefits of ECMO ➼*Rationale:* Evaluates child's and family's understanding of the procedure and provides a gauge for ongoing education.
- Respiratory assessment, including breath sounds, chest movement, PO_2, SaO_2, and SvO_2 ➼*Rationale:*. Assessment of lung function is of primary concern during ECMO. Initially, breath sounds and chest movement are diminished or absent. Reduced flow causes decreases in arterial and mixed venous oxygen saturations. Breath sounds and chest movement become more notable as the child's condition improves.
- Cardiovascular assessment, including mean arterial pressure, arterial waveform, peripheral pulses, perfusion, SvO_2, and SaO_2 ➼*Rationale:* Cardiovascular assessment is key to monitoring the child's overall condition and the ability of the ECMO circuit to meet the child's need. Rising SaO_2 with a falling SvO_2 can indicate cardiac dysfunction.
- Fluid balance assessment, including fluid intake, urine output, blood loss, severity of edema, and body weight ➼*Rationale:* With the initiation of ECMO, fluid shifts are significant. Fluctuation in urine output changes the amount of heparin excreted in the urine and can alter the circulating heparin and influence activated clotting times.
- Hemostasis assessment, including activated clotting time, heparin consumption, platelet count, fibrinogen level, prothrombin time, activated partial thromboplastin time, fibrin split products, and blood loss ➼*Rationale:* Clotting factor consumption in the ECMO circuit can result in decreased clotting factor levels, prolonged clotting times, and increased risk of bleeding.

CHILD AND FAMILY EDUCATION

Individualized, developmentally appropriate education is provided to the family and to the child based on desire for knowledge, readiness to learn, and overall neurologic and psychosocial state.

- Explain ECMO therapy, including the purpose, steps, and rationale ➼*Rationale:* Providing information decreases

fear and anxiety and reassures the family that further stress on the heart and lungs has been reduced and that healing may begin to occur.

- Describe the cause of increased edema and reinforce that the problem is temporary and will resolve as healing progresses ➼*Rationale:* Providing information decreases fear and anxiety. Changes in the child's physical appearance are upsetting to the family.
- Describe the reason for blood product transfusions; reinforce the overall low risk of transfusion-acquired disease and the increased risk of complications if transfusions are not given as needed ➼*Rationale:* Anxiety over transfusion-acquired disease is common.
- Explain to the family the specific changes in the child's status that indicate recovery ➼*Rationale:* Knowledge of what factors are assessed to indicate recovery helps the family to ask informed questions about the child's condition.
- Describe the relationship between the primary diagnosis and the expected duration of ECMO ➼*Rationale:* A time frame may help to decrease anxiety during the recovery process.
- Explain the potential complications of ECMO and how they are treated ➼*Rationale:* The family can ask informed questions about the child's status and be reassured that most complications are not life threatening.
- Encourage questions and answer questions as they arise ➼*Rationale:* Reinforcement of information is needed during periods of stress.

EQUIPMENT

- Personal protective equipment, including eye protection, mask, and gown
- Stethoscope
- Manual ventilation device: Flow or self-inflating with appropriately sized mask connected to an oxygen/air source
- Appropriately sized mask
- Appropriately sized disposable suction catheters
- Suction source (wall regulator or portable machine) with collection container and tubing
- Resuscitation medications: Epinephrine, sodium bicarbonate, calcium gluconate
- Crystalloid solution, as ordered for hypotension
- X-ray plate
- Pain and sedation medication, as ordered
- Neuromuscular blocking agent, as ordered
- Heparin loading dose, as ordered
- Blood products for ECMO circuit priming
- Dressing material: Sterile gauze, occlusive dressing
- Cardiorespiratory monitor
- Pulse oximetry (SpO_2) and mixed venous oxygen saturation (SVo_2) monitor

Procedure	for Assisting during ECMO Cannulation	
Steps	**Rationale**	**Considerations**
1. Ensure child and family understand procedure and questions are answered.	Evaluates and reinforces understanding of previously taught information.	Developmental, cognitive, and anxiety levels determine approach to and effectiveness of teaching. A complete explanation may be delayed depending on the child's condition and the urgency of the procedure.
2. Gather needed equipment and supplies.	Facilitates completion of task in a timely manner.	
3. Remove all unnecessary equipment and furniture from the child's room.	Creates space for the surgical team and the ECMO circuit.	
4. Ensure cardiorespiratory monitoring is in place. *(Level II*)*	Assesses cardiorespiratory status during procedure.	Verify the ET and monitoring leads are secure before the child is draped for surgery.
5. Wash hands and put on personal protective equipment, including eye protection; mask, and a gown, as indicated.	Reduces transmission of infection. Protects personnel health.	
6. Assist the surgical team with positioning the child for cannulation.	The child or the bed may have to be moved to allow the surgeon access to the cannulation site.	
7. Place an x-ray plate under the child's chest before cannulation.	Facilitates post procedure film for verification of cannula position while the child remains draped.	The surgeon must secure the cannulas while the film is removed.
8. Ensure that the manual resuscitation bag is removed from the bed before the child is draped for surgery. *(Level VI*)*	Potential explosion hazard if material in the oxygen-enriched area under drapes is ignited by spark from the electrosurgical unit.	
9. Administer medication for pain and sedation, as ordered.	Surgical procedure.	Monitor blood pressure closely.
10. Administer neuromuscular blockade, as ordered.	Surgical procedure.	
11. Administer heparin loading dose, as ordered.	Prevents clotting in the cannulas before initiation of ECMO support.	
12. Monitor blood pressure closely as ECMO support is initiated. Treat as ordered. *(Level VI*)*	Children can have either hypertension or hypotension in the first minutes with ECMO.	Children undergoing veno-venous ECMO who have severe hypotension may need emergent conversion to V-A support.
13. Wean ventilator settings, as appropriate.	Lung rest can begin as soon as adequate ECMO support has been achieved.	
14. Apply occlusive dressing to the cannulation site.	Cannula insertion site is dressed as a central line.	The dressing for transthoracic cannulation is applied and maintained by the surgical team. A neck dressing is typically non-occlusive (dry, sterile gauze).
15. Monitor arterial blood gases as ordered until condition is stable.	Blood gases are needed to determine the proper level of ECMO sweep gas flow rate and oxygen concentration.	

Procedure continues on following page

---

* Level II: Theory-based; no research data to support recommendations; recommendations from expert consensus group may exist
  Level VI: Clinical studies in a variety of patient populations and situations to support recommendations

Procedure for Assisting during ECMO Cannulation—*Continued*

Steps	Rationale	Considerations
16. Adjust bed height as requested by the ECMO specialist.	Venous drainage to the circuit is gravity dependent.	The bed may have to be changed if height adjustment is inadequate.
17. Remove protective items and wash hands.	Reduces transmission of infection. Protects personnel health.	

Expected Outcomes / Unexpected Outcomes

Expected Outcomes	Unexpected Outcomes
• Improvement in oxygen delivery	• Inadequate oxygenation
• Decreased ventilation support	
• Cannulation site is free of bleeding	• Excessive bleeding at cannulation site
• Maintenance of coagulation balance	• Intracranial bleeding
	• Excessive hemolysis
	• Coagulopathy
	• Hemorrhage
	• Thrombocytopenia
• Child remains infection free	• Infection
• Improvement in systemic perfusion	• Hemodynamic instability
• The ECMO equipment is fully functional with adequate venous drainage	• Mechanical failure
	• Pneumothorax
	• Hemothorax
	• Inadequate fluid volume
• Child has acceptable level of comfort	• Unmanaged pain and agitation

Monitoring and Care of the Child

Activities and Interventions	Rationale	Reportable Conditions
1. Respiratory assessment.	Indicates the adequacy of ECMO in supporting respiratory function and providing lung rest.	• Sudden decrease in breath sounds • Decreased SaO_2/PaO_2 • Decreased mixed SvO_2 • Sudden increase or decrease in chest tube drainage
2. Cardiovascular assessment.	Change in cardiovascular performance may indicate a deterioration in the child's clinical condition or inadequate functioning of the ECMO circuit. Children undergoing V-A ECMO may have reduced cardiac output. Deterioration in cardiac function may alter the need for conversion from V-V ECMO to V-A ECMO.	• Loss of pulsatility on arterial line tracing • Decreased mean arterial pressure • Diminished heart sounds • Decreased peripheral pulses • Decreased SvO_2 • Increased serum lactate levels
3. Neurologic assessment.	Changes in neurologic status may be related to evolving intracranial bleeding or other injury.	• Decrease in responsiveness • Change in pupil size or responsiveness • Abnormal movement or posturing
4. Skin integrity.	Position changes may be restricted by cannula placement.	• Signs of pressure-related injury, including skin redness, breakdown, necrosis, or ulcerations
5. Cannulation site assessment.	Sutures can dislodge over time Site can become infected. Bleeding from site is possible Pressure from cannula may cause skin breakdown.	• Signs of wound infection • Significant bleeding • Loose or dislodged sutures

Monitoring and Care of the Child—Cont'd

Activities and Interventions	Rationale	Reportable Conditions
6. Monitor fluid balance.	Delivery of adequate ECMO flow depends on maintenance of normal intravascular volume. Capillary leak and third-space fluid loss reduces intravascular volume.	• Decreased urine output • Increased body weight or edema • The ECMO pump cuts out
7. Monitor bleeding and related coagulation factors. Administer blood products as indicated.	Bleeding from systemic heparinization is a major concern. Blood products are necessary to maintain adequate blood volume and provide needed coagulation factors.	• Signs of coagulopathy • Thrombocytopenia • Hemolysis • Hemorrhage
8. Provide adequate nutrition.	Promotes healing and recovery.[17]	• Indications of feeding intolerance • Indication of changes in body composition
9. Assess comfort and provide appropriate interventions.	Early identification of the child's comfort allows for immediate attention.	• Report of unresolved pain and discomfort

Documentation

- Hourly activated clotting time
- Heparin consumption (units/kg/h)
- The ECMO pump flow rate (mL/kg/min)
- The ECMO sweep gas FIO_2 and flow rate
- Cardiorespiratory and neurologic assessment results
- Findings of skin assessment
- Additional interventions needed before, during, and after procedure
- Comfort assessment and any specific interventions provided
- Child and family education
- Unexpected outcomes and related treatment

References

1. Hazinski MF, et al, editors: *Pediatric advanced life support provider manual,* Dallas, 2002, American Heart Association
2. Thompson A: Pediatric airway management. In Fuhrman B, Zimmerman J, editors: *Pediatric critical care,* ed 3, Philadelphia, 2006, Elsevier.
3. McCance K, Huether S: *Pathophysiology: the biologic bases for disease in adults and children,* Philadelphia, 2002, Mosby.
4. Thibodeau G, Patton K, editors: *Anatomy and physiology,* ed 5, Philadelphia, 2003, Mosby.
5. Extracorporeal Life Support Organization: ELSO guidelines for neonatal consultation, from http://www.elso.umich.edu.
6. Dalton H: Extracorporeal life support. In Fuhrman B, Zimmerman J, editors: *Pediatric critical care,* ed 2, Philadelphia, 2005, Mosby.
7. Fortenberry J, et al: Extracorporeal life support for posttraumatic acute respiratory distress syndrome at a children's medical center, *J Pediatr Surg* 38:1211-1226, 2003.
8. Thiagarajan R, et al: Extracorporeal membrane oxygenation as a bridge to cardiac transplantation in a patient with cardiomyopathy and hemophilia A, *Intens Care Med* 29:985-988, 2003.
9. Seib PM, et al: Blade and balloon atrial septostomy for left heart decompression in patients with severe ventricular dysfunction on extracorporeal membrane oxygenation, *Catheterization Cardiovasc Intervent* 46:179-186, 1999.
10. Chaturvedi R, et al: Cardiac ECMP for biventricular hearts after paediatric open heart surgery, *Heart* 90:545-551, 2004.
11. Chan YS, et al: Insertion of percutaneous ECMO cannula, *Am J Emerg Med* 18:184-185, 2000.
12. Pranikoff T and Hines MH: Vascular access for extracorporeal support. In Van Meurs K, Lally K, Peek G and Zwischenberger J, ed: *Extracorporeal cardiopulmonary support in critical care,* ed 3, 2005, ELSO.
13. Fortenberry JD, et al: Neutrophil and cytokine activation with neonatal extracorporeal membrane oxygenation, *J Pediatr* 128:670-678, 1996.
14. Arnold P, Jackson S, Wallis J, et al: Coagulation factor activity during neonatal extracorporeal membrane oxygenation, *Intens Care Med* 27: 1395-1400, 2001.
15. Zwischenberger JB, Bowers RM, Pickens GJ: Tension pneumothorax during extracorporeal membrane oxygenation, *Ann Thorac Surg* 47:868-871, 1989.
16. Van Meurs KP, et al: Maximum blood flow rates for arterial cannulae used in neonatal extracorporeal membrane oxygenation, *ASAIO Transactions* 36:M679-681, 1990.
17. Scott L, et al: Early enteral feedings in adults receiving venovenous extracorporeal membrane oxygenation, *JPEN* 28:295-300, 2004.

Additional Reading

Sheehan A: Bedside nursing care and ECMO specialist responsibilities. In Van Meurs K, editor: *ECMO specialist training manual,* Ann Arbor, 1999, Extracorporeal Life Support Organization.

High Frequency Oscillatory Ventilation

P U R P O S E : High frequency oscillatory ventilation is a method of ventilation in which alveolar gas exchange is maintained with supraphysiologic respiratory rates with small tidal volumes superimposed on a continuous positive pressure

Roberta L. Hales

PREREQUISITE KNOWLEDGE

- Child development as it relates to clinical assessment and implications for high frequency oscillatory ventilation (HFOV)
- Anatomy and physiology of the pediatric pulmonary system, including structural characteristics specific to the infant and child[1-4]
- Signs and symptoms of inadequate oxygenation and ventilation[2]
- Mastery of pediatric advanced life support competencies, including indications for an artificial airway and other adjuncts used to support ventilation[1]
- Endotracheal tube suctioning and care (see Procedure 2)
- Use of manual ventilation device (see Procedure 27)
- Definitions of essential terms
  - ❖ Frequency (F): Mechanical rate measured in hertz; 1 Hz = 60 breaths per minute (bpm)
  - ❖ Mean airway pressure (mPaw): Mean pressure delivered over time
  - ❖ Amplitude: Change in pressure (ΔP) generated across the mean airway pressure and measured within the circuit
  - ❖ Anatomic dead space: Volume of gas in the conducting airways, trachea to terminal bronchioles, where no gas exchange occurs
  - ❖ Attenuation: Lessening the force or magnitude of the pressures that are delivered to the child
  - ❖ Bias flow: Continuous flow of fresh gas to replenish the oxygen and remove the carbon dioxide (CO_2) from the child circuit[5-7]

- ❖ Chest wiggle factor (CWF): The body wiggle or vibration caused by high frequency ventilation (HFV)
- ❖ Power: The electrical current control that displaces the diaphragm-sealed piston. As the piston is displaced in a forward and backward square-wave pattern, amplitude pressure fluctuations are superimposed on mPaw.[6,7]
- ❖ Tidal volume (Vt): Volume of gas for each breath
- ❖ Alveolar ventilation: $(Vt)^2 \times (F)$[8,9]
- A near linear relationship exists between lung volume and surface area.[10]
- High frequency ventilation is defined by the US Food and Drug Administration as frequencies greater than 150 bpm or 2.5 Hz.[11] HFV delivers small Vts usually less than or equal to anatomic dead space volume during conventional ventilation (CV). A decoupling of oxygenation and CO_2 elimination occurs as long as the lung is inflated.[12]
- Alveolar recruitment continues for several hours after HFV therapy begins and partial pressure of CO_2 ($PaCO_2$) values may initially climb.
- Gas exchange is enhanced by additive mechanisms to the bulk flow and molecular diffusion of conventional ventilation. The exact mechanisms of gas exchange vary for different modes.[13] Suggested mechanisms include convection (bulk flow), asymmetric velocity, Taylor dispersion, pendelluft, molecular diffusion, and cardiogenic mixing (Figure 26-1).[5,8,9,13-16] Except for molecular diffusion, each mechanism involves generation of convective fluid motion.[16]
- Although study results are mixed, HFV has been used safely and effectively to reduce lung disease and mortality

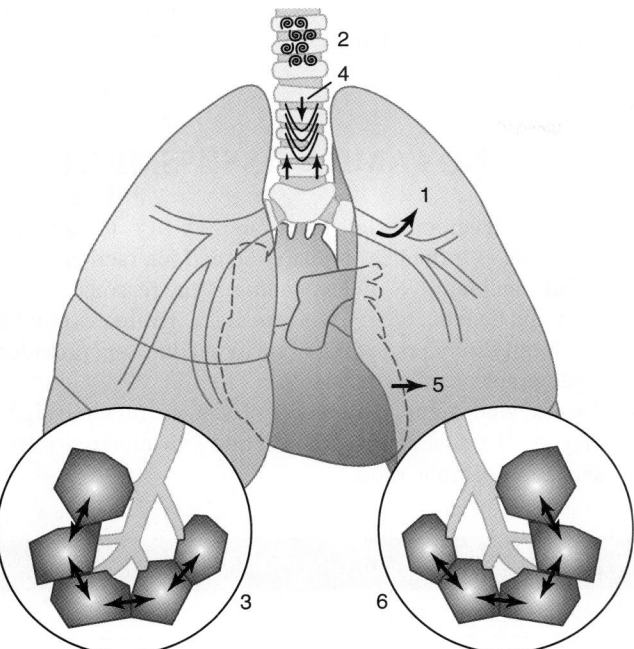

FIGURE 26-1 Mechanisms of Gas Exchange. *1,* Direct bulk convection: Provides fresh gas flow to alveoli closest to primary airways, which causes ventilation with Vt less than or equal to anatomic dead space. *2,* Taylor (longitudinal) dispersion: Radial diffusion of gas molecules across concentration gradient between center and periphery of airways. *3,* Pendeluft: High frequencies cause pressure differences in adjacent alveolar units. Movement of gas across adjacent alveolar units occurs because of inequalities of time constants and pressure gradients. *4,* Asymmetric velocity (gas) profiles: Gas in center accelerates at greater velocity and is propelled length of airway, whereas gas on periphery of airway diffuses radially. *5,* Cardiogenic mixing: Cardiac contractions may support peripheral gas mixing by causing flow within adjacent parenchymal regions. *6,* Molecular diffusion: Diffusion of gas across alveolar capillary membrane.[5,8,9,15]

rates in some groups of children and adults.[17-19] HFV has been clinically applied to children and adults with the following conditions:

* Diffuse alveolar disease, including hyaline membrane disease, acute respiratory distress syndrome (systemic inflammatory response syndrome),[20,21] and pneumonia
* Airleak syndromes, including pulmonary interstitial emphysema and persistent pneumothoraces[22,23]
* Congenital diaphragmatic hernia and pulmonary hypoplasia
* Nonhomogeneous disease, including focal pneumonia and meconium aspiration
* Failure of CV to provide adequate ventilatory support
* Several HFV modes are available. Modes are described by the delivery method and classified by the exhalation mechanism (active or passive). The most common method of HFV is HFOV.
  * High frequency oscillatory ventilation is produced by a piston pump or a diaphragm with ventilation at a frequency of 900 to 3600 cycles per second.[13] The main controls of HFOV are mPaw, driving pressure (also

known as the power), bias flow, frequency, and inspiratory time. The piston-driven devices have a piston-centering control mechanism.[13] Oxygenation is primarily controlled by mPaw and fraction of inspired oxygen concentration (FiO$_2$). The mPaw is created by resistance to the bias flow and can be adjusted with a change in the bias flow or the mPaw adjust control. The continuous mPaw sustains an "open lung" concept that optimizes lung recruitment and oxygenation.[13,20,22]

* In HFOV, inspiration and expiration are active. The gas is pushed in and out of the lungs by the piston or oscillating diaphragm. The active nature of exhalation may be an essential mechanism in prevention of gas trapping.[20]
* The HFOV power adjusts the electrical current to displace the piston, which causes pressure fluctuation (ΔP) to produce stroke volume.
* Oscillatory amplitude is the result of the ΔP produced by the forward and backward displacement of the piston to create volume displacement.[5,9,15] The ETT and respiratory system attenuate and misshape the pressure into a triangular pattern.[6,7,15,24] The smaller the ETT, the greater the attenuation, which causes smaller pressure waveforms in the alveoli. The larger the ETT, the greater the pressure waveforms, which can enhance ventilation.[5-7,15]
* During HFOV, the child exhibits a chest wiggle factor. A wiggle that extends to the umbilicus for infants, the iliac crest for children, and the mid thigh for adolescents is recommended.[25]
* Potential complications of HFOV include:
  * Hemodynamic compromise
    * Decreased venous return from increased intrapulmonary pressure
  * Barotrauma
    * Excessive air trapping (hyperinflation)[9,24,26]
    * Necrotizing tracheobronchitis and shearing of alveolar regions from high gas flow velocities
  * Inadequate humidification
    * High gas flows can cause inadequate delivery of humidity.
  * Intraventricular hemorrhage in the neonate
    * Increased intrapulmonary pressure can cause a decrease of venous blood flow back to the heart.
  * ETT obstruction
    * A sudden rise in PaCO$_2$
    * Stoppage of the HFOV from increased pressure in the system (less likely in the Sensormedics 3100B; Viasys Healthcare)
    * Loss of circuit pressure from disconnection, rupture of diaphragms in circuit, and piston/magnet dysfunction
* Initial therapeutic strategies and interventions can be guided by the child's underlying condition
  * Diffuse alveolar disease
    * A mPaw 4 to 8 cm H$_2$O higher than CV
    * Frequency set according to guidelines
    * Power/amplitude 4.0 adjust to appropriate CWF
  * Pulmonary interstitial emphysema

- ○ Set mPaw equal or less that CV
- ○ Higher frequency
- ○ Adjust power/amplitude to achieve minimal chest wall wiggle
- ❖ Gross air leak syndrome
  - ○ Initial strategy is the same as with diffuse alveolar disease.
  - ○ Achievement of adequate oxygenation as evidenced by FiO_2 of less than 60%; decrease the mPaw and power/amplitude
  - ○ SaO_2 85% to 90%
  - ○ Hypercarbia with a blood pH of more than 7.25
- ❖ Nonhomogeneous lung disease (diffuse haziness)
  - ○ A mPaw 2 to 4 cm H_2O higher than CV
  - ○ Lower frequency: 6 to 10 Hz
  - ○ Power/amplitude 4.0 adjust to appropriate CWF

- The HFOV treatment strategy recommendations differ on the basis of clinical indicators and needs of the child (Table 26-1).

CHILD AND FAMILY ASSESSMENT

- Child's developmental level and ability to interact ➥*Rationale:* Influences preparation and interaction.
- Child's and family's understanding of the reasons for and risks and benefits of HFOV ➥*Rationale:* Evaluates child's and family's understanding of the procedure and provides a gauge for ongoing education.
- Assess vital signs ➥*Rationale:* Changes in vital signs may be the first indication of child's awareness, tolerance, and complications.

TABLE 26-1	Summary Treatment Strategies	
Clinical Indicators	**Therapeutic Intervention**	**Treatment Rationale**
FiO_2 > 0.60		
High PaCO$_2$ with:		
PaO$_2$ = okay	Increase ΔP	Increase ΔP to achieve optimal PaCO$_2$
PaO$_2$ = low	Increase mPaw, ΔP, FiO$_2$	Adjust mPaw and FiO$_2$ to improve O$_2$ delivery
PaO$_2$ = high	Increase ΔP; decrease	Decrease FiO$_2$ to minimize O$_2$ exposure
FiO_2 > 0.60		
Normal PaCO$_2$ with:		
PaO$_2$ = okay	No action	No action
PaO$_2$ = low	Increase mPaw, FiO$_2$	Adjust mPaw and FiO$_2$ to improve O$_2$ delivery
PaO$_2$ = high	Decrease FiO$_2$	Decrease FiO$_2$ to minimize O$_2$ exposure
FiO_2 > 0.60		
Low PaCO$_2$ with:		
PaO$_2$ = okay	Decrease ΔP	Decrease ΔP to achieve optimal PaCO$_2$
PaO$_2$ = low	Increase mPaw, FiO$_2$; decrease ΔP	Adjust mPaw and FiO$_2$ to improve O$_2$ delivery
PaO$_2$ = high	Decrease FiO$_2$, ΔP	Decrease FiO$_2$ to minimize O$_2$ exposure
FiO_2 < 0.60		
High PaCO$_2$ with:		
PaO$_2$ = okay	Increase ΔP	Increase ΔP to achieve optimal PaCO$_2$
PaO$_2$ = low	Increase FiO$_2$; increase ΔP	Increase FiO$_2$ to improve PaO$_2$
PaO$_2$ = high	Increase ΔP; decrease mPaw	Decrease mPaw to reduce PaO$_2$
FiO_2 < 0.60		
Normal PaCO$_2$ with:		
PaO$_2$ = okay	No action	No action
PaO$_2$ = low	Increase FiO$_2$	Increase FiO$_2$ to improve PaO$_2$
PaO$_2$ = high	Decrease mPaw, FiO$_2$	Decrease mPaw to reduce PaO$_2$
FiO_2 < 0.60		
Low PaCO$_2$ with:		
PaO$_2$ = okay	Decrease ΔP	Decrease ΔP to achieve optimal PaCO$_2$
PaO$_2$ = low	Increase FiO$_2$; decrease ΔP	Increase FiO$_2$ to improve PaO$_2$
PaO$_2$ = high	Decrease mPaw; decrease ΔP	Decrease mPaw

From Viasys Healthcare, Inc., Conshohocken, PA.

FiO$_2$=Fraction of inspired oxygen; ΔP=change in pressure; PAW=mean airway pressure; PaO$_2$=Partial pressure oxygen.

- Assess respiratory status →*Rationale:* Recognition of a change in respiratory function could prevent further complications.
- Assess cardiovascular stability →*Rationale:* Inadequate mean arterial pressure results in hemodynamic instability, which causes decreased cardiac output and tissue/organ perfusion.
- Level of child's consciousness →*Rationale:* Child should be comfortable and without awareness.
- Assess intravascular volume status →*Rationale:* Volume status is increased to a central venous pressure (CVP) of approximately 10 to 15 mm Hg to handle the increase in intrapulmonary pressure.
- Observe child for signs of pain and anxiety →*Rationale:* Inadequate management of pain and anxiety can result in interference with HFOV, which may cause insufficient oxygenation and ventilation.
- Note baseline blood pH before initiation of HFOV →*Rationale:* A blood pH of less than 7.25 is buffered before initiation of oscillation. The $PaCO_2$ commonly rises for the first 2 hours after initiation of HFOV.
- Evaluate chest radiograph (CXR) before initiation of HFOV →*Rationale:* Preoscillatory CXR establishes baseline lung volumes.

CHILD AND FAMILY EDUCATION

Individualized, developmentally appropriate education is provided to the family and to the child based on desire for knowledge, readiness to learn, and overall neurologic and psychosocial state.

- Explain HFOV, including the purpose and risks to the child →*Rationale:* Providing information decreases fear and anxiety.
- Explain the assessments necessary during HFOV →*Rationale:* Knowledge that the child's condition is continuously monitored may decrease anxiety and fear.
- Provide family with descriptions and explanations of equipment alarms →*Rationale:* Increased awareness of alarms decreases fear and anxiety for the family.
- Encourage questions and answer questions as they arise →*Rationale:* Reinforcement of information is needed during periods of stress.

EQUIPMENT

- Sensormedics 3100A or 3100B
  - ❖ 3100A (Figure 26-2)
  - ❖ 3100B, size greater than 35 kg (Figure 26-3)
- Ventilator circuit, appropriately sized
- Humidifier and sterile water
- Pulse oximetry (SpO_2) monitor
- Transcutaneous CO_2 ($TcCO_2$) monitor
- Cardiorespiratory monitor
- Suction
- Oxygen and air source
- Manual ventilation device: Flow or self-inflating with appropriately sized mask
- Rubber stopper
- Intravenous fluids: Normal saline solution (NSS) or lactated Ringer's (LR) solution
- Medication: Sedation and neuromuscular blockade, as indicated

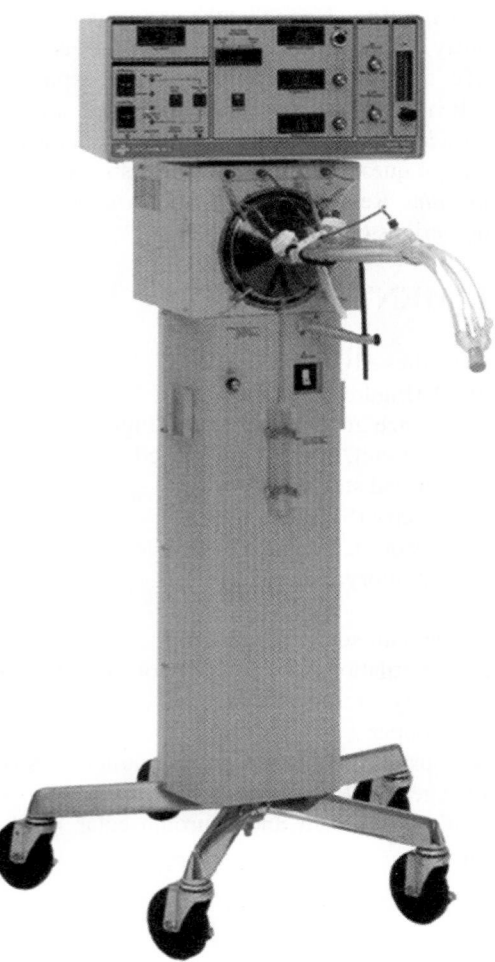

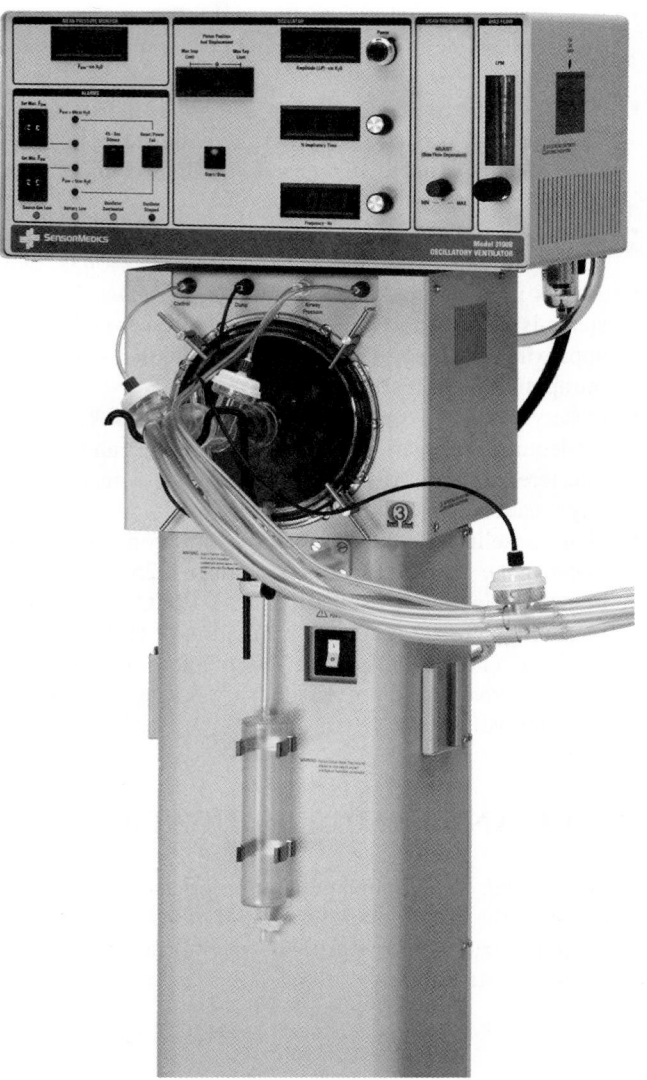

FIGURE 26-2   Sensormetics 3100A. Specifications include: bias flow, 40 lpm; max ΔP, approximately 105 cm H_2O; safety dump pressure, 50 cm H_2O; safety dump alarm delay, no delay; circuit length, 25 inches; mPaw limit, manual (approximately 10 to 45 cm H_2O); piston centering, manual; visual set maximum mPaw alarm, red LED (nonlatching); cooling gas flow, 10 lpm. *Lpm,* Liters per minute.

FIGURE 26-3   Sensormetics 3100B. The 3100B ventilator is based on technology of 3100A but features slight change to some subsystems to provide enhanced performance, safety, and reliability for its intended applications. Specifications include: bias flow, 60 lpm; max ΔP, approximately 130 cm H_2O; safety dump pressure, 60 cm H_2O; safety dump alarm delay, 1.5-second delay; circuit length, 51 inches; mPaw limit, automatic (linked to max mPaw alarm; piston centering, automatic; visual set maximum mPaw alarm, red LED (latching); cooling gas flow, 25 lpm. *Lpm,* Liters per minute.

Procedure for High Frequency Oscillatory Ventilation

Steps	Rationale	Considerations
1. Ensure child and family understand procedure and questions are answered.	Evaluates and reinforces understanding of previously taught information.[16]	Developmental, cognitive, and anxiety levels determine approach to and effectiveness of teaching.
2. Wash hands.	Reduces transmission of micro-organisms.	
3. Apply cardiorespiratory monitor, including $TcCO_2$ and SpO_2 monitors. *(Level II*)*	Indicates adequacy of ventilation and signs and symptoms of complications. Allows the practitioner to immediately respond to slight changes in CO_2 and oxygenation levels.[27]	The recommended temperature of the $TcCO_2$ monitor probe is 43°C to 43.5°C, with the site changed every 3 to 4 hours. Correlate $TcCO_2$ with arterial blood gases (ABGs).
4. The prescribing practitioner orders ventilator settings on basis of appropriate guidelines for HFOV (Table 26-2).	A practitioner's order is required for the application of mechanical ventilation.	
5. Gather needed equipment and supplies.	Facilitates completion of task in a timely manner.	Use the appropriate size circuit for the ventilator (see Figures 26-2 and 26-3).
6. Prepare delivery system for administration of intravenous fluids.	Preparation prevents delay in care. Increased intrapulmonary pressure may decrease venous return to the right heart and cause systemic hypotension.	Normal saline solution or LR solution is typically used.
7. Suction child's ETT before initiation of therapy.	Suctioning provides a mechanism of airway clearance for children with artificial airways.	Suctioning should not occur in the first 24 hours of therapy, unless it is clinically indicated.
8. Prepare appropriate medication dose for sedation and neuro-muscular blockade.	Preparation prevents delay in care.	Neuromuscular blockade may not always be necessary.
9. Administer and titrate sedation and neuromuscular blockade.[28]	Sedation and neuromuscular blockade should be adjusted to adequate levels before initiation of HFOV.	Administer the minimal dose of paralytic agent necessary to achieve the desired effect.[29]
10. Calibrate circuit and complete performance verification.	Proper function of the ventilator must be shown before initiation. Do not attempt to use another circuit configuration because this could	A rubber stopper is needed to occlude the circuit for calibration and performance procedures. Be sure the stopcock on the water trap is closed.

Procedure continues on following page

* Level II: Theory-based; no research data to support recommendations; recommendations from expert consensus group may exist

TABLE 26-2	High Frequency Oscillatory Ventilation: Setting Guidelines			
	Premature to Term Infant	**Small Child**	**Large Child**	**Adolescent**
Bias flow (lpm)	8–15	15–25	20–30	
Frequency (Hz)	15–10	10–8	8–6	6–5
Power/amplitude (ΔP)*	2 (initial setting)	2 (initial setting)	4 (initial setting)	4 (initial setting)
Inspiratory time	33%	33%	33%	33%

*Adjust power/amplitude according to good CWF.
Data from *Operators' manual 3100A high frequency oscillatory ventilator*, 2002, Sensormedics Corporation; *Operators' manual 3100B high frequency oscillatory ventilator*, 1999, Sensormedics Corporation; Viasys Healthcare, Inc., Conshohocken, PA.
Lpm, Liters per minute.

Procedure for High Frequency Oscillatory Ventilation—*Continued*

Steps	Rationale	Considerations
	result in injury to the child or operator or damage to the equipment.[6,7]	Do not use the equipment if circuit calibration or ventilator performance failure is seen.
11. Initiate ventilator settings after review of order. a. Set bias flow.	Start/stop button activates and deactivates the oscillator. Bias flow provides fresh gas to the circuit and enhances CO_2 clearance. Bias flow works interchangeably with the mPaw; adjust knob to establish the set mPaw pressure.	A green light emitting diode (LED) signifies the oscillator is enabled. If the bias flow is less than the oscillatory flow, CO_2 clearance is inadequate, reducing the ventilation affect while increasing the pressure differential to high levels (amplitude). If bias flow is greater than oscillatory flow, CO_2 clearance may be impeded. Remember to readjust the mPaw after changes in bias flow.
b. Set mPaw and increase by 1 to 2 cm H_2O every 5 minutes until oxygenation is established with SpO_2 of 90% to 93% (see Table 26-1). c. Set frequency.	The goal is maximum alveolar recruitment without overdistension of the lungs. The mPaw pressure is adjusted to maintain optimal lung volume. Frequency is the secondary control for ventilation. Frequency is dependent on the Child's size (weight).	The mPaw can fluctuate with temperature and humidity changes. Lung volumes equilibrate slowly to changes in ventilator pressures. Frequency usually needs no adjustment once the rate has been established. Frequency is not weaned as in conventional ventilation. A decrease in frequency causes an increase in volume displacement, which would decrease the $PaCO_2$ level. Too high of a frequency may cause an elevated $PaCO_2$ because of small volume displacement (less than anatomic dead space).
d. Set power control changing amplitude/ΔP and adjust by increments of 5 cm H_2O for CWF.	Adjustment of the power control changes the piston displacement, which results in a ΔP (amplitude). Amplitude/ΔP is the primary control for ventilation.	Attenuation varies according to the size of ETT. Observation of adequate CWF is the means to establish ΔP/amplitude.
e. Set inspiratory time.	The use of an I:E of 1:2 has been shown to minimize the risk of air trapping.[24]	Increasing the inspiratory time percentage is a maneuver used with the large pediatric patient when ΔP (amplitude) and frequency do not work. Caution should be used with children who have increased airway resistance.
f. Set FiO_2 and wean for SpO_2 of 90% to 93% or more unless goal is permissive hypoxemia ($SpO_2 \geq 85\%$).	Adjust FiO_2 to lowest possible level.	Inability to wean FiO_2 by 10% in the first 24 hours may constitute poor lung expansion or HFOV failure. At FiO_2 of 40% or less, reevaluate lung volume for the possibility to decrease mPaw.

Procedure for High Frequency Oscillatory Ventilation—*Continued*		
Steps	**Rationale**	**Considerations**
g. Set manual piston centering (3100A only).	Improper positioning of the piston could limit the oscillatory motion.	The 3100B automatically centers the piston.
h. Set humidification to achieve proximal airway temperature of 36°C to 37°C.	The use of heat and humidity with mechanical ventilation is necessary to prevent damage to the mucosa of the respiratory system.	High flow heated humidifiers provide variable ranges of temperature and humidity. Heated wire circuits provide heat to the gas inside the circuit.
i. Set ventilator alarms (Figure 26-4).	Ventilator alarms protect the child from injury and equipment damage. An SpO$_2$ of more than 95% may be indicative of overinflation that necessitates a decrease in the mPaw.	Set SpO$_2$ alarms at a narrow range. Loss of pressure in the circuit causes an audible and visual alarm.
j. Position child and circuit to avoid pressure areas, prevent pulling on tubing, and promote ventilator function.	Reduces the risk for skin breakdown from immobilization. Airway stability.	Avoid air mattresses because they affect the resonant frequency of the chest.[30] Angle the circuit so humidity drains to the water trap below the diaphragm.

❖ **Warning Alarms:** indicated by visual red light and audible tone
  ▪ Minimum mPaw: automatically reset with resolution of condition
  ▪ mPaw limit: automatically reset with resolution of condition
❖ **Safety Alarms:** indicated by a visual red light and audible tone.
  ▪ mPaw exceeds > 50 cmH$_2$0 (3100B: > 60 cmH$_2$0): oscillator stops and must be manually reset after resolution of condition.
  ▪ If disabled:
    • The start/stop button must be enabled (green light).
    • Push the reset button until airway pressure increases in the system.
  ▪ mPaw < 20% of Set Max mPaw on 3100A, 3100B <5 cm H$_2$0, automatically resets with resolution of low pressure condition.
  ▪ If disabled:
    • The start/stop button must be enabled (green light).
    • Push the reset button until airway pressure increases in the system.
❖ **Power Failure:** loss of power is indicated by a visual red light and audible tone
  ▪ Push the reset button
  ▪ To restart the oscillator you must push the Start/stop switch
❖ **Caution Alarms:** activate a visual yellow light with no audible. Alarms can only be reset with correction of the condition.
  ▪ Battery low
  ▪ Source gas low
  ▪ Oscillator overheated
❖ **Oscillator Stopped Alarm:** activates a visual red light and audible alarm
  ▪ Activation occurs when the ΔP is < 5-7 cmH$_2$0
  ▪ The oscillator may continue to operate under these conditions.
  ▪ Resets automatically when condition is resolved
  ▪ Note: if Start/stop was pushed to stop the oscillator the alarm is inactivated.
❖ **Thermal Cutout Safety System:** yellow caution light prior to shut down of oscillator
  ▪ This alarm is activated secondary to overheating of the oscillator.

FIGURE 26-4 HFOV safety features and alarms. *Data from Operators' manual 3100A high frequency oscillatory ventilator, 2002, Sensormedics Corporation;* Operators' manual 3100B high frequency oscillatory ventilator, *1999, Sensormedics Corporation.*

Expected Outcomes	Unexpected Outcomes
• Adequate ventilation and oxygen delivery and consumption • Improved alveolar recruitment as evidenced by improved lung expansion • Respiratory muscle rest • Hemodynamic stability and adequate blood flow to the heart • Child remains infection free • Adequate airway humidification • High frequency oscillatory ventilation instituted without injury to airway, lungs, or skin	• Inadequate ventilation and oxygenation • Lung overinflation or air leak syndrome: pneumothorax, pneuomomediastinum, pneumoperitoneum, subcutaneous emphysema • Hemodynamic compromise • Intraventricular hemorrhage (neonatal and newborn population) • Ventilator-associated pneumonia • Tenacious sputum • ETT obstruction • Barotrauma • Necrotizing tracheitis • Disruption in skin integrity

Monitoring and Care of the Child

Activities and Interventions	Rationale	Reportable Conditions
1. Review CXR within the first 4 hours, then every 12 hours for 24 hours, then every 24 hours. Do not stop the piston during the CXR.	Assists in evaluation of lung volume. Inadequate lung volume inhibits optimal gas exchange.	• Inadequate lung volume as evidenced with CXR
2. Monitor and adjust ventilator settings on basis of treatment strategies (see Table 26-1).	Maintain appropriate ventilatory support. Assists in evaluation of lung volume.	• Changes in ordered ventilator settings • Significant changes in mPaw
3. Evaluate CWF (especially important after the child's position is changed).	Evaluation of CWF alerts the clinician of changes in the child's lung compliance. Changes in CWF may indicate mucous plugging, dislocation of the endotracheal tube, or pneumothorax.	• Significant changes in CWF
4. Assess physiologic stability, including cardiac function (heart sounds, heart rate, blood pressure, and perfusion). To complete an adequate assessment of heart sounds, stop the piston by disenabling the start/stop button.	Provides information about the child's hemodynamic status. The child is especially at risk for hypotension when mPaw pressures are high and hypovolemia or cardiac dysfunction is present.	• Tachycardia • Hypotension • Poor perfusion, including cool extremities and changes in color
5. Monitor respiratory status, including work of breathing and chest auscultation, to assess the symmetry of lung sounds and note the intensity of the piston.	Changes in the symmetry of the chest or intensity of the piston could indicate changes in lung compliance, mucous plugging, endotracheal tube dislodgement, or pneumothorax.	• Signs of hypoxia, including decreased level of consciousness, tachypnea and tachycardia, increased work of breathing, cyanosis, and a decreased oxygen saturation level • Significant changes in chest sounds and intensity of piston
6. Evaluate ABGs after the first hour of initiation, then every 2 hours for 8 hours, then every 4 hours and as needed with change in clinical condition or ventilator parameters.	The ABG analysis provides quantitative measurements of CO_2 and oxygen levels.	• Significant changes from previous ABG levels
7. Continuous noninvasive respiratory monitoring, including $TcCO_2$ and SpO_2.	Noninvasive monitoring provides continuous evaluation of oxygenation and ventilation. Weaning the FiO_2 is often based on the SpO_2.	• Significant changes in $TcCO_2$ and SpO_2

Monitoring and Care of the Child—Cont'd

Activities and Interventions	Rationale	Reportable Conditions
8. Monitor TcCO$_2$ probe site. Initially evaluate and rotate site after 2 hours, then increase by 1-hour intervals to 3-hour to 4-hour schedule. If site appears reddened, decrease time interval and reevaluate.	Rotate probe site to prevent burning of the skin.	• Skin discoloration or breakdown at probe site
9. Suction ETT (see Procedure 2). If a closed suction system is used, stop the piston during the procedure and then restart. Do not disconnect the child from the HFOV.	Suctioning establishes airway patency and removes secretions.	• Inability to clear secretions • Deteriorating respiratory status
10. Note child's level of comfort and provide appropriate sedation and neuromuscular blockade.	Early identification of the child's discomfort allows for immediate attention. Adequate sedation is necessary with a neuromuscular blockade.	• Unresolved pain and discomfort • Continued irritability
11. Reposition child as tolerated.	Children are at risk for skin breakdown from immobilization.	• Any noted breakdown of skin integrity
12. Monitor humidity to ensure adequate airway humidification.	Adequate humidification is necessary to prevent mucosal damage. Inadequate humidification can cause problems with mucous plugging and decreased CWF, which decreases ventilation.	• Mucous plugs that result in decreased ventilation

Documentation

- Cardiorespiratory assessment, including vital signs, chest sounds, TcCO$_2$, SvO$_2$, and ABGs
- Date and time HFOV initiated
- Ventilator settings, including FiO$_2$, mode, frequency, mPaw, power, amplitude, Ti and bias flow (every 2 to 4 hours and with changes)
- Assessment of CWF
- Characteristics of ETT secretions
- Condition of skin at probe site
- Additional interventions and child's response
- Comfort assessment and any specific interventions provided
- Child and family education
- Unexpected outcomes and related treatment

References

1. Hazinski MF, et al, editors: *Pediatric advanced life support provider manuel,* Dallas, 2002, American Heart Association.
2. Curley MAQ, Thompson J: Oxygenation and ventilation. In Curley MAQ, Moloney-Harmon P, editors: *Nursing care of critically ill infants and children,* ed 2, Philadelphia, 2001, Saunders.
3. Thompson A: Pediatric airway management. In Fuhrman B, Zimmerman J, editors: *Pediatric critical care,* ed 3, Philadelphia, 2006, Mosby.
4. McCance K, Huether S: *Pathophysiology: the biologic bases for disease in adults and children,* Philadelphia, 2002, Mosby.
5. Durand DJ, Asselin JM: High Frequency ventilation: theory and clinical strategy, Division of Neonatology and the Department of Respiratory Therapy, Children's Hospital of Oakland. Unpublished manuscript.
6. Operators' manual 3100A high frequency oscillatory ventilator, 2002, Sensormedics Corporation, Yorba Linda, CA.
7. Operators' manual 3100B high frequency oscillatory ventilator, 1999, Sensormedics Corporation, Yorba Linda, CA.
8. Chan V, Greenough: The effect of frequency on carbon dioxide levels during high frequency oscillation, *J Perinat Med* 22L: 103-106, 1994.

9. Priebe GP, Arnold JH: High frequency oscillatory ventilation in pediatric patients, *Respir Care Clin North Am* 7,4:633-645, 2001.

10. Null D, Perlman N: High frequency oscillatory ventilation: disease specific clinical management strategies, *Critical care review current applications and economics, Sensormedics Corporation,* 1-4, 1999.

11. Office of Device Evaluation, US Food and Drug Administration, Office of Device Recognized Consensus Standards: *Part B Supplementary information ASTM F1100-90 standard specification for ventilators intended for use in critical care,* retrieved July 5, 2006, from http://www.access-data.fda.gov/scripts/cdrh/cfdocs/cfStandards/search.cfm.

12. Duval ELIM, Maarkhorst DG, et al: High frequency oscillatory ventilation in pediatric patients, *Neth J Med* 56:177-185, 2000.

13. Venkataraman ST: Mechanical ventilation and respiratory care. In Fuhrman B, Zimmerman J, editors: *Pediatric critical care,* Philadelphia, 2006, Elsevier.

14. Chang HK: Mechanisms of gas transport during ventilation by high-frequency oscillation, *J Appl Physiol* 56:3,553-563, 1984.

15. Johnson J: *HFOV slide show.* Unpublished material. 2002.

16. Pillow JJ: High frequency oscillatory ventilation: mechanisms of gas exchange and lung mechanics, *Crit Care Med* 33(10 Suppl):S135-S141, 2005.

17. Hynes-Gay P, MacDonald R: Using high frequency oscillatory ventilation to treat adults with acute respiratory distress syndrome, *Crit Care Nurs* 21(5):38-46, 2001.

18. Bollen C, et al: Cumulative metaanalysis of high-frequency versus conventional ventilation in premature neonates, *Am J Respir Crit Care Med* 168:1150-1155, 2003.

19. Courtney SE, et al: High frequency oscillatory ventilation versus conventional mechanical ventilation for very-low-birth-weight infants, *N Eng J Med* 347:643-652, 2002.

20. Chan K, Stewart T: Clinical use of high-frequency oscillatory ventilation in adult patients with acute and respiratory distress syndrome, *Crit Care Med* 33(3 Suppl):S170-S174, 2005.

21. Mehta S, et al: High frequency oscillatory ventilation in adults: the Toronto experience, *Chest* 126:518-527, 2004.

22. Froese A, Kinsella J: High frequency oscillatory ventilation: lessons from the neonatal/pediatric experience, *Crit Care Med* 33(3 Suppl):S115-S121, 2005.

23. Pokora T, et al: Neonatal high-frequency jet ventilation, *Pediatrics* 72:27-32, 1983.

24. Grenier B, Thompson J: High-Frequency oscillatory ventilation in pediatric patients, *Resp Care Clin North Am* 2,4:545-557, 1996.

25. Sweeney A-M, Lyle J, Ferguson N: Nursing and infection control issues during high-frequency oscillatory ventilation, *Crit Care Med* 33(3 Suppl):S204-S208, 2005.

26. Beamer WC, et al: High frequency jet ventilation produces auto-PEEP, *Crit Care Med* 12:734-735, 1984.

27. Berkenbosh JW, Tobias JD: Transcutaneous carbon dioxide monitoring during high frequency oscillatory ventilation in infants and children, *Crit Care Med* 30(5):1024-1027, 2002.

28. Sessler C: Sedation, analgesia and neuromuscular blockage for high frequency oscillatory ventilation, *Crit Care Med* 33(3 Suppl):S209-S216, 2005.

29. Marraro GA: Innovative practices of ventilatory support with pediatric patients, *Pediatr Crit Care Med* 4(1):8-20, 2003.

30. Curley MAQ, Molengraft J: Care of the child supported on high frequency oscillatory ventilation, *AACN Clin Iss* 5(1):49-58, 1994.

Additional Readings

Arnold JH, et al: High frequency ventilation in pediatric respiratory failure, *Crit Care Med* 21:272-278, 1993.

Arnold JH: High frequency oscillatory ventilation: theory and practice in paediatric patients, *Paed Anaest* 6:437-441, 1996.

Arnold JH, et al: Prospective randomized comparison of high frequency oscillatory ventilation and conventional mechanical ventilation in pediatric respiratory failure, *Crit Care Med* 22:1530-1539, 1994.

Avila K, et al: High frequency oscillatory ventilation: a nursing approach to bedside care, *Neonatal Network* 13(5):23-30, 1994.

Clark RH: High frequency ventilation in pediatric respiratory failure: a multicenter experience, *Crit Care Med* 28(12):3941-3942, 2000.

Dobyns E, et al: Interactive effects of high frequency ventilation and inhaled nitric oxide in acute hypoxemic respiratory failure in pediatrics, *Crit Care Med* 30(11):2425-2429, 2002.

Gerstman DR, et al: The provo multicenter early high frequency oscillatory ventilation trial: improved pulmonary and clinical outcome in respiratory distress syndrome, *Pediatrics* 98:1044-1057, 1996.

Gutierriz JA, et al: Hemodynamic effects of high frequency oscillatory ventilation in severe pediatric respiratory failure, *Intens Care Med* 21:505-510, 1995.

Hales R, et al: Early Intervention with HFOV and APRV for a pediatric patient with aspiration pneumonitis: a case study [abstract], *Respir Care* 47(9):1035, 2002.

Kemp J: Nursing care of the baby receiving high frequency ventilation: the importance of familiarity with the ventilation technique, *Neonatal Nurs* 3(2):31-35, 1997.

Krishman JA, Brower RG: High frequency ventilation for acute lung injury and ARDS, *Chest* 118(3):795-807, 2000.

MacIntyre N, Branson R: Humidification and aerosol therapy during mechanical ventilation. *Mechanical ventilation,* Philadelphia, 2001, Saunders.

MacIntyre N, Branson R: High frequency ventilation. *Mechanical ventilation,* Philadelphia, 2001, Saunders.

Moromisato DY, et al: Mercury inhalation poisoning and acute lung injury in a child, *Chest* 105:613-615, 1994.

Papazian L, et al: Comparison of prone positioning and high frequency oscillatory ventilation in patients with acute respiratory distress syndrome, *Crit Care Med* 33(10):2162-2171, 2005.

Rosenberg RB, et al: High frequency ventilation for acute pediatric respiratory failure, *Chest* 104:1216-1221, 1993.

Sarnaik RP, et al: Predicting outcome in children with severe acute respiratory failure treated with high frequency ventilation, *Crit Care Med* 24:1396-1402, 1996.

Schexnayder SM, et al: High frequency oscillatory ventilation as a bridge to extracorporeal membrane oxygenation in pediatric respiratory failure, *Resp Care* 40:44-47, 1995.

Thome U, et al: Ventilation strategies and outcomes in randomized trials of high frequency ventilation, *Arch Dis Childhood Fetal Neonatal* 90:F466-F473, 2005.

Touch SM, Greenspan JS: High frequency ventilation. In Festa CJ, editor: *Clinical guidelines for mechanical ventilation,* Newtown, PA, 2002, Handbooks in Health Care Co.

Van Genderingen HR, et al: Reduction of oscillatory pressure along the endotracheal tube is indicative for maximal respiratory compliance during high frequency ventilation: a mathematical model study, *Pediatr Pulmon* 31:458-463, 2001.

Venegas JG, et al: Understanding the pressure cost of ventilation: why does high frequency work? *Crit Care Med* (9):S49-57, 1994.

Manual Ventilation Devices

PURPOSE: A manual ventilation device is used to provide manual ventilation for a child in whom spontaneous ventilation is impaired or absent and for suctioning or emergency situations in children with artificial airways

Laurie S. Finger

PREREQUISITE KNOWLEDGE

- Child development as it relates to clinical assessment and procedure
- Anatomy and physiology of the pediatric pulmonary system, including structural characteristics specific to the infant and child[1,3]
    - The airway diameter of the infant and young child is smaller than that of an adult (see Figure 1-1 in Procedure 1). Circumferential edema narrows an infant's airway by 75% (as opposed to 40% in the adult) and produces a 16-fold rise in resistance to airflow that leads to a substantial increase in the infant's work of breathing.[1,3]
    - The tongue of the infant is relatively larger in the oropharynx as compared with the adult's tongue. Therefore, the tongue occupies more space in the mouth and becomes the primary obstruction in an unconscious infant. Appropriate head position is crucial to opening the airway.[1,3]
    - The larynx of the infant and young child is more anterior and cephalad than the adult's, and the epiglottis is longer and floppier.[1,3]
    - The chest wall of the infant and young child is more compliant, and the chest wall muscles are less developed than in the adult, which makes sustaining high respiratory rates for long periods of time more difficult (see Figure 23-1 in Procedure 23). Children simply tire more quickly than do adults.[1,3]
    - Because of an increase in metabolic rate, the child's oxygen consumption is high. In a respiratory

crisis, the child becomes hypoxemic earlier than an adult.[3]

- Infants and young children are more at risk for respiratory failure from upper and lower respiratory infections, obstructions, and foreign bodies than are adults because of anatomic and physiologic differences in the airways and lungs.
- Mastery of pediatric advanced life support competencies[1]
- Signs and symptoms of inadequate oxygenation and ventilation.
- Endotracheal tube (ETT) suctioning and care (see Procedure 2)
- An appropriately sized mask provides a tight seal and fits so that it extends from the bridge of the nose to the cleft of the chin, encompassing the mouth and nose. Care must be taken to avoid placement of the mask too high over the eyes or too low over the chin (see Figure 8-1 in Procedure 8).[1,3,4]
- The two basic types of manual ventilation devices are self-inflating and flow-inflating devices (Figure 27-1).
    - Self-inflating devices: The standard self-inflating bag consists of mask or ETT connector, a thick plastic reservoir bag for fresh gas, a valve system to control air flow, and sometimes a distal port for oxygen and oxygen reservoir bag.[1,5]
        - Self-inflating devices expand spontaneously (independent of gas flow) after compression, drawing in either ambient air or oxygen through a one-way intake valve. During bag compression, the valve closes and a second valve opens to force gas into the child's airway. When the bag is released, an

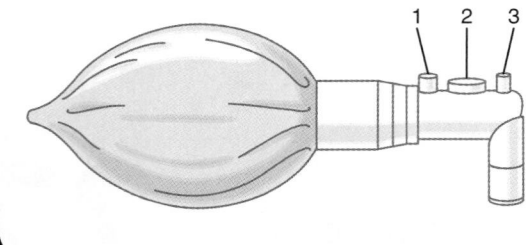

A

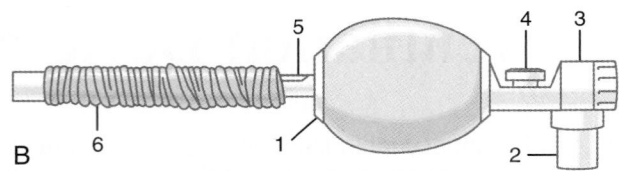

B

FIGURE 27-1   Manual Ventilation Devices. **A,** Flow-inflating manual ventilation device. *1,* Oxygen inlet; *2,* flow-control valve; *3,* pressure manometer attachment site. **B,** Self-inflating manual resuscitation devices. *1,* Oxygen inlet; *2,* patient outlet; *3,* one-way valve assembly; *4,* pressure-relief (pop-off) valve; *5,* air inlet; *6,* optional oxygen reservoir.

outlet valve permits the exhaled gases to be vented to the atmosphere and the bag self inflates.

- A self-inflating bag delivers only room air unless supplementary oxygen is attached.[6]
- A pediatric bag requires a minimum of 10 to 15 L/min and an adult bag requires at least 15 L/min for the inflow rate to maintain adequate volume in the reservoir. The concentration of oxygen delivered depends on the liter flow and the tidal volume (Vt) and peak inspiratory flow rate. With 10 L/min delivered, the concentration of oxygen varies from 30% to 80%. For delivery of a higher oxygen concentration between 60% and 95%, an oxygen reservoir must be attached and an oxygen flow of 10 to 15 L/min into a reservoir is required.[6,7,8,9]
- A pressure release valve is often a part of these bags to limit the impact of barotrauma. In emergency situations, a bag without a pop-off valve should be used to ensure adequate tidal volume.[1]
- Self-inflating devices are available in at least three sizes: neonatal, pediatric, and adult. A pediatric self-inflating bag with a volume of 450 to 500 mL is recommended because smaller bags may not deliver an effective Vt or the inspiratory times needed by full-term infants.[10-12] For larger children and young adults, the adult devices provide volumes of greater than 750 mL.[1,3,4]
- The advantages of self-inflating devices include the ability to use the device without an external oxygen source, the ability to refill spontaneously after being squeezed, the technical ease of use of this device over the flow-inflating device, and the availability of a pressure-release "pop-off" valve to prevent overinflation when too much pressure is applied to the device.[1,3,4]

- The disadvantages of a self-inflating device include the ability to refill with or without a tight seal with a mask on the child's face, the requirement of a reservoir to deliver 100% oxygen, inability to provide 100% free-flow (blow-by) oxygen, and the difficulty of providing high-inflating pressures (that may be needed to adequately inflate a child's lungs) unless the "pop-off" valve is occluded or disabled.[1,3,4]
- ❖ Flow-inflating devices: A flow-inflating manual ventilation system is made up of a soft reservoir bag, a pressure monitoring port, a pressure relief (expiratory) valve, and an oxygen outlet for the gas flow needed to inflate the bag.[5,6,9]
  - When oxygen flows into a flow-inflating manual ventilation device, the gas continues out through the patient outlet without inflating the reservoir bag unless the outlets are occluded. To support inhalation and inflate the reservoir bag, the patient outlet (with mask attached) is properly sealed on the child's face, the flow-control valve is open to allow continuous flow of compressed gases (from the oxygen source), either the pressure manometer attachment site is attached to a manometer or the exhalation valve is partially closed, and the device has no leaks or tears.[1,3,4,5,8]
  - Manual flow-inflating bags generally require more expertise because of the need to adjust the air flow and adjust the outlet control valve to manage the volume of gas in the reservoir.
  - An inline manometer is recommended to monitor volume of collected gas and its resulting pressure to prevent barotrauma.[2] The manometer also helps to assess breath-to-breath inflation consistency.
  - At least 250 mL/kg/min is needed for the bag to inflate.[1] If the valve is too far opened, the gas escapes, resulting in collapse of the bag. If the exhalation valve is closed too much, the bag overinflates and produces high airway pressures. If the valve is too tight, unsatisfactory washout of exhaled gases may lead to rebreathing of exhaled air and hypercapnia.[8] In addition, the bag may refill too slowly to ensure an adequate quantity of gas for the next breath.
  - The volume of the reservoir bag is based on the size of the child. A 500-mL bag can be used for an infant, a 600-mL to 1000-mL bag can be used for a child, and a 1500-mL to 2000-mL bag can be used for an adult.[1]
  - The advantages of a flow-inflating device include the ability to administer 100% oxygen at all times, the added consistency (over self-inflating bags) in delivering gas,[2] the ability to more easily assess the seal of the face mask (with the degree of bag inflation), and the added capacity to assess lung compliance by an experienced practitioner.[1,3,4]
  - The disadvantages of a flow-inflating device are the requirement of an external oxygen source and a tight seal with the face mask to make the bag inflate, the additional practice needed for effective use, and the usual absence of a pressure release valve.[1,3,4]

- Minute ventilation is determined by the Vt and ventilation rate. Only the inspiratory force and TV needed to cause the chest to rise visibly are used.[10] Excessive force and TV may cause overinflation of the lungs, impeding venous return, and inflation of the stomach, leading to vomiting and aspiration.[1,3,4]
- Manual ventilation devices may be used in a one-practitioner or two-practitioner technique.
  - ❖ The one-practitioner technique requires the practitioner to tilt the child's head back with the heal of one hand, holding the mask and applying downward pressure with the thumb and index finger and placing the three remaining fingers along the angle of the jaw to elevate the jaw while squeezing the manual ventilation device with the other hand (Figure 27-2).[1]
  - ❖ When two people are available, one practitioner uses both hands to open the airway and apply a firm seal with the mask on the face and the second practitioner squeezes the manual ventilation device. The two-practitioner technique may be more effective than the one-practitioner technique. This technique provides a better seal and may be necessary in children with increased airway resistance or noncompliant lungs (Figure 27-3).[1,11,16]

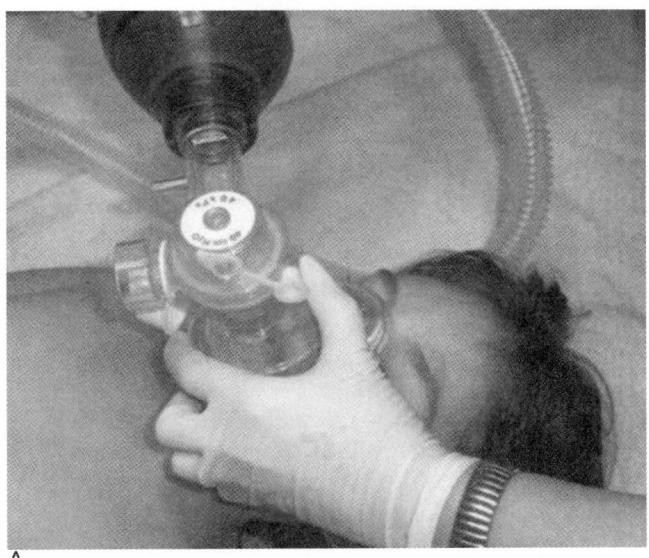

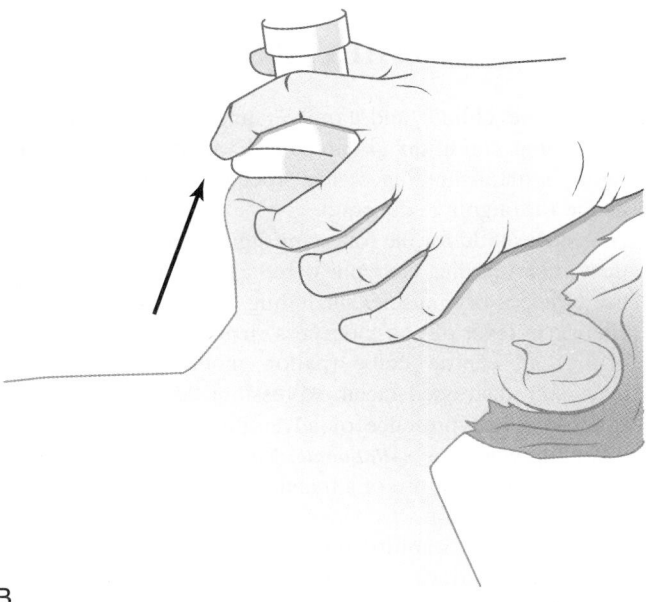

A   B

FIGURE 27-2   Proper Technique for One-Person Manual Ventilation. **A,** *Top view:* Mask is held in place with thumb and forefinger forming a C. **B,** *Side view:* Fingers form "E" to lift jaw and avoid soft tissues of neck to prevent laryngeal tracheal compression.

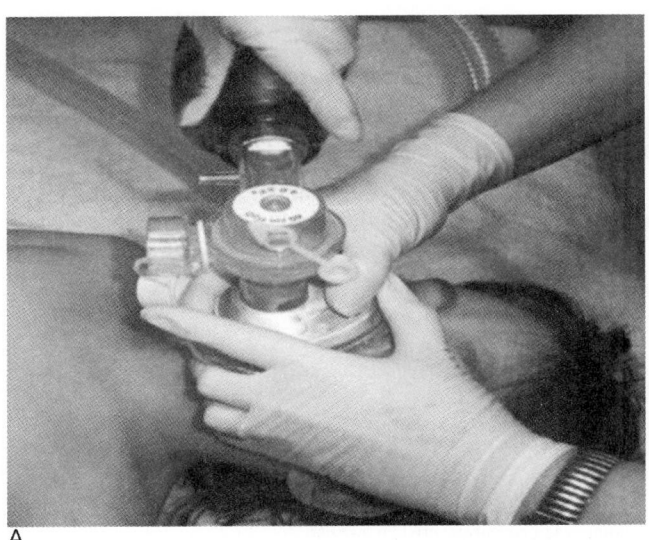

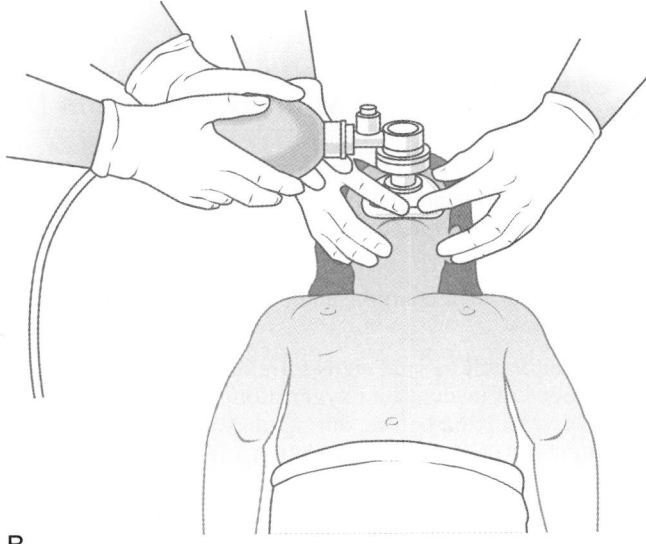

A   B

FIGURE 27-3   Proper Technique for Two-person Manual Ventilation. **A,** *Top view:* First person holds mask and second person compresses ventilation bag. **B,** *Side view:* Both hands of first person are used to open airway and maintain tight seal of face mask.

- In children with artificial airways, manual ventilation devices are used with attachment of the device to the end of the airway and compression of the bag with enough TV and force to raise the chest wall.
- A risk of gastric inflation from spillover of gases exists with manual ventilation. The gastric distention that results may interfere with effective ventilation and cause vomiting and aspiration. Several strategies can be used to minimize gastric inflation including avoiding excessive peak inspiratory pressures, applying cricoid pressure (only used in nonresponsive children) during intubation and by using a nasogastric or orogastric tube for decompression.[10,11,13]

CHILD AND FAMILY ASSESSMENT

- Assess the child's and family's understanding of the underlying condition ➛**Rationale:** Evaluates child's and family's understanding of the procedure and provides a gauge for ongoing education.
- Assess the child for the following signs of respiratory distress: tachycardia; tachypnea; retractions; nasal flaring; use of accessory muscles, including grunting and stridor; change in level of consciousness (irritable to obtunded); change in central color (pallor, mottling, duskiness, cyanosis); distressed facial expression; decreased breath sounds; or the presence of adventitious breath sounds, including wheezing ➛**Rationale:** Respiratory status determines the need for use of a manual ventilation device and further intervention.
- Assess the child's ability to maintain cardiac and respiratory stability during manual ventilation ➛**Rationale:** Determines the need for a second person to perform hyperoxygenation/hyperventilation.

CHILD AND FAMILY EDUCATION

Individualized, developmentally appropriate education is provided to the family and to the child based on desire for knowledge, readiness to learn, and overall neurologic and psychosocial state.

- In nonemergent situations, such as before suctioning and during transportation, explain to the child and family the necessity and purpose of the manual ventilation device ➛**Rationale:** Knowledge improves the child's and family's understanding of the procedure, deceases fear and anxiety, and increases cooperation with the plan of care.
- After emergent use for resuscitation and intubation, explain to the family the necessity and purpose of the manual ventilation device ➛**Rationale:** Knowledge improves the family's understanding of the plan of care for the child and decreases fear and anxiety.
- Encourage questions and answer questions as they arise ➛**Rationale:** Reinforcement of information is needed during periods of stress.

EQUIPMENT

- Manual self-inflating or flow-inflating ventilation device
- Face mask of appropriate size, as indicated
- Oxygen source and tubing, as indicated
- Oxygen analyzer and blender when child needs fractional amounts of oxygen (FiO_2)
- Positive end-expiratory pressure (PEEP) valve, depending on child's need for PEEP of more than 5 cm H_2O
- Pressure manometer to gauge peak inspiratory pressures, as indicated
- Stethoscope, as needed
- Clean gloves, including personal protective equipment as indicated, such as eye protection and mask

Procedure for a Manual Ventilation Device

Steps	Rationale	Considerations
1. Ensure child and family understand procedure and questions are answered.	Evaluates and reinforces understanding of previously taught information.	Developmental, cognitive, and anxiety levels determine approach to and effectiveness of teaching.
2. Gather needed equipment and supplies.	Facilitates completion of task in a timely manner.	
3. Monitor child's vital signs for indications of inadequate oxygenation and ventilation before, during, and after use of a manual ventilation device. (*Level II**)	Identifies adequacy of ventilation and signs and symptoms of complications.	

* Level II: Theory-based; no research data to support recommendations; recommendations from expert consensus group may exist

Procedure	**for a Manual Ventilation Device**—*Continued*	
Steps	**Rationale**	**Considerations**
4. Wash hands and put on clean gloves and personal protective equipment, including eye protection; mask, and gown (as indicated). *(Level VI*)*	Reduces transmission of infection. Protects personnel health from exposure to microbial pathogens and body fluids.	
5. Assess lung sounds.	Indicates adequacy of ventilation. Comparison for postprocedural auscultation.	
6. Assess the manual ventilation device for proper functioning. If an oxygen source is necessary, assure the manual ventilation device is connected and sufficient flow of oxygen exists to maintain the reservoir's inflation (Figure 27-4).	Helps to ensure adequate ventilation during use. Helps to ensure the child receives an adequate amount of oxygen during manual ventilation. Flow-inflating devices only fill if attached to an external source of oxygen.[1,3,4]	May need to adjust flow from oxygen source and exhalation valve before use. The appropriate amount of inflation can be achieved by setting the flow meter between 5 and 10 L/min, assuming an adequate seal.[4] A self-inflating manual ventilation device may be used without an oxygen source, but ideally, during resuscitation and suctioning, oxygen should be used.[1,3,4] *(Level V*)* The self-inflating device delivers 21% oxygen if no external oxygen source is available.

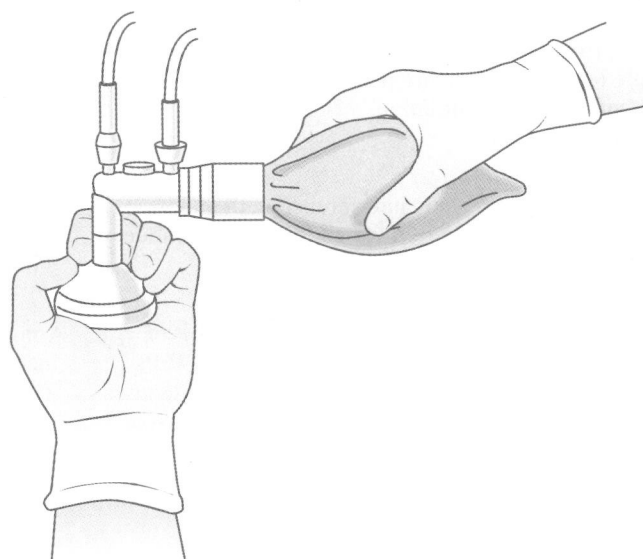

FIGURE 27-4   Testing of flow-inflating manual device. Test for sufficient flow of oxygen to maintain reservoir's inflation.

7. When the child needs a face mask: a. Attach the appropriately sized mask to the end of the manual ventilation device.	An appropriately sized mask provides a tight seal; otherwise, oxygen escapes around the mask and the child may receive inadequate ventilation. The appropriately sized mask also prevents injury to the child's face.[1,3,4]	

Procedure continues on following page

* Level V: Clinical studies in more than one or two patient populations and situations to support recommendations
Level VI: Clinical studies in a variety of patient populations and situations to support recommendations

Procedure for a Manual Ventilation Device—*Continued*

Steps	Rationale	Considerations
b. Position the child to optimally open and align the airway (see Figure 15-4 in Procedure 15).[1,3,4] *(Level V*)* c. Apply appropriately sized mask to the child's face (see Figure 8-1 in Procedure 8).[1,4]	Positioning aligns the posterior pharynx, larynx, and trachea, allowing easy air entry.[1,4] *(Level V*)*	Exact positioning depends on the age and disposition of the child (see Figure 15-4 in Procedure 15). Hyperextension of the neck may restrict air entry.[1,4]
8. When child has an artificial airway: a. Remove child from ventilator or other oxygen delivery device. b. Attach manual ventilation device to airway at patient outlet.	The device must be attached directly to the artificial airway for ventilation to take place.	
9. Compress the manual ventilation device, with only enough Vt and inspiratory force to see the child's chest rise gently.[1,3,4] *(Level V*)*	Use of excess inspiratory force or Vt may cause barotrauma and stomach insufflation.	For self-inflating bags, depressing or disabling the "pop-off" valve may lead to excess inspiratory pressure.[1,3,4]
10. If needed for adequate ventilation, adjust the pressure delivered and inflation of the reservoir at either the flow meter on the oxygen source or the flow-control valve.[4]	Ensures adequacy of inspiratory pressure and Vt.	An overinflated device may deliver excessive pressure to the child, and an underinflated device may collapse completely, taking too long to refill between breaths.[1,4]
11. Ventilate at a rate that maintains adequate oxygenation and ventilation. *(Level V*)* Use appropriate Vt and inspiratory time to allow lungs to fully expand and sufficient expiratory time to allow for escape of carbon dioxide (CO_2).	Ventilation rates vary according to the child's age and clinical needs. Sufficient inspiratory and expiratory time are needed for adequate ventilation.[1,3]	In addition to chest rise, oxygen saturations, heart rate, and adequate aeration noted during auscultation are used to assess the adequacy of ventilatory breaths.
12. In the presence of spontaneous breathing, attempt to synchronize manual ventilations with the child's own ventilatory efforts.[16]	Prevents interference with and enhances the child's own ventilatory efforts.	Overriding of the child's respiratory rate may be needed depending on child's condition and intrinsic rate.
13. With use of a PEEP valve or pressure manometer, provide the same PEEP and peak inspiratory pressures (PiP) as the child receives from HV ventilation.	Children on more than a PEEP of 5 cm H_2O or who have high PiPs need continuation of these pressures during manual ventilation to avoid atelectasis and maintain ventilation and oxygenation.[3]	A higher PEEP or PiP may be necessary depending on the child's condition.
14. For the child with an artificial airway, reattach the ventilator or other oxygen delivery device to the artificial airway.		
15. Remove personal protective equipment and wash hands.	Reduces transmission of infection.	

* Level V: Clinical studies in more than one or two patient populations and situations to support recommendations

Expected Outcomes	Unexpected Outcomes
• Appropriate oxygen, PEEP, and PiP are provided to meet the child's needs	• Overinflation or underinflation of the lungs • Inadequate oxygenation and ventilation • Hypoxemia • Barotrauma, pneumothorax • Atelectasis
• Hemodynamic stability • Equipment is fully functional before, during, and after procedure • Adequate seal of face mask maintained	• Hemodynamic instability • Equipment failure • Accidental extubation • Inability to maintain an adequate seal with the face mask
• Child maintains an acceptable level of comfort	• Unmanaged pain and irritability

Monitoring and Care of the Child

Activities and Interventions	Rationale	Reportable Conditions
1. Assess respiratory status and the need for manual ventilation. 2. Evaluate the effectiveness and functionality of the manual ventilation device during use.	Provides indications for manual ventilation. Determines the ability of the manual device to ventilate the child.	• Deteriorating respiratory status • Inability to manually ventilate child despite proper airway, seal, and equipment • Lack of chest rise with appropriate TV and inspiratory force
3. Physiologic stability, including vital signs, oxygen saturations, and clinical condition during and after use of the manual ventilation device.	Change in vital signs and clinical appearance may indicate inadequate oxygenation and ventilation.	• Hemodynamic instability, including sudden tachycardia, bradycardia, and hypotension that do not respond to the use of the manual ventilation device • Significant changes in oxygenation saturation and arterial/venous blood gases • Increased work of breathing, including nasal flaring, accessory muscle use, and retractions
4. Assess comfort and provide appropriate interventions.	Early identification of the child's discomfort allows for immediate attention.	• Report of unresolved pain and discomfort

Documentation

- Impetus for manual ventilation, including respiratory assessment
- Date, time, and frequency of procedure
- Child's response to manual ventilation, including postprocedure respiratory assessment
- Additional interventions needed before, during, and after procedure
- Comfort assessment and any specific interventions provided
- Child and family education
- Unexpected outcomes and related treatment

References

1. Hazinski MF, Zaritzky AL, Nadkarni V, et al, editors: *Pediatric advanced life support provider manuel,* Dallas, 2002, American Heart Association.

2. Hussey S, Ryan C, Murphy B: Comparison of three manual ventilation devices using an intubated mannequin, *Arch Dis Childhood Fetal Neonatal* 89(6):F490-493, 2004.

3. Curley MAQ, Thompson JF: Oxygenation and ventilation. In Curley MAQ, Moloney-Harmon PA, editors: *Critical care nursing of infants and children,* ed 2, Philadelphia, 2001, Saunders.

4. *Textbook of neonatal resuscitation,* ed 4, 2000, American Academy of Pediatric and American Heart Association.

5. Escobedo M, Engle W, Myers T: Positive pressure ventilation devices for neonatal resuscitation, PowerPoint Presentation NRP, Current Issues Seminar, retrieved July 1, 2006, from *http://www.aap.org/nrp/pdf/PositivePressure Ventilation.pdf.*

6. American Heart Association: Guidelines for cardiopulmonary resuscitation and emergency cardiovascular care part 11: pediatric basic life support, *Circulation* 112(Suppl 24):156-166, 2005.

7. Finer NN, Barrington KJ, Al-Fadley F, et al: Limitations of self-inflating resuscitators, *Pediatrics* 77:417-420, 1986.

8. Trimble T: *Using anesthesia bags,* Emergency Nursing World, 2005, retrieved July 1, 2006, from http://www.enw.org/A-Bags.htm.

9. Thompson A: Pediatric airway management. In Fuhrman B, Zimmerman J, editors: *Pediatric critical care,* ed 3, Philadelphia, 2006, Elsevier.

10. American Heart Association: Guidelines for cardiopulmonary resuscitation and emergency cardiovascular care part 12: pediatric advanced life support, *Circulation* 112(Suppl 24):167-187, 2005.

11. Jesudian MC, Harrison RR, Keenan RL, et al: Bag-valve-mask ventilation; two rescuers are better than one: preliminary report, *Crit Care Med* 13:122-123, 1985.

12. Terndrup TE, Kanter RK, Cherry RA: A comparison of infant ventilation methods performed by prehospital personnel, *Ann Emerg Med* 18:607-611, 1989.

13. Field D, Milner AD, Hopkin IE: Efficiency of manual resuscitators at birth, *Arch Dis Child* 61:300-302, 1986.

14. Berg MD, Idris AH, Berg RA: Severe ventilatory compromise due to gastric distention during pediatric cardiopulmonary resuscitation, *Resuscitation* 36:71-73, 1998.

15. Moynihan RJ, Brock-Utne JG, Archer JH, et al: The effect of cricoid pressure on preventing gastric insufflation in infants and children, *Anesthesiology* 78:652-656, 1993.

16. Burns S: Manual self-inflating resuscitation manual ventilation device. In Lynn-McHale D, Carlson K, editors: *AACN procedure manual for critical care,* ed 4, Philadelphia, 2001, Saunders.

Mechanical Ventilation: Conventional Modes

PURPOSE: Conventional modes of mechanical ventilation provide positive pressure ventilation for improvement in oxygenation and ventilation, airway protection, and physiologic support of a critically ill child

Holly F. Webster

PREREQUISITE KNOWLEDGE

- Child development as it relates to clinical assessment and implications for conventional modes of mechanical ventilation
- Anatomy and physiology of the pediatric pulmonary system, including structural characteristics specific to the infant and child[1-3]
- Signs and symptoms of inadequate oxygenation and ventilation[1]
- Mastery of pediatric advanced life support competencies, including indications for an artificial airway and other adjuncts used to support ventilation[2]
- Endotracheal tube (ETT) suctioning and care (see Procedure 2)
- Use of manual ventilation device (see Procedure 27)
- The mechanism of inspiration and expiration in the spontaneously breathing child occurs with contraction of the diaphragm, which flattens and expands the volume of the chest cavity. The structures of the thoracic cavity create a force that holds back lung inflation; therefore, a certain amount of force is needed to overcome the natural impedance that the structures generate.[4] In turn, increased *negative* intrapleural pressure is generated and causes gas to flow inward. Exhalation is passive, created by the elastic recoil of the lung (Figure 28-1).
- Resistance, compliance, functional residual capacity (FRC), and closing capacity (CC) may be altered by

pulmonary conditions and are mediated by specific ventilatory interventions.
- In infants and small children (<6 years of age), CC is greater than FRC, which accounts for the susceptibility of infants and young children to atelectasis.[4]
- Airway resistance spreads evenly between the upper and lower airways in infants; as children age, the upper airways encounter more of the airway resistance.[4]
- Physiologic concepts of lung mechanics that interface with the ventilator[3] (Box 28-1)
- Lung volumes and capacities (Figure 28-2)
- Differences in lung volumes for infants and adults (Figure 28-3)
- Tidal volume (Vt) is the volume of gas that flows to the alveoli during inspiration. A normal Vt value is 6 to 8 mL/kg, regardless of age, dependant on age and size of the child. Part of this volume remains in the upper airways where no gas exchange occurs and is referred to as deadspace ventilation (VD). VD values average 1 to 2 mL/kg and comprise approximately 25% to 30% of the Vt. The deadspace may be increased in lung disease, most commonly from ventilation/perfusion (V/Q) mismatching. With the addition of an ETT, deadspace is augmented.
- Interface between volume and pressure for the thorax, lungs, and chest wall for the adult, infant, and infant with decreased compliance (Figure 28-4)
- Mechanical ventilation that provides positive pressure initiates inspiration with application of pressure, which

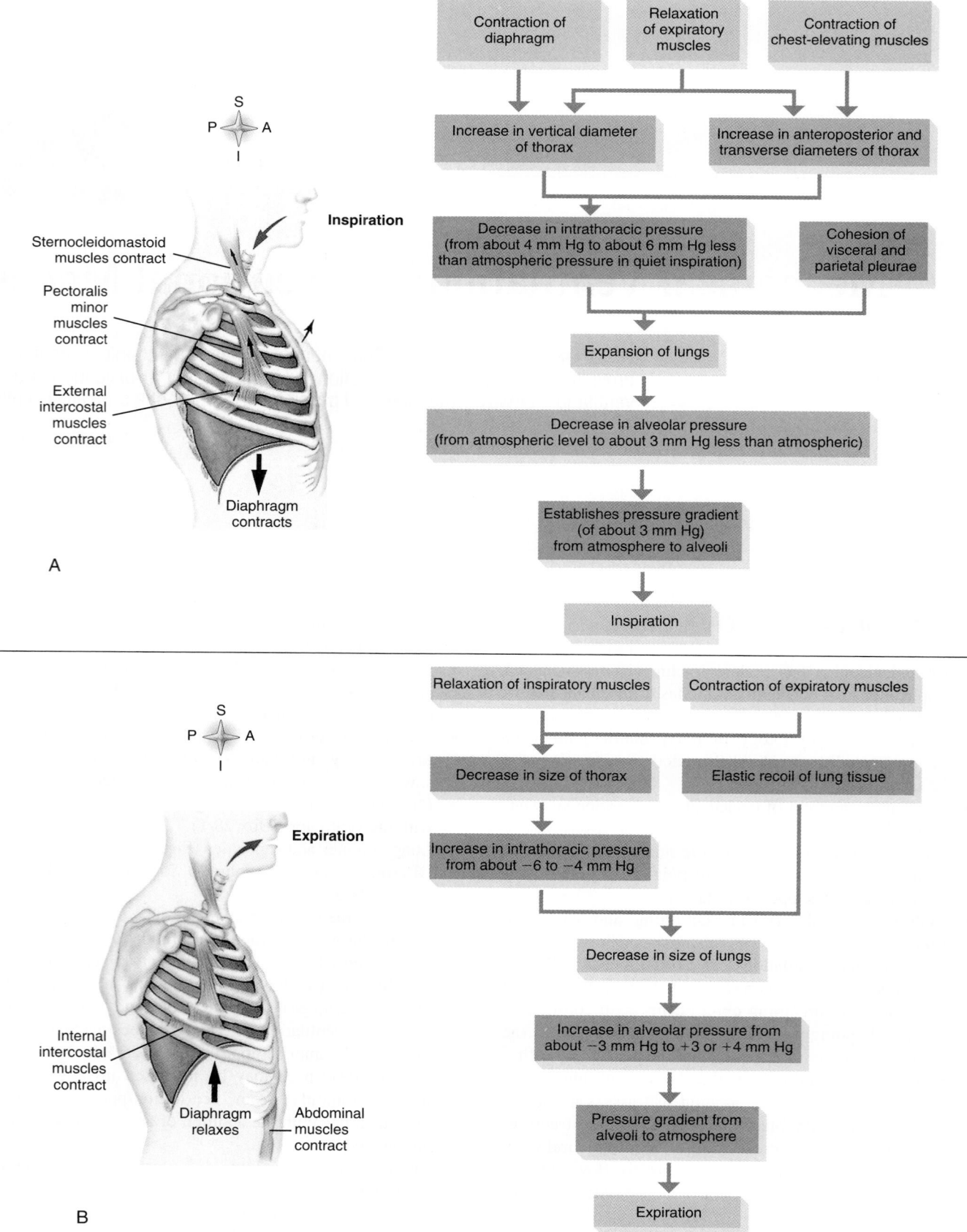

FIGURE 28-1   Mechanism of Inspiration and Expiration. **A,** Mechanism of inspiration. As thoracic volume increases, pressure in lungs decreases and draws air inward. **B,** Mechanism of expiration. As thoracic volume decreases, lung pressure increases and pushes air outward. *From Thibodeau G, Patton K, editors:* Anatomy and physiology, *ed 5, Philadelphia, 2003, Mosby.*

- **Compliance:** a measure of lung "stiffness" Compares the change in Volume : Pressure; $\Delta V / \Delta P$. A "stiff" lung requires $\uparrow$ pressure to deliver volume

- **Resistance:** obstruction to airflow. May be inspiratory resistance (bronchospasm) or expiratory resistance (air trapping).

- **Vital Capacity (Vc):** the volume of air measured after a forced inspiration and forced exhalation. Vc ~ 60 ml/kg

- **Functional Residual Capacity (FRC):** the volume of gas remaining in the lung at the end of a normal tidal volume breath. FRC = Closing volume + residual volume + expiratory volume. FRC ~ 30 ml/kg

- **Closing Capacity (CC):** the point at which the distal airways begin to collapse. CC = Closing volume + Residual volume. Normally, CC < FRC.

- **Tidal Volume (Vt):** the volume of air inspired in one breath. A spontaneously breathing person will generate 4-8 cc/kg of Vt, the lower end associated with small infants and neuromuscular weakness.

- **Deadspace Ventilation (V$_D$):** the volume of gas which does not participate in gas exchange. Under normal conditions, V$_D$ accounts for 2 cc/kg, approximately one-third of the Vt, occurring in the upper airways. With pulmonary abnormalities V$_D$ may be increased to du intrapulmonary shunting (ventilation-perfusion-VQ mismatching).

- **Minute Ventilation (V$_E$):** defined as the volume of gas inspired over a one-minute period. V$_E$ = Vt x Respiratory Rate

BOX 28-1   Definition of Lung Mechanics.

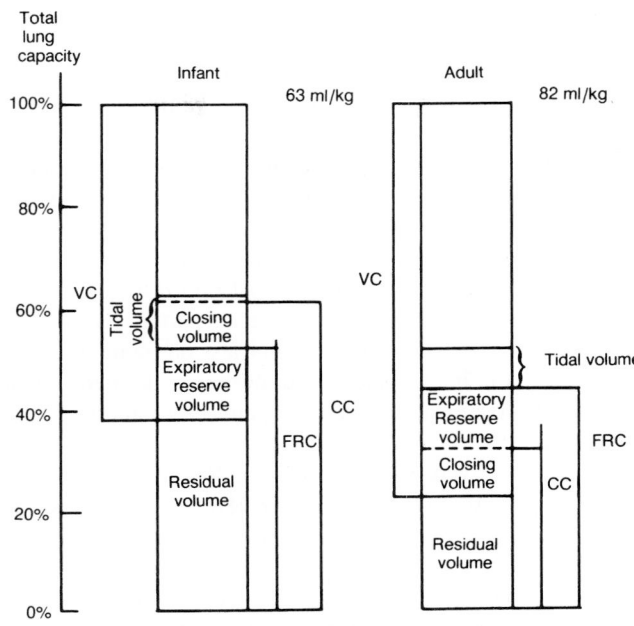

FIGURE 28-3 Lung Volumes of Infants and Children. Breathing of infant takes place in range of closing capacity. *CC,* Closing capacity; *VC,* vital capacity; *FRC,* functional residual capacity. *From Curley MAQ, Thompson JE: Oxygenation and ventilation. In Curley MAQ, Moloney-Harmon PA, editors: Critical care nursing of infants and children, ed 2, Philadelphia, 2001, Saunders.*

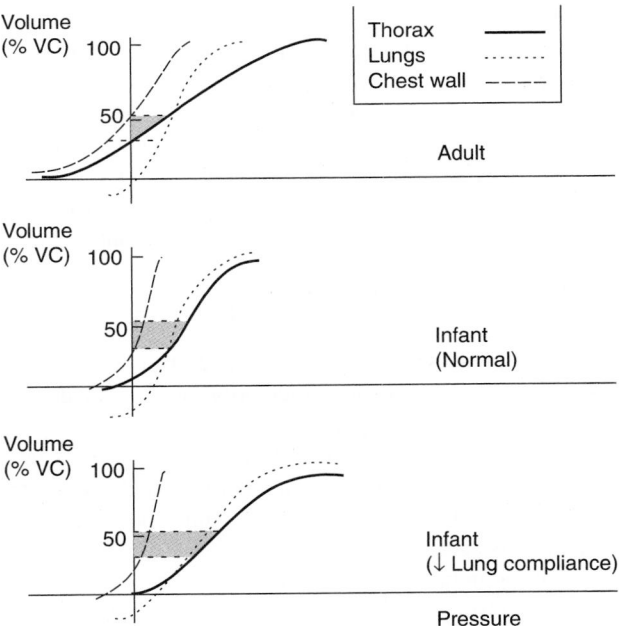

FIGURE 28-4 Representation of Volume Pressure Relationships of Thorax, Lungs, and Chest Wall. Representation of volume pressure relationships of thorax, lungs, and chest wall in adult, normal infant, and infant with decreased lung compliance. Volume-pressure relationships of lungs are similar in adult and normal infant. Volume pressure relationship of chest wall is steeper in infant and indicates greater chest wall compliance. *VC,* Vital capacity. *From Fuhrman B, Zimmerman J: Pediatric critical care, ed 3, Philadelphia, 2006, Mosby.*

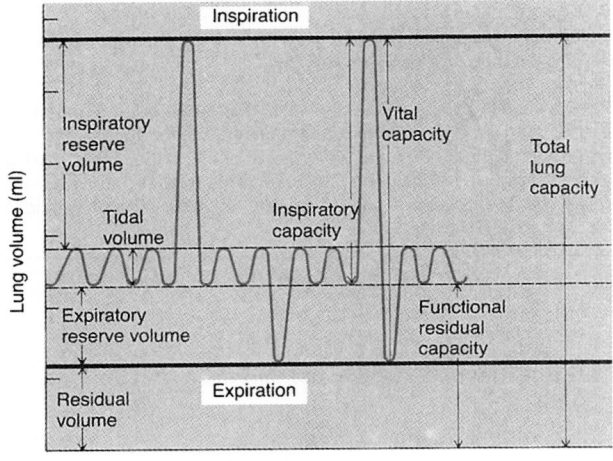

FIGURE 28-2 Lung Volumes and Capacities. *From Curley MAQ, Thompson JE: Oxygenation and ventilation. In Curley MAQ, Maloney-Harmon PA, editors: Critical care nursing of infants and children, ed 2, Philadelphia, 2001, Saunders.*

delivers a flow of gas into the lungs. Positive pressure ventilators raise the mean airway pressure (mPaw) above intrapleural pressure, thus reversing the intrathoracic pressure dynamics from spontaneous breathing.[3]

- Indications for positive pressure ventilation (PPV) include:
  - Ventilatory failure from apnea or pulmonary disease defined as a partial pressure of carbon dioxide ($PaCO_2$) of more than 60 mm Hg (or 20 mm Hg over baseline) or inadequate ventilation as indicated by a vital capacity (Vc) of less than 15 mL/kg
  - Hypoxemia defined as an arterial partial pressure of oxygen (PaO_2) of 80 mm Hg or less on room air at sea level or inadequate ventilation as defined by a PaO_2–fractional inspired oxygen (FiO_2) ratio of less than 300
  - Loss of airway reflexes, including loss of gag and swallow reflexes, from changes in level of consciousness (Glasgow Coma Score of 8 or less) or specific neurologic deficits
  - Cardiovascular failure (e.g., cardiogenic shock, sepsis) that results in decreased cardiac output (CO) and therefore, decreased oxygen delivery (DO_2)
  - Management of increased intracranial pressure (ICP) with regulation of $PaCO_2$ to control cerebral blood flow
- The challenge in defining an optimal ventilatory strategy is in matching pulmonary characteristics to ventilator functions. In reality, no child has homogenous lung disease that allows predetermined ventilator settings for optimal oxygenation and ventilation.
- Oxygenation is determined by the altitude (barometric pressure), FiO_2, and mPaw.
- The mPaw is the average airway pressure over one respiratory cycle. Factors that determine mPaw include: inspiratory flow (F), peak inspiratory pressure (PIP), inspiratory time (T_I), peak end-expiratory pressure (PEEP), and respiratory rate (RR). The two most significant determinants of mPaw are PIP and PEEP.

$$mPaw = F + PIP + T_I + EEP + RR$$

- Positive pressure ventilation is needed if a child is unresponsive to oxygen supplementation or if an inadequate ventilatory effort or apnea exists.
- Mechanical ventilators include an input power, a drive system, a control system, a cycling mechanism, and a method of providing PEEP, with humidifier and oxygen blender as accessories.[4]
- Common modes of ventilation (Box 28-2)
- The "control" variable initiates and regulates inspiration.[5] In a view of ventilation from the control variable, the two primary ventilator strategies are pressure-regulated (controlled) ventilation and volume-regulated (controlled) ventilation (Table 28-1).
- The pressure-regulated ventilator delivers a breath for a specific time until a preset pressure limit is achieved. With each breath, Vt varies based on the set pressure limit, compliance of the lung, and synchrony between the

CMV: Controlled Mandatory Ventilation. Used with volume control or pressure controlled ventilation. All variables in the ventilator cycle are pre-determined. Child cannot breath spontaneously from the circuit and does not exert any effort, which can lead to muscle weakness (or, "de-conditioning").

A/C: Assist Control. All variables are predetermined. If the child attempts to initiate a breath the ventilator will complete the breath at predetermined settings. If the child's effort interferes with the timing of the ventilator rate, the child's effort may not be recognized, or it may be preempted, causing asynchrony.

SIMV: Synchronized Intermittent Mandatory Ventilation. A breaths/minute rate (IMV) is set, with other variables preset according to the control variable (volume or pressure) and desired phase variables. The child can breathe spontaneously off the circuit in between the ventilator breaths, with or without pressure support. If child initiates a breath within a predetermined time prior to the next ventilator-timed breath, the ventilator will recognize this as a trigger to complete the breath.

MMV: Mandatory Minute Ventilation. The preset minute ventilation (VE) is based on child's ideal weight. The child can breathe spontaneously or assisted, while the ventilator tracks the tidal volume (Vt) and respiratory rate (RR). In some ventilators, the V_T and the RR are compared to internal targets and adjustments are made to either or both to achieve the preset V_E, with a targeted V_t, and a calculated target RR (which varies). The ventilator can be pre-set to provide pressure support (PS) with each breath, or in some ventilators, the PS is variable, based on internal ventilator measurements of the child's resistance and compliance. Some ventilators use MMV with SIMV. Other ventilators will allow total spontaneous breathing and provide breaths only if the child is apneic to achieve the targeted V_E.

PRVC: Pressure Regulated Volume Control (Dual Control Mode). An SIMV-mode with preset Vt and IMV. The ventilator monitors the child's lung compliance and airway resistance, and continuously adjusts the PIP to deliver the Vt (variable PIP) at the lowest possible pressure. PS can be added to assist the child's spontaneous breathing.

PSV: Pressure Support Ventilation. A mechanism which augments a spontaneous breath to a predetermined airway pressure to allow the child to achieve desired Vt. Appropriate PS minimizes the resistance of the ET tube. The mechanism is flow-cycled, ie, the child can draw as much flow with variable inspiratory time Ti, but when the child's flow demands drop to a pre-set level, the ventilator terminates inspiration. PSV, alone, does not incorporate a back-up rate

CPAP: Continuous Positive Airway Pressure. Spontaneous breathing occurs with preset end expiratory pressure. There is no back-up rate if the child becomes apneic.

APRV: Airway Pressure Release Ventilation. A pressure-controlled mode of ventilation. Spontaneous or assisted breathing for a pre-set time (eg 3 seconds) occurs at a high level of CPAP/PEEP (eg 30 cm H_2O pressure); periodically the CPAP/PEEP is released to a low level (eg, to 5 cm H_2O pressure) for 1-2 seconds to allow greater exhalation (CO_2 removal).

Box 28-2　Modes of Ventilation.

breaths initiated by the child and those that are provided by the ventilator.[2]

- The volume-regulated ventilator provides a preset Vt with each breath, and when the volume is reached, inspiration is terminated. With volume ventilation, the child's upper airway and lung compliance influences the peak pressure needed to achieve the prescribed Vt.[2]

TABLE 28-1	Comparison of Volume-Controlled and Pressure-Controlled Ventilation	
Variable	**Volume Control**	**Pressure Control**
Cycle	Volume	Time or flow
Trigger	Child and machine	Child and machine
Limit	Flow	Pressure
Tidal volume	Constant	Variable
Peak pressure	Variable	Constant
Advantages	Constant Vt	Avoids excessive PIP
	V_E increases linearly with ΔVt	Decreases barotraumas
Disadvantages	Risks barotrauma with $\downarrow C_L$	Vt variability risks atelectasis or lung collapse

C_L, Lung compliance; Vt, tidal volume; V_E, minute ventilation; PIP, peak inspiratory pressure.

- When the end of expiration is controlled by the mechanical ventilator, the breath is identified as a mandatory breath. The child does not control the mandatory breath. It is determined by a preset time, pressure, or volume. A mandatory breath may be initiated by the ventilator with a present frequency or minute ventilation, or it can be initiated by the child. The characteristics of inspiration and expiration are the same whether the breath is started by mechanical means or by the child.

- In assist control mode, the child's prescribed ventilatory rate is achieved by the mechanical breaths the child receives from the ventilator and the number of breaths triggered by the child.

- A spontaneous breath is defined as a breath initiated and terminated by the child. A spontaneous breath can be supported or assisted by a mechanical breath, which occurs when the inspiratory pressure is greater than the expiratory pressure.

- For an assisted breath, the ventilator is triggered to supply a positive pressure breath with either pressure or flow after the child initiates a breath. A mechanical ventilator that has a preset pressure, volume, or flow can initiate inspiration, but the child must assert some effort for inspiration to be triggered by pressure or flow. Sensors that measure the child's effort include *pressure* sensors and *flow* sensors. Flow sensors are generally more sensitive to the child's effort; the child needs to displace a minimal volume of gas to access flow from the circuit. A pressure sensor measures the amount of negative pressure the child exerts, which then opens a valve. This method may increase work of breathing and distress.

- For the termination of inspiration and the start of expiration, a cycling variable is also necessary and can be predetermined by a preset pressure, volume, or time.[4]

- Volume-cycled ventilation indicates that when a preset Vt is achieved, inspiration ends. Volume control assures that a preset Vt is delivered, but it is achieved with preset time (time-cycled) or preset flow (flow-cycled) mode.[4]

- Time-cycled ventilators provide a preset T_I, and inspiration is terminated when that preset time has occurred.[4]

- One method of understanding PPV characterizes mode, control, and phase variables (Figure 28-5).

- Pressure support ventilation (PSV) facilitates comfort and achieves more stable minute ventilation (V_E), with or without spontaneous intermittent ventilation (SIMV). Guidelines for *minimal* PSV support for children with adequate strength can be based on ETT size[6]:

ETT Size	PSV
3.0–3.5	10
4.0–4	5–8
>5.0	6

- Pressure support ventilation suggests that this is a "pressure-controlled" strategy; however, the pressure delivered to support a spontaneous breath is created by flow and terminated when the child's demand for flow falls to a preset level. Therefore, PSV is a flow-cycled pressure-regulated mode.

- During preset pressure ventilation, any alterations in PIP or PEEP change the Vt, unless both are adjusted equally in the same direction. For example, if PIP is 30 and PEEP is 10, the pressure change (ΔP) is 20; if the PIP is decreased to 26 (a decrease of 4), to preserve Vt (mirrored by the ΔP), the PEEP must be decreased (by 4) to 6: $\Delta P = 26 - 6 = 20$.

- Dual-control ventilation is becoming more available and allows both Vt and PIP ventilation simultaneously, with time-cycling to terminate inspiration.

- Ventilator adjustments to improve oxygenation and ventilation (Figure 28-6)

- An important aspect of caring for a child on PPV is use of lung protective strategies, which include low Vt (6 mL/kg), controlled plateau pressures of 30 or less, and early and aggressive PEEP.[7-9] The recommendations from ARDSnet[9] include strategies for improving oxygenation with FiO_2 and PEEP (Table 28-2). An open-lung model with stepwise progression of PEEP to recruit atelectatic lung segments in children with restrictive lung disease, such as acute lung injury, is suggested.

- PEEP is based on child's disease process. For children with ventilation for general physiologic support, a minimal PEEP of 4 to 5 is adequate. For children with pulmonary disease, the PEEP is adjusted according to underlying pathophysiology.

- With restrictive lung disease, such as ARDS, PEEP is increased in stepwise increments to recruit collapsed lung segments with the goal of a FiO_2 of 0.5 or less and an oxygen saturation (SaO_2) of 88% or more. For obstructive disease, such as asthma, PEEP should be increased with great caution because this condition is characterized by overdistention of alveoli (although may be mixed with atelectasis).

- PEEP may reduce the ΔP during the opening and closing of alveoli, which can cause sheer injury. With alveoli stinted open at end expiration, the force of inspiratory

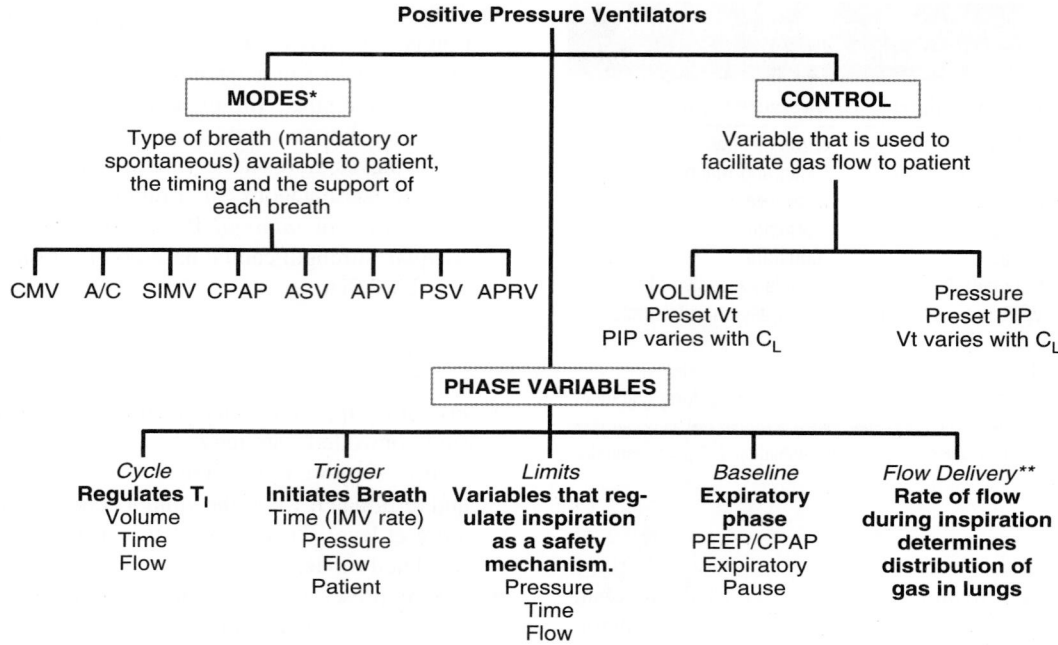

FIGURE 28-5   Positive Pressure Ventilators. Positive pressure ventilation can be characterized by mode, control, and phase variables.

Oxygenation: ↑ FiO$_2$
    ↑ mPaw   ↑ PEEP
        ↑ Ti
        ↑ Flow
        ↑ PIP[1]

Ventilation: ↑ IMV[2]
    ↑V$_E$ ↑ Vt
        ↑ Expiratory time
        ↓ Dead Space

FIGURE 28-6   Ventilator Adjustments to Improve Oxygenation and Ventilation. PIP works only in pressure-controlled ventilation. Auscultate breath sounds before increasing IMV. If IMV rate is too high, inadequate expiratory time may exist. *Mpaw,* Mean airway pressure; *PEEP,* positive end expiratory pressure; *T$_I$,* inspiratory time; *PIP,* peak inspiratory pressure; *IMV,* intermittent mandatory ventilation; *V$_E$,* minute ventilation; *Vt,* tidal volume.

TABLE 28-2	Improvement of Oxygenation with FiO$_2$ and PEEP						
FiO$_2$	0.3	0.4	0.4	0.5	0.5	0.6	0.6	0.7
PEEP	5	5	8	8	10	10	12	12
FiO$_2$	0.7	0.8	0.8	0.9	0.9	1.0	1.0	1.0
PEEP	14	14	16	16	18	20	22	24

From NIH National Heart, Lung Blood Institute ARDS Clinical Network: *Mechanical ventilation protocol summary,* 2005, retrieved from www.ardsnet.org.

distention is less. At high levels of PEEP, which increases mPaw, often the Vt can be reduced for lung protection.

- Various flow delivery patterns are available, such as "decelerating flow" or "square wave" flow. The choice in flow delivery depends on the resistance and compliance of the lung.
- Complications of mechanical ventilation (Box 28-3)
- With significant changes in oxygenation and ventilation (when the child is already on PPV), disconnect the child

---

Mechanical Malfunction: Loss of gas flow secondary to circuit disconnection, loss of air or oxygen (O_2) supply or internal malfunction of ventilator.
Indications: Child does not receive adequate Vt and may struggle, become cyanotic and/or develop dysrhythmias.

Airway: The endotracheal tube (ETT) may become dislodged or obstructed due to a kink or secretions. Tracheal inflammation and/or erosion may lead to tracheal stenosis.
Indications: The presence of an air leak around the ETT should be confirmed at least once/day; optimally an air leak is present at a positive inspiratory pressure (PIP) of $\leq$ 20-25 mm Hg. A higher PIP suggests airway edema.

Airleak: An increased tidal volume (Vt) or PIP may predispose the child to a pneumothorax, pneumomediastinum or pneumopericardium.
Indications: Deterioration in arterial oxygen saturation (SaO_2) and/or hemodynamic instability with alterations in breath sounds suggests the need for immediate intervention. The presence of subcutaneous emphysema, recognized by a crackling noted by palpation on chest wall or neck may also accompany an air leak.

Infection: An infection, especially ventilator-associated pneumonia (VAP) is associated with increased morbidity and mortality. The child is at risk for infection secondary to circuit condensation or contamination, aspiration of abdominal contents, and interruption of both the ventilator circuit and other invasive lines often used in children on PPV.
Indications: Fever, increased or decreased white blood cell (WBC) count with a shift in WBC indices, as well as hemodynamic instability provides evidence of the presence of an infection.

Hemodynamic Instability: High intrathoracic pressure may cause decreased venous return, decreased cardiac output (CO) and intrapulmonary shunting.
Indications: For a child on positive pressure ventilation (PPV) symptoms of high intrathoracic pressure including decreased CO, tachycardia, decreased perfusion, pale-to-cyanotic color, decreased mentation, require immediate intervention.

Box 28-3   Complications of Mechanical Ventilation.

---

from the ventilator, increase the child's FiO_2 and hand bag the child with a manual ventilation device. If the child's condition does not improve, consider troubleshooting with the mnemonic:

DOPE = Displacement **O**bstruction **P**neumothorax **E**quipment failure

CHILD AND FAMILY ASSESSMENT

- Child's developmental level and ability to interact ⇥*Rationale:* Influences preparation and interaction.
- Child's and family's understanding of the reasons for and risks and benefits of conventional modes of mechanical ventilation ⇥*Rationale:* Evaluates child's and family's understanding of mechanical ventilation and provides a gauge for ongoing education.
- Assess vital signs ⇥*Rationale:* Changes in vital signs may be the first indication of child tolerance and complications.
- Assess for signs and symptoms of ventilatory failure, including increased $PaCO_2$, and symptoms of hypercarbia, such as decreased mental status, tachycardia, hypertension, and dilated pupils ⇥*Rationale:* Recognition of a change in respiratory function may indicate further intervention is needed and prevent complications.
- Assess for signs and symptoms of hypoxemia, including decreased SaO_2, pale or cyanotic color, tachycardia or bradycardia (late), tachypnea, agitation or decreased mental status (late), increased work of breathing (retractions), and acidosis ⇥*Rationale:* Recognition of a change in respiratory

function may indicate further intervention is needed and prevent complications.
- Assess cardiovascular stability ⇥*Rationale:* Inadequate mean arterial pressure results in hemodynamic instability, which causes decreased cardiac output and tissue/organ perfusion.
- Observe child for signs of pain and anxiety ⇥*Rationale:* Inadequate management of pain and anxiety can result in interference with mechanical ventilation, which may cause insufficient oxygenation and ventilation.

CHILD AND FAMILY EDUCATION

Individualized, developmentally appropriate education is provided to the family and to the child based on desire for knowledge, readiness to learn, and overall neurologic and psychosocial state.

- Explain the reasons for, and purpose and risks of PPV therapy ⇥*Rationale:* Anticipatory explanations may decrease fear and anxiety, foster trust, and facilitate cooperation.
- Discuss sensory information, including the sound of the ventilator, the sensation of lung inflation, and coughing ⇥*Rationale:* Awareness of the sensations may reduce anxiety.
- Provide family with descriptions and explanations of equipment alarms ⇥*Rationale:* Increased awareness of alarms decreases fear and anxiety for the family.

- Discuss relaxation methods that can be incorporated in the child's care, including reading to the child, providing quiet distractions, and facilitating rest ➤➤*Rationale:* Relaxation promotes improved oxygenation and ventilation.
- Identify a method of communication between the child and family and the health care providers ➤➤*Rationale:* Understanding the child's needs may reduce anxiety and frustration.
- Provide assurance that the family can still be present and involved in the child's care ➤➤*Rationale:* The goal is to alleviate anxiety and minimize the fear of ventilator-controlled breathing.

- Discuss the need for suctioning the ETT at regular intervals and the expected coughing sensation ➤➤*Rationale:* Suctioning is always uncomfortable and sometimes painful. The anxious appearance of the child and observing airway secretions can be upsetting. Repeating of instructions before each suctioning attempt may help to alleviate anxiety.
- Encourage questions and answer questions as they arise ➤➤*Rationale:* Reinforcement of information is needed during periods of stress.

Procedure for Mechanical Ventilation: Conventional Modes

Steps	Rationale	Considerations
1. Ensure child and family understand procedure and questions are answered.	Evaluates and reinforces understanding of previously taught information.	Developmental, cognitive, and anxiety levels determine approach to and effectiveness of teaching.
2. Wash hands.	Reduces transmission of microorganisms.	
3. Ensure cardiorespiratory monitor is in place, including end tidal CO_2 (ETCO$_2$) and SpO_2 if indicated. *(Level II*)*	Provides information on the adequacy of ventilation and signs and symptoms of complications. Allows the practitioner to immediately respond to physiologic status.	
4. The prescribing practitioner orders ventilator settings.	A medical order is required for the application of mechanical ventilation.	
5. Gather needed equipment and supplies.	Facilitates completion of task in a timely manner.	
Volume-Controlled Ventilation		
6. Mode of ventilation is selected.	The choice of mode must be individualized to the child.	If the child is awake and able to tolerate breathing spontaneously, the mode should allow comfortable spontaneous breathing with enough support to guarantee the desired Vt or V_E. A/C modes are not preferred in awake children because of relative discomfort.
7. Initial Vt is set to produce an effective Vt of 8 to 10 mL/kg.	The Vt is individualized to the child and disease state. A higher Vt is associated with lung injury, and an effective Vt of larger than 18 mL/kg is not recommended.[4,7]	For confirmation of adequate aeration, observe chest excursion and auscultate lung sounds.

* Level II: Theory-based; no research data to support recommendations; recommendations from expert consensus group may exist

Procedure	**for Mechanical Ventilation: Conventional Modes**—*Continued*	
Steps	**Rationale**	**Considerations**
8. The cycle mechanism (volume, time, or flow) is set.	Individualized to the child and capabilities of the ventilator used. Determines the termination of inspiration.	Children with hypoxemia may benefit from a longer controlled T_I, and time-cycled mode may be preferred over flow or volume cycled.
9. Intermittent mandatory ventilation (IMV) is set. May adjust IMV based on $PaCO_2$, with assumption that the Vt is held constant. New IMV rate = $$\frac{PaCO_2 \text{ (child)} \times IMV \text{ (set)}}{\text{Desired } PaCO_2}$$	The IMV is set to achieve appropriate minute ventilation with $V_E =$ Vt × RR. The IMV setting depends on how much mandatory ventilation is desired.	Initially, V_E can be estimated as 200 mL/kg. For complete control, the calculated IMV is used. For spontaneous breathing, a lower rate is chosen and then adjusted by $PaCO_2$. When permissive hypercapnia is desired for lung protection, pH (rather than $PaCO_2$) drives changes in IMV.
10. T_I: expiratory time (T_E) ratio (typically, 1:≥2) is set.	Consider that T_I influences oxygenation and T_E influences ventilation ($PaCO_2$).	For children with restrictive lung disease, a longer T_I may be useful. For obstructive disease, a longer expiratory time may be necessary.
11. The PEEP is selected.	The PEEP is based on child's lung function and disease process. Normal glottic closure at end exhalation is prevented when an ETT is present; therefore, a minimal amount of PEEP ($\cong 4$ cm) maintains physiologic FRC in all children. For children with pulmonary disease, the PEEP is adjusted according to underlying pathophysiology. One goal for use of PEEP is to reduce FiO_2 to less toxic levels ($FiO_2 \leq 0.5$).	For children on higher levels of PEEP, interruption of the ventilator circuit (e.g., suctioning) may cause a significant loss of FRC.
12. Other considerations: *Trigger sensitivity:* The ventilator is triggered when either a pressure sensor or flow sensor recognizes the child's effort. *Flow rate and pattern:* The circuit may provide either continuous flow or demand flow.	Adjust the trigger sensitivity to affect the required effort of the child to access flow from the circuit. For children with new ventilation, the trigger and sensitivity should be adjusted to provide complete comfort and rest. Tailor flow rate and pattern to meet child's needs.	The initial flow can be delivered quickly or in a more uniform fashion (as in spontaneous breathing). Infants may not be strong enough to open the valve on a demand flow circuit.
13. Set appropriate alarms and limits.	High and low pressure, T_I, and Vt limits are set depending on the cycling mechanism chosen. Low pressure alarms are used to detect disconnection in the system. High pressure alarms are used for notification of increased pressure in the system.	In the volume-controlled mode, the child's lung compliance may cause variable PIP. Conventionally, the high pressure alarm is set 8 to 10 mm Hg above the child's PIP to protect the lungs from sudden changes in resistance or compliance.

Procedure continues on following page

Procedure	**for Mechanical Ventilation: Conventional Modes**—*Continued*	
Steps	**Rationale**	**Considerations**
14. To set mandatory minute ventilation (MMV), set V_E as a percentage (100% = 100% of calculated V_E). Consider starting with a normal (calculated) V_E (see Figure 28-7).	Calculated to provide adequate support to minimize work of breathing.	The child's ideal body weight is used to calculate V_E. The V_E is set at "100%." Depending on the specific ventilator, the IMV rate, T_I, Vt, and PIP/PSV may be either preset or variable. This mode of ventilation may be difficult to maintain in children with large air leaks and profuse secretions. Tachypnea may cause diminished Vt because the ventilator is preset to ensure the target V_E (Vt × RR). A rapid rate causes the ventilator to maintain V_E by reducing the Vt, which may lead to atelectasis.
15. To set PSV, if required	Set a pressure level to provide enough pressure support to achieve a targeted Vt.	With initiation of PSV, consider comfort and a target Vt. Used with or without SIMV. Higher initial PSV levels may be needed by some children depending on disease and strength of the child.
Pressure-Controlled Ventilation		
16. Select the mode of ventilation.	Selected for children that a ventilation is focused on maintaining an exact PIP-PEEP (ΔP) ratio.	The ΔP is proportionate to Vt; therefore, changes in ΔP cause proportional changes in Vt. For pressure-controlled/limited mode, A/C or SIMV are the most commonly used APV/APRV pressure regulate each cycle but with a pre-set Vt.
17. Adjust the PIP and PEEP to achieve the targeted Vt.	Set parameters based on previous ventilator settings or "best guess."	The initial settings may be arbitrary. One method is to set the desired PEEP and then adjust the PIP upward until the desired Vt is achieved.
18. The cycle mechanism is set.	Determines the termination of inspiration with a preset T_I, V_t, or flow.	Commonly, a time-cycled method is used with pressure-limited ventilation. On some ventilators, additional choices are flow and volume cycled. In pressure-controlled ventilation, the set PIP is controlled throughout inspiration but does not terminate inspiration.
19. The IMV rate, trigger, I:E, and PEEP are set (as described in volume-controlled section).	Individualized to the child and disease state. Required for this mode of ventilation.	The mPaw and V_E are closely monitored as the IMV and I:E are adjusted.

Procedure for Mechanical Ventilation: Conventional Modes—*Continued*

Steps	Rationale	Considerations
20. For pressure-regulated volume control (PRVC): A targeted Vt and an appropriate T_I are set.	The goal is to set the ventilator to deliver the target Vt with the least amount of pressure, which may be preset or variable (with a high limit). Size and condition of child guide T_I. Often instituted to provide a protective lung strategy approach.	The PRVC is usually time cycled. The Vt is established by the ventilator measuring resistance and compliance and is controlled with variable flow ($Vt = T_I \times Flow$). Ventilators with these modes often have a five-breath "learning curve" to adjust to the child's resistance and compliance. Occasionally, the child may struggle during those five breaths, especially with lower IMV rates. If the high limit is alarming, the child may either need suctioning or have progressive lung disease, with decreasing compliance.
21. The IMV rate, I:E ratio, trigger, and PEEP are preset (as described in volume-controlled section).	Settings are according the child's age and condition.	After the PEEP is set, the PIP is calculated *above* the PEEP. If the PEEP is set at 5 and the child requires 15 cm PIP, the resulting PIP is 20.
22. Set and activate low and high alarms.	Alarms are set depending on the cycling mechanism chosen. Low pressure alarms are used to detect disconnection in the system. High pressure alarms are used for notification of increased pressure in the system.	

Expected Outcomes

- Adequate oxygenation and ventilation
- Maintenance of adequate pH and $PaCO_2$
- Support work of breathing
- Ventilation without lung injury
- Hemodynamic stability
- Maintenance of skin integrity
- Airway in correct position
- Child remains infection free
- Mobilization and removal of secretions
- Adequate airway humidification
- Acceptable level of comfort

Unexpected Outcomes

- Inadequate ventilation and oxygenation (hypoxemia, hypercarbia, acidosis, alkalosis)
- Lung overinflation, air leak syndrome: pneumothorax, pneumomediastinum, pneumoperitoneum, subcutaneous emphysema
- Acute lung injury: volutrauma or progression of lung disease
- Hemodynamic instability
- Skin breakdown or pressure ulcer
- Unplanned extubation or malpositioned ETT
- Ventilator-associated pneumonia
- Tenacious sputum
- ETT obstruction
- Unmanaged pain and agitation

Monitoring and Care of the Child

Activities and Interventions	Rationale	Reportable Conditions
1. Ensure that a manual ventilation bag, mask, and suction are immediately available and connected at child's bedside.	Equipment is necessary for sudden changes in the child's condition.	• Absent or poorly functioning equipment
2. Monitor signs and symptoms of changes in oxygenation/ventilation, including lung sounds and aeration of lung segments, vital signs, oxygen saturation, $ETCO_2$/transcutaneous CO_2 ($TcCO_2$), and arterial/venous blood gases; cyanosis, work of breathing, adequacy of chest excursion, and chest radiograph findings.	To determine changes in respiratory status, effectiveness of therapy, and need for additional intervention.	• Tachypnea • Diminished breath sounds • Significant changes in oxygenation saturation, $ETCO_2$/$TcCO_2$, and arterial/venous blood gases • Cyanosis • Increased work of breathing • Poor chest excursion • Adverse chest radiograph findings

3. Assess physiologic stability, including cardiac function and hemodynamic changes (heart sounds, heart rate, blood pressure, and perfusion).	Increased intrathoracic positive pressure may reduce venous return and cardiac output. Likewise, positive pressure may cause a pneumothorax, which can also decrease CO.	• Hypotension
		  ❖ Poor perfusion, including cool extremities and changes in skin color
		  ❖ Tachycardia
		  ❖ Decreased breath sounds SvO_2 or SaO_2
		  ❖ Tracheal shift
		  ❖ Asymmetry of chest
		  ❖ Sudden increase in PIP or mPaw

4. Observe for child-ventilator synchrony.	Asynchrony causes increased work of breathing and distress Asynchrony in a small child is commonly associated with flow regulation; access to flow and speed of delivery ("pramp") influence the child's ability to breathe comfortably.	• Agitation • Decreased SaO_2 • Increased $PaCO_2$
5. Ventilator checks every 1 to 2 hours, including FiO_2, PIP, Vt, PEEP, mPaw, and other relevant ventilator settings, including temperature of inspired gas (maintain at 35°C to 37°C). Ensure activation of all alarms each shift.	Drift in oxygen may occur from oxygen source; auto-PEEP may also occur. Body temperature can be significantly altered by the temperature of inspired gas. Patient safety.	• Changes in settings that deviate from prescribed settings • Inappropriate alarming • Drift of humidifier temperature greater than 0.5°C
6. Provide additional ventilatory support, including manual breaths and adjustments in mechanical ventilation as indicated by signs of hypoxemia, hypercarbia, and hemodynamic instability.	Early intervention when inadequate ventilatory support and hemodynamic instability occur may prevent added clinical deterioration.	• Continued hypoxemia, including decreased SaO_2 or PaO_2, cyanosis, decreased mental status, tachypnea, tachycardia, or bradycardia (late) • Continued signs of hypercarbia, including increased blood pressure, dilated pupils, decreased mental status, shallow or irregular RR, tachycardia • Unresolved hemodynamic instability
7. Monitor and adjust ventilator settings based on treatment strategies.	Changes in lung compliance may change PIP/Vt.	• Inability to resolve etiology of the alarm

Monitoring and Care of the Child—Cont'd

Activities and Interventions	Rationale	Reportable Conditions
8. Monitor ventilator alarms and changes from prescribed settings, including an increased PIP or change in Vt.	An alarm indicating an increase in PIP or change in Vt may be associated with a need for suctioning or airway obstruction. Low pressure alarm may indicate that ventilator tubing is disconnected.	• Continued alarms despite routine interventions
9. Ensure ETT is secure and stabilized. • Consider attaching circuit to bed or device to ensure security while allowing movement of the child. • Replace loosened tape quickly.	Reduces risk of extubation. Eliminates undue pressure on skin from ETT and tubing.	• Unplanned extubation • Skin redness and ulceration
10. Suction ETT as indicated (see Procedure 2) and note characteristics of secretions.	Maintain airway patency and remove secretions.	• Inability to pass suction catheter • Inability to clear secretions • Change in quantity and characteristics of secretions • Change in SaO_2 (indicative of derecruitment) • Intolerance to suctioning
11. Minimize ventilator sources of infection by minimal interruption to circuit and emptying condensation in tubing.	Ventilator-assisted pneumonia (VAP) is a significant cause of morbidity in children with ventilation.[10,11]	• Fever or temperature instability • Change in white blood cell count • Change in character of secretions • Inability to maintain circuit free of condensation
12. Note child's level of comfort and provide appropriate sedation and neuromuscular blockade; paralytics should be used sparingly.[8] • Provide daily "drug holidays" or neurostimulation monitors for those children on paralytic therapy.	Early identification of the child's comfort allows for immediate attention. May be necessary to achieve ventilator synchrony. Paralytics mask the child's underlying neurologic state.	• Unresolved pain and discomfort • Continued irritability • Unresolved child-ventilator asynchrony
13. Consider keeping head of bed at 30 degrees	Elevating the head of bed reduces incidence rate of aspiration.[10]	
14. Assess skin every 2 to 4 hours, including pressure areas of nose/mouth (in contact with the ETT) and other areas of pressure to the body, with particular attention paid to bony prominences. Keep skin clean and dry.	Impaired skin integrity increases the risk for infection.	• Areas of skin breakdown
15. Reposition child (including head) every 1 to 2 hours.	To alleviate pressure points and prevent skin breakdown.	• Skin breakdown • Mucosal bleeding
16. Provide interventions to maintain oral integrity and hygiene, including brushing teeth, gums, and tongue at least twice a day and moisturizing lips every 2 to 4 hours.	Oral care reduces inflammation.[12] *(Level IV*)* Dental plaque provides a median for infection that has been shown to be responsible for VAP.[4,13] *(Level IV*)* Dental plaque can be removed with brushing.	• Excessive plaque build up • Necrosis • Ulcerations • Trauma to lungs, tongue, roof of mouth

* Level IV: Limited clinical studies to support recommendations

Continued

Monitoring and Care of the Child—Cont'd

Activities and Interventions	Rationale	Reportable Conditions
17. Monitor gastric insufflation and remove air from the stomach as indicated.	Positive pressure ventilation can lead to increased gas flow to the stomach. Decompression of the stomach decreases the risk of aspiration.[8]	• Inability to empty stomach
18. Ensure a method of communication has been established with the child. For small children, simple picture boards can be used. Older children may need more sophisticated picture boards or perhaps a dry-erase board.	Decreases anxiety and fear, enhances assessment, and includes child in care.	• Change in ability to communicate
19. Provide distraction with television, books, and toys.	May enhance child cooperation and enhance ability to adequately ventilate the child.	• Irritability that interferes with ventilation

Documentation

- Cardiorespiratory assessment, including vital signs, lung sounds, work of breathing, arterial blood gases, pulse oximetry, and $ETCO_2$ or $TcCO_2$ monitoring
- Date and time of initiation of ventilator assistance
- Record of ventilator settings, including FiO_2, mode, Vt, IMV, PIP, rate, and PEEP (every 2 to 4 hours and with changes)
- Timing of suctioning and characteristics of ETT secretions
- Additional interventions and child's response
- Comfort assessment and any specific interventions provided
- Child and family education
- Unexpected outcomes and related treatment

References

1. Curley MAQ, Thompson JE: Oxygenation and ventilation. In Curley MAQ, Moloney-Harmon P, editors: *Critical care nursing of infants and children,* ed 2, Philadelphia, 2001, Saunders.
2. Hazinski MF, et al, editors: *Pediatric advanced life support provider manual,* Dallas, 2002, American Heart Association.
3. Venkataraman ST: Mechanical ventilation and respiratory care. In Fuhrman B, Zimmerman J, editors: *Pediatric critical care,* ed 3, Philadelphia, 2006, Mosby.
4. American Association of Critical Care Nurses: *Practice alert: oral care of the critically ill,* 2006, retrieved August 16, 2006, from http://www.aacn.org/AACN/practiceAlert. nsf/vwdoc/PracticeAlertMain.
5. Campbell RS, Davis BR: Pressure-control versus volume-control ventilation: does it matter? *Respir Care* 47(4): 416-424, 2002.
6. Randolph AG, et al: Effect of mechanical ventilator weaning protocols on respiratory outcomes in infants and children, *J Am Med Assoc* 288(20):2561-2568, 2002.
7. The Acute Respiratory Distress Syndrome Network: Ventilation with lower tidal volumes as compared with traditional tidal volume for acute lung injury and the acute respiratory distress syndrome, *N Engl J Med* 342(18):1301-1308, 2000.
8. Bolton CF: Critical illness polyneuropathy and myopathy, *Crit Care Med* 29(12):2388-2390, 2001.
9. National Heart, Lung and Blood Institute ARDS Clinical Trials Network: Higher versus lower positive end expiratory pressures in patients with acute respiratory distress syndrome, *N Engl J Med* 351:327-336, 2004.
10. Elward A: Pediatric ventilator-associated pneumonia, *Pediatr Infect Dis J* 22(5):445, 2003.
11. Torres A, Ewig S: Diagnosing ventilator-associated pneumonia, *N Engl J Med* 350(5):433-435, 2004.
12. Fitch J, Munro C, Glass C, et al: Oral care in the adult intensive care unit, *Am J Crit Care* 8:314-318, 1999.
13. Fourrier F, Duvivier B, Boutigny H, et al: Colonization of dental plaque: a source of nosocomial infections in intensive care unit patients, *Crit Care Med* 26:301-308, 1998.

Additional References

Goldsmith JP, Karotkin EH: *Assisted ventilation of the neonate,* Philadelphia, 2003, Saunders.
Grant MJ, Webster HF: Pulmonary system. In Slota M, editor: *Core curriculum for pediatric critical care nursing,* Philadelphia, 2005, Saunders.
Hazinski MF: Pulmonary disorders. In Hazinski MF, editor: *Manual of pediatric critical care,* St Louis, 1999, Mosby.
Thibodeau G, Patton K, editors: *Anatomy and physiology,* ed 5, Philadelphia, 2003, Mosby.

Negative Pressure Ventilation

PURPOSE: Negative pressure ventilation is used for noninvasive support in children with acute and chronic respiratory insufficiency

Roberta L. Hales

PREREQUISITE KNOWLEDGE

- Child development as it relates to clinical assessment and implications for negative pressure ventilation (NPV)
- Anatomy and physiology of the pediatric pulmonary system, including structural characteristics specific to the infant and child
- With institution of NPV, intact airway reflexes should be present to decrease the risk of aspiration.
- Intermittent and continuous NPV exposes the exterior surface of the chest wall to subatmospheric pressure.[1-4]
- Indications for NPV include:
  - ❖ Mild to moderate acute respiratory distress[5]
  - ❖ Subacute or chronic respiratory failure
    - ○ Central hypoventilation
    - ○ Neuromuscular disease or weakness (muscular dystrophy, spinal muscle atrophy, spinal cord injury)
    - ○ Chest wall disorders or deformities
  - ❖ Cardiovascular disorders[1]
    - ○ Congenital heart disease with passive flow shunts (Fontan)
    - ○ Phrenic nerve palsy
- Contraindications to NPV include:
  - ❖ Gastrointestinal bleeding
  - ❖ Fixed upper airway obstruction[6]
  - ❖ Abdominal surgery
  - ❖ Unstable thorax: rib fractures, chest trauma, flail chest
- Advantages of NPV include[1-4,7,8]:
  - ❖ Reduced cardiovascular compromise
  - ❖ Reduced airway complications

- ❖ Decreased need for sedation
- ❖ Preservation of physiologic functions: speech, cough, swallowing
- Disadvantages of NPV include:
  - ❖ In use, NPV is noisy, bulky, and cumbersome
  - ❖ Limitation of easy access to the child
  - ❖ Difficulty with achievement of adequate seal to optimize ventilation
  - ❖ Potential discomfort and musculoskeletal pain
  - ❖ In children with bulbar dysfunction or weakness, natural airway is unprotected[1]
- The two components of NPV ventilators are an airtight chamber to cover the thorax and abdomen and a pump to generate negative pressure.[2,3]
- Several types of negative pressure ventilators are available, including:
  - ❖ Tank ventilator, Porta Lung, Emerson JH, Cambridge, Mass (Figure 29-1)
  - ❖ Cuirass
  - ❖ Jacket Pulmo Wrap, Life Care International, Inc, Lafayette, CO
  - ❖ Poncho-wrap, Emerson JH
  - ❖ Hayek oscillator, Breasy Medical Equipment, Inc, Stanford, CT
- Types of pumps include the bellow pump and rotary pump
- Modes of negative pressure ventilation include[1-3]:
  - ❖ Cyclic negative pressure: Intermittent preset negative pressure to assist inspiration with a passive exhalation; the most common mode.
  - Negative/positive pressure: Same as cyclic negative pressure except a positive pressure is applied to the

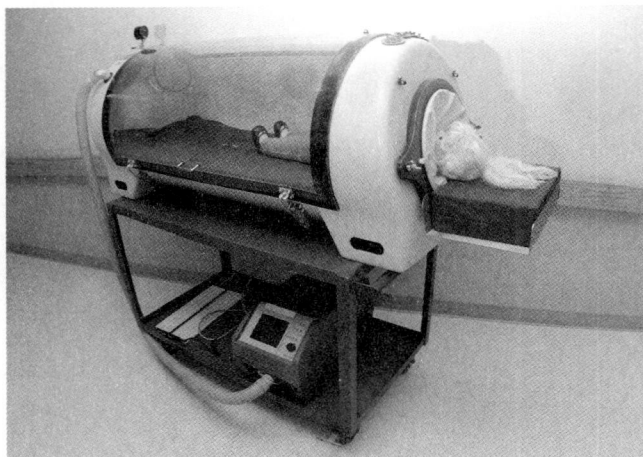

FIGURE 29-1 Tank ventilator, Porta Lung. *Courtesy of Michael Duff, RRT-NPS, Respiratory Care Department, Children's Hospital of Philadelphia.*

chamber during the expiratory phase; the active expiratory phase, assist cough, may promote airway clearance of sputum.[2,6]

❖ Continuous negative pressure (CNEP): Continuous negative pressure is applied throughout the respiratory cycle; children breathe spontaneously around CNEP.

❖ Cyclic negative pressure with negative end expiratory pressure (NEEP): Intermittent preset negative pressure to assist inspiration with a continuous negative pressure applied during expiration.

❖ Secretion clearance mode (Hayek oscillator): Oscillations around a negative baseline followed by an artificial cough; artificial cough has a prolonged inspiratory phase followed by a forced short expiratory phase.[6]

CHILD AND FAMILY ASSESSMENT

- Child's developmental level and ability to interact ➣*Rationale:* Influences preparation and interaction.
- Child's and family's understanding of the reasons for and risks and benefits of NPV ➣*Rationale:* Evaluates child's and family's understanding of the procedure and provides a gauge for ongoing education.
- Information about the child's disease and current status ➣*Rationale:* Complete analysis before the initiation of therapy assists the clinicians with goals and plans.
- Assess for upper airway patency ➣*Rationale:* Upper airway obstruction interferes with airflow during NPV.
- Assess child's protective airway reflexes ➣*Rationale:* Children with bulbar dysfunction or weakness are at increased risk for aspiration.
- Assess vital signs ➣*Rationale:* Baseline vital signs assist the bedside clinician in evaluation of tolerance of NPV.

- Assess cardiovascular stability ➣*Rationale:* Children with labile blood pressures undergo evaluation before negative pressure ventilation.
- Assess child's ventilatory status: spontaneous tidal volume, end tidal carbon dioxide ($EtCO_2$), pulse oximetry (SpO_2), respiratory rate, breath sounds, and negative inspiratory force ➣*Rationale:* Evaluating ventilatory status before initiation of therapy provides baseline parameters for comparison during NPV.

CHILD AND FAMILY EDUCATION

Individualized, developmentally appropriate education is provided to the family and to the child based on desire for knowledge, readiness to learn, and overall neurologic and psychosocial state.

- Describe the negative pressure device and demonstrate application to child and family ➣*Rationale:* Providing information decreases anxiety and fear.
- Explain the necessary assessments while the child receives NPV ➣*Rationale:* Knowledge that the child will be continuously monitored decreases anxiety and fear.
- Discuss appropriate expected outcomes of NPV ➣*Rationale:* Family and healthcare team can formulate similar goals and expectations.
- Teach and support the family in use of distraction techniques (i.e., reading a book, visuals, etc) ➣*Rationale:* Increases child's cooperation.
- Encourage questions and answer questions as they arise ➣*Rationale:* Reinforcement of information is needed during periods of stress.

EQUIPMENT

- Negative pressure ventilator (tank ventilator, Porta Lung [see Figure 29-1]; Cuirass; Jacket Pulmo Wrap; Ponchowrap; Hayek oscillator)
- Bellow pump or rotary pump (33-CR, Emerson JH; NEV-100, Respironics, Inc, Murrysville, Pa; Maxivent Mallincrodt, Pleasantville, CA)[4]
- Nasal cannula for assist device with NPV
- Cardiorespiratory monitor
- Pulse oximeter
- An $EtCO_2$ monitor
- Transcutaneous carbon dioxide ($TcCO_2$; optional)
- Suction
- Oxygen
- Low pressure alarm

Procedure for Negative Pressure Ventilation

Steps	Rationale	Considerations
1. Ensure child and family understand procedure and questions are answered.	Evaluates and reinforces understanding of previously taught information.	Developmental level, cognitive ability, and anxiety level determine approach to and effectiveness of teaching.
2. Assemble equipment and supplies.	Preparation prevents delay of procedure.	
3. Wash hands.	Reduces transmission of micro-organisms.	
4. Before initiation, child should void.	Voiding prevents stoppage of NPV.	
5. Obtain arterial blood gas values before the initiation of therapy and correlate with $EtCO_2$ measured via a nasal cannula.	Use of $EtCO_2$ monitoring assists the clinician with ventilator adjustments.	
6. Review prescribing practitioner's order.	Medical order is needed for the initiation of mechanical ventilation.	
7. Place child in the ventilator. With use of a Pulmo Wrap, place the child on a firm mattress (without water) and elevate the head of the bed no greater than 30 degrees. *(Level V*)*	Selection of the appropriate device according to the child's size and degree of ventilation.	
8. Adjust the air-tight seals. *(Level V*)*	The ability of the ventilator to deliver an adequate tidal volume is dependent on the integrity of the seal.	Be careful not to make the seal too tight because this causes discomfort and increases the risk of skin integrity. Extra padding may be needed for comfort of the child.
9. Select and set mode. *(Level V*)*	Selection of mode is variable depending on the goal of the therapy.	Controlled NPV achieves respiratory muscle rest. Assist control NPV results in reduction of diaphragm exertion.[2]
10. Select and set mechanical rate. *(Level V*)*	Mechanical rate is selected when the child is placed in cyclic negative pressure, negative/positive pressure, and cyclic negative pressure with NEEP.	Use of the nasal cannula assist device can aid in the synchronization of the ventilator.
11. Gradually increase the negative pressure from 0 cm H_2O to the prescribed negative pressure. *(Level II)*	A gradual increase allows the child time to acclimate to the new therapy.[7,9]	Coaching and encouragement are needed at this stage. Vocalization during the inspiratory phase indicates inadequate negative pressure to provide diaphragm rest.[7] Adjust negative pressure and mechanical rate to exceed the child's spontaneous minute ventilation by 10% to 20%.[7,9]
12. Increase prescribed continuous negative expiratory pressure when used. *(Level IV*)*	Continuous negative pressure increases residual lung volume.	The degree of negative pressure may vary during the respiratory cycle.

Procedure continues on following page

* Level II: Theory-based; no research data to support recommendations; recommendations from expert consensus group may exist
Level IV: Limited clinical studies to support recommendations
Level V: Clinical studies in more than one or two patient populations and situations to support recommendations

Procedure for Negative Pressure Ventilation—*Continued*

Steps	Rationale	Considerations
13. Titrate supplemental oxygen as per prescribing practitioner's order. (*Level VI**)	Application of supplemental oxygen may be necessary to achieve acceptable oxygen levels.	Dual nasal cannula may be used to monitor $EtCO_2$ and deliver supplemental oxygen. Nasal cannula supplemental oxygen, dependent on liter flow, may interfere with the nasal cannula assist device.
14. Set and activate low pressure alarms.	Safety alarms identify disconnection or inadequate delivery of set pressures.	The addition of an external alarm may be necessary on some of the NPV pumps.

* Level VI: Clinical studies in a variety of patient populations and situations to support recommendations

Expected Outcomes

- Maintenance of normal alveolar ventilation
- Reduction in respiratory muscle work
- Decrease in the level of carbon dioxide retention
- Improved lung volume evidenced with chest radiograph
- Avoidance of airway intubation
- Respiratory and cardiovascular stability
- Maintenance of skin integrity
- Child has an acceptable level of comfort

Unexpected Outcomes

- Signs of inadequate oxygenation and ventilation
- Increased work of breathing
- Child-ventilator asynchrony
- Upper airway obstruction
- Aspiration
- Intubation
- Increasing cardiovascular and respiratory compromise
- Skin breakdown
- Unmanaged pain and anxiety

Monitoring and Care of the Child

Activities and Interventions	Rationale	Reportable Conditions
1. Child synchrony with the machine.	To ensure delivery of set pressures, decrease child anxiety and tachypnea.	• Child-ventilator asynchronization
2. Assess signs and symptoms of changes in oxygenation and ventilation indices, including monitoring of oxygen saturation, nasal $EtCO_2$, and evaluation of arterial blood gases (ABG), if arterial line is present.	Identifies changes in effectiveness of NPV.	• Diminished breath sounds • Significant changes in oxygenation saturation and arterial or venous blood gases • Increased work of breathing, including nasal flaring, accessory muscle use, and retractions
3. Evaluation of cardiac function, including heart rate and blood pressure.	Monitoring of heart rate and blood pressure provides information about the child's hemodynamic status. Whole body exposure to NPV could potentially lower blood pressure as a result of venous pooling. Chest wall apparatuses have been shown to decrease intrathoracic pressure, so right atrial pressure becomes more negative, enhancing venous return.[2]	• Dysrhythmias, including tachycardia to bradycardia • Hypertension to hypotension
4. Skin assessment of areas in contact with air tight seals.	Impaired skin integrity increases the risk for infection and decreases child's tolerance of NPV.	• Altered skin integrity

Documentation

- Ventilator settings (every 2 to 4 hours), including mode, negative inspiratory pressure, negative expiratory pressure, inspiratory time, mechanical rate, alarm functional, and oxygen flow (FiO_2)
- Respiratory status, including work of breathing, chest wall expansion, synchronous versus asynchronous breathing, lung sounds, pulse oximeter reading, $EtCO_2$, and $TcCO_2$
- Vital signs
- Skin assessment of areas that are sealed: neck, arms, and waist
- Comfort assessment and any specific interventions provided
- Additional interventions necessary
- Child and family education
- Unexpected outcomes and related treatment

References

1. Ayad O: Negative pressure ventilation. In Festa C, editor: *Clinical guidelines for mechanical ventilation,* Newtown, PA, 2002, Handbooks in Health Care Co.
2. Corrado A, Gorini M: Long-term negative pressure ventilation, *Resp Care Clin* 8(4):545-557, 2002.
3. Sivan Y, et al: Assisted ventilatory support and oxygen treatment. In Taussig L and Landau L, editors: *Pediatric respiratory medicine,* St Louis, 1999, Mosby.
4. Smith IE, et al: Choosing a negative pressure ventilation pump: are there any important differences, *Eur Respir J* 8:1792-1795, 1995.
5. Corrado A, Gorini M: Negative pressure ventilation in the treatment of acute respiratory failure: an old noninvasive technique reconsidered, *Eur Resp J* 9(7):1531-1544, 1996.
6. Klonin H, Bowman B, et al: Negative pressure ventilation via chest cuirass to decrease ventilator-associated complications in infants with acute respiratory failure: a case series, *Resp Care* 45(5):486-490, 2000.
7. Lyons WS: Negative pressure ventilation, *JAMA* 289(8):983, 2003.
8. Thomson A: The role of negative pressure ventilation, *Arch Dis Child* 77(5):454-458, 1998.
9. Previtera J: Negative pressure ventilation: operating procedure, 2003, from http://www.nemc.org/RespCare/npv.htm. Retrieved 2/16/06.

Additional Readings

Bach JR: A historical perspective on the use of noninvasive ventilatory support alternatives, *Respir Care Clin North Am* 2:161-181, 1996.

Bach JR: Noninvasive respiratory muscle aids and intervention goals. In Bach JR, editor: *Noninvasive mechanical ventilation,* Philadelphia, 2002, Hanley and Belfus, Inc.

Cirignotta F, Schiavina M, et al: Central alveolar hypoventilation treated with negative pressure ventilation, *Mon Arc Chest Dis* 51(1):22-26, 1996.

Corrado A, Confalonieri M, et al: Iron lung vs. mask ventilation in the treatment of acute on chronic respiratory failure in COPD patients: a multicenter study, *Chest* 121(1):189-195, 2002.

Cropp A, DiMarco AF: Effects of intermittent negative pressure ventilation on respiratory muscle function in patients with severe chronic obstructive pulmonary disease, *Am Rev Respir Dis* 135(5):1056-1061, 1987.

Cvetnic WG, Cunningham MD, et al: Reintroduction of continuous negative pressure ventilation in neonates: two year experience, *Pediatr Pulmon* 8:245-253, 1990.

Gappa M, Costeloe K, et al: Effect on continuous negative extrathoracic pressure on respiratory mechanics and timing in infants recovering from neonatal respiratory distress syndrome, *Pediatr Res* 36:364-372, 1994.

Gorini M, Villella G, et al: Effects of assist negative pressure ventilation by microprocessor-based iron lung on breathing effort, *Thorax* 57:258-262, 2002.

Heulitt M: The use of negative pressure ventilation in infants with acute respiratory failure: old technology, new idea, *Resp Care* 45(5):479, 2000.

Hill NS: Negative pressure ventilation for facilitation of weaning from mechanical ventilation-back to the future? *Resp Care* 39:19-20, 1994.

Hill NS: Clinical applications of body ventilators, *Chest* 90:897-905, 1986.

Leung P, Jubran A, et al: Comparison of assisted ventilator modes on triggering, patient effort and dyspnea, *Am J Resp Crit Care Med* 155:1940-1948, 1997.

Pierce JM, Jenkins IA, et al: The successful use of continuous negative extrathoracic pressure in a child with glenn shunt and respiratory failure, *Intens Care Med* 21:766-768, 1995.

Samuels M, Southall D: The role of negative pressure ventilation, *Arch Dis Child* 79(1):94, 1998.

Sanna A, Veriter C: Upper airway obstruction induced by negative pressure ventilation in awake healthy subjects, *J Appl Physiol* 75:546-552, 1993.

Shekerdemian LS, Bush A, et al: Cardiopulmonary interactions in healthy children and children after simple cardiac surgery: the effects of positive and negative pressure ventilation, *Heart* 78(6): 587-593, 1997.

Shoptaugh M, Cvetnic WG, et al: Pulmonary mechanics generated by positive end expiratory and continuous negative pressure, *J Perinatol* 13:341-348, 1993.

Splaingard ML, Frates RC Jr, et al: Home negative pressure ventilation: report of 20 years of experience in patients with neuromuscular disease, *Arch Phy Med Rehabil* 66:239-242, 1985.

Torelli L, Zoccali G, et al: Comparative evaluation of the haemodynamic effects of continuous negative external pressure (CNEP) and positive end expiratory pressure (PEEP) in mechanically ventilated trauma patients, *Intens Care Med* 21:67-70, 1995.

Noninvasive Positive Pressure Ventilation

PURPOSE: To support the ventilation of children with acute and chronic respiratory failure with noninvasive positive pressure measures and to minimize the need for endotracheal intubation

Roberta L. Hales and Eileen Briening

PREREQUISITE KNOWLEDGE

- Child development as it relates to clinical assessment and implications for noninvasive positive pressure ventilation (NPPV)
- Anatomy and physiology of the pediatric pulmonary system, including structural characteristics specific to the infant and child[1,2]
- Mastery of pediatric advanced life support competencies[2]
- Signs and symptoms of inadequate oxygenation and ventilation[1]
- Bag mask ventilation (see Procedure 27)
- Knowledge of terms and modes of NPPV (Figure 30-1)
- The purpose of NPPV is to improve oxygenation, decrease left ventricular afterload, reduce atelectasis, and minimize the need for endotracheal intubation.[3] The principle advantage of NPPV is avoidance of an artificial airway, which decreases the risk of nosocomial infections and the incidence rate of chronic lung disease and other complications.[4]
- With initiation of NPPV, an intact cough and gag reflex decreases the risk of aspiration.
- A variety of nasal prong and mask interfaces are available for NPPV (Figure 30-2). The choice is highly individualized and based on the ability to provide sufficient positive pressure to adequately ventilate the child and to optimize the child's comfort. The choice of mask or nasal prongs and the related head gear for stabilization is often done with trial and error. Standard adult small nasal prongs (Figure 30-3) and child-size nasal prongs (Figure 30-4) have been used and generally are more comfortable

for wear. Nasal prongs systems, however, create leaks around the prongs and resistance across the narrow orifices, reducing or eliminating the child's ability to trigger the bilevel machine.[5] Full face masks (Figure 30-5) and nasal masks (Figure 30-6) are available and have the main advantage of an improved seal. Head gear is available in a cap style (see Figure 30-6) or with a tube configuration (see Figure 30-3).

- Continuous positive airway pressure (CPAP) provides continuous positive pressure in the airway throughout the respiratory cycle (inspiratory and expiratory phase).
  - ❖ Nasal CPAP can be delivered via nasal mask or prongs and is most useful in infants because they are obligatory nose breathers.[6] The loss of pressure in the hypopharynx results in a variation in the actual CPAP delivered to the trachea. Thick secretions are more likely to impede gas flow from nasal prongs; therefore, adequate humidification and frequent suctioning are necessary with use.[6] Experience with use of nasal CPAP appears to improve efficacy.[7]
  - ❖ Mask CPAP requires an appropriately sized mask that provides a tight seal. A full face mask fits to extend from the bridge of the nose to the cleft of the chin, encompassing the mouth and nose. A nasal mask may cause less claustrophobia and allows the child to talk and vomit without aspiration.[3] Care must be taken to avoid placement of the mask too high over the eyes because this creates a leak in the system and a potential complication of eye irritation.
  - ❖ Improvements in rate of bronchopulmonary dysplasia and an increase in average daily weight gain have

Common Terms and Modes

<u>Terms:</u>

Inspiratory Positive Airway Pressure (IPAP): Positive airway pressure applied during inspiration

Expiratory Positive Airway Pressure (EPAP): Positive airway pressure applied during expiration

Mechanical Breath Rate: Preset number of breaths per minute

Inspiratory Time Percentage: Percentage of time (seconds) of the respiratory cycle for the inspiratory phase

Rise Time: The amount of time it takes to reach to peak inspiratory flowrate.

Ramp: Gradual increase of pressure to set IPAP and EPAP over time/breaths.

Interface: Device used to provide noninvasive positive pressure ventilation (e.g. mask, nasal prongs)

<u>Modes:</u>

Spontaneous Mode (S): Patient- triggered breaths are supported with bi-level positive airway pressures. Patient determines the respiratory rate.

Spontaneous Timed Mode (S/T): Patient-triggered breaths are supported with bi-level positive airway pressures. If patient does not breath, or the ventilator does not detect triggering, the ventilator delivers a preset mechanical rate at the preset bi-level positive airway pressures.

Timed (T): The ventilator cycles a preset mechanical rate and inspiratory time at the preset bi-level positive airway pressures.

FIGURE 30-1   Common Terms and Modes. *From Chiefetz IM: Invasive and noninvasive pediatric mechanical ventilation,* Resp Care *48(4):442-453, 2003.*

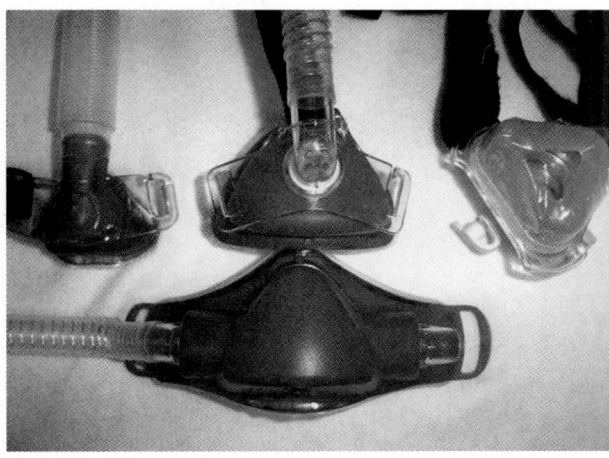

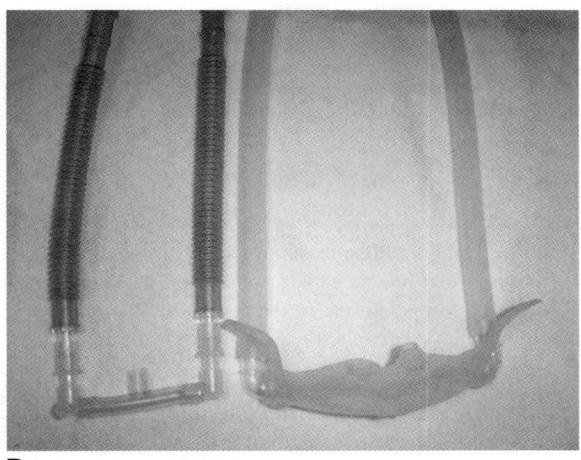

A   B

FIGURE 30-2   **A,** Standard pediatric nasal interfaces: MiniMe nasal mask (SleepNet Corp, Manchester, NH); small child's mask (Respironics, Murrysville, Penn); Profile Lite small mask (Respironics); small, medium, and large Infant Nasal CPAP Cannulae (Hudson RCI, Temecula, Calif). *Image courtesy of H. Panich.* **B,** Nasal CPAP cannulae (Hudson RCI).

been reported in early use of nasal CPAP in low–birth weight infants.[7]

• Bilevel positive airway pressure (BiPAP) uses both CPAP and a patient-triggered volume of positive inspiratory pressure delivered via a nasal or full face mask.[8,9] BiPAP has the advantage of providing added positive pressure during inspiration, but patient-ventilator asynchrony becomes an important issue.[8]

• Indications for NPPV[8,10]:
  ❖ Acute respiratory failure, including those children with mild to moderate respiratory distress associated with alveolar hypoventilation, postextubation or

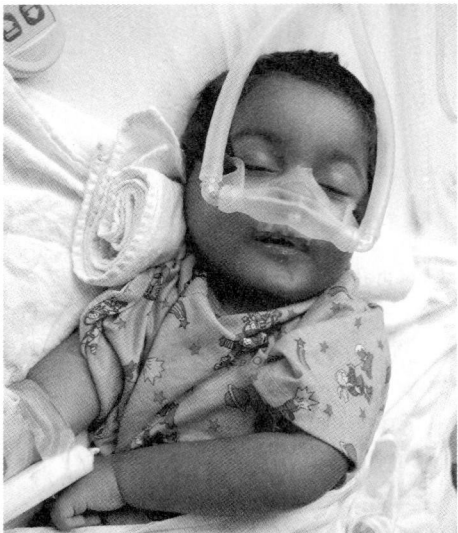

FIGURE 30-3   Standard adult small nasal interface with tubing head gear (SNAPP nasal interface, Tiara Medical Systems, Lakewood, Ohio). *Image courtesy of H. Panich.*

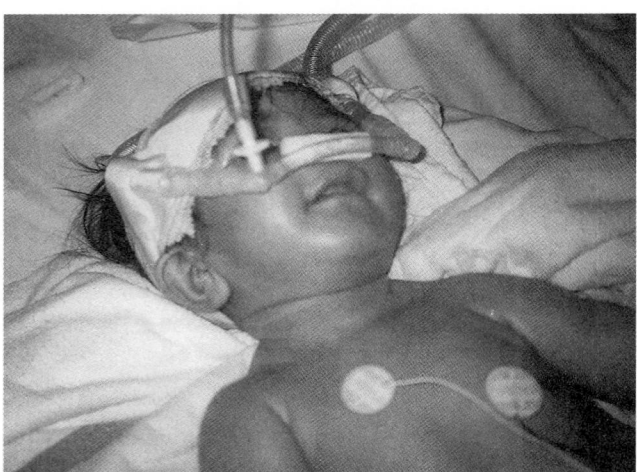

FIGURE 30-4   Infant with spinal muscle atrophy with use of nasal CPAP prongs as interface. *From Bach J, Niranjan V: Noninvasive ventilation in children. In Bach J, editor: Noninvasive mechanical ventilation, Philadelphia, 2002, Hanley and Belfus.*

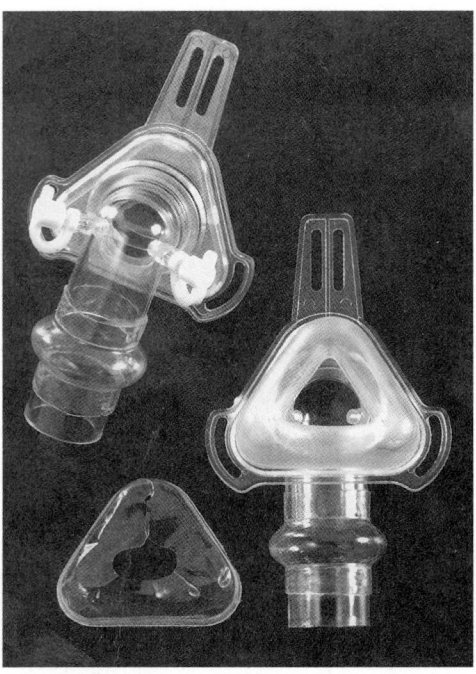

FIGURE 30-5   Respironics small child mask/comfort flap, front and back views. *From Bach J, Niranjan V:* Noninvasive ventilation in children. In Bach J, editor: *Noninvasive mechanical ventilation, Philadelphia, 2002, Hanley and Belfus.*

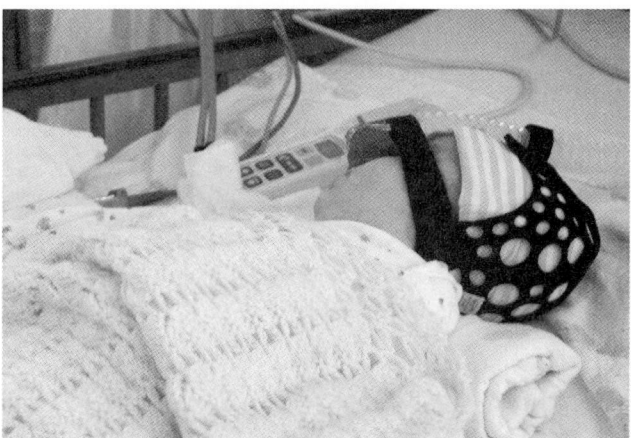

FIGURE 30-6   MiniMe nasal mask secured with petite headgear (SleepNet Corp). *Image courtesy of H. Panich.*

chronic stridor associated with laryngomalacia, and significant or symptomatic atelectasis

- ❖ Subacute or chronic lung disease, including bridge to transplant, obstructive sleep apnea, home ventilation, neuromuscular disease/weakness, chronic obstructive pulmonary disease, and chest wall disorders or deformities
- Contraindications for NPPV include[3,11,12]:
  - ❖ Absolute: Cardiovascular instability or cardiopulmonary arrest, apnea, facial burns or trauma, gastrointestinal bleeding, choanal stenosis/atresia, inability to protect airway
  - ❖ Relative: Inability to clear secretions, agitation, inability to trigger machine
- Potential complications of NPPV[13-17]

- ❖ Interface issues, including loss of skin integrity, especially over bony prominences of the nasal bridge; eye irritation; and improper fixation of mask or nasal prongs, resulting in leaks
- ❖ Air pressure and flow issues, such as nasal discomfort, including dryness, congestion, and pain; gastric insufflation; aspiration; and pneumothorax, hyperinflation, and air trapping
- ❖ Impedance of speech

CHILD AND FAMILY ASSESSMENT

- Child's developmental level and ability to interact
  ➤*Rationale:* Influences preparation and interaction.

- Child's and family's understanding of the reasons for and risks and benefits of NPPV ➤➤*Rationale:* Evaluates child's and family's understanding of the procedure and provides a gauge for ongoing education.
- Patency of the upper airway, including nasal passages ➤➤*Rationale:* Nasal obstruction (i.e., choanal atresia, congenital anomalies) can interfere with successful application of the mask interface.
- Signs and symptoms of airway secretions and inadequate oxygenation and ventilation, including visible secretions from the airway, inspiratory wheezes, expiratory crackles, diminished breath sounds, tachypnea, shallow respirations, tachycardia or bradycardia, hypertension/hypotension, and cyanosis ➤➤*Rationale:* Changes in cardiorespiratory status may indicate that NPPV is ineffective in providing adequate ventilatory support. An increase in intrapulmonary pressure could decrease venous return to the heart.
- Child's ability to protect the natural airway with the gag and cough reflex ➤➤*Rationale:* NPPV increases the risk for aspiration from the positive pressure.
- Level of child's consciousness, level of anxiety, and cognitive ability ➤➤*Rationale:* Uncooperative and semiconscious children are at increased risk for aspiration from decreased airway protective reflexes.
- Any pertinent medical history or condition that predisposes the child to added difficulty with ventilation and oxygenation ➤➤*Rationale:* Certain medical conditions interfere with and increase the risk of NPPV.
- Pressure areas and skin around and under mask ➤➤*Rationale:* Reduction of skin breakdown and elimination of potential source for infection.
- Oral cavity, including plaque builds ➤➤*Rationale:* Cleaning of the oral cavity and removal of plaque remain essential to prevent infection.[18,19]

CHILD AND FAMILY EDUCATION

Individualized, developmentally appropriate education is provided to the family and to the child based on desire for knowledge, readiness to learn, and overall neurologic and psychosocial state.

- Explain NPPV, including purpose, steps, rationale, and risks to the child and family ➤➤*Rationale:* Open communication decreases anxiety and fear for the child and family.
- Discuss appropriate expected outcomes of NPPV ➤➤*Rationale:* Allows family and health care team to formulate similar goals and expectations.
- Explain the necessary assessments while the child undergoes supplemental oxygen therapy ➤➤*Rationale:* Knowing that the child will be continuously monitored decreases anxiety and fear.
- Explain alarms to the child and family ➤➤*Rationale:* Providing information about alarms may allay anxiety and fear.
- Encourage questions and answer questions as they arise ➤➤*Rationale:* Reinforcement of information is needed during periods of stress.

EQUIPMENT

- Appropriately sized mask/nasal prongs with complementing head gear
- Machine with appropriate capabilities (Table 30-1)
- Tubing and exhalation valve
- Humidifier, as indicated
- Low pressure alarm
- Pulse oximetry
- Cardiorespiratory monitor
- Suction
- Oxygen
- Appropriate protective equipment

TABLE 30-1	Noninvasive Positive Pressure Ventilators				
Ventilator	**Modes**	**Pressure Range**	**Sensitivity**	**Ramp/Delay**	**Alarms**
Respironics ST/D	CPAP, S, S/T, T	4 -20 cm H_2O	Flow	None	None
Respironics Vision	S/T, CPAP	4 -40 cm H_2O	Flow	None	Yes
Respironics Biflex	S S	3 -20 cm H_2O	Flow	Yes	Yes
Respironics Synchrony	CPAP, S, S/T,T	4 -30 cm H_2O	Flow	Yes	Yes
Sullivan VPAP II	CPAP, S	2 -25 cm H_2O	Flow	Yes	Yes
Sullivan VPAP II ST	CPAP, S, S/T, T	2 -25cm H_2O	Flow	Yes	Yes
PuritanBennett Knight Star	A/C , I/E, CPAP	3 -30 cm H_2O	Flow	Yes	Yes

CPAP, Continuous positive airway pressure; *S,* spontaneous mode; *S/T,* spontaneous timed mode; *T,* timed mode; *A/C,* assist control mode; *I/E,* inspiratory to expiratory ratio.
Respironics, Murrysville, PA; Sullivan (Resp Med Inc., Northridge Australia); Puritan Bennett (Pleasanton, CA).

Procedure for NPPV

Steps	Rationale	Considerations
1. Ensure child and family understand procedure and questions are answered.	Evaluates and reinforces under standing of previously taught information.[4]	Developmental, cognitive, and anxiety levels determine approach to and effectiveness of teaching.
2. Collect all necessary equipment and supplies.	Preparation ensures completion of procedure safely and without delays.	
3. Measure and select appropriate interface, head gear, and ventilator (see Figures 30-2 to 30-6). *(Level V*)*	Inappropriate interface and head gear reduce the effectiveness of NPPV and may increase complications and decrease compliance.[20,21] Head gear is needed to stabilize the interface. The ventilator is chosen based on the intent of therapy and functionality of the device.	Because of the limited availability of smaller mask sizes, consider use of nasal prongs for children less than 1 year of age. Attention to excessive leaks and triggering problems is especially necessary with use of nasal prongs. Evaluation of machine capabilities assists with appropriate selection (see Table 30-1). An exhalation valve is necessary with use of a single limb circuit to provide adequate clearance of expiratory gases and prevent rebreathing of carbon dioxide (CO_2).
4. Wash hands and put on personal protective equipment as indicated.	Reduces transmission of infection. Protects personnel health.	
5. Apply selected interface to child and connect to ventilator. *(Level V*)*	For effective ventilation, the interface must be fitted to the child's face/nose.	Initiation of therapy might require short intervals or trials with mask or nasal prongs before continuous application of NPPV. Noninvasive positive pressure ventilation, especially delivered via mask, is often applied at intervals to allow for breaks in skin pressure.
6. Initiate therapy at prescribed ventilatory settings.	A prescribing practitioner's order is necessary for the application of mechanical ventilation.	
7. Select and set mode (see Figure 30-1). *(Level IV*)*	Selection of mode is variable depending on the goal of therapy and child's spontaneous breathing effort.	Spontaneously timed mode (S/T) is often used to provide guaranteed minimal minute ventilation for respiratory support.

8. Select and set mechanical rate. Consider:
  Infants: 25 to 30 breaths per minute (bpm)
    Small children: 15 to 20 bpm
    Adolescents: 10 to 12 bpm[22]
(Level IV)*
	Mechanical rate is selected with the S/T mode or timed mode (T). Rate selection should be made on basis of the minimal minute ventilation for the child.	For facilitation of synchronization in children unable to trigger the machine, S/T mode is used with slightly higher back-up rates.

9. Select and set inspiratory positive airway pressure (IPAP). Consider 6 to 18 cm H_2O. *(Level IV*)*	The IPAP pressures are adjusted to achieve good chest wall excursion with a resolution of tachypnea and hypercapnia.[22]	Monitoring of pressures with manometer is recommended for verification of delivery of preset pressure.

* Level IV: Limited clinical studies to support recommendations
  Level V: Clinical studies in more than one or two patient populations and situations to support recommendations

Procedure for NPPV—*Continued*

Steps	Rationale	Considerations
	A direct correlation is found between pressure differential and tidal volume exchange.	With higher mechanical rates, IPAP pressures may need lowering to guarantee delivery of pressure at the shorter inspiratory time.
10. Select and set expired positive airway pressure (EPAP). Consider 4 to 6 cm H_2O. *(Level IV*)*	The EPAP levels are set to maintain adequate expiratory flow. Children with severe hypoxemia or air trapping may need higher levels of EPAP to increase the mean airway pressure to improve oxygenation or counter elevated levels of intrinsic positive end expiratory pressure (PEEP).[22]	Monitoring of pressures with manometer is recommended for verification of delivery of preset pressure. Lower EPAP pressures may be effective in young children, but adolescents need higher pressures, similar to adults.[12]
11. Titrate the liter flow of oxygen (L/min) or fractional inspired oxygen (FiO_2). *(Level IV*)*	Supplemental oxygen may be necessary after the initiation of NPPV to keep oxygen saturations at more than 90%.	Oxygen can be added to the side port on the mask or directly into the inspiratory circuit.
12. Select and set inspiratory time (Ti).	Required for the T mode.	
13. Adjust rise time. *(Level IV*)*	The time to reach peak inspiratory flow impacts the efficacy of NPPV, especially the child's tolerance with an adjustment in flow pattern during the inspiratory phase.	Children with high respiratory rates and resistance may need a quicker rise time to provide synchronization.
14. Activate ramp. *(Level II*)*	Ramps can be used to increase tolerance during initiation of NPPV. Gradual increases of pressure over time may enhance the child's acceptance of therapy.	
15. Adjust humidifier. *(Level II*)*	Humidification is used with NPPV ventilation to thin secretions and humidify the airway.	Heated humidification is usually used on children less than 3 years of age. Use of a passover humidifier is usually adequate, but children with thick or tenacious secretions may need the added benefit of heated humidification.[9] NPPV initiated only at night is less likely to need humidification.
16. Set and activate low pressure or flow alarms.	Low pressure alarms are used to detect disconnection in the system. High pressure alarms are used for notification of increased pressure in the system. Flow alarms measure the leak in L/min and are activated when the leak increases above the preset flow alarm.	Not all noninvasive ventilators come with internal alarms, so an external alarm may need to be added.
17. Remove any personal protective equipment and wash hands.	Reduces transmission of infection. Protects personnel health.	

* Level II: Theory-based; no research data to support recommendations; recommendations from expert consensus group may exist
Level IV: Limited clinical studies to support recommendations

Expected Outcomes[13]

- Improved oxygenation and ventilation
- Improved lung volume as indicated on chest x-ray (CXR)
- Reduction in work of breathing
- Child-ventilator synchrony

- Prevent intubation and invasive ventilation
- Maintain effective gastrointestinal function

- Ability to clear secretions
- Maintain skin integrity

- Child has acceptable level of comfort

Unexpected Outcomes

- Hypoxemia
- Hypercarbia
- Respiratory muscle fatigue
- Respiratory effort that is asynchronous with the ventilator
- Hyperinflation/air trapping
- Pneumothorax
- Intubation and invasive ventilation
- Gastric insufflation
- Aspiration
- Decreased ability to cough and clear secretions
- Skin breakdown or pressure ulcers
- Abrasion and pressure injury, including to the eye
- Nasal discomfort, congestion, and pain
- Unmanaged pain and agitation

Monitoring and Care of the Child

Activities and Interventions	Rationale	Reportable Conditions
1. Assess signs and symptoms of changes in oxygenation/ventilation, including lung sounds, vital signs, oxygen saturation, and work of breathing.	Determines changes in respiratory status and effectiveness of therapy.	• Diminished breath sounds • Significant changes in oxygenation saturation and arterial/venous blood gases • Increased work of breathing
2. Patterns of breathing, including synchrony with machine.	Ensures delivery of set pressures. Adequate support decreases rapid and shallow breathing pattern and promotes a slower and deeper pattern.	• Ventilatory asynchrony
3. Check and maintain the proper fit of the child's NPPV device. Monitor leaks around the interface.	Ensures that the child receives desired ventilatory support.	• Inappropriately fit mask that affects the delivery of adequate pressures
4. Monitor for gastric insufflation and decompress stomach as needed.	Noninvasive positive pressure ventilation can lead to increased gas flow to the stomach. Decompression of the stomach decreases the risk of aspiration.[4]	• Inability to empty stomach
5. Consider humidification with delivery of NPPV.	Thin secretions are more easily mobilized.	• Thick secretions that cannot be cleared
6. Oral and nasal airway suctioning as needed.	Increased secretions may impede ventilation.	• Change in amount and character of secretions[11]
7. Assess skin in contact with interface every 2 to 4 hours and as necessary, with particular attention paid to bony prominences. Keep skin clean and dry.	Impaired skin integrity increases the risk for infection. Bridge of nose and cheeks are prone to skin breakdown.	• Areas of skin breakdown
8. Provide distraction with television, books, toys, or games.	May enhance child's cooperation with application of noninvasive interface.	• Irritability that interferes with ventilation
9. Reposition child (including head) every 1 to 2 hours.	Alleviates pressure points and prevents skin breakdown.	• Skin breakdown

Documentation

- Date and time therapy is initiated and stopped
- Type of mask/nasal prongs used for therapy
- Child's tolerance of therapy
- Assessment of skin integrity, including skin assessment, eye irritation, and nasal irritation
- Ventilator settings, including mode, rate (set/actual), IPAP, EPAP, Ti, oxygen flow (FiO_2), rise time, ramp (if used), humidifier temperature and water level, and alarms functional
- Assessment of cardiorespiratory status, including vital signs, lung sounds, chest wall expansion, work of breathing, synchrony with ventilator, pulse oximetry, and end tidal CO_2 or transcutaneous CO_2 monitoring
- Unexpected outcomes
- Additional interventions needed before, during, and after NPPV
- Comfort assessment and any specific interventions provided
- Child and family education

References

1. Curley MAQ, Thompson JF: Oxygenation and ventilation. In Curley MAQ, Moloney-Harmon PA, editors: *Critical care nursing of infants and children,* ed 2, Philadelphia, 2001, Saunders.
2. Hazinski MF, et al, editors: *Pediatric advanced life support provider manual,* Dallas, 2002, American Heart Association.
3. Stoltzfus S: The role of noninvasive ventilation, *Dimens Crit Care Nurs* 25(2):66-70, 2006.
4. Chieifetz IM: Invasive and noninvasive pediatric mechanical ventilation, *Resp Care* 48(4):442-453, 2003.
5. Panitch HB: Respiratory issues in the management of children with neuromuscular disease, *Resp Care* 51(8):885-893, 2006.
6. Venkataraman ST: Mechanical ventilation and respiratory care In Fuhrman B, Zimmerman J, editors: *Pediatric critical care,* ed 3, Philadelphia, 2006, Mosby.
7. Aly H, et al: Does the experience with the use of nasal continuous positive airway pressure improve over time in extremely low birth weight infants? *Pediatrics* 114(3):697-702, 2004.
8. Essouri S, et al: Noninvasive positive pressure ventilation in infants with upper airway obstruction: comparison of continuous and bilevel positive pressure, *Intens Care Med* 31:574-580, 2005.
9. Mador MJ, et al: Effect of heated humidication on compliance and quality of life in patients with sleep apnea using nasal continuous positive airway pressure, *Chest* 128:2151-2158, 2005.
10. Durning S, Hales RL: Every breath you take, *Nurs Manage* 36-38, 2003.
11. Pelosi P, Severginni P, et al: Non-invasive ventilation by conventional interfaces and helmet in the emergency department, *Eur J Emer Med* 10(2):79-86, 2003.
12. Teague WG: Pediatric application of noninvasive ventilation, *Resp Care* 42(2):414-423.
13. Hill NS: Complications of noninvasive mask ventilation, *Resp Care* 42(2):432-442, 1997.
14. Morley C: Continuous distending pressure, *Arch Dis Child Fetal Neonatal Ed* 81:F152-F156, 1999.
15. Robertson NJ, et al: Nasal deformities resulting from flow driver continuous positive airway pressure, *Arch Dis Child Fetal Neonatal Ed* 75:F209-F212, 1996.
16. Millet V, et al: Necrosis of the nasal columella secondary to nasal continuous positive airway pressure, *Arch Pediatr* 5:485, 1997.
17. Buettiker V, et al: Advantages and disadvantages of different nasal CPAP systems in newborns, *Intens Care Med* 30:926-930, 2004.
18. Fourrier F, et al: Colonization of dental plaque, a source of nosocomial infections in intensive care patients, *Crit Care Med* 26:432-437, 1998.
19. American Association of Critical Care Nurses: (2006) *Practice alert: oral care of the critically ill,* 2006, retrieved August 16, 2006, from http://www.aacn.org/AACN /practiceAlert.nsf/vwdoc/PracticeAlertMain.
20. Gregoretti C, et al: Evaluation of patient skin breakdown and comfort with a new facemask for non-invasive ventilation: a multi-center study, *Intens Care Med* 28(3):278-284, 2002.
21. Turner R: NPPV: face versus interface, *Resp Care* 42(4):389-393, 1997.
22. Bach J, Niranjan V: Noninvasive ventilation in children. In Bach J, editor: *Noninvasive mechanical ventilation,* Philadelphia, 2002, Hanley and Belfus, Inc.

Additional Readings

Bach JR: *Noninvasive mechanical ventilation,* Philadelphia, 2002, Hanley and Belfus.

Bourke SC, Williams TL, et al: Non-invasive ventilation in motor neuron disease: current UK practice, *Amyotroph Lateral Scler Other Motor Neuron Disord* 3(3):145-149, 2002.

British Thoracic Society Standards of Care Committee: Non-invasive ventilation in acute respiratory failure, *Thorax* 57(3):192-211, 2002.

Calderini E, Confalonieri M, et al: Patient-ventilator asynchrony during noninvasive ventilation, *Intens Care Med* 25:662-667, 1999.

Elliott MW: Non-invasive ventilation-mechanisms of benefit, *Medizinisehe Klinik* 94:Sondemr:2-6, 1999.

Evans TW: Non-invasive positive pressure ventilation in acute respiratory failure, *Intens Care Med* 27:166-178, 2001.

Fortenberry JD, Del Toro J, et al: Management of pediatric acute hypoxemic respiratory insufficiency with bi-level positive pressure (BIPAP) nasal mask ventilation, *Chest* 108(4):1059-1064, 1995.

Girault C, Daudenthum I, et al: Noninvasive ventilation as a systematic extubation and weaning technique in acute-on-chronic respiratory failure, *Am J Respir Crit Care Med* 160:86-92, 1999.

Gregoretti C, Confalonieri M, et al: Evaluation of patient skin breakdown and comfort with a new facemask for non-invasive ventilation: a multi-center study, *Intens Care Med* 28:278-284, 2002.

Keenan S, Powers C, et al: Noninvasive positive pressure ventilation for post extubation respiratory distress, *JAMA* 287:3238-3244, 2002.

MacIntyre N, Branson R: *Mechanical ventilation,* Philadelphia, 2001, Saunders.

Mehta S, Hill NS: Noninvasive ventilation, *Am J Respir Crit Care Med* 163:540-577, 2001.

Pierson DJ: Noninvasive positive pressure ventilation, *Resp Care* 42(2):370-379, 1997.

Sanchez E: CPAP and BiPAP: support modes for the spontaneously breathing patient. In Festa C, Bigos D, Baumgart S, editors: *Clinical guidelines for mechanical ventilation,* Newtown, PA, 2002, Handbooks in Health Care Co.

Simonds AK: Nocturnal ventilation in neuromuscular disease-when and how? *Monaldi Arch Chest Dis* 57(5-6):273-276, 2002.

Teague WG, Fortenberry JD: Noninvasive ventilatory support in pediatric respiratory failure, *Resp Care* 40(1):86-96, 1995.

Teague WG, Kervin L, et al: Nasal bi-level positive airway pressure acutely improves ventilation and oxygen saturation in children with upper airway obstruction [abstract], *Am Rev Respir Dis* 143(4, Part 2):505A, 1991.

Waters K, Everett FM, et al: Use of nasal CPAP instead of tracheostomy for palliative care in two children, *J Paediatr Child Health* 30(2):179-181, 1994.

Wunderink RG, Jennings SG: Noninvasive ventilation. In MacIntyre NR, Branson RD, editors: *Mechanical ventilation,* Philadelphia, 2001, Saunders.

Pronation Therapy

P U R P O S E : Prone positioning is used as supportive therapy to improve gas exchange in pediatric patients with acute lung injury or acute respiratory distress syndrome

Eileen Briening

PREREQUISITE KNOWLEDGE

- Child development as it relates to clinical assessment and procedure
- Anatomy and physiology of the pediatric pulmonary system, including structural characteristics specific to the infant and child[1-3]
- Signs and symptoms of inadequate oxygenation and ventilation, including the physiologic symptoms of respiratory distress
- Mastery of pediatric advanced life support competencies, including use of artificial airways, oxygen delivery systems, and tracheal suctioning[4]
- An understanding of the pathophysiology of acute lung injury (ALI) and acute respiratory distress syndrome (ARDS)
  - ❖ In ALI/ARDS infection, blood loss or traumatic and inhalation injury damages the capillaries in the lungs or alveoli, causing fluid to leak from the capillaries into the alveoli. Some alveoli fill with fluid and other alveoli collapse, which leads to poor gas exchange and decreased lung compliance.[5]
- Prone positioning is thought to be an inexpensive and noninvasive method to improve ventilation.[5] Several studies have shown that pronation therapy improves oxygenation in patients with acute respiratory failure.[6-11] Most researchers, however, have not found an improvement in survival rates or a reduction in ventilator days.[12-15]
- The exact mechanism of improved oxygenation with prone positioning is not clearly understood. Computerized tomographic scan studies have shown that patients with ARDS have an uneven distribution of alveolar collapse.[9] Prone positioning appears to affect regional inflation/ventilation of the lung and recruit more of the atelectatic posterior lung regions.[9,10,16,17] The shifting of fluid from the dorsal lung may allow undamaged lung regions to be recruited and oxygenated, thereby enhancing ventilation.[18] Other possible suppositions for improved oxygenation include a decrease in abdominal compression of the chest and improved mobilization and removal of secretions.[9,19]

- Contraindications to prone positioning include unresolved increased intracranial pressure, unstable spine, uncontrolled hemodynamic instability, open chest or unstable chest wall, and unstable long bone or pelvic fractures[6,7,10,18]

- Response to therapy may occur immediately or up to 6 to 12 hours after prone positioning.[10] Responders have been described as those patients with improvement in the partial pressure of oxygen/fractional concentration of oxygen in inspired gas (PaO_2/FiO_2) ratio by 15% to 20% or with an increase in PaO_2 of greater than 10 mm Hg.[7,10,16,18]

- A trial of prone positioning is recommended for assessment of the child's level of response. The amount of time the child is in the prone position is highly variable and is dependent on the child's response to therapy. A schedule of every 4 to 6 hours has been recommended by some investigators, although others suggest that patients maintain a longer period of time in the prone position (12 to 20 hours).[10,11,17]

- If the child responds to therapy but does not continue to have improved oxygen saturation (SaO_2) in the supine position, consideration is given to more frequent prone positioning, with the time supine or lateral limited for 1 hour.[10,18]

- With prone positioning of a child, oxygen saturations may initially decrease but typically return to baseline within 5 minutes. If oxygen saturations do not return to baseline or the child's condition becomes hemodynamically unstable, consideration is given to a return to the supine position.[10]
- Discontinuation of therapy is considered if the child has adverse reactions or does not show a positive response.

CHILD AND FAMILY ASSESSMENT

- Child's developmental level and ability to interact ➡*Rationale:* Influences preparation and interaction.
- Child's and family's understanding of the reasons for and risks and benefits of prone positioning ➡*Rationale:* Evaluates child's and family's understanding of the procedure and provides a gauge for ongoing education.
- Signs and symptoms of inadequate oxygenation and ventilation ➡*Rationale:* Indicates effective pulmonary function.
- Level of anxiety, consciousness, and hemodynamic stability ➡*Rationale:* Determines the need for additional support and the ability to tolerate the prone position.
- Note skin diseases, nutrition deficits, bone deformities, and height and weight of the child ➡*Rationale:* Prevents areas of pressure and potential breakdown, maintain functional positioning of joints, and prevent accidental extubation.
- Presence of increased intracranial pressure, unstable spine, uncontrolled hemodynamic instability, or unstable long bone fractures ➡*Rationale:* Contraindications to prone positioning.
- Assess security of the endotracheal tube (ETT), feeding tube, intravascular lines, and monitoring devices ➡*Rationale:* Decreases risk of accidental extubation or line/tube displacement during turning. Supports continued therapy and monitoring.
- Assess level of sedation and neuromuscular blockade ➡*Rationale:* Indicates potential risk for accidental extubation and loss of arterial/venous line access and access of other tubes.
- Assess need for suctioning ➡*Rationale:* Pronation therapy often increases tracheal and oral secretions.

CHILD AND FAMILY EDUCATION

Individualized, developmentally appropriate education is provided to the family and to the child based on desire for knowledge, readiness to learn, and overall neurologic and psychosocial state.

- Explain pronation therapy, including the purpose, steps, rationale, and risks to the child ➡*Rationale:* Providing information decreases fear and anxiety.
- Discuss appropriate expected outcomes of the procedure ➡*Rationale:* Allows family and medical team to formulate similar goals and expectations.
- Encourage questions and answer questions as they arise ➡*Rationale:* Reinforcement of information is needed during periods of stress.

EQUIPMENT

- Neuromuscular blocking agents, as indicated
- Sedative agents, as indicated
- Pillows, small blankets, and gel pads
- Draw sheets
- Personal protective equipment

Procedure for Pronation Therapy

Steps	Rationale	Considerations
1. Ensure child and family understand procedure and questions are answered.	Evaluates and reinforces understanding of previously taught information.[7]	Developmental level, cognitive ability, and anxiety level determine approach to and effectiveness of teaching.
2. Collect all necessary equipment and supplies.	Preparation ensures completion of procedure safely and in a timely manner.	Individual cushions with egg crate material for head, chest, pelvic area, and extremities may be helpful.[20] Verify that intubation equipment, including appropriately sized tubes, face mask, ventilation bag, and intubation medications are in the room in case of accident extubation. Have fluids on hand and ready to administer for a significant drop in blood pressure. May consider placement of a transpyloric feeding tube or discontinuation of feedings 1 hour before changing child to prone position.[10,20]

Procedure	**for Pronation Therapy**—*Continued*

Steps	Rationale	Considerations
3. Wash hands and put on personal protective equipment as indicated.	Reduces transmission of infection. Protects personnel health.	
4. Monitor child's vital signs and indications of inadequate oxygenation and ventilation before, during, and after procedure. *(Level II*)* • Remove anterior electrocardiographic (ECG) leads and replace ECG electrodes on back, shoulders, or sides of child.	Identifies adequacy of ventilation and signs and symptoms of complications. Prevents skin irritation and pressure injury from ECG electrodes or cables. Allows for easier access to electrodes and continued monitoring during turn.[18]	Pulse oximetry (SaO$_2$) and capnography (ETCO$_2$) are recommended to ensure continuous monitoring of oxygenation and ventilation.
5. If child is receiving a paralytic, provide eye lubrication and consider patching or taping eyelids closed.[10,18]	Helps prevent corneal drying and eye injury.	Depends on the disposition and clinical condition of the child.
6. Reinforce and secure all tubes (such as ETT, feeding tubes) and empty drainage bags (Foley, ileostomy).	Decreases risk of accidental extubation or line/tube displacement during turning.	Consider need to suction child's artificial airway and oropharynx before turning. Consider inflating the cuff of the ETT or tracheostomy.[20]
7. Administer appropriate medications to the child as indicated.	Provides comfort to child and reduces risk of accidental extubation or loss of arterial/venous line access.	Sedation might need to be increased for turning.[18]
8. Assemble appropriate number of assistants.	The number of assistants needed is dependent on the age, size, and condition of the child.[11]	A minimum of two nurses and a respiratory therapist should be present at the bedside, with one person at the head and two additional assistants on each side of the child. A prescribing practitioner should be readily available.
9. Temporarily cap all nonessential vascular lines.[21]	Minimizes risk of dislodgement during pronation process. Reduces the risk of aspiration.[22]	
10. Position all lines and tubes inserted above the waist towards the head of the bed, with sufficient slack allowed (e.g., subclavian lines, upper extremity vascular lines, or nasogastric tubes; Figure 31-1).	Minimizes tangling, kinking, or disconnection during the pronation process.	Carefully drape ventilator tubing above the head.
11. Position chest tubes and lines (e.g., femoral lines, Foley catheter tubing) below waist towards the end of the bed.		Place drainage systems at end of the bed with tubing along the child's side. The respiratory therapist may need to move the ventilator to the opposite side of the bed.
12. Confirm correct number of participants and ensure all participants clearly understand their role.	Facilitates ease of prone positioning; communicates responsibilities to each individual.	Individuals may be assigned specific lines or tubes to monitor. For prevention of injury, all individuals who assist with turning the child must use a wide base of support during pronation procedure.[10]

Procedure continues on following page

Procedure continues on following page

---

* Level II: Theory-based; no research data to support recommendations; recommendations from expert consensus group may exist

Procedure	**for Pronation Therapy**—*Continued*	
Steps	**Rationale**	**Considerations**

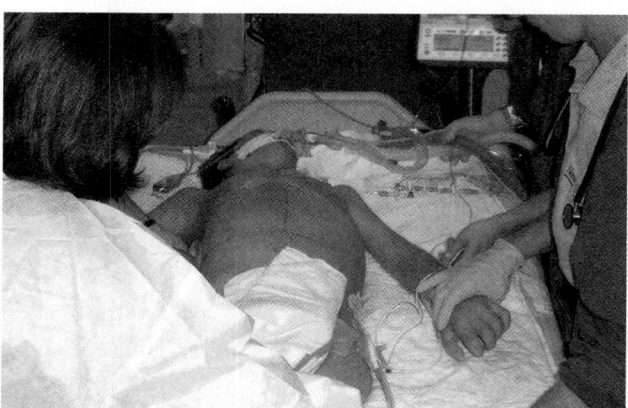

FIGURE 31-1   Preparation of Child for Prone Positioning. Position all lines and tubes inserted above waist towards head of bed, with sufficient slack allowed. Position chest tubes and lines placed below waist towards end of bed.

Steps	Rationale	Considerations
13. One person stands at the head of the bed, lifts the head, and controls the position of ETT and ventilator tubing.[10,18] *(Level IV*)*	The health care provider assigned to the head of the bed manages the airway and head position.	
14. For a larger child: a. Use a draw sheet to move the child to the side of the bed furthest from the ventilator. b. Place arms close to the body. Carefully tuck the child's lower arm and hand nearest the ventilator under the buttocks (palm up). c. Place the outer leg (the side to be rotated) on top of the inner leg. Cross the legs at the ankle. *(Level IV*)*	Provides sufficient room to rotate the body safely.[22] Draw sheet assists with patient alignment. Protects the arm from injury during turning.[18]	An alternative is to place a draw sheet over the child, position chest and pelvic cushions, cover with full sheet, and tuck in edges of sheet under child, creating a mummy effect.[20] An infant or toddler may be lifted up and turned prone without additional linens and then lifted again for placement of cushions under child.[20] One individual, closest to the child, maintains close contact with the bed to maintain patient safety. If using Vollman Prone Positioner (Hill-Rom, Inc, Batesville, Inc.), follow specific directions.[10]
15. On the count of the person responsible for the airway, turn the child to prone position. Consider a half turn, pause, and reassess, especially for patients with transient hemodynamic instability (Figure 31-2).	Better success has been noted by some with a full turn to prone.[18] Turning to the lateral position for an initial period may be prudent for the child.[10]	Avoid sudden and unexpected forward and backward rotation.[18] Keep the child's head in alignment with the body.
16. Briefly assess child's clinical condition and patency and security of all lines/tubes and reposition as necessary.	Supports ongoing therapy.	Any lines/tubes that were capped should be uncapped and reattached.[21]
17. Ensure child's head is turned to side, with head and ear well cushioned, high enough off the bed for proper alignment with the spine.[18] Place an absorbent pad under nose and mouth.	Supports body alignment. Minimizes the risk of pressure injury and skin breakdown to the head and ear. Pad helps to absorb secretions.	

* Level IV: Limited clinical studies to support recommendations

Procedure for **Pronation Therapy**—*Continued*

Steps	Rationale	Considerations

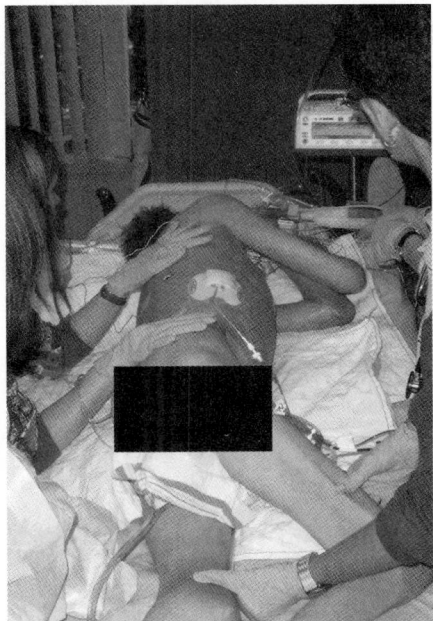

FIGURE 31-2 Turning Child to Prone Position. On count of person responsible for airway, turn child to prone position. Consider half turn, pause, and reassess, especially for those patients with transient hemodynamic instability.

Steps	Rationale	Considerations
18. Place arms in a comfortable position, ensuring good extremity alignment. Typically, arms are positioned at sides with elbows slightly flexed and palms down.	Keeps the shoulders and elbows in natural alignment.[10]	Other positions of comfort can also be used (such as the "swim" position with one arm up and one arm down).[10]
19. Place blankets or gel pads under bony prominences.	Prevents pressure injury to skin. Allows for correct body alignment.	Minor adjustments may be necessary to obtain proper alignment (Figure 31-3).

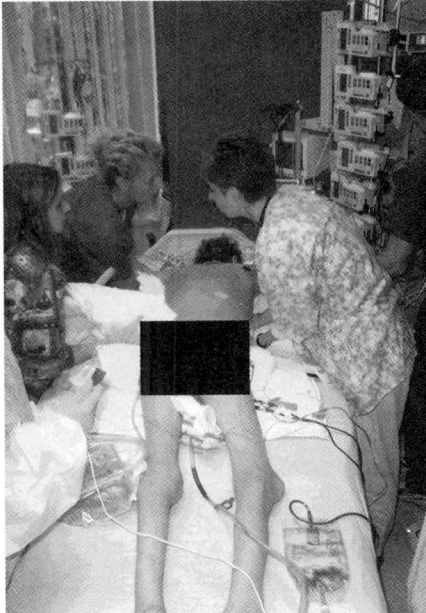

FIGURE 31-3 Positioning of Child. Adjust cushions and child to obtain proper alignment.

Procedure continues on following page

Procedure	for Pronation Therapy—*Continued*	
Steps	**Rationale**	**Considerations**

- Position knees and feet with appropriately sized rolls. A support or pillow under the distal femur and lower leg is recommended (Figure 31-4).[20]

The upper chest and hips may be supported with foam pad or rolled blankets so the abdomen protrudes. *(Level IV*)*
Consider use of hydrocolloid dressing over areas where pressure or skin injuries are likely to appear (i.e., elbows, knees, bony prominences of the pelvis).[10] *(Level I*)*

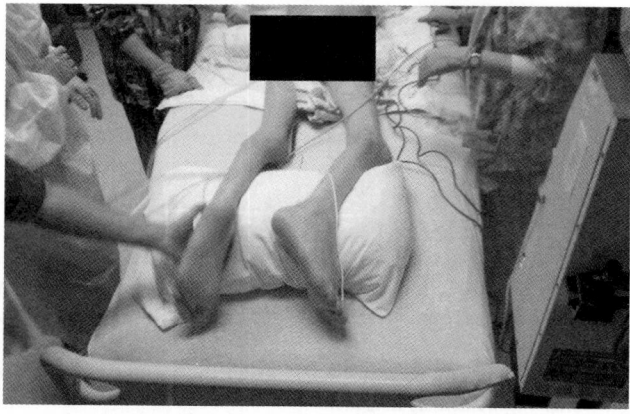

FIGURE 31-4   Cushions for Lower Legs. Support or pillow under distal femur and lower leg is recommended.

Steps	Rationale	Considerations
20. Recalibrate pressure systems.	Continued monitoring is necessary.	
21. Reassess child's clinical condition.[18]	Ensure stability.	Consider drawing arterial blood gas (ABG) 30 minutes after turning.[10,18] Administer fluids and inotropes as necessary to support blood pressure.
22. Wash hands and remove any personal protective equipment.	Reduces transmission of micro-organisms.	
23. Leave child in the prone position for 4 to 18 hours or as tolerated.[6] *(Level V*)*	Timeframe varies depending on the child's condition, effectiveness of therapy, and institutional guidelines.	Frequently monitor pressure areas, such as bony prominences, including ears and tops of feet. Check vascular access sites for bleeding.
24. Alter child's position slightly at least every 1 to 2 hours.[10]	Maintains skin integrity.	The face and ears are most vulnerable because of limited structural padding.[10]
Return Child to Supine Position		
25. Prepare the child for turning.	Preparation ensures the child and family understand the procedure and that procedure is done safely and without delays.	Sedation might need to be increased for turning.[18]

* Level I: Manufacturer's recommendations only
Level IV: Limited clinical studies to support recommendations
Level V: Clinical studies in more than one or two patient populations and situations to support recommendations

Procedure for Pronation Therapy—*Continued*

Steps	Rationale	Considerations
26. Gather appropriate number of assistants and ensure all understand their roles.	The number of assistants needed is dependent on the age, size, and condition of the child.	A minimum of two nurses and a respiratory therapist should be present at the bedside, with one person at the head and two additional assistants on each side of the child. A prescribing practitioner should be readily available.
27. Wash hands and put on personal protective equipment, as indicated.	Reduces transmission of infection.	
28. Arrange ventilator tubing and other tubes and lines for sufficient length and mobility to avoid pulling.[10]	Minimizes tangling, kinking, or disconnection during the pronation process.	Tubes and lines placed above the waist are moved toward the head; tubes and lines below the waist and chest tubes are placed at the foot.
29. Remove pillows and supports.[10]	Preparation ensures completion of procedure safely and in a timely manner.	
30. a. Align child at edge of bed closest to the ventilator.[10] b. Bring arms to either side of head.[10] c. For larger children, cross the leg closest to the edge of the bed over the opposite leg at ankle. Use draw sheet to lift the child as needed.[10]	Provides sufficient room to rotate the body safely.[22] Draw sheet assists with turning and maintaining patient alignment. Protects the arm from injury during turning [18]	An alternative to placing a draw sheet is to cover the child with full sheet and tuck in edges of sheet under child, creating a mummy effect.[20] An infant or toddler may be lifted up and turned supine without additional linens and then lifted to place cushions under child.[20]
31. On the count of the person responsible for the airway, turn the child to supine or lateral position (as predetermined by the team) toward the center of the bed and away from the ventilator.	Coordination is essential. Protects airway and ensures body alignment.	All participants assist in ensuring that lines and tubes remain in place.
32. Once turn is complete, reposition the child, with consideration for comfort and proper body alignment.	Supports body alignment. Minimizes the risk of pressure injury and skin breakdown.	
33. Reassess the child's clinical condition. Replace ECG electrodes and all vascular access lines and tubing. Recalibrate pressure systems.	Ensures stability. Continued monitoring is necessary.	
34. Wash hands and remove any personal protective equipment.	Reduces transmission of infection.	

Expected Outcomes

- Improved oxygenation and ventilation
- Increased recruitment of atelectatic posterior lung areas
- Improved mobilization and removal of secretions
- Maintenance of all lines and tubes

- Child has acceptable level of comfort
- Maintain skin integrity

- Hemodynamic stability

Unexpected Outcomes

- No improvement in oxygenation and ventilation

- Dislodgement of endotracheal tube that results in hypoxemia
- Removal of vascular access lines that results in hemorrhage
- Pneumothorax from chest tube dislodgement
- Accidental removal of other tubes or lines
- Unmanaged pain and agitation
- Skin breakdown or pressure ulcers
- Abrasion and pressure injury, including to the eye
- Hemodynamic instability

Monitoring and Care of the Child

Activities and Interventions	Rationale	Reportable Conditions
1. Assess cardiorespiratory status, including respiratory rate, work of breathing, heart rate, blood pressure, SaO_2, $ETCO_2$. • Consider arterial blood gas 30 minutes after position change and note PaO_2/FiO_2 ratio.	Assess tolerance and response to procedure. Ensure airway security and other therapies (i.e., inotropes) continue to provide adequate support.	• Failure to return to baseline respiratory rate and effort, heart rate, and blood pressure[10] • Airway displacement • Hypoxemia, poor peripheral perfusion, hemodynamic instability
2. Assess child for pain control and sedation.	Prone position may be uncomfortable for child.	• Unresolved pain or agitation
3. Monitor skin and bony prominences for signs of redness and breakdown. Consider placement of hydrocolloid dressing over areas where shearing and friction injuries are likely to occur (i.e., elbows, knees, bony prominences of the pelvis).[10]	Maintenance of skin integrity and reduction of pressure, shear, and friction injuries.	• Areas of breakdown
4. Reposition child (including head) slightly every 1 to 2 hours.	Alleviates pressure points and prevents skin breakdown.	• Skin breakdown
5. Oral and airway suctioning as needed.	Increased mobilization of secretions may occur and necessitate more frequent suctioning of oropharynx or endotracheal tube.	• Change in amount and character of secretions[10]

Documentation

- Cardiorespiratory status, including SaO_2, $ETCO_2$, heart rate, and blood pressure, before, during, and after pronation therapy
- Skin assessment
- Length of time in prone position
- Any complications noted during turning or while child is in prone position
- Additional interventions necessary before, during, and after pronation therapy
- Color, amount, consistency, and odor of tracheal secretions
- Child's response to pronation therapy
- Comfort assessment and any specific interventions provided
- Child and family education
- Unexpected outcomes and related treatment

References

1. Thompson A: Pediatric airway management. In Fuhrman B, Zimmerman J, editors: *Pediatric critical care,* ed 3, Philadelphia, 2006, Mosby.
2. McCance K, Huether S: *Pathophysiology: the biologic bases for disease in adults and children,* Philadelphia, 2002, Mosby.
3. Curley MAQ, Thompson JE: Oxygenation and ventilation. In Curley MAQ, Moloney-Harmon PA, editors: *Critical care nursing of infants and children,* ed 2, Philadelphia, 2000, Saunders.
4. Hazinski MF, et al, editors: *Pediatric advanced life support provider manual,* Dallas, 2002, American Heart Association.
5. Murray N: *Textbook of respiratory medicine,* ed 3, Philadelphia, 2002, Saunders.
6. Anderson MR: Update on pediatric acute respiratory distress syndrome, *Resp Care* 48(3):261-279, 2003.
7. Curley MAQ, Thompson JE, Arnold JH: The effects of early and repeated prone positioning in pediatric patients with acute lung injury, *Chest* 118:156-163, 2000.
8. Gattinoni L, et al: Effect of prone positioning on the survival of patients with acute respiratory failure, *N Engl J Med* 345:568-573, 2001.
9. Kornecki A, et al: Randomized trial of prolonged prone positioning in children with acute respiratory failure, *Chest* 119(1):211-218, 2001.
10. Vollman K: Pronation therapy. In Lynn-McHale Wiegand DJ, Carlson K, editors: *AACN procedure manual for critical care,* ed 5, Philadelphia, 2005, Elsevier.
11. Balas MC: Prone positioning in patients with acute respiratory distress syndrome: applying research to practice, *Crit Care Nurs* 20:24-36, 2000.
12. Curley MA, et al: Effect of prone positioning on clinical outcomes in children with acute lung injury: a randomized controlled trial, *JAMA* 294(2):229-237, 2005.
13. Main E: Prone positioning does not reduce the ventilation period or mortality in paediatric acute lung injury, *Aus J Physiotherapy* 52(1):63, 2006.
14. Gattinoni L, et al: Decrease in $PaCO_2$ with prone position is predictive of improved outcome in acute respiratory distress syndrome, *Crit Care Med* 31:2804-2805, 2003.
15. Guerin C, et al: Effects of systematic prone positioning in hypoxemic acute respiratory failure, *JAMA* 292:2379-2387, 2004.
16. Pelosi P, et al: Prone position in ARDS, *Eur Respir J* 20:1017-1028, 2002.
17. Pelosi P, et al: Effects of the prone position on respiratory mechanics and gas exchange during acute lung injury, *Am J Resp Crit Care Med* 157:387-393, 1998.
18. Marion BS: A turn for the better: "prone positioning" of patients with ARDS, *AJN* 101(5):26-34, 2001.
19. Albert RK: Prone position in ARDS: what do we know, and what do we need to know, *Crit Care Med* 27(11):2574-2575, 1999.
20. Curley MAQ, et al: Clinical trial design: Effects of pediatric prone positioning on clinical outcomes in infants and children with acute respiratory distress syndrome. *Journal of Crit Care* 21(1), 23-32, 32-37.
21. Grant MJ, Curley MAQ: Pulmonary critical care problems. In Curley MAQ, Moloney-Harmon PA, editors: *Critical care nursing of infants and children,* ed 2, Philadelphia, 2001, Saunders.
22. Vollman KM: What are the practice guidelines for prone positioning of acutely ill patients? *Crit Care Nurs* 21:84-86, 2001, 2005.

Additional Readings

Breiburg AN, et al: Efficacy and safety of prone positioning for patients with acute respiratory distress syndrome, *J Adv Nurs* 32:922-999, 2000.

Murray TA, Patterson LA: Prone positioning of trauma patients with acute respiratory distress syndrome and open abdominal incisions, *Crit Care Nurs* 22:52-56, 2002.

Oczenski W, et al: Recruitment maneuvers during prone positioning in patients with acute respiratory distress syndrome, *Crit Care Med* 33(1):54-62, 2005.

Sawhney A, Puliyel JM: Prone to survive. [comment], *Crit Care Med* 33(10):2448-2449, 2005.

Weaning from Mechanical Ventilation

P U R P O S E : To ensure safety and efficiency in weaning children from invasive positive pressure ventilation to a successful extubation

Holly F. Webster

PREREQUISITE KNOWLEDGE

- Child development as it relates to clinical assessment and implications for weaning from mechanical ventilation
- Anatomy and physiology of the pediatric pulmonary system including structural characteristics specific to the child[1,2]
- Signs and symptoms of inadequate oxygenation and ventilation.[3]
- Mastery of pediatric advanced life support competencies including indications for an artificial airway and other adjuncts used to support ventilation.[2]
- Endotracheal tube (ETT) suctioning and care (see Procedure 2)
- Use of manual ventilation device (see Procedure 27)
- Use of conventional modes of mechanical ventilation (see Procedure 28)[1]
- Procedure for negative inspiratory force (NIF) measurements (see Procedure 21)
- Weaning from positive pressure ventilation (PPV) involves three stages: identifying criteria for weaning, the weaning phase, and extubation.
- The success of weaning depends upon the reason for intubation, which may include: hypoxemia, hypoventilation, general physiologic support and airway protection.
- Causes of delayed or unsuccessful weaning (Table 32-1)
- Tailoring the weaning method to the child and having a plan are important factors for successful weaning. The duration of weaning can be minimized with strict adherence to a plan or protocol.[3] Weaning by spontaneous breathing trials (with minimal pressure support) has been successful for some children.[4]
- Knowledge and skills related to airway management including recognition of inadvertent tube dislodgement, suctioning, intubation procedures with appropriate medications, and blood gas interpretation

TABLE 32-1	Causes of Delayed or Unsuccessful Weaning
Hypoxemia (or Impaired Oxygen Delivery)	**Hypercarbia (Respiratory Pump Failure)**
Hypoventilation	Hypoventilation
Impaired pulmonary exchange	Neurologic impairment
V/Q mismatching	Depressed CNS due to sedation
Diffusion defect	Cervical spine injury
Shunt	Phrenic nerve dysfunction
Increased work of breathing	Respiratory muscle function
Increased VO_2	Atrophy from disuse
Severe anemia	Fatigue
Decreased cardiac output	Abdominal distention
Fever	Malnutrition
Seizures	Ca+, Mg+, phosphorus deficiency
	Increase CO_2 production
	Fever
	Excess carbohydrate intake
	Muscle activity-agitation, seizure, shivering

V/Q = ventilation perfusion; VO_2 = oxygen consumption; CNS = Central Nervous System; Ca+ = calcium; Mg = magnesium; CO_2 = carbon dioxide.

- The heart and lungs are physiologically intertwined in the oxygen delivery (DO_2) system. If a baseline abnormality exists in one, it will impact the other system.
- Work of breathing (WOB) is defined as: WOB = Pressure (force) × Volume (displacement). *Pressure* (force) is generated to overcome airway resistance and the elastic properties of the lung and chest wall. *Volume* is the movement of gas flow into and out of the lungs during respiration. In the child, two-thirds of the WOB is determined by tissue elasticity and compliance and one-third is due to airway resistance. Airway resistance becomes a proportionately smaller factor in older children and adolescents because of increasing airway diameter.
- The normal WOB in infants and small children is 20-25% of the total oxygen consumption (VO_2).[5] VO_2 is increased with fever, musculoskeletal movement, neurogenic hyperventilation, imposed impediments such as ETT (increased airway resistance), abdominal distention (causing reduced diaphragmatic excursion) and intolerance of ventilator mode. Efforts to reduce VO_2 are important in facilitating weaning.
- The child's current ventilatory support including type of flow delivery (continuous vs. demand) and the trigger sensor employed
- Standard criteria for readiness to wean (Box 32-1). Meeting all of the criteria does not guarantee a successful course of weaning.[10] Abnormalities in more than one variable may be useful negative predictors and may influence the method and duration of weaning.
- The rate of failed extubation varies (2.7%–22%) depending on institution.[6] Several studies have concluded that infants less than 24 months on mechanical ventilation for longer than 48 hours are at higher risk for extubation failure.[6,7]
- Weaning techniques for small infants and those who are chronically ventilated often differ from those methods used for older children and those who have been intubated less than 48 hours.

Box 32-1 Assessment for Readiness to Wean

Spontaneous Vt ≥ 5 ml/kg
FiO_2 ≤ .40
PEEP ≤ 5 cm H_2O
PIP ≤ 25 cm H_2O
Vc >15 ml/kg
NIF >20 cm H_2O
PCO_2 normal or at child's baseline; pH: normal
Normal work of breathing
Hemodynamically stable
Adequate body strength/tone
Effective gag and cough reflexes
Pain control achieved without excessive sedation
Normal respiratory drive
Good aeration throughout lung fields

Vt, tidal volume; FiO_2, fraction of inspired oxygen; PIP, peak inspiratory pressure; NIF, negative inspiratory force; Vc, vital capacity; PEEP, peak end expiratory pressure; PCO_2, partial pressure of expired CO_2.

- Children who have been on mechanical ventilation for a long duration will likely need a period of time for improving strength and endurance of the respiratory muscles.
- Signs of weaning intolerance (Box 32-2)
- Infants may appear to be "quietly resting" and exhibit *very* discreet signs of intolerance. Therefore, best observation is with an infant's chest exposed.
- The initiation and frequency of trials is influenced by age, duration of intubation and tolerance of preceding trials. Generally, however, a period of 4-6 hours with baseline respiratory support is allowed to provide for rest and recovery.
- To facilitate successful weaning trials, the child should be well rested, without unnecessary discomfort, and physiologically stable.
- In infants and young children who normally require routine naps, it may be difficult to discern the difference between a "routine nap" and hypercarbia secondary to exhaustion from weaning.
- The process of weaning includes gradually reducing PPV, with the child assuming a greater proportion of minute ventilation (V_E). Guidelines for target rates include infants: 8-10 breaths per min (bpm); children: 6-8 bpm, and adolescent: 0-4 bpm
- Weaning is based on measurements of oxygenation and ventilations including pulse oximetry (SaO_2), end-tidal CO_2 ($ETCO_2$) and transcutaneous CO_2 ($TcCO_2$) and arterial blood gases (ABG) as well as the clinical appearance of the child.
- Infants and small children respond to increased WOB by increasing respiratory rate (RR), at the expense of Vt, to maintain minute ventilation (V_E).
- A smaller ETT imposes a higher resistance to inspiration. Suggested minimum pressure support ventilation (PSV) for various ETT sizes are as follows[4]:

ETT Size	PSV
3.0 to 3.5	10
4.0 to 4.5	8
≥5.0	6

- The two factors with the greatest lung toxicity are O_2 and inspiratory volume. Peak inspiratory pressure (PIP) limits the inspiratory volume directly; therefore, decreasing PIP will decrease Vt.

CHILD AND FAMILY ASSESSMENT

- Child's developmental level and ability to interact
  ➸*Rationale:* Influences preparation and interaction.

Box 32-2 Weaning Intolerance Criteria

Respiratory rate >1.5-2 × Child's baseline (early)
Decreased respiratory rate (late)
Increased WOB evidenced by increased use of accessory muscles
Pale, gray or cyanotic
General fatigue

- Child's and family's understanding of the reasons for and risks and benefits of weaning from mechanical ventilation ➥*Rationale:* Evaluates child's and family's understanding of the procedure and provides a gauge for ongoing education.
- Prior to weaning trial, reassess for readiness-to-wean. ➥*Rationale:* In the interval between planning and implementation, the child's condition may change.
- Review signs of weaning intolerance *before* initiating a trial ➥*Rationale:* Preparation and recognition of a change in respiratory function will direct further intervention and prevent complications.
- Note clinical exam findings that indicate hypercarbia including sleepiness, hypertension and dilated pupils. ➥*Rationale:* Recognition of a change in respiratory function will direct further intervention and prevent complications.
- Monitor vital signs including SaO_2, $ETCO_2$ or $TcCO_2$, and ABG during the weaning process ➥*Rationale:* Supports stability and readiness to wean. Pulse oximetry, $ETCO_2$ and $TcCO_2$ measurements provide a continuous assessment of oxygenation during weaning. Although not essential, a blood gas may be drawn prior to initiating weaning trials for final confirmation of readiness to wean.
- Assess the child's level of fatigue, pain and sedation, nutrition and fluid status, and the presence or absence of parents ➥*Rationale:* Preparation and addressing these issues may aid in successful weaning. It is important to avoid fatigue, which may cause regression in the weaning process.

CHILD AND FAMILY EDUCATION

Individualized, developmentally appropriate education is provided to the family and to the child based on desire for knowledge, readiness to learn, and overall neurologic and psychosocial state.

- Explain the reasons, purpose and risks of weaning from mechanical ventilation ➥*Rationale:* Anticipatory explanations may decrease fear and anxiety, foster trust and facilitate cooperation.
- Discuss the possible experiences of the child during ventilator changes including short periods of shortness of breath ➥*Rationale:* Withdrawal of PPV may cause anxiety or discomfort and anticipatory information fosters trust and facilitates cooperation.
- Reassure child and family that weaning will be done slowly allowing for breaks during the weaning process, especially for children who have been ventilated for long periods of time ➥*Rationale:* Diminishing PPV support can cause great anxiety and impede the weaning process.
- Reassure child and family of the continued presence of a caregiver during weaning ➥*Rationale:* The goal is to alleviate anxiety and minimize the fear, harm, or unnecessary discomfort during the weaning process.
- Discuss relaxation methods that can be incorporated in the child's care, including reading to the child, providing quiet distractions, and facilitating rest ➥*Rationale:* Relaxation will promote improved oxygenation and ventilation and positively impact weaning process.
- Encourage questions and answer questions as they arise. ➥*Rationale:* Reinforcement of information is needed during periods of stress.

EQUIPMENT

- Pressure manometer for NIF measurements (see Procedure 21)
- Spirometer for Vc measurements
- Tracheotomy collar or T-piece adapters
- Weaning protocol or documented plan
- Intubation equipment and supplies (see Procedure 15)

Procedure for Weaning from Mechanical Ventilation		
Steps	**Rationale**	**Considerations**
1. Ensure child and family understand procedure and questions are answered.	Evaluates and reinforces understanding of previously taught information.	Developmental level, cognitive ability, and anxiety level will determine approach to and effectiveness of teaching.
2. Review criteria for identifying weaning tolerance *prior* to initiating weaning (see Box 32-2).	A clear understanding of the weaning criteria is necessary to ensure early identification of weaning intolerance.	
3. Wash hands.	Reduces transmission of microorganisms.	
4. Ensure adequate cardiorespiratory monitoring. *(Level II*)*	Provides information on weaning tolerance. Allows the practitioner to immediately respond to physiologic status.	

* Level II: Theory-based; no research data to support recommendations; recommendations from expert consensus group may exist

Procedure for **Weaning from Mechanical Ventilation**—*Continued*		
Steps	**Rationale**	**Considerations**
5. Minimize sedation while providing adequate comfort measures.	A minimum level of adequate analgesia will support successful weaning.	Adequate analgesia is possible without depressing respiratory effort and is not contraindicated in weaning or extubation. Assistance from pain specialists can be useful especially for children with high pain scores.
6. Determine the weaning plan with the health care team.	A clear plan or protocol is essential to ensure efficiency of weaning.	Weaning trials are ideally done during day time hours, to allow complete rest for 8-12 hours at night. If the child has been on PPV for a short duration (~ <48 hrs), extubation at the earliest opportunity may better serve the child than delaying until the following day.
Spontaneous Intermittent Mandatory Ventilation (IMV)		
7. Define the target IMV rate and the frequency of changes. *(Level II*)*	The efficiency of weaning depends upon a clear plan which may be subject to alterations secondary to special considerations.	The IMV rate from which a child will be extubated is somewhat arbitrary, and age-dependent. In addition, the frequency of changes may be influenced by the duration of intubation.
8. Note type of flow delivery (continuous vs demand) and the sensor used to trigger the ventilator.	The child must have an ability to breathe through the circuit. Opening a demand valve may increase WOB	Flow sensors are generally more sensitive to effort than pressure sensors. In addition, unlike a circuit with continuous flow the demand flow circuit requires the child to entrain a set amount of flow to open the valve which requires greater strength.
9. Monitor signs of weaning intolerance including RR and Vt. Notify prescribing practitioner as indicated.	Recognition of a change in respiratory function will direct further intervention and prevent complications. A rapid RR and Vt < 5 ml/kg may cause atelectasis.	Infants and small children respond to increased WOB by increasing RR, at the expense of Vt, to maintain V_E.
10. If indicated, return the child to a previous setting or give complete rest on the ventilator.	Modification of the weaning plan is based on individual needs.	
Pressure Support Ventilation		
7. Consider an initial decrease in PSV of 1-2 cm increments every 2-6 hours.	Adjustments are made to ensure that the child achieves a target Vt (≥5 mL/kg) with minimal increased WOB.[4,8] *(Level IV*)*	The intent of PSV is to offset the WOB imposed by the resistance of the ETT.
8. Continue to wean the child until the lowest appropriate PSV level has been achieved for the tube size, with a Vt ≥5 mL/kg.	Weaning the child to minimal but adequate support prior to extubation may promote success.	Although target PSV goals have been suggested, the final target and duration of spontaneous breathing must be individualized. In some cases, however, prolonging a spontaneous trial may impose greater WOB, tiring the child.

Procedure continues on the following page

---

* Level II: Theory-based; no research data to support recommendations; recommendations from expert consensus group may exist
Level IV: Limited clinical studies to support recommendations

Procedure for **Weaning from Mechanical Ventilation**—*Continued*

Steps	Rationale	Considerations
9. Observe the child for positive indicators of successful extubation for 2-4 hours (or longer, as indicated) before final evaluation of readiness-to-extubate is determined (see Box 32-1).	Intubations of <48 hours often do not require a prolonged observation period; however, for children who have been intubated for a long duration, a longer observation period may be required.	

Pressure Support Ventilation/ Spontaneous Intermittent Mandatory Ventilation (SIMV)

Steps	Rationale	Considerations
7. *Option 1:* • Wean the IMV to a targeted rate with the PSV level continually adjusted to ensure a Vt ≥ 5 ml/kg. • Wean PSV (as outlined in previous section). *Option 2:* • Alternately, wean IMV and PSV with each step for a predefined frequency and duration of changes.	Weaning strategy varies depending upon the size of the child and the duration of intubation. As IMV is weaned, PS can be adjusted to reduce work of breathing and support further weaning of IMV. An alternating strategy may accomplish gentle "muscle conditioning."	Children with long duration PPV are likely the best candidates for PSV + SIMV-mode weaning. For infants, a ventilator capable of volume ventilation with small Vt, continuous flow, and a flow sensor at the child interface minimizes WOB during weaning. Newer ventilators incorporate modes which allow variable PS with a preset IMV rate. With these ventilators IMV is actively weaned while the PS is automatically adjusted to guarantee a Vt of approximately 6-7 ml/kg.

Time-cycled, Pressure Limited Mode

Steps	Rationale	Considerations
7. Wean FiO_2 to < 4.[8]	High FiO_2 risk lung toxicity.	The frequency of changes is predetermined by the prescribing practitioner based on clinical assessment and measurements of oxygenation/ventilation (ABG, $TiCO_2$, $ETCO_2$, SaO_2). If the circuit provides continuous flow, the child can breathe spontaneously between breaths to ensure that V_E requirement is being met. If PSV is not available, the spontaneous breaths may be shallow, which puts the child at risk for atelectasis. If the child has been in the assist-control mode (rather than SIMV) switching to SIMV first to allow spontaneous breathing may improve success of weaning.
8. Wean PIP by 1-2 cm increments until $PaCO_2$ is > 40 mm Hg and/or PIP < 15 cm Hg. Decreases in PIP should not precede if Vt is < 5 ml/kg.	Weaning PIP only is acceptable until the $PaCO_2$ rises or the PaO_2 falls. Maintaining a Vt of 5cc/kg will reduce the WOB that may occur with lower a RR.	With a Vt of approximately 7 ml/kg, weaning PIP only will decrease Vt.
9. Decrease PEEP in 1 cm H_2O increments to a level of 4-5 cm H_2O ensuring a PaO_2 > 80 mmHg.	Weaning PEEP independently or concurrently with PIP is individualized to the needs of the child	Consider concurrent weaning of PEEP with PIP. This option facilitates maintenance of Vt/V_E without burden to the child.
10. Wean IMV rate.	When the target PIP/PEEP has been achieved with acceptable Vt/V_E, the child can be weaned from the IMV rate.	

Procedure	**for Weaning from Mechanical Ventilation**—*Continued*	
Steps	**Rationale**	**Considerations**

Spontaneous Breathing Trials

Steps	**Rationale**	**Considerations**
7. Define the duration and time intervals for spontaneous breathing as well as the method for resting the child with baseline ventilatory support between trials.	Duration and time intervals are individualized to the child. The goals of spontaneous trials are to either confirm readiness to extubate or to provide respiratory muscle conditioning.	Caution is used with children who have been pharmacologically paralyzed, or have underlying neuromuscular weakness.
8. *Choose a weaning method:* T-piece circuit or CPAP and/or PSV	The choice of method is individually determined, based on availability of equipment, local practice standard, and the needs of the child. The T-piece offers very little resistance to gas flow; there are no valves to open nor are there circuits to clear.[9]	For older children, the resistance imposed by the ETT is thought to mimic the WOB that is necessary for successful extubation. Infants may have difficulty tolerating spontaneous breathing without added CPAP and PSV.
9. *Consider timing of weaning intervals:* • For children ventilated <24 hours consider one 30 minute to 1 hour trial. • For children ventilated for longer periods of time consider several trials/day for 24 to 48 hour.	Children who are on PPV < 48 hours should not lose significant strength during this time. Other children may require repeated trial periods or "muscle conditioning" to regain sufficient strength.	Vt must be monitored at all times. Use the criteria in Table 32-2 for on-going assessment during the trial period.

TABLE 32-2	**Risk of Reintubation**	
Variable	**Low-risk**	**High-risk**
$Vt_{spontaneous}$ (ml/kg)	≥6.5	≤3.5
FiO_2	≤.30	>.40
mPaw (cm H_2O)	<5	>8.5
Oxygen index	≤1.4	≥4.5
FrVe (%)	≤20	≥30
Mean inspiratory flow (ml/kg/sec)	>14	<8

Adapted from Venkataraman ST: Mechanical ventilation and respiratory care. In Fuhrman B and Zimmerman J, editors: *Pediatric critical care,* ed 3, Philadelphia, 2006, Mosby.

Vt = Tidal volume; FiO_2 = fraction of inspired oxygen; Paw = mean airway pressure; FrVe = fraction of total minute ventilation provided by the ventilator.

Expected Outcomes	Unexpected Outcomes
• Efficient and successful extubation • Adequate oxygenation and ventilation • Child remains injury free • Hemodynamic stability • Acceptable level of comfort	• Fatigue causing delay of further weaning • Hypercapnia or hypoxemia • Atelectasis • Tracheal injury • Hemodynamic instability • Unmanaged pain and agitation

Monitoring and Care of the Child

Activities and Interventions	Rationale	Reportable Conditions
1. Evaluate child stability, including the factors that identify readiness to wean before and during the weaning process.	Premature attempts at weaning or failure to recognize interfering factors may cause significant compromise to the child.	• Both pulmonary-related changes and system changes are reported in a timely fashion
2. Ensure that a manual ventilation bag, mask, and suction are immediately available and connected at child's bedside.	Equipment is necessary for sudden changes in the child's condition.	• Absent or poorly functioning equipment
3. Continuously observe and monitor child including vital signs, Vt, ABG, SaO$_2$, ETCO$_2$, or TCO$_2$, and signs of increased WOB.	Pediatric patients exhibit more subtle clinical signs of fatigue. Regardless of strategy, vigilance is important in monitoring fatigue. Increased WOB leading to fatigue may occur in a short time frame with final *decompensation* occurring abruptly.	• Use of accessory muscles, nasal flaring or increased RR (1.5-2x baseline) • Changes in monitoring parameters
4. Elevate the head of the bed as child's condition permits, to allow the diaphragm to "drop," facilitating excursion.	The principal muscle which supports respiration in infants and young children is the diaphragm. Any factor which impedes diaphragm excursion will compromise the child.	• Abdominal distention in infants
5. Note child's level of comfort and provide appropriate sedation.	Early identification of the child's discomfort allows for immediate attention.	• Unresolved pain and discomfort • Continued irritability
6. Provide adequate nutrition.	Consideration must be given to the potential increases in energy expenditure.	• Poor growth

Documentation

- Cardiorespiratory assessment including vital signs, lung sounds, work of breathing, ABGs, pulse oximetry, and ETCO$_2$ or TcCO$_2$ monitoring.
- As weaning progresses record ventilator settings including FiO$_2$, mode, Vt, IMV, PIP, rate and PEEP (every 2-4 hours and with changes)
- Signs of weaning intolerance
- Unexpected outcomes
- Additional interventions and child's response
- Comfort assessment and any specific interventions provided
- Child and family education

References

1. Thibodeau G, Patton K: *Anatomy and Physiology,* ed 5, Philadelphia, 2003, Mosby.
2. Hazinski, MF et al, editors: *Pediatric Advanced Life Support Provider Manual,* Dallas, 2002, American Heart Association.
3. MacIntyre NR, et al: Evidence-based guidelines for weaning and discontinuing ventilatory support. *Chest* 120(suppl6): 375S-395S, 2001.
4. Randolph AG, et al.: Effect of mechanical ventilator weaning protocols on respiratory outcomes in infants and children. *JAMA* 288(20), 2561-2568, 2002.
5. Curley MAQ, Thompson JE: Oxygenation and ventilation. In Curley MAQ, Moloney-Harmon, PA, editors: *Critical care nursing of infants and children,* ed 2, Philadelphia, 2001, Saunders.
6. Kurachek SC, et al: Extubation failure in pediatric intensive care: A multiple-center study of risk factors and outcomes. *Crit Care Med,* 31(11), 2657-2664, 2003.
7. Edmunds S, et al: Extubation failure in a large pediatric ICU population. *Chest* 119(3), 897-899, 2001.
8. Spitzer AR, et al: Positive-pressure ventilation. In: Goldsmith JP, Karotkin EH, editors: *Assisted ventilation of the neonate,* ed 4, Philadelphia, 1996, Saunders.
9. Straus C, et al: Contribution of the endotracheal tube and the upper airway to breathing workload. *Am J Respir Crit Care Med* 157(1), 23-30, 1998.
10. Venkataraman, ST et al: Validation of predictors of extubation success and failure in mechanically ventilated infants and children. *Critical Care Medicine,* 28(8), 2991-2995, 2000.
11. Venkataraman ST: Mechanical ventilation and respiratory care. In Fuhrman B and Zimmerman J, editors: *Pediatric critical care,* ed 3, Philadelphia, 2006, Mosby, pp. 683-718.

Additional Readings

Hubble CL, et al: Deadspace to tidal volume ratio predicts successful extubation in infants and children. *Crit Care Med* 28(6), 2034-2040, 2000.

Luyt K et al: Compared with specialist registrars, experienced staff nurses shorten the duration of weaning neonates from mechanical ventilation. *Ped Crit Care Med* 3(4), 351-354, 2002.

Manczur TI, et al: Comparison of predictors of extubation from mechanical ventilation in children. *Ped Crit Care Med* (1)1, 28-32, 2000.

Schultz TR: Weaning children from mechanical ventilation: a prospective randomized trial of protocol-directed versus physician-directed weaning. *Resp Care* 46(8), 772-780, 2001.

Thoracic Cavity Management

Chest Tube Placement: Assist

P U R P O S E :   Chest tubes are inserted to evacuate air, fluid, and blood from the intrapleural or mediastinal space and to facilitate reexpansion of the lung. Chest tubes can also be used to instill fibrinolytic agents for the treatment of pleural empyema.

Kerry Shields

PREREQUISITE KNOWLEDGE

- Child development as it relates to clinical assessment and assistance with chest tube placement
- Anatomy and physiology of the pediatric pulmonary system, including mechanics of breathing[1,2]
  - ❖ Negative pressure exists in the pleural space. This potential space is between the visceral pleura (con-

nected to the lungs) and the parietal pleura (connected to the ribcage Figure 33-1).
- ❖ During the inspiratory phase of breathing, the diaphragm drops and the external intercostal muscles and sternocleidomastoid muscles expand the rib cage. When the rib cage moves, the lungs move with it.
- ❖ As the chest expands, the gas pressure decreases in the alveoli and the pleural pressure becomes more

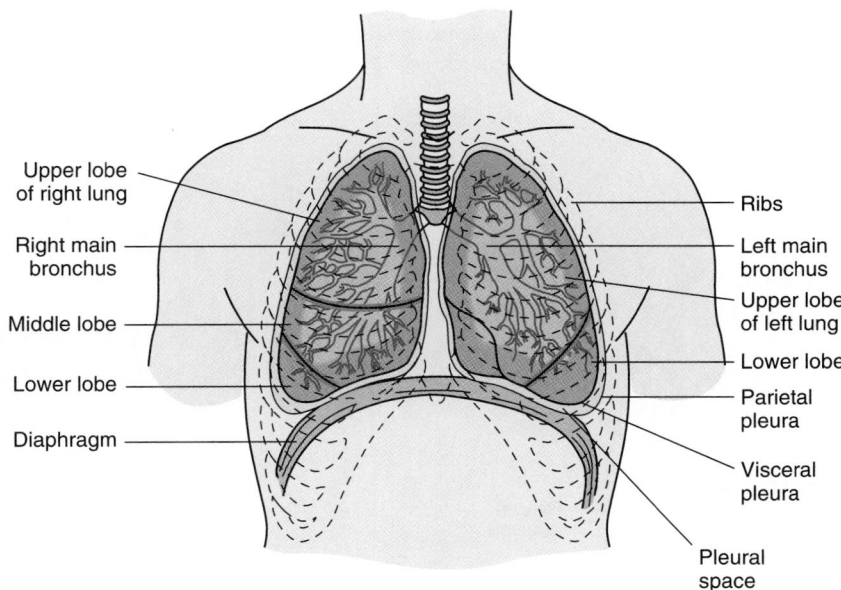

Upper lobe of right lung

Right main bronchus

Middle lobe

Lower lobe

Diaphragm

Ribs

Left main bronchus

Upper lobe of left lung

Lower lobe

Parietal pleura

Visceral pleura

Pleural space

FIGURE 33-1   Anatomy of the Chest. *From Huffstutler SY: Assessment of the respiratory system. In Phipps WJ, Monahan FD, et al, editors:* Medical-surgical nursing: health and illness perspectives, *ed 7, St. Louis, 2003, Mosby.*

negative. Air enters the lung at atmospheric pressure.[1,2]

- Chest tube size is determined by the size of the child and the intended use[3] (Table 38-1). Chest tubes inserted for drainage of blood tend to be larger than chest tubes inserted for evacuation of air. Pigtail catheters are as effective as large-bore chest tubes for pneumothoraces.[4-6]
- Understanding of the clinical indication for placement of the chest tube
- While the penetrated lung heals, chest tubes, also called thoracotomy tubes, are inserted into the pleural space to restore negative pressure and allow lung expansion.
- Indications for a chest tube[2-4,7,8]
  - ❖ Pneumothorax: Air in the pleural space (Figure 33-2)
  - ❖ Pleural effusion (Figure 33-3)
  - ❖ Hemothorax: Blood in the pleural space (Figure 33-4)
  - ❖ Empyema: Pus in the pleural space
  - ❖ Tension pneumothorax (Figure 33-5)
  - ❖ Chylothorax: Chyle from the thoracic duct in the pleural space

- ❖ Thoracotomy, specifically postcardiac surgery in which pleural and mediastinum have been entered (placed during surgery)
- ❖ Instillation of fibrinolytic agents for treatment of empyema
- ❖ Penetrating chest trauma
- Blunt trauma, penetrating trauma, positive pressure ventilation, and iatrogenic causes may alter the negative pressure in the pleural space and cause a pneumothorax.[4,6]
- A closed pneumothorax occurs when the chest wall is intact. The pleural space alone has been penetrated. Air is able to enter the pleural space but is not able to escape. Cystic fibrosis and positive pressure ventilation may result in a closed pneumothorax (Figure 33-2, *A*).[4]
- An open pneumothorax occurs when both the chest wall and the pleural space are penetrated. Air is able to enter and escape the pleural space through the penetration. Stab wounds or surgical trauma may result in an open pneumothorax (Figure 33-2, *B*).[4]

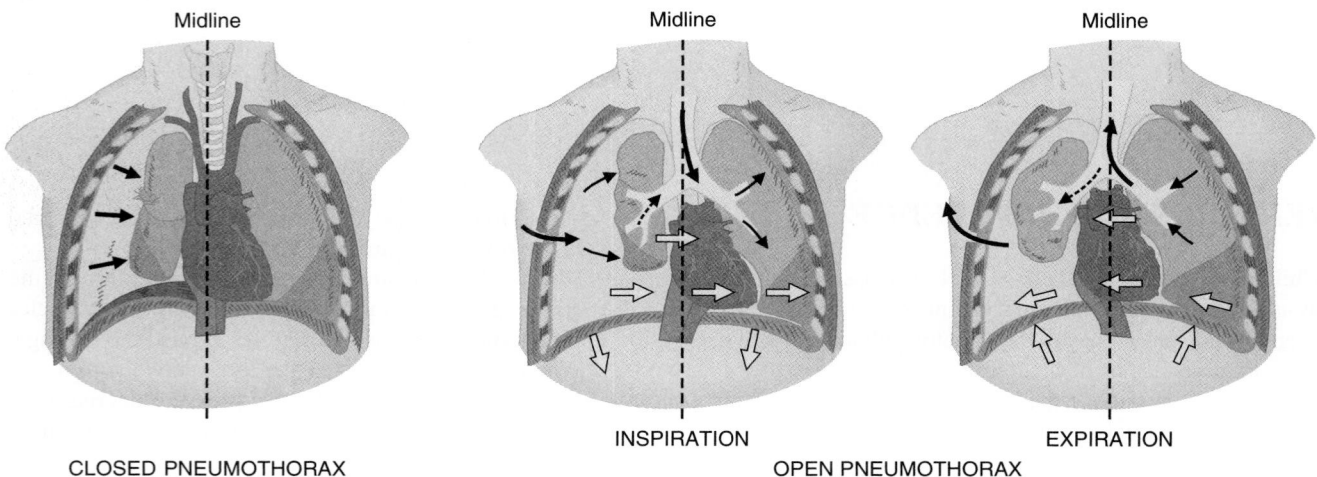

FIGURE 33-2   Pneumothorax. *White AH: Management of clients with acute pulmonary disorders. In Black JM, Hawks JH, editors:* Medical-surgical nursing: clinical management for positive outcomes, *ed 7, Philadelphia, 2005, Saunders.*

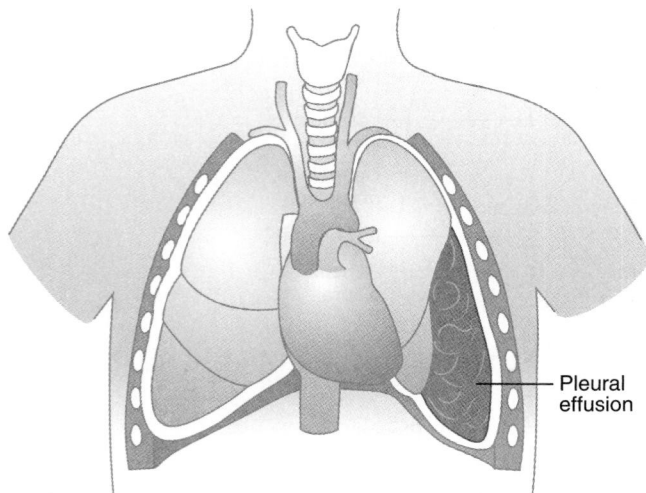

FIGURE 33-3   Pleural Effusion.

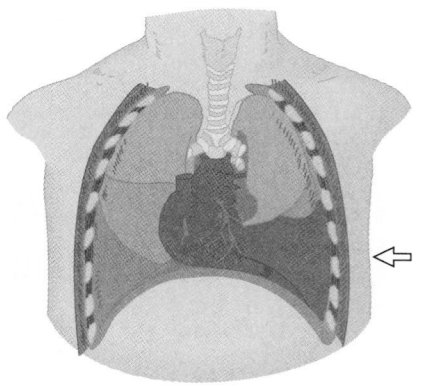

FIGURE 33-4   Hemothorax. *White AH: Management of clients with acute pulmonary disorders. In Black JM, Hawks JH, editors:* Medical-surgical nursing: clinical management for positive outcomes, *ed 7, Philadelphia, 2005, Saunders.*

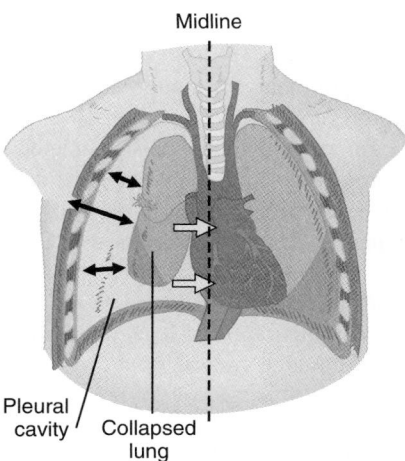

Midline

Pleural
cavity
Collapsed
lung

FIGURE 33-5   Tension Pneumothorax. *Modified from White AH: Management of clients with acute pulmonary disorders. In Black JM, Hawks JH, editors:* Medical-surgical nursing: clinical management for positive outcomes, *ed 7, Philadelphia, 2005, Saunders.*

- A tension pneumothorax occurs when air accumulates in the pleural space and cannot escape. As air flows into the affected side of the lung, an increase in pressure occurs and shifts the trachea, heart, and other midline structures to the unaffected side. This event is an emergent situation because the pressure can decrease venous return and compress the heart, which decreases cardiac output and eventually may lead to the collapse of the unaffected lung (Figure 33-5).[8]
- Typical signs and symptoms of pneumothorax include tachypnea, decreased breath sounds on the affected side, increased work of breathing, unequal chest rise, decreased oxygen saturation, tachycardia, hypotension, and possible dysrhythmias.
- Signs of tension pneumothorax include grunting, tachypnea, retractions, dyspnea, agitation, hypoxia, decreased to absent breath sounds on the affected side, tympany to percussion, tracheal shift to the unaffected side, subcutaneous emphysema, muffled heart sounds, and neck vein distention.[8]
- Crepitus (subcutaneous emphysema) can indicate that holes of the chest tube are outside of the pleural space and air is leaking into the subcutaneous tissue.
- Chest tube site placement is determined by the indication. Tubes placed to drain air are typically placed anterior toward the apex. Tubes placed to drain fluid, blood, or pus are typically placed inferior and posterior.[6]
- The point of entry for chest tubes into the pleural space is typically the third to fifth intercostal space in the mid to anterior axillary line, usually at the level of the nipple. An incision is made one intercostal space below the insertion point (usually at the sixth rib) and dissected with a hemostat until the rib is reached. The chest tube is placed in a clamp and guided through the entry site. The tube is then sutured in place, and an occlusive dressing is applied (see Figure 38-4).[3,7]
- No absolute contraindications to placement of a chest tube exist if the child is in respiratory distress from a closed pneumothorax or has a tension pneumothorax.

The risks outweigh the benefits when the lung needs to be expanded. Careful consideration must be given with anticoagulant medications, coagulopathy, and skin infections at the insertion site.[4]
- Multiple chest tubes may be necessary to evacuate additional locations or causes of collection.
- Mediastinal tubes are placed to drain effusions and to evacuate blood and fluid after cardiac surgery, which may collect around the heart and result in compression and cardiac tamponade. Mediastinal tubes are placed anterior or posterior.
- Knowledge of institutional closed chest drainage systems, the availability of wall or portable suction, and the need for adapters
- Informed consent is required unless procedure is emergent.

CHILD AND FAMILY ASSESSMENT

- Child's developmental level and ability to interact **➤➤Rationale:** Influences preparation and interaction.
- Child's and family's understanding of the reasons for and risks and benefits of chest tube placement **➤➤Rationale:** Evaluates child's and family's understanding of the procedure and provides a gauge for ongoing education.
- Desire of family members to be present during the procedure **➤➤Rationale:** The presence of family may provide comfort and support; although family members should have the choice not to remain with the child.
- Cardiopulmonary assessment, including vital signs, visual inspection of breathing patterns and chest wall movement, auscultation of lung fields, and signs of inadequate oxygenation and ventilation, such as decreased arterial oxygen saturation, increased work of breathing, supplemental oxygen requirement, cyanosis, changes in heart rate and blood pressure, anxiety, and agitation **➤➤Rationale:** Evaluating cardiopulmonary status provides valuable information in determining the child's need for and ability to tolerate the procedure and influences the type of anesthetics and sedation prescribed.
- Review of last chest x-ray results **➤➤Rationale:** Location of pleural air, blood, or fluid.
- Assess recent serum laboratory results, including complete blood count, platelet count, prothrombin time, and partial thromboplastin time **➤➤Rationale:** Determines the risk of bleeding.
- Assessment of skin integrity at the insertion site **➤➤Rationale:** Avoidance of active skin lesions or infection at the insertion site.
- History of reactions or allergies to medication (betadine, lidocaine, anesthetics, or sedatives) and tape **➤➤Rationale:** Prevention of harm.

CHILD AND FAMILY EDUCATION

Individualized, developmentally appropriate education is provided to the family and to the child based on desire for knowledge, readiness to learn, and overall neurologic and psychosocial state.

- Explain the procedure for chest tube placement, including the indication, procedure, and rationale ➤➤*Rationale:* Providing information decreases fear and anxiety.
- Explain the chest tube apparatus and drainage system, and if time permits, allow the family to view the drainage system ➤➤*Rationale:* Information decreases fear and anxiety.
- Explain that during the insertion of the needle the child may feel pressure at the insertion site ➤➤*Rationale:* Providing information helps prepare the child for events during the procedure, thus reducing anxiety.
- Begin teaching interventions for assistance in lung expansion, including frequent turning, cough and deep breathing, chest physiotherapy, and incentive spirometry ➤➤*Rationale:* Interventions can be an adjunct to chest tubes to expand the lung and prevent further collapse.
- Discuss ways to decrease pain and anxiety during the procedure, and explain plan for pain assessment and treatment for the duration of the chest tube placement ➤➤*Rationale:* Decreasing anxiety about pain and adequate pain control can facilitate coughing, deep breathing, and chest physiotherapy.
- Explain how the child can assist with the procedure ➤➤*Rationale:* The child is provided with an opportunity to participate in or assist with the procedure.
- Explain the importance of facilitation of drainage with the tubing kept free of kinks ➤➤*Rationale:* This effort may assist in prevention of accumulation of intrapleural process.
- Encourage questions and answer questions as they arise ➤➤*Rationale:* Reinforcement of information is needed during periods of stress.

EQUIPMENT

- Emergency equipment, including manual ventilation bag, mask, and oxygen supply
- Cardiorespiratory monitor and pulse oximeter, as indicated
- Personal protective equipment as indicated, including sterile gloves, sterile gown, mask, and goggles
- Systemic pain medication and local 1% lidocaine, as ordered
- 25-gauge 5/8-inch needle and syringe for lidocaine
- Syringe for administration of local anesthetic
- Closed chest drainage system
- Suction source
- Tubing and connectors
- Chest tube equipment: chest tube, two Kelly clamps, scalpel, needle holder, gauze, hemostats, and sterile gauze
- Pigtail catheter equipment: pigtail catheter, pigtail catheter kits, sterile three-way stopcock, needleless access device, No. 11 blade, 30-mL syringe (if substituted for a chest tube)
- Betadine or chlorhexidine, if not included in chest tube tray
- Sterile water
- Sterile towels
- Hemostats
- Tape
- Sutures
- Suture scissors
- Dressing materials, including petroleum dressing, dry gauze, tape, and occlusive dressing

Procedure   for Chest Tube Placement: Assist

Steps	Rationale	Considerations
1. Ensure child and family understand procedure and questions are answered. Ensure informed consent has been obtained by practitioner performing the procedure.	Evaluates and reinforces understanding of previously taught information. In many situations, informed consent is necessary before chest tube insertion. Ensures medical-legal compliance as supported by the JCAHO.	Developmental level, cognitive ability, and anxiety levels determine approach and effectiveness of teaching. For emergencies, refer to institution-specific protocol for assumption of consent.
2. Gather equipment and supplies. Ensure emergency equipment is present and in working order.	Preparation facilitates completion of the procedure in a timely manner.	Volume replacement and intubation equipment may be needed if child becomes hypotensive or needs a secure airway. Consider child's allergies to adhesive tape.
3. Ensure adequate cardiorespiratory monitoring.	Children may have decompensation during the procedure.	Consider an increase in volume on the pulse oximeter or cardiac monitor to allow an auditory signal and visual monitoring during procedure.

Procedure	**for Chest Tube Placement: Assist**—*Continued*	
Steps	**Rationale**	**Considerations**
4. Conduct final patient verification process (e.g., "Time Out") per institution-specific protocol.	Confirms correct child, procedure, and site; prevents unnecessary medical procedures (JCAHO requirement).	The bedside nurse's familiarity with child's chest x-ray results is helpful.
5. Ensure child has undergone premedication for procedure and that a plan for pain control is in place. *(Level VI*)*	Chest tube placement is a painful procedure. Pain and anxiety control helps child maintain position.[9]	The medication dose is dependent on child's weight, previous experience with pain, and other concurrent conditions. Intravenous morphine is the typical pain medication used during chest tube insertion.[9,10] *(Level V*)*
6. Set up the closed chest drainage system per manufacturer's recommendations (see Procedure 35).	An evacuation system is necessary to drain the pleural space.	
7. Wash hands and put on protective equipment.	Reduces transmission of microorganisms. Protects personnel health.	Ensure that child does not have a latex allergy when decisions are made on gloves and equipment.
8. Position child supine with affected side slightly up[8] (Figure 33-6). *(Level V*)*	Allows access to the insertion site.	The sitting position is an alternative for those children who are unable to lay flat because of respiratory distress.

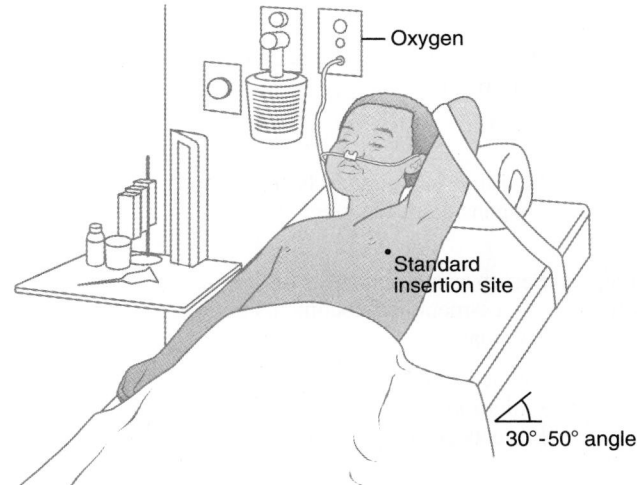

FIGURE 33-6 Positioning for Chest Tube Placement. *Modified from Roberts JR, Hedges JR: Clinical procedures in emergency medicine, ed 4, Philadelphia, 2004, Saunders.*

9. Assist practitioner with opening chest tube kit and preparing site.	Allows practitioner to maintain sterile technique.	
10. Provide emotional support and coping behaviors to child throughout procedure.	Increases comfort and maintains a calm atmosphere.	Examples of support or coping behaviors: distraction, diversion, relaxation, and guided imagery. Respect expressions of emotion.

Procedure continues on following page

---

* Level V: Clinical studies in more than one or two patient populations and situations to support recommendations
Level VI: Clinical studies in a variety of patient populations and situations to support recommendations

Procedure for Chest Tube Placement: Assist—*Continued*

Steps	Rationale	Considerations
11. Once chest tube is placed, remove cap from the end of connection tubing and sterilely attach it to end of chest tube. The child's side of tubing is connected to collection chamber (to right when looking at the front of the system).	Creates a closed system for drainage and restoring negative pressure.	Additional chest tubes may be connected to the same suction source via "Y" type connections.
12. Assist with suturing the chest tube in position.	Secures tube to prevent dislodging.	Note whether "purse string" sutures are used.
13. Place chest tube to the ordered amount of negative pressure. The suction side of tubing is connected to suction side of unit (to the left when looking at front of the system).	Gravity restores negative intrapleural pressure. Additional negative pressure may be ordered to further evacuate intrapleural space.	Attach system to child before placing the unit to desired suction.
14. Secure closed chest drainage system below chest level and secure drainage system and connection points in the tubing.[11,12] *(Level V*)*	Assists with gravity drainage and decreases the potential for an air leak in the system via connections.	Pieces of tape placed horizontally over connections can also be used. Nylon bands have been used to provide added security for connection tubing. Unlike a water seal chamber, a dry control drain continues to provide a secure closed system if overturned.
15. Apply occlusive petroleum dressing, cover with dry gauze, and secure with occlusive dressing or tape.[13] *(Level V*)*	Prevents air leakage at site of insertion.	
16. Obtain chest x-ray results and assess child after procedure.[3,11] *(Level V*)*	Identifies location of chest tube and expansion of the lung.	
17. Observe insertion site and initial drainage into the closed collection system.	Serves as a baseline for further assessment and documents initial drainage.	
18. Dispose of equipment and wash hands.	Reduces transmission of microorganisms. Protects personnel health.	

* Level V: Clinical studies in more than one or two patient populations and situations to support recommendations

Expected Outcomes	**Unexpected Outcomes**
• Negative pressure is restored • Re-expansion of the affected lung • Improved oxygenation and ventilation • Complication-free insertion of chest tube • Site remains infection free • Child has an acceptable level of comfort	• Improper placement of chest tube • Lung does not respond • Equipment or suction malfunction • Laceration of diaphragm, spleen, or liver • Pulmonary contusion • Infection • Unmanaged pain and anxiety

Monitoring and Care of the Child

Activities and Interventions	Rationale	Reportable Conditions
1. Monitor respiratory, cardiovascular, and neurologic status before, during, and after the procedure.	Ongoing assessment is necessary for evaluation of the effectiveness of therapy. Changes in vital signs and physical assessment alert the caregiver to unexpected outcomes.	• Respiratory distress (grunting, tachypnea, retractions, dyspnea, agitation, hypoxia) • Decreased to absent breath sounds • Subcutaneous emphysema • Tracheal shift to the unaffected side • Cardiovascular collapse • Anxiety, restlessness, or feeling of doom • Tachycardia • Hypotension • Chest pain
2. Obtain a chest radiograph after completion of the procedure.	Confirms placement of the chest tube and drainage of pleural space.	• Pneumothorax • Enlarging pleural effusion • Improperly placed chest tube
3. Monitor the insertion site.	Any open wound is at risk for infection and bleeding. Air leak can occur from the insertion site.	• Excessive bleeding or draining from the site • Signs of infection, including fever, tenderness, inflammation, and redness at the insertion site • Subcutaneous emphysema • Tube dislodgement
4. Evaluate chest tube drainage, including amount, color, and consistency.	An increase in drainage may indicate increased bleeding and may necessitate transfusion. A decrease in drainage may indicate clotting of the chest tube.	• Continued excessive sanguineous bleeding • Change in character of the drainage • Abrupt cession of drainage
5. Assess system for air leaks.	Air leak can indicate that the lung is not healing properly or that the system is not airtight.	• Persistent or new air leak
6. Assess pain status.	Evaluate pain management and sedation plan.	• Pain unrelieved with pain management plan • Pain interfering with interventions to expand lung

Documentation

- Date, time, and length of procedure
- Correct site, correct procedure, and correct person verification, including consent
- Indication for insertion of chest tube
- Assessment findings before and after chest tube placement (breath sounds and signs of oxygenation and ventilation)
- Name and credentials of individual placing tube
- Size of tube, location of insertion, and whether a "purse string" suture is used
- Amount, color, and consistency of drainage
- Local anesthetic or systemic anesthetic used and child's response
- Amount of negative pressure suction
- Chest radiograph obtained
- Site assessment and type of dressing used
- Comfort assessment and any specific interventions
- Additional interventions necessary
- Child and family education
- Unexpected outcomes and related treatment

References

1. Fuhrman B, Zimmerman J: *Pediatric critical care*, St. Louis, 2005, Mosby.
2. Thibodeau G, Patton K: *Anatomy and physiology,* St. Louis, 2003, Mosby.
3. Gunn V, Nechyba C: *The Harriet Lane handbook,* Philadelphia, 2002, Mosby.
4. Lawrence D, Carlson K: Procedure 19: chest tube placement (assist). In Lynn-McHale DJ, Carlson K: *AACN procedure manual for critical care,* Philadelphia, 2005, Elsevier.
5. Dull K, Fleisher G: Pigtail catheters versus large-bore chest tubes for pneumothoraces in children treated in the emergency department, *Pediatr Emerg Care* 18(4):265-267, 2002.
6. Moloney-Harmon P, Czerwinski: *Nursing care of the pediatric trauma patient,* Philadelphia, 2003, Saunders.
7. Hazinski MF et al: *Pediatric advanced support provider manual,* Dallas, 2002, American Heart Association.
8. Roberts JR, Hedges JR: *Clinical procedures in emergency medicine,* ed 4, Philadelphia, 2004, Saunders.
9. Kaplin R, Yang C: Sedation and analgesia in pediatric patients for procedures outside the operating room, *Anesthesiol Clin North Am* 20:181-194, 2002.
10. Baumann MH: Management of spontaneous pneumothorax: An American college of chest physicians delphi consensus statement, *Chest* 119(2):590-602, 2001.
11. Allibone L: Nursing management of chest drains, *Nurs Stand* 17(22):45-56, 2003.
12. Carroll P: Exploring chest drain options, *RN* 63(10):50-54, 56, 2000.
13. Taeusch H, et al: *Pediatric and neonatal tests and procedures,* Philadelphia, 1996, Saunders.

Additional Reading

Valenzuela R, Rosen D: Topical lidocaine-prilocaine cream (EMLA) for thoracostomy tube removal, *Anesthesia Analgesia,* 88(5):1107-1108, 1999.

Chest Tube Removal: Assist

P U R P O S E : Chest tubes are removed when the reason for placement has been resolved, including resolution of expected surgical drainage, pneumothorax, or hemothorax

Kerry Shields

PREREQUISITE KNOWLEDGE

- Child development as it relates to clinical assessment and assistance with chest tube removal
- Anatomy and physiology of the pediatric pulmonary system including mechanics of breathing[1] (see Figure 33-1)
- Understanding of initial clinical indication for placement of chest tube
  - ❖ Chest tubes are placed for the drainage of air (pneumothorax), fluid (pleural effusion), blood (hemothorax), pus (empyema), and chyle (chylothorax).[2,3]
  - ❖ Mediastinal chest tubes are usually placed in the operating room by the surgeon after cardiothoracic surgery.
- Indications of readiness for chest tube removal[4-9]:
  - ❖ No air leak on water seal for 24 hours (pneumothorax); this is assessed with observation of the water seal or air leak chamber for bubbling.
  - ❖ Drainage of less than 2 mL/kg total pleural fluid drainage in 24 hours
  - ❖ Pneumothorax of less than 10% or complete resolution per chest x-ray results
  - ❖ Resolution of underlying process
  - ❖ Lung is re-expanded
  - ❖ Improved respiratory status
  - ❖ The chest tube is nonfunctional
- Depending on the child's condition and ventilatory requirements, a chest tube may need to remain in place despite removal indications.

- Level IV data indicate that complications after chest tube removal are not affected by the use of maximal inspiration versus expiration. Most studies use a maximal inspiration intervention in procedures.[4,5,10]
- Significant differences are found in the protocols for evaluation and removal of a chest tube. Care must be taken to follow the protocol of the individual institution, with respect to current practices and the child's clinical condition.
  - ❖ In some institutions, chest tubes are clamped for 4 hours after the last evidence of air leak before discontinuation of the chest tube.
  - ❖ Mediastinal chest tubes placed after cardiothoracic surgery are often removed 24 to 36 hours after surgery when the drainage has become minimal and progressed to serous from sanguineous.
  - ❖ Chest tubes can be safely removed after thoracic surgery without a water seal trial, which allows for earlier chest tube removal, decreased pain, and decreased hospital cost.[11]
  - ❖ Chest tubes sutured with a "purse sting" suture need two individuals for chest tube removal. One removes the drain, and the second promptly ties the purse string suture (see Figure 39-1).
- Pharmacologic (mechanism of action, dosing, side effects, and contraindications) knowledge about systemic or local anesthetics used for procedural analgesia during chest tube removal[9,12]
  - ❖ Chest tube removal is a painful procedure.

CHILD AND FAMILY ASSESSMENT

- Child's developmental level and ability to interact ➻*Rationale:* Influences preparation and interaction.
- Child's and family's understanding of the reasons for and risks and benefits of removal of the chest tube ➻*Rationale:* Evaluates child's and family's understanding of the procedure and provides a gauge for ongoing education.
- Desire of family members to be present during the procedure ➻*Rationale:* The presence of family may provide comfort and support, although family members should have the choice not to remain with the child.
- Thorough cardiopulmonary assessment, including vital signs, visual inspection of breathing patterns and chest wall movement, auscultation of lung fields, and signs of oxygenation and ventilation ➻*Rationale:* This assessment ensures the child's readiness for chest tube removal and provides a comparison for post removal assessment.
- Assess presence of air leak (bubbling in the water chamber) and amount and appearance of drainage ➻*Rationale:* Assesses child's readiness for chest tube removal.
- Review of last chest x-ray results ➻*Rationale:* Radiologic evidence of resolution of pneumothorax, effusion, or hemothorax.
- History of reactions or allergies to medication (betadine, lidocaine, anesthetics, or sedatives) and tape ➻*Rationale:* Prevention of harm.
- Assess skin integrity at insertion site ➻*Rationale:* Assesses signs of infection or inflammation.

CHILD AND FAMILY EDUCATION

Individualized, developmentally appropriate education is provided to the family and to the child based on desire for knowledge, readiness to learn, and overall neurologic and psychosocial state.

- Explain the procedure for chest tube removal, including the indication, procedure, and rationale ➻*Rationale:* Providing information increases knowledge, and preparation helps reduces anxiety, which increases the child's ability to cooperate during the procedure. Information increases parental satisfaction.
- Review the original clinical indication for chest tube placement and criteria for removal ➻*Rationale:* Assesses child's

and family's understanding of chest tubes and reinforcement of original teaching.
- Explain how the child can assist with the procedure ➻*Rationale:* The child is provided with an opportunity to participate or assist with the procedure, which may limit introduction of air into the pleural space.
- Review the plan for lung expansion techniques after chest tube removal, including ambulation, frequent position change, cough, deep breathing, and incentive spirometry ➻*Rationale:* The planned techniques decrease the risk of further pneumothorax by increasing lung expansion and the removal of secretions. Information increases knowledge and provides the opportunity for the child to participate in the interventions that are a part of the recovery process.
- Review signs of fluid and air accumulation, including shortness of breath, chest pain, and dyspnea and instruct the child and family to report these symptoms immediately ➻*Rationale:* Prompt recognition of signs of re-accumulation and respiratory distress facilitates early intervention.
- Review the plan for pain control, including pain scale, use of medications, and implications of splinting of the affected side ➻*Rationale:* Pain control facilitates mobility, deep breathing and coughing, positioning, and recovery.
- Encourage questions and answer questions as they arise ➻*Rationale:* Reinforcement of information is needed during periods of stress.

EQUIPMENT

- Personal protective equipment as indicated, including gloves, gown, mask, and goggles
- Cardiorespiratory monitor and pulse oximeter, as indicated
- Emergency equipment, including manual ventilation bag, mask, and oxygen source
- Clamps, as indicated
- Additional 4×4 gauze
- Suture removal kit (scissors, tweezers)
- Pain medication
- Dressing (petrolatum gauze and occlusive dressing or tape)
- Absorbent pad
- Sterile specimen collection cup, as indicated

Procedure for Chest Tube Removal: Assist

Steps	Rationale	Considerations
1. Ensure that child and family understand procedure and questions are answered.	Reinforces understanding of previously taught information.	Developmental, cognitive, and anxiety levels determine approach and effectiveness of teaching.
2. Gather all necessary equipment and supplies, and ensure that emergency equipment is present and in working order.	Preparation facilitates completion of procedure in a timely manner.	
3. Ensure adequate cardiopulmonary monitoring.	Children may decompensate during procedure.	
4. Ensure child has undergone premedication as indicated for the procedure and that a plan for pain control is in place.[9,12] *(Level IV*)*	Removal of chest tubes is a painful procedure. Pain and anxiety control helps child maintain position.	Medication dose is dependent on child's weight and previous experience with pain and on other concurrent conditions. *(Level V*)*
5. Wash hands and put on clean gloves.	Reduces transmission of microorganisms. Protects personnel health.	Ensure that child does not have a latex allergy in your decision on gloves and equipment.
6. Conduct final patient verification process (e.g., "Time out") per institution-specific protocol.	Confirms correct patient, procedure, and site, and prevents unnecessary medical procedures (JCAHO requirement).	The bedside nurse's familiarity with child's chest x-ray results is helpful.
7. Position child to permit easy access to chest tube with an absorbent pad underneath. *(Level III*)*	Ensures accessibility to insertion site.	Ensure that child can tolerate a position change.
8. Ensure other chest tubes connected with a Y connector to chest tube being removed are separated before removal. *(Level III*)*	Prevents introduction of air into pleural space.	When child has more than one chest tube, be sure that each chest tube is labeled correctly and that proper chest tube is removed. If chest tube has previously been placed to water seal, this step may not be necessary. Some institutions may recommend clamping chest tube during removal.
9. Provide emotional support and coping behaviors to child throughout procedure.	Increases comfort and maintains a calm atmosphere.	Examples of support or coping behaviors: distraction, diversion, relaxation, and guided imagery. Respect expressions of emotion.
10. Assist with opening suture removal kit and opening packaging for the petroleum gauze, dry gauze, and dressing.	This is not a sterile procedure, although aseptic technique is necessary to prevent infection. Petroleum gauze must be ready immediately on removal of chest tube to decrease introduction of air into the pleural space.	
11. Assist in loosening dressing over insertion site.	Allows for access to chest tube.	This step can be done by individual removing the chest tube or by the individual assisting.

Procedure continues on following page

---

* Level III: Laboratory data; no clinical data to support recommendations
  Level IV: Limited clinical studies to support recommendations
  Level V: Clinical studies in more than one or two patient populations and situations to support recommendations

Procedure   for Chest Tube Removal: Assist—*Continued*

Steps	Rationale	Considerations
12. If suture is *not* a purse string suture, assist with cutting the sutures.		This step can be done by individual removing the chest tube or by the individual assisting.
13. If a purse string suture *is* present, assisting individual ties purse string suture promptly after removal of drain[4] (Figure 39-1). *(Level III*)*	Closes insertion site.	Suture can typically be removed 5 to 7 days after tube removal. *(Level III*)*
14. Instruct child to take a deep breath and hold or to exhale and hold.[5,10] *(Level V*)*	Creates positive pressure in pleural space and helps to limit introduction of air into pleural space.	Removal of chest tube at the end of inspiration or at end of expiration results in similar incident rates of recurrent pneumothoraces.[5,10] If child is receiving mechanical ventilation, chest tubes are typically removed at the end of inspiratory phase of the mandatory breath.[5,8] *(Level III*)* Consider child's age and developmental level in instruction of child.
15. After tube is removed, immediately apply petroleum dressing over site. *(Level III*)*	Prevents introduction of air into pleural space.	If purse string sutures are present or wound is fully closed, this step may be unnecessary. *(Level III*)*
16. Secure dry gauze dressing and occlusive dressing or tape over petroleum dressing. *(Level III*)*	Absorbs excess drainage and secures dressing.	Dressing is typically removed 2 days after tube removal. *(Level III*)*
17. Dispose of equipment in a biohazard bag and wash hands.	Reduces transmission of microorganisms. Protects personnel health.	
18. Evaluate cardiorespiratory status and obtain a chest x-ray as indicated.[2,4,5,7,8,10,13] *(Level V*)*	Evaluate expansion of lung. Clinical signs identify a child with a pneumothorax.	A chest x-ray is recommended immediately to 8 hours after chest tube removal,[2,4,5,7,8,10,14] 24 hours after chest tube removal, and when signs of respiratory distress or decompensation occur.[7] *(Level IV*)*

* Level III: Laboratory data; no clinical data to support recommendations
Level IV: Limited clinical studies to support recommendations
Level V: Clinical studies in more than one or two patient populations and situations to support recommendations

Expected Outcomes	Unexpected Outcomes
• Child has adequate oxygenation and ventilation	• Respiratory decompensation during or after the procedure
• No re-accumulation of fluid or air in the pleural or mediastinal space	• Re-accumulation of fluid or air in the pleural or mediastinal space
• Thoracostomy site is infection free	• Site infection
• Secure exit wound with minimal drainage	• Air leak
	• Excessive bleeding or drainage from site
• Child has adequate pain control during the procedure	• Unmanaged pain and anxiety

Monitoring and Care of the Child

Activities and Interventions	Rationale	Reportable Conditions
1. Monitor respiratory, cardiovascular, and neurologic status before, during, and after the procedure.	Ongoing assessment is necessary to evaluate the effectiveness of therapy. Changes in vital signs and physical assessment alert the caregiver to unexpected outcomes.	• Respiratory distress (grunting, tachypnea, retractions, dyspnea, agitation, and hypoxia) • Decreased to absent breath sounds • Subcutaneous emphysema • Tracheal shift to the unaffected side • Cardiovascular collapse • Anxiety, restlessness, or feeling of doom • Tachycardia • Hypotension • Chest pain
2. Assess pain during and after chest tube removal.	Unmanaged pain can interfere with deep breathing and full lung expansion.	• Pain unrelieved with pain management plan • Pain interfering with interventions to expand lung
3. Obtain and review chest radiographic results.	Post procedural follow-up. Air could be introduced accidentally during the procedure.	• Pneumothorax • Re-accumulation of fluid, blood, pus, or chyle
4. Assess the chest tube insertion site for signs and symptoms of infections	An increased risk of infection is seen with invasive tubes. Prolonged chest tube placement increases the risk for infection.	• Fever • Site redness or warmth • Site tenderness • Purulent drainage
5. Assess the chest tube insertion site for air leak, bleeding, or drainage.	Air can leak from the insertion site. Continual bleeding could indicate vessel injury. The chest tube may have tamponaded the internal artery or vein.	• Excessive persistent bleeding not controlled with direct pressure
6. If a purse string suture exists, assess the site for necrosis.	A tightly pulled suture may restrict blood flow to the site.	• Dark, purple, or dusky skin at site

Documentation

- Date and time of procedure and use of purse string suture
- Child's response to procedure
- Assessment findings before and after chest tube removal (breath sounds and signs of oxygenation and ventilation)
- Chest radiographic results obtained
- Local anesthetic or systemic anesthetic used and child's response
- Assessment of site and presence of bleeding
- Comfort assessment and any specific interventions
- Additional interventions necessary before, during, and after chest tube removal
- Child and family education
- Unexpected outcomes and related treatment

References

1. Kanter RK: Control of breathing and acute respiratory failure. In Fuhrman B, Zimmerman J, editors: *Pediatric critical care,* Philadelphia, 2005, Elsevier.
2. Allibone L: Nursing management of chest drains, *Nurs Stand* 17(22):45-56, 2003.
3. Baumann MH: Management of spontaneous pneumothorax: an American College of Chest Physicians delphi consensus statement, *CHEST* 119(2):590-602, 2001.
4. Adrales G, et al: A thoracostomy tube guideline improves management efficiency in trauma patients, *J Trauma* 52(2): 210-216, 2002.
5. Bell R, et al: Chest tube removal: end-inspiration or end-expiration? *J Trauma* 50(4):674-677, 2001.
6. Marshall M, et al: Suction vs. water seal after pulmonary resection: a randomized prospective study, *CHEST* 121(3): 831-835, 2002.

7. Pacanowski JP, et al: Is routine roentgenography needed after closed tube thoracostomy removal? *J Trauma* 48(4):684-688, 2000.

8. Pizano L, et al: When should a chest radiograph be obtained after chest tube removal in mechanically ventilated patients? A prospective study, *J Trauma* 53(6):1073-1077, 2002.

9. Kirkwood P: Chest tube removal: perform. In Lynn-McHale Wiegand DJ, Carlson K: *AACN procedure manual for critical care,* ed 5, Philadelphia, 2005, Elsevier.

10. Martino K, et al: Prospective randomized trial of thoracostomy removal algorithms, *J Trauma* 46(3):369-373, 1999.

11. Waldhausen J, et al: Removal of chest tubes in children without water seal after elective thoracic procedures: a randomized prospective study, *J Am College Surg* 194(4):411-415, 2002.

12. Rosen D, et al: Analgesia for pediatric thoracostomy tube removal, *Anesthesia Analgesia* 90(5):1025-1028, 2000.

13. Baumann M: What drainage system is ideal? And what other chest tube management questions, *Current Opinion Pulmon Med* 9(4):276-281, 2003.

Additional Readings

Carroll P: Exploring chest drain options, *RN* 63(10):50-54, 2000.

Gallin A: Pneumothorax, *Nurs Stand* 13(10):35-39, 1998.

Kaplan R, Yang C: Sedation and analgesia in pediatric patients for procedures outside the operating room, *Anesthesiol Clin North Am* 20:181-194, 2002.

Sahn S, Heffner J: Primary care, *N Engl J Med* 342(12):868-874, 2000.

Valenzuela R, Rosen D: Topical lidocaine-prilocaine cream (EMLA) for thoracostomy tube removal, *Anesthesia Analgesia* 88(5):1107-1108, 1999.

Closed Chest Drainage System: Set Up and Management

P U R P O S E : Closed chest drainage systems are used to help restore negative pressure by evacuating air, blood, fluid, and other drainage from the intrapleural or mediastinal space and to facilitate reexpansion of the lung

Kerry Shields

PREREQUISITE KNOWLEDGE

- Anatomy and physiology of the pediatric pulmonary system
- Understanding of negative pressure and the mechanics of breathing[1]
- Understanding of clinical indications for chest tube
  - ❖ Chest tubes are placed for the drainage of air, blood, or fluid from the pleural or mediastinal space on the basis of the child's symptoms with clinical correlation of the radiographic findings.
  - ❖ Chest tubes are placed after cardiovascular surgery for evacuation of air that enters the pleural space during the procedure or removal of blood or fluid from the operative area.[2]
- Typical signs and symptoms of pneumothorax include tachypnea, decreased breath sounds on the affected side, increased work of breathing, decreased oxygen saturation, tachycardia, hypotension, and possible dysrhythmias.
- Signs of tension pneumothorax include grunting, tachypnea, retractions, dyspnea, agitation, hypoxia, decreased to absent breath sounds on the affected side, unequal chest rise, tympany to percussion, tracheal shift to the unaffected side, subcutaneous emphysema, muffled heart sounds, and neck vein distention.
- Normal intrapleural pressure is approximately -4 cm H_2O pressure, and at the end of exhalation, the pressure decreases to -8 cm H_2O[3].

- Knowledge of the type of drainage system used by the institution
  - ❖ Traditional wet suction units are three-chamber units, which use water for desired suction level, water seal chamber, and collection chamber (Figure 35-1).

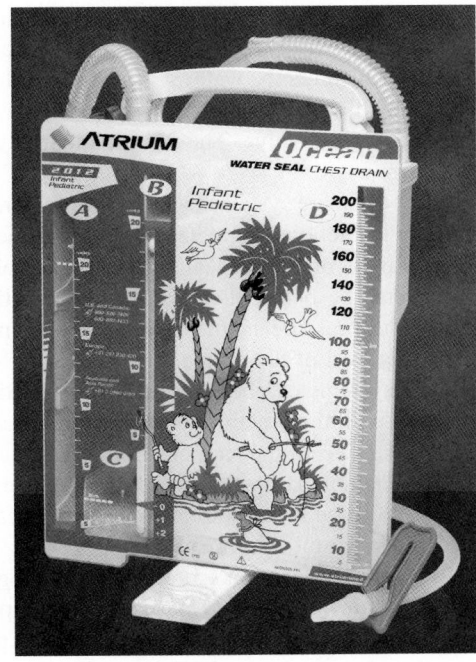

FIGURE 35-1 Wet Suction Drainage Unit. *Courtesy of Atrium Medical Corporation.*

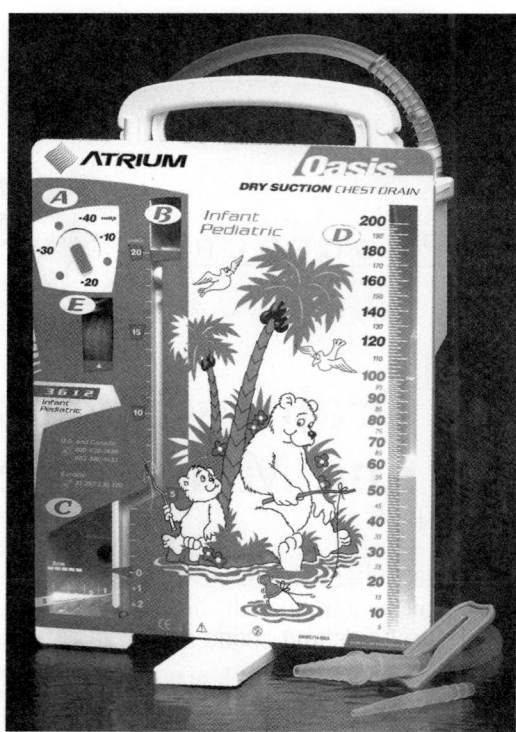

FIGURE 35-2   Dry Suction Drainage Unit. *Courtesy of Atrium Medical Corporation.*

❖ Dry suction units use a regulator or restricted orifice mechanism for the desired level of suction, water seal chamber, and collection chamber (Figure 35-2).

❖ Dry suction/dry valve units use a regulator or restricted orifice mechanism for the desired level of suction, vacuum protection valve, optional air leak indicator, and collection chamber.

• In all disposable closed chest drainage systems, the tubing from the child enters first into the collection chamber; it then enters the water seal or air leak detection chamber, which prevents backflow of air via water or one-way mechanical valve. The last chamber is the suction chamber.

• Closed chest drainage systems can be placed to gravity or water seal or to suction for greater air or fluid evacuation.

❖ When gravity or water seal is used, the collection system must be below the level of the insertion site because the pressure in the thoracic cavity must be greater than that of the drainage unit.

❖ Drainage systems can be converted from suction and water seal with the practitioner's order by disconnecting the tubing from the suction source. This tubing is left open and not clamped. Occluding the tubing could cause an increase in intrathoracic pressure because air is unable to exit the system.

• In children with spontaneous breathing, tidaling is the term used when the water rises with inspiration (increased negative pressure) and falls with expiration (decreased negative pressure). This tidaling provides a continuous manometer of the pressure changes in the pleural space and indicates overall respiratory effort. The absence of tidaling suggests obstruction in drainage.[2,4]

• Stripping of pleural chest tubes is not recommended because it can cause large fluctuations in intrathoracic pressure.[5,6]

• Because of the risk of tension pneumothorax, clamping of the chest tube is typically contraindicated unless it is done for brief periods of time.[2,4,7]

• A mediastinal tube is placed in the mediastinum just below the sternum and prevents blood fluid from accumulating around the heart. No tidaling is seen because the tube is not in the lung cavity and does not reflect interpleural pressures.[8]

• When traveling with a child with chest tubes, the chest tube drainage system must be below the child's thoracic level.

CHILD AND FAMILY ASSESSMENT

• Child's developmental level and ability to interact ➤*Rationale:* Influences preparation and interaction.

• Child's and family's understanding of the reasons for and risks and benefits of the procedure ➤*Rationale:* Evaluates child's and family's understanding of the procedure and provides a gauge for ongoing education.

• Cardiopulmonary assessment, including vital signs, visual inspection of breathing patterns and chest wall movement, auscultation of lung fields, and signs of inadequate oxygenation and ventilation, such as decreased arterial oxygen saturation, increased work of breathing, supplemental oxygen requirement, cyanosis, increased heart rate and blood pressure, anxiety, and agitation ➤*Rationale:* Prompt recognition of an accumulation of fluid or air facilitates early intervention.

• Examination of the entire length of tubing and connections from the insertion site to the drainage system and avoidance of dependent loops of tubing ➤*Rationale:* Air leaking from connections interrupts the closed system, and dependent loops impede gravity drainage.

CHILD AND FAMILY EDUCATION

Individualized, developmentally appropriate education is provided to the family and to the child based on desire for knowledge, readiness to learn, and overall neurologic and psychosocial state.

• Review of the closed chest tube drainage system and the need for the drainage system to remain lower than the insertion site ➤*Rationale:* Review increases child and family cooperation and understanding.

• Review of interventions for opening lung fields, including ambulation, frequent turning, cough and deep breathing, chest physiotherapy, and incentive spirometry ➤*Rationale:* This review increases child and family cooperation with lung conditioning exercises.

- Review of plan for pain management and assessment and use of age-appropriate and developmentally appropriate pain assessment scale ➥*Rationale:* Adequate management of the child's pain encourages greater cooperation with lung conditioning interventions and decreases shallow "splinting" breathing.
- Review of signs of air or fluid accumulation in the pleural or mediastinal space and chest tube malfunction ➥*Rationale:* Prompt recognition of accumulation or respiratory distress can facilitate early intervention.
- Encourage questions and answer questions as they arise ➥*Rationale:* Reinforcement of information is needed during periods of stress.

EQUIPMENT

- Emergency equipment, including manual ventilation bag, appropriately sized mask, oxygen source, clamps, and occlusive dressing
- Suction source
- Clean gloves
- Second drainage system available if collection system malfunctions or collection chamber is full
- Pen (to mark drainage level and time)
- Sterile water or sterile saline (per institution-specific protocol)

Procedure for Closed Chest Drainage System: Set Up and Management

Steps	Rationale	Considerations
Set Up		
1. Ensure child and family understand closed drainage system and questions are answered.	Evaluates and reinforces understanding of previously taught information.	Developmental, cognitive, and anxiety levels determine approach and effectiveness of teaching.
2. Ensure emergency equipment is at bedside and is properly functioning.	Respiratory decompensation may occur or the tube may become dislodged and emergency equipment must be accessible.	
3. Ensure adequate cardiorespiratory monitoring.	Tube may become dislodged or may not provide adequate evacuation of air or fluid.	
4. Wash hands and put on clean gloves.	Reduces transmission of microorganisms. Protects personnel health.	Ensure that child does not have a latex allergy in decisions on gloves and equipment.
5. Set up closed chest drainage system.	Consider manufacturer's instructions.	Institutions may use more than one type of closed chest drainage system.
Wet suction system:	Water acts as a one-way valve as child breathes.[5]	
a. Fill water seal with sterile water (or normal saline solution) to the 2-cm line (as indicated by manufacturer and hospital policy; Figure 35-3). *(Level I*)*		Do not overfill chamber. A fluid level of 2 cm or greater in water chamber makes breathing more difficult for child.[3,5] If chamber is overfilled, a needle with a syringe can be used to aspirate excess water. On some models, the front-faced grommet can be used. If a stop cock is present, it must be in the "open" position (parallel to the tubing). Normal saline solution may cause foaming in the pressure chamber.
b. Fill suction control to ordered suction pressure (typically −20 cm water). *(Level I*)*	The water regulates amount of suction of the unit.	Water suction of −10 cm may be adequate for neonates. A gentle continuous bubbling is all that is needed for suction; bubbling at a higher intensity does not correlate with greater suction strength.

Procedure continues on following page

* Level I: Manufacturer's recommendations only

Procedure	**for Closed Chest Drainage System: Set Up and Management**—*Continued*	
Steps	**Rationale**	**Considerations**

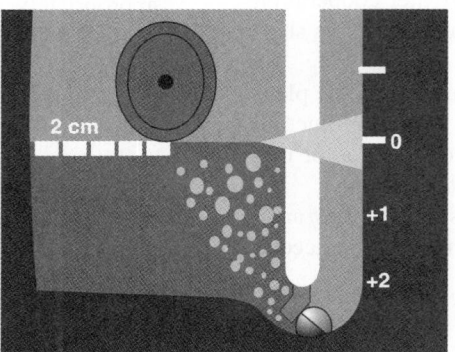

FIGURE 35-3   Water Seal Chamber. Air leak is indicated by bubbling from right to left.
Courtesy of Atrium Medical Corporation.

		If suction source cannot be adjusted and system uses a stopcock, stopcock can be gradually closed (turned horizontal to tubing) to limit vacuum flow into the chest drain and regulate bubbling if necessary.[5]
Dry suction system: a. Fill water seal chamber with sterile water (or normal saline solution) per hospital protocol and manufacturer's recommendations. b. Set negative pressure with dial on the front of drainage system. An indicator appears when desired level of suction is achieved.	Dry suction systems also use water in water seal chamber. Dry suction units have either a regulator or a restricted orifice mechanism that acts as the one-way valve for air escape.	**Do not set suction before connecting to child.** Dry suction can achieve suction levels of −40 cm water of negative pressure.
Dry suction/dry valve system: a. Fill air leak indicator with water as per manufacturer's recommendations. b. Set negative pressure with dial on front of the drainage system. An indicator appears when desired level of suction is achieved.		**Do not set suction before connecting to the child.** A dry control drain retains the one-way valve even if it is inadvertently knocked over. Air leak indicator does not fluctuate with spontaneous breathing as does the water seal system.
6. Connect the system to the child (see Procedure 33).		
7. Apply suction as appropriate for the type of suction system.		
Management 8. Ensure proper level of suction is applied to unit. a. **Wet suction** system	Suction is determined by column of water and not by amount of external suction.	Because of evaporation, wet suction systems need to be refilled periodically. Suction is typically set at −20 cm water.[2] *(Level V*)* Suction source is set to −80 mm Hg or higher for desired unit suction of −20 cm water or greater.[2] *(Level I*)*

Procedure	**for Closed Chest Drainage System: Set Up and Management**—*Continued*	
Steps	**Rationale**	**Considerations**
b. **Dry suction** system	Suction is determined by dry suction dial; an indicator appears when desired negative pressure is obtained.	Dry suction can maintain a suction level of up to −40 cm water. A negative pressure greater than −40 cm water is not recommended.[3]

9. Observe for air leak.
  a. Check for secure connections.
  b. Clamp the tubing at the chest wall.
    • If bubbling stops, the leak is in the lung.
    • If bubbling continues, the leak is between clamp and collection unit.
  c. Sequentially clamp tubing until reaching the chamber to discover location of the leak.[3] *(Level III*)*
	Bubbles move from right to left to indicate air leak. The water acts as a one-way valve.	Bubbling occurs during exhalation if child is breathing spontaneously. In children with mechanical ventilation and positive end expiratory pressure (PEEP), constant bubbling is seen. Air leak is expected when chest tube is initially placed as the pneumothorax is evacuated.

10. To sample drainage, use a 20-gauge or smaller needle and insert it directly at dependent loop. *(Level I*)*	Samples may be required for testing.	
11. To withdraw excess water in water seal or set suction, insert a 20-gauge or smaller needle in front-faced grommet. *(Level I*)*	An excess level of water in water seal chamber can increase child's work of breathing.[5]	Larger sized needles can damage self-sealing quality of the grommet.
12. If system is inadvertently knocked over, place it upright and assess water level in water seal chamber.	If a significant amount of drainage has entered water seal chamber, changing the system is advisable.	Many systems have "knock over protection" that retains the proper water seal when system is not upright.

13. To change the system:
  a. Briefly clamp tube to the child.
  b. Replace it with sterile technique with a new set up tubing.
  c. Ensure connections are air tight.
  d. Unclamp tube immediately on new connection. *(Level I*)*
	System is changed when collection chamber is filled or drainage has entered water seal chamber.	Prolonged clamping of tubing places child at risk for tension pneumothorax.

14. If the tube is dislodged, place petroleum gauze dressing over the insertion site. *(Level I*)*	Prevents air from entering the pleural cavity.	If the child has an active air leak, occlusive dressing does not permit escape of air from the affected lung. This may cause tension pneumothorax.
15. If tubing comes apart from chest tube or if drainage collection system breaks place end of chest tube in a container of sterile water until a new collection system can be obtained.[9] *(Level III*)*	Allows air or fluids to leave pleural space and prevents room air from entering tube and causing a possible pneumothorax.	Clamping chest tube is not safe if lung has not reinflated. This may cause tension pneumothorax.
16. When child is put in prone position, system is hung at the foot of the bed. Tubing is placed along child's side parallel to insertion site.[9] *(Level III*)*	Decreases risk of dislodging chest tube with turning.	Be vigilant about chest tube compression when child is prone positioned. Having child well supported can prevent chest tube compression.[10]

* Level I: Manufacturer's recommendations only
  Level III: Laboratory data; no clinical data to support recommendations

Expected Outcomes

- Negative pressure is restored
- Equipment functions effectively
- Reexpansion of the affected lung
- Improved oxygenation and ventilation
- Drainage of air, fluid, pus, or blood as per initial clinical indication and gradual reduction

- Gradual cessation of air leak/tidaling in water seal
- Site remains infection free
- Child has an acceptable level of comfort

Unexpected Outcomes

- Misplaced tube or dislodgement of tube
- Clotting of chest tube
- Tension pneumothorax

- Re-accumulation of fluid or air in the pleural or mediastinal space
- Excessive bleeding
- New or persistent air leak in system
- Infection
- Unmanaged pain and anxiety

Monitoring and Care of the Child

Activities and Interventions	Rationale	Reportable Conditions
1. Monitor respiratory, cardio-vascular, and neurologic status.	Ongoing assessment is necessary to evaluate the effectiveness of therapy. Assess for re-accumulation of air or fluid in the pleural or mediastinal space.	• Respiratory distress (grunting, tachypnea, retractions, dyspnea, agitation, hypoxia) • Decreased to absent breath sounds • Subcutaneous emphysema • Tracheal shift to the unaffected side • Cardiovascular collapse • Anxiety, restlessness, or feeling of doom • Tachycardia • Hypotension • Chest pain
2. Monitor insertion site.	Any open wound is at risk for infection and bleeding. Air leak can occur from the insertion site.	• Excessive bleeding or draining from the site Signs of infection, including fever, tenderness, inflammation, and redness at the insertion site • Crepitus • Tube dislodgement
3. Monitor drainage output from the chest tube (amount, color, and consistency).	An increase in drainage may indicate increased bleeding and may necessitate transfusion. A decrease in drainage may indicate clotting of the chest tube. After ambulation an increase in drainage may occur.	• Continued excessive sanguineous bleeding (<2 mL/kg/h) • Abrupt cession of drainage
4. Assess the system for air leaks.	Air leak can indicate that the lung is not properly healing or that the system is not airtight.	• Persistent or new air leak
5. Check water seal and suction level at least once per shift.	Assessment ensures that the system is working properly and that negative intrapleural pressure is maintained.	
6. Observe for tidaling in the water seal chamber.	Indicates tube patency. Tidaling may cease when lung is expanded. Water rises during expiration and falls during inspiration with positive pressure ventilation.	• Tidaling ceases
7. Assess pain.	Evaluate pain management and sedation plan. Unmanaged pain can interfere with deep breathing and full lung expansion.	• Pain unrelieved with pain management plan • Pain interfering with interventions to expand lung

Documentation

- Amount of suction
- Chest tube drainage amount and color
- Cardiorespiratory assessment findings (breath sounds and signs of adequate oxygenation and ventilation)
- Presence of an air leak
- Site assessment
- Chest x-ray obtained and results
- Lung expansion techniques (chest physiotherapy, cough and deep breathing, incentive spirometry, and ambulation)
- Comfort assessment and any specific interventions
- Additional interventions necessary
- Child and family education
- Unexpected outcomes and related treatment

References

1. Kanter RK: Control of breathing and acute respiratory failure. In Fuhrman B, Zimmerman J, editors: *Pediatric critical care,* Philadelphia, 2005, Elsevier.
2. Allibone L: Nursing management of chest drains, *Nurs Stand* 17(22):45-56, 2003.
3. Pickett J: Closed chest tube drainage systems. In Lynn-McHale DJ, Carlson K, editors: *AACN procedure manual for critical care,* ed 5, Philadelphia, 2005, Saunders.
4. Carroll P: Chest tubes made easy, *RN* 58(12):46-56, 1995.
5. Carroll P: Chest drainage competency manual, Hudson, NH, 2001, Atrium Medical Corporation.
6. Duncan C, Erickson R: Pressure associated with chest tube stripping, *Heart Lung* 11(2):166, 1982.
7. Golden P, Norton J, Merrell R: Redefining chest tube management: analysis of the state of practice, *Dimensions Crit Care Nurs* 14:6-13, 1995.
8. Perry AG, Potter P: *Clinical nursing skills and techniques,* ed 5, St. Louis, 2004, Elsevier.
9. Shuster PM: Chest tubes: to clamp or not to clamp, *Nurse Educator* 23(3):9, 13, 1998.
10. Marion BS: A turn for the better: prone positioning of patients with ARDS: a guide to the physiology and management of this effective, underused intervention, *Am J Nurs* 101(5):26-34, 2001.

36

Pleural Catheter: Care

P U R P O S E : Pleural catheters remove air, fluid, and blood from the pleural space and restore negative pressure for reexpansion of the lung and improvement in oxygenation and ventilation

Judith A. Mulloney

PREREQUISITE KNOWLEDGE

- Child development as it relates to clinical assessment and pleural catheter care
- Anatomy and physiology of the pediatric pulmonary system including mechanics of ventilation[1]
- Principles of closed chest drainage systems
- The negative intrapleural pressure present in the thoracic cavity must remain negative to keep the lungs fully expanded.
- Under normal circumstances, the thoracic cavity is a closed airtight gap between the lung and the chest wall. Any disruption causes a loss of negative pressure within the intrapleural space.[2]
- Understanding of the clinical indication for the child's pleural catheter
- Indications for a pleural catheter[2,3]
  - ❖ Pneumothorax: Air in pleural space (see Figure 33-2)
  - ❖ Pleural effusion (see Figure 33-3)
  - ❖ Hemothorax: Blood in pleural space (see Figure 33-4)
  - ❖ Empyema: Pus in pleural space
  - ❖ Tension pneumothorax (see Figure 33-5)
  - ❖ Chylothorax: Chyle from the thoracic duct in the pleural space
  - ❖ Instilling fibrinolytic agents for the treatment of pleural empyema
- A percutaneously placed pigtail catheter may be used in place of a thoracostomy tube.

- Typical signs and symptoms of pneumothorax include tachypnea, decreased breath sounds on the affected side, increased work of breathing, unequal chest rise, decreased oxygen saturation, tachycardia, hypotension, and possible dysrhythmias.
- Signs of tension pneumothorax include grunting, tachypnea, retractions, dyspnea, agitation, hypoxia, decreased to absent breath sounds on the affected side, tympany to percussion, tracheal shift to the unaffected side, subcutaneous emphysema, muffled heart sounds, and neck vein distention.[4]
- Placement is determined by the indication. Catheters placed to drain air are typically placed anterior toward the apex. Catheters placed to drain fluid, blood, or pus are typically placed inferior and posterior.[2]
- Crepitus (subcutaneous emphysema) can indicate that holes of the chest tube are outside of the pleural space and that air is leaking into the subcutaneous tissue.[3]
- Pain medication should be provided before the insertion, during maintenance of the pleural catheter, and before removal.
- When traveling with a child with chest tubes, ensure that the pleural catheter drainage system is below the child's thoracic level.
- Suction is not turned on until after the child is connected to the pleural catheter. A suction pressure of 15 to 20 cm H_2O pressure is typically used.[3]
- Bubbling in the water seal chamber indicates that a leak is present. A fluctuation in the level of the water seal

chamber of 5 to 10 cm (rising with inspiration and falling with expiration) is observed with spontaneous respiration. This process is called tidaling. If the child is mechanically ventilated, the pattern is the opposite. If suction is being applied, it should be temporarily stopped to assess for fluctuations in the water seal chamber.

- Knowledge of institutional closed chest drainage systems, the availability of wall or portable suction, and the need for adapters

CHILD AND FAMILY ASSESSMENT

- Child's developmental level and ability to interact ➤*Rationale:* Influences preparation and interaction.
- Child's and family's understanding of the reasons for and risks and benefits of having a pleural catheter ➤*Rationale:* Evaluates child's and family's understanding of the procedure and provides a gauge for ongoing education.
- Desire of family members to be present during procedures ➤*Rationale:* The presence of family may provide comfort and support, although family members should have the choice not to remain with the child.
- Cardiopulmonary assessment, including vital signs, visual inspection of breathing patterns and chest wall movement, auscultation of lung fields, and signs of inadequate oxygenation and ventilation, such as decreased arterial oxygen saturation, increased work of breathing, supplemental oxygen requirement, cyanosis, increased heart rate and blood pressure, anxiety, and agitation ➤*Rationale:* Evaluating cardiopulmonary status provides valuable information in determining the child's need for and ability to tolerate the procedure.
- Review of chest x-ray results ➤*Rationale:* Radiologic evidence of resolution of pneumothorax, effusion, and hemothorax.
- Noted fluctuations in water seal chamber and air leak indicator ➤*Rationale:* Evaluates air leak and functionality of pleural catheter.
- Examination of the entire length of tubing and connections from the insertion site to the drainage system and avoidance of dependent loops of tubing ➤*Rationale:* Air

leaking from connections interrupts the closed system, and dependent loops impede gravity drainage.
- Assessment of skin integrity at the insertion site ➤*Rationale:* Assesses for signs of infection or inflammation.

CHILD AND FAMILY EDUCATION

Individualized, developmentally appropriate education is provided to the family and to the child based on desire for knowledge, readiness to learn, and overall neurologic and psychosocial state.

- Explain the indication, procedure, and rationale for the pleural catheter ➤*Rationale:* Providing information decreases fear and anxiety.
- Explain the pleural catheter apparatus ➤*Rationale:* Information decreases fear and anxiety.
- Explain interventions to assist in lung expansion, including frequent turning, cough and deep breathing, chest physiotherapy, and incentive spirometry ➤*Rationale:* Interventions can be an adjunct to pleural catheters to expand the lung and prevent further collapse.
- Review signs of air or fluid accumulation in the pleural space and catheter malfunction ➤*Rationale:* Prompt recognition of accumulation or respiratory distress can facilitate early intervention.
- Explain the plan for pain assessment and treatment for the duration of the pleural catheter placement ➤*Rationale:* Decreasing anxiety about pain and adequate pain control can facilitate coughing, deep breathing, and chest physiotherapy.
- Encourage questions and answer questions as they arise ➤*Rationale:* Reinforcement of information is needed during periods of stress.

EQUIPMENT

- Clamps as indicated
- Tape and pins as indicated
- Dressing materials, including petroleum dressing, dry gauze, tape, and occlusive dressing as needed
- Medication for pain discomfort as ordered by the prescribing practitioner

Procedure for Pleural Catheter: Care

Steps	Rationale	Considerations
1. Ensure child and family understand purpose of pleural catheter and questions are answered.	Evaluates and reinforces understanding of previously taught information.	Developmental, cognitive, and anxiety levels determine approach and effectiveness of teaching.
2. Gather equipment and supplies.	Preparation facilitates completion of procedure in a timely manner.	If child does not have a secure artificial airway, have emergency airway equipment at bedside.
3. Ensure all connections in chest drainage system are securely taped. *(Level V*)*	Taping prevents accidental disconnection of tube and prevents air from reentering chest.	
4. Ensure pleural catheter is secured.	Prevents side-to-side movement of pleural catheter and accidental dislodgement.	Care is taken in securing pleural catheter; pinning catheter to clothing or bed may lead to sudden dislodgement. Pigtail catheters have a higher incidence of dislodgment, kinking and disconnection especially in neonates.[6]
5. Ensure suction is set according to prescribed orders.	Suction is often necessary to assist in drainage.[7,8]	Suction should not be turned on until the system is connected to the child.
6. Ensure drainage tubing has a straight flow to drainage collection device and does not have any dependent loops or kinks. *(Level V*)*	If fluid collects in a dependent loop between child and collection system at a height greater than suction control unit, tube becomes sealed, which may lead to a collapsed lung because air and fluid collect again in the pleural space.[8]	
7. Administer pain medication as prescribed and ensure that a plan for pain control is in place. *(Level VI*)*	Pain medication ensures that child is comfortable.	The medication dose is dependent on child's weight and previous experience with pain and on other concurrent conditions. Some studies have reported a lower incidence rate of pain with a pigtail catheter compared with larger bore thoracostomy tubes.[9]
8. Ensure clamps are kept at the bedside.	Clamps may be necessary to replace drainage system or may be used to determine source of an air leak if bubbling occurs in water seal compartment.	Child is at risk for a tension pneumothorax when clamps are used and air or fluid cannot escape. Clamps are not used for transportation of child or when child is getting out of bed.
9. Troubleshoot problems that may arise with system or with child (Table 36-1).	Immediate attention to problems minimizes child's chance of complications.	

* Level V: Clinical studies in more than one or two patient populations and situations to support recommendations
  Level VI: Clinical studies in a variety of patient populations and situations to support recommendations

TABLE 36-1	**Pleural Catheter Care: Troubleshooting**	
Problem	**Possible Causes**	**Intervention**
1. Water level in water seal chamber does not rise and fall with breathing	Clot in catheter tubing or child's chest	Gently pinch tubing around clot and gingerly milk fluid to move it into collection chamber; repeat as necessary. Unless absolutely necessary, do not strip tubing because this creates high negative pressure and can damage lung tissue.
	Dependent loop or kink in patient tube with fluid occlusion	Straighten catheter and tubing along its length to its connection with collection device.
	Dislodgment of catheter from child Disconnection of tube from chest tube connector	If tube accidentally pulls out, insertion site should be immediately sealed with sterile petroleum gauze dressing to prevent air from entering pleural cavity; notify physician immediately.
	Tube clamp may be closed	Always keep tube clamp for each tube at bedside. Quickly clamp tube to prevent sucking air injury and notify prescribing practitioner immediately.
	Chest drain is not positioned sufficiently below child's chest	Clamp only when indicated; otherwise, leave tube open. Lower drainage system to allow for gravity drainage.
	Inline connectors not properly secured, allowing for air leak	Ensure that inline connectors are properly secured and sealed at all times; check for loose connections periodically.
2. Constant bubbling is seen in water seal chamber	Confirms air leak is present	To determine source of air leak, momentarily clamp tube to drain and observe water seal. If bubbling stops, air leak may be from catheter connections or child's chest. Check catheter connections and child's dressing for partially withdrawn catheter. If catheter is dislodged, follow procedure as previously mentioned. If bubbling continues after temporarily clamping child's tube, system leak is indicated and necessitates system replacement.
3. Overfilled water seal level (water >2 cm limit line) or overfilled suction control chamber	Too much water was added to chamber	Press and hold negative-pressure relief valve at top of drainage system to vent excess negative pressure in water seal chamber. Release valve when level of water returns to 2-cm mark. To remove water from suction control chamber, insert syringe and withdraw excess.
4. Not enough water in water seal or suction control chamber	Evaporation versus underfill or spillage	Add additional water to suction control chamber by temporarily turning off suction source, removing rubber stopper, and adding water to desired level. Additional water may be added to water seal chamber with syringe by quickly and temporarily clamping child's tube and injecting water to desired level.
5. Suction control chamber is not bubbling or is bubbling too vigorously	Check suction source for disconnection or too much suction source pressure in system	Ensure that suction tubing is connected and suction source is turned on. Constant gently bubbling is normal. Vigorous bubbling causes quicker evaporation. Adjust suction control source for gentle bubbling.
6. Chest drainage system has been accidentally knocked over	Human error	Set system upright and check fluid levels in water seal and suction control chambers for proper volumes. Adjust accordingly. Most units have baffle system that prevents fluid from mixing between chambers, allowing for proper function after setting upright again.
7. Child must be transported or leave unit	As situation indicates (e.g., computed tomographic scan, surgery)	Do not clamp catheter tubing; disconnect suction tubing from suction source. System continues to collect fluid (by gravity) or air (by water seal).
8. Specimen collection necessary	Prescribing practitioner's orders for laboratory analysis	Remove fluid with needle and syringe from self-sealing portion of drainage tubing after following hospital policy for cleaning tubing fluid collection site.

Herberg A: Chest tubes. In Bowden VR, Greenberg CS, editors: *Pediatric nursing procedures,* Philadelphia, Lippincott Williams & Wilkins.

Expected Outcomes

- Air, fluid, or blood is removed from the pleural space with gradual reduction in amount of drainage
- Equipment is fully functional
- Reexpansion of the affected lung
- Improved oxygenation and ventilation
- Gradual cession of air leak or tidaling in the water seal
- Site remains infection free
- Child maintains an acceptable level of comfort

Unexpected Outcomes

- Equipment or suction malfunction
- Clotting of the catheter or tubing
- Tension pneumothorax
- Reaccumulation of air, fluid, or blood in the pleural space
- New or persistent air leak in system
- Infection
- Unmanaged pain and anxiety

Monitoring and Care of the Child

Activities and Interventions	Rationale	Reportable Conditions
1. Monitor respiratory, cardio-vascular, and neurologic status.	Ongoing assessment is necessary to evaluate effectiveness of therapy. Changes in vital signs and physical examination results alert the caregiver to unexpected outcomes.	• Respiratory distress (grunting, tachypnea, retractions, dyspnea, agitation, or hypoxia) • Decreased to absent breath sounds • Muffled heart tones • Subcutaneous emphysema • Tracheal shift • Anxiety, restlessness, or feeling of doom • Tachycardia • Dysrhythmias • Hypotension • Fever
2. Check water seal for bubbling and fluctuation every 4 hours or more often as indicated by child's condition.	Fluctuation of water in water seal compartment shows a normal reflection of pressure changes in pleural cavity during respiration. Bubbling indicates that air is draining, which is normal for a child with a pneumothorax. If the child is on a ventilator with positive end expiratory pressure (PEEP), continuous bubbling is present.	• Changes in bubbling and fluctuation of the water seal
3. Monitor insertion site and surrounding skin for presence of infection or subcutaneous air every day or with each dressing change.	Skin integrity is affected by the insertion of a pleural catheter. Any open wound is at risk for infection and bleeding. Air leak can occur from insertion site.	• Excessive bleeding or purulent drainage from the site • Signs of infection, including fever, tenderness, inflammation, or redness at the insertion site • Subcutaneous emphysema • Catheter dislodgement
4. Monitor drainage output (amount, color, and consistency).	An increase in drainage may indicate increased bleeding and may necessitate transfusion. A decrease in drainage may indicate an obstruction in the tubing or kinking.[10,11]	• Continued, excessive sanguineous bleeding (>2 mL/kg/hr) • Abrupt cessation of drainage
5. Assess the system for air leaks, including the integrity of the pleural catheter and drainage tubing every 2 to 4 hours or as often as the child's condition indicates.	Assessment makes certain that the system is intact and prevents kinks or dependent loops from forming. Air leak can indicate that the system is not air tight.	• Persistent or new air leak

Monitoring and Care of the Child—Cont'd

Activities and Interventions	Rationale	Reportable Conditions
6. Assess pain status and administer pain medication as indicated. *(Level VI*)*	Evaluate pain management and sedation plan. Unmanaged pain can interfere with the child's ability to move, take deep breaths, and change positions, impeding full lung expansion.	• Pain unrelieved with pain management plan • Pain interfering with interventions to expand lung

* Level VI: Clinical studies in a variety of patient populations and situations to support recommendations

Documentation

- Assessment findings, including breath sounds and signs of oxygenation and ventilation
- Size and type of catheter
- Amount, color, and consistency of drainage
- Amount of water seal suction, prescribed water level for suction, and presence of air leak
- Chest radiograph obtained and results
- Laboratory specimen analysis results
- Site assessment results
- Comfort assessment and any specific interventions
- Additional interventions necessary
- Child and family education
- Unexpected outcomes and related treatment

References

1. Kanter RK: Control of breathing and acute respiratory failure. In Fuhrman B, Zimmerman J, editors: *Pediatric critical care,* Philadelphia, 2006, Elsevier.
2. Lawrence D, Carlson K: Procedure 19: Chest tube placement (assist). In Lynn-McHale Wiegand DJ, Carlson K, editors: *AACN procedure manual for critical care,* Philadelphia, 2005, Elsevier.
3. Allibone L: Nursing management of chest drains, *Nurs Stand* 17(22):45-56, 2003.
4. Baumann MH: Management of spontaneous pneumothorax: an American College of Chest Physicians delphi consensus statement, *Chest* 119(2):590-602, 2001.
5. Carroll P: Exploring chest drain options, *RN* 63(10):50-54, 56, 2000.
6. Robert JS, et al: Efficacy and complications of percutaneous pigtail catheters for thoracostomy in pediatric patients, *Chest* 114(4):1116-1121, 1998.
7. Cerfolio R, et al: Prospective randomized trial compares suction versus water seal for air leaks, *Ann Thorac Surg* 71:1613-1617, 2001.
8. Colt HG, et al: Evaluation of patient-related and procedure related factors contributing to pneumothorax following thoracentesis, *Chest* 116:134-138, 1999.
9. Dull KE, Fleisher GR: Pigtail catheters versus large-bore chest tubes for pneumothoraces in children treated in the emergency department, *Pediatr Emerg Care* 18:265-267, 2002.
10. Laronga C, et al: A treatment algorithm for pneumothoraces complicating central venous catheter insertion, *Am J Surg* 180:523-527, 2000.
11. Padman R: Pleural space disease in pediatric patients: a retrospective analysis, *Del Med J* 73:333-338, 2001.

Additional Readings

Aru G, et al: Selective use of chest tubes in thoracotamies for congenital cardiovascular problems, *Ann Thorac Surg* 68:1376-1379, 1999.

Carroll P: Chest tubes made easy, *RN* 58(12):46-56, 1995.

Carroll P: *Chest drainage competency manual,* Hudson, NH, 2001, Atrium Medical Corporation.

Gunn V, Nechyba C: *The Harriet Lane handbook,* Philadelphia, 2002, Mosby.

Pierrepoint MJ, et al: Pigtail catheter drain in the treatment of empyema thoracis, *Arch Dis Child* 87:331-332, 2002.

Thoracentesis: Assist

PURPOSE: Thoracentesis is performed to drain pleural fluid for diagnostic or therapeutic purposes or to evacuate a tension pneumothorax

Deb Templin

PREREQUISITE KNOWLEDGE

- Child development as it relates to clinical assessment and the procedure
- Anatomy and physiology of the pediatric pulmonary system [1,2]
- The primary indication for a thoracentesis is pleural effusion (see Figure 33-3). Other indications include tension pneumothorax (see Figure 33-2), hemothorax (see Figure 33-4) and empyema.
- Thoracentesis is typically an elective procedure and is used as a diagnostic tool to obtain pleural fluid. A therapeutic thoracentesis is also done to relieve symptoms caused by a pleural effusion.
- A pleural effusion can either be an exudate or a transudate. Exudates are usually cloudy or contain pus and result from pleural inflammation or an irregularity in lymphatic flow. The fluid of a transudate is typically serous and light yellow and forms because of factors that affect the rate of formation or absorption of pleural fluid[3] (see Table 41-1).
- Signs and symptoms of a pleural effusion include dull percussion on the affected side, absence or decrease in breath sounds, dyspnea, increased work of breathing and tactile fremitus.[3] Small pleural effusions can be asymptomatic.
- Ultrasound scan–guided thoracentesis has reduced complications.[3] Consider this approach for children with paralyzed hemidiaphragms, therapy with high levels of positive end-expiratory pressure (PEEP), small pleural effusions, pleural adhesions (e.g., empyema), previous tuberculosis, and multiple previous thoracentesis or thoracostomy tubes.
- No absolute contraindications to a thoracentesis exist when the child is in respiratory distress or has a tension pneumothorax. Relative contraindications for a thoracentesis include anticoagulant medication, bleeding disorders, and insertion through an area of infection.
- Knowledge of the mechanism of action, dosing, side effects, and contraindications for anesthetics or sedatives used for procedural sedation[3]

CHILD AND FAMILY ASSESSMENT

- Child's developmental level and ability to interact **➤➤Rationale:** Influences preparation and interaction.
- Child's and family's understanding of the reasons for and risks and benefits of the procedure **➤➤Rationale:** Evaluates child's and family's understanding of the procedure and provides a gauge for ongoing education.
- Desire of family members to be present during the procedure **➤➤Rationale:** The presence of family may provide comfort and support, although family members should have the choice not to remain with the child.
- Cardiopulmonary assessment, including vital signs, visual inspection of breathing patterns and chest wall movement, auscultation of lung fields, and signs of inadequate oxygenation and ventilation, such as decreased

arterial oxygen saturation, increased work of breathing, supplemental oxygen requirement, cyanosis, increased heart rate and blood pressure, anxiety, and agitation ➤*Rationale:* Evaluating cardiopulmonary status provides valuable information in determining the child's need for and ability to tolerate the procedure. Assessment influences the type of anesthetics or sedative prescribed and the swiftness of the procedure.

- History of reactions or allergies to medication (betadine, lidocaine, anesthetics, or sedatives) ➤*Rationale:* Prevention of harm.
- History of bleeding disorders or anticoagulants or antiplatelet medication ➤*Rationale:* These disorders may increase the risk of complications.
- History of previous thoracentesis ➤*Rationale:* Previous thoracentesis may have caused scarring, which can make this procedure more difficult.
- Previous experience or reaction to an invasive procedure ➤*Rationale:* The child's previous experience may affect how this event is perceived.
- Review of chest x-ray and ultrasound scan findings (if indicated) ➤*Rationale:* Location of pleural air, blood, or fluid. An anterior posterior chest radiograph may be adequate for significant fluid accumulations. A lateral chest x-ray may, however, be necessary. A lateral decubitus radiograph should be obtained if a smaller loculated fluid is suspected. Ultrasound scan may also confirm liquid versus solid lesion.[4]
- Assessment of recent serum laboratory results, including complete blood count, platelet count, prothrombin time, and partial thromboplastin time ➤*Rationale:* Determines the risk of bleeding.
- Assessment of skin integrity at the insertion site ➤*Rationale:* Avoidance of active skin lesions or infection at the insertion site.

CHILD AND FAMILY EDUCATION

Individualized, developmentally appropriate education is provided to the family and to the child based on desire for knowledge, readiness to learn, and overall neurologic and psychosocial state.
- Explain the procedure and the reason for the thoracentesis, including risks and benefits ➤*Rationale:* Providing information increases knowledge, and preparation helps reduce anxiety. This explanation increases the child's ability to cooperate during the procedure. Providing information increases parental satisfaction.
- Discuss ways to decrease pain and anxiety during the procedure and explain plan for pain assessment and treatment for the duration of the chest tube placement ➤*Rationale:* Decreasing anxiety about pain and adequate pain control can facilitate coughing, deep breathing, and chest physiotherapy.
- Explain that during the insertion of the needle (small opening) the child may feel pressure at the insertion site ➤*Rationale:* Providing information helps prepare the child for events during the procedure and reduces anxiety.
- Explain how the child can assist with the procedure ➤*Rationale:* Provides the child with an opportunity to participate or assist with the procedure.
- Encourage questions and answer questions as they arise ➤*Rationale:* Reinforcement of information is needed during periods of stress.

EQUIPMENT

- Emergency equipment, including manual ventilation bag, mask, and oxygen supply
- Cardiorespiratory monitor or pulse oximeter as indicated
- Personal protective equipment as indicated, including sterile gloves, sterile gown, mask, and goggles
- Medication, including systemic pain medication and local 1% lidocaine as ordered
- Sterile drapes/towels
- 25-gauge 5/8-inch needle
- Syringe (for local)
- Antiseptic solution (chloraprep/betadine)
- Sterile gauze
- 18-gauge to 22-gauge needle[5]
- Sterile 10-mL and 20-mL syringe
- Collection bag or additional syringes
- Sterile three-way stopcock
- Band-Aid or adhesive dressing
- Containers for laboratory studies
- Anaerobic and aerobic media bottles for culture
- Laboratory requests

Procedure for Thoracentesis: Assist

Steps	Rationale	Considerations
1. Ensure child and family understand procedure and the reason for thoracentesis, including risks and benefits. Ensure consent has been obtained.	Evaluates and reinforces understanding of previously taught information. In many situations, informed consent is required before chest tube insertion. Informed consent is a process where the child and family acknowledge their understanding of indications for the procedure, the procedure itself, and its risks.	Developmental, cognitive, and anxiety levels determine approach and effectiveness of teaching.[6]
2. Assist in gathering all supplies and equipment necessary to complete the procedure.	Organization and preparation assist in efficient completion of the procedure.	
3. Wash hands.	Reduces transmission of microorganisms. Protects personnel health.	
4. Conduct final patient verification process (e.g., "Time Out") per institution-specific protocol (Joint Commission Requirement).	Confirms correct patient, procedure, and site and prevents unnecessary medical procedures.	
5. Ensure adequate cardiorespiratory monitoring.	Children may decompensate during the procedure. Anesthetics and sedation can alter child's vital signs, respiratory pattern and effort, level of consciousness/mental status, and oxygen requirements.	Consider whether child has a secure airway or is becoming hypotensive. The availability of volume replacement and intubation equipment may be important. Consider increasing the volume on the pulse oximeter or cardiac monitor to allow an auditory signal and visual monitoring during the procedure.
6. Administer systemic anesthetics or sedative medication as ordered.[3] (*Level VI**)	Thoracentesis is a painful procedure. Pain and anxiety control help the child maintain position.	Pain assessment/score is reflective of the effectiveness of the anesthetics.
7. Assist the practitioner in drawing up local anesthetic (1% lidocaine) to anesthetize the skin and rib periosteum. (*Level II**)	Thoracentesis is a painful procedure.	Topical lidocaine-prilocaine cream (EMLA) and local anesthetic can be used if time allows.
8. Position child supine with the head of bed elevated. The affected side is slightly rotated. Place arm of the affected side above child's head (see Figure 33-6). (*Level II**)	Air rises to the apex. The arm is immobilized during procedure so that the arm is out of procedure area to allow easier access to the intercostal spaces and to decrease chances to contaminate the sterile site.	Sitting position is an alternative. Sitting is believed to be the ideal position for adults and older children who can tolerate this position[2] (see Figure 41-1).
9. Assist with preparing the site with antiseptic solution and draping the sterile area.	Removes microorganisms from the skin and reduces risk of infection.	
10. Provide emotional support and coping behaviors to the child throughout the procedure.	Increases comfort and maintains a calm atmosphere.	Examples of support or coping behaviors: distraction, diversion, relaxation, and guided imagery. Respect expressions of emotion.
11. After fluid removal fill specimen tubes with pleural fluid or cap syringe. Send pleural fluid to laboratory.	Laboratory analysis is used for diagnostic reasons.	Laboratory studies to consider for pleural fluid include: protein, culture and gram stain, differential white blood cell count, amylase, specific

*   Level II: Theory-based; no research data to support recommendations; recommendations from expert consensus group may exist
    Level VI: Clinical studies in a variety of patient populations and situations to support recommendations

Procedure for Thoracentesis: Assist—*Continued*

Steps	Rationale	Considerations
		gravity, protein, pH, lactate dehydrogenase, and glucose.[4] Triglyceride levels if chylothorax is suspected.
12. Place an occlusive dressing over the puncture site. *(Level II*)*	Prevents pneumothorax or leakage of pleural fluid.	
13. Remove arm immobilizer and place child in a comfortable position.	Arm is immobilized for the procedure.	
14. Obtain chest radiograph, as indicated. *(Level VI*)*	Evaluates pleural effusion and ensures no pneumothorax exists.	
15. Dispose of equipment, remove needles, sharp objects, and wash hands.	Reduces transmission of microorganisms. Protects personnel health.	

* Level II: Theory-based; no research data to support recommendations; recommendations from expert consensus group may exist
Level VI: Clinical studies in a variety of patient populations and situations to support recommendations

Expected Outcomes

- Unresolved pleural effusion or air within the pleural space
- Continued signs and symptoms of inadequate oxygenation and ventilation
- Evacuation of pleural effusion
- Reexpansion of the affected lung
- Improved oxygenation and ventilation
- Complication-free procedure

- Remains infection free

- Acceptable level of comfort

Unexpected Outcomes

- Laceration of spleen or liver
- Pulmonary contusion
- Iatrogenic pneumothorax
- Hemothorax
- Bleeding from puncture of the intercostal vessels
- Pleural infection
- Site infection
- Unmanaged pain and anxiety

Monitoring and Care of the Child

Activities and Interventions	Rationale	Reportable Conditions
1. Monitor respiratory, cardiovascular, and neurologic status before, during, and after the procedure.	Ongoing assessment is necessary to evaluate the effectiveness of therapy. Changes in vital signs and physical assessment results alert the caregiver to unexpected outcomes.	- Respiratory distress (grunting, tachypnea, retractions, dyspnea, agitation, and hypoxia) - Decreased to absent breath sounds - Subcutaneous emphysema - Tracheal shift to the unaffected side - Cardiovascular collapse - Anxiety, restlessness, or feeling of doom - Tachycardia - Hypotension - Chest pain
2. Assess pain status during and after thoracentesis.	Evaluation of pain management and sedation plan.	- Pain unrelieved with pain management plan - Pain that interferes with interventions to expand lung

Documentation

- Description of the procedure, including date, time, and length of procedure
- Correct site, correct procedure, and correct person verification, including consent
- Indications for procedure
- Assessment findings before and after thoracentesis (breath sounds and signs of oxygenation and ventilation)
- Name and credentials of the individual who performed the procedure
- Local anesthetic or systemic anesthetic used and the child's response
- Description of the pleural fluid
- Site assessment and type of dressing used
- Chest radiograph obtained and results
- Laboratory studies sent
- Comfort assessment and any specific interventions
- Additional interventions necessitated
- Child and family education
- Unexpected outcomes and related treatment

References

1. Thibodeau G, Patton K: *Anatomy and physiology,* St. Louis, 2003, Mosby.
2. Fuhrman B, Zimmerman J, editors: *Pediatric critical care,* 3rd ed. Philadelphia, 2006, Elsevier.
3. Roberts JR, Hedges JR: *Clinical procedures in emergency medicine,* ed 4, Philadelphia, 2004, Saunders.
4. Carlson K: Thoracentesis (assist). In Lynn-McHale Wiegand DJ, Carlson K, editors: *AACN procedure manual for critical care,* Philadelphia, 2005, Elsevier.
5. Kaplan R, Yang C: Sedation and analgesia in pediatric patients for procedures outside the operating room, *Anesthesiol Clin North Am* 20:181-194, 2002.
6. Boyer D: Evaluation and management of a child with a pleural effusion, *Pediatr Emerg Care* 21(1):63-68, 2005.
7. Taeusch H, et al: *Pediatric and neonatal tests and procedures,* Philadelphia, 1996, Saunders.
8. Gaynard L, et al: *Psychosocial care of children in hospitals: a clinical practice manual,* Rockville, MD, 1998, Child Life Council.
9. Bryant R, Salmon C: Pleural empyema, *Clin Infect Dis* 22:747-764, 1996.

Additional Readings

Behrman R, Kliegman R, Jenson H: *Nelson textbook of pediatrics,* ed 17, Philadelphia, 2004, Saunders.
Dresser S, Melnyk BM: The effectiveness of conscious sedation on anxiety, pain, and procedural complications in young children, *Pediatr Nurs* 29(4):320-323, 2003.
Efrati O, Barak A: Pleural effusions in the pediatric population, *Pediatr Rev* 23:417-425, 2002.
Murray J, Nadel J: *Textbook of respiratory medicine,* ed 3, Philadephia, 2000, Saunders.
Stephens BK, et al: Techniques to comfort children during stressful procedures, *Adv Mind-Body Med* 15(1):49-60, 1999.

Chest Tube Placement: Perform

P U R P O S E : Chest tubes are inserted to evacuate air, fluid, and blood from the intrapleural or mediastinal space and to facilitate reexpansion of the lung. Chest tubes can also be used to instill fibrinolytic agents for the treatment of pleural empyema.

Deb Templin

PREREQUISITE KNOWLEDGE

- Child development as it relates to clinical assessment and assistance with chest tube placement
- Anatomy and physiology of the pediatric pulmonary system including mechanics of breathing[1,2]
- Chest tubes, also called thoracotomy tubes, are inserted into the pleural space to restore negative pressure and allow lung expansion.
- Indications for a chest tube[3-5]
  ❖ Pneumothorax: Air in the pleural space (see Figure 33-2)
  ❖ Pleural effusion (see Figure 33-3)
  ❖ Hemothorax: Blood in the pleural space (see Figure 33-4)
  ❖ Empyema: Pus in the pleural space
  ❖ Tension pneumothorax (see Figure 33-5)
  ❖ Chylothorax: Chyle from the thoracic duct in the pleural space
  ❖ Thoracotomy, specifically after cardiac surgery in which pleural and mediastinum have been entered (placed during surgery)
  ❖ Instillation of fibrinolytic agents for empyema
  ❖ Penetrating chest trauma

- Chest tube size is determined by the size of the child and the intended use (Table 38-1).
- Chest tubes inserted for drainage of blood tend to be larger than chest tubes inserted for evacuation of air.
- Pigtail catheter size generally is the same regardless of the child's size.
- Pigtail catheters are as effective as large-bore chest tubes for pneumothoraces.[4,6,7]
- Blunt trauma, penetrating trauma, positive pressure ventilation, and iatrogenic causes may alter the negative pressure in the pleural space and cause a pneumothorax.[4,8]
  ❖ An open pneumothorax occurs when both the chest wall and the pleural space are penetrated. Air is able to enter and escape the pleural space through the penetration. Stab wounds or surgical trauma may result in an open peumothorax.[2]

TABLE 38-1	Chest Tube Size
Age	**Chest Tube Size**
Newborn	10F to 12F
Infant	10F to 12F
1-year-old	16F to 20F
3-year-old	16F to 20F
6-year-old	20F to 28F
10-year-old	28F to 32F
Adolescent	32F to 42F

Data from Gunn VL, Nechyba C, editors: *The Harriet Lane handbook,* ed 16, St. Louis, 2002, Mosby.

❖ A closed pneumothorax occurs when the chest wall is intact. The pleural space alone has been penetrated. Air is able to enter the pleural space but is not able to escape. Cystic fibrosis and positive pressure ventilation may result in a closed pneumothorax.[4]

❖ A tension pneumothorax occurs when air accumulates in the pleural space and cannot escape. As air flows into the affected side of the lung, an increase in pressure occurs and shifts the trachea, heart, and other midline structures to the unaffected side. Tension pneumothorax is an emergent situation because the pressure can decrease venous return; compress the heart, which decreases cardiac output; and eventually lead to the collapse of the unaffected lung.[3]

- Typical signs and symptoms of pneumothorax include tachypnea, decreased breath sounds on the affected side, increased work of breathing, unequal chest rise, decreased oxygen saturation, tachycardia, hypotension, and possible dysrhythmias.

- Signs of tension pneumothorax include grunting, tachypnea, retractions, dyspnea, agitation, hypoxia, decreased to absent breath sounds on the affected side, tympany to percussion, tracheal shift to the unaffected side, subcutaneous emphysema, muffled heart sounds, and neck vein distention.[3]

- Chest tube site placement is determined by the indication. Tubes placed to drain air are typically placed anteriorly toward the apex. Tubes placed to drain fluid, blood, or pus are typically placed inferior and posterior.[6,9]

- Crepitus (subcutaneous emphysema) can indicate that holes of the chest tube are outside of the pleural space and air is leaking into the subcutaneous tissue.

- Multiple chest tubes may be necessary to evacuate additional locations or causes of collection.

- Mediastinal tubes are placed to drain effusions and after cardiac surgery to evacuate blood and fluid that may accumulate around the heart and cause compression and cardiac tamponade. Mediastinal tubes are placed anterior or posterior.

- No absolute contraindications to placement of a chest tube exist if the child is in respiratory distress from a closed pneumothorax or has a tension pneumothorax. The risks outweigh the benefits when the lung needs to be expanded. Careful consideration must be given when the child is undergoing anticoagulant therapy, has a coagulopathy, or has a skin infection at the insertion site.[4]

- Knowledge of the mechanism of action, dosing, side effects, and contraindications for anesthetics or sedatives used for procedural sedation.[10]

CHILD AND FAMILY ASSESSMENT

- Child's developmental level and ability to interact ➺*Rationale:* Influences preparation and interaction.

- Child's and family's understanding of the reasons for and risks and benefits of chest tube placement ➺*Rationale:* Evaluates child's and family's understanding of the procedure and provides a gauge for ongoing education.

- Desire of family members to be present during the procedure ➺*Rationale:* The presence of family may provide comfort and support, although family members should have the choice not to remain with the child.

- Cardiopulmonary assessment, including vital signs, visual inspection of breathing patterns and chest wall movement, auscultation of lung fields, and signs of inadequate oxygenation and ventilation, such as decreased arterial oxygen saturation, increased work of breathing, supplemental oxygen requirement, cyanosis, changes in heart rate and blood pressure, anxiety, and agitation ➺*Rationale:* Evaluating cardiopulmonary status provides valuable information in determining child's need for and ability to tolerate the procedure and influences the type of anesthetics or sedative prescribed.

- History of reactions or allergies to medication (betadine, lidocaine, anesthetics, or sedatives) and tape ➺*Rationale:* Prevents harm.

- History of bleeding disorders or anticoagulant or antiplatelet therapy ➺*Rationale:* These disorders and therapies may increase the risk of complications.

- History of problems with anesthetics or sedated procedures ➺*Rationale:* Determines appropriate anesthetics or sedative.

- History of previous chest tubes ➺*Rationale:* Previous thoracentesis may have caused scarring, which can make this procedure more difficult.

- Previous experience or reaction to an invasive procedure ➺*Rationale:* Child's previous experience may affect how this event is perceived.

- Review of chest x-ray findings ➺*Rationale:* Location of pleural air, blood, or fluid.

- Assess recent serum laboratory results, including complete blood count, platelet count, prothrombin time, and partial thromboplastin time ➺*Rationale:* Determines the risk of bleeding.

- Assessment of skin integrity at the insertion site ➺*Rationale:* Avoids active skin lesions or infection at the insertion site.

CHILD AND FAMILY EDUCATION

Individualized, developmentally appropriate education is provided to the family and to the child based on desire for knowledge, readiness to learn, and overall neurologic and psychosocial state.

- Explain the procedure for chest tube placement, including the indication, procedure, and rationale ➺*Rationale:* Providing information decreases fear and anxiety.

- Explain the chest tube apparatus and drainage system and, if time permits, allow the family to view the drainage system ➺*Rationale:* Providing information decreases fear and anxiety.

- Discuss ways to decrease pain and anxiety during the procedure and explain the plan for pain assessment and treatment for the duration of the chest tube placement ➺*Rationale:* Decreasing anxiety about pain and adequate pain control can facilitate coughing, deep breathing, and chest physiotherapy.

- Explain that during the insertion the child may feel pressure at the insertion site ➤➤*Rationale:* Providing information helps prepare the child for events during the procedure, reducing anxiety.
- Explain how the child can assist with the procedure ➤➤*Rationale:* The child is provided with an opportunity to participate or assist with the procedure.
- Explain the importance of facilitating drainage by keeping the tubing free of kinks ➤➤*Rationale:* The explanation may assist in prevention of accumulation of intrapleural process.
- Encourage questions and answer questions as they arise ➤➤*Rationale:* Reinforcement of information is needed during periods of stress.

EQUIPMENT

- Emergency equipment, including manual ventilation bag, mask, and oxygen supply
- Cardiorespiratory monitor and pulse oximeter, as indicated
- Personal protective equipment as indicated, including sterile gloves, sterile gown, mask, and goggles

- Systemic pain medication and local 1% lidocaine
- 25-gauge 5/8-inch needle and syringe for lidocaine
- Closed chest drainage system
- Suction source
- Tubing and connectors
- Chest tube
- Chest tube insertion tray (if available)
- Syringe for administration of local anesthetic
- Chest tube equipment: chest tube, Kelly clamps (two), scalpel, needle holder, gauze, hemostats, and sterile gauze
- Pigtail catheter equipment: pigtail catheter, pigtail catheter kits, sterile three-way stopcock, needleless access device, No. 11 blade, 30-mL syringe if substituted for a chest tube
- Betadine or chlorhexidine if not included in the chest tube tray
- Sterile water
- Sterile towels
- Tape
- Sutures
- Suture scissors
- Dressing materials, including petroleum dressing, dry gauze, tape, and occlusive dressing

Procedure for Chest Tube Placement: Perform

Steps	Rationale	Considerations
1. Ensure child and family understand procedure and questions are answered. Acquire informed consent unless procedure is emergent.	Evaluates and reinforces understanding of previously taught information. In many situations, informed consent is required before chest tube insertion. Ensures medical-legal compliance as suggested by the Joint Commission of Accredited Healthcare Organization.	Developmental, cognitive, and anxiety levels determine approach and effectiveness of teaching. For emergencies refer to institution-specific protocol for assumption of consent.
2. Gather equipment and supplies. Ensure emergency equipment is present and in working order.	Preparation facilitates completion of procedure in a timely manner.	Availability of volume replacement and intubation equipment may be important if child becomes hypotensive or needs a secure airway. Consider child's allergies to adhesive tape.
3. Ensure adequate cardiorespiratory monitoring.	Children may decompensate during procedure.	Consider increasing volume on pulse oximeter or cardiac monitor to allow an auditory signal and visual monitoring during procedure.
4. Conduct final patient verification process (e.g., time out) per institution-specific protocol.	Confirms correct child, procedure, and site and prevents unnecessary medical procedures (JCAHO requirement).	

Procedure continues on following page

Procedure | **for Chest Tube Placement: Perform**—*Continued*

Steps	Rationale	Considerations
5. Ensure child is premedicated for procedure and that a plan for pain control is in place. *(Level VI*)*	Chest tube placement is a painful procedure.[10] Pain and anxiety control helps child maintain position.	Medication dose is dependent on child's weight and previous experience with pain and on other concurrent conditions.
6. Position child supine with affected side slightly rotated up. Place arm of affected side above child's head[3] (see Figure 33-5). *(Level II*)*	Arm may be immobilized with soft restraint during procedure, which allows arm to be out of procedure area and easier access to intercostal spaces and decreases chance to contaminant sterile site.	Sitting position is an alternative for those children who are unable to lay flat because of respiratory distress.
7. Wash hands and put on protective equipment, including sterile gloves.	Reduces transmission of micro-organisms. Protects personnel health.	Ensure that child does not have a latex allergy in decision on gloves and equipment.
8. Prepare supplies and equipment necessary to complete procedure: a. Attach needle holder to suture. b. Attach Kelly clamp or hemostat to distal end of chest tube if using large bore tube (Figure 38-1). c. Prepare lidocaine syringe. *(Level II*)*	Organization and preparation assist in procedure performance.	
9. Locate site to start subcutaneous tunnel. The sixth rib (generally two ribs below nipple) is used. Follow rib laterally to midaxillary line[5] (Figure 38-2).		Alternatively, second intercostal space at mid-clavicular line can be used (see Figure 38-2).

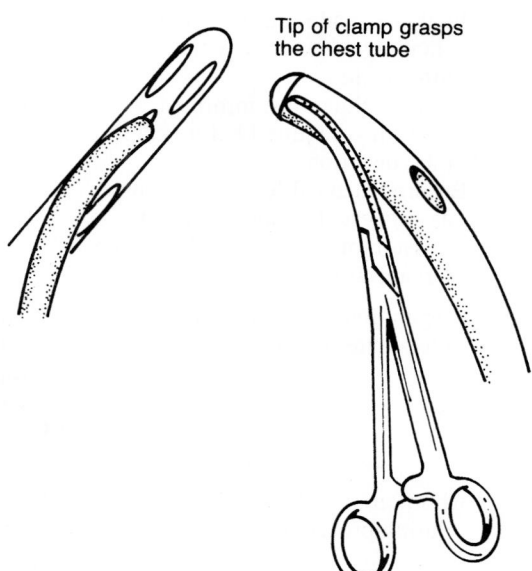

Tip of clamp grasps the chest tube

FIGURE 38-1   Tube is grasped with curved clamp, with tube tip protruding from jaws. *From Roberts JR, Hedges JR: Clinical procedures in emergency medicine, ed 4, Philadelphia, 2004, Saunders.*

* Level II: Theory-based; no research data to support recommendations; recommendations from expert consensus group may exist
  Level VI: Clinical studies in a variety of patient populations and situations to support recommendations

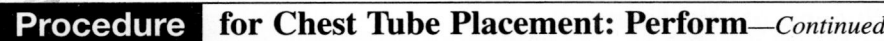

Procedure	**for Chest Tube Placement: Perform**—*Continued*	
Steps	**Rationale**	**Considerations**

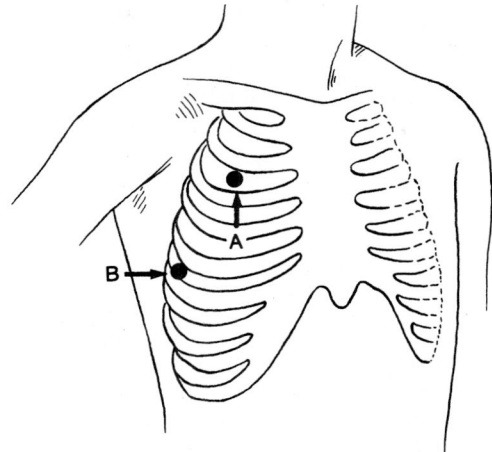

FIGURE 38-2 Standard Sites for Tube Thoracostomy. *A,* Fourth or fifth intercostal space, midaxillary line. *B,* Second intercostal space, midclavicular line. *Roberts JR, Hedges JR:* Clinical procedures in emergency medicine, *ed 4, Philadelphia, 2004, Saunders.*

10. Prepare site with antiseptic solution and drape area with sterile drape.	Removes microorganisms from skin, which reduces risk of infection.	Prepare site from clavicle to abdomen; axillary line to anterior chest.
11. Reidentify landmarks and insertion site.	Ensures proper placement of chest tube.	Skin incision is usually one rib below thoracic wall entry (sixth rib). The thoracic wall entry is at fourth or fifth intercostal space, midaxillary line (level of the nipple).[5]
12. Anesthetize skin at level of incision, subcutaneous tissue, muscle (in a track above the incision), and rib periosteum with local anesthetic (liberally using buffered 1% lidocaine without epinephrine; Figure 38-3). *(Level VI*)*	Chest tube insertion is painful.	Always aspirate during insertion to prevent lidocaine from being instilled into a blood vessel. Use local anesthetic generously.

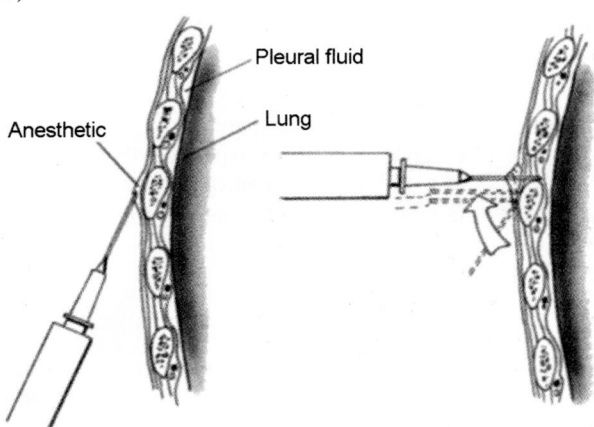

Pleural fluid

Lung

Anesthetic

FIGURE 38-3 Administration of Local Anesthetics. Begin with incision site and extend superiorly to pleural entry site. *Roberts JR, Hedges JR:* Clinical procedures in emergency medicine, *ed 4, Philadelphia, 2004, Saunders.*

Procedure continues on following page

* Level VI: Clinical studies in a variety of patient populations and situations to support recommendations

Procedure for Chest Tube Placement: Perform—*Continued*		
Steps	**Rationale**	**Considerations**

13. **Chest tube insertion**
    - Large bore tube
      - a. Make a 1-cm to 3-cm transverse skin incision into subcutaneous tissue directly over rib (Figure 38-4). *(Level II*)*

Allows for introduction of Kelly clamp and chest tube.

Incision must be large enough to admit a finger.
The incision is directed over the superior aspect of the rib to prevent neurovascular injury.

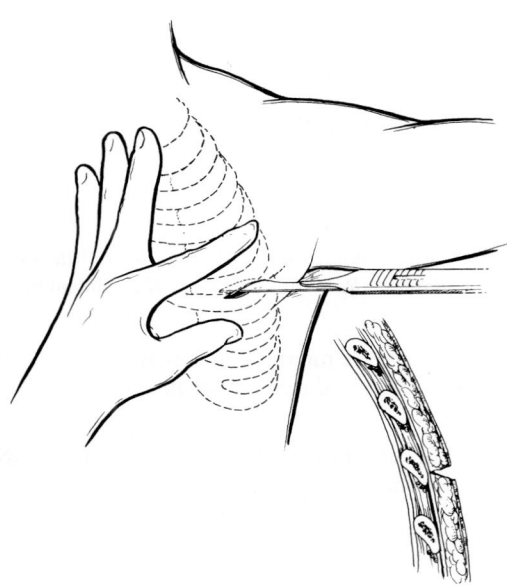

FIGURE 38-4   Transverse skin incision is made directly inferior of anesthetized rib down to subcutaneous tissue. *Dumire SM, Paris P:* Atlas of emergency procedures, *Philadelphia, 1994, Saunders.*

b. Place curved Kelly clamp into skin incision with the tips directed away from chest wall. Dissect a track one rib space above incision site (Figure 38-5, *A*). *(Level II*)*	Creates a tract to facilitate tube placement and prevent infection and air entry when chest tube is removed.[3,11]	Dissection is accomplished with use of the Kelly clamp in an open and spreading manner.
c. Turn closed Kelly clamp and aim toward superior aspect of rib (Figure 38-5, *B*) puncture through parietal pleura into pleural space cavity with tip of the Kelly clamp (Figure 38-5, *C*). *(Level II*)*	Ensure that pleural space is entered on superior aspect of rib to avoid injury to neurovascular bundle (nerve, artery, and vein).	Puncturing pleural space may require force because of resistance; although resistance decreases once pleura is entered. The child may have an increase in pain during this time until pleura is entered. Enter pleura cautiously, not more than 1 cm.[7]
d. Widen hole by opening and spreading Kelly clamp and insert a gloved finger to dilate track and hole in the pleura. Mark entry site with your gloved finger. *(Level II*)*	Ensure that hole is large enough for chest tube.	Caution should be used to avoid injury if a rib is fractured.

* Level II: Theory-based; no research data to support recommendations; recommendations from expert consensus group may exist

Procedure for Chest Tube Placement: Perform—*Continued*

Steps	Rationale	Considerations

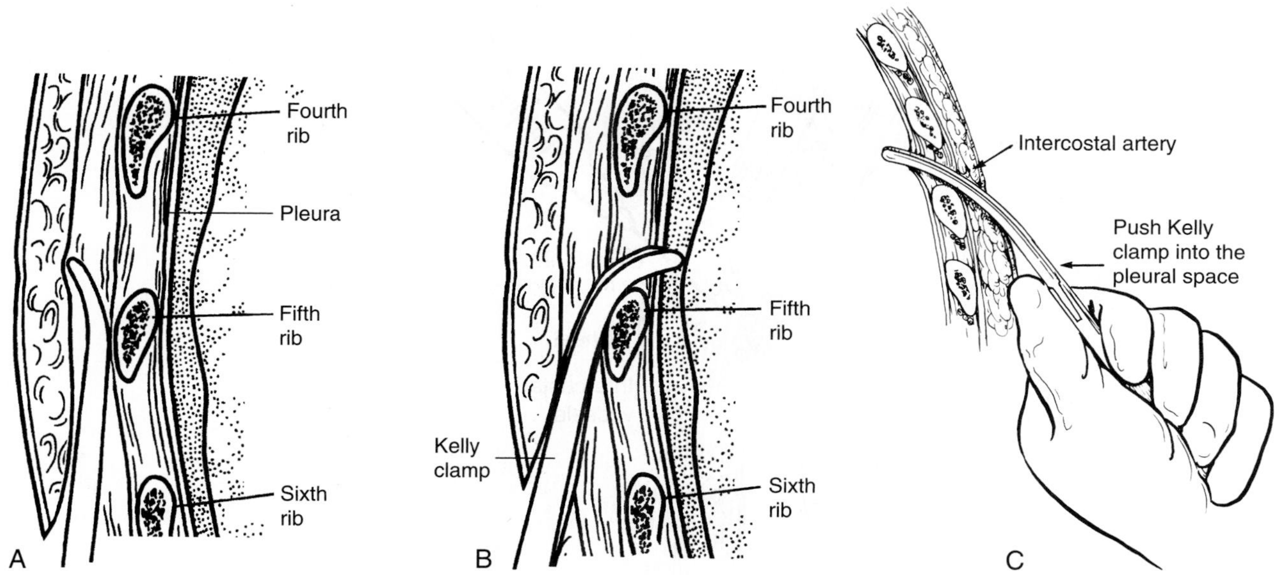

FIGURE 38-5 Dissection for Tube Thoracostomy. **A,** Introduce clamp with tip pointed away from pleura. **B,** Turn clamp and dissert through pleura at point above rib. **C,** Push closed clamp with steady pressure into pleura. *Dieckmann R, et al, editors:* Pediatric emergency and critical care procedures, *St. Louis, 1997, Mosby. Dumire SM, Paris P:* Atlas of emergency procedures, *Philadelphia, 1994, Saunders.*

Steps	Rationale	Considerations
e. With the attached Kelly clamp to the distal end of chest tube, insert the chest tube back into hole identified by gloved finger. Guide chest tube into pleural space. The chest tube is advanced until all holes are inside pleural space. *(Level II*)*	Assists with proper placement of the chest tube.	Air collects in nondependent areas (anterior), and fluid collects in dependent areas (posterior). To drain fluid, direct the chest tube posterior. To drain air, direct the tube anterior.[3,8]
Proceed to step 14.		
• **Pigtail catheter**		
a. Insert needle with a syringe attached. Aspirate while advancing needle toward the superior aspect of rib. When rib is encountered, "walk over" rib until pleural space is entered (Figure 38-6). *(Level II*)*	Application of negative pressure (aspirating) prevents a pneumo thorax and identifies whether a blood vessel has been entered. Intercostal vessels are located on the inferior surface of rib.	

Procedure continues on following page

* Level II: Theory-based; no research data to support recommendations; recommendations from expert consensus group may exist

AP This procedure should be performed only by physicians, advanced practice nurses, and other health care professionals (including critical care nurses) with additional knowledge, skills, and demonstrated competence per professional licensure or institutional standard.

Procedure **for Chest Tube Placement: Perform**—*Continued*

Steps	Rationale	Considerations

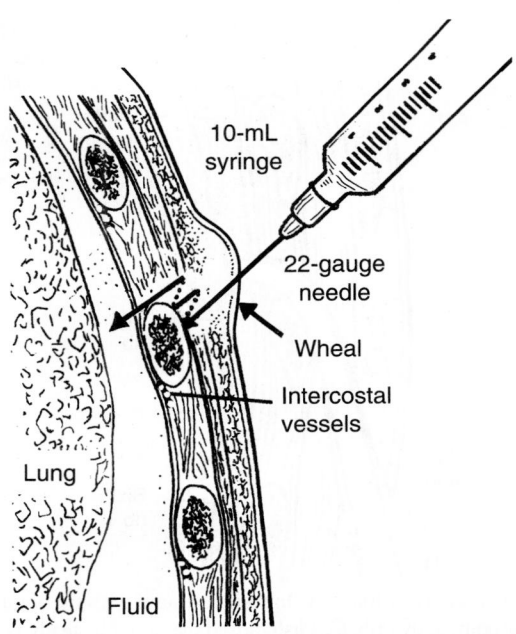

FIGURE 38-6   Needle is "walked" over rib into pleural space. *Dieckmann R, et al, editors:* Pediatric emergency and critical care procedures, *St. Louis, 1997, Mosby.*

b. Insert guide wire through needle into pleural space. Withdraw needle (Figure 38-7, *A* and *B*). *(Level I*)*

Use of Seldinger's technique.

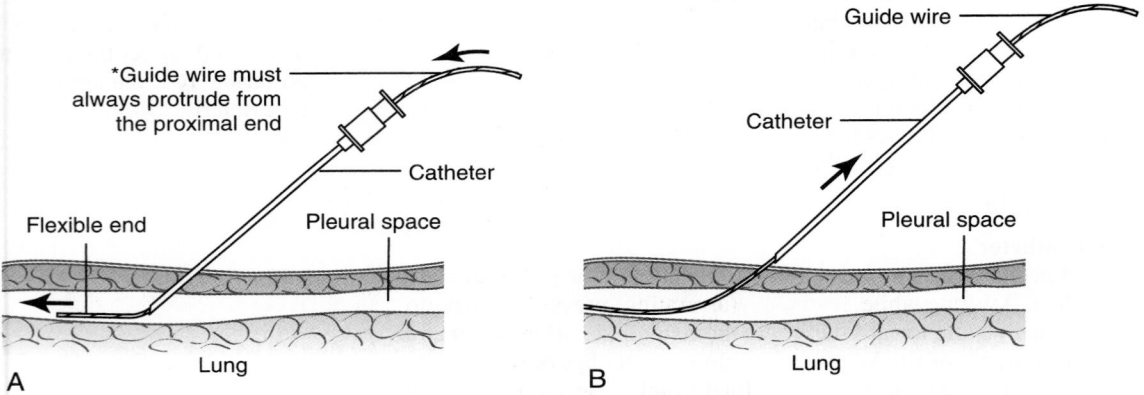

FIGURE 38-7   **A,** Guide wire is passed over rib into pleural space. **B,** Needle is withdrawn, leaving wire in pleural space.

c. With use of a blade, make a small incision and insert the dilator/introducer over the guide wire into the skin and subcutaneous tissue. Remove the dilator/introducer (Figure 38-7, *C*). *(Level I*)*

Ensure that the hole is large enough for the chest tube.

* Level I: Manufacturer's recommendations only

Procedure for Chest Tube Placement: Perform—*Continued*

Steps	Rationale	Considerations
d. Thread catheter over guide wire into pleural space. Advance to ensure that all holes are in pleural space (Figure 38-7, *D*). Remove guide wire (Figure 38-7, *E*). (*Level I**)	Use of Seldinger's technique.	A twisting motion can be helpful.
e. Apply three-way stopcock and attach syringe to remove contents in pleural space.	Allows for aspiration of fluid or instillation of fluid or medication.	

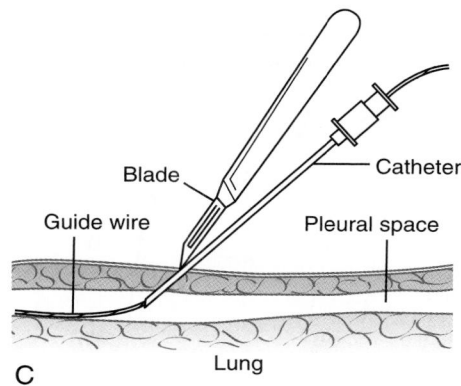

C

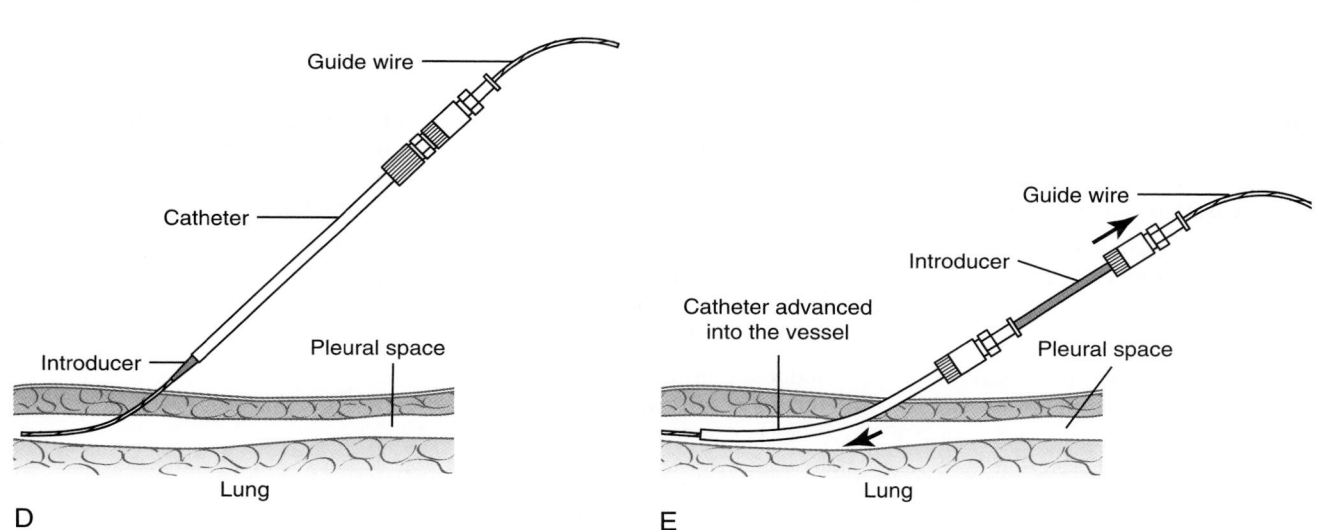

D   E

FIGURE 38-7, CONT'D **C,** Small incision is made in skin and dilator/introducer is inserted over guide wire. **D,** Catheter is threaded over guide wire into pleural space. **E,** Guide wire and introducer are removed. *From Roberts, R. Hedges J. (1998).* Clinical procedures in emergency medicine, *ed 3, Philadelphia, Saunders.*

Procedure continues on following page

* Level I: Manufacturer's recommendations only

Procedure | for Chest Tube Placement: Perform—*Continued*

Steps	Rationale	Considerations
14. Connect tube securely to pleural drainage system with suction (see Procedure 35).	Creates a closed system for evacuation of pleural contents (air, fluid, blood, or pus) and restores negative pressure.	Ensure that all connections between chest tube and pleural drainage system are secure.
15. Secure chest tube to the skin with sutures.[12] Wrap the free end of suture around the tube. Tie ends of the suture snugly around the top of tube (Figure 38-8). *(Level II*)*	Secures tube to prevent tube dislodgement.	The method of securing tube is dependent on the individual practitioner. A purse string suture permits the incision to be closed when chest tube is removed.

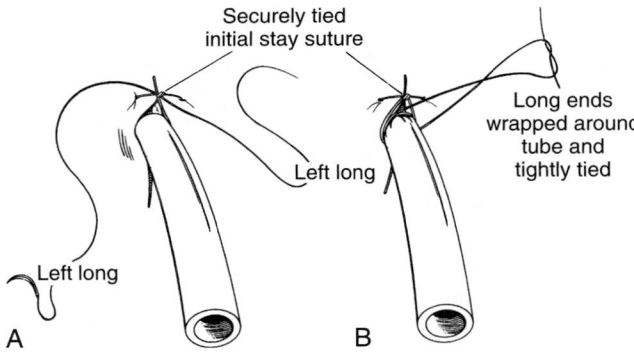

FIGURE 38-8   Stay Suture is Placed Next to Tube to Close Skin Incision. **A,** Knot is tied securely, and ends, which subsequently wrap around chest tube, are left long. **B,** Ends of suture are wound twice about tube and tied securely. *Roberts JR, Hedges JR:* Clinical procedures in emergency medicine, *ed 4, Philadelphia, 2004, Saunders.*

Steps	Rationale	Considerations
16. Apply occlusive petroleum dressing at the level of skin, cover with dry gauze, and secure with occlusive dressing or tape.[11] *(Level V*)*	Petroleum gauze prevents air from entering chest cavity.	In general, a petroleum dressing is usually not necessary to pigtail catheters because the wound at insertion point is small.
17. Obtain a chest x-ray and assess child after procedure.[6,11,12] *(Level VI*)*	Confirms location of chest tube and expansion of the lung. Evaluates level of sedation and impact of the procedure.	Breath sounds may not be immediately changed after insertion.
18. Dispose of equipment, remove needles and sharp objects, and wash hands.	Reduces transmission of microorganisms. Protects personnel health.	

* Level II: Theory-based; no research data to support recommendations; recommendations from expert consensus group may exist
Level V: Clinical studies in more than one or two patient populations and situations to support recommendations
Level VI: Clinical studies in a variety of patient populations and situations to support recommendations

Expected Outcomes	Unexpected Outcomes
• Equipment functions effectively	• Equipment or suction malfunction
• Negative pressure is restored	• Lung does not respond
• Reexpansion of the affected lung	• Continued signs and symptoms of inadequate oxygenation and ventilation
• Improved oxygenation and ventilation	• Laceration of the diaphragm, spleen, or liver
• Procedure completed without complications	• Pulmonary contusion
	• Improper placement of the chest tube
	• Hemothorax
	• Bleeding from puncture of the intercostals vessels
• Site remains infection free	• Infection
• Child has an acceptable level of comfort	• Unmanaged pain and anxiety

Monitoring and Care of the Child

Activities and Interventions	Rationale	Reportable Conditions
1. Monitor respiratory, cardio-vascular, and neurologic status before, during, and after the procedure.	Ongoing assessment is necessary for evaluation of the effectiveness of therapy. Changes in vital signs and physical examination results alert the caregiver to unexpected outcomes.	• Respiratory distress (grunting, tachypnea, retractions, dyspnea, agitation, and hypoxia) • Decreased to absent breath sounds • Subcutaneous emphysema • Tracheal shift to the unaffected side • Cardiovascular collapse • Anxiety, restlessness, or feeling of doom • Tachycardia • Hypotension • Chest pain
2. Obtain chest radiograph after completion of the procedure.	Confirms placement of the chest tube and drainage of the pleural space.	• Pneumothorax • Hemothorax • Enlarging pleural effusion • Improperly placed chest tube
3. Monitor the insertion site.	Any open wound is at risk for infection and bleeding. Air leak can occur from insertion site.	• Excessive bleeding or draining from the site • Signs of infection, including fever, tenderness, inflammation, and redness at the insertion site • Crepitus • Tube dislodgement
4. Evaluate chest tube drainage (amount, color, and consistency).	An increase in drainage may indicate increased bleeding and may necessitate transfusion. A decrease in drainage may indicate clotting of the chest tube.	• Continued excessive sanguineous bleeding • Change in character of the drainage • Abrupt cession of drainage
5. Assess the system for air leaks.	Air leak can indicate that the lung is not properly healing or that the system is not airtight.	• Persistent or new air leak
6. Assess pain status.	Evaluate pain management and sedation plan.	• Pain unrelieved with pain management plan • Pain interfering with interventions to expand lung

Documentation

- Date, time, and length of procedure
- Correct site, correct procedure, and correct person verification, including consent
- Indication for chest tube insertion
- Assessment findings before and after chest tube placement (breath sounds and signs of oxygenation and ventilation)
- Size of tube, location of insertion, and whether a "purse string" suture was used
- Amount, color, and consistency of drainage
- Local anesthetic or systemic anesthetic used and child's response
- Amount of negative pressure suction
- Chest radiograph ordered and results
- Site assessment and type of dressing used
- Comfort assessment and any specific interventions
- Additional interventions necessary
- Child and family education
- Unexpected outcomes and related treatment

References

1. Thibodeau G, Patton K: *Anatomy and physiology,* St. Louis, 2003, Mosby.
2. Fuhrman B, Zimmerman J, editors: *Pediatric critical care,* 3rd ed, Philadelphia, 2006, Elsevier.
3. Roberts JR, Hedges JR: *Clinical procedures in emergency medicine,* ed 4, Philadelphia, 2004, Saunders.
4. Lawrence D: Chest tube placement (perform), In Lynn-McHale DJ, Carlson K, editors: *AACN procedure manual for critical care,* ed 5, Philadelphia, 2005, Saunders.
5. Hazinski MF et al: *Pediatric advanced life support provider manual,* Dallas, 2002, American Heart Association.
6. Dull K, Fleisher G: Pigtail catheters versus large-bore chest tubes for pneumothoraces in children treated in the emergency department, *Pediat Emerg Care* 18(4):265-267, 2002.
7. Gunn V, Nechyba C: *The Harriet Lane handbook,* Philadelphia, 2002, Mosby.
8. Moloney-Harmon P, Czerwinski: *Nursing care of the pediatric trauma patient,* Philadelphia, 2003, Saunders.
9. Gaynard L, et al: *Psychosocial care of children in hospitals: a clinical practice manual,* Rockville, MD, 1998, Child Life Council.
10. Kaplan R, Yang C: Sedation and analgesia in pediatric patients for procedures outside the operating room, *Anesthesiol Clin North Am* 20:181-194, 2002.
11. Taeusch H, et al: *Pediatric and neonatal tests and procedures,* Philadelphia, 1996, Saunders.
12. Allibone L: Nursing management of chest drains, *Nurs Stand* 17(22):45-56, 2003.

Additional Readings

Dieckmann R, et al, editors: *Pediatric emergency and critical care procedures,* St. Louis, 1997, Mosby.
Roberts J, et al: Efficacy and complications of percutaneous pigtail catheters for thoracostomy in pediatric patients, *Chest* 114:1116-1121, 1998.

AP
Chest Tube Removal: Perform

PURPOSE: Chest tube removal from the pleural or mediastinal space is performed when the chest tube is no longer necessary or functioning

Deb Templin

PREREQUISITE KNOWLEDGE

- Child development as it relates to clinical assessment and the procedure
- Anatomy and physiology of the pediatric pulmonary system including mechanics of breathing[1,2]
- Understanding of the initial clinical indication for the placement of the child's chest tube
  - Chest tubes are placed in the pleural or mediastinal space to drain air, fluid (chylothorax, pus, transudate/exudate), or blood.[3]
  - Mediastinal chest tubes are usually placed in the operating room by the surgeon after cardiothoracic surgery
- Indications of readiness for chest tube removal.[4-9]
  - No air leak on the water seal for 24 hours (pneumothorax), assessed with observation of the water seal/air leak chamber for bubbling
  - Drainage of less than 1-2 mL/kg total pleural fluid drainage in 24 hours
  - Pneumothorax of less than 10% or completely resolved per chest x-ray results
  - Resolution of underlying process
  - Improved respiratory status
  - Lung reexpanded
  - Nonfunctional

- Depending on the child's condition and ventilatory requirement, chest tubes may need to remain in place despite the removal indications being met.
- Chest tubes sutured with a "purse sting" suture require two individuals for chest tube removal. One removes the drain, and the second promptly ties the purse string suture (Figure 39-1).
- Personnel and equipment need to be readily available for reinsertion of a new chest tube if it becomes necessary.
- Level IV data indicate that complications after chest tube removal are not affected by the use of maximal inspiration

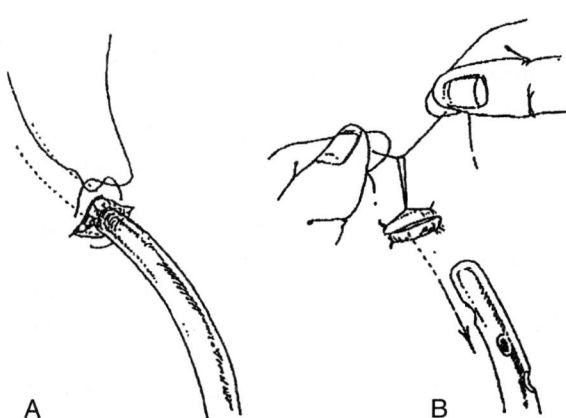

A   B

FIGURE 39-1 **A,** Removal of chest tube with purse-string suture. First throw of knot is mattress suture. **B,** Removal of chest tube and typing of purse-string suture. *Leonar S, Nikaidoh H: Thoracentesis and chest tube insertion. In Levin D, Morriss F, editors:* Essentials of pediatric intensive care, *St Louis, 1990, Quality Medical Publishing.*

versus expiration. Most studies use a maximal inspiration intervention in their procedures.[4,5,10]

- Mediastinal chest tubes placed after cardiothoracic surgery are often removed 24 to 36 hours after surgery when the drainage has become minimal and progressed to serous from sanguineous.
- Chest tubes can be safely removed without a water seal trial after thoracic surgery, which allows for earlier chest tube removal, decreased pain, and decreased hospital cost.[11]
- Chest tube removal is a painful procedure.
- Pharmacologic (mechanism of action, dosing, side effects, and contraindications) knowledge about systemic or local anesthetics used for procedural analgesia during chest tube removal[12,13]
- Removal of the chest tube is done swiftly to prevent introduction of air into the pleural space.

CHILD AND FAMILY ASSESSMENT

- Child's developmental level and ability to interact ➤➤*Rationale:* Influences preparation and interaction.
- Child's and family's understanding of the reasons for and risks and benefits of removal of the chest tube ➤➤*Rationale:* Evaluates the child's and family's understanding of the procedure and provides a gauge for ongoing education.
- Desire of family members to be present during the procedure ➤➤*Rationale:* The presence of family may provide comfort and support, although family members should have the choice not to remain with the child.
- Thorough cardiopulmonary assessment, including vital signs, visual inspection of breathing patterns and chest wall movement, auscultation of lung fields, and signs of oxygenation and ventilation ➤➤*Rationale:* Child's readiness for chest tube removal is ensured, and comparison for postremoval assessment is provided.
- History of bleeding disorders or anticoagulants or antiplatelet therapy ➤➤*Rationale:* Disorders or therapies may increase the risk of complications (i.e., bleeding).
- Assess presence of air leak (bubbling in the water chamber) and amount and appearance of drainage ➤➤*Rationale:* Assesses child's readiness for chest tube removal.
- Review of last chest x-ray results ➤➤*Rationale:* Radiologic evidence of resolution of pneumothorax, effusion, or hemothorax.
- History of reactions or allergies to medication (tape, anesthetics, or sedatives) ➤➤*Rationale:* Prevents harm.
- History of problems with anesthetics or sedated procedures ➤➤*Rationale:* Determines appropriate anesthetics or sedative.
- Assess skin integrity at the insertion site ➤➤*Rationale:* Assesses for signs of infection or inflammation.

CHILD AND FAMILY EDUCATION

Individualized, developmentally appropriate education is provided to the family and to the child based on desire for knowledge, readiness to learn, and overall neurologic and psychosocial state.

- Explain the procedure for chest tube removal, including the indication, procedure, and rationale ➤➤*Rationale:* Providing information increases knowledge, and preparation helps reduce anxiety, which increases the child's ability to cooperate during the procedure. Information increases parental satisfaction.
- Discuss ways to decrease pain and anxiety during the procedure ➤➤*Rationale:* Pain and anxiety control help the child maintain position.
- Explain that during the removal of the chest tube the child may feel pain or discomfort ➤➤*Rationale:* Specific information helps prepare the child for events during the procedure and reduces anxiety.
- Explain how the child can assist with the procedure ➤➤*Rationale:* The child is provided with an opportunity to participate or assist with the procedure, and introduction of air into the pleural space may be limited.
- Review plan for lung expansion techniques after chest tube removal, including ambulation, frequent position change, cough, deep breathing, and incentive spirometry ➤➤*Rationale:* Decreased risk of further pneumothorax by increased lung expansion and the removal of secretions. Information increases knowledge and provides opportunity for the child to participate in the interventions that are part of the recovery process.
- Review signs of fluid and air accumulation, including shortness of breath, chest pain, and dyspnea and instruct the child and family to report these symptoms immediately ➤➤*Rationale:* Prompt recognition of signs of reaccumulation and respiratory distress facilitates early intervention.
- Review the plan for pain control after removal, including pain scale, use of medications, and implications of splinting of the affected side ➤➤*Rationale:* Pain control facilitates mobility, deep breathing and coughing, positioning, and recovery.
- Encourage questions and answer questions as they arise ➤➤*Rationale:* Reinforcement of information is needed during periods of stress.

EQUIPMENT

- Personal protective equipment as indicated, including gloves, gown, mask, and goggles
- Cardiorespiratory monitor and pulse oximeter, as indicated
- Emergency equipment, including manual ventilation bag, mask, and oxygen source
- Clamps, as indicated
- Additional 4×4 gauze
- Suture removal kit (scissors, tweezers)
- Pain medication
- Dressing (petroleum gauze and occlusive dressing)
- Absorbent pad
- Sterile specimen collection cup, as indicated

Procedure   for Chest Tube Removal: Perform

Steps	Rationale	Considerations
1. Ensure child and family understand procedure and questions are answered.	Reinforces understanding of previously taught information.	Developmental, cognitive, and anxiety levels determine approach and effectiveness of teaching. Chest tube removal is a painful procedure.[14]
2. Gather all necessary equipment and supplies, and ensure that emergency equipment is present and in working order.	Preparation facilitates completion of the procedure in a timely manner.	
3. Ensure adequate cardiopulmonary monitoring.	Children may decompensate during procedure.	
4. Prescribe systemic anesthetics or sedative medication as indicated.[12,13] *(Level VI*)*	Removal of chest tubes is a painful procedure. Pain and anxiety control help child maintain position.	
5. Wash hands and put on clean gloves and protective equipment.	Reduces transmission of microorganisms. Protects personnel health.	
6. Conduct final patient verification process (e.g., "Time Out") per institution-specific protocol)	Confirms correct patient, procedure, and site and prevents unnecessary medical procedures (JCAHO requirement).	
7. Position child to permit easy access to chest tube with an absorbent pad underneath.	Ensures accessibility to insertion site.	When child has more than one chest tube, be sure that each chest tube is labeled correctly and that the proper chest tube is removed.
8. Prepare supplies and equipment necessary to complete the procedure. Open the sterile removal kit. Prepare petroleum gauze.	This is not a sterile procedure, although aseptic technique is necessary to prevent infection. Petroleum gauze must be ready immediately on removal of chest tube to decrease introduction of air into pleural space.	Petroleum gauze is used in removal of a large-bore chest tube. Ensure that other chest tubes connected with a Y connector to the chest tube being removed are separated before removal. *(Level III*)*
9. Discontinue suction to drainage system. *(Level II*)*	Prevents tissue aspiration into the chest tube during the removal process.	
10. Remove dressing covering the chest tube entry site.	Allows access to the chest tube.	
11. Remove the suture that secures the chest tube to the skin. If a purse string suture is present, ensure that a loose throw is found in it. *(Level II*)*	Frees the chest tube from the skin. The purse string suture should be ready to tie.	
12. Instruct child to take a deep breath and hold or exhale and hold.[4,5,7,15] *(Level V*)*	Creates positive pressure in the pleural space and helps to limit the introduction of air into the pleural space.	Removal of chest tube at the end of inspiration or at the end of expiration results in a similar incident rate of recurrent pneumothoraces.[4,5,9,15]

Procedure continues on following page

* Level II: Theory-based; no research data to support recommendations; recommendations from expert consensus group may exist
  Level III: Laboratory data; no clinical data to support recommendations
  Level V: Clinical studies in more than one or two patient populations and situations to support recommendations
  Level VI: Clinical studies in a variety of patient populations and situations to support recommendations

Procedure   for Chest Tube Removal: Perform—*Continued*

Steps	Rationale	Considerations
		If child has mechanical ventilation, the chest tubes are typically removed at the end of the inspiratory phase of the mandatory breath.[4,8] *(Level III*)*
13. Remove chest tube quickly at end of inspiration or at the end of expiration. *(Level V*)*	Prevents air from entering pleural space.	If chest tube is removed during inspiration, air enters the pleural space. An assistant is helpful with removal of the chest tube or placement of the dressing over the site. Ensure that entire chest tube is removed.
14. Immediately place folded gauze over the chest tube entry site. *(Level II*)*	Prevents air from entering the pleural space.	If a purse string suture is present, hold the sutures during chest tube removal.
15. Tie down the purse string suture if present. *(Level II*)*	Closes chest tube entry site.	Tissue necrosis can occur if sutures are pulled too tightly.
16. Apply occlusive dressing to the chest tube entry site. *(Level II*)*	Prevents air from entering pleural space.	Use petroleum gauze over chest tube site if no purse string suture is present or with a large-bore chest tube.
17. Dispose of equipment, remove needles, sharp objects, and wash hands.	Reduces transmission of microorganisms. Protects personnel health.	
18. Evaluate cardiorespiratory status and obtain chest radiograph if indicated.[18,19] *(Level V*)*	Evaluates expansion of lung. Clinical symptoms identify child with pneumothoraces.[18,19]	

* Level II: Theory-based; no research data to support recommendations; recommendations from expert consensus group may exist
  Level III: Laboratory data; no clinical data to support recommendations
  Level V: Clinical studies in more than one or two patient populations and situations to support recommendations

Expected Outcomes

- Child has adequate oxygenation and ventilation

- No reaccumulation of fluid or air in the pleural or mediastinal space
- Thoracostomy site is infection free
- Secure exit wound with minimal drainage

- Adequate pain control during procedure

Unexpected Outcomes

- Respiratory decompensation during or after procedure
- Reaccumulation of fluid or air in the pleural or mediastinal space
- Site infection
- Air leak
- Excessive bleeding or drainage from site
- Unmanaged pain and anxiety

Monitoring and Care of the Child

Activities and Interventions	Rationale	Reportable Conditions
1. Monitor respiratory, cardiovascular, and neurologic status before, during, and after procedure.	Ongoing assessment is necessary for evaluation of effectiveness of therapy. Changes in vital signs and physical assessment alert the caregiver to unexpected outcomes.	• Respiratory distress (grunting, tachypnea, retractions, dyspnea, agitation, and hypoxia) • Decreased to absent breath sounds • Subcutaneous emphysema • Tracheal shift to the unaffected side • Cardiovascular collapse • Anxiety, restlessness, or feeling of doom • Tachycardia • Hypotension • Chest pain

Monitoring and Care of the Child—Cont'd

Activities and Interventions	Rationale	Reportable Conditions
2. Assess pain during and after chest tube removal.	Unmanaged pain can interfere with deep breathing and full lung expansion.	• Pain unrelieved with pain management plan • Pain interfering with interventions to expand lung
3. Obtain and review chest radiograph results.	Postprocedural follow up. Air could be introduced accidentally during the procedure.	• Pneumothorax • Reaccumulation of fluid, blood, pus, or chyle
4. Assess chest tube insertion site for signs and symptoms of infection.	Increased risk of infection with invasive tubes. Prolonged chest tube placement increases the risk for infection.	• Fever • Site redness or warmth • Site tenderness • Purulent drainage
5. Assess chest tube insertion site for air leak, bleeding, or drainage.	Air can leak from insertion site. Continual bleeding could indicate vessel injury. Chest tube may have tamponaded the internal artery or vein.	• Excessive persistent bleeding not controlled with direct pressure
6. If "purse string" suture is used, assess site for necrosis.	A tightly pulled suture may restrict blood flow to the site.	• Dark, purple, or dusky skin at the site

Documentation

- Date, time, length of procedure, and use of purse strings
- Child's response to procedure
- Assessment findings before and after chest tube removal (breath sounds and signs of oxygenation and ventilation)
- Results of follow-up chest radiograph, if applicable
- Systemic anesthetic used and child's response
- Assessment of site and presence of bleeding
- Comfort assessment and any specific interventions
- Additional interventions necessary before, during, and after chest tube removal
- Child and family education
- Unexpected outcomes and related treatments

References

1. Thibodeau G, Patton K: *Anatomy and physiology,* St. Louis, 2003, Mosby.
2. Fuhrman B, Zimmerman J: *Pediatric critical care,* 3rd ed., 2006, Philadelphia, Elsevier.
3. Allibone L: Nursing management of chest drains, *Nurs Stand* 17(22):45-56, 2003.
4. Bell R, et al: Chest tube removal: end-inspiratory or end-expiratory? *J Trauma* 50(4):674-677, 2001.
5. Adrales G, et al: A thoracostomy tube guideline improves management efficiency in trauma patients, *J Trauma* 52(2):210-216, 2002.
6. Marshall M, et al: Suction vs water seal after pulmonary resection: a randomized prospective study, *CHEST* 121(3):831-835, 2002.
7. Pacanowski JP, et al: Is routine roentgenography needed after closed tube thoracostomy removal? *J Trauma* 48(4):684-688, 2000.
8. Pizano L, et al: When should a chest radiograph be obtained after chest tube removal in mechanically ventilated patients? a prospective study, *J Trauma* 53(6):1073-1077, 2002.
9. Kirkwood P: Chest tube removal: Perform. In Lynn-McCale Wiegand DJ, Carlson K, editors: *AACN procedure manual for critical care,* ed 5, 2005, Philadelphia, Saunders.
10. Martino K, et al: Prospective randomized trial of thoracostomy removal algorithms, *J Trauma* 46(3):369-373, 1999.
11. Waldhausen J, et al: Removal of chest tubes in children without water seal after elective thoracic procedures: a randomized prospective study, *J Am College Surg* 194(4):411-415, 2002.
12. Rosen D, et al: Analgesia for pediatric thoracostomy tube removal, *Anesthesia Analgesia* 90(5):1025-1028, 2000.
13. Kaplan R, Yang C: Sedation and analgesia in pediatric patients for procedures outside the operating room, *Anesthesiol Clin North Am* 20:181-194, 2002.
14. Gaynard L, et al: *Psychosocial care of children in hospitals: a clinical practice manual,* Rockville, MD, 1998, Child Life Council.

15. Baumann M: What drainage system is ideal? And what other chest tube management questions, *Curr Opin Pulmon Med* 9(4): 276-281, 2003.

16. Valenzuela R, Rosen D: Topical lidocaine-prilocaine cream (EMLA) for thoracostomy tube removal, *Anesthesia Analgesia* 88(5):1107-1108, 1999.

17. Baumann MH: Management of spontaneous pneumothorax: an American college of chest physicians delphi consensus statement, *CHEST* 119(2):590-602, 2001.

18. McCormick J: The use of routine chest X-ray films after chest tube removal in postoperative cardiac patients, *Ann Thoracic Surg* 74(6):2161-2164, 2002.

19. Pacharn P, et al: Are chest radiographs routinely necessary following thoracostomy tube removal? *Pediatr Radiol* 32(2):138-142, 2002.

Additional Reading

Stephens BK, et al: Techniques to comfort children during stressful procedures, *Adv Mind-Body Med* 15(1):49-60, 1999.

AP
Needle Thoracostomy: Perform

PURPOSE: Needle thoracostomy is used to decompress a tension pneumothorax and is a temporary intervention that is followed by placement of a thoracostomy tube

Deb Templin

PREREQUISITE KNOWLEDGE

- Child development as it relates to clinical assessment and the procedure
- Anatomy and physiology of the pediatric pulmonary system[1,2]
- A needle thoracostomy is performed in children with a tension pneumothorax. With a needle placed in the pleural space for removal of air, tension is relieved and the mediastinal structures shift back toward center.
- A tension pneumothorax occurs when air enters the pleural space (during inspiration) and is unable to escape (during exhalation). The air trapped in the pleural space accumulates during each breath, increasing intrapleural pressure and causing the lung to collapse. In addition, the accumulated air causes the mediastinum structures to shift toward the unaffected lung, which results in reduced venous return and ultimately decreases cardiac output.[3,4] A tension pneumothorax is a medical emergency, and treatment is immediate needle compression (Figure 40-1).
- Signs of tension pneumothorax include grunting, tachypnea, retractions, dyspnea, agitation, hypoxia, decreased to absent breath sounds on the affected side, tympany to percussion, tracheal shift to the unaffected side, subcutaneous emphysema, muffled heart sounds, and neck vein distention.[3,5]

- Knowledge of the mechanism of action, dosing, side effects, and contraindications for anesthetics or sedatives used for procedural sedation[6]

CHILD AND FAMILY ASSESSMENT

- Child's developmental level and ability to interact **➤➤Rationale:** Influences preparation and interaction.
- Child's and family's understanding of the reasons for and risks and benefits of the procedure **➤➤Rationale:** Evaluates child's and family's understanding of the procedure and provides a gauge for ongoing education.
- Desire of family members to be present during the procedure **➤➤Rationale:** The presence of family may provide comfort and support, although family members should have the choice not to remain with the child.
- Cardiopulmonary assessment, including vital signs, visual inspection of breathing patterns and chest wall movement, auscultation of lung fields, and signs of inadequate oxygenation and ventilation, such as decreased arterial oxygen saturation, increased work of breathing, supplemental oxygen requirement, cyanosis, changes in heart rate and blood pressure, anxiety, and agitation **➤➤Rationale:** Evaluating cardiopulmonary status provides valuable information in determining the child's need for and ability to tolerate the procedure and influences the type of anesthetics or sedative prescribed.
- History of reactions or allergies to medication (betadine, lidocaine, anesthetics, or sedatives) and tape **➤➤Rationale:** Prevents harm.

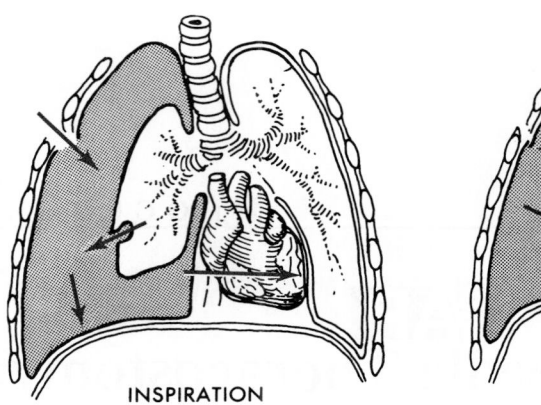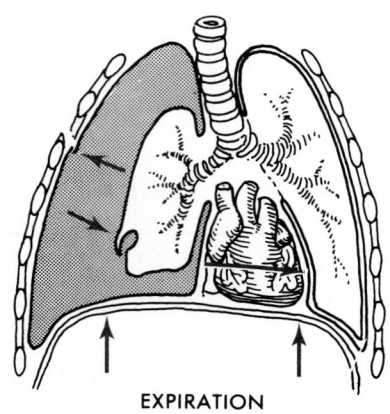

INSPIRATION   EXPIRATION

FIGURE 40-1   Tension Pneumothorax. Right pneumothorax under tension, total collapse of right lung, and shift of mediastinal structures to left are seen. *Marx J, et al:* Rosen's emergency medicine: concepts and clinical practice, *ed 5, St. Louis, 2002, Mosby.*

- History of bleeding disorders or anticoagulant or antiplatelet therapy ➦*Rationale:* Disorders or therapies may increase the risk of complications (i.e., bleeding).
- Previous experience or reaction to an invasive procedure ➦*Rationale:* Child's previous experience may effect how this event is perceived.
- Assessment of skin integrity at the insertion site ➦*Rationale:* Avoidance of active skin lesions or infection at insertion site.

CHILD AND FAMILY EDUCATION

Individualized developmentally appropriate education is provided to the family and to the child based on desire for knowledge, readiness to learn, and overall neurologic and psychosocial state.

- Explain the procedure and the reason for needle thoracentesis, including risks and benefits ➦*Rationale:* Providing information increases knowledge, and preparation helps reduce anxiety, which increases the child's ability to cooperate during the procedure. Information increases parental satisfaction.
- Discuss ways to decrease pain and anxiety during the procedure ➦*Rationale:* Pain and anxiety control help the child maintain position.
- Explain that during the insertion of the needle the child may feel pressure at the insertion site ➦*Rationale:*

Providing specific information helps prepare the child for events during the procedure, reducing anxiety.
- Explain how the child can assist with the procedure ➦*Rationale:* The child is provided with an opportunity to participate or assist with the procedure.
- Encourage questions and answer questions as they arise ➦*Rationale:* Reinforcement of information is needed during periods of stress.

EQUIPMENT

- Cardiorespiratory monitor or pulse oximeter as indicated
- Emergency equipment, including manual ventilation bag, mask, and oxygen supply
- Personal protective equipment as indicated, including sterile gloves, sterile gown, mask, and goggles
- Sterile drapes/towels
- Antiseptic solution (chloraprep/betadine)
- Sterile gauze
- Local anesthetic (1% lidocaine) if condition allows
- 25-gauge 5/8-inch needle
- 3-mL syringe (for local)
- 18-gauge to 20-gauge over-the-needle catheter or needle[3]
- Sterile 10-mL or 20-mL syringe
- Sterile three-way stopcock
- Band-Aid or adhesive dressing

Procedure | for Needle Thoracostomy: Perform

Steps	Rationale	Considerations
1. Ensure child and family understand procedure and reason for the thoracostomy, including risks and benefits. Obtain informed consent, if applicable.	Evaluates and reinforces understanding of previously taught information. In many situations, informed consent is required before needle thoracostomy. Informed consent is a process in which child and family acknowledge their understanding of indications for procedure, the procedure itself, and its risks.	Developmental, cognitive, and anxiety levels determine approach and effectiveness of teaching.[7]
2. Administer oxygen and ventilate as indicated.	Treats hypoxia and hypercapnia.	
3. Gather all supplies and equipment necessary to complete the procedure.	Organization and preparation assist in procedure performance.	
4. Wash hands.	Reduces transmission of microorganisms. Protects personnel health.	
5. Conduct final patient verification process (e.g., time out) per institution-specific protocol	Confirms correct patient, procedure, and site and prevents unnecessary medical procedures (JCAHO requirement).	
6. Ensure adequate cardiorespiratory monitoring.	Children may decompensate during procedure.	Consider whether child has a secure airway or is becoming hypotensive. The availability of volume replacement and intubation equipment may be important. Consider increasing volume on pulse oximeter or cardiac monitor to allow an auditory signal and visual monitoring during procedure.
7. If child is responsive, prescribe systemic anesthetics or sedative medication as indicated.[6] *(Level VI*)*	Pain and anxiety control help the child maintain position.	
8. Position child supine. Place arm of the affected side above child's head[5] (see Figure 33-6). *(Level II*)*	Air rises to the apex. Arm is immobilized during procedure, which allows the arm to be out of procedure area and easier access to the intercostal spaces and decreases the chance to contaminate sterile site.	
9. Put on gloves and protective equipment.	Reduces transmission of microorganisms. Protects personnel health.	
10. Locate second intercostal space at midclavicular line on the side of the suspected pneumothorax (see Figure 38-2).		Alternative is the fifth intercostal space in the anterior auxiliary line.[5]

Procedure continues on following page

* Level II: Theory-based; no research data to support recommendations; recommendations from expert consensus group may exist
  Level VI: Clinical studies in a variety of patient populations and situations to support recommendations

AP This procedure should be performed only by physicians, advanced practice nurses, and other health care professionals (including critical care nurses) with additional knowledge, skills, and demonstrated competence per professional licensure or institutional standard.

Procedure for Needle Thoracostomy: Perform—*Continued*

Steps	Rationale	Considerations
11. Prepare chest at the level of second intercostal space, midclavicular line on affected side, with antiseptic solution and drape.	Removes microorganisms from skin, reducing the risk of infection. Identifies landmark for needle thoracostomy.	Prepare alternative site if used.
12. If child is responsive, anesthetize the skin and rib periosteum (see Figure 38-3). *(Level II*)*	Anesthetizes area that can cause pain when needle is inserted.	Done only if time and conditions permit. Always aspirate during insertion to prevent instillation of lidocaine into a blood vessel.
13. Reidentify intercostal space.	Identifies landmark for needle thoracostomy.	
14. Insert over-the-needle catheter or needle with syringe attached through the skin and onto the rib. Once the rib is encountered, "walk over" superior aspect of inferior rib, with continued negative pressure/aspiration until pleural space is entered (Figure 40-2). *(Level II*)*	Intercostal vessels are located on inferior surface of rib.	Often when pleural space has been entered, a "pop" or a rush of air occurs. An immediate improvement should be seen in respiratory and cardiac status.

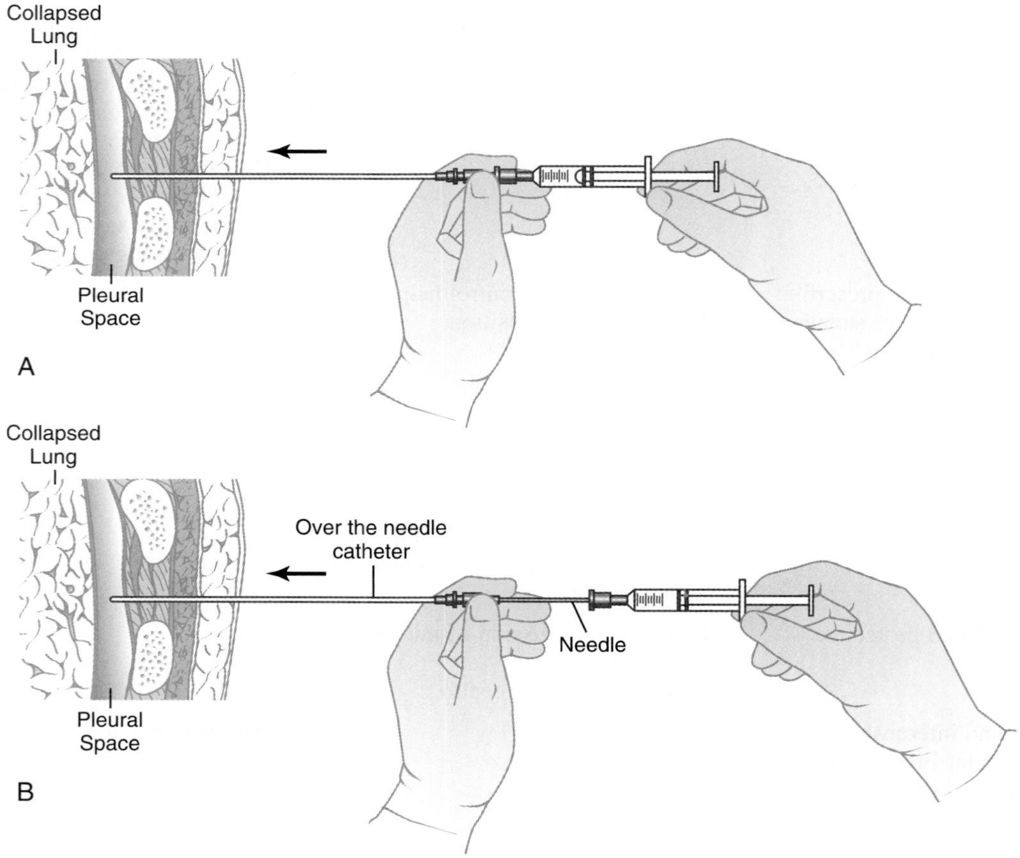

FIGURE 40-2   Needle Placement for Needle Thoracostomy. **A,** Advance needle into pleural space during aspiration of air. **B,** With over-the-needle catheter, thread it over needle into pleural space and remove needle. *From Roberts J, Hedges J:* Clinical procedures in emergency medicine, *ed 4, Philadelphia, 2004, Saunders.*

* Level II: Theory-based; no research data to support recommendations; recommendations from expert consensus group may exist

Procedure	**for Needle Thoracostomy: Perform**—*Continued*	
Steps	**Rationale**	**Considerations**
15. Aspirate all air that is present.	Reduces tension pneumothorax to a pneumothorax.	If an over-the-needle catheter is used, the needle/stylette is removed and then air is aspirated. The catheter can be left in place until chest tube is placed.
16. When air is evacuated and etiology resolved, remove needle and place dressing as indicated.	Air is evacuated so needle is no longer necessary.	Definitive treatment of a tension pneumothorax is to place a chest tube after emergency needle decompression.
17. Dispose of equipment in appropriate biohazard container and wash hands.	Reduces transmission of micro-organisms. Protects personnel health.	

Expected Outcomes

- Negative pressure is restored
- Reexpansion of affected lung
- Improved oxygenation and ventilation
- Reduction of tension pneumothorax to a simple pneumothorax
- Complication-free procedure

- Child remains infection free

- Child has an acceptable level of comfort

Unexpected Outcomes

- Lung does not respond
- Continued signs and symptoms of inadequate oxygenation and ventilation

- Laceration of diaphragm, spleen, or liver
- Pulmonary contusion
- Iatrogenic pneumothorax
- Hemothorax
- Bleeding from puncture of intercostal vessels
- Pleural infection
- Site infection
- Unmanaged pain and anxiety

Monitoring and Care of the Child

Activities and Interventions	**Rationale**	**Reportable Conditions**
1. Monitor respiratory, cardiovascular, and neurologic status before, during, and after needle thoracostomy.	Provides baseline assessment. Changes in vital signs and physical examination results alert the caregiver to unexpected outcomes. Permits recognition of a new pneumothorax or reaccumulation of tension pneumothorax before chest tube can be placed.	• Respiratory distress (grunting, tachypnea, retractions, dyspnea, agitation, and hypoxia) • Decreased to absent breath sounds • Subcutaneous emphysema • Tracheal shift to the unaffected side • Cardiovascular collapse • Anxiety, restlessness, or feeling of doom • Tachycardia • Hypotension • Chest pain
2. Obtain chest radiograph after completion of procedure.	Confirms evacuation of fluid/air.	• Pneumothorax, hemothorax • Other deleterious findings
3. Assess pain status during and after needle thoracostomy.	Evaluate pain management strategy.	• Pain unrelieved with pain management plan • Pain that interferes with interventions to expand lung
4. Monitor insertion site.	Any wound risks infection and bleeding.	• Excessive bleeding and drainage from site

Documentation

- Description of procedure, including date, time, and length of procedure (include needle size and amount of air/fluid aspirated)
- Correct site, correct procedure, and correct person verification
- Indications for procedure
- Assessment findings before and after procedure (breath sounds and signs of oxygenation and ventilation)
- Local anesthetic or systemic anesthetic used, if applicable, and child's response
- Site assessment and type of dressing used
- Results of follow-up chest radiograph
- Comfort assessment and any specific interventions
- Additional interventions necessary
- Child and family education
- Unexpected outcomes and related treatment

References

1. Thibodeau G, Patton K: *Anatomy and physiology,* St. Louis, 2003, Mosby.
2. Fuhrman B, Zimmerman J, editors: *Pediatric critical care,* ed 3, Philadelphia, 2006, Elsevier.
3. Roberts JR, Hedges JR: *Clinical procedures in emergency medicine,* ed 4, Philadelphia, 2004, Saunders.
4. Goodrich C: Needle thoracostomy (perform). In Lynn-McHale Wiegand DJ, Carlson K, editors: *AACN procedure manual for critical care,* ed 5, Philadelphia, 2005, Elsevier.
5. Hazinski, MF et al: *Pediatric life support provider manual,* Dallas, 2002, American Heart Association.
6. Kaplan R, Yang C: Sedation and analgesia in pediatric patients for procedures outside the operating room, *Anesthesiol Clin North Am* 20:181-194, 2002.
7. Gaynard L, et al: *Psychosocial care of children in hospitals: a clinical practice manual,* Rockville, MD, 1998, Child Life Council.

Additional Reading

Dieckmann R, et al, editors: *Pediatric emergency and critical care procedures,* St. Louis, 1997, Mosby.

AP
Thoracentesis: Perform

P U R P O S E : Thoracentesis is performed to drain pleural fluid for diagnostic or therapeutic purposes or to evacuate a tension pneumothorax

Deb Templin

PREREQUISITE KNOWLEDGE

- Child development as it relates to clinical assessment and the procedure
- Anatomy and physiology of the pediatric pulmonary system[1,2]
- The primary indication for a thoracentesis is pleural effusion (see Figure 33-3). Other indications include tension pneumothorax (see Figure 33-5) hemothorax (see Figure 33-4), and empyema.[3]
- Thoracentesis is typically an elective procedure and is used as a diagnostic tool to obtain pleural fluid. A therapeutic thoracentesis is also done to relieve symptoms caused by a pleural effusion.[4]
- A pleural effusion can either be an exudate or a transudate. Exudates are usually cloudy or contain pus and result from pleural inflammation or an irregularity in lymphatic flow. The fluid of a transudate is typically serous and light yellow and forms because of factors that affect the rate of formation or reabsorption of pleural fluid (Table 41-1).[5,6]
- Signs and symptoms of a pleural effusion include dull percussion on the affected side, absence or decrease in breath sounds, dyspnea, increased work of breathing and tactile fremitus.[5] Small pleural effusions can be asymptomatic.

TABLE 41-1	Evaluation of Exudate and Transudate Pleural Fluid	
Measurement	**Exudate**	**Transudate**
pH	<7.3	>7.4
Protein (g/dL)	<3.0	> 3.0
Fluid:serum ratio	>0.5	<0.5
LDH (IU)	>200 (2/3 serum level)	<200 (2/3 serum level)
Pleural fluid:serum: LDH ratio	>0.6	<0.6
Pleural fluid:serum protein ratio	<0.5	>0.5
WBCs	>1000/mm³	<1000/mm³
RBCs	>5000	<5000
Glucose	Less than serum	Same as serum
Specific gravity	>1.016	<1.016

LDH, Lactate dehydrogenase; *RBCs,* red blood cells; *WBCs,* white blood cells.
Adapted from Gunn VL, Nechyba C, editors: *The Harriet Lane handbook,* ed 16, St Louis, 2002, Mosby and Boyer D: Evaluation and management of a child with a pleural effusion, *Pediatr Emerg Care* 21(1):63-68, 2005.

- Ultrasound scan–guided thoracentesis has reduced complications.[5] Consider this approach for children with paralyzed hemidiaphragms, with high levels of positive end-expiratory pressure (PEEP) therapy, small pleural effusions, pleural adhesions (e.g., empyema), previous tuberculosis, and multiple previous thoracentesis or thoracostomy tubes.
- No absolute contraindications to a thoracentesis exist when the child is in respiratory distress or has a tension

AP This procedure should be performed only by physicians, advanced practice nurses, and other health care professionals (including critical care nurses) with additional knowledge, skills, and demonstrated competence per professional licensure or institutional standard.

pneumothorax. Relative contraindications for thoracentesis include anticoagulant medication, bleeding disorders, and insertion site infection.

- Knowledge of the mechanism of action, dosing, side effects, and contraindications for anesthetics or sedatives used for procedural sedation[7]

CHILD AND FAMILY ASSESSMENT

- Child's developmental level and ability to interact ➥*Rationale:* Influences preparation and interaction.
- Child's and family's understanding of the reasons for and risks and benefits of the thoracentesis ➥*Rationale:* Evaluates child's and family's understanding of the procedure and provides a gauge for ongoing education.
- Desire of family members to be present during the procedure ➥*Rationale:* The presence of family may provide comfort and support, although family members should have the choice not to remain with the child.
- Cardiopulmonary assessment, including vital signs, visual inspection of breathing patterns and chest wall movement, auscultation of lung fields, and signs of inadequate oxygenation and ventilation, such as decreased arterial oxygen saturation, increased work of breathing, supplemental oxygen requirement, cyanosis, increased heart rate and blood pressure, anxiety, and agitation ➥*Rationale:* Evaluating cardiopulmonary status provides valuable information in determining the child's need for and ability to tolerate the procedure and influences the type of anesthetics or sedative prescribed and the swiftness of the procedure.
- History of reactions or allergies to medication (betadine, lidocaine, anesthetics, or sedatives) ➥*Rationale:* Prevents harm.
- History of bleeding disorders or anticoagulant or antiplatelet therapy ➥*Rationale:* These disorders and therapies may increase the risk of complications.
- History of previous thoracentesis ➥*Rationale:* Previous thoracentesis may have caused scarring, which can make this procedure more difficult.
- Previous experience or reaction to an invasive procedure ➥*Rationale:* The child's previous experience may effect how this event is perceived.
- Review of chest x-ray findings and ultrasound scan results (if indicated) ➥*Rationale:* Location of pleural air, blood, or fluid. An anterior posterior chest radiograph may be adequate for significant fluid accumulations. A lateral decubitus radiograph is obtained if a smaller loculated fluid is suspected.[4] Ultrasound scan results may also confirm liquid versus solid lesion.[5]
- Assess recent serum laboratory results, including complete blood count, platelet count, prothrombin time, and partial thromboplastin time ➥*Rationale:* Determines risk of bleeding.

- Assess skin integrity at the insertion site ➥*Rationale:* Avoidance of active skin lesions or infection at the insertion site.

CHILD AND FAMILY EDUCATION

Individualized, developmentally appropriate education is provided to the family and to the child based on desire for knowledge, readiness to learn, and overall neurologic and psychosocial state.

- Explain the procedure and the reason for thoracentesis, including risks and benefits ➥*Rationale:* Providing information increases knowledge, and preparation helps reduce anxiety, which increases the child's ability to cooperate during the procedure. Information increases parental satisfaction.
- Discuss ways to decrease pain and anxiety during the procedure and explain the plan for pain assessment and treatment during the procedure ➥*Rationale:* Pain and anxiety control help the child maintain position.
- Explain that during the insertion of the needle the child may feel pressure at the insertion site ➥*Rationale:* Providing specific information helps prepare the child for events during the procedure, reducing anxiety.
- Explain how the child can assist with the procedure ➥*Rationale:* The child is provided with an opportunity to participate or assist with the procedure.
- Encourage questions and answer questions as they arise ➥*Rationale:* Reinforcement of information is needed during periods of stress.

EQUIPMENT

- Cardiorespiratory monitor or pulse oximeter as indicated
- Emergency equipment, including manual ventilation bag, mask, and oxygen supply
- Personal protective equipment as indicated, including sterile gloves, sterile gown, mask, and goggles
- Anesthetics or sedation medication and syringes for administration
- Local anesthetic (1% lidocaine) if condition allows
- 25-gauge 5/8-inch needle
- Sterile drapes/towels
- Antiseptic solution (chloraprep/betadine)
- Sterile gauze
- Syringe (for local anesthetic)
- 18-gauge to 22-gauge over-the-needle catheter or needle[7]
- Sterile 10-mL or 20-mL syringe
- Collection bag or additional syringes
- Sterile three-way stopcock
- Band-Aid or adhesive dressing
- Containers for laboratory studies
- Anaerobic and aerobic media bottles for culture
- Laboratory requests

Procedure for Thoracentesis: Perform

Steps	Rationale	Considerations
1. Ensure child and family understand procedure and reason for thoracentesis, including risks and benefits. Obtain informed consent.	Evaluates and reinforces understanding of previously taught information. In many situations, informed consent is required before thoracentesis. Ensures medical-legal compliance as suggested by Joint Commision of Accreditation of Healthcare Organizations.	Developmental, cognitive, and anxiety levels determine approach and effectiveness of teaching.[7] For emergencies refer to institution-specific protocol for assumption of consent.
2. Gather all supplies and equipment necessary to complete the procedure.	Organization and preparation assist in procedure performance.	
3. Wash hands.	Reduces transmission of micro-organisms. Protects personnel health.	
4. Conduct final patient verification process (e.g., time out) per institution-specific protocol.	Confirms correct child, procedure, and site and prevents unnecessary medical procedures (JCAHO requirement).	
5. Ensure adequate cardiorespiratory monitoring.	Children may decompensate during the procedure. Anesthetics and sedation can alter child's vital signs, respiratory pattern and effort, level of consciousness/mental status, and oxygen requirements.	Consider whether the child has a secure airway and is at risk for blood pressure instability. The availability of volume replacement and intubation equipment may be important. Consider increasing the volume on the pulse oximeter or cardiac monitor to allow an auditory signal and visual monitoring during the procedure.
6. Prescribe systemic anesthetics or sedative medication.[8] (Level VI*)	Pain and anxiety control help the child maintain position.	
7. Position child supine and elevated with the affected side slightly rotated. Place arm of affected side above child's head (see Figure 33-6). (Level II*)	Air rises to the apex. Arm is immobilized during procedure, which allows the arm to be out of procedure area and allows easier access to the intercostal spaces and decreases the chance to contaminant the sterile site.	A sitting position is recommended for adults and children who are able to tolerate this position[2] (Figure 41-1).
8. Identify correct intercostal space for needle insertion.	Evaluates the site for thoracentesis.	Site depends on the approach. Identify the highest point of the pleural fluid and choose one intercostal space below this point.[2]
9. Put on gloves and protective equipment.	Reduces transmission of micro-organisms. Protects personnel health.	
10. Prepare equipment and supplies, including lidocaine.	Thoracentesis is a painful procedure.	Lidocaine and Prilocaine (Emla) can be used topically, if time allows injectable anesthetic for rib periosteum is still necessary.

Procedure continues on following page

* Level II: Theory-based; no research data to support recommendations; recommendations from expert consensus group may exist
  Level VI: Clinical studies in a variety of patient populations and situations to support recommendations

Procedure **for Thoracentesis: Perform**—*Continued*

Steps	Rationale	Considerations

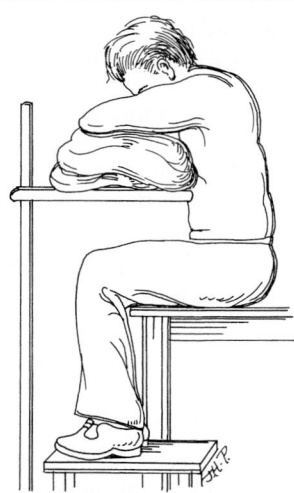

FIGURE 41-1   Sitting Position for Thoracentesis. *Carlson K: Procedure 24 thoracentesis (perform). In Lynn-McHale Wiegand DJ, Carlson K, editors:* AACN *procedure manual for critical care, ed 5, Philadelphia, 2005, Elsevier.*

Steps	Rationale	Considerations
11. Prepare the chest with antiseptic solution and drape.	Removes microorganisms from the skin and reduces risk of infection.	
12. Anesthetize the skin and rib periosteum (see Figure 38-3). *(Level II*)*	Anesthetize the area that can cause pain when the needle is inserted.	Always aspirate during insertion to prevent instillation of lidocaine into a blood vessel.
13. Reidentify correct intercostal space. Insert needle with a syringe attached. Advance needle (while applying negative pressure and aspirating) toward the superior aspect of the rib.[6]	Application of negative pressure (aspirating) identifies whether a blood vessel has been entered.	
14. When the rib is encountered, "walk over" the superior aspect of the rib with continued negative pressure and aspiration until the pleural space is entered (see Figure 38-6). *(Level II*)*	Intercostal vessels are located on the inferior surface of the rib.	
15. Obtain pleural fluid for analysis. With removal of the syringe, place thumb over the opening and then attach a stopcock with the syringe to remove remaining pleural fluid. *(Level II*)*	Prevents air from entering the pleura and reduces the chance of pneumothorax.	
16. When fluid is obtained or drainage completed, remove the needle and place occlusive dressing over the site.	The needle is no longer necessary. Prevents pneumothorax or leakage of pleural fluid.	
17. Remove arm immobilizer and place child in a comfortable position.	Arm is immobilized for the procedure.	

* Level II: Theory-based; no research data to support recommendations; recommendations from expert consensus group may exist

Procedure for Thoracentesis: Perform—*Continued*

Steps	Rationale	Considerations
18. Order laboratory studies.	Laboratory analysis is used for diagnostic reasons.	Laboratory studies for pleural fluid including: protein, culture and gram stain, differential white blood cell count, amylase, specific gravity, protein, pH, lactate dehydrogenase, and glucose.[3] Triglyceride level if chylothorax is suspected.
19. Obtain chest radiograph, as indicated. *(Level VI*)*	Follow up pleural effusion and rule out pneumothorax.	
20. Dispose of equipment, remove needles, sharps objects, and wash hands.	Reduces transmission of microorganisms. Protects personnel health.	

* Level VI: Clinical studies in a variety of patient populations and situations to support recommendations

Expected Outcomes

- Evacuation of air or fluid
- Reexpansion of the affected lung
- Improved oxygenation and ventilation
- Procedure completed without complications

- Remains infection free

- Acceptable level of comfort

Unexpected Outcomes

- Lung does not respond
- Continued signs and symptoms of inadequate oxygenation and ventilation
- Laceration of spleen or liver
- Pulmonary contusion
- Iatrogenic pneumothorax
- Hemothorax
- Bleeding from puncture of the intercostal vessels
- Pleural infection
- Site infection
- Unmanaged pain and anxiety

Monitoring and Care of the Child

Activities and Interventions	Rationale	Reportable Conditions
1. Monitor respiratory, cardiovascular, and neurologic status before, during, and after the procedure.	Ongoing assessment is necessary for evaluation of the effectiveness of therapy. Changes in vital signs and physical examination results alert the caregiver to unexpected outcomes.	• Respiratory distress (grunting, tachypnea, retractions, dyspnea, agitation, and hypoxia) • Decreased to absent breath sounds • Subcutaneous emphysema • Tracheal shift to the unaffected side • Cardiovascular collapse • Anxiety, restlessness, or feeling of doom • Tachycardia • Hypotension • Chest pain
2. Assess pain status during and after thoracentesis.	Evaluate pain management strategy.	• Pain unrelieved with pain management plan • Pain that interferes with interventions to expand lung
3. Obtain and review chest radiograph results.	Post-procedural followup.	• Unresolved evacuating air or fluid
4. Assess insertion site.	Any wound increases infection risk.	• Excessive bleeding or drainage

Documentation

- Description of the procedure, including date, time, and length of procedure (include patient position and needle size)
- Correct site, correct procedure, and correct person verification, including consent
- Description of pleural fluid, including amount aspirated
- Indications for the procedure
- Assessment findings before and after the procedure (breath sounds and signs of oxygenation and ventilation)
- Local anesthetic or systemic anesthetic used and child's response
- Site assessment and type of dressing used
- Laboratory studies ordered and results
- Chest radiograph obtained and results
- Comfort assessment and any specific interventions
- Additional interventions necessary
- Unexpected outcomes and related treatment
- Child and family education

References

1. Thibodeau G, Patton K. *Anatomy and physiology,* St. Louis, 2003, Mosby.
2. Fuhrman B, Zimmerman J: *Pediatric critical care,* ed 3, Philadelphia, 2006, Elsevier.
3. Roberts JR, Hedges JR: *Clinical procedures in emergency medicine,* ed 4, Philadelphia, 2004, Saunders.
4. Carlson K: Thoracentesis (assist). In Lynn-McHale Wiegand DJ, Carlson K, editors: *AACN procedure manual for critical care,* ed 5, Philadelphia, 2005, Elsevier.
5. Boyer D: Evaluation and management of a child with a pleural effusion, *Pediatr Emerg Care* 21(1):63-68, 2005.
6. Gunn V, Nechyba C: *The Harriet Lane handbook.* Philadelphia, 2002, Mosby.
7. Taeusch H, et al: *Pediatric and neonatal tests and procedures,* Philadelphia, 1996, Saunders.
8. Kaplan R, Yang C: Sedation and analgesia in pediatric patients for procedures outside the operating room, *Anesthesiol Clin North Am* 20:181-194, 2002.
9. Gaynard L, et al: *Psychosocial care of children in hospitals: a clinical practice manual,* Rockville, MD, 1998, Child Life Council.
10. Bryant R, Salmon C: Pleural empyema, *Clinical Infectious Disease,* 22, 747-764, 1996.

P R O C E D U R E **42**

Emergency Medication Preparation and Administration

P U R P O S E : To ensure appropriate and safe preparation and administration of medications in an emergent situation

Julie Creaden

PREREQUISITE KNOWLEDGE

- Activation of emergency alert system
- Child's medical and surgical history, including allergies
- Mastery of pediatric basic and advanced life support competencies
- Appropriate pediatric dosing of emergency medications, indications for use, method of action, and adverse reactions
- Ability to accurately calculate, draw up, and administer medications on the basis of child's weight and available drug concentration
- Ability to accurately calculate, correctly mix, and administer prescribed doses of continuous infusions of cardiac medications
- Solution and medication compatibility and drug interactions
- Aseptic technique
- Alternative methods of delivery of emergency medications (i.e., intraosseous, endotracheal)
- Normal infant, child, and adolescent heart rates, blood pressures, and respiratory rates
- Basic and advanced electrocardiographic (ECG) interpretation

CHILD AND FAMILY ASSESSMENT

- History of chronic diseases, such as congenital heart disease, cardiac arrhythmias, syncope, past surgical or catheterization procedures, and previous electrophysiologic complications ➥*Rationale:* These conditions can impact the types of medication selected and the location at which they are administered during an emergency situation. This information can also assist with determination of the most effective treatment options for cardiopulmonary support.
- Hemodynamic status before the emergency situation ➥*Rationale:* This information can aid in identification of the cause of the life-threatening event.
- History of prior ECGs ➥*Rationale:* Establishes preadmission/preevent baseline rhythm.
- Medication history, including use of herbal supplements, drug exposure, acid-base balance, and electrolyte levels ➥*Rationale:* Drug therapy and electrolyte or acid-base abnormalities could impede the response to medications. Certain medications, herbal supplements, or drug exposures may be implicated as the cause of the life-threatening event.
- History of previous response to anesthesia or conscious sedation ➥*Rationale:* Influences the type of sedation used during the emergency situation to safely achieve desired results.
- Knowledge of family's understanding of the child's condition and prognosis and their goals for the child's treatment ➥*Rationale:* This knowledge aids in anticipating and ascertaining family needs, available support systems, and degree of involvement.
- Desire of family to be present during the resuscitation ➥*Rationale:* The option to be with the child during a

life-threatening event reassures the family that the child is receiving optimal care, legitimizes the child's condition, and may provide some sense of comfort and control, but the family should also have the choice not to remain with the child.[1]

CHILD AND FAMILY EDUCATION

Individualized, developmentally appropriate education is provided to the child and to the family based on desire for knowledge, readiness to learn, and overall neurologic and psychosocial state. Simple explanations are most effective during an emergency situation. Anticipate that information needs to be repeated.[1]

- Review the child's medical condition and rationale for emergency intervention with the family ➻*Rationale:* Information helps to decrease the family's anxiety level and offers reassurance during an extremely stressful period in their lives.
- Communicate regularly with the family during the emergency situation or resuscitation ➻*Rationale:* Communication aids in assessing the family's need for support and initiation of social and spiritual services.[1,2]
- Assure the family that medication is administered to keep the child comfortable during intubation and resuscitation ➻*Rationale:* Providing information to the family helps decrease stress and anxiety, and assuring the family that pain will be managed may decrease the family's fears.

- Allow the family the opportunity to be present during resuscitation efforts with assigned support personnel and per institutional protocol ➻*Rationale:* Research shows that family presence during resuscitation efforts may assist the family with coping if the child dies and that viewing the efforts of the health care team during an emergency is reassuring to the family. Family presence can help reduce anxieties of the unknown course of events.[2]

EQUIPMENT

- Cardiorespiratory monitoring, including ECG recorder
- Electrocardiographic patches and leads
- Skin preparation
- Alcohol swabs
- Various size syringes to draw up individual medication doses
- Needles or needleless access devices
- Intravenous (IV) supplies
- 0.9% sterile saline solution flushes
- Intubation equipment, including sedation and muscle relaxant medications, individualized to the child's history and institution-specific protocols
- Emergency cart
- Defibrillator
- Resuscitation sheet
- Emergency medication sheet with medications and dosages calculated based on the child's weight

---

Procedure | for Emergency Medication Preparation and Administration

Steps	Rationale	Considerations
1. Perform rapid assessment of child and environment. (*Level VI**)	Assists in identification of factors that contribute to deterioration in health status.	Knowledge of the child's diagnosis provides background for the child's response to certain medications and may identify the underlying reason for deterioration in condition. Determines likelihood that environmental factors, such as equipment failure, accidental trauma, and foreign body aspiration, may have contributed to hemodynamic deterioration.
2. Assess the family's desire to be at the bedside during the resuscitation. This step occurs simultaneously with Step 1 as part of the provider assessment of the child and environment.	Family may feel supported when allowed to remain during resuscitation efforts; it provides them with a better understanding of what is being done for the child.[2]	Family presence during resuscitation should be offered per institution-specific protocol with a health care team member available to support the family during the resuscitation.
3. Position the child supine and ensure the airway is open. (*Level VI**)	Proper positioning provides full access to the child for complete assessment and support of the ABCs of resuscitation (see Step 4).	

* Level VI: Clinical studies in a variety of patient populations and situations to support recommendations

Procedure for Emergency Medication Preparation and Administration—*Continued*

Steps	Rationale	Considerations
4. Initiate support of **A**irway, **B**reathing, and **C**irculation as necessary. *(Level VI*)*	The length of time child is without a pulse is directly associated with morbidity and mortality.	Follow Pediatric Advanced Life Support (PALS) guidelines.
5. Activate the emergency alert system and notify appropriate staff per institution-specific protocol. *(Level VI*)*	Sufficient help optimizes outcomes for the child.	Follow institution-specific protocols for initiation of a resuscitation or activation of emergency response.
6. Gather necessary supplies and equipment, including emergency cart and defibrillator.	Ensures that all equipment is at the bedside to facilitate resuscitation without delays.	Children with pacemakers need further assessment of pacemaker malfunction and underlying rhythm.
7. Ensure that the child is properly connected to the cardiopulmonary monitor, noninvasive blood pressure or arterial line monitoring, and pulse oximetry. *(Level II*)*	Monitors hemodynamic response to resuscitation efforts.	Goals for hemodynamic parameters should take into consideration child's age, weight, and medical history.
8. Wash hands and put on clean gloves. *(Level VI*)*	Standard precautions; reduces transmission of microorganisms.	
9. If necessary, establish IV access.	Facilitates administration of emergency medications.	Before IV access is established, consider history of vascular compromise (i.e., history of Blalock-Taussig shunt); the child's nurse should assist with the identification of optimal IV access sites. Multiple IV sites should be established if possible.
10. If IV placement is unsuccessful, proceed to placement of intraosseous (IO) catheter; for the child in cardiac arrest, immediate IO access is recommended if IV access is not already in place.[3] *(Level II*)* (See Procedures 145 and 154 for further information). *(Level VI*)*	The PALS guidelines recommend IO placement if reliable IV access is not established quickly.[3] IO access can be quickly achieved in an emergency.[3]	Intraosseous placement allows administration of all emergency medications.[3,4] Drugs administered via the intraosseous route must be followed by a sterile saline solution flush of at least 5 mL, which ensures drug delivery to the central circulation. Fluids should be given with a pressure bag or pump.[3] Bone marrow toxic drugs are not given via the intraosseous route.
11. Secure IV access.	Prevents accidental dislodgement of IV access during emergency situation.	Avoid air in IV lines because of risk of cerebral/pulmonary emboli, especially in children with systemic to pulmonary or right to left shunts.[5,6]
12. If unable to establish IV or IO access or if access procedure is prolonged or interrupted, epinephrine, atropine, lidocaine, and naloxone can be given to intubated children or children with tracheostomies via the endotracheal route. IV or IO access is always preferred.[3] *(Level V*)*	Provides an alternate route for emergency medication administration if needed.	PALS recommendations for endotracheal administration of Atropine, 0.03 mg/kg Naloxone, <5 years or ≤ 20 kg, 0.1 mg/kg ≥5 years or > 20 kg, 2 mg Lidocaine 2-3 mg Absorption via this route is variable. The recommended initial endotracheal dose of epinephrine is 0.1 mg/kg of 1:1000 solution.

Procedure continues on following page

---

* Level II: Theory-based; no research data to support recommendations; recommendations from expert consensus group may exist
Level V: Clinical studies in more than one or two patient populations and situations to support recommendations
Level VI: Clinical studies in a variety of patient populations and situations to support recommendations

Procedure	for Emergency Medication Preparation and Administration—*Continued*		
Steps	**Rationale**	**Considerations**	
		Dilute drug with 0.9% saline to a volume of 5 mL and administer directly into the endotracheal tube or tracheostomy tube. Follow endotracheal administration with 5 positive pressure ventilation breaths.[3] Stop chest compressions briefly while giving meds.[3]	
13. Calculate medication doses according to the recommended dose for child's weight and age; dose calculation should be independently verified by a second qualified health care provider. If available, use individualized emergency medication sheet.[3] Table 42-1 provides medication recommendations per PALS protocols.	Minimizes risk for medication error.	Knowledge of the child's age, weight, height, and allergies is imperative in preparation of appropriate emergency medications for administration. A length-based resuscitation tape may be used to estimate weight if needed.[3]	
14. Draw each medication dose up into an individual syringe.	Avoids potential overdosing when small volumes of medication are necessary.	Medication doses are individualized to the child based on weight. One prefilled emergency medication syringe can provide multiple doses. Stopcocks or needleless access devices can be used to draw multiple medication doses from the prefilled syringe.	
15. Label all medications with the name of the drug, dose, and concentration before administration.[7] *(Level V*)*	Assures that the correct medication and dose is prepared and administered.		
16. Announce medication to be given before administration; include the number of doses the child has received with this dose (e.g., "second dose of epinephrine is in"). *(Level II*)*	Ensures that all team members are aware of the amount of medication received by the child and serves as a "repeat back" of the order to prescribing practitioner.		
17. Ensure "five rights" of medication administration: right patient, right medication, right dose, right route, and right time. *(Level V*)*	Minimizes the risk for medication errors.	All children should have an identification band to facilitate patient identification. .	
18. Order and deliver emergency medications in accordance with PALS guidelines. *(Level V*)*	Medications have specific administration guidelines to ensure safe and rapid delivery and to attain the desired response.	Delivery considerations for specific medications: Calcium chloride: Administer slowly; central venous administration is preferred. Epinephrine dose: IV/IO administration, 0.01 mg/kg (0.1 mL/kg of 1:10,000 concentration). Endotracheal administration, 0.1 mg/kg (0.1 mL/kg of 1:1000).	

*　Level II: Theory-based; no research data to support recommendations; recommendations from expert consensus group may exist
　Level V: Clinical studies in more than one or two patient populations and situations to support recommendations

Procedure **for Emergency Medication Preparation and Administration**—*Continued*

Steps	Rationale	Considerations
		Prostaglandin E1: Monitor for apnea, hypotension, hypoglycemia, and hypocalcemia. Sodium bicarbonate: Infuse slowly and only if ventilation is adequate.[3]
19. Flush medication in with 5 mL of 0.9% saline solution.[3]	Ensures medication reaches the central circulation.	
20. Monitor child's response to medication administration.	Ongoing monitoring of response to medications and interventions directs the next step of care.	Patients with heart transplant have denervated hearts and do not respond to atropine.[8] If response to adenosine is not immediate, consider administration of a second dose to assure delivery in the rapid manner necessary to convert to normal sinus rhythm. A higher dose may be needed when given peripherally.[3]
21. Ensure that multiple rounds of single dose emergency medications, fluid boluses, and saline solution flushes are prepared, labeled, and available for immediate administration.[3,7,9] *(Level V*)*	In an emergency situation, team members must prepare additional doses of emergency medications to facilitate immediate treatment of changes in the child's hemodynamic status without delay.	
22. Prepare continuous infusion of vasoactive drugs. Titrate to desired effect (see Table 42-1 for vasoactive drug infusion recommendations per PALS protocol). *(Level V*)*	The goal of continuous infusions is to maintain adequate blood pressure, heart rate, and perfusion.	Use of standard concentrations for continuous infusions is recommended to decrease medication errors.
23. Monitor results of blood samples sent for chemistry and gas exchange. *(Level VI*)*	Electrolyte and acid-base imbalance may negatively impact effects of resuscitation medications. *(Level VI*)*	Children in the immediate postoperative period need special attention to fluid status, maintenance of normothermia, acid base balance, electrolyte disturbance, and rhythm issues.[5,6]
24. Provide family with regular updates on the status of the child during resuscitation if they are not at the bedside. *(Level V*)*	May facilitate family coping; aids in assessment of family's need for support and initiation of social and spiritual services.[1,2] May provide some reassurance that child is receiving optimal care.	Address the child and family at a developmentally appropriate level; when speaking with the family, refer to the child by name.

* Level V: Clinical studies in more than one or two patient populations and situations to support recommendations
  Level VI: Clinical studies in a variety of patient populations and situations to support recommendations

TABLE 42-1	Drugs Used in Pediatric Advanced Life Support	
Drug	**Dosage (Pediatric)**	**Remarks**
Adenosine	0.1 mg/kg (maximum 6 mg) 0.2 mg/kg for second dose	Rapid IV push Maximum first dose: 6 mg Maximum single dose: 12 mg Follow immediately with ≥ 5 mL 0.9% saline flush
Amiodarone for refractory VF, Pulseless VT/VF	5 mg/kg rapid IV/IO	Maximum: 15 mg/kg/24 hours IV Maximum single dose: 300 mg

Amiodarone for perfusing ventricular
  and supraventricular arrhythmias
	Loading dose: 5 mg/kg IV/IO over 20 to 60
	  minutes (maximum single dose 300 mg)
		Repeat to maximum of 15 mg/kg/day IV

Atropine sulfate	0.02 mg/kg IV/IO; may double this dose for second IV/IO dose	Minimum single dose: 0.1 mg
Can be given via endotracheal tube		Maximum doses: Child single dose: 0.5 mg Child total dose: 1 mg Adolescent single dose: 1 mg Adolescent total dose: 2 mg Endotracheal administration: 0.03 mg/kg

Calcium chloride 10% = 100 mg/mL= 27.2
  mg/mL elemental calcium
	20 mg/kg (0.2 mL/kg of 10% solution)
	  slow IV/IO push
		Give slowly
		Central venous administration preferred if available
		Adult dose: 5-10 mL

Dobutamine hydrochloride	2 to 20 mcg/kg/minute	Titrate to desired effect May produce or exacerbate hypotension May produce tachyarrhythmias

Dopamine hydrochloride	2 to 20 mcg/kg/min	If infusion dose >20 mcg/kg/minute is required
		  consider using alternative adrenergic agent
		  (e.g., epinephrine)
		Extravasation may cause tissue injury

Epinephrine for symptomatic bradycardia	All IV/IO doses: 0.01 mg/kg (0.1 mL/kg of 1:10,000 standard concentration)	
Can be given via endotracheal tube	All endotracheal doses: 0.1 mg/kg (0.1 mL/kg 1:1000 high concentration)	

Epinephrine for asystolic or pulseless
  arrest
	IV/IO dose: 0.01 mg/kg (0.1 mL/kg of
	  1:10,000 standard concentration)
		Maximum dose 1 mg IV/IO; 10 mg endotracheal

Can be given via endotracheal tube	Administer every 3-5 minutes during arrest.
	All endotracheal doses: 0.1 mg/kg (0.1
	  mL/kg of 1:1000 high concentration)
	Administer every 3-5 minutes of arrest
	  until IV/IO access achieved; then begin
	  with first IV dose	

Epinephrine continuous infusion	Begin with rapid infusion, then titrate to
	  response. Typical initial infusion 0.1-1
	  mcg/kg/minute
	Higher doses may be effective
		Titrate to desired effect
		High dose infusions may produce vasoconstriction,
		  may compromise perfusion; low doses may
		  decrease renal and splanchnic blood flow

Glucose	IV/IO infusion: 0.5 to 1 g/kg (maximum
	  recommended IV/IO concentration, 25%;
	  can prepare by mixing 50% dextrose
	  1:1 with sterile water)
	50% dextrose (0.5 g/mL); give 1-2 mL/kg
	25% dextrose (0.25 g/mL); give 2 to
	  4 mL/kg
	10% dextrose (0.1 g/mL); give 5 to 10 mL/kg
	5% dextrose (0.05 g/mL); give 10 to
	  20 mL/kg if volume tolerated
		Use bedside glucose test to confirm hypoglycemia;
		  hyperglycemia may worsen neurologic outcome of
		  cardiopulmonary arrest or trauma; do not
		  administer routinely during resuscitation.
		Maximum concentration for newborn administration,
		  12.5% (0.125 g/mL)

Lidocaine
  Can be given via endotracheal tube
	Bolus IV/IO therapy: 1 mg/kg rapid IV/IO
	  push (maximum dose; 100 mg)
	Continuous IV/IO Infusion; 20 to 50 mcg/kg/
	  minute; administer bolus dose (1 mg/kg)
	  when infusion is initiated if bolus has not
	  been given within previous 15 minutes.
	Endotracheal dose 2-3 mg/kg
		Reduce infusion dose if severe CHF or low cardiac
		  output is compromising hepatic and renal blood flow
		Contraindicated for wide-complex ventricular
		  escape beats associated with bradycardia

TABLE 42-1	Drugs Used in Pediatric Advanced Life Support—Cont'd	

Drug	Dosage (Pediatric)	Remarks
Magnesium sulfate	25 to 50 mg/kg IV/IO over 10 to 20 minutes; faster in torsades For asthma: 25-50 mcg/kg (maximum dose 2 gm) over 10 to 20 minutes	Maximum dose: 2 g Contraindicated in renal failure Possible hypotension and bradycardia with rapid bolus
Milrinone	Loading: 50 to 75 mcg/kg IV/IO over 10-60 minutes (longer infusion times reduce risk of hypotension) Infusion: 0.5 to 0.75 mcg/kg/minute IV/IO	Monitor for hypotension during loading dose, particularly in volume depleted patients

Naloxone
  Can be given by IV/IO/IM/SQ
  Endotracheal route possible; other routes preferred
	<5 years old or ≤20 kg: 0.1 mg/kg IV/IO/ET
	≥5 years old or >20 kg: 2 mg IV/IO/ET
	Continuous IV/IO infusion: 0.04 to 0.16 mg/kg/hour
		If total reversal is not required (e.g. respiratory depression), smaller doses (1 to 5 mcg/kg) may be used; titrate to effect.

Norepinephrine	Begin at rates of 0.1 to 2 mcg/kg/minute IV/IO; adjust infusion rate to achieve desired change in blood pressure and systemic perfusion	May produce hypertension, organ ischemia, and arrhythmias. Extravasation may cause tissue necrosis (treat with phentolamine)
Prostaglandin E_1	Begin at 0.05 to 0.1 mcg/kg/minute IV/IO infusion; titrate to effect	Monitor for apnea, hypotension, hypoglycemia, seizures, hyperpyrexia, hypocalcemia
Sodium bicarbonate	1 mEq/kg per dose IV/IO	Infuse slowly preceeded and followed by adequate ventilation Do not mix with any resuscitation drugs. Flush IV tubing with 0.9% saline before and after administration
Sodium nitroprusside	Children ≤40 kg: 1 to 8 mcg/kg/minute IV/IO infusion Children > 40 kg: 0.1 to 5 mcg/kg/minute IV/IO infusion Mix in 5% dextrose in water	May cause hypotension, particularly with hypovolemia Titrate to desired effect Light sensitive; cover drug reservoir with opaque material or use specialized administration set Typically change the solution every 24 hours.

$$\text{Continuous infusion rate (mL/h)} = \frac{\text{Weight (kg)} \times \text{desired dose (mcg/kg/min)} \times 60 \text{ min/h}}{\text{Concentration (mcg/mL)}}$$

VT= ventricular tachycardia; VF=ventricular fibrillation; CHF= congestive heart failure
* For tracheal administration, dilute drug with 0.9% saline to volume of 5 mL and follow with 5 positive-pressure ventilations.
Adapted from:
American Heart Association Emergency Cardiovascular Care Committee, Subcommittee on Pediatric Resuscitation. Pediatric advanced life support. In: Field JM, Hazinski MF, Gilmore D, eds. *Handbook of Emergency Cardiovascular Care for Healthcare Providers*. South Deerfield, MA: Channing Bete Company, 2006:74-97.
American Heart Association Emergency Cardiovascular Care Committee, Subcommittee on Pediatric Resuscitation. Part 12: Pediatric advanced life support. Circulation. 2005; 112(24, supplement 4):IV-171.
Reproduced with permission: *Pediatric Advanced Life Support*, 2005, 2006, Copyright American Heart Association.

Expected Outcomes

- The PALS guidelines are followed for emergency medication dosing and administration
- Child receives the prescribed dose of medication

- Medications are readily available and rapidly administered as prescribed
- Medication doses are given via the most effective available route of administration
- Child has desired response to administered medications, and vital signs stabilize

Unexpected Outcomes

- Inappropriate medications or medication doses are ordered during resuscitation
- Child receives the wrong dose or medication, or the medication is administered via the wrong route
- Delay in preparation and administration of emergency medications
- Additional doses of medication are administered with little or no effect
- Child continues to have decompensation and does not survive the event

Monitoring and Care of the Child

Activities and Interventions	Rationale	Reportable Conditions
1. Continuously monitor vital signs and the child's response to therapy.	Accurate monitoring of vital signs helps in assessment of response to administered medications.	• Adverse reaction to medication administration • No improvement with medication administration
2. Continuously monitor ECG findings and assess changes in heart rhythm and perfusion in response to medication administration and interventions.	Indicates response to interventions.	• Arrhythmias/asystole after medication administration
3. Monitor IV access throughout the resuscitation to ensure patency.	Ensures that medications are delivered into the central circulation and prevents complications of infiltration.	• Inability to administer medications or fluids through vascular access • Infiltration of medications into subcutaneous tissue or muscle
4. Ensure real time documentation of medications ordered and administered.	Appropriate documentation of course of events, including vital signs at the time of medication administration, chronicles response and possibly dictates the next appropriate medication to be administered.	• Incorrect dosing or delivery of medications • Inability to retrieve information on medication administration during the resuscitation event

Documentation

- Description of procedure, including date, time, and length of procedure (include needle size and amount of air aspirated)
- Correct site, correct procedure, and correct person verification
- Indications for procedure
- Assessment findings before and after procedure (breath sounds and signs of oxygenation and ventilation)
- Local anesthetic or systemic anesthetic used, if applicable, and child's response
- Site assessment and type of dressing used
- Results of follow-up chest radiograph
- Comfort assessment and any specific interventions
- Additional interventions necessary
- Child and family education
- Unexpected outcomes and related treatment

References

1. Haddad A: Ethics in action: family presence during codes, *RN* 65(11);31-34, 2002.
2. McGahey PR: Family presence during pediatric resuscitation: a focus on staff, *Crit Care Nurse* 22(6):29-34, 2002.
3. American Heart Association Emergency Cardiovascular Care Committee, Subcommittee on Pediatric Resuscitation. Pediatric advanced life support. In: Field JM, Hazinski MF, Gilmore D, eds. *Handbook of emergency cardiovascular care for healthcare providers.* South Deerfield, MA: Channing Bete Company, 2006:74.
4. American Heart Association Emergency Cardiovascular Care Committee, Subcommittee on Pediatric Resuscitation Vascular access. In Hazinski MF, Zarisky AL, Nadkami VM, Hickey RW, Schexnayder SM, Berg RA (eds): *PALS provider manual*, Dallas, 2002, American Heart Association
5. Creaden JA, Kohr LM: The nurse practitioner's role in patient management. In Mavroudis C, Backer CL, editors: *Pediatric cardiac surgery*, ed 3, Philadelphia, 2003, Mosby.
6. Cardiovascular disorders. In Hazinski MF, editor: *Nursing care of the critically ill child,* 2nd ed, St. Louis, 1992, Mosby, pp. 117-194
7. Tilleul P, et al: Intravenous drug preparation practices: a survey in a French university hospital, *Pharmacy World Sci* 25(6):276-279, 2003.
8. Wade CR, et al: Postoperative nursing care of the cardiac transplant recipient, *Crit Care Nurs Q* 27(1):17-28, 2004.
9. Shah AN, et al: Effect of an intervention standardization system on pediatric dosing and equipment size determination: a crossover trial involving simulated resuscitation events, *Arch Pediatr Adolesc Med* 157(3):229-236, 2003.

Open Sternotomy: Assist

P U R P O S E : To alleviate compression of the heart from cardiac tamponade and to identify potential sources of bleeding

Melissa Mullen, Terie Pearl, and Gail Keyser

PREREQUISITE KNOWLEDGE

- Sterile technique
  - ❖ Open sternotomy is a sterile procedure done emergently at the bedside of a child, often in unstable condition. All members of the team involved should be skilled in and should practice sterile technique.
  - ❖ The goal is creation of a sterile environment that mimics that of the operating room in the confines of the nursing unit.
- Cardiac anatomy and physiology
- Pediatric postoperative cardiac surgical care and possible complications of cardiac surgery
- The child's congenital heart disease and specific repair
- Signs and symptoms of cardiac tamponade: tachycardia with narrowing pulse pressure followed by hypotension, elevated filling pressures, altered mental status, distant heart sounds, jugular venous distention, decreased cardiac output with cool extremities, and diminished peripheral pulses[1]
- Pathophysiology and management of cardiac tamponade[1]
  - ❖ Bleeding is a postoperative complication that can and does occur after open heart surgery; generally drainage tubes are placed during surgery to drain blood away from the heart. If the blood is not drained away, blood accumulates around the heart.
  - ❖ Cardiac tamponade is a collection of fluid or blood that accumulates around the heart and impairs cardiac output, it is a surgical emergency.

- ❖ Tamponade is of particular concern in the early postoperative period when active bleeding occurs; however, tamponade can occur at any time.
  - ○ When intracardiac lines or temporary pacing wires are removed, bleeding and cardiac tamponade is a real risk and the child must be monitored appropriately.
- Emergent bedside reexploration is indicated when the child's condition is unstable or the child is at risk for imminent arrest or in cardiac arrest and the suspected cause is tamponade.[1,2]
- Indications for reexploration may include:
  - ❖ Active hemorrhage that must be repaired
  - ❖ A mediastinal chest tube that does not drain effectively because of clot or the position of the tube in relation to the accumulation of blood or fluid
  - ❖ Echocardiographic evidence of a pericardial effusion
  - ❖ Enlarged cardiac silhouette on chest radiograph
- Mastery of pediatric advanced life support competencies
- Skill in setting up and providing internal cardiac defibrillation
- Mechanical ventilation, sedation/anesthesia, and paralysis are prerequisites to an emergent open sternotomy.[2]
- Responsibilities of each member of the health care team who participates in the procedure
  - ❖ Bedside Nurse
    - ○ Monitors the child
    - ○ Establishes sterile area
    - ○ Opens the sterile drape pack and instruments
    - ○ Assists the surgeon if operating room (OR) staff are not available

- Ensures that necessary blood products are available at bedside
- Documents
  - ❖ Critical Care or Anesthesia Practitioner
    - Provides analgesia/anesthesia
    - Provides airway management
    - Provides resuscitation
  - ❖ Surgeon or Surgical Fellow/Physician's Assistant/Nurse Practitioner
    - Prepares and drapes the child
    - Obtains informed consent from the family as time and situation permits
    - Opens and closes the chest
  - ❖ Charge Nurse
    - Facilitates notification of surgeon, OR team, blood bank, and other resources and services as needed
    - Assists the bedside nurse
    - Provides crowd control
    - Assists with documentation
    - Notifies and updates the family
  - ❖ Patient Care Assistant
    - Obtains necessary equipment/supplies
    - Obtains necessary blood products
  - ❖ Operating Room Nurse (when available)
    - Opens sterile supplies and instruments
    - Sets up sterile field
    - Assists surgeon with procedure
- Open sternotomy is usually performed emergently; if time and circumstances permit, informed consent should be obtained from the family.
- Institution-specific protocol/procedure in place for assumption of consent

CHILD AND FAMILY ASSESSMENT

- Child's developmental level and ability to interact ➻*Rationale:* These factors influence preparation of the child and interaction; ability to interact may be an indication of adequacy of cerebral perfusion.
- Signs and symptoms of tamponade ➻*Rationale:* Cardiac tamponade is a surgical emergency; early recognition facilitates prompt treatment.
- Child's laboratory data, including complete blood count (CBC), prothrombin time (PT), partial thromboplastin time (PTT), and fibrinogen ➻*Rationale:* Thrombocytopenia and abnormal coagulation studies are potential causes of bleeding and should be evaluated and treated. Tracking trends in hemoglobin and hematocrit indicate the extent of blood loss.
- Need for type and cross match and blood products ➻*Rationale:* The child may need emergent blood product replacement in the face of active bleeding, and during the procedure, damage to structures may necessitate emergent transfusion.
- Chest tube patency and amount and character of drainage ➻*Rationale:* Tamponade can occur from hemorrhage after cardiac surgery that necessitates repair, coagulation abnormalities, or malfunctioning chest drainage devices.

Active bleeding with chest drainage of more than 3 mL/kg/h should be watched carefully. Chest tube drainage that suddenly decreases or stops warrants careful investigation.[1]

- Medical history of allergies and coagulation abnormalities and preoperative status ➻*Rationale:* Provides a baseline for assessment of change in status or potential complications.
- Chest radiograph (CXR) findings ➻*Rationale:* CXR findings consistent with tamponade and bleeding include widened mediastinum and enlarged cardiac silhouette. Symptoms may also be related to a hemothorax or pleural effusion that necessitates a chest tube, not an open sternotomy.
- Transthoracic echocardiogram (ECHO) findings ➻*Rationale:* The ECHO is an important diagnostic tool that can indicate whether a collection of fluid or blood is impairing cardiac output.
- Family availability or contact information ➻*Rationale:* The family may not be at the bedside or in the nursing unit. The family must be notified as soon as possible by the staff; location of the family physically or by telephone and notification of ongoing events is imperative. Communication, even the communication of frightening information, is crucial in a trustful relationship.
- Possibility of preprocedure consent and teaching ➻*Rationale:* If the procedure must be performed emergently, detailed teaching and consent may not be possible. Teaching and time for questions must be provided to the family after the procedure.
- Family's understanding of the urgency and indications for the procedure ➻*Rationale:* Although detailed discussions may need to occur after the procedure because of the emergent nature of the procedure, the family should have an understanding of the indications for this procedure.

CHILD AND FAMILY EDUCATION

Individualized, developmentally appropriate education is provided to the family and to the child based on desire for knowledge, readiness to learn, and overall neurologic and psychosocial state.

- Explain the reason for the procedure and the expected outcome; review risks of the procedure as presented by the surgical team ➻*Rationale:* Reinforcement and repeating of information facilitates understanding during stressful events.
- Detailed teaching and information may not be possible until after the procedure is completed ➻*Rationale:* Open sternotomy is generally an emergency procedure; time for family teaching usually occurs after the procedure.
- Encourage questions and answer questions as they arise ➻*Rationale:* Reinforcement of information is needed during periods of stress. This is especially important given the emergent nature of the procedure.

EQUIPMENT

- Blood products per prescribing practitioner's order or unit-specific or institution-specific protocol
- Chest tubes and chest tube drainage device
- Nonsterile equipment
  - Electrocautery unit (Bovie®, Bovie Medical, St. Petersburg, FL)
  - Grounding pad
  - Light source
  - Surgical headlight
  - Metal table for instruments
  - Hats and masks for everyone at the bedside or in the room
  - Surgeon's loops
  - Defibrillator with appropriately sized external and sterile internal paddles
- Medications
  - Emergency resuscitation medications
  - Anesthetic, sedative, and neuromuscular blockade medications per anesthesiologist or prescribing practitioner responsible for sedation and airway during the procedure
  - Antibiotic for irrigation; generally vancomycin, unless the child has a known allergy
  - Sterile 0.9% saline solution for irrigation
- Sterile drape pack
  - Sterile towels/drapes
  - Half sheets (two) or pediatric lap sheet
  - Sterile 4×4 sponges
  - Sterile lap sponges
- Cautery handpiece
- Sterile suction tubing
- Povidone-iodine (2-oz bottle)
- No. 15 and 11 surgical blades
- 2-0 silk ties
- Suture for vessels (Prolene 5-0)
- Suture for closing skin
- Suture shods
- Sterile gloves of appropriate sizes
- Sterile gowns
- Hemaclips (small, medium, large)
- Sterile instruments
  - Knife handles (two)
  - Forceps (Debakey and Adsen)
  - Scissors (Metz-curved, and Mayo-straight)
  - Wire cutters
  - Suction tips (small Pinchon and Pump)
  - Mosquitos, curved (six) and straight (six)
  - Schnidts (four)
  - Tubing clamps (four)
  - Needle holders (four)
  - Vascular needle holders (two)
  - Vascular clamps (variety of curved and straight)
  - Vein retractors (two)
  - Sternal retractors (various sizes)
  - Chest retractors
  - Rummel tourniquets
  - Weitlaner retractor
  - Hemaclip appliers (small, medium, large)
  - Sponge stick (two)
  - Towel clips (six)

Procedure for Open Sternotomy: Assist

Steps	Rationale	Considerations
1. As time permits, ensure family understands procedure and questions are answered.	Evaluates and reinforces understanding of previously taught information.	Developmental level, cognitive function, and anxiety levels determine timing of, approach to, and effectiveness of teaching.
2. Notify surgeon and surgical team.	The OR team may be needed at the bedside or to set up the OR.	If the OR team is not available, their roles are assumed by the bedside nurse and charge nurse.
3. Provide family a place or area near procedure location to wait and provide ongoing upates during the procedure.	Ongoing and interactive communication helps the family cope during a frightening and stressful time.	
4. If time permits, confirm that consent for the procedure has been obtained.	Ensures medical-legal compliance as suggested by the Joint Commission on Accreditation of Healthcare Organizations (JCAHO).	Generally this is an emergency procedure and time to obtain consent is not available; refer to institution-specific protocol for assumption of consent.
5. Reduce the number of personnel at the bedside to only the essential needed.	This is a sterile procedure; the goal is to create as sterile an environment as possible.	If personnel do not have a role, they should vacate the sterile area but be available to obtain supplies and equipment and to support the family.

Procedure continues on following page

Procedure for Open Sternotomy: Assist—*Continued*

Steps	Rationale	Considerations
6. Provide all personnel at bedside with hats and masks.	This is a sterile procedure; use of barrier devices reduces transmission of microorganisms.	
7. Wash hands with institution-approved antiseptic soap.	Standard precautions; reduces transmission of microorganisms.	
8. Obtain all necessary supplies and equipment, including emergency medications and equipment.	Time is critical in an emergency. Ensures availability of equipment and supplies as needed.	Many institutions have drape and instrument carts set up with all needed equipment and supplies available at all times.
9. Place child supine, with head of the bed flat.	Facilitates access to the sternal incision.	
10. Ensure medications for pain/anesthesia, sedation, and neuromuscular blockade are available.	Ensures adequate pain management and visualization of the surgical area.	
11. As time and situation permits, identify child with appropriate patient/procedure verification process (e.g., "Time out").	Confirms correct patient, procedure, and site as recommended by JCAHO.	Verification process and documentation is institution specific. Use active communication techniques.
12. Open the supplies with sterile technique.	Decreases the risk of infection.	
13. Apply a grounding pad for the electrocautery unit.	The cautery unit is an electrical device; safe use necessitates that the child is grounded for prevention of electrical shock.	
14. Wash hands with institution-approved antiseptic soap. Surgeon and assistants should perform a surgical scrub.	Decreases transmission of microorganisms.	Alcohol-based hand gel may be used in some institutions; refer to institution-specific protocol.
15. Put on sterile gown and gloves and assist the surgeon and assistants in putting on sterile gown and gloves.	Maintains sterile environment.	
16. Clean the chest with betadine solution with 4×4 gauze from the drape pack and a sponge stick from the instrument tray.	Decreases skin flora and infection risk.	Solution used for skin antisepsis may vary among institutions; refer to institution-specific protocol.
17. Block off the surgical area with sterile towels and secure with towel clips.	Provides a sterile field; reduces transmission of microorganisms.	
18. Place the pediatric lap sheet over the towels so the opening is over the site of the incision.	Secures the area of the sternum for opening.	
19. Place the cautery pencil and sterile suction tubing on the lap sheet and secure with a towel clamp.	Suction is used to remove fluid; cautery is used to control bleeding.	

Procedure for Open Sternotomy: Assist—*Continued*

Steps	Rationale	Considerations
20. Carefully pass off one end of the suction tubing and the non-working end of the cautery to be connected to the suction canister and cautery machine.	Maintains sterile field.	
21. Load No. 15 and 11 blades on the knife handles.	The knife is used to incise the skin.	
22. Connect Pinchon suction tip to the suction tubing.	The incision is small; a regular suction tip may not fit.	
23. Give the surgeon the No. 15 knife.	Necessary for skin incision.	
24. Have sponge and forceps ready; give to the assistant when requested.	Forceps may be needed to remove clot.	
25. Have Metz scissors ready; give to the surgeon or assistant when requested.	Used to cut sutures.	
26. Have wire scissors available; give to the surgeon or assistant when requested.	Tamponade may be relieved by opening sub xyphoid only; if further exposure is necessary, the sternal wires must be cut.	
27. Have vein retractor available; give to the surgeon or assistant when requested.	Used to retract the skin and muscle.	
28. Inquire what type drain the surgeon prefers; give to the surgeon or assistant when requested.	Mediastinal drain is placed to facilitate drainage of blood and fluid after surgery.	
29. Warm sterile 0.9% saline solution with antibiotic added for irrigation and give to the surgeon or assistant when requested.	Used to irrigate the surgical field; decreases risk of infection.	
30. Have closing suture ready; give to the surgeon or assistant when requested.	Used to close the incision.	If the sternum is to be left open, a strut or gortex and additional supplies may be necessary per the surgeon's preference.
31. Apply sterile dressing.	Protects wound and collects drainage.	
32. Dispose of used supplies and equipment appropriately, including sharps.	Reduces transmission of micro-organisms. Protects personnel health.	Some equipment may need to be returned for sterile processing and reuse.
33. Remove protective garb and wash hands.	Standard precautions; reduces transmission of microorganisms.	
34. If emergency procedure cart was used, restock the cart per unit-specific or institution-specific protocol.	Ensures equipment is readily available when needed.	

Expected Outcomes	Unexpected Outcomes
• Cardiac tamponade is resolved	• Cardiac arrest or need for extracorpeal membrane oxygenation (ECMO) • Unresolved tamponade that leads to death
• Bleeding is controlled and blood product requirements are decreased	• Continued bleeding
• Chest drains effectively drain surgical area	• Coagulapathies
• Cardiac output improved, resulting in improved tissue perfusion	• Decreased or absent drainage from chest drains • Dysrhythmias, including heart block
• Child is free from lung injury	• Ventricular dysfunction • Pneumothorax • Hemothorax
• Child is free from infection	• Wound infection • Sepsis
• The ECHO findings indicate pericardial effusion is resolved; CXR shows stable cardiac silhouette	• Fluid reaccumulation • Recurrence of tamponade
• Child has acceptable level of comfort	• Unmanaged pain

Monitoring and Care of the Child

Activities and Interventions	Rationale	Reportable Conditions
1. During the procedure, monitor heart rate, rhythm, blood pressure, pulse oximetry, urine output; ideally the child has central line access and arterial blood pressure monitoring.	Open sternotomy is a surgical procedure, often an emergency. Adequate monitoring of the child during and after the procedure is imperative for patient safety.	• Rhythm changes, including asystole, bradycardia, tachycardia, heart block, and ventricular or atrial arrhythmias • Hypotension that may necessitate blood or fluid replacement and escalation of inotropic support • Hypertension that may necessitate escalation of vasopressor medications • Arterial blood gas abnormalities that may necessitate medication administration or change in mechanical ventilation settings • Decreased or no urine output • Narrowed pulse pressure • Elevated filling pressures as indicated by transduced right atrial line or central venous pressure monitoring line
2. Monitor coagulation and hematology laboratory results before, during, and after the procedure (CBC, PT, international normalized ratio [INR], PTT, and fibrinogen).	Anemia, thrombocytopenia, and coagulation abnormalities can exist before or result from the procedure. These abnormalities may necessitate treatment.	• Hemoglobin 1 g/dL less than baseline • Platelets less than 50,000 • Elevated coagulation studies • Ongoing bleeding
3. Analgesia and sedation monitoring and documentation per institution-specific protocol.	This is a surgical procedure that necessitates sedation, analgesia, and neuromuscular blockade of the child; appropriate monitoring facilitates prompt identification of side effects, complications, or inadequate sedation or analgesia.	• Changes in level of consciousness • Pupil changes • Pain or agitation

Monitoring and Care of the Child—Cont'd

Activities and Interventions	Rationale	Reportable Conditions
4. Monitor chest tube drainage and patency carefully every 15 minutes for 1 hour, then every 30 minutes for 1 hour, then every hour.	Determines blood loss before, during, and after the procedure. Excessive bleeding should resolve. The chest tube can clot or malfunction and inadequately drain.	• Abrupt cessation of chest tube drainage • Abrupt increase of chest tube drainage • Bleeding of more than 3 mL/kg/h • Clots present in chest tube and drainage system that impair drainage
5. Obtain CXR after procedure.	Confirms placement of any new chest tubes or drainage devices; confirms absence of hemothorax, pneumothorax, and enlarged cardiac silhouette after the procedure.	• Pneumothorax • Hemothorax • Pleural effusion • Enlarged cardiac silhouette
6. Obtain echocardiogram at completion of procedure.	Evaluates cardiac function and resolved accumulation of fluid, blood, or clot in pericardial space.	• Diminished cardiac function that necessitates additional or increased inotropic support • Ongoing fluid accumulation or hematoma

Documentation

- Procedure performed, date, time of initiation and completion, person performing procedure, and individuals assisting
- Presence of informed consent, if obtained
- Indications for the procedure
- Estimated blood loss
- Personnel notified
- Patient/procedure verification process
- Vital signs and other assessments throughout the procedure
- Medications administered
- Fluids administered
- Child's response and outcome of procedure
- Child and family education
- Blood products administered
- Chest tube output at completion of procedure
- Unexpected outcome and related treatment

References
1. Curley MAQ, Moloney-Harmon P, editors: *Critical care nursing of infants and children,* ed 2, Philadelphia, 2001, Saunders.
2. Wessel DL, Laussen P: Cardiac intensive care. In Fuhrman BP, Zimmerman J, editors: *Pediatric critical care,* ed 3, Philadelphia, 2006, Mosby.

Additional Reading
Chang AC, Hanley FL, et al: *Pediatric cardiac intensive care,* Baltimore, 1998, Williams & Wilkins.

Pericardiocentesis: Assist

P U R P O S E : A catheter is inserted into the pericardial space to evacuate pericardial fluid for diagnostic or therapeutic management of effusions and cardiac tamponade

Kerri Oates and Ruth M. Lebet

PREREQUISITE KNOWLEDGE

- Child development as it relates to clinical assessment
- Mastery of pediatric advanced life support competencies
- Appropriate pediatric dosing of analgesics
- Appropriate management of the child undergoing procedural sedation
  - ❖ Ketamine has been suggested as an appropriate agent for this procedure because it is less likely to cause hypoventilation and hypotension and because it increases cardiovascular sympathetic tone.[1]
- Principles of aseptic technique
- Anatomy and physiology of the heart
- Signs and symptoms of cardiac tamponade, including elevated venous pressures, neck vein distension, hypotension not responsive to fluid resuscitation, muffled heart sounds, pulsus paradoxus of more than 10 mm Hg, and narrow pulse pressure. Neck vein distension, pulsus paradoxus, and muffled heart sounds are difficult to identify in the infant and small child.[1-4]
  - ❖ A few small studies in children have reported that significant falls in the peak of the pulse oximetry waveform with inspiration were associated with pulsus paradoxus.[5] *(Level V*)*
- Signs and symptoms of pericarditis, including tachycardia, fever, cough, chest pain, distant heart sounds, hepatomegaly, and friction rub[1-3]

- Causes of pericardial effusion, including viral or idiopathic pericarditis, malignant disease, Kawasaki disease, rheumatic fever, late effects of some chemotherapeutic agents, bleeding at the surgical site after cardiac surgery, postpericardiotomy syndrome, chest trauma, HIV, and systemic lupus erythematosis.[1,2,4]
- Diagnostic procedures for identification or localization of effusion[1-3,6]
  - ❖ Chest x-ray: this image does not distinguish cardiomegaly from effusion; a second imaging study is needed to confirm effusion
  - ❖ Echocardiogram (echo)
  - ❖ A study of 73 pediatric patients undergoing percutaneous echocardiographically guided pericardiocentesis found that this technique resulted in fewer complications than traditional blind pericardiocentesis.[6] *(Level IV*)*
  - ❖ Benefits of echo-guided pericardiocentesis are: rapid confirmation of the presence of an effusion; accurate location of the effusion
  - ❖ Magnetic resonance imaging (MRI)
  - ❖ Computed tomography (CT) scan
- Complications of pericardiocentesis, including myocardial injury, laceration of a coronary artery, arrhythmias, pneumothorax, hemopericardium, liver laceration, and infection[1,4]
- Except in an emergency, informed consent is necessary before pericardiocentesis

---

* Level V: Clinical studies in more than one or two patient populations and situations to support recommendations

* Level IV: Limited clinical studies to support recommendations

CHILD AND FAMILY ASSESSMENT

- Child's developmental level and ability to interact ➸*Rationale:* These factors influence preparation of the child and interaction.
- History of congenital heart defect ➸*Rationale:* Presence of a congenital heart defect may complicate placement of the pericardial catheter.
- History of cardiac surgery and date and type of surgery performed ➸*Rationale:* More ectopy may be expected in children with recent surgery.
- History of recent infection or fever ➸*Rationale:* Determines need for cultures of fluid obtained during the procedure and the need for an infectious disease consultation.
- Time since last oral intake ➸*Rationale:* If the child is to undergo sedation or anesthesia, information is need for implementation of fasting guidelines per institution-specific protocol.
- Child's and family's understanding of the reasons for and risks and benefits of pericardiocentesis ➸*Rationale:* Evaluates child's and family's understanding of the procedure and provides a guide for ongoing education.
- Desire of family members to be present during the procedure ➸*Rationale:* Family members may provide support and comfort measures to the child but should have the choice not to remain with the child.

CHILD AND FAMILY EDUCATION

Individualized, developmentally appropriate education is provided to the family and to the child based on the desire for knowledge, readiness to learn, and overall neurologic and psychosocial state.

- Provide information on the cause of the pericardial effusion and reasons to evacuate the fluid ➸*Rationale:* Providing information decreases anxiety and fear, allows the family's participation in decision making, and facilitates informed consent.
- Review the steps involved to evacuate the fluid, including the sedation/analgesia/anesthesia strategy, and review how the child will be sedated and will feel after the sedation ➸*Rationale:* Review of the steps involved prepares the older child to know what to expect, and the family's anxiety and concern that the child will have pain or anxiety may be decreased.
- Explain that the drainage tube may be left in place to allow for additional drainage if a large amount of fluid or evidence of continued fluid accumulation is found ➸*Rationale:* Advance knowledge of events facilitates coping of the family and child.
- Encourage questions and answer questions as they arise ➸*Rationale:* Reinforcement of information is needed during periods of stress and is especially important given the emergent nature of this procedure.

EQUIPMENT

- A 3-inch 22-gauge spinal needle (infant)
- A 4-inch to 6-inch, 16-gauge to 18-gauge spinal needle (older child or adolescent)
- Syringes (5-mL, 10-mL, 20-mL, and 50-mL)
- Electrocardiogram (ECG) machine with alligator clip
- Echo machine (in the Emergency Department or Intensive Care Unit [ICU] setting)
- Fluoroscopy (in the cardiac catheterization laboratory)
- Appropriate skin antiseptic: chlorhexidine for children 2 months or older; povidone-iodine for infants less than 2 months
- Sterile gloves, gowns, and masks
- Appropriately sized pigtail catheter: 5F, 6F, 7F, or 7.5F, with dilator and introducer
- Three-way stopcock
- Suture
- Blade
- Culture tubes
- Tape or transparent dressing to secure catheter
- Sterile saline solution
- 1% lidocaine for tissue infiltration with appropriately sized needle and syringe
- Topical anesthetic cream (EMLA [Asta-Zeneca, LP, Wilmington, DE]; Ela-Max [Ferndale Laboratories, Inc., Ferndale, MI], lidocaine hydrochloride: topical)
- Gauze
- Band-aid

Procedure for Pericardiocentesis: Assist

Steps	Rationale	Considerations
1. Ensure child and family understand procedure and questions are answered.	Evaluates and reinforces understanding of previously taught information.	Developmental and cognitive levels and degree of anxiety determine teaching approach and influence effectiveness.
2. Document time of child's last oral intake.	If the child is to undergo sedation or anesthesia; compliance with fasting guidelines minimizes the risk of aspiration.	Refer to institution-specific fasting guidelines for infants and children.

Procedure continues on following page

Procedure **for Pericardiocentesis: Assist**—*Continued*

Steps	Rationale	Considerations
3. Confirm that signed informed consent has been obtained.	Ensures medical-legal compliance as suggested by the Joint Commission on Accreditation of Healthcare Organizations (JCAHO).	For emergency situations, the organization may have a protocol/procedure in place for assumption of consent. Refer to institution-specific protocols.
4. Ensure cardiorespiratory monitoring, including blood pressure monitoring, is in place and that the child has functioning venous access.	Continuous cardiorespiratory monitoring allows continuous assessment of the child's status. Hypotension is an anticipated complication of this procedure. Functioning venous access is necessary for administration of emergency medications or sedation/ analgesia as needed.	Alarm limits set should be individualized to the child.
5. Gather needed equipment and supplies.	Facilitates completion of the procedure in a timely manner.	
6. Administer prescribed sedation and numbing cream to site at least 30 minutes before the procedure. In some situations, anesthesia is provided by an anesthesiologist or certified registered nurse anesthetist (CRNA).	Allow time for the sedatives to take effect and time for the cream to numb the skin. Critically ill children may not tolerate conscious sedation and may need a general anesthetic.	Numbing cream is placed at the subxiphoid process. In emergency situations, this step is omitted.
7. Wash hands.	Standard precautions.	
8. Position child supine with the head elevated at a 30-degree angle. *(Level II*)*	Allows the heart to drop down in the chest for access.	Lowers the diaphragm and abdominal organs, which allows blood to pool in the apex of the heart.
9. Identify child with appropriate patient/procedure verification process (e.g., "time out").	Confirms correct patient, procedure, and site as recommended by the Joint Commission for Accreditation of Healthcare Organizations (JCAHO) and prevents unnecessary medical procedures.	Verification process and documentation is institution specific. Use active communication techniques.
10. Clean skin around the xiphoid area with chlorhexidine or povidone-iodine; sterile drapes are placed.	Prepares sterile environment; reduces transmission of microorganisms.	
11. The individual who performs the procedure and others who are in the procedure area put on masks, gowns, and gloves.	Promotes aseptic environment and reduces the transmission of microorganisms.	
12. Subxiphoid area is injected with local anesthetic, most often 1% lidocaine.	Provides additional pain relief during and after the procedure.	Used when procedural sedation is provided (as opposed to anesthesia).
13. In a sterile fashion, provide the appropriately sized syringe (20-mL or 50-mL is recommended) partially filled with sterile saline solution and attached to the needle. A stopcock and a second syringe with saline solution may also be necessary if echo is used.	If a question of position of the needle remains once fluid is aspirated into the syringe, 5 mL of agitated saline solution may be injected into the pericardial space to provide a contrast study of microbubbles seen on echo.	

* Level II: Theory-based; no research data to support recommendations; recommendations from expert consensus group may exist

Procedure for Pericardiocentesis: Assist—*Continued*

Steps	Rationale	Considerations
14. With an alligator clip, attach a precordial electrocardiographic lead to the needle hub if the procedure is to be done without echo or fluoroscopic guidance.[1]	If needle is advanced through the pericardium and contacts wall of the ventricle, an injury pattern (wide QRS, marked ST-T wave changes) or ventricular ectopy is noted on ECG trace.	
15. The needle is inserted inferior and to the left of the xiphoid process and advanced at a 45-degree angle toward the left scapular tip with continuous aspiration until fluid is obtained. This is optimally done with echo or fluoroscopic guidance. If the procedure is done blind, immediately notify the individual performing the procedure if ECG changes are seen.	Echo or fluoroscopic guidance provides visualization of the placement of the needle into the pericardial space, which minimizes complications. *(Level IV*)*	The needle is removed slowly if ECG changes are seen. If echo is used, the needle may be inserted in the left chest where the effusion has been localized.[6]
16. If child's condition is hemodynamically stable, 25 to 50 mL of fluid can be removed initially. *(Level IV*)*	Fluid is removed in small aliquots to maintain hemodynamic stability. Removal of large volumes has been reported to result in cardiogenic shock.[7]	The size of child should be considered; removal of large amounts of fluid relative to the child's total blood volume may necessitate fluid replacement.
17. After fluid removal, if a catheter is to be left in place for continued drainage, a guide wire is passed through the needle and the needle is removed.	The catheter is threaded over the guide wire and placed in the pericardial space. The catheter allows ongoing drainage of fluid from the pericardial space.	
18. A skin incision is made at the insertion site, and a vessel dilator is threaded over the guide wire. The dilator is removed, and an introducer is threaded over the guide wire; the guide wire is removed, and a pigtail catheter is threaded through introducer and positioned along left heart border. The introducer is removed.	Dilation facilitates placement of the catheter with minimal trauma.	
19. The catheter is sutured in place, and a transparent dressing is applied over the site.	Secures the catheter and guards against inadvertent dislodgement of the catheter.	
20. Connect the pigtail catheter to a sterile collection unit for continuous drainage or place a sterile cap on the end of the catheter for intermittent drainage.	Maintains sterility of system and allows drainage and measurement of fluid.	Intermittent drainage of the pigtail catheter has been associated with less catheter obstruction.[6] *(Level IV*)*
21. If specimens have been collected, label them immediately at the bedside and send them to the laboratory. Use two patient identifiers on the specimen label.	Allows for a "double-check" and prevents the possibility of sending the wrong specimen or mislabeling the specimen.	Refer to institution-specific protocols for obtaining and sending laboratory specimens and appropriate patient identifiers.

Procedure continues on following page

* Level IV: Limited clinical studies to support recommendations

Procedure for Pericardiocentesis: Assist—*Continued*

Steps	Rationale	Considerations
22. Dispose of used supplies and equipment in appropriate receptacle; ensure that sharps are disposed of appropriately.	Standard precautions; reduces transmission of microorganisms. Protects personnel.	
23. Remove gown, gloves, and mask and dispose of appropriately; wash hands.	Standard precautions; reduces transmission of microorganisms.	
24. Obtain chest x-ray or repeat echocardiogram.	Confirms catheter placement and drainage of fluid.	

Expected Outcomes

- Needle or pigtail catheter is located in the pericardial space; fluid is removed
- Procedure is completed without complications; hemodynamic status remains stable or improves

- Catheter remains patent
- Child has acceptable level of comfort

Unexpected Outcomes

- Inability to locate effusion or remove fluid

- Laceration of coronary arteries that leads to hemopericardium or tamponade
- Pneumothorax
- Arrhythmias that result from myocardial injury
- Death from myocardial perforation
- Hemodynamic compromise/hypotension during and after the procedure
- Inability to drain fluid through the catheter
- Unmanaged pain

Monitoring and Care of the Child

Activities and Interventions	Rationale	Reportable Conditions
1. Monitor child's tolerance of fluid removal.	Children with hemodynamically compromised conditions may need fluid boluses of 10 to 15 mL/kg until the condition is stable.	• Hemodynamic compromise • Unresponsiveness to fluid bolus
2. Vital signs are obtained every 5 minutes during the procedure, every 15 minutes for 1 hour after the procedure is completed, and then every hour for 4 hours.	Allows assessment of the child's tolerance of the procedure; deterioration in vital signs after procedure completion may indicate fluid has reaccumulated.	• Unstable or deteriorating vital signs
3. Assess effectiveness of pain management strategy and provide appropriate interventions. Allow the family to assist with nonpharmacologic means to comfort and support the child.	Early identification of the child's discomfort allows for immediate attention.	• Report of unresolved pain and discomfort • Continued irritability or changes in physiologic condition

Documentation

- Child and family education
- Size of catheter placed and individual who placed the catheter
- Volume of fluid drained
- Specimens collected
- Medications administered
- Child's response to the evacuation of fluid
- Patient/procedure verification process
- X-ray confirmation of catheter placement
- Comfort assessment and any specific interventions provided
- Unexpected outcomes and related treatment

References

1. Scarfone RJ, et al: Cardiac tamponade complicating post-pericardiotomy syndrome, *Pediatr Emerg Care* 19(4):268-271, 2003.
2. Altman C: Pericarditis and pericardial disease. In Garson Jr A, Bricker J, Fisher D, et al, editors: *The science and practice of cardiology*, ed 2, Baltimore, 1998, Williams & Wilkins.
3. Behrman RE, et al: *Nelson textbook of pediatrics*, ed 17, Philadelphia, 2004, Elsevier.
4. Spodick DH: Pathophysiology of cardiac tamponade, *Chest* 113(5):1372, 1998.
5. Tamburro RF, et al: Detection of pulsus paradoxus associated with large pericardial effusions in pediatric patients by analysis of the pulse-oximetry waveform, *Pediatrics* 109(4):673-677, 2002.
6. Tsang TS, et al: Percutaneous echocardiographically guided pericardiocentesis in pediatric patients: evaluation of safety and efficacy, *J Am Soc Echocardiograph* 11(11):1072-1077, 1998.
7. Tsang TS, et al: Echocardiographically guided pericardiocentesis: evolution and state-of-the-art technique, *Mayo Clinic Proc* 73(7):647-652, 1998.

Additional Readings

Lanros NE, Barber JM: Chest trauma: damage to the heart, pericardium, and aortic arch. In Lanros NE, Barber JM, editors: *Emergency nursing: with certification preparation & review*, ed 4, Stamford, CT, 1997, Appleton & Lange.

Metules TJ: Iatrogenic injuries: cardiac tamponade, 1999, *RNWeb*, from http://www.rnweb.com/rnweb/.

Tsang TS, et al: Rescue echocardiographically guided pericardiocentesis for cardiac perforation complicating catheter-based procedures: the Mayo Clinic experience, *J Am Coll Cardiol* 32(5):1345, 1998.

Zaglaniczny K, Acker J: Anatomy and physiology of the pediatric population. In Zaglaniczny K, Acker J, editors: *Clinical guide to pediatric anesthesia*, Philadelphia, 1999, Saunders.

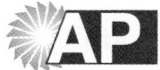

Cardioversion

P U R P O S E : To terminate a rapid rhythm that causes cardiovascular compromise with timed delivery of energy (shock) to the heart

Mary Rummell

PREREQUISITE KNOWLEDGE

- Child development as it relates to clinical assessment and synchronized cardioversion
- Anatomy and physiology of the heart, specifically the conduction system
- Basic electrocardiographic (ECG) interpretation
- Identification and classification of arrhythmias in the pediatric patient with knowledge of the effect of the rhythm on pulse, heart rate, and systemic perfusion
- Tachyarrhythmias treated with synchronized cardioversion include supraventricular tachycardia (SVT), ventricular tachycardia (VT) with a pulse, and atrial flutter. Synchronized cardioversion is the treatment of choice in children with hemodynamic compromise with SVT or VT with a pulse.[1-3] Treatment of atrial flutter is usually elective and should be planned to provide for adequate sedation and pain management.[4]
- Cardiovascular assessment of the infant and child, including normal infant, child, and adolescent heart and respiratory rates
- Mastery of pediatric advanced life support competencies
- Electrical safety considerations

- Mechanical and safety features of the defibrillator, including the ability to switch between paddles and multifunction defibrillator electrode pads and adult and pediatric paddles
- Appropriate pediatric dosing of analgesics and competency in procedural sedation

CHILD AND FAMILY ASSESSMENT

- Child's developmental level and ability to interact **➟Rationale:** These factors influence preparation of the child and interaction.
- History of illness, fever, hypoxemia, hypovolemia, metabolic stress, drugs/poisons/toxins, and pain or anxiety **➟Rationale:** Determines all potential causes for the tachycardia. Sinus tachycardia (ST) is caused by the previous conditions, and the underlying cause of the ST should be treated. ST does not respond to synchronized cardioversion.[4,5]
- Vital signs, including heart rate, blood pressure, color, work of breathing, pulses, and systemic perfusion **➟Rationale:** Identifies the infant or child with hemodynamic compromise to determine urgency of the situation and to develop a plan of care that incorporates the most appropriate therapies and support systems to ensure optimal outcomes.[3-5]
- Electrocardiographic results for SVT or VT **➟Rationale:** Differentiates between ST and SVT because treatment differs. Evaluates VT and the presence or absence of pulses.[4]

- Family's understanding of arrhythmia, severity of child's cardiovascular status, and cardioversion procedure, including risks and benefits ➤➤*Rationale:* The family should understand the seriousness of the child's condition and the urgency of the procedure.[2,4]
- Desire of family members to remain with the child during the procedure ➤➤*Rationale:* Family may provide support to the child after the procedure but may not be comfortable being present during the procedure; family members should have the choice not to remain with the child. A designated health care team member should be identified to provide the family with support and updates during the procedure.[2,4]

CHILD AND FAMILY EDUCATION

The decision to use synchronized cardioversion is made when the child has an unstable tachyarrhythmia. Rapid evaluation is necessary for determination of the history, the rhythm, and the effect on systemic perfusion. Education is provided to the family and the child as the assessment and the decision for synchronized cardioversion are made. Short simple explanations are most effective during an emergency situation. Anticipate that information needs to be repeated.

- Assess the family's understanding of the etiology of child's instability ➤➤*Rationale:* Assessment provides the basis for identification of educational needs and development of an educational plan.
- Review the child's medical condition and rationale for emergency intervention with the family ➤➤*Rationale:*

Providing information helps to decrease the family's anxiety level and offers reassurance during a time of extreme stress; concrete information, such as review of the rhythm strip, may facilitate learning.
- Explain the procedure to the family and the child at an appropriate developmental level for child ➤➤*Rationale:* Providing information helps to decrease anxiety.
- Encourage questions and answer questions as they arise ➤➤*Rationale:* Reinforcement of information is needed during periods of stress and is especially important given the emergent nature of the procedure.

EQUIPMENT

- Defibrillator/monitor capable of delivering a synchronized shock
- Pediatric paddles (for use in infants less than 1 year of age or 10 kg or less) and adult paddles
- Conduction/electrode paste, prepackaged gelled conduction pads, or multifunctional defibrillator electrode pads
  ❖ Multifunction defibrillator electrode pads are available in pediatric and adult sizes. Refer to the manufacturer's recommendations for appropriate sizing.
- Electrocardiographic electrodes and cable for defibrillator
- Emergency pediatric resuscitation equipment/medications
- Appropriately sized bag-valve-mask resuscitation bag
- Blankets to position the infant
- Clean gloves

Procedure **for Cardioversion**		
Steps	**Rationale**	**Considerations**
1. As time permits, ensure child and family understand procedure and questions are answered.	Evaluates and reinforces understanding of previously taught information.	Developmental level, cognitive ability, and anxiety level determine approach to and effectiveness of teaching.
2. Bring defibrillator/monitor and emergency equipment cart to the bedside.	Ensures availability of emergency equipment.	
3. Wash hands and put on clean gloves.	Standard precautions; reduces transmission of microorganisms.	
4. Attach ECG electrodes to periphery of the chest. Place on shoulders or lateral chest surfaces. Ground lead may be on the abdomen or thigh (Figure 45-1).[4] (*Level VI**)	Allows evaluation of the chest, ability to perform cardiac compressions if necessary, and placement of paddles/multifunction defibrillator electrodes.	Follow specific directions on defibrillator/monitor. ECG input to monitor may come from the bedside monitoring equipment through a cable that plugs into the input jack on the defibrillator/ monitor. Input may also come from the multifunction pediatric defibrillator electrode pads (Figure 45-2).

Procedure continues on following page

* Level VI: Clinical studies in a variety of patient populations and situations to support recommendations

Procedure | **for Cardioversion**—*Continued*

Steps	Rationale	Considerations

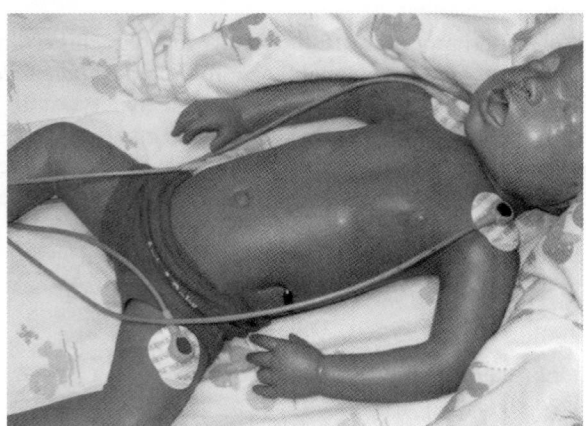

FIGURE 45-1   Placement of ECG leads on infant before cardioversion.

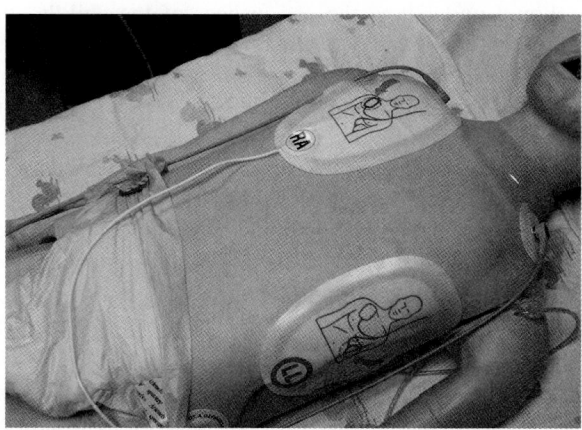

FIGURE 45-2   Use of multifunction defibrillator electrode pads on child.

Steps	Rationale	Considerations
		ECG input from the paddles is not recommended because artifact from movement of the paddles may simulate an R wave and result in inappropriate discharge of energy.
5. Select a defibrillator/monitor lead that displays an R wave of sufficient amplitude to be counted by the tachometer and a T wave that is not counted. Be sure that artifact does not interfere with the conduction. *(Level VI*)*	Provides a clear ECG recording that facilitates synchronization and prevents energy delivery on the T wave.	Select one of the leads in the lead select position. Do *not* use the paddle position. Adjust the gain as necessary to adequately display the R wave.
6. Activate the synchronization mode by pressing the sync button on the defibrillator/monitor.	The R wave must be identified and marked by the defibrillator/monitor to provide the synchronization. The marker must be only on the R wave. This reduces the possibility of delivering energy on the T wave (the vulnerable period) that may precipitate ventricular fibrillation and cardiac arrest (Figure 45-3).[1,4,6] *(Level VI*)*	The defibrillator monitor displays a cue when sync mode is activated, such as the word "sync" displayed at the bottom of the monitor screen or the sync button may light up.
7. Select the desired energy dose. *(Level VI*)*	Currently, for both monophasic and biphasic defibrillators, the American Heart Association recommends an initial dose for synchronized cardioversion in both infants and children of 0.5 to 1 J/kg. If the tachyarrhythmia persists, the dose is doubled to 1 to 2 J/kg.[1,3,4,7]	If the SVT persists after two attempts at cardioversion, reevaluate the rhythm for ST.[4]
8. Select the appropriately sized paddles.[3,4,8] *(Level VI*)*	Select the paddles or electrode pads to provide the lowest transthoracic impedance and the greatest current flow.	Transthoracic impedance is decreased with use of the largest sized paddles or pads that provide good contact with the chest but do not touch each other. The pediatric paddles should be used for infants 1 year of age or less and 10 kg or less.[3,4,6,8]

* Level VI: Clinical studies in a variety of patient populations and situations to support recommendations

Procedure **for Cardioversion**—*Continued*

Steps	Rationale	Considerations

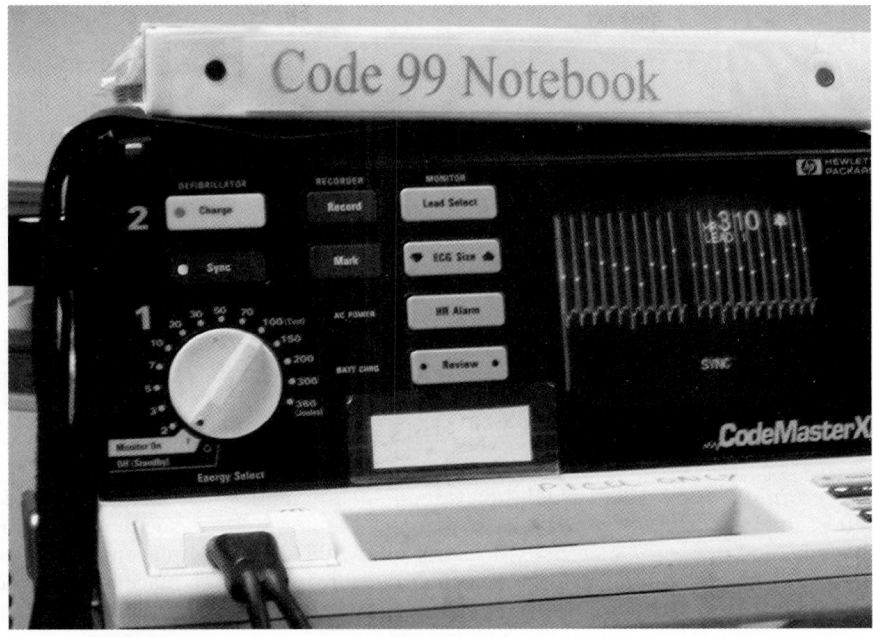

FIGURE 45-3 Supraventricular tachycardia on defibrillator/monitor set in sync mode. Note marking on each of R waves, light activated on sync button, and "sync" displayed on screen.

Steps	Rationale	Considerations
9. Apply electrode cream/gel to both paddle surfaces. Take care not to get gel on hands. May also use prepackaged gelled conduction pads. *(Level VI*)*	Improves the delivery of current.	Do *not* rub paddles together to spread the gel. This may cause a discharge between the paddles. Do *not* use saline solution–soaked pads because they may cause an arc between paddles. Do *not* use alcohol because it raises impedance and can cause skin burns. Sonographic gels are not good conductors. May use multifunction pediatric defibrillator electrode pads. Do *not* cut the electrodes for any reason.[4]
10. Place the paddles on the chest so that the heart is between the paddles/multifunction electrode pads. *(Level VI*)* *Anterior chest position:* One paddle on the upper right chest below the clavicle, the other on the left chest, left of the nipple at the anterior axillary line (Figure 45-4).	Cardioversion requires the flow of current through the myocardium a millisecond after depolarization and before repolarization. This countershock terminates the tachycardia and restores a stable rhythm.[4] If the paddles/pads are incorrectly placed, the energy does not travel through the heart and fails to terminate the tachycardia.	Choose the largest paddle/pad size that allows for good contact with the skin without touching each other. A space of 1 inch is recommended between the pads to prevent arcing from one pad to the other. If this spacing is not possible, then paddles must be used.

Procedure continues on following page

* Level VI: Clinical studies in a variety of patient populations and situations to support recommendations

Procedure | **for Cardioversion**—*Continued*

Steps	Rationale	Considerations

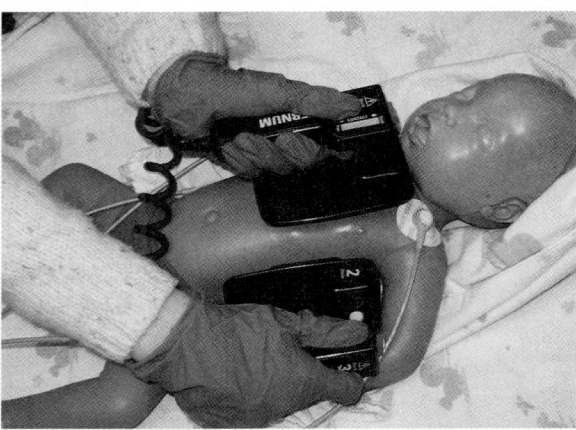

FIGURE 45-4   Correct placement of pediatric paddles on anterior chest of infant.

Anterior-posterior position: One paddle/pad just left of the sternum, the other on the back behind the heart (Figure 45-5).

The paddles/pads require sufficient space between them so that the electricity does not follow the course of least resistance from one paddle to the other instead of through the heart.[4,6,9]

If the paddles/pads are too large for adequate skin contact with standard placement, the anterior-posterior placement should be used.[3,4,8,10] Blanket rolls can be used to support the infant.

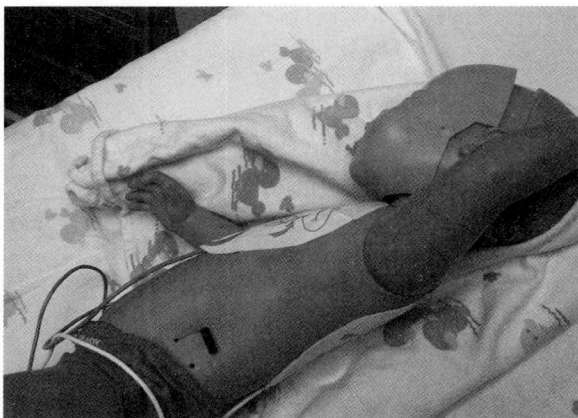

FIGURE 45-5   Correct placement of pediatric multifunction defibrillator electrode pads in anterior-posterior position on infant. Infant in photo is lying on side. Infant may also be positioned on back.

Permanent pacemaker: Paddles/pads should not be placed directly over a permanent pacemaker generator.

Temporary pacemaker: Disconnect the pacing wires from the temporary generator. Cover the wire tips with the attached cap or clean powder-free glove to prevent conduction from the defibrillator.

Place the paddles/pads 10 to 15 cm away from generator site. Transmission of electricity through the generator prevents the full energy dose from reaching the heart and may damage or reset the generator.[4,6]

Transmission of current along temporary pacemaker wires may damage heart muscle.[6]

Procedure for Cardioversion—*Continued*

Steps	Rationale	Considerations
11. Apply firm pressure to each paddle/pad.	Provides optimal contact with skin and decreases transthoracic impedance. Improves flow of electrical current through the heart.	
12. Charge paddles/pads per instructions from the manufacturer.	Paddles usually have a charge button on the right-hand paddle. A charge button is also found on the front of the defibrillator/monitor.	
13. Ensure safety of child and colleagues.[4,9] One: I am clear. Two: You are clear. Three: Oxygen is clear. Four: Everyone is clear.	Electrical current is dangerous to anyone in contact with the child and anything touching the child. Oxygen from respiratory devices presents a fire hazard if a spark occurs with arcing during delivery of the energy.[3,4,9]	Oxygen must be removed completely out of the field of electrical current because of the possibility of combustion.
14. Verify that the defibrillator is in the synchronous mode with accurate marking of the R wave. Verify the energy dose selected. Verify that everyone is clear of the child.	Ensures appropriate dose, timing of dose, and safety of child and colleagues.	Dose: 0.5 to 1 J/kg body weight. Pediatric and adult sized paddles should be available.
15. Depress buttons on both paddles or on the defibrillator/monitor control panel and hold until charge is delivered.	The monitor/defibrillator only discharges after identification of the R wave. This may necessitate the recognition of two to three QRS complexes. The buttons *must* be held until the energy is discharged.	With use of pads, select PADS from the ECG source button, use an electrode adaptor cable, and attach pads to the cable. The discharge buttons are on the adaptor cable. Each defibrillator/monitor has unit-specific information.
16. Observe the monitor for: Conversion of the tachyarrhythmia to a slower single-focus rhythm. Continuation of the tachyarrhythmia. Ventricular fibrillation (VF).	Delivery of energy should result in depolarization of the myocardial muscle cells, resulting in a single-focus rhythm (sinus rhythm).	If the tachyarrhythmia continues, reset the Joules to 1 to 2 J/kg, reset the synchronization, and attempt again. If still not successful after the second attempt, reevaluate the rhythm.[4,6] VF may occur. If VF occurs, reset the defibrillator/ monitor and proceed with defibrillation (see Procedure 46 for further information).
17. Continue to monitor the child after successful cardioversion for recurrence of the tachyarrhythmia.	Child may have conversion back into tachyarrhythmia unless the underlying cause is identified and treated.	
18. Clean defibrillator, remove residual conduction gel from paddles, and discard used supplies.	Standard precautions; reduces transmission of microorganisms.	
19. Remove gloves and wash hands.	Standard precautions.	

Expected Outcomes

- Appropriate functioning of defibrillator
- Conversion of the tachyarrhythmia to a single-source rhythm (sinus rhythm)
- Improved cardiac output

- Stable respiratory status
- Skin integrity remains intact
- Child has acceptable level of comfort

Unexpected Outcomes

- Missing equipment or equipment failure
- Persistent tachyarrhythmias
- Ventricular fibrillation
- Asystole
- Indications of shock including weak or absent peripheral pulses, delayed capillary refill time, mottled skin tones, cool extremities, and decreased level of consciousness
- Respiratory failure or arrest
- Skin burns
- Unmanaged pain or anxiety

Monitoring and Care of the Child

Activities and Interventions	Rationale	Reportable Conditions
1. Evaluate cardiorespiratory status before, during, and after cardioversion.	Ensure adequate oxygenation and ventilation before and throughout procedure. Provide ongoing evaluation of cardiac output. May need to change to defibrillation from synchronized cardioversion.[4]	• Decreased oxygen saturation • Increased work of breathing • Apnea • Hypotension • Poor perfusion • Loss of pulses • Deterioration in neurologic status
2. Continuous monitoring and evaluation of ECG.	Assess results of cardioversion attempts. Perfusing rhythm may degenerate into nonperfusing rhythm. Tachyarrhythmia may reoccur after successful cardioversion.[4,6]	• Ventricular fibrillation • Asystole • Tachyarrhythmia (SVT, VT, atrial flutter) • No change in rhythm with cardioversion attempts
3. Ensure that child has venous access.	Intravenous antiarrhythmics may be necessary for ongoing treatment for arrhythmia.	• Unsuccessful intravenous (IV) placement
4. Assess the skin for the presence of burns.	Skin burns may occur from local hyperthermia and increased sensitivity of the skin of infants and young children.	• Skin burns
5. Evaluate child's response to cardioversion and the effectiveness of pain management strategy. Provide appropriate interventions. Encourage the family to assist. with nonpharmacologic means to comfort and support the child.	Procedure is frightening and painful, especially to a child who does not have the developmental ability to understand procedure. Early identification of discomfort. promotes prompt attention.	• Unresolved pain and discomfort (document with age-appropriate pain scale). See Procedure 173. • Continued irritability
6. Evaluate response of family and child to diagnosis and understanding of pathophysiology of tachyarrhythmia.	Tachyarrhythmias may necessitate pharmacotherapy or radiofrequency ablation and may reoccur. Compliance with management is necessary.	• History of noncompliance with medical management • Lack of understanding of mechanism of tachyarrhythmia

Documentation

- Assessment of airway, breathing, and circulation
- Cardiac rhythm with printout of ECG before, during, and after cardioversion
- Joules used and number of attempts for conversion
- Child's response to cardioversion
- Printout from defibrillator if available
- Comfort assessment and any specific interventions provided
- Child and family education
- Unexpected outcomes and related treatment

References
1. Atkins DL, Chameides L, Fallat ME, et al: Resuscitation science of pediatrics, *Ann Emerg Med* 37(4 Suppl):S41-S48, 2001.
2. Brown K, Bocock J: Update in pediatric resuscitation, *Emerg Med Clin North Am* 20(1):1-26, 2002.
3. Castle N: Paediatric resuscitation: advanced life support. *Emerg Nurs* 10(1):31-38, 2002.
4. Hazinski MF: *PALS provider manual,* Dallas, 2002, American Heart Association.
5. Hazinski MF: *Manual of pediatric critical care,* St. Louis, 1999, Mosby.
6. Hambach C: Cardioversion. In Lynn-McHale DJ, Carlson K, editors: *AACN procedure manual for critical care,* ed 4, Philadelphia, 2001, Saunders.
7. Mair M: Emergency: monophasic and biphasic defibrillators, *AJN* 103(8):58-60, 2003.
8. Pilcher J: *Pocket guide to neonatal EKG interpretation,* Petaluma, CA, 1998, NICU INK Book Publishers.
9. Cook L: Staying current on defibrillator safety, *Nursing* 33(11):44-46, 2003.
10. Samson RA, Berg RA, Bingham R, et al: Use of automated external defibrillators for children: an update, *Circulation* 107(25):3251-3262, 2003.

AP

Defibrillation: External

P U R P O S E : To restore an organized perfusing rhythm with the sudden depolarization of myocardial cells to stop pulseless ventricular tachycardia and ventricular fibrillation and allow the activity of the natural organized pacemaker of the heart to resume

Mary Rummell

PREREQUISITE KNOWLEDGE

- Anatomy and physiology of the heart, specifically the conduction system
- Basic interpretation of an electrocardiogram (ECG)
- Identification of abnormal rhythms in the pediatric patient, specifically ventricular tachycardia and ventricular fibrillation
- Cardiovascular assessment of the infant and child with emphasis on systemic perfusion and peripheral pulses
- Mastery of pediatric basic and advanced life support competencies, including CPR and airway management techniques
- Defibrillation occurs with a sudden depolarization of a mass of myocardium by an electric current passing through the heart.[1,2] This current stops the electrical activity for a brief period reflected as asystole on the cardiac monitor. The intrinsic cardiac rhythm then follows if adequate stores of high-energy phosphates responsible for the automaticity of the myocardium are seen.[1]
- Electrical safety considerations
- Mechanical and safety features of the defibrillator

CHILD AND FAMILY ASSESSMENT

- Perform a rapid cardiopulmonary assessment for identification of abnormal rhythm and treatment of potential causes of the life-threatening arrhythmia ➡️*Rationale:* The primary cause of cardiorespiratory arrest in infants and children is unknown. The arrest may be related, but not limited to, asphyxia, submersion, sepsis, sudden infant death, or ingestion of toxins. Most cardiac arrests result from hypoxia that progresses to hypercarbia, respiratory arrest, and bradycardia. If no intervention occurs, asystole follows. In adults, the primary cause is cardiac in origin.[1,3,4]
- Repeated cardiopulmonary assessment after 1 minute of CPR and at regular intervals thereafter ➡️*Rationale:* Prompt rescue breathing and compressions have shown improved outcomes in the restoration of spontaneous circulation.[1,3-6]
- ECG results for ventricular fibrillation (VF) or ventricular tachycardia (VT) ➡️*Rationale:* Identifies life-threatening arrhythmia facilitates immediate intervention.
- Assess the child for the presence of vascular access ➡️*Rationale:* Emergency medication administration most likely is necessary; identifies available routes for medication administration or need to obtain vascular access. See Procedure 42.
- The family's understanding of the severity of the child's cardiovascular status and the desire to remain with the child during the resuscitation and defibrillation procedures ➡️*Rationale:* Surveys show that family members feel supported when allowed to stay with the child. They also feel comfort by remaining at the bedside even if the resuscita-

tion attempts fail.[1,5] A designated health care team member should be assigned as the support person for the family.

CHILD AND FAMILY EDUCATION

The decision to perform defibrillation is made when the child has a nonperfusing rhythm. Because the resumption of a perfusing rhythm is necessary for life, little time is available for education to the family before the procedure. If the family remains with the child, the support person should also provide education. Short simple explanations are most effective during an emergency situation. Anticipate that information needs to be repeated.

- Rapid assessment of the etiology of the child's unstable rhythm and the family's understanding of events leading up to the situation ➤➤*Rationale:* Assessment provides the basis for education.
- Explanation of the procedure by the support person as it occurs, if the family wishes to remain with the child ➤➤*Rationale:* The family may wish to witness the process and to understand what is done to support the child. If the family is unable or does not wish to be present during the resuscitation, the support person provides regular updates and support during the resuscitation.[1,7]

- Provide information as to next steps in the plan of care at the conclusion of the procedure ➤➤*Rationale:* Regardless of outcome, the family is operating in crisis mode and needs help and direction for next steps in this unfamiliar situation.
- Encourage questions and answer questions as they arise ➤➤*Rationale:* Reinforcement of information is needed during periods of stress and crisis and is especially important given the emergent nature of the procedure.

EQUIPMENT

- Defibrillator/monitor, defibrillator/monitor/automated external defibrillator (AED), or automated external defibrillator (AED) equipped with pediatric adaptor and pads
- Pediatric paddles (for use in infants less than 1 year of age or 10 kg or less) and adult paddles
- Conduction/electrode paste, prepackaged gelled conduction pads, or multifunction pediatric defibrillator electrode pads
- Emergency pacing equipment
- Emergency pediatric resuscitation, intubation equipment, and medications
- Appropriately sized bag-valve-mask resuscitation device
- Clean gloves

Procedure | for Defibrillation: External

Steps	Rationale	Considerations
1. Bring defibrillator/monitor and emergency equipment cart to the bedside.	Necessary for management of emergent situation and provision of defibrillation.	Effective CPR should be in process and continued throughout the defibrillation procedure, except during the period when the energy is discharged.
2. Wash hands and put on clean gloves.	Reduces transmission of microorganisms.	
3. Select the appropriately sized paddles.[1,3,5,8-10] *(Level VI*)*	Select the paddles or electrode pads that provide the lowest transthoracic impedance and the greatest current flow.	Transthoracic impedance is decreased with use of the largest sized paddles or pads that provide good contact with the chest but do not touch each other. A 1-inch space is recommended between the pads to prevent arcing. Pediatric paddles should be used for infants 1 year of age or less and 10 kg or less.[1,5,8,11,12] The use of a stand alone AED with a pediatric adaptor and pediatric electrode pads is approved for children older than 1 year with no signs of circulation.[3,4,9,10] If pediatric pads are not available, you may use adult pads as long as the pads do not touch.[11]

Procedure continues on following page

* Level VI: Clinical studies in a variety of patient populations and situations to support recommendations

Procedure for Defibrillation: External—*Continued*

Steps	Rationale	Considerations
		CPR should be provided for 1 minute before the AED is attached.
4. Apply electrode cream/gel to both paddle surfaces; take care not to get the gel on hands. May also use prepackaged gelled conduction pads. *(Level VI*)*	Improves the delivery of current.	Do *not* rub paddles together to spread gel. This may cause a discharge between the paddles. Do *not* use saline solution–soaked pads because they may cause an arc between paddles. Do *not* use alcohol because it raises impedance and can cause skin burns. Sonographic gels are not good conductors. Do not cut multifunction pediatric defibrillator electrode pads for any reason.[1]
5. Turn on the defibrillator; select the desired energy dose. *(Level VI*)*	Currently, for both monophasic and biphasic defibrillators, the American Heart Association recommends an initial dose of 2 J/kg. If the life-threatening arrhythmia persists after one shock and 5 cycles of CPR, the dose is increased to 4 J/kg and repeated followed by 5 cycles of CPR; if the shockable rhythm persists the dose of 4 J/kg is repeated followed by 5 cycles of CPR.[1,5,7,11,12]	The dose may need to be rounded (either up or down) to the closest energy dose setting available on the defibrillator.[1,5]
6. Place the paddles on the chest so that the heart is between the paddles/ multifunction electrode pads. *(Level VI*)* *Anterior chest:* One paddle is on upper right chest below the clavicle, the other on the left chest, left of the nipple at the anterior axillary line (Figure 46-1).	If paddles/pads are incorrectly placed, the energy does not travel through the heart and fails to briefly stop the electrical activity. The paddles/pads require sufficient space between them so that the electricity does not follow the course of least resistance from one paddle to the other instead of through the heart.[1,2,8,11-14]	Choose the largest paddle/pad size that allows for good contact with the skin without the paddles/pads touching each other. If the paddles/pads are too large for adequate skin contact, the anterior-posterior placement should be used.[1,5,8,9,15]

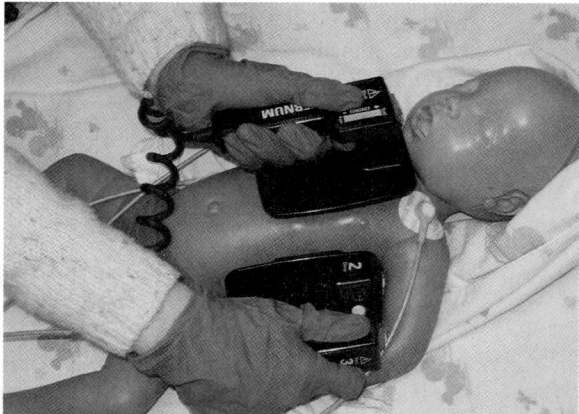

FIGURE 46-1   Correct placement of pediatric paddles of anterior chest of infant 10 kg or less or 1 year of age or less.

Procedure **for Defibrillation: External**—*Continued*

Steps	Rationale	Considerations
Anterior-posterior: One paddle/pad just left of the sternum, the other on the back behind the heart (Figure 46-2).	Place the paddles/pads 10 to 15 cm away from generator site. Transmission of electricity through the generator prevents the full energy dose from reaching the heart and may damage or reset the generator.[1,12]	

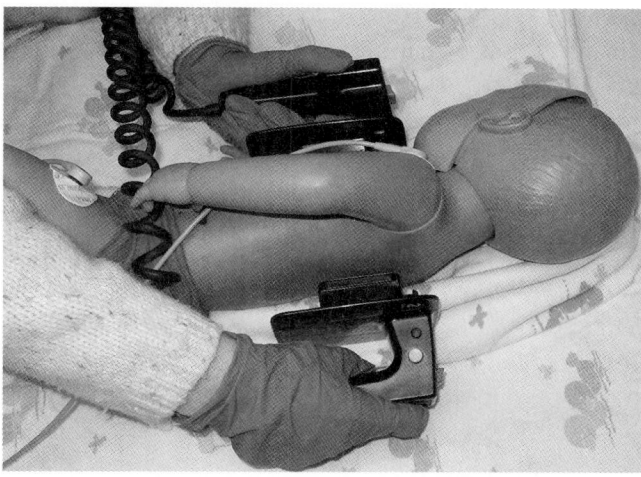

FIGURE 46-2 Correct position of pediatric paddles in anterior-posterior position. Blankets help to support infant on side and maintain open airway.

Permanent pacemaker: Paddles/pads should not be placed directly over a permanent pacemaker generator.	Transmission of current along temporary pacemaker wires may damage heart muscle.[1]	
Temporary pacemaker: Disconnect the pacing wires from the temporary generator. Cover the wire tips with the attached cap or clean glove to prevent conduction from the defibrillator.		
7. Apply firm pressure to each paddle/pad.	Provides optimal contact with the skin and decreases transthoracic impedance. Improves flow of electrical current through the heart.	
8. Charge the paddles/pads according to instructions from the manufacturer.	Paddles usually have a charge button on the right-hand paddle. A charge button is also found on the front of the defibrillator/monitor. The charge button is on the cable connector with the multifunction defibrillator electrodes.	With use of an AED, the AED interprets the rhythm, charges the pads, and delivers the energy.[1,15]

Procedure continues on following page

AP This procedure should be performed only by physicians, advanced practice nurses, and other health care professionals (including critical care nurses) with additional knowledge, skills, and demonstrated competence per professional licensure or institutional standard.

Procedure for Defibrillation: External—*Continued*

Steps	Rationale	Considerations

9. Ensure the safety of the child and colleagues.[1,13]
    One: I am clear.
    Two: You are clear.
    Three: Oxygen is clear.
    Four: Everyone is clear.
	Electrical current is dangerous to anyone in contact with the child and anything touching the child. Oxygen from respiratory devices presents a fire hazard if a spark occurs with arcing during delivery of the energy.[1,5,14]	

10. Verify the rhythm. Verify the energy dose selected. Verify that everyone is clear of child.	Ensure the appropriate dose and safety to the patient and colleagues.	
11. Depress the discharge buttons on both paddles or on the defibrillator/monitor control panel.	Delivers energy.	With use of pads, select PADS from the ECG source button, use an electrode adaptor cable, and attach pads to cable. The discharge buttons are on the adaptor cable. Each defibrillator/monitor has unit-specific information; refer to the manufacturer's information. With combination monitor/defibrillator/AED equipment, the use of pediatric pads does NOT automatically decrease the joules in the AED mode. The manual mode must be used for all pediatric patients ≤8 years.[11]
12. Observe monitor for restoration of perfusing rhythm or continuation of VF/VT. Assess peripheral pulses and perfusion.	Delivery of energy should result in depolarization of the myocardial muscle cells, resulting in a pause (asystole) and then restoration of a perfusing rhythm.	
13. If VF/VT continues, resume compressions and ventilations, and reset the joules to 4 J/kg and deliver the second shock. If still not successful, resume compressions and ventilations, and reset at 4 J/kg and deliver a third shock.[1,5,11]	Early defibrillation is critical to convert VF/VT. The combination of defibrillation and compressions/ventilation minimizes "no flow" time and improves outcomes.[11]	Each shock should be followed by 5 cycles (about 2 min) of CPR.[11]
14. If the third shock is unsuccessful, resume CPR for 1 minute and then give epinephrine per Pediatric Advanced Life Support (PALS) protocol. *(Level VI*)*	Any additional increase in the energy delivered may damage heart muscle. The administration of epinephrine may increase the response to additional shocks.[1,5]	
15. Attempt to identify and treat reversible causes of VT/VF per PALS protocol.	Treatment of reversible causes of VT/VF may assist with termination of tachycardia.	
16. If successful in converting to perfusing rhythm, continue to monitor rhythm and hemodynamic status.	Assesses child's response to defibrillation. Monitor pulses to determine perfusing rhythm.	
17. Clean the defibrillator, remove residual conduction gel from the paddles, and discard used supplies.	Standard precautions; reduces transmission of microorganisms.	
18. Remove gloves and wash hands.	Standard precautions; reduces transmission of microorganisms.	

* Level VI: Clinical studies in a variety of patient populations and situations to support recommendations

Expected Outcomes	Unexpected Outcomes
• Restoration of an organized perfusing rhythm	• Persistent unorganized rhythm that leads to asystole or death
• Improved hemodynamic stability	• Ongoing hemodynamic instability
• Identification of precipitating event	• Inability to identify precipitating event that results in inability to convert rhythm
• Child has adequate oxygenation and ventilation	• Respiratory collapse
	• Inability to oxygenate or ventilate the child
	• Cerebral hypoxia and brain death
• If child's condition is paced, pacemaker remains functional	• Pacemaker dysfunction
• Skin integrity remains intact	• Skin burns
• Appropriate functioning of defibrillator	• Missing equipment or equipment failure

Monitoring and Care of the Child

Activities and Interventions	Rationale	Reportable Conditions
1. Provide continuous evaluation of respiratory and cardiorespiratory function.	Adequate oxygenation, ventilation, and circulation are necessary for the myocardium to respond to defibrillation.	• Decreased oxygen saturation • Difficult ventilation • Ineffective CPR
2. Provide continuous ECG monitoring during and after defibrillation.	Arrhythmias may develop after a successful response to defibrillation.	• Arrhythmias • Pulseless rhythm
3. Monitor electrolyte levels.	Abnormal electrolyte levels may contribute to VT/VF or may result from hypoxia and/or acidosis.	• Abnormal electrolyte levels, blood gases
4. Ensure functioning vascular access.	Intravenous fluids, continuous vasoactive medications, and IV antiarrhythmia medications may be necessary.	• Inability to obtain vascular access
5. Evaluate the skin for burns.	Skin burns may occur after defibrillation from local hyperthermia and the increased sensitivity of the skin of infants and children.	• Skin burns
6. Ensure and provide ongoing information and support to the family.	Provision of regular information during an emergency situation facilitates the family's coping. Frightening life-threatening situations necessitate psychosocial and educational support.	• Inability to access support systems • Inability of family to cope with the critical condition of child

Documentation

- Precipitating events
- Initial assessment of airway, breathing, and circulation; initiation of CPR
- Child's response to defibrillation
- Cardiac rhythm with printout of ECG results before, during, and after defibrillation
- Number of defibrillation attempts and joules used with each attempt
- Printout from defibrillator if available
- Education provided to family
- Unexpected outcomes and related treatment

References

1. Hazinski MF: *PALS provider manual*, Dallas, 2002, American Heart Association.
2. Wilson V: Defibrillation (external). In Lynn-McHale Wiegand DJ, Carlson K, editor: *AACN procedure manual for critical care*, ed 4, Philadelphia, 2001, Saunders.
3. Samson RA, et al: Use of automated external defibrillators for children: an update–an advisory statement from the Pediatric Advanced Life Support Task Force, International Liaison Committee of Resuscitation, *Pediatrics* 112(1):163-168, 2003.
4. Weil MH, et al: Cardiopulmonary resuscitation: one size does not fit all, *Circulation* 107:794, 2003.
5. Castle N: Pediatric resuscitation: advanced life support, *Emerg Nurs* 10(1):31-38, 2002.
6. Hazinski MF: *Manual of pediatric critical care*, St. Louis, 1999, Mosby.
7. Brown K, Bocock J: Update in pediatric resuscitation, *Emerg Med Clin North Am* 20(1):1-26, 2002.
8. Pilcher J: *Pocket guide to neonatal EKG interpretation*, Petaluma, CA, 1998, NICU INK Book Publishers.
9. Samson RA, et al: Use of automated external defibrillators for children: an update, *Circulation* 107(25):3251-55, 2003.
10. Samson RA, et al. In Jun, K (editor): Use of AEDs for children age 1 to 8: evidence for safe use now sufficient, *Curr Emerg Cardiovasc Care/Am Heart Assoc* Fall: 11, 2003.
11. Hazinski, MF, Nolan, J: International Liaison Committee on Resuscitation. 2005 International consensus on cardiopulmonary resuscitation and emergency cardiovascular care science with treatment recommendations. *Circulation* 112(22):17-25, 73-100, 2005.
12. Deboer S, et al: Pediatric defibrillation: concerns and opportunities, *Pediatr Emerg Care* 18(6):466-468, 2002.
13. Atkins DL, Chameides L, Fallat ME, et al: Resuscitation science of pediatrics, *Ann Emerg Med* 37(4 Suppl):S41-48, 2001.
14. Cook L: Staying current on defibrillator safety, *Nursing* 33(11):44-46, 2003.
15. Mair M: Emergency: monophasic and biphasic defibrillators, *AJN* 103(8):58-60, 2003.

Cardiac Pacemakers

Atrial Electrogram

P U R P O S E : To assist in differentiation of cardiac rhythms by revealing atrial activity that might be obscured on the surface electrocardiogram or to establish optimal positioning of a transesophageal atrial pacing catheter

Debra Hanisch

PREREQUISITE KNOWLEDGE

- Child development as it relates to clinical assessment and obtaining an atrial electrogram (AEGM)
- Normal cardiac anatomy and physiology, including the principles of cardiac conduction
- Child's congenital heart disease and associated short-term and long-term electrophysiologic complications
- Child's medical and surgical history, including placement of internal pacemaker or internal defibrillator
- Indications for obtaining an atrial electrogram include:
  - ❖ Evaluation of rhythms when atrial activity is not clearly discernible on the surface electrocardiogram (ECG), supraventricular tachycardia (SVT), atrial flutter with 2:1 atrioventricular (AV) block, junctional rhythms, wide-complex tachycardias
  - ❖ Positioning of a transesophageal pacing catheter
- Atrial arrhythmias are frequently misdiagnosed in children. The adjunctive use of an AEGM significantly improves the accuracy of rhythm diagnoses.[1]
- Connection of the atrial leads to the right arm (RA) and left arm (LA) ECG leads (lead I), the right arm (RA) and left leg (LL) leads (lead II), or the V lead produces an isolated atrial electrogram in that respective lead.
- Normal infant, child, and adolescent heart rates
- Basic and advanced ECG and cardiac arrhythmia interpretation

- Familiarity with electrophysiologic terminology (see Box 51-1)
- Clinical assessment and interpretation of hemodynamic monitoring
- Mastery of pediatric advanced life support competencies
- Activation of the emergency alert system when a complication is detected

CHILD AND FAMILY ASSESSMENT

- Child's developmental level and ability to interact ➧*Rationale:* These factors influence preparation of the child and interaction and affect the child's ability to cooperate with instructions or assist with the procedure by remaining still.
- Child's and family's understanding of the reasons for and risks and benefits of obtaining an AEGM ➧*Rationale:* Evaluates child's and family's understanding of the procedure and provides a gauge for ongoing education.
- History of congenital heart disease, cardiomyopathy, cardiac arrhythmias, syncope, cardiac surgical or catheterization procedures, electrophysiologic complications, and projected cardiac surgery requirements ➧*Rationale:* These conditions impact the placement of the pacing wires and the type of arrhythmias the child may experience and aid in anticipatory planning for future interventions.

- Baseline assessment of cardiac rhythm and documentation of a rhythm strip ➥*Rationale:* Determines the child's initial heart rate and rhythm.
- Assess the child for presence of atrial epicardial pacing wires, which typically exit to the right of the sternum ➥*Rationale:* These wires are connected to a multichannel ECG machine or bedside monitor to obtain the AEGM.
- Assess the child's hemodynamic status: blood pressure, peripheral perfusion, oxygen saturation, and any reported symptomatology ➥*Rationale:* Baseline assessment is done to compare with subsequent assessments done during and after pacing, if instituted.
- Family's desire to be present during the procedure ➥*Rationale:* The family may provide support and comfort measures to the child but should have the choice not to remain with the child.

CHILD AND FAMILY EDUCATION

Individualized, developmentally appropriate education is provided to the child and family based on desire for knowledge, readiness to learn, and overall neurologic and psychosocial state.

- Provide information on the child's medical condition and reasons for AEGM ➥*Rationale:* Educationally appropriate information helps to decrease the child's and family's anxiety levels and offers reassurance.

- If developmentally appropriate, demonstrate the placement of equipment to be used and provide an explanation of the equipment function immediately before initiation of the procedure ➥*Rationale:* Visual examples can decrease fear and anxiety.
- For older children who will remain conscious throughout the procedure, describe what will be experienced and what will be expected of them ➥*Rationale:* Information provided in advance promotes coping and encourages the child's cooperation and compliance.
- Encourage questions and answer questions as they arise ➥*Rationale:* Reinforcement of information is needed during periods of stress.

EQUIPMENT

- Cardiorespiratory monitor
- Electrocardiographic patches and recorder
- A 12-lead or 15-lead ECG machine or bedside monitor with recorder
- Temporary atrial epicardial pacing wires or transesophageal pacing catheter (see Procedure 53 for further information)
- Alligator clips for ECG leads or AEGM-modified lead wires (Figure 47-1)
- Emergency cart
- Defibrillator

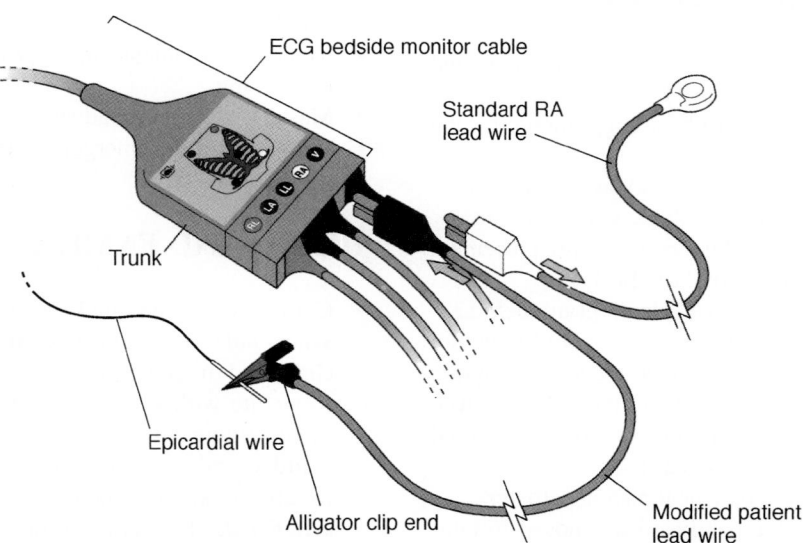

FIGURE 47-1   Modified AEGM lead with alligator clip may be used with ECG bedside monitor cable to connect to epicardial wire or transesophageal pacing catheter. *From Preuss T, Lynn-McHale DJ: Atrial electrogram. In Lynn-McHale DJ, Carlson KK, editors:* AACN procedure manual for critical care, *ed 4, Philadelphia, 2001, Saunders. Drawing by Todd Sargood.*

Procedure for Obtaining an Atrial Electrogram

Steps	Rationale	Considerations
1. Ensure child and family understand procedure and questions are answered.	Evaluates and reinforces understanding of previously taught information.	Developmental level, cognitive ability, and anxiety level determine approach to and effectiveness of teaching.
2. Gather needed supplies and equipment, including emergency cart and defibrillator.	Facilitates completion of the procedure without delays and allows rapid emergency response if necessary.	
3. Wash hands and put on clean gloves.	Standard precautions; reduces transmission of microorganisms. Microfractures in epicardial pacing wires may not be visible. Use of gloves protects staff from receiving microshocks during handling of pacing wires.	Use latex-free gloves in children allergic to latex.
4. Position child on a flat surface with the head of bed elevated 30 to 45 degrees. *(Level II[*])*	Proper positioning can decrease the incidence of equipment malfunction and alligator clip dislodgment and may decrease the child's anxiety.	Proper positioning can also facilitate airway stability.
5. Ensure child is properly connected to cardiorespiratory monitoring, including noninvasive blood pressure or arterial line monitoring and pulse oximetry.[1,2] Cardiac monitor or ECG machine should have at least two simultaneously recordable channels. *(Level II[*])*	Child's rhythm should be monitored throughout procedure. Having at least two channels enables comparison of surface ECG with AEGM.	Documentation should include recorded rhythm strips of the surface ECG and AEGM.
6. Identify temporary atrial epicardial pacing wires and expose ends in preparation for connection to the ECG machine or monitor. *(Level II[*])*	Differentiation of atrial from ventricular epicardial wires is important.	Atrial epicardial wires are usually located to the right of the sternum and ventricular wires to the left (Figure 47-2). However, the presence of complex congenital heart defects may necessitate deviation from typical epicardial wire exit sites.[3]
7. Remove any insulation from the ends of the wires.	Necessary for establishment of an electrical connection.	
8. If a transesophageal pacing catheter is to be used in lieu of epicardial wires, refer to Procedure 53 for information on placement of a transesophageal pacing catheter.	Electrodes of the transesophageal pacing catheter must be positioned in esophagus behind the left atrium to obtain an AEGM. *(Level II[*])*	The AEGM is used to help optimize the pacing catheter's position (Figure 47-3).[4]
9. For a bipolar AEGM, unclip the RA and LA leads from the child and connect the two atrial epicardial wires or the two connector pins on the transesophageal pacing catheter to the RA and LA lead inputs. *(Level II[*])*	Connections to both of the wires or both pins must be established to obtain a bipolar AEGM.	The AEGM-modified patient lead wires with alligator clips may be needed to facilitate the electrical connection (see Figure 47-1).[2] Avoid the use of adhesive tape to secure tips of epicardial wires because it may prohibit good contact and result in an inability to obtain adequate tracing.

Procedure continues on following page

Procedure for Obtaining an Atrial Electrogram—*Continued*

Steps	Rationale	Considerations

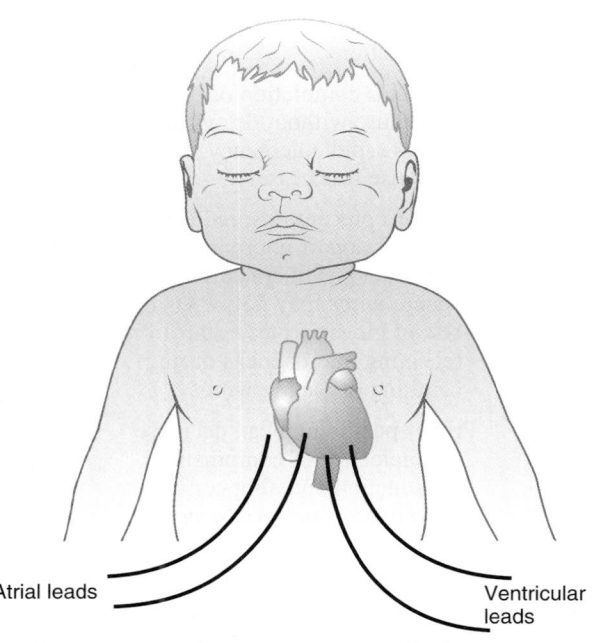

FIGURE 47-2 Diagram depicts typical location of temporary atrial and ventricular epicardial leads. Note that atrial leads exit to right and ventricular leads to left of median sternotomy.

Steps	Rationale	Considerations
10. Record lead I along with at least one V-lead on the multichannel recorder. *(Level II*)*	Lead I detects electrical activity between the RA and LA electrodes, producing a pure AEGM. The simultaneous V lead provides a surface ECG to use for comparison. Use of additional leads may further enhance the data.	Leads II, III, aVR, aVL, and aVF represent combinations of the AEGM and surface ECG. As an alternative, the RA and LL leads can be used, in which case lead II displays the pure AEGM.
11. For a unipolar AEGM, connect the V lead input to one of the atrial epicardial wires with the alligator clip. *(Level II*)*	The chest lead detects electrical activity in a unipolar configuration.	A unipolar AEGM is a useful approach when only one atrial epicardial wire is available.
12. Analyze rhythm strips with comparison of the pure AEGM with the surface ECG(s). *(Level II*)*	The AEGM helps to delineate atrial activity that might be obscured on the surface ECG.	The atrial activity on the AEGM has a larger signal amplitude than ventricular activity (Figures 47-4 and 47-5).
13. If atrial overdrive pacing is to be attempted, disconnect the atrial wires from ECG input leads and connect to the preamplifier and pacing stimulator. *(Level II*)*	Pacing activity creates significant artifact on the AEGM if the connection is maintained.	Occasionally, a switch box is used to change the connection back and forth between the AEGM and the pacing stimulator.[5]
14. At completion of procedure, disconnect lead wires from the ECG machine or monitor and reconnect to child's monitor.	Resumes cardiac monitoring.	Continue to wear gloves whenever handling the unprotected ends of the pacing wires or catheter to avoid the potential for microshock.[6]
15. Dispose of supplies and used equipment appropriately and wash hands.	Standard precautions; decreases transmission of microorganisms.	

Procedure | **for Obtaining an Atrial Electrogram**—*Continued*

Steps	Rationale	Considerations

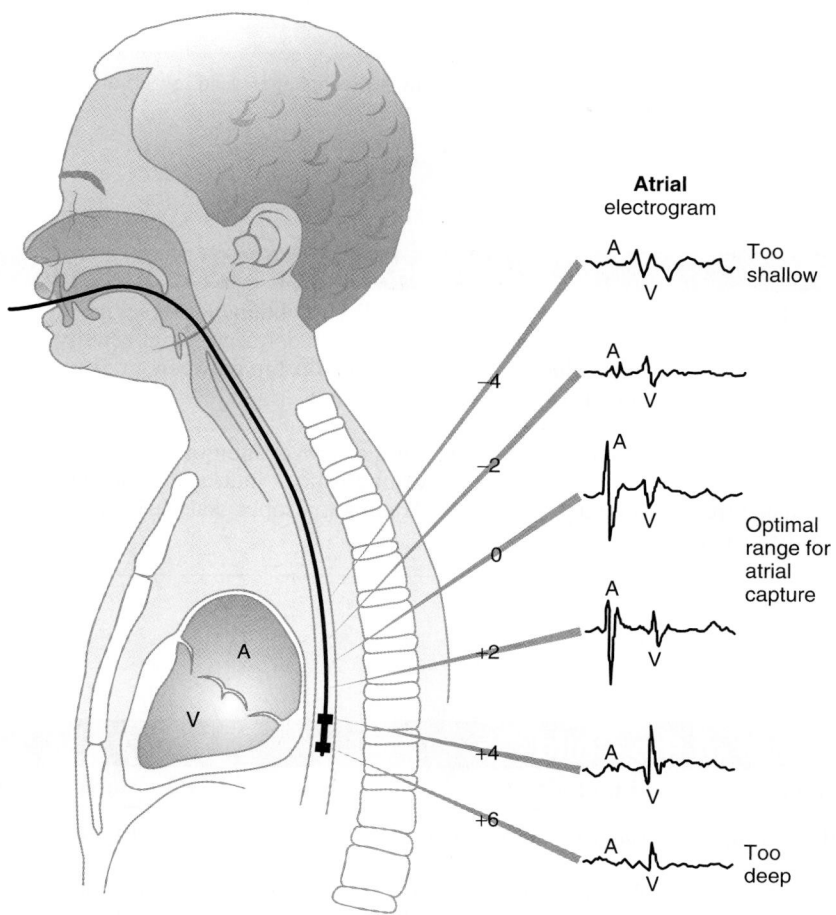

FIGURE 47-3 The AEGM is used to guide proper positioning of transesophageal pacing catheter. Maximal atrial signal amplitude corresponds to optimal position for atrial pacing. *Diagram modified with permission from CardioCommand, Inc, www.CardioCommand.com.*

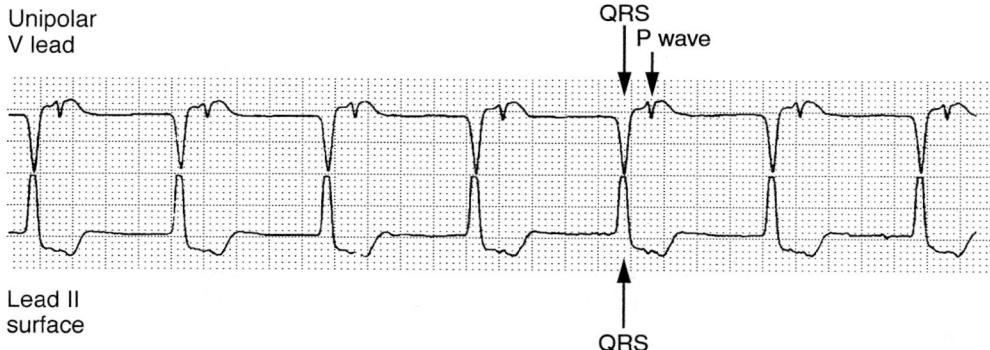

FIGURE 47-4 Bipolar atrial electrogram in lead I is compared with surface ECG in V lead. Note prominence of atrial signal in AEGM in comparison with diminutive ventricular signal. *From From Preuss T, Lynn-McHale DJ: Atrial electrogram. In Lynn-McHale DJ, Carlson K, editors:* AACN procedure manual for critical care, *ed 4, Philadelphia, 2001, Saunders.*

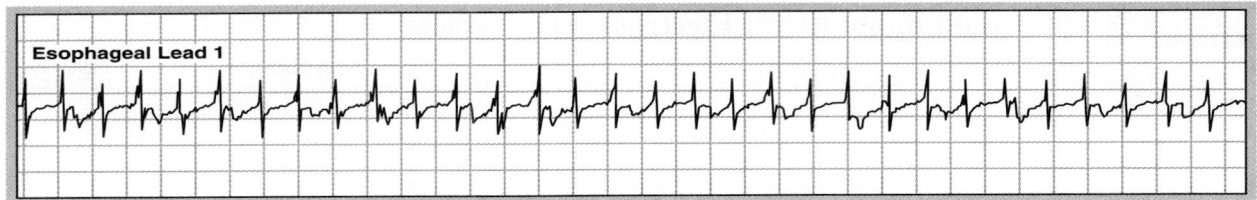

FIGURE 47-5   Bipolar atrial electrogram from transesophageal lead reveals atrial flutter.

Expected Outcomes

- Clear tracing is obtained
- Identification of atrial activity
- The relationship between atrial and ventricular activity is determined and the rhythm diagnosis is confirmed
- Significant arrhythmias are recognized and managed appropriately
- Esophageal mucosa remains free from injury if a transesophageal catheter is used

Unexpected Outcomes

- Inability to obtain clear tracing
- Inability to delineate atrial activity
- The relationship between atrial and ventricular activity is unclear
- Further provocation of arrhythmias from manipulation or microshock induction of a tachyarrhythmia
- Trauma to esophageal mucosa

Monitoring and Care of the Child

Activities and Interventions	Rationale	Reportable Conditions
1. Monitor cardiac rhythm throughout the procedure.	Early identification of arrhythmias.	• Arrhythmias
2. Monitor vital signs and level of consciousness.	Assess for hemodynamic instability associated with the child's heart rhythm.	• Alteration in hemodynamic status or level of consciousness
3. Evaluate and treat arrhythmias if indicated.	Goal is to improve the child's hemodynamic status.	• Failure to adequately manage arrhythmias
4. Monitor epicardial wire exit sites per institution-specific protocol.	Monitor for indications of exit site infection.	• Signs of infection, including drainage, warmth, redness, and tenderness

Documentation

- Child and family education
- Child's vital signs and response to the procedure
- Procedure note, including any medications given, paced settings (if used), and findings or results
- Electrocardiogram and AEGM strips obtained
- Unexpected outcomes and related treatment

References

1. Humes R, et al: Utility of temporary atria epicardial electrodes in postoperative pediatric cardiac patients, *Mayo Clin Proc* 64:516-521, 1989.
2. Preuss T, Lynn-McHale DJ: Atrial electrogram. In Lynn-McHale DJ, Carlson K, editors: *AACN procedure manual for critical care*, ed 4, Philadelphia, 2001, Saunders.
3. Knick BJ, Saul JP: Immediate arrhythmia management. In Zeigler VL, Gillette PC, editors: *Practical management of pediatric cardiac arrhythmias*, Armonk, NY, 2001, Futura Publishing Co, Inc.
4. www.CardioCommand.com. CardioCommand, Inc., The Adjustable Heart, 2001, Accessed originally on 2/10/04, most recently on 4/24/06.
5. Saul JP: Transesophageal atrial recording and pacing. In Walsh EP, Saul JP, Triedman JK, editors: *Cardiac arrhythmias in children and young adults with congenital heart disease*, Philadelphia, 2001, Lippincott Williams & Wilkins.
6. Hickey CS, Baas LS: Temporary cardiac pacing, *AACN Clin Issues Crit Care Nurs* 2:107-117, 1991.

Additional Readings

Baas LS, et al: Care and safety of pacemaker electrodes in intensive care and telemetry nursing units, *Am J Crit Care* 6:302-311, 1997.

Bumgarner LI: Diagnostic uses of epicardial electrodes after cardiac surgery, *Prog Cardiovasc Nurs* 7:21-24, 1992.

Dziadulewicz L, Lang R: The use of atrial electrograms in the diagnosis of supraventricular dysrhythmias, *AACN Clin Issues* 3:203-208, 1992.

Atrial Overdrive Pacing

P U R P O S E : To terminate abnormal atrial rhythms

Karen Kilian

PREREQUISITE KNOWLEDGE

- Child development as it relates to clinical assessment and atrial overdrive pacing
- Mastery of pediatric advanced life support competencies
- Appropriate pediatric dosing of analgesics and competency in procedural sedation
- Normal cardiac anatomy and physiology, including the principles of cardiac conduction
- Normal infant, child, and adolescent heart rates
- Child's congenital heart disease and associated short-term and long-term electrophysiologic complications
- Child's medical history, including upper airway problems and surgical history, which includes placement of an internal pacemaker or internal defibrillator
- Atrial overdrive pacing is performed to treat atrial tachycardia that causes hemodynamic instability; the patient may or may not have a history of atrial tachycardia. The atrial tachycardia may be new onset or refractory to medications.
- This procedure is typically performed on an emergent basis with anesthesia or sedation. Some children may need intubation. Aspiration risk related to a full stomach is increased for children undergoing overdrive pacing with esophageal lead wire.
- Patients in atrial fibrillation are predisposed to blood clots in the atrium. Ideally, children should undergo anticoagulation therapy before conversion to sinus rhythm with the therapy maintained for 2 to 3 months after conversion. An echocardiogram should be performed before the procedure to rule out structural issues and presence or absence of blood clots in the heart.

- If transesophageal echocardiography is necessary because of poor windows or if overdrive pacing with esophageal lead wire is planned, institution of overdrive pacing may occur in either the operating room or the intensive care unit per institution-specific protocol.
- Mastery of basic and advanced electrocardiogram (ECG) and cardiac arrhythmia interpretation
- Ability to differentiate between mechanical and electrical capture
- Familiarity with electrophysiologic (EP) terminology. (see Box 51-1)
- Assessment of hemodynamic response to pacing therapy
- Familiarity with chosen method of overdrive pacing (esophageal, transvenous, or use of epicardial wires)
- Signs and symptoms of complications associated with transvenous pacing lead placement
- Informed consent is generally necessary before atrial overdrive pacing

CHILD AND FAMILY ASSESSMENT

- Developmental level and ability to interact ➤➤***Rationale:*** These factors influence preparation of the child, interaction, and the child's ability to cooperate with instructions or assist with the procedure by remaining still.
- Child's and family's understanding of the reasons for and risks and benefits of the procedure ➤➤***Rationale:*** Evaluates child's and family's understanding of the procedure and provides a gauge for ongoing education.
- History of congenital heart disease, cardiomyopathy, cardiac arrhythmias, syncope, cardiac surgical or catheterization procedures, electrophysiologic complications, and

projected cardiac surgery requirements ➤➤*Rationale:* These conditions can impact the type of atrial overdrive pacing used, assist with anticipatory planning for optimal treatment of potential complications, and determine best course of pharmacotherapy after rhythm is terminated.

- History of upper airway or esophageal anomalies ➤➤*Rationale:* These conditions may preclude passage of an esophageal lead; this information also facilitates development of an effective airway management plan.
- Current hemodynamic status ➤➤*Rationale:* Initiation of inotropic support may be necessary to stabilize the child's condition before, during, or after the procedure.
- History of ECGs ➤➤*Rationale:* Establishes prior baseline rhythm.
- Medication history, including use of herbal supplements or anticoagulation therapy, drug exposure, acid-base balance, and electrolyte levels ➤➤*Rationale:* Drug therapy and electrolyte or acid-base abnormalities could impede pacing ability. Certain medications or drug exposures may be implicated as the cause for the tachycardia. Anticoagulation history assists in determination of risk of atrial clot formation.
- History of previous response to anesthesia or procedural sedation ➤➤*Rationale:* This history may influence the type of sedation used for the procedure to safely achieve desired results.
- Family's desire to be present during procedure ➤➤*Rationale:* The family may provide support and comfort measures to the child but should have the choice not to remain with the child.

CHILD AND FAMILY EDUCATION

Individualized, developmentally appropriate education is provided to the family and to the child based on desire for knowledge, readiness to learn, and overall neurologic and psychosocial state.

- An individualized educational plan should be developed that includes information on the child's medical condition and rationale for atrial overdrive pacing ➤➤*Rationale:* Educationally appropriate information helps to decrease the child's and family's anxiety levels and offers reassurance during an extremely stressful period in their lives.
- If possible and developmentally appropriate, describe the procedure with visual aids ➤➤*Rationale:* Visual examples can decrease fear and anxiety.
- Explain the type of overdrive atrial pacing to be used, the location where the procedure will be done, and the rationale for preprocedural echocardiography and possible anticoagulation therapy ➤➤*Rationale:* Providing infor-

mation to the child and family decreases fear and anxiety and can increase compliance with the plan of care.

- Provide developmentally appropriate information on the pacing process, postprocedure care, and goals of therapy ➤➤*Rationale:* Providing information to the child and family decreases fear and anxiety and can increase compliance with the plan of care.
- Provide information to the child and family about the type of sedation and pain medication to be administered during the procedure because atrial overdrive pacing is uncomfortable, especially when an esophageal lead wire is used, and the child will need pain medication and sedation ➤➤*Rationale:* Knowing that anticipated pain will be preemptively treated decreases fear and anxiety of the child and family.
- Inform the child (if appropriate) and family about potential complications, such as the development of ventricular tachycardia necessitating defibrillation or cardioversion ➤➤*Rationale:* For the child and family to give informed consent, they must be aware of the benefits and risks associated with the procedure. This information prepares the child and family for future necessary therapies.
- Inform the child and family that intubation may be necessary if esophageal pacing is used as a means of ensuring a stable airway and allowing for maximum sedation to be used during the procedure ➤➤*Rationale:* Providing information in advance promotes successful coping of the child and family.
- Encourage questions and answer questions as they arise ➤➤*Rationale:* Reinforcement of information is needed during periods of stress and is especially important given the usually emergent nature of this procedure.

EQUIPMENT

- Cardiopulmonary monitor
- Electrocardiographic patches, leads, and recorder
- 12-lead or 15-lead ECG machine
- Atrial overdrive pacemaker
- Clean gloves
- Transvenous pacing catheter, if appropriate
- Echocardiogram machine
- Transesophageal probe, if appropriate
- Local anesthetic spray for throat
- Lubricant (preferably with local anesthetic) for nasal insertion
- Skin preparation
- Intravenous (IV) supplies
- Airway management supplies
- Emergency cart
- Defibrillator

Procedure | for Atrial Overdrive Pacing

Steps	Rationale	Considerations
1. Ensure child and family have met with prescribing practitioner who will perform procedure and that consent for procedure has been obtained.	Ensures purpose and procedural risks have been addressed; ensures medical-legal compliance as suggested by the Joint Commission on Accreditation of Healthcare Organizations (JCAHO).	The child (if developmentally appropriate) and legal guardian must be included in the discussion. For emergency situations, the organization may have a protocol/procedure in place for assumption of consent.
2. Ensure child and family understand procedure and questions are answered.	Evaluates and reinforces understanding of previously taught information.	This procedure may be performed under emergent conditions that may preclude preprocedural teaching.
3. Ensure fasting guidelines have been implemented per institution-specific protocol.	Minimizes risk of complications related to aspiration of stomach contents.	The NPO time is related to the child's age and type of sedation to be administered; in emergency situations, follow specific institution-specific protocol.
4. Wash hands and put on clean gloves. *(Level IV*)*	Standard precautions; reduces transmission of microorganisms.	
5. Position child supine; for esophageal overdrive pacing, the head is placed in a neutral position. *(Level II*)*	Proper positioning facilitates insertion of esophageal probe and decreases the incidence rate of equipment dislodgment and, for child receiving anesthesia, prevents tissue or nerve injury.	Proper positioning can facilitate airway stability.
6. Ensure appropriate cardiorespiratory monitoring, including noninvasive blood pressure (NIBP) or arterial line monitoring and pulse oximetry.[1-3] *(Level II*)*	Monitors for hemodynamic compromise before, during, and after procedure.	Child may have decompensation or need initiation of inotropic agents or another intervention before or during procedure.
7. Obtain 12-lead ECG. *(Level II*)*	Documents rhythm before intervention.	
8. Echocardiogram is obtained.[1,2] *(Level II*)*	Rules out presence of atrial thrombus.	A transesophageal echocardiogram may be necessary if child has a history of multiple cardiac surgeries and poor windows. If thrombus is present, consider delaying procedure and institute anticoagulation therapy.
9. Method of overdrive pacing is selected.	Choices are limited on the basis of child's size, medical history, and current pacing status (i.e., presence of pacemaker or atrial epicardial leads).[1,4]	
10. Gather supplies and equipment, including emergency cart and defibrillator.	Ensures that all equipment is at the bedside for the procedure and facilitates completion of the procedure without delay; emergency equipment is readily available if needed.	Necessary supplies and equipment depend on type of pacing to be used and location of procedure (intensive care unit [ICU] versus operating room).
11. Identify child with appropriate patient/procedure verification process (e.g., "time out").	Confirms correct patient, procedure, and site as recommended by JCAHO; prevents unnecessary medical procedures.	Verification process and documentation is institution specific. Use active communication techniques.

* Level II: Theory-based; no research data to support recommendations; recommendations from expert consensus group may exist
  Level IV: Limited clinical studies to support recommendations

Procedure	for Atrial Overdrive Pacing—*Continued*	
Steps	**Rationale**	**Considerations**
12. Wash hands and put on clean gloves.	Standard precautions; decreases transmission of microorganisms.	
13. If not present, establish IV access. *(Level VI*)*	Intravenous access is established for sedation and cardiac medication administration if child's hemodynamic status remains unstable despite conversion to sinus rhythm.	Before IV access is established, consider any history of vascular compromise (i.e., history of Blalock-Taussig shunt).
14. Sedation or anesthesia is administered per institution-specific.	Atrial overdrive pacing is uncomfortable and can be painful. Sedation and anesthesia decrease anxiety, alleviate discomfort, and decrease movement of child during the procedure. *(Level VI*)*	The type of sedation/anesthesia used is dependent on child's prior experience with these medications and drug allergy history. Monitor carefully for respiratory depression in children without intubation. A decision may be made to electively intubate to ensure the airway is secure during the procedure, especially in infants and young children. In rare instances, an esophageal probe can compress the airway; additional sedation may be necessary for transesophageal pacing.
15. Assist with insertion of pacing leads if transvenous or transesophageal pacing is selected.	Pacing electrodes must be in place to perform the procedure.	If present, ensure that epicardial atrial leads are able to capture appropriately. If transesophageal pacing is used, vigilant monitoring of airway is mandatory. Use of local anesthetic spray on the throat and lubrication of the probe facilitates advancement. *(Level II*)*
16. Ensure that pacing wire connections to pacemaker are secure and attached to appropriate input sites. *(Level I*)*	Nonsecure or inappropriate connections can lead to capture failure.	
17. Initiate rhythm strip.	Allows documentation of response to the procedure and analysis of rhythm.	
18. Turn on pacemaker and place in atrial pacing mode (AAI). *(Level I*)*	Senses current atrial activity.	Rapid atrial pacing mode may be used, depending on type of atrial overdrive pacemaker used.
19. Set milliamps at 10 to 20.[1,3] *(Level II*)*	Ensures enough energy to capture atrium.	If child has undergone pacing in the recent past, the amount of energy necessary to capture may be unchanged; use that setting if known.
20. Heart rate is gradually increased on the pacemaker until pacemaker rate is 10 to 30 bpm over child's atrial rate with capture obtained. *(Level II*)*	Abrupt changes may precipitate untoward rhythm disturbances.[1,3] Captures atrium with the goal of "resetting" cardiac rhythm cycle, terminating abnormal rhythm.[1]	Dependent on the type of pacemaker system used; check the manufacturer and institution-specific guidelines.
21. Overdrive pacing rate is maintained for approximately 30 seconds. *(Level I*)*	Suppresses rhythm disturbance and interrupts the reentry circuit of abnormal rhythm.	

Procedure continues on following page

* Level I: Manufacturer's recommendations only
  Level II: Theory-based; no research data to support recommendations; recommendations from expert consensus group may exist
  Level VI: Clinical studies in a variety of patient populations and situations to support recommendations

Procedure for Atrial Overdrive Pacing—*Continued*

Steps	Rationale	Considerations
22. Rate on pacemaker is gradually reduced to the point where it senses only.[1] *(Level II[*])*	Abrupt reduction may result in return of rhythm disturbance.	Pacing can be stopped once sinus rhythm is obtained.
23. Obtain 12-lead ECG.	Verifies current rhythm.	May help identify underlying pathology, such as Wolff-Parkinson-White syndrome.[1,2]
24. Dispose of supplies and used equipment appropriately; remove gloves and wash hands.	Standard precautions; reduces transmission of microorganisms.	

[*] Level II: Theory-based; no research data to support recommendations; recommendations from expert consensus group may exist

Expected Outcomes	Unexpected Outcomes
• Termination of abnormal rhythm	• Reoccurrence of abnormal rhythm focus or degeneration into ventricular tachycardia or ventricular fibrillation
• Neurologic status is stable or improved	• Signs of cerebral embolic stroke after conversion to sinus rhythm
• Stable hemodynamic status	• Low cardiac output with normal sinus rhythm
• Stable respiratory status	• Respiratory compromise that necessitates supplemental oxygen, bilevel positive airway pressure (BIPAP), or intubation
• Return to presedation or anesthesia status within expected time frame	• Child remains sedated or anesthetized for a prolonged period
	• Paradoxic agitation
• Acceptable level of comfort	• Unmanaged pain

Monitoring and Care of the Child

Activities and Interventions	Rationale	Reportable Conditions
1. During procedure, monitor vital signs per institution-specific protocol for procedural sedation, or more often if indicated.	Allows early identification of complications from procedure or sedation/anesthesia.	• Significant change in vital signs • Indications of airway compromise
2. Monitor for abnormal rhythm disturbances, including premature conducted beats.	Allows identification of complications from the procedure, such as recurrent atrial tachycardia and new onset ventricular tachycardia. If pharmacologic measures have been used, bradycardia may result.[1] Early recognition of abnormal beats/rhythm allows earlier pharmacologic therapy if indicated.	• Premature atrial contractions • Runs of supraventricular tachycardia • Ventricular tachycardia
3. Monitor use of inotropic agents with current administration.	Inotropic agents may enhance ectopic beats and rhythms. Use lowest amount of inotrope necessary to achieve desired effects.	• A need to increase inotropic support because of a change in hemodynamic status
4. Monitor hemodynamic status	Many pharmacologic agents are negative inotropes; monitor for signs of low cardiac output. Pacing may be necessary to maintain an acceptable heart rate if child's condition becomes bradycardic with symptoms of low cardiac output.[3,4]	• Bradycardia below age-appropriate guidelines with symptomatic hypotension and low urine output

Monitoring and Care of the Child—Cont'd

Activities and Interventions	Rationale	Reportable Conditions
5. Monitor respiratory status.	Allows detection of complications, such as airway compromise.[1]	• Respiratory distress or failure • Airway compromise
6. Monitor neurologic status.	Allows identification of signs of embolic event.[1] History of atrial fibrillation predisposes child to clots in the atrium.	• Deterioration of neurologic status, including weakness or decreased movement of limbs, slurred speech for verbal children, and seizure activity
7. Monitor level of sedation/analgesia during the procedure.	Ensures adequate comfort and sedation levels. Decreases child's and family's anxiety level.	• Unmanaged pain • Inadequate or excessive sedation • Level of consciousness that is inappropriate for the degree of medical therapy
8. Monitor recovery from sedation/anesthesia.	Monitors for return to baseline and full recovery.	• Delayed recovery from sedation/anesthesia; untoward reactions to sedation/anesthesia. such as nausea and vomiting
9. During recovery, assess effectiveness of pain management strategy and provide appropriate interventions. Encourage family to assist with nonpharmacologic means to comfort and support the child.	Early identification of discomfort allows for immediate attention.	• Unresolved pain and discomfort • Continued irritability or changes in physiologic condition

Documentation

- Consent for procedure
- Pertinent medical history, including history of anticoagulation therapy and results of preprocedural echocardiogram
- Procedural note with description of procedure, type of pacing leads used, settings used for overdrive pacing, child's response, and tolerance
- 12-Lead ECG results before and after conversion
- Child's hemodynamic and respiratory status after conversion
- Neurologic status before and after conversion
- Vital signs throughout the procedure and recovery per institution-specific protocol
- Sedation/anesthesia necessary for procedure and response
- Comfort assessment and any specific interventions provided
- Child and family education
- Unexpected outcomes and related treatment

References
1. Zeigler VL, Gillette PG: *Practical management of pediatric cardiac arrhythmias,* Armonk, NY, 2001, Future Publishing Company, Inc.
2. Takeda M, et al: Use of temporary atrial pacing in management of patients after cardiac surgery, *Cardiovasc Surg* 4(5):623-627, 1996.
3. Wu JM, et al: Atrial overdrive pacing for conversion of atrial flutter in children, *Acta Paed Sin* 32(1):1-7, 1991.
4. Maginot K, et al: Applications of pacing strategies in neonates and infants, *Progress Pediatr Cardiol* 11(1):65-75, 2000.

Additional Reading
Gregoratos G, Abrams J, Epstein A, et al: ACC/AHA/NASPE 2002 guideline update for implantation of cardiac pacemakers and antiarrhythmia devices. a report of the American College of Cardiology/American Heart Association Task Force on Practice Guidelines, Bethesda, MD, 2002, American College of Cardiology Foundation Resource Center & American Heart Association.

Electrocardiogram: Obtaining and Monitoring a 12-Lead Electrocardiogram

P U R P O S E : Continuous electrocardiographic (ECG) monitoring provides a baseline assessment of cardiac rhythm and monitors heart rate. The 12-lead ECG is a noninvasive tool that permits the diagnosis of cardiac arrhythmias and identification of coronary artery disease, cardiomyopathy, chamber hypertrophy, and enlargement.

Sarah S. LeRoy

PREREQUISITE KNOWLEDGE

- Child development as it relates to clinical assessment and ECG monitoring, including child anxiety management techniques, such as attention diversion or medical play
- Basic anatomy and physiology of the conduction system
- The normal cardiac cycle as it relates to the ECG tracing
- In contrast to cases in adults, most pediatric cardiac emergencies are the result of respiratory failure; thus, cardiorespiratory (CR) monitoring is a vital component for monitoring children at risk, with or without a positive cardiac history.
- Continuous ECG monitoring systems typically use three or five leads on the chest, but this monitoring is not generally used as a diagnostic tool because lead placement is not standardized.
- Indications for continuous cardiorespiratory monitoring and for obtaining a 12-lead ECG in the pediatric patient:
  - ❖ Continuous cardiorespiratory monitoring is indicated in children with jeopardized health status or conditions that are potentially unstable (e.g., during conscious sedation, severe respiratory infection, or perioperatively).
- Indications for obtaining a 12-lead ECG include:
  - ❖ Known or suspected congenital or acquired heart disease (CHD)

- ❖ Known or suspected arrhythmia
- ❖ Monitoring of response to antiarrhythmia medications
- ❖ To assess for cardiac evidence of severe electrolyte abnormalities, including hypokalemia/hyperkalemia and hypocalcemia/hypercalcemia
- ❖ To assess for ischemic changes
- ❖ To assess for pacemaker functioning
- ❖ To evaluate for pericarditis
- Normal cardiac anatomy and chest landmarks for proper electrode placement
- Cardiac diagnoses and conditions that necessitate modification of electrode placement or affect ECG interpretation
- Use of available CR monitoring systems and available 12-lead ECG machine
- Normal pediatric ECG tracings and ability to identify abnormal tracings that result from errors in lead position or artifact
- Expected alterations in ECG tracing for a child who is undergoing pacing
  - ❖ Child with a ventricular pacemaker that is sensing and pacing has a vertical pacemaker spike that initiates ventricular depolarization with a wide complex QRS. The pacemaker spike has no fixed relationship to atrial activity, so no P wave may be seen in front of the spike.
  - ❖ Child with an atrial pacemaker that is sensing and pacing has a pacemaker spike followed by an atrial

complex. If atrioventricular (AV) conduction is normal, a normal QRS complex follows.
  ❖ Child with an AV sequential pacemaker has two sets of pacemaker spikes: one before the P wave and one before the wide QRS complex.
- An electrocardiogram records the sum of the myocardial electrical forces from the surface of the chest wall; a 12-lead ECG looks at these forces in a variety of planes.
- Quality of a 12-lead ECG is affected by the expertise of the individual who obtains the study, especially related to lead placement.
- Rule of 300 for calculation of heart rate:
  ❖ Use this method only when the heart rate is regular
  ❖ Locate an R wave that falls on a heavy grid line
  ❖ Count the number of large boxes on the ECG paper between this R wave and the next R wave
  ❖ Divide 300 by the number of large boxes (this can be an approximate number; e.g., 1.5 or 1.75)

CHILD AND FAMILY ASSESSMENT

- Child's developmental level and ability to interact ➥*Rationale:* These factors influence preparation of the child and interaction.
- Child's and family's understanding of the purpose and means of ECG monitoring to be used ➥*Rationale:* Assuring children and families understand the purpose of medical testing facilitates trust and rapport and helps engage parents as active partners in the child's care.
- Child's anxiety level related to the monitoring equipment ➥*Rationale:* Some children become fearful when the electrodes are attached to the lead wires, which may result in significant movement artifact that limits tracing interpretation. Allowing the child to manipulate (play) with the lead wires and place electrodes on a parent's arm, to show that the monitoring does not hurt, may increase the child's sense of control and thus facilitate participation.
- Factors specific to the child that may affect lead placement or tracing interpretation ➥*Rationale:* Alternate electrode placement may be indicated in specific situations, including paced rhythm or dextrocardia. Patient factors that affect pediatric ECG interpretation include age, cardiac diagnosis, pacing, and whether the pacemaker was inhibited to obtain the tracing. Other significant patient factors include chest abnormalities, such as severe pectus excavatum or kyphoscoliosis. Infant respiratory patterns (e.g., abdominal breathing versus chest breathing) guides effective electrode placement and lead choice.

CHILD AND FAMILY EDUCATION

Individualized, developmentally appropriate education is provided to the family and to the child based on desire for knowledge, readiness to learn, and overall neurologic and psychosocial state.

- Explain the purpose, method, and duration of ECG monitoring. If a 12-lead ECG is performed, discuss the length of the procedure and when test results are available. Use of complex medical terminology should be limited, and potentially threatening words should be replaced with words that are neutral and age-appropriate (e.g., stickers versus electrodes). ➥*Rationale:* Information given in an age-appropriate manner permits child's and family's understanding regarding the purpose of the test and how it will personally impact/benefit them, which is anticipated to promote collaboration and trust between the family and health care provider. Use of age-appropriate neutral language can help avoid unnecessary child anxiety.
- Explain the steps involved in obtaining an ECG tracing. If a 12-lead ECG is needed, explain to the child the need to lay still and flat for 5 to 10 minutes while the electrodes (stickers) are placed and that the skin will be cleaned with something that may feel cold but that nothing will hurt (no "owies" or "boo-boos"). ➥*Rationale:* Information helps to decrease the child's and caregiver's anxiety levels and offers reassurance during an extremely stressful period.
- Explain the benefits and limitations of continuous CR monitoring. Include the relatively high frequency of false alarms that can be caused by movement or electrode dislodgement. Explain how alarms are assessed by the staff (e.g., if telemetry is available at a central station) and that, in general, if the child's condition appears to be stable (e g., no significant change in consciousness, responsiveness, or energy levels), the alarm is most likely false. Assure family that all alarms are evaluated. ➥*Rationale:* CR monitoring frequently results in false alarms that can create unnecessary parental anxiety. If telemetry is available, the family should be informed of the ability to perform distance monitoring and determine, in most instances, whether an alarm is false. This information may decrease parental anxiety and avoid parental dissatisfaction associated with perceived delay in alarm response time by the caregivers.
- Encourage questions and answer questions as they arise ➥*Rationale:* Reinforcement of information is needed during periods of stress.

EQUIPMENT

- Electrocardiographic recording device (either 12-lead machine or cardiorespiratory monitor)
- Electrocardiographic patches and leads
- Electrocardiographic recording paper specific to available recording device
- Supplies to clean skin at the electrode site per institution-specific protocol
- Scissors in case of significant chest hair (optional)
- Video or DVD player, puppets, or other diversionary activities

Procedure for ECG Monitoring/Obtaining a 12-Lead ECG

Steps	Rationale	Considerations
1. Ensure child and family understand procedure and questions are answered.	Evaluates and reinforces understanding of previously taught information.	Developmental level, cognitive ability, and anxiety level determine approach to and effectiveness of teaching.
2. Gather needed equipment and supplies.	Facilitates completion of the task in a timely manner.	
3. Identify child with two patient identifiers per institutional protocol.	Ensures the procedure is performed on the correct child and avoids unnecessary tests and procedures.	
4. Turn on ECG monitor and enter necessary data into the system (bedside monitor, central monitoring station, ECG machine).	Computerized ECG analysis normal values are age dependent. Other information, such as gender and current medications, may be necessary for a 12-lead ECG.	If a machine other than child's bedside monitor is used to record a 12-lead ECG, patient information must be entered into the system, including name, age, medical record number, and whether or not the child is currently undergoing pacing. Artifact from paced ECGs can often be minimized by accessing ECG machine specific features; refer to the manufacturer's instructions.
5. Wash hands. *(Level VI*)*	Standard precautions; reduces transmission of microorganisms.	
6. Provide for appropriate privacy; position child comfortably in supine position. *(Level II*)*	Accurate electrode placement generally necessitates exposure of the chest. Supine positioning provides optimal access for electrode placement. Alternative positioning may be necessary for the child who is extremely anxious, developmentally delayed, or wheelchair bound.	Privacy is an important consideration for school-aged children and adolescents. If necessary, a 12-lead ECG can be adequately performed in a semireclining position, in a parent's lap or in a wheelchair. Use child anxiety management techniques if needed.[1]
7. Identify electrode sites on the basis of the type of monitoring necessary.[1,2]	Site depends on the type of monitoring necessary (e.g., 12-lead versus 3-lead or 5-lead CR monitoring at the bedside).	Neonatal leads come as small karaya pads with loose wires that are color coded red, black, and white and are plugged directly into the appropriate receptacle in the end of the monitoring cable.
8. Prepare sites per electrode manufacturer's instructions. Use scissors to clip chest hair if necessary. *(Level VI*)*	Cleaning and drying the skin before electrode application may improve adherence of the electrode. Quality of tracing obtained depends on intact skin-electrode interface. Shaving the hair on the chest is not recommended because it may cause microabrasions and provide an entry portal for microorganisms.	Rubbing the site with gauze before placement of electrodes may improve electrode adherence.

* Level II: Theory-based; no research data to support recommendations; recommendations from expert consensus group may exist
  Level VI: Clinical studies in a variety of patient populations and situations to support recommendations

Procedure	**for ECG Monitoring/Obtaining a 12-Lead ECG**—*Continued*	
Steps	**Rationale**	**Considerations**
9. Place electrodes as appropriate for necessary monitoring (Figure 49-1, for chest lead placement for 12-lead ECG).	Ensures that an accurate recording is obtained.	Ensure that electrodes with gel have not passed the expiration date and that the gel is not dried out because electrodes that have dried out do not conduct the signal effectively.

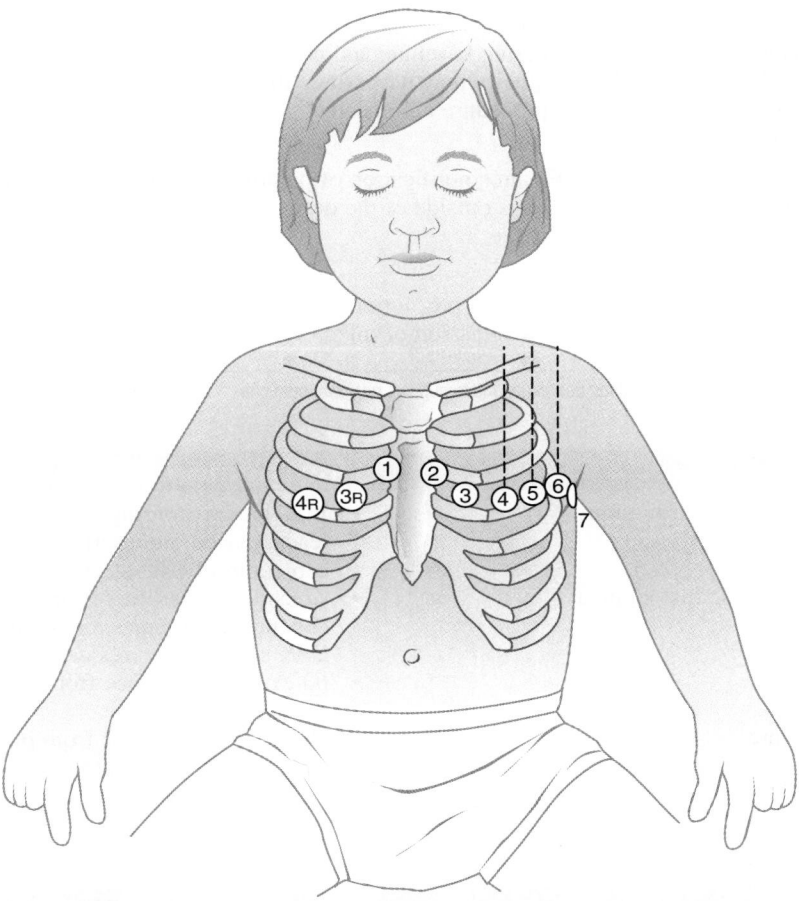

FIGURE 49-1   Positioning of precordial leads for 12-lead pediatric ECG. V1 is placed in fourth intercostal space immediately to right of sternum; V4 is placed in fifth intercostal space, left midclavicular line; V3 is midway between V2 and V4; V5 and V6 are at same level as V4; V5 is at anterior axillary line; and V6 is at midaxillary line. Additional precordial leads may be used, including V7 (level of V6 at posterior axillary line), V4R (fifth right intercostal space; midclavicular line), and V3R (midway between V1 and V4R).

10. Attach lead wires to the monitor cable. *(Level I*)*	Nonsecure or inappropriate connections can lead to incomplete tracings or inability of the monitor to pick up tracing.	Consider obtaining a 15-lead ECG or add V_3R or V_4R chest leads to evaluate the neonate with significant RV forces or to identify the risk of ischemia.[3]

Procedure continues on following page

Procedure for ECG Monitoring/Obtaining a 12-Lead ECG—*Continued*

Steps	Rationale	Considerations
11. Ensure 12-lead ECG machine is set at a standard recording speed of 25 mm/sec.[4] *(Level VI*)*	Standard recording speed allows the use of the rule of 300, the easiest method for estimation of the heart rate when the rhythm is regular.[4]	Temporarily slowing the recording speed can allow for more accurate evaluation of abnormal rhythms, such as atrial tachycardia.[4]
12. Record tracing.	Verifies current rhythm.	
13. If a 12-lead ECG has been obtained, review recording to ensure good quality before removal of electrodes. If recording is acceptable, remove electrodes and clean the skin.	Problems such as artifact, wandering baseline, and poor signal quality may necessitate that procedure be repeated.	
14. If continuous CR monitoring is necessary, activate the appropriate alarm parameters.	Ensures notification of parameters outside of the desired range.	Verify that the alarm parameters are safe and acceptable for the child at the beginning of each shift or with any patient hand-off.
15. Dispose of supplies and used equipment appropriately; wash hands.	Standard precautions; reduces transmission of microorganisms.	

* Level VI: Clinical studies in a variety of patient populations and situations to support recommendations

Expected Outcomes

- Accurate recording of electrocardiogram

- Minimal artifact or electrode dislodgment

- Child tolerates procedure

Unexpected Outcomes

- Inaccurate recording as a result of misplacement of leads, inaccurate insertion of lead wires into patient cable, out-of-date electrodes, or excessive artifact[4]
- Considerable artifact from improper skin preparation, concurrent therapies, or conditions that are unavoidable, such as seizures or high-frequency ventilation
- 60-cycle interference from electrical/mechanical equipment
- High level of distress from inadequate preparation, hurried personnel, vulnerable age (stranger anxiety), or prior negative hospital experience

Monitoring and Care of the Child

Activities and Interventions	Rationale	Reportable Conditions
1. Skin integrity, particularly for prolonged CR monitoring or with evidence of skin sensitivity to electrode gel or adhesive.	Electrode materials may cause irritation of the skin; consider switching to another type of electrode or using skin preparation to protect the skin.	• Skin breakdown
2. Quality of tracing obtained.	Identifies need to relocate or replace electrodes. Allows appropriate monitoring.	• Persistent equipment malfunction
3. Perform rhythm analysis with assessment of at least five parameters, including P waves, QRS width, A-V synchrony, rate, and rhythm.[1,4]	Evaluates tracing for presence of abnormalities. If child is undergoing pacing, assesses functioning of pacemaker.	• Change in rate, rhythm, or other parameters that indicates potential complications • Presence of lethal arrhythmias
4. Heart rate or respiratory rate falls outside of set parameters.	Notifies clinician to evaluate child's status and intervene as appropriate.	• Significant changes in heart or respiratory rate
5. Presence of arrhythmia.	Facilitates appropriate treatment and interventions.	• Hemodynamically significant arrhythmia

---

Documentation

- Indications for ECG monitoring or 12-lead ECG
- Initiation or continuation of ECG monitoring with appropriate alarms specified and activated or successful completion of 12-lead ECG
- For 12-lead ECG, document any alternative lead placement used and the reason for alternative placement
- Any abnormal tracings with examples included in the medical record
- Prescribing practitioner notification of significant arrhythmia
- Child and family education
- Unexpected outcomes and related treatment

References

1. Garson A: *The electrocardiogram in infants and children: a systematic approach,* Philadelphia, 1983, Lea & Febiger.
2. Park MY, Guntheroth WG: *How to read pediatric ECGs,* St Louis, 1992, Mosby.
3. Mowery B, Suddaby EC: ECG interpretation: what is different in children? *Pediatr Nurs* 27(3):227-314, 2001.
4. Hanisch D: Pediatric arrhythmias, *J Pediatr Nurs* 16(5): 351-362, 2001.

Additional Readings

Adams MG, Drew BJ: Body position effects on the ECG: implication for ischemia monitoring, *J Electrocardiol* 30:285-291, 1997.
Booker KJ, et al: Lead wire reversal during 12-lead ECG monitoring, *Prog Cardiovasc Nurs* 16:35-35, 2001.
Drew BJ, et al: Accuracy of the EASI 12 lead electrocardiogram compared to the standard 12-lead electrocardiogram for diagnosing multiple cardiac abnormalities, *J Electrocardiol* 32s:38-47, 1999.
Schijvenaars B, et al: Effect of electrode positioning on ECG interpretation by computer, *J Electrocardiol* 30:247-256, 1997.

PROCEDURE 50

Implanted Cardioverter/Defibrillator

PURPOSE: An implantable cardioverter defibrillator (ICD) functions by monitoring the heart rhythm and delivering corrective electrical therapy when indicated for the child who is at risk for sudden arrhythmic death

Kathleen Hinoki and Laurene Fry

PREREQUISITE KNOWLEDGE

- Child development as it relates to clinical assessment and pediatric ICD placement
- Normal anatomy and physiology of the heart[1]
- Conduction pathway of the heart[1]
- Electrophysiology (EP) terminology, such as bradycardia pacing, sensing, and defibrillation (see Box 51-1)
- Mastery of pediatric advance life support competencies
- Principles of aseptic technique
- Appropriate pediatric dosing of analgesics and competency in procedural sedation
- Ability to monitor and interpret paced and intrinsic electrocardiograms (ECGs)
- Implantable cardioverter defibrillators are implanted under the skin in the upper chest (transvenous) or in the abdomen (epicardial).
- Implantable cardioverter defibrillators also contain a single-chamber or dual-chamber pacemaker.
- Depending on the type of device selected, insertion may be done in the operating room or the cardiac catheterization suite.
- Informed consent is necessary before placement of an ICD.

CHILD AND FAMILY ASSESSMENT

- Child's developmental level and ability to interact ➻*Rationale:* These factors influence preparation and interaction.
- Body image concerns and concerns about lifestyle and activity changes[2] ➻*Rationale:* Children and adolescents with ICDs may have concerns about body image because the ICD device may be visible as a large bump under the skin of the chest or abdomen. Adolescents may have concerns about being "different" from peers because of limitations in activity.
- Child's and family's fears and concerns related to the need for the device and the ability to provide emergency care (e.g., CPR, activating emergency response system) ➻*Rationale:* Identification of fears and concerns facilitates development of an effective teaching plan.
- History of congenital heart disease, cardiomyopathy, cardiac arrhythmias, syncope, surgery, and projected future cardiac surgery[3] ➻*Rationale:* These conditions influence the type of device or leads and the implantation approach that is selected.
- History of previous sedation and anesthesia experiences ➻*Rationale:* History may influence the type of sedation or anesthesia that is used.

- Desire of family members to be present at the hospital during the procedure ➥*Rationale:* Family should be available because of anesthesia and surgical risks and also for provision of support and comfort measures for the child.

CHILD AND FAMILY EDUCATION

Individualized, developmentally appropriate education is provided to the family and to the child based on desire for knowledge, readiness to learn, and overall neurologic and psychosocial state.

- Provide information on the child's medical condition and need for the device ➥*Rationale:* Providing information decreases anxiety and fear.[2]
- If possible, show the child and family an actual device ➥*Rationale:* A visual learning experience enhances the understanding of the procedure and the informed consent process.
- If available and appropriate for the family, provide the family with educational materials available from the ICD manufacturer ➥*Rationale:* These materials may augment the education provided and may contain device-specific information helpful to the family.
- Provide information on the implantation process, postoperative care, follow-up, activity restrictions, and safety issues, including electromagnetic interference (EMI)[3,4] ➥*Rationale:* Postoperative incisional infections or inappropriate or inadequate ICD therapy may occur if instructions are not followed.
- Explain to the child and family that hospitalization for battery replacement is necessary periodically ➥*Rationale:* Providing information in advance facilitates coping and decreases anxiety.
- Discuss with the child and family how the device works and describe the sensation associated with firing of the device[3,4] ➥*Rationale:* Providing information to the child and family reduces fear and anxiety associated with the device.[2]

- Educate the child and family on restrictions associated with the implantation of a pacemaker, such as the avoidance of magnetic resonance imaging (MRI), precautions regarding exposure to radiofrequency devices or power-generating equipment, and the safe use of items such as cellular phones as discussed in the device manufacturer's patient manual ➥*Rationale:* Providing information to the child and family reduces fear and increases compliance with discharge instructions.
- Promote, advocate, and facilitate completion of medical alert jewelry application ➥*Rationale:* All children with an ICD should wear a medical alert identification to alert care providers and to prevent serious injury from exposure to harmful treatments or diagnostic tests, such as MRIs.
- Encourage questions and answer questions as they arise ➥*Rationale:* Reinforcement of information is needed during periods of stress.

EQUIPMENT

- Device/ICD leads
- Skin preparation tray
- Sterile instrument tray
- Sterile drapes or towels
- Sterile sutures and dressing
- Sterile gloves, gowns, masks, and hats
- Cardiorespiratory monitor
- Sterile sleeve for telemetry
- Pacing cables
- Grounding pad
- Lead introducer
- Cautery
- Intravenous (IV) supplies
- Emergency cart
- Programmer specific to selected device or magnet

Procedure	for Implanted Cardioverter/Defibrillator	
Steps	**Rationale**	**Considerations**
1. Ensure child and family have met with implantation practitioner.	Discussion of purpose and surgical risks needs to be addressed.	Child, as developmentally appropriate, and family should be active participants in conversation.
2. Ensure child and family understand procedure and questions are answered.	Evaluates and reinforces understanding of previously taught information.	Developmental level, cognitive ability, and anxiety level determine approach to and effectiveness of teaching.
3. Ensure fasting guidelines have been implemented per institution-specific protocol. (*Level VI**)	Prevents complications related to emesis or aspiration can be achieved.	The NPO time is related to the child's age and type of diet.

Procedure continues on following page

* Level VI: Clinical studies in a variety of patient populations and situations to support recommendations

Procedure for Implanted Cardioverter/Defibrillator—*Continued*

Steps	Rationale	Considerations
4. Confirm that consent for the procedure has been obtained.	Ensures medical-legal compliance as suggested by the Joint Commission on Accreditation of Healthcare Organizations (JCAHO).	The legal guardian must provide consent.
5. Gather necessary equipment and supplies.	Preparation and presence of all materials facilitate completion of the procedure without delay.	Device placed is dependent on the child's anatomy and the practitioner's preference.
6. Wash hands.	Standard precautions; reduces transmission of microorganisms.	
7. If not present, establish IV access. *(Level VI*)*	IV is established for sedation and medication administration.	Before IV access is established, consider any history of vascular compromise (i.e., history of Blalock-Taussig shunt).
8. Administer prescribed sedation per institution-specific protocol. *(Level VI*)*	Sedation often helps decrease a child's anxiety level and promotes easier separation from family.	Type of sedation should consider child's weight and allergy history.
9. Wash hands and put on hat, mask, sterile gown, and sterile gloves per institutional protocol for procedure area.	Standard precautions; protective garb reduces the risk of infection.	
10. Position child on procedural table.	Proper positioning prevents nerve and tissue injuries while the child is anesthetized or immobile.	Use of positioning aids may be necessary.
11. Ensure appropriate cardiorespiratory monitoring and place grounding pad on the child. *(Level III*)*	Children may have decompensation during the procedure. Inappropriate shocks should be avoided.	Vigilance is particularly necessary when ventricular fibrillation is induced.[5]
12. Identify the child with appropriate patient and procedure verification process (e.g., "time out").	Confirms correct patient, procedure, and site as recommended by JCAHO; prevents unnecessary medical procedures.	Verification process and documentation is institution specific. Use active communication techniques.
13. Ensure prescribed IV antibiotics are administered before and after implantation. *(Level IV*)*	Antibiotic administration within 20 minutes of the surgical incision decreases the risk of a postoperative infection.	Consideration should be given to child's drug allergy history.
14. Prepare child's chest or abdomen with antibacterial agent per institution-specific protocol. *(Level IV*)*	Cleaning the skin decreases the risk of a postoperative infection.	
15. Cover child with sterile drapes or towels; establish sterile field.	Allows manipulation of sterile equipment and supplies without contamination; decreases the risk of infection.	
16. Leads are placed by cardiologist or cardiac surgeon; generator is inserted.[5] *(Level I*)*	Lead placement must be documented with fluoroscopy to ensure optimal function of pacemaker.	Lead placement depends on the size of child and type of device.
17. Ensure continuous ECG monitoring and emergency preparedness during pacemaker insertion.[6] *(Level IV*)*	The pacemaker is deactivated during implantation to avoid injury to surgical personnel. *(Level I*)*	Cardiopulmonary resuscitation should be initiated in the event of a lethal arrhythmia. The device is activated and deactivated by exposure to a large magnet.

* Level I: Manufacturer's recommendations only
  Level III: Laboratory data; no clinical data to support recommendations
  Level IV: Limited clinical studies to support recommendations
  Level VI: Clinical studies in a variety of patient populations and situations to support recommendations

Procedure for Implanted Cardioverter/Defibrillator—*Continued*

Steps	Rationale	Considerations
18. Pacemaker is activated and a dry sterile pressure dressing is placed over insertion site.	Sterile pressure dressing decreases the chance of infections and swelling.	
19. Transport child to postanesthesia/recovery area per institution-specific protocol.	Allows continued monitoring after the procedure.	Length of time in the hospital is typically less than 24 hours after implant.
20. Dispose of used supplies and equipment, including sharps, appropriately; wash hands.	Standard precautions; reduecs transmission of microorganisms.	
21. Ensure postimplant x-ray is obtained. *(Level II*)*	Verifies proper lead position.	

* Level II: Theory-based; no research data to support recommendations; recommendations from expert consensus group may exist

Expected Outcomes

- Implantable cardioverter defibrillator device and leads remain in proper position
- Acceptable sensing and pacing thresholds are achieved
- Implantable cardioverter defibrillator effectively detects rhythm disturbances and delivers therapy as programmed
- Return to presedation or anesthesia status within expected time frame
- Surgical site is free from infection
- Child has acceptable level of comfort

Unexpected Outcomes

- Lead displacement
- Unable to achieve acceptable sensing and pacing thresholds
- Implantable cardioverter defibrillator does not detect rhythm disturbances or fires inappropriately
- Child remains sedated or anesthetized for a prolonged period
- Paradoxic agitation
- Infection at surgical site
- Unmanaged pain

Monitoring and Care of the Child

Activities and Interventions	Rationale	Reportable Conditions
1. Monitor vital signs throughout procedure and during recovery per institution-specific protocol.	Allows early identification of complications from procedure or anesthesia/sedation.	• Unstable vital signs • Respiratory compromise • Significant blood loss
2. Monitor cardiac rhythm throughout procedure and recovery.	Allows identification of arrhythmias and child's response to device activation.	• Arrhythmias • Failure of device to function after activation
3. Monitor level of sedation or analgesia during procedure.	Ensures adequate comfort and sedation levels. Decreases child's and family's anxiety level.	• Unmanaged pain • Inadequate sedation • Level of consciousness is inappropriate for degree of medical therapy
4. Monitor recovery from sedation or anesthesia.	Monitors for return to baseline and full recovery.	• Delayed recovery from sedation or anesthesia • Untoward reactions to sedation or anesthesia, such as nausea and vomiting or paradoxic agitation

Continued

Monitoring and Care of the Child—Cont'd

Activities and Interventions	Rationale	Reportable Conditions
5. During recovery, assess effectiveness of pain management strategy and provide appropriate interventions. Encourage family to assist with nonpharmacologic means to comfort and support the child.	Early identification of discomfort allows for immediate attention.	• Report of unresolved pain and discomfort • Continued irritability and changes in physiologic condition
6. Evaluate incision site approximately 1 week after implant. 7. Monitor child's ICD at regular intervals, every 1 to 6 months.[3]	Allows identification of infection at the incision site. Routine evaluations are needed to monitor for rhythm disturbances, what therapies have been delivered and whether they were effective, and battery status.	• Redness, swelling, or drainage from incision site • If child receives a shock but feels fine afterwards, family should call in to inform ICD team of event • If child receives multiple shocks or does not feel well after receiving a shock, immediate medical attention is advised

Documentation

- Consent for procedure
- Compliance with fasting guidelines
- Patient and procedure verification process
- Vital signs throughout procedure and recovery per institution-specific protocol
- Sedation or anesthesia necessary for procedure and response
- Child's response to device activation
- Device implantation record
- X-ray interpretation after implantation
- Procedural note
- Comfort assessment and any specific interventions provided
- Child and family education
- Unexpected outcomes and related treatment

References

1. Allen HD, et al: *Moss and Adams' heart disease in infants, children, and adolescents,* vol 1, Philadelphia, 2000, Lippincott Williams & Wilkins.
2. DeMaso DR, et al: Psychosocial factors and quality of life in children and adolescents with implantable cardioverter-defibrillators, *Am J Cardiol* 93(1):582-587, 2004.
3. Dougherty C, et al: Description of a nursing intervention program after an implantable cardioverter defibrillator, *Heart Lung* 33(3):183-190, 2004.
4. Rao BH, Saksena S: Implantable cardioverter-defibrillators in cardiovascular care: technologic advances and new indications, *Curr Opin Crit Care* 9:362-368, 2003.
5. Reiffel JA, Dizon J: The implantable cardioverter-defibrillator patient perspective, *Circulation* 105(9):1022-1024, 2002.
6. Wolbrette DL, Naccarelli GV: Management of implantable cardioverter defibrillator patients: role of predischarge electrophysiologic testing and proper patient instruction before hospital discharge, *Curr Opin Cardiol* 16(1):72-75, 2001.

Additional Readings

Berul CI: Cardiac arrhythmias and device therapy: results and prospectives for the new century, Armonk, NY, 2000, Futura Publishing Company, Inc.

Pinski SL, Trohman RG: Interference in implantable cardiac devices, part I, *Pacing Clin Electrophysiol* 25(9):1367-1381, 2002.

Pinski SL, Trohman RG: Interference in implanted cardiac devices, part II. *Pacing Clin Electrophysiol* 25(10):1496-1509, 2002.

Sears SF, et al: Young at heart: understanding the unique psychosocial adjustment of young implantable cardioverter defibrillator recipients, *Pacing Clin Electrophysiol* 24(7):1113-1117, 2000.

Serwer GA, Dorostkar PC, Leroy SS: Clinical cardiac pacing and defibrillation, Philadelphia, 2000, Saunders.

Walsh EP, et al: *Cardiac arrhythmias in children and young adults with congenital heart disease*, Philadelphia, 2001, Lippincott Williams & Wilkins.

Permanent Pacemaker: Assessing Function

P U R P O S E : To assess functioning of a newly placed or established permanent pacemaker

Maggie Fischer

PREREQUISITE KNOWLEDGE

- Child development as it relates to clinical assessment and permanent pacemaker assessment
- Mastery of pediatric advanced life support competencies
- Normal cardiac anatomy and physiology, including the principles of cardiac conduction[1]
- An understanding of the child's congenital heart disease and associated short-term and long-term electrophysiologic complications
- Permanent pacemakers are implanted in children with:
  - ❖ Symptomatic bradycardia
  - ❖ Advanced atrioventricular (AV) block with syncope, dizziness, exercise intolerance, or heart failure
  - ❖ Congenital or acquired heart block
  - ❖ Postoperative heart block that persists longer than 7 to 10 days
  - ❖ Bradycardia-dependent ventricular tachycardia (Long QT syndrome)
- Specific indications for permanent pacemaker implantation in the child

- Ability to monitor and interpret paced and intrinsic electrocardiograms (ECGs) See Figure 51-1, for examples of paced ECGs.
- Ability to differentiate between mechanical and electrical capture
- Ability to assess and interpret child's response to pacing therapy
- Familiarity with North American Society of Pacing and Electrophysiology (NASPE) generic pacemaker code (Table 51-1)
- Appropriate heart rate ranges for children
- Magnet application to initiate nonsensing function and events that necessitate magnet use
- Familiarity with activation of the emergency alert system
- Concepts related to permanent pacemakers (Box 51-1, for a glossary of pacemaker terminology)
  - ❖ Permanent pacemakers may be placed with a transvenous or epicardial approach
  - ❖ Permanent pacing systems may have an atrial lead, a ventricular lead, or both. Pacing mode programming may include AAI(R), VVI(R), DDD(R), DVI, and VDD (Table 51-2).[2-4]

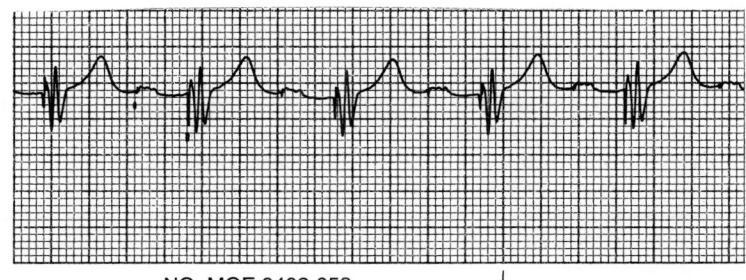

NO. MQE 9402-053

A: AV Pacing

FIGURE 51-1 Examples of Paced ECG Tracings.

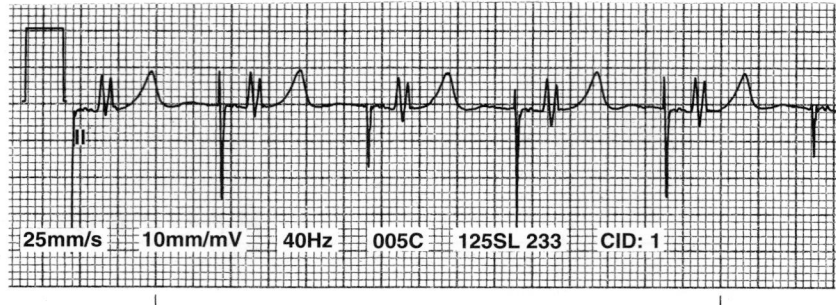

B: AAI pacing

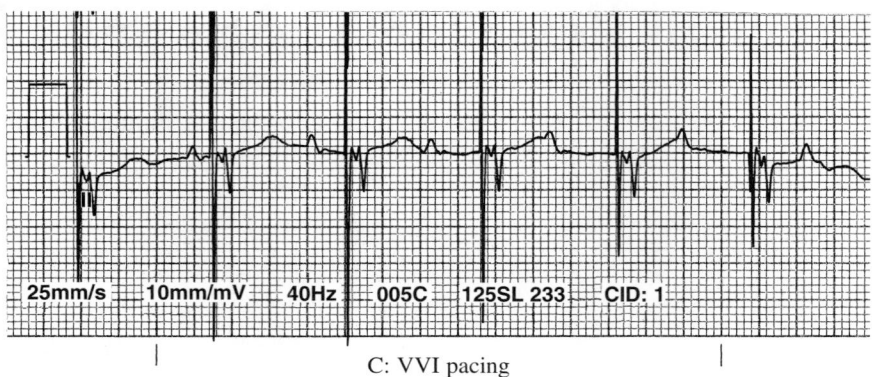

C: VVI pacing

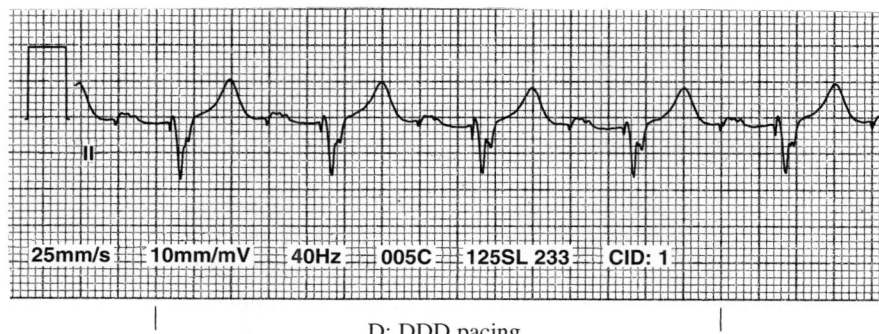

D: DDD pacing

FIGURE 51-1 CONT'D   Examples of Paced ECG Tracings.

TABLE 51-1	North American Society of Pacing and Electrophysiology-British Pacing and Electrophysiology Group (NASPE-BPEG) Generic Pacemaker Code

Letter I: Chamber Paced	Letter II: Chamber Sensed	Letter III: Response to Sensed Event	Letter IV: Programmability/ Rate Response	Letter V: Antitachycardic Functions
O: None	O: None	O: None	O: None	O: None
A: Atrium	A: Atrium	I: Inhibit	P: Simple programmable	P: Antitachycardiac pacing
V: Ventricle	V: Ventricle	T: Triggered	M: Multiprogrammable	S: Shock
D: Dual (A + V)	D: Dual (A + V)	D: Dual (I + T)	C: Communicating	D: Dual (P + S)
			R: Rate modulation	

From Bernstein D, Camm AJ, Flether RD, et al: The NASPE/BPEG generic pacemaker code for anti-bradyarrhythmia and adaptive-rate pacing and anti-tachyarrhythmia devices, *Pacing Clin Electrophysiol PACE* 10:794-799, 1987.

Box 51-1	**Glossary of Pacing Terminology**

Asynchronous (Fixed-Rate): Paced events occur at the programmed rate regardless of the intrinsic heart rate. Sensing does not occur so the pacemaker competes with the intrinsic heart rhythm. An example of this type of mode is: AOO, VOO, DOO.

Antitachycardia Pacing: Involves the delivery of one to several paced stimuli to the atrium or ventricle in an attempt to terminate tachycardia. Typically done to terminate ventricular tachycardia; most implantable cardioverter defibrillators (ICDs) have this capability.

Atrial Pacing: Single-chamber pacing in which atrium is paced at a set rate.

Atrial Overdrive Pacing: Atrial pacing at rates of more than 200 impulses/min used to terminate atrial tachycardia, atrial flutter, or atrial fibrillation. This is typically done via temporary pacing with epicardial wires after cardiac surgery. Newer dual-chamber pacemakers have this capability.

Atrial Refractory Period: The length of time when the atrial channel cannot respond to ventricular incoming signals.

Atrial Tracking: State of dual-chamber pacing, when sensed atrial activity triggers a ventricular paced beat at the end of a programmed AV interval.

Atrioventricular (AV) Interval: The length of time during dual-chamber pacing between a sensed or paced atrial beat and the delivery of a ventricular paced beat. The AV interval is programmed in milliseconds (ms), where an AV interval of 120 ms is equal to a PR interval of 0.12 seconds. Many pacemakers have an adaptive feature that allows the AV interval to be shortened when the intrinsic atrial rate is increased to mimic physiologic responses to heart rate acceleration.

Base Rate: Lower rate pacemaker setting at which pacemaker paces when no intrinsic heart rate is present.

Biventricular Pacing (Cardiac Resynchronization Therapy): Mode of pacing that provides atrial-synchronized biventricular pacing with standard dual-chamber pacing technology in addition to the placement of a special third lead that is implanted via the coronary sinus and positioned in a cardiac vein to sense or pace the left ventricle. After a sensed atrial contraction or atrial-paced event, both ventricles are stimulated to synchronize their contraction. Biventricular pacing results in reduced mitral regurgitation, optimal left ventricular filling, and improved cardiac function. Cardiac resynchronization therapy (CRT) is a proven treatment for patients with heart failure–induced conduction disturbances and ventricular dyssynchrony.[1]

Blanking Period: Brief period during dual-chamber pacing when the ventricle is unable to respond to any stimulus. This occurs simultaneously with every atrial paced beat to prevent the ventricle channel from sensing the paced atrial beat and misinterpreting it as a ventricular event (also known as crosstalk) and therefore inhibiting the ventricular paced beat.

Capture: Ability of pacemaker to depolarize chamber being paced. On ECG, appropriate atrial pacing is seen when an atrial spike is followed by a P wave and appropriate ventricular pacing is seen as a ventricular spike followed by a wide QRS.

Demand Pacing: Setting at which pacing occurs only when the intrinsic heart rate falls below the programmed pacemaker rate.

Dual-Chamber Pacing: Type of pacing where both atria and ventricles can be programmed to be paced, establishing AV synchrony.

Escape Interval: Period of time between a sensed cardiac event and the next paced beat, which is typically equal to the programmed paced rate.

Fusion Beat: Occurs when an intrinsic depolarization occurs at the same time as a paced beat. This typically occurs in the ventricle.

Hysteresis: Programmable feature that allows the pacing interval after the paced beat (escape interval) to be longer than the basic pacing interval, allowing for more intrinsic cardiac activity.

Inhibited Response: Demand pacing where pacing is inhibited when an intrinsic beat is sensed.

Magnet Mode: Denotes the occurrence when a magnet is placed over the pulse generator. The generator response differs among manufacturers, but the pacemaker essentially goes into a preset asynchronous mode at a preset rate and in a preset manner. A change in magnet-induced pacing rate usually indicates that the generator is at end of life (needs replacement).

Output: Electrical stimulus delivered by the pacemaker defined by the pulse amplitude and the pulse width.

Oversensing: Inappropriate sensing of electrical signals that results in inhibition of paced beat; causes include crosstalk, electromagnetic interference, T waves, and cardiac muscle movement (myocardial potentials).

Pacing Interval: Time between two consecutive paced events; measured in milliseconds (ms).

Postventricular Atrial Refractory Period (PVARP): Dual-chamber pacemaker programmable setting that is part of the total atrial refractory period. This parameter is used to prevent the atrial channel from inappropriately sensing far-field ventricular signals, such as T waves and myocardial potentials. It can also be used to avoid pacemaker-mediated tachycardia by preventing the atrial channel from sensing retrograde signals.

Rate Modulation/Rate Response: Dual-chamber pacemaker parameter that allows the pacemaker to increase the pacing rate in response to increased physical activity. The pacemaker contains an accelerometer or piezoelectric crystal that is activated by either vibration/motion or minute ventilation. This sensor allows for continuous adjustments to the programmed rate.

Refractory Period: The length of time after a sensed or paced event when the pacemaker does not respond to incoming signals.

Sensing: The pacemaker's ability to recognize and respond to an intrinsic cardiac depolarization.

Sensing Threshold: The smallest amount (measured in millivolts) of intrinsic atrial or ventricular signal that can be consistently sensed by the pacemaker.

Stimulation Threshold (Capture or Pacing Threshold): The least amount of voltage necessary to consistently capture the heart.

Undersensing: Failure of the pacemaker to appropriately sense intrinsic cardiac depolarizations, which can result in competition between the pacemaker and the intrinsic rhythm.

Ventricular Pacing: Single-chamber pacemaker that only paces the ventricle.

Ventricular Refractory Period: The length of time after a ventricular sensed or paced beat during which the ventricle channel cannot respond to incoming signals.

From Jacobson C, Gerity D: Pacemakers and implantable defibrillators. In Woods S, Sivarajan Froelicher E, Underhill Motzer S, editors: *Cardiac nursing,* ed 4, Philadelphia, 2000, Lippincott Williams & Wilkins. http://www.medtronic.com/physician/hf/treatment.html.

TABLE 51-2	Dual-Chamber Pacing Modes		
Mode	Chambers Paced	Chambers Sensed	Response to Sensing
DVI	Dual (A + V)	Ventricle	Ventricular sensing inhibits A and V pacing
VDD	Ventricle	Dual (A + V)	A sensing triggers V pacing
			V sensing inhibits V pacing
DDI	Dual (A + V)	Dual (A + V)	A sensing inhibits A pacing
			V sensing inhibits V pacing
DDD	Dual (A + V)	Dual (A + V)	A sensing inhibits A pacing, triggers V pacing
			V sensing inhibits A and V pacing

A, Atrium; *V,* ventricle.

From Jacobson C, Gerity D: Pacemakers and implantable defibrillators. In Woods S, Sivarajan Froelicher E, Underhill Motzer S, editors: *Cardiac nursing,* ed 4, Philadelphia, 2000, Lippincott Williams & Wilkins.

- Concepts related to transvenous pacemakers
  - ❖ Transvenous implantation is the method of choice in most adult and adolescent patients with access with the cephalic, subclavian, jugular, or axillary veins.
  - ❖ The transvenous pacemaker pocket is developed in the pectoral area (usually on the nondominant left side)
- Concepts related to epicardial pacemakers
  - ❖ Implantation is performed through a xyphoid approach.
  - ❖ Method of choice in a neonate or a small child (<25 kg) or when the transvenous approach is not possible (e.g., after a Fontan operation or because of anatomic limitations)
  - ❖ The pacemaker pocket for epicardial implants is made in the epigastric or abdominal cavity.
- Complications of permanent pacemaker placement
  - ❖ Complications with the transvenous approach include lead dislodgment, perforation of the heart with risk of tamponade, supraventricular or ventricular arrhythmias, and pacemaker pocket infection or hematoma.[5]
  - ❖ Complications with an epicardial approach include lead fracture and laceration of the heart.[5]
  - ❖ Development of twiddler's syndrome: Unconscious repeated rotation by the patient of a subcutaneous pacemaker generator that causes the leads to loop and wrap around the generator, which results in lead dislodgement or fracture.[1] Children may be more susceptible to twiddler's syndrome because they have thinner subcutaneous tissue and may not fully comprehend the consequences of their actions if recognized.
  - ❖ Development of pacemaker syndrome: Initially described in patients with ventricular pacemakers; related to nonphysiologic timing of atrial and ventricular contractions, which may occur in a variety of pacing modes. Pacemaker syndrome represents the clinical consequences of loss of AV synchrony, retrograde ventriculoatrial (VA) conduction, and absence of rate response to physiologic need.[6] Presenting symptoms include pulsations in the neck or abdomen, headache, cough or jaw pain from cannon a waves (atrial contraction against closed AV valves), and pulmonary and hepatic venous congestion from increased left and right atrial pressure. Other symptoms include extremely pro-

longed first degree AV block or a nodal rhythm that is faster than the atrial rate.[6]

CHILD AND FAMILY ASSESSMENT

- History of dizziness, sweating, palpitations, chest pain, shortness of breath, lethargy, or loss of consciousness ➡*Rationale:* These conditions may indicate pacemaker complications.
- Child's developmental level and ability to interact ➡*Rationale:* These factors influence preparation of the child and interaction.
- Child's and family's understanding of the reasons for and risks and benefits of the procedure ➡*Rationale:* Evaluates child's and family's understanding of the procedure and provides a gauge for ongoing education.
- Child's type of pacemaker and pacing mode ➡*Rationale:* This information is necessary for assessment of whether the pacemaker is functioning correctly.
- If the pacemaker is newly placed, child's comfort level ➡*Rationale:* Child may have incisional pain; prompt identification allows for effective treatment.
- Family's desire to be present during the procedure ➡*Rationale:* The family may provide support and comfort to the child during the procedure but should have the option not to remain with the child.

CHILD AND FAMILY EDUCATION

Individualized, developmentally appropriate education is provided to the family and to the child based on desire for knowledge, readiness to learn, and overall neurologic and psychosocial state.

- Explain the need to remain flat in bed for 8 hours after the implant to prevent lead dislodgment or fracture ➡*Rationale:* A lead revision may be necessary if dislodgment or fracture with subsequent noncapture occurs.
- Explain the need to wear an arm sling on the operative side for 2 to 4 weeks for children with a new transvenous system ➡*Rationale:* Ipsilateral shoulder movement should be minimized for the first month to prevent dislodgement of the pacing lead.

- Reinforce and educate the child and family on monitoring for signs and symptoms that may indicate pacemaker malfunction, lead failure, undersensing or oversensing; provide information on activity restrictions, safety precautions with regards to electromagnetic interference, and follow-up requirements, including the telephone transmission schedule and who to call with questions or concerns[5] ➤➤*Rationale:* Pacemaker malfunction or inadequate therapy may occur if instructions are not followed.
- Educate the family as to the life expectancy of the generator and leads ➤➤*Rationale:* The family and child are provided with information needed to monitor the child for indications that the generator or pacemaker is not working appropriately, which decreases fear and anxiety related to the device.
- Inform the family of signs and symptoms of incisional infection ➤➤*Rationale:* The child and family are informed of reasons to notify the health care team, which allows prompt assessment and intervention and encourages active participation in care by the family and child.
- Explain the child's activity restrictions: no contact sports or heavy lifting ➤➤*Rationale:* Protects the implanted device and child's safety. Providing the rationale for restrictions promotes compliance with the restrictions.
- Educate the child and family about safety precautions with regard to electromagnetic interference, such as magnets, powerful electrical equipment, and cellular phones[7] ➤➤*Rationale:* Family and child are alerted to situations and circumstances that should be avoided to promote the child's safety.
- Ensure that the family understands follow-up instructions: when and who to call with concerns or questions, timing of telephone transmissions, and scheduled appointments ➤➤*Rationale:* The family is provided with information needed to safely care for the child at home.
- If available, provide written educational material to the child and family related to the pacemaker ➤➤*Rationale:* Written material permits the family to refer to a source of information that reinforces verbal teaching. Educational materials for reference can help to reduce anxiety and fear.
- Ensure that the child wears medical alert identification. If the pacemaker has just been inserted, advocate for and facilitate the application process to obtain the medical alert identification; have child or family member keep the company-issued pacemaker identification card in a wallet. ➤➤*Rationale:* All children with a pacemaker should possess some form of medical alert identification to notify health care personnel and dentists in the case of an emergency and to prevent serious harm to the child from exposure to therapy, devices, or equipment that may cause injury or interfere with pacemaker function.
- Encourage questions and answer questions as they arise ➤➤*Rationale:* Reinforcement of information is needed during periods of stress.

EQUIPMENT

- Stethoscope
- Calipers
- Electrocardiogram machine/ECG patches (available as needed)
- Telemetry equipment with printing capability
- Defibrillator readily available on the unit
- Child's pacemaker settings and parameters
- Programmer specific to selected device or magnet
- Crash cart readily available on the unit

Procedure for Permanent Pacemaker: Assessing Function

Steps	Rationale	Considerations
1. Ensure child and family understand procedure and questions are answered.	Evaluates and reinforces understanding of previously taught information.	Developmental level, cognitive ability, and anxiety level determine approach to and effectiveness of teaching.
2. Gather needed equipment and supplies; ensure that all monitoring equipment is functioning properly. Confirm that the printer is working and that the paper supply is adequate.	Ensures that all equipment necessary for the procedure is at bedside and functioning properly to facilitate completion of procedure without delays.	Ensure that telemetry monitoring has correct patient information. Make sure the "Pace ON" feature is activated in telemetry system to ensure recognition of pacemaker spikes.
3. Wash hands. *(Level VI*)*	Standard precautions; reduces transmission of microorganisms.	
4. Identify child with two patient identifiers per institution-specific protocol.	Ensures correct patient and correct procedure as recommended by the Joint Commission for Accreditation of Healthcare Organizations (JCAHO).	Promotes patient safety.

Procedure continues on following page

* Level VI: Clinical studies in a variety of patient populations and situations to support recommendations

Procedure | for Permanent Pacemaker: Assessing Function—*Continued*

Steps	Rationale	Considerations
5. Position child supine.[4] *(Level II*)*	Supine positioning provides optimal access for electrode placement. Alternative positioning may be necessary for the child who is extremely anxious, developmentally delayed, or wheelchair bound.	Allow family members to remain at the bedside to provide support and comfort to the child.
6. Place ECG patches and connect to cardiac/telemetry monitor. *(Level I*)*	Nonsecure or inappropriate connections can lead to incomplete tracings or inability of monitor to pick up tracing.	After surgery, all patients with pacemakers and new leads should be on telemetry or a monitor for at least 24 to 48 hours per institution-specific protocol.[3,4]
7. Run rhythm strip. *(Level II*)*	Verifies current rhythm.	A rhythm strip should always be obtained if a patient has dizziness, palpitations, chest pain, shortness of breath, presyncope, or symptoms of pacemaker sydrome[3,4,6]; these are symptoms experienced with pacemaker malfunction. *(Level IV*)*
8. Verify pacing parameters: pacing mode and heart rate parameters, output, pulse width, postventricular atrial refractory period (PVARP), and AV intervals. *(Level I*)*	Verifies that programmed parameters are appropriate for child and confirms that settings match the implant printout. The PVARP may be preset on many models, as can pulse width, and cannot be determined without interrogation.[2]	Parameters can be ascertained from implant printout or progress note and verified by pacemaker interaction with intrinsic rhythm on ECG results.
9. Verify that pacemaker is capturing appropriately (presence of a spike on paced beats). *(Level II*)*	Assesses for lead and pacemaker malfunction. The most common complication of transvenous pacing is lead dislodgment.[5]	Atrial capture occurs when a pacer spike immediately precedes a P wave.[2,3] Ventricular capture occurs when a pacer spike immediately precedes a QRS complex.[2,3]
10. Verify that appropriate sensing is present. *(Level II*)*	Assesses for lead and pacemaker malfunction. Sensing function may be lost before pacing function.	If pacemaker undersensing is present, paced beats may be shorter than paced cycle length. If oversensing is present, paced beats may be longer than the paced cycle length.
11. Evaluate incision for signs of edema, drainage, or erythema. *(Level IV*)*	Assess for signs of complication at insertion site (hematoma, seroma, or infection).	For epicardial implants, incision and pacemaker pockets are in epigastric or abdominal area. For transvenous implants, incision and pacemaker pockets are in left or right pectoral area.
12. Obtain a chest x-ray.	Confirms lead placement and evaluates for complications such as lead fracture, lead dislodgement, or cardiac tamponade.[2,5] If the transvenous system is new, evaluate for pneumothorax.	Only necessary with a new pacing system or lead revision. Obtain a chest x-ray if symptoms are suspicious of lead dysfunction to rule out twiddler's syndrome, lead dislodgement, or lead fracture.[1]
13. Child should remain flat in bed after pacemaker implant per institution-specific protocol. *(Level III*)*	Early complications may include lead dislodgement or fracture, perforation of the heart, tamponade, or arrhythmias.[2,5]	The child can be allowed to ambulate once a chest x-ray and pacemaker check have been completed.

* Level I: Manufacturer's recommendations only
  Level II: Theory-based; no research data to support recommendations; recommendations from expert consensus group may exist
  Level III: Laboratory data; no clinical data to support recommendations
  Level IV: Limited clinical studies to support recommendations

Procedure for Permanent Pacemaker: Assessing Function—*Continued*		
Steps	**Rationale**	**Considerations**
14. If child has a transvenous system, immobilize arm or shoulder on the side in which generator has been implanted. *(Level III*)*	Prevents lead dislodgement or fracture from repeated overextension of the arm and shoulder.[5]	The time frame for use is institution specific; generally, use of sling is recommended for 2 to 4 weeks.
15. Dispose of supplies and used equipment appropriately; wash hands.	Standard precautions; reduces transmission of microorganisms.	

* Level III: Laboratory data; no clinical data to support recommendations

Expected Outcomes

- Incision site and pacemaker pocket are free from hematoma, seroma, or infection
- Rhythm strip shows appropriate pacemaker function
- Appropriate pacemaker sensing

- Rhythm is regular

- Pacemaker lead remains intact and functioning
- Child's hemodynamic status remains stable

- Child has acceptable level of comfort

Unexpected Outcomes

- Hematoma, seroma, or infection present around the incision site or pacemaker pocket
- Pacemaker noncapture
- Undersensing or oversensing noted with rates slower than or faster than the paced rate
- Rhythm irregularity with atrial or ventricular arrhythmias present
- Lead dislodgement or fracture
- Cardiac arrhythmia
- Cardiac tamponade
- Unmanaged pain

Monitoring and Care of the Child

Activities and Interventions	**Rationale**	**Reportable Conditions**
1. Monitor child's heart rate and rhythm via telemetry, rhythm strip, and palpation of pulse.	Documents effectiveness of pacing therapy and assists in determination of whether the programmed settings are appropriate for child.	• Heart rate drops below the programmed settings • Rhythm irregularity
2. Assess for appropriate pacemaker capture and sensing.	Assists in determination of whether pacing thresholds are appropriate for child.	• Pacemaker noncapture (pacer spike without a corresponding P wave or QRS complex)
3. Monitor for presence of palpitations, dizziness, shortness of breath, or chest pain.	These symptoms may indicate pacemaker malfunction or rhythm disturbance.	• Undersensing: Paced beats that are faster than the set low rate • Oversensing: Paced beats that are slower than the set low rate
4. Assess condition of incision site.	Evaluates for signs of hematoma, seroma, or infection.	• Fever or erythema • Edema • Drainage at the incision site
5. Assess child's and family's understanding of pacemaker teaching and follow-up care.	Ensures compliance with the follow-up plan and decreases fear and anxiety related to device.	• Child or parent reports inability to comply with follow-up plan • Family or child unable to comprehend pacemaker instructions
6. Assess effectiveness of pain management strategy and provide appropriate interventions. Encourage family to assist with nonpharmacologic means to comfort and support child.	Early identification of pain facilitates prompt treatment.	• Unresolved pain or discomfort • Continued irritability or changes in physiologic condition

Documentation

- Heart rate and rhythm
- Evidence of inappropriate pacemaker activity (undersensing, oversensing, noncapture, or failure to pace)
- Any reported symptoms of pacemaker syndrome or chest pain, palpitations, dizziness, shortness of breath, or presyncope
- Condition of the incision site with new pacemaker implantation
- Verification of pacemaker mode, rate, output, pulse width, and sensing values
- Child and family education
- Corrective action taken to fix inappropriate pacemaker activity
- Comfort assessment and any specific interventions provided
- Unexpected outcomes and related treatment

References

1. Abrams S, Peart I: Twiddler's syndrome in children: an unusual cause of pacemaker failure, *Br Heart J* 73:190-192, 1995.
2. Berul C, Cecchin F: Indications and techniques of pediatric cardiac pacing, *Expert Rev Cardiovasc Ther* 1(2):165-176, 2003.
3. Deal B, et al: *Current concepts in diagnosis and management of arrhythmias in infants and children,* New York, 1998, Futura Publishing Co., Inc.
4. Furman S, et al: *A practice of cardiac pacing,* ed 3, New York, 1993, Futura Publishing Co., Inc.
5. Thomson J, et al: Pacing activity, patient and lead survival over 20 years of permanent epicardial pacing in children, *Ann Thorac Surg* 77:1366-1370, 2004.
6. Horenstein MS, Karpawich PP: Pacemaker syndrome in the young: do children need dual chamber as the initial pacing mode? *Pacing Clin Electrophysiol.* 27(5):600-605, 2004.
7. Hekmat K, et al: Interference by cellular phones with permanent implanted pacemakers: an update, *Europace* 6(4):363-369, 2004.

Additional Reading

Park M: *Pediatric cardiology for practitioners,* ed 3, St. Louis, 1996, Mosby.

Transcutaneous Pacing: Initiation and Monitoring

P U R P O S E : To provide ventricular pacing on an emergent basis when an immediate increase in heart rate is necessary to maintain adequate hemodynamics.

Karen Kilian

PREREQUISITE KNOWLEDGE

- Normal cardiac anatomy and physiology, including the principles of cardiac conduction
- An understanding of children with acquired or congenital heart disease and associated short-term and long-term electrophysiologic complications
- Familiarity with the child's medical and surgical history, including placement of permanent internal pacemaker or internal defibrillator
- Temporary transcutaneous pacing supports cardiac output in children who need emergent pacing to increase the heart rate. Temporary transcutaneous pacing may also be indicated on an elective or stand-by basis when the child is at risk for rhythm disturbances that could create hemodynamic compromise (i.e., cardioversion, replacement of a permanent pacemaker, or drug-induced brady-dysrhythmia).[1-3]
- Emergent temporary transcutaneous pacing is accomplished with placement of pacing pads in the subclavicular area and left lower sternal border regions and attachment of the cables to an external pacemaker. Infants and obese childern should have pacing patches placed in the anterior/posterior position.[2-4] Refer to manufacturer-specific packaging for exact placement reference when applying pads (see Figure 45-5 for the anterior/posterior pad position in an infant).
- Pediatric pads should be used for children up to 15 kg.[3,5,6]
- Adult pads should be used for children more than 15 kg.[3,5,6]

- Institution of temporary pacing may occur in any location where continuous cardiopulmonary monitoring is available. The child should then be transferred to the intensive care unit for further management of the underlying medical condition. Once the condition is stabilized, children are usually scheduled for permanent pacemaker placement.
- Clinical studies have shown that continuous temporary transcutaneous pacing can be efficacious for up to 14 hours.[2]
- Normal infant, child, and adolescent heart rates
- Basic and advanced electrocardiographic (ECG) and cardiac arrhythmia interpretation
- Ability to differentiate between intrinsic and paced beats with capture on ECG
- Familiarity with electrophysiologic terminology (see Procedure 51 for a glossary of pacing terminology)
- Assessment of hemodynamics in response to pacing therapy
- Familiarity with activation of the emergency alert system
- Mastery of pediatric advanced life support competencies

CHILD AND FAMILY ASSESSMENT

- History of congenital heart disease, cardiomyopathy, cardiac arrhythmias, syncope, cardiac surgical or catheterization procedures, previous electrophysiologic complications, and projected cardiac surgery requirements (permanent pacing device or automated implanted cardioverter/defibrillator) **»»Rationale:** These conditions can impact the placement of the pacing pads; knowledge of projected cardiac surgery requirements assists with anticipatory planning for optimal long-term treatment.[3,7]

- Current hemodynamic status **»»Rationale:** Initiation of inotropic support may be necessary to stabilize the child's condition before, after, or during the procedure.[1]
- History of 12-lead ECGs **»»Rationale:** Establishes prior baseline rhythm.
- Medication history, including herbal supplements, street and over-the-counter drug use, current acid-base balance, and electrolyte levels **»»Rationale:** Drug therapy and electrolyte or acid-base abnormalities could impede the ability to pace the child. Certain medications or drug exposures may be implicated as the cause for the dysrhythmia.[7]
- Child's developmental level and ability to interact **»»Rationale:** These factors influence preparation of the child and interaction and determine the child's ability to cooperate with instructions.
- History of response to anesthesia or conscious sedation **»»Rationale:** Previous response may influence the type of sedation used for the procedure to safely achieve desired results.
- Child's and family's understanding of the reasons for and risks and benefits of the procedure **»»Rationale:** Evaluates family's and child's understanding of the procedure and provides a gauge for ongoing education.
- Family's desire to be present during the procedure **»»Rationale:** The family may provide support and comfort measures to the child during the procedure but should have the choice not to remain with the child.

CHILD AND FAMILY EDUCATION

Individualized, developmentally appropriate education is provided to the family and to the child based on desire for knowledge, readiness to learn, and overall neurologic and psychosocial state.

- Provide information on the child's medical condition and rationale for temporary pacing **»»Rationale:** Educationally appropriate information helps to decrease the child's and family's anxiety levels and offers reassurance during a stressful period.
- Inform the family that temporary transcutaneous pacing is used to stabilize the child's condition until a permanent pacemaker can safely be placed **»»Rationale:** Information about the plan of care assists in preparing the child and family for future procedures and decreases anxiety and fear.[5]
- If time permits, demonstrate the placement of the pacing pads and provide an explanation of the procedure immediately before initiation of the procedure **»»Rationale:** Visual examples can decrease fear and anxiety.
- Provide developmentally appropriate information on the pacing process, postprocedural care, and activity restriction requirements **»»Rationale:** Providing information to the child and family decreases fear and anxiety and may increase compliance with plan of care.
- Inform the child and family that medication will be administered to keep the child comfortable during pacing therapy as appropriate **»»Rationale:** Transcutaneous pacing is uncomfortable; the child will need analgesia or sedation.
- Encourage questions and answer questions as they arise **»»Rationale:** Reinforcement of information is needed during periods of stress and is especially important given the usually emergent nature of this procedure.

EQUIPMENT

- Cardiopulmonary monitor
- Electrocardiographic patches and recorder
- 12-lead or 15-lead ECG machine
- Transcutaneous pacemaker device
- Pacing pads
- Pacing cable
- Supplies to clean the skin (optional)
- Intravenous (IV) supplies (if access not established)
- Medications for sedation per prescribing practitioner's order
- Emergency cart
- Defibrillator

Note: Defibrillator may be used for monitoring and pacing the child; refer to specific manufacturer's instructions regarding unit set up and utilization.

Procedure for Transcutaneous Pacing

Steps	Rationale	Considerations
1. As time and situation permits, facilitate a meeting of child and family with the practitioner who will perform procedure.	Facilitates discussion of reasons for and risks and benefits of the procedure.	If situation and time permit, informed consent is obtained from the child's legal guardian. In emergent conditions, if legal guardians are not available, informed consent may be waived until after child's condition is stabilized; refer to institution-specific protocol.

Procedure for Transcutaneous Pacing—*Continued*

Steps	Rationale	Considerations
2. Ensure child and family understand procedure and questions are answered.	Evaluates and reinforces understanding of previously taught information.	This procedure may be performed in emergent conditions that may preclude preprocedural teaching.
3. If sedation is planned, provide fasting guidelines per institution-specific protocol.	Prevents complications related to aspiration while the child is sedated.	Fasting time is related to the child's age and type of sedation to be administered.
4. Gather needed equipment and supplies, including emergency cart and defibrillator.	Ensures that all equipment is at the bedside; facilitates completion of the procedure without delays.	An extra set of pacing pads should always be available in case of equipment malfunction.
5. Wash hands.	Standard precautions; reduces transmission of microorganisms.	
6. Position child on a flat surface with the head of bed elevated 30 to 45 degrees. *(Level II*)*	Proper positioning may decrease the incidence rate of equipment malfunction and pad dislodgment and may decrease child's anxiety.	Proper positioning also facilitates airway stability.
7. Ensure that child is properly connected to cardiopulmonary, non-invasive blood pressure (NIBP), or arterial line monitoring and pulse oximetry.[1,2,7] *(Level II*)*	Allows monitoring for hemodynamic compromise before, during, and after the procedure.	The child may need initiation of inotropic agents or other medical intervention before or during the procedure.
8. Obtain 12-lead ECG. *(Level II*)*	Documents rhythm before intervention.	If the child's condition is unstable or 12-lead ECG has been obtained, skip this step.
9. If necessary and time permits, establish IV access. *(Level VI*)*	Intravenous access should be established for sedation and cardiac medication administration if the child's hemodynamic status continues to necessitate support despite transcutaneous pacing.[1]	Before IV access is established, take into consideration history of vascular compromise (i.e., history of Blalock-Taussig shunt).
10. Ensure a stable airway and administer sedation per prescribing practitioner's order and institution-specific to keep the child comfortable.[2]	Transcutaneous pacing is uncomfortable and can be painful. Sedation decreases anxiety, alleviates discomfort, and decreases movement of child during the procedure.[2,3] *(Level VI*)*	Monitor for respiratory depression in children without intubation. Consider intubation/mechanical ventilation with infants and young children because transcutaneous pacing may cause breathing difficulty from skeletal muscle stimulation from the pacing.
11. Ensure that area where pads will be placed is clean, dry, and intact. *(Level II*)*	Any residue on skin may increase the chance of burns to the skin.[4]	A minimum of 1 inch should be maintained between pads to prevent arcing, which is especially important in infants and children because of the small size of the chest.[5,6]
12. Place transcutaneous pacing pads on child's chest per anatomic guidelines and without having the patches in such proximity to each other that they are touching. The subclavicular and lower left sternal border is the correct placement for most children. *(Level II*)*	Proper pad placement ensures flow of electrical current through the ventricles as opposed to from patch to patch.[2,3]	Small infants and obese children should have patches placed anteriorly and posteriorly for maximal effect.[5,6] Children with dextrocardia should have pads placed either in the anterior-posterior or in the anterior-anterior position but with the apex patch on the right.[7]

Procedure continues on following page

---

* Level II: Theory-based; no research data to support recommendations; recommendations from expert consensus group may exist
  Level VI: Clinical studies in a variety of patient populations and situations to support recommendations

Procedure	**for Transcutaneous Pacing**—*Continued*	
Steps	**Rationale**	**Considerations**
		Do not place patches over an internal pacemaker or internal defibrillator.[5]
13. Attach pacing pads to the pacing cables. Connect the pacing cables to the pacemaker unit and turn the unit on; default settings are automatically engaged. *(Level I*)*	Default settings start the emergency pacing at high-energy output in an attempt to capture the heart mechanically.[2]	Default settings are based on adult heart rates; the output is set at the maximal amount of milliamps. Refer to manufacturer's guidelines for specifics of attaching pads to pacing cable and initiating pacing.
14. Set heart rate per the prescribing practitioner's order or age-appropriate guidelines; a typical starting rate is 100 bpm.[2] *(Level II*)*	Default settings tend to be those appropriate for an adult (i.e., 60 bpm); increase the heart rate as needed to ensure adequate cardiac output.[2] Heart rate selected is based on the age of child to optimize cardiac output and avoid additional stress on the heart.[2]	Children under stress may need a higher than normal heart rate to maintain an adequate cardiac output.[2]
15. Verify presence or absence of a pulse.[1-3]	Electrical capture does not ensure mechanical capture.[2] *(Level VI*)*	If child has an arterial line, a pressure tracing should be present with mechanical capture. Bedside ultrasound scan has been used to confirm mechanical capture in emergency transcutaneous pacing. Validation of mechanical capture with hemodynamic monitoring may be difficult because of weak pulse volume or interference from skeletal muscle contractions. Ultrasound scan can assist in differentiation between causes of persistent hypotension despite successful pacing.[8]
16. Determine the pacemaker mode of VVI (ventricular demand) versus VOO (asynchronous ventricular pacing). *(Level II*)*	Mode of VVI is preferred because the pacemaker senses the child's intrinsic rate and does not fire; VOO is asynchronous and paces regardless the of child's own heart rate.[1,2,7]	In an emergency situation, VOO may be the most appropriate mode. Change to VVI when the child's condition has been stabilized.[7] *(Level II*)*
17. Adjust milliamps (mA) to determine the point at which electrical capture occurs; then increase mA to 1.5 times the point of capture. *(Level I*)*	Adjusting mA to 1.5 times the amount that captures the heart ensures an adequate safety margin.[2,3,7]	
18. Obtain 12-lead ECG.	Documents paced rhythm.	
19. Dispose of used supplies and equipment; wash hands.	Standard precautions; reduces transmission of microorganisms.	

* Level I: Manufacturer's recommendations only
  Level II: Theory-based; no research data to support recommendations; recommendations from expert consensus group may exist
  Level VI: Clinical studies in a variety of patient populations and situations to support recommendations

Expected Outcomes	Unexpected Outcomes
• Correct placement of transcutaneous pacing pads	• No electrical capture or mechanical capture because of incorrectly placed pads
• Electrical and mechanical capture ensures adequate cardiac output; child's pulse is strong and regular	• Electrical capture without mechanical capture
• Adequate heart rate achieved, with improvement in cardiac output	• Inability to provide adequate cardiac output with pacing
• Hemodynamic status is stabilized, permitting placement of permanent pacing device	• Inability to stabilize child's condition for placement of either a transvenous or epicardial pacing system
• Child's skin under pacing pads remains intact	• Skin breakdown or burns in area where pads were applied
• Child has acceptable level of comfort	• Unmanaged pain

Monitoring and Care of the Child

Activities and Interventions	Rationale	Reportable Conditions
1. Verify that mechanical capture is in synchrony with electrical capture.	Electrical capture (pacing spikes and QRS complexes) can occur without mechanical capture (palpable pulse and blood pressure).[4,6]	• Weak, thready, or absent pulse • Signs of low cardiac output
2. Monitor hemodynamic response to paced rhythm.	Child may need adjustments to transcutaneous pacemaker settings on the basis of hemodynamic response.[1] Failure to improve cardiac output may indicate the need for an adjustment in transcutaneous pacemaker settings.[2,5] Child may need further medical intervention if condition continues to deteriorate.	• Signs of low cardiac output • Continued deterioration in status
3. Change pads every 8 hours or according to manufacturer's recommendations and assess skin for abrasions or burn injury from pacing pads.	Burns may occur under the pads, especially if the transcutaneous system is used for extended periods.[2]	• Abrasions or burns with blister formation
4. Monitor child's response to and recovery from sedation per institution-specific protocol.	Administration of moderate sedation necessitates careful monitoring as child recovers.	• Respiratory compromise related to sedation • Extended sedation
5. Assess effectiveness of pain management strategy and provide appropriate interventions. Encourage the family to assist with non-pharmacologic means to comfort and support the child as appropriate.	Transcutaneous pacing is painful.[2,3] Regular assessment of pain allows early identification and prompt treatment.	• Child reports pain or discomfort; use age-appropriate pain scale to quantify (see Procedure 173) • Signs and symptoms of pain, including tearing, grimacing, sweating, and rapid shallow breathing • Adverse reactions to sedation

Documentation

- Child and family education
- Consent for procedure
- Verification of pulse and blood pressure with initiation of pacing
- Child's response to pacing therapy
- Child's response to sedation during procedure and recovery, per institution-specific protocol
- Time and date pacing was started
- 12-Lead ECG results before and after pacing was initiated
- Time, date, and location of pacing pad application
- Pacemaker parameters; rate, mA, and pacing mode
- Resolution of dysrhythmia
- Medications administered
- Appearance of skin after pacing patch removal
- Pain assessment and any specific interventions provided
- Unexpected outcomes and related treatment

References

1. Hazinski MF: *PALS provider manual,* Dallas, 2002, American Heart Association.
2. Gammage M: Temporary cardiac pacing, *Heart* 83:715-720, 2000.
3. Jacobson C, Gerity D: Pacemakers and implantable defibrillators. In Woods S, Sivarajan Froelicher E, Underhill Motzer S, editors: *Cardiac nursing,* ed 4, Philadelphia, 2000, Lippincott Williams & Wilkins.
4. Gregoratos G, et al: ACC/AHA/NASPE 2002 guideline update for implantation of cardiac pacemakers and antiarrhythmia devices: a report of the American College of Cardiology/American Heart Association task force on practice guidelines, *J Am College Cardiol* 40(9):1703-1719, 2002.
5. Maginot KR, et al: Applications of pacing strategies in neonates and infants, *Progress Pediatr Cardiol* 11(1): 65-75, 2000.
6. Rein AJT, et al: Noninvasive external pacing in the newborn, *Pediatr Cardiol* 20:290-292, 1999.
7. Zeigler VL, Gillette PG: *Practical management of pediatric cardiac arrhythmias*, New York, 2001, Futura Publishing Co., Inc.
8. Holger JS, et al: Use of ultrasound to determine ventricular capture in transcutaneous pacing, *Am J Emerg Med* 23(2):197-198, 2005.

Additional Readings

Ettin D, Cook T: Using ultrasound to determine external pacer capture, *J Emerg Med* 17(6):1007-1009, 1999.
Hatlestad D: The benefits of electricity: transcutaneous pacing in EMS, *Emerg Med Services* 31(9):38-40, 42, 44-45, 2002.

Transesophageal Pacing: Assist

P U R P O S E :   To temporarily increase the atrial rate to treat bradycardia, perform atrial overdrive pacing to convert atrial tachyarrhythmias, record atrial electrograms to aid in diagnosis of complex arrhythmias, or perform transesophageal electrophysiology studies

Debra Hanisch

PREREQUISITE KNOWLEDGE

- Normal cardiac anatomy and physiology, including the principles of cardiac conduction
- Child's congenital heart disease and associated short-term and long-term electrophysiologic complications
- Familiarity with the child's medical history, including upper airway problems, and surgical history, including placement of internal pacemaker or internal defibrillator
- Indications for transesophageal atrial pacing include emergency atrial pacing for bradycardia in the absence of atrioventricular (AV) block, pace overdrive suppression of atrial tachyarrhythmias (supraventricular tachycardia, atrial flutter), evaluation of electrophysiologic mechanisms in supraventricular tachycardia, and assessment of antiarrhythmic drug therapy efficacy.[1-3]
- Institution of transesophageal atrial pacing typically occurs in the intensive care unit.
- Transesophageal atrial pacing is for short-term use only.
- The left atrium lies in close proximity to the esophagus, which enables effective pacing of the atria by way of a transesophageal catheter.[4]
- This procedure is typically performed on an emergent basis with anesthesia and sedation. Some children may need intubation. Because NPO time may not be adequate, a risk for aspiration does exist.[3]
- Technical skill in oral-gastric and nasal-gastric tube placement
- Appropriate pediatric dosing of analgesics and competency in procedural sedation

- Mastery of pediatric advanced life support competencies
- Knowledge of normal infant, child, and adolescent heart rates
- Skills in basic and advanced electrocardiographic (ECG) and cardiac arrhythmia interpretation
- Familiarity with electrophysiologic terminology (see Procedure 51 for a glossary of pacing terminology)
- Clinical assessment and interpretation of hemodynamic monitoring
- Ability to activate the emergency alert system
- Child development as it relates to clinical assessment and transesophageal pacing
- Informed consent is generally necessary before atrial overdrive pacing.

CHILD AND FAMILY ASSESSMENT

- Child's and family's understanding of the reasons for and risks and benefits of the procedure ➤➤*Rationale:* Evaluates child's and family's understanding of the procedure and provides a gauge for ongoing education.
- History of congenital heart disease, cardiomyopathy, cardiac arrhythmias, syncope, cardiac surgical or catheterization procedures, electrophysiologic complications, and projected cardiac surgery requirements ➤➤*Rationale:* These conditions can assist with anticipatory planning for optimal treatment of potential complications and determination of the best course of pharmacotherapy after rhythm is terminated.
- History of upper airway or esophageal anomalies[1] ➤➤*Rationale:* These conditions may preclude passage of an

esophageal lead, and history identifies factors that may necessitate modification of airway management plans.

- Current hemodynamic status ➳*Rationale:* Assessments are done before, during, and after transesophageal pacing for determination of tolerance of the procedure.[1,3]
- History of ECGs ➳*Rationale:* Establishes prior baseline rhythm.
- Medication history, including use of herbal supplements or anticoagulation therapy, drug exposure, acid-base balance, and electrolyte levels ➳*Rationale:* Drug therapy, electrolyte, or acid-base abnormalities could impede pacing ability. Certain medications or drug exposures may be implicated as the cause for the tachycardia.
- Child's developmental level and ability to interact ➳*Rationale:* These factors influence preparation of the child and interaction, determine the child's ability to cooperate with instructions, and identify the need for sedation.
- History of adverse response to anesthesia or conscious sedation ➳*Rationale:* Adverse response may influence the type of sedation used for the procedure to safely achieve desired results.
- Family's desire to be present during the procedure ➳*Rationale:* The family may provide support and comfort measures to the child but should have the choice not to remain with the child.

CHILD AND FAMILY EDUCATION

Individualized, developmentally appropriate education is provided to the family and to the child based on desire for knowledge, readiness to learn, and overall neurologic and psychosocial state.

- Provide information on the child's medical condition and the need for the procedure ➳*Rationale:* Educationally appropriate information helps to decrease the child's and family's anxiety levels and offers reassurance during an extremely stressful period.

- If developmentally appropriate, show the child and family the transesophageal pacing catheter and explain the placement procedure ➳*Rationale:* Visual examples decrease anxiety and fear.
- Provide information on the pacing process and postprocedural care ➳*Rationale:* Providing information to the child and the family decreases fear and anxiety and can increase compliance with plan of care.
- Provide information to the child and family about sedation medication administered during pacing therapy to manage anxiety and discomfort associated with placement of the transesophageal pacing wire[1] ➳*Rationale:* Assures child and family that pain and anxiety will be managed appropriately, decreases fears related to the procedure and promotes compliance.
- Provide information regarding postprocedural activity level, follow-up, activity restrictions, and safety issues. Allowable activity level is dependent on cardiopulmonary stability and the ability of the child to cooperate with restrictions. For an older child who might remain conscious throughout the procedure, describe what the experience will be and what will be expected of the child. ➳*Rationale:* Child's and family's cooperation and compliance are encouraged.
- Encourage questions and answer questions as they arise ➳*Rationale:* Reinforcement of information is needed during periods of stress.

EQUIPMENT

- Cardiopulmonary monitor
- Electrocardiographic patches and recorder
- Alligator clips on ECG leads or atrial electrogram (AEGM)–modified lead wires (see Figure 47-1 for an image of a lead wire)
- Transesophageal pacing stimulator (Figure 53-1)
- Preamplifier (see Figure 53-1)
- Transesophageal pacing catheter; any of the following are suitable[1]:

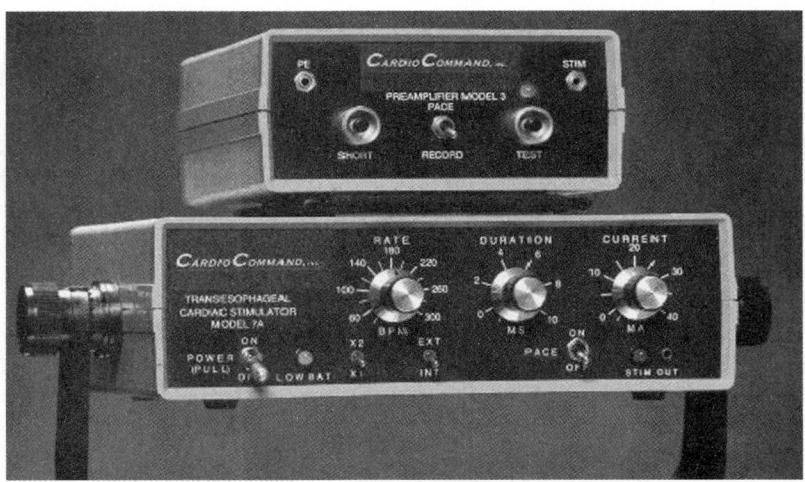

FIGURE 53-1 Preamplifier and pacing stimulator for transesophageal pacing. *Photo courtesy of CardioCommand, Inc, www.CardioCommand.com.*

- ❖ Transesophageal pacing catheter (TAPCATH 205, Tampa, FL CardioCommand, Inc; 5F, 13-mm electrode spacing) (Figure 53-2)
- ❖ Transvenous pacing catheter (4F to 5F, 10-mm electrode spacing)
- ❖ Coronary sinus electrode catheter (4F to 6F, variable electrode spacing)
- ❖ Pill electrode for transesophageal atrial pacing/recording (bipolar electrode encased in a gelatin capsule with 8-mm electrode spacing; no longer commercially available) (Figure 53-3)
- Switch box for switching between recorder and stimulator (dependent on type of system used)

- Multichannel ECG machine or bedside monitor with recorder
- Transesophageal probe
- Echocardiogram machine
- Local anesthetic spray for throat
- Lubricant (preferably with local anesthetic for nasal insertion)
- Skin preparation
- Clean gloves
- Intravenous (IV) supplies
- Airway management supplies
- Emergency cart
- Defibrillator

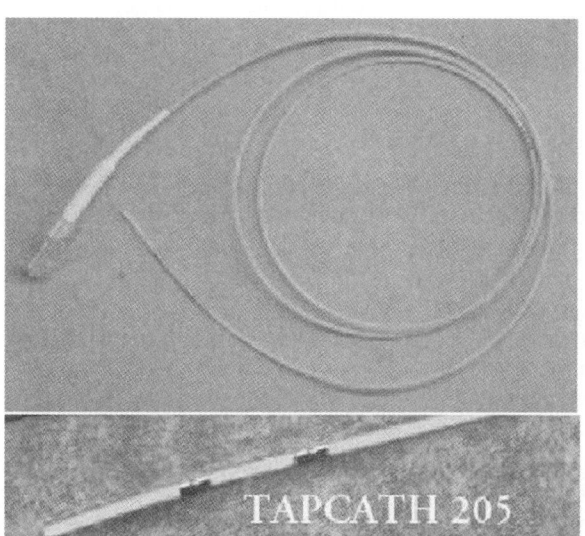

FIGURE 53-2 A 5F TAPCATH 205 bipolar transesophageal pacing catheter with "phone jack" end to plug into CardioCommand, Inc, preamplifier. *Photo courtesy of CardioCommand, Inc, www. CardioCommand.com.*

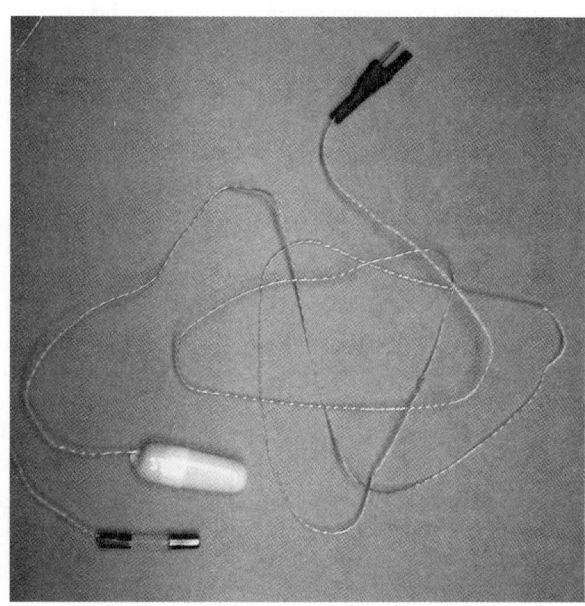

FIGURE 53-3 "Pill electrode" for transesophageal pacing shown with and without gelatin capsule. Formerly sold by Arzco, Chicago, Ill, this product is no longer commercially available. *Photo by D. Hanisch.*

Procedure for Transesophageal Pacing: Assist

Steps	Rationale	Considerations
1. Ensure signed informed consent has been obtained.	Ensures discussion of purpose and procedural risks with family and child as appropriate.	Ensures medical-legal compliance as suggested by the Joint Commission on Accreditation of Healthcare Organizations. (JCAHO)
2. Ensure child and family understand procedure and questions are answered.	Evaluates and reinforces understanding of previously taught information.	This procedure may be performed in emergent conditions that may preclude preprocedural teaching.
3. Implement fasting guidelines per institution-specific protocol.	If the child is to receive sedation or anesthesia, prevents complications related to aspiration. *(Level IV*)*	Fasting guidelines are related to the child's age and type of sedation to be administered.

Procedure continues on following page

* Level IV: Limited clinical studies to support recommendations

Procedure for Transesophageal Pacing: Assist—*Continued*

Steps	Rationale	Considerations
4. Gather needed equipment and supplies, including the emergency cart and defibrillator.	Facilitates completion of the procedure in a timely manner.	Cardioverter-defibrillator should be readily accessible.
5. Wash hands and put on clean gloves *(Level IV*)*	Standard precautions; reduces transmission of microorganisms	Use nonlatex gloves; esophageal pacing catheters are latex free.
6. Position the child on a flat surface with the head of the bed elevated 30 to 45 degrees. *(Level II*)*	Proper positioning can decrease the incidence rate of equipment dislodgement and prevent tissue nerve injury.[4]	Proper positioning facilitates airway stability.
7. Ensure child is properly connected to cardiopulmonary, noninvasive blood pressure (NIBP), or arterial line monitoring and pulse oximetry.[1,4,5] ECG machine should provide at least two simultaneously recordable channels. *(Level II*)*	Monitor for hemodynamic compromise before, during, and after the procedure.[1-3]	Documentation should include recorded rhythm strips before, during, and after pacing.
8. Identify child with appropriate patient/procedure verification process (e.g., "time out").	Confirms correct patient, procedure, and site as recommended by JCAHO and prevents unnecessary medical procedures.	Verification process and documentation are institution specific. Use active communication techniques.
9. If not present, establish IV access. *(Level VI*)*	Intravenous access should be established for sedation and cardiac medication administration in the event child's hemodynamic status deteriorates.[1,3]	Before IV access is established, take into consideration history of vascular compromise (i.e., Blalock-Taussig shunt).
10. Ensure a stable airway and administer sedation per prescribing practitioner's order or institution-specific protocol to ensure that child is comfortable.[2,5]	Transesophageal pacing wire placement is uncomfortable and can be painful. Sedation decreases anxiety, alleviates discomfort, and decreases movement of child during the procedure.[1] *(Level VI*)*	Type of sedation/anesthesia used is dependent on the child's prior experience with these medications and drug allergy history. Watch for respiratory depression in children who are not intubated. Use of transesophageal probe may (rarely) compress the airway. Additional sedation may be necessary for this procedure.

11. Calculate depth of catheter insertion (in centimeters)[4,5]:
    Oral: Child's height (cm)/5
    Nasal: Add an additional 3 to 4 cm to oral length
    In infants and small children, measure from the nares to the xiphoid.
    Add an additional 3 to 4 cm and mark the catheter with tape.
	Initially, electrode tip of the catheter needs to be inserted in esophagus just beyond the level of left atrium and then adjusted with slow withdrawal of catheter back to optimal position.[4] *(Level I*)*	Consider use of the graph from Benson et al[4] to estimate depth of insertion on the basis of height (Figure 53-4). *(Level III*)*

* Level I: Manufacturer's recommendations only
Level II: Theory-based; no research data to support recommendations; recommendations from expert consensus group may exist
Level III: Laboratory data; no clinical data to support recommendations
Level IV: Limited clinical studies to support recommendations
Level VI: Clinical studies in a variety of patient populations and situations to support recommendations

Procedure	for Transesophageal Pacing: Assist—*Continued*	
Steps	**Rationale**	**Considerations**

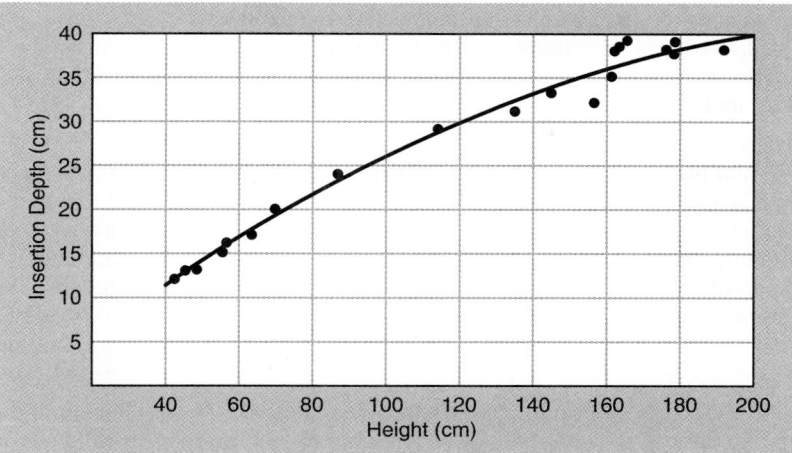

FIGURE 53-4   Estimated depth of insertion of transesophageal pacing catheter from nares or mouth to point of lowest atrial pacing threshold. *From Benson DW Jr, et al: Transesophageal atrial pacing threshold: role of inter-electrode spacing, pulse width and catheter insertion depth,* Am J Cardiol 53:63-67, 1984.

12. Spray pharyngeal area with a topical anesthetic.	Minimizes discomfort associated with procedure.	Avoid anesthetic or sedation agents that may affect conduction or inducibility with a transesophageal electrophysiology study.
13. Lubricate distal tip of pacing catheter with anesthetic gel.	Facilitates passage of catheter and minimizes mucosal irritation and discomfort associated with the procedure.[1] *(Level VI*)*	
14. Insert pacing catheter either transorally or transnasally to predetermined depth. Flex head forward to facilitate insertion. If child is conscious, have child remain upright and swallow while catheter is advanced. *(Level I*)*	Flexion and swallowing facilitate passage of catheter into esophagus rather than the trachea.	Use only water-soluble lubricants. Sips of water may be given to encourage swallowing. If the child is uncooperative, consider sedation. An oral airway may be needed if a transoral approach is used to prevent the child from biting down on the catheter.
15. Connect pacing catheter to obtain an AEGM.	An AEGM is used to aid positioning of electrode catheter within the esophagus behind left atrium.[2] The AEGM can be diagnostic as well.[1]	See Procedure 47 for further discussion of AEGM.
16. Withdraw slowly and then advance the pacing catheter as needed to optimize the atrial signal on the electrogram.	Atrial signal is maximal when electrodes are in closest proximity to left atrium (see Figure 47-3).[4,5]	Fluoroscopy may be used adjunctively to aid in positioning the catheter.[4,5]
17. With skin preparation and tape, tape pacing catheter securely in place.	Reduces risk of dislodgement once optimal positioning has been achieved.	If atrial pacing is to be used, optimal positioning of electrodes enables one to pace atrium effectively with capture without excessive output from the pacing stimulator. If catheter is positioned too low and a high output is used, ventricular pacing, though rare, is possible.[1]

Procedure continues on following page

* Level I: Manufacturer's recommendations only
Level VI: Clinical studies in a variety of patient populations and situations to support recommendations

Procedure for Transesophageal Pacing: Assist—*Continued*

Steps	Rationale	Considerations
18. Assist with transesophageal pacing (TAP) as needed. To perform TAP, connect the pacing catheter to preamplifier and pacing stimulator.	Establishes connection to enable transesophageal pacing.	
19. Initial pace settings should be programmed at desired atrial pacing rate and output levels set to a current of 10 milliamperes (mA) at a pulse duration of 10 milliseconds (ms).[3] *(Level I[*])*	Ensures safe delivery of desired pacing pulses.	Follow manufacturer's instructions for proper connectivity. Do not use a temporary pacemaker intended for transvenous pacing because the output settings tend to be too low (maximum pulse width, 2 ms; current, 20 to 25 mA) to achieve successful TAP.[2]
20. Initiate pacing and adjust the current to a level approximately 50% above minimal amount that produces atrial capture (capture threshold).[1] *(Level II[*])*	Child's discomfort correlates with amount of pacing current delivered. Most children have "heartburn" or chest discomfort between 8 and 12 mA.[1]	Pacing rate to be used depends on child's arrhythmia and indication for pacing. Failure to capture at 20 mA should prompt catheter repositioning.[3]
21. When finished, carefully withdraw pacing catheter.	Minimizes child's discomfort.	Injury to esophageal mucosa may occur if duration of pacing exceeds 1 hour. *(Level III[*])*
22. Discard used supplies and equipment. Remove gloves and wash hands.	Standard precautions; reduces transmission of microorganisms.	

* Level I: Manufacturer's recommendations only
 Level II: Theory-based; no research data to support recommendations; recommendations from expert consensus group may exist
 Level III: Laboratory data; no clinical data to support recommendations

Expected Outcomes

- Child receives safe and effective short-term transesophageal pacing
- Child's condition remains hemodynamically stable during and after procedure
- Child has sensation of "slight heartburn"
- Esophageal mucosa is free from injury
- Child has minimal or no gagging, choking, or nausea
- Child's respiratory status remains stable throughout procedure and recovery

Unexpected Outcomes

- Further provocation of arrhythmias or induction of ventricular arrhythmias
- Hypotension
- Cardiac arrest
- Child has severe discomfort
- Trauma to esophageal mucosa
- Severe coughing, gagging, or vomiting
- Respiratory failure or distress
- Airway compromise that necessitates intervention

Monitoring and Care of the Child

Activities and Interventions	Rationale	Reportable Conditions
1. Ensure cardiac monitoring during and after procedure.	Monitors for arrhythmias.	• Arrhythmias
2. Monitor vital signs and level of consciousness.	Assesses for hemodynamic instability associated with the child's heart rhythm.[3]	• Alteration in child's hemodynamic status or level of consciousness
3. Monitor for complications of procedure and for full recovery from procedure and sedation.	Tachycardia may return; if pharmacologic measures have been used, bradycardia may result.[4] Ensures full recovery from sedation/anesthesia. Child may need pacing to maintain acceptable heart rate if bradycardia with symptoms of low cardiac output[1,2] occurs after transesophageal pacing.	• Recurrent atrial tachycardia • New onset ventricular tachycardia • Respiratory distress or failure • Airway compromise • Signs of embolic event[5] • Delayed recovery from sedation
4. Evaluate and treat arrhythmias if indicated.	Goal is to improve child's hemodynamic status.[1-3]	• Failure to adequately manage arrhythmias
5. Assess effectiveness of pain management strategy and provide appropriate interventions. Encourage the family to assist with nonpharmacologic means to comfort and support the child.	Early identification of pain allows immediate intervention.	• Persistent esophageal pain • Continued irritability or changes in physiologic condition

Documentation

- Child and family education
- Consent for TAP procedure
- Vital signs and response to the procedure
- Electrocardiogram/AEGM strips: baseline, during pacing, and final ECG tracings
- Procedure note with medications given, paced settings used, and findings or results
- Comfort assessment and any specific interventions provided
- Documentation of procedural sedation per institution specific protocol
- Unexpected outcomes and related treatment

References

1. Saul JP: Transesophageal atrial recording and pacing. In Walsh EP, et al, editors: *Cardiac arrhythmias in children and young adults with congenital heart disease,* Philadelphia, 2001, Lippincott Williams & Wilkins.
2. Knick BJ, Saul JP: Immediate arrhythmia management. In Zeigler VL, Gillette PC, editors: *Practical management of pediatric cardiac arrhythmias,* Armonk, NY, 2001, Futura Publishing Co, Inc.
3. Winslow AT, et al: Acute treatment of arrhythmias. In Gillette PC, Garson A, editors: *Clinical pediatric arrhythmias,* ed 2, Philadelphia, 1999, Saunders.
4. Benson DW Jr, et al: Transesophageal atrial pacing threshold: role of interelectrode spacing, pulse width and catheter insertion depth, *Am J Cardiol* 53:63-67, 1984.
5. www.CardioCommand.com. CardioCommand, Inc., The Adjustable Heart, 2001, Accessed originally on 2/10/04, most recently on 4/24/06.

Additional Reading

Benson DW Jr, et al: Transesophageal cardiac pacing: history, application, technique, *Clin Prog Pacing Electrophysiol* 2:360-372, 1984.

Transvenous and Epicardial Pacing: Monitoring

P U R P O S E : To monitor the effectiveness of temporary transvenous or epicardial pacing

Maggie Fischer

PREREQUISITE KNOWLEDGE

- Normal cardiac anatomy and physiology, including the principles of cardiac conduction
- An understanding of pediatric acquired or congenital heart disease and associated short-term and long-term electrophysiologic complications
- Familiarity with the child's medical and surgical history, including placement of permanent internal pacemaker or internal defibrillator
- Child development as it relates to clinical assessment and temporary pacemaker monitoring
- Indications for temporary transvenous or epicardial pacing
  - ❖ Congenital heart block
  - ❖ Advanced second-degree or third-degree heart block caused by certain drugs, myocarditis, or myocardial infarction
  - ❖ Second-degree or third-degree heart block from heart surgery
  - ❖ Tachycardia in selected children for evaluation of termination of arrhythmias
- Temporary transvenous and epicardial pacing is instituted to increase the heart rate to support cardiac output in children who have congenital or acquired heart block. Temporary transvenous and epicardial pacing may also be indicated on an elective or stand-by basis when the child is at risk for rhythm disturbances that could create hemodynamic compromise (i.e., cardioversion, replace-

ment of a permanent pacemaker, or patients with a drug-induced bradydysrhythmia).[1-3]
- Institution of temporary transvenous and epicardial pacing may occur in any location where continuous cardiopulmonary monitoring is available. The child should then be transferred to a telemetry unit or the intensive care unit for further monitoring and management of the underlying medical condition.[1,4]
- Temporary pacemakers
  - ❖ Temporary pacemaker lead placement may be performed with a transvenous or epicardial approach. Typically, implantation occurs in the catheterization laboratory, intensive care unit, or operating room with echocardiographic or fluoroscopic guidance. The child's hemodynamic status, age, and pacing history determine the urgency with which pacing is necessary and the approach chosen.
  - ❖ The type of analgesia and anesthesia used for the procedure is dependent on the child's hemodynamic status and the clinical setting.
  - ❖ Temporary pacing systems may have an atrial lead, a ventricular lead, or both. Pacing mode programming may include AAI, VVI, DVI, VDD, or DDD.[3-5]
  - ❖ Temporary pacemaker wires are intended to be used for 7 to 14 days (until the heart block has resolved or a permanent system is implanted).
- Transvenous approach
  - ❖ Transvenous access for temporary pacing systems is possible using sites that include the subclavian,

internal or external jugular, brachial, and femoral veins.[5]

❖ Transvenous leads may be inserted by the physician at the bedside. The transvenous pacing catheter should be immobilized as much as possible. The entry site should be covered with a self-adhesive transparent dressing.

- Epicardial approach
  ❖ Temporary epicardial pacing systems are placed in children undergoing cardiac surgery in whom atrioventricular (AV) block develops. In addition to pacing for bradycardia, epicardial systems can be used in selected children to evaluate and treat tachycardia.[5-7]
  ❖ Epicardial leads are placed at the end of an open heart procedure. Single or paired epicardial wires are put on the atrium and the ventricle. The temporary epicardial wires are sutured loosely onto the epicardium and brought out through the chest wall. The atrial wires are generally brought out through the right side of the chest. The ventricular wires are brought out through the left side of the chest.[5,6]
  ❖ One or more ground wires may also be placed and used for epicardial unipolar pacing. The ground wire is placed in the positive terminal of the pulse generator, and the epicardial wire is placed in the negative terminal.[6]
  ❖ The leads should be fixed to the skin to prevent traction or displacement.
  ❖ When not in use, the exposed ends of the pacing wires must be protected with caps or gauze; the wires are then secured to the child's chest.
  ❖ When the child is undergoing pacing, the external pulse generator should be pinned to the child's gown so it cannot be moved away from the child. All connections and cables should be checked regularly.
- Complications of temporary pacing systems
  ❖ Lead dislodgement
  ❖ Heart perforation
  ❖ Arrhythmias
- Normal infant, child, and adolescent heart rates
- Skill in basic and advanced electrocardiographic (ECG) and cardiac arrhythmia interpretation
- Ability to differentiate between intrinsic and paced rhythm on ECG
- Familiarity with the North American Society of Pacing and Electrophysiology (NASPE) generic pacemaker code and basic electrophysiologic terminology (see Tables 51-1 and 51-2 for a glossary of pacemaker-related terminology)
- Assessment of hemodynamics in response to pacing therapy
- Ability to activate the emergency alert system
- Mastery of pediatric advanced life support competencies

CHILD AND FAMILY ASSESSMENT

- History of congenital heart disease, cardiomyopathy, cardiac arrhythmias, pacing therapy, syncope, cardiac surgical or catheterization procedures, electrophysiologic complications, and projected cardiac surgery requirements[6] ➠*Rationale:* These conditions impact the place-

ment of the pacing wires and the type of arrhythmias the child may experience and aids in anticipatory planning for future interventions.

- Medication history, including herbal supplements, street and over-the-counter drug use, and current acid-base balance and electrolyte levels[3] ➠*Rationale:* Drug therapy and electrolyte or acid-base abnormalities could impede pacing ability. Certain medications or drug exposures may be implicated as the cause for dysrhythmias.
- Baseline assessment of cardiac rhythm and document a rhythm strip ➠*Rationale:* Determination of the child's baseline heart rate and rhythm.
- Child's hemodynamic status (blood pressure, peripheral perfusion, oxygen saturation) and associated symptoms that reflect altered cardiac output and tolerance of pacing therapy[5,7] ➠*Rationale:* Baseline assessment is performed and compared with subsequent assessments done during and after pacing. Initiation of inotropic support may be necessary to stabilize the child's condition during the procedure.
- Type of pacing wires available. Epicardial atrial wires typically exit to the right of the sternum, whereas ventricular wires exit to the left of the sternum. A ground wire may also be used for epicardial unipolar pacing. ➠*Rationale:* Type of available pacing wires determines the type of pulse generator and pacing mode used.
- Child's developmental level and ability to interact ➠*Rationale:* These factors influence preparation and interaction.
- Level of consciousness and cognitive ability ➠*Rationale:* Determines the child's ability to cooperate with instructions or assist with the procedure by remaining still.
- History of response to anesthesia or conscious sedation ➠*Rationale:* Response may influence type of sedation used for procedure to safely achieve desired results.
- Child's and family's understanding of the reasons for and risks and benefits of transvenous or epicardial pacing ➠*Rationale:* Evaluates child's and family's understanding of the procedure and provides a gauge for ongoing education.
- Family's desire to be present during the procedure ➠*Rationale:* The family may provide support and comfort measures to the child but should have the choice not to remain with the child.

CHILD AND FAMILY EDUCATION

Individualized, developmentally appropriate education is provided to the family and to the child based on desire for knowledge, readiness to learn, and overall neurologic and psychosocial state.

- Provide developmentally appropriate information on the child's medical condition, the indications for temporary pacing, and the length of therapy. The explanation should include information that this type of therapy is used to stabilize the child's condition until either sinus rhythm returns or a permanent pacemaker can be placed (typically within 7 to 14 days).[5] ➥*Rationale:* Information helps to decrease the child's and family's anxiety levels and assists in preparing the child and family for future procedures.

- Provide an explanation of the pacing process and the steps involved in evaluating and monitoring for the effectiveness of the pacing therapy ➥*Rationale:* Information on the plan of care assists in decreasing the child's and family's anxiety levels and offers reassurance that the child is being closely monitored.
- Show the child (when appropriate) and family the pacing wires and pacemaker ➥*Rationale:* Visual examples can decrease fear and anxiety and increase understanding.
- Provide information on the plan of care, including the activity restrictions necessary during temporary pacing. Explain the need to avoid tension on the pacing wires or leads to prevent lead dislodgment and the pulse generator to prevent cable disconnection from the device or the pacing leads. ➥*Rationale:* Information on the activity restrictions necessary during temporary pacing increases compliance and decreases the complications associated with pacemaker noncapture.
- Encourage questions and answer questions as they arise ➥*Rationale:* Reinforcement of information is needed during periods of stress.

EQUIPMENT

- Cardiopulmonary monitor
- Electrocardiographic patches
- Two batteries: Standard 9-V alkaline or lithium batteries, depending on generator model; one inserted into the pacemaker and an extra back-up battery taped to the box
- Temporary pulse generator; any of the following are suitable depending on the type of pacing desired:
  - ❖ Single-chamber pulse generator
    - ○ Modes: VVI, VOO, AAI, and AOO
    - ○ Medtronic Model 5375 (alligator clips may be necessary with this model[8]; Figure 54-1, Medtronic, Redmond, WA)
      - ○ Basic pacing rates, 30 to 180 ppm, continuously adjustable
      - ○ Output amplitude, 0.1 to 20 mA, continuously adjustable
      - ○ Sensitivity, 1.5 to 20 mV
    - ○ Medtronic Model 5348[8] (Figure 54-2)
      - ○ Basic pacing rates, 30 to 180 ppm, continuously adjustable
      - ○ Rapid atrial pacing rates:
        - ○ 80 to 380 ppm (5 ppm increments)
        - ○ 380 to 540 ppm (10 ppm increments)
        - ○ 540 to 800 ppm (20 ppm increments)
        - ○ Output amplitude, 0.1 to 20 mA, continuously adjustable
        - ○ Pulse width, 1.8 ms
        - ○ Sensitivity, 0.5 to 20 mV
        - ○ Refractory, 250 mS
        - ○ Blanking: pace, 125 ms; sense, 75ms

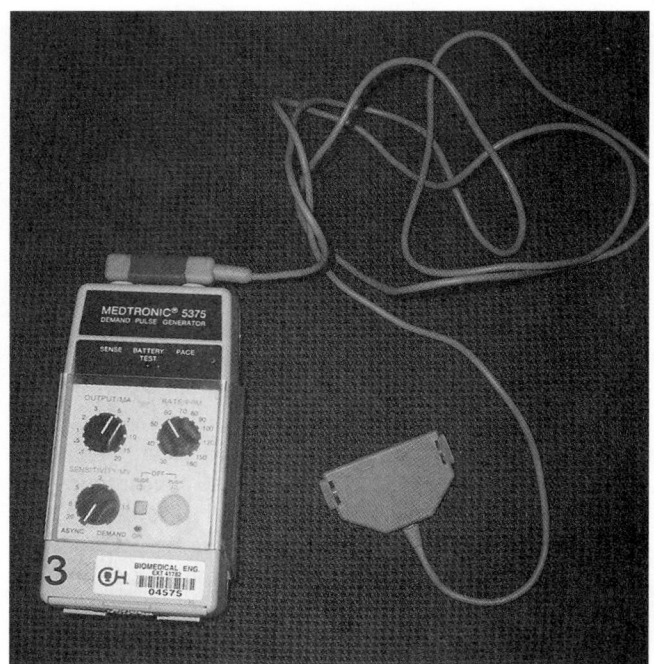

FIGURE 54-1 Single-chamber pulse generator, Medtronic model 5375. *Photo courtesy of Medtronic USA, Inc.*

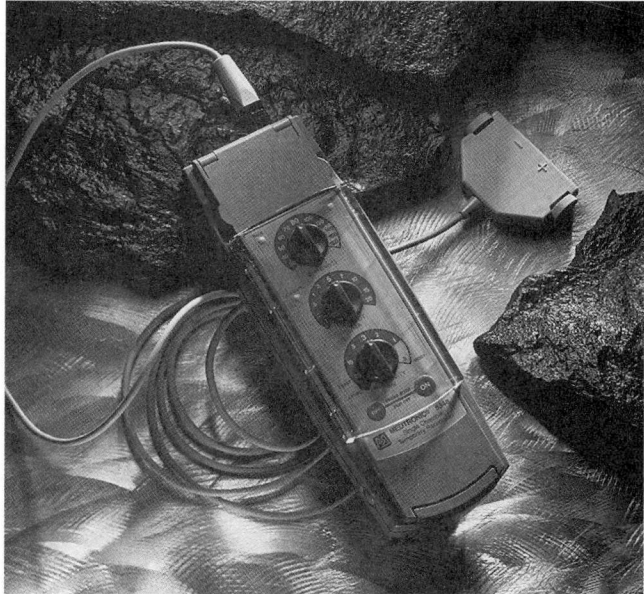

FIGURE 54-2 Single-chamber pulse generator, Medtronic model 5348. *Photo courtesy of Medtronic USA, Inc.*

- ❖ Dual-chamber pulse generator
  - ○ Modes: DDD, VDD, DVI, DOO, VVI, VVT, VOO, AAI, AAT, and AOO
  - ○ Medtronic Model 5346[8]
    - ○ Basic pacing rates, 30 to 180 ppm, continuously adjustable
    - ○ Rapid atrial pacing rates, 72 ppm and 100 to 800 ppm (10 ppm increments, ±5%)
    - ○ Output amplitude: atrial, 0.1to 20 mA; ventricular, 0.1 to 25 mA

- Pulse width: atrial, 1.0 ms; ventricular, 2 ms; emergency mode, 2 ms
- Sensitivity: atrial, 0.5 to 15 mV; ventricular, 1 to 15 mV
- Atrial-ventricular (A-V) interval, 6 and 20 to 300 ms
- Refractory period:
  - Atrial, 150 to 500 ms; AAT mode, 325 – 750 m
  - Ventricular, 250 ms; VVT mode, varies according to rate
- Safety pace, 110 ms
- Blanking, 100 ms (26 ms in ventricular channel at atrial pace in DVI and DDD modes)

❖ Medtronic Model 5388[8] (Figure 54-3)
  - Basic pacing rates, 30 to 200 ppm, continuously adjustable
  - Upper pacing rates, 80 to 230 ppm
  - Rapid atrial pacing rates, 80 to 800 ppm
  - Output amplitude: atrial, 0.1 to 20 mA; ventricular, 0.1 to 25 mA
  - Pulse width: atrial, 1.0 ms; ventricular, 1.5 ms
  - Sensitivity: atrial, 0.4 to 10 mV; ventricular, 0.8 to 20 mV
  - A-V Interval, 20 to 300 ms
  - Refractory period:
    - Atrial, 150 to 500 ms
    - Ventricular, 250 ms
  - Ventricular blanking: pace, 125 ms; sense, 75 ms
- Gauze, tape, transparent dressing
- Stethoscope
- Calipers

- Telemetry equipment with printing capability
- Defibrillator (available on unit)
- Child's pacemaker settings/parameters

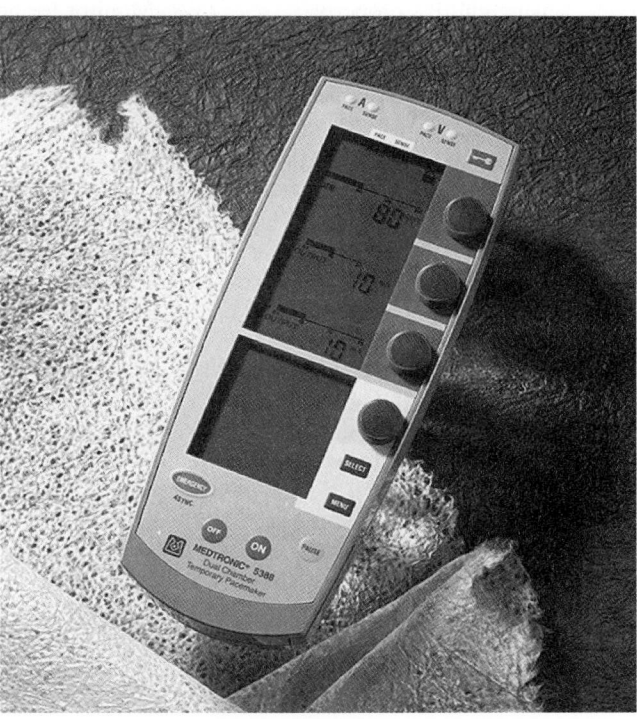

FIGURE 54-3 Dual-chamber pulse generator, Medtronic model 5388. *Photo courtesy of Medtronic USA, Inc.*

Procedure for Transvenous and Epicardial Pacing: Monitoring

Steps	Rationale	Considerations
1. Ensure child and family understand procedure and questions are answered.	Evaluates and reinforces understanding of previously taught information.	This procedure may be performed in emergent conditions that may preclude preprocedural teaching.
2. Collect necessary supplies and equipment, including generator battery and paper for ECG printout.	Ensures that all equipment for the procedure is at the bedside to facilitate completion of procedure without delays.	Always have an extra pulse generator and battery at bedside in case of equipment malfunction.
3. Wash hands and put on clean gloves.	Standard precautions; reduces transmission of microorganisms. Epicardial leads may have microfractures in the wire insulation that are not visible. Use of gloves protects child and personnel from microshocks during handling of pacing wires.	Use nonlatex gloves for children who are allergic to latex.
4. Position child on a flat surface with the head of bed elevated 30 to 45 degrees. *(Level II*)*	Proper positioning can decrease the incidence rate of equipment malfunction and may decrease the child's anxiety.	Proper positioning can also facilitate airway stability.

Procedure continues on following page

* Level II: Theory-based; no research data to support recommendations; recommendations from expert consensus group may exist

Procedure | for Transvenous and Epicardial Pacing: Monitoring—*Continued*

Steps	Rationale	Considerations
5. Ensure child is properly connected to cardiopulmonary monitoring, blood pressure monitoring, and pulse oximetry.[1,2] *(Level II*)*	Monitor for hemodynamic compromise during the procedure. The current pacemaker settings may need to be adjusted to optimize cardiac output.	Child may need the initiation of inotropic agents or other medical intervention during procedure.
6. Compare pacemaker settings with the prescribing practitioner's orders (mode, rate, output, pulse width, and A-V interval). *(Level II*)*	Ensures that pacemaker settings have not been inadvertently altered without knowledge of the medical team. The pacemaker may revert to default settings if equipment malfunctions; default settings are based on adult population.	Newer generator models have a security feature that "locks in" settings. Settings should be based on age and hemodynamic status of child to optimize cardiac output and avoid additional stress on the heart.[5]
7. Verify that patient connector cables are secured into appropriate receptacles (marked "A" for atrium or "V" for ventricle). *(Level II*)*	For optimization of capture, pacing wires must be correctly and securely inserted into the pulse generator.	Atrial epicardial wires are usually located to the right of the sternum, and ventricular wires to the left of the sternum. However, presence of complex congenital heart defects may necessitate deviation from the typical exit sites.[4] A ground wire may be used for epicardial unipolar temporary pacing. Ground wires may be located on either side of the sternum. When used, the ground wire should be inserted into the positive terminal of the pulse generator.[6]
8. Ensure telemetry monitoring is functioning and obtain an ECG printout.	Verifies that atrial or ventricular pacemaker capture is present.	Be sure that the "pace on" feature is activated in telemetry system to ensure recognition of the pacemaker spikes. Atrial capture occurs when a pacer spike immediately precedes a P wave. Ventricular capture occurs when a pacer spike immediately precedes a QRS complex. If child's intrinsic rhythm is dominant, the paced rate is increased by 10 bpm above the intrinsic rate to ensure capture.[2]
9. Assess for atrial or ventricular noncapture. If present, increase milliampere (mA) output settings. Any increase in threshold values should be documented and reported. *(Level II*)*	The mA output should be programmed to two to three times the capture threshold. Increases in threshold indicate that more output is needed to pace the heart. This increase is inversely related to lead function longevity.[4]	Increase the output until atrial or ventricular capture is confirmed on telemetry or an ECG (mA output ranges are 5 to 20 mA).[4,5,8] The minimal increase in mA output should be used to minimize scar tissue development, which can result in a need for an increase in output.[6] Monitor for presence of abdominal muscle stimulation (with epicardial system) or pectoral muscle stimulation (with transvenous system).

* Level II: Theory-based; no research data to support recommendations; recommendations from expert consensus group may exist

Procedure for Transvenous and Epicardial Pacing: Monitoring—*Continued*

Steps	Rationale	Considerations
10. Verify that appropriate sensing is present. If **undersensing** is occurring, the atrial or ventricular sensitivity should be decreased. If **oversensing** is occurring, the atrial or ventricular sensitivity should be increased. *(Level I*)*	Assesses effectiveness of current pacemaker settings. If pacemaker undersensing is present, paced beats may be early; if oversensing is present, paced beats may be late.	**Undersensing:** Lowest number (in millivolt) for sensitivity is the most sensitive setting (sensitivity ranges, 0.4 mV to 20 mV). The number should be *decreased* to make the pacemaker *more sensitive*.[4] Causes of undersensing are: lead dislodgement, poor lead position, lead insulation defect, and low-amplitude cardiac signal. **Oversensing:** Highest number (in millivolt) for sensitivity is the *least sensitive* setting (sensitivity ranges, 0.4 mV to 20 mV). The number should be *increased* to make pacemaker *less sensitive*.[4] Causes of oversensing are: lead fracture and lead disconnection.[9]
11. Assess pacing wire exit site for signs of infection or possible lead/catheter tension.	Careful attention to the exit site reduces potential for infection or wire fracture.	Leads or catheter should be fixed to the skin to prevent traction or displacement. Pulse generator should be pinned to the bed or the child's gown to prevent tension and disconnection.
12. Place a cap or gauze over exposed ends of the catheter (transvenous system) or lead tips (epicardial system). The tip of a rubber glove may be used to cover the exposed catheter or lead tip, which is then taped down to the chest wall.	Prevents injury to the exposed ends of the catheter (transvenous system) or lead tips (epicardial system) when not attached to a temporary pulse generator.	Avoid use of powdered gloves or adhesive to prevent residue from interfering with conduction between the wires and the pulse generator.
13. Evaluate capture thresholds daily with medical staff present. The output (in volts) is gradually decreased until capture is lost. Document point at which capture is lost. *(Level II*)*	Determines level of pacemaker dependency by identifying the minimum amount of output necessary to consistently capture the chamber being paced.	The output (in mA) should be programmed at two to three times the threshold value to allow for a margin of safety.[2]
14. Evaluate child's underlying or intrinsic rhythm daily with the medical staff present. The underlying rhythm is documented, and the pacemaker low rate may be adjusted.	Evaluates need for continued therapy. Facilitates adjustment of pacing parameters on the basis of hemodynamic status, and determines duration of pacing requirement.	The paced rate is gradually reduced until the underlying rhythm is revealed. The paced rate setting may be decreased to allow for more intrinsic activity. The pause button may also be used on certain pacemaker models to permit a pause in pacing with subsequent restoration of previous settings after 10 seconds. A permanent pacemaker may be indicated if heart block persists for more than 10 days or with severe bradycardia.[5,7] The defibrillator should be nearby.
15. Remove gloves and wash hands.	Reduces the transmission of microorganisms.	

---

* Level I: Manufacturer's recommendations only

Level II: Theory-based; no research data to support recommendations; recommendations from expert consensus group may exist

TABLE 54-1	Descriptions of Abnormal Pacemaker Functioning

	Sample ECG Appearance	Some Possible Clinical Consequences	Some Possible Causes	Corrective Measures
Undersensing Device fails to detect existing cardiac depolarizations, therefore competes with the native rhythm	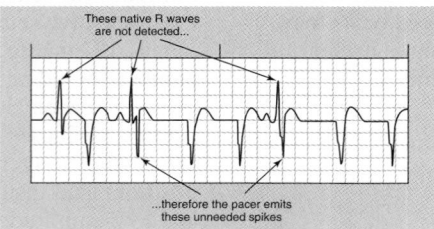 These native R waves are not detected... ...therefore the pacer emits these unneeded spikes	Competition with a native rhythm Stimulation of dysrhythmias ("R-on-T")	Lead disconnected from pacer or from viable myocardium Sensitivity set too low Lead fracture Low battery	Check connection of lead to pacer Increase sensitivity (turn sensing control to a SMALLER number) 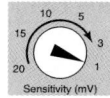 Reposition or change lead Change battery
Oversensing Device detects noncardiac electrical events and interprets them as cardiac depolarizations, therefore is wrongly inhibited from pacing	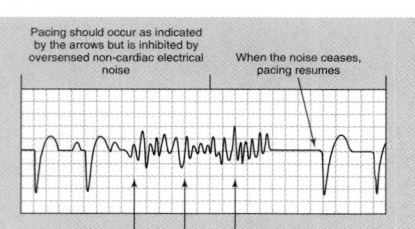 Pacing should occur as indicated by the arrows but is inhibited by oversensed non-cardiac electrical noise. When the noise ceases, pacing resumes.	Pacemaker-dependent patients receive no stimuli from the pacemaker, producing a pause in rhythm and reduction in cardiac output	Electrical potential caused by noncardiac muscle contraction (especially pectorals) is detected and misinterpreted by the device Interference from electrical sources (ungrounded equipment, short circuits) is detected and misinterpreted by the device Sensitivity set too high	Decrease sensitivity (turn sensing control to a LARGER number) 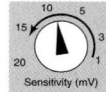 Remove all ungrounded electrical equipment or have it evaluated by hospital engineers
Noncapture Device emits stimuli, which fail to depolarize the myocardium	This dual chamber device paces and captures in the atrium and ventricle for the first two beats. Ventricular capture is then lost; the ventricular pacing spikes are not followed by depolarizations. Fortunately, ventricular escape begins.	Pacemaker-dependent patients receive no stimuli from the pacemaker, producing a pause in rhythm and reduction in cardiac output	Lead disconnected from pacer or from viable myocardium Output set too low in the noncaptured chamber Lead fracture High pacing threshold resulting from medication or metabolic changes Low battery	Check connection of lead to pacer Increase output in the noncaptured chamber Reposition or change lead Change battery Alter medication regimen, correct metabolic changes

From Witherell CL: Cardiac rhythm control devices, *Crit Care Nurs Clin North Am* 6(1):85-101, 1994.

Expected Outcomes

- Appropriate pacemaker capture and function; child's pulse is strong and regular

- Appropriate sensing and inhibition of intrinsic activity
- Adequate heart rate achieved with improvement in cardiac output
- Heart rate and rhythm are regular

Unexpected Outcomes

- Pacemaker noncapture or failure to pace (no spike generated)
- Poor cardiac output as evidenced by poor perfusion, cool extremities, prolonged capillary refill, and decreased urine output
- Pacemaker undersensing or oversensing
- Arrhythmias present
- Inability to provide adequate cardiac output with pacing

Monitoring and Care of the Child

Activities and Interventions	Rationale	Reportable Conditions
1. Monitor child's heart rate and rhythm.	Inability to maintain set heart rate or stable rhythm may indicate equipment malfunction, lead failure, or a change in child's condition, warranting changes in pacing parameters.	• Heart rate less than lower rate of pacemaker • Rhythm irregularity • Pacemaker competing with intrinsic rhythm, not corrected with altered sensitivity
2. Verify that mechanical capture is in synchrony with electrical capture.	Electrical capture (pacing spikes and QRS complex) may be present without mechanical capture (pulse and blood pressure).	• Weak, thready, or absent pulse • Signs of low cardiac output
3. Assess for appropriate sensing.	Undersensing or oversensing may result in ineffective pacing therapy.	• Undersensing (failure of pacemaker to see intrinsic activity resulting in inappropriate pacing) • Oversensing (inappropriate inhibition by pacemaker resulting in pauses or slower than expected lower rates)
4. Monitor for presence of symptoms (palpitations, dizziness, shortness of breath, or chest pain). Run an ECG strip when child has symptoms and verify the heart rate by palpating child's pulse.[3,4]	Changes in child's condition may indicate complications with pacemaker or rhythm.	• Palpitations • Dizziness • Shortness of breath • Chest pain
5. Monitor hemodynamic response to paced rhythm.	Failure to improve cardiac output may indicate need for adjustment in pacemaker settings.	• Signs of low cardiac output
6. Perform epicardial wire exit site care or transvenous catheter exit site care per institution-specific protocol.	Minimizes risk of infection and potential for wire fracture.	• Signs of infection • Wire fracture • Fever

Documentation

- Education of child and family
- Time and date pacing started and stopped
- Child's response to pacing therapy
- Heart rate and rhythm interpretation (paced and intrinsic rhythm)
- Verification of pacemaker mode, rate, output, and sensing values
- Evidence of inappropriate pacemaker activity (undersensing, oversensing, noncapture)
- Underlying rhythm and capture thresholds and any corrective action taken based on these findings
- Condition of wire exit site and connector/ lead sites
- Battery changes
- Any reported symptoms during pacing therapy (chest pain, palpitations, or dizziness)
- Unexpected outcomes and related treatment

References

1. Berul C, Cecchin F: Indications and techniques of pediatric cardiac pacing, *Expert Rev Cardiovasc Ther* 1(2):165-176, 2003.
2. Craig J, et al: Tissue perfusion. In Curley MAQ, Moloney-Harmon P, editors: *Critical Care Nursing of infants and children,* ed 2, Philadelphia, 2001, Saunders.
3. Deal B, et al, editors: *Current concepts in diagnosis and management of arrhythmias in infants and children,* Armonk, NY, 1998, Futura Publishing Co, Inc.
4. Furman S, et al, editors: *A practice of cardiac pacing,* ed 3, Armonk, NY, 1993, Futura Publishing.
5. Gammage M: Temporary cardiac pacing, *Heart* 83:715–720, 2000.

6. Jacobson C, Gerity D: Pacemakers and implantable defibrillators. In Woods S, et al, editors: *Cardiac nursing*, ed 4, Philadelphia, 2003, Lippincott Williams & Wilkins.

7. Maginot KR, et al: Applications of pacing strategies in neonates and infants, *Progress Pediatr Cardiol* 11(1): 65–75, 2000.

8. www.medtronic.com/ brady/ clinician/ medtronicpacing. Medtronic, Inc., Medtronic web site, 2005. Accessed 5/9/06

9. Witherall CL: Cardiac rhythm control devices. *Critical Care Nursing Clinics of North America*, 1996; 6:95–102.

Additional Readings

American Heart Association: *Pediatric advanced life support provider manual*, Dallas, 2002, American Heart Association.

Deal B, et al: Surgical therapy of cardiac arrhythmias. In Mavroudis C, Backer C, editors: *Pediatric cardiac surgery*, ed 3, Philadelphia, 2003, Mosby.

Gregoratos G, et al: ACC/ AHA/ NASPE 2002 guideline update for implantation of cardiac pacemakers and antiarrhythmia devices. a report of the American College of Cardiology/ American Heart Association Task Force on practice guidelines, *J Cardiovasc Electrophysiol* 13(1):1183–1199, 2002.

Park M: *Pediatric cardiology for practitioners*, 3 ed, St. Louis, 1996, Mosby.

AP

Epicardial Pacing Wire Removal: Perform

PURPOSE: To remove temporary epicardial pacing wires, placed during cardiac surgery for the diagnosis and treatment of postoperative arrhythmias

Patricia O'Brien

PREREQUISITE KNOWLEDGE

- Anatomy and physiology of the conduction system and congenital heart defects
- Ability to interpret electrocardiographic (ECG) tracings
- Types of temporary wires and wire placement
  - ❖ Children may have ventricular leads (placed on the left side of the chest) or atrial leads (placed on the right side of the chest) or both.
  - ❖ Leads are placed on the heart at the end of the operation before chest closure. The ends of the pacing leads are then brought through the skin and secured to the skin with either a suture or a knot created with the wire.
  - ❖ Epicardial wires are covered in a colored plastic casing.
  - ❖ If a ground wire is used, the gray metal wire is looped through the skin and is not attached to the heart.[1]
- Child's specific cardiac defect and repair performed
- Contraindications to wire removal: presence of second-degree or third-degree heart block with compromised hemodynamics, pacemaker dependency, and coagulopathy[1]
- Complications of wire removal and related signs and symptoms: graft injury, bleeding, tamponade, hemothorax, and ventricular dysrhythmias[2,3]
- Mastery of pediatric advanced life support competencies
- Child development as it relates to clinical assessment and removal of epicardial pacing wires

CHILD AND FAMILY ASSESSMENT

- History of postoperative arrhythmias and rationale for temporary pacing requirement ➧➧*Rationale:* These conditions may necessitate further studies for determination of readiness for pacing wire removal.[4]
- History of heart surgery or postoperative bleeding and length of time wires have been in place ➧➧*Rationale:* These factors may increase the difficulty of wire removal.
- Function of conduction pathway ➧➧*Rationale:* Presence of sinus rhythm or a stable rhythm is necessary before pacing wire removal.
- Anticoagulation status ➧➧*Rationale:* The presence of coagulopathy necessitates treatment before pacing wire removal for prevention of bleeding during and after the procedure.
- Readiness for hospital discharge ➧➧*Rationale:* For discharge in a timely manner, the pacing wires should be removed at least 4 hours before discharge to allow monitoring for complications.
- Child's and family's understanding of the reasons for and risks and benefits of the procedure ➧➧*Rationale:* Evaluates child's and family's understanding of the procedure and provides a gauge for ongoing education.
- Child's developmental level and ability to interact ➧➧*Rationale:* These factors influence preparation of child and interaction.
- Level of consciousness and cognitive ability ➧➧*Rationale:* Determines whether the child is able to follow instructions to assist with the procedure.
- Desire of family members to be present during the procedure ➧➧*Rationale:* Family may provide support and

comfort measures to the child but should have the choice not to remain with the child.

CHILD AND FAMILY EDUCATION

Individualized, developmentally appropriate education is provided to the family and to the child based on desire for knowledge, readiness to learn, and overall neurologic and psychosocial state.

- Provide information about epicardial pacing wire removal, including reassurance that the child no longer needs the use of the wires and the steps involved in removal ➥*Rationale:* Information decreases fear and anxiety.
- If developmentally appropriate, explain how the child can assist with the procedure (lie still against a solid surface, breathing exercises) ➥*Rationale:* The procedure is safer, easier, and less painful when child is cooperative.
- When developmentally appropriate, prepare the child for sensation of mild pain or discomfort associated with wire removal ➥*Rationale:* Complete information can enhance a trusting relationship with the caregiver and offer the

opportunity to use distraction techniques to decrease discomfort associated with the procedure.

- Explain the rationale for cardiac monitoring requirement after pacing wire removal and the discharge delay for approximately 4 hours (or per institution-specific protocol) ➥*Rationale:* Complete information optimizes compliance with hospital policy to monitor for the development of bleeding or arrhythmias after pacing wire removal.
- Encourage questions and answer questions as they arise ➥*Rationale:* Reinforcement of information is needed during periods of stress.

EQUIPMENT

- Suture removal kit or #11 straight scalpel blade
- Skin cleanser (typically povidone-iodine and alcohol wipes) per institution-specific protocol
- Sterile 2×2 gauze
- Band-Aids
- Sterile gloves
- Cardiac monitoring
- Defibrillator and code cart immediately available

Procedure for Epicardial Pacing Wire Removal: Perform

Steps	Rationale	Considerations
1. Ensure child and family understand procedure and questions are answered.	Evaluates and reinforces understanding of previously taught information.	Developmental level, cognitive ability, and anxiety level determine approach to and effectiveness of teaching.
2. Check coagulation study results if child is undergoing anticoagulation therapy or has a positive history for coagulopathy. *(Level II*)*	Normalize coagulation studies when possible before removal of pacing wires to avoid the risk of bleeding.	Consider removing the pacing wires before initiation of anti-coagulation therapy. Caution must be taken when removing pacing wires in children who are receiving heparin, Lovenox, coumadin, Plavix, asprin or those who have a history of thrombocytopenia or bleeding. Consult with the attending physician for the acceptable range for coagulation studies and whether clotting factors should be given prior to pacing wire removal. Acceptable ranges for pacing wire removal include an international normalized ratio (INR) less than INR 1.6 and a platelet count > 50,000. Heparin therapy is usually stopped for 3 to 4 hours before the procedure and then restarted after the procedure.[4]

* Level II: Theory-based; no research data to support recommendations; recommendations from expert consensus group may exist

Procedure for Epicardial Pacing Wire Removal: Perform—*Continued*

Steps	Rationale	Considerations
		Normalization of coagulation studies may be contraindicated in children's mechanical aortic or mitral valves or history of emboli.
3. Coordinate timing of procedure with availability of surgeon.	Small risk of bleeding leading to tamponade or cardiac arrest, both requiring surgical intervention.[4]	Wire removal should only occur during daytime hours when surgical staff is available in hospital.
4. Check availability of nursing assistance.	A support person can assist with ensuring that child remains still during procedure and can provide distraction techniques to decrease discomfort and anxiety associated with procedure.	
5. Plan location of the procedure. (*Level VI**)	Avoid performing procedure in child's "safe zone" to decrease anxiety and stress of hospitalization.	Follow institution-specific protocol regarding safe zones, such as patient rooms, and use a treatment room for all procedures. In certain circumstances, the child may choose the setting.
6. Ensure availability of appropriate cardiopulmonary monitoring and defibrillator on the nursing unit. (*Level IV**)	Assists with assessment and treatment of procedural complications, including arrhythmias and cardiac tamponade.	
7. Gather all necessary equipment and supplies.	Preparation and availability of all materials facilitate completion of the procedure without delay.	
8. Wash hands.	Reduces transmission of microorganisms.	
9. Put on sterile gloves.	Standard precaution for removal of invasive lines.	
10. Provide for appropriate privacy; position the child flat or at a 30-degree to 45-degree angle on a solid surface.	Facilitates safe removal of pacing wires. Wire removal requires exposure of the chest.	In general, the semiupright position is preferred by children and is associated with less anxiety. Lying on a flat solid surface minimizes the natural tendency to pull backward during the procedure and assists in immobilizing child during procedure.[4] Privacy is an important consideration for school-aged children and adolescents.
11. Remove all tape and dressings from around the pacing wires and disconnect the pacing wires from the temporary pacemaker if applicable.	Allows for complete visualization of the pacing wire insertion site and knot or suture securing placement of the pacing wire.	

Procedure continues on following page

* Level IV: Limited clinical studies to support recommendations
 Level VI: Clinical studies in a variety of patient populations and situations to support recommendations

Procedure for Epicardial Pacing Wire Removal: Perform—*Continued*

Steps	Rationale	Considerations
12. Assess wire insertion site for redness, drainage, or swelling. *(Level VI*)*	Alerts caregiver to a potential source of infection.	If site appears to be infected and child has fever, consider obtaining a white blood cell count (WBC), blood culture, and culture of the drainage from the site. Consider starting child on antibiotic therapy appropriate to treat gram-positive organisms.[1]
13. Clean insertion sites and surrounding area with skin antiseptic agents. *(Level II*)*	Reduces risk of infection.	Institution-specific protocol determines the antiseptic agent used, most commonly chlorhexidine or povidone-iodine.
14. Determine method used to secure temporary pacing wire in place. a. If sutures are used to secure wire to skin, cut the sutures with a scissors or straight scalpel blade and pull out the sutures from the skin. b. If the knot method was used, hold knot securely with pickups and identify which end of wire is attached to heart versus connects to temporary pacemaker. *(Level II*)*	Confirms correct method for releasing the wire from skin to avoid a retained wire in the chest.	If the knot method was used and the incorrect end of wire is cut, child may need to return to the operating room for wire removal per institution-specific protocol.
15. Remove the portion of wires connected to the heart with a steady downward motion and cover insertion site with dry sterile gauze. *(Level II*)*	Steady downward motion follows the angle of wires in the chest and the least amount of resistance to removal is encountered.	Wires can become adherent to the chest wall and become more difficult to remove. This difficulty is more likely to occur in children with previous heart surgery or a history of postoperative bleeding and is associated with length of time the pacing wires have been in place.[3,5]
16. If removal of pacing wire is unsuccessful, attempt to wiggle the wire to loosen, and then leave wire taped to child's skin under some tension for a period of time. If the second attempt at wire removal is unsuccessful, consult with surgeon to discuss management. Depending on institution-specific protocol, some wires may be cut at the level of the skin and left in place if they cannot be removed.	Wires may be adherent to the chest wall and become difficult to remove. Gentle back and forth movement or application of tension to the wire may assist in loosening. Temporary pacing wires left in the mediastinum carry a slight risk of late infection, migration, or foreign body reaction.[5]	If the pacing wires will be cut and left in place: • Put on sterile gloves. • Cleanse the wire and surrounding area with skin antiseptic. • With pickups, put gentle tension on the wire to pull it taut. • Cut wire with sterile scissors at the exit site from the skin. The opposite end of wire retracts back under skin. • Cover the site with a band-aid.

*   Level II: Theory-based; no research data to support recommendations; recommendations from expert consensus group may exist
   Level VI: Clinical studies in a variety of patient populations and situations to support recommendations

Procedure for Epicardial Pacing Wire Removal: Perform—*Continued*

Steps	Rationale	Considerations
In some situations, the surgeon reattempts wire removal; if unsuccessful, schedule child for wire removal in the operating room because of risks associated with temporary pacing wire retention.		If the plan is to surgically remove wires, follow institution-specific protocol to prepare child and family for surgery. Educate family about the procedure, recovery time, and discharge. Institute NPO orders, obtain surgical consents, and set up for blood. Under general anesthesia, a small incision is made in the chest wall to remove the wire. The wire is removed, anesthesia is reversed, and the child is observed for at least 4 hours before discharge.[2,3,5]
17. Clean site with sterile gauze and then apply band-aid.	Cover area until the insertion site has healed to prevent infection.	
18. Examine extracted wires for breaks, pieces of tissue, or drainage. *(Level II*)*	Determines the risk of migration, wire fragment retention, bleeding, or infection.	
19. Dispose of used supplies and equipment appropriately.	Standard precautions; reduces transmission of microorganisms.	
20. Remove gloves and wash hands.	Standard precautions.	
21. Observe child for possible complications for at least 4 hours after wire removal. *(Level II*)*	Rarely, serious adverse events that result in hemodynamic compromise may occur, such as ventricular fibrillation or significant bleeding.	It is recommended that children be monitored for a period of at least 4 hours after pacing wire removal prior to discharge. Removal of pacing wires 1 day before discharge is preferable. If complications do occur, immediately begin appropriate measures to stabilize child's condition, including CPR if indicated, and notify the surgeon immediately. An echocardiogram may be indicated if cardiac tamponade is suspected. *(Level IV*)*

* Level II: Theory-based; no research data to support recommendations; recommendations from expert consensus group may exist
Level IV: Limited clinical studies to support recommendations

Expected Outcomes

- Temporary epicardial pacing wires are removed without incident

- Child's condition is hemodynamically stable

- Child is free from infection

Unexpected Outcomes

- Severe bleeding causing cardiac tamponade or hemothorax from injury to the heart or coronary arteries[2,3]
- Bleeding at insertion site after wire removal
- Inability to remove pacing wire[6]
- Tissue noted on extracted pacing wire
- Cardiac compression from malposition of the pacing wires being wrapped around the heart[5]
- Development of a hemodynamically significant arrhythmia (ventricular tachycardia or fibrillation)[4]
- Purulent drainage at the insertion site
- Fever

Monitoring and Care of the Child

Activities and Interventions	Rationale	Reportable Conditions
1. Monitor child's hemodynamic status.	Changes in child's condition may indicate the development of complications associated with the procedure.	• New onset of arrhythmias • Hemodynamically significant tachycardia • Signs of decreased cardiac output: hypotension, increased irritability, anxiety, lethargy, pallor, diaphoresis, or emesis[1]

2. If bleeding develops from the pacing wire insertion site, apply firm pressure for several minutes until drainage stops.
    Apply pressure dressing if necessary.
    If the bleeding does not respond to these measures, notify the surgeon or prescribing practitioner, review coagulation status, ensure availability of blood products, and consider diagnostic studies.
	Small amounts of bleeding may occur at the pacing wire exit site as a result of trauma to the skin but should immediately stop with pressure.	• Significant bleeding at the insertion site
		• Bleeding persists after firm pressure applied for several minutes

3. If purulent drainage is noted on the pacing wire or at the insertion site, obtain a culture of the site, cleanse the site, and place a dry sterile dressing; assess the child for further signs of infection. Consider obtaining a complete blood cell count (CBC) and blood culture. Discuss the need for antibiotics or topical management with prescribing practitioner.	Purulent drainage at the pacing wire site may be indicative of a localized or deep sternal infection.	• Signs of infection
4. Assess the effectiveness of pain management strategy and provide appropriate interventions. Encourage family to assist with nonpharmacologic means to comfort and support child.	The child should have only minimal pain with the procedure; early identification of unexpected pain or discomfort allows for immediate attention to the child's pain.	• Unresolved pain and discomfort • Continued irritability or changes in physiologic condition

Documentation

- Child and family education
- Recent prothrombin time (PT), partial thromboplastin time (PTT), and INR, with anticoagulation therapy or positive history of coagulopathy, and the plan of care before pacing wire removal
- Procedure, including individual performing procedure, number of wires removed, and child's response
- Unexpected outcomes and related treatment
- Comfort assessment and any specific interventions provided

References

1. Jacobson C, Gerity D: Pacemakers and implantable defibrillators. In Woods S, et al, editors: *Cardiac nursing*, ed 4, Philadelphia, 2000, Lippincott Williams & Wilkins.
2. Carroll KC, et al: Risks associated with removal of ventricular pacing wires after cardiac surgery, *Am J Crit Care* 7(6):444-449, 1998.
3. Johnson LG, et al: Complications of epicardial pacing wire removal, *J Cardiovasc Nurs* 7(2):32-40, 1993.
4. Dahlberg S, Mooradd M: Temporary cardiac pacing. In Irwin R, et al, editors: *Procedures and techniques in intensive care medicine*, ed 3, Philadelphia, 2003, Lippincott Williams & Wilkins.
5. Bolton JWR, Mayer JE: Unusual complications of temporary pacing wires in children, *Ann Thorac Surg* 54(4): 769-70, 1992.
6. Manion PA: Temporary epicardial pacing in the postoperative cardiac surgical patient, *Crit Care Nurs* 13(2)30-38, 1993.

Additional Reading

Deal B, et al: Surgical therapy of cardiac arrhythmias. In Mavroudis C, Backer C, editors: *Pediatric cardiac surgery*, ed 3, Philadelphia, 2003, Mosby.

AP

Transvenous Pacemaker Insertion: Perform

P U R P O S E :   To provide temporary cardiac pacing in children with an inadequate heart rate until a permanent solution is in place or to terminate a dysrhythmia in children with hemodynamic compromise

Constance E. Cephus

PREREQUISITE KNOWLEDGE

- Normal cardiac anatomy and physiology, including the conduction pathway
- Child's congenital heart disease, if present, or acquired heart disease and associated short-term and long-term electrophysiologic complications
- Child's medical and surgical history, including placement of internal pacemaker or internal defibrillator
- Temporary transvenous pacing is performed to provide emergent support of cardiac output in children who require pacing leads in direct contact with the myocardium to achieve an adequate heart rate or to terminate a dysrhythmia.[1]
- Temporary transvenous pacing is accomplished with central venous access via the femoral, jugular, or subclavian vein and then advancement of a balloon-tipped ventricular pacing lead through the vena cava and right atrium into the right ventricle.[2]
- Institution of temporary pacing typically occurs in the cardiac catheterization laboratory with fluoroscopy guidance for pacing lead placement. If the child's hemodynamic condition is unstable, the procedure may occur in the intensive care unit or emergency department with electrocardiogram (ECG) or ultrasound guidance for lead placement.[3,4] Moderate sedation or general anesthesia is

administered depending on situation and institution-specific protocol.
- After initiation of transvenous pacing, the child should be transferred to the intensive care unit. Once the condition is stabilized, permanent pacemaker placement is usually scheduled to occur within 72 hours.[2,5]
- Normal infant, child, and adolescent heart rates
- Basic and advanced ECG and cardiac arrhythmia interpretation
- Components of a transvenous pacing catheter
- Understanding of pulse generator use, including selection of appropriate settings
- Ability to differentiate between mechanical and electrical capture
- Familiarity with electrophysiologic terminology (see Tables 51-1 and 51-2 for a glossary of terminology)
- Ability to assess hemodynamic response to pacing therapy
- Common venous access routes for transvenous lead placement and familiarity with child's history of vascular access
- Complications associated with transvenous pacing lead placement (right ventricle perforation, lead dislodgement, infection, thrombus formation, venous obstruction, catheter-induced arrhythmias, vessel or valve damage) and related signs and symptoms
- Mastery of pediatric advanced life support competencies
- Child development as it relates to clinical assessment and transvenous pacemaker insertion
- Principles of aseptic technique
- Appropriate pediatric dosing of analgesics and competency in procedural sedation

- In a non-emergent situation, informed consent is necessary before placement of a transvenous pacemaker.

CHILD AND FAMILY ASSESSMENT

- History of congenital heart disease, cardiomyopathy, cardiac arrhythmias, syncope, cardiac surgical or catheterization procedures, surgical electrophysiologic complications, and projected future cardiac surgery requirements ➤*Rationale:* These conditions may limit the options for venous access and assist with anticipatory planning for optimal treatment of potential complications and the type of permanent pacemaker implanted.[5,6]
- Current hemodynamic status ➤*Rationale:* Initiation of inotropic support may be necessary to stabilize the child's condition before, during, or after the procedure. The child's hemodynamic status determines the emergent nature of the procedure.[6]
- History of ECGs ➤*Rationale:* Establishes prior baseline rhythm.
- Medication history, including use of herbal supplements, drug exposures, acid-base balance, and electrolyte levels ➤*Rationale:* Drug therapy and electrolyte or acid-base abnormalities could impede pacing ability. Certain medications or drug exposures may be implicated as the cause for the dysrhythmia.[2]
- Child's developmental level and ability to interact ➤*Rationale:* These factors influence preparation and interaction.
- Level of consciousness and cognitive ability ➤*Rationale:* Determines the child's ability to cooperate with instructions or assist with the procedure by remaining still.
- Child's and family's understanding of the reasons for and risks and benefits of the procedure ➤*Rationale:* Evaluates the child's and family's understanding of the procedure and provides a gauge for ongoing education.
- History of response to anesthesia or conscious sedation ➤*Rationale:* Response may influence the type of sedation used for the procedure to safely achieve desired results.[5]
- Family's desire to be present during the procedure ➤*Rationale:* The family may provide support and comfort measures to the child but should have the choice not to remain with the child. If the procedure is performed emergently, support staff should be with the family throughout the procedure.

CHILD AND FAMILY EDUCATION

Individualized, developmentally appropriate education is provided to the family and to the child based on desire for knowledge, readiness to learn, and overall neurologic and psychosocial state.

- Provide information on the child's medical condition and the need for device placement ➤*Rationale:* Appropriate information helps to decrease the child's and family's anxiety levels and offers reassurance during an extremely stressful period.
- As time permits, show the child and family an actual lead and pacemaker device ➤*Rationale:* Visual examples decrease anxiety and fear and may facilitate understanding.
- Provide information on the pacing process, post-procedural care, and activity restriction requirements necessary to ensure the device remains in place and functional ➤*Rationale:* Providing information to the child and family decreases fear and anxiety and can increase compliance with plan of care.
- Provide information to the child and family on how the pacing catheter is placed and the complications that may occur[7,8] ➤*Rationale:* Providing information to the child and family decreases fear and anxiety regarding the procedure and assists in preparation for future interventions.
- Provide information to the child and family about the sedation and pain medication administered during transvenous pacing wire insertion ➤*Rationale:* Transvenous pacing wire insertion is painful; the child will need pain control and sedation.[5] When the family and child know that pain will be managed, anxiety is decreased.
- Provide information regarding post-procedural activity level, follow-up, activity restrictions, and safety issues. Allowable activity level is dependent on cardiopulmonary stability and the ability of the child to cooperate with restrictions. ➤*Rationale:* Compliance with activity restrictions is improved when the child and family understand the rationale and related safety issues.
- Encourage questions and answer questions as they arise ➤*Rationale:* Reinforcement of information is needed during periods of stress.

EQUIPMENT

- Introducer kit (appropriate for the pacing lead size), which includes:
  - ❖ Local anesthetic
  - ❖ Percutaneous introducer needle
  - ❖ Guidewire
  - ❖ Introducer sheath with dilator
- Heparinized saline solution flush
- Syringes
- Needles
- 3-0 silk sutures with needle
- Sterile needle holder and scissors
- Pacing catheter: 3F, 4F, or 5F (Figure 56-1)
- Sterile accordion sleeve as appropriate to pacing catheter
- Pacing cable (Figure 56-2)
- Pulse generator with new battery
- Skin preparation tray
- Skin antiseptic (usually chlorhexidine or povidone-iodine)
- Sterile towels, gowns, gloves, and masks
- Dressing supplies
- Cardiopulmonary monitoring
- Electrocardiographic patches and recorder
- 12-lead or 15-lead ECG machine
- Emergency equipment, including defibrillator immediately available
- Fluoroscopy or echocardiography as requested

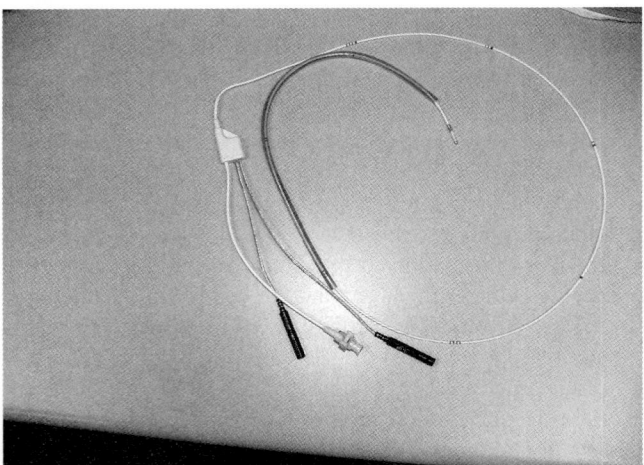

FIGURE 56-1   Transvenous pacing catheter.

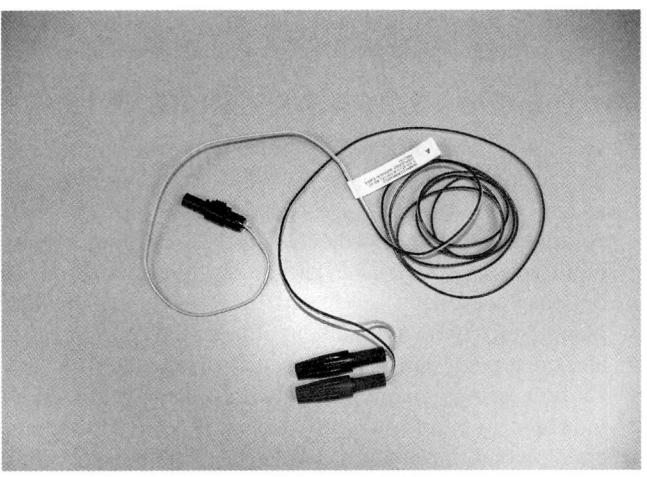

FIGURE 56-2   Pacing cable used to connect transvenous pacing catheter to pulse generator.

Procedure for Transvenous Pacemaker Insertion: Perform

Steps	Rationale	Considerations
1. Ensure child and family understand procedure and questions are answered.	Evaluates and reinforces understanding of previously taught information.	Developmental level, cognitive ability, and anxiety level determine approach to and effectiveness of teaching.
2. Obtain consent from legal guardian per institution-specific protocol.	Ensures medical-legal compliance as suggested by the Joint Commission on Accreditation of Health Care Organizations (JCAHO).	For emergency situations, the organization may have a protocol in place for assumption of consent.
3. Ensure fasting guidelines have been implemented per institution-specific protocol.	Prevents complications related to emesis/aspiration.	Fasting time is related to child's age.
4. Obtain necessary pre-procedural laboratory tests.	Electrolyte and acid-base imbalance may negatively impact the ability to achieve optimal pacing capability. A type and cross may be obtained as a precaution in case of bleeding.[1] *(Level VI*)*	If venous access is difficult or unavailable or if child's condition is unstable, consider obtaining necessary blood samples and administering antibiotic therapy immediately after venous access has been established for the procedure.[5,6]
5. If the situation permits, administer antibiotics 30 minutes before the procedure.	Antibiotics should be administered to decrease the risk of procedural-related infection.	Subacute bacterial endocarditis (SBE) prophylaxis as recommended by the American Heart Association should be administered to children with a history of congenital heart disease.[2] *(Level VI*)*

* Level VI: Clinical studies in a variety of patient populations and situations to support recommendations

Procedure for Transvenous Pacemaker Insertion: Perform—*Continued*

Steps	Rationale	Considerations
6. Gather needed equipment and supplies.	Ensures that all equipment for the procedure is at the bedside to facilitate completion of procedure without delays. Aids in immediate intervention for unexpected events.	Device selected is dependent on the child's cardiac anatomy and arrhythmia history.
7. Wash hands. *(Level VI[*])*	Standard precautions; reduces transmission of microorganisms.	
8. Identify child with appropriate patient and procedure verification process (e.g., "time out").	Confirms correct patient, procedure, and site as recommended by JCAHO; prevents unnecessary medical procedures.	Verification process and documentation are institution specific. Use active communication techniques.
9. Position child flat or as appropriate for central line insertion. *(Level VI[*])*	Proper position prevents nerve or tissue injury.	Use of soft restraints may be necessary.
10. Ensure child is properly connected to cardiopulmonary monitor, blood pressure monitoring, and pulse oximetry.[1] *(Level II[*])*	Monitors for hemodynamic compromise before, during, and after the procedure.[1]	The child may need initiation of inotropic agents or other interventions because of a change in hemodynamic status.[6]
11. Connect ECG machine and record the 12-lead ECG for baseline rhythm. *(Level II[*])*	Documents rhythm before intervention.	Interpretation of ECG results is based on lead placement and underlying heart condition (e.g., dextrocardia).
12. Ensure a stable airway; sedation/anesthesia is administered by a second individual, per institution-specific protocol.	Sedation and anesthesia decrease anxiety, alleviate discomfort, and decrease movement of child during the procedure.[5] *(Level VI[*])*	Paralytic agents may be necessary in addition to anxiolytics and analgesics.
13. Test the functioning of pulse generator after a new battery is inserted. *(Level I[*])*	Assesses function of the pulse generator.[8]	If a malfunction is detected, obtain a replacement pulse generator in a timely fashion.
14. The person who performs the procedure and the assistant put on gowns, hats, masks, and sterile gloves. *(Level VI[*])*	Instituting sterile conditions assists with decreasing the incidence rate of infection.[5,7]	
15. Cleanse insertion site with skin antiseptic solution per institution-specific protocol. *(Level VI[*])*	Reduces the incidence rate of catheter-related blood stream infection.	The skin antiseptic used is institution specific.
16. Cover site with sterile drapes.	Provides a sterile field, reduces the incidence rate of contamination of sterile supplies, and prevents infection.	
17. With the introducer set, obtain central venous access (see Procedure 153).	Central venous access is the route used for transvenous lead placement.[5,6]	If central venous access has previously been established, obtain a chest x-ray to document catheter position before the start of the procedure. Children with a history of central venous access may need prior computed tomography (CT) or angiography to assess the patency of the subclavian vein.[5,6]

Procedure continues on following page

* Level I: Manufacturer's recommendations only
Level II: Theory-based; no research data to support recommendations; recommendations from expert consensus group may exist
Level VI: Clinical studies in a variety of patient populations and situations to support recommendations

Procedure for Transvenous Pacemaker Insertion: Perform—*Continued*

Steps	Rationale	Considerations
18. If an accordion sleeve is used, attach the sterile accordion sleeve to the introducer.	The sleeve maintains the sterility of the pacing catheter if manipulation of the pacing catheter is necessary.	
19. Insert pacing catheter through the diaphragm of the introducer catheter.	The pacing catheter is introduced into the central vein by way of the introducer catheter. The introducer diaphragm seals around the pacing catheter, which prevents blood loss or introduction of air.	If a sterile sleeve is used, the pacing catheter is threaded through the sleeve and then through the introducer.
20. Inflate the balloon when tip of the pacing catheter is in vena cava. *(Level I*)*	Balloon is inflated to facilitate passage of the catheter from the right atrium into the right ventricle as a result of venous blood flow.	Reduces the risk of atrial tachy-arrhythmias during passage through the right atrium and the risk of trauma to the tricuspid valve leaflets during passage into the right ventricle.[3,5] *(Level II*)*
21. Monitor and record the ECG results while steadily advancing the pacing catheter through the right atrium and into the right ventricle. *(Level II*)*	The catheter may induce ventricular tachycardia.	Changes in the ECG pattern document progress from the vena cava to the right atrium to the right ventricle.[5,7] Echocardiography guidance or fluoroscopy may be used for ventricular lead placement.[3,4]
22. Deflate balloon when pacing catheter is properly positioned. *(Level I*)*	Balloon is no longer necessary when the catheter is advanced into the ventricle.	The catheter is correctly positioned when the electrodes make contact with the ventricular myocardium.
23. Disconnect ECG machine and connect pacing cable to the pacing catheter pins. *(Level I*)*	Electricity travels from the pulse generator to the myocardium via the pacing cable and pacing catheter.	All connections must be secure to ensure proper sensing and capture and to prevent accidental disconnection.[7]
24. Initiating pacing; ensure that capture is obtained and that the settings selected are appropriate.	Presence of capture ensures the pacing catheter is in contact with the myocardium.	If capture is not obtained, the catheter must be repositioned.
25. Secure the pacing catheter in place per institution-specific protocol.	Aids in prevention of accidental dislodgement or catheter migration.	The depth of insertion of the pacing catheter should be noted and documented.
26. Apply sterile dressing. *(Level VI*)*	Prevents infection.	
27. Secure the pacer connecting cable and generator.	Aids in prevention of accidental dislodgement, or disconnection.[5-7]	
28. Obtain 12-lead ECG and chest x-ray results. *(Level VI*)*	Documents paced rhythm and catheter position.[1]	
29. Dispose of the supplies and used equipment appropriately, including sharps.	Standard precautions; reduces transmission of microorganisms. Protects personnel health.	
30. Remove gown, mask, hat, and gloves; wash hands.	Standard precautions.	

* Level I: Manufacturer's recommendations only
  Level II: Theory-based; no research data to support recommendations; recommendations from expert consensus group may exist
  Level VI: Clinical studies in a variety of patient populations and situations to support recommendations

Expected Outcomes	**Unexpected Outcomes**
• Lead placed in the right ventricle	• Inability to position the pacing catheter in the right ventricle
• Electrocardiogram shows capture and ventricular pacing consistent with the pulse generator settings	• Inability to achieve ventricular capture
	• Inappropriate sensing that results in inappropriate pacing
• Chest x-ray shows the pacing catheter in the appropriate position	• Lead is not in the right ventricle
• Pacing results in hemodynamic improvement	• Child's hemodynamic status does not improve or worsens
• Child is free from procedure-related complications	• Pericardial effusion with or without tamponade; result of right ventricular perforation during the procedure
	• Hemothorax or pneumothorax; result of puncture or tear during the procedure
	• Catheter-induced arrhythmias
	• Thrombus formation
	• Bleeding
	• Pulmonary embolism
	• Venous obstruction
	• Lead dislodgement
	• Lead fracture
	• Cellulitis or infection
• Child returns to pre-sedation or pre-anesthesia level of consciousness	• Adverse response to sedation or analgesia
• Child has acceptable level of comfort	• Unmanaged pain

Monitoring and Care of the Child

Activities and Interventions	Rationale	Reportable Conditions
1. Monitor the ECG pattern.	Proper pacemaker function results in an ECG pattern that is consistent with the pulse generator settings.[5] Allows for quick recognition of return of normal cardiac rhythm or cardiac dysrhythmias.[5,6] Changes in ECG pattern may indicate catheter migration.[5,7]	• Inconsistent sensing • Inappropriate sensing • Loss of capture • Competitive pacing • Dysrhythmias
2. Monitor the hemodynamic response to paced rhythm.	Determines achievement of the therapeutic goal, which is improvement in cardiac output.[1,2]	• Poor systemic perfusion as evidenced by cool extremities, poor peripheral pulses, capillary refill of more than 3 seconds, or urine output of less than 1 mL/kg/hr • Hypotension
3. Monitor for signs and symptoms of complications.	Allows for the prompt recognition and treatment of complications to optimize outcomes.[7]	• Signs and symptoms of: tamponade, pulmonary embolism, pneumothorax, hemothorax, infection, or bleeding complications
4. Assess the effectiveness of pain management/analgesia strategy and provide appropriate interventions. Encourage the family to assist with nonpharmacologic means to comfort and support the child.	Ensures that child's comfort level is adequate.[5] Ensures that the activity level is managed to protect pacing catheter position and prevent dislodgement or loss of capture.	• Inability to relieve the child's discomfort • Inappropriate level of consciousness for the degree of medical therapy • Increase in child's activity level, with catheter position at risk

Continued

Monitoring and Care of the Child—Cont'd

Activities and Interventions	Rationale	Reportable Conditions
5. Change the dressing per institution-specific protocol. 6. Ensure the pulse generator settings and all connections are checked every shift.	Reduces the incidence rate of infection.[5] Ensures proper pacing.	• Signs and symptoms of phlebitis, cellulitis, or infection • Problems with the locking mechanism on the pulse generator • Inability to maintain tight connections • Pulse generator settings other than those prescribed

Documentation

- Consent for procedure
- Education of the child and family
- Electrocardiographic strips obtained before, during, and after the procedure
- Lead implantation record, including time and date of initiation of pacing and the pacing catheter and introducer sizes used during the procedure
- Pulse generator settings
- Vital signs and hemodynamics
- Level of consciousness and pain scale rating per institution-specific sedation/analgesia protocol
- Medications given during the procedure and the child's response
- Assessment of the insertion site
- Time and date the pulse generator was placed on standby
- Time and date the pacing catheter was removed
- Unexpected outcomes and related treatment

References

1. Knick BJ, Saul JP: Immediate arrhythmia management. In Zeigler VL, Gillette PC, editors: *Practical management of pediatric cardiac arrhythmias*, Armonk, NY, 2001, Futura Publishing Co, Inc.
2. Craig J, et al: Tissue perfusion. In Curley MAQ, Moloney-Harmon P, editors: *Critical care nursing of infants and children*, ed 2, Philadelphia, 2001, Saunders.
3. Riley D, Bania T: Ultrasound-guided transvenous pacing as an educational tool in emergency medicine, *Acad Emerg Med* 8(5):467, 2001.
4. Aguilera PA, et al: Emergency transvenous cardiac pacing placement using ultrasound guidance, *Ann Emerg Med* 36(3):224-227, 2000.
5. Dahlberg S, Mooradd M: Temporary cardiac pacing. In Irwin R, Rippe J, Curley F, et al, editors: *Procedures and techniques in intensive care medicine*, ed 3, Philadelphia, 2003, Lippincott Williams & Wilkins.
6. Jacobson C, Gerity D: Pacemakers and implantable defibrillators. In Woods S, et al: *Cardiac nursing*, ed 4, Philadelphia, 2000, Lippincott Williams & Wilkins.

7. Betts TR: Regional survey of temporary transvenous pacing procedures and complications, *Postgrad Med J* 79:463-465, 2003.
8. Overbay D, Criddle L: Mastering temporary invasive cardiac pacing, *Crit Care Nurs*. 24(3):25-32, 2004.

Additional Readings

Gregoratos G, et al: ACC/AHA/NASPE 2002 guideline update for implantation of cardiac pacemakers and antiarrhythmia devices: a report of the American College of Cardiology/American Heart Association Task Force on practice guidelines, *J Cardiovasc Electrophysiol* 13(1):1183-1199, 2002.
Hanseus K, et al: Emergency pacing and subsequent permanent pacemaker implantation in a premature infant of 1770 g with a follow-up of 6 years, *Pediatr Cardiol* 21:470-473, 2000.
Pinto N: Temporary transvenous pacing with an active fixation bipolar lead in children: a preliminary report, *PACE* 26:1519-1522, 2003.

Circulatory Assist Devices

PROCEDURE **57**

Intraaortic Balloon Pump: Management

PURPOSE: Intraaortic balloon pump (IABP) therapy is used to increase systemic perfusion, decrease myocardial workload, decrease afterload, and increase coronary artery perfusion

Desiree Fleck

PREREQUISITE KNOWLEDGE

- Anatomy and physiology of the cardiovascular system
- Principles of hemodynamic monitoring, electrophysiology, dysrhythmias, and coagulation
- Clinical and technical competence related to the use of the IABP
- Mastery of pediatric advanced life support competencies
- Principles of aseptic technique
- Appropriate pediatric dosing of analgesics and sedatives
- Child development as it relates to clinical assessment and IABP
- Indications for IABP therapy are as follows[1]:
  - ❖ Cardiogenic shock
  - ❖ Right or left ventricular failure or low cardiac output unresponsive to maximal pharmacologic support
  - ❖ Severe persistent and progressive metabolic acidosis
  - ❖ Preoperative management of congenital heart lesions, such as ventricular septal defects (VSDs), atrioventricular canals, and left-sided heart tumors
  - ❖ Inability to wean from cardiopulmonary bypass
  - ❖ Bridge to cardiac transplantation, ventricular assist device, or total artificial heart
  - ❖ Cardiac injury, including contusion and coronary artery tears
  - ❖ Septic shock
- Contraindications to IABP therapy include:
  - ❖ Weight of less than 2.0 kg[2]
  - ❖ Brain death
  - ❖ Unlikely survival

- ❖ Moderate to severe aortic insufficiency
- ❖ Dissecting aortic aneurysm
- ❖ Patent ductus arteriosus
- ❖ Severe coagulopathy
- Intraaortic balloon pump therapy is an acute short-term therapy for children with reversible left or right ventricular failure or is an adjunct to other therapies for irreversible heart failure. Cardiac assistance with the IABP is performed to improve myocardial oxygen supply and reduce cardiac workload. Intraaortic balloon (IAB) pumping is based on the principles of counterpulsation (Figure 57-1).
  - ❖ The events of the cardiac cycle provide the stimulus for balloon function, and the movement of helium gas between the balloon and the control console gas source produces inflation and deflation of the balloon.
  - ❖ Recognition of the R wave or the QRS complex on the electrocardiogram (ECG) is the most commonly used trigger source. However, recognition may be difficult with severe tachycardia.
  - ❖ Inflation occurs during ventricular diastole and causes an increase in aortic pressure, which displaces blood proximally to the coronary arteries and distally to the rest of the body. The result is an increase in myocardial oxygen supply and subsequent improvement in cardiac output.
  - ❖ Deflation occurs just before ventricular systole or ejection. The pressure decreases within the aortic root and reduces afterload and cardiac workload.
  - ❖ In children and infants, echocardiography may be more helpful in timing because of high heart rates.[3]

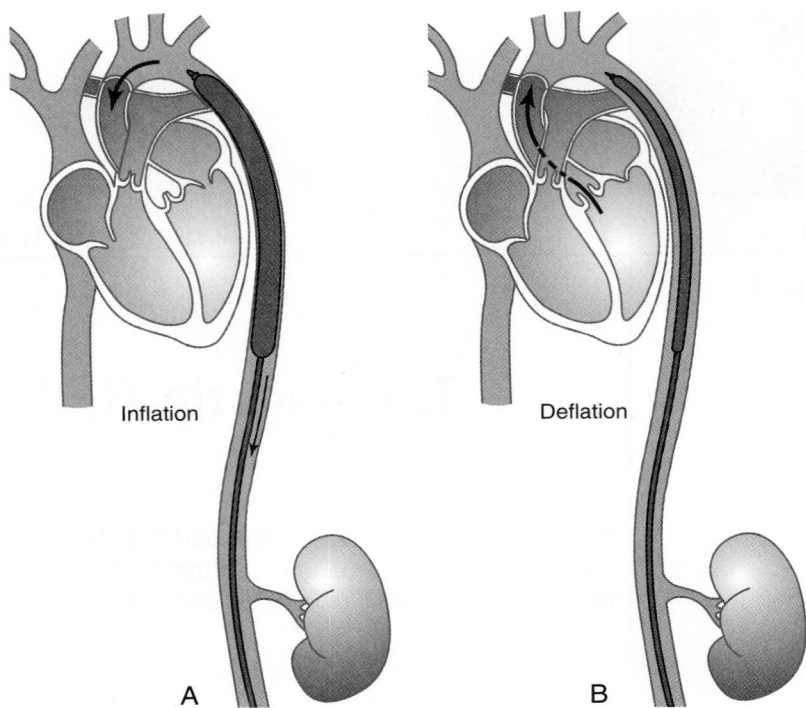

FIGURE 57-1   Principles of Counterpulsation. Intraaortic balloon is inflated in diastole (**A**) and deflated during systole (**B**). *Reproduced with permission from Quaal SJ:* Comprehensive intraaortic balloon pumping, *St. Louis, 1993, Mosby.*

* ❖ Because of the size of the vessels in children, meticulous attention to circulation is essential to decrease complications; IABP is limited.
* Insertion and placement verification proceed as follows:
  * ❖ The IAB catheter is commonly placed in the femoral artery via arteriotomy with a Gortex or Dacron side arm in the operating room.
  * ❖ Placement in adolescents may be done in the cardiac catheterization laboratory.
  * ❖ The IAB catheter lies just below the subclavian artery and superior to the renal arteries. This position allows for maximal balloon effect without occlusion of other arterial supplies (Figure 57-2).
  * ❖ The IAB should not fully occlude the aorta during inflation, but the aorta should be 40% to 60% occluded.
  * ❖ Fluoroscopy may be used to aid in proper IAB catheter positioning, especially for children with a tortuous aorta.
  * ❖ Correct catheter position is verified via radiography if fluoroscopy is not used during catheter insertion.
* Timing methods of IABP therapy vary slightly from manufacturer to manufacturer. With the traditional or conventional method, the IAB deflates before isovolumetric contraction. With the real-time method, the inflation of the IAB extends throughout diastole.[4,8]
* The mechanics of the IABP control console vary from manufacturer to manufacturer.
* Specific information concerning controls, alarms, troubleshooting, and safety features is available from each

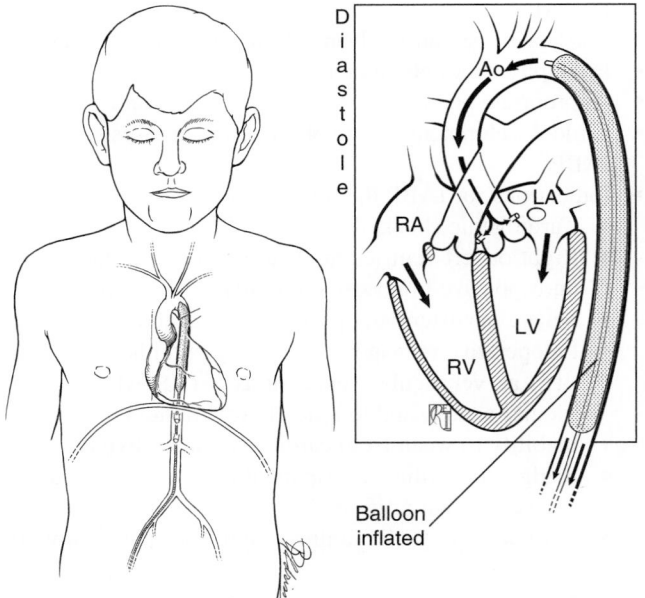

FIGURE 57-2   Correct position of intraaortic balloon pump in aorta just below subclavian artery and above renal arteries. *Reprinted with permission from Jacobs J: Pediatric mechanical circulatory support. In Mavroudis C, Backer CL, editors:* Pediatric cardiac surgery, *Philadelphia, 2003, Mosby.*

manufacturer and should be read thoroughly by the nurse before use of the equipment.

- Removal of the IABP catheter in children and infants occurs in the operating room, with repair of the femoral artery.
- Placement and removal of the IABP catheter requires informed consent.

CHILD AND FAMILY ASSESSMENT

- Child's developmental level and ability to interact ➡*Rationale:* These factors influence preparation of the child and interaction.
- Child's and family's understanding of the reasons for and risks and benefits of the procedure ➡*Rationale:* Evaluates the child's and family's understanding of the procedure and provides a gauge for ongoing education.
- Child's medical history, specifically related to competency of the aortic valve, aortic disease, congenital defects, or peripheral vascular disease ➡*Rationale:* Identifies baseline data regarding cardiac functioning and provides contraindications to IABP therapy.
- Child's cardiovascular, hemodynamic, peripheral vascular, and neurovascular status ➡*Rationale:* Provision of baseline data.
- Assessment of the extremity selected for IABP catheter placement for quality and strength of femoral, popliteal, dorsalis pedis, and posterior tibial pulses ➡*Rationale:* Identifies concerns related to perfusion of the extremity.
- Child's current laboratory profile, including complete blood count (CBC), platelet count, prothrombin time (PT), partial thromboplastin time (PTT), bleeding time, and international normalized ratio (INR) ➡*Rationale:* Baseline coagulation studies are helpful in determination of the risk for bleeding. Platelet function may be affected by the mechanical trauma from balloon inflation and deflation.
- Assessment of signs and symptoms of cardiac failure that necessitate IABP therapy, including the following:
  - ❖ Heart rate greater than 160 bpm
  - ❖ Systolic blood pressure (SBP) less than 70 mm Hg + (2 × age) with vasopressor support in child older than 1 year of age
  - ❖ Cardiac index less than 2.0 despite inotropic support
  - ❖ Central venous pressure (CVP) greater than 18 mm Hg
  - ❖ Pulmonary artery wedge pressure (PAWP) or left atrial pressure (LAP) greater than 18 mm Hg
  - ❖ Decreased mixed venous oxygen saturation
  - ❖ Severe persistent acidosis
  - ❖ Severe hypoxemia
  - ❖ Inadequate peripheral perfusion
  - ❖ Urine output less than 0.5 mL/kg/hr
  - ❖ Assess for thrombocytopenia

  ➡*Rationale:* Physical signs and symptoms result from the heart's inability to adequately contract and from inadequate systemic perfusion.

CHILD AND FAMILY EDUCATION

Individualized, developmentally appropriate education is provided to the family and to the child based on desire for knowledge, readiness to learn, and overall neurologic and psychosocial state.

- Assess the child's and family's understanding of IABP therapy and the reason for its use ➡*Rationale:* Clarification or reinforcement of information is an expressed family need during times of stress and anxiety.
- Explain the standard care to the child and family, including the insertion procedure, IABP sounds, frequency of assessment, alarms, dressings, need for immobility of the affected extremity, expected length of therapy, and parameters for discontinuation of therapy ➡*Rationale:* Information reduces anxiety and facilitates coping and encourages the child and family to ask questions and voice specific concerns about the procedure.
- After catheter removal, instruct the child and family to report any warm or wet feeling on the leg and any dizziness or lightheadedness ➡*Rationale:* These sensations may indicate bleeding at the insertion site.
- Encourage questions and answer questions as they arise ➡*Rationale:* Reinforcement of information is needed during periods of stress and is especially important given the emergent nature of the procedure.

EQUIPMENT

- Intraaortic balloon pump and gas supply
- Electrocardiogram and arterial pressure monitoring supplies
- Intraaortic balloon catheter (size range, 2.5F to 7.0F; a larger size may be considered in teenagers; balloon catheters vary in balloon volumes from 2.5 to 20 mL). Volume should be 40% to 60% of estimated stroke volume (Table 57-1).[1]
- Pediatric safety chamber and tubing
- One sterile cut-down tray, including sterile drape and #10 and #15 blades
- Antiseptic solution
- Caps, goggles, masks, sterile gowns, gloves, and drapes
- Sterile dressing supplies
- 1% lidocaine without epinephrine: one 30-mL vial
- Sterile stopcocks: one two-way and one three-way
- One Luer-lock plug
- One sterile 60-mL syringe (supplied with 20.0-mL balloon)
- One sterile 20-mL syringe (supplied with all balloons except 20.0-mL)
- Two 18-inch (46-cm) lengths of sterile umbilical tape
- One sterile 3-inch (7.6-cm) section of 6-mm or smaller prosthetic graft
- One basin filled with sterile saline solution
- Vascular sutures
- Skin sutures (0-silk)
- Single pressure transducer system

TABLE 57-1	Pediatric IAB Sizing					
Age	Weight	IAB Volume	Catheter Size	Catheter Length	IAB Diameter	IAB Preload
<1 y	3 to 8 kg	2.5 mL	4.5F	10.7 cm	6 mm	6 mL
1 to 2.5 y	8 to 13 kg	5.0 mL	5.5F	12.8 cm	8 mm	10 mL
2.5 to 5 y	13 to 18 kg	7.0 mL	5.5F	14.2 cm	9 mm	12 mL
5 to 12 y	18 to 40 kg	12 mL	7.0F	17.8 cm	10 mm	17 mL
>12 y	>40 kg	20 mL	7.0F	19.4 cm	12 mm	26 mL
Teenagers	Similar to adult height and weight		May consider adult IAB: 25 mL or 34 mL			

Adapted from Veasy LG, Webster HF, McGough EC: Intraaortic balloon pumping, adaptation for pediatric use, *Crit Care Clin* 2:237-249, 1986.

Additional equipment to have available depending on the child's status:

- Analgesics and sedatives per prescribing practitioner's order
- Lead apron (needed if the procedure is performed with fluoroscopy)
- Intravenous (IV) solutions per prescribing practitioner's order
- Emergency medications and resuscitation equipment
- Vasopressors per prescribing practitioner's order
- Antibiotics per prescribing practitioner's order
- Heparin infusion or dextran if prescribed

Procedure   for Assisting with IAB Catheter Insertion

Steps	Rationale	Considerations
1. Ensure child and family understand procedure and questions are answered; reinforce information as needed.	Evaluates and reinforces understanding of previously taught information.	Developmental level, cognitive ability, and anxiety level determine approach to and effectiveness of teaching.
2. Validate that informed consent form has been signed.	Protects the rights of child and family and makes a competent decision possible for the child and family; ensures medical-legal compliance as suggested by the Joint Commission on Accreditation of Healthcare Organizations (JCAHO).	In emergency situations, the organization may have a protocol or procedure in place for assumption of consent.
3. Ensure patency and adequacy of central and peripheral venous access.	Central access is needed for vasopressor administration; peripheral access is acceptable for fluid administration.	
4. Gather needed equipment and supplies.	Facilitates completion of task in a timely manner; facilitates maintenance of a sterile field.	
5. Identify child with appropriate patient and procedure verification process (e.g., "Time out").	Confirms correct patient, procedure, and site as recommended by JCAHO; prevents unnecessary medical procedures.	
6. Place child in a supine position and prepare identified insertion site with an antiseptic solution.	Prepares intended access site and positions child for IAB insertion.	
7. Wash hands and don caps, goggles, masks, sterile gowns, and gloves for all health care personnel involved in the procedure.	Standard precautions; reduces transmission of microorganisms and body secretions and helps to maintain a sterile environment.	

Procedure for Assisting with IAB Catheter Insertion—*Continued*

Steps	Rationale	Considerations
8. Turn on the helium gas. *(Level I*)*	Activates the gas that drives the balloon pump.	Follow the manufacturer's recommendations.
9. Use sedation or anesthesia as needed; the affected extremity may need to be restrained.	Movement of lower extremity may inhibit insertion of the catheter or contribute to catheter kinking once the IAB is in place.	A sheet placed over the affected leg and tucked in or a knee immobilizer may minimize movement of the affected leg. An arm board may be needed in an infant or small child.
10. Establish ECG input to IABP console and obtain an ECG configuration with optimal R wave amplitude and absence of artifact. Indirect ECG input can be obtained via "slave" of the bedside ECG to the IABP console. Follow manufacturer's instructions.	The R wave is preferred trigger signal from which the IABP can reference systole and diastole and therefore establish inflation and deflation points.	A secondary ECG source is desirable in the event of lead disconnection or loss of trigger. Review the manufacturer's instructions for selection of the appropriate trigger control. If the patient has a pacemaker, the trigger should be set to reject the pacemaker artifact. However, the rate may be too high to ensure adequate timing.
11. Assist with placement of hemodynamic monitoring lines if not already present.	Hemodynamic monitoring is necessary for assessment and management of the child who needs IABP therapy.	A radial arterial line is commonly inserted. The arterial line tracing is used to assess and optimize timing and also may be used as a trigger source.
12. Prepare the graft as directed.	Maintains sterility and eases insertion.	
13. Complete IABP console preparation. Refer to instruction manual. Turn off auto fill switch. *(Level I*)*	Ensures adequate functioning of the IABP device.	Pump console models vary; a review of the manufacturer's instructions is recommended.
14. Select most appropriate size of balloon catheter (see Table 57-1).[1,9-11]	Ensures adequate volume to achieve optimal hemodynamic effects from IABP therapy.	Catheters vary in balloon volumes.
15. Remove IAB catheter from the sterile packing and place catheter and insertion tray on a sterile field.	Makes supplies available and maintains sterility.	
16. Administer a heparin bolus as directed, per the prescribing practitioner's order (may not be necessary in postoperative cases).	Anticoagulation therapy may decrease the incidence rate of thromboemboli related to the indwelling IAB catheter.	Systemic anticoagulation therapy may not be used in all patients (especially after cardiac surgery).[12]
17. Attach the supplied one-way valve to the luer tip of the distal end of the balloon lumen.	Creates a device for air removal from the balloon catheter.	Maintains the wrap of the balloon for insertion.
18. Pull back slowly on syringe until all air is aspirated.	Removes air from the balloon, which creates a vacuum.	
19. Disconnect the syringe only.	Prevents air entry back into the balloon.	Leave the one-way valve in place.
20. Lubricate the IAB catheter with sterile saline solution.	Decreases "drag" on the catheter during insertion.	
21. Flush the inner lumen of the IAB catheter with heparinized saline solution before insertion.	Removes air from the central lumen.	If the catheter is not flushed before insertion, allow backflow of arterial blood before connection to the flush system.

Procedure continues on following page

Procedure for Assisting with IAB Catheter Insertion—*Continued*

Steps	Rationale	Considerations
22. The graft is prepared and attached by the surgeon before insertion of the balloon catheter.	Prepares for balloon catheter entry.	
23. Assist with balloon catheter insertion.	Catheter placement is a necessary part of the IAB setup.	Some IABs are inserted without a sheath. If the IAB is inserted via the sheathless method, only the dilator is used.[13]
24. Assist with removal of the one-way valve according to the manufacturer's recommendations. *(Level I*)*	Releases vacuum and readies the balloon for counterpulsation.	
25. Attach pediatric safety chamber.	Ensures safety in pediatric patients.	Balloon male luer attaches to the female luer-lock of the safety chamber. All junctions must be leak free. Refer to the manufacturer's instructions.
26. If the inner lumen of a double-lumen catheter is used to monitor arterial pressure, attach a three-way stopcock with a continuous heparinized flush and transducer to the monitor. Set alarms.	Monitors arterial pressure.	The inner lumen, if used, must be attached to an alarm system because undetected disconnection could result in life-threatening hemorrhage. Refer to institution-specific protocol regarding the use of a heparinized flush system. Note that the proximal tip of the inner-lumen used for arterial pressure monitoring is at the level of the left subclavian artery, *not* at the aortic arch; therefore, this is *not* the same location as a "central" line placed at the aortic root.[8]
27. Attach balloon-lumen tubing to the safety chamber and to the IABP console.	Attachment is necessary because the console programs and operates balloon counterpulsation.	
28. Adjust the console so that safety chamber is lowest point in the balloon catheter.	Prevents collection of condensed water vapor and decreases pull or traction on the IAB catheter.	
29. Preload IAB for filling.	Prevents overfilling of the IAB based on body surface area.	See Table 57-1 for appropriate balloon size and amount. The auto-fill module should not be used. The system must be reconfigured for manual filling.
30. Follow manufacturer's steps for timing, troubleshooting, and patient monitoring. *(Level I*)*	Provides for appropriate operation of counterpulsation.	Many IABP consoles have features for automatic timing. Refer to specific manufacturer instructions.
31. Level the air-fluid interface of the stopcock and zero the hemodynamic monitoring system.[14]	Ensures accurate arterial pressure measurement.	Refer to specific manufacturer's instructions. See Procedure 137 for further information on leveling and zeroing transducer.
32. Obtain a portable chest x-ray as soon as possible.	Correct IAB catheter position must be confirmed to prevent complications associated with the interference of the arterial blood supply.	If fluoroscopy is used for insertion of the catheter, an x-ray immediately after placement is not necessary.

* Level I: Manufacturer's recommendations only

Procedure for Assisting with lAB Catheter Insertion—*Continued*

Steps	Rationale	Considerations
33. Apply a sterile dressing to the catheter insertion site.	Allows for aseptic management.	
34. Discard the used supplies and equipment in the appropriate container.	Standard precautions; reduces transmission of microorganisms.	
35. Remove and discard personal protective equipment; wash hands.	Standard precautions; reduces transmission of microorganisms.	

Procedure for Timing of the lABP

Steps	Rationale	Considerations
1. Select an ECG lead that optimizes the R wave.	The R wave is usually used to trigger the balloon.	An alternate trigger can be used if necessary.
2. Time the IABP with the arterial waveform. *(Level I*)*	The arterial waveform assists in identification of accurate IAB inflation and deflation.	Refer to specific manufacturer's instructions for automatic timing. This may need to be turned off in infants and children because of rapid heart rates.[15] Transthoracic echocardiography has been shown to be useful in timing of IABP in infants and children because of tachycardia.[3]
3. Set the augmentation level low and increase slowly.	Allows the assessment of the optimal level.	
4. Set the IABP frequency to the every-other-beat setting (1:2 or 50%; Figure 57-3)	A comparison can be made between the assisted and unassisted arterial waveforms.	

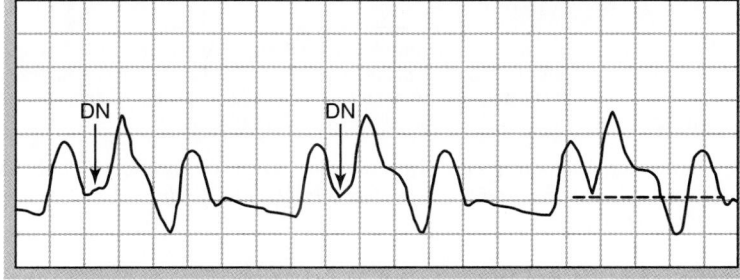

FIGURE 57-3   Intraaortic balloon pump frequency of 1:2. *Reprinted with permission from Quaal SJ: Comprehensive intraaortic balloon pumping, St. Louis, 1993, Mosby.*

5. Inflation		
a. Identify the dicrotic notch of the assisted systolic waveform (see Figure 57-3).	The dicrotic notch represents closure of aortic valve.	
b. Adjust the inflation later to expose the dicrotic notch of the unassisted systolic waveform.	Identifies the landmark for accurate inflation.	

Procedure continues on following page

* Level I: Manufacturer's recommendations only

Procedure | for Timing of the lABP—*Continued*

Steps	Rationale	Considerations
c. Slowly adjust the inflation earlier until the dicrotic notch disappears and a sharp V wave forms (see Figure 57-3).	Balloon augmentation should occur after the aortic valve closes.[16]	A sharp V wave may not be seen in children with low systemic vascular resistance.
d. Compare the augmented pressure with the child's unassisted systolic pressure.	Balloon augmentation should be equal to or greater than the child's unassisted systolic blood pressure. Look for an optimal decrease in presystolic pressure and the greatest decrease in peak systolic pressure.[15]	If balloon augmentation is less than the child's systolic pressure, consider that the balloon is positioned too low, that the child is hypovolemic or tachycardic, or that the balloon volume is set too low.[17]
e. Adjust inflation if needed.	Necessary to achieve optimal diastolic augmentation.	The timing of inflation varies slightly depending on the location of the arterial line. *Radial:* Inflate 40 to 50 ms before the dicrotic notch. *Femoral:* Inflate 120 ms before the dicrotic notch (Figure 57-4). Because of the distance[16] of the radial and femoral arteries from the actual closure of the aortic valve, the arterial waveforms are delayed.[18]

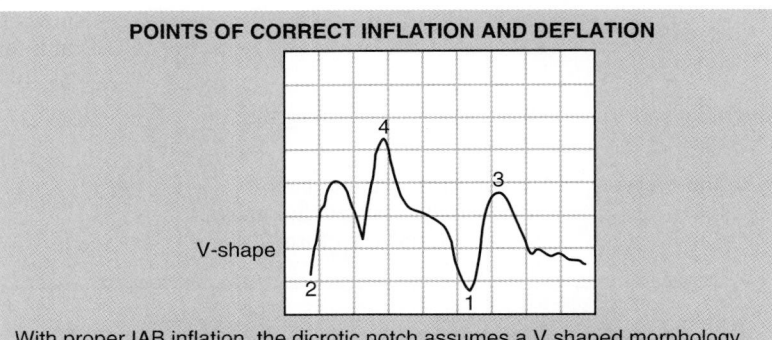

POINTS OF CORRECT INFLATION AND DEFLATION

V-shape

With proper IAB inflation, the dicrotic notch assumes a V shaped morphology. With proper deflation, BAEDP (1) is lower than UAEDP (2) and assisted systole (3) is lower, or at least equal to, unassisted systole (2). Balloon inflation raises diastolic pressure (4).

FIGURE 57-4 Intraaortic balloon pump with dicrotic notch of assisted systolic waveform. *Quaal SJ: Conventional timing using the arterial pressure waveform. In Quaal SJ, editor:* Comprehensive intraaortic balloon pumping, *St. Louis, 1993, Mosby.*

Steps	Rationale	Considerations
6. Deflation		
a. Identify the assisted and unassisted aortic end-diastolic pressures and the assisted and unassisted systolic pressures (see Figure 57-3).[6]	These landmarks are important in determination of accurate IAB deflation.	The IABP frequency is set at 1:2 (50%).
b. Set the balloon to deflate so that the balloon-assisted aortic end-diastolic pressure is as low as possible (lower than the child's unassisted diastolic pressure) while still maintaining optimal diastolic augmentation and not impeding on the next systole (the assisted systole).	The assisted systolic pressure is less than the unassisted systolic pressure as a result of a decrease in afterload, which thus reduces the myocardial workload.[19]	Reduction of afterload decreases energy needed by the heart during systole. Afterload reduction is important to achieve without diminishment of diastolic augmentation.

Procedure | **for Timing of the lABP**—*Continued*

Steps	Rationale	Considerations
7. Set the IABP frequency to 1:1 (100%; Figure 57-5).	Ensures that each heartbeat is assisted.	

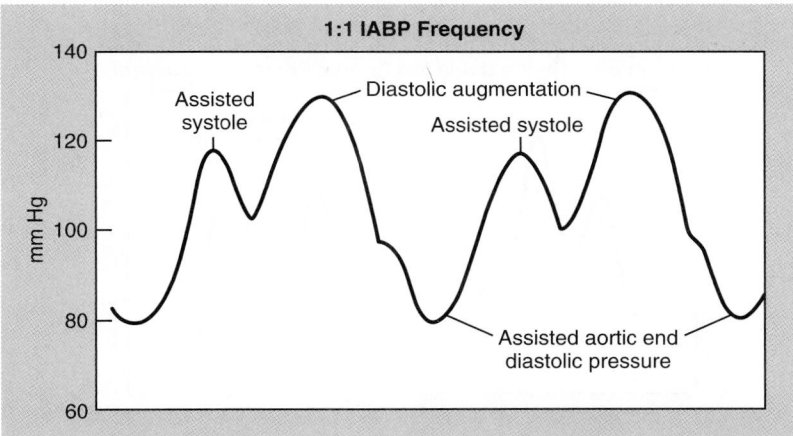

FIGURE 57-5   Intraaortic balloon pump timing of 1:1. *From* Seminar in Intraaortic Balloon Pumping, *Montvale, NJ, Datascope Corp.*

8. Assess timing every hour and whenever the heart rate changes by more than 10 bpm or the rhythm changes. *(Level I*)*	Inappropriate timing prevents effective IABP therapy.	The computerized IABPs vary in the degree of adjustment to changes in heart rate and rhythm. Refer to the specific manufacturer's guidelines for automatic timing adjustment, which may be difficult because of placement of IABP and arterial lines.
9. Assess and intervene to correct inappropriate timing.	Ensures accurate timing and optimal functioning of the IABP.	Assess for decreased heart rate and improvements in the child's condition (i.e., urine output, mixed venous oxygenation, peripheral pulses, and capillary refill).[11,20,21]
a. Problem: Early inflation (Figure 57-6). Intervention: Move inflation later.	Inflation occurs before closure of the aortic valve, leading to premature aortic valve closure, increased left ventricular volume, and decreased stroke volume.	

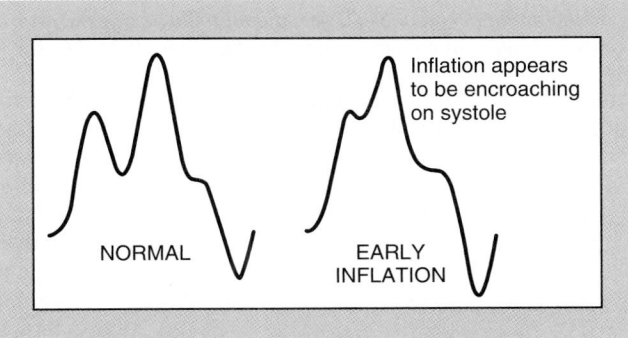

FIGURE 57-6   Early inflation. *From Quaal SJ: Conventional timing using the arterial pressure waveform. In Quaal SJ, editor:* Comprehensive intraaortic balloon pumping, *St. Louis, 1993, Mosby.*

Procedure continues on following page

Procedure for Timing of the lABP—*Continued*

Steps	Rationale	Considerations

b. Problem: Late inflation (Figure 57-7). Intervention: Adjust inflation earlier.

A delay in inflation leads to a decrease in coronary artery perfusion.

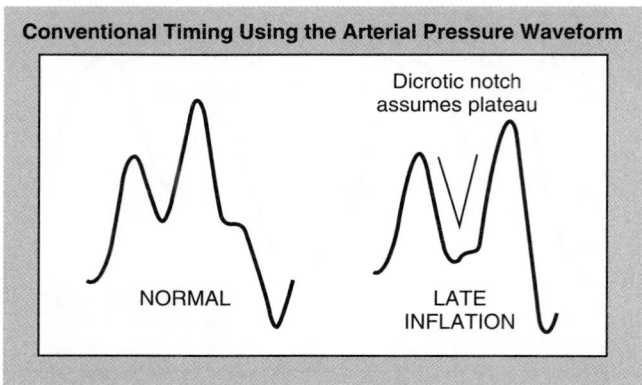

FIGURE 57-7   Late inflation. *From Quaal SJ: Conventional timing using the arterial pressure waveform. In Quaal SJ, editor: Comprehensive intraaortic balloon pumping, St. Louis, 1993, Mosby.*

c. Problem: Early deflation (Figure 57-8). Intervention: Adjust deflation later.

Deflation occurs before the aortic valve opens, which leads to decreased balloon augmentation and less or no afterload reduction; coronary artery perfusion may also be decreased.

Note the sharp diastolic wave after augmentation and the increase in the assisted systolic pressure.

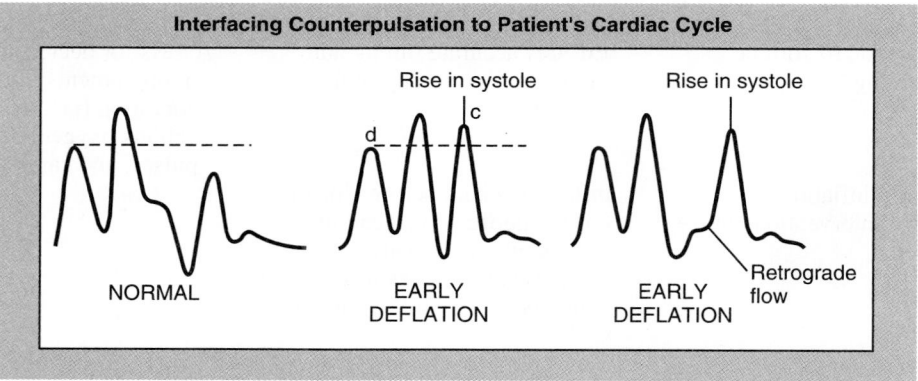

FIGURE 57-8   Early deflation. *From Quaal SJ: Conventional timing using the arterial pressure waveform. In Quaal SJ, editor: Comprehensive intraaortic balloon pumping, St. Louis, 1993, Mosby.*

d. Problem: Late deflation (Figure 57-9). Intervention: Adjust deflation earlier.

Deflation occurs after the aortic valve has opened, which leads to an increase in the aortic end-diastolic pressure and an increase in afterload.

Note the delayed diastolic wave after augmentation and the diminished assisted systole.
If the real-time method of timing is used, late deflation is not identified with changes in the aortic end-diastolic pressure but is identified with a diminished assisted systolic pressure, an increase in heart rate, an increase in filling pressures, and a decrease in cardiac output and cardiac index.[4-6,13,22]

Procedure for Timing of the lABP—*Continued*

Steps	Rationale	Considerations

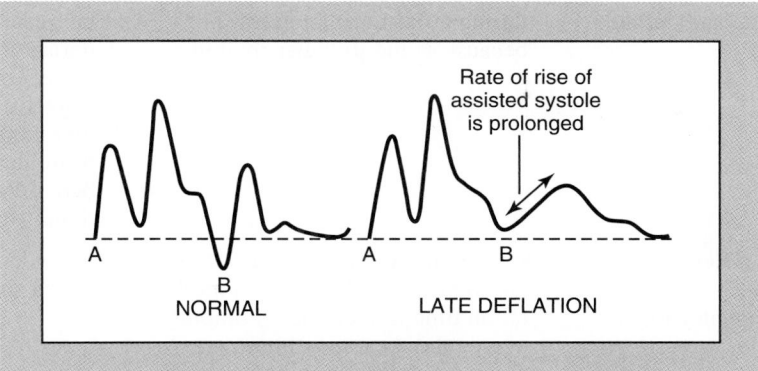

FIGURE 57-9 Late deflation. *From Quaal SJ: Conventional timing using the arterial pressure waveform. In Quaal SJ, editor:* Comprehensive intraaortic balloon pumping, *St. Louis, 1993, Mosby.*

Procedure for Preloading/Filling IAB

Steps	Rationale	Considerations
1. Remove adult safety disk and install the pediatric adapter.	Allows pediatric pumping.	
2. Attach a three-way stopcock and the supplied syringe to side port luer fitting of the safety chamber.	Needed to fill and preload the IAB.	
3. Press the IAB fill key and hold until "manual fill IAB" message appears on the screen.	Allows for filling of gas for operation of the IAB.	
4. Open the stopcock and withdraw the contents of the safety chamber until a strong resistance is felt.	Ensures adequate pumping of the IAB.	
5. Close the stopcock to the safety chamber.	The chamber should be empty.	
6. Attach the filled syringe to the safety chamber and open the stopcock between the syringe and the safety chamber.	Allows for filling of gas.	
7. Press the IAB fill key for 1 second. *(Level I*)*	Contents are pulled into the safety chamber.	Do not inject the gas into the safety chamber.
8. Close the stopcock off to safety chamber.	Ensures the adequate volume of IAB to work appropriately.	
9. Press assist/standby key to initiate pumping.	Initiates pumping.	

* Level I: Manufacturer's recommendations only

Procedure for Troubleshooting

Steps	Rationale	Considerations
1. Atrial fibrillation Set the IABP to inflate and deflate most of child's beats.	IABP therapy is not 100% effective during atrial fibrillation (AF) because of the irregular rhythm.	The underlying cause of AF should be treated. IABPs automatically deflate the balloon on the R wave. Use the atrial fibrillation trigger mode or the R wave deflation mode. The real-time method of timing may track dysrhythmias better than traditional or conventional IABP timing.[4,6]
2. Tachycardia (heart rate [HR], >160 bpm) Change the IABP frequency to 1:2.[15]	Because diastole is shortened during tachycardia, the balloon augmentation time is shortened. Pumping every other beat may improve mean arterial pressure (MAP).	The underlying cause of the tachycardia should be treated.
3. Asystole a. Switch the trigger to arterial pressure.	This trigger can be used with at least a 15–mm Hg rise in arterial pressure.	Refer to manufacturer's manual for this information because the minimal value of millimeters of mercury needed to use this feature varies.
b. Set inflation to provide diastolic augmentation and set deflation to occur before upstroke of the next systole. *(Level IV*)*	Programs the machine for appropriate preset timing.	Preliminary research suggests that when used during cardiopulmonary resuscitation, IAB counterpulsation increases cerebral and coronary perfusion.[19]
c. If chest compressions do not provide an adequate trigger: • Turn to the internal trigger. • Set the rate at 60 to 80 bpm. Set the IABP frequency to 1:2. Turn the balloon augmentation down to 50%.	The internal trigger keeps the IAB catheter moving so that clot formation is minimized. Maintains consistent movement of the IAB catheter. The 1:2 frequency is adequate to prevent thrombus formation on the IAB catheter. Slight inflation and deflation of the IAB catheter prevents clot formation.	
4. Ventricular tachycardia or ventricular fibrillation a. Ensure personnel are cleared from the child and equipment before cardioversion or defibrillation.	Prevents spread of energy to health care personnel; maintains electrical safety.	
b. Use cardioversion or defibrillation as necessary; see Procedures 45 and 46.	Converts rhythm.	The IABP console is electrically isolated.
5. Loss of vacuum or IABP failure a. Check and tighten connections on pneumatic tubing.	A loose connection may contribute to a loss of vacuum.	
b. Check the compressor power source.	Ensures that power is available to drive the helium.	
c. Hand inflate and deflate the balloon every 5 minutes with half the total balloon volume if necessary.	Prevents clot formation along the dormant balloon.	

* Level IV: Limited clinical studies to support recommendations

Procedure for Troubleshooting—*Continued*

Steps	Rationale	Considerations
d. Reload the system.	The amount of preload decreases during normal operation.	Follow the preload operation according to the manufacturer's instructions.
e. Change the IAB console.	Establishes a power source and effective IABP therapy.	
6. Suspected balloon perforation a. Observe for loss of augmentation.	Gas may be gradually leaking from the balloon catheter.	Always set the alarms so the alarm sounds with a 10–mm Hg drop in diastolic augmentation.
b. Check for blood in catheter tubing.	Blood in the tubing indicates that the balloon has perforated and that arterial blood is present.	A balloon leak can be self-sealing as a result of surface tension between the inside and outside of the IAB membrane. Self-sealing may be evidenced by the presence of dried blood in the catheter tubing. The dried blood may appear as a brownish coffee-ground–like substance.
c. Assess for changes or lack of normal balloon pressure waveform.	The balloon pressure waveform may be absent if the balloon is unable to retain gas, or the pressure plateau may gradually decrease if the IAB is leaking gas.	
7. Balloon perforation a. Place the IABP on standby mode.	Prevents further IAB pumping and continued gas exchange.	Some IABP consoles automatically shut off if a leak is detected. The IAB catheter should be removed within 15 to 30 minutes.
b. Clamp IAB catheter.	Prevents arterial blood back up.	
c. Disconnect IAB catheter from the IABP console.	Prevents blood from backing up into the IABP console.	
d. Notify prescribing practitioner.	The IAB catheter needs to be removed or replaced immediately.	An IAB leak that has sealed itself off may result in entrapment of the IAB in the vasculature. Surgical removal may be necessary.
e. Prepare for IAB catheter removal or replacement.	The IAB catheter should not lie dormant for longer than 30 minutes.	Removal is generally done in the operating room.
f. Discontinue anticoagulation therapy.	Clotting occurs more readily if anticoagulation therapy is stopped (necessary with removal of the catheter)	

Procedure for Weaning and IAB Catheter Removal

Steps	Rationale	Considerations
1. Wash hands; put on gloves and protective eyewear as appropriate.	Standard precautions; reduces transmission of microorganisms and body secretions.	
2. Assess clinical readiness for weaning.	Optimal clinical and hemodynamic parameters validate readiness for weaning.	The child's hemodynamic status should be optimal before weaning of IABP therapy. Signs of clinical readiness include the following: heart rate less than 140 bpm, SBP greater than 70 mm Hg with minimal or no vasopressor support, PAWP less than 18 mm Hg, CVP less than 12 mm Hg, cardiac index greater than 2.4, mixed venous oxygen saturation between 60% and 80%, capillary refill less than 2 seconds, and urine output greater than 0.5 mL/kg/hr.
3. Change the assist ratio to 1:2 (50%) and monitor the child's response for 1 to 6 hours or as noted per institution-specific protocol.	Length of time necessary to wean from IABP therapy depends on the hemodynamic response of the patient and the length of time the patient has undergone IABP therapy.[23,24]	
4. If hemodynamic parameters remain satisfactory, further change the ratio from 1:3 to 1:8 (depending on the child and the balloon console assist frequencies, or as prescribed).	IABP consoles vary in assist ratios.	Refer to institution-specific protocol on weaning procedures.
5. Discontinue heparin or dextran administration 4 to 6 hours before IAB catheter removal or reverse heparin administration with protamine as prescribed just before catheter removal.	Discontinuation decreases the likelihood of bleeding after balloon removal.	
6. Turn the IABP to standby or off mode.	Ensures deflation of the IAB catheter.	
7. Assist prescribing practitioner with removal of the percutaneous balloon.	Facilitates removal.	
8. Disconnect IAB from safety chamber. Pull a vacuum on the IAB with the syringe and the three-way stopcock. The snares are removed from the graft.		Ensure that hemostasis is obtained.
9. Assess the insertion site for signs of bleeding or hematoma formation before application of a sterile pressure dressing.	Assists in the detection of bleeding.	
10. Apply a pressure dressing to the insertion site for 2 to 4 hours.	Minimizes bleeding from the insertion site.	
11. Monitor vital signs and hemodynamic parameters every 15 minutes for four times, every 30 minutes for two times, and then every hour as the child's condition warrants.	Validates stability or identifies hemodynamic compromise.	

Procedure for Weaning and IAB Catheter Removal—*Continued*

Steps	Rationale	Considerations
12. Assess the quality of perfusion to the decannulated extremity immediately after removal and every hour for two times, then every 2 hours.	Removal of the IAB catheter may dislodge thrombi on the catheter and lead to arterial occlusion.	
13. Maintain immobility of decannulated extremity and bedrest with the head of the bed no greater than 30 degrees for 8 hours.	Promotes healing and decreases stress at the insertion site.	
14. Discard the used supplies and equipment in the appropriate receptacle; remove personal protective equipment and wash hands.	Standard precautions; reduces transmission of microorganisms and body secretions.	

Expected Outcomes

- Increased myocardial oxygen supply

- Decreased myocardial oxygen demands
- Increased cardiac output
- Increased tissue perfusion, including cerebral, renal, and peripheral circulation
- Appropriate IABP placement
- Child has acceptable level of comfort
- Coagulation status remains within normal limits
- Balloon remains intact
- Child remains free from infection
- Aorta remains free from injury
- Extremity in which the IAB is inserted remains warm and well perfused

Unexpected Outcomes

- No improvement in myocardial oxygen supply
- Cardiac arrhythmias
- Persistent elevated myocardial oxygen demands
- Difficulty with timing IABP
- Impaired perfusion to mesenteric, renal, cerebral, or peripheral circulation
- Inappropriate IAB placement
- Unmanaged pain
- Bleeding or coagulation disorders
- Balloon perforation
- Local or systemic infection
- Aortic dissection
- Impaired circulation to extremity in which the IAB is inserted

Monitoring and Care of the Child

Activities and Interventions	Rationale	Reportable Conditions
1. Perform systematic cardiovascular, peripheral vascular, and hemodynamic assessments every 15 to 60 minutes as the child's status necessitates.		
2. Level of consciousness (note: the child may be sedated or paralyzed during IABP therapy).	Assesses for adequate cerebral perfusion; thrombi may develop and dislodge during IABP therapy or the IAB may migrate, decreasing blood flow to the carotid arteries.	• Deterioration in level of consciousness
3. Vital signs, central venous pressures, and left atrial pressures.	Shows the effectiveness of IABP therapy.	• Unstable vital signs and significant changes in hemodynamic pressures • Lack of response to IABP therapy
4. Arterial catheter and IAB waveforms.	Ensures the effectiveness of IABP timing and therapy	• Difficulty in achieving effective IABP therapy
5. Cardiac output, cardiac index, and systemic vascular resistance determinations if pulmonary artery catheter is present.	Shows the effectiveness of IABP therapy.	• Abnormal cardiac output, cardiac index, and systemic vascular resistance values

Continued

Monitoring and Care of the Child—Cont'd

Activities and Interventions	Rationale	Reportable Conditions
6. Circulation to extremities, including pulses, limb temperature, color, and capillary refill. Circulation to abdominal arteries.	Validates adequate peripheral perfusion. If reportable conditions are found, they may indicate catheter or embolus obstruction of perfusion to the extremity. Specifically, decreased perfusion to the left arm may indicate misplacement of the IAB catheter.[18]	• Capillary refill greater than 2 seconds • Diminished or absent pulses (e.g., antecubital, radial, popliteal, tibial, pedal) • Color pale, mottled, or cyanotic • Diminished or absent sensation • Pain in extremities or abdomen • Diminished or absent movement • Extremities cool or cold to touch • Abdominal distention • Diarrhea
7. Urine output.	Validates adequate perfusion to the kidneys.	• Urine output of less than 0.5 mL/kg/h
8. Assess heart and lung sounds every 4 hours and as needed.	Abnormal heart and lung sounds may indicate the need for additional treatment. ***Special note:*** When the child's condition permits, place the IABP on standby mode to accurately auscultate heart and lung sounds because IABP therapy creates extraneous sounds and impairs heart and lung sound assessment.	• Abnormal heart and lung sounds
9. Maintain the head of the bed flat; the bed may be tilted.	Prevents kinking of the IAB catheter and migration of the catheter.	• Because of the child's size, flexion of the affected hip must be avoided.[19]
10. Monitor for signs of inappropriate IAB placement.	The IAB catheter may be positioned too high or too low, thus occluding the left subclavian, celiac, inferior or superior mesenteric, or renal arteries.	• Diminished or absent antecubital or radial pulse • Color of left arm pale, mottled, or cyanotic • Diminished or absent sensation to the left arm • Dampened radial arterial pressure waveform • Diminished or absent movement of the left arm • Diminished or absent bowel sounds • Increased abdominal girth • Abdomen firm to touch • Tympany • Abdominal pain • Decreased urine output, less than 0.5 mL/kg/hr • Increased urine osmolality • Increased blood urea nitrogen or creatinine levels • Reduced IABP augmentation
11. Monitor for signs of balloon perforation.	In the event of balloon perforation, a small amount of helium is released into the aorta, potentially causing an embolic event.	• Blood or brown flecks in tubing • Loss of IABP augmentation • Control console alarm activation (e.g., gas loss)
12. Maintain accurate IABP timing.	If timing is not accurate, cardiac output may decrease rather than increase.	• Inability to time IABP or maintain IABP timing
13. Refill the IAB every 45 to 60 minutes.	If the IAB is not filled appropriately, cardiac output may decrease.	• Inability to refill IAB

Monitoring and Care of the Child—Cont'd

Activities and Interventions	Rationale	Reportable Conditions
14. Log roll child every 2 hours. Prop pillows to support the child and to maintain alignment. Consider the use of pressure-relief devices. *(Level V[*])*	Promotes comfort and skin integrity and prevents kinking of the IAB catheter. ***Special note:*** Logrolling may not be tolerated in children with severe hemodynamic compromise; low-pressure beds are necessary for these children and can decrease the occurrence of pressure ulcers in children who need IABP therapy.[4,24]	• Skin breakdown or altered skin integrity
15. Immobilize the cannulated extremity with a draw sheet tucked under the mattress or with a soft ankle restraint, a knee immobilizer, or IV arm board.	Prevents dislodgment and migration of the IAB catheter. ***Special note:*** Assess skin integrity and perfusion distal to the immobilization device every hour.	• Dislodgement or migration of IAB catheter
16. Initiate passive and active range-of-motion exercises every 2 hours to extremities that can be mobilized.	Prevents venous stasis and muscle atrophy.	• Decrease in range of motion
17. Assess the area around the IAB catheter insertion site every 2 hours and as needed for evidence of hematoma or bleeding.	The IAB catheter inflation and deflation traumatizes red blood cells and platelets. Anticoagulation therapy may alter hemoglobin, hematocrit, and coagulation values.[12]	• Bleeding at insertion site • Hematoma at insertion site
18. Provide psychologic support to the family and child. Reassure the child constantly and provide explanations frequently.[1,11]	Children are frequently intubated, sedated, and paralyzed but may be fully aware of what is occurring.	• Unmanaged agitation
19. Maintain anticoagulation therapy as prescribed and monitor coagulation study results.	Prophylactic anticoagulation therapy may be used to prevent thrombi and emboli development.	• Abnormal coagulation studies
20. Monitor child for systemic evidence of bleeding or coagulation disorders.	Hematologic and coagulation profiles may be altered as a result of blood loss during balloon insertion, as a result of anticoagulation therapy, and as a result of platelet dysfunction from mechanical trauma by balloon inflation and deflation.[12]	• Bleeding from IAB insertion site • Bleeding from incisions or mucous membranes • Petechiae or ecchymoses • Guiac-positive nasogastric aspirate or stool • Hematuria • Decreased hemoglobin or hematocrit • Decreased filling pressures • Increased heart rate • Retroperitoneal hematoma • Pain in the lower abdomen, flank, thigh, or lower extremity
21. Change the IAB catheter site dressing every 24 hours. Cleanse the site with normal saline solution. Cleanse the site with an antiseptic solution.	Decreases the incidence rate of infection and allows an opportunity for site assessment.	• Signs or symptoms of infection

[*] Level V: Clinical studies in more than one or two patient populations and situations to support recommendations

Continued

Monitoring and Care of the Child—Cont'd

Activities and Interventions	Rationale	Reportable Conditions
Allow time for the antiseptic solution to dry. Apply a sterile dressing and label with the date, time, and nurse's initials.		
22. Assess for balloon entrapment.[26-28]	Entrapment is the inability to remove the IAB because of the presence of a large hardened mass of blood within the IAB. As a result, the IAB is entrapped somewhere in the aortoiliac system or possibly in the abdominal aorta. A pinhole leak or tear in the IAB allows blood to be sucked into the IAB, and a clot forms. Blood dries and becomes dehydrated because of the repeated passage of helium through the IAB.	• Flecks of blood within the catheter or bright red blood
23. Assess for balloon migration.	The IAB should be positioned just below the left subclavian artery just above the renal arteries. If the IAB migrates proximally, it may occlude the subclavian or carotid artery. If the IAB migrates too low, it could occlude the renal or mesenteric arteries.	• Signs of possible subclavian artery occlusion: unequal or absent radial pulse and dampening or loss of the arterial pressure waveform in the ipsilateral radial artery • Signs of possible carotid artery occlusion: change in level of consciousness and orientation or unilateral neurologic deficit • Signs of renal artery occlusion: oliguria or anuria, hematuria, back or flank pain, nausea, and anorexia • Signs of mesenteric occlusion: abdominal pain, diarrhea, nausea, and decreased bowel sounds
24. Monitor for parameters that show clinical readiness to wean from IABP therapy.	Close observation of the child's tolerance to weaning procedures is necessary to ensure that the body's oxygen demands can be met. The presence of these reportable conditions indicates that consideration should be given to weaning the child from the IABP.	• Good peripheral pulses • Heart rate less than 150 bpm • Absence of lethal or unstable dysrhythmias • A SBP greater than 70 mm Hg with little or no vasopressor support • A LAP less than 18 mm Hg • A CVP less than 12 mm Hg • Cardiac index greater than 2.4 • Mixed venous O_2 between 60% and 80% • Capillary refill less than 3 seconds • Urine output greater than 0.5 mL/kg/h

---

Documentation

- Child and family education
- Site, procedure, and patient verification process
- Insertion site assessment
- Insertion of the IAB catheter (including size of catheter used and balloon volume and fill volume)
- Hemodynamic status
- Peripheral pulses and neurovascular assessment of the affected extremity
- The IABP pressures (unassisted end-diastolic pressure, unassisted systolic pressure, balloon augmented pressure, assisted systolic pressure, assisted end-diastolic pressure, and MAP)
- Any difficulties with insertion
- The IABP frequency
- Child's response to the procedure and to IABP therapy
- Confirmation of placement of the IAB (e.g., chest x-ray results)
- Comfort assessment and any specific interventions provided
- Unexpected outcomes and related treatment

References

1. Veasy LG, Webster HF, McGough EC: Intra-aortic balloon pumping; adaptation for pediatric use, *Crit Care Clin* 2:237-249, 1986.
2. del Nido PJ, Swan PR, Benson LN, et al: Successful use of intraaortic balloon pumping in a 2-kilogram infant, *Ann Thorac Surg* 46:574-576, 1998.
3. Minich L, Tani LY, McGough EC, et al: A novel approach to pediatric intraaortic balloon pump timing using M-Mode echocardiography, *Am J Cardiol* 80(3):367-369, 1998.
4. Cadwell CA, Tyson G: Real timing. In Quaal SJ, editor: *Comprehensive intraaortic balloon counterpulsation,* ed 2, St. Louis, 1993, Mosby Yearbook.
5. Cadwell CA, Hobson KS, Petis S, et al: Clinical observations with real timing, *Crit Care Nurs Clin North Am* 8(4):357-370, 1996.
6. Joseph DL, Spadoni SM: Timing waveform analysis, *Crit Care Nurs Clin North Am* 8(4):349-356, 1996.
7. Quaal SJ: Caring for the intra-aortic balloon pump patient: most frequently asked questions, *Crit Care Nurs Clin North Am* 8:471-476, 1996.
8. Quaal SJ: Intra-aortic balloon pumping timing: an overview, *Critical Care Int* January-February:12-14, 1997.
9. Booker PD: Intra-aortic balloon pumping in young children, *Paediatr Anaest* 7:501-507, 1997.
10. Pinkney KA, Minich L, Tani LY, et al: Current results with intraaortic balloon pumping in infants and children, *Ann Thorac Surg* 73:887-891, 2002.
11. Webster JF, Veasy LG: Intra-aortic balloon pumping in children, *Heart Lung J Crit Care* 14:548-555, 1985.
12. Vanderheide RH, Thadhani R, Kufer DJ: Association of thrombocytopenia with the use of intra-aortic balloon pumps, *Am J Med* 105:27-32, 1998.
13. Diver D: Sheathless balloon insertion. In Quaal SJ, editor: *Comprehensive intraaortic balloon counterpulsation,* ed 2, St. Louis, 1993, Mosby Yearbook.
14. Quaal SJ: Interactive hemodynamics of IABC. In Quaal SJ, editor: *Comprehensive intraaortic balloon counterpulsation,* ed 2, St. Louis, 1993, Mosby Yearbook.
15. Wojner AW: Assessing the five points of the intra-aortic balloon pump waveform, *Crit Care Nurs* 14:45-52, 1994.
16. Quaal SJ: Conventional timing using the arterial pressure waveform. In Quaal SJ, editor: *Comprehensive intra-aortic balloon counterpulsation,* ed 2, St. Louis, 1993, Mosby Yearbook.
17. Pantalos GM, Minich LL, Tani LY, et al: Estimation of timing errors for intra-aortic balloon pump use in pediatric patients, *ASIA OJ* 45:166-171, 1999.
18. Quaal SJ: Interpreting the arterial pressure waveform in the intra-aortic balloon pumped patient, *Prog Cardiovas Nurs* 15:116-118, 2001.
19. Anella J, McCloskey A, Vieweg C: Nursing dynamics of pediatric intraaortic balloon pumping, *Crit Care Nurs* 10(4):24-37, 1995.
20. Geiger J, Hall T, Breeze E, et al: Intra-aortic balloon pumps in children: a small-nursing-team approach, *Crit Care Nurs* 17(3):79-86, 1997.
21. Anonymus: Intra-aortic balloon pumps, *Health Devices* 26(5):184-216, 1997.
22. Arafa OE, Pedersen TH, Svennebig JL, et al: Vascular complications of the intra-aortic balloon pump in patients undergoing open-heart operations: 15 year experience, *Ann Thoracic Surg* 67:645-651, 1999.
23. Hanlon-Pena PM, Ziegler JC, Stewart R: Management of the intra-aortic balloon pump patient, *Crit Care Nurs Clin North Am* 8:389-408, 1996.
24. Sitzer VA, Atkins PJ: Developing and implementing a standard of care for intra-aortic balloon counterpulsation, *Crit Care Nurs Clin North Am* 8(4):451-457, 1996.
25. Brodie BR, Stuckey TD, Hansen C, et al: Intra-aortic balloon counterpulsation before primary percutaneous transluminal coronary angioplasty reduces catheterization laboratory events in high-risk patients with acute myocardial infarction, *Am J Cardiol* 84:18-23, 1999.
26. Chaus N, Babounashvilli A, Doundoua D, et al: *Intra-aortic balloon counterpulsation in high risk coronary angioplasty,* Athens, Greece, 2000, presented at 1st World Conference on Intra-aortic Balloon Counterpulsation.
27. Stavarski DH: Complications of intra-aortic balloon pumping: preventable or not preventable? *Crit Care Nurs Clin North Am* 8(4):409-421, 1996.
28. Spadoni S: Preoperative intra-aortic balloon counterpulsation in high-risk coronary patients, *Can Perfusion Canadienne* 10:30-33, 2000.

Additional Readings
Akomea-Agyin C, Kejriwal NK, Franks R, et al: Intraaortic balloon pumping in children, *Ann Thorac Surg* 67:1415-1420, 1999.

Anderson RD, Ohman EM, Holmes DR Jr, et al: Use of intra-aortic balloon counterpulsation in patients presenting with cardiogenic shock: observations from the GUSTO-I study, *J Am Coll Cardiol* 30:708-715, 1997.

Arafa OE, Geiran OR, Anderson K, et al: Intra-aortic balloon pumping for predominantly right ventricular failure after heart transplantation, *Ann Thorac Surg* 70:1587-1593, 2000.

Bates ER, Stomel RJ, Hochman JS, et al: The use of intra-aortic balloon counterpulsation as an adjunct to reperfusion therapy in cardiogenic shock, *J Cardiol* 65(suppl 1):S37-S42, 1998.

Blusch T, Sirbu H, Zenker D, et al: Vascular complications related to intra-aortic balloon conterpulsation: an analysis of ten years experience, *Thoracic Cardiovasc Surg* 45:55-59, 1997.

Castelli P, Condemi A, Munsari M, et al: Intra-aortic balloon counterpulsation outcome in cardiac surgical patients, *J Cardiovasc Vasc Anesth* 15:700-703, 2001.

Cook L, Pillar B, McCord G, et al: Intra-aortic balloon pump complications: a five-year retrospective study of 283 patients, *Heart Lung* 28:195-202, 1999.

Flewelling-Goran: Vascular complications of the patient undergoing intra-aortic balloon pumping, *Crit Care Nurs Clin North Am* 459:459-468, 1989.

Garrett K, Grady KL: Intra-aortic balloon pumping through the common iliac artery: management of the ambulatory intra-aortic balloon pump patient, *Prog Cardiovasc Nurs* 15:14-20, 2000.

Hazinski MF: Cardiovascular disorders. In Hazinski MF, editor: *Manual of pediatric critical care*, St. Louis, 1999, Mosby.

Jacobs J: Pediatric cardiac assist devices. In Mavroudis C, Backer CL, editors: *Pediatric cardiac surgery*, Philadelphia, 2003, Mosby.

Jensen C, Hill CS: Mechanical support for congestive heart failure in infants and children, *Crit Care Nurs Clin North Am* 6(1):165-174, 1994.

Kalina J: Use of the balloon pressure waveform in conjunction with the augmented arterial pressure waveform. In Quaal SJ, editor: *Comprehensive intra-aortic balloon counterpulsation,* ed 2, St. Louis, 1993, Mosby Yearbook.

Kang N, Edwards M, Larbalestier R: Preoperative intra-aortic balloon pumps in high-risk patients undergoing open-heart surgery, *Ann Thoracic Surg* 72:54-57, 2001.

Low R: Intra-aortic balloon counterpulsation in acute myocardial infarction: too few or too many? *JACC* 41:1946-1947, 2003.

Mertlich GB, Quaal SJ, Borgmeier PR, et al: Effect of increased intra-aortic balloon pressure on catheter volume: relationship to changing attitude, *Crit Care Med* 20:297-303, 1992.

Mouloupolos SD: Intra-aortic balloon counterpulsation in the treatment of cardiogenic shock: hemodynamic effects and clinical challenges, *Cardiol Clin Updates*, retrieved May 24, 2001, from http://www.medscape.com/viewprogram607/pmt.

Pollock J, Charlton, MC, Williams WB, et al: Intraaortic balloon pumping in children, *Ann Thorac Surg* 29:522-528, 1980.

Quaal SJ: Conventional timing using the arterial pressure waveform. In Quall SJ, editor: *Comprehensive intra-aortic balloon counterpulsation,* ed 2, St. Louis, 1993, Mosby Yearbook.

Quaal SJ: Physiological and clinical analysis of the arterial pressure waveform in the IABP patient, *Can Perfusion Canadienne* 10:6-13, 2000.

Stone GW, Ohman E, Miller M, et al: Contemporary utilization and outcomes of intra-aortic balloon counterpulsation in acute myocardial infarction, *JACC* 41:1940-1947, 2003.

Torchiana DF, Hirsch G, Buckley MJ, et al: Intra-aortic balloon pumping for cardiac support: trends in practice and outcome, *J Thoracic Cardiovasc Surg* 114:758-764, 1997.

Veasy LG, Blalock RC, Orth JL, et al: Intra-aortic balloon pumping in infants and children, *Circulation* 68:1095-1100, 1983.

Ventricular Assist Device: Management

P U R P O S E : A ventricular assist device (VAD) is an extra-corporeal pump that can take over part or all of the pumping function of the left or right ventricle. A VAD is used in situations of life-threatening reversible ventricular failure or as a bridge to transplant in the event that cardiac function does not recover

Rosita Y. Maley

PREREQUISITE KNOWLEDGE

- Anatomy and physiology of the cardiac and pulmonary systems
- Principles of oxygen delivery to tissues
- Principles of hemodynamic monitoring, cardiopulmonary bypass, electrophysiology and dysrhythmias, and coagulation
- Care and management of the child after cardiac surgery
- Medications used to support cardiac output
- Clinical and technical competence related to the specific VAD in use
- A VAD can be placed in the intensive care unit (ICU) or operating room. Specific information concerning controls, alarms, troubleshooting, and safety features is available from the manufacturer; the institution-specific protocol should be read thoroughly before use of the equipment. Refer to the operator's manual for the specific VAD used for more detail.[1]
- A VAD may be placed for right ventricle support (RVAD), left ventricle support (LVAD), or biventricular support (BVAD).
- The VADs approved for use in children in the United States are generally one of two types[2,3]:
  - ❖ Centrifugal pump, such as the Biomedicus (Medtronic-Biomedicus, Minneapolis, MN), which can be used in neonates, infants, and children
  - ❖ Pulsatile VADs, such as the Thoratec LVAD (Thoratec Laboratories Corp., Pleasanton, CA), which has been used in children of more then 20 kg with a body surface area (BSA) of more than 0.8 m²

- Several manufacturers have VADs in development, with the goal of development of a device that can be used with children of all sizes with minimal complications; several clinical trials are in process.[4-6]
- Assessment and management of complications of VAD therapy include, but are not limited to: bleeding, renal dysfunction, infection, embolism, and cardiac tamponade.
- Identification and management of mechanical system failure
- Management of cardiovascular emergencies (i.e., tamponade)
- Indications for VAD therapy
  - ❖ Inability to wean from cardiopulmonary bypass
  - ❖ Hypoxemia and pulmonary hypertension
  - ❖ Cardiomyopathy
  - ❖ Cardiac arrest
  - ❖ Bridge to transplantation
  - ❖ Destination
- Relative contraindications of VAD therapy
  - ❖ Severe dysfunction of other organ systems (especially central nervous system)
  - ❖ Extreme prematurity
  - ❖ Sepsis
- Some pediatric studies indicate that congenital heart disease is a significant risk factor in the use of VAD therapy.[2,3,7,8]
- Mastery of pediatric advanced life support competencies
- Principles of aseptic technique
- Child development as it relates to clinical assessment and use of a VAD
- Informed consent is required if placement of the VAD is a planned procedure.

CHILD AND FAMILY ASSESSMENT

- History of congenital cardiac disease, invasive cardiac procedures, or cardiac surgery, with attention to competency of the cardiac valves, atrial or ventricular septal defects, and pulmonary hypertension ⇢*Rationale:* Provides baseline data related to cardiac function and facilitates decision making regarding the type of VAD inserted and postoperative management. Previous experiences can alter the child's and family's response.
- Cardiovascular, hemodynamic, neurovascular, neurologic, and psychosocial assessment and infectious suitability for VAD therapy ⇢*Rationale:* Provides baseline data and helps with determining the type of VAD to be used.
- Child's age, body mass index, and BSA ⇢*Rationale:* Provides baseline data and helps with determine the type of VAD to be used.
- Current laboratory profile, including complete blood count, platelet count, prothrombin time, partial thromboplastin time (PTT), international normalized ratio (INR), fibrinogen, Thromboelastogram (TEG), blood chemistry, blood urea nitrogen (BUN), creatinine, lactate, arterial blood gas, mixed venous oxygen saturation, and B-type natriuretic peptide (BNP) ⇢*Rationale:* Provides baseline data and potential indication of end-organ dysfunction related to low cardiac output state. Predicts the risk for bleeding or coagulation issues. BNP is a hormone secreted by the ventricle in response to wall stress from pressure or volume overload and has diuretic and vasorelaxant properties; elevated BNP levels correlate with worsening heart failure in adult studies and are used as an adjunct in diagnosis, treatment, and risk stratification.[9]
- Skin assessment with the Modified Braden Q Pressure Ulcer Risk Assessment Tool (See Procedure 125) or institution-specific protocol ⇢*Rationale:* Determines the degree of risk and facilitates implementation of interventions to prevent skin breakdown.
- Developmental level of child and family ⇢*Rationale:* Developmental level influences preparation, interaction, and compliance.
- Level of consciousness and cognitive ability ⇢*Rationale:* Determines how to include the child in the postimplantation teaching plan.
- Neurologic system with physical examination and head ultrasound scan for infants with open fontanel[10] ⇢*Rationale:* Provides baseline data and helps determine suitability of type of VAD selected.
- Function of immunologic system ⇢*Rationale:* Child is at risk for sepsis from multiple invasive sites and debilitated nutritional state.
- Child's and family's available emotional and spiritual support ⇢*Rationale:* Assesses need for additional resources from a multidisciplinary team to provide support until recovery, transplant, or withdrawal of support.
- If no opportunity for preprocedural teaching occurs, the teaching starts with family updates. The family's and child's understanding of the current situation, rationale for use of the device, and expected outcomes are evaluated ⇢*Rationale:* Assessment of family's understanding allows development of an individualized teaching plan. Previous experiences and developmental level of family affect family's response.

CHILD AND FAMILY EDUCATION

Individualized, developmentally appropriate education is provided to the family and to the child based on desire for knowledge, readiness to learn, and overall neurologic and psychosocial state.

- Provide information about the VAD, including the reason for the VAD and an explanation of steps provided in the daily monitoring of a child with a VAD ⇢*Rationale:* Clarification or reinforcement of information is an expressed need of the child and family during times of stress and anxiety.
- Provide information about the environment and the expected plan of care to the child and family, including frequency of assessments, function of equipment, sounds and alarms, dressings, mobility limitations, and parameters to discontinue therapy. A picture book about other children with VADs and their families or a meeting with a child with a VAD and the family, if both families are agreeable, may be helpful. ⇢*Rationale:* The communication and visual stimulation provides information and encourages the child and family to ask questions or voice concerns or fears of the therapy. Meeting another family with a VAD provides social support.
- If developmentally appropriate, explain how the child can assist with activities of daily living (ADLs) while living with a VAD ⇢*Rationale:* Providing information decreases anxiety and fear and increases compliance and promotes the child's participation in care.
- Develop an individualized teaching plan for the child and family if the urgency of the child's condition and need for a VAD does not permit teaching and education before implantation of the VAD ⇢*Rationale:* Providing information decreases anxiety and fear and increases compliance. The severity of the child's condition may make preoperative teaching impossible. As soon as the child's condition improves, teaching should begin.
- Encourage questions and answer questions as they arise ⇢*Rationale:* Reinforcement of information is needed during periods of stress and is especially important if the procedure is emergent.

EQUIPMENT

- Equipment and supplies specific to the type of VAD in use
- Hemodynamic monitoring equipment
- Anticoagulation monitoring equipment
- Pressure relieving devices for the skin
- Thermoregulation equipment
- Skin care supplies
- Wound care and dressing supplies
- Emergency equipment and supplies

Procedure for Ventricular Assist Device: Management

Steps	Rationale	Considerations
1. If time and circumstances permit, ensure that child and family understand procedure and that questions are answered.	Evaluates and reinforces understanding of previously taught information.	Developmental level, cognitive ability, and anxiety level determine approach to and effectiveness of teaching.
2. Gather needed equipment and supplies.	Facilitates completion of procedure in a timely manner.	
3. If VAD is to be placed as a scheduled procedure, confirm that consent for procedure has been obtained.	Ensures medical-legal compliance as suggested by the Joint Commission on Accreditation of Healthcare Organizations (JCAHO).	In emergency situations, refer to institution-specific protocol for assumption of consent.
4. Use two patient identifiers to identify the child.	Promotes patient safety and ensures that the correct child receives correct therapy.	Two patient identifiers should be used for identification of the child per institution-specific protocol; most commonly, name and medical record number are used in inpatient settings.
5. Review emergency procedures specific to the VAD in use.	Certain conditions, such as loss of power, VAD failure, inadvertent cannula removal, or tubing disconnection, may be life threatening to the child and necessitate immediate recognition and management.	Management of power loss or VAD failure varies greatly between devices; review the manufacturer's instructions in detail before caring for the child with a VAD.
6. As appropriate for the specific VAD, confirm that settings match prescribing practitioner's order.	Settings that can be adjusted vary among VADs.	
7. Observe atrial monitor pressure readings and waveforms.	Atrial monitor reflects emptying of the ventricle, wall stress, and the possibility of myocardial recovery.[10]	
8. Obtain neurologic assessment every hour or per institution-specific protocol; assist with daily head ultrasound scans for infants. (*Level V**)	Cerebrovascular accidents, hemorrhages, and seizures are a major source of morbidity for the child with VAD support.[11]	Seizures may not be detected in a child who is sedated and chemically paralyzed.
9. Obtain temperature measurements every 2 to 4 hours or per institution-specific protocol. (*Level IV**)	A significant blood volume may be extracorporeal, and the child may need large volumes of fluid administration, which puts the child at risk for hypothermia, especially during the initial 24 hours.[12]	The VAD and child may need separate thermoregulation interventions.
10. Administer anticoagulant therapy as prescribed or per institution-specific protocol. (*Level V**)	Blood moving through artificial devices is prone to clotting or thrombus formation; most VADs necessitate anticoagulation therapy for the child.	Each VAD necessitates different levels of anticoagulation[13]; refer to the manufacturer's recommendations.
11. Provide nutritional support as prescribed.	Adequate nutrition is necessary to meet increased metabolic needs and promote wound healing.	Transpyleroric enteral nutrition or parenteral nutrition can be used to provide goal calories of 80 to 100 kcal/kg/d.

Procedure continues on following page

---

* Level IV: Limited clinical studies to support recommendations
  Level V: Clinical studies in more than one or two patient populations and situations to support recommendations

Procedure for Ventricular Assist Device: Management—*Continued*

Steps	Rationale	Considerations
12. Use measures to maintain skin integrity, such as: ambulation if permitted based on the type of VAD used; slight turning to minimize pressure points; skin care; passive range of motion and repositioning of extremities; use of hand rolls; mouth care; placement on a preventive surface, such as a low air-loss bed; and use of gel pillows.	Hypervigilance is needed to prevent skin breakdown, especially if the VAD used necessitates that the child be relatively immobile.	Risk of skin breakdown can be evaluated with a tool such as the modified Braden Q Pressure Ulcer Risk Assessment Tool; the appropriate skin care algorithm can be identified and implemented. See Procedure 125 for further information. *(Level V*)*
13. Provide wound care and dressing changes with aseptic technique according to the manufacturer's recommendations or institution-specific protocol. *(Level I*)*	Manufacturer's recommendations vary based on the type of access inserted; some substances may harm tubing or reservoirs of a particular VAD.	
14. Inspect tubing, valves, and VAD chambers as appropriate to the specific VAD, per manufacturer's recommendations or institution-specific protocol. *(Level I*)*	Identifies thrombus formation and inadequate emptying of chambers.[1]	
15. Inspect all connections to ensure a tight fit; if appropriate, inspect tubing for kinks.	Loose connections may result in exsanguinations; kinks in tubing prevent blood flow.	
16. Secure and stabilize cannula during procedures that necessitate movement of the child, such as chest x-ray, dressing change, linen change, or ambulation if permitted with the VAD in use.	Inadvertent dislodgement of cannula is a life-threatening event.	
17. Use all appropriate pharmacologic and nonpharmacologic techniques for pain management. *(Level IV*)*	The child will have pain from VAD placement and limited mobility.	Pain and anxiety can be managed with continuous or scheduled infusions of opioids and benzodiazepines and various nonpharmacologic techniques.
18. Ensure VAD is plugged into emergency power outlets with generator backup.	Ensures that electrical power is available from a back-up source in the event of a power outage.	

* Level I: Manufacturer's recommendations only
Level IV: Limited clinical studies to support recommendations
Level V: Clinical studies in more than one or two patient populations and situations to support recommendations

Expected Outcomes	Unexpected Outcomes
• Child has improved cardiac output	• Hypotension
	• Cardiac output does not improve or deteriorates
• Child's respiratory status remains stable or improves	• Respiratory failure
• End organs are adequately perfused	• Renal dysfunction
	• Hepatic dysfunction
	• Seizures
• The VAD provides a bridge to transplantation or recovery	• Withdrawal of support
• Child is free from complications of anticoagulation therapy	• CVA
	• Bleeding

Expected Outcomes	Unexpected Outcomes
• Child is free from complications related to VAD	• Thrombus • Hemolysis • Pump malfunction or mechanical failure • Circuit dysfunction • Air embolus • Infection • Cardiac tamponade • Hypothermia
• Child's skin is free from injury related to immobility	• Skin breakdown • Foot drop
• Child has an acceptable level of comfort	• Unmanaged pain

Monitoring and Care of the Child

Activities and Interventions	Rationale	Reportable Conditions
1. Perform cardiovascular and hemo-dynamic assessment, including atrial pressures as available, every 60 minutes and with changes in child's status.	Heart rate, arterial pressure, right atrial and left atrial pressures, and venous oxygen saturation (SVO_2) show effectiveness of VAD therapy. Atrial pressures reflect emptying of the ventricle, wall stress, and the possibility of myocardial recovery.[9]	• Bradycardia • Hypotension • Right atrial or left atrial pressures outside the desired parameters
2. Monitor oxygen delivery.	Mixed venous oxygen saturation, arterial blood gas analysis, and serum lactate values are indicators of effective oxygenation.	• Decrease in SVO_2 • Increased serum lactate level
3. Monitor urine output and serum creatinine level.	Adequate urine output and serum creatinine levels within normal limits are indicators of adequate perfusion of the kidneys.	• Urine output less than 1 mL/kg/h or less than the desired parameters • Rising serum creatinine levels
4. Monitor indicators of nutritional status, including weight and total protein, serum albumin, and pre-albumin values.	Assesses effectiveness of nutritional support.	• Inability to provide prescribed calories • Nausea or vomiting • Abnormal laboratory values
5. Monitor anticoagulation status per manufacturer's recommendations and institution-specific protocol.	Recommendations for anticoagulation therapy are specific to the type of VAD in use.	• Bleeding • Thrombus formation
6. Monitor neurologic status frequently.	Hemorrhage, CVA, and seizures are associated with the use of VADs.	• Seizures • Deterioration in neurologic status
7. Monitor safety and security of cannula at all times.	Inadvertent cannula removal is a life-threatening event.	• Unsecure cannula • Inadvertent cannula removal
8. Monitor for indications of systemic or local infection.	Multiple sources of infection associated with prolonged ICU stay, central lines, mechanical ventilation, open chest, and wound sites.	• Fever • Laboratory study results that indicate infection • Changes in hemodynamic status • Redness, drainage, or swelling at the cannula insertion site
9. Monitor skin integrity.	Child is at risk for skin breakdown from relative immobility that may be necessary.	• Skin breakdown

Continued

Monitoring and Care of the Child—Cont'd

Activities and Interventions	Rationale	Reportable Conditions
10. Monitor child's pain level with a pain scale appropriate to child's developmental level (see Procedure 173 for further information). Determine the effectiveness of pain management strategies.	The child will have pain related to VAD placement and limited mobility; assessment for the presence of pain on a regular basis ensures prompt and effective treatment. Pain management strategy many be ineffective and need modification.	• Unmanaged pain
11. Monitor for readiness to wean from VAD support.	Assesses effectiveness of therapies.	• Improvement in vital signs • Improvement in mixed venous oxygen saturation • Improvement in cardiac ejection seen with adequate arterial line tracing with decreasing flows

Documentation

- Child and family education
- Type of VAD in use
- VAD settings
- Neurologic status
- Child's response to therapy
- Laboratory values
- Pain assessment
- Assessment of incision and drive line site
- Confirmation of placement
- Hemodynamic status
- Skin integrity
- Anticoagulation status
- Unexpected outcomes and related treatment

References

1. Fleck DA, Hargraves J: Ventricular assist devices. In Lynn-McHale Wiegand DJ, Carlson K, editors: *AACN procedure manual for critical care,* ed 5, Philadelphia, 2005, Saunders.
2. Reinhartz O, et al: Multicenter experience with the thoratec ventricular assist device in children and adolescents, *J Heart Lung Transplant* 20(4):439-448, 2001.
3. Undar A, et al: Outcomes of congential heart surgery patients after extracorporeal life support at Texas Children's Hospital, *Artificial Organs* 28(10):963-966, 2004.
4. Duncan BW: *Mechanical support for cardiac and respiratory failure in pediatric patients,* New York, 2001, Marcel Dekker Inc.
5. Lietz K, Miller LW: Left ventricular assist devices: evolving devices and indications for use in ischemic disease, *Curr Opin Cardiol* 19(6):613-618, 2004.
6. Morales DLS, et al: Lessons learned from the first application of the DeBakey VAD child: an intracorporeal ventricular assist device for children, *J Heart Lung Transplant* 24:331-337, 2005.
7. Reinhartz O, et al: Thoratec ventricular assist devices in children with less than 1.3 m² of body surface area, *Am Soc Artificial Internal Organs J* 49:727-730, 2003.

8. Stiller B, et al: Consumption of blood products during mechanical circulatory support in children: comparison between ECMO and a pulsatile ventricular assist device, *Intens Care Med* 30:1814-1820, 2004.
9. Lin N, et al: Relation of age, severity of illness, and hemodynamics with brain natriuretic peptide levels in patients <20 years of age with heart disease, *Am J Cardiol* 96(6):847-850, 2005.
10. Seib PM, : Blade and balloon atrial septostomy for left heart decompression in patients with severe ventricular dysfunction on extracorporeal membrane oxygenation, *Catheterization Cardiovasc Intervent* 46(2):179-186, 1999.
11. Gannon CM, et al: When combined, early bedside head ultrasound and electroencephalography predict abnormal computerized tomography or magnetic resonance brain imaging obtained after extracorporeal membrane oxygenation treatment, *J Perinatol* 21(7): 451-455, 2001.
12. Jacobs JP, et al: Rapid cardiopulmonary support for children with complex cardiac heart disease, *Ann Thorac Surg* 70(3):742-50, 2000.
13. Biswas AK, et al: Aprotonin in the management of life-threatening bleeding during extracorporeal life support, *Perfusion* 15(3):211-216, 2000.

Additional Readings

Canody CM, Savage L: The left ventricular assist device, *Am J Nurs* May(Suppl):15-20, 1999.

Chang AC, Hanley FL, et al: *Pediatric cardiac intensive care,* Baltimore, 1998, Williams & Wilkins.

Chang AD, McKenzie ED: Myocardial dysfunction, extracorporeal membrane oxygenation, and ventricular assist devices. In Fuhrman BP, Zimmerman JZ, editors: *Pediatric critical care,* ed 3, Philadelphia, 2006, Mosby.

Curley MAQ, Moloney-Harmon P, editors: *Critical care nursing of infants and children,* ed 2, Philadelphia, 2001, Saunders.

PROCEDURE **59**

Flow-Directed Pulmonary Artery Catheter: Cardiac Output Measurement

P U R P O S E : The pulmonary artery catheter is used to measure pulmonary artery systolic, diastolic, and mean pressure along with pulmonary capillary wedge pressure. When a cardiac output measurement is performed, true cardiac output, cardiac index, systemic vascular resistance, and pulmonary vascular resistance are assessed. This information is then used to guide fluid management and inotropic and vasoactive support in the critically ill child. Proper technique in obtaining a thermodilutional cardiac output is critical to ensure accurate measurements

Dan Graves

PREREQUISITE KNOWLEDGE

- Anatomy and physiology of the great vessels and heart
- Understanding of pediatric congenital heart defect anatomy if the child has a defect
- Understanding of hemodynamic pressure monitoring transducer assembly and function; see Procedure 63
- Pulmonary artery (PA) catheter anatomy (see Figure 60-1)
- Ability to identify transduction waveforms of the right atrium (RA), right ventricle (RV), PA, and pulmonary capillary wedge (PCW) (see Figure 60-2)
- Ability to identify basic arrhythmias is mandatory when caring for a child with a PA catheter
- Normal values for RA, PA, and PCW pressures
- Mastery of pediatric advanced life support competencies
- Pharmacology of inotropic and vasoactive medications
- Terminology for cardiovascular function[1]
  - ❖ Preload: The amount of blood that is to be ejected from the left ventricle just before systole. An increase in the preload causes stretch receptors in the myocardium to increase the cardiac output, up to a

certain point. At the point at which the preload increases beyond the capacity of the ventricle, the cardiac output begins to decrease, which is the basis for the Frank-Starling law of the heart.
  - ❖ Afterload: The amount of pressure that the left ventricle has to overcome to eject blood into the aorta, which is directly related to the systemic vascular resistance.
  - ❖ Contractility: The intrinsic ability of the myocardium to pump unrelated to the factors of preload or afterload, which is related to the strength of myocardial muscle shortening. Sympathetic nervous system innervation is the primary control mechanism for contractility.
  - ❖ Cardiac output (CO): The quantity of blood that is ejected into the aorta each minute by the left ventricle. A normal cardiac output in a healthy adult male averages 5.6 L/min. The equation for cardiac output is: heart rate × stroke volume.
  - ❖ Cardiac index (CI): A method for relation of cardiac output to body surface area (BSA), which allows comparison of values between children of various

ages and sizes. CI is calculated by dividing the CO by the BSA.

❖ Systemic vascular resistance (SVR): The impedance to arterial blood flow as it perfuses into the peripheral vasculature. This parameter can be identified with Poiseuille's equation. The components of this equation include vessel radius, length of the vessel, and pressure lost along the vessel distance.

❖ Pulmonary vascular resistance (PVR): Similar concept to the SVR relating directly to the pulmonary vasculature

❖ Stroke volume (SV): The end diastolic left ventricular volume minus the end systolic left ventricular volume. SV is the amount of blood ejected in one single systole. In adults, a constant of 80 is used for calculation of cardiac output, however, in pediatrics the SV is variable for infants and children depending on size and age.

❖ Heart rate (HR): The number of systoles during 1 minute that is normally controlled by the automaticity of the sinus atrial node. The stretching of the wall of the right atrium above preload causes an increase in heart rate by 10% to 15%. This stretch also activates the Bainbridge reflex, which causes an increase in heart rate.

❖ Mixed venous oxygen saturation: The oxygen saturation within the pulmonary artery, which is a reflection of the body's uptake of oxygen during perfusion through the arterial to venous blood system

❖ Table 59-1 is a reference of pediatric normal values and formulas for hemodynamic parameters[1,2]

• Output can be measured through the use of thermodilution calculation.

• Thermodilution CO is calculated after a room temperature injectate is infused through the proximal port. A measurement of time to temperature change at the thermistor probe, which is located at the most distal portion of the PA catheter, is used to calculate CO.[1]

• The temperature change of the injectate forms a curve; the area under the curve is used to calculate the CO. Different clinical conditions affect the appearance of the curve. Figure 59-1 has examples of CO curves.

• Injectate volumes range from 5 mL to 10 mL, depending on size of the child

• Every PA catheter comes with a reference chart in the packaging. This reference lists the known computation constant to use based on the type and size of the PA catheter and the volume and temperature of the injectate. This constant is programmed into the monitor used to calculate the CO.

• Some PA catheter systems have the ability to monitor a continuous CO. This type of catheter includes a filament that heats the blood in the pulmonary artery and calculates the change in temperature to obtain the continuous measurements.[1]

• Injectate temperatures are determined by institution-specific protocol. Room temperature injectate is commonly used. Iced injectate has been shown to cause dysrhythmias.[1,2]

CHILD AND FAMILY ASSESSMENT

• A complete cardiovascular assessment should be performed just before CO measurement ➤➤*Rationale:* This assessment correlates the clinical assessment with the thermodilution CO calculated with the monitor.

• Assess intracardiac waveforms before the thermodilution CO is obtained ➤➤*Rationale:* Confirms correct position of the PA catheter.

• Height and weight are obtained to calculate BSA ➤➤*Rationale:* The BSA is used to calculate CI.

• Child's and family's understnding of the reasons for and risks and benefits of the procedure ➤➤*Rationale:* Evaluates child's and family's understanding and provides a gauge for ongoing education.

TABLE 59-1	Pediatric Hemodynamic Reference Values and Formulas	
Parameter	**Formula**	**Normal Range**
Cardiac output (CO)	$CO = HR \times SV$	4 to 8 L/min*
Cardiac index (CI)	$CI = CO/BSA$	3.3 to 6 L/min/m^2
Stroke volume (SV)	$SV = CO \times 1000/HR$	60 to 100 mL/beat*
Stroke volume index (SVI)	$SVI = SV/BSA$	30 to 60 mL/m^2
Systemic vascular resistance (SVR)	$SVR = MAP - CVP/CO \times 80$	900 to 1600 dyne/s/cm^{-5}*
Systemic vascular resistance index (SVRI)	$SVRI = MAP - CVP/CI \times 79.9$	800 to 1600 dyne-s/cm^5/m^2
Pulmonary vascular resistance (PVR)	$PVR = PAM - PAWP/CO \times 80$	155 to 255 dyne/s/cm^{-5}*
Pulmonary vascular resistance index (PVRI)	$PVRI = PAM - PAWP/CI \times 79.9$	80 to 240 dyne-s/cm^5/m^2

* Adult reference; use index references to normalize to pediatric patients.
Adult values referenced from Lynn-McHale and Carlson.[1]
Pediatric values referenced from Fuhrman and Zimmerman.[2]
MAP, Mean arterial pressure; *PAM,* pulmonary artery mean; *PAWP,* pulmonary artery wedge pressure.
Data from Lynn-McHale DJ, Carlson KK, editors: *AACN procedure manual for critical care,* ed 5, Philadelphia, 2005, Saunders; and Fuhrman BP, Zimmerman JJ, editors: *Pediatric critical care,* ed 3, Philadelphia, 2006, Mosby.

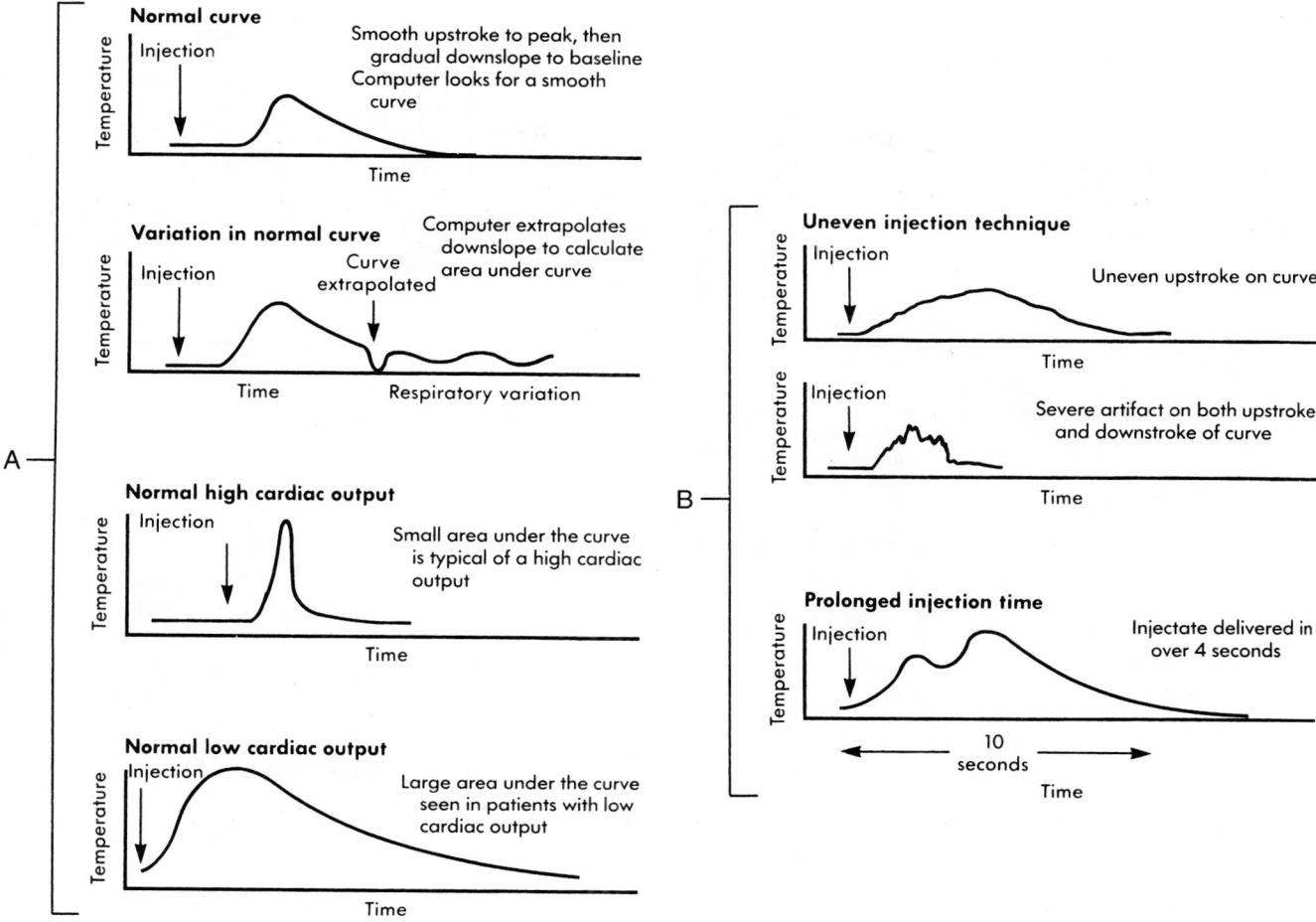

FIGURE 59-1   **A,** Variations in normal cardiac output curve seen in certain clinical conditions. **B,** Abnormal cardiac output curves that produce erroneous cardiac output value. *From Thelan LA, et al:* Textbook of critical care nursing: diagnosis and management, *St. Louis, 1998, Mosby.*

CHILD AND FAMILY EDUCATION

Individualized, developmentally appropriate education is provided to the child and family based on desire for knowledge, readiness to learn, and overall neurologic and psychosocial state.

- Provide the family, and child if appropriate, with information about the reasons for thermodilutional CO measurement and the steps in the procedure ➣**Rationale:** Providing information decreases anxiety and fear.
- If developmentally appropriate, the child should be informed when an injection of fluid through the proximal line is performed ➣**Rationale:** Some children have a feeling of coldness during the injection.
- The child and family should be provided with information about the frequency of CO measurements ➣**Rationale:** Information may decrease stress related to frequent interventions.

- Encourage questions and answer questions as they arise ➣**Rationale:** Reinforcement of information is needed during periods of stress.

EQUIPMENT

- Electrocardiogram (ECG) monitor
- Pulmonary artery and central venous pressure (CVP) monitoring lines transduced with appropriate waveforms and confirmed correct position
- Thermistor line connected to the CO monitor
- A closed system of prescribed intravenous (IV) fluid for injection attached to a three-way stopcock and then attached to the proximal injectate line (Figure 59-2)
- External temperature probe from the CO monitor attached to the closed IV fluids system. Some systems have an in-line temperature probe, and others need placement and securing of a thermometer against the IV bag.
- Pulmonary artery catheter insert with information relating to computation constant and injectate temperature and volume

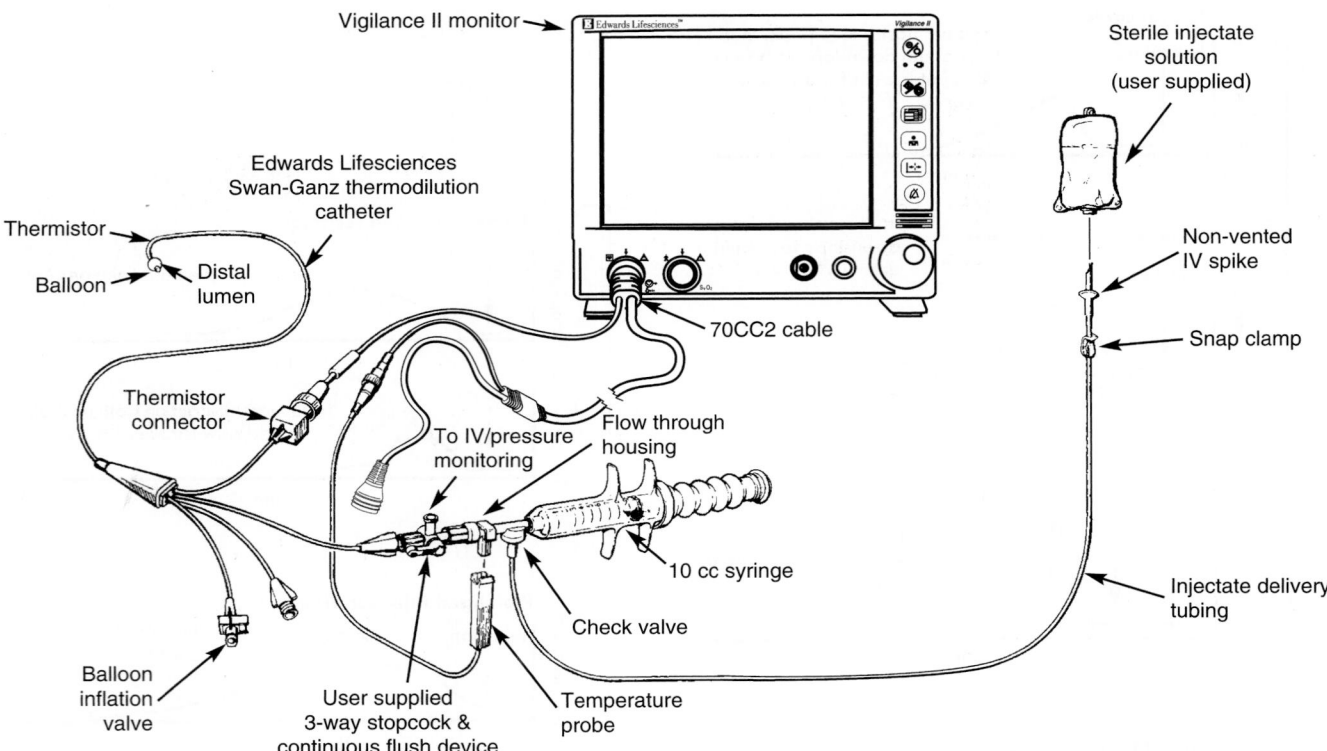

FIGURE 59-2   Cardiac output set preparations for cardiac output measurement. Room temperature injectate preparation. *From Edwards Lifesciences, LLC, Irvine, Calif.*

Procedure | for Pulmonary Artery Catheter: Cardiac Output Measurement

Steps	Rationale	Considerations
1. Ensure child and family understand procedure and questions are answered.	Evaluates and reinforces understanding of previously taught information.	Developmental level, cognitive ability and anxiety level will determine approach to and effectiveness of teaching.
2. If not previously done, obtain height and weight of child.	Data needed for calculation of BSA.	Body surface area is used in the calculation of CI, a measure that allows comparison of data between patients.
3. Place child in supine position with the head flat or elevated no more than 20 degrees. *(Level IV*)*	Facilitates accurate measurement.	
4. Wash hands and use standard precautions.	Reduces transmission of microorganisms.	
5. Ensure child is attached to a continuous ECG monitor.	Arrhythmias are commonly seen in children who have PA catheters in place.	
6. Ensure pressure transducer monitoring lines are appropriately set up and zeroed and have expected waveforms.	Ensures that the catheter is positioned correctly and that the data used in CO calculations are correct.	

* Level IV: Limited clinical studies to support recommendations

Procedure | **for Pulmonary Artery Catheter: Cardiac Output Measurement**—*Continued*

Steps	Rationale	Considerations
7. Identify child with two patient identifiers.	Confirms the correct procedure and correct patient as recommended by the Joint Commission on Accreditation of Health Care Organizations.	Verification process and documentation is institution specific. Use active communication techniques.
8. Connect thermistor probe to CO monitor or computer. *(Level I*)*	Necessary for calculations.	
9. Attach the prescribed IV fluids to the proximal injectate port with a three-way stopcock and aseptic technique (Figure 59-2 for set up diagram).	Use of a closed system decreases the possible introduction of bacteria into the bloodstream, which is essential because three injections will be done for each CO measurement.	
10. Connect external thermometer to the injectate source, as appropriate for the system in use. *(Level I*)*	Allows the CO monitor to calculate the initial injectate temperature.	Some systems have an in-line thermometer, and others need attachment to the side of the IV fluid bags.
11. With aseptic technique, attach a 10-mL syringe to the three-way stopcock.	Prevents introduction of bacteria into the bloodstream.	
12. Initiate set up of the CO monitor; select the appropriate module to start the process.	Depending on the system being used, begin set up to start the thermodilution procedure.	Set up varies among cardiac monitor manufacturers. Refer to the specific instructions for the monitor being used.
13. Determine PA catheter's computational constant and enter this number into the monitor. *(Level I*)*	This constant sets up the monitor for the specific size and type of PA catheter being used, which is necessary to obtain an accurate CO measurement.	Skipping this step can result in inaccurate CO measurements.
14. Note the displayed pulmonary artery temperature along with the injectate temperature.	The injectate temperature should be at least 10°F lower than the core body temperature to obtain an accurate CO.[1]	Without a temperature gradient, the thermistor is not able to calculate a CO.
15. Confirm that volume and temperature selected correlate with the computational constant previously entered into the CO monitor.	The constant should correlate with the catheter type, temperature, and volume of injectate to obtain accurate data.	
16. Withdraw prescribed volume of injectate into a 10-mL syringe.	Withdrawal is achieved by turning the stopcock off to the child and drawing from the IV fluid bag, which is part of the closed system.	
17. Depress the start button on the monitor.	Attempt to time the injection with the end expiration to maximize the accuracy of cardiac output measurement.[1]	
18. Quickly inject entire volume in the syringe into the proximal injectate line.	Total fluid volume should be injected in less than 4 seconds. *(Level IV*)*	Slow injections may cause inaccurate results.
19. Observe the CO waveform.	The waveform should correlate with Figure 59-1.	

Procedure continues on following page

* Level I: Manufacturer's recommendations only
Level IV: Limited clinical studies to support recommendations

Procedure for Pulmonary Artery Catheter: Cardiac Output Measurement—*Continued*

Steps	Rationale	Considerations
20. Repeat steps 14 to 19 a total of three times.	An average of three attempts increases the accuracy of the reading.	
21. Average the results of the three CO measurements.[1]	Discard any injection in which the waveform was abnormal or the value obtained was more than 10% different than the middle value.	A 10% difference is considered standard error. Values that fall outside this range should be discarded. The two remaining values may be averaged or a fourth measurement may be obtained.[1,2]
22. Enter necessary data into the hemodynamic calculation menu of the CO monitor.	Typically monitors need the child's weight and height. The CO measurement is automatically entered.	
23. Confirm that monitor performed the hemodynamic calculations. CI is usually calculated by the CO monitor (CO divided by BSA).	Cardiac index calculation takes into consideration variability based on the child's size. Manual performance of the calculations is often recommended as a double check of the monitor.	Hemodynamic calculations should match the child's clinical condition. If the numbers do not match, the calculations should be redone.
24. Remove the three-way stopcock from the proximal injectate line.	Prevents inadvertent fluid administration to the child.	
25. Resume previous infusion/fluids through the proximal injectate line.	The patency of the proximal line is assured with continuous fluid infusion or appropriate flushing schedule.	
26. Discard any disposable equipment in the appropriate trash receptacle and wash hands.	Standard precautions; reduces transmission of microorganisms.	
27. Document the data obtained in the medical record.	Captures the data for comparison with previous values.	
28. Inform the medical team of the results of the hemodynamic calculations.	Prevents unnecessary usage of the PA catheter if feedback is provided after each calculation.	The PA catheter should be discontinued when the information obtained is no longer useful in the medical management of the critically ill child.
29. Update family of child's status as appropriate.	Informed families tend to cope with hospitalization more successfully.	

Expected Outcomes

- An accurate thermodilution CO measure is obtained

- The child's cardiovascular function is assessed and appropriate treatment is provided

- The PA catheter remains sealed in a sterile field

- The PA catheter remains patent and CO is obtained

- The child remains free from dysrhythmias
- The thermodilution CO and subsequently calculated CI are used to evaluate other hemodynamic parameters, such as SVR and PVR

Unexpected Outcomes

- A thermodilution CO is unobtainable
- False measurement is obtained because of improper technique
- Deterioration in cardiovascular function is not identified or appropriate treatment is not administered
- Air embolism
- Introduction of bacteria into the bloodstream from poor aseptic technique
- The PA catheter is not patent and measurements cannot be obtained
- Ventricular dysrhythmias
- Inability to evaluate hemodynamic parameters

Monitoring and Care of the Child

Activities and Interventions	Rationale	Reportable Conditions
1. Perform assessment before and after CO measurements are obtained. This examination should include a cardiovascular, respiratory, and neurologic examination.	Allows for a baseline assessment to compare clinical condition with obtained thermodilution CO.	• Failure to obtain a CO with the thermodilution procedure • Change in clinical condition from baseline
2. Assess the insertion site for signs of bleeding, integrity of the dressing and sleeve, and catheter position.	Prevents complications of catheter insertion.	• Rupture of the sterile accordion sleeve • Change in the depth of catheter insertion, especially after movement of the child
3. Confirm placement of the PA catheter by observing PA waveform.	Confirms correct catheter placement before the thermodilution cardiac output is performed.	• Change in position of the PA catheter as evidenced by change in waveform appearance
4. Assess the functioning of the distal and proximal catheter ports.	Ensures that catheter lumens are patent.	• Inability to flush injectate into proximal injectate line or withdraw blood
5. Monitor core temperature.	Confirms placement and function of thermistor probe.	• Inability to obtain core temperature
6. Evaluate CO curve obtained with each measurement to evaluate reliability of value reported.	Abnormal curves suggest improper technique or change in clinical status (see Figure 59-1 for a diagram of a normal curve).	• Abnormal or dramatic change from trended CO
7. Monitor the child's tolerance of the procedure.	Ensures adequate pain and sedation management in the critically ill child.	• Ventricular arrhythmias • Inadequate pain control or sedation

Documentation

- CO measurements and individual who performed the thermodilution measurements
- Hemodynamic parameters calculated after CO was obtained
- Injectate volume and temperature
- Patient identification
- Clinical assessment associated with CO measurement
- Print-out of hemodynamic parameters placed in medical record
- Changes in medical management based on results of CO measurement obtained
- Family education and comprehension
- Child's tolerance of the procedure
- Waveform identification
- Intracardiac pressure readings obtained
- Child's status before and after the procedure
- Assessment of the insertion site
- Unexpected outcomes and related treatment

References
1. Lynn-McHale Wiegand DJ, Carlson K, editors: *AACN procedure manual for critical care,* ed 5, Philadelphia, 2005, Saunders.
2. Fuhrman BP, Zimmerman JJ, editors: *Pediatric critical care,* ed 3, Philadelphia, 2006, Mosby.

Additional Readings
Bullock BA, Henze RL, editors: *Focus on pathophysiology,* Philadelphia, 2000, Lippincott.

Dieckmann RA, et al, editors: *Illustrated textbook of pediatric emergency & critical care procedures,* St. Louis, 1997, Mosby.

Duke J. *Anesthesia secrets,* ed 2, Philadelphia, 2000, Hanley & Belfus, Inc.

Guyton AC, Hall JE, editors: *Textbook of medical physiology*, ed 10, Philadelphia, 2000, Saunders.

Ivanov R, et al: The incidence of major morbidity in critically ill patients managed with pulmonary artery catheters: a meta-analysis, *Crit Care Med* 28(3):615-618, 2000.

Morgan GE, et al, editors: *Clinical anesthesiology,* ed 3, New York, 2002, Lange Medical Books/McGraw-Hill.

Pollack MM: Bedside pulmonary artery catheterization in pediatrics, *J Pediatr* 96(2):274-276, 1980.

Roizen MG: Practice guidelines for pulmonary artery catheterization: an updated report by the American Society of Anesthesiologist Task Force on Pulmonary Artery Catheterization, *Anesthesiology* 99(4): 2003

Salm TJV, et al, editors: *Atlas of bedside procedures*, ed 2, Boston, 1988, Little, Brown and Company.

Truwit JD: The pulmonary artery catheter in the ICU, part 1: technique and measurements, *J Crit Illness* 18(1):9-18, 2003.

Flow-Directed Pulmonary Artery Catheter: Insertion Assist

PURPOSE: A thermodilutional catheter is inserted into the main pulmonary artery for measurement of pulmonary artery systolic, diastolic, mean, and pulmonary capillary wedge pressures and cardiac output. This information is then used to guide fluid management and vasoactive and inotropic drug support in the critically ill child.

Dan Graves

PREREQUISITE KNOWLEDGE

- Anatomy and physiology of the great vessels and heart
- An understanding of pediatric congenital heart defect anatomy is a prerequisite if the child has a defect.
- Understanding of hemodynamic transducer assembly and function (see Procedure 63)
- Pulmonary artery (PA) catheter anatomy (Figure 60-1)
- PA catheters available include the following[1]:
  - ❖ 5F PA catheter, which consists of four channels: a central venous pressure (CVP) port, a distal port, a thermistor port, and a balloon port
  - ❖ 7F PA catheter, which consists of four channels: a CVP port, a distal port, a thermistor port, and a balloon port
  - ❖ 7.5F PA catheter, which consists of five channels: a CVP port, a right ventricle (RV) port, a thermistor port, a distal port, and a balloon port
- The 5F PA catheter needs 0.5 mL of air to inflate the balloon. Most manufacturers supply a syringe that limits the amount of air used to inflate the balloon to 0.5 mL.
- The 7F and 7.5F PA catheters need 1.5 mL of air to inflate the balloon. Most manufacturers supply a syringe that limits the amount of air used to inflate the balloon to 1.5 mL.
- Ability to establish and maintain a sterile environment
- Ability to identify transduced waveforms of the right atrium (RA), RV, PA, and pulmonary capillary wedge (Figure 60-2)[2]
- Flow-directed PA catheters allow assessment of true cardiac output (CO), cardiac index (CI), systemic vascular resistance (SVR), and pulmonary vascular resistance (PVR)
- The pulmonary capillary wedge pressure (PCWP) is a reflection of left atrial (LA) pressure
- Pulmonary end diastolic pressure is slightly less than the PCWP. This knowledge allows LA pressure estimation without wedging the balloon.
- The identification of basic arrhythmias is imperative in assisting with PA catheter insertion and placement
- Knowledge of normal values for RA pressure, PA pressure, and PCWP
- Mastery of pediatric advanced life support competencies
- Indications for PA catheter placement include the following[1]:
  - ❖ Children with low CO whose conditions are not responsive to standard treatments

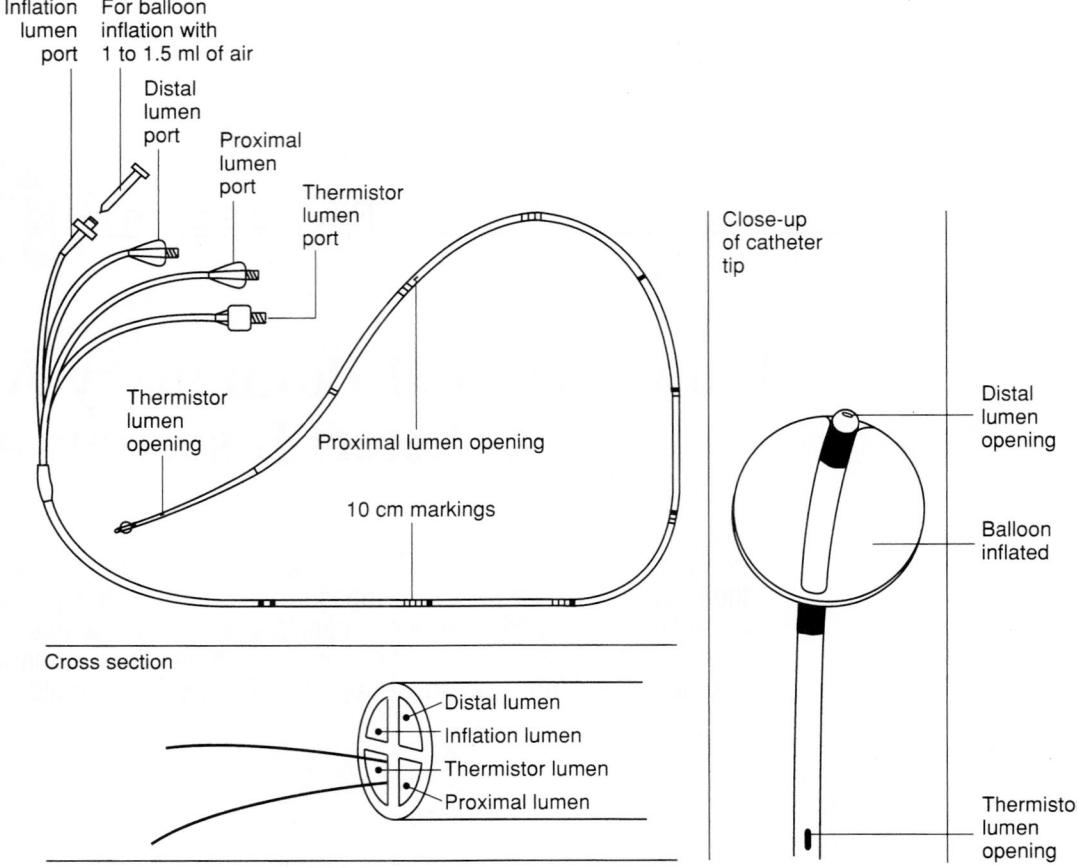

FIGURE 60-1   Anatomy of pulmonary artery (PA) catheter. PA catheter contains four lumens. Black markings are found on catheter, in 10-cm increments and beginning at distal end, and can be used to note length of catheter insertion. At distal end of catheter is latex rubber balloon of 0.5-mL to 1.5-mL capacity, which, when inflated, extends slightly beyond tip of catheter without obstructing it. Balloon inflation cushions tip of catheter and prevents contact with right ventricular wall during insertion. Balloon also acts to float catheter into position and allows measurement of pulmonary artery wedge pressure. *From Lynn-McHale, Carlson K, editors:* AACN procedure manual for critical care, *ed 4, Philadelphia, 2001, Saunders.*

- ❖ Children with adult respiratory distress syndrome (ARDS) with high peak end expiratory pressures
- ❖ Children with elevated PVR
- • No absolute contraindications to PA catheter insertion exist. Relative contraindications to PA catheter placement include[1]:
  - ❖ Intracardiac shunting lesions that might result in inaccurate hemodynamic readings or improper line placement
  - ❖ Tricuspid or pulmonary valve dysfunction
  - ❖ Ventricular arrhythmias that may worsen with PA catheter placement
  - ❖ Children with RV to PA discontinuity or placement of an RV to PA conduit to establish continuity
- • Complications of PA catheters
  - ❖ Infection
  - ❖ Pneumothorax or hemothorax
  - ❖ External hemorrhage
- • Complications directly related to PA catheter insertion

- ❖ Arrhythmias
- ❖ Pulmonary embolism
- ❖ Unrecognized PA occlusion
- ❖ Pulmonary hemorrhage
- ❖ Perforation of tricuspid or pulmonary valve
- ❖ Air embolism
- • The use of PA catheters to guide treatment in critically ill patients has been shown to reduce morbidity rates.[3]

CHILD AND FAMILY ASSESSMENT

- • Assessment of the family for determination of understanding of risks versus benefits of the PA catheter placement ➥*Rationale:* Assesses the family's understanding of the risks of PA catheter placement allows evaluation of whether informed consent has been obtained for the procedure.
- • Child's developmental level and ability to interact ➥*Rationale:* These factors influence preparation of the child and interaction.

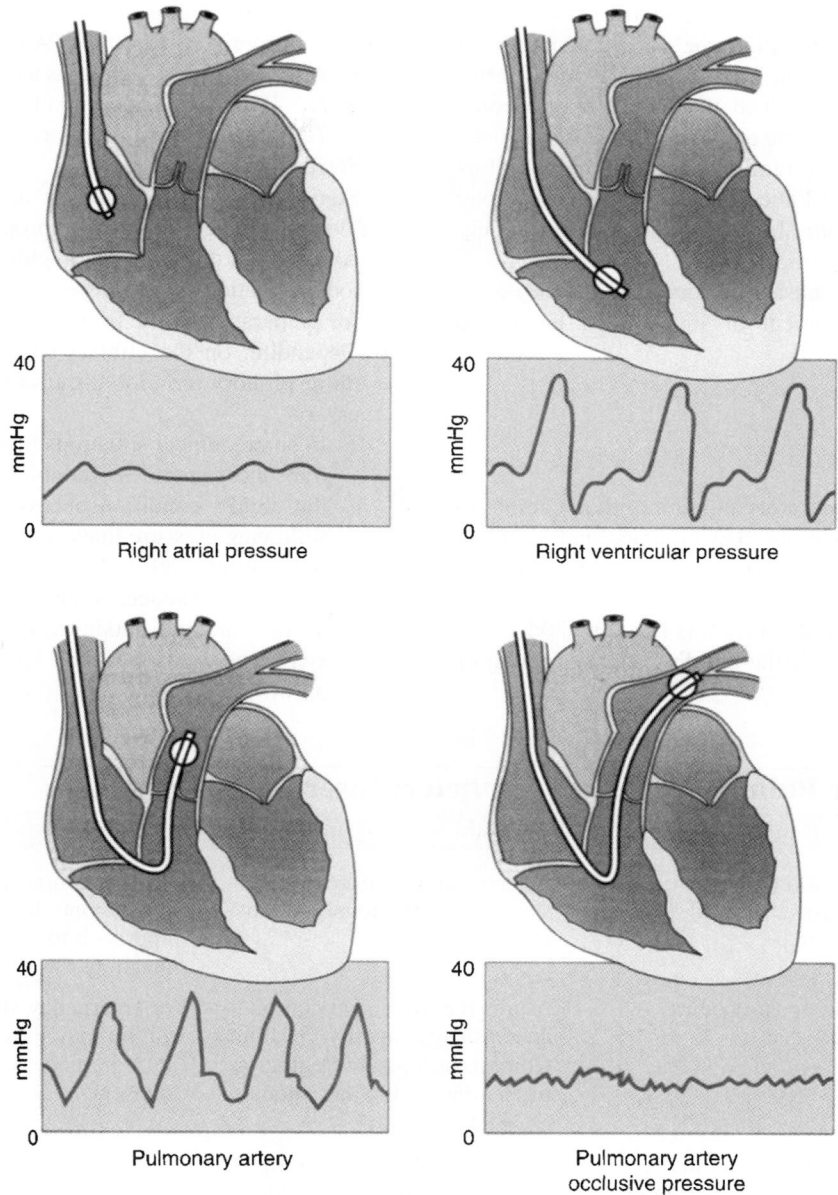

FIGURE 60-2   Catheter advancing through heart with appropriate waveforms. *From Lynn-McHale DJ, Carlson K, editors:* AACN procedure manual for critical care, *ed 4, Philadelphia, 2001, Saunders.*

- Identification of the presence of cardiac defects and repairs ➛➛*Rationale:* Cardiac defects and repairs may affect the ability to insert and use the catheter.
- Identification of preexisting cardiac arrhythmias ➛➛*Rationale:* Arrhythmias are a frequently seen complication during insertion of a PA catheter.
- Identification and correction of electrolyte and acid-base abnormalities before placement of the PA catheter ➛➛*Rationale:* A normal electrolyte and acid-base balance lowers the risk for prolonged arrhythmias.
- Child's level of sedation ➛➛*Rationale:* Appropriate sedation of the child prevents undue stress or pain during the procedure and facilitates insertion.
- Presence of functioning intravenous (IV) access ➛➛*Rationale:* Functioning IV access is necessary for

administration of emergency medications or sedation or analgesia as needed during the procedure.

CHILD AND FAMILY EDUCATION

Individualized, developmentally appropriate education is provided to the family and to the child based on desire for knowledge, readiness to learn, and overall neurologic and psychosocial state.

- Explain to the family and child (if appropriate) that medications will be used to keep the child comfortable and quiet during the procedure ➛➛*Rationale:* The explanation may decrease anxiety and fear of the family and child.

- Provide information about the reason for placement of the PA catheter and a timeframe for performing the procedure ➤➤*Rationale:* The time necessary for catheter insertion may be lengthy, and the family may become anxious. Providing a realistic time frame decreases anxiety.
- Explain to the child and family that additional monitoring lines will be placed and that additional alarms may be activated ➤➤*Rationale:* Information decreases anxiety and fear
- Encourage questions and answer questions as they arise ➤➤*Rationale:* Reinforcement of information is needed during periods of stress.

EQUIPMENT

- Appropriate cardiorespiratory monitor with the ability to display electrocardiographic (ECG) trace and to transduce and display pressure readings and waveforms
- Flow-directed PA catheter:
  - ❖ 5F, 70 cm if the child's weight is less than 20 kg
  - ❖ 7F or 7.5F, 110 cm if the child's weight is 20 kg or more[4]

- Cordis introducer catheter (Cordis Corporation, Miami, FL) appropriately sized for PA catheter
  - ❖ A 6F introducer catheter is used for the 5F PA catheter
  - ❖ A 7.5F or 8F introducer catheter is used for the 7F and 7.5F PA catheters, respectively
- Sterile catheter sleeve
- Sterile drapes, gowns, gloves, surgical masks, and caps
- Two transducer lines with appropriate monitor cables
- Antiseptic solution, such as chlorhexidine or povidone-iodine solution, depending on institution-specific protocol for preparation of the insertion site
- Depending on the clinical situation and available cardiorespiratory monitor, a transducer bridge may be necessary
  - ❖ In some clinical situations, the limit to the number of transducer modules available is reached. For instance, the child's condition necessitates monitoring of the following pressure lines: arterial, intracranial pressure monitoring, CVP and PA ports, which require the use of four transducer monitors. If the monitor only allows for three modules, a bridge can be set up to switch between CVP and PA port monitoring, which allows for spot checks of the CVP.

Procedure for Pulmonary Artery Catheter: Insertion Assist		
Steps	**Rationale**	**Considerations**
1. Ensure family and child (if appropriate) understand procedure and questions are answered.	Evaluates and reinforces understanding of previously taught information.	Developmental level, cognitive ability and anxiety level will determine approach to and effectiveness of teaching.
2. Confirm that consent for procedure has been obtained.	Ensures medical-legal compliance as suggested by the Joint Commission on Accreditation of Healthcare Organizations (JCAHO).	For emergency situations, the organization may have a protocol or procedure in place for assumption of consent.
3. Ensure that ECG monitoring is in place and that the child has functioning secondary venous access.	Continuous ECG monitoring is necessary during PA catheter insertion to monitor for arrhythmias. Functioning venous access is necessary for administration of emergency medications or sedation or analgesia as needed.	
4. Assemble equipment.	The presence of all materials facilitates completion of procedure in a timely manner.	
5. Provide for appropriate privacy; position the child to facilitate insertion of the catheter.	Promotes child's privacy and a sterile environment. Facilitates catheter insertion.	
6. Wash hands.	Standard precautions; reduces transmission of microorganisms.	
7. Prepare and prime transducer lines with appropriate fluid. Check all connections for security. See Procedure 63.	Transducer lines are used to transmit pressure readings and waveforms. Secure connections of system prevent air embolism.	Fluids used to prime lines may be premixed or prepared according to institution specific protocol.

Procedure for **Pulmonary Artery Catheter: Insertion Assist**—*Continued*		
Steps	**Rationale**	**Considerations**
8. Assess each transducer line to ensure correlating movement of the transduced waveforms displayed on the bedside monitor.	Ensures functioning of the system before the procedure.	
9. Zero each line according to manufacturer's recommendations at the phlebostatic axis.	Assures accurate pressure readings.	See Figure 137-2 for location of the phlebostatic axis.
10. Identify the child with appropriate patient and procedure verification process (e.g., "Time out").	Confirms correct patient, procedure, and site as recommended by the JCAHO; prevents unnecessary medical procedures.	The verification process and documentation are institution specific. Use active communication techniques.
11. After hand washing, caps, masks, gowns, and gloves are donned by operator (individual who inserts catheter) and by individuals who are participating in the procedure.	Decreases the risk of infection.	
12. Establish a sterile field.	Allows manipulation of sterile equipment and supplies without contamination; decreases the risk of infection.	
13. Assist with placement of the introducer catheter into a central vein.	The introducer provides a site to insert the PA catheter. The catheter is placed through a diaphragm in the introducer.	The right internal jugular or left subclavian vein is the preferred site of insertion. The right internal jugular vein produces a direct path into the right atrium. Rarely is the femoral vein usedbecause of difficulty in advancing the catheter into the right atrium.[5] See Procedure 140 for additional information.
14. Confirm the placement of the introducer with x-ray.	Ensures the correct placement of the introducer, which is necessary for correct insertion of the PA catheter.	Analysis of a blood sample as a secondary method of confirmation shows a CO_2 level consistent with a venous blood gas sample.
15. Prime lumens of PA catheter with appropriate sterile fluid.	Ensures patency of lumens and removes air from lumens, which prevents inadvertent air embolism.	Heparinized saline or 0.9% saline solution may be used to prime the catheter lumens, on the basis of operator and institution-specific preferences. Children with known sensitivity to heparin should only receive a saline solution prime.
16. Evaluate transducer lines for the presence of air bubbles.	Air bubbles should be removed to prevent air embolism.	An air embolism can be devastating for a child with an intracardiac shunt, which allows the embolism to travel to the brain.
17. Assist the operator with removal of the PA catheter from the packaging in a sterile manner.	The assistant should handle the port side of the catheter without contaminating the sterile packaging.	
18. Connect the distal port and the CVP port to transducer lines.	Allows waveforms to be displayed during catheter insertion.	On some catheters, the CVP port may be identified as the proximal port.

Procedure continues on following page

Procedure for Pulmonary Artery Catheter: Insertion Assist—*Continued*

Steps	Rationale	Considerations
19. If not previously done, connect the transducers to the bedside monitor.	Required for display of wave forms and numeric values.	
20. Secure transducers and zero them at the level of the phlebostatic access.	Ensures accurate pressure readings.	This establishes atmospheric pressure as the reference point with which obtained measurements are compared.
21. Adjust the scale of displayed transducer waveforms to obtain an optimum waveform.	An optimum scale allows the transduced waveform to be visualized during placement of the PA catheter.	The scale is dependent on the child's condition. A child with known pulmonary hypertension needs a larger scale to see the entire waveform.
22. Inflate PA catheter balloon.	Tests balloon's integrity before insertion.	This test should not be performed more than once to prevent dysfunction of the balloon. Avoid placing direct pressure on the balloon during inflation to prevent balloon rupture.
23. Gentle movement of catheter tip by the operator should reveal waveform changes on the monitor tracing.	This confirms that the transducer tracing works when catheter is in place.	
24. A sterile accordion sleeve is placed over the PA catheter before the PA catheter is inserted into the introducer.	The accordion sleeve allows for the minute movement of the PA catheter while maintaining sterility of the catheter.	
25. The catheter is inserted by the operator through the self-sealing valve in the introducer.	Seats the catheter in the vein prior to threading catheter.	
26. As the catheter is advanced, monitor the waveform displayed. Notify the operator when a right atrial waveform is noted.	The RA waveform will show minimal variation with a mean pressure consistent with CVP.	
27. At the direction of the operator, inflate PA catheter balloon to the appropriate volume as recommended by the package insert.	Inflating the balloon assists in "floating" the PA catheter into position.	The balloon should always be deflated when the catheter is withdrawn.
28. The operator advances the PA catheter with a constant steady motion until a wedge waveform appears (Figure 60-3). Notify the operator of ectopy as it occurs.	Note the progression in the change of the waveform as the catheter passes into the RV, the PA, and eventually the wedge position.	Ventricular ectopy is common when the PA catheter is passing through the RV. The practitioner should be aware of the ectopy and should be expeditious in movement through the RV.
29. Record a graphic wedge pressure for the medical record.	The PCWP is a reflection of the LA pressure in the absence of mitral stenosis or regurgitation.	The balloon should be wedged for no longer than 15 seconds to prevent ischemia in the distal pulmonary vasculature.
30. Deflate balloon.	The balloon should deflate fully and should only be wedged for a limited period of time.	Blood flow is negligible downstream from the PA when the balloon is inflated.
31. Note a pulsatile waveform with the balloon deflated.	Confirms that the catheter is no longer wedged, thus occluding a distal pulmonary arteriole.	The PA catheter should always have a pulsatile waveform when the balloon is not inflated.
32. The sterile accordion sleeve is connected to the introducer, which creates a seal.	Allows for small manipulations of the catheter within the sleeve without introducing bacteria into the bloodstream.	The catheter may migrate forward into a wedged position or backward into the RV. Either situation necessitates manipulation of the catheter.

Procedure	**for Pulmonary Artery Catheter Insertion: Assist**—*Continued*	
Steps	**Rationale**	**Considerations**

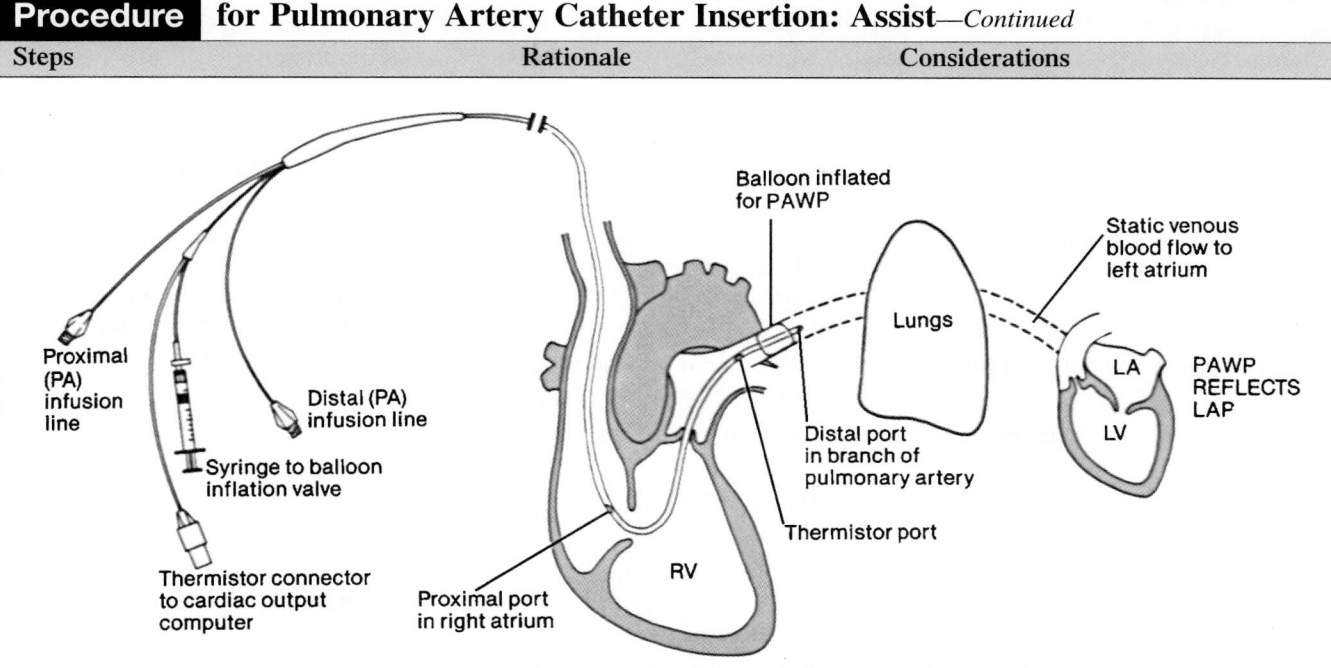

FIGURE 60-3   Pulmonary artery (PA) catheter location within heart. Pulmonary artery wedge pressure (PAWP) is indirect measure of left atrial and left ventricular end-diastolic pressure. *From Lynn-McHale DJ, Carlson KK, editors:* AACN procedure manual for critical care, *ed 4, Philadelphia, 2001, Saunders.*

Steps	Rationale	Considerations
33. Place a sterile dressing over the introducer.	Prevents insertion site infections.	Dressings should be changed and maintained according to institution-specific protocol.
34. Ensure that alarms are appropriately set and activated.	Properly set and functioning alarms provide notification of situations such as tubing disconnection or wedged catheter.	Alarm limits are set on the basis of parameters specific to the individual child.
35. Obtain a chest x-ray.	Verifies correct placement of the PA catheter. Radiographic abnormalities such as a pneumothorax are identified.	
36. Dispose of used equipment, including sharps, appropriately.	Standard precautions, reduces transmission of microorganisms. Protects personnel health.	
37. Cleanse child of any blood or excessive preparation solution.	If povidone-iodine is used to clean the skin, care should be taken to remove all visible povidone-iodine to prevent a burn.	
38. Remove gloves; wash hands.	Standard precautions.	

Procedure for PA Cathether Removal

Steps	Rationale	Considerations
1. Ensure family understands procedure and questions are answered.	Reinforces and evaluates previously taught information.	Developmental level, cognitive ability and anxiety level will determine approach to and effectiveness of teaching.
2. Place child in a supine position.	Allows for easy access and facilitates removal of PA catheter.	Institution-specific protocol or State Nurse Practice Act directs which individuals may remove PA catheters. Consult appropriate resources.
3. Wash hands and put on clean gloves.	Standard precautions; reduces risk of infection.	
4. Remove dressing from insertion site.	Necessary for access to the catheter.	
5. Discontinue all fluids running through PA catheter lumens.	Prevents fluid spills.	
6. Turn off the alarms for the PA and CVP waveforms.	Prevents false alarms.	The ECG alarm should remain on because ectopy may occur during catheter removal.
7. Deflate balloon completely and open balloon port to air.	Ensures complete deflation of the balloon, which prevents damage to structural components of the heart when catheter is removed.	
8. Secure introducer catheter with one hand and begin to remove the PA catheter with a continuous motion.	The ECG monitor should be observed for arrhythmias during the removal of the PA catheter, especially as it migrates through the RV.	If resistance is noted, *do not* proceed; contact the prescribing practitioner immediately. The catheter may be knotted or adhered, and forceful removal could damage cardiovascular structures.
9. After removal, inspect the catheter tip to ensure that it is intact.	Ensures removal of the entire catheter.	
10. Dispose of supplies and used equipment appropriately.	Standard precautions; reduces transmission of microorganisms.	
11. Remove gloves, wash hands.	Standard precautions; reduces risk of infection.	
12. After PA catheter is removed, a decision is made as to whether the introducer will remain in place. If introducer will remain, replace sterile dressing over introducer catheter.	Some introducer catheters leak unless a cap, obturator or occlusive dressing is placed over the diaphragm portion. An open diaphragm may result in infection, air embolism, or bleeding.	

Expected Outcomes	Unexpected Outcomes
• PA catheter tip is positioned in a distal pulmonary artery • Transducer waveforms are visible and monitored at all times • Child remains free from catheter complications • Child remains free from cardiac arrhythmias • Catheter ports and tip remain intact and balloon remains functional • Catheter is removed without difficulty	• Incorrect positioning of the PA catheter: aorta, subclavian artery, RV, or wedged position • Waveforms are not displayed • Monitor malfunction • Infection and sepsis • Pneumothorax or hemothorax • Hemorrhage • Local hematoma • Pericardial effusion • Infarction of the pulmonary artery • Pulmonary hemorrhage • Frequent ectopy • Catheter balloon rupture or failure • Air embolism • Knotting of the PA catheter • Inability to remove the PA catheter

Monitoring and Care of the Child

Activities and Interventions	Rationale	Reportable Conditions
1. Perform an assessment of child before and after the procedure that includes a cardiovascular, respiratory, and neurologic examination.	Allows for a baseline assessment for comparison of clinical changes during and after insertion of the PA catheter.	• Deterioration in cardiovascular, respiratory or neurological exam
2. Monitor cardiac rhythm continuously during catheter insertion and after insertion of the PA catheter.	Arrhythmias are common during placement and maintenance of PA catheters. Early identification and treatment of arrhythmias decrease detrimental effects.	• Ventricular arrhythmias (may be caused by migration of the catheter into the RV) • Sudden change in intracardiac pressures (may be caused by cardiac tamponade or pulmonary hypertensive crisis)
3. Monitor blood pressure at least every 5 minutes during procedure.	Identifies deterioration in status during placement of the PA catheter. Arterial line monitoring is preferred.	• Hypotension
4. Monitor waveforms continuously.	Allows early recognition of a displaced catheter.	• Wedged or RV waveform • Failure to occlude the pulmonary artery during balloon inflation • Lack of a pulsatile waveform when the balloon is deflated
5. Assess insertion site for signs of bleeding or infection. Maintain sterile integrity of the dressing.	Assures early recognition of treatable complications.	• Excessive bleeding around the insertion site • Rupture of the sterile accordion sheath (breeches sterility of the catheter)
6. Monitor catheter marking at level of introducer diaphragm.	Allows identification of change in depth of insertion, especially after patient movement, which may indicate migration of the PA catheter.	• Change in catheter marking at level of introducer diaphragm
7. Regularly assess the functioning of all catheter lumens.	Allows identification of a nonfunctioning catheter lumen.	• Inability to withdraw blood from port or inability to flush a port on the PA catheter (may be indicative of an occluded line)

Continued

Monitoring and Care of the Child—Cont'd

Activities and Interventions	Rationale	Reportable Conditions
8. Review chest x-ray results after placement of PA catheter.	Allows detection of a pneumothorax or hemothorax. Proper catheter position is verified.	• Increased respiratory distress or deterioration in blood gas values • Incorrect catheter tip placement • Knotting of catheter • Unresolved pain • Pain level greater than 5/10
9. Monitor levels of pain before, during, and after insertion of PA catheter using pain scale appropriate to child's age or developmental level; see Procedure 173: Pain Assessment Scales.	Ensures adequate analgesia and guides pain management in a critically ill child.	

Documentation

- Introducer size and location
- Institution specific documentation of patient/procedure verification process
- Name and certification of individual who inserted the catheter
- PA catheter size and centimeter marking at introducer diaphragm
- Presence of signed consent for procedure
- Chest x-ray results
- Child and family education
- Child's tolerance of the procedure
- Waveform identification with graphic trends placed in the permanent medical record
- Intracardiac pressure readings
- Assessment of insertion site
- Child's status before and after procedure
- Unexpected outcomes and related treatment

References

1. Fuhrman BP, Zimmerman JJ, editors: *Pediatric critical care,* ed 3, Philadelphia, 2006, Mosby.
2. Lynn-McHale Wiegand DJ, Carlson K, editors: *AACN procedure manual for critical care,* ed 5, Philadelphia, 2005, Saunders.
3. Ivanov R, et al: The incidence of major morbidity in critically ill patients managed with pulmonary artery catheters: a meta-analysis, *Crit Care Med* 28(3):615-618, 2000.
4. Dieckmann RA, et al, editors: *Illustrated textbook of pediatric emergency & critical care procedures,* St Louis, 1997, Mosby.
5. Truwit JD: The pulmonary artery catheter in the ICU, part 1: technique and measurements, *J Crit Illness* 18(1):9-18, 2003.

Additional Readings

Pollack MM: Bedside pulmonary artery catheterization in pediatrics, *J Pediatr* 96(2):274-276, 1980.
Roizen MG: Practice guidelines for pulmonary artery catheterization. An updated report by the American Society of Anesthesiologist Task Force on Pulmonary Artery Catheterization, *Anesthesiology* 99(4): 2003.
Salm TJV, et al: *Atlas of bedside procedures,* ed 2, Boston, 1988, Little, Brown and Company.

Heart Rate and Blood Pressure: Obtaining an Accurate Measurement

P U R P O S E : Heart rate (HR) and noninvasive blood pressure (NIBP) measurements are essential elements of the pediatric physical assessment. Correct measurement technique is imperative to ensure accurate values.

Andrea Torzone

PREREQUISITE KNOWLEDGE

- Heart rate and NIBP are physiologic parameters. In addition to physical assessment, HR and NIBP values are a basis for major diagnostic and therapeutic decisions; therefore, measurements must be correct and reproducible.[1]
- Heart rate and NIBP values that fall out of the expected range warrant further physical examination, investigation, and notification of the prescribing practitioner.
- Blood pressure (BP) evaluation should be included as part of a complete physical assessment of the pediatric patient.[2]
  - ❖ Auscultation is the preferred method of BP measurement.[3,4]
  - ❖ Repeated measurements over time, rather than a single isolated determination, are necessary for establishment of consistent and significant observations.[2]
  - ❖ Elevated BP values in children correlate with hypertension in early adulthood.[3]
- Heart rate should be measured for a full minute, by listening on the chest to the apical pulse at the apex of the heart and by palpating the peripheral pulse (Table 61-1 shows age-specific heart rates).
- Blood pressure values obtained with noninvasive methods can be reliable and consistent if recorded in standardized conditions with a well-functioning measurement device.[2]
- Blood pressure can be noninvasively measured with the auscultatory method (sphygmomanometer), oscillomet-

TABLE 61-1	Age-Specific Heart Rates
Age	**Heart Rate (bpm)**
<1 d	93 to 154
1 to 2 d	90 to 150
3 to 6 d	90 to 165
1 to 3 wk	105 to 180
1 to 2 mo	120 to 180
3 to 5 mo	105 to 185
6 to 11 mo	110 to 170
1 to 2 y	90 to 150
3 to 4 y	73 to 140
5 to 7 y	65 to 130
8 to 11 y	60 to 130
12 to 15 y	60 to 120

Table adapted from information in Craig J, Smith JB, Fineman L: Tissue perfusion. In Curley MAQ, Moloney-Harmon PA, editors: *Critical care nursing of infants and children*, ed 2, Philadelphia, 2001, Saunders, and Gunn VL, Nechyba C: *Johns Hopkins: The Harriet Lane handbook: a manual for pediatric house officers*, ed 16, Philadelphia, 2002, Mosby.

ric devices, or palpation. Oscillometric devices are electronic units that provide accurate systolic BP readings in infants and children in whom auscultatory measurements are difficult to obtain.[2]

- ❖ In sphygmomanometry, the pressure necessary to collapse the artery in the arm or leg is determined with inflation of the cuff. As the cuff is deflated, the pressure is noted as sounds produced by the arterial pulse waves (Korotkoff's sounds) appear and disappear again as flow through the artery resumes.[1]

❖ Korotkoff's sounds
  ○ K1: First appearance of clear, repetitive, tapping sounds, which coincides with reappearance of a palpable pulse. The pressure at which this occurs corresponds to systolic blood pressure.
  ○ K2: Sounds are softer and longer, with the quality of an intermittent murmur
  ○ K3: Sounds become crisper and louder
  ○ K4: Sounds are muffled, less distinct, and softer
  ○ K5: Disappearance of Korotkoff's sounds. K5 is a reliable measure of diastolic BP for children.[1,3]

• Automated devices are useful in situations in which auscultation is difficult, such as in infants and in the intensive care setting, where frequent BP measurements are necessary. Automated devices use oscillometric methods for measurement of BP, with detection of oscillations on the walls of the occluded artery as the cuff is deflated. Systolic and mean BP values are measured, but diastolic BP is a derived value and therefore may not be accurate.[1,4,5] In most circumstances, the recommended method of BP measurement in children is auscultation.[3]

• In situations in which NIBP is unobtainable with auscultation or oscillometric device, an approximation of systolic pressure may be obtained with palpation of the radial pulse, with rapid inflation of the cuff until the pulse is no longer felt and then slow deflation of the cuff until the pulse is felt again. This method is not preferred because it provides only an approximation of systolic pressure.[6]

❖ In a modification of this technique, a Doppler sensor is placed over the artery and the pulse signal is identified. The cuff is rapidly inflated until the sound is lost and then slowly deflated until the pulse signal is heard again. This method is not preferred because it provides only an approximation of systolic pressure.

❖ Systole: Contraction of the heart, especially of the ventricles, by which the blood is driven through the aorta and pulmonary artery to traverse the systemic and pulmonary circulations, respectively; its occurrence is indicated physically by the first sound of the heart heard on auscultation, by the palpable apex beat, and by the arterial pulse

❖ Diastole: Normal postsystolic dilation of the heart cavities, during which they fill with blood; diastole of the atria precedes that of the ventricles, and diastole of either chamber alternates rhythmically with systole or contraction of that chamber

• Body size is the most important determinant of BP in childhood and adolescence.[3] BP measurements vary with the size of a child. Current charts for BP values in children are based on gender, age, and height, which allow consideration of different levels of growth and body size in evaluation of BP.

• Normal BP is defined as systolic and diastolic BP less than the 90th percentile for age and gender.[3] Tables 61-2 and 61-3 show normal values.

• Prehypertensive BP is defined as average systolic or diastolic BP greater than or equal to the 90th percentile but less than the 95th percentile.[3]

| TABLE 61-2 | BP Levels for Boys by Age and Height Percentile |

		SBP, mm Hg							DBP, mm Hg						
		Percentile of Height							Percentile of Height						
Age, yr	BP Percentile	5th	10th	25th	50th	75th	90th	95th	5th	10th	25th	50th	75th	90th	95th
1	50th	80	81	83	85	87	88	89	34	35	36	37	38	39	39
	90th	94	95	97	99	100	102	103	49	50	51	52	53	53	54
	95th	98	99	101	103	104	106	106	54	54	55	56	57	58	58
	99th	105	106	108	110	112	113	114	61	62	63	64	65	66	66
2	50th	84	85	87	88	90	92	92	39	40	41	42	43	44	44
	90th	97	99	100	102	104	105	106	54	55	56	57	58	58	59
	95th	101	102	104	106	108	109	110	59	59	60	61	62	63	63
	99th	109	110	111	113	115	117	117	66	67	68	69	70	71	71
3	50th	86	87	89	91	93	94	95	44	44	45	46	47	48	48
	90th	100	101	103	105	107	108	109	59	59	60	61	62	63	63
	95th	104	105	107	109	110	112	113	63	63	64	65	66	67	67
	99th	111	112	114	116	118	119	120	71	71	72	73	74	75	75
4	50th	88	89	91	93	95	96	97	47	48	49	50	51	51	52
	90th	102	103	105	107	109	110	111	62	63	64	65	66	66	67
	95th	106	107	109	111	112	114	115	66	67	68	69	70	71	71
	99th	113	114	116	118	120	121	122	74	75	76	77	78	78	79
5	50th	90	91	93	95	96	98	98	50	51	52	53	54	55	55
	90th	104	105	106	108	110	111	112	65	66	67	68	69	69	70
	95th	108	109	110	112	114	115	116	69	70	71	72	73	74	74
	99th	115	116	118	120	121	123	123	77	78	79	80	81	81	82
6	50th	91	92	94	96	98	99	100	53	53	54	55	56	57	57

TABLE 61-2	**BP Levels for Boys by Age and Height Percentile—Cont'd**

		SBP, mm Hg							DBP, mm Hg						
		Percentile of Height							Percentile of Height						
Age, yr	BP Percentile	*5th*	*10th*	*25th*	*50th*	*75th*	*90th*	*95th*	*5th*	*10th*	*25th*	*50th*	*75th*	*90th*	*95th*
	90th	105	106	108	110	111	113	113	68	68	69	70	71	72	72
	95th	109	110	112	114	115	117	117	72	72	73	74	75	76	76
	99th	116	117	119	121	123	124	125	80	80	81	82	83	84	84
7	50th	92	94	95	97	99	100	101	55	55	56	57	58	59	59
	90th	106	107	109	111	113	114	115	70	70	71	72	73	74	74
	95th	110	111	113	115	117	118	119	74	74	75	76	77	78	78
	99th	117	118	120	122	124	125	126	82	82	83	84	85	86	86
8	50th	94	95	97	99	100	102	102	56	57	58	59	60	60	61
	90th	107	109	110	112	114	115	116	71	72	72	73	74	75	76
	95th	111	112	114	116	118	119	120	75	76	77	78	79	79	80
	99th	119	120	122	123	125	127	127	83	84	85	86	87	87	88
9	50th	95	96	98	100	102	103	104	57	58	59	60	61	61	62
	90th	109	110	112	114	115	117	118	72	73	74	75	76	76	77
	95th	113	114	116	118	119	121	121	76	77	78	79	80	81	81
	99th	120	121	123	125	127	128	129	84	85	86	87	88	88	89
10	50th	97	98	100	102	103	105	106	58	59	60	61	61	62	63
	90th	111	112	114	115	117	119	119	73	73	74	75	76	77	78
	95th	115	116	117	119	121	122	123	77	78	79	80	81	81	82
	99th	122	123	125	127	128	130	130	85	86	86	88	88	89	90
11	50th	99	100	102	104	105	107	107	59	59	60	61	62	63	63
	90th	113	114	115	117	119	120	121	74	74	75	76	77	78	78
	95th	117	118	119	121	123	124	125	78	78	79	80	81	82	82
	99th	124	125	127	129	130	132	132	86	86	87	88	89	90	90
12	50th	101	102	104	106	108	109	110	59	60	61	62	63	63	64
	90th	115	116	118	120	121	123	123	74	75	75	76	77	78	79
	95th	119	120	122	123	125	127	127	78	79	80	81	82	82	83
	99th	126	127	129	131	133	134	135	86	87	88	89	90	90	91
13	50th	104	105	106	108	110	111	112	60	60	61	62	63	64	64
	90th	117	118	120	122	124	125	126	75	75	76	77	78	79	79
	95th	121	122	124	126	128	129	130	79	79	80	81	82	83	83
	99th	128	130	131	133	135	136	137	87	87	88	89	90	91	91
14	50th	106	107	109	111	113	114	115	60	61	62	63	64	65	65
	90th	120	121	123	125	126	128	128	75	76	77	78	79	79	80
	95th	124	125	127	128	130	132	132	80	80	81	82	83	84	84
	99th	131	132	134	136	138	139	140	87	88	89	90	91	92	92
15	50th	109	110	112	113	115	117	117	61	62	63	64	65	66	66
	90th	122	124	125	127	129	130	131	76	77	78	79	80	80	81
	95th	126	127	129	131	133	134	135	81	81	82	83	84	85	85
	99th	134	135	136	138	140	142	142	88	89	90	91	92	93	93
16	50th	111	112	114	116	118	119	120	63	63	64	65	66	67	67
	90th	125	126	128	130	131	133	134	78	78	79	80	81	82	82
	95th	129	130	132	134	135	137	137	82	83	83	84	85	86	87
	99th	136	137	139	141	143	144	145	90	90	91	92	93	94	94
17	50th	114	115	116	118	120	121	122	65	66	66	67	68	69	70
	90th	127	128	130	132	134	135	136	80	80	81	82	83	84	84
	95th	131	132	134	136	138	139	140	84	85	86	87	87	88	89
	99th	139	140	141	143	145	146	147	92	93	93	94	95	96	97

The 90th percentile is 1.28 SD, the 95th percentile is 1.645 SD, and the 99th percentile is 2.326 SD over the mean.

Blood Pressure Level for Boys by Age and Height Percentile From National High Blood Pressure Education Program Working Group on High Blood Pressure in Children and Adolescents: The fourth report on the diagnosis, evaluation, and treatment & high blood pressure in children and adolescents, *Pediatrics* 114:555-576, 2004.

TABLE 61-3	BP Levels for Girls by Age and Height Percentile

Age, yr	BP Percentile	SBP, mm Hg							DBP, mm Hg						
		Percentile of Height							Percentile of Height						
		5th	*10th*	*25th*	*50th*	*75th*	*90th*	*95th*	*5th*	*10th*	*25th*	*50th*	*75th*	*90th*	*95th*
1	50th	83	84	85	86	88	89	90	38	39	39	40	41	41	42
	90th	97	97	98	100	101	102	103	52	53	53	54	55	55	56
	95th	100	101	102	104	105	106	107	56	57	57	58	59	59	60
	99th	108	108	109	111	112	113	114	64	64	65	65	66	67	67
2	50th	85	85	87	88	89	91	91	43	44	44	45	46	46	47
	90th	98	99	100	101	103	104	105	57	58	58	59	60	61	61
	95th	102	103	104	105	107	108	109	61	62	62	63	64	65	65
	99th	109	110	111	112	114	115	116	69	69	70	70	71	72	72
3	50th	86	87	88	89	91	92	93	47	48	48	49	50	50	51
	90th	100	100	102	103	104	106	106	61	62	62	63	64	64	65
	95th	104	104	105	107	108	109	110	65	66	66	67	68	68	69
	99th	111	111	113	114	115	116	117	73	73	74	74	75	76	76
4	50th	88	88	90	91	92	94	94	50	50	51	52	52	53	54
	90th	101	102	103	104	106	107	108	64	64	65	66	67	67	68
	95th	105	106	107	108	110	111	112	68	68	69	70	71	71	72
	99th	112	113	114	115	117	118	119	76	76	76	77	78	79	79
5	50th	89	90	91	93	94	95	96	52	53	53	54	55	55	56
	90th	103	103	105	106	107	109	109	66	67	67	68	69	69	70
	95th	107	107	108	110	111	112	113	70	71	71	72	73	73	74
	99th	114	114	116	117	118	120	120	78	78	79	79	80	81	81
6	50th	91	92	93	94	96	97	98	54	54	55	56	56	57	58
	90th	104	105	106	108	109	110	111	68	68	69	70	70	71	72
	95th	108	109	110	111	113	114	115	72	72	73	74	74	75	76
	99th	115	116	117	119	120	121	122	80	80	80	81	82	83	83
7	50th	93	93	95	96	97	99	99	55	56	56	57	58	58	59
	90th	106	107	108	109	111	112	113	69	70	70	71	72	72	73
	95th	110	111	112	113	115	116	116	73	74	74	75	76	76	77
	99th	117	118	119	120	122	123	124	81	81	82	82	83	84	84
8	50th	95	95	96	98	99	100	101	57	57	57	58	59	60	60
	90th	108	109	110	111	113	114	114	71	71	71	72	73	74	74
	95th	112	112	114	115	116	118	118	75	75	75	76	77	78	78
	99th	119	120	121	122	123	125	125	82	82	83	83	84	85	86
9	50th	96	97	98	100	101	102	103	58	58	58	59	60	61	61
	90th	110	110	112	113	114	116	116	72	72	72	73	74	75	75
	95th	114	114	115	117	118	119	120	76	76	76	77	78	79	79
	99th	121	121	123	124	125	127	127	83	83	84	84	85	86	87
10	50th	98	99	100	102	103	104	105	59	59	59	60	61	62	62
	90th	112	112	114	115	116	118	118	73	73	73	74	75	76	76
	95th	116	116	117	119	120	121	122	77	77	77	78	79	80	80
	99th	123	123	125	126	127	129	129	84	84	85	86	86	87	88
11	50th	100	101	102	103	105	106	107	60	60	60	61	62	63	63
	90th	114	114	116	117	118	119	120	74	74	74	75	76	77	77
	95th	118	118	119	121	122	123	124	78	78	78	79	80	81	81
	99th	125	125	126	128	129	130	131	85	85	86	87	87	88	89
12	50th	102	103	104	105	107	108	109	61	61	61	62	63	64	64
	90th	116	116	117	119	120	121	122	75	75	75	76	77	78	78
	95th	119	120	121	123	124	125	126	79	79	79	80	81	82	82
	99th	127	127	128	130	131	132	133	86	86	87	88	88	89	90
13	50th	104	105	106	107	109	110	110	62	62	62	63	64	65	65
	90th	117	118	119	121	122	123	124	76	76	76	77	78	79	79
	95th	121	122	123	124	126	127	128	80	80	80	81	82	83	83
	99th	128	129	130	132	133	134	135	87	87	88	89	89	90	91
14	50th	106	106	107	109	110	111	112	63	63	63	64	65	66	66
	90th	119	120	121	122	124	125	125	77	77	77	78	79	80	80
	95th	123	123	125	126	127	129	129	81	81	81	82	83	84	84

TABLE 61-3	BP Levels for Girls by Age and Height Percentile—Cont'd

		SBP, mm Hg							DBP, mm Hg						
		Percentile of Height							Percentile of Height						
Age, yr	BP Percentile	*5th*	*10th*	*25th*	*50th*	*75th*	*90th*	*95th*	*5th*	*10th*	*25th*	*50th*	*75th*	*90th*	*95th*
	99th	130	131	132	133	135	136	136	88	88	89	90	90	91	92
15	50th	107	108	109	110	111	113	113	64	64	64	65	66	67	67
	90th	120	121	122	123	125	126	127	78	78	78	79	80	81	81
	95th	124	125	126	127	129	130	131	82	82	82	83	84	85	85
	99th	131	132	133	134	136	137	138	89	89	90	91	91	92	93
16	50th	108	108	110	111	112	114	114	64	64	65	66	66	67	68
	90th	121	122	123	124	126	127	128	78	78	79	80	81	81	82
	95th	125	126	127	128	130	131	132	82	82	83	84	85	85	86
	99th	132	133	134	135	137	138	139	90	90	90	91	92	93	93
17	50th	108	109	110	111	113	114	115	64	65	65	66	67	67	68
	90th	122	122	123	125	126	127	128	78	79	79	80	81	81	82
	95th	125	126	127	129	130	131	132	82	83	83	84	85	85	86
	99th	133	133	134	136	137	138	139	90	90	91	91	92	93	93

The 90th percentile is 1.28 SD, the 95th percentile is 1.645 SD, and the 99th percentile is 2.326 SD over the mean.

Blood Pressure Level for Boys by Age and Height Percentile From National High Blood Pressure Education Program Working Group on High Blood Pressure in Children and Adolescents: The fourth report on the diagnosis, evaluation, and treatment & high blood pressure in children and adolescents, *Pediatrics* 114:555-576, 2004.

- Hypertension is defined as average systolic or diastolic BP greater than or equal to the 95th percentile for age and gender measured on at least three separate occasions[3]
- Hypertension in children has many causes, including renal artery thrombosis or stenosis, congenital renal malformations, renal parenchymal diseases, coarctation of the aorta, and bronchopulmonary dysplasia, in addition to primary hypertension[2]

CHILD AND FAMILY ASSESSMENT

- Child's developmental level and ability to interact ➻*Rationale:* These factors influence preparation and interaction.
- Diagnosis and reason for obtaining HR and BP ➻*Rationale:* Diagnosis or other considerations may affect method and location selected to obtain HR or BP.
- Child's level of anxiety ➻*Rationale:* Evaluates anxiety and fear; child's apprehension may affect HR and BP values.
- Child's and family's understanding of the reasons for and risks and benefits of the procedure ➻*Rationale:* Evaluates the child's and family's understanding of the procedure and provides a gauge for ongoing education.

CHILD AND FAMILY EDUCATION

Individualized, developmentally appropriate education is provided to the child and to the family based on desire for knowledge, readiness to learn, and overall neurologic and psychosocial state. Answer questions as they arise and reinforce information as needed.

- Explain the reason for obtaining HR and BP values to the family and child, if developmentally appropriate ➻*Rationale:* Education and information reduce fear of the unknown. Anxiety and fear may alter values obtained; explanation of the procedure may calm the child and provide a more accurate measurement.
- If developmentally appropriate, explain how the child can help during HR and BP measurement (i.e., quietly sitting still) ➻*Rationale:* Measurement may be affected by the child's movement, crying, or apprehension.
- Inform the child that the cuff squeezes or "hugs" the arm and that this sensation lasts only a short time ➻*Rationale:* Sensory information about a procedure before the procedure is performed to help children tolerate and cooperate with the procedure.

EQUIPMENT

- Alcohol pad
- Stethoscope
- Sphygmomanometer
- Cuff of appropriate size for child with sphygmomanometer or automated device for oscillometric measurement

Procedure for HR and BP: Obtaining an Accurate Measurement

Steps	Rationale	Considerations
1. Ensure child and family understand procedure and questions are answered.	The procedure is easier to complete when child and family understand it.	The child's and family's understanding of the procedure is influenced by developmental levels.
2. Select appropriate size of BP cuff. Estimate with inspection or measure the circumference of the bare upper arm at the midpoint between the shoulder and elbow and select an appropriate size cuff. The bladder width should be approximately 40% of the arm circumference. The bladder inside cuff should encircle 80% to 100% of the circumference of the arm in children less than 13 years old (Figure 61-1).[3] *(Level II*)*	Proper cuff size is crucial for accurate BP measurement. To measure BP in children 3 years of age, cuff sizes available should include: Three pediatric cuffs of varying sizes Standard adult cuff Oversized cuff Thigh cuff for leg BP measurement[2,3]	Use of a smaller cuff than appropriate leads to falsely high BP readings; use of a cuff that is wider or larger than appropriate may produce falsely low readings. Neonatal and infant cuffs are available in a variety of sizes.

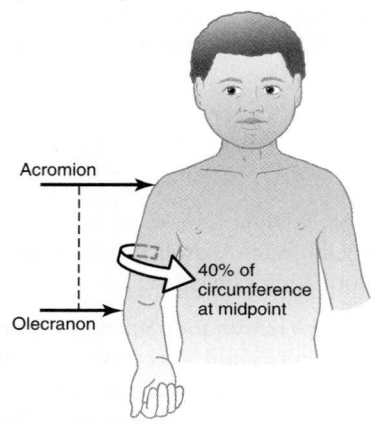

A. Determination of proper cuff size: step 1. The cuff bladder width should be approximately 40% of the circumference of the arm measured at a point midway between the olecranon and acromion

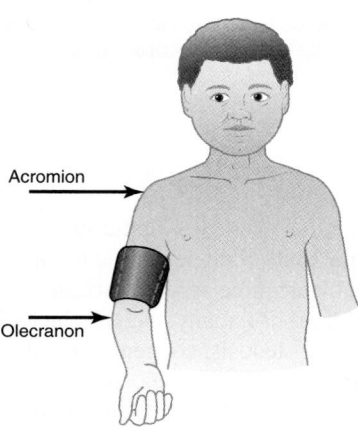

B. Determination of proper cuff size: step 2. The cuff bladder should cover 80% to 100% of the circumference of the arm.

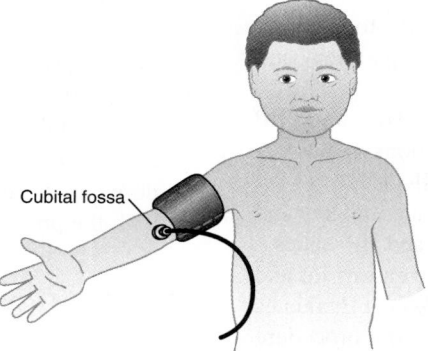

C. Blood pressure measurement: Blood pressure should be measured with cubital fossa at heart level. The arm should be supported. The stethoscope bell is placed over the brachial artery pulse, proximal and medial to the cubital fossas, below the bottom edge of the cuff.

FIGURE 61-1   Determination of Proper Cuff Size for the Child. *Redrawn from National High Blood Pressure Education Program Working Group on Hypertension Control in Children and Adolescents: Update on the 1987 Task Force Report on High Blood Pressure in Children and Adolescents: a working group report from the National High Blood Pressure Education Program, Pediatrics 98:651, 1996.*

* Level II: Theory-based; no research data to support recommendations; recommendations from expert consensus group may exist

Procedure for HR and BP: Obtaining an Accurate Measurement—*Continued*

Steps	Rationale	Considerations
3. Collect additional equipment needed.	Correct equipment ensures that accurate readings are obtained.	
4. Provide a quiet examination area. Calm and reassure the child. Allow time to recover from recent activity or apprehension.	Facilitates accurate reading.	Accurate HR and BP values are difficult to obtain in the moving or agitated child. Being held by a parent may calm an infant and increase a young child's comfort.
5. Wash hands.	Standard precautions; reduces the transmission of microorganisms.	
6. Position child to allow access to chest and arm. When child is comfortable and quiet, listen with stethoscope to the apical pulse on chest for 1 full minute to obtain heart rate. Palpate child's pulse (brachial for infants; radial for child) for 1 full minute and compare the values.	Auscultation of HR combined with palpation of pulse for a full minute allows identification of arrhythmias and discrepancies between heart sounds and pulse.	Ensure that the child is calm and comfortable in the selected position.

To Obtain a BP Value with Auscultation:

Steps	Rationale	Considerations
7. To obtain a BP value, position child sitting or infant supine. BP should be measured after at least 3 to 5 minutes of rest, with midpoint of the arm supported at heart level.[3] *(Level II*)*	The sitting position ensures that midpoint of arm is at the level of the heart.	Sitting upright is the optimal position for BP measurement, but critically ill children should remain in a position to maintain hemodynamic stability.
8. Palpate brachial artery and place cuff so that the midline of the bladder is over arterial pulsation and then wrap and secure the cuff snugly around child's bare upper arm.	Proper cuff application improves the accuracy of measurement.	Clothing with sleeves should be removed. Rolling up a sleeve may cause a tourniquet effect around the upper arm. Use of alternate locations to obtain a BP measurement, such as calf or thigh, may be necessary.
9. Place the earpieces of the stethoscope in the ears, angled forward.	Proper positioning of the earpieces allows the best sound transmission.	A quiet room allows for easier listening to Korotkoff's sounds.
10. Gently place bell of stethoscope over the brachial artery pulsation, just above the antecubital fossa but below the lower edge of cuff (see Figure 61-1).	The bell, or low-frequency filter, of stethoscope allows more accurate auscultation of Korotkoff's sounds than does the diaphragm. Excessive pressure on brachial artery may affect Korotkoff's sounds.	
11. Palpate radial pulse. Inflate cuff rapidly to 20 mm Hg above the point where radial pulse disappears. Partially open valve and deflate bladder at 2 mm Hg/second and while listening to the brachial pulsation.	Once radial pulse is no longer palpated, the fingers may be removed from site to deflate the valve easily.	Deflating the cuff too rapidly may cause inaccurate BP measurements.
12. As pressure in cuff decreases, note the pressure reading on the manometer for first appearance of tapping Korotkoff's sounds (K1).[1]	K1 indicates systolic BP.[1] *(Level II)*	

Procedure continues on following page

Procedure	for HR and BP: Obtaining an Accurate Measurement—*Continued*	
Steps	**Rationale**	**Special Considerations**
13. Note pressure reading when the Korotkoff's sounds muffle (K4) and when sounds disappear (K5).[1]	Korotkoff's sounds can often be heard through entire period of cuff deflation; K5 (absence of sounds) denotes diastolic BP in children less than 13 years of age.[1] *(Level II*)*	
14. After the last Korotkoff's sounds are heard, completely deflate the cuff.		
15. Immediately record systolic and diastolic values, rounded upwards to the nearest 2 mm Hg. When sounds are heard until a level of 0 mm Hg, phase K4 value should be recorded also.	Record measurements immediately so as not to forget.	
16. Repeat measurement after at least 30 seconds and average the two readings.	BP value varies widely from physiologic variables; BP values should be measured at least twice and averaged.	
17. Record site used to obtain the measurement, cuff size, and child's position.	Allows reproduction of measurement in the same location, with the same cuff, in the same position. Differences in BP measurements in extremities may signal pathology and warrant further evaluation.	Hypertension in upper extremities with a lower BP value in lower extremities may signal coarctation of the aorta, which necessitates further investigation.
18. Wash hands.	Standard precautions; reduces the transmission of microorganisms.	
To obtain a BP value with an oscillometric device:		
19. Ensure device is functioning correctly and that a safety inspection has been completed appropriately.	Ensures accurate readings; promotes patient safety.	
20. Ensure device is set for a mode appropriate for child's size and type of cuff being used.	Ensures accurate readings and prevents unnecessarily high inflation of the cuff that causes excessive discomfort to child.	
21. To obtain BP value, position child sitting or the infant supine. BP should be measured after at least 3 to 5 minutes of rest, with the midpoint of the arm supported at heart level.[3] *(Level II*)*	The sitting position ensures that the midpoint of the arm is at the level of the heart.	Sitting upright is an optimal position for BP measurement, but critically ill children should remain in a position to maintain hemodynamic stability.
22. Palpate the brachial artery and place the cuff so that midline of the bladder is over the arterial pulsation and then wrap and secure the cuff snugly around child's bare upper arm.	Proper cuff application improves the accuracy of measurement.	Clothing with sleeves should be removed. Rolling up a sleeve may cause a tourniquet effect around the upper arm. Use of alternate locations, such as calf or thigh, may be necessary to obtain a BP measurement.
23. Activate the device to initiate the BP measurement.	Initiates measurement.	

* Level II: Theory-based; no research data to support recommendations; recommendations from expert consensus group may exist

Procedure for HR and BP: Obtaining an Accurate Measurement—*Continued*

Steps	Rationale	Special Considerations
24. Record measurements displayed for systolic, diastolic, and mean measurements.	Documents measurements obtained.	
25. Record site used to obtain measurement, cuff size, and child's position.	Allows reproduction of measurement in the same location, with the same cuff, in the same position. Differences in BP measurements in extremities may signal pathology and warrant further evaluation.	Hypertension in the upper extremities with a lower BP value in the lower extremities may signal coarctation of the aorta, which necessitates further investigation.
26. If device is to be used for ongoing BP monitoring, set and activate appropriate alarms.	Notifies nurse of abnormal values and promotes patient safety.	

Expected Outcomes

- Accurate values for HR and BP are obtained and recorded

- Child tolerates the procedure with minimal discomfort

Unexpected Outcomes

- Inaccurate HR and BP values obtained due to various factors, including incorrect procedure; inappropriate cuff size; anxious, agitated, or crying children; noise in examination room that makes Korotkoff's sounds difficult to hear; and small size of infants
- Child is unable to tolerate the procedure

Monitoring and Care of the Child

Activities and Interventions	Rationale	Reportable Conditions
1. Calm the patient before measurement of HR and BP.	Agitation, movement, or crying may lead to inaccurate HR and BP measurements.	• Heart rate or BP values that are higher or lower than expected or vary significantly from baseline values for the specific child • Differences of more than 10 mm Hg between upper and lower extremity BP values
2. Monitor child's ability to tolerate the procedure.	Heart rate and BP values are obtained frequently in acute and critical care setting.	• Inability to obtain BP value because of agitation or other factors

Documentation

- Blood pressure measurement, including date and time, position of the child, and limb and cuff size used
- Prescribing practitioner notified in the case of unexpected or abnormal HR or BP value and related treatment
- Heart rate measurement
- Child's response to the procedure
- Child and family education

References

1. Perloff D, et al: Human blood pressure determination by sphygmomanometry, *Circulation* 88:2460-2467, 1993.
2. Task Force on Blood Pressure Control in Children: Report of the Second Task Force on Blood Pressure Control in Children—1987, From the National Heart, Lung, and Blood Institute, Bethesda, MD, *Pediatrics* 79:1-24, 1987.
3. National High Blood Pressure Education Program Working Group on Hypertension Control in Children and Adolescents: Update on the 1987 Task Force Report on High Blood Pressure in Children and Adolescents: a working group report from the National High Blood Pressure Education Program, *Pediatrics* 98:649-658, 1996.
4. National High Blood Pressure Education Program Working Group on High Blood Pressure in Children and Adolescents: The fourth report on the diagnosis, evaluation, and treatment of high blood pressure in children and adolescents, *Pediatrics* 114:555-576, 2004.
5. Park M, et al: Comparison of auscultatory and oscillometric blood pressures, *Arch Pediatr Adolesc Med* 155:50-53, 2001.
6. Craig J, et al: Tissue perfusion. In Curley MAQ, Moloney-Harmon PA, Editors: *Critical care nursing of infants and children,* Philadelphia, 2001, Saunders.

Additional Reading

Bates B: *A guide to physical examination and history taking,* ed 6, Philadelphia, 1995, JB Lippincott Company.

Left Atrial Intracardiac Line: Care and Management

P U R P O S E : In the operating room, a left atrial intracardiac catheter is inserted following an intracardiac surgical procedure before the discontinuation of cardiopulmonary bypass, and is used to obtain data regarding pulmonary venous pressure and saturation; left ventricular preload, afterload, and function; intracardiac shunting; and systemic intravascular volume status in the intraoperative and postoperative periods

Dorothy M. Beke and Patricia Lincoln

PREREQUISITE KNOWLEDGE

- Normal cardiac anatomy and physiology
- Familiarity with postoperative care requirements of infants and children after cardiac surgery and ability to identify which types of cardiac defects warrant the use of left atrial (LA) pressure monitoring
- The individual child's congenital heart defect and the surgical procedure performed
- In the operating room left atrial catheters (LACs) or lines are placed in infants and children undergoing open heart surgery, whose postoperative management is influenced by data regarding pulmonary venous pressure and saturation, left ventricular preload, afterload, and function, intracardiac shunting and intravascular volume status.[1-5]
- LACs are inserted directly into the left atrium and anchored to the heart by a suture. The catheter typically exits the skin more left and laterally than does the right atrial catheter (RAC).[3,4]
- Appropriate setup, use, and troubleshooting of hemodynamic monitoring systems; refer to Procedure 63: Pressure Transducer Systems for further information
- The LAC is connected to a stopcock and then to pressure tubing and a transducer. The transducer is connected to a continuous infusion pump to maintain patency and avoid thrombus and emboli formation and a monitor that displays the LA waveform and a numeric value.[1,6]
- To obtain an accurate numeric LA measurement, the transducer must be positioned at the phlebostatic axis or reference point located at the fourth intercostal space–midaxillary line.[2,4,5] See Procedure 137, Figure 137-2, for instructions on locating the phlebostatic axis.
- An understanding of hemodynamic monitoring and LA waveform analysis
- Normal LA pressures are 4 to 12 mm Hg.[3,4]
  - ❖ Low pressures indicate pulmonary venous obstruction, decreased preload or reduced afterload.[3,4]
  - ❖ Elevated pressures indicate increased left ventricular afterload, depressed left ventricular function, mitral valve stenosis, or regurgitation.[3,4]
- Normal LA waveform consists of five deflections: a, c, x, v, and y (Figure 62-1)
  - ❖ The a wave reflects the pressure rise produced by atrial systole.
  - ❖ The c wave reflects the slight increase in intra-atrial pressure that is associated with opening of the aorta and closure of the mitral valve leaflets and can appear as a separate positive deflection, a notch on the a wave. In the infant or child, it may be absent altogether due to the distensibility of the atria.

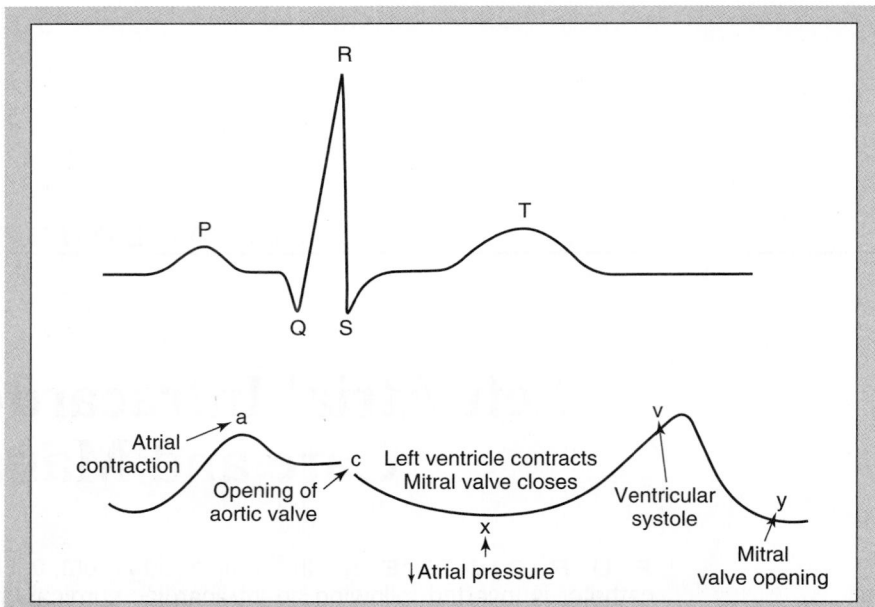

FIGURE 62-1   ECG and left atrial pressure waveform. *Drawing courtesy Dorothy M. Beke, 2004.*

❖ The x wave reflects mitral valve closure with a decrease in atrial pressure.

❖ The v wave is produced by the contraction of the ventricles causing the atrioventricular valve leaflets to bulge into the atria during atrial diastole.

❖ The y wave reflects the mitral valve opening.[1]

- Ability to interpret electrocardiogram (ECG) tracings and correlate findings with LA waveform

- Ability to analyze and interpret abnormal LA waveforms

  ❖ Cannon a waves are associated with cardiac rhythm abnormalities (i.e., junctional or dissociated rhythm).[1]

  ❖ Elevated a waves may be indicative of left ventricular dysfunction or enlargement, pulmonary hypertension, or mitral stenosis.

  ❖ Absence of a waves may occur with atrial fibrillation.

  ❖ Exaggerated a waves may be indicative of mitral stenosis.

  ❖ Exaggerated v waves may be indicative of mitral regurgitation.

  ❖ Elevated a and v waves are associated with cardiac tamponade.[1,6]

- Ability to recognize and determine the causes of over- or under-damped waveforms, abnormal waveform tracings, and/or numeric findings[2,4,7,8]

- Prevent air infusion in to the left atrium, which may predispose the child to stroke or other end organ dysfunction[2,4,8,9]

- Aseptic technique with dressing changes and accessing of LAC is crucial to avoid sepsis.[10,11]

- Mastery of pediatric advanced life support competencies

- Child development as it relates to clinical assessment and use of an LAC

CHILD AND FAMILY ASSESSMENT

- Type of congenital heart disease, previous cardiac medical and surgical interventions and the results of recent echocardiographic, cardiac catheterization laboratory, and medical imaging data ➤➤*Rationale:* The type of congenital heart defect, associated cardiac surgeries, and preoperative data determines the rationale for LAC use.

- Components of current surgical repair, intraoperative findings including direct measurements, surgical times (cardiopulmonary bypass, cross-clamp, and deep hypothermic arrest), intraoperative complications, and intraoperative transesophageal echocardiographic findings ➤➤*Rationale:* This information influences the expected and acceptable pressure measurements obtained by the LAC.

- Current hemodynamic status ➤➤*Rationale:* Perfusion status should correlate with LAC pressure measurement.

- Current heart rhythm, medication history, chest radiographic and laboratory findings ➤➤*Rationale:* Drug therapy, electrolyte and/or acid-base abnormalities, and presence of arrhythmias impact the LAC waveform and pressure measurements.

- Child's developmental level and ability to interact ➤➤*Rationale:* These factors influence preparation of the child and interaction.

- Child's level of sedation and comfort ➤➤*Rationale:* Pain and agitation can lead to accidental line dislodgement.

- Child's and family's understanding of the cardiac lesion, indication for surgical procedure, and reasons, risks, and benefits of LAC use ➤➤*Rationale:* Evaluates child's and family's understanding of information and provides a gauge for ongoing education.

CHILD AND FAMILY EDUCATION

Individualized, developmentally appropriate education is provided to the family and to the child based on desire for knowledge, readiness to learn, and overall neurologic and psychosocial state.

- Provide information regarding indications, function and management of LAC and monitoring including waveform display, use of alarms and approximate time catheter will remain in place ➥*Rationale:* Information provided may increase the child's and family's knowledge base and decrease anxiety.
- Explain to family and child (when age appropriate) rationale for bed rest and sedation use related to the presence of an indwelling LAC. Parents must be informed about inability to pick up and hold child to prevent LAC dislodgement ➥*Rationale:* Avoids potential LAC dislodgement, damage, or leakage.
- Show family and child (when appropriate) the actual catheter and insertion site. Point out areas where line is secured to child's body and explain need for frequent assessment of insertion site and catheter setup ➥*Rationale:* Providing information may decrease the incidence and/or degree of line complications by increased compliance with line care guidelines.
- Encourage questions and answer questions as they arise ➥*Rationale:* Reinforcement of information is needed during periods of stress.

EQUIPMENT

- Continuous heparin flush solution (1 unit/mL or per institution-specific protocol) to maintain patency and prevent blood back-up into the monitoring system
- Pressure transducer system including transducer, pressure tubing, and cable specific to cardiorespiratory monitor in use
- Leveling device
- Labeling tape
- Infusion pump or pressure bag for fluid administration via LAC
- Cardiorespiratory monitor for continual assessment of left atrial waveform, heart rate, and arterial blood pressure
- Intravenous tubing and inline micron filter (per institution-specific protocol) if line is used for continuous infusion other than heparin-containing solution
- Stopcock placed between infusion tubing and left atrial catheter for line access, per institution-specific protocol
- Syringes
- Alcohol pads
- Equipment for line repair (per institution-specific protocol)
  - ❖ 23 or 25 Fr butterfly needle
  - ❖ Gauze
  - ❖ Tongue blade
  - ❖ Tape
- Occlusive, transparent sterile dressing
- Clean gloves

Procedure for Left Atrial Intracardiac Line: Care and Management

Steps	Rationale	Considerations
1. Ensure child and family understand procedure and questions are answered.	Evaluates and reinforces understanding of previously taught information.	Developmental level, cognitive ability, and anxiety level will determine approach to and effectiveness of teaching.
2. Gather needed equipment and supplies; review prescribing practitioner's order or institution-specific protocol for flush solution to be administered via the LAC.	Facilitates completion of procedure in a timely manner. Ensures correct fluid is administered.	Setup should be primed and at the bedside ready for hook-up to facilitate transfer back from the operating room and assessment of LAC without delays.
3. Select an appropriate monitoring scale. (Level II*)	Allows accurate LAC waveform interpretation.	0 to 25 mm Hg is scale generally used.
4. Wash hands and put on clean gloves.	Standard precautions; reduces transmission of microorganisms.	Latex-free gloves are generally used.
5. Prime or flush entire pressure transducer system with prescribed fluid; for further information on pressure transducer system setup, refer to Procedure 63. (Level VI*)	Removes air bubbles; air bubbles introduced into LAC can cause air embolism. Air bubbles within the tubing will dampen the waveform.[6]	

Procedure continues on following page

---

* Level II: Theory-based, no research data to support recommendations: recommendations from expert consensus group may exist
  Level VI: Clinical studies in a variety of patient populations and situations to support recommendations

Procedure for Left Atrial Intracardiac Line: Care and Management—*Continued*

Steps	Rationale	Considerations
6. On child's arrival from operating room, assess blood return of LAC. *(Level II*)*	Blood return demonstrates that catheter has not migrated outside the vascular space.	Blood from LAC is generally brighter red than venous blood because the left atrium receives oxygenated pulmonary venous return. Presence of decreased left atrial saturation may be indicative of a right to left shunt at the atrial level, LAC displacement, or pulmonary venous desaturation and lung pathology.[4] If unable to obtain blood return, try using a smaller-volume syringe. If still unsuccessful, notify prescribing practitioner and check placement of LAC on chest film.
7. Locate the phlebostatic reference point by identifying the phlebostatic axis based on child's position; level transducer to phlebostatic axis. Refer to Figure 137-2 in Procedure 137. *(Level VI*)*	Ensures transducer system's zeroing interface is maintained at the level of the phlebostatic axis, for accurate readings. If interface is above the phlebostatic axis, LA pressures will be falsely low; if interface is below the phlebostatic axis, LA pressures will be falsely high.	Consider marking the phlebostatic axis on the child's chest to ensure consistent readings. When the child moves from supine to a position in which the head of the bed is elevated, the phlebostatic reference point should be rechecked and the transducer re-leveled. In some institutions the transducer is placed next to the child parallel to the phlebostatic axis; refer to institution-specific protocol.
8. Connect LAC to transducer system by flushing into stopcock to ensure no air is present or introduced and zero at the phlebostatic axis. *(Level I*)*	Required for accurate LA pressure monitoring.	LA pressure in the postoperative child is usually 4 to 12 mm Hg.[12,13]
9. Assess LA waveform. *(Level II*)*	Confirms placement of LAC and accuracy of pressure reading.	If damping of the waveform is noted, LAC should be checked for blood return and the line assessed for presence of air or clot. If resistance is noted when attempting to check for blood return, notify prescribing practitioner immediately.
10. Correlate LA pressure reading with clinical findings and diagnostic studies. *(Level V*)*	Determines accuracy of numeric measurement.	Elevation in LA pressure may be indicative of poor left ventricular function, left ventricular hypertrophy, mitral stenosis, mitral regurgitation, intracardiac left to right shunting at the atrial level, left atrial hypoplasia, pulmonary hypertension, dysrhythmias, fluid overload, or cardiac tamponade.[4] Artifactual causes include the

* Level I: Manufacturer's recommendations only
Level II: Theory-based, no research data to support recommendations: recommendations from expert consensus group may exist
Level V: Clinical studies in more than one or two patient populations and situations to support recommendations
Level VI: Clinical studies in a variety of patient populations and situations to support recommendations

Procedure	for Left Atrial Intracardiac Line: Care and Management—*Continued*

Steps	Rationale	Considerations
		LAC not in correct position (not in LA, wedged, or in ventricle), pressure transducer below the level of the heart or the pressure transducer improperly zeroed.[4] Decreased LA pressures may be due to intravascular volume depletion or inadequate preload.[4] Artifactual causes include LAC malfunction due to a clot or crack in the catheter, the pressure transducer above the level of the heart, or the pressure transducer being improperly zeroed.[4]
11. Obtain chest x-ray before using the information obtained from the left atrial tracing. *(Level V*)*	Verifies placement of LAC in the left atrium to ensure accurate data.[1,11,15]	LAC is usually placed via the right superior pulmonary vein into the left atrium[3,7,10] (Figure 62-2), and in some cases, via the left atrial appendage.[15] LAC may not be readily visible on the x-ray of a larger patient.

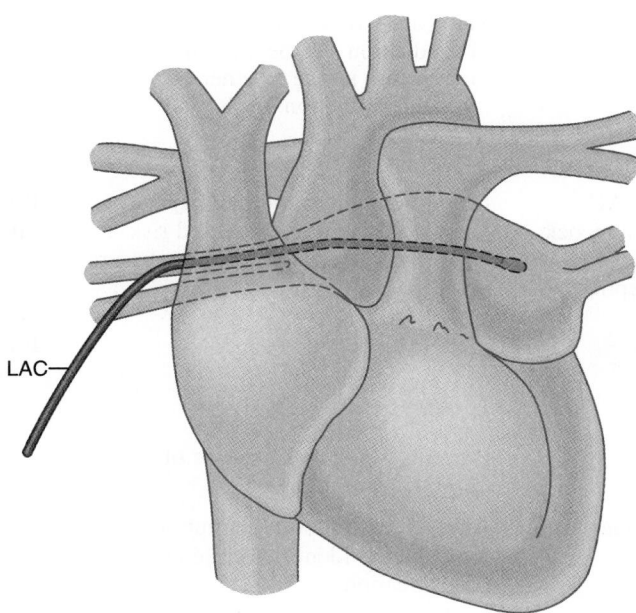

FIGURE 62-2 Left atrial catheter placement via right superior pulmonary vein. *Drawing courtesy Dorothy M. Beke, 2004.*

Procedure continues on following page

* Level V: Clinical studies in more than one or two patient populations and situations to support recommendations

Procedure	for Left Atrial Intracardiac Line: Care and Management—*Continued*	
Steps	**Rationale**	**Considerations**
12. Set monitor alarms on the basis of the child's current clinical status and hemodynamic values. *(Level II*)*	Alerts care provider to changes in child's hemodynamic status and dynamic changes of LAC that may require intervention.	Promotes patient safety.
13. Continuously monitor LA waveform and pressure while LAC is in place. *(Level II*)*	Assesses for changes in child's hemodynamic status. Changes in LA waveforms should correlate with ECG or blood pressure changes, and other variation in hemodynamics.[4,7,12,14]	The a wave usually occurs during the PR interval. The c wave correlates with the RS-T interval, and the v wave is generally noted during the TP interval of the ECG[4,14] (see Figure 62-1). Malposition of the LAC in to the ventricle may cause dysrhythmias.[4]
14. Continuously infuse solution via LAC. *(Level II*)*	Maintains LAC patency; decreases potential emboli and/or thrombus formation.[10]	A solution of 1 unit of heparin per 1 mL of 0.9% saline, D5W or D10W may assist in preventing thrombus formation.[15] Change infusion fluid every 24 hours and line setup every 48 hours or per institution-specific protocol.
15. Avoid medication infusions or any situation that may introduce air and/or emboli into the LAC. *(Level II*)*	Medication infusion or air emboli introduction via the arterial circuit may cause stroke or other end organ dysfunction.[6]	Avoid infusion of vasoactive medications. In emergency situations, the LAC may be used for medication administration per institution-specific protocol.
16. Monitor for disruption of LAC system integrity; evaluate stopcock connection for cracks; replace cracked stopcock using aseptic technique.	Disruption of system integrity may result in bleeding, increased risk of infection, and inaccurate pressure readings.	If blood is noted to be backing up in the LAC, check all connections for tightness and evaluate for a crack in the LAC at the stopcock connection. If a crack is noted in the LAC, the line must be repaired immediately.
LAC Repair		
17. Clamp off line to child.	Prevents blood loss because of high LA pressures.	
18. Notify prescribing practitioner.	Alerts practitioner to disruption in catheter. Identifies child at risk for infection.	
19. Gather needed equipment and supplies.	Facilitates completion of task in a timely manner.	
20. Prepare sterile field; place needed supplies on field.	Aseptic technique is used during line repair.	
21. Put on sterile gloves and eyewear if appropriate.	Aseptic technique; standard precautions.	
22. Clean LAC with alcohol, and cut immediately above the disruption site using sterile scissors.	Aseptic technique; removes segment of catheter that is damaged.	

* Level II: Theory-based, no research data to support recommendations: recommendations from expert consensus group may exist

Procedure	for Left Atrial Intracardiac Line: Care and Management—*Continued*	
Steps	**Rationale**	**Considerations**
23. Carefully thread a butterfly needle (size 23 or 25 Fr) into the LAC.	Required to connect LAC to stopcock.	
24. Secure LAC to a tongue blade using sterile gauze and tape.	Prevents further kinking or line disruption.	
25. Dispose of used supplies and equipment, including sharps, in appropriate receptacle.	Standard precautions; reduces transmission of microorganisms. Protects personnel health.	
26. Remove personal protective equipment; wash hands.	Standard precautions; reduces transmission of microorganisms.	

Expected Outcomes

- LAC position is confirmed in LA by chest x-ray and blood return
- Accurate LA pressure and waveform obtained and findings as expected for child based on surgical intervention

- Child is free from complications related to LAC

- LAC insertion site is free from signs of infection

- LAC remains in place until electively removed
- Child demonstrates acceptable level of comfort

Unexpected Outcomes

- Unable to visualize catheter in LA on chest x-ray
- Unable to obtain blood return
- Abnormal waveform
- Abnormal LA pressure
- Inaccurate waveform and/or pressure related to incorrect leveling of transducer, failure to zero system
- Thrombosis
- Uncontrolled bleeding
- Air embolus
- Dysrhythmias related to catheter migration into left ventricle
- Signs of infection at LAC insertion site
- LAC-associated sepsis
- Unplanned catheter removal
- Unmanaged pain or agitation that threatens catheter placement

Monitoring and Care of the Child

Activities and Interventions	Rationale	Reportable Conditions
1. Continuously monitor LA pressure and waveform.	Allows monitoring of hemodynamic parameters and detection of potential postoperative problems.	- Abnormalities in left atrial pressure or waveform
2. Assess LAC for line integrity and presence of air every hour.	Reduces risk of infection, bleeding, and stroke.	- Cracks in LAC or connections - Inability to remove air from the line
3. Obtain daily chest x-ray while LAC is in place.	Monitors for line migration.	- Line dislodgment/ incorrect location - Lack of blood return
4. Maintain dry, occlusive, sterile dressing over LAC insertion site. Change every 24 hours or per institution-specific protocol.	Reduces risk of LAC dislodgement and sepsis.	- Inadvertent removal of LAC - Leakage of blood or fluid from LAC or LAC insertion site - Erythema, edema or drainage at insertion site

5. Zero transducer:
  • During initial setup.
  • If disconnection occurs between the transducer and the monitor cable.
  • When values obtained do not fit clinical picture.
  • Routinely every shift or per institution-specific protocol.
	Ensures accuracy of hemodynamic monitoring system.	- Unable to perform zero
		- Pressure readings do not correspond to child's clinical picture despite transducer zeroing and calibration (as appropriate)

Continued

Monitoring and Care of the Child—Cont'd

Activities and Interventions	Rationale	Reportable Conditions
6. Ensure all connections are tight and stopcock is closed to air. Place sterile caps on all stopcocks.	Loose connections or open stopcocks will cause a decrease in pressure within the fluid-filled system and blood may exert a back pressure into the pressure tubing. Stopcocks may be a source of contamination.	• Contamination of system
7. Ensure infusion pump is turned on and infusing or pressure bag is inflated to 300 mm Hg.	Low pressure in pressure bag or pump failure will result in blood back-up with possible clotting of catheter, inaccurate readings, or thrombus formation.	• Unable to flush catheter • Unable to obtain blood return from catheter
8. Ensure alarms are set appropriately and are on at all times.	Alerts caregiver to pressure changes outside of the desired range and disconnections in the pressure monitoring system.	• Pressures outside of desired range
9. Change pressure transducer system and flush solution based on manufacturer's recommendations and/or institution-specific protocol.	The Centers for Disease Control and Prevention (CDC) recommend that flush solution and disposable transducer systems can be used safely for 72 hours.[16]	• Tubing or flush solution not changed as recommended • Signs and symptoms of infection
10. Assess effectiveness of comfort management strategy and provide appropriate interventions. Encourage family to assist in using nonpharmacologic means to comfort and support the child.	Agitation and restlessness may result in inadvertent LAC removal. Early identification of pain or agitation facilitates prompt treatment.	• Unresolved pain or agitation • Inadvertent catheter removal • Continued irritability, changes in physiologic condition

Documentation

- Child and family education
- Alarm limit settings
- Left atrial waveform
- Left atrial waveform pressure readings
- Dressing change
- LAC insertion site appearance
- Blood return from LAC confirming patency
- Infusion fluid and rate
- X-ray confirmation of LAC in left atrium
- Fluid, tubing, and transducer change
- Zeroing and calibration at beginning of each shift and as indicated
- Comfort assessment and specific interventions provided
- Unexpected outcomes and related treatment

References

1. Darovic G: Cardiovascular anatomy and physiology. In Darovic GO, editor: *Hemodynamic monitoring: invasive and non-invasive clinical application*, ed 3, Philadelphia, 2002, Saunders.
2. Flori HR, et al: Transthoracic intracardiac catheters in pediatric patients recovering from congenital heart defect surgery: associated complications and outcome, *Crit Care Med* 28(8):2997-3001, 2000.
3. Johnston LJ, McKinley DF: Cardiac tamponade after removal of atrial intracardiac monitoring catheters in a pediatric patient: case report, *Heart Lung* 29(4):256-261, 2000.
4. Roth SJ: Postoperative care. In Chang AC, et al, editors: *Pediatric cardiac intensive care*, Baltimore, 1998, Williams & Wilkins.
5. Santini F, et al: Routine left atrial catheterization for the postoperative management of cardiac surgical patients: is the risk justified? *Eur J Cardiothorac Surg* 16:218-221, 1999.
6. Craig J, et al: Cardiovascular critical care problems. In Curley MAQ, Moloney-Harmon P, editors: *Critical care nursing of infants and children*, ed 2, Philadelphia, 2001, Saunders.
7. Akl BF, et al: Brief communications: unusual complication of direct left atrial pressure monitoring line, *J Thorac Cardiovasc Surg* 88:1033-1037, 1984.
8. Leitman BS, et al: The left atrial catheter: its uses and complications, *Radiology* 185(2):611-612, 1992.
9. Gold JP, et al: Transthoracic intracardiac monitoring lines in pediatric surgical patients: a ten-year experience, *Ann Thorac Surg* 42:185-191, 1986.
10. Freeman R, et al: Catheter tip cultures on open-heart surgery patients: associations with site of catheter and age of patients, *Thorax* 36:355-359, 1981.
11. Lincoln P: Policy 2.10: intracardiac line dressing. In Children's Hospital, Boston, editor: *Children's Hospital, Boston ICU nursing policy and procedure manual*, Boston, 2003, Children's Hospital.
12. Bridges E: Hemodynamic monitoring. In Woods S, et al, editors: *Cardiac nursing*, ed 5, Baltimore, 2005, Lippincott Williams & Wilkins.
13. Castaneda A, et al: Perioperative care. In *Cardiac surgery of the neonate and infant*, Philadelphia, 1994, Saunders.
14. Craig J, et al: Tissue perfusion. In Curley MAQ, Moloney-Harmon PA, editors: *Critical care nursing of infants and children*, ed 2, Philadelphia, 2001, Saunders.
15. Johnson AB, Lincoln P: Policy 2.2: removal of intracardiac line. In Children's Hospital, Boston, editor: *Children's Hospital, Boston ICU nursing policy and procedure manual*, Boston, 2003, Children's Hospital.
16. Centers for Disease Control and Prevention: Guidelines for the prevention of intravascular catheter related infections, *MMWR Morbid Mortal Wkly Rep* 51(No. RR-10):1-29, 2002.

Additional Readings

Ceyran H, et al: Benefit of using triple-lumen catheter to monitor left atrial pressure, *Acta Anaesthesiol Scand* 47:430-432, 2003.

Zahorec R, Holoman M: Transatrial access for left atrial pressure monitoring in cardiac surgery. *Eur J Cardiothorac Surg* 11:379-380, 1997.

Pressure Transducer Systems

PURPOSE: To provide a catheter-to-monitor interface so that intravascular and intracardiac pressures can be measured. The transducer detects the physical energy of a pressure and converts it to an electrical signal that is amplified and displayed as a waveform and numeric value.

Peggy Dorr

PREREQUISITE KNOWLEDGE

- Understanding of the normal anatomy and physiology of the cardiovascular system
- Normal pressure values and waveforms for all sites measured (see Procedures 59, 62, 64, 65, and 137)
- For measurement of arterial blood pressure or central venous pressure, a catheter is placed into an artery or large vein, respectively
- Intracardiac pressures can be measured via a thermodilution catheter floated into the pulmonary artery with central venous pressure (CVP), right atrial (RA) pressure, pulmonary artery (PA) pressure, or pulmonary capillary wedge pressure (PCWP) monitored and displayed or via transthoracic catheters placed during cardiac surgery. These catheters can be placed to obtain RA, PA, or left atrial (LA) pressures.
- Disposable transducers are most commonly used because they are cost effective, durable, and highly accurate. They do not drift with time or temperature and are calibrated to within ±2% or 1 mm Hg, whichever is greater.[1] Disposable transducers also eliminate the risks of infection more commonly seen with reusable systems.[2]
- For ensured accuracy of the hemodynamic monitoring system, correct positioning of the transducer at the phlebostatic axis and zeroing of the system are extremely important. Calibration is no longer necessary given the advanced technology of today's monitoring systems.[1] Figure 137-2 shows instructions for locating the phlebostatic axis.
  - ❖ Positioning of the transducer level with the phlebostatic axis positions the transducer at the level of the atrium to eliminate the effects of hydrostatic pressure[3]
- In addition to arterial, venous, and intracardiac pressures, pressure transducer systems may also be used to measure intracranial, bladder, and compartment pressures (see Procedures 76, 97, and 124)
- Principles of aseptic technique
- Child development as it relates to clinical assessment and use of pressure transducer systems
- Ability to use and troubleshoot a unit-specific or institution-specific hemodynamic monitoring system

CHILD AND FAMILY ASSESSMENT

- Child's developmental level and ability to interact ➤➤*Rationale:* These factors influence preparation before and interaction during the procedure.
- Child's and family's understanding of the reasons for and risks and benefits of pressure monitoring ➤➤*Rationale:* Evaluates the child's and family's understanding of the procedure and provides a gauge for ongoing education.

- Pressures being transduced ➤➤*Rationale:* Needed for determination of the number of transducers necessary, identification of expected waveform, and selection of the appropriate alarm limits and monitoring scale.
- Factors unique to the child that may cause alterations in waveforms or in values obtained for parameters being transduced and monitored ➤➤*Rationale:* Surgical repairs, unusual anatomy, and disease process are factors unique to the child that may affect pressures or waveforms.
- History of heparin-induced thrombocytopenia (HITT) or heparin sensitivity or allergy ➤➤*Rationale:* If heparin sensitivity, allergy, or history of HITT is known, avoid the use of heparin in the line.

CHILD AND FAMILY EDUCATION

Individualized, developmentally appropriate education is provided to the family and to the child based on desire for knowledge, readiness to learn, and overall neurologic and psychosocial state. The goals of giving information are to promote a sense of mastery of the events to occur, to facilitate the child's and family's understanding of the purpose of these events, and to correct misinformation.[4]

- Provide information about the purpose of hemodynamic monitoring and the information to be gained from this monitoring ➤➤*Rationale:* An understanding of this invasive technique is facilitated, allowing for acceptance and decreased anxiety.

- Explain and demonstrate the procedure and the results of hemodynamic monitoring, including catheter placement, dressings, intravenous (IV) tubing, and waveforms ➤➤*Rationale:* The child and family are prepared for what to expect at the bedside and possible changes in the child's appearance; anxiety may be decreased.
- Encourage questions and answer questions as they arise ➤➤*Rationale:* Reinforcement of information is needed during periods of stress.

EQUIPMENT

- Noncompliant pressure tubing with institution-specific transducer system
- Intravenous tubing to be placed from the syringe or fluid bag to the pressure transducer set-up
- Syringe pump or pressure bag (depending on the child's size and unit-specific or institution-specific protocols)
- Premixed bag of heparinized saline solution or a bag of normal saline solution and heparin vial
- Sterile dead-end caps
- Stopcock (per unit-specific or institution-specific protocol)
- Monitoring system
- Pressure monitoring cable
- Syringe with saline solution or heparin flush per the prescribing practitioner's order or institution-specific protocol
- Clean gloves
- Carpenter's level or other leveling device
- Transducer holder for the IV pole (optional)

Procedure for Pressure Transducer Systems

Steps	Rationale	Considerations
1. Ensure child and family understand procedure and questions are answered.	Evaluates and reinforces understanding of previously taught information.	Developmental level, cognitive ability, and anxiety level determine approach to and effectiveness of teaching.
2. Review prescribing practitioner's order or institution-specific protocol for flush solution to be used.	Flush solution establishes fluid column necessary for pressure to be correctly transmitted to transducer and maintains patency of the catheter.	
3. Gather needed equipment and supplies.	Facilitates completion of task in a timely manner and aids in maintaining asepsis.	
4. Wash hands.	Standard precautions; reduces transmission of microorganisms.	
5. Obtain a premixed flush solution or prepare flush solution. Commercially prepared flush solution is available as one unit of heparin per milliliter of fluid	A heparinized solution is generally used to prevent coagulation of blood within the catheter because most sites that are	Depending on the site of hemodynamic monitoring, type of flush solution may vary (i.e., arterial line solutions and LA lines almost always

Procedure continues on following page

Procedure for Pressure Transducer Systems—*Continued*

Steps	Rationale	Considerations
volume or 2 units of heparin per milliliter of fluid volume; refer to institution-specific protocols. *(Level II*)*	monitored with a pressure transducer system are low-flow systems.[5]	use a 0.9% saline solution; CVP, RA, or PA flush solutions may be dextrose based if necessary to increase parenteral caloric intake). Refer to institution-specific protocols for fluid standards. Refer to institution-specific protocols for the amount of heparin added per milliliter of flush solution (usually 1 to 3 units/mL); some institutions do not use heparin.
6. Draw up a syringe of flush solution or connect bag of flush solution to IV tubing; tubing may be a straight set or tubing used with a syringe pump.	A syringe pump system should be used for infants and children; use of a straight set with a pressure bag should be reserved for adolescents. The syringe pump set-up ensures constant delivery of a set smaller volume of fluid (1 to 2 mL/h), whereas a pressure bag set at 300 mm Hg delivers approximately 3 mL/h through a fast-flush valve system. *(Level III*)*	Although the pressure tubing may prohibit unrestricted flow of fluid, a transducer that is unexpectedly opened allows a large volume of fluid to flow into the child, which can be dangerous to the smaller child. Other potential risks associated with fast-flush systems include the dislodgement of a thrombus from the cannula tip and retrograde embolization of flush solution into the central arteries or cerebral circulation. The risk also exists of local arterial vasospasm and transient elevation of arterial, intracranial, or atrial pressures with rapid flushing.[6] Continuous flush systems decrease the incidence rate of distal embolization and carry a lower rate of nosocomial infections than intermittently flushed catheters.[7]
7. Connect pressure tubing to syringe or the end of the tubing from the infusion bag. If a closed blood draw system is not used, a stopcock at the end of pressure tubing facilitates laboratory draws.	Pressure tubing is necessary to obtain accurate readings. Air filters cannot be placed between the catheter and the pressure tubing because they affect the accuracy of the pressure reading.	Use of wide-bore high-pressure (noncompliant) tubing of length less than 48 inches improves accuracy of the waveform and numeric reading.[3]
8. Flush fluid through the entire system, including all stopcock sites, ensuring that all air bubbles are removed from the tubing.	Air bubbles interrupt fluid column and result in underestimation of systolic pressure and overestimation of diastolic pressure.[1,3]	
9. After system is flushed with fluid and all air bubbles are removed, clamp the system closed.	Prevents accidental free flow of fluid into the child when the system is connected to the catheter.	
10. Replace vented stopcock caps with nonvented closed caps. Do not place excess stopcocks in the system; use no more than necessary to facilitate blood draws.	If the stopcock is accidentally turned such that it is open to the child and the stopcock port, a nonvented cap prevents blood loss.	Stopcocks can be a source of infection.[2]

* Level II: Theory-based; no research data to support recommendations; recommendations from expert consensus group may exist
  Level III: Laboratory data; no clinical data to support recommendations

Procedure	for Pressure Transducer Systems—*Continued*	
Steps	**Rationale**	**Considerations**
11. Ensure syringe or bag and tubing are labeled per institution-specific protocol.	Identifies date that tubing and syringe or bag should be changed.	
12. Connect pressure cable specific to the transducer and monitor in use to the primed tubing or transducer set-up.	Necessary for signal to be transmitted from transducer to monitor.	Ensure a snug fit of all cables. Loose connections interfere with the transmission of data, negating any waveform or pressure measurement.
13. Connect pressure cable to the monitor, turn monitor on, and label the pressure to be monitored appropriately.	Correct labeling of pressures is necessary for accurate identification and interpretation of multiple waveforms and pressure readings.	
14. On the monitor display, select appropriate scale for pressure being measured.	If scale on the monitor is inaccurate (too high or low) for the pressure being read, the waveform is substandard and can possibly be misinterpreted.	
15. Position air-fluid interface of the transducer at phlebostatic axis, using a level to ensure the transducer is in line with the right atrium (estimated with the phlebostatic axis); see Figure 137-2 for instructions on locating the phlebostatic axis. *(Level VI*)*	Transducer must be accurately positioned to obtain accurate pressure measurements. If the transducer is above the level of the RA, the displayed pressure reading is lower than the actual pressure. If the transducer is below the level of the RA, the displayed pressure reading is higher than the actual pressure.[1,3]	The phlebostatic axis is defined as the level of the right atrium, which can be found by locating the intersection of the fourth intercostal space and the midaxillary line.[3,8] A plastic transducer holder that fits on an IV pole can be used to position transducers, which allows all transducers to be aligned at the phlebostatic axis and to be easily moved up or down based on changes in child's position. Transducers can be placed directly on the bed, but they must be elevated to the midaxillary line for an accurate reading.
16. Turn the stopcock at the transducer off to child and remove the cap, maintaining asepsis; open system to air.	Allows monitor to use atmospheric pressure as a reference for zero.[1,3]	
17. Zero the system at monitor. Observe display to ensure that it displays a value of zero.	Watching the monitor display is important to ensure that the line goes to baseline and the numeric reading displays zero.	This step can be done before the pressure system is connected to the child.
18. Replace cap on stopcock with aseptic technique; turn stopcock back so that system is open to child and flush system, off to nonvented cap.	Closes system when zeroing is complete; reinstitutes pressure monitoring.	If desired, dynamic response testing (DRT) may be performed at this point. DRT is done to determine whether a hemodynamic monitoring system will accurately reproduce a patient's cardiovascular pressures.[3] Because of the volume of fluid infused and the fast-flush necessary during this test, DRT should only be performed in older children or adolescents. Refer to institution-specific protocols; the steps of the procedure can be referenced in Lynn-McHale

Procedure continues on following page

* Level VI: Clinical studies in a variety of patient populations and situations to support recommendations

Procedure | for Pressure Transducer Systems—*Continued*

Steps	Rationale	Considerations
		Wiegand DJ, Carlson K, editors: *AACN procedure manual for critical care,* ed 5, Philadelphia, 2005, Saunders;[9] or McGhee and Bridges.[3]
19. Set limits on monitor as appropriate for child's age and baseline hemodynamic status.	Promotes patient safety by providing notification of system disconnect, inadvertent catheter removal, changes in vital signs, and other potentially hazardous situations.	Ensure that at least one monitor alarm is on for arterial pressure systems at all times, as a safety precaution (disconnect alarm).
20. Put on clean gloves.	Standard precautions; prevents blood exposure.	
21. Attach transducer system to catheter (arterial, CVP, RA, LA, PA); open all clamps. Attach a 5-mL or larger syringe, half filled with saline flush solution, to stopcock at the transducer if one is present. Draw back slightly, observing the fluid or blood aspirated for any air bubbles; remove all air bubbles.	If air is infused into the child, it can lead to pulmonary emboli, strokes, seizures, or other end-organ damage, especially in children with intracardiac shunts.[1,8]	If a stopcock is not included in system, ensure that no air is present in the catheter or pressure transducer system before making connection.
22. After all air has been removed from tubing and catheter, slowly flush to clear tubing of blood.	If blood is left in the tubing, it can act as a medium for organism growth. Blood in the system also alters pressure readings.[1]	
23. Observe waveform and displayed numeric values and compare with expected waveform and values.	Assesses accuracy of data.	
24. Dispose of used supplies and equipment in appropriate receptacle.	Standard precautions; reduces transmission of microorganisms.	
25. Remove gloves; wash hands.	Standard precautions.	

Expected Outcomes	Unexpected Outcomes
• Pressure transducer system is set up and maintained aseptically	• Contamination of fluid or tubing that results in infection • Loose connections within the pressure monitoring system
• Transducer is leveled at phlebostatic axis and monitor is zeroed at appropriate intervals	• Transducer is incorrectly leveled, resulting in inaccurate pressures • Transducer is not zeroed, resulting in inaccurate pressures
• Appropriate waveform and pressure readings are displayed on monitor	• Infusion pump is not on or pressure bag is not inflated correctly • Air bubbles or blood are noted within the system

Monitoring and Care of the Child

Activities and Interventions	Rationale	Reportable Conditions
1. Check catheter insertion sites every hour for signs of infiltration or leaks.	Early recognition of site problems may prevent long-term complications.	• Blanching of the skin above or below the level of an arterial catheter that occurs with routine flushing
2. Evaluate and document waveforms and pressures every 1 to 2 hours (see Procedures 60, 62, 64, and 65 for discussions of specific pressure waveforms).	Changes in hemodynamic waveforms may indicate either hemodynamic changes in the child or catheter-related problems.	• Dampened or flat waveforms or abnormal pressure readings (including those that read negative numbers)
3. Administration set-up for central and arterial lines should be changed no more frequently than at 72-hour intervals.[2] (Level IV*)	Three well-controlled studies provided data that revealed replacing administration sets no more frequently than 72 hours after initiation is safe and cost effective.[2]	• If any tubing was used to administer blood, blood products, or lipid emulsions, the administration set must be changed within 24 hours.[2]

* Level IV: Limited clinical studies to support recommendations

Documentation

- Child and family education
- Date and time of hemodynamic monitoring system set-up
- Assessment of insertion site and surrounding tissue
- Type of flush solution and rate of infusion
- Unexpected outcomes and related treatment

References

1. Craig J, et al: Tissue perfusion. In Curley MAQ, Moloney-Harmon PA, editors: *Critical care nursing of infants and children,* ed 2, Philadelphia, 1996, Saunders.
2. O'Grady NP, et al: Guidelines for the prevention of intravascular catheter related infections, *MMWR* 51(No.RR-10): 1-29, 2002.
3. McGhee BH, Bridges MEJ: Monitoring arterial blood pressure: what you may not know, *Crit Care Nurs* 22(2):60-79, 2002.
4. LeRoy S, et al: Recommendations for preparing children and adolescents for invasive cardiac procedures, *Circulation* 108:2550-2564, 2003.
5. Clark SL: Arterial lines: an analysis of good practice, *J Child Health Care* 3(1):23-27, 1999.
6. Weiss M, et al: Arterial fast bolus flush systems used routinely in neonates and infants cause retrograde embolization of flush solution into the central arterial and cerebral circulation, *Can J Anesthesia* 50:386-391, 2003.
7. Heitmiller ES, Nyhan D: Perioperative monitoring. In Nichols DG, et al, editors: *Critical heart disease in infants and children,* St Louis, 1995, Mosby.
8. Callow L, et al: Cardiovascular system. In Slota MC, editor: *Core curriculum for pediatric critical care nursing,* Philadelphia, 1998, Saunders.
9. Preuss T, Lynn-McHale Wiegand DJ: Single- and multiple-pressure transducer systems. In Lynn-McHale Wiegand DJ, Carlson K, editors: *AACN procedure manual for critical care,* ed 5, Philadelphia, 2005, Saunders.

Pulmonary Artery Intracardiac Line: Care and Management

P U R P O S E : Transthoracic pulmonary artery intracardiac catheters are placed directly into the pulmonary artery in children undergoing cardiac surgery who may be at risk for postoperative pulmonary artery hypertension or pulmonary hypertensive crisis to directly measure the pulmonary artery systolic, diastolic, and mean pressures

Louise Callow

PREREQUISITE KNOWLEDGE

- Cardiovascular anatomy and physiology
- Pulmonary anatomy and physiology
- The individual child's congenital heart defect and the surgical procedure preformed
- Principles of aseptic technique
- Normal values for intracardiac pressures related to the individual child's specific cardiac defect, physiology, and age
- Normal waveforms for right ventricular (RV) and pulmonary artery (PA) pressure tracings
- Mastery of pediatric advanced life support competencies
- Understanding of the location of the PA catheter in the heart and PA and the insertion technique in the operating room (Figure 64-1)
- Indications for PA catheter use[1-6]
  - ❖ Aid in the diagnosis of complications after reparative or palliative surgery for congenital heart disease including tamponade
  - ❖ Management during the postoperative period of children at high risk undergoing cardiac surgical procedures
  - ❖ Determine etiology of hypotensive state, such as hypovolemia, sepsis, heart failure, and cardiac tamponade

- ❖ Hemodynamic monitoring and evaluation after surgery of children with organ dysfunction who need fluid management and infusion of vasoactive medications
- ❖ Hemodynamic monitoring and evaluation of children with pulmonary artery hypertension (PAH) from elevated pulmonary vascular resistance (PVR), pulmonary venous hypertension, residual cardiac lesions or low cardiac output after surgery, or pulmonary hypertensive crisis
- ❖ Calculation of intracardiac left to right shunt fractions
- ❖ Measurement of mixed venous oxygen saturation
- ❖ Infusion of vasoactive medications, blood products, total parenteral nutrition (TPN), electrolyte replacements, and routine medication administration
- Appropriate set-up, use, and troubleshooting of hemodynamic monitoring systems (see Procedure 63 for further information)
- A PA catheter can not be used in the child with right ventricular to pulmonary artery discontinuity. Placement of a RV to PA conduit to establish continuity between the RV and PA is a relative contraindication to the use of a transthoracic PA catheter.[2,5]
- Pulmonary artery pressure (PAP) may be elevated because of pulmonary artery hypertension, pulmonary disease, mitral valve disease, left ventricular failure,

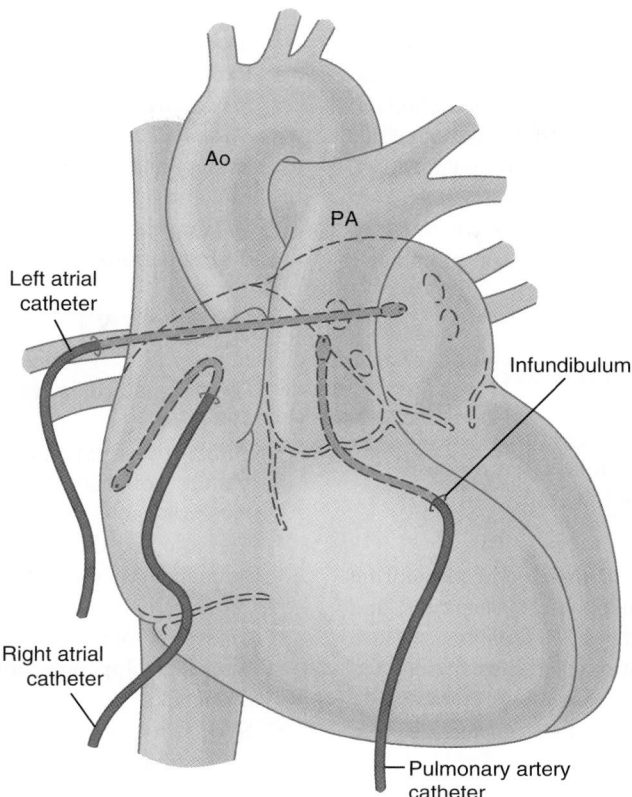

FIGURE 64-1 Drawing of Transthoracic Intracardiac PA Catheter Placement. Catheter is placed intraoperatively through right ventricular outflow tract into main PA. *From Allen HD, Clark EB, Gutgesell HP, et al, editors: Moss and Adams' heart disease in infants, children and adolescents, ed 6, Philadelphia, 2000, Lippincott Williams & Wilkins.*

atrial or ventricular left to right shunts, pulmonary emboli, hypervolemia, primary pulmonary hypertension, cardiac tamponade, or pulmonary process (pneumonia, effusion, or pneumothorax).[1-3,5]
- The PAP may be decreased because of hypovolemia or vasodilation.[1-5]
- The PA diastolic pressure is an indirect measurement of left ventricular end diastolic pressure (LVEDP), except in cases of pulmonary hypertension, acute respiratory distress syndrome (ARDS), tachycardia, pulmonary embolus, or anomalies of the pulmonary veins.[1-5]
- Child development as it relates to clinical assessment and use of a PA catheter.

CHILD AND FAMILY ASSESSMENT

- Child's developmental level and ability to interact ➡️***Rationale:*** These factors influence preparation of the child and interaction.
- Child's baseline hemodynamic and cardiovascular status ➡️***Rationale:*** Provides data for comparison.
- Child's baseline pulmonary status. If the child has mechanical ventilation, notation of the ventilator mode, the presence or absence of positive end-expiratory pressure (PEEP), the oxygen concentration, and use of additional inhaled gas ➡️***Rationale:*** The presence of mechanical ventilation, use of hyperoxygenation or hyperventilation, or use of inhaled nitric oxide alters PA pressures.
- Child's cardiac surgical history related to repair or palliation of the congenital heart defect and currently used medications related to problems with cardiovascular or pulmonary anatomy or physiology. Assessment of preoperative cardiac catheterization data when available. ➡️***Rationale:*** Previous surgical reconstruction or preoperative medications can affect PA pressure. Preoperative catheterization data can identify children at increased risk for elevation in pulmonary artery pressure or pulmonary vascular resistance or those at risk of pulmonary hypertensive crisis after surgery.
- Child's current laboratory profile, including electrolyte, arterial blood gas and lactate, and coagulation studies ➡️***Rationale:*** Identifies abnormalities that may affect cardiac or pulmonary function and alter PAP; identifies coagulation abnormalities that may result in bleeding from the insertion site.
- Vasoactive medications currently used to alter the child's PA pressures ➡️***Rationale:*** Identifies medications (oral or intravenous) that alter PAP.
- Patency of the mediastinal chest tube ➡️***Rationale:*** Bleeding associated with line removal is evacuated via

the chest tube. Blood that is not evacuated may result in cardiac tamponade.

- Child's and family's understanding of the reasons for and risks and benefits of PA catheter use ➤➤*Rationale:* Evaluates the child's and family's understanding of PA catheter use and provides a gauge for ongoing education.
- Child's level of sedation and comfort ➤➤*Rationale:* Pain and agitation can lead to accidental line dislodgement or an increase in PA pressures, resulting in pulmonary hypertensive crisis.

CHILD AND FAMILY EDUCATION

Individualized, developmentally appropriate education is provided to the family and to the child based on desire for knowledge, readiness to learn, and overall neurologic and psychosocial state.

- Provide information about the catheter and monitoring system, including waveform display, use of alarms, and approximate time the catheter will remain in place ➤➤*Rationale:* Providing information decreases anxiety and fear.
- Provide information regarding the PA catheter location, reason for placement, and information provided by the PA catheter ➤➤*Rationale:* Providing information about why a

PA catheter is helpful and how it will help the child; decreases the family's and child's anxiety.

- Explain the use of the PA catheter for blood sampling procedures and infusion of medications and fluids ➤➤*Rationale:* Explanations regarding these uses reduce anxiety and keep the family and child informed.
- Encourage questions and answer questions as they arise ➤➤*Rationale:* Reinforcement of information is needed during periods of stress.

EQUIPMENT

- Gloves and protective eyewear
- 4×4 gauze
- Antibiotic ointment and dressing
- Waterproof absorbent pads
- Pressure cables for interface with monitor
- Pressure transducer system, including flush solutions recommended per institution-specific protocol
- Pressure bag or syringe pump
- Pressure tubing with flush device and transducer
- Luer lock stopcock caps
- Stopcocks
- Syringes: 1-mL and 5-mL
- Tubes and syringes for blood samples
- Specimen labels

Procedure	for Pulmonary Artery Intracardiac Line: Care and Management	
Steps	**Rationale**	**Considerations**
Pressure Monitoring Set-Up		
1. Ensure child and family understand procedure and questions are answered.	Evaluates and reinforces understanding of previously taught information.	Developmental level, cognitive ability, and anxiety level determine approach to and effectiveness of teaching.
2. Gather needed equipment and supplies.	Facilitates completion of procedure in a timely manner.	
3. Wash hands. *(Level VI*)*	Standard precautions; reduces transmission of microorganisms.	
4. Review prescribing practitioner's order or institution-specific protocol for flush solution to be administered through the PA catheter; generally a heparinized solution is used.[1,3,6] *(Level II*)*	Heparinized solutions minimize thrombus and fibrin deposits on catheters that might lead to thrombosis or bacterial colonization of the catheter.	Although heparinized solutions are standard for line patency, heparin may cause thrombocytopenia.
5. Prime or flush entire pressure transducer system with prescribed fluid; for further information on pressure transducer system set-up, see Procedure 63. *(Level VI*)*	Removes air bubbles; air bubbles introduced into child's circulation may cause air embolism. Air bubbles within the tubing dampen the waveform.[1,4]	Air is more easily removed when the system is not under pressure.
6. Use two patient identifiers to verify correct patient.	Promotes patient safety; ensures that heparinized flush is administered to the correct child.	Two patient identifiers should be used for patient identification per institution-specific protocol; most com-

---

* Level II: Theory-based; no research data to support recommendations; recommendations from expert consensus group may exist
Level VI: Clinical studies in a variety of patient populations and situations to support recommendations

Procedure | **for Pulmonary Artery Intracardiac Line: Care and Management**—*Continued*

Steps	Rationale	Considerations
		monly, name and birth date or name and medical record number are used.
7. Connect hemodynamic flush system to PA catheter stopcock port, ensuring that no air is introduced.	Ensures that air is not introduced during PA connection.	
8. Connect pressure cable from PA transducer to bedside monitor.	Connects PA catheter to bedside monitoring system, allowing waveform and numeric display.	
9. Set scales as appropriate for pressure tracing.	Permits numeric and waveform analysis.	PA scale is commonly 40 mm Hg. Scales are adjusted based on the child's PA pressure.[1]
10. Secure system to a pole mount and level to the phlebostatic axis (see Figure 137-2 for instructions on locating the phlebostatic axis). *(Level VI*)*	Ensures that air-fluid zeroing interface (stopcock) is maintained at the level of the phlebostatic axis. If air-fluid interface is above the phlebostatic axis, PA pressures are falsely low. If air-fluid interface is below the phlebostatic axis, PA pressures are falsely high.	In some institutions, the transducer is placed next to child parallel to the phlebostatic axis; refer to institution-specific protocol.
11. Zero the PA monitoring system according to monitoring system manufacturer's instructions. *(Level I*)*	Ensures accuracy of readings by compensating for zero drift.	
12. Observe waveform and pressure readings.	Ensures that system is correctly assembled and that PA catheter is in the correct location.	Improper positioning of PA catheters increases child's risk for pulmonary infarction and pulmonary artery rupture.
13. Set alarms; upper and lower limits are set on the basis of the child's current clinical status and hemodynamic values.	Activates bedside and central monitoring alarm system; promotes patient safety.	
14. Position child in supine position with the head of bed at 0 to 45 degrees.[7,8] *(Level V*)*	Studies have shown PA pressure measurements to be accurate up to a 45-degree angle.	Accuracy of pressure measurements in the lateral position has not been determined.
15. Measure systolic and diastolic and mean PAP consistently at the end of expiration.[1,3,5,6]	Measurements obtained at end expiration are most accurate because the effects of pulmonary pressures are minimized (see Figure 64-2).	A discrete difference is seen between PAPs during spontaneous and mechanical ventilation. In spontaneous ventilation, intrathoracic pressure varies with inspiration (pressure decreases) and expiration (pressure increases). During mechanical ventilation, the application of peak end expiratory pressure alters the native intrathoracic pressure readings.[1,6]
16. Determine end expiration by observing rise and fall of the chest during breathing and correlating with graphic hemodynamic, respiratory, or continuous airway pressure waveforms.	Aids in accurate identification of end expiration.	

Procedure continues on following page

* Level I: Manufacturer's recommendations only
Level V: Clinical studies in more than one or two patient populations and situations to support recommendations
Level VI: Clinical studies in a variety of patient populations and situations to support recommendations

Procedure **for Pulmonary Artery Intracardiac Line: Care and Management**—*Continued*

Steps	Rationale	Considerations

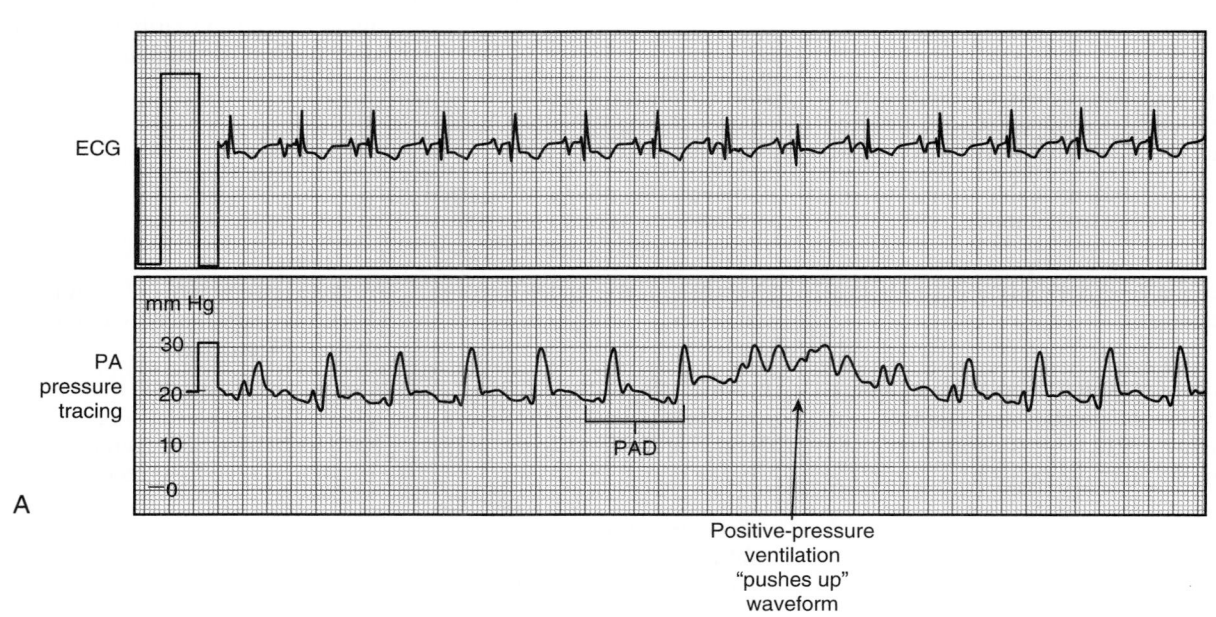

Positive-pressure
ventilation
"pushes up"
waveform

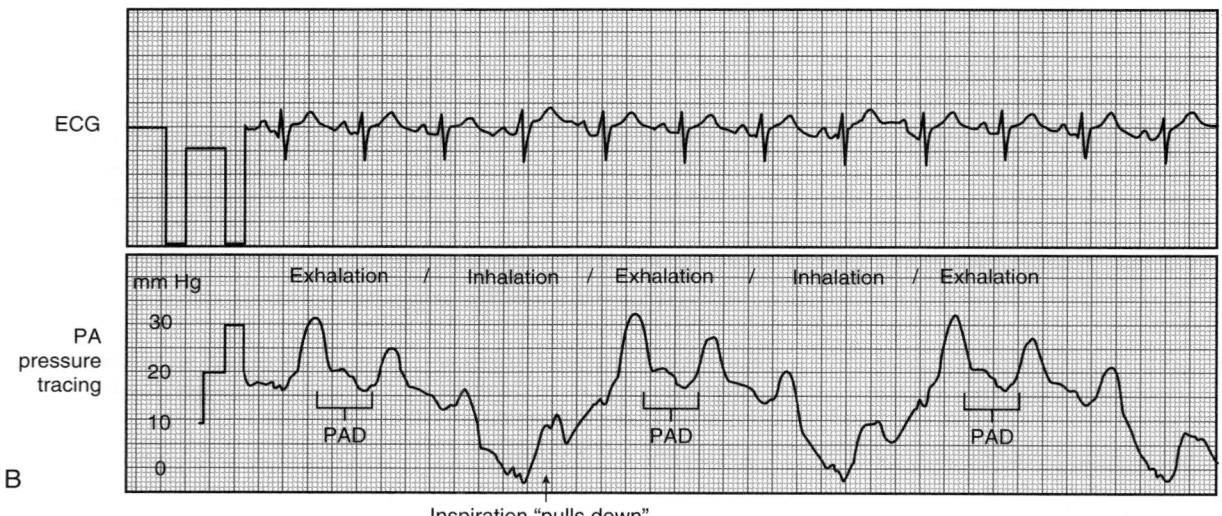

Inspiration "pulls down"
PA pressure waveform
in a spontaneously
breathing patient

FIGURE 64-2   Pulmonary artery waveform alterations with respiratory cycle. For accuracy, PA pressure readings are read at end expiration. **A,** Positive pressure ventilation increases intrathoracic pressure, falsely elevating PAP. **B,** With spontaneous breathing, normal inhalation decreases intrathoracic pressure and creates falsely low reading. *From Thelan LA, Urden LD, Lough ME, et al: Critical care nursing: diagnosis and management, ed 3, St Louis, 1998, Mosby.*

Obtaining Blood Specimen

Steps	Rationale
1. Ensure child and family understand procedure and questions are answered.	Evaluates and reinforces understanding of previously taught information.
2. Gather needed equipment and supplies, including appropriate laboratory tubes.	Facilitates completion of task in a timely manner.

Procedure for Pulmonary Artery Intracardiac Line: Care and Management—*Continued*

Steps	Rationale	Considerations
3. Use two patient identifiers to verify correct patient.	Promotes patient safety; ensures that blood specimens are drawn on the correct patient.	
4. Wash hands; put on clean gloves.	Standard precautions; reduces transmission of microorganisms.	
5. Silence monitor alarms.	Prevents unnecessary alarm activation during sampling procedure.	
6. Label syringe to be used for drawing "discard." *(Level II*)*	Prevents blood in discard syringe from being sent to the laboratory for analysis.[9]	
7. Clean stopcock port site or needleless access site with an alcohol wipe or antiseptic swab.	Reduces transmission of microorganisms.	Refer to institution-specific protocol for antiseptic solution used for cleaning port or needleless access site.
8. Turn stopcock so that "off" arm is toward child ("off to the patient" position) and if necessary, remove occlusive cap.	Closes port oriented toward child; prevents backflow of blood from PA line when sampling port is opened.	PA waveform will be lost. Needleless access caps should not be removed.
9. Attach labeled discard syringe to the stopcock or insert syringe with needleless access device into needleless access site.	Discard volume necessary depends on the type of flush system and the size and length of tubing.	Dead space volume must be accurately determined to ensure that the samples are free of contaminants (heparin or crystalloids). In general, recommended discard volume is at least three times the dead space volume.[9,10] *(Level IV*)*
10. Rotate stopcock so that "off" arm of stopcock is toward transducer ("off to the transducer" position).	Allows withdrawal of discard volume by opening the patient and sampling ports.	
11. Aspirate line and slowly draw discard.	Ensures an accurate blood sample free of contaminates such as heparin or crystalloids.	Refer to institution-specific protocol regarding amount of waste or discard to be drawn before drawing blood sample.
12. If a needleless access site is being used, remove the syringe with discard volume. If syringe is directly attached to the stopcock, rotate stopcock so that the "off" arm of stopcock is off to the syringe, child, and transducer.	Prevents excess blood withdrawal and contamination of the transducer. Prevents backflow of blood from PA line when stopcock port is opened.	Remove the syringe with the discard volume and place to the side. Care must be taken to prevent mistaking the discard specimen from the actual specimens to be sent to the laboratory, which is prevented by labeling the discard syringe.[2]
13. Attach blood gas (BG) syringe or an appropriately sized syringe for the amount of blood to be sampled via the needleless access port; attach directly	Syringe or Vacutainer must be securely attached to prevent leakage of blood from stopcock and tubing.	If appropriate, discard excess heparin from BG syringe before attaching to the stopcock port. Determine the minimal amount of

Procedure continues on following page

* Level II: Theory-based; no research data to support recommendations; recommendations from expert consensus group may exist
  Level IV: Limited clinical studies to support recommendations

Procedure	for **Pulmonary Artery Intracardiac Line: Care and Management**—*Continued*	
Steps	**Rationale**	**Considerations**
to the stopcock or attach a collection tube to the Vacutainer (Becton, Dickinson and Co., Franklin Lakes, NJ®).		blood necessary for laboratory analysis before sampling to prevent nosocomial anemia.
14. If needed, rotate stopcock to the "open to the patient" position; slowly withdraw desired amount of blood.	Stopcock must be open to the patient for specimen collection.	Do not pull on the syringe plunger if resistance is felt.
15. Rotate the stopcock to the "off to the syringe" position and remove the syringe.	Ensuring that stopcock is turned "off to the syringe" prevents inadvertent blood loss from the system.	
16. Place blood in appropriate specimen tubes.	Needed to transport specimens to the laboratory.	Specimen collection tubes are determined by the institution.
17. Reinfusion of the discard volume to the child is not recommended.[9,10] If discard is to be returned to the child, replace syringe with discard onto stopcock. Rotate stopcock to the "off to the transducer" position; aspirate slightly to evacuate air bubbles; slowly reinfuse the blood in syringe and then rotate stopcock to "off to the syringe" position.	Reinfusion of discard reduces the blood loss that occurs when multiple specimens are obtained over several hours or days.	Reinfuse discard volume if this is consistent with institution-specific protocol. Concerns with reinfusing discard volume include possible contamination of the discard syringe, potential that discard volume contains clots, and exposure of clinician to blood.[9,10] Assess ease of reinfusion; do not force.
18. Manually flush the PA line at the stopcock with syringe or at the transducer with the fast flush device, using quick bursts.	Clears line of residual blood; prevents clot formation.	If heparin is used in the flush, use only the amount of flush necessary to clear line to avoid potential complications associated with heparin use.
19. If occlusive cap was removed, recap port with a sterile cap and ensure that stopcock is in "off to the syringe" position.	Minimizes risk of contamination of system and ensures resumption of accurate monitoring.	
20. If a closed blood sampling system is used, refer to Procedure 138 for information on use of a closed blood sampling system.	Closed blood sampling systems decrease exposure of healthcare workers to blood and decrease nosocomial anemia when frequent blood draws are necessary. *(Level II*)*	
21. Observe for return of pressure waveform and reading.	Assures that line is in functioning order, that stopcocks are turned correctly, and that line is free of air.	
22. Reactivate monitor alarms.	Provides for notification of PA pressures at an unacceptable level or of inadvertent disconnection of line.	Alarm ranges are set per institution-specific protocol or patient status.
23. Label specimens at bedside and complete laboratory paperwork per institution-specific protocol.	Promotes patient safety; ensures accurate and efficient processing of specimen.	Expel any air bubbles from the BG syringe. Place BG syringe on ice if required by institution-specific protocol. Follow institution-specific protocols for handling and labeling laboratory specimens.

* Level II: Theory-based; no research data to support recommendations; recommendations from expert consensus group may exist

Procedure | for Pulmonary Artery Intracardiac Line: Care and Management—*Continued*

Steps	Rationale	Considerations
24. Discard used supplies and equipment in appropriate receptacle.	Standard precautions; reduces transmission of microorganisms.	
25. If PA catheter is used to infuse medications, flush medication through the stopcock.	Flushing PA catheter prevents air embolus when infusing medications.	Infusion of medications through the PA catheter should be the last resort for access. Assure that medications are compatible to prevent precipitation and occlusion of the catheter.
26. Turn stopcock to provide pressure monitoring and waveform with infusion.	The waveform is dampened and pressure measurements inaccurate while medications are actively infusing.	To obtain accurate pressure readings, turn infusion off and read the pressure then resume the medication infusion.
27. Remove gloves, wash hands.	Standard precautions; reduces transmission of microorganisms.	

Expected Outcomes

- Child is free from PA catheter-related infection

- PA catheter remains in place until electively removed
- Child is free from complications related to the PA catheter

- Accurate PA waveforms and pressures are obtained

- Accurate placement of the pulmonary artery catheter

- Ability to obtain accurate information about response to treatment and to guide treatment of pulmonary artery hypertension
- Early recognition of acute elevations in pulmonary artery pressure that may represent a pulmonary hypertensive crisis
- Adequate blood specimen obtained with minimal blood loss
- Specimens are placed in correct sample tubes, labeled appropriately, and sent to laboratory in the appropriate time frame

Unexpected Outcomes

- Local infection at catheter insertion site
- Infection from PA catheter that results in sepsis
- Unplanned catheter removal
- Thrombosis
- Tamponade
- Hemothorax
- Uncontrolled bleeding
- Venous air emboli
- Pulmonary infarction
- Pulmonary artery rupture
- Inaccurate waveforms and pressures related to incorrect leveling of transducer, excess tubing in monitoring system, or zero of system not done
- Catheter migrates into the right ventricle (RV); ventricular dysrhythmias
- Catheter is wedged
- Information obtained is equivocal and does not provide clear information about effectiveness of treatment
- Acute PA pressure elevation is not recognized

- Inadequate, diluted, or hemolyzed blood specimen
- Excessive blood volume removed
- Specimens are mislabeled, placed in incorrect sample tubes, or not sent to laboratory in a timely fashion

Monitoring and Care of the Child

Activities and Interventions	Rationale	Reportable Conditions
1. Monitor PA systolic and diastolic pressure readings continuously. Obtain hemodynamic values hourly and as necessary with condition changes.	Pulmonary hypertensive crisis results in an acute rise in PAP. Alterations in ventilation, vasoactive medications, or child's responsiveness may result in elevations in PAP.	• Elevated PA pressures • Deterioration of child's status after titration of medications • Significant changes in hemodynamics

Continued

Monitoring and Care of the Child—Cont'd

Activities and Interventions	Rationale	Reportable Conditions
2. Monitor configuration of the PA catheter waveform (Figure 64-3).	Damped waveform may indicate thrombus formation in the catheter lumen. Catheter may migrate into right ventricle or become wedged.	• Dampened PA waveform • Waveform suggests catheter is wedged • Waveform suggests catheter is in RV • Ventricular arrhythmia

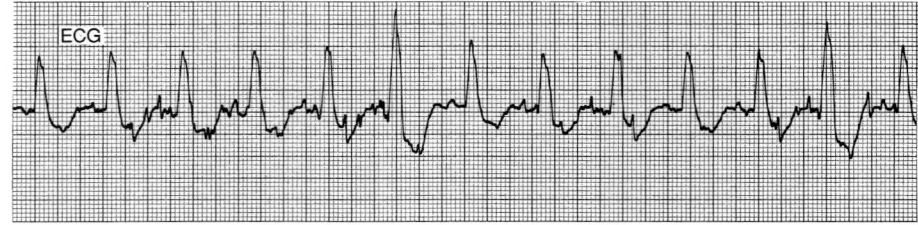

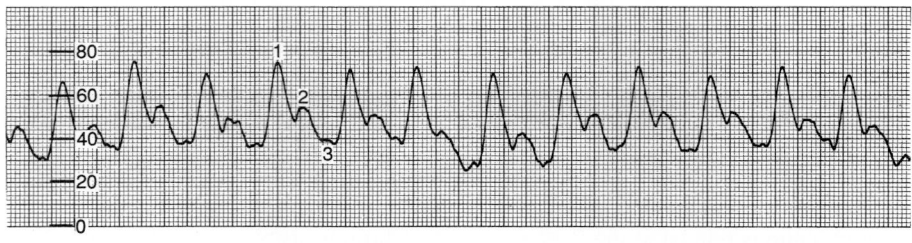

FIGURE 64-3   Pulmonary artery waveform with components. *1*, PA systole; *2*, dicrotic notch; *3*, PA diastole. *From Preuss T, Lynn-McHale Wiegand D: Pulmonary artery catheter and pressure lines, troubleshooting. In Lynn-McHale Wiegand DJ, Carlson K, editors:* AACN procedure manual for critical care, *ed 5, Philadelphia, 2005, Saunders.*

Activities and Interventions	Rationale	Reportable Conditions
3. Date and time when the initial dressing was applied in operating room.	Indicates when dressing was placed and when it is due to be changed.	• Dressing change does not occur when required
4. Monitor the child and site for signs of infection.	Infection can develop because of the invasive nature of the catheter. The PA catheter should be removed at the first sign of infection if it is considered to be the source.[11]	• Redness, swelling, or drainage at the catheter insertion site
5. Zero the transducer During initial set-up: • If disconnection occurs between transducer and monitoring cable. • If disconnection occurs between monitoring cable and monitor. • When values obtained do not fit the clinical picture • Routinely every shift. Follow manufacturer recommendations for disposable and reusable systems. *(Level I*)*	Ensures accuracy of hemodynamic monitoring system; minimizes the risk of contamination of the system.	• Inability to zero line • Pressure readings do not correspond to the child's clinical picture despite transducer zeroing and calibration
6. Ensure that all connections are tight and that all stopcocks are closed to air. Place sterile dead-end caps on all stopcocks. Replace with new sterile caps whenever the caps are removed.	Loose connections or open stopcocks cause a decrease in pressure within the fluid-filled system and blood may exert a back pressure into the pressure tubing. Stopcocks can be a source of contamination. Stopcocks that are part of the initial setup are commonly vented; vented caps must be replaced with non-	• System is contaminated

Monitoring and Care of the Child—Cont'd

Activities and Interventions	Rationale	Reportable Conditions
	vented caps to maintain sterility and closed system.	
7. Ensure that the pressure bag is inflated to 300 mm Hg (greater than 20 kg) or that the infusion pump is turned on and infusing.	Low pressure from the bag or infusion pump failure results in blood back-up with possible clotting of the catheter and inaccurate readings or thrombus formation.	• Inability to flush catheter • Inability to withdraw blood from catheter
8. After use of the PA catheter for blood sampling, flush the entire line to remove blood and air from the system. *(Level III*)*	Blood can become a medium for bacterial growth.[11] Prevents clot formation within the monitoring system. Prevents air embolus into the PA. Prevents dampening of the pressure tracing and inaccurate pressure measurements.	• Inability to flush catheter • Inability to withdraw blood from catheter • Dampened waveform that does not improve with flushing
9. Pressures alarms should be set based on the child's normal levels and turned on at all times.	Signals pressure changes outside of the desired range and disconnections in the pressure monitoring system.	• Pressures outside of the desired range
10. Change reusable transducer systems based on manufacturer recommendations and institution-specific protocol. Change the flush solution based on institution-specific protocol.	The Centers for Disease Control and Prevention (CDC) recommend that the flush system can be used safely for 72 hours. This recommendation is based on research conducted with disposable pressure monitoring systems used for peripheral and central lines.[11] *(Level IV*)*	• Tubing or flush solution not changed as recommended • Signs and symptoms of infection
11. Label tubing with date and time the system was prepared.	Identifies when the system needs to be changed.	• Tubing not labeled
12. Use aseptic technique when zeroing, flushing, or obtaining blood samples from the catheter. *(Level VI*)*	Prevents bacterial contamination of the system.[11]	
13. Follow institution-specific protocol for frequency of dressing change and type of dressing applied, including application of antimicrobial ointment to catheter.	Decreases the risk of infection at the catheter site. The CDC has made no recommendation for the frequency of routine PA catheter dressing change but recommends replacing dressing when the dressing becomes damp, loosened, or soiled or when inspection of the site is necessary.[11] *(Level II*)* Routine use of antimicrobial ointment at central venous catheter insertion sites is not recommended.	• The PA catheter dressing becomes saturated quickly after a dressing change, which may indicate catheter fracture, other type of leakage, or change in the catheter tip location • Indications of infection at the PA catheter insertion site
14. Monitor results of the specimens obtained.	Monitors child's status; facilitates identification of possible errors in obtaining the specimens (e.g., inadequate discard volume drawn results in erroneous results).	• Abnormal laboratory values

* Level II: Theory-based; no research data to support recommendations; recommendations from expert consensus group may exist
  Level III: Laboratory data; no clinical data to support recommendations
  Level IV: Limited clinical studies to support recommendations
  Level VI: Clinical studies in a variety of patient populations and situations to support recommendations

Documentation

- Child and family education
- Catheter insertion site assessment
- Pulmonary artery pressures
- Pulmonary artery waveforms
- Solutions infused into catheter and rate
- Date and time of dressing change
- Date and time of monitoring system tubing and flush solution change
- Date and time of blood sampling and specimens obtained
- Results of laboratory studies obtained; practitioner notified of critical laboratory values
- Waveform assessment after any catheter manipulation (blood drawing, flushing)
- Child's hemodynamic status
- Unexpected outcomes and related treatment

References

1. Craig J, et al: Cardiovascular critical care problems. In Curley MAQ, Moloney-Harmon P, editors: *Critical care nursing of infants and children,* ed 2, Philadelphia, 2001, Saunders.
2. Gold JP, et al: Transthoracic intracardiac monitoring lines in pediatric surgical patients: a ten-year experience, *Ann Thorac Surg* 42(2):185-191, 1986.
3. Johnston LJ, McKinley DF: Cardiac tamponade after removal of atrial intracardiac monitoring catheters in a pediatric patient: case report, *Heart Lung* 29(4):256-261, 2000.
4. Lindberg L, et al: How common is severe pulmonary hypertension after pediatric cardiac surgery? *J Thorac Cardiovasc Surg* 123(6):1155-1163, 2002.
5. Wessel DC, Laussen PC: Cardiac intensive care. In Fuhrman BP, Zimmerman J, editors: *Pediatric critical care,* ed 3, Philadelphia, 2006, Mosby.
6. Roth SJ: Postoperative care. In Chang AC, et al, editors: *Pediatric cardiac intensive care,* Baltimore, 1998, Williams and Wilkins.
7. Cason CL, et al: Effects of backrest elevation and position on pulmonary artery pressures, *Cardiovasc Nurs* 26:1-5, 1990.
8. Chulay M, Miller T: The effect of backrest elevation on pulmonary artery and pulmonary capillary wedge pressures in patients after cardiac surgery, *Heart Lung* 131:38-40, 1984.
9. Frey AM: Drawing blood samples from vascular access devices: evidence-based practice, *J Infusion Nurs* 26(5):285-293, 2003.
10. Dech ZF, Szaflarski NL: Nursing strategies to minimize blood loss associated with phlebotomy, *AACN Clin Issues* 7(2):277-287, 1996.
11. Pearson ML: Hospital infection control practices advisory committee: guideline for prevention of intravascular device-related infections, *Infection Control Hospital Epidemiol* 17:438-473, 1996.

Additional Readings

Ahrens TS, Taylor LA: *Hemodynamic waveform analysis,* Philadelphia, 1992, Saunders.

Castaneda AR, et al: *Cardiac surgery of the neonate and infant,* Philadelphia, 2002, Saunders.

Hazinski MF: *Manual of pediatric critical care,* ed 2, Philadelphia, 1999, Mosby.

Mavroudis C, Backer CL, editors: *Pediatric cardiac surgery,* ed 3, Philadelphia, 2003, Mosby.

Rogers MC, Nichols DG, editors: *Textbook of pediatric intensive care,* ed 3, Baltimore, 1996, Williams and Wilkins.

Singh NC, editor: *Manual of pediatric critical care,* Philadelphia, 1997, Saunders.

Right Atrial Intracardiac Line: Care and Management

P U R P O S E : Right atrial (RA) intracardiac lines are placed in infants and children following open heart surgery to monitor the intracardiac pressure of the right atrium as an indicator of cardiac filling and function. In addition, these lines provide vascular access and a site for monitoring venous oxygenation.

Aimee Jennings

PREREQUISITE KNOWLEDGE

- Normal cardiac anatomy and physiology
- Proper care and management of the right atrial catheter (RAC) is essential to optimizing the function and utility of the catheter.
- Familiarity with postoperative care requirements of infants and children after cardiac surgery
- The individual child's congenital heart defect and the surgical procedure performed
- Rationale for RA intracardiac line (catheter) monitoring is to provide information on the child's hemodynamic status including information on preload, intravascular volume status, right ventricular compliance, tricuspid valve disease, and atrial shunting.[1] In addition, these lines provide vascular access and a site for monitoring venous oxygenation.
- Children undergoing any intracardiac surgery may have an RAC placed in the operating room. The catheter tip is placed in the RA, anchored to the heart, and then brought through the chest wall, where it is attached to a pressure transducer and tubing.
- Familiarity with RAC pressure tracing waves and ability to distinguish normal variations in waveform from abnormal wave patterns.[1-3]
- Appropriate setup, use, and troubleshooting of hemodynamic monitoring systems. Refer to Procedure 63.

- Familiarity with troubleshooting equipment related to alterations in pressure readings: decreased wave amplitude, loss of waveform.[1-4] RAC should be recalibrated to atmospheric pressure at the phlebostatic axis at least every 8 to 12 hours, following repositioning of the child, and as needed.[1-3,5,6] Refer to Procedure 137, Figure 137-2 for instructions on locating the phlebostatic axis.
- Diligent monitoring for potential RAC-related complications is mandatory, and appropriate interventions should be taken in the event of complications.[4,6,7]
- Recognize RA pressure and waveform changes and understand the implications for care regarding the child's hemodynamic or pulmonary status.[1-4,6,7]
- Normal RA pressures are 1 to 6 mm Hg.[6]
- Post-operative parameters for RA pressure after cardiac surgery may be 6 to 12 mm Hg or higher depending on cardiovascular physiology.
  - ❖ Elevated RA pressures may reflect decreased right ventricular compliance, abnormal ventricular systolic or diastolic function, right ventricular hypertrophy, right ventricular volume overload, tricuspid valve disease, left ventricular to right atrial shunt, intravascular volume overload, cardiac tamponade, or tachyarrhythmia.[6]
  - ❖ Artifactual causes of elevated RA pressure include incorrect position of the catheter, either in the ventricle or wedged, the pressure transducer being located

below the level of the heart, or the pressure transducer being improperly calibrated or zeroed.[6]

- ❖ Reduced RA pressures may reflect low intravascular volume status or inadequate preload.
- ❖ Artifactual causes of reduced RA pressures include catheter malfunction either due to clot or cracking of the catheter, the pressure transducer being located above the level of the heart, or the pressure transducer improperly calibrated or zeroed.[6]
- Maintenance fluids and medications may be infused through the RAC. A heparinized solution should be infused through the line to maintain patency and prevent clot formation.[1,4,8] Infusion fluids and rates vary according to institution-specific protocol.
- Meticulous aseptic technique should be used when accessing the RAC or changing intravenous fluids, pressure transducers, and tubing.[4,6,9] Care must be taken to prevent air from entering the RAC.[5,10]
- Normal infant, child, and adolescent heart rates and blood pressures
- Skills for basic and advanced electrocardiogram (ECG) and cardiac arrhythmia interpretation
- Mastery of pediatric advanced life support competencies
- Child development as it relates to clinical assessment and use of RAC

CHILD AND FAMILY ASSESSMENT

- History of congenital heart disease, cardiomyopathy, cardiac dysrhythmias, and cardiac surgical and/or catheterization procedures ➧➧*Rationale:* These conditions affect the rationale for RAC placement and may contribute to elevated or decreased RA pressure readings.
- Current hemodynamic status ➧➧*Rationale:* An understanding of baseline hemodynamic status is needed for appropriate assessment of changes in RA pressures.
- Current heart rhythm, medication history, chest radiographic and laboratory findings ➧➧*Rationale:* Drug therapy, electrolyte and/or acid-base abnormalities, presence of dysrhythmias, and RAC placement affect the RAC waveform and pressure measurements.
- Child's level of sedation and comfort ➧➧*Rationale:* Pain and agitation can lead to accidental line dislodgement and falsely elevated RA pressure.
- Medical history associated with use of sedation and comfort measures ➧➧*Rationale:* Sedation and comfort measures may be used to ensure compliance with activity restrictions.
- Child's developmental level and ability to interact ➧➧*Rationale:* These factors influence preparation of the child and interaction, and guide strategies to ensure security of the RAC.
- Level of consciousness and cognition ➧➧*Rationale:* Determine child's ability to cooperate with activity restrictions or need for soft restraints.
- Child's and family's understanding of the cardiac lesion, indications for surgical procedure, and reasons for and risks and benefits of RAC use ➧➧*Rationale:* Evaluates

child's and family's understanding of the procedure and provides a gauge for ongoing education.
- Family's desire to be present at child's bedside ➧➧*Rationale:* Family may provide support and comfort measures to their child but should have the choice not to remain with the child.

CHILD AND FAMILY EDUCATION

Individualized, developmentally appropriate education is provided to the family and to the child based on desire for knowledge, readiness to learn, and overall neurologic and psychosocial state.

- Provide information on the child's medical condition and the need for RAC monitoring ➧➧*Rationale:* Providing educationally appropriate information helps to decrease the child's and family's anxiety levels and offers reassurance during an extremely stressful period in their lives.
- As circumstances permit, before surgery provide the child and family with information about the purpose for RAC monitoring and the components involved in routine care ➧➧*Rationale:* Explaining the purpose for RAC monitoring and routine care helps to decrease anxiety about the presence of a catheter in the heart.
- During the preoperative intensive care unit (ICU) tour and/or once the child has been stabilized during the immediate postoperative period, describe for the child and the family the location of the line and the corresponding tubing. In simple terms explain how the system works and reinforce the purpose of the RAC[1,3,5,6] ➧➧*Rationale:* Providing educationally appropriate information helps to decrease anxiety about equipment, especially in the highly technical ICU.
- Explain the risks associated with RAC use and the types of interventions that may be required to stabilize the child, including fluid administration, blood transfusion, or emergent sternotomy[4,5-7] ➧➧*Rationale:* Providing information, including a discussion of the benefits and risks associated with the procedure, potential complications, and the required associated interventions help prepare families and decrease anxiety.
- Explain activity restrictions related to child repositioning and family assistance with activities to avoid tension on RAC lines with potential dislodgement[4,9] ➧➧*Rationale:* Explaining the rationale for the restriction aids in the family's understanding and may increase compliance with plan of care.
- Explain to child and family the potential need for sedation and/or soft restraints while RAC is present to prevent inadvertent RAC dislodgement ➧➧*Rationale:* Providing information about need for these measures can reduce the child's and family's anxiety and may increase compliance with the plan of care, decreasing the likelihood of inadvertent RAC line removal, dislodgement, or compromise from repositioning or line tension.
- Encourage family members to comfort and console the child to reduce agitation and movements, decreasing the

potential for RAC line dislodgement ➤*Rationale:* Alternative approaches to providing comfort may help reduce the need for sedation and medical mobilization.

- Encourage questions and answer questions as they arise ➤*Rationale:* Reinforcement of information is needed during periods of stress.

EQUIPMENT

- Continuous heparin flush solution (2 unit/mL or per institution-specific protocol) to maintain patency and prevent blood back-up into the monitoring system
- Pressure transducer system including transducer, pressure tubing, and cable specific to cardiorespiratory monitor in use
- Leveling device
- Labeling tape
- Infusion pump or pressure bag for fluid administration via RAC
- Cardiorespiratory monitor for continual assessment of RA waveform, heart rate, and arterial blood pressure
- Intravenous tubing and inline air filter (per institution-specific protocol) if line is used for continuous infusion other than heparin-containing solution
- Stopcock placed between infusion tubing and RAC for line access, per institution-specific protocol
- Syringes
- Alcohol pads
- Dressing supplies: gauze and tape or transparent semipermeable dressing
- Clean gloves

Procedure	for Right Atrial Intracardiac Line: Care and Management		
Steps	**Rationale**		**Considerations**
1. Ensure child and family understand procedure and questions are answered.	Evaluates and reinforces understanding of previously taught information.		Developmental level, cognitive ability, and anxiety level will determine approach to and effectiveness of teaching.
2. Gather needed equipment and supplies; review prescribing practitioner's order or institution-specific protocol for flush solution to be administered via RAC.	Facilitates completion of procedure in a timely manner. Ensures correct fluid is administered.		Setup should be primed and at the bedside ready for hook-up to facilitate transfer back from the operating room and assessment of RAC without delays.
3. Wash hands.	Standard precautions; reduces transmission of microorganisms.		RAC care and management require aseptic technique.[4,8,9]
4. Assemble RAC monitoring system that includes a transducer, an extension of nondistensible pressure tubing and a stopcock and prime it with heparinized fluid per prescribing practitioner's order or institution-specific protocol.[3,5,8] *(Level VI*)*	Prevents air from remaining in system. Nondistensible pressure tubing maintains the fluid oscillation in the monitoring system facilitating waveform analysis.[3,8]		A stopcock placed between the monitoring system and the RAC provides a port for removing air bubbles and withdrawing blood samples.[3,8] For further information on pressure transducer setup, refer to Procedure 63.
5. Inflate pressure bag or program infusion pump for designated rate of fluid administration per institution-specific protocol.[3]	Regulates infusion of intracardiac monitoring fluid.		Standard pressure bags are inflated to 200 to 300 mm Hg; follow manufacturer recommendations.
6. Connect monitor cable to monitoring system with transducer and inspect the system for the presence of air.[1,3,4,8]	Connects transducer to monitor so that signal is displayed. Prevents air from entering the system.		If air is detected in the system, it should be evacuated immediately or it may result in the development of a pulmonary embolism or cerebrovascular event.[4,5]

Procedure continues on following page

---

* Level VI: Clinical studies in a variety of patient populations and situations to support recommendations

Procedure	for Right Atrial Intracardiac Line: Care and Management—*Continued*	
Steps	**Rationale**	**Considerations**
7. Wash hands; put on clean gloves.	Standard precautions; reduces transmission of microorganisms.	
8. On arrival from operating room, ensure child is flat in bed.[2-5] *(Level VI*)*	Proper positioning optimizes measurement accuracy.	Right atrial pressure reference point changes with change in child's position.[8]
9. Ensure that child is properly connected to cardiopulmonary monitor, and appropriate parameters are monitored.[11] *(Level II*)*	Facilitates accurate assessment of child's current hemodynamic status.	Correlate RA pressure waveform and numeric value with clinical findings and other hemodynamic data.[6]
10. Connect monitoring system with transducer and stopcock to the RAC, ensuring that both the monitoring system and the intracardiac line are completely fluid filled. *(Level II*)*	Prevents air in the system, ensures accurate pressure measurement.	Strategies to prevent air in the line include having another nurse flush the monitoring line simultaneously while the monitoring line and RAC are connected and/or establishing a meniscus of fluid bulging above the rims of the monitoring line and RAC.[5]
11. Withdraw blood from RAC using the stopcock and gently flush the RAC. *(Level II*)*	Evaluates for the presence of air and line patency or occlusion.	Caution must be taken when flushing the RAC due to the potential for clot of air embolism.[4] Report and document if resistance is encountered when flushing RAC or attempting to draw back from the RAC.
12. Close all ports with sterile caps. *(Level II*)*	Prevents infection.	Meticulous care must be taken to maintain a closed system keeping all connections and stopcock ports sterile.[1,3,4,8]
13. Mount the monitoring system securely at the bedside and level transducer with the child's phlebostatic axis using leveling device (see Figure 137-2). *(Level VI*)*	Ensures transducer system's interface is maintained at the level of the phlebostatic axis, for accurate readings.	The phlebostatic axis is the halfway point between the anterior and posterior diameter of the chest intersecting with the 4th intercostal space.[1] Use leveling device to ensure proper alignment of transducer. Consider marking the phlebostatic axis on the child's chest to ensure consistent readings.
14. Zero the RAC to atmospheric pressure by opening a port at the transducer with the stopcock positioned "off" to the child, open to the transducer and zeroing transducer per manufacturer's instructions. *(Level VI*)*	Opening the port at the level of the transducer establishes atmospheric pressure at that level. Zeros to atmospheric pressure.	Avoid incorrect stopcock position when calibrating where transducer is open to the child and off to the transducer. This may allow air to enter the system or blood loss from backflow from the RAC.[5]
15. Evaluate RAC waveform with ECG tracing (Figure 65-1).[1-6] *(Level II*)*	Confirm placement of RAC and accuracy of pressure readings.	Evaluate RA pressure waveform for the following components: **a wave** = atrial contraction, associated with PR interval.

* Level II: Theory-based, no research data to support recommendations: recommendations from expert consensus group may exist
  Level VI: Clinical studies in a variety of patient populations and situations to support recommendations

Procedure for Right Atrial Intracardiac Line: Care and Management—*Continued*

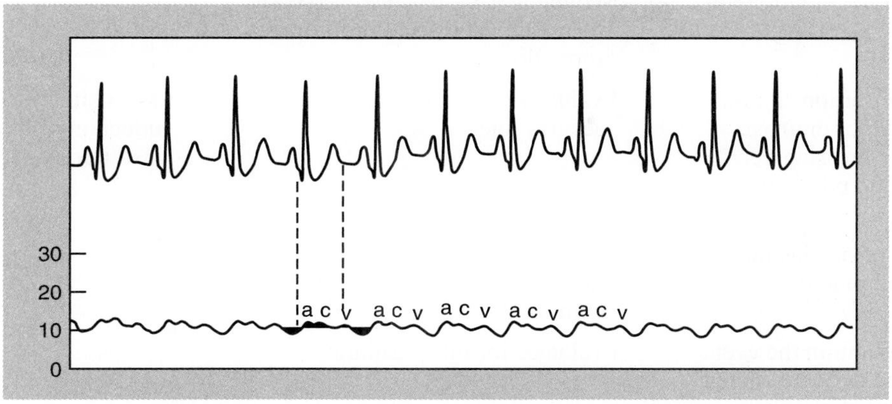

Steps	Rationale	Considerations

FIGURE 65-1 Correlation of RAP waveform with ECG tracing. *From Gardner PE: Pulmonary artery pressure monitoring,* AACN Clin Issues *4[1]:103, 1993.*

Steps	Rationale	Considerations
		c wave = closure of the tricuspid valve, associated with QRS. **v wave** = filling of the atrium during systole, associated with T wave.[3]
16. Correlate RA pressure reading with clinical findings and diagnostic studies. *(Level VI*)*	Validates accuracy of RA pressure readings.	Elevated RA pressures may be due to tip of the catheter being in the ventricle or wedged, the transducer being below the level of the heart, or the transducer improperly zeroed.[6] Decreased RA pressures may be due to the catheter being cracked or clotted, the transducer being located above the heart, or the transducer improperly zeroed.[6]
17. Record mean RA pressure. *(Level VI*)*	Documentation facilitates evaluation of trends over time.	Elevated RA pressure readings may reflect decreased right ventricular compliance, right ventricular volume overload, tricuspid valve disease, left ventricular to right atrial shunt, intravascular volume overload, cardiac tamponade, or artifact.[6] Decreased RA pressure readings may reflect low intravascular volume, inadequate preload, or artifact.[6]
18. Set monitor alarms on the basis of child's current clinical status and hemodynamic values. *(Level II*)*	Alerts care provider to changes in child's hemodynamic status and dynamic changes that may require intervention.	Promotes patient safety.
19. Continuously monitor RA waveform and pressure while RAC is in place. *(Level II*)*	Assess for changes in child's hemodynamic status.	Changes in RA waveforms should correlate with ECG changes, blood pressure changes, and other variations in hemodynamics.

Procedure continues on following page

* Level II: Theory-based, no research data to support recommendations; recommendations from expert consensus group may exist
  Level VI: Clinical studies in a variety of patient populations and situations to support recommendations

Procedure   for Right Atrial Intracardiac Line: Care and Management—*Continued*

Steps	Rationale	Considerations
20. Continuously infuse solution via RAC.	Maintains RAC patency; decreases potential emboli and/or thrombus formation.	
21. Evaluate RAC insertion site for erythema, edema, or drainage and apply sterile dressing per institution-specific protocol. *(Level VI*)*	Evaluates for signs of infection and secures line.	Assess site every hour for signs of infection or bleeding per institution-specific protocol.[5,9]
22. Ensure patency of mediastinal chest tube(s) and monitor drainage. *(Level II*)*	May assist with the prevention or identification of RAC-related complications.[4,7]	
23. Troubleshoot system in the event of an unexpected or acute change in RA pressure readings or abnormal waveform tracing.	Evaluates for false readings.	
24. Obtain chest x-ray on return from surgery and daily while RAC is in place per institution-specific protocol.[10] *(Level II*)*	Evaluates for line placement.	Chest x-rays can assist with the identification of line migration and the development of intracardiac line–related complications.[5,10]
25. Dispose of used supplies and equipment in appropriate receptacle.	Standard precautions; reduces transmission of microorganisms.	
26. Remove gloves; wash hands.	Standard precautions.	

* Level II: Theory-based, no research data to support recommendations; recommendations from expert consensus group may exist
 Level VI: Clinical studies in a variety of patient populations and situations to support recommendations

Expected Outcomes	Unexpected Outcomes
• Accurate RA pressure and waveform obtained and findings as expected for child based on surgical intervention and underlying cardiac defect	• Abnormal waveform • Abnormal RA pressure • Inaccurate waveform and/or pressure related to incorrect leveling of transducer or failure to zero system
• RA catheter integrity and placement maintained until elective removal	• Dysrhythmias or cardiac tamponade caused by catheter migration or dislodgement • Unplanned catheter removal
• Child is free from complications related to RAC	• Blood transfusion requirement due to exsanguination from loose connections within the RAC monitoring system • Air embolism from loose connections in the RAC fluid system • Embolus from clot or vegetation formed on the intracardiac line
• RAC insertion site is free from signs of infection	• Erythema, edema, and/or drainage noted at insertion site • RAC associated sepsis
• Chest x-ray demonstrates RAC in RA and no significant change in cardiac silhouette	• Chest x-ray demonstrates RAC in right ventricle or elsewhere, or increased cardiac silhouette possibly associated with cardiac tamponade related to dislodged RAC
• Child demonstrates acceptable level of comfort	• Unmanaged pain or agitation that threatens catheter placement

Monitoring and Care of the Child

Activities and Interventions	Rationale	Reportable Conditions
1. Continuously monitor hemo-dynamic indicators and clinical status.	Continuous monitoring aids in directing child's care and management, with the ability to rapidly change treatment if indicated.	• Changes in RA pressure that reflect significant changes in child's status
2. Assess RAC every hour and as needed for integrity of the system and presence of air in the system.	Loss of intracardiac line integrity alters RA pressure readings, and can lead to air embolism, bleeding from or clotting of the line.[4,7]	• Compromised line integrity • Air embolism • Clot in the system that cannot be removed
3. Continuously monitor RA pressure and waveform.	Allows monitoring of hemodynamic parameters and detection of potential postoperative problems.	• Abnormalities in RA pressure or waveform despite recalibration (see Figure 65-1)
4. Assess catheter insertion site every hour and change dressing every 24 hours or per institution-specific protocol.[4,9]	Assesses for loss of catheter integrity and/or signs of infection.	• Bleeding at site • Fluid leakage at site • Signs of infection (redness, drainage, tenderness at site, fever, or elevation in white blood cell count)
5. Evaluate chest tube drainage every hour or per institution-specific protocol.	Change in chest tube drainage color, amount, and consistency may reflect a RAC complication.	• Changes in chest tube drainage color, amount, or character with changes in RAC, line function, or child's status

6. Zero transducer:
  • During initial setup.
  • If disconnection occurs between the transducer and the monitor cable.
  • When values obtained do not fit clinical picture.
  • Routinely every shift or per institution-specific protocol.
	Ensures accuracy of hemodynamic monitoring system.	• Unable to perform zero procedure
		• Pressure readings do not correspond to child's clinical picture despite transducer zeroing and calibration (as appropriate)

7. Ensure infusion pump is turned on and infusing or pressure bag is inflated to 300 mm Hg.	Low pressure in pressure bag or pump failure will result in blood back-up with possible clotting of catheter, inaccurate readings, or thrombus formation.	• Unable to flush catheter • Unable to obtain blood return from catheter
8. Change pressure transducer system and flush solution based on manufacturer's recommendations and/or institution-specific protocol.	The Centers for Disease Control and Prevention (CDC) and research findings recommend that flush solution and disposable transducer systems can be used safely for 72 hours.[12]	• Tubing or flush solution not changed as recommended • Signs and symptoms of infection
9. Assess effectiveness of comfort management strategy and provide appropriate interventions. Encourage family to assist in using nonpharmacologic means to comfort and support the child.	Agitation and restlessness may result in inadvertent RAC removal. Early identification of pain or agitation facilitates prompt treatment.	• Unresolved pain or agitation • Inadvertent catheter removal • Continued irritability, changes in physiologic condition

Documentation

- Child and family education
- RA pressure readings
- RA waveform
- Sedation/analgesia or medical immobilization device (if used)
- Infusion fluid and rate
- Disruption of line integrity, repair of RAC, and prescribing practitioner notification
- Comfort assessment and specific interventions provided
- Dressing change and appearance of catheter insertion site
- Confirmation of RAC placement by chest x-ray
- Fluid, tubing, and transducer change
- Zeroing and calibration (as required) at beginning of shift and as indicated
- Alarm limit settings
- Unexpected outcomes and related treatment
- RAC removal (refer to Procedure 68)

References

1. Arnone M: Central venous/right atrial pressure line removal. In Lynn-McHale DJ, Carlson K, editors: *AACN procedure manual for critical care,* ed 4, Philadelphia, 2001, Saunders.
2. Arnone M: Central venous/right atrial pressure line site care. In Lynn-McHale DJ, Carlson K, editors: *AACN procedure manual for critical care,* ed 4, Philadelphia, 2001, Saunders.
3. Arnone M: Central venous/right atrial pressure monitoring. In Lynn-McHale DJ, Carlson K, editors: *AACN procedure manual for critical care,* ed 4, Philadelphia, 2001, Saunders.
4. Bridges E: Hemodynamic monitoring. In Woods S, et al, editors: *Cardiac nursing,* ed 4, Philadelphia, 2000, Lippincott.
5. Clarian Health Partners: Left atrial pressure monitoring: pediatric. In Clarian Health Partners, editors: *Pediatric patient care policy manual,* Indianapolis, 2002, Clarian Health Partners.
6. Craig J, et al: Cardiovascular critical care problems. In Curley MAQ, Moloney-Harmon P, editors: *Critical care nursing of infants and children,* ed 2, Philadelphia, 2001, Saunders.
7. Flori HR, et al: Transthoracic intracardiac catheters in pediatric patients recovering from congenital heart defect surgery: associated complications and outcomes, *Crit Care Med* 28(8):2997-3001, 2000.
8. Gardner PE: Pulmonary artery pressure monitoring, *AACN Clin Issues* 4(1):98-119, 1993.
9. Indiana University School of Medicine Department of Surgery, Section of Cardiothoracic Surgery: Right atrial line removal. In Indiana University School of Medicine Department of Surgery, Section of Cardiothoracic Surgery, editors: *Pediatric nurse practitioner procedures,* Indianapolis, 1999, Indiana University School of Medicine.
10. Johnston LJ, McKinley DF: Cardiac tamponade after removal of atrial intracardiac monitoring catheters in a pediatric patient: case report, *Heart Lung* 29(4):256-261, 2000.
11. Roth SJ: Postoperative care. In Chang AC, et al, editors: *Pediatric cardiac intensive care,* Baltimore, 1998, Williams & Wilkins.
12. Centers for Disease Control and Prevention: Guidelines for the prevention of intravascular catheter related infections, *MMWR Morbid Mortal Wkly Rep* 51(No. RR-10):1-29, 2002.

Additional Readings

Bridges EJ: Monitoring pulmonary artery pressures: just the facts, *Crit Care Nurse* 20(6):59-76, 2000.

Castaneda A, et al: Perioperative care. In *Cardiac surgery of the neonate and infant,* Philadelphia, 1994, Saunders.

McGhee BH, Bridges MEJ: Monitoring arterial blood pressure: what you may not know, *Crit Care Nurse* 22(2):60-79, 2002.

66

Left Atrial Intracardiac Line Removal: Perform

PURPOSE: To safely remove a left atrial catheter inserted in the operating room following an intracardiac surgical procedure once the necessary data are obtained from the left atrial intracardiac line, and it is no longer needed

Dorothy M. Beke and Patricia Lincoln

PREREQUISITE KNOWLEDGE

- Normal cardiac anatomy and physiology
- Familiarity with postoperative care requirements of infants and children after cardiac surgery and ability to identify which types of cardiac defects warrant the use of left atrial (LA) pressure monitoring
- In the operating room left atrial intracardiac catheters (LACs) or lines are placed in children undergoing open heart surgery and whose postoperative management is influenced by data regarding pulmonary venous pressure and saturation, left ventricular preload, afterload, and function, intracardiac shunting and intravascular volume status.[1-4]
- LACs are inserted directly into the LA and anchored to the heart by a suture. The catheter typically exits the skin more left and laterally to the right atrial catheter.[4,5]
- Familiarity with LAC pressure tracing waves and ability to distinguish normal variations in waveform from abnormal wave patterns

- A heparinized solution should be infused through the line to maintain patency and prevent clot formation.[6]
- Ability to identify rationale for LAC removal, which may include improvement in the child's medical condition so that LAC monitoring is no longer required, line malfunction, or infection.[2]
- An alternative intravenous (IV) access route must be available before LAC removal.[2,5]
- Type-specific or O-negative packed red blood cells must be available in blood bank or on the unit prior to initiation of the procedure.[2,5]
- Effects of prothrombin time (PT), partial thromboplastin time (PTT), and International Normalized Ratio (INR) on hemostasis and indications for treatment of abnormal levels. Hemoglobin, hematocrit, and platelet count should also be within an acceptable range before line removal to reduce the risk of sequelae and optimize outcomes.[2,4-7]
- Risks associated with LAC removal, including bleeding, entrapment, and dysrhythmias[2-5,7]
- Ability to recognize signs and symptoms of cardiac tamponade and implement appropriate interventions to decrease morbidity and mortality.[3,5,8]
- Aseptic technique is required for care and removal of an LAC.[2]
- Knowledge of normal infant, child, and adolescent heart rates and blood pressures

- Basic and advanced electrocardiogram (ECG) and cardiac dysrhythmias interpretation
- Mechanism to activate the emergency alert system when a complication is detected
- Mastery of pediatric advanced life support competencies
- Child development as it relates to clinical assessment and LAC removal
- Appropriate pediatric dosing of sedatives and analgesics
- Knowledge of state nurse practice act and institution-specific protocol regarding LAC removal; this procedure is performed by a licensed practitioner with advanced training

CHILD AND FAMILY ASSESSMENT

- Child's and family's understanding of indications for LAC removal as well as the risks and benefits of the procedure ➤*Rationale:* Improves child's and family's cooperation and understanding; provides a gauge for ongoing education.
- Ensure all required data are obtained from LAC before removal ➤*Rationale:* LA monitoring provides information regarding pulmonary venous pressure, left ventricular function, intravascular volume and intracardiac shunting. Premature removal of the LAC may result in inability to collect crucial information.[4]
- Review chest x-ray before LAC removal ➤*Rationale:* Verifies LAC position and identifies potential problems with removal.
- Evaluate results of recent PT, PTT, INR, hemoglobin, hematocrit, and platelet count ➤*Rationale:* Assesses for bleeding risk during and after LAC removal; facilitates treatment of abnormal values as appropriate before LAC removal.
- Appearance of LAC insertion site ➤*Rationale:* Assesses for signs of infection. A culture of the LAC tip may be warranted if bacteremia is suspected or present.
- Presence and patency of alternate vascular access sites[2,5,8,9] ➤*Rationale:* Because of the severity of potential complications with LAC removal, alternate vascular access is essential for the rapid administration of fluid boluses or blood transfusion.
- Child's developmental level[2] ➤*Rationale:* Developmental level influences preparation of the child.
- Level of consciousness and cognition[6] ➤*Rationale:* Determines child's ability to cooperate with instructions. LAC removal is often performed during a phase in the postoperative course when the child continues to receive sedatives and analgesics. Children may not comprehend instructions while sedated, thereby potentially increasing fear and anxiety.

- Family's desire to be present during the procedure ➤*Rationale:* Family may support and comfort the child during the procedure but should have the choice not to remain with the child.

CHILD AND FAMILY EDUCATION

Individualized, developmentally appropriate education is provided to the family and to the child based on desire for knowledge, readiness to learn, and overall neurologic and psychosocial state.

- Provide information regarding LAC removal including potential complications and their associated interventions ➤*Rationale:* Providing information may increase the child's and family's knowledge base, improve cooperation, and decrease anxiety.
- Provide reassurance and rationale to the family and child as to why LAC monitoring is no longer required ➤*Rationale:* Children and families feel anxious about no longer having the additional information provided on the monitor; providing reassurance that LAC monitoring is no longer needed helps to decrease anxiety about the procedure.
- Explain that the child may feel a sensation of mild pulling in the chest. This procedure may be uncomfortable, but should not be painful ➤*Rationale:* The sensation associated with LAC removal can be very disconcerting for children. An explanation of the sensation helps to decrease anxiety during LAC removal.
- Encourage questions and answer questions as they arise ➤*Rationale:* Reinforcement of information is needed during periods of stress.

EQUIPMENT

- Cardiopulmonary, arterial blood pressure, and noninvasive blood pressure monitoring
- Pulse oximetry
- Stethoscope
- Clean gloves
- Surgical blade (#11) or suture removal kit
- Sterile gauze (2×2 or 4×4)
- Dressing supplies or adhesive bandage, per institution-specific protocol
- Unit of type-specific or emergency O-negative red blood cells on standby in blood bank or on the unit, per institution-specific protocol
- Colloid or crystalloid fluid immediately available at child's bedside

Procedure for Left Atrial Intracardiac Line Removal: Perform

Steps	Rationale	Considerations
1. If indicated, consult with prescribing practitioner to ensure all possible data has been obtained from LAC before removal; if LAC is to be removed by RN, review prescribing practitioner's order for LAC removal. *(Level II*)*	Data obtained from the LAC assist with managing the child's hemo-dynamic status; premature catheter removal results in inability to obtain key data.[2,6,10]	Cardiac surgeon, mediastinal tray and emergency equipment should be readily available in the case of complications requiring emergent treatment.
2. Review chest x-ray; locate LAC and assess for abnormal LAC placement or "kinks" in catheter. *(Level II*)*	Confirms placement of LAC.	LAC may not be readily visible on the chest x-ray of a larger child. LAC is usually placed via the right superior pulmonary vein to the left atrium[1,7,10] (refer to Figure 62-1 in Procedure 62).
3. Assess and document current PT, PTT, INR, hemoglobin, hematocrit, platelet count, and child's current medications. *(Level II*)*	Bleeding is an adverse compli-cation of LAC removal.[1,2,4-6,8,10] Abnormal values may increase risk of bleeding with LAC removal either at the site or in the peri-cardial space, which may lead to cardiac tamponade. *(Level VI*)*	Coagulopathies must be evaluated, and treatment considered before discontinuing LAC to avoid complications of cardiac tamponade, excessive blood loss, and hypovolemia.[1,2] Medication(s) that alter platelet function or coag-ulation studies may cause bleed-ing with LAC removal. Consult with prescribing practitioner before LAC removal if child is receiving such medication.
4. Ensure availability of a unit of type-specific or O-negative packed red blood cells before procedure. *(Level II*)*	In situations of excessive bleeding with LAC removal, blood must be readily available for replace-ment to avoid hypovolemia and low hematocrit.[2,3,5]	Review institution-specific protocol regarding Jehovah's Witness patients.
5. Ensure the availability of a functional alternative IV access route. *(Level II*)*	Provides IV access in case of complication such as bleeding or tamponade requiring inter-vention.[2,3,5]	
6. Administer IV sedation and/or anal-gesia as appropriate; refer to pres-cribing practitioner's order.	Physiologic responses of an agitated, anxious, or combative child may contribute to a rise in LA pressure and increase risk of potential complications.[1,2,4,10]	Administer sedation and/or analgesia in timely manner. Perform procedure during peak effect of medication. Monitor child for tolerance of medication and procedure.
7. Ensure child and family understand procedure and questions are answered.	Evaluates and reinforces under-standing of previously taught information.	Developmental level, cognitive ability, and anxiety level will determine approach to and effec-tiveness of teaching.

Procedure continues on following page

* Level II: Theory-based, no research data to support recommendations; recommendations from expert consensus group may exist
  Level VI: Clinical studies in a variety of patient populations and situations to support recommendations

Procedure	**for Left Atrial Intracardiac Line Removal: Perform**—*Continued*	
Steps	**Rationale**	**Considerations**
8. Gather needed equipment and supplies.	Facilitates completion of procedure in a timely manner.	
9. Assess and document vital signs (heart rate, blood pressure, atrial pressure, oxygen saturation) before removal of LAC.[4,10] *(Level II*)*	Baseline values assist with assessment of changes in hemodynamic status which may require intervention.[4,6]	
10. Ensure and document patency of chest tube(s) before LAC removal. *(Level IV*)*	Patent chest tube(s) facilitates evacuation of rapid accumulation of blood in the pericardial space after LAC removal, avoiding cardiac tamponade and potential cardiac arrest.[2,5]	If bleeding occurs, chest tube(s) may need to be milked to prevent thrombus formation in tube(s) and potential cardiac tamponade.
11. Wash hands and put on clean gloves. *(Level II*)*	Standard precautions; reduces transmission of microorganisms.	If splashing of blood is anticipated, gown and eye/face protection should be worn.
12. Provide for appropriate privacy; position the child comfortably and such that LAC removal is facilitated.	LAC removal requires exposure of the chest. Proper positioning of the child ensures child's comfort and facilitates completion of the procedure.	Privacy is an important consideration for school-aged children and adolescents.
13. Identify child using appropriate patient/procedure verification process (e.g., timeout) before LAC line removal.	Confirms correct patient, procedure and site as recommended by the Joint Commission on Accreditation of Healthcare Organizations (JCAHO); prevents unnecessary medical procedures.	Differentiate position and location of LAC from other intracardiac lines, if present, on chest x-ray. Verification process and documentation is institution specific. Use active communication techniques.
14. Remove occlusive dressing over LAC insertion site. Use sterile scissors or surgical blade to cut suture and remove suture from skin. *(Level II*)*	Prepares for removal of LAC. *(Level IV*)*	If using a blade, avoid manipulating blade toward the child.
15. Steadily and slowly withdraw LAC while observing waveform on monitor. Stop pulling if moderate resistance is encountered. *(Level II*)*	LAC retention is a risk of LAC removal.[1-3,6,7,9-11] Increased resistance may indicate LAC entrapment. *(Level VI*)*	The LAC should come out with minimal resistance. If resistance is noted, the surgeon should be notified immediately.
16. Examine catheter tip upon removal. *(Level V*)*	Frayed tip may indicate entrapment of residual portion of LAC or catheter embolization.[2,3,7,11]	Notify surgeon immediately if LAC entrapment or catheter embolization is suspected.
17. Assess and monitor child for changes in vital signs or signs of bleeding. *(Level II*)*	Agitation, tachycardia, increased intracardiac filling pressure, hypotension, narrowed pulse pressure, decreased peripheral perfusion, muffled heart sounds,	

* Level II: Theory-based, no research data to support recommendations; recommendations from expert consensus group may exist
Level IV: Limited clinical studies to support recommendations
Level V: Clinical studies in more than one or two patient populations and situations to support recommendations
Level VI: Clinical studies in a variety of patient populations and situations to support recommendations

Procedure **for Left Atrial Intracardiac Line Removal: Perform**—*Continued*

Steps	Rationale	Considerations
	dyspnea, pulsus paradoxus, and/or sudden cessation of chest tube drainage may indicate cardiac tamponade.[2,5]	
18. Use gauze to wick away blood collecting at insertion site. *(Level II*)*	Prevents excessive bleeding from LAC tract.	Consider weighing gauze to measure blood loss following LAC removal, especially in small infants.
19. Gently milk chest tube(s) if indicated.	Ensures patency of chest tube(s) and may prevent tamponade.[5,7,8]	Monitor color and amount of chest tube drainage. In the event of significant bleeding, LAC entrapment, or line fragmentation, notify prescribing practitioner. Transfusion of blood products or surgical intervention may be required.
20. Cover site with adhesive bandage or dressing per institution-specific protocol.	May reduce incidence of infection.	
21. Obtain chest x-ray per institution specific protocol. *(Level II*)*	Evaluates for the presence of tamponade or bleeding due to line removal.[3,5] Chest x-ray may assist in identifying retained LAC fragment.[9]	An echocardiogram should be obtained if an increase in cardiac size or haziness in lung fields is noted on chest x-ray.
22. Dispose of used supplies and equipment, including sharps, in appropriate receptacle.	Standard precautions; reduces transmission of microorganisms. Protects personnel health.	
23. Remove personal protective equipment and wash hands.	Standard precautions.	

* Level II: Theory-based, no research data to support recommendations; recommendations from expert consensus group may exist

Expected Outcomes	Unexpected Outcomes
• LAC removed intact without resistance or signs of catheter fraying	• Fragmented or entrapped LAC
	• Unable to remove LAC because of resistance; surgical procedure required for removal
• Stable hemodynamics without bleeding or cardiac tamponade	• Excessive bleeding requiring transfusion of blood products
	• Cardiac tamponade.
• Chest x-ray unchanged following LAC removal	• Enlarged heart on chest x-ray
• Child demonstrates acceptable level of comfort	• Unmanaged pain or anxiety

Monitoring and Care of the Child

Activities and Interventions	Rationale	Reportable Conditions
1. Monitor child's hemodynamic status before, during, and after LAC removal.	Unstable hemodynamics may indicate complications.	• Hemodynamic instability
2. Monitor ease of LAC removal and status of LAC on removal.	Resistance during LAC removal attempt may indicate LAC entrapment.	• Inability to remove LAC due to resistance • Fragmented LAC
3. Assess PT, PTT, International Normalized Ratio (INR), hemoglobin, and platelet count before procedure.	Abnormal values should be corrected before procedure to decrease risk of bleeding associated with line removal.	• Platelets <50,000/mm^3 • Abnormal values for PT, PTT, or INR • Modest to significantly decreased hematocrit for child's age and underlying heart defect
4. Continually monitor dressing site and chest tube output for the first 15 minutes after LAC removal, then assess every 15 minutes for 1 hour.[7]	Assesses for bleeding from LAC insertion site.	• Continuous or copious bleeding at catheter insertion site • Continuous or copious bleeding from chest tubes
5. Assess effectiveness of pain and anxiety management strategies and provide appropriate interventions. Encourage family to assist in using nonpharmacologic means to comfort and support the child.	Early identification of pain and anxiety facilitates prompt treatment.	• Unresolved pain, anxiety, or discomfort • Inability to perform procedure due to child's level of anxiety or pain • Continued irritability, changes in physiologic condition

Documentation

- Child and family education
- Hemodynamic status before, during, and after LAC removal
- PT, PTT, platelet count, and hematologic values
- Date and time of procedure
- Individual performing the procedure
- Amount of bleeding from LAC insertion site and from chest tubes following procedure
- Condition of LAC tip on removal and ease of LAC removal
- Appearance of LAC insertion site
- Chest x-ray findings after LAC removal
- Blood transfusion or fluid bolus administration required as a result of LAC removal
- Unexpected outcomes and related treatment

References

1. Flori HR, et al: Transthoracic intracardiac catheters in pediatric patients recovering from congenital heart defect surgery: associated complications and outcomes, *Crit Care Med* 28(8):2997-3001, 2000.
2. Johnson AB, Lincoln P: Policy 2.2: removal of intracardiac line. In Children's Hospital, Boston, editors: *Children's Hospital, Boston ICU nursing policy and procedure manual,* Boston, 2003, Children's Hospital.
3. Leitman BS, et al: The left atrial catheter: its uses and complications, *Radiology* 185(2):611-612, 1992.
4. Roth SJ: Postoperative care. In Chang AC, et al, editors: *Pediatric cardiac intensive care,* Baltimore, 1998, Williams & Wilkins.
5. Johnston LJ, McKinley DF: Cardiac tamponade after removal of atrial intracardiac monitoring catheters in a pediatric patient: case report, *Heart Lung* 29(4): 256-261, 2000.
6. Craig J, et al: Tissue perfusion. In Curley MAQ, Moloney-Harmon PA, editors: *Critical care nursing of infants and children,* ed 2, Philadelphia, 2001, Saunders.
7. Akl BF, et al: Brief communications: unusual complication of direct left atrial pressure monitoring line, *J Thorac Cardiovasc Surg* 88:1033-1037, 1984.
8. Santini F, et al: Routine left atrial catheterization for the post-operative management of cardiac surgical patients: is the risk justified? *Eur J Cardiothorac Surg* 16:218-221, 1999.

9. Yeo TC, et al: Retained left atrial catheter: an unusual cardiac source of embolism identified by transesophogeal echocardiography, *J Am Soc Echocardiogr* 11(1):66-70, 1998.
10. Gold JP, et al: Transthoracic intracardiac monitoring lines in pediatric surgical patients: a ten-year experience, *Ann Thorac Surg* 42:185-191, 1986.
11. Ford SE, Manley PN: Indwelling cardiac catheters, an autopsy study of associated endocardial lesions, *Arch Pathol Lab Med* 106(7):314-317, 1982.

Additional Readings

Ceyran H, et al: Benefit of using triple-lumen catheter to monitor left atrial pressure, *Acta Anaesthesiologica Scandin* 47(4):430-432, 2003.
Zahorec R, Holoman M: Transatrial access for left atrial pressure monitoring in cardiac surgery, *Eur J Cardiothorac Surg* 11:379-380, 1997.

AP
Pulmonary Artery Intracardiac Line Removal: Perform

P U R P O S E : To safely remove a transthoracic pulmonary artery catheter when invasive intracardiac pressure monitoring is no longer necessary, to avoid risk of complications associated with the catheter, or when the catheter is no longer needed to infuse medication

Louise Callow

PREREQUISITE KNOWLEDGE

- Normal cardiac anatomy and physiology
- Pulmonary anatomy and physiology
- Impact of child's specific congenital heart disease on cardiac and pulmonary anatomy and physiology
- Surgical reconstruction performed specific to the individual child
- Rationale for pulmonary artery (PA) monitoring is to provide information on intracardiac pressures and oxygen saturations. PA catheters are useful in identifying residual left to right shunts following ventricular septal defect closures, right ventricular outflow tract (RVOT) obstruction during PA pullback with catheter removal, and in children at risk for postoperative pulmonary hypertension
- PA intracardiac catheters are placed in the operating room during open heart surgery. The catheter is inserted into the RVOT and threaded up in the main PA. The end of the catheter exits through and is anchored to the heart, and then brought through the chest wall, where it is attached to a pressure transducer and tubing.[1]

- A heparinized solution should be infused through the PA catheter to maintain patency and prevent clot formation. Infusion fluids and rates vary according to institution-specific protocol
- Indications for removal of PA catheter[2-5]
  - The child's condition is improved sufficiently that measurement of the PA pressure is no longer necessary to guide therapy
  - A risk of complications from the presence of the PA catheter exists
  - The catheter is no longer needed to infuse medication directly into the pulmonary bed
  - A risk of infection is associated with the prolonged use of the catheter
- Normal values for intracardiac pressures related to the child's specific cardiac defect and physiology
- Normal prothrombin time (PT), partial thromboplastin time (PTT), International Normal Ratio (INR) valves
- Venous access routes available in the event of patient compromise related to complications of PA catheter removal
- Normal waveforms for right ventricular (RV) and PA pressure tracings
- Potential complications of PA catheter removal:[3,4,6]
  - Venous air embolus
  - Uncontrolled bleeding
  - Thrombosis

❖ Cardiac tamponade
❖ Inability to percutaneously remove PA catheter
❖ PA catheter knotting
- Ability to recognize signs of complications associated with PA catheter removal and appropriate interventions required to decrease morbidity and mortality
- Appropriate timing of PA catheter removal is determined in collaboration with the cardiac surgeon.
- Cardiac surgeon should be available when the catheter is removed because catheter breakage or bleeding may occur, necessitating emergent operative intervention.[3]
- Type-specific or O-negative packed red blood cells must be available in blood bank or on the unit before initiating the procedure.
- Contraindications to removal of the PA catheter:[3,4]
  ❖ Child's coagulation values (PT, PTT, INR) are prolonged
  ❖ Child's platelet count is less than 50,000
  ❖ Hemoglobin (Hgb) and/or hematocrit (Hct) are not within acceptable range
  ❖ Child's sternal incision is open
  ❖ Resistance is met during the removal of the PA catheter
- Principles of aseptic technique
- Mastery of pediatric advanced life support competencies
- Appropriate pediatric dosing of sedatives and competency in procedural sedation
- Child development as it relates to clinical assessment and removal of a PA catheter
- Knowledge of state Nurse Practice Act and institution-specific protocol regarding PA catheter removal; this procedure is performed by a licensed practitioner with advanced training

CHILD AND FAMILY ASSESSMENT

- Child's and family's understanding of the reasons for and risks and benefits of the procedure ➥*Rationale:* Evaluates the child's and family's understanding of the procedure and provides a gauge for ongoing education.
- Electrocardiographic (ECG) results and vital signs, including PA pressures before catheter removal ➥*Rationale:* Provides baseline data; identifies the catheter is no longer necessary.
- Recent chest x-ray results ➥*Rationale:* Verifies placement of the PA catheter and identifies potential complications if PA catheter has migrated.
- Recent laboratory study results including type and screen, coagulation status (Hgb and Hct), and platelet count ➥*Rationale:* If the child has abnormal coagulation study results or a low platelet count, correction may be required or hemostasis may be difficult to achieve after catheter removal. A current type and screen ensures availability of blood.

- Integrity of the PA catheter ➥*Rationale:* Identifies obvious defects that could cause breakage of the catheter during removal.
- Presence and patency of mediastinal chest tubes ➥*Rationale:* Drainage of blood from the mediastinum is facilitated should bleeding occur after catheter removal.
- Presence and patency of alternate vascular access sites ➥*Rationale:* Because of the severity of potential complications with PA catheter removal, alternative vascular access is essential for rapid administrations of fluid boluses or blood.
- Child's developmental level and ability to interact ➥*Rationale:* These factors influence preparation of the child and interaction.
- Child's level of sedation ➥*Rationale:* If the child is active or crying, the PA pressure rises and potentially increases bleeding, which makes hemostasis more difficult to achieve.
- Child's allergies and previous adverse reactions to sedation ➥*Rationale:* Identifies possible complications of sedation medications.
- Desire of family members to be present during the procedure ➥*Rationale:* The family may provide comfort and support to the child during the procedure but should have the choice not to remain with the child.

CHILD AND FAMILY EDUCATION

Individualized, developmentally appropriate education is provided to the family and to the child based on desire for knowledge, readiness to learn, and overall neurologic and psychosocial state.

- Explain the procedure and the reason for catheter removal ➥*Rationale:* Providing information decreases anxiety.
- Explain the importance of the child lying still during catheter removal; review the plan for the use of medications for sedation ➥*Rationale:* Child and family compliance is ensured, and safe catheter removal is facilitated.
- Instruct the child and family to report any bleeding from the insertion site after catheter removal ➥*Rationale:* Assists with identification and prompt treatment of bleeding.
- Encourage questions and answer questions as they arise ➥*Rationale:* Reinforcement of information is needed during periods of stress.

EQUIPMENT

- Cardiopulmonary and blood pressure (BP) monitoring
- Pulse oximetry (SpO₂) monitoring
- Stethoscope

- Clean gloves and protective eyewear
- Sterile 4×4 gauze
- Waterproof absorbent pads
- Suture removal kit or surgical blade
- Dressing supplies or adhesive bandage per institution-specific protocol

- Sterile specimen container (needed if culture of the catheter tip is obtained)
- Unit of type-specific or O-negative packed red blood cells on standby per unit- or institution-specific protocol
- Colloid or crystalloid fluid immediately available at child's bedside

Procedure for Pulmonary Artery Intracardiac Line Removal: Perform		
Steps	**Rationale**	**Considerations**
1. Ensure child and family understand procedure and questions are answered.	Evaluates and reinforces understanding of previously taught information.	Developmental level, cognitive ability, and anxiety level determine approach to and effectiveness of teaching.
2. Ensure one unit of type-specific or O-negative packed red blood cells is available in blood bank or on the unit before catheter removal.[3] *(Level II*)*	Ensures that blood is immediately available for urgent transfusion if bleeding occurs with catheter removal.	Refer to institution-specific protocol for requirements for blood product availability.
3. Review platelet count and coagulation study results; verify Hgb and Hct levels before catheter removal.[3] *(Level II*)*	If values are abnormal, transfusion of products can be given before catheter removal for prevention of bleeding and possible tamponade.	Coagulopathies must be evaluated and treatment considered before removing the PA catheter in order to avoid complications of cardiac tamponade, excessive blood loss, and hypovolemia. Medications that alter coagulation studies or platelet function should be held prior to PA catheter removal.
4. Review chest x-ray; locate PA catheter and assess for abnormal placement or kinks in catheter.	Confirms placement of PA catheter.	
5. Ensure availability of cardiac surgeon during catheter removal.[3] *(Level II*)*	Catheter breakage or excessive bleeding during catheter removal may occur and necessitate emergent operative intervention.	Cardiac surgeon, mediastinal tray and emergency equipment should be readily available in case of complications requiring emergent treatment.
6. Ensure the availability of functional alternative IV access. *(Level II*)*	Ensures IV access in case of complications, such as bleeding or tamponade, requiring intervention.	
7. Ensure the child has received prescribed medications for sedation and is appropriately sedated.	Reduces the incidence and severity of complications such as hemorrhage or tamponade.	
8. Assess and document all required data (HR, BP, PA pressure, SpO$_2$) before removal of PA catheter. *(Level II*)*[2]	Data obtained from PA catheter assists with management of the child's hemodynamic status before removal of the catheter. Premature catheter removal results in inability to obtain key data.	Use of intraoperative transesophageal echocardiogram (TEE) has significantly decreased the need for PA catheter use.
9. Gather needed equipment and supplies.	Facilitates completion of task in a timely manner.	

* Level II: Theory-based; no research data to support recommendations; recommendations from expert consensus group may exist

Procedure for Pulmonary Artery Intracardiac Line Removal: Perform—*Continued*		
Steps	**Rationale**	**Considerations**
10. Wash hands. *(Level VI*)*	Standard precautions; reduces transmission of microorganisms.	
11. Identify the child using two patient identifiers.	Confirms correct patient and procedure as recommended by the Joint Commission for Accreditation of Healthcare Organizations (JCAHO).	Verification process is institution specific; name and medical record number are generally recommended for inpatients.
12. Ensure and document patency of chest tube(s) before PA catheter removal. *(Level IV*)*	Facilitates the evacuation of blood from the mediastinum after intracardiac line removal.[2]	If chest tubes are present but not draining well, it is recommended that the fibrin clot limiting drainage out of the chest tubes be evacuated before PA catheter removal.
13. Place child flat in bed in the supine position.	Facilitates drainage of mediastinal blood should bleeding occur after catheter removal.	
14. Place waterproof absorbent pad under the child's torso. Provide appropriate privacy.	Contains any bloody drainage associated with removal and serves as a receptacle for the PA catheter.	
15. Ensure the child is positioned so that PA catheter is readily visible.	Facilitates visualization of catheter and access to catheter insertion site; facilitates catheter removal.	
16. Discontinue intravenous (IV) solutions infusing into PA catheter or transfer to another IV site.	Fluids are no longer needed; ensures a closed system and prevents air from entering the system.	If PA pull-back is to be done, pressure transducer system must remain attached to allow continued pressure and waveform monitoring.
17. Open and prepare supplies and equipment.	Prepares for removal; ensures that all equipment and supplies needed are available.	
18. Wash hands; put on clean gloves and protective eyewear.	Standard precautions; reduces transmission of microorganisms.	
19. If stopcocks are attached to the PA catheter, turn them off to the child.	Prepares for catheter removal.	If PA pull-back is to be done, do not turn stopcock off to the child; this would prevent monitoring of pressures and waveforms.
20. Remove dressing.	Allows visualization of insertion site and assessment for signs of wound infection.	Signs of infection may determine the need to send a culture of the catheter tip, culture blood from the catheter before removal, or culture the insertion site.[5] Consider child's temperature and white blood cell count with differential as indicators of infection.
21. Clip and remove sutures.	Frees PA catheter; facilitates removal.	

Procedure continues on following page

* Level IV: Limited clinical studies to support recommendations
   Level VI: Clinical studies in a variety of patient populations and situations to support recommendations

Procedure	**for Pulmonary Artery Intracardiac Line Removal: Perform**—*Continued*	
Steps	Rationale	Considerations
22. Pull catheter steadily through skin insertion site until end of catheter clears the skin surface.	Prevents clotting of blood at catheter tip and introduction of air.	If concerns of a residual RVOT obstruction exist, a measurable gradient can be obtained when the PA catheter is pulled back into the right ventricle (RV) (PA pull-back). The mean pressure change from the PA to the RV yields the gradient across the RVOT.
23. Do not continue to remove the catheter if resistance is met; notify the cardiac surgeon immediately.[2,3] (*Level II**)	Excessive tension on the catheter during removal may cause catheter fracture with a portion of the catheter remaining in the heart, which creates the risk of catheter embolus.[3]	
24. Place PA catheter on sterile 4×4 gauze pad and check to be sure that the entire catheter was removed.	Assessment of the catheter assures removal of entire catheter.	
25. Place tip of the PA catheter in a sterile container if catheter is to be sent for culture.	Verifies the presence or absence of organism growth on the catheter.	
26. Place 4×4 gauze over insertion site. Observe for bleeding, but do not apply pressure. Allow to drain on the gauze, and change the gauze as necessary until bleeding stops.	Prevents blood, if present, from collecting in the mediastinal cavity after catheter removal. Ensures hemostasis.	
27. Observe and drain the chest tubes; measure volume of blood loss that occurs through the chest tubes. (*Level II**)	Identifies excessive blood loss and need for transfusion.	
28. Once bleeding has stopped, place an adhesive bandage or small occlusive dressing over the catheter insertion site wound per institution-specific protocol.	May reduce the risk of infection at catheter insertion site wound.	Use of antimicrobial ointment at site is institution specific; refer to institution-specific protocol. Per institution-specific protocol, site may be left uncovered.
29. Dispose of used equipment and supplies, including sharps, in appropriate receptacle; wash hands.	Standard precautions; reduces transmission of microorganisms. Protects personnel health.	
30. Remove gloves and protective eyewear; wash hands.	Standard precautions.	
31. Obtain chest x-ray. (*Level II**)	Evaluates for the presence of tamponade or bleeding due to line removal; may assist in identifying retained PA catheter fragment.	An echocardiogram should be obtained if an increase in cardiac size or haziness in lung fields is noted on chest x-ray.

* Level II: Theory-based; no research data to support recommendations; recommendations from expert consensus group may exist

Expected Outcomes	Unexpected Outcomes
• PA catheter is easily removed without complications	• Venous air embolus
	• Uncontrolled bleeding
	• Thrombosis
	• Inability to percutaneously remove PA catheter
	• PA catheter knotting
• Hemodynamics remain at baseline after catheter removal	• Hypotension
	• Bradycardia or tachycardia
• Blood is evacuated through the catheter insertion site or chest tubes	• Tamponade
	• Thrombosis
• Child remains free from infection	• PA catheter–related infection
• Child tolerates procedure with minimal anxiety	• Excessive agitation or anxiety
• Chest x-ray is unchanged following PA catheter removal	• Cardiomegaly
	• Effusion
	• Cardiac tamponade

Monitoring and Care of the Child

Activities and Interventions	Rationale	Reportable Conditions
1. Date, time, and initial the wound dressing; monitor site for redness, swelling, or drainage.	Indicates when dressing was placed and when it is due to be changed. Monitors for indications of wound infection, ongoing bleeding at site.	• Purulent or foul-smelling draining from catheter insertion wound • Erythema or swelling at catheter insertion wound • Significant amount of bleeding at insertion site
2. Monitor central venous pressure (CVP), BP, pulse pressure, perfusion, and HR and rhythm before, during and at least every 15 minutes for 30 minutes after removal of the catheter for possible signs of tamponade.[3,6]	Facilitates rapid recognition and intervention in the event of a complication. Bleeding or tamponade can develop late after catheter removal from leakage of blood through the PA catheter insertion site. Reduces risk of complication from unrecognized tamponade.	• Abnormal vital signs • Decreased peripheral perfusion • Bleeding from the site • Increased chest tube output • Change in character of chest tube drainage (appears bloody) • Respiratory compromise • Signs of cardiac tamponade: increased HR, decreased BP, widened pulse pressure
3. Monitor electrolyte levels, complete blood count, and results of coagulation studies as indicated.	Abnormal laboratory results may indicate bleeding or infection.	• Laboratory results that indicate acidosis or increased lactate value • Decreasing Hgb or Hct levels, altered coagulation studies • Increased white blood cell count
4. Continuously monitor chest tube output after PA catheter removal.	Bleeding can continue after removal of PA catheter through catheter insertion site.	• Continuous or copious sanguineous drainage from chest tubes.[2]

Documentation

- Child and family education
- Date and time of catheter removal
- Practitioner who performed catheter removal
- Approximate blood loss from insertion site and chest tubes during procedure and any blood products administered
- Medications administered for the procedure and child's response
- Hemodynamic status of child before and after removal of PA catheter
- Appearance of PA catheter insertion site
- PT, PTT, INR, platelet count, and hematologic values before and after procedure as relevant to child's clinical status
- Condition of PA catheter tip on removal and ease of PA catheter removal
- Results of chest x-ray following procedure
- Child's response to procedure
- Unexpected outcomes and related treatment

References

1. Roth SJ: Postoperative care. In Chang AC, et al, editors: *Pediatric cardiac intensive care,* Baltimore, 1998, Williams & Wilkins.
2. Boggs RL, et al: *AACN procedure manual for critical care,* Philadelphia 1993, Saunders.
3. Johnston LJ, McKinley DF: Cardiac tamponade after removal of atrial intracardiac monitoring catheters in a pediatric patient: case report, *Heart Lung* 29(4):256-61, 2000.
4. Wadas TM: Pulmonary artery catheter removal, *Crit Care Nurs* 14:62-72, 1994.
5. Pearson ML: Guideline for prevention of intravascular device-related infections: Hospital Infection Control Practices Advisory Committee, *Infect Control Hosp Epidemiol* 17(7):438-73, 1996.
6. Craig J, et al: Cardiovascular critical care problems. In Curley MAQ, Moloney-Harmon P, editors: *Critical care nursing of infants and children,* ed 2, Philadelphia, 2001, Saunders.

Additional Readings

Ahrens TS, Taylor LA: *Hemodynamic waveform analysis,* Philadelphia, 1992, Saunders.
Darovic GO: *Hemodynamic monitoring: invasive and noninvasive clinical application,* ed 3, Philadelphia, 2002, Saunders.

AP

Right Atrial Intracardiac Line Removal: Perform

P U R P O S E : To safely remove a right atrial intracardiac line when invasive intracardiac pressure monitoring is no longer necessary, the line is no longer functioning as a source of pressure monitoring and/or venous access, the line is infected or malpositioned or central venous access is no longer needed

Aimee Jennings

PREREQUISITE KNOWLEDGE

- Normal cardiac anatomy and physiology
- Familiarity with postoperative care requirements of infants and children after cardiac surgery
- Rationale for right atrial intracardiac catheter (RAC) or line monitoring is to provide information about the child's hemodynamic status including information on preload, intravascular volume status, right ventricular compliance, tricuspid valve disease, and atrial shunting.[1] In addition, these lines provide vascular access and a site for monitoring venous oxygenation.
- Children undergoing intracardiac surgery may have an RAC placed in the operating room. The catheter tip is placed in the RA, anchored to the heart, and then brought through the chest wall, where it is attached to a pressure transducer and tubing.
- A heparinized solution should be infused through the RAC to maintain patency and prevent clot formation.[1-3] Infusion fluids and rates vary according to institution-specific protocol.

- Maintenance fluids and medications may be infused through RAC.[2-6] Potassium, magnesium, and calcium levels should be within normal limits prior to RAC removal. If institution-specific protocol does not support infusion of magnesium, calcium and potassium via a peripheral intravenous line, replacement therapy should be administered via RAC prior to removal.
- An alternative intravenous (IV) access route must be identified for medication infusion before RAC removal.[7,8] IV access is necessary in the event of patient compromise related to complication of RAC removal.
- Type-specific or O-negative packed red blood cells must be available in blood bank or on the unit before initiating the procedure.[4,5,8]
- Effects of prothrombin time (PT), partial thromboplastin time (PTT), and International Normalized Ratio (INR) on hemostasis and indications for treatment of abnormal levels. Hemoglobin, hematocrit, and platelet count should also be within an acceptable range before line removal to reduce the risk of sequelae and optimize outcomes.[3,6,8,9]
- Familiarity with RAC pressure waveforms and ability to distinguish normal variations in waveform from abnormal wave patterns (refer to Figure 65-1 in Procedure 65)
- Indications for RAC removal: improvement in the child's medical condition such that RAC monitoring or

additional venous access is no longer required, line malfunction, or infection. RAC requires aseptic technique for care and removal.[2,3,6,7]

- Ability to recognize signs of complications associated with RAC removal and the appropriate interventions required to decrease morbidity and mortality.[3,5,10]
- Normal infant, child, and adolescent heart rates and blood pressures
- Basic and advanced electrocardiogram (ECG) and cardiac dysrhythmias interpretation
- Mechanism to activate the emergency alert system when a complication is detected
- Mastery of pediatric advanced life support competencies
- Child development as it relates to clinical assessment and RAC removal
- Appropriate pediatric dosing of sedatives and analgesics
- Knowledge of state nurse practice act and institution-specific protocol regarding RAC removal; this procedure is performed by a licensed practitioner with advanced training

CHILD AND FAMILY ASSESSMENT

- Child's and family's understanding of indications for RAC removal as well as the risks and benefits of the procedure ➥*Rationale:* Evaluates child's and family's understanding of the procedure and provides a gauge for ongoing education.
- History of congenital heart disease, ventricular dysfunction, pulmonary hypertension, cardiac dysrhythmias, hepatologic or hematologic problems, and cardiac surgical and/or catheterization procedures ➥*Rationale:* These conditions affect the potential for the development of complications.
- Current medication history ➥*Rationale:* Use of anticoagulation or nonsteroidal medications may result in the development of complications such as bleeding.
- Recent laboratory specimen results and availability of a type and screen ➥*Rationale:* Elevated coagulation panel or prolonged bleeding times may delay RAC removal until corrected. A current type and screen is needed for blood to be available for RAC removal or for treatment of the coagulopathy.
- Recent chest x-ray results ➥*Rationale:* Verifies placement of the RAC and identifies potential complications such as ectopy or dysrhythmias if RAC has migrated.
- Current hemodynamic status ➥*Rationale:* An understanding of hemodynamic monitoring is needed for appropriate recognition of changes in hemodynamic status during and after RAC removal.[1,3,6,7,9]
- Appearance of RAC insertion site ➥*Rationale:* Assesses for signs of infection. A culture of the line tip may be warranted if bacteremia is suspected or present.
- Relocate medications or fluids infusing via the RA that will be continued to a different infusion site[3,11] ➥*Rationale:* Abrupt discontinuation of fluid and medica-

tion infusions could negatively affect the child's cardiac output.

- Presence and patency of alternate vascular access sites[3,7,9] ➥*Rationale:* Because of the severity of potential complications with RAC removal, alternate vascular access is essential for the rapid administration of fluid boluses or blood transfusion. Alternate vascular access may also be necessary for infusion of fluid or medication previously infused via the RAC.
- Child's developmental level[7] ➥*Rationale:* Developmental level influences preparation of the child.
- Level of consciousness and cognition[7] ➥*Rationale:* Determines child's ability to cooperate with instructions. RAC removal is often performed during a phase in the postoperative course when the child continues to receive sedatives and analgesics. Children may not comprehend instructions while sedated, thereby potentially increasing the child's fear and anxiety.
- Family's desire to be present during the procedure ➥*Rationale:* Family may support and comfort the child during the procedure but should have the choice not to remain with the child.

CHILD AND FAMILY EDUCATION

Individualized, developmentally appropriate education is provided to the child and to the family based on desire for knowledge, readiness to learn, and overall neurologic and psychosocial state.

- Explain to the family and child, if developmentally appropriate, the steps involved in RAC removal and provide the rationale for line removal ➥*Rationale:* Providing educationally appropriate information helps to decrease the child's and family's anxiety level and offers reassurance during an extremely stressful period.
- Provide reassurance and rationale to the family and child on the reasons that RAC monitoring is no longer required ➥*Rationale:* Child and family may feel anxious about no longer having the additional information provided on the monitor. Providing reassurance that RAC monitoring is no longer needed helps decrease anxiety about the procedure.
- Explain that the child may feel a sensation of mild pulling in the chest. This procedure may be uncomfortable, but should not be painful ➥*Rationale:* The sensation associated with RAC removal can be very disconcerting for children. An explanation of the sensation helps to decrease anxiety during RAC removal.
- Explain the common occurrence of bleeding at the catheter insertion site and/or bleeding through chest tubes (mediastinal chest tubes are often present)[3,7,8,10] ➥*Rationale:* The child or family may become anxious at the sight of blood. Preparing the child for this may decrease anxiety.

- Explain the relatively low incidence of complications associated with RAC removal such as excessive bleeding and/or compromised cardiac and respiratory status that require intervention[3,6,7,9,10] ➤*Rationale:* Complications from RAC removal rarely happen when the procedure is performed by a trained practitioner. However, when complications occur, they are often significant and require immediate intervention. Educating the child and family about the risks and treatments may decrease anxiety.
- In the event of a complication, explain the complication and the interventions required to stabilize the child.[3,6,7,9,10] ➤*Rationale:* Children and families have the right to be informed about the complications and necessary interventions related to RAC removal.
- Encourage questions and answer questions as they arise ➤*Rationale:* Reinforcement of information is needed during periods of stress.

EQUIPMENT

- Cardiopulmonary, arterial blood pressure, and/or noninvasive blood pressure monitoring
- Pulse oximetry
- Clean gloves
- Dressing supplies or adhesive bandage per institution-specific protocol
- Stethoscope.
- Suture removal kit or #11 surgical blade
- Sterile gauze (2×2 or 4×4)
- Sterile culture container for the catheter tip (if indicated)
- Unit of type-specific or O-negative packed red blood cells on standby in the blood bank or on the unit per institution-specific protocol[8]
- Colloid or crystalloid fluid immediately available at child's bedside[3,8,9]

Procedure for Right Atrial Intracardiac Line Removal: Perform

Steps	Rationale	Considerations
1. If indicated, review prescribing practitioner's order for RAC removal and consult with prescribing practitioner to ensure all required data are obtained from RAC before removal. *(Level II*)*	Data obtained from the RAC assist with managing the child's hemodynamic status before removal of the catheter; premature catheter removal results in inability to obtain key data.[4,6-8,10]	Cardiac surgeon and mediastinal tray and equipment should be readily available in the case of complications requiring emergent treatment.
2. Review chest x-ray; locate RAC, and assess for abnormal placement or kinks in catheter. *(Level II*)*	Confirms placement of RAC.	
3. Assess and document current PT, PTT, INR, hemoglobin, hematocrit, platelet count, and child's current medications. *(Level II*)*	Bleeding is an adverse complication of RAC removal.[3,6-10] Abnormal values may increase risk of bleeding with RAC removal either at the site or in the pericardial space, which may lead to cardiac tamponade.	Coagulopathies must be evaluated, and treatment considered before discontinuing the RAC in order to avoid complications of cardiac tamponade, excessive blood loss, and hypovolemia.[6,9] Medications that alter coagulation studies or platelet function should be held before RAC removal. Consult with prescribing practitioner before RAC removal if child is receiving such medication.
4. Ensure availability of a unit of type-specific or O-negative packed red blood cells before procedure. *(Level II*)*	In situations of excessive bleeding with RAC removal, blood must be readily available for replacement to avoid hypovolemia and low hematocrit.[3,6,8-10]	Review institution-specific protocol regarding Jehovah's Witness patients.

Procedure continues on following page

* Level II: Theory-based, no research data to support recommendations: recommendations from expert consensus group may exist

Procedure	**for Right Atrial Intracardiac Line Removal: Perform**—*Continued*	
Steps	**Rationale**	**Considerations**
5. Ensure the availability of functional alternative IV access. *(Level II*)*	Provides IV access in case of complication such as bleeding or tamponade requiring intervention.[6,9]	Medications infusing through RAC should be switched to alternative IV site; ensure the concentration of the medications is appropriate for peripheral administration if the IV is peripheral. Replace magnesium, calcium, and/or potassium as needed prior to RAC removal if institution-specific protocol does not support infusion of replacement therapy via a peripheral IV line.
6. Ensure child and family understand procedure and questions are answered.	Evaluates and reinforces understanding of previously taught information.	Developmental level, cognitive ability, use of sedation and/or analgesia, and anxiety level will determine approach to and effectiveness of teaching.
7. Administer IV sedation and/or analgesia as appropriate; refer to prescribing practitioner's order.	Reduces RA pressure and decreases the incidence and severity of complications such as hemorrhage and tamponade.[6,9]	Monitor child's response to medications. Family can aid in comforting, consoling, and distracting child.
8. Gather needed equipment and supplies.	Facilitates completion of procedure without delays.	
9. Wash hands. *(Level VI*)*	Standard precautions; reduces transmission of microorganisms.	Procedure requires aseptic technique.[7,8,10,11]
10. Assess and document vital signs before removal of RAC.	Baseline values assist with assessment of changes in hemodynamic status that may require intervention.[6,11]	
11. Ensure and document patency of chest tube(s) before RAC removal.[2,6,8] *(Level IV*)*	Facilitates the evacuation of blood from the mediastinum after intracardiac line removal.[9]	If chest tubes are present but not draining well, it is recommended that the fibrin clot limiting drainage out the tubes to be evacuated before RAC removal.
12. Provide appropriate privacy; position child supine with head of bed (HOB) elevated between 0 and 30 degrees. *(Level II*)*	RAC removal requires exposure of the chest. Provides best position for access to and monitoring of child. HOB at 30 degrees may be more comfortable for the child than positioning flat or upright at more than 60 degrees.	Trendelenburg position is not required for this procedure; air embolism is unlikely. RACs differ from central venous catheters in that RACs have a smaller diameter and course through more tissue planes before entering the vascular system. Furthermore, a purse string suture is often present at the myocardial insertion site of the RAC[3,8]; if present, this suture helps close the myocardium after RAC removal. Privacy is an important consideration for school-aged children and adolescents.
13. Ensure that child is properly connected to monitoring devices.[10] *(Level II*)*	Aids in the assessment of complications from RAC removal, allowing for prompt intervention and treatment.	Children with RAC lines have limited reserve when compromised because of their postoperative status.

* Level II: Theory-based, no research data to support recommendations: recommendations from expert consensus group may exist
Level IV: Limited clinical studies to support recommendations
Level VI: Clinical studies in a variety of patient populations and situations to support recommendations

Procedure	for Right Atrial Intracardiac Line Removal: Perform—*Continued*

Steps	Rationale	Considerations
14. Remove dressing, put on clean gloves, and clean RAC insertion site before line removal. *(Level II*)*	Reduces possible transmission of microorganisms related to RAC removal.	Refer to institution-specific protocol for cleaning RAC insertion site. Splashing of blood can be anticipated, gown and eye/face protection should be worn.
15. Assess RAC insertion site (Figure 68-1).[3,10,11] *(Level VI*)*	Evaluates for the signs of infection or indications that catheter may not be intact, requiring intervention.	Report and document suspicious or unexpected findings.

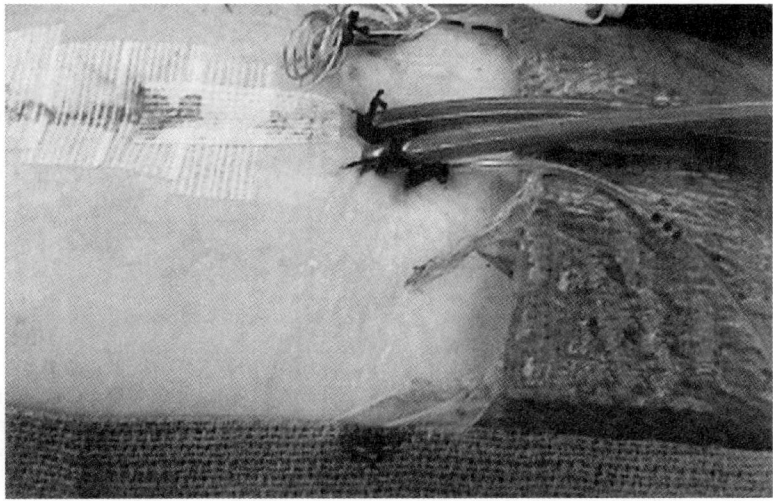

FIGURE 68-1 Photograph illustrating right atrial catheter (RAC) insertion site beneath mediastinal chest tube insertion sites; note suture around RAC at insertion. This photo illustrates a fiberoptic RAC.

Steps	Rationale	Considerations
16. Identify child using appropriate patient/procedure verification process (e.g., timeout) before RAC line removal.	Confirms correct patient, procedure, and site as recommended by the Joint Commission on Accreditation of Healthcare Organizations (JCAHO); prevents unnecessary medical procedures.	Differentiate position and location of RAC from other intracardiac lines if present on chest x-ray. Verification process and documentation is institution specific. Use active communication techniques.
17. Discontinue RAC infusion; turn stopcock nearest child to "off" position. *(Level II*)*	Discontinues the flow of fluid through RAC.	Leaving the stopcock off to the child will promote clotting of the RAC.
18. Silence RAC monitor alarm.	Alarm sounding can be disruptive and anxiety producing for child and family.	Monitoring alarms for other parameters should remain on.
19. Use sterile scissors or surgical blade to cut skin sutures present; remove suture from skin.	Prepares for removal of RAC.	If using blade, avoid manipulating blade toward child.

Procedure continues on following page

* Level II: Theory-based, no research data to support recommendations: recommendations from expert consensus group may exist
Level VI: Clinical studies in a variety of patient populations and situations to support recommendations

Procedure	for **Right Atrial Intracardiac Line Removal: Perform**—*Continued*	
Steps	**Rationale**	**Considerations**
20. Gently grasp RAC and steadily and slowly withdraw RAC in the direction of the child's umbilicus (caudal);[8] stop pulling if moderate resistance encountered. *(Level II*)*	Decreases risk of complications related to RAC removal.[8] RAC retention is a risk of RAC removal; increased resistance may indicate RAC entrapment.[6,7,10,11]	RAC should come out with minimal resistance; if resistance is noted, the surgeon should be notified immediately. Abruptly pulling the line, or pulling at an acute angle to the insertion site increases the risk of line breakage, pain, line retention, and myocardial stress.[8]
21. After removal of RAC, wick away blood collecting at insertion site with gauze. *(Level II*)*	Application of pressure at the insertion site may promote the formation of a subcutaneous hematoma and/or promote cardiac tamponade.[8,9]	In small infants, measure amount of bleeding from insertion site by weighing gauze.
22. Assess RAC tip for line integrity; send tip for culture if indicated.[3] *(Level II*)*	Frayed RAC tip may indicate fracture of the catheter.	Suspicion of a retained line should be reported to the surgeon. Chest x-ray should be used to evaluate presence and position of a retained intracardiac line.[3,8]
23. Once bleeding has stopped, place an adhesive bandage or small occlusive dressing over the RAC insertion site, per institution-specific protocol. *(Level II*)*	May prevent infection at insertion site.	Monitor dressing for excessive bleeding after RAC removal.
24. Assess and monitor child for changes in vital signs or signs of bleeding.[3,8,10]	Indications of compromise are generally present within 20 minutes of line removal.	Monitor color and amount of chest tube drainage. In the event of significant bleeding, RAC entrapment or line fragmentation, notify prescribing practitioner; transfusion of blood products or surgical intervention may be required.
25. Obtain chest x-ray. *(Level II*)*	Evaluates for the presence of tamponade or bleeding due to line removal. Chest x-ray may assist in identifying retained RAC fragment.	An echocardiogram should be obtained if an increase in cardiac size or haziness in lung fields is noted on chest x-ray.
26. Dispose of used supplies and equipment, including sharps, in appropriate receptacle.	Standard precautions; reduces transmission of microorganisms. Protects personnel health.	
27. Remove personal protective equipment and wash hands.	Standard precautions.	

* Level II: Theory-based, no research data to support recommendations: recommendations from expert consensus group may exist

Expected Outcomes

- RAC is removed intact without resistance or signs of catheter fraying

- Stable hemodynamic parameters, minimal or mild bleeding at insertion site and/or into mediastinal chest tubes[8,10]

- Isolated premature atrial contraction or premature ventricular contraction
- RAC insertion site clean and dry; child is free from signs of infection
- Chest x-ray unchanged following RAC removal

- Child demonstrates acceptable level of comfort

Unexpected Outcomes

- Unable to remove RAC because of resistance; surgical procedure required for removal
- RAC integrity is disrupted [3,9,10]
- Excessive bleeding requiring transfusion of blood products
- Cardiac tamponade from blood trapped in mediastinal space[3,9,10]
- Persistent or significant cardiac dysrhythmias

- Insertion site with erythema, edema, discharge
- Purulent drainage noted on catheter tip
- Enlarged heart on chest x-ray could correlate with cardiac tamponade
- Unmanaged pain or anxiety

Monitoring and Care of the Child

Activities and Interventions	Rationale	Reportable Conditions
1. Assess recent platelet count, hemoglobin, PT, PTT, and International Normalized ratio (INR); correct abnormalities as indicated.	These lab values are used as indicators of potential bleeding/clotting abnormalities that may increase the risk for bleeding after RAC removal.[3,7-10]	• Platelets <50,000/mm^3 • Moderate to significantly decreased hematocrit for child's age and condition • Abnormal values for PT, PTT, INR

2. Monitor child's hemodynamic status before, during, and after procedure.	Facilitates rapid recognition and intervention in the event of a complication.[1,3,6,9,10]	• Signs of cardiac tamponade:
		   Increased heart rate
		   Decreased blood pressure
		   Widened pulse pressure
		• Respiratory compromise

3. Continually monitor dressing site and chest tube output after RAC removal. [10]	Assesses for bleeding from RAC insertion site.	• Significant amount of bleeding at insertion site. • Continuous or copious sanguineous drainage from chest tubes[3,6,9]
4. Keep dressing clean, dry, and intact.[11]	Prevents infection.	• Signs of infection: redness, drainage, tenderness, fever, or elevation in white blood cell count
5. Until healed, change dressing and assess insertion site at least every 24 hours for infection or improper healing or per institution-specific protocol.	Infection and improper healing can present even several days following line removal.[3,8]	• Signs of infection • Abnormal or delayed healing
6. Assess effectiveness of pain and anxiety management strategies and provide appropriate interventions. Encourage family to assist in using nonpharmacologic means to comfort and support the child.	Early identification of pain and anxiety facilitates prompt treatment.	• Unresolved pain, anxiety, or discomfort • Unable to perform procedure due to child's level of anxiety or pain • Continued irritability, changes in physiologic condition

Documentation

- Child and family education
- Child's tolerance of the procedure
- Appearance of RAC insertion site
- PT, PTT, platelet count, and hematologic values before and after procedure as is relevant to child's clinical status
- Hemodynamic status before, during, and after RAC removal
- Amount of bleeding from RAC insertion site and from chest tubes following procedure
- Date and time of RAC removal
- Individual performing the procedure
- Condition of RAC tip on removal, and ease of RAC removal
- Hemodynamics before, during, and after the procedure
- Results of chest x-ray following procedure
- Hemodynamic and physiologic response to sedation and/or analgesia administered
- Blood transfusion or fluid bolus administration required as a result of RAC removal
- Unexpected outcomes and related treatment

References

1. Bridges E: Hemodynamic monitoring. In Woods S, et al, editors: *Cardiac nursing,* ed 4, Philadelphia, 2000, Lippincott.
2. Clarian Health Partners: Left atrial pressure monitoring: pediatric. In Clarian Health Partners, editors: *Pediatric patient care policy manual,* Indianapolis, 2002, Clarian Health Partners.
3. Flori HR, et al: Transthoracic intracardiac catheters in pediatric patients recovering from congenital heart defect surgery: associated complications and outcomes, *Crit Care Med* 28(8):2997-3001, 2000.
4. Arnone M: Central venous/right atrial pressure monitoring. In Lynn-McHale DJ, Carlson K, editors: *AACN procedure manual for critical care,* ed 4, Philadelphia, 2001, Saunders.
5. Gardner PE: Pulmonary artery pressure monitoring, *AACN Clin Issues* 4(1):98-119, 1993.
6. Roth SJ: Postoperative care. In Chang AC, et al, editors: *Pediatric cardiac intensive care,* Baltimore, 1998, Williams & Wilkins.
7. Craig J, et al: Cardiovascular critical care problems. In Curley MAQ, Moloney-Harmon P, editors: *Critical care nursing of infants and children,* ed 2, Philadelphia, 2001, Saunders, pp. 624-626.
8. Indiana University School of Medicine Department of Surgery, Section of Cardiothoracic Surgery: Right atrial line removal. In Indiana University School of Medicine Department of Surgery, Section of Cardiothoracic Surgery, editors: *Pediatric nurse practitioner procedures,* Indianapolis, 1999, Indiana University School of Medicine.
9. Johnston LJ, McKinley DF: Cardiac tamponade after removal of atrial intracardiac monitoring catheters in a pediatric patient: case report, *Heart Lung* 29(4):256-261, 2000.
10. Arnone M: Central venous/right atrial pressure line removal. In Lynn-McHale DJ, Carlson K, editors: *AACN procedure manual for critical care,* ed 4, Philadelphia, 2001, Saunders.
11. Arnone M: Central venous/right atrial pressure line sitecare. In Lynn-McHale DJ, Carlson K, editors: *AACN procedure manual for critical care,* ed 4, Philadelphia, 2001, Saunders.

Additional Readings

Bridges EJ: Monitoring pulmonary artery pressures: just the facts, *Crit Care Nurse* 20(6):59-76, 2000.

Castaneda A, et al: Perioperative care. In *Cardiac surgery of the neonate and infant,* Philadelphia, 1994, Saunders.

McGhee BH, Bridges MEJ: Monitoring arterial blood pressure: what you may not know, *Crit Care Nurse* 22(2):60-79, 2002.

PROCEDURE **69**

Arterial and Venous Sheath Removal

P U R P O S E : Arterial and venous sheaths are placed during diagnostic and interventional cardiac catheterizations. Proper removal of these sheaths aids in achieving and maintaining hemostasis and maximizing the child's comfort.

Peggy Dorr

PREREQUISITE KNOWLEDGE

- Technical and clinical competence in removal of arterial and venous sheaths is necessary; refer to institution-specific protocol and state-specific Nurse Practice Act regarding individuals permitted to remove arterial and venous sheaths
- Child development as it relates to clinical assessment and procedure
- Mastery of pediatric advanced life support competencies
- Principles of aseptic technique
- Although these sheaths are typically removed in the cardiac catheterization laboratory, they may occasionally be left in and removed in the recovering unit.
- Knowledge of the anatomy of the femoral artery and vein and of the technique for the percutaneous approach to the insertion of arterial and venous sheaths
- Knowledge of the anticoagulation therapy used during the procedure and any reversal of remaining anticoagulant after the procedure is completed
  - ❖ Heparin is typically used during catheterization procedures because of its short duration.
- Knowledge of appropriate tests used to measure coagulation status and child's target anticoagulation level for removal of sheaths
  - ❖ Partial thromboplastin time (PTT) assesses anticoagulation from heparinization.

  - ❖ An activate clotting time (ACT) is a quick test that can be done at the bedside if the equipment is available.
- Sheath removal can be associated with many complications, including:
  - ❖ External bleeding at the site
  - ❖ Internal bleeding at the site (i.e., retroperitoneal)
  - ❖ Vascular complications (hematoma, arteriovenous fistula, pseudoaneurysm, thrombus, or embolus)
  - ❖ Several studies have documented an increased incidence rate of arterial complications, such as loss of pulse, with interventions that involved balloon dilation of systemic obstructions.[1,2]
  - ❖ Studies of the efficacy of heparin infusions, streptokinase, urokinase, and tissue-type plasminogen activator (t-PA) for the treatment of loss of pulse have shown positive results with reestablishment of arterial patency.[2-4]
- Most complications are seen in children of 5 kg or less during and after a cardiac catheterization and include lower extremity hypoperfusion after arterial access and blood loss that necessitates transfusion.[5]
- Manual compression devices and collagen plugs are not approved for use in children. The amount of pressure delivered and the length of the device necessary to deliver the plug are inappropriate for the pediatric population.
- A patch (SyvekPatch, Marine Polymer Technologies, Inc., Danvers, Massachusetts) coated with a polymer that

accelerates the coagulation process at multiple levels has been approved by the US Food and Drug Administration (FDA) as an "external device to control bleeding from vascular access sites and percutaneous catheters."[6] Several studies have documented the efficacy of this product in accelerating the hemostasis process, which allows mobility or ambulation sooner than the typical 4 to 6 hours and a tendency toward earlier discharge in children after a catheterization.[7]

CHILD AND FAMILY ASSESSMENT

- Developmental level of the child ➻*Rationale:* Understanding the stages of cognitive development in children is imperative to understanding their perceptions of health-related events.[8] The child's developmental level influences the preparation necessary before sheath removal, including the need for boarding or sedation to ensure safety and hemostasis.
- History of cardiac disease, previous surgeries, reason for catheterization, and an understanding of any interventions performed during the cardiac catheterization ➻*Rationale:* Cardiac and disease history is important during assessment for increased risk associated with abnormal anatomy, coagulation disorder, or interventions. A large study on the risks of cardiac catheterization found that "relative to diagnostic procedures, interventional catheterizations were independently associated with a greater risk of complication."[1]
- Assess PTT or ACT ➻*Rationale:* Coagulation study results should be within normal limits to decrease the risk of bleeding after sheath removal. A normal ACT is 70 to 120 seconds,[9] but hemostasis is attainable with manual pressure and a higher ACT. If an ACT or PTT is extremely elevated, a dose of protamine sulfate may be given to neutralize the anticoagulant activity of the heparin. Other laboratory values that may need assessment are calcium and platelets, especially if hemostasis is difficult to obtain.
- Assess electrocardiographic (ECG) rhythm and rate, respiratory rate, and blood pressure ➻*Rationale:* Establishes baseline data. If blood pressure value is above normal for the child's age, medications (antihypertensives or anxiolytics/analgesics, on the basis of the child's history and current status) should be considered to lower the blood pressure into the normal range to achieve and maintain hemostasis.
- Desire of family members to be present during the procedure ➻*Rationale:* Family members may provide support and comfort measures to the child but should have the choice not to remain with the child.

CHILD AND FAMILY EDUCATION

Individualized, developmentally appropriate education is provided to the family and to the child based on desire for knowledge, readiness to learn, and overall neurologic and psychosocial state. The goals of information given are to promote a sense of mastery of the events to occur, to facilitate the child's and family's understanding of the purpose of these events, and to correct misinformation.[8]

- Explain the procedure to the family and child, including sensations felt with sheath removal and the need for extended (5 to 10 minutes) manual compression of the area ➻*Rationale:* A thorough understanding of the procedure provides information, may help ease anxiety, and may enable the family to provide greater support to the child.
- Explain the possible changes in color, temperature, and sensation of the lower extremity with manual compression ➻*Rationale:* Awareness of the visible changes that may occur may prevent increased fear or anxiety from the family and child.
- Explain the importance of bed rest with the head of bed no greater than 30 degrees and the need to keep the lower extremities straight for a specific period of time. Infants and small children may need to be placed on leg boards to assure hemostasis and prevent complications such as hematoma formation or external bleeding. ➻*Rationale:* Providing information may prevent increased fear or anxiety and promote compliance.
- Encourage questions and answer questions as they arise ➻*Rationale:* Reinforcement of information is needed during periods of stress.

EQUIPMENT

- Cardiorespiratory monitoring system with pulse oximetry and blood pressure capability
- Clean and sterile gloves
- Sterile gauze
- SyvekPatch (if available)
- Povidone-iodine swabstick or solution
- Suture removal kit (if sutures remain)
- Tincture of benzoin swabstick or solution
- Pressure dressing tape
- Personal protective equipment, including protective eye wear and gown
- Appropriate pediatric emergency equipment, medications, fluid, and infusion pumps readily available
- Laboratory services, including the ability to perform an ACT test or obtain appropriate laboratory studies (PTT, calcium, platelets)

Procedure for Arterial and Venous Sheath Removal

Steps	Rationale	Considerations
1. Ensure child and family understand procedure and questions are answered.	Evaluates and reinforces understanding of previously taught information. *(Level VI*)*	Developmental level; cognitive ability and anxiety level determine approach to and effectiveness of teaching
2. Gather all necessary equipment and supplies.	Preparation and presence of all materials facilitate completion of procedure without delays.	
3. Ensure appropriate cardiorespiratory monitoring.	Children may decompensate during the procedure, especially if a sedative or narcotic was administered.	Consider child's neurologic and hemodynamic status in selection of appropriate level of monitoring.
4. Administer analgesic or anxiolytic before sheath removal, if necessary.	Facilitates pain or anxiety management, ensuring vital signs remain within normal limits and reduction of movement when the child is comfortable.	Consider timing of most recent analgesic or anxiety medication before giving another dose of same or similar medications.
5. Provide for appropriate privacy; position child to facilitate removal of the sheaths.	Respects child's rights. Facilitates sheath removal.	Privacy is an important consideration for school-aged children and adolescents.
6. Wash hands and put on clean gloves.	Standard precautions; reduces transmission of microorganisms.	
7. Put on personal protective equipment (eye protection, gown).	Standard precautions; reduces transmission of microorganisms.	
8. Remove any dressing over existing arterial and venous sheaths.	Prepares for sheath removal.	
9. Discard clean gloves and put on sterile gloves.	Maintains asepsis of site.	
10. Clean site around and on the catheter sheaths with povidone-iodine solution.	Ensures an aseptic field and reduces transmission of microorganisms.	
11. Remove any sutures that may have been left in place.	Prepares for sheath removal.	
12. Fold a gauze patch in half and place on top of sheath entry sites. Fingers should be placed with one above entry site, one on entry site, and one below entry site. *(Level IV*)*	Vessel puncture sites are superior and medial to actual skin puncture site. The sheaths are inserted at a 45-degree angle to the vessels.[10]	If a SyvekPatch is available, remove patch and hold with paper-like side face down. Allow a few drops of blood to escape from the sheath site after removal to activate the polymer. Hold patch over insertion site as described and continue with direct pressure.
13. While holding pressure over site, slowly and smoothly remove the arterial sheath only.	Removal of both sheaths simultaneously increases the risk for development of an arteriovenous fistula.[10]	
14. After 30 seconds, remove the venous sheath. Maintain consistent pressure on the sites throughout this process.	Pressure should be applied where the vessel, not the skin, was punctured. Compression should only be forceful enough to prevent bleeding, which can usually be achieved while still maintaining an arterial pulse in the foot.[10]	

Procedure continues on following page

* Level IV: Limited clinical studies to support recommendations

Level VI: Clinical studies in a variety of patient populations and situations to support recommendations

Procedure for **Arterial and Venous Sheath Removal**—*Continued*

Steps	Rationale	Considerations
15. Maintain manual pressure on both sites for a minimum of 10 minutes.	Pressure is necessary to ensure the bleeding stops and hemostasis is achieved.	Pressure must not be released anytime during these initial 10 minutes. Do not lift to check the site until the entire time has elapsed.
16. After 10 minutes, slowly roll the fingers up off of the site and assess for bleeding.	If the motion is sharp or jerky, clot formation and hemostasis may be disrupted.	
17. If bleeding is noted, return pressure to site for another 5 to 10 minutes.	Most vessels stop bleeding within 20 minutes.[10]	If bleeding appears to be brisk, consider giving another dose of protamine. If bleeding is delayed or slow, continuation of applied pressure should be adequate.
18. After bleeding has stopped, place a fresh small square of sterile gauze immediately over the puncture wound sites.	Gauze helps apply direct pressure at the wound site.	If SyvekPatch is used, do not remove the patch. Apply tincture of benzoin around the patch and a pressure dressing directly over the patch.
19. While maintaining pressure, have another staff member swab the area around the site with tincture of benzoin.	Tincture of benzoin helps ensure the integrity of the dressing over the wound for an extended period of time.	
20. Apply two to three strips of pressure dressing tape over the site. Strips should begin at hip level and be pulled tight over the wounds and secured on the inside of leg.	Pressure from the adhesive dressing helps maintain hemostasis and prevent bleeding.	
21. Dispose of supplies and used equipment in an appropriate receptacle.	Standard precautions; decreases transmission of microorganisms.	
22. Remove personal protective equipment and wash hands.	Reduces transmission of microorganisms; protects personnel health.	
23. Keep bandaged area exposed for continuous visual observation.	If sites are covered and bleeding occurs, a significant amount of blood loss could occur before the bleeding is noticed by the health care team.	
24. Maintain leg boards on small children and assist all children to keep supine and fairly calm for 4 to 6 hours. *(Level IV*)*	With legs kept straight, the clot is maintained, ensuring hemostasis.	Small infants and toddlers may need sedation to help them stay still, whereas older children should engage in diversionary activities such as videos, music, or TV. Reports from facilities that use the SyvekPatch have shown shorter immobilization times with a small incidence rate of complications, such as bleeding or hematoma.[11]

* Level IV: Limited clinical studies to support recommendations

Expected Outcomes	Unexpected Outcomes
• Hemostasis at site; no external or internal bleeding noted • Pulses are palpable distal to site; extremity is pink and warm, with brisk capillary refill • Child is comfortable and able to lie still and supine for required length of time	• Clot does not form at site; child continues to bleed without direct pressure • Absence of distal pulses; cool pale extremity • Palpable "thrill" over insertion site after hemostasis achieved • Child is anxious or scared, crying or irritable, and unable to lie still or keep legs straight

Monitoring and Care of the Child

Activities and Intervention	Rationale	Reportable Conditions
1. Vital signs, including affected extremity pulse, color, and temperature, obtained every 15 minutes for 1 hour, every 30 minutes for 1 hour, and every 1 hour for 2 hours; then routine assessment based on institution-specific or unit-specific protocols. (Level II*)	Frequency of vital sign documentation can decrease over time because the longer clot hemostasis is maintained, the less chance there is for disruption of the clot. Alterations in arterial patency are detected with checking the extremity for pulse and color, whereas a significant change in heart rate or blood pressure could indicate a retroperitoneal bleed.[12]	• Abnormal vital signs • Cool extremity; weak pulse or loss of pulse in extremity • If the affected extremity is pulseless after sheath removal, DeGiovanni[3] suggests administration of an initial heparin dose of 100 U/kg, followed by an infusion at 20 U/kg/h[3] • If the affected extremity remains pulseless 4 hours after sheath removal, fibrinolytic therapy must be considered immediately
2. Assess site for bleeding on the same schedule as vital signs.	Bleeding can occur at the site with no initial changes in vital signs or distal perfusion. The actual area must be observed for active bleeding.	• Active bleeding
3. Assess effectiveness of pain management strategy and provide appropriate interventions. Encourage family to assist with nonpharma-cologic means to comfort and support the child.	Early identification of child's pain allows for immediate attention.	• Report of unresolved pain and discomfort • Continued irritability, changes in physiologic condition

* Level II: Theory-based; no research data to support recommendations; recommendations from expert consensus group may exist

Documentation

• Vital signs, including extremity pulses, color, temperature, sensation
• Presence or absence of bleeding at wound site
• Medications or aids used to promote hemostasis (protamine, SyvekPatch)
• Duration of pressure application
• Child's ability to sit up and ambulate after 4 to 6 hours with no disruption to clot hemostasis
• Fluid intake
• Comfort assessment and any specific interventions provided
• Date, time, and name of individual who performs sheath removal
• Status of sheath when removed
• Unexpected outcomes and related treatment
• Child and family education

References

1. Vittiello R, et al: Complications associated with pediatric cardiac catheterization, *J Am Coll Cardiol* 32(5):1433-1440, 1998.
2. Zeevi B, et al: Acute complications in the current era of therapeutic cardiac catheterization for congenital heart disease, *Cardiol Young* 9(3):266-272, 1999.
3. DeGiovanni JV: Management of an absent pulse following arterial catheterization, *Images Paediatr Cardiol* 13:19-21, 2002.
4. Balaguru D, et al: Early and late results of thrombolytic therapy using tissue-type plasminogen activator to restore arterial pulse after cardiac catheterization in infants and small children, *Am J Cardiol* 19(7):908-910, 2003.
5. Rhodes JF, et al: Impact of low body weight on frequency of pediatric cardiac catheterization complications, *Am J Cardiol* 86(11):1275-1278, 2000.
6. Weiner B, et al: Hemostasis in the era of the chronic anticoagulated patient, *J Invas Cardiol* 15(11):669-674, 2003.
7. Madhok A, et al: Use of SyvekPatch® in children undergoing cardiac catheterization, *Pediatr Cardiol Today* Oct:6-8:2004.
8. LeRoy S, et al: Recommendations for preparing children and adolescents for invasive cardiac procedures, *Circulation* 108:2550-2564, 2003.
9. Jacobs DS, et al: *Laboratory test handbook,* Hudson, OH, 2003, Lexi-Comp, Inc.
10. Perry SB: Manual techniques of cardiac catheterization: vessel entry and catheter manipulation. In Lock JE, Keane JF, Perry SB, editors: *Diagnostic and interventional catheterization in congenital heart disease,* Boston, 2000, Kluwer Academic Publishers.
11. Nader RG, et al: Clinical evaluation of the SyvekPatch® in consecutive patients undergoing interventional, EPS and diagnostic cardiac catheterization procedures, *J Invas Cardiol* 14(6):305-307, 2002.
12. Pigula FA, et al: Management of retroperitoneal arterial injury after heart catheterization in children, *Soc Thorac Surg* 69(5):1582-1584, 2000.

Additional Reading

Lin PH, et al: Surgical intervention for complications caused by femoral artery catheterization in pediatric patients, *J Vasc Surg* 34(6):1071-1078, 2001.

Pericardial Catheter: Management

PURPOSE: A pericardial catheter is placed and maintained in the pericardial space for continuous or intermittent drainage of effusion

Michele J. Borisuk

PREREQUISITE KNOWLEDGE

- Normal anatomy and physiology of the cardiac system
- Specific cardiac anatomy of the child with a pericardial effusion
- Principles of aseptic technique
- Mastery of pediatric advanced life support competencies
- Child development as it relates to clinical assessment and pericardial catheter management
- Appropriate pediatric dosing of analgesics
- A pericardial effusion is a collection of fluid in the pericardial space.
  - ❖ Fluid can be serous, serous sanguinous, chylous (leaking from thoracic duct), purulent, blood, or occasionally medications if surgically placed intracardiac lines have become dislodged to the pericardial space.
- Causes of pericardial effusion include congestive heart failure, effusion after cardiac surgery, overhydration, hypoproteinemia, pericardial injury and inflammation, tumors, uremia, radiation, aneurysms, trauma, or coagulation defects. If the thoracic duct is draining into the pericardial space, the effusion is chylous.[1,2]
- Normally, the pericardial space contains 15 to 50 mL of pericardial fluid.[1]
- Recognition of signs and symptoms of tamponade: elevated venous pressures, neck vein distension, hypotension not responsive to fluid resuscitation, muffled heart sounds, pulsus paradoxus of more than 10 mm Hg, and narrow pulse pressure. Identification of neck vein distension, pulsus paradoxus, and muffled heart sounds is difficult in the infant and small child.[3-6]

- ❖ A few small studies in children have reported that a significant fall in the peak of the pulse oximetry waveform with inspiration was associated with pulsus paradoxus.[7] *(Level V*)*
- The first structures to be affected are usually those of the right heart. A pericardial effusion leads to tamponade, when the diastolic pressure within the chambers of the heart equals the pressure exerted by the pericardial fluid thus interfering with filling pressures, systemic venous congestion, and right heart failure.[8]
- Pericardiocentesis may be necessary for diagnostic purposes or when medical management fails and tamponade is a concern (see Procedure 44 for further information).
- Depending on the clinical situation, the catheter may be left in place for continuous or intermittent drainage for several days as needed.[2] The insertion of an indwelling pericardial catheter for continuous or intermittent drainage avoids the need for repeated pericardiocentesis and may be the treatment of choice for some children.[1,2]
  - ❖ When left in place, the catheter is attached to a closed drainage system or to a closed capped system for intermittent drainage.
  - ❖ A capped intermittent drainage system may be flushed with 2 to 3 mL of heparin (10 units/mL) or 0.9% saline solution for catheter maintenance.[1,2]
  - ❖ Use of intermittent drainage may be associated with a decreased incidence rate of catheter obstruction as compared with continuous drainage[2] *(Level IV*)*

---

* Level IV: Limited clinical studies to support recommendations
  Level V: Clinical studies in more than one or two patient populations and situations to support recommendations

❖ The indwelling pericardial catheter is usually removed when effusion fluid drainage has dropped below 10 to 30 mL/24 h and the effusion is resolved as shown with echocardiography. No data define the timing of pericardial catheter removal; it is usually dependent on prescribing practitioner preference and the child's clinical status.[1,2]

CHILD AND FAMILY ASSESSMENT

- Child's developmental level and ability to interact ➤*Rationale:* These factors influence preparation of the child and interaction.
- Child's and family's understanding of the reasons for and risks and benefits of pericardial catheter placement and maintenance ➤*Rationale:* Evaluates child's and family's understanding of the procedure and provides a gauge for ongoing education.
- Child's coping mechanisms ➤*Rationale:* Child's ability to cope with perceived pain and procedures should be assessed; measures to assist the child with coping are then pursued.
- Child's cardiovascular and hemodynamic status: heart rate, electrocardiographic (ECG) results, respiratory rate, blood pressure, pulse pressure, presence of pulsus paradoxus (inspiratory fall in systolic), heart sounds, perfusion, and peripheral pulses ➤*Rationale:* Evaluates hemodynamic status monitors for evidence of instability and tamponade.
- Pericardial drainage for amount, acute change in amount of drainage, change in color, and consistency ➤*Rationale:* Assessing catheter drainage assists in evaluation of complications, catheter patency, and degree of ongoing effusion.
- Indications of catheter occlusion or dislodgement with evaluation for acute cessation of drainage, evidence of hemodynamic instability, tamponade, and catheter length at insertion site ➤*Rationale:* Catheter occlusion or dislodgement may result in hemodynamic instability.
- Family's ability to function as a support system for the child during the procedure ➤*Rationale:* Family members are generally an effective support system for the child during potentially stressful situations. If the family is not comfortable with support for the child during the procedure, alternative support staff such as Child Life Therapy should be accessed.

CHILD AND FAMILY EDUCATION

Individualized, developmentally appropriate education is provided to the family and to the child based on desire for knowledge, readiness to learn, and overall neurologic and psychosocial state.

Note: Support services, such as Child Life Specialists, should be used to assist in teaching the child about the procedure when age appropriate.

- Describe pericardial effusion and the need for indwelling pericardial catheter to family members and the child as appropriate ➤*Rationale:* Providing information to the child and family decreases anxiety and meets the need for information.
- Describe the drainage method (intermittent or continuous) to the child and family ➤*Rationale:* Promotes child's and family's understanding of the procedure and the plan of care, which allows for child and family involvement in care.
- Describe the need for continuous monitoring and any activity restrictions while the pericardial catheter is in place ➤*Rationale:* Providing information to the child and family decreases anxiety, meets the need for information, and promotes cooperation.
- Describe the need for possible diagnostic testing (i.e., echocardiography, chest radiographs) in evaluation of the effusion and catheter placement ➤*Rationale:* Prepares the child and family for ongoing evaluation and facilitates understanding of plan of care.
- Explain that the catheter may be uncomfortable, especially at the insertion site after insertion; assure the child and family that pain medication will be administered to promote comfort ➤*Rationale:* Effective pain management reduces child and family anxiety.
- Describe infection risks and encourage child and family adherence to good hygiene ➤*Rationale:* Educates the child and family concerning the risk of infection; promotes cooperation with plan of care.
- Discuss the need for the catheter to be well secured to prevent dislodgement and the importance of monitoring catheter security with movement of the child ➤*Rationale:* Prevents accidental dislodgement of the catheter.
- Encourage questions and answer questions as they arise ➤*Rationale:* Reinforcement of information is needed during periods of stress.

EQUIPMENT

To empty the drainage bag:

- Clean gloves
- Container for fluid collection

For intermittent aspiration:

- Sterile gloves
- Syringes (20-mL to 60-mL) for aspiration
- Alcohol swabs or other antiseptic swabs per institution-specific protocol
- Sterile 0.9% saline solution for irrigation
- Heparinized saline solution (10 to 30 units/mL) per prescribing practitioner's order
- Sterile end cap if needleless access port is not used

Procedure for Pericardial Catheter Management

Steps	Rationale	Considerations
Empty Drainage/Collection Bag		
1. Ensure child and family understand procedure and questions are answered. Procedural support staff such as Child Life Specialist should be present as needed.	Evaluates and reinforces understanding of previously taught information.	Developmental level, cognitive ability, and anxiety level determine approach to and effectiveness of teaching.
2. Gather needed equipment and supplies.	Facilitates completion of task in a timely manner.	
3. Identify child with two patient identifiers per institution-specific protocol.	Promotes patient safety; ensures right patient and right procedure.	
4. Wash hands. *(Level VI*)*	Standard precautions; reduces transmission of microorganisms.	
5. Obtain vital signs and cardiorespiratory assessment results.	Provides a baseline assessment, which allows comparison with subsequent assessments.	
6. Wash hands; put on clean gloves. *(Level VI*)*	Use of aseptic technique minimizes incidence of infection.	
7. Turn stopcock off to child.[9]	Prevents pneumopericardium.	Child may need family and staff support during drainage process because of fear of procedures.
8. Open emptying port of drainage collection bag.[1]	Allows fluid to be emptied from collection bag.	
9. Empty the pericardial drainage into a collection container; close emptying port.	Allows fluid volume to be measured. Closing of port closes the system and prevents leaking of fluid.	
10. Turn stopcock off to emptying port; open to drainage catheter.	Allows fluid to drain from pericardial space to collection bag.	
11. Measure and document amount of drainage.	Monitors system patency and output.	
12. Discard used supplies and equipment in appropriate container.	Standard precautions; reduces transmission of microorganisms.	
13. Remove gloves; wash hands.	Standard precautions.	
Intermittent Aspiration		
1. Ensure child and family understand procedure and questions are answered. Procedural support staff such as Child Life Specialist should be present as needed.	Evaluates and reinforces understanding of previously taught information.	Developmental level, cognitive ability, and anxiety level determine approach to and effectiveness of teaching.
2. Gather needed equipment and supplies.	Facilitates completion of task in a timely manner.	
3. Identify child with two patient identifiers per institution-specific protocol.	Promotes patient safety; ensures right patient and right procedure.	
4. Review prescribing practitioner's order for frequency of fluid aspiration (e.g., daily, twice a	Identifies frequency of fluid aspiration.	Follow institution-specific protocol regarding personnel permitted to aspirate pericardial catheters.

Procedure continues on following page

* Level VI: Clinical studies in a variety of patient populations and situations to support recommendations

Procedure for Pericardial Catheter Management—*Continued*

Steps	Rationale	Considerations
day, or more frequently if clinically indicated).		Intermittent aspiration may be used for evaluation of effusion accumulation within the pericardium over a certain period of time (i.e,. 24 hours) for better prediction of ability to remove catheter without reoccurrence of effusion.[2] *(Level IV[*])*
5. Wash hands. *(Level VI[*])*	Standard precautions; reduces transmission of microorganisms.	
6. Obtain vital signs and cardio-respiratory assessment results.	Provides a baseline assessment, which allows comparison with subsequent assessments.	
7. Uncoil catheter and extension tubing as necessary to access stopcock port.	Facilitates access to stopcock for fluid removal.	
8. Wash hands and put on sterile gloves.[1,9]	Use of aseptic technique minimizes incidence of infection.	
9. If stopcock is capped, remove cap from the three-way stopcock; this step is not necessary if needleless access port is present.	Allows access to stopcock port for fluid aspiration.	
10. Clean the infusion port/needle-less access cap of the three-way stopcock with an alcohol swab or antiseptic swab per institution-specific protocol.[1,9]	Use of aseptic technique minimizes incidence rate of infection.	
11. Attach sterile 60-mL syringe to three-way stopcock directly or with needleless access device.	Syringe is used to collect fluid aspirated.	
12. Turn stopcock so it is open to the syringe and child.	Opens drainage system for removal of fluid.	
13. Gently aspirate pericardial fluid.[1,9]	Removes accumulated fluid from pericardial space; gentle aspiration minimizes pericardial injury from acute pressure changes.[1,9]	Child may need to be placed in alternating side lying positions during aspiration of pericardial fluid to promote drainage.
14. Turn stopcock off to syringe port and remove syringe with aspirated fluid.	Fluid is measured and discarded.	Pericardial fluid samples may be collected for diagnostic tests (e.g., protein, glucose, hematocrit, white blood cell count, bacterial or fungal cultures).
15. Attach syringe with sterile flush solution per prescribing practitioner's order and gently flush catheter.[1,2,9]	Flushing clears pericardial catheter and decreases likelihood that catheter will become occluded.	Monitor vital signs and ECG while flushing catheter. Catheter should flush smoothly with minimal resistance. Do not forcefully flush catheter; if unable to flush catheter, notify prescribing practitioner. A 2-mL to 3-mL dose of heparinized (10 units/mL) saline solution or 0.9% saline solution is usually used to flush catheter.[1,2,9]
16. Turn stopcock off to syringe port; remove syringe.	Prevents pericardial fluid from backing into catheter and forming	

Procedure for Pericardial Catheter Management—*Continued*		
Steps	**Rationale**	**Considerations**
	blockage; maintains a closed system; prevents pneumopericardium.	
17. Close stopcock port with a new sterile cap if cap was initially removed for stopcock access.[1,8]	Maintains closed sterile system; decreases risk of infection.	
18. Coil catheter and tubing; secure to child.	Prevents inadvertent catheter removal.	Per institution-specific guidelines and the child's status, child may be out of bed for play and socialization.
19. Discard drainage and used supplies in appropriate receptacles; remove gloves and wash hands.	Standard precautions; reduces transmission of microorganisms.	

Management of Pericardial Catheter Occlusion

1. Determine whether the drainage system is lower than catheter insertion point and reposition as needed.[1,8]	Facilitates drainage by gravity.	
2. Assess whether external mechanical cause of pericardial catheter blockage exists; if present, correct.	Relieves mechanical obstruction to flow of pericardial fluid.	Mechanical obstruction may be from tubing kinks or tubing compressed under the child. Turning child to side facilitates the fluid to pool inferiorly in the pericardium for drainage.
3. Ensure tubing is not disconnected and reconnect with aseptic technique if necessary.[1,9]	Ensures intact drainage system.	
4. Determine whether the stopcock is in the incorrect position; correct if needed.	Stopcock may have been turned during patient care, activity, or manipulation by child.	

If catheter remains blocked:

5. Gather needed supplies and equipment.	Facilitates completion of procedure in a timely manner.	Follow institution-specific protocol regarding personnel permitted to aspirate pericardial catheters.
6. Wash hands; put on sterile gloves.	Use of aseptic technique reduces incidence rate of infection.	
7. Turn stopcock off to drainage bag.	Allows access to pericardial catheter.	
8. Remove sterile cap from infusion port of stopcock.	Allows syringe to be attached.	
9. Clean infusion port of stopcock with alcohol swab or antiseptic swab per institution-specific protocol.	Reduces microorganisms.	
10. Flush the pericardial catheter with 2 to 5 mL of heparinized (10 units/mL) 0.9% sterile saline solution or fluid as prescribed (i.e., 30 units of heparin per mL of 0.9% sterile saline solution).[1,9]	Attempts to clear pericardial catheter; heparinized saline solution is used if the drainage is serous or fibrous in consistency.	
11. Turn stopcock off to the infusion port to allow drainage into drainage bag; remove syringe.	Allows drainage of flush and pericardial fluid; assesses patency of drainage system after manipulation.	

Procedure continues on following page

Procedure for Pericardial Catheter Management—*Continued*

Steps	Rationale	Considerations
12. Close stopcock infusion port with a new sterile cap if cap was initially removed for stopcock access.	Maintains closed sterile system; decreases risk of infection.	
13. If the previous measures do not remove the catheter blockage, consider changing the pericardial drainage tubing or allowing heparinized saline solution to dwell in catheter for 15 minutes and again attempt gentle aspiration.[1,9]	Allowing heparinized saline solution to dwell may break down material causing catheter occlusion.	If measures do not remove the catheter blockage, notify prescribing practitioner.
14. Discard used supplies and equipment in appropriate receptacles; remove gloves and wash hands.	Standard precautions; reduces transmission of microorganisms.	

Expected Outcomes

- Pericardial effusion is drained
- Drainage system remains patent and intact

- Child's condition remains hemodynamically stable during placement of catheter and during and after manipulation of catheter
- Child remains free from infection while catheter is in place
- Child has acceptable level of comfort
- Catheter remains in place until elective removal

Unexpected Outcomes

- Reaccumulation of pericardial effusion
- Catheter occlusion or fracture
- Catheter does not drain
- Inability to flush catheter
- Disruption of closed system
- Cardiac tamponade
- Dysrhythmia
- Indications of inadequate peripheral perfusion
- Local infection at insertion site
- Indications of sepsis
- Unmanaged pain
- Accidental dislodgement of the catheter

Monitoring and Care of the Child

Activities and Intervention	Rationale	Reportable Conditions
1. Place child in comfortable position in bed with head of bed raised no greater than 30 degrees.[1,2,9]	Reduces anxiety; allows fluid to pool inferiorly in the pericardium, facilitating drainage.	• Child is unable to maintain desired position because of agitation or increased activity
2. Ensure that all connections throughout drainage system are secure.	Maintains closed secure system for drainage and decreases risk of infection.	• Inadvertent disruption of closed system
3. Maintain drainage/collection bag securely at a lower level than catheter entry site.[1,9]	Promotes drainage flow and prevents catheter occlusion.	• No drainage from pericardial catheter
4. After placement or manipulation of catheter, a systematic cardiovascular and hemodynamic assessment should be performed every 60 minutes and as child's status necessitates.[1,9]	Monitors for signs and symptoms of cardiac tamponade and pericardial catheter-related problems.	• Signs of cardiac tamponade: dyspnea, tachypnea, tachycardia, hypotension, increased jugular venous pressure, pulsus paradoxus, muffled heart sounds, precordial dullness to percussion, altered level of consciousness, dysrhythmias

Monitoring and Care of the Child—Cont'd

Activities and Intervention	Rationale	Reportable Conditions
5. Assess patency of pericardial catheter drainage system every hour and as needed.	Pericardial catheter blockage predisposes the child to reaccumulation of pericardial fluid that may lead to cardiac tamponade.	• Cessation of pericardial drainage • Signs and symptoms of cardiac tamponade
6. Assess amount and type of fluid drainage from the pericardial catheter hourly and as needed.	Monitors type and amount of pericardial fluid drainage.	• Change in amount or color of pericardial drainage from child's baseline
7. Change the pericardial dressing according to institution-specific protocol and when the dressing becomes damp, loosened, or soiled; monitor for indications of local infection at insertion site.[1,9]	Assesses for signs and symptoms of infection. Infective pericarditis is associated with high mortality and morbidity rates.	• Elevated white blood cell count • Temperature elevation greater than 38.5°C • Signs and symptoms of infection at the insertion site (pain, erythema, drainage)
8. Change pericardial tubing and drainage bag every 72 hours or according to institution-specific protocol.[1,9]	Reduces the incidence rate of infection.	• Inability to disconnect tubing or drainage bag from catheter
9. Assess effectiveness of pain management strategy and provide appropriate interventions. Encourage family to assist with nonpharmacologic means to comfort and support the child.	Child may have chest pain or pleuritic type pain while the pericardial catheter is in place.	• Inadequate pain relief with analgesics • Continued irritability or changes in physiologic condition
10. Monitor parameters that show clinical readiness for removal of the pericardial catheter.	Facilitates early removal of the pericardial catheter; decreases infection risk.	• Pericardial drainage less than 25 to 30 mL over the previous 24 hours[1,2,9] • Hemodynamic stability as evidenced by stable systolic blood pressure within the normal range for child's age, no pulsus paradoxus, vital signs within normal range for child's age • Absence of pericardial effusion shown on echocardiogram

Documentation

- Baseline physical assessment results
- Description of catheter entry site
- Signs and symptoms of infection
- Patency of pericardial catheter
- Description of and volume of drainage
- Cardiorespiratory assessment results and vital signs after each manipulation of catheter
- Medication administration
- Child and family education
- Pain assessment and any specific interventions provided
- Unexpected outcomes and related treatment

References
1. Hamel WJ: Care of patients with an indwelling pericardial catheter, *Crit Care Nurs* 18(5):40-45, 1998.
2. Tsang TSM, et al: Percutaneous echocardiographically guided pericardiocentesis in pediatric patients; evaluation of sagety and efficacy, *J Am Soc Echocardiog* 11(11):1072-1077, 1998.
3. Scarfone RJ, et al: Cardiac tamponade complicating postpericardiotomy syndrome, *Pediatr Emerg Care* 19(4):268-271, 2003.
4. Altman C: Pericarditis and pericardial disease. In Garson A Jr, Bricker J, Fisher D, et al, editors: *The science and practice of cardiology,* ed 2, Baltimore, 1998, Williams & Wilkins.

5. Behrman RE, et al: *Nelson textbook of pediatrics,* ed 17, Philadelphia, 2004, Elsevier.
6. Spodick DH: Pathophysiology of cardiac tamponade, *Chest* 113(5):1372, 1998.
7. Tamburro RF, et al: Detection of pulsus paradoxus associated with large pericardial effusions in pediatric patients by analysis of the pulse-oximetry waveform, *Pediatrics* 109(4):673-677, 2002.
8. McCance KL, Huether S: *Pathophysiology: the biology basis for disease in adults and children,* ed 2, St. Louis, 1994, Mosby.
9. McCloy K: Pericardial catheter management. In Lynn-McHale DJ, Carlson K, editors: *AACN procedure manual for critical care,* ed 4, Philadelphia, 2001, Saunders.

Pulmonary Hypertension: Management

P U R P O S E : To avoid life-threatening exacerbations of pulmonary hypertension

Jo Ann Nieves

PREREQUISITE KNOWLEDGE

- Normal anatomy and physiology of the cardiopulmonary system
- The management of pulmonary hypertension (PHTN) is frequently necessary in children with idiopathic pulmonary venous obstruction or specific cardiac lesions, in children undergoing cardiovascular surgery, and in premature infants.
- The child's congenital or acquired heart disease and its impact on the pulmonary vasculature
- Risk factors for the development of PHTN (Table 71-1)
- Term neonates have elevated pulmonary vascular resistance and PHTN for the first 2 to 6 weeks of life.[1] Other

TABLE 71-1	Risk Factors for Pulmonary Hypertension
Risk Factor	**Condition**
Age	Neonates possess highly reactive pulmonary beds[1]
Chromosomal abnormalities	Down syndrome: potential development of accelerated progression and severity of pulmonary arterial damage[3-5,7,9]
Congenital or acquired heart disease	AVC, large VSD, large PDA
Acyanotic systemic to pulmonary artery shunts under high pressure Increased pulmonary venous pressure	TAPVR, LV failure, severe MS, pulmonary vein obstruction
Cyanotic congenital heart disease	TGA, truncus arteriosus, univentricular heart with high flow
Adults with congenital heart disease and left to right shunts	ASD
Eisenmenger's syndrome	VSD, Patient who has developed irreversible pulmonary arteriolar damage in which PVR is more than SVR; child is cyanotic[7] Waterson shunt, Potts shunt, central shunts[9]
Presence of long-standing systemic to pulmonary artery to systemic shunt	
Pretransplant recipient with long-standing cardiac dysfunction	Dilated cardiomyopathy, LV failure
Cardiac surgery	Cardiopulmonary bypass and hypothermia may result in endothelial cell injury, release of vasoconstrictor agents, impaired nitric oxide production, and formation/exposure to microemboli and atelectasis[2,3,5,6]

AVC, Atrioventricular canal defect; *VSD,* ventricular septal defect; *PDA,* patent ductus arteriosus; *TAPVR,* total anomalous pulmonary venous return; *LV,* left ventricle; *MS,* mitral stenosis; *TGA,* transposition of the great arteries; *ASD,* atrial septal defect

TABLE 71-2	Assessment of Pulmonary Hypertension

Parameter	Range
Normal Pulmonary Artery Pressures (PAP)	
Systolic pulmonary artery pressure	15 to 25 mm Hg
Diastolic pulmonary artery pressure	8 to 15 mm Hg
Mean pulmonary artery pressure	10 to 20 mm Hg
Pulmonary Hypertension	
Systolic pulmonary artery pressure	>1/2 systemic (arterial blood pressure)
Mean pulmonary artery pressure	>25 mm Hg at rest
Pulmonary Vascular Resistance Index	
Normal	1 to 3 index units
Elevated	>4 index unit

children at risk for development of progressive pulmonary vessel changes and PHTN include:

❖ Children with large left to right shunts under high pressure

❖ Children with chronically elevated left atrial pressure or obstructed pulmonary venous drainage

❖ Children with cyanotic conditions

❖ Children undergoing cardiac surgery[2]

- Pulmonary vascular disease can develop within the first year of life.[3]

- Children at risk for Eisenmenger's syndrome include children with an unrepaired left to right intracardiac shunt that over time causes irreversible pulmonary arteriolar damage in which pulmonary vascular resistance (PVR) exceeds systemic vascular resistance (SVR). These children develop cyanotic conditions from the reversal of the intracardiac shunt. Medical care is directed at supportive measures, including pulmonary vasodilators, supplemen-

tal oxygen, and anticongestive therapy. Exacerbation of PVR and drops in SVR can result in worsening cyanosis and coronary perfusion.[3,4-7]

- Normal pulmonary vascular pressures[8] (Table 71-2)
- Ability to differentiate between a pulmonary hypertensive event and pulmonary hypertensive crisis (Table 71-3)
- Pulmonary hypertension can be identified with echocardiography or cardiac catheterization.[3,6,8,9]
- Ability to interpret cardiac catheterization data to identify children at risk for PHTN. Assessment with cardiac catheterization is the most reliable method of determination of risk for PHTN. It provides specific pulmonary pressure and resistance parameters and response to pharmacologic treatments, including oxygen.[3,8-10]
- Factors that can provoke PHTN include alveolar hypoxia, endotracheal suctioning, hypercarbia, painful stimuli, acidosis, and hypothermia that results in acute pulmonary vasoconstriction with subsequent right ventricular failure and poor cardiac output.[3,6-7,10-11]
- Management of PHTN includes:
  ❖ Use of 100% oxygen; however, it must be used with caution in children with single ventricle physiology
  ❖ Controlled ventilation
  ❖ Intravenous vasodilators (can result in systemic hypotension)
  ❖ Nitric oxide
  ❖ Prostacyclin
  ❖ Sildenafil, which is currently being investigated for use in children[12-14]
- Familiarity with intracardiac and central venous line assessment and monitoring (see Procedures 62, 64, and 65)
- Signs and symptoms of complications in children with PHTN associated with routine nursing care
- Mastery of pediatric advanced life support competencies
- Appropriate pediatric dosing of analgesics, sedatives, and emergency medications
- Activation of emergency alert system when a complication is detected

TABLE 71-3	Pulmonary Hypertensive Event Versus Pulmonary Hypertensive Crisis	
Condition	**Pulmonary Hypertensive Event**	**Pulmonary Hypertensive Crisis**
Definition	Acute rise in pulmonary arterial pressure to 75% of systemic pressure with stable arterial blood pressure	Paroxysmal event where pulmonary artery systolic pressures match or exceed systemic pressures, resulting in right ventricular failure and immediate fall in left atrial preload, systemic blood pressure
Parameters:		
Heart rate	Elevated	Elevated
Arterial blood pressure	Stable	Decreased
Oxygen saturation	Stable or decreased	Decreased
Central venous/right atrial pressure	Stable or elevated	Elevated
Pulmonary artery pressure	Elevated	Elevated
Left atrial pressure	Stable	Decreased
Cardiac output	Decreased	Severely decreased
Systemic perfusion	Decreased	Severely decreased

CHILD AND FAMILY ASSESSMENT

- Child's developmental level and ability to interact ➤➤*Rationale:* These factors influence preparation of the child, interaction, and type of nonpharmacologic comfort tools used, and determine the child's ability to follow instructions and comply with treatment regimen.
- History of hospitalizations, cardiac disease, or prematurity ➤➤*Rationale:* Identifies children who are at higher risk for development of PHTN; cardiac outputs of children undergoing bidirectional Glenn-type or Fontan-type procedures are dependent on low or normal pulmonary vascular resistance.[10,15-17]
- Results of diagnostic studies that evaluate pulmonary vascular resistance ➤➤*Rationale:* Early identification and treatment of PHTN can optimize outcomes.
- Presence of acute or chronic respiratory illness, including respiratory syncytial virus (RSV), bronchopulmonary dysplasia (BPD), asthma, and chronic airway obstruction ➤➤*Rationale:* Identifies children who are at higher risk for development of acute pulmonary vasoconstriction.[6,18]
- Current health status, including the presence of alveolar hypoxia, hypercarbia, acidosis, atelectasis, hypothermia, pain, or agitation ➤➤*Rationale:* These conditions can provoke pulmonary vasoconstriction.[16,19]
- Child's and family's understanding of child's condition and expected interventions ➤➤*Rationale:* Evaluates child's and family's understanding of condition and interventions and provides of a gauge for ongoing education.

CHILD AND FAMILY EDUCATION

Developmentally appropriate education is provided to the family and to the child based desire for knowledge, readiness to learn, and overall neurologic and psychosocial state.

- Provide basic information about the child's medical condition and risk factors for development of PHTN ➤➤*Rationale:* Providing information decreases fear and anxiety.
- Describe the expected hospital course and long-term care requirements, including home oxygen therapy as appropriate ➤➤*Rationale:* Providing information regarding the potential expected course of care can decrease the child's and family's anxiety and enhance cooperation.
- Provide information on the hemodynamic and clinical parameters used to diagnose PHTN ➤➤*Rationale:* Providing information regarding the assessment and monitoring used to diagnose PHTN may increase child's and family's understanding of the treatment regimen and decrease anxiety.
- Provide information on invasive monitoring lines in use, including central venous pressure (CVP), right atrial pressure (RA), left atrial pressure (LA), pulmonary artery pressure (PAP), and arterial line ➤➤*Rationale:* Providing information can decrease the child's and family's anxiety and enhance cooperation.
- Explain the management strategies that may be used to treat PHTN, including mechanical ventilation, supplemental oxygen after extubation, sedation, neuromuscular blockade, analgesics for pain control, intravenous vasodilator drugs, and inhaled pulmonary vasodilators ➤➤*Rationale:* Providing information may increase child's and family understanding of the treatment regimen and decrease fear and anxiety.
- Encourage questions and answer questions as they arise ➤➤*Rationale:* Reinforcement of information is needed during periods of stress.

EQUIPMENT

- Oxygen saturation monitor
- Stethoscope
- Cardiopulmonary monitor
- Monitor and transducer system for intracardiac or central venous lines as appropriate
- Manual resuscitation device with appropriately sized face mask and 100% oxygen source
- Oxygen blender (for child with single ventricle physiology)
- Medications as appropriate: sedation, analgesia, neuromuscular blocking agents
- Nonpharmacologic comfort tools (pacifier, music, etc)
- Intravenous or inhaled pulmonary vasodilators (nitric oxide, prostacyclin)
- Emergency cart with emergency medications

Procedure	for Pulmonary Hypertension: Management	
Steps	**Rationale**	**Considerations**
1. Ensure child and family understand procedure and questions are answered.	Evaluates and reinforces understanding of previously taught information.	Developmental level, cognitive ability, and anxiety level determine approach to and effectiveness of teaching.
2. Evaluate results of diagnostic studies to determine baseline PVR.	Early identification and treatment of PHTN events or crisis can minimize morbidity and mortality rates.[1,3,6,8,10,16,17,20,21]	

Procedure continues on following page

Procedure | for **Pulmonary Hypertension: Management**—*Continued*

Steps	Rationale	Considerations
3. Ensure necessary supplies and equipment are readily available at the bedside. *(Level II*)*	Aids in providing immediate intervention for the management of a PHTN event or crisis.	Children with preoperative PHTN may have acute rises in pulmonary artery pressure and resistance followed by right ventricular failure and low cardiac output at any time.[15,16,21]
4. Wash hands. *(Level VI*)*	Standard precautions; reduces transmission of microorganisms.	
5. Connect child to noninvasive and invasive monitoring per prescribing practitioner's order or institution-specific protocol.	Assists with the identification of slow or acute rises in PAP, right ventricular failure, and low cardiac output from PHTN.[15,16,21]	
6. Determine acceptable hemodynamic and laboratory parameters specific to the child, on basis of age, diagnosis, current health status, and medical history. *(Level VI*)*	Facilitates early recognition of PHTN events or crisis on basis of deviations from predetermined individualized hemodynamic and clinical parameters.	Acceptable ranges for the following should be determined to guide care: • Ratio of PAP to arterial blood pressure (ABP) • Right atrial pressure (RAP) or CVP • Arterial oxygen saturation • Mixed venous oxygen saturation • Arterial oxygen level when weaning fraction of inspired oxygen (FIO_2) • Arterial blood gas results • Serum lactate value
7. Monitor for signs and symptoms of PHTN event or crisis. *(Level VI*)*	A PHTN event or crisis may develop in response to routine management.	See Table 71-3.
8. Promote adequate gas exchange and oxygenation. *(Level VI*)*	Suboptimal gas exchange results in pulmonary vasoconstriction and elevated pulmonary vascular resistance.	Alveolar hypoxia is a potent trigger for vasoconstriction.[2,21]
9. Premedicate and hyperventilate with 100% oxygen before suctioning.[19,20,22] *(Level VI*)*	Endotracheal suctioning has been identified as a strong stimulus provoking acute pulmonary vasoconstriction.[11,19,23] Oxygen is a potent pulmonary vasodilator.	Hyperventilation and oxygen therapy must be used with caution in the child with single ventricle physiology because excessive pulmonary vasodilation could result in systemic hypoperfusion.[19,24] Consider use of an in-line suctioning system; suction with two people if no in-line system is available.
10. Adjust ventilatory parameters to achieve desired blood gas surevalues. *(Level VI*)*	Use of oxygen and controlled ventilation promotes pulmonary vasodilation and assists with stabilizing PAP.[10,14,19,21-22]	Goals: • Hypocarbia (~30 mm Hg partial pressure of carbon dioxide in arterial blood [$PaCO_2$]) • Alkalosis (pH >7.45 to 7.50)[10,14,18,19] • Infusion of alkaline solution (sodium bicarbonate) may be used to induce a metabolic alkalosis[18] • Gradual weaning of oxygen therapy/ ventilation (partial pressure of oxygen in arterial blood [PaO_2], >100 mm Hg)[21] • Excessive hyperventilation can lead to a reduction in cerebral blood flow, arrhythmias, and a decrease in cardiac index[22]

* Level II: Theory-based; no research data to support recommendations; recommendations from expert consensus group may exist
Level VI: Clinical studies in a variety of patient populations and situations to support recommendations

Procedure	for Pulmonary Hypertension: Management—*Continued*	
Steps	**Rationale**	**Considerations**
11. Provide adequate sedation, analgesia, and neuromuscular blockade. *(Level V*)*	Agitation and pain exacerbate pulmonary vasoconstriction.[16,19]	Bolus doses of analgesics or sedatives administered before suctioning and painful procedures can blunt stress response.[11] Implement nonpharmacologic measures to provide comfort/distraction.
12. Administer pulmonary vasodilator therapy per prescribing practitioner's order; use two patient identifiers before medication administration. *(Level VI*)*	Causes pulmonary vasodilation, which results in lower pulmonary vascular resistance and pulmonary pressures that in turn decrease the workload of the right ventricle and increase cardiac output.[3,5-7,9,12,13,25]	Intravenous and oral vasodilators can cause both systemic and pulmonary vasodilation; as a precautionary measure have 0.9% saline available at the bedside before initiation of new medication. Selective pulmonary vasodilators, such as inhaled nitric oxide, do not cause systemic hypotension.
13. Obtain radiographic studies and blood samples for arterial blood gas (ABG), venous blood gas (VBG), complete blood cell count (CBC), and chemistry analysis per prescribing practitioner's order; use two patient identifiers when obtaining and labeling laboratory samples and radiographic studies. *(Level VI*)*	Facilitates identification and treatment of conditions that can exacerbate PHTN; avoids potential toxicity associated with pulmonary vasodilators. Use of two patient identifiers promotes patient safety.	Conditions that can result in pulmonary vasoconstriction and elevated PVR include alveolar hypoxia, microatelectasis, hypercarbia, respiratory and metabolic acidosis, hypothermia, pain, agitation, elevated hematocrit, low cardiac output, and decreased coronary perfusion.[16,19,23]
14. Cluster care when possible. *(Level II*)*	Pulmonary hypertension can be exacerbated by routine care events or during changes in child's management.	A PHTN event or crisis may develop during weaning of: • Mechanical ventilation Sedation/analgesia/ neuromuscular blockade • Vasodilator therapy • Pulmonary hypertension may also be exacerbated by an increase in catecholamine agents[10,13,14,16]
15. Wean mechanical support and all inhaled and intravenous medications slowly, including oxygen.[3,14,16] *(Level VI*)*	Prevents rebound PHTN effect caused by attempt to wean medications, inhaled nitric oxide or ventilatory support too rapidly.[2,6,13,14,21,25]	Inhaled nitric oxide is a selective direct pulmonary vasodilator. Dosing is 1 to 20 ppm. Effects include lower PAP and PVR with stable blood pressure (BP), improved cardiac output and index measurements, and improved arterial saturations and PaO_2.[2,6,10,17,22,23] Monitor methemoglobin every 6 to 12 hours if inhaled nitric oxide is used; must report if level is more than 5%.[22]
16. Communicate response to treatment and procedures to members of health care team.	Facilitates communication among health care providers and assists with developing strategies to optimize tolerance of procedures and avoid exacerbation of PHTN events and crises.	The PHTN symptoms may include an acute elevation in PAP with an initially stable left arterial pressure, (LAP) which then begins to fall and elevated CVP and heart rate, with decreased oxygen saturations and systemic perfusion.[19,20]

* Level II: Theory-based; no research data to support recommendations; recommendations from expert consensus group may exist
Level V: Clinical studies in more than one or two patient populations and situations to support recommendations
Level VI: Clinical studies in a variety of patient populations and situations to support recommendations

Expected Outcomes

- Child has stable hemodynamics with adequate perfusion
- Child has adequate gas exchange and oxygenation
- Child weans successfully from sedation, analgesia, and mechanical ventilation
- Child weans successfully from pulmonary vasodilator therapy
- Nursing interventions show promotion of pulmonary vasodilation
- Child has acceptable level of comfort

Unexpected Outcomes

- Pulmonary hypertensive crisis with systemic hypotension
- Hypoventilation and hypoxia that result in unstable hemodyamics and poor systemic perfusion
- Hypoventilation that results in pulmonary event or crisis
- Rebound effect from rapid wean of therapy
- Alveolar hypoxia and pain/agitation with suctioning
- Unmanaged pain or agitation

Monitoring and Care of the Child

Activities and Interventions	Rationale	Reportable Conditions
1. Monitor hemodynamic parameters and perfusion status on an ongoing basis. *(Level VI*)*	Assists in recognizing PHTN events and facilitates implementation of appropriate treatment. Improved pulmonary vasodilation is indicated by: lower PAP and PVR, improved cardiac output/cardiac index measurement, resolving tachycardia, improved arterial saturations and mixed venous saturations, serum lactate levels less than 2.2, and improved signs of systemic perfusion. Elevation in pulmonary artery pressures and resistance can produce right ventricular (RV) failure, low cardiac output, and sudden systemic hypotension.	• Tachycardia • Lower arterial oxygen saturations or PaO_2 • Elevation in CVP/RAP or pulmonary artery pressure • Worsening perfusion status • Lower venous oxygen saturation (SVO_2) • Acidosis • Rising serum lactate level • Systemic hypotension
2. Monitor respiratory status and arterial blood gases.	Optimal ventilation minimizes occurrence of PHTN events. Child may have failure to tolerate weaning from oxygen, ventilatory support, systemic vasodilators, sedation, chemical paralysis, or narcotics, which can precipitate pulmonary vasoconstriction.	• Elevation of $Paco_2$ • End-tidal (ET) CO_2 >40 • Drop in Pao_2 more than 10 mm Hg from baseline (or < 100 mm Hg) • pH <7.40 • Arterial saturation <90% (or 5% less than baseline)
3. Identify PHTN events and crises.	An acute rise of pulmonary artery pressure to more than 75% of systemic pressure with stable arterial BP. An event turns into a crisis when arterial blood pressure falls.	• Pulmonary hypertension events/crisis symptoms (see Table 71-3)
4. Monitor for potential toxicity to inhaled nitric oxide.	Toxicity with use of inhaled nitric oxide is rare but possible.	• Methemoglobin >5% • Nitrogen dioxide >5 ppm
5. Assess effectiveness of pain management strategy and provide appropriate interventions. Encourage family to assist with nonpharmacologic means to comfort and support the child.	Early identification of inadequate pain or agitation management allows prompt treatment.	• Unresolved pain or agitation • Continued irritability or changes in physiologic condition

* Level VI: Clinical studies in a variety of patient populations and situations to support recommendations

Documentation

- Child and family education
- Child's clinical response to initiation or weaning of oxygen, sedation, vasodilators, and mechanical ventilatory support
- Ongoing clinical assessment
- Results of radiologic and laboratory testing, including ABG, VBG, chemistry, lactate, and CBC
- Child's response to suctioning
- Medications, treatments, and fluids administered
- Comfort assessment and any specific interventions provided
- Unexpected outcomes and related treatment

References

1. Fineman JR, et al: Fetal and postnatal circulations: pulmonary and persistent pulmonary hypertension of the newborn. In Allen HC, et al, editors: *Moss and Adams' heart disease in infants, children and adolescents including the fetus and young adult,* ed 6, vol 1, Baltimore, 2001, Williams & Wilkins.
2. Roberts JD, et al: Inhaled nitric oxide in congenital heart disease, *Circulation* 87(2):447-453, 1993.
3. Barst R: Clinical management of patients with pulmonary hypertension. In Allen HC, Clark EM, et al, editors: *Moss and Adams' heart disease in infants, children and adolescents including the fetus and young adult,* ed 6, vol 2, Baltimore, 2001, Williams & Wilkins.
4. Yamaki S, et al: Inoperable pulmonary vascular disease in infants with congenital heart disease, *Ann Thorac Surg* 66(5):1565-1570, 1998.
5. Christensen DD: Initial experience with bosentan therapy in patients with Eisenmenger's Syndrome, *Pediatr Cardiol Today* 1(4):1-2, 2003.
6. Ivy D: Diagnosis and treatment of severe pediatric pulmonary hypertension, *Cardiol Rev* 9(4):227-237, 2001.
7. Rashid A, Ivy D: Severe paediatric pulmonary hypertension: new management strategies, *Arch Dis Child* 90:92-98, 2005.
8. Coe PF: Managing pulmonary hypertension in heart transplantation: meeting the challenge, *Crit Care Nurs* 20(2):22-28, 2000.
9. Gaine S: Pulmonary hypertension, *JAMA* 284(24):3160-3168, 2000.
10. Rabinovitch M: Pathophysiology of pulmonary hypertension. In Allen HC, et al, editors: *Moss and Adams' heart disease in infants, children and adolescents including the fetus and young adult,* ed 6, vol 2, Baltimore, 2001, Williams & Wilkins.
11. Hickey PR, et al: Blunting of stress responses in the pulmonary circulation of infants by Fentanyl, *Anesthesia Analgesia* 64:1137-1142, 1985.
12. Atz AM, et al: Sildenafil augments the effect of inhaled nitric oxide for postoperative pulmonary hypertensive crises, *J Thorac Cardiovasc Surg* 124(3):628-629, 2002.
13. Atz AM, Wessel DL: Sildenafil ameliorates effects of inhaled nitric oxide withdrawal, *Anesthesiology* 91(1):307-310, 1999.
14. Tulloh R: Management and therapeutic options in pulmonary hypertension. *Expert Review of Cardiovascular Therapy.* 4(3):361-374, 2006
15. Lindberg L, et al: How common is severe pulmonary hypertension after pediatric cardiac surgery? *J Thorac Cardiovasc Surg* 123(6):1155-1163, 2002.
16. Wessel D: Managing low cardiac output syndrome after congenital heart surgery, *Crit Care Med* 29(10):S220-S230, 2001.
17. Gamillscheg A, et al: Inhaled nitric oxide in patients with critical pulmonary perfusion after Fontan-type procedures and bidirectional Glenn anastomosis, *J Thorac Cardiovasc Surg* 113(3):435-442, 1997.
18. Boyer KM: RSV and timing of surgery for congenital heart disease, *Crit Care Med* 27(9):2065-2066, 1999.
19. Hazinski MF: Cardiovascular disorders. In *Manual of pediatric critical care,* St. Louis, 1999, Mosby.
20. Bando K, et al: Pulmonary hypertension after operations for congenital heart disease: analysis of risk factors and management, *J Thorac Cardiovasc Surg* 112(6):1600-1609, 1996.
21. Hopkins RA, et al: Pulmonary hypertensive crisis following surgery for congenital heart defects in young children, *Eur J Cardiothorac Surg* 5:628-634, 1991.
22. Morris K, et al: Comparison of hyperventilation and inhaled nitric oxide for pulmonary hypertension after repair of congenital heart disease, *Crit Care Med* 8(20):2974-2978, 2000.
23. Miller OI, et al: Inhaled nitric oxide and prevention of pulmonary hypertension after congenital heart surgery: a randomized double blind study, *Lancet* 356:1464-1469, 2000.
24. Hoffman GM, et al: Venous saturation and the anaerobic threshold in neonates after the Norwood procedure for hypoplastic left heart syndrome, *Ann Thorac Surg* 70:1515-1521, 2000.
25. Ivy DD, et al: Dipyridamole attenuates rebound pulmonary hypertension after inhaled nitric oxide withdrawal in postoperative congenital heart disease, *J Thorac Cardiovasc Surg* 115(4):875-882, 1998.

Additional Readings

Beke DM, et al: Management of the pediatric postoperative cardiac surgery patient. *Crit Care Nurs Clin North Am,* 17:405-416, 2005.

Chang AC, et al: *Pediatric cardiac intensive care,* Baltimore, 1998, Williams & Wilkins.

Humbert M, et al: Treatment of pulmonary arterial hypertension. *N Engl J Med,* 351:1425-1436, 2004.

Kouchoukos NT, et al: Post-operative care. In Kirklin, Barrett-Boyes, editors: *Cardiac surgery: morphology, diagnostic criteria, natural history, techniques, results, and indications,* ed 3, Salt Lake City, 2003, Churchill Livingstone.

Merle C: Nursing considerations in the neonate with congenital heart disease, *Clin Perinatol* 28(1):223-233, 2001.

O'Brien P, Boisvert JT: Current management of infants and children with single ventricle anatomy, *J Pediatr Nurs* 16(5):338-350, 2001.

Staple Removal

PURPOSE: To remove surgical staples, placed to add support to an incision, when the incision has healed

Michele J. Borisuk

PREREQUISITE KNOWLEDGE

- Anatomy and physiology of the integumentary system
- An understanding of the healing inhibitors in children who have undergone a surgical procedure that necessitates closure of the incision with surgical staples
- Signs and symptoms of infection or impaired incision healing
- Surgical staples are usually removed 7 to 10 days after wound closure.
- The healing process of a surgical wound varies from person to person; therefore, alternating staples may be removed to maintain integrity of the incision until further healing takes place. Once the incision is healed, the remaining staples are removed.
- Complications of staple placement and removal include erythema, drainage, failure of wound closure, infection, and retention of part of a staple under the skin.
- Removal of surgical staples may be uncomfortable.
- An incision has only 5% of its normal tensile strength at the time of suture removal.[1]
- Principles of aseptic technique
- Recognition of the child's developmental and emotional status and routine coping mechanisms during hospitalization

CHILD AND FAMILY ASSESSMENT

- Child's developmental level and ability to interact ➡*Rationale:* These factors influence preparation of the child and interaction.

- Child's and family's understanding of the reasons for and risks and benefits of staple removal ➡*Rationale:* Evaluates the child's and family's understanding of the procedure and provides a gauge for ongoing education.
- Status of the integument and intactness of the surgical incision to establish the ability to maintain an intact incision when the surgical staples are removed ➡*Rationale:* Surgical staples are placed to support the incision until the skin is healed and intact. Variation in the healing process is a possibility, and the removal of all staples at one time may not be indicated. Removal of alternating staples can maintain incision integrity until further healing takes place. Once the incision is healed, the remaining staples are removed.
- Presence of factors that impair healing, such as infection risks, nutritional status, and hygiene issues ➡*Rationale:* The presence of risk factors may impair wound healing; keeping the incision clean and dry can prevent infection.
- Signs or symptoms of incision infection ➡*Rationale:* Infection can break down the integrity of the surgical wound, resulting in failure of the wound to close.
- The child's coping mechanisms ➡*Rationale:* The child's ability to cope with perceived pain and procedures should be assessed; measures to assist the child with coping are then pursued.
- The family's ability and desire to function as a support system for the child during the procedure ➡*Rationale:* Family members are generally an effective support system for the child during incision care and potentially stressful situations. If the family member is not

comfortable with support for the child during the procedure, alternative support staff, such as Child Life Therapy, should be used.

CHILD AND FAMILY EDUCATION

Individualized, developmentally appropriate education is provided to the family and to the child based on desire for knowledge, readiness to learn, and overall neurologic and psychosocial state.

Note: Support services, such as Child Life Specialists, should be used to assist in teaching the child about the procedure when age appropriate.

- Describe the process of surgical staple removal to the family and to the child as appropriate ➤*Rationale:* Providing information to the child and family decreases anxiety and meets the need for information.

- Explain that the removal of the staples may be uncomfortable and that analgesics may be administered if necessary to promote comfort ➤*Rationale:* The child and family understand that pain will be managed; the explanation decreases anxiety and promotes comfort.
- Encourage questions and answer questions as they arise ➤*Rationale:* Reinforcement of information is needed during periods of stress.

EQUIPMENT

- Sterile single-use surgical staple remover
- Povidone-iodine pads
- Sterile gloves
- Alcohol swabs
- Sterile 2×2 or 4×4 gauze pads
- Steri-strips
- Tape

Procedure for Removal of Surgical Staples

Steps	Rationale	Considerations
1. Ensure that child and family understand procedure and that questions are answered.	Evaluates and reinforces understanding of previously taught information.	Developmental level, cognitive ability, and anxiety level determine approach to and effectiveness of teaching.
2. Gather needed supplies and equipment.	Facilitates completion of the procedure in a timely manner.	
3. Consider enlisting an assistant to help with the procedure.	Young or uncooperative children may have difficulty remaining quiet and cooperative during the procedure.	Family members may prefer not to assist with immobilization and it should not be an expectation of the family.
4. Identify child with two patient identifiers per institution specific protocol.	Confirms correct patient and procedure as recommended by the Joint Commission on Accreditation of Healthcare Organizations; prevents unnecessary medical procedures.	Promotes patient safety.
5. Wash hands. *(Level VI*)*	Standard precautions; reduces the transmission of microorganisms.	
6. Provide for appropriate privacy.	Removal of staples may require exposure of the chest.	Privacy is an important consideration for school-aged children and adolescents.
7. Place child in a comfortable position in bed with the surgical incision in full view.	Promotes child's comfort and allows full view examination of the surgical incision.	May need to permit child to reposition during the procedure to minimize fear and anxiety. The child should, however, maintain a position so that the practitioner has a full view of the surgical incision.
8. Remove dressings from the incision if present and assess the integrity of the entire surgical incision.	Ensures complete evaluation of incision integrity to establish that	Every other staple, every third staple, or staples in areas of

Procedure continues on following page

* Level VI: Clinical studies in a variety of patient populations and situations to support recommendations

Procedure for Removal of Surgical Staples—*Continued*

Steps	Rationale	Considerations
	the incision is healed adequately to support the removal of the staples.	delayed healing may need to be left in place to promote complete incision healing.
9. Observe for signs and symptoms of infection (redness, pain, swelling, drainage from the incision, increased skin temperature, or fever). *(Level IV*)*	Ensures that the incision is healed or healing without infection.	
10. Clean entire incision with alcohol with aseptic technique; remove all debris. *(Level II*)*	Allows for thorough examination of the incision and decreases the risk of secondary infection.	
11. With a sterile surgical staple remover, insert the teeth of staple remover between the staple and skin. Squeeze levers of the staple remover together, crimping the staple in the center so the two lateral sides rise. *(Level I*)*	Bends the staple, straightening the staple ends so that it is easily removed from the skin.	Do not lift the remover while squeezing the levers together because this causes tension on the skin.[2] Follow recommendations of the manufacturer of the specific staple remover used.
12. Gently ease the staple out of the skin. Place removed staple in a receptacle to be discarded in an appropriate receptacle.	Removes staple; facilitates inspection of the incision.	Inspect staple to ensure that entire staple has been removed.
13. Assess surgical incision before and after each staple is removed for skin integrity and healing.	Assures integrity of incision.	If incision edges separate, stop staple removal and notify the prescribing practitioner.[2]
14. Repeat the process until all staples are removed; clean the incision a second time with povidone-iodine and allow to air dry.	Removes residue; allows a final inspection of the entire surgical incision.	
15. Apply adhesive strips as needed to assure skin integrity.	Provides support to the incision.	
16. Discard used supplies and equipment in an appropriate receptacle.	Standard precautions; staples should be discarded in a biohazardous waste receptacle.	
17. Remove gloves; wash hands.	Standard precaution; reduces transmission of microorganisms.	

* Level I: Manufacturer's recommendations only
Level II: Theory-based; no research data to support recommendations; recommendations from expert consensus group may exist
Level IV: Limited clinical studies to support recommendations

Expected Outcomes	Unexpected Outcomes
• Incision heals in expected time frame • Incision is free from infection and complications	• Delayed wound healing • Wound infection • Erythema • Drainage from staple sites
• Staples are removed without complications • Incision edges remain well approximated after staple removal • Child has an acceptable level of comfort during and after staple removal	• Portion of staple retained in incision • Separation of incision edges before, during, or after staple removal • Unmanaged pain or anxiety

Monitoring and Care of the Child

Activities and Interventions	Rationale	Reportable Conditions
1. Assess the incision for signs or symptoms of infection before, during, and after staple removal	Infections may compromise the integrity of the incision	• Redness, pain, swelling, drainage from the incision, increased skin temperature, or fever
2. Assess incision edge approximation and stability before, during, and after staple removal	Identifies incision healing status; determines whether all staples should be removed or whether only alternating or every third staple should be removed	• Incision edges are not well approximated • Incision edges separate after staple removal is initiated or completed
3. Assess the need for pain medication before suture removal and encourage the family to assist with nonpharmacologic means to comfort and support the child	The procedure may be uncomfortable; some children may benefit from administration of a mild analgesic before staple removal	• Excessive pain associated with staple removal

Documentation

- Incision assessment, including healing process of the surgical wound
- Signs and symptoms of infection
- Areas of incision reopening
- Number of staples removed
- Number of staples remaining and the date when the incision should be reassessed for removal of remaining staples
- Comfort assessment and any specific interventions provided
- Child and family education
- Unexpected outcomes and related treatment

References
1. Autio L, et al: The four s's of wound management: staples, suturing, steri-strips and sticky stuff, *Holistic Nurs Pract* 16(2):80-88, 2002.
2. Pullen RL Jr: Removing sutures and staples, *Nursing* 33(10):18, 2003.

Additional Reading
Johnson RG, et al: Cutaneous closure after cardiac operations: a controlled, randomized, prospective comparison of intradermal versus staple closures, *Ann Surg* 226(5):606-612, 1997.

AP

Pleural Pigtail Catheter: Insertion

PURPOSE: A pleural pigtail catheter is inserted into the pleural space to drain accumulated fluid or air that compromises the child's cardiorespiratory status

Erika Lynne Speier

PREREQUISITE KNOWLEDGE

- Anatomy and physiology of the cardiopulmonary system
- Ability to identify anatomic landmarks used in insertion of the catheter
- Postulated benefits of the pigtail catheter compared with a conventional "stiff" chest tube, include: decreased trauma with insertion, decreased pain that results in increased mobility of the child, a smaller scar from the small size of the tube, and improved safety[1]
- Complications of pleural pigtail catheter insertion and maintenance: hemothorax, pneumothorax, failure to drain air or effusion, inadvertent cannulation of a vessel, catheter dislodgement, kinking of the catheter, disconnection of the drainage device[1]
- Indications of patency of the catheter and knowledge of the drainage system attached to the catheter
- Pigtail catheters used to drain air or fluids are inserted into the pleural cavity.
- An 8F pigtail catheter is typically used for drainage of pleural effusions or pneumothoraces. Pigtail catheters are available in a variety of sizes, including 5F, 6F, 7F, 8F, and 8.5F.
- After placement, the catheter is sutured in place and covered with a sterile transparent dressing.

AP This procedure should be performed only by physicians, advanced practice nurses, and other health care professionals (including critical care nurses) with additional knowledge, skills, and demonstrated competence per professional licensure or institutional standard.

- Pigtail catheters are not typically intended for drainage of empyemas or suspected viscous fluid because the small diameter of the catheter may become plugged with thick drainage.
- Laboratory studies for diagnosis of the pleural fluid for exudate or transudate should be sent on placement of the pigtail catheter.
- Mastery of pediatric advanced life support competencies
- Appropriate pediatric dosing of analgesics and competency in procedural sedation
- Child development as it relates to clinical assessment and pigtail catheter insertion
- Informed consent is required before placement of a pleural pigtail catheter.

CHILD AND FAMILY ASSESSMENT

- Child's developmental level ➤➤*Rationale:* Child's developmental level influences preparation and interaction.
- Child's (as appropriate) and family's understanding of reasons for placement of the pigtail catheter ➤➤*Rationale:* The family and child should be assessed to determine understanding of the risks versus benefits of catheter placement.
- Child's (as appropriate) and family's understanding of the benefits and risks associated with catheter placement ➤➤*Rationale:* Assesses the family's ability to give informed consent for the procedure.
- History of abnormal anatomy, recent surgical procedures of the chest, and altered coagulation studies ➤➤*Rationale:* The placement technique may need modification.

- Child's cardiorespiratory status →*Rationale:* The sedation and analgesia plan for the procedure may need modification if cardiorespiratory compromise is present.
- Allergies →*Rationale:* Drug allergies may necessitate modification of the sedation and analgesia plan or use of topical anesthetic.
- Desire of family members to be present during the procedure →*Rationale:* Family may provide comfort measures and support during the procedure, but they should have the choice not to remain with the child.

CHILD AND FAMILY EDUCATION

Individualized, developmentally appropriate education is provided to the child and to the family based on desire for knowledge, readiness to learn, and overall neurologic and psychosocial state.

- Provide information to the child (as appropriate) and family regarding the need for placement of the pigtail catheter →*Rationale:* Providing information decreases anxiety and fear.
- Provide information about pleural fluid and causes of accumulation, including the rationale to drain the fluid to improve the child's cardiopulmonary status →*Rationale:* Providing information enables participation in the child's medical management and decreases fear and anxiety.
- Explain the risks related to placement of the pigtail catheter, including unexpected bleeding and inappropriate placement of the catheter that could compromise the child's status, necessitating increased medical therapy and intervention. Relief of large effusion could necessitate volume resuscitation if hemodynamic instability occurs. →*Rationale:* The family is provided with information about and indications for the procedure, facilitating informed consent.
- Explain to the family and child (if appropriate) that medications will be used to keep the child comfortable during the procedure, which include local anesthetics, sedation, or pain medications that include opioids →*Rationale:* Providing information decreases anxiety and fear.
- Explain the need for a chest x-ray once the catheter is inserted because radiographic imaging of the chest determines the appropriate placement of the chest tube and drainage of the air or fluid →*Rationale:* Providing information decreases the family's anxiety about repeated x-rays.
- Explain the need to send the fluid for analysis for determination of fluid consistency because analysis may alter the treatment plan (e.g., if the fluid is high in protein/triglyceride count and is milky in color, a chylothorax is suspected and the child's nutrition should be changed to maximize resolution by changing formula or diet to low-fat/nonfat) →*Rationale:* Providing information decreases anxiety and promotes compliance with the plan of care.
- Encourage questions and answer questions as they arise →*Rationale:* Reinforcement of information is needed during periods of stress.

EQUIPMENT

- Appropriately sized pigtail catheter set (7F to 8.5F Fuhrman Pigtail Catheter, Cook Critical Care, Bloomington, IN) set is frequently used) that contains:
  - ❖ Needle
  - ❖ Dilator
  - ❖ Pigtail catheter
  - ❖ Introducer wire
  - ❖ Stopcock
  - ❖ Chest tube attachment
- Chlorhexidine or povidone-iodine antiseptic solution
- Sterile towels or sterile sheet
- A 10-mL syringe
- Three 4×4 gauze dressings
- 1% Lidocaine
- Small-gauge needle and appropriately sized syringe for lidocaine administration
- Transparent sterile dressing
- 3-0 silk suture with needle
- Sterile scissors
- Sterile needle driver
- Sterile gloves and sterile gown, cap, and mask
- Chest drainage system
- Wall suction and suction tubing

Procedure	**for Pleural Pigtail Catheter: Insertion**	
Steps	**Rationale**	**Considerations**
1. Ensure family and child (if appropriate) understand procedure and questions are answered.	Evaluates and reinforces understanding of previously taught information.	Developmental level, cognitive ability, and anxiety level determine approach to and effectiveness of teaching.
2. Obtain informed consent.	Ensures medical-legal compliance as suggested by the Joint Commission on Accreditation of Healthcare Organizations (JCAHO).	For emergency situations, the organization may have a protocol in place for assumption of consent.

Procedure continues on following page

AP This procedure should be performed only by physicians, advanced practice nurses, and other health care professionals (including critical care nurses) with additional knowledge, skills, and demonstrated competence per professional licensure or institutional standard.

Procedure for Pleural Pigtail Catheter: Insertion—*Continued*

Steps	Rationale	Considerations
3. Ensure that electrocardiographic (ECG) monitoring is in place and that child has functioning venous access.	Continuous ECG monitoring allows monitoring of child's status. Functioning venous access is necessary for administration of emergency medications or sedation and analgesia as needed.	Consider child's underlying diagnosis before selection of appropriate sedative and analgesic.
4. Assemble equipment.	Having all materials present facilitates completion of procedure in a timely manner.	
5. Ensure that appropriate sedatives and analgesics have been administered before beginning procedure. *(Level IV*)*	Sedatives and analgesics facilitate completion of procedure, decrease pain during insertion of catheter, and minimize the risk of inappropriate placement or complications.	Medication and dose is dependant on child's weight, current level of sedation, and cardiovascular status.
6. Position child supine, with the head of bed slightly elevated. Raise arm above the head to improve access to the insertion site. *(Level II*)*	Allows the best visualization of insertion site, facilitates catheter insertion, and maintains appropriate position.	This may be achieved with an assistant holding child or with soft restraints.
7. Identify child with appropriate patient and procedure verification process (e.g., "Time out")	Confirms correct patient, procedure, and site as recommended by the JCAHO; prevents unnecessary medical procedures.	The verification process and documentation are institution-specific. Use active communication techniques.
8. After hand washing, put on cap, mask, eyewear, sterile gown, and sterile gloves. *(Level II*)*	Decreases the risk of infection.	The hat, mask, and eyewear should be put on before the sterile gown and sterile gloves.
9. Establish a sterile field.	Allows manipulation of sterile equipment and supplies without contamination; decreases the risk of infection.	
10. Scrub area with chlorhexidine or povidone-iodine solution.	Minimizes risk of infection.	Chlorhexidine is not recommended for use in children under 2 months of age. Follow institution-specific protocol for preparation of insertion site.
11. Administer 1% lidocaine with a small-bore needle in the skin, periosteum of the rib, and parietal pleura.	Local anesthetic; decreases pain.	
12. When local anesthesia has been achieved, insert the needle and advance over the superior surface of the rib, aspirating to confirm pleural fluid or air[1,2] (Figure 73-1).	Identifies desired location for catheter placement.	For pneumothorax, insert the catheter along the midclavicular line or more laterally between the third to fifth intercostal space. For fluid, insert the catheter between the fifth to seventh intercostal space at the midaxillary line.[3]

* Level II: Theory-based; no research data to support recommendations; recommendations from expert consensus group may exist
   Level IV: Limited clinical studies to support recommendations

Procedure **for Pleural Pigtail Catheter: Insertion**—*Continued*

Steps	Rationale	Considerations

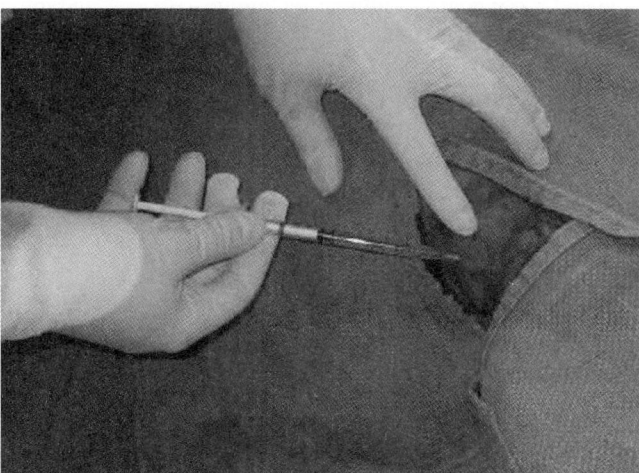

FIGURE 73-1   Small needle with attached syringe is advanced into pleural space.

Steps	Rationale	Considerations
13. Once fluid or air has been confirmed, remove needle.	Ensures that location selected is appropriate to drain the fluid or air collection.	If no fluid or air is retrieved, ultrasound scan or repeat chest film may be necessary for better localization of the pneumothorax or pleural effusion.
14. Using needle supplied in the pigtail catheter set, attach a 10-mL syringe to the needle and reintroduce this needle in the already anesthetized skin. Advance over superior surface of the rib, aspirating until fluid or air is retrieved[1,2] (Figure 73-2).		

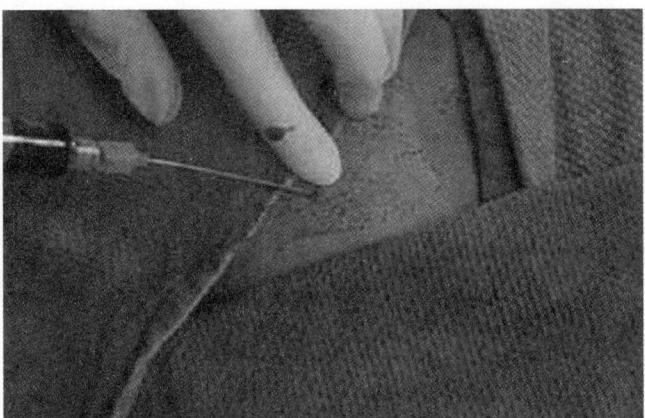

FIGURE 73-2   Needle from pigtail catheter set is introduced into pleural space, with aspiration of fluid.

Procedure continues on following page

Procedure	**for Pleural Pigtail Catheter: Insertion**—*Continued*	
Steps	**Rationale**	**Considerations**
15. Detach syringe from the needle and introduce the wire through needle hub (Seldinger technique). Once wire is advanced past the tip of the needle and is secure, remove needle over the wire, leaving the wire in place[1,2] (Figure 73-3).	Standard Seldinger technique; allows the dilator to be advanced over the wire.	Stabilize tip of the needle to prevent further advancement of the needle into the chest cavity.

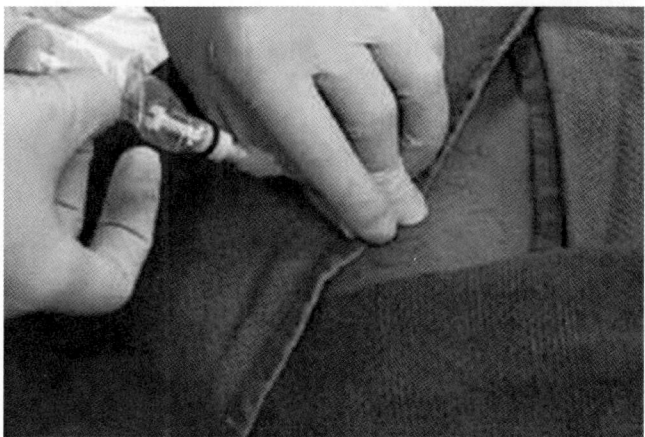

FIGURE 73-3   Guide wire is advanced through needle hub.

16. Holding wire in place, introduce the dilator over wire and dilate the skin and subcutaneous tissue (Figure 73-4). *(Level II*)*	Standard technique; the dilator opens a tract that facilitates insertion of pigtail catheter.	

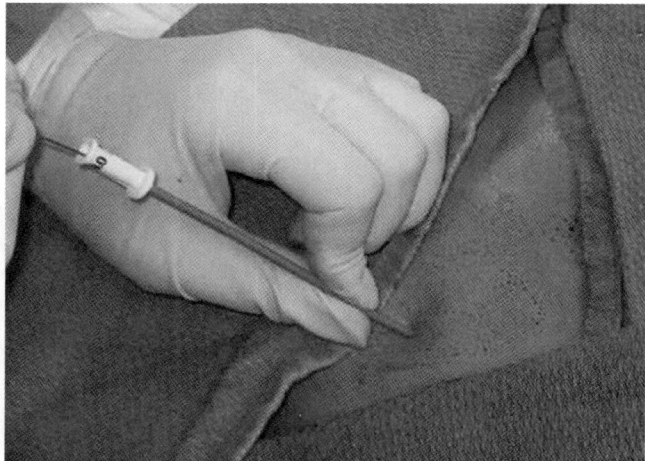

FIGURE 73-4   Dilator is placed over guide wire.

17. Remove dilator, keeping the wire in place. Introduce the pigtail catheter over the wire and insert catheter into chest wall cavity; observe for drainage of fluid or air (Figure 73-5).	Appropriate placement of the chest tube allows fluid or air to be drained and promotes improvement of cardiorespiratory status.	

* Level II: Theory-based; no research data to support recommendations; recommendations from expert consensus group may exist

Procedure for **Pleural Pigtail Catheter: Insertion**—*Continued*

Steps	Rationale	Considerations

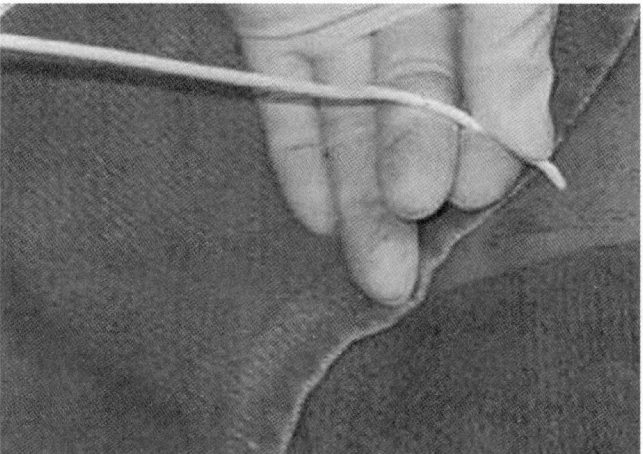

FIGURE 73-5 Pigtail catheter is placed over guide wire.

18. Attach pigtail catheter to a closed sterile drainage system at 15 to 20 cm of wall suction. *(Level II*)* — Attachment to a closed drainage system maintains sterility of the procedure and ongoing monitoring of fluid or air drainage. — Use of any closed drainage system is appropriate. *(Level I*)*

19. Suture catheter in place with 3-0 silk suture (Figure 73-6). — Allows for secure placement without dislodgement. — The size of suture is dependant on weight and age of child.

20. Apply a transparent dressing over chest tube. — Prevents dislodgement and minimizes the risk of contamination at insertion site. Allows visualization of insertion site.

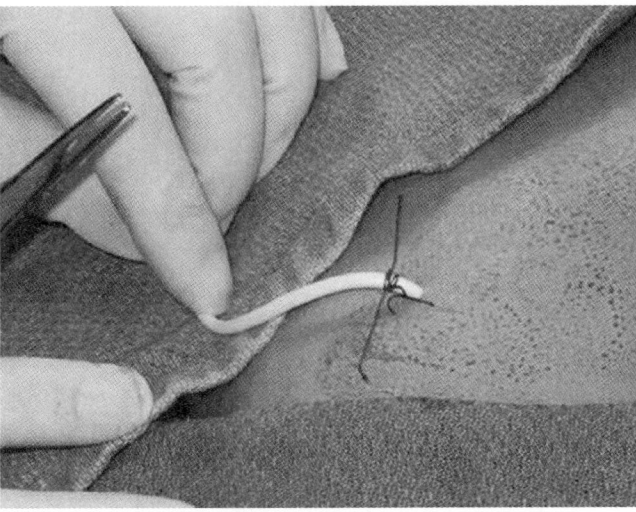

FIGURE 73-6 Catheter is sutured in place.

Procedure continues on following page

* Level I: Manufacturer's recommendations only
  Level II: Theory-based; no research data to support recommendations; recommendations from expert consensus group may exist

AP This procedure should be performed only by physicians, advanced practice nurses, and other health care professionals (including critical care nurses) with additional knowledge, skills, and demonstrated competence per professional licensure or institutional standard.

Procedure	**for Pleural Pigtail Catheter: Insertion**—*Continued*	
Steps	**Rationale**	**Considerations**
21. Discard used supplies and equipment in appropriate receptacles. Ensure that sharps are properly disposed of. Remove gloves. Wash hands.	Standard precautions; reduces the transmission of microorganisms. Promotes staff and patient safety.	
22. Obtain a chest x-ray.	Confirms appropriate placement of catheter.	
23. Send pleural fluid for studies to confirm diagnosis. *(Level VI*)*	Treatment depends on type of fluid drained.	Obtain appropriate sterile tubes to send fluid to the chemistry/microbiology laboratory before starting the procedure.
24. Document procedure in medical record.	Allows retrieval of pertinent information.	

* Level VI: Clinical studies in a variety of patient populations and situations to support recommendations

Expected Outcomes	**Unexpected Outcomes**
• Appropriate placement of pleural pigtail catheter	• Inappropriate placement of the catheter • Inadvertent placement of the pigtail catheter into the abdominal cavity or layers of the diaphragm • Injury to the lung or heart with incorrect placement
• Removal of air or fluid from pleural cavity • Improved cardiorespiratory status	• Fluid or air is unable to be drained • Cardiorespiratory compromise with worsening of status or decreased breath sounds on the side of the chest tube • Pneumothorax or hemothorax
• Child tolerates the procedure with minimal pain and anxiety	• Unmanaged pain or anxiety

Monitoring and Care of the Child

Activities and Interventions	**Rationale**	**Reportable Conditions**
1. Monitor intactness and patency of catheter and drainage system.	A dislodged catheter may result in cardiorespiratory compromise and the need for reinsertion of the chest tube.	• Catheter dislodgement • Failure of the catheter to drain
2. Monitor child's hemodynamic status.	Increased tachypnea, tachycardia, or blood pressure (BP) instability may be a result of inappropriate catheter placement, poor pain control, or hemodynamic fluctuations with removal of large volumes of fluid or air.	• Cardiorespiratory compromise
3. Monitor child's cardiopulmonary examination.	Complications affect the quality and equality of breath sounds and heart tones.	• Absent or decreased breath sounds • Presence of pericardial rub

---

Documentation

- Informed consent
- Patient and side or site verification process
- X-ray findings and the child's hemodynamic status before the procedure
- Hemodynamic status after catheter placement
- Procedure details, including the size of pigtail catheter placed, the name of the individual who placed the catheter, and laboratory studies sent
- Volume of fluid or air removed and consistency and color
- Child's tolerance of the procedure
- X-ray findings after the procedure
- Sedation and analgesia provided
- Unexpected outcomes and related treatment

References

1. Roberts JS, et al: Efficacy and complications of percutaneous pigtail catheters for thoracostomy in pediatric patients, *Chest* 114:1116-1121, 1998.
2. Fuhrman BP, Zimmerman JJ, editors: *Pediatric critical care,* ed 2, St. Louis, 1998, Mosby.
3. Curley MAQ, Moloney-Harmon P, editors: *Critical care nursing of infants and children,* ed 2, Philadelphia, 2001, Saunders.

Additional Readings

Furhman BP, et al: Pleural drainage using modified pigtail catheters, *Crit Care Med* 14:575-576, 1986.

LeDoux D: Cardiac surgery. In Woods SL, et al, editors: *Cardiac nursing,* ed 3, Philadelphia, 1995, Lippincott.

Leonard S, Nikaidoh H: Thoracentesis and chest tube insertion. In Levin D, Morriss F, editors: *Essentials of pediatric intensive care,* St Louis, 1990, Quality Medical Publishing.

Robinson CF: Thoracic cavity management. In Boggs RL, Wooldridge-King M, editors: *AACN procedure manual for critical care,* ed 3, Philadelphia, 1993, Saunders.

Siefert PC: *Cardiac surgery,* St Louis, 1994, Mosby–Year Book Inc.

PROCEDURE **74**

Cerebral Tissue Oxygenation Monitoring: Insertion Assist, Monitoring, and Care

P U R P O S E : Continuous monitoring of brain tissue oxygenation (PbtO$_2$) allows the practitioner to identify cerebral hypoxia and target interventions to prevent cerebral ischemia and secondary head injury

Wallis Halperin Wallis

PREREQUISITE KNOWLEDGE

- Pediatric neuroanatomy and physiology
- Principles of aseptic technique
- The net balance of cerebral oxygen supply and the body's metabolic demand is reflected in brain tissue oxygenation (PbtO$_2$).
- The cranium is an enclosed box that consists of three components: brain, cerebral spinal fluid (CSF), and blood.
  - ❖ Normally, when a rise in one of these components occurs, the brain compensates with autoregulation, shunting of CSF, and compliance to maintain the balance of the brain, blood, and CSF.
  - ❖ Loss of autoregulation results in increased intracranial pressure (ICP), which causes a decrease in cerebral blood flow and results in decreased cerebral tissue oxygenation.
- Traditionally, cerebral monitoring of children with acute intracranial disorders has consisted of monitoring cerebral perfusion pressure (CPP): mean arterial pressure (MAP) minus ICP.
  - ❖ When the CPP was kept at an age-appropriate value (Table 74-1), the brain was thought to be adequately perfused and oxygenated. Multiple studies[1-6] have shown that ICP and CPP monitoring alone do not accurately reflect tissue oxygenation in the injured

brain. Monitoring of PbtO$_2$ along with ICP allows the CPP to be individualized and optimized for each child.
- Currently, two cerebral, or brain, tissue oxygenation monitors are on the market. The monitor primarily used in the pediatric critical care arena is LICOX (Integra NeuroSciences/GMS, Plainsboro, NJ; Figures 74-1 and 74-2). This procedure refers to the LICOX brain tissue

TABLE 74-1	Age-Specific Optimal Cerebral Perfusion Pressures (mm Hg)		
Age (yr)	**Goal CPP***	**Normal BP range**	**Normal MAP**
0-1	40-50	75/40–105/66	52–80
2-4	50-60	87/53–105/66	64–80
5-8	60	97/57–112/71	70–85
8-17	70	112/80–128/80	90–96

* Note: Individual patient's optimal CPP must be determined with goal CPP, PbtO$_2$ more than 20 mm Hg and ICP less than 15 mm Hg. For example, 75-year-old with CPP of 45, PbtO$_2$ of 25, and ICP of 25 does not have an adequate level and CPP may need to be increased. Alternatively, 9-year-old with CPP of 55, PbtO$_2$ of 25, and ICP of 12 may have CPP measurement and no further increase in CPP needs to take place.

BP, Blood pressure.

Reproduced with permission from Children's Hospital of Orange County at Mission, Mission Hospital. Care of the traumatic brain injured patient less than 30 kg procedure, *CHOC at Mission procedure manual,* Mission Viejo, CA, 2004, Children's Hospital of Orange County at Mission.

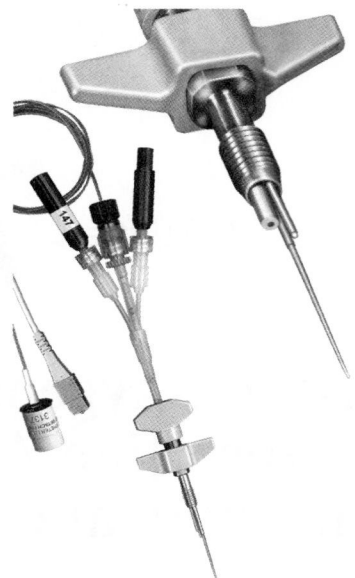

FIGURE 74-1   LICOX Bolt with Comboprobe. Copyright ©
2006 by *Integra LifeSciences Corporation. Compliments of Integra
LifeSciences.*

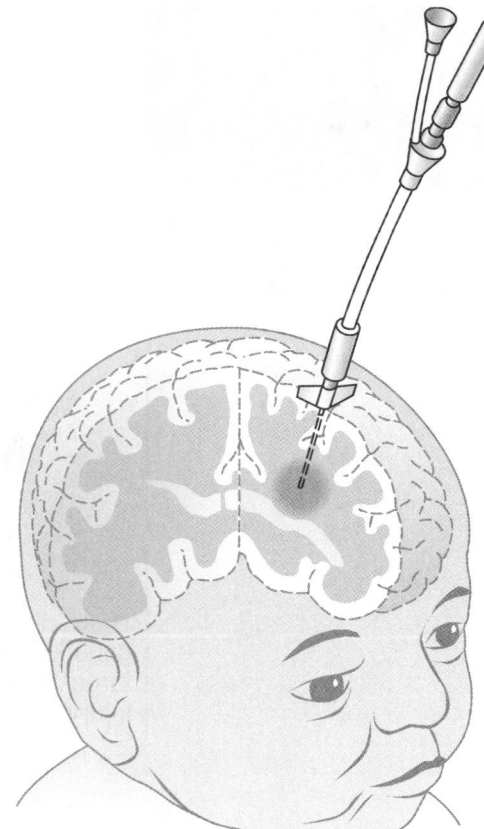

FIGURE 74-3   LICOX catheter placement. Copyright © 2006
by *Integra LifeSciences Corporation. Compliments of Integra
LifeSciences.*

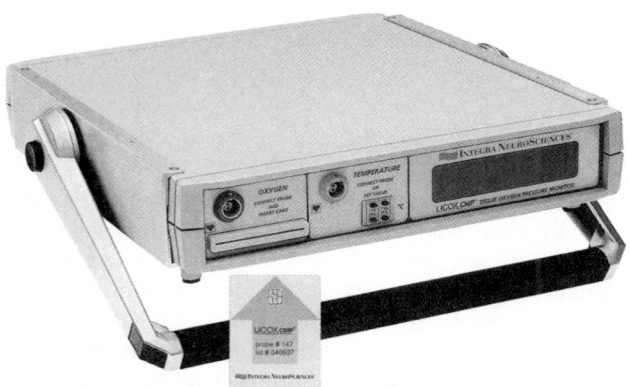

FIGURE 74-2   LICOX monitor system with smart card.
Copyright © 2006 by *Integra LifeSciences Corporation.
Compliments of Integra LifeSciences.*

oxygenation monitor. The Paratrend system (Diametrics
Medical, Roseville, MN) is another brain tissue
monitor less frequently used in pediatrics due to it's
limited area of oxygen sensing which produces a
greater variability of $PbtO_2$ measurements in comparison to the LICOX system which has a larger oxygen
sensing area.[7]

- The LICOX brain oxygenation and temperature probe is
a catheter that measures oxygen partial pressure (mm Hg)
in the interstitial space in the brain tissue. The LICOX
system has been used since the 1980s to monitor tissue
oxygenation. A minimally invasive catheter microprobe
is implanted directly into the white matter of the brain to
a predetermined depth and is connected to the LICOX

monitor by an electrical cable (Figure 74-3). The system
is calibrated with a "smart card" that is inserted into the
LICOX monitor before use.
- Debate exists on optimal placement site of the catheter,
with pros and cons identified for both areas.[1-2,4-6,8-10]
  ❖ Placement of the probe in the penumbra of an injury
  allows for more detailed information on cerebral oxygenation in the area of the brain that is at most risk
  (Figure 74-4).
  ❖ Placement of the probe in a relatively healthy part of
  the brain reflects global cerebral oxygenation (Figure
  74-5).
- The practitioner placing the probe will determine the
optimal intraparenchymal placement after review of the
brain computerized tomography (CT) scan.[11]
- The position of the catheter should be assessed by CT
scan after placement.[7]
- Indications for $PbtO_2$ monitoring are:
  ❖ Children with increased ICP
  ❖ Potential compromise in cerebral perfusion
  ❖ Conditions that lead to cerebral ischemia
- Contraindication to LICOX catheter placement: consid-
erable coagulopathy and an insertion site infection.
- Risks of LICOX catheter placement are development of a
small hematoma and infection.[1-6] Multiple studies found

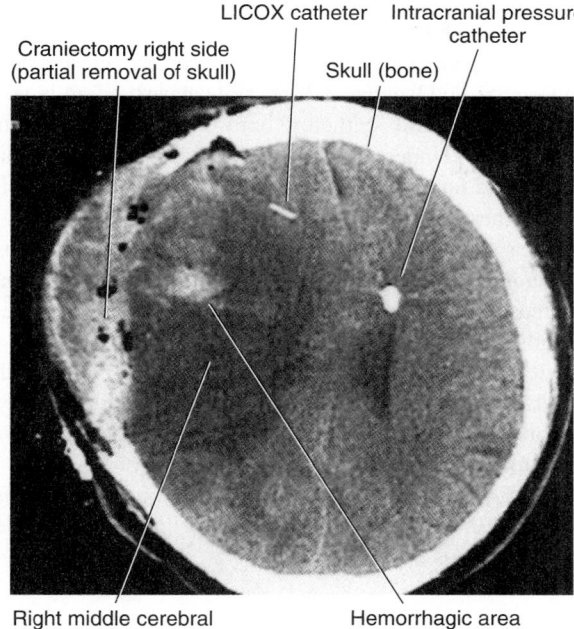

FIGURE 74-4   Computed tomographic scan shows placement of LICOX catheter in penumbral area of infarct in brain. Note small white LICOX catheter in right side of brain. Placement of LICOX probe in right hemisphere near injury allows detection of regional oxygen status. *From Littlejohns LR, Bader MK, March K: Brain tissue oxygen monitoring in severe brain injury, 1: research and usefulness in critical care, Crit Care Nurs 23(4):20, 2003.*

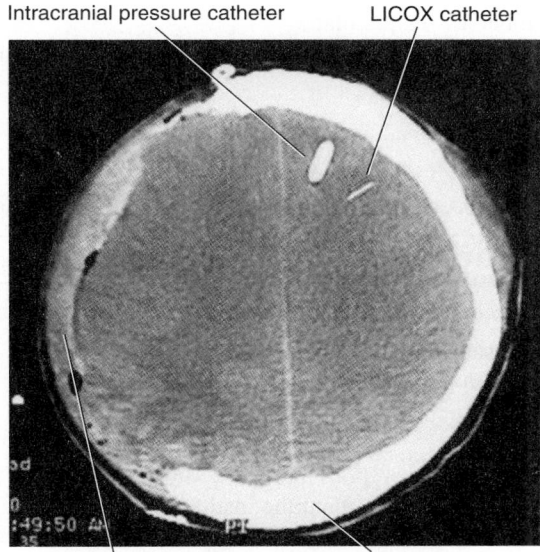

FIGURE 74-5   Contrast-enhanced computed tomographic scan shows placement of LICOX catheter in cerebral hemisphere contralateral to injury. Placement in left hemisphere allows detection of global oxygen status. *From Littlejohns LR, Bader MK, March K: Brain tissue oxygen monitoring in severe brain injury, 1: research and usefulness in critical care, Crit Care Nurs 23(4):20, 2003.*

TABLE 74-2	**Factors that Affect Brain Tissue Oxygenation**
Increases $PbtO_2$	**Decreases $PbtO_2$**
100% FIo_2	Arterial hypoxia
Hypercapnia	Hypocapnia
Optimization of CPP by increasing MAP with fluids and vasopressors if needed	Hypotension
Lowering of ICP with setting head of bed at 30 degrees, drainage of CSF, normothermia, sedation, and mannitol	Increased ICP
Increased O_2 content with transfusion of packed red blood cells (PRBC)	Anemia
Decrease in metabolic demands with maintenance of normothermia and treatment of pain and anxiety	Increased metabolic demands, such as fever, pain, and anxiety

CPP = Cerebral perfusion pressure; MA = mean arterial pressure; ICP = intracranial pressure.

no infection and no sequelae from the small hematomas, if they occurred.[1,2,5,6,12] *(Level IV*)*

- Many factors affect $PbtO_2$, such as oxygen, carbon dioxide, and temperature (Table 74-2).
- Numeric values with the LICOX system[2,6,8]:
  - ❖ With placement in noninjured tissue, normal values of $PbtO_2$ are between 20 and 35 mm Hg.
  - ❖ Treatment goal is usually a $PbtO_2$ of 20 mm Hg or higher.
  - ❖ Intervention with targeted therapies is indicated when the $PbtO_2$ is less than 15 mm Hg.
  - ❖ Episodes of $PbtO_2$ of less than 10 mm Hg for more than 30 minutes were associated with a poor neurological outcome.[10]
  - ❖ A consensus exists that low $PbtO_2$ (less than 15 mm Hg for longer than 30 minutes or less than 10 mm Hg for 10 minutes) is predictive of a high risk of death.[10]
- Child development as it relates to neurologic assessment and $PbtO_2$ monitoring
- Mastery of pediatric advanced life support competencies
- Appropriate pediatric dosing of analgesics and sedatives
- Informed consent is required before placement of a LICOX catheter

CHILD AND FAMILY ASSESSMENT

- Child's complete neurologic status ➙*Rationale:* Baseline neurologic data facilitate recognition of changes that may occur as a result of oxygenation probe insertion.
- Child's medical history, including history of present illness and known allergies ➙*Rationale:* Promotes understanding of cause of, or potential for, alterations in $PbtO_2$; prevents exposure of the child to medications known to cause an allergic reaction.

* Level IV: Limited clinical studies to support recommendations

- Current laboratory profile, including complete blood count (CBC), platelet count, prothrombin time (PT), partial thromboplastin time (PTT), bleeding time, and international normalized ratio (INR) ➤*Rationale:* Baseline coagulation studies are necessary to determine bleeding risk during probe insertion. A platelet count of less than 50,000 is a contraindication to the procedure.
- Child's (as appropriate) and family's understanding of the reasons for and risks and benefits of the procedure ➤*Rationale:* Evaluates child's and family's understanding of previously taught information and provides a gauge for ongoing education.
- Child's developmental level and ability to interact ➤*Rationale:* These factors influence preparation of the child and interaction and selection of an appropriate pain scale (see Procedure 173 for further information).
- Previous pain and sedation experiences of child and family and the child's and family's identification of pain and anxiety management strategies that have been helpful in the past ➤*Rationale:* Identifies pain management strategies likely to be successful or previous difficulties with sedation.

CHILD AND FAMILY EDUCATION

Individualized, developmentally appropriate education is provided to the family and to the child based on desire for knowledge, readiness to learn, and overall neurologic and psychosocial state.

- Provide the child (as appropriate) and family with information about the brain tissue oxygenation monitor, the purpose of brain tissue oxygenation monitoring and that a CT scan of brain will be done following placement to ensure proper placement of the probe ➤*Rationale:* Providing information may reduce family's and child's anxiety and fear and provide the child and family with an opportunity to ask questions.
- Provide explanation of insertion, monitoring, alarm system, and care of $PbtO_2$ catheter. If possible, have the family view the monitor and catheter before insertion and use ➤*Rationale:* Understanding is improved and may allay child's and family's anxiety and enhance cooperation with further therapies.
- Discuss expected outcomes of the $PbtO_2$ catheter use ➤*Rationale:* Child's and family's stress and anxiety may decrease if they are aware of goals, duration, and expectations of $PbtO_2$ catheter use.
- Review the pain and anxiety management plan for the child ➤*Rationale:* Providing information decreases anxiety and fear and reassures the child and family that pain and anxiety will be managed appropriately.
- Encourage questions and answer questions as they arise ➤*Rationale:* Reinforcement of information is needed during periods of stress.

EQUIPMENT

- LICOX CMP monitor and connecting cables
- Interface box to bedside monitor
- Clean and sterile gloves
- Gowns, hats, masks, and eye protection as indicated for bolt placement
- Cranial access kit
- Intracranial bolt system with introducer kit
- PMO LICOX or $PbtO_2$ probe of choice
- Clippers or razor
- Antiseptic solution
- Number 11 scalpel blade
- Sterile occlusive dressing of choice, preferably transparent.

Procedure for Cerebral Tissue Oxygenation Monitoring

Steps	Rationale	Considerations
1. Ensure child and family understand procedure and questions are answered.	Evaluates and reinforces understanding of previously taught information.	Developmental level, cognitive ability, and anxiety level determine approach to and effectiveness of teaching.
2. Confirm presence of informed consent.	Ensures medical-legal compliance as suggested by the Joint Commission of Accreditation of Healthcare Organizations (JCAHO).	For emergency situations, implement the institution-specific protocol for assumption of consent.
3. Gather needed equipment and supplies.	Facilitates completion of task in a timely manner.	
4. Wash hands.	Standard precautions; reduces transmission of microorganisms.	

Procedure for Cerebral Tissue Oxygenation Monitoring—*Continued*		
Steps	**Rationale**	**Considerations**

5. Assemble necessary equipment for procedure.
    Check LICOX CMP monitor to assure all cables are connected.
    Switch CMP monitor *off* before connecting or disconnecting the LICOX bus connector or power supply connector.
    Connect the low voltage output cable of the LICOX power supply to socket provided at the rear of the LICOX CMP.
    Connect the blue PbtO$_2$ probe cable to the appropriate blue port of the front of the LICOX monitor.
    Connect the green temperature cable to the LICOX CMP if a brain temperature probe will be placed by the neurosurgeon.
    Connect blue/green cables to the combined Y-cable with oxygen and temperature combo PMO probe.
    Connect the ground connector at the rear of the instrument to the ground system if needed. *(Level I*)*
	Assembling and checking all equipment before procedure prevents delays in procedure and monitoring as a result of equipment failure or missing equipment.	If the neurosurgeon does not place the brain temperature probe, then the brain temperature must be manually dialed in for accurate readings of PbtO$_2$.[9]

6. Gather bolt introducer kit, bolt kit, PbtO$_2$ probe, ICP bolt, and sterile supplies. Obtain drill bit.[9]	Monitoring probes are placed through introducer.	
7. Assess child's pain with appropriate pain scale; administer preprocedural analgesia and sedation as indicated and per prescribing practitioner's order. *(Level II*)*	Treatment of pain and anxiety is a vital part of providing optimal care. Pain management is an important component in the management and prevention of increased ICP.	Identify child with two patient identifiers per institution-specific protocol before medication administration.
8. Identify child with appropriate patient/procedure verification process (e.g., "Time out").	Confirms correct patient, procedure, and site as recommended by JCAHO; prevents unnecessary medical procedures.	Verification process and documentation is institution specific. Use active communication techniques.
9. Put on personal protective equipment as indicated for procedure.	Standard precautions; reduces transmission of microorganisms.	
10. Assist neurosurgeon with preparing the area and with procedure as indicated.	Neurosurgeon places bolt introducer, PbtO$_2$ probe, temperature probe, and tissue ICP probe. Aseptic technique is necessary.	The neurosurgeon prepares the area as follows: shave, prepare with povidone-iodine, infiltrate skin with lidocaine, drape area.
11. Remove the PbtO$_2$ probe protector and packaging from probe. Save the "smart" card from package insert. *(Level I*)*	Prepares probe for insertion. "Smart" card is needed for the LICOX monitor to function.	Check that the serial numbers match on the PbtO$_2$ probe and the "smart" card to ensure accurate calibration.
For Dual Lumen with PMO Combo Probe 12. Do not disconnect the extension.	Extension serves to connect the probe and introducer.	

Procedure continues on following page

---

* Level I: Manufacturer's recommendations only
  Level II: Theory-based; no research data to support recommendations; recommendations from expert consensus group may exist

Procedure	for Cerebral Tissue Oxygenation Monitoring—*Continued*	
Steps	**Rationale**	**Considerations**
13. Insert the probe into the introducer and advance it as far as possible.	Sets probe to correct depth.	
14. Rotate the threaded cap of the catheter's male Luer-type connector onto the female Luer-type connector of the introducer.	Secures catheter to introducer.	
15. Hold the extension tube of the catheter by the Luer-type catheter when securing Luer-type fittings. *(Level I*)*	Prevents rotation of catheter.	
For Original Licox Probe		
16. Insert the $PbtO_2$ probe into introducer as far as possible in one of the two smaller channels on the three-way introducer. *(Level I*)*	Placing probe to predetermined depth places the probe in the white matter. Probe is used for $PbtO_2$ monitoring.	
17. Insert the temperature probe as far as possible in the opposite of the two smaller channels on the three-way introducer. *(Level I*)*	Placing probe to predetermined depth places the probe in the white matter. Probe is used for brain temperature monitoring.	Brain temperature was found to be one to two degrees higher than rectal and bladder temperatures in most studies.[4,8]
18. Place ICP sensor into ICP port if parenchymal ICP is to be monitored. If ICP monitoring is already in place via ventriculostomy, cap off the ICP port on the three-way introducer. *(Level I*)*	Required for ICP monitoring via LICOX system. Capping unused port maintains a closed system.	
19. Tighten compression seal to secure $PbtO_2$, temperature, and ICP sensors. *(Level I*)*	Tightening the compression seal once all probes are in place adds stability and security.	
20. Ensure power cord is connected in the rear of the monitor. *(Level I*)*	LICOX does not have a battery source.	
21. Ensure blue oxygen and green temperature cables are connected on the front panel. *(Level I*)*	Necessary to establish brain tissue and brain oxygenation monitoring.	
22. Turn on monitor. *(Level I*)*	Powers up device.	On/off switch is on the back of machine.
23. Insert the "smart" card from the $PbtO_2$ probe introducer package into the slot on the front panel until it snaps into position. *(Level I*)*	Probe calibration data are stored in the "smart" card; monitor does not function without the smart card.	The metallic contact pads on the card face downward. The arrow on the card shows the direction of insertion.
24. Connect oxygen probe to the blue LICOX cable. *(Level I*)*	Necessary to establish brain tissue oxygen monitoring.	
25. Connect temperature probe to the green LICOX cable. In the event a temperature probe is not placed in the parenchyma, the brain temperature must be manually entered on the front panel of the monitor. *(Level I*)*	Necessary to establish brain tissue temperature monitoring. The temperature coefficient is needed to calculate $PbtO_2$ values.	

* Level I: Manufacturer's recommendations only

Procedure	for Cerebral Tissue Oxygenation Monitoring—*Continued*	
Steps	**Rationale**	**Considerations**
26. Wait approximately 10 to 120 minutes to begin recording PbtO$_2$ values. *(Level I*)*	Equilibration of tissue may take up to 120 minutes after insertion.	Normal range of white matter PbtO$_2$ is 20 to 30 mm Hg. *(Level IV*)*
To Connect LICOX Monitor to Bedside Monitor		
27. Gently disconnect patient oxygen and temperature probes from blue and green cables. Connect LICOX monitor to ICU bedside monitor. Insert "smart" card into LICOX monitor. Wait 1 minute for reading on LICOX to stabilize, then press "zero" on the bedside monitor. Both monitors should now display 0 mm Hg. Reconnect oxygen and temperature probes to blue and green cables. Both monitors should now display the same value. *(Level I*)*	Allows LICOX readings to be displayed on the bedside monitor. Gentle removal of cables from probes helps to prevent dislodgement of probes.	In the event the child must be transported, disconnect the LICOX probes at the patient end. Do not twist or torque the probes. Gently pull the blue and green connectors straight out, disconnecting from the actual probes. Refer to bedside monitor guidelines for specific information.
28. Discard used supplies and equipment, including sharps, in appropriate receptacles; wash hands.	Standard precautions; reduces transmission of microorganisms. Protects personnel health.	
29. Do not discard the fluid-filled protection tube of the brain oxygenation probe. Follow manufacturer's instructions if an after-measurement check is to be completed. *(Level I*)*	Necessary if the tissue probe is to be tested later for function of the probe.	This test is performed after the probe is removed from the brain.
30. When monitoring is completed, catheter is removed by the neurosurgeon. Oxygen and temperature probes should be removed first, followed by the introducer. After the introducer is removed, the bolt can be removed from the skull.[9] *(Level I*)*	Ensures correct device removal.	
31. Refer to operations manual for troubleshooting guidelines. *(Level I*)*	Troubleshooting guidelines facilitate management of monitor-related problems.	

Adapted with permission from Children's Hospital of Orange County at Mission, Mission Hospital. LICOX procedure: *CHOC at Mission procedure manual*, Mission Viejo, CA, 2004, Children's Hospital of Orange County at Mission.
* Level I: Manufacturer's recommendations only
  Level IV: Limited clinical studies to support recommendations

Expected Outcomes

- Reliable and accurate brain tissue oxygenation and temperature values are obtained
- Preservation and maximization of balance between cerebral perfusion, cerebral oxygenation, and cerebral metabolic demand with stabilization of ICP
- Early detection of compromised cerebral perfusion and impaired cerebral oxygenation
- Precise prompt management of impaired cerebral perfusion or compromised cerebral oxygenation
- Catheter is inserted without complications
- Catheter insertion site is free from infection
- Child has acceptable level of comfort

Unexpected Outcomes

- Values obtained appear unreliable
- Inability to obtain readings
- Inability to preserve balance between cerebral perfusion, oxygenation, and metabolic demand
- The ICP continues to increase
- Deteriorations in cerebral perfusion and cerebral oxygenation are not identified
- Delay in management of impaired cerebral perfusion or oxygenation
- Hemorrhage in the area of implantation (rare)
- Infection at catheter insertion site
- Unmanaged pain

Monitoring and Care of the Child

Activities and Interventions	Rationale	Reportable Conditions
1. Initial monitoring and management of child should include: 　• Maintain oxygen saturation (SpO$_2$) 100% 　• Optimize MAP 　• Maintain PbtO$_2$ greater than 20 mm Hg 　• Maintain normothermia 　• Maintain ICP less than 20 mm Hg *(Level IV*)*	Increasing inspired oxygen tension increases PbtO$_2$ levels[9,13,14] (see Table 74-1 for optimal age-dependent MAP and CPP levels).[15] See Table 74-2 for interventions to increase PbtO$_2$ levels and decrease ICP levels. Table 74-3 shows team interventions used to manage PbtO$_2$.	• PbtO$_2$ level less than 15 mm Hg not responding to interventions; PbtO$_2$ level less than 15 mm Hg that lasts for extended periods correlates with a greater chance of death[2,5,6,12,13] • Sustained increase in ICP because this further compromises PbtO$_2$ levels • Increased temperature not responding to standard interventions
2. After insertion of catheter (or on return from operating room), test position of LICOX 　• Increase fraction of inspired oxygen (FIo$_2$) to 100% to assess that PbtO$_2$ increases as well 　• If PbtO$_2$ does not increase, assess position of catheter with computerized tomographic (CT) scan	LICOX catheter placement should be confirmed with CT scan to ensure accurate placement. When the LICOX catheter is not placed in the white matter of the brain, the measures of brain tissue oxygenation are inaccurate; if anticipated response is not seen, the catheter may be placed in dead tissue.[9,10,13,16]	• LICOX catheter not functional after testing • Results of CT scan show incorrect catheter position
3. Monitor child's neurologic status, including pupillary response to light, motor response, PbtO$_2$, ICP, MAP, CPP, and vital signs hourly and as needed.	Hourly neurologic assessment along with continuous ICP monitoring validates clinical observations, correlates findings, and guides interventions.[2,13,16]	• Changes in neurologic status • Inability to obtain ICP value
4. Provide a safe environment to prevent inadvertent dislodgement of catheter with repeated explanations appropriate to the child's age and developmental level, sedation, analgesia, and family assistance as appropriate. Encourage family to use methods appropriate to the child's developmental level to comfort and support the child.	Prevention of dislodgement of catheter is critical because dislodgement can result in inaccurate PbtO$_2$ readings. If protective/restraint devices are necessary, assessment for use of least restrictive device, care, and documentation must follow institution-specific protocol to ensure a safe environment for the child[10,15] (see Procedure 200 for further information).	• Device dislodgement

* Level IV: Limited clinical studies to support recommendations

TABLE 74-3	Team Interventions and PbtO$_2$

Factors that Decrease PbtO$_2$	Interventions to Increase PbtO$_2$
Tissue hypoxia	Increase fraction of inspired oxygen delivered
Decreasing Paco$_2$	Increase Paco$_2$ by decreasing ventilator rate or tidal volume
Decreased CPP related to decreased MAP	Increase CPP by giving fluids (albumin or 0.9% saline solution); maintain CVP at 5 to 15 mm Hg, PCWP at 10 to 15 mm Hg
	With euvolemic condition, add vasopressors as needed to increase MAP
Low hemoglobin and hematocrit levels, which equal decreased oxygen content	Transfuse with PRBC until hemoglobin is 11 gm/dL, hematocrit is 33%
Increased ICP	Drain cerebrospinal fluid until ICP is less than 20 mm Hg
	Administer sedatives and analgesics to ensure child is adequately sedated (goal of bispectral index monitor [BIS] readings of 10 to 20)
	Administer mannitol 0.25 mg to 1 gram/kg as an intravenous bolus (be prepared to administer more fluid if excessive diuresis occurs and MAP falls)
	Consider administration of pentobarbital for refractory increases in ICP
Increased body temperature	Decrease body temperature with cooling measures (acetaminophen, cooling fan, etc)
Systemic Causes	
Pulmonary	Evaluate and treat disease states that cause a decrease in pulmonary oxygenation (pneumonia, acute respiratory distress syndrome, pulmonary edema, pleural effusions)
Cardiac/hemodynamic	Evaluate hemodynamic profile and treat parameters to maximize cardiac output
	Check preload: CVP or PCWP
	Check afterload: Distal pulses, perfusion, or systemic vascular resistance
	Check stroke volume/left ventricular stroke work index for contractility
	Consider echocardiogram for children without a pulmonary artery (PA) catheter
	Check cardiac enzyme levels, troponin level, 12-lead electrocardiogram

CVP, Central venous pressure; *PCWP,* pulmonary capillary wedge pressure.
Adapted with permission from Bader MK, Littlejohns LR, March K: Brain tissue oxygen monitoring in severe brain injury, II, *Crit Care Nurs* 23(4):34, 2003.

Documentation

- Child and family education, including mode and level of learning
- Hourly documentation of PbtO$_2$, brain and body temperature, ICP, CPP, PCWP and cardiac index (if pulmonary artery catheter is used), central venous pressure, and oxygen saturation
- Values for previous parameters outside of desired range and descriptions of specific interventions provided to treat deviations
- Date, time, individual who performed insertion of PbtO$_2$ catheter, and difficulties or abnormalities during insertion
- Verification that catheter tip lies in desired position (brain CT scan to verify placement)
- Medications administered and child's response to medications
- Child's tolerance of insertion procedure and ongoing catheter presence and any specific interventions provided
- Unexpected outcomes and related treatments

References

1. Dings J, et al: Brain tissue P0$_2$ monitoring: catheter stability and complications, *J Neurological Residency* 19:241-245, 1997.
2. Dings J, et al: Clinical experience with 118 brain tissue oxygen partial pressure catheter probes, *Neurosurgery* 43(5):1082-1095, 1998.
3. Haitsma LK, Maas AL: Advanced monitoring in the intensive care unit: brain tissue oxygen tension, *Curr Opin Crit Care* 8:115-120, 2002.
4. Rumana C, et al: Brain temperature in head injured patients. Presented at 10th International Symposium on Intracranial Pressure and Neuromonitoring in Brain Injury, May 25-29, 1997, Williamsburg, VA.
5. Valadka AB, et al: Relationship of brain tissue P0$_2$ to outcome after severe head injury, *Crit Care Med* 26(9):1576-1581, 1998.
6. van den Brink WA, et al: Brain oxygen tension in severe head injury, *Neurosurgery* 46(4):868-876, 2000.
7. Bader, MK: Recognizing and treating ischemic insults to the brain: The role of brain tissue oxygen monitoring, Critical Care Nursing Clinics of North America (18)243-246, 2006.
8. Henker RA, et al: Comparison of brain temperature with bladder and rectal temperatures in adults with severe head injury, *Neurosurgery* 42:1071-1075, 1998.
9. Integra Neurosciences: *LICOX CMP brain oxygenation monitoring system operations manual,* Plainsboro, NJ, 2000, Integra Neurosciences.

10. Littlejohns LR, et al: Brain tissue oxygen monitoring in severe brain injury, I: research and usefulness in critical care, *Crit Care Nurs* 23(4):17-25, 2003.

11. Maloney-Wilensky E, Bloom S : Brain Tissue Oxygen Monitoring: Insertion (Assist) Care, and Troubleshooting. In Lynn-McHale Wiegand DJ, Carlson K, editors: *AACN procedure manual for critical care,* ed 5, Philadelphia, 2005, Saunders.

12. Sarrafzadeh AS, et al: Cerebral oxygenation in contusioned vs. nonlesioned brain tissue: monitoring of PbtO$_2$ with LICOX and Paratrend, *Acta Neurochir* 71:186-189, 1998.

13. Bader MK, et al: Brain tissue monitoring in severe brain injury, II: implications for critical care teams and case study, *Crit Care Nurs* 23(4):29-43, 2003.

14. Menzel M, et al: Cerebral oxygenation in patients after severe head injury: monitoring and effects of arterial hyperoxia on cerebral blood flow, metabolism, and intracranial pressure, *J Neurosurg Anesthesiol* 11(4):240-251, 1999.

15. Suzuki K: The changes of regional cerebral blood flow with advancing age in normal children, *Nagoya Med J* 34:159-170, 1990.

16. American Association of Neuroscience Nurses: Technology. In Bader MK, Littlejohns LL, editors: *AANN core curriculum for neuroscience nursing,* ed 4, Philadelphia, 2004, Saunders.

Additional Readings

Bond AE, et al: Needs of family members of patients with severe traumatic brain injury: implications for evidence-based practice, *Crit Care Nurs* 23(4);63-72, 2003.

Brain Trauma Foundation, American Association of Neurological Surgeons, Joint Section on Neurotrauma and Critical Care: Guidelines for the management of severe traumatic brain injury, *J Neurotrauma* 17(6/7):451-553, 2000.

Palmer S, et al: The impact on outcomes in a community hospital setting of using the AANS traumatic brain injury guidelines, *J Trauma Injury Infection Crit Care* 50:657-664, 2001.

Intracranial/Intraparenchymal Catheter: Insertion Assist, Set-up, and Care

PURPOSE: An intracranial/intraparenchymal catheter is inserted as part of the management of a child with increased intracranial pressure to continuously monitor intracranial pressure, calculate cerebral perfusion pressure, and provide information on cerebral compliance and autoregulation. This information is used to guide therapeutic interventions and present the clinician with prognostic data related to the child's clinical status.

Antoinette DeSalis and Kelly Keefe Marcoux

PREREQUISITE KNOWLEDGE

- Normal anatomy and physiology of the pediatric brain
- Neurologic assessment of the infant, child, and adolescent, including cranial nerve assessment and Glasgow Coma Scale (GCS)
- Principles of hemodynamic monitoring
- Concepts related to intracranial pressure (ICP) monitoring and intracranial dynamics, including:
  - ❖ Monro-Kellie doctrine
  - ❖ Autoregulation
  - ❖ Compensation
  - ❖ Normal ICP measurements
  - ❖ Intracranial hypertension
  - ❖ See Procedure 76 for a thorough discussion of this topic.
- Not all children with increased ICP are appropriate candidates for ICP monitoring (e.g., near drowning)
- Indications for ICP monitoring in children:
  - ❖ A GCS of less than 8 in severe traumatic brain injury (TBI)[1]
  - ❖ Clinical signs of increasing ICP
  - ❖ Neurodiagnostic test results indicative of high probability of increased ICP (e.g., cerebral edema; traumatic mass lesion; intracerebral bleed)

- ❖ Moderate TBI with inability to monitor child's neurologic status because of sedation, neuromuscular blockade, or anesthesia
- ❖ Other neurologic disorders (e.g., slit ventricle syndrome)

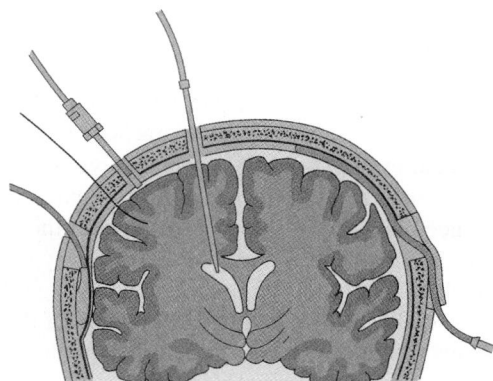

FIGURE 75-1 Methods of intracranial pressure monitoring: sites used for monitoring device placement. *From Kerr M, Crago EA: Nursing management: acute intracranial problems. In O'Brien PG, Giddens JF, Bucher L, editors:* Medical-surgical nursing: assessment and management of clinical problems, *St Louis, 2004, Mosby.*

- Methods of ICP monitoring (Figure 75-1)
  - ❖ Intraventricular catheter
    - ○ Gold standard[2,3]
    - ○ Most accurate
    - ○ Catheter is inserted into the frontal portion of lateral ventricle through a twist drill hole anterior to the coronal sutures
    - ○ Only method that allows cerebrospinal fluid (CSF) drainage
  - ❖ Intraparenchymal catheter
    - ○ Catheter placed directly into brain tissue
    - ○ Usually placed ipsilateral to major intracerebral injury
  - ❖ Subdural/subarachnoid device
    - ○ An ICP "bolt"
    - ○ Usually placed ipsilateral to major intracerebral injury
    - ○ Inserted through a twist drill hole into the subarachnoid or subdural space
    - ○ May not be accurate if ICP is increased
  - ❖ Epidural catheter/sensor
    - ○ No dural penetration
    - ○ Low risk of infection
    - ○ Inaccurate ICP measurement
- Types of ICP monitoring catheters and transducers
  - ❖ Intracranial (catheter tip) transducer (Figures 75-2 and 75-3)
    - ○ Zeroed once, before insertion; does not require leveling for ICP measurement
    - ○ Can be placed directly into brain parenchyma or intraventricular, epidural, or subdural/subarachnoid space
    - ○ Transducer located at tip of catheter
    - ○ Types include fiberoptic sensor (e.g., Camino or Ventrix [Integra Lifesciences Corp., Plainsboro, NJ]) or microprocessor/microchip sensor (i.e., Codman & Shurtleff monitor [Codman & Shurtleff, Inc., Raynham, MA])
    - ○ Advantages: Avoids artifact from occlusion by air bubbles or debris
    - ○ Disadvantages: Mechanical failure; inability to recalibrate in situ
  - ❖ Extracranial transducer
    - ○ Fluid-coupled device; can be connected to intraventricular, subdural, or subarachnoid catheter
    - ○ Requires use of external strain-gauge transducer
    - ○ Requires leveling of transducer to external reference point approximating the level of the foramen of Monro (e.g., top of external auditory meatus)
- Although ICP monitoring is used mainly to guide therapy, it also allows observation and trending of the height and shape of the waveforms, which may predict cerebral perfusion and cerebrovascular status.
- Normal and abnormal ICP waveforms
- Cerebral perfusion pressure calculation
- Current recommendations in the management of increased ICP[4] (management varies per prescribing practitioner and institution-specific protocol)
  - See Procedure 76 for a thorough discussion of this topic.

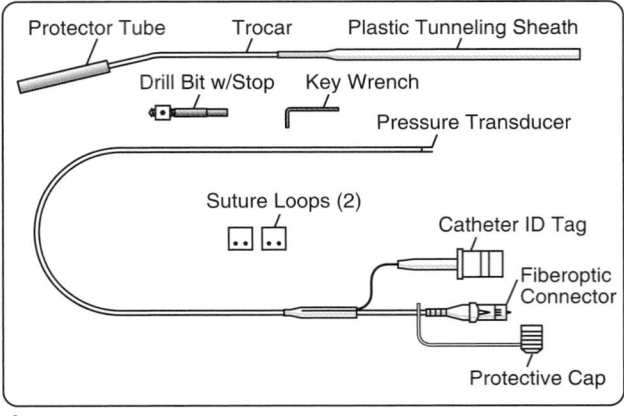

A

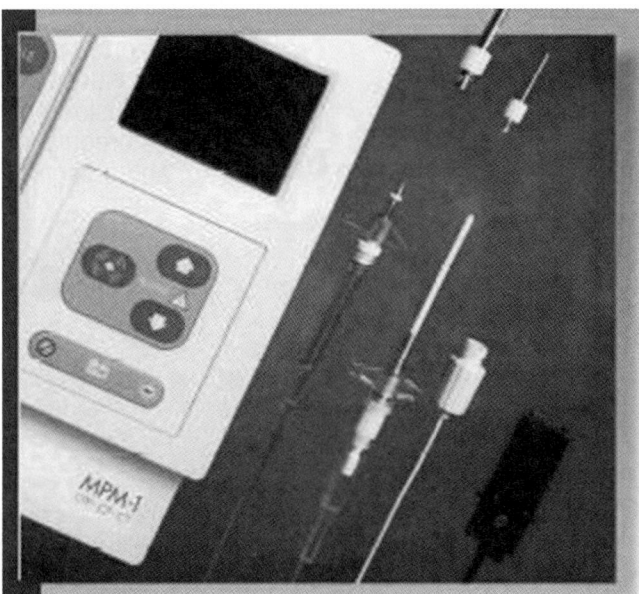

FIGURE 75-2   Fiberoptic transducer tip catheter and monitoring system. Copyright © 2006 by *Integra LifeSciences Corporation. Compliments of Integra Lifesciences.*

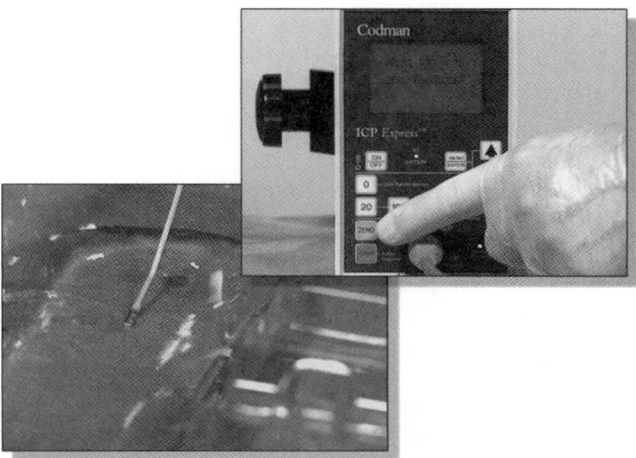

FIGURE 75-3   Microprocessor/microchip catheter and monitoring system. *Courtesy of Codman & Shurtleff, Inc, Raynham, MA.*

- ICP devices must be securely sutured in place to prevent accidental dislodgement or migration and must be covered with a dry sterile occlusive dressing. A bolt may not be sutured in place, but must be secured well to prevent accidental dislodgement.
- Complications of intracranial/intraparenchymal catheter insertion include infection, hemorrhage, breakage, malfunction of device, difficulty with placement, and dislodging of device.[5]
- Principles of aseptic technique
- Child and family development as it relates to clinical assessment and intracranial/intraparenchymal catheter insertion
- Informed consent is required before placement of an intracranial/intraparenchymal catheter.
- Mastery of pediatric advanced life support competencies
- Appropriate pediatric dosing of analgesics and competency in procedural sedation
- Selection and use of developmentally appropriate pain scale (see Procedure 173 for more information)

CHILD AND FAMILY ASSESSMENT

- History of child's present injury or illness ➥*Rationale:* Sudden illness or traumatic injuries can influence the ability of the family to understand procedures because of related stress. The child's neurologic injury may affect the ability to understand procedure.
- Vital signs ➥*Rationale:* Vital signs are an essential part of a complete assessment of the child.
- Child's current baseline neurologic status ➥*Rationale:* Provides a baseline assessment to determine any change in neurologic status during placement of the ICP monitor.
- Child's developmental level and ability to interact ➥*Rationale:* These factors provide important information as to current variation from child's usual baseline and also influence preparation of the child and interaction.
- Indications of increased ICP (see Procedure 76) ➥*Rationale:* If child has signs of increased ICP, this procedure becomes a medical emergency.
- Current laboratory profile, including complete blood count (CBC), prothrombin time (PT), and partial thromboplastin time (PTT) ➥*Rationale:* Establishes baseline values and identifies abnormalities before procedure.
- Family's and child's (as appropriate) understanding of the reasons for and risks and benefits of the procedure ➥*Rationale:* Evaluates family's and child's understanding of the procedure and provides a gauge for ongoing education.

- Family members desire to remain with the child during procedure ➥*Rationale:* If institution-specific protocol allows family presence, the family should have the choice to remain with the child in order to provide comfort and support.

CHILD AND FAMILY EDUCATION

Individualized, developmentally appropriate education is provided to the family and to the child based on desire for knowledge, readiness to learn, and overall neurologic and psychosocial state.

- Provide the family with information about ICP catheter placement, including the reason for placement, basic functions, and necessary precautions related to ICP catheter/transducer system, including activity limitations ➥*Rationale:* Providing information may decrease fear and anxiety and promote compliance with plan of care.
- Describe appearance of the ICP catheter after insertion ➥*Rationale:* Providing information may decrease fear and anxiety, and information provided in advance promotes successful coping.
- Provide the family with information about the monitoring system, including alarms, and assure the family that alarm status is monitored at all times ➥*Rationale:* The family is assured that alarms are monitored and responded to quickly, which may decrease anxiety.
- Discuss the signs and symptoms of increased ICP with family ➥*Rationale:* The family is prepared for potential acute changes in the child's neurologic status and the need for immediate intervention; the family is encouraged to participate in plan of care.
- Encourage questions and answer questions as they arise ➥*Rationale:* Reinforcement of information is needed during periods of stress and is especially important if catheter insertion must be performed emergently.
- If the family desires to stay with the child during the procedure and institution-specific protocol permits family presence, provide the family with accurate information regarding the procedure, family's role, and expectations ➥*Rationale:* Presence of family may provide support and comfort to the child, and clearly defined institution-specific protocol for family presence facilitates this; however, family members should also have the choice not to remain with the child.

Box 75-1	Example of Cranial Access Kit Contents

Preparation Components:
A. Double-edged razor (1)
B. Povidone-iodine, 30-mL package (2; not included in catalog no. 82-6616)
C. Povidone-iodine (PVP) swabs, package/3 (1; not included in catalog no. 82-6616)
D. Gauze sponges, 4×4, 12-ply (10)
E. Medicine cup, 2-oz, 60-mL (2)

Cranial Access Preparation:
F. Ruler, 6-inch (1)
G. Marking pen (1)
H. Fenestrated drape with barrier, 15×15 (1)
I. Absorbent towel, 15×21 (3)

Cranial Access:
J. Xylocaine, 1% with epinephrine 30-mL ampule (1)
K. Sodium chloride, 0.9%, 10-mL ampule (2)
L. Syringe, 12-mL (2)
M. Needle, 18-gauge × 1½-inch (2)
N. Needle, 25-gauge × 5/8-inch (1)
O. Spinal needle, 18-gauge × 3½-inch (1)
P. Ventricular needle, 12-gauge × 3½-inch (1)
Q. Scalpel, #15 (1)
R. Scalpel, #11 (1)
S. Retractor, blunt (1)
T. Hand crank drill (1)
U. 2.7-mm drill bit with stop and wrench (1)
V. 5.8-mm drill bit with stop and wrench (1)
W. Bone wax (1)
X. Mosquito forceps, curved (2)
Y. Culture tube with screw cap (1)

Wound Closing/Dressing:
Z. 2.0 Silk suture (1)
AA. 3.0 Nylon suture (1)
BB. Needle holder, serrated (1)
CC. Adson forceps (1)
DD. Adson forceps with teeth (1)
EE. Suture scissors (1)
FF. Nonwoven sponges, 2×2, 4-ply (4)

Contents of the CODMAN Cranial Access Kit. *Courtesy of Codman & Shurtleff, Inc, Raynham, MA.*

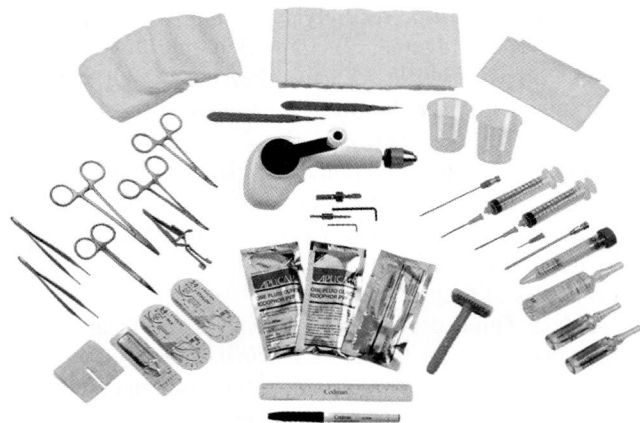

FIGURE 75-4   Sample cranial access kit. Copyright © 2006 by *Integra LifeSciences Corporation. Compliments of Integra Lifesciences.*

EQUIPMENT

- Sterile gloves, gowns, drapes, and towels
- Surgical caps and masks
- Protective eyewear
- Disposable razor or clippers
- Povidone-iodine solution
- Topical anesthetic (1% lidocaine)
- Cranial access kit (see Box 75-1 and Figure 75-4)

- Hand drill
- Scalpel
- Scalp retractor
- Needle holder
- Suture

Fluid-Coupled System with Extracranial Transducer

- Intracranial catheter
- Noncompliant pressure tubing
- Three-way stopcock
- Preservative-free 0.9% saline solution (NS)
- External strain gauge transducer
- Transducer cable
- Tape
- "No-flush" transducer set-up (stopcock on end, primed with preservative-free NS)

Fiberoptic Catheter or Microprocessor System with Intracranial Transducer

- An ICP catheter
- Microprocessor/ICP monitor
- Preamp connector cable
- Cable to connect microprocessor/ICP monitor to bedside monitor
- Intracranial pressure monitor
- Bedside monitor with capability to monitor ICP
- Sterile occlusive dressing (bioocclusive transparent dressing or 4×4 gauze pad and tape)
- Emergency cart with emergency medications and airway equipment

Procedure	for Intracranial/Intraparenchymal Catheter: Insertion Assist, Set-up, and Care	
Steps	**Rationale**	**Considerations**
1. Ensure child and family understand procedure and questions are answered.	Evaluates and reinforces understanding of previously taught information.	Developmental level, cognitive ability, and anxiety level determine approach to and effectiveness of teaching.
2. Confirm presence of informed consent.	Ensures medical-legal compliance as suggested by the Joint Commission on Accreditation of Healthcare Organizations (JCAHO).	In emergency situations, follow institution-specific protocol/ procedure for assumption of consent.
3. Wash hands.	Standard precautions; reduces transmission of microorganisms.	
4. Gather and prepare needed equipment and supplies.	Facilitates procedure completion in a timely manner.	
5. Ensure appropriate cardiorespiratory and hemodynamic monitoring is in place with appropriate alarm limits set and alarms activated.	Child may decompensate during procedure.	Observe bedside monitor and obtain frequent vital signs during procedure. Emergency equipment should be readily available.
6. Identify child with appropriate patient/ procedure verification process (e.g., "Time out"). *(Level II*)*	Confirms correct patient, procedure, and site as recommended by JCAHO; prevents unnecessary medical procedures.	Verification process and documentation is institution specific. Use active communication techniques.
7. Put on clean gloves and personal protective equipment as appropriate.	Standard precautions; reduces transmission of microorganisms.	Garb required of individuals in the room during catheter insertion varies from institution to institution; refer to institution-specific protocol.
8. Assess child's pain with pain scale appropriate to child's age and developmental level. Administer pain or sedation medications as appropriate and per prescribing practitioner's order.	Promotes child's comfort during procedure; facilitates completion of procedure.	
9. Assist practitioner who is inserting catheter with establishing sterile field and preparing equipment.	Aseptic technique protects child from exposure to microorganisms and contamination of the surgical site, reducing likelihood of infection.	
10. Assist practitioner who is inserting catheter with preparing child for catheter placement, including administration of local anesthetic; maintain sterile field.	Aseptic technique protects child from exposure to microorganisms and contamination of the surgical site, reducing likelihood of infection.	
For Fluid Coupled System:		
11. Assemble transducer and tubing; flush with preservative free NS.	Removes air, which causes dampened waveform, from tubing and transducer system.	Air that is not cleared may delay the procedure because it causes system malfunction.

Procedure continues on following page

* Level II: Theory-based; no research data to support recommendations; recommendations from expert consensus group may exist

Procedure for Intracranial/Intraparenchymal Catheter: Insertion Assist, Set-up, and Care—*Continued*

Steps	Rationale	Considerations
12. Place sterile closed cap on transducer after flush is instilled or clamp transducer tubing if NS syringe is left attached. If syringe is left in place, ensure syringe is appropriately labeled. *(Level II*)*	Dead-end cap or labeling of fluid and clamp closure must be used to prevent inadvertent flushing of the fluid-filled system into the intracranial space.[5]	
13. Once catheter is inserted, connect transducer tubing to intracranial catheter.	Establishes fluid column that transmits signal to monitor to display waveform.	
14. Review prescribing practitioner's order and level air fluid interface of external transducer to specified reference point. *(Level II*)*	Levels transducer to foramen of Monro, reference point for intracranial pressure, ensuring accurate pressure reading.[4,5]	Landmarks used to locate the foramen of Monro include the outer canthus of the eye, tragus of the ear, or external auditory meatus. Regardless of reference point used, the same reference point must be consistently used to level the child's transducer.[5,6]
15. Open transducer to atmospheric pressure and zero to monitor per manufacturer's instructions. *(Level IV*)*	Zeroing to atmospheric pressure is necessary to ensure accurate pressure reading.[5]	
For an Intracranial Catheter Tip Transducer:		
16. Turn on ICP monitor specific to the catheter being inserted.	Catheter must be used with brand-specific monitor. Confirms monitor is functioning.	
17. Assist practitioner who is inserting catheter with connection of monitor to fiberoptic/microprocessor catheter.	Allows practitioner to maintain sterility without interruption of sterile field.	Maintain monitor cable away from sterile field during remainder of procedure. Catheter is fragile; avoid kinking catheter.
18. Zero catheter according to manufacturer's instructions before insertion. *(Level I*)*	Catheter must be zeroed to atmospheric pressure before insertion into cranium to ensure accuracy of ICP readings.[5]	Catheter with intracranial transducer is zeroed once *before* insertion. It does not need, or allow for, repeated zero procedures after insertion.
19. If technology is available, connect intracranial pressure monitor to bedside monitor.	Allows waveform and numeric display, correlation of ICP data with other hemodynamic measurements, and tracking of data via bedside and central monitor.	Bedside monitor must have ICP monitoring capability specific to intracranial catheter tip transducer in use.
20. Calibrate the ICP monitor to the bedside monitor according to manufacturer's directions. *(Level I*)*	Necessary for accurate data transmission to bedside monitor from catheter tip transducer monitor; ensures ICP readings and cerebral perfusion pressure (CPP) calculations from bedside monitor are correct.	Calibration can be performed at any time but at a minimum of each shift. Calibration should also be done when any disconnection of the two monitors occurs. Because of multiple available pressure monitors, calibration should be done according to manufacturer's directions.

* Level I: Manufacturer's recommendations only
  Level II: Theory-based; no research data to support recommendations; recommendations from expert consensus group may exist
  Level IV: Limited clinical studies to support recommendations

Procedure	for Intracranial/Intraparenchymal Catheter: Insertion Assist, Set-up, and Care—*Continued*		
Steps	**Rationale**	**Considerations**	
21. If available, turn on CPP parameter of bedside monitor.	The ICP and mean arterial pressure (MAP) data are used to automatically calculate CPP.	Arterial line is necessary for automatic calculation of CPP.	
22. Assist practitioner who is inserting catheter with identification of optimal catheter placement.	Placement is usually preferred in the nondominant hemisphere unless contraindicated.	Presence of skull fracture, postoperative site, or etiology of cerebral insult may limit placement options.	
23. Assist practitioner with insertion of catheter.	Facilitates procedure completion.	Depth of insertion varies depending on desired intracranial placement and age of child.	
24. Assess ICP waveform on monitor display, including waveform morphology.	Presence of a good waveform ensures that the pressure monitor has been placed accurately in the cranial vault.	See Figures 76-1, 76-2, and 76-3 in Procedure 76 for ICP waveforms.	
25. Apply sterile occlusive dressing and complete head dressing if indicated.	Sterile dressing is necessary to prevent contamination of surgical site.	Complete head dressing may be necessary to support catheter and prevent catheter damage.	
26. Note and document opening pressure displayed on ICP monitor.	Documentation of opening pressure is important for management of increased ICP and trending of readings.	Intracranial pressure monitor immediately displays data; the bedside monitor may have a delay in ICP display.	
27. Document CPP.	Provides indirect information regarding cerebral perfusion.	If invasive blood pressure monitoring is not available, CPP is calculated using the MAP from noninvasive blood pressure and the ICP (CPP = MAP − ICP).	
28. Discard used supplies and equipment, including sharps, in appropriate receptacles.	Standard precautions; reduces transmission of microorganisms. Protects personnel health.		
29. Remove personal protective equipment; wash hands.	Standard precautions.		

Expected Outcomes

- Intracranial/intraparenchymal catheter is correctly placed without difficulty

- Accurate reliable ICP data, including appropriate waveform, ICP value, and CPP calculation are obtained

- Aseptic technique maintained throughout procedure

- Neurologic examination results remain stable throughout procedure
- Child has acceptable level of comfort throughout procedure

Unexpected Outcomes

- Catheter is incorrectly placed
- Procedure is prolonged because of difficulty with catheter placement
- Intraparenchymal hemorrhage
- Equipment failure, including damaged catheter
- For fluid-coupled system, incorrect placement of external transducer results in inaccurate values
- For fluid-coupled system, damped waveform from air in system
- Break in aseptic technique
- Local infection or infection of central nervous system develops
- Intracranial or intraparenchymal hemorrhage results in deterioration of neurologic examination
- Unmanaged pain or agitation

Monitoring and Care of the Child

Activities and Interventions	Rationale	Reportable Conditions
1. Monitor child's neurologic status, including pupillary response to light; motor response; and vital signs before, during, and after procedure. *(Level II*)*	Identifies changes in neurologic condition that occur during procedure; facilitates prompt response.[1,4,7-9]	• Changes in neurologic status

2. Obtain and document ICP every hour.
    Hourly charting should include documentation of highest ICP for that hour and the mean ICP at the time of vital sign assessment.
    Specify whether abnormal ICP reading occurs only with stimulation (e.g., suctioning). *(Level II*)*
	ICP is a critical component of a complete neurologic assessment.
	Trending of ICP over time is more significant than any one reading.
	Evaluation of trends allows for identification of pressure waves and evaluation of therapeutic modalities.[4,7-10]
	ICP reading should be correlated with child's clinical status.
		• Elevation, abnormalities, or deviations of ICP
		• Sustained ICP readings greater than 20 mm Hg or a predetermined level based on child's status

3. Observe ICP waveform trends at baseline, hourly, and as needed.
    Assess ICP waveform for normal morphology.
    Note any abnormal waveforms.
    Observe for dampening of waveform.
    Print and document baseline and abnormal ICP waveforms.
	See Figures 76-1, 76-2 and 76-3 for more information and figures of abnormal waveforms.
	Dampening of ICP waveform in fluid-coupled monitoring system may indicate air bubbles.
	
	Dampening in a fiberoptic catheter may indicate malfunction of the catheter or significant change in cerebral compliance.
		• P2 elevations
		• A or B waveform trends
		• No numeric display on transducer tip catheter monitor
		• Dislodgement of ICP catheter
		• No waveform after trouble shooting

4. Calculate and record CPP every hour and as needed.	Cerebral blood flow is indirectly measured with the CPP. Refer to age-related variables when determining the critical threshold for CPP because MAP values are dependent on age (see Table 76-2 in Procedure 76).[1,2,4,7,8,10,11]	• The CPP parameters for reporting are dependent on child's age, etiology of neurologic injury, individual child's status, and practitioner preference • A CPP that is less than the critical threshold of 40 to 70 mm Hg in children can lead to cerebral ischemia
5. Set appropriate alarm limits for ICP and CPP based on child's baseline, prescribing practitioner's order, and institution-specific protocol.	The ICP limits should default to normal age values (e.g., 0 to 15 mm Hg) but should be adapted based on child's average ICP reading.	• Values outside identified parameters
6. Check integrity, stability, and sterility of intracranial catheter at least hourly and with position changes.	Regular hourly assessment of system ensures reliability and safety of ICP monitoring and prevents contamination by microorganisms leading to infection. All connections on the extracranial fluid-coupled ICP system should be clamped and secured with tape to prevent inadvertent instillation of NS into the intracranial compartment.	• Loss of integrity of ICP monitoring system • Inadvertent instillation of NS into intracranial compartment
7. Fluid-coupled system: level and maintain transducer at the anatomic reference point for the foramen of Monro.	Correct leveling of the transducer ensures accurate readings.[5]	• Incorrect leveling of transducer that results in inaccurate readings

* Level II: Theory-based; no research data to support recommendations; recommendations from expert consensus group may exist

Monitoring and Care of the Child—Cont'd

Activities and Interventions	Rationale	Reportable Conditions
8. Fluid-coupled system: zero transducer at frequency indicated in institution-specific protocol and after repositioning of the child or the external transducer; calibrate monitor if necessary. *(Level IV*)*	Zeroing uses atmospheric pressure as the zero reference point for the monitor and ensures the accuracy of ICP readings. Periodic zeroing minimizes the effect of zero drift.[5]	• Inability to zero system
9. Assess integrity of occlusive insertion site dressing and optional full head dressing regularly.	Allows direct visualization of insertion site. Prevents contamination of insertion site by wet, soiled, or loose dressing.	• Considerable drainage at ICP monitor insertion site or on head dressing (may indicate bleeding, leakage of CSF, or infection) • Contamination of ICP monitor insertion site • Device dislodgement • Agitation unresponsive to interventions
10. Prevent inadvertent dislodgement of ICP catheter with repeated age-appropriate explanations, sedation, analgesia, and parental assistance as appropriate. Encourage family to use developmentally appropriate measures to support and comfort child.	Dislodgement of intraventricular catheter may result in need for additional procedure, infection, or pneumoencephaly.	

* Level IV: Limited clinical studies to support recommendations

Documentation

- Child and family education
- Presence of informed consent
- Patient and procedure verification process
- Date, time, type of intracranial pressure monitoring catheter placed, and individual who placed catheter
- Pain, sedation, and local anesthetic medications given and child's tolerance
- Pain assessment before, during, and after procedure
- Opening ICP and initial waveform
- Neurologic assessment before and after ICP monitoring catheter placement, including pupil light reflex, motor response; age-appropriate GCS, and vital signs, including MAP
- Documentation of hourly ICP, CPP, and ICP waveform assessment
- Appearance of dressing and insertion site
- Unexpected outcomes and related treatment

References

1. Adelson PD, et al: Indications for intracranial pressure monitoring in pediatric patients with severe traumatic brain injury; guidelines for the acute medical management of severe traumatic brain injury in infants, children, and adolescents, *Pediatr Crit Care Med* 4(3 suppl):s19-s24, 2003.
2. Adelson PD, et al: Intracranial pressure monitoring technology; guidelines for the acute medical management of severe traumatic brain injury in infants, children, and adolescents, *Pediatr Crit Care Med* 4(3 suppl):s28-s32, 2003.
3. Kirkness CJ, et al: Intracranial pressure waveform analysis; clinical and research applications, *J Neurosci Nurs* 32(5):271-277, 2000.
4. Bader MK, et al: Ventriculostomies and intracranial pressure monitoring: in search of a 0% infection rate, *Heart Lung* 24(2):166-172, 1995.
5. March K: Intracranial pressure monitoring: why monitor? *AACN Clin Iss* 16(4):456-475, 2005.
6. Vernon-Levett P: Intracranial dynamics. In Curley MAQ, Moloney-Harmon PA, editors: *Critical care nursing of infants and children,* ed 2, Philadelphia, 2001, Saunders.
7. Sullivan J: Intracranial bolt insertion (assist), monitoring, care, troubleshooting, and removal. In Lynn-McHale DJ, Carlson K, editors: *AACN procedure manual for critical care,* ed 4, Philadelphia, 2001, Saunders.
8. American Association of Neuroscience Nurses: Intracranial pressure monitoring. In Bader MK, Littlejohns LL, editors: *AANN core curriculum for neuroscience nursing,* ed 4, Philadelphia, 2004, Saunders.
9. Adelson PD, et al: Threshold for treatment of intracranial hypertension; guidelines for the acute medical management of severe traumatic brain injury in infants, children, and adolescents, *Pediatr Crit Care Med* 4(3 suppl):s25-s30, 2003.

10. Czosnka M, et al: Hemodynamic characterization of intracranial pressure plateau waves in head-injury patients, *J Neurosurg* 91(1):11-19, 1999.

11. Bader MK: What is the recommended external reference point for zeroing an intracranial pressure monitoring system at the foramen of Monro? *Crit Care Nurs* 19(6):92-93, 1999.

Additional Readings

Adelson PD, et al: Critical pathway for the treatment of established intracranial hypertension in pediatric traumatic brain injury, *Pediatr Crit Care Med* (4)3:s65-s67, 2003.

Hlatky R, Robertson CS: Multimodality monitoring in severe head injury, *Curr Opin Anaesthesiol* 15(5):489-493, 2002.

Markovitz B, et al., editors: picuBOOK: an online resource for pediatric critical care, PedsCCM, retrieved May 5, 2006, from http://pedsccm.wustl.edu/All-Net/main.html.

76

Intracranial Pressure Monitoring

P U R P O S E : Intracranial pressure monitoring provides crucial information regarding the dynamic relationship between the intracranial contents and the pathophysiology that results with a critical rise in one of these contents without a commensurate decrease in another. This monitoring is used mainly to guide therapy.

Wallis Halperin Wallis and Kelly Keefe Marcoux

PREREQUISITE KNOWLEDGE

- Normal anatomy and physiology of the pediatric brain
- Neurologic assessment of the infant, child, and adolescent, including cranial nerve assessment
- Principles of hemodynamic monitoring
- Intracranial pressure (ICP) monitoring with prompt treatment of intracranial hypertension is associated with the best clinical outcomes in children.[1]
- Cerebrospinal fluid (CSF) comprises 7% to 10% of the intracranial volume (see Procedure 79 for a review of CSF flow, rate, distribution, and characteristics).
- The Monro-Kellie doctrine states that the intracranial vault is a closed system composed of three components: the brain tissue (~80%), the CSF (7% to 10%), and the blood (7% to 10%). Any increase in one or more of these compartments necessitates a decrease in one or more of the other compartments for the total cranium volume to remain fixed.
- Compensatory mechanisms to lower cerebral blood volume include the expulsion of CSF from the ventricular space through the foramen magnum and into the spinal subarachnoid space, increased CSF absorption, decreased CSF production, and increased venous return via the jugular veins.

- Autoregulation is the maintenance of a constant cerebral blood flow (CBF) through vasodilation and vasoconstriction despite changes in systemic blood pressure. The tone and resistance in the cerebral arteries are constantly adjusted in response to local tissue biochemical changes and arterial pressure. Factors that control cerebral blood flow include[2,3]:
  - ❖ Blood pressure: Constant blood flow is maintained despite a change in arterial blood pressure.
  - ❖ Metabolic changes: Local blood flow is increased to match increased local metabolic needs (e.g., fever).
  - ❖ Arterial carbon dioxide tension: Increase in tension of arterial carbon dioxide ($Paco_2$) leads to vasodilatation, which leads to increased cerebral blood flow.
  - ❖ Arterial oxygen tension: Cerebral blood flow increases when the arterial oxygen tension (Pao_2) falls below 50 to 55 mm Hg.
  - ❖ Biochemical alterations: Cerebral blood flow increases in response to an increase in potassium, calcium, hydrogen ions, cytokines, adenosine, and nitric oxide.
  - ❖ Blood viscosity: Blood flow may be decreased with polycythemia.
- Compensation is time limited; ultimately, loss of autoregulation results in intracranial hypertension.[4]
- The ICP is the total pressure exerted by the blood, brain, and CSF in the intracranial vault.

- Increased ICP occurs with an increase in one compartment without a compensatory decrease in one or more of the other compartments.
- Normal ICP measurements (1 mm Hg = 1.36 cm H_2O)
  - ❖ Infant: 1.5 to 6 mm Hg
  - ❖ Young child: 3 to 7 mm Hg
  - ❖ Older child/adult: 0 to 10 mm Hg
- Intracranial hypertension is defined as ICP greater than 20 mm Hg for more than 5 minutes or increased ICP unresponsive to traditional management (see subsequent discussion).
- Conditions that may lead to increased ICP
  - ❖ Cerebral edema (interstitial, vasogenic, or cytotoxic)
  - ❖ Mass lesion (brain tumor, abscess, etc)
  - ❖ Traumatic head injury
  - ❖ Hypoxic brain injury
  - ❖ Epidural hematoma, subdural hematoma, subarachnoid hemorrhage
  - ❖ Arteriovenous malformation (AVM)
  - ❖ Hydrocephalus
  - ❖ Intracranial infections (meningitis, encephalitis)
  - ❖ Congenital or developmental disorders (Arnold-Chiari malformation, myelomeningocele, craniosynostosis)
  - ❖ Metabolic disorders (syndrome of antidiuretic hormone [SIADH], hypoxia, hypercapnia, acidosis)
  - ❖ Idiopathic (pseudotumor cerebri)
  - ❖ Seizures
  - ❖ Valsalva's maneuver
  - ❖ Noxious stimuli
- Not all children with increased ICP are appropriate candidates for ICP monitoring (e.g., near drowning).
- Indications for ICP monitoring in children
  - ❖ Glasgow Coma Scale (GCS) of less than 8 in severe traumatic brain injury (TBI)[1]
  - ❖ Clinical signs of increasing ICP
  - ❖ Neurodiagnostic test results indicative of high probability of increased ICP (e.g., cerebral edema; traumatic mass lesion; intracerebral bleed)
  - ❖ Moderate TBI with inability to monitor child's neurologic status because of sedation, neuromuscular blockade, or anesthesia
  - ❖ Other neurologic disorders (e.g., slit ventricle syndrome)
- The presence of an open fontanel or sutures in an infant does not prevent the occurrence of intracranial hypertension and does not exclude the value of ICP monitoring.[1]
- Methods of ICP monitoring
  - ❖ Intraventricular catheter
    - ○ Gold standard[5,6]
    - ○ Most accurate
    - ○ Catheter is inserted into the frontal portion of lateral ventricle through a twist drill hole anterior to the coronal sutures
    - ○ Only method that allows CSF drainage
  - ❖ Intraparenchymal catheter
    - ○ Catheter placed directly into brain tissue, usually placed ipsilateral to major intracerebral injury
  - ❖ Subdural/subarachnoid device
    - ○ An ICP "bolt"

- ○ Inserted through a twist drill hole into the subarachnoid or subdural space
- ○ May not be accurate if increased ICP
- ❖ Epidural catheter/sensor
  - ○ No dural penetration
  - ○ Low risk of infection
  - ○ Inaccurate ICP measurement
- All ICP devices must be securely sutured to prevent accidental dislodgement or migration and covered with a dry sterile occlusive dressing.
- Types of ICP monitoring catheters and transducers
  - ❖ Intracranial (catheter tip) transducers
    - ○ Only need to be zeroed before insertion; do not need leveling for ICP measurement
    - ○ Can be placed directly into brain parenchyma or intraventricular, epidural, or subdural/subarachnoid space
    - ○ Transducer is at tip of catheter
    - ○ Fiberoptic: A light sensor is used to correlate to ICP waveform; a beam of light travels down the catheter, and ICP is determined by the distortion of the light beam produced by the pressure on the catheter tip; can be placed directly into brain parenchyma or intraventricular (e.g., Camino or Ventrix, Integra Lifesciences Corp, Plainsboro, NJ).
    - ○ Microprocessor/microchip: Correlates atmospheric pressure to ICP; can be placed directly into brain parenchyma or intraventricular (i.e. Codman & Shurtleff monitor, Codman & Shurtleff, Inc, Raynham, MA)
    - ○ Advantages: Ease of placement; solid state (as compared with fluid-filled); allows measurement of ICP intraparenchymally in children with compressed ventricles; avoids artifact from occlusion by air bubbles or debris
    - ○ Disadvantages: Mechanical failure (e.g., sensor failure); inability to recalibrate in situ
  - ❖ Extracranial transducer
    - ○ Can be used with intraventricular subdural/subarachnoid monitoring device
    - ○ Fluid-coupled device
    - ○ Requires use of external strain-gauge transducer
    - ○ Requires "leveling" of transducer to external reference point approximating the level of the foramen of Monro (e.g., top of ear, external auditory meatus, tragus of the ear)
- Intracranial pressure monitoring is used mainly to guide therapy, but it also allows for observation and trending of the height and shape of the waveforms, which may predict cerebral perfusion and cerebrovascular status.
- The ICP waveforms must be monitored with the appropriate scale on the bedside monitor to accurately assess waveform morphology (scales of 0 to 18 or 0 to 30 are sufficient if the ICP is within normal range); scale must be adjusted according to child's ICP readings.
- Normal ICP waveforms: The waveform reflects the pulsation of cerebral vessels and has three important peaks (Figures 76-1).

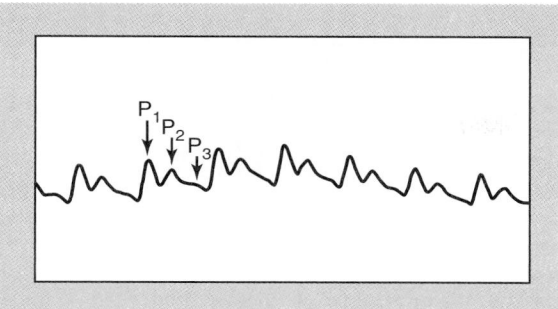

FIGURE 76-1 Components of the normal intracranial pressure waveform: P1, P2, and P3. *From Kirkness CJ, et al: Intracranial pressure waveform analysis: clinical and research implication,* J Neurosci Nurs *32(5):272, 2000.*

❖ P1 (percussion wave): Tallest; originates from pulsations of intracranial arteries; consistent amplitude
❖ P2 (tidal wave): Lower amplitude with more variations; ends with dicrotic notch; reflects cerebral compliance; P2 elevations may signify loss of cerebral compliance (Figure 76-2)
❖ P3 (dicrotic wave): Lowest amplitude; returns to baseline; originates from venous pulsations of the brain; falls immediately after the dicrotic notch on the arterial waveform
• Abnormal ICP waveforms (Figure 76-3)
  ❖ These "waves" are graphic representations of ICP values trended over time (minutes to hours).
  ❖ A waves: Plateau-like; "pressure waves"; occur with ICP more than 50 to 100 mm Hg from an already increased ICP baseline; last 5 to 20 minutes; indicates decreased cerebral compliance
  ❖ B waves: Occur approximately every 2 minutes; may reach 50 mm Hg; correspond to change in respiratory pattern (i.e., Cheyne-Stokes); may increase if compliance decreases
  ❖ C waves: Rhythmic oscillations without known clinical relevance; may occur every 4 to 8 minutes
  ❖ Flat wave: Indicative of brain death; cerebral perfusion pressure (CPP) = ICP (no cerebral blood flow (CBF)
• CPP is an indirect measure of cerebral blood flow calculated by measuring the difference between the mean arterial pressure (MAP) and ICP; CPP = MAP − ICP.
• The CPP must be maintained above a certain value to prevent cerebral ischemia.

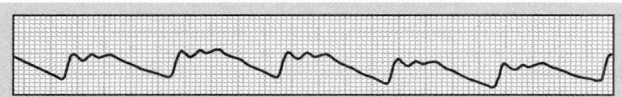

FIGURE 76-2 Example of intracranial waveform with decreased compliance. From March K: Application technology in the treatment of traumatic brain injury, *Crit Care Nurs Q* 23(3):28, 2000.

❖ Accepted normal values
  ○ Adults: CPP > 70 mm Hg
  ○ Children: CPP > 50 to 60 mm Hg
  ○ Infants/toddlers: CPP > 40 to 50 mm Hg
• A CPP less than the age-appropriate range indicates hypoperfusion of the brain.[7]
• Management of increased ICP includes prevention of secondary injury, such as cerebral ischemia and cerebral edema.
• Current recommendations in the management of increased ICP[8] (management varies as per practitioner and institution)
  ❖ Decrease cerebral volume
    ○ Surgical intervention
      • Evacuation of mass lesion to decrease mass effect
      • Decompressive craniectomy (often reserved for refractory intracranial hypertension)
    ○ Osmolar therapy
      • Mannitol boluses 0.25 gram to 1 gram/kg repeated as needed until upper limit (serum osmolality > 320 mOsm) is reached to maintain ICP < 20 mm Hg; or before ICP monitoring if signs of neurologic deterioration or herniation are present
      • Hypertonic saline solution–continuous drip 0.1 to 1 mL/kg/hr titrated to maintain ICP < 20 mm Hg)[10]; serum osmolality of 360 mOsm/L appears to be well tolerated[10] with hypertonic saline, as is serum sodium as high as 160 mEq/L[9]
  ❖ Ventriculostomy to drain CSF
  ❖ Maintain adequate arterial oxygenation
  ❖ Maintain age-appropriate CPP
    ○ Consider vasopressor support (e.g., neosynephrine) to maintain age-appropriate MAP
  ❖ Decrease cerebral blood flow
    ○ Maintain head of bed (HOB) elevated 30 degrees
    ○ Maintain head in midline position to promote venous drainage
  ❖ Maintain normocarbia (PaCO$_2$ ~35 mm Hg)
    ○ Consider mild hyperventilation (PaCO$_2$ 30 to 35 mm Hg)
    ○ No *prophylactic* hyperventilation; hyperventilation only for acute transient significant ICP elevations or impending herniation
  ❖ Decrease cerebral metabolic rate
    ○ Prevent hyperthermia; control fever
    ○ Provide adequate sedation and analgesia with or without neuromuscular blockade
    ○ Prevent and treat seizure activity
      • Consider seizure prophylaxis in the first week after head injury; treat if evidence of seizure activity or temporal mass lesion
  ❖ For refractory intracranial hypertension, consider
    ○ Hyperventilation (PaCO$_2$ < 30 mm Hg)
    ○ Moderate hypothermia (32°C to 34°C)
    ○ Lumbar drain

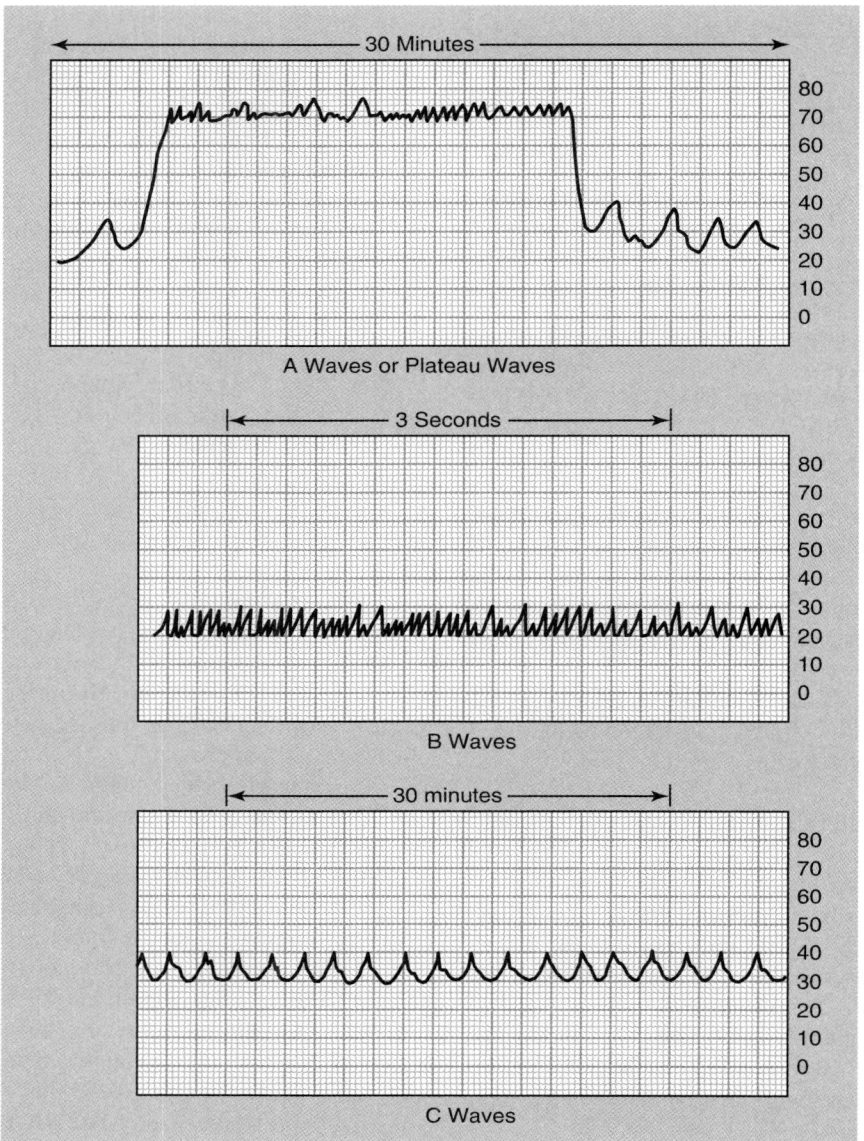

FIGURE 76-3   Abnormal ICP waveforms. A waves or plateau waves, are sustained plateau elevations in intracranial pressure; when pressure falls, it does not return to baseline preceding plateau wave. B waves are steep rapid elevations in intracranial pressure that are brief and are not as high as A waves. C waves, or Lundberg waves, show smaller increase in intracranial pressure and reflect arterial blood pressure changes. *From Pollack-Latham CL: Intracranial pressure monitoring: part II; patient care, Crit Care Nurs 7(6):54, 1987.*

- ○ Decompressive craniectomy
- ○ High-dose barbiturate therapy
- See Procedures 75 and 77 for further information.

CHILD AND FAMILY ASSESSMENT

- Obtain vital signs ➥*Rationale:* Vital signs are an essential part of a complete assessment of the child.
- Child's baseline neurologic status ➥*Rationale:* Provides a baseline assessment to determine any change in neurologic status during placement of the ICP monitor.

- Child's developmental level and ability to interact ➥*Rationale:* These factors provide important information as to current variation from child's baseline and also influence preparation of the child and interaction.
- Signs of increased ICP
  - ❖ *Infant:* Increased head circumference, full fontanel, engorged scalp veins, cranial nerve VI palsy, irregular respirations, apnea, seizure, setting sun sign (upward gaze palsy), hyperreactive reflexes, decreased reactivity of pupils, pupil asymmetry
  - ❖ *Older child/adolescent:* Headache, nausea, vomiting, ataxia, drowsiness, blurred vision, decreased reactivity of pupils, pupil asymmetry

❖ *Late signs:* Bradycardia, hypertension, irregular respirations (Cushing's triad); nonreactive pupils ➤*Rationale:* If child has signs of increased ICP, this procedure becomes a medical emergency.

- Current laboratory profile, including complete blood count (CBC), prothrombin time (PT), and partial thromboplastin time (PTT) ➤*Rationale:* Establishes baseline values for identification of abnormalities before procedure.

- Child's (as appropriate) and family's understanding of the reasons for and risks and benefits of the procedure ➤*Rationale:* Evaluates child's and family's understanding of the procedure and provides a gauge for ongoing education.

- Child's known allergies ➤*Rationale:* Prevents exposure of the child to medications or substances known to be allergens for the child.

CHILD AND FAMILY EDUCATION

Individualized, developmentally appropriate education is provided to the family and to the child based on desire for knowledge, readiness to learn, and overall neurologic and psychosocial state.

- Explain and reinforce the rationale for monitoring of ICP and CSF to the child and family as developmentally appropriate ➤*Rationale:* Family's and child's anxiety and fear of the unknown are reduced, and an opportunity is given to ask questions.

- Explain the basic function and care of the ICP monitoring system to the child and family as appropriate ➤*Rationale:* Providing information decreases anxiety and fear and encourages compliance with planned interventions.

- Discuss the signs and symptoms of increased ICP with the family ➤*Rationale:* The family is prepared for potential acute changes in the child's neurologic status and the need for immediate intervention.

- Encourage the family to assist in activities of daily living as appropriate (e.g., bathing, range of motion, reading to the child) ➤*Rationale:* The family may provide support and reassurance to the child and should be encouraged to participate in appropriate care activities if it is not detrimental to the ICP.

- Encourage questions and answer questions as they arise ➤*Rationale:* Reinforcement of information is needed during periods of stress and is especially important if the procedure is performed emergently.

EQUIPMENT

- Extracranial transducer/fluid-coupled system
  - ❖ ICP catheter
  - ❖ Noncompliant pressure tubing
  - ❖ Three-way stopcock
  - ❖ Preservative-free 0.9% saline solution (NS)
  - ❖ External strain gauge transducer
  - ❖ Transducer cable
  - ❖ Tape
  - ❖ "No-flush" transducer set-up (stopcock on end, primed with preservative-free NS)
- Intracranial transducer/fiberoptic catheter or sensor system
  - ❖ ICP catheter
  - ❖ Microprocessor/ICP monitor
  - ❖ Preamp connector cable
  - ❖ Cable to connect microprocessor/ICP monitor to bedside monitor
- Bedside monitor
- Cranial access kit
- External drainage bag if ventriculostomy is placed
- Bright light
- Pupillometer[12] (optional)
- Emergency cart with emergency medications and airway equipment

Procedure	**for ICP Monitoring: Assessment, Monitoring, and Waveform Interpretation**	
Steps	**Rationale**	**Considerations**
1. Ensure child and family understand procedure and questions are answered.	Evaluates and reinforces understanding of previously taught information.	Developmental level, cognitive ability, and anxiety level determine approach to and effectiveness of teaching.
2. Gather needed equipment and supplies.	Facilitates completion of task in a timely manner.	
3. Wash hands.	Standard precautions; reduces transmission of microorganisms.	

4. Confirm the integrity of the system setup:
    Assess all connections and tubing for continuity and security.
    For fluid-coupled system: Assess for air bubbles in pressure tubing and remove if possible.
    Adjust any malfunction of ICP monitoring devices according to manufacturer's guidelines and institution-specific protocol.
    If unable to rectify problem, notify neurosurgeon for possible change of ICP monitoring system. *(Level IV*)*
	Cables and connecting devices that are not secure can lead to mechanical failure.
	Fluid-coupled systems may develop air bubbles or a leak that interferes with accurate readings and requires either the flushing of the pressure tubing or external strain gauge transducer or changing the tubing. Loose connections may also lead to invasion by microorganisms.
	Fiberoptic or sensor system catheters may become damaged or dislodged and may need to be replaced.
	All ICP monitoring devices may become occluded with blood or brain tissue, resulting in a dampened waveform.
	Catheter occlusion may require manipulation, flushing, or replacement.[5,9,13]
		Notify prescribing practitioner promptly for intervention if unable to repair with suggested interventions.
		Ensure a "no-flush" system is connected to transducer when using a fluid-coupled system to prevent inadvertent instillation of NS into ventricles.
		Prevention of infection is paramount for children with an ICP monitoring device in place.
		Manipulation or flushing of the catheter is usually performed by the neurosurgeon or prescribing practitioner; refer to institution-specific protocol and State Nurse Practice Act.

5. Assess ICP waveform (see Figures 76-1, 76-2, and 76-3).	Unanticipated changes in ICP readings or waveform changes require prompt assessment of catheter placement and reliability of connections.	Notify prescribing practitioner immediately if loss of waveform or abnormal waveform persists after troubleshooting.
6. Level extracranial transducer of fluid-coupled system to foramen of Monro.	This reference point can be best estimated by drawing an imaginary line between the top of the ear and the outer canthus of the eye.[14]	Other reference points include the outer canthus of the eye, the tragus of the ear, or the external auditory meatus. Regardless of the reference point used, the same reference point must be consistently used to level the child's transducer.
7. For fluid-coupled system, zero transducer at frequency indicated in institution-specific protocol and calibrate monitor if required. *(Level IV*)*	Zeroing uses atmospheric pressure as the zero reference point for the monitor and ensures the accuracy of ICP readings.[13] Fluid-coupled devices must be rezeroed periodically, with position changes and whenever dampening of the waveform occurs. Fiberoptic and sensor devices are zero calibrated before insertion	See Procedure 63 for more information on zeroing and calibration of fluid-coupled systems. Newer transducers and monitoring systems do not require calibration.

* Level IV: Limited clinical studies to support recommendations

Procedure	for ICP Monitoring: Assessment, Monitoring, and Waveform Interpretation—*Continued*		
Steps	**Rationale**	**Considerations**	
	and do not require any further zeroing.		
8. Assess ICP monitor for mechanical failure.	Ensures correct functioning of equipment. Fiberoptic catheters that have excessively high readings, such as 888 or 999, usually indicate damaged fibers and require replacement of the catheter.[5,6,9,13]	Notify prescribing practitioner promptly if unable to rectify inaccurate readings or waveforms because catheter may need to be replaced.	
9. Assess device insertion site. *(Level IV*)*	Direct visualization of the insertion site ensures catheter is in place and dressing is intact.[9,13]	An occlusive dressing should be applied to insertion site. Frequency of dressing change and provision of local site care vary considerably by institution; refer to institution-specific protocol.	
10. Assess stability of the device. *(Level IV*)*	The device must be stable and imbedded in the skull to provide reliable data.[9,13]	When moving child and providing care, the ICP device must be secured at all times.	
11. For ventriculostomy: Assess patency of CSF drainage system by ensuring unobstructed flow of CSF through the system to the drainage bag. If no drainage is present, a catheter flush or change of CSF drainage system with aseptic technique may be necessary; refer to State Nurse Practice Act and institution-specific protocol for further guidance on flushing ICP monitoring catheter. *(Level IV*)*	Brain tissue, blood clots, or sediment may occlude drainage system.[6,9,13]	Notify prescribing practitioner if substantial amount of blood, brain tissue, or sediment is noted in intraventricular catheter or drainage system because it may indicate additional pathologic conditions.	
12. Wash hands.	Standard precautions.		

* Level IV: Limited clinical studies to support recommendations

Expected Outcomes

- Accurate reliable ICP waveforms, data, and CPP calculations are obtained

- Prompt identification and management of acute changes in ICP or abnormal ICP waveform

- Prompt identification and management of acute change in CPP; particularly a decrease in CPP, which may indicate cerebral ischemia

- The ICP monitor remains in place until electively removed
- The ICP monitor insertion site is free from infection

- Child has acceptable level of comfort

Unexpected Outcomes

- Inaccurate data
- Poor waveform
- Fiberoptic catheter is inoperable because of catheter breakage
- Fluid-coupled system is occluded
- Wedging or displacement of sensor catheter
- Delayed response to increased ICP or abnormal waveform
- Malfunctioning equipment is not identified
- Inaccurate calculation of CPP results in unrecognized cerebral ischemia
- Incorrectly leveled fluid-coupled system results in incorrect CPP value
- Inadvertent displacement or removal of ICP monitor
- Cerebrospinal fluid leakage or infection at ICP monitor insertion site
- Unmanaged pain or agitation

Monitoring and Care of the Child

Activities and Interventions	Rationale	Reportable Conditions
1. Monitor child's neurologic status, including pupillary response to light, motor response, and vital signs hourly and as needed.	Hourly neurologic assessments along with continuous ICP monitoring validate clinical observations, correlate findings, and guide interventions.[9,13,15]	• Changes in neurologic status
2. Obtain and document ICP every hour and with significant increases. Hourly charting should identify the highest pressure for the hour. Average for the hour is used to calculate CPP.	The ICP is a critical component of a complete neurologic assessment. Trending of ICP over time is more significant than any one reading. Evaluation of trends allows identification of pressure waves and evaluation of therapeutic modalities.[4,6,9,13,15] When documenting ICP data, take into consideration that a certain amount of "zero drift" may occur each day an intracranial transducer catheter remains in situ.[5]	• Elevation, abnormalities, or sudden drop of ICP • Sustained ICP readings greater than 20 mm Hg or threshold set by prescribing practitioner
3. Observe ICP waveform trends at baseline, at least hourly and as needed. Print and document baseline and abnormal ICP waveforms.	Facilitates identification of abnormal ICP. Table 76-1 shows comparison of ICP pressure trends with clinical signs and symptoms.[6,13,16,17]	• P2 elevations and A or B wave-form trends • No waveform after trouble-shooting
4. Calculate and record CPP every hour and as needed.	A CPP that is less than the critical threshold of 40 to 70 in children may indicate cerebral ischemia. Cerebral blood flow is indirectly measured with the CPP; refer to age-related variables when determining the critical threshold for CPP because MAP values are dependent on age.[6,7,9,13,15,18] (Table 76-2 shows normal MAP values.)	• CPP values outside parameters set by prescribing practitioner • Hypotension
5. Check integrity, stability, and sterility of intracranial or intra-ventricular catheter at least hourly and with position changes.	Regular assessment of system ensures reliability and safety of ICP monitoring and prevents contamination by microorganisms leading to infection. All ports on the extracranial fluid-coupled ICP system should be clamped and secured with tape to prevent inadvertent instillation of NS into the intracranial cavity. Whenever the child's position changes, the possibility of disruption of the system exists.[5,13,14,19]	• Loss of integrity of ICP monitor-ing system • Cerebrospinal fluid leaking around ventriculostomy • Cerebrospinal fluid becomes blood tinged
6. For fluid-coupled systems, ensure transducer is maintained at the anatomic reference point for the foramen of Monro (i.e., top of external auditory canal) to ensure accurate reliable data.	Leveling of the transducer is necessary to ensure accurate readings (see Procedure 63 for further information).	• Inaccurate values obtained because of incorrect leveling of transducer
7. Fluid-coupled system requires zeroing of external transducer periodically and after any repositioning of the child or the external transducer.	The monitor is periodically zeroed to ensure accurate readings and prevent zero drift; see Procedure 63 for further information.	• Inability to zero system

Monitoring and Care of the Child—Cont'd

Activities and Interventions	Rationale	Reportable Conditions
8. For ventriculostomy, assess drainage, position of tubing and catheter, level of drainage system, security of stopcock and connections, and absence of CSF leak at least every hour.	Observation at regular intervals is necessary to accurately assess the position of the drainage system, amount of CSF drainage, and any complications.	• CSF drainage that exceeds parameters identified in prescribing practitioner's order • Sudden inadvertent change in level of drainage system with significant drainage
9. Assess integrity of occlusive insertion site dressing and optional full head dressing regularly. Change insertion site dressing and head dressing per prescribing practitioner's order or institution-specific protocol.	Allows direct visualization of insertion site. Prevents contamination of insertion site by wet, soiled, or loose dressing. Responsibility for changing dressings and site care varies among institutions; follow institution-specific protocol.	• Considerable drainage at ICP monitor insertion site or on head dressing (may indicate bleeding, leakage of CSF, or infection) • Contamination of ICP monitor insertion site • Fever
10. Monitor child's vital signs, pain, and comfort levels.	Significant vital sign changes may indicate pain or agitation or an unexpected consequence, such as herniation, increased ICP, bleeding, or infection.	• Sustained deterioration in vital signs • Unmanaged pain or agitation • Bradycardia, hypertension, abnormal respirations, ICP more than 20 mm Hg, decreased pupil reactivity
11. Prevent inadvertent dislodgement of ICP catheter with repeated age-appropriate explanations, sedation, analgesia, and parental assistance as appropriate. Encourage family to use developmentally appropriate measures to support and comfort child.	Dislodgement of intraventricular catheter may result in excessive CSF drainage or pneumocephaly.	• Device dislodgement • Agitation unresponsive to interventions
12. For fluid-coupled systems, change ICP monitoring and drainage system with aseptic technique according to manufacturer's instructions and institution-specific protocol.	Limits risk of infection at insertion site and within ventricular system. Recommendations for optimal frequency for changing ICP monitoring system vary widely, from not interrupting the integrity of the system at all to changing ICP monitoring setup every 24, 48, or 72 hours; refer to institution-specific protocol.[13,19]	• Device dislodgement during system change • Monitoring and drainage system not changed per institution-specific protocol • Contamination of monitoring and drainage system
13. Per prescribing practitioner's order or institution-specific protocol, obtain routine CSF specimens with aseptic technique from intraventricular catheter, with use of sampling port on CSF drainage system, and send for laboratory analysis of culture and sensitivity, gram stain, cell count, glucose, and protein or studies required per institution-specific protocol or prescribing practitioner's order; refer to State Nurse Practice Act for guidelines on drawing samples from intraventricular catheters.	Assessment of CSF is crucial in the diagnosis of possible infection. Insufficient data exist to support frequency of routine CSF sampling and evaluation. Following institution-specific protocol is recommended concerning frequency of routine CSF sampling.[4,12,13,19] *(Level II*)*	• Elevated CSF WBC count • Elevated CSF protein • Decreased CSF glucose • Abnormal gram stain and culture or identification of specific organism

*Level II: Theory-based; no research data to support recommendations; recommendations from expert consensus group may exist

TABLE 76-1	Comparison of ICP Pressure Trends	
Description	Pressure (mm Hg)	Clinical Signs and Symptoms
A waves	50–100	Abnormal changes in respiratory patterns; pupil dilation or abnormal pupillary responses; sweating; flushing; changes in vital signs, such as bradycardia, headache, vomiting
B waves	20–50	Decreased level of consciousness, agitation, headache, posturing, respiratory compromise
C waves	4–20	No accepted clinical significance
Normal	4–15	Normal

Data compiled from Vernon-Levett P: Intracranial dynamics. In Curley MAQ, Moloney-Harmon PA, editors: *Critical care nursing of infants and children,* ed 2, Philadelphia, 2001, Saunders.

TABLE 76-2	Normal Mean Arterial Blood Pressures by Age	
Age	Normal Blood Pressure Range in mm Hg	Normal Mean Arterial Pressure in mm Hg
Birth to 1 yr	70/40–105/66	50–80
2 to 4 yr	87/53–105/66	64–80
5 to 8 yr	97/57–112/71	70–85
8 to 17 yr	112/70–128/80	84–96

Information compiled from American Heart Association: Recognition of respiratory failure and shock. In Hazinski MF, editor: *PALS provider manual,* Dallas, 2002, American Heart Association.

Craig J, Smith JB, Fineman L: Tissue Perfusion. In Curley MAQ, Moloney-Harmon, PA. editors: *Critical care nursing of infants and children,* ed 2, Philadelphia, 2001, Saunders.

National High Blood Pressure Education Program Working Group on High Blood Pressure in Children and Adolescents: The fourth report on the diagnosis, evaluation, and treatment of high blood pressure in children and adolescents, *Pediatrics* 114:555-576, 2004.

Documentation

- Type of ICP monitor (i.e., intraparenchymal, intraventricular)
- Hourly assessment of ICP reading and calculation of CPP
- Hourly neurologic assessment, including pupil light reflex, motor response; age-appropriate GCS, and vital signs, including MAP
- Pain and agitation scores; effectiveness of interventions to manage pain and agitation
- Assessment of head dressing
- If applicable, level of transducer and external drainage bag
- Hard copy of ICP waveform trends (including A and B waveform trends)
- Abnormal ICP and CPP values and interventions taken to treat ICP and CPP deviations
- Amount and characteristics of CSF drainage every hour or per prescribing practitioner's order or institution-specific protocol
- ICP waveform morphology, including autoregulation and cerebral compliance
- Child's response to interventions aimed at decreasing elevated ICP
- Child's neurologic status before and after troubleshooting a problem and the interventions taken to resolve the problem, including manipulation of monitoring device or catheter
- Child and family education
- Unexpected outcomes and related treatment

References

1. Adelson PD, et al: Indications for intracranial pressure monitoring in pediatric patients with severe traumatic brain injury; guidelines for the acute medical management of severe traumatic brain injury in infants, children, and adolescents, *Pediatr Crit Care Med* 4(3 supp):s19-s24, 2003.
2. Vernon-Levett P. Intracranial dynamics. In Curley MAQ, Moloney-Harmon PA, editors: *Critical care nursing of infants and children,* ed 2, Philadelphia, 2001, Saunders
3. Hickey JV: Intracranial hypertension: theory and management of increased intracranial pressure. In Hickey JV, editor: *The clinical practice of neurological and neurosurgical nursing,* ed 5, Philadelphia, 2003, Lippincott, Williams & Wilkins.
4. Hazinski MF, et al: Neurologic disorders. In Hazinski MF, editor: *Manual of pediatric critical care,* St Louis, 1999, Mosby.
5. Adelson PD, et al: Intracranial pressure monitoring technology; guidelines for the acute medical management of

severe traumatic brain injury in infants, children, and adolescents, *Pediatr Crit Care Med* 4(3 supp):s28-s32, 2003.

6. Bullock R, et al: Guidelines for the management of severe traumatic brain injury, *J Neurotrauma* 17:451-553, 2000.

7. Adelson PD, et al: Cerebral perfusion pressure; guidelines for the acute medical management of severe traumatic brain injury in infants, children, and adolescents, *Pediatr Crit Care Med* 4(3 supp):s31-s33, 2003.

8. Adelson PD, et al: Critical pathway for the treatment of established intracranial hypertension in pediatric traumatic brain injury; guidelines for the acute medical management of severe traumatic brain injury in infants, children, and adolescents, *Pediatr Crit Care Med* 4(3supp):s65-67, 2003.

9. American Association of Neuroscience Nurses: Intracranial pressure monitoring. In Bader MK, Littlejohns LL, editors: *AANN core curriculum for neuroscience nursing,* ed 4, Philadelphia, 2004, Saunders.

10. Adelson PD, et al: Use of hyperosmolar therapy in the management of severe traumatic brain injury; guidelines for the acute medical management of severe traumatic brain injury in infants, children, and adolescents, *Pediatr Crit Care Med* 4(3 supp):s40-s44, 2003.

11. Khanna S, et al: Prolonged hypernatremia controls elevated intracranial pressure in pediatric head injury patients [abstract], *Crit Care Med* 26:421-422, 2000.

12. Taylor WR, et al: Quantitative pupillometry, a new technology: normative data and preliminary observations in patients with acute head injury, *J Neurosurg* (98):205-213, 2003.

13. Sullivan J, Severeance-Lossin, L: Intraventricular catheter insertion (assist) monitoring, care, troubleshooting and removal. In Lynn-McHale Wiegand DJ, Carlson K, editors: *AACN procedure manual for critical care,* ed 5, Philadelphia, 2005, Saunders.

14. Bader MK: What is the recommended external reference point for zeroing an intracranial pressure monitoring system at the foramen of Monro? *Crit Care Nurs* 19(6):92-93, 1999.

15. Adelson PD, et al: Threshold for treatment of intracranial hypertension; guidelines for the acute medical management of severe traumatic brain injury in infants, children, and adolescents, *Pediatr Crit Care Med* 4(3 supp):s25-s30, 2003.

16. Czosnka M, et al: Hemodynamic characterization of intracranial pressure plateau waves in head-injury patients, *J Neurosurg* 91(1):11-19, 1999.

17. Kirkness CJ, et al: Intracranial pressure waveform analysis; clinical and research applications, *J Neurosci Nurs* 32(5):271-277, 2000.

18. Hlatky R, Robertson CS: Multimodality monitoring in severe head injury, *Curr Opin Anaesthesiol* 15(5):489-493, 2002.

19. Bader MK, Littlejohns L, Palmer S: Ventriculostomies and intracranial pressure monitoring: in search of a 0% infection rate, *Heart Lung* 24(2):166-172, 1995.

Additional Readings

Brain Trauma Foundation, American Association of Neurological Surgeons, Joint Section on Neurotrauma and Critical Care: Guidelines for the management of severe traumatic brain injury, *J Neurotrauma* 17(6/7):451-553, 2000.

Brain Trauma Foundation, American Association of Neurological Surgeons, Joint Section on Neurotrauma and Critical Care: Intracranial pressure treatment threshold, *J Neurotrauma* 17(6-7):493-495, 2000.

Brain Trauma Foundation, American Association of Neurological Surgeons, Joint Section on Neurotrauma and Critical Care: Guidelines for cerebral perfusion pressure, *J Neurotrauma* 17(6-7):507-511, 2000.

Downard C, et al: Relationship between cerebral perfusion pressure and survival in pediatric brain-injured patients, *J Trauma* 49(4):654-658, 2000.

Jensen RL, et al: Risk factors of intracranial pressure monitoring in children with fiberoptic devices: a critical review, *Pediatr Neurosurg* 47:16-22, 1997.

Intraventricular Catheter: Insertion Assist, Monitoring, and Care

P U R P O S E : An intraventricular catheter is inserted into the lateral ventricle and is used for drainage of cerebrospinal fluid, monitoring of intracranial pressure, calculation of cerebral perfusion pressure, and assessment of cerebral compliance and autoregulation. Cerebrospinal fluid drainage via a ventriculostomy may be an integral component of increased intracranial pressure management.

Heidi Martin and Kelly Keefe Marcoux

PREREQUISITE KNOWLEDGE

- Neuroanatomy and physiology
- An intraventricular catheter (IVC) is inserted into the anterior horn of the lateral ventricle through the nondominant cerebral hemisphere via a burr hole (Figure 77-1).[1,2]
- An IVC may be used for[1-3]:
  - ❖ Drainage of cerebral spinal fluid (CSF)
  - ❖ Monitoring of intracranial pressure (ICP)
  - ❖ Calculation of cerebral perfusion pressure (CPP)
  - ❖ Assessment of cerebral compliance and auto regulation
- An IVC is placed directly into the lateral ventricle with sterile technique by a neurosurgeon or other practitioner with specialty training.
  - ❖ Landmarks used are approximately 1 cm anterior to the coronal suture, 2 to 3 cm from the midline, in the line of the pupil in the nondominant hemisphere.
  - ❖ If the child is less than 3 years old and nondominant hemisphere has not yet been identified, the catheter is generally placed on the right.[1]
  - ❖ The IVC is sutured in place at the insertion site, and the area is covered with an occlusive dressing.
- Advantages of IVC placement include[1-4]:

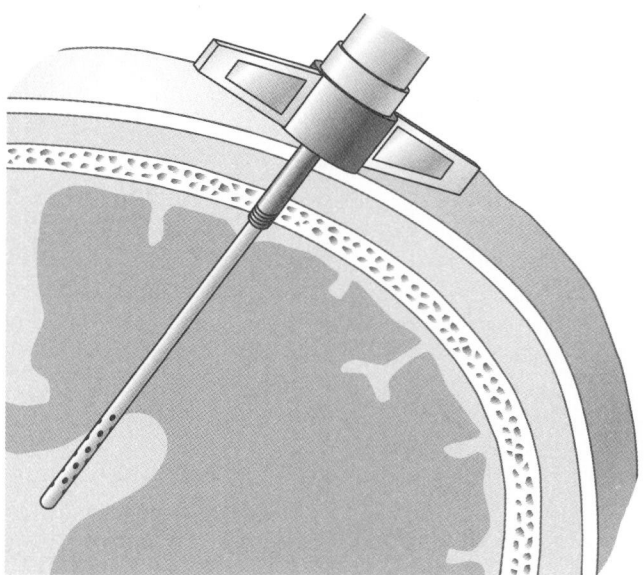

FIGURE 77-1 Intraventricular Catheter Placement. Note tip of catheter in lateral ventricle and fenestrations in catheter tip. Copyright © 2006 by *Integra Lifesciences Corporation. Compliments of Integra LifeSciences.*

- ❖ Accuracy
- ❖ Ability to drain CSF
- ❖ Ability to obtain CSF for laboratory analysis
- ❖ Ability to identify rapid changes in ICP
- ❖ Potential to identify changes in compliance
- Complications of IVC placement include:
  - ❖ Hemorrhage
  - ❖ Difficulty with placement in the presence of small or shifted ventricles
  - ❖ Infection
- An IVC attached to a drainage system is a closed sterile system that allows CSF to drain into a graduated flow chamber that can be adjusted to a prescribed resistance level, usually referenced to the foramen of Monro (see Figure 80-1 in Procedure 80).[1,2,4]
- The height of the drip chamber determines the pressure at which CSF drains from the ventricles into the collection chamber.
  - ❖ The level of the drainage system determines the amount of resistance to CSF flow within the system. The prescribed level for the drainage system may be indicated as cm H_2O or mm Hg (note: 1 mm Hg = 1.36 cm H_2O).
  - ❖ If the drip chamber is set at 15 cm H_2O or 12 mm Hg above the foramen of Monro, CSF should drain when the ICP is approximately 12 mm Hg.
  - ❖ If the level of the drainage system is suddenly lowered, rapid drainage of CSF from the ventricles may occur, resulting in ventricular collapse and the potential for development of a subdural hematoma.[5] Drainage systems generally have a safety mechanism to prevent sudden change in level of the drainage system.
- The prescribing practitioner may order intermittent or continuous drainage of CSF, depending on the child's condition and the type of ventriculostomy used. One study in children with traumatic brain injury showed increased CSF removal with continuous drainage.[3,6]
- If CSF is ordered to drain continuously, the ICP should never exceed the level at which the drainage system is set (e.g., if the drip chamber is set at 20 cm H_2O, then the ICP should not exceed approximately 15 mm Hg).
- The type of IVC used varies based on the clinical situation (i.e., size of child's ventricles and the need for ICP monitoring). It may be a fluid-coupled device, fiberoptic transducer tipped catheter, or microprocessor device.
  - ❖ Fluid-coupled system: The IVC is connected to an external transducer if ICP monitoring is indicated.
    - ○ Simultaneous ICP monitoring and CSF drainage is *not possible* with fluid-coupled systems
    - ○ Options for ICP monitoring and CSF drainage for this type of system include:
      - • Continuous CSF drainage with intermittent ICP monitoring
      - • Continuous ICP monitoring with intermittent CSF drainage
  - ❖ Fiber optic catheters or catheters with a microprocessing unit are stiff fragile IVCs that have a sensor on the tip of the catheter for ICP monitoring. Fiberoptic

IVCs allow simultaneous measurement of ICP and CSF drainage.
- Normal ICP ranges from 0 to 15 mm Hg (or 0 to 20 cm H_2O).[1]
- CSF comprises 7% to 10% of the intracranial volume (see Procedure 79 for a review of CSF flow, rate, distribution, and characteristics).
- See Procedure 76 for a review of the following concepts:
  - ❖ Monro-Kellie doctrine
  - ❖ Compensatory mechanisms to maintain a stable ICP
  - ❖ Autoregulation
  - ❖ Normal ICP measurements in the infant, young child, and adolescent
  - ❖ Intracranial hypertension
  - ❖ Conditions that increase ICP
  - ❖ Indications for ICP monitoring in children
  - ❖ Methods of ICP monitoring
  - ❖ Types of ICP monitoring catheters and transducers
  - ❖ Normal and abnormal ICP waveforms
  - ❖ Recommendations for the management of increased ICP
- Cerebral perfusion pressure is the difference between the mean arterial pressure (MAP) and the ICP and is calculated with the following formula: CPP = MAP − ICP.
- The CPP must be maintained above a certain level to prevent cerebral ischemia. Accepted normal values are[1,2,4,7]:
  - ❖ Adults: CPP > 70 mm Hg
  - ❖ Children: CPP > 50 to 60 mm Hg
  - ❖ Infants/toddlers: CPP > 40 to 50 mm Hg
- A CPP less than the age-appropriate range indicates hypoperfusion of the brain.
- The goals of management of increased ICP are to:
  - ❖ Maintain effective cerebral perfusion through maintenance of adequate systemic perfusion and control of ICP
  - ❖ Preserve cerebral function
  - ❖ Prevent secondary injury to the brain
- Child development as it relates to clinical assessment and IVC placement
- Principles of aseptic technique
- Informed consent is required before placement of an IVC
- Mastery of pediatric advanced life support competencies
- Appropriate pediatric dosing of analgesics and competency in procedural sedation
- Selection and use of developmentally appropriate pain scale (see Procedure 173 for more information)

CHILD AND FAMILY ASSESSMENT

- Baseline vital signs ➟*Rationale:* Baseline vital signs are essential to detect changes that may occur.
- Child's baseline neurologic status, including signs of increased ICP (see Procedure 76) ➟*Rationale:* Establishes a baseline level before procedure. Children are at risk for intracranial hypertension and herniation. If the child has signs of increased ICP, this procedure becomes a medical emergency.

- Child's baseline developmental level and ability to interact ➤*Rationale:* Identifies current variation from child's usual baseline; influences preparation of the child and interaction.
- Signs of infection: Temperature >38.5°C; complete blood count (CBC; particularly white blood cell [WBC] and differential) ➤*Rationale:* Child is at risk for development of infection because of breakdown in normal barrier defense mechanism.
- Current laboratory profile, including CBC, prothrombin time (PT), and partial thromboplastin time (PTT) ➤*Rationale:* Establishes baseline values and identifies abnormalities before procedure.
- Child's and family's (as appropriate) understanding of the reasons for and risks and benefits of the procedure ➤*Rationale:* Evaluates child's and family's understanding of the procedure and provides a gauge for ongoing education.
- Desire of family members to remain with the child during procedure ➤*Rationale:* Family's presence may provide support and comfort to the child during the procedure if institution-specific protocol facilitates family presence; family members should also have the choice not to remain with the child.

CHILD AND FAMILY EDUCATION

Individualized, developmentally appropriate education is provided to the child and to the family based on desire for knowledge, readiness to learn, and overall neurologic and psychosocial state.

- Provide the family with information about IVC placement, including the reason for placement, basic functions, and care of the IVC ➤*Rationale:* Providing information decreases anxiety and fear.
- Explain the importance of preventing any disconnection of the IVC/drainage system or movement of child above or below the predetermined height of the CSF drainage system ➤*Rationale:* Moving the child above the CSF drainage system or disconnection of the system causes rapid drainage of CSF from the ventricular system. Moving the child below predetermined level for the drainage system prevents CSF from draining.
- Explain the need to assess the child's neurologic status frequently and the expected outcome of IVC placement ➤*Rationale:* Providing information decreases the child's and family's anxiety and fear.
- Provide the family with information about the monitoring system, including alarms; assure the family that alarm status is monitored by staff at all times ➤*Rationale:* Assuring the family that alarms are monitored and responded to quickly may decrease anxiety.

- Reassure the child and family that adequate pain relief is provided throughout the procedure ➤*Rationale:* Providing information may decrease family's fears related to inadequate pain control.
- If family desires to stay during procedure and institution-specific protocol permits family presence, provide family with accurate information regarding procedure, family's role, and expectations ➤*Rationale:* The family is prepared and clearly defined guidelines and expectations are provided.
- Encourage questions and answer questions as they arise ➤*Rationale:* Reinforcement of information is needed during periods of stress and is especially important if IVC placement is performed emergently.

EQUIPMENT

- Local anesthetic (lidocaine 1%)
- Intracranial access kit (see Procedure 75, Figure 75-4, and Box 75-1 for cranial access kit contents)
- External CSF drainage system
- Pole mount bracket
- Intravenous (IV) pole
- Sterile gloves and surgical gowns
- Surgical caps and masks
- Sterile occlusive dressing (sterile 4×4 gauze pads)
- Emergency cart with emergency medications and airway equipment
- If monitoring ICP:
  ❖ Bedside monitor
  ❖ For fluid-coupled system with extracranial transducer:
    ○ Ventricular catheter
    ○ Noncompliant pressure tubing
    ○ Three-way stopcock
    ○ Preservative-free 0.9% saline solution (NS)
    ○ External strain gauge transducer
    ○ Transducer cable
    ○ "No-flush" transducer set-up (stopcock on end, primed with preservative-free NS)
  ❖ For fiberoptic transducer tipped catheter or sensor system with intracranial transducer:
    ○ Ventricular catheter
    ○ Microprocessor/ICP monitor
    ○ Preamp connector cable
    ○ Cable to connect microprocessor/ICP monitor to bedside monitor
  Note: Depending on manufacturer and institution-specific equipment, kits may come assembled with all necessary supplies.

Procedure for Intraventricular Catheter: Insertion Assist, Monitoring, and Care

Steps	Rationale	Considerations
1. Ensure child and family understand procedure and questions are answered.	Evaluates and reinforces understanding of previously taught information.	Developmental level, cognitive ability, and anxiety level determine approach to and effectiveness of teaching.
2. Confirm presence of informed consent. *(Level II*)*	Ensures medical-legal compliance as suggested by the Joint Commission on Accreditation of Healthcare Organizations (JCAHO).	In emergency situations, follow institution-specific protocol for assumption of consent.
3. Wash hands. *(Level VI*)*	Standard precautions; reduces transmission of microorganisms.	
4. Ensure appropriate cardiorespiratory and hemodynamic monitoring is in place with appropriate alarm limits set and alarms activated.	Child may decompensate during procedure.	Observe bedside monitor and obtain frequent vital signs during procedure. Emergency equipment should be readily available.
5. Assemble necessary equipment and supplies.	Facilitates completion of procedure in a timely fashion.	
6. Identify child with appropriate patient and procedure verification process (e.g., "Time out") *(Level II*)*	Confirms correct patient, procedure, and site as recommended by JCAHO; prevents unnecessary medical procedures.	Verification process and documentation is institution specific. Use active communication techniques.
7. Put on personal protective equipment as appropriate; wash hands, put on clean or sterile gloves as indicated.	Standard precautions; reduces transmission of microorganisms.	Garb required of individuals in the room during catheter insertion varies from institution to institution; refer to institution-specific protocol.
8. Assess child's pain with pain scale appropriate to child's age and developmental level. Administer pain or sedation medications as appropriate and per prescribing practitioner's order.	Promotes child's comfort during procedure; facilitates completion of procedure.	
9. Assist practitioner who is inserting catheter with establishing sterile field and preparing equipment.	Aseptic technique protects child from exposure to microorganisms and contamination of the surgical site, reducing likelihood of infection.	
10. Assist practitioner with preparing child for catheter placement, including administration of local anesthetic; maintain sterile field.	Aseptic technique protects child from exposure to microorganisms and contamination of the surgical site, reducing likelihood of infection.	
If ICP is to be Measured with a Fluid-Coupled System:		
11. Assemble transducer and tubing; flush with preservative-free NS to remove all air; label appropriately. *(Level II*)*	Preservative-free NS must be used to prevent damage to nervous system tissue.[1]	Air in the transducer system can delay the procedure as a result of malfunction. Heparin is not used because of risk of intracranial bleeding.

Procedure continues on following page

* Level II: Theory based, no research data to support recommendations; recommendations from expert consensus group may exist
  Level VI: Clinical studies in a variety of patient populations and situations to support recommendations

Procedure   for Intraventricular Catheter: Insertion Assist, Monitoring, and Care—*Continued*

Steps	Rationale	Considerations
12. Place sterile cap on transducer after flush is instilled or clamp transducer tubing if NS bag or syringe is left attached. If syringe is left in place, ensure syringe is appropriately labeled. *(Level II*)*	Dead-end cap must be placed on tubing to prevent air from entering the system, which can dampen the waveform.[1,2,4] Dead-end cap or labeling of fluid and clamp closure must be used to prevent inadvertent flushing of the fluid-filled system into the ventricular space.	Leaving NS bag connected is not generally recommended because inadvertent administration of fluid into the ventricle may result in increased ICP or bleeding.[2]
13. Once catheter is inserted, connect transducer tubing to IVC.	Establishes fluid column, which transmits signal to monitor to display waveform and pressure reading.	
14. Level air-fluid interface per institution-specific protocol or prescribing practitioner's order (e.g., external auditory meatus)[1,2,4] *(Level IV*)*	Levels transducer to foramen of Monro, reference point for ICP, ensuring accurate pressure readings.	Landmarks used to locate the formen of Monro include the outer canthus of the eye, tragus of the ear, and external auditory meatus. Regardless of reference point used, the same reference point must be consistently used to level the ICP transducer.[1,2] Level of the transducer must be readjusted with each position change to ensure accurate ICP readings.
15. Open transducer to atmospheric pressure and zero to monitor per manufacturer's instructions. *(Level IV*)*	Zeroing to atmospheric pressure is necessary to ensure accurate pressure reading.[2]	

If ICP is to be Measured with a Catheter Tip Transducer:

Steps	Rationale	Considerations
16. Turn on ICP monitor specific to the catheter being inserted.	Catheter must be used with brand-specific monitor. Confirms monitor is functioning.	
17. Assist practitioner who is inserting catheter with connection of monitor to fiberoptic/microprocessor catheter.	Allows practitioner to maintain sterility without interruption of sterile field.	Maintain monitor cable away from sterile field during remainder of procedure. Catheter is fragile; avoid kinking catheter.
18. Zero catheter before insertion according to manufacturer's instructions. *(Level I*)*	Catheter must be zeroed to atmospheric pressure before insertion into cranium to ensure accuracy of ICP readings.[1,2]	Catheter with intracranial transducer is zeroed once, before insertion. It does not need, or allow, repeated zero procedures after insertion.
19. If technology is available, connect intracranial pressure monitor to bedside monitor.	Allows waveform and numeric display, correlation of ICP data with other hemodynamic measurements, and tracking of data via bedside and central monitor.	Bedside monitor must have ICP monitoring capability specific to intracranial catheter tip transducer in use.
20. Calibrate the ICP monitor to the bedside monitor according to manufacturer's directions. *(Level I*)*	Required for accurate data transmission to bedside monitor from catheter tip transducer monitor; ensures ICP readings and CPP calculations from bedside monitor are correct.	Calibration can be performed at any time but at a minimum of each shift. Calibration should also be done when any disconnection of the two monitors occurs.

* Level I: Manufacturer's recommendations only

Level II: Theory based, no research data to support recommendations; recommendations from expert consensus group may exist

Level IV: Limited clinical studies to support recommendations

Procedure | **for Intraventricular Catheter: Insertion Assist, Monitoring, and Care**—*Continued*

Steps	Rationale	Considerations
21. If available, turn on CPP parameter of bedside monitor.	The ICP and MAP data are used to automatically calculate CPP.	Arterial line is required for automatic calculation of CPP.
22. Assist practitioner with identification of optimal area for IVC placement.	Placement is usually preferred in the nondominant hemisphere unless contraindicated.	
23. Assist practitioner with IVC placement.	Facilitates procedure completion.	The IVC is usually sutured in place.
24. Assist practitioner with or apply sterile occlusive dressing over catheter insertion site. *(Level II*)*	Prevents contamination of insertion site by wet, soiled, or loose dressing.	
25. If IVC is to be connected to external drainage system, review prescribing practitioner's order for level of drip chamber. Note: A typical order is to place the drip chamber 10 cm H$_2$O above the external auditory meatus or other consistent reference point (e.g., outer canthus of eye, phlebostatic axis).	Proper leveling of the drip chamber in relation to the child's catheter is essential to prevent overdrainage or underdrainage of CSF.	The level of the drip chamber must be readjusted with each position change to prevent underdrainage or overdrainage of CSF.
26. Prepare the external drainage system. Prime the system using sterile technique with sterile NS from the patient stopcock through to the drip chamber. Verify absence of leaks and that the fluid flows freely to the drainage bag; assist practitioner to connect drainage system to the IVC.	Verify that all connections are secure (e.g., stopcocks).	CSF leakage can occur if connections are not secured.
27. Assess for presence of CSF drainage. See Procedure 80.	Assesses patency and functioning of system.	CSF drainage may not be present in the case of small or slit ventricles.
28. Connect to ICP monitoring system; for external transducer system, orient stopcocks to provide drainage per prescribing practitioner's order (continuous or intermittent drainage).	Required to monitor ICP and display waveform. If continuous drainage is ordered, stopcock is open to child, and drainage system off to transducer. If intermittent drainage is ordered, stopcock is open to child and transducer, off to drainage system.	See Procedure 80 for further discussion of this topic.
29. Obtain opening ICP. *(Level IV*)*	Initial ICP reading determines need to institute immediate management of increased ICP. Provides baseline and facilitates trending of ICP readings.	
30. Assess ICP waveform, including morphology.	Presence of ICP waveform and CSF drainage indicates adequate placement of IVC.	See Figures 76-1, 76-2, and 76-3 in Procedure 76 for ICP waveform assessment and interpretation.
31. If measuring ICP, calculate CPP and record every hour.	Evaluates cerebral perfusion.	
32. Consider application of whole head dressing per institution-specific protocol or inserting practitioner's preference.	Protects catheter and insertion site.	

Procedure continues on following page

* Level II: Theory-based; no research data to support recommendations; recommendations from expert consensus group may exist
  Level IV: Limited clinical studies to support recommendations

Procedure for Intraventricular Catheter: Insertion Assist, Monitoring, and Care—*Continued*

Steps	Rationale	Considerations
33. Discard used supplies and equipment, including sharps, in appropriate receptacles.	Standard precautions; reduces transmission of microorganisms. Protects personnel health.	
34. Remove personal protective equipment; wash hands.	Standard precautions.	
35. Evaluate child's neurological examination results.	Identifies changes that occurred during procedure.	

Expected Outcomes

- CSF is drained appropriately (if drainage is instituted)

- The IVC remains in place until electively removed
- The ICP remains within desired range of 0 to 15 mm Hg; CPP remains at more than 50 mm Hg
- Accurate reliable ICP data, including appropriate waveform, ICP value, and CPP calculation obtained

- Child's neurologic examination remains stable throughout procedure
- Child remains free from complications of IVC placement

- Child has acceptable level of comfort throughout procedure
- Prompt management of any acute changes in ICP

Unexpected Outcomes

- Minimal or excessive CSF drainage due to improper position of external drainage system
- CSF does not drain because of improper IVC placement
- CSF does not drain because IVC is plugged with brain tissue or sediment
- Inadvertent dislodgement of IVC
- The ICP is consistently more than 20 mm Hg with CPP less than 50 mm Hg
- Equipment failure, including damaged catheter
- For fluid-coupled system, incorrect placement of external transducer results in inaccurate values
- For fluid-coupled system, dampened waveform from air in system
- Deterioration of neurologic examination

- Infection from break in aseptic technique during IVC insertion
- Hemorrhage
- Herniation
- Unmanaged pain or agitation

- Acute changes in ICP are not recognized and treated

Monitoring and Care of the Child

Activities and Interventions	Rationale	Reportable Conditions
1. Monitor child's neurologic status, including pupillary response to light, motor response, and vital signs before, during, and after procedure.	Identifies changes in neurologic condition occurring during procedure; facilitates prompt response.	• Changes in neurologic status
2. Maintain child's position with head of bed elevated to 30 degrees and head midline.	Facilitates cerebral blood drainage.	• Elevated ICP despite appropriate head position
3. Assess ICP hourly. Hourly charting should include documentation of highest ICP for that hour and the mean ICP at the time of vital sign assessment. Specify whether abnormal ICP reading occurs only with stimulation (e.g., suctioning). (*Level II**)	The ICP is a critical component of a complete neurologic assessment. Maintenance of ICP at less than 20 mm Hg or at specified value per prescribing practitioner's order is important to prevent further intracranial injury.	• Elevated ICP or ICP reading deviating from child's "normal" values • Sustained ICP at more than 20 mm Hg or predetermined level

* Level II: Theory-based; no research data to support recommendations; recommendations from expert consensus group may exist

Monitoring and Care of the Child—Cont'd

Activities and Interventions	Rationale	Reportable Conditions
4. Assess ICP waveform trends at least hourly and as needed; assess waveform for: Normal morphology Dampening of waveform Abnormal waveforms	Identifies abnormal waveforms. Dampening of the ICP waveform in a fluid-coupled system may indicate an air bubble in the system or malposition of the catheter. Dampening in a fiberoptic catheter may indicate malfunction or significant change in cerebral compliance. See Figures 76-1, 76-2 and 76-3 in Procedure 76 for more information and figures of abnormal wave forms.	• P2 elevations • A or B waveform trends • No numeric display on transducer tip catheter monitor • No waveform after troubleshooting
5. Calculate and record CPP hourly and as needed.	The CPP indirectly measures cerebral blood flow and is dependent on an adequate MAP to maintain adequate cerebral perfusion. Because MAP values vary with age, maintenance of a CPP appropriate for age is important.	• CPP less than 40 to 70 mm Hg or per prescribing practitioner's order
6. Check integrity, stability, and sterility of IVC and dressing at least hourly and with position changes.	All IVCs require hourly assessment of system to ensure accuracy and safety of ICP monitoring and prevent contamination by microorganisms leading to infection. All connections on the extracranial fluid-coupled IVC system should be clamped and secured with tape to prevent inadvertent instillation of NS into the ventricular system. Whenever the child's position changes, the possibility of disruption of system exists.[1,2,4]	• Loss of integrity of ICP monitoring system • CSF leaking around IVC • Fluid instilled into ventricles
7. Fluid-coupled system: Level and maintain transducer at the anatomic reference point for the foramen of Monro *(Level II*)*	Correct leveling of the transducer ensures accurate readings.[1,2]	• Incorrect leveling of transducer resulting in inaccurate readings
8. Fluid-coupled system: Zero transducer every 8 hours or at frequency indicated in institution-specific protocol and after repositioning of the child or external transducer; calibrate monitor if necessary. *(Level IV*)*	Zeroing uses atmospheric pressure as the zero reference point for the monitor and ensures the accuracy of ICP readings. Periodic zeroing minimizes the effect of zero drift.[2]	• Inability to zero system
9. Monitor volume and character of CSF drainage hourly or as indicated. Ensure stopcocks that regulate drainage are correctly oriented; if stopcock is temporarily closed to drainage for intermittent ICP reading, ensure it is reopened; if stopcock is temporarily opened to drainage bag for intermittent drainage, ensure it is reclosed.	CSF drainage may be ordered continuously or intermittently. Any significant change in amount of CSF drainage, particularly no drainage, could indicate a change in the child's status. Brain tissue, blood clots, or sediment may occlude drainage system.[8-10]	• Volume of CSF drained exceeds desired hourly volume per notification parameters in prescribing practitioner's order • Drainage system appears blocked, does not drain • Cerebrospinal fluid becomes blood-tinged • Substantial amount of blood, brain tissue, or sediment noted in IVC or drainage system
10. Assess integrity of occlusive site dressing or head dressing.	Prevents dislodgement and contamination of insertion site by wet, soiled, or loose dressing.	• Drainage at IVC site or on head dressing

---

* Level II: Theory-based; no research data to support recommendations; recommendations from expert consensus group may exist
Level IV: Limited clinical studies to support recommendations

Continued

Monitoring and Care of the Child—Cont'd

Activities and Interventions	Rationale	Reportable Conditions
Change insertion site dressing and head dressing per institution-specific protocol or prescribing practitioner's order.	Responsibility for changing dressings and site care varies depending on institution.	
11. With aseptic technique, change CSF drainage system per institution-specific protocol or prescribing practitioner's order.	Limits risk of infection at insertion site and within ventricular system. No data identify optimal frequency for changing ICP monitoring system. Recommendations vary from not interrupting the integrity of the system at all to changing ICP monitoring setup every 24, 48, or 72 hours.[7,11]	• IVC dislodgement • Full CSF drainage bag
12. Obtain CSF specimens for specified laboratory evaluation from CSF drainage system per institution-specific protocol or prescribing practitioner's order (see Procedure 83).	Assessment of CSF is important in the diagnosis of possible infection. Insufficient data exist to support frequency of routine CSF sampling and evaluation; recommendations are to follow institution-specific protocol concerning frequency of routine CSF sampling.[1,2,4,11]	• Results of CSF indicative of infection (elevated white blood cell count, elevated protein, and decreased glucose) • Abnormal gram stain and culture
13. Set appropriate alarm limits for ICP and CPP based on child's baseline, prescribing practitioner's order, or institution-specific protocol.	ICP limits should default to normal age values (e.g., 0 to 15 mm Hg) but should be adapted based on child's average ICP readings. Provides notification of CSF collection chamber being dropped.	• Values outside identified parameters • Alarm activation from drop in position of CSF drainage system and increased CSF drainage
14. Prevent inadvertent dislodgement of IVC with repeated age-appropriate explanations, sedation, analgesia, and family assistance as appropriate. Encourage family to use developmentally appropriate measures to support and comfort the child.	Dislodgement of IVC may result in need for additional procedure, infection, or pneumocephaly.	• Device dislodgement • Agitation unresponsive to interventions

Documentation

- Child and family education
- Patient and procedure verification process per institution-specific protocol
- Date and time of IVC insertion, type of catheter placed (e.g., fiberoptic), and individual who placed IVC
- Description of the color, clarity, and characteristics of CSF
- Opening pressure and waveform description at time of IVC insertion
- Type of dressing applied
- Level of transducer and external drainage bag, as applicable
- Child's tolerance of procedure
- Interventions to decrease ICP and child's response to therapy
- Hourly assessment of CSF drainage; volume, color, and clarity
- Hourly assessment of ICP reading and CPP
- Hourly assessment of child's neurologic examination
- Comfort assessment and any specific interventions provided
- Routine assessment of integrity of dressing
- Dressing and tubing changes
- Protective/restraint devices in use and associated assessments per institution-specific protocol
- Date, time of IVC removal, and individual who removed IVC
- Unexpected outcomes and related treatment

References

1. Vernon-Levett P: Intracranial dynamics. In Curley MAQ, Moloney-Harmon PA, editors: *Critical care nursing of infants and children,* ed 2, Philadelphia, 2001, Saunders.
2. March K: Intracranial pressure monitoring: why monitor? *AACN Clin Iss* 16(4):456-475, 2005.
3. Adelson PD, et al: The role of cerebrospinal fluid drainage in the treatment of severe pediatric traumatic brain injury, *Pediatr Crit Care Med* (4)3:s38-s39, 2003.
4. Hickey JV: Intracranial hypertension: theory and management of increased intracranial pressure. In Hickey JV, editor: *The clinical practice of neurological and neurosurgical nursing,* ed 5, Philadelphia, 2003, Lippincott Williams & Wilkins.
5. Tasker RC, Czosnyka M: Intracranial hypertension and brain monitoring. In Fuhrman BP, Zimmerman J, editors: *Pediatric critical care,* ed 3, Philadelphia, 2006, Mosby.
6. Shore PM, et al: Continuous versus intermittent cerebrospinal fluid drainage after sever traumatic brain injury in children: effect on biochemical markers, *J Neurotrauma* 21(9):1113-1122, 2004.
7. Adelson PD, et al: Cerebral perfusion pressure, *Pediatr Crit Care Med* (4)3:s31-s33, 2003.
8. Adelson PD, et al: Use of hyperosmolar therapy in the management of severe traumatic brain injury; guidelines for the acute medical management of severe traumatic brain injury in infants, children, and adolescents, *Pediatr Crit Care Med* 4(3 supp):s40-s44, 2003.
9. Adelson PD, et al: Threshold for treatment of intracranial hypertension; guidelines for the acute medical management of severe traumatic brain injury in infants, children, and adolescents, *Pediatr Crit Care Med* 4(3 supp):s25-s30, 2003.
10. American Association of Neuroscience Nurses: Intracranial pressure monitoring. In Bader MK, Littlejohns LL, editors: *AANN core curriculum for neuroscience nursing,* ed 4, Philadelphia, 2004, Saunders.
11. Sullivan J: Intracranial bolt insertion (assist), monitoring, care, troubleshooting, and removal. In Lynn-McHale DJ, Carlson KK, editors: *AACN procedure manual for critical care,* ed 4, Philadelphia, 2001, Saunders.

Jugular Venous Saturation Monitoring: Insertion Assist, Monitoring, and Care

P U R P O S E : Jugular venous catheters and the monitoring of jugular venous oxygen saturation (Sjvo$_2$) are used to monitor cerebral blood flow and cerebral metabolism. This information is used to direct care after injury to cerebral tissue and to treat the ensuing sequelae.

Andrea J. Velasco

PREREQUISITE KNOWLEDGE

- Knowledge of pediatric neuroanatomy and physiology
- Knowledge of intracranial pressure (ICP) monitoring and management of increased ICP
- Principles of hemodynamic monitoring
- Secondary injury to brain tissue is caused by hypoxemia and ischemia.
- Damage to brain tissue causes dysfunction in the autoregulatory mechanisms of the brain, which maintain and control cerebral perfusion, and thereby increases the chances of secondary injury.[1]
- The area of the jugular vein just below the skull is bulbous and contains drained cerebral blood. Placement of a catheter into this area allows for measurement of the oxygen saturation after cerebral perfusion has occurred and is an indicator of cerebral oxygenation.[2]
- Jugular venous oxygen saturation monitoring may be helpful in children with increased ICP, potential for cerebral ischemia, or impairment of cerebral perfusion.[3]
- The Sjvo$_2$ catheter is placed in the right jugular vein, which usually drains most of the cerebral blood, or ipsilateral to the site of injury.[4,5] The catheter is inserted in a retrograde fashion, and placement is verified radiographically. The ideal placement of the tip of the catheter is just below the jugular foramen in the bulbous region; hence, the term "jugular bulb" (Figure 78-1).[2] Placement is

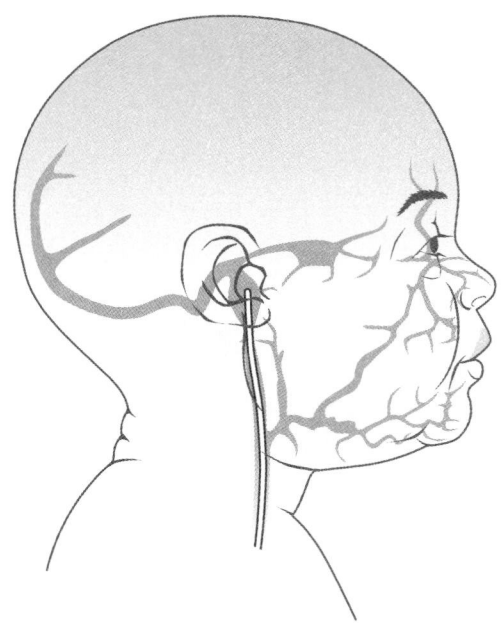

FIGURE 78-1 Placement of Jugular Bulb Venous Catheter. Note tip of catheter is located in jugular bulb. *From Kidd KC, Criddle L: Using jugular venous catheters in patients with traumatic brain injury,* Crit Care Nurs *21(6):18, 2001.*

confirmed via head or neck x-ray; the catheter tip should be above C1, just posterior to the mastoid process.[3-5]

- Catheters used to measure $Sjvo_2$ are available with or without fiberoptic capabilities and are available as small as 3F. $Sjvo_2$ can be monitored intermittently or continuously with an oximetry catheter and a system such as the Vigilance or Explorer monitor (Edwards Lifesciences, Irvine, CA).
- $Sjvo_2$ indicates global perfusion and does not indicate areas of focal injury.[3-5]
- $Sjvo_2$ is not an absolute indicator of cerebral perfusion, and changes in saturation should be validated with other clinical means (i.e., physical assessment, ICP monitoring) to ensure complete and accurate management of increased ICP and the related sequelae.[3-5]
- $Sjvo_2$ measurements are used to estimate the amount of oxygen the brain tissue extracts and the amount of blood the brain tissue receives. The measurement technique is analogous to the way in which a pulmonary artery catheter is used to estimate cardiac output.[2,4]
- The currently accepted normal range of $Sjvo_2$ is 55% to 70%.[4-6]
- Increases in $Sjvo_2$ above 70% warrant investigation and may indicate an increase in cerebral blood flow or a decrease in cerebral oxygen demand (i.e., hypertension, increased tension of arterial carbon dioxide ($Paco_2$), brain tissue death).[4-6]
- Decreases in $Sjvo_2$ below 55% warrant investigation and may indicate a decrease in cerebral blood flow or an increase in cerebral oxygen demand (i.e., hypovolemia, decreased $Paco_2$, hypoxemia, increased ICP, fever, seizure activity, agitation).[4-6]
- The $Sjvo_2$ value is determined with arterial oxygen content saturation (Cao_2), cerebral blood flow, and cerebral oxygen consumption.
- Cerebral oxygen uptake can be indirectly measured with the cerebral extraction of oxygen (Ceo_2) and the arteriovenous jugular oxygen content difference ($AVjDo_2$).
  - ❖ Cerebral oxygen extraction ratio is expressed as $Ceo_2 = (Sao_2 - Sjvo_2)/Sao_2$. The normal ratio is 0.4, which means the brain extracts 40% of the oxygen that is delivered. If the saturation of blood delivered is 100%

and the brain extracts 40% of that oxygen, the returning blood (jugular venous blood) should have a saturation of 60%.[2]
  - ❖ The $AVjDo_2$ calculation necessitates both arterial and jugular blood gas analysis: $AVjDo_2$ (mL/dL) = arterial oxygen content saturation (Cao_2) − jugular venous oxygen content saturation ($Cjvo_2$).
  - ❖ An increase in $AVjo_2$ or Ceo_2 indicates increased oxygen uptake in the brain.
  - ❖ A decrease in $AVjo_2$ or Ceo_2 indicates decreased oxygen uptake in the brain.
  - ❖ Table 78-1 has further information.
- To ensure accuracy of oxygen saturation measurements, blood should be withdrawn slowly from the catheter at a rate of 1 mL/min. This technique avoids contamination of the sample from extracranial blood that also drains into the jugular vein.[1,3,4]
- Rotation of the child's head or neck or improper position of the catheter within the jugular vein may result in inaccurate measurements. Other factors that may affect accuracy include hemoglobin concentration, systemic arterial oxygen saturation, core temperature, and CO_2 levels. Verification of accuracy of catheter readings is important before intervention.[3-5]
- Contraindications to placement of an $Sjvo_2$ catheter include local neck infection at insertion site, impaired venous drainage, jugular venous occlusion or malformation, and local neck trauma. Relative contraindications include coagulopathy, brain stem injury, cervical spine injury, and presence of tracheostomy.[4,5]
- Complications of placement of an $Sjvo_2$ catheter include pneumothorax, carotid artery puncture, nerve injury, thrombosis, infection, and increased ICP from obstruction of venous return.[3-5]
- Principles of aseptic technique
- Child development as it relates to clinical assessment and $Sjvo_2$ monitoring
- Appropriate dosing of pediatric analgesia and competency in procedural sedation
- Mastery of pediatric advanced life support competencies
- Informed consent is required for placement of an $Sjvo_2$ catheter.

TABLE 78-1	Normal and Abnormal Measurements of $Sjvo_2$ Monitoring	
Measurement	**Normal Values**	**Abnormal Values**
$Sjvo_2$	55% to 70%	<55%: Indicates cerebral hypoperfusion >70%: Indicates "luxury perfusion"
$AVjDo_2$	3.5 to 8.1 mL/dL	Increased value indicates increase in oxygen uptake by cerebral cells Decreased value indicates decrease in oxygen uptake by cerebral cells
Ceo_2	24% to 42%	Increased value indicates increase in oxygen uptake by cerebral cells Decreased value indicates decrease in oxygen uptake by cerebral cells

Adapted from Sullivan J: Jugular bulb oxygenation monitoring. In Lynn-McHale DJ, Carlson K, editors: *AACN procedure manual for critical care*, ed 4, Philadelphia, 2001, Saunders.

CHILD AND FAMILY ASSESSMENT

- Child's neurologic status, including ICP ➤➤*Rationale:* Provides a baseline assessment used to determine effects of the procedure or placement of catheter. Provides information used to determine appropriate preparation of the child and need for sedation or analgesia.
- Child's and family's understanding of the reasons for and risks and benefits of the procedure ➤➤*Rationale:* Evaluates child's and family's understanding of the procedure and provides a gauge for ongoing education; facilitates informed consent.
- Condition of area for catheter insertion and surrounding structures for signs of trauma or infection ➤➤*Rationale:* Infection and neck trauma are contraindications for catheter placement.
- Obtain laboratory data, including complete blood count (CBC), platelet count, prothrombin time (PT), partial thromboplastin time (PTT), bleeding time, and international normalized ratio (INR) ➤➤*Rationale:* Presence of coagulopathies is a contraindication for catheter placement; abnormal values warrant close observation once catheter is placed.
- Desire of family members to remain with the child during procedure ➤➤*Rationale:* Family may provide support and comfort to the child during the procedure if institution-specific protocol facilitates family presence, however, family should have the choice not to remain with the child.

CHILD AND FAMILY EDUCATION

Individualized, developmentally appropriate education is provided to the family and to the child based on desire for knowledge, readiness to learn, and overall neurologic and psychosocial state.

- Provide information concerning the purpose for and expected outcomes of the jugular catheter ➤➤*Rationale:* Providing information decreases fear and anxiety.
- Explain the process involved with insertion, monitoring, and care of the catheter ➤➤*Rationale:* Explanation of the process and open communication provide opportunities for questions and clarification and understanding of plan of care.

- Describe appearance of the catheter after insertion ➤➤*Rationale:* Providing information may decrease fear and anxiety; information provided in advance promotes successful coping.
- Provide the family with information about the monitoring system, including alarms; assure the family that alarm status is monitored at all times ➤➤*Rationale:* Assuring family that alarms are monitored and responded to quickly may decrease anxiety.
- If family desires to stay with the child during the procedure and institution-specific protocol permits family presence, provide family with accurate information regarding procedure, family's role, and expectations ➤➤*Rationale:* Presence of family may provide support and comfort to the child, and clearly defined institution-specific protocol for family presence facilitates this.
- Encourage questions and answer questions as they arise ➤➤*Rationale:* Reinforcement of information is needed during periods of stress.

EQUIPMENT

- Surgical caps and gowns
- Sterile gloves
- Sterile drapes and towels
- Masks and protective eye wear
- 2% Chlorhexidine gluconate solution[3] or institution-specific skin antiseptic solution
- Local anesthetic: 1% or 2% lidocaine without epinephrine
- Three Luer lock 5-mL syringes
- Needle for withdrawal of lidocaine from vial
- 23-gauge or 25-gauge needle for administration of lidocaine
- Catheter to be inserted; generally 3F or 4F, with or without fiberoptic capabilities per inserting practitioner's preference
- Central venous catheter insertion tray, if supplies are not provided with catheter
- Optical module and associated cable and oximetric monitor if fiberoptic catheter used
- Flush solution per prescribing practitioner's order or institution-specific protocol
- Pressure tubing system with transducer
- Sterile occlusive central venous catheter dressing

Procedure | for Jugular Venous Saturation Monitoring: Insertion Assist

Steps	Rationale	Considerations
1. Ensure child and family understand procedure and questions are answered.	Evaluates and reinforces understanding of previously taught information.	Developmental level, cognitive ability, and anxiety level determine approach to and effectiveness of teaching.
2. Gather needed equipment and supplies.	Facilitates completion of task in a timely manner.	Determine whether catheter requested is to have fiberoptic capabilities for continuous monitoring of Sjvo$_2$.
3. Confirm that consent for procedure has been obtained.	Ensures medical-legal compliance as suggested by the Joint Commission on Accreditation of Healthcare Organizations (JCAHO).	For emergency situations, implement institution-specific protocol for assumption of consent.
4. Wash hands.	Standard precautions; reduces transmission of microorganisms.	
5. Prepare pressure monitoring system using aseptic technique. Prime tubing with heparinized 0.9% saline solution or flush solution per institution-specific protocol. Connect to monitoring cable and system.	Ensures that system is available and functioning before catheter insertion. Aseptic technique ensures sterility of system.	Assess pressure monitoring tubing for air bubbles and remove any air to prevent possible air emboli. See Procedure 137 for further information on priming transducer set-up.
6. If indicated, prepare oximetric monitor; turn on power and calibrate according to manufacturer's instructions.	Assures proper functioning and set-up of monitor before procedure.	Not all catheters require calibration before catheter insertion; care should be taken to follow manufacturer's instructions to ensure proper catheter functioning.
7. Ensure appropriate cardiorespiratory and hemodynamic monitoring is in place with appropriate alarm limits set and alarms activated.	Child may decompensate during procedure.	Observe bedside monitor and obtain frequent vital signs during procedure. Emergency equipment should be readily available.
8. Identify child with appropriate patient and procedure verification process (e.g., "Time out"). *(Level II*)*	Confirms correct patient, procedure, and site as recommended by JCAHO; prevents unnecessary medical procedures.	Verification process and documentation is institution specific. Use active communication techniques.
9. Place the child's head midline with the head of bed elevated to 30 degrees.[7] *(Level IV*)*	Ensures optimal positioning of jugular vasculature, allowing proper drainage of cerebral blood.	
10. Document vital signs after placing head in midline position. Include blood pressure, ICP, and cerebral perfusion pressure (CPP).	Provides a baseline to compare significant changes during positioning, sedation, and catheter placement.	
11. Assess child's pain with age-appropriate and developmentally appropriate pain scale; administer analgesia or sedation per prescribing practitioner's order.	Ensures maximum comfort for child during procedure.	See Procedure 173 for further information.
12. Turn child's head away from the insertion site in a lateral direction. Note vital signs and ICP after repositioning.	Places child in optimal position for catheter insertion; identifies effect positioning has on ICP.	If the child is in a cervical collar or cervical traction, head should remain midline. Catheter placement is possible without optimal positioning.

Procedure continues on following page

Procedure for Jugular Venous Saturation Monitoring: Insertion Assist—*Continued*

Steps	Rationale	Considerations
13. Assist practitioner who is inserting catheter with putting on sterile garb.	Ensures aseptic technique for catheter placement.	Institution-specific protocol indicates appropriate garb for all individuals in the room during catheter placement. See Procedure 140 for more information.
14. Assist with cleansing of insertion 2% chlorhexidine gluconate or other antiseptic solution per institution-specific protocol. *(Level VI*)*	Decreases skin flora at site before drape placement; reduces the chance of microorganism contamination.	Centers for Disease Control and Prevention (CDC) recommend chlorhexidine in children more than 2 months old because it has been shown to decrease risk of catheter-related blood stream infections.
15. Assist with placement of drapes to create sterile field.	Facilitates aseptic technique.	
16. Open sterile insertion tray; practitioner removes sterile tray and places on sterile field. Aseptically place catheter onto sterile field. Aseptically provide sterile flush solution needed for catheter before insertion.	Maintains sterility of field.	Each practitioner has a particular technique for obtaining flush solution for the catheter. Regardless of technique used, aseptic technique is vital.
17. Assist as needed throughout procedure.	Facilitates catheter placement.	See Procedure 140 for more information.
18. Monitor child's vital signs and neurologic status throughout the procedure.	Identifies need for intervention for pain or agitation or change in neurologic status.	When the child's head is placed in a lateral position, an increase in ICP may occur from decreased venous drainage.
19. After catheter has been secured to the skin, flush the catheter; attach the pressure monitoring system to the catheter.	Ensures patency of catheter and proper functioning of system.	Catheter should be flushed slowly as the flow is directed toward the brain.
20. Cover insertion site and catheter with transparent occlusive dressing.[8] *(Level VI*)*	Maintains sterility of insertion site; prevents infection of site and catheter.	Change dressing according to institution-specific protocol. CDC recommendation for transparent occlusive dressing is every 7 days or whenever the dressing is visibly soiled or no longer intact.[8]
21. Level and zero pressure monitoring system; assess waveform.	Leveling and zeroing ensures accurate values are obtained; waveform assessment assists in identification of catheter location.	See Procedure 63 for more information.
22. Set monitor alarms to appropriate settings and activate alarms.	Facilitates prompt identification of abnormal values or problems with system.	
23. Discard used supplies and equipment, including sharps, in appropriate receptacles.	Standard precautions; reduces transmission of microorganisms. Protects personnel health.	
24. Remove protective garb; wash hands.	Standard precautions.	
25. Obtain a lateral head and neck x-ray.[3-5] *(Level II*)*	Verifies proper placement of catheter.	Ideal placement is in the jugular bulb of the internal jugular vein.
26. Obtain a jugular venous blood gas and follow manufacturer's instructions for in vivo calibration of oximetric monitor.[2] *(Level VI*)*	Ensures reliability of $SjvO_2$ monitoring.	All oximetric systems require in vivo calibration.

* Level II: Theory-based; no research data to support recommendations; recommendations from expert consensus group may exist
Level VI: Clinical studies in a variety of patient populations and situations to support recommendations

Expected Outcomes	Unexpected Outcomes
• Accurate and reliable Sjvo$_2$ readings are obtained, allowing accurate analysis of cerebral blood flow	• Inability to obtain readings because of catheter or monitor failure
	• Catheter is not in the internal jugular vein
• Early detection of and intervention for compromise in cerebral blood flow or oxygen delivery	• Compromise in cerebral blood flow or oxygen delivery is undetected
• Child is free from catheter-related complications	• Catheter or insertion site infection
	• Hemorrhage or hematoma at insertion site
	• Jugular venous thrombosis
	• Air embolism
• Catheter is placed without complications	• Puncture of carotid artery
	• Pneumothorax
	• Nerve damage
• Child has acceptable level of comfort throughout procedure	• Unmanaged pain or agitation

Monitoring and Care of the Child

Activities and Interventions	Rationale	Reportable Conditions
1. Monitor and record vital signs and neurologic status immediately after procedure, followed by continuous monitoring.	Provides a baseline; can be used to determine any impedance of cerebral drainage related to catheter. An increase in ICP after Sjvo$_2$ catheter placement may indicate impaired jugular venous outflow.	• ICP values sustained at more than 20 mm Hg for more than 5 minutes • Changes in neurologic status, vital signs, or ICP
2. Monitor and record baseline Sjvo$_2$ after in vivo calibration, followed by continuous monitoring.	Provides a baseline, allowing determination of changes, and may provide direction for treatment.	• Decrease in Sjvo$_2$ below 55% • Increase in Sjvo$_2$ above 70%
3. Level and zero pressure monitoring system per institution-specific protocol.	Ensures accuracy of pressure waveform and pressure monitoring.	• Loss of or change in pressure waveform or dramatic increase or decrease in pressure reading
4. Calibrate Sjvo$_2$ at interval indicated in manufacturer's instructions or when questionable readings are obtained; recommended calibration interval varies significantly among catheter brands.[4,5] *(Level II*)*	Catheter may be lodged against a vessel, or light at end of catheter may malfunction.[4]	• Sjvo$_2$ value outside desired parameters
5. Monitor for Sjvo$_2$ desaturations.	Sjvo$_2$ desaturations indicate decreased cerebral oxygenation and the need for immediate interventions to improve cerebral oxygen delivery and blood flow. Verify desaturation with blood gas analysis.	• Sjvo$_2$ value of less than 55%
6. Monitor insertion site hourly for signs of infection, infiltration, or bleeding.	Ensures early detection of possible complications.	• Excessive bleeding at insertion site • Hematoma • Drainage or redness at insertion site
7. Assess catheter integrity and stability hourly.	Ensures catheter remains in correct location.	• Inadvertent catheter dislodgement
8. Ensure security of tubing and flush system; change tubing and flush solution every 72 hours or per institution-specific protocol. *(Level VI*)*	Minimizes breaks in system; decreases risk of infection.	• Contamination of flush system or fluid

* Level II: Theory-based; no research data to support recommendations; recommendations from expert consensus group may exist
Level VI: Clinical studies in a variety of patient populations and situations to support recommendations

Continued

Monitoring and Care of the Child—Cont'd

Activities and Interventions	Rationale	Reportable Conditions
9. Protect catheter with the use of repeated age-appropriate explanations, sedation, analgesia, and family assistance as appropriate. Encourage family to use developmentally appropriate measures to support and comfort the child. If necessary, implement medical immobilization or restraint devices.	Prevents inadvertent dislodgement of catheter, which may result in hemorrhage or infection; prevents loss of monitoring mechanism.	• Device dislodgement • Agitation unresponsive to interventions

Documentation

- Child and family education
- Presence of informed consent
- Patient and procedure verification process
- Date and time of catheter insertion and individual who placed catheter
- Type and size of catheter placed and insertion site
- Catheter position with x-ray
- Catheter patency and waveform
- Type and amount of flush infused
- Sedation or analgesia administered and child's response
- Baseline and hourly $SjvO_2$ reading
- Assessment of catheter insertion site and dressing
- Neurologic assessment and ICP reading before, during, and after procedure
- Child's tolerance to procedure, including pain assessment before, during, and after procedure
- Hourly neurologic assessment, vital signs, and ICP recording
- Use of medical immobilization/restraint devices and appropriate documentation per institution-specific protocol
- Unexpected outcomes and related treatment

References

1. Clay H: Validity and reliability of the $SjvO_2$ catheter in neurologically impaired patients: a critical review of the literature, *J Neurosci Nurs* 32(4):194-204, 2000.
2. Kidd KC, Criddle L: Using jugular venous catheters in patients with traumatic brain injury, *Crit Care Nurs* 21(6):16-22, 2001.
3. Coplin WM, O'Keefe GE, Grady MS, et al: Accuracy of continuous jugular bulb oximetry in the intensive care unit, *Neurosurgery* 42(3):533-540, 1998.
4. Stevens WJ: Multimodal monitoring: head injury management using $SjvO_2$ and LICOX, *J Neurosci Nurs* 36(6):332-339, 2004.
5. White H, Baker A: Continuous jugular venous oximetry in the neurointensive care unit: a brief review, *Can J Anesthesia* 49(6):623-629, 2002.
6. Perez A, et al: Jugular venous oxygen saturation or arteriovenous difference of lactate content and outcome of children with severe traumatic brain injury, *Pediatr Crit Care Med* 4:33-38, 2003.
7. Adelson PD, et al: Critical pathway for the treatment of established intracranial hypertension in pediatric traumatic brain injury, *Pediatr Crit Care Med* (4)3:s65-67, 2003.
8. Centers for Disease Control and Prevention: Guidelines for the prevention of intravascular catheter related infections, *MMWR* 51(No.RR-10):1-29, 2002.

Additional Readings

Chieregaot A, et al: Normal jugular bulb oxygen saturation, *J Neurol Neurosurg Psychiatr* 74(6):784, 2003.

Haun S, Segeleon JE: Increased intracranial pressure/intracranial pressure monitoring. In Tobias J, editor: *Pediatric critical care: the essentials*, Armonk, NY, 1999, Futura.

Kim M, et al: Estimation of jugular venous O_2 saturation from cerebral oximetry or arterial O_2 saturation during isocapnic hypoxia, *J Clin Monitoring Computing* 16:191-199, 2000.

Pellicer A., et al: Noninvasive continuous monitoring of the effects of head position on brain hemodynamics in ventilated infants, *Pediatrics* 109(3):434-441, 2002.

Souter MJ, Andrews PJD: Validation of the Edslab dual lumen oximetry catheter for continuos monitoring of jugular bulb oxygen saturation after severe head injury, *Br J Anaesthesia* 76:744-746, 1996.

Special Neurologic Procedures

Cerebrospinal Fluid Drainage: Assessment

PURPOSE: Cerebrospinal fluid may be obtained in a variety of situations, such as from a lumbar puncture, a cerebrospinal fluid (CSF) leak, or from an external ventricular drain or catheter. Assessment of the fluid obtained identifies abnormalities and helps direct the child's care.

Bridget Connolly

PREREQUISITE KNOWLEDGE

- Pediatric neuroanatomy and physiology
- Characteristics of normal CSF: Clear odorless fluid that is produced by the choroid plexus of the ventricular system at a rate of 20 to 30 mL/h in adults and 20 mL/h in children; adults have 90 to 150 mL of CSF circulating at any one time, and infants have approximately 50 mL.[1,2]
- CSF bathes the brain and spinal cord and helps to protect them from injury by providing a cushion.
- Normal production and flow of CSF: CSF is produced by the choroid plexus and then flows from the lateral ventricles through the foramen of Monro into the third ventricle. The fluid then flows through the aqueduct of Sylvius into the fourth ventricle located in the area of the pons and medulla. CSF leaves the ventricular system through the foramen of Magendie and foramen of Luschka and fills the subarachnoid space around the brain and spinal cord (Figure 79-1). Most of the CSF produced is reabsorbed by the arachnoid villi.
- Certain situations such as shunt malfunctions, increased intracranial pressure (ICP), infections, or wound leaks, necessitate external drainage of CSF. If prolonged drainage is necessary, a lumbar drain or an external ventricular drain (EVD) is usually placed. However, if only a small amount of CSF is needed for diagnostic purposes or temporary relief of ICP, a lumbar puncture (LP), ventriculoperitoneal shunt tap, or direct ventricular tap may be performed as appropriate. See Procedures 77, 80, 81, 82, and 83 for further information.

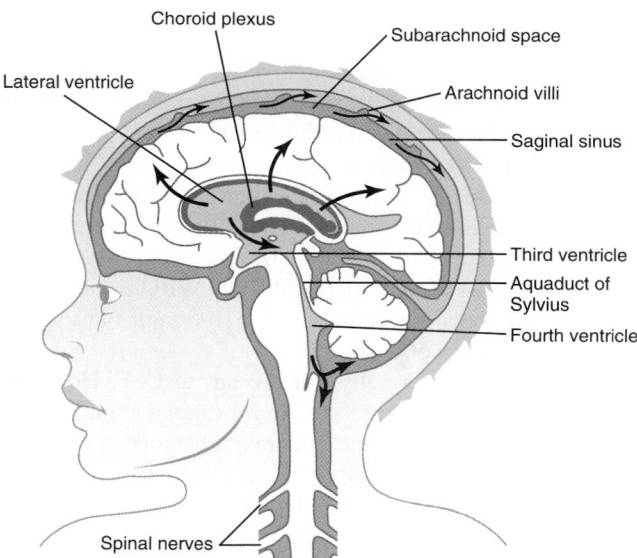

FIGURE 79-1 Flow of Cerebrospinal Fluid (CSF). *Illustration © Lynne Larson, Biovisual Communications, Menlo Park, CA, 2004.*

- A complete evaluation of CSF is essential for diagnosis of meningitis, encephalitis, ventriculitis, or a subarachnoid hemorrhage. Evaluation of CSF is also helpful in monitoring the efficacy of antimicrobial therapy during treatment of a central nervous system (CNS) infection. Information can also be obtained for demyelinating, degenerative, and collagen vascular diseases.[1]

- Summary of indications for CSF drainage for a particular child
  - ❖ Diagnosis of infection or various disease processes
  - ❖ Treatment of increased intracranial pressure (ICP)
  - ❖ Diversion of CSF
  - ❖ Intraventricular hemorrhage
  - ❖ Access for treatment of ventriculitis
  - ❖ After resection of mass lesion
  - ❖ Hydrocephalus not amenable to placement of in situ shunt
- CSF analysis
  - ❖ Color and consistency
    - ○ The term "xanthrochromia" is used to describe a yellowish discoloration of the CSF usually caused by lysis of red blood cells, hyperbilirubinemia, carotenemia, or an elevated protein level (>150 mg/dL).[1,3,4]
    - ○ The CSF may appear pink in color because of bleeding; brownish-gray because of CNS melanoma; or greenish because of leukemic meningeal infiltration.[2]
    - ○ The fluid may appear cloudy or turbid if microorganisms are present or if the white blood cell (WBC) count is elevated.[2]
    - ○ Blood-tinged CSF may be present after a traumatic lumbar puncture or ventricular tap but usually clears as sequential tubes are collected; however, if the fluid is persistently bloody, a subarachnoid hemorrhage should be suspected.
  - ❖ Cell count
    - ○ A cell count, including WBC and red blood cell (RBC), should be performed. Normal WBC counts in CSF may be up to 5 WBC/mm³ in adults and up to 15 WBC/mm³ in newborns.[1,3-5]
    - ○ In cases of bacterial meningitis, 87% of patients have a WBC count of more than 1000/mm³ and 99% have a WBC count of more than 100/mm³.[3,4]
    - ○ In cases of viral meningitis, the WBC count is usually much lower at less than 100/mm³ but may be as high as 500/mm.[3,4,6]
    - ○ RBC are normally not present in CSF. However, RBCs may be present after a traumatic tap or may be indicative of an intracranial hemorrhage.[1-6]
  - ❖ The WBC differential
    - ○ A typical WBC differential consists of 70% lymphocytes and 30% monocytes.[4]
    - ○ In children, the presence of polymorphonuclear (PMN) cells is considered abnormal. However, CSF in neonates may contain 1 to 2 PMN cells.[1] An elevated PMN cell count usually suggests bacterial meningitis or an early phase of viral or aseptic meningitis.[1,3] However, the presence of PMN cells in CSF cannot be the sole criterion for distinguishing between bacterial and viral meningitis because children with viral meningitis may have elevated PMN counts in the early phase of the illness and for the duration of the illness.[5]
    - ○ Cerebrospinal fluid lymphocytosis may be indicative of viral, tuberculous, or fungal meningitis; demyelin-ating diseases; brain tumor; spinal cord tumor; immunologic diseases; or chemical irritation.[1,3]
- Protein
  - ❖ Normal CSF protein levels range from 18 to 58 mg/dL in adults and 10 to 40 mg/dL in children.[1]
  - ❖ Neonatal CSF protein can be as high as 120 mg/dL; however, it usually reaches the normal childhood range by 3 months of age.[1]
  - ❖ Elevated protein levels may indicate an infection, intracranial hemorrhage, multiple sclerosis, Guillain-Barré syndrome, malignant disease, or other immunologic and degenerative conditions.[1,3,4]
  - ❖ Low protein levels may result from immunologic, vascular, or degenerative disorders; malignant diseases, such as brain and spinal cord tumors; or unintended loss of CSF from a dural leak, frequent lumbar punctures, or a lumbar drain.[1,2]
- Glucose
  - ❖ Normal glucose levels in CSF are usually about 60% of the serum glucose in the adult, 60% of the serum glucose in a child, and about 80% of the serum glucose in the neonate.[1-3]
  - ❖ For an accurate measurement, the serum glucose should be obtained approximately 1 to 2 hours before sampling the CSF.
  - ❖ A low CSF glucose level may be the result of bacterial meningitis, diffuse meningeal disease, certain viral meningitides, subarachnoid hemorrhage, serum hypoglycemia, or fungal infections.[1-3] In cases of viral infections, the CSF glucose is typically within normal range.[3]
- Microbiology
  - ❖ Both a gram stain and a culture should be performed on the CSF sample. Gram stain results are usually available within 24 hours. Cultures are not finalized until 72 hours. Gram stains yield positive results in approximately 60% to 80% of cases of untreated bacterial meningitis and 40% to 60% of cases of partially treated bacterial meningitis.[3,4,7]
  - ❖ The most common organisms that cause meningitis in 1-month-old to 2-month-old infants are *group B streptococcus, Escherichia.coli,* and *Listeria monocytogenes.*
  - ❖ *Haemophilus influenzae,* meningococcus, and pneumococcus are most common in 3-month-olds to 5-year-olds.
  - ❖ Meningococcus and pneumococcus are most common in older children, adolescents, and adults.[3]
  - ❖ As new vaccines become widely available, the common causative organisms may change.
  - ❖ Once an organism is identified, drug sensitivities are tested so that an appropriate antibiotic is selected for treatment of the infection.
  - ❖ Polymerase chain reaction (PCR). This test has a high sensitivity and specificity for many CNS infections and is especially useful in the diagnosis of viral meningitis caused by herpes simplex virus (HSV), Epstein-Barr virus, and enteroviruses. The PCR is the test of choice for HSV-I.[7]
  - ❖ Table 79-1 is a summary of CSF findings in bacterial and viral meningitides.

TABLE 79-1	Summary of CSF Findings In Bacterial and Viral Meningitides		
Parameter	**Normal**	**Bacterial Meningitis**	**Viral Meningitis**
Color and consistency	Clear, colorless	Cloudy, turbid	May be cloudy, turbid
WBC count (cells/mm^3)	0-5 (up to 15 in newborns)	1000-10,000 Range <100-20,000	<500 Range <100-500
Protein (mg/dL)	Children 10-40 Newborns up to 120	Elevated	Normal
Glucose (mg/dL)	60% serum glucose (80% of serum glucose in neonates)	<60% of serum glucose	Normal
Culture	Normal	Positive for an organism	May be positive for virus (PCR test is more definitive)

Information compiled from Behrman RE, et al, editors: *Nelson textbook of pediatrics*, ed 17, Philadelphia, 2004, Saunders.
Negrini B, et al: Cerebrospinal fluid findings in aseptic versus bacterial meningitis, *Pediatrics* 105(2):316-319, 2000.
Seehusen DA, et al: Cerebrospinal fluid analysis, *Am Family Physician* 68(6):1103-1108, 2003.
Zunt JR, Marra CM: Cerebrospinal fluid testing for the diagnosis of central nervous system infection, *Neurologic Clin* 17(4):675-689, 1999.

- Order of obtaining samples, if several specimens of various types are obtained (e.g., virology, microbiology, chemistry studies)
- Appropriate containers for specimens to be collected and minimum fluid volumes required for those specimens
- Specimen labeling requirements
- Specimen handling requirements
- Child development as it relates to clinical assessment and CSF drainage assessment
- Principles of aseptic technique

CHILD AND FAMILY ASSESSMENT

- Baseline vital signs ➤➤*Rationale:* Vital signs are an essential part of a complete assessment of the child and may also be used to aid in a diagnosis.
- Neurologic assessment of the child ➤➤*Rationale:* A change in neurologic examination results may indicate a problem and can support the diagnosis of infection, intracranial hypertension, or shunt malfunction.
- Signs of meningeal irritation (irritability, photophobia, headache, nuchal rigidity) or signs of increased ICP (irritability, lethargy, headache, vomiting, change in mental status) ➤➤*Rationale:* These signs may be used to support a diagnosis of CNS infection or increased ICP possibly resulting from a shunt malfunction.
- Child's developmental level and ability to interact ➤➤*Rationale:* These factors influence preparation of the child and interaction.
- Child's and family's understanding of the reasons for and risks and benefits of CSF drainage assessment ➤➤*Rationale:* Evaluates child's and family's understanding of the procedure and provides a gauge for ongoing education.
- Desire of family members to be present during the procedure ➤➤*Rationale:* Family may provide support and comfort measures to the child, but they should have the choice not to remain with the child during the procedure.

CHILD AND FAMILY EDUCATION

Individualized, developmentally appropriate education is provided to the family and to the child based on desire for knowledge, readiness to learn, and overall neurologic and psychosocial state.

- Provide information about CSF, including the therapeutic reasons for drainage ➤➤*Rationale:* Providing information decreases anxiety and fear.
- Explain how the family and child, depending on developmental level, can assist in ensuring proper care and safety of the drainage system ➤➤*Rationale:* If the drainage system remains intact, complications such as leakage and infection from dislodgement or disconnection can be prevented.
- Review signs and symptoms of CNS infection, meningeal irritation, increased ICP, or any other pertinent information ➤➤*Rationale:* Recognition of appropriate signs and symptoms can empower the child and family and help aid in diagnosis.
- Explain the importance of hourly nursing assessment of the drainage system and area of CSF leakage ➤➤*Rationale:* Providing information decreases anxiety and fear.
- Encourage questions and answer questions as they arise ➤➤*Rationale:* Reinforcement of information is needed during periods of stress.

EQUIPMENT

- Clean gloves
- Appropriate specimen tubes
- Specimen labels that contain two patient identifiers
- Appropriate laboratory requisitions
- Special supplies or equipment necessary for specimen handling

Procedure for Cerebrospinal Fluid Drainage: Assessment

Steps	Rationale	Considerations
1. Ensure child and family understand procedure and questions are answered.	Evaluates and reinforces understanding of previously taught information.	Developmental level, cognitive ability, and anxiety level determine approach to and effectiveness of teaching.
2. Gather needed supplies and equipment.	Facilitates completion of task in a timely manner.	
3. Wash hands.	Standard precautions; reduces transmission of microorganisms.	
4. Utilize two patient identifiers to verify correct child. *(Level II*)*	Promotes patient safety; ensures specimens are obtained from the correct child.	Compare information on specimen labels with child's identification band or use mechanism described in institution-specific protocol.
5. Perform complete neurologic assessment.	Establishes baseline.	A change in the neurologic examination results may be the result of excessive CSF drainage.
6. Put on clean gloves. *(Level VI*)*	Standard precautions; reduces transmission of microorganisms.	
7. Obtain or assist with obtaining CSF sample and place in appropriate specimen tube.	Use of appropriate specimen tube ensures valid results are obtained.	Appropriate specimen collection tubes are institution specific; refer to institution-specific laboratory instructions.
8. Label specimens at the bedside and complete laboratory paperwork per institution-specific protocol. *(Level II*)*	Promotes patient safety; ensures accurate and efficient processing of specimen.	Follow institution-specific protocols for handling and labeling laboratory specimens.
9. Send specimens to laboratory promptly. *(Level VI*)*	Delay in transporting specimens to laboratory may alter results obtained.	
External Drainage System (Steps 10 and 11)		
10. Examine the entire length of tubing from child to drainage chamber; note appearance of fluid in the tubing. *(Level II*)*	Identifies fluid that is an abnormal color or contains debris.	The presence of brain tissue and blood clots may interfere with flow of CSF.
11. Observe CSF inside collection chamber and note the amount, color, and consistency of the fluid.	Identifies abnormalities in volume, color, and consistency of fluid; abnormalities may indicate infection or hemorrhage.	The presence of WBC or fibrin can cause the CSF to look turbid or cloudy. A change in CSF color from clear to bloody may indicate sudden hemorrhage and necessitate immediate notification of a neurosurgeon.
12. Discard used supplies and equipment in an appropriate receptacle.	Standard precautions; reduces transmission of microorganisms.	
13. Remove gloves; wash hands.	Standard precautions.	

* Level II: Theory-based; no research data to support recommendations; recommendations from expert consensus group may exist
  Level VI: Clinical studies in a variety of patient populations and situations to support recommendations

Expected Outcomes

- Neurologic examination results remain stable
- The CSF specimen for analysis is collected without difficulty
- The CSF specimens are placed in correct specimen tubes, labeled appropriately, and sent to the laboratory in the appropriate time frame
- Results are available in a reasonable time

- Identification of CSF leak

- The CSF drain functions properly

Unexpected Outcomes

- Change in neurologic examination results
- Inability to obtain sufficient fluid volume for evaluation
- Specimens are mislabeled
- Specimens are placed in incorrect sample tubes
- Delay in sending specimens to laboratory
- Delay in laboratory reporting
- Specimen is lost or unusable
- The CSF leak is not identified, with subsequent development of CNS infection
- Drain malfunction

Monitoring and Care of the Child

Activities and Interventions	Rationale	Reportable Conditions
1. Monitor neurologic status before and after specimen collection and as indicated.	Provides data for ongoing diagnosis and treatment.	• Change in neurologic status
2. Monitor for signs and symptoms of meningitis and increased ICP.	Signs and symptoms of meningitis or increased ICP may indicate the need for further testing and evaluation.	• Change in level of consciousness • Irritability • Lethargy • Vomiting • Change in vital signs • Temperature greater than 38.5°C or per prescribing practitioner's notification guidelines • Photophobia • Nuchal rigidity • Headaches • Seizure
3. Check laboratory reports for results of CSF studies, including gram stain, WBC count, RBC count, glucose, and protein.	Prompt identification of abnormal results facilitates rapid treatment, which improves outcome. Values of cell count, glucose, and protein may indicate an infectious process; gram stain results can give a preliminary etiology. Final culture result is usually reported after 72 hours.	• Laboratory report of lost or unusable specimens • Results not available in a reasonable time frame • Elevated WBC count • Elevated RBC count • Low glucose level • Elevated protein level • Bacteria on gram stain • Positive culture with identification of organism

Documentation

- Child and family education
- Child's neurologic status before and after collection
- Color, amount, and consistency of CSF
- Date, time, and amount of drainage collected for evaluation
- Area from which CSF drainage flows (i.e., type of drain or site of leakage)
- Condition of drainage system
- Unexpected outcomes and related treatment

References

1. Behrman RE, et al, editors: *Nelson textbook of pediatrics,* ed 17, Philadelphia, 2004, Saunders.
2. Goetz CG: *Textbook of clinical neurology,* ed 2, Philadelphia, 2003, Saunders.
3. Ravel R: *Clinical laboratory medicine,* ed 6, New York, 1995, Mosby-Year Book, Inc.
4. Seehusen DA, et al: Cerebrospinal fluid analysis, *Am Family Physician* 68(6):1103-1108, 2003.
5. Negrini B, et al: Cerebrospinal fluid findings in aseptic versus bacterial meningitis, *Pediatrics* 105(2):316-319, 2000.
6. Shpritz DW: Neurodiagnostic studies, *Nursing Clin North Am* 34(3):593-606, 1999.
7. Zunt JR, Marra CM: Cerebrospinal fluid testing for the diagnosis of central nervous system infection, *Neurologic Clin* 17(4):675-689, 1999.

Additional Readings

Gertz SD: *Liebman's neuroanatomy made easy and understandable,* ed 5, Gaithersberg, MD, 1996, Aspen Publishers.
Guyton AC: *Textbook of medical physiology,* Philadelphia, 1981, Saunders.
Hickey JV: *The clinical practice of neurological and neurosurgical nursing,* ed 4, Philadelphia, 1997, Lippincott.
Slota MC, editor: *Core curriculum for pediatric critical care nursing,* Philadelphia, 1998, Saunders.

Externalized Ventricular Shunts and Drains: Catheter Management

PURPOSE: An intraventricular catheter is externalized and connected to a drainage system to divert cerebrospinal fluid, decrease intracranial pressure, drain blood from an intraventricular bleed or surgery, or treat ventriculitis from a shunt infection. The catheter may be inserted via a ventriculostomy, or an existing ventricular shunt may be externalized.

Amy Carnall-Grogan and Kelly Keefe Marcoux

PREREQUISITE KNOWLEDGE

- Anatomy and physiology of the pediatric brain
- Developmentally appropriate neurologic assessment techniques
- Physiology of cerebrospinal fluid (CSF) flow (see Procedure 79)
- Purpose of a ventriculoperitoneal (VP) shunt (see Procedure 82)
- Average rates of CSF production[1,2]
  - ❖ Newborn: Approximately 1 mL/h
  - ❖ Child: Approximately 10 to 20 mL/h (250 to 500 mL/d)
  - ❖ Adult: Approximately 20 to 30 mL/h (500 mL/d)
- Total volume of CSF in ventricles[1,2]
  - ❖ Newborn: Approximately 5 mL
  - ❖ Infant: 40 to 60 mL
  - ❖ Child: 60 to 120 mL
  - ❖ Adult: Approximately 150 mL
- Normal CSF pressure inside the ventricles is 110 mm H_2O (11 cm H_2O).[1,2] Water pressure is frequently used as the unit of measure, although millimeters of mercury (mm Hg) are used if intracranial pressure (ICP) is also monitored. Note: Conversion for centimeters of H_2O to millimeters of mercury is 1 mm Hg = 1.36 cm H_2O.

- In the acutely injured pediatric brain, ventricular volumes and CSF flow may be altered depending on the insult (e.g., intraventricular bleed leading to decreased CSF reabsorption; cerebral edema compressing ventricular space).[1,2]
- Signs of increased ICP from hydrocephalus[1,2]
  - ❖ Infant: Increased head circumference, full fontanel, engorged scalp veins, Macewen's sign, cranial nerve VI palsy, irregular respirations, apnea, seizure, setting sun sign (upward gaze palsy), hyperreactive reflexes
  - ❖ Older child/adolescent: Headache, nausea, vomiting, ataxia, drowsiness, blurred vision, papilledema
  - ❖ Late signs: Bradycardia, hypertension, and irregular respirations (Cushing's triad)
- An externalized ventricular drain (EVD) may be:
  - ❖ A drain inserted into the ventricle via a ventriculostomy
  - ❖ An externalized shunt that is the externalization of an existing internal ventricular shunt. Ventricular shunts are most commonly ventriculoperitoneal (VP); other commonly used shunts are ventriculoatrial (VA) or ventriculopleural.[3]
  - ❖ This distinction is important because care of the drain varies depending on whether or not it is a straight

drainage system without a valve or whether it has a valve in situ (i.e., an externalized VP shunt).

- EVDs are closed sterile systems that allow CSF to drain into a sliding graduated flow chamber that can be adjusted to a prescribed level.
- An EVD may be used in the place of an infected shunt.[3]
  - ❖ In some situations, the VP shunt is externalized and the CSF flow control valve left in place. If this is the case, less of a concern exists for maintaining the external pressure with the flow chamber because the flow rate of CSF is regulated by the valve, preventing overdrainage of CSF.
  - ❖ Alternatively, the VP shunt may be removed entirely and an intraventricular catheter (IVC) placed (see Procedure 77). This system does not have a valve, and overdrainage of CSF is a potential complication.
- Externalization of a ventricular drain or insertion of an IVC is generally performed with sterile technique by a neurosurgeon.
- An IVC may be placed or a VP shunt may be externalized emergently in the critically ill child who has increased ICP from a distal shunt malfunction, peritonitis, or ventricular bleed, etc. This procedure may be done at the bedside in an emergency.
- Indications for externalization of VP shunt or placement of an IVC for CSF drainage include[2,3]:
  - ❖ VP shunt infection
  - ❖ Peritonitis from infected VP shunt
  - ❖ Ventricular hemorrhage
  - ❖ Increased ICP
  - ❖ Postoperative CSF diversion
  - ❖ Drainage of excess CSF
- Potential complications with externalized drainage of CSF[2]
  - ❖ Overdrainage
  - ❖ Underdrainage
  - ❖ Infection
  - ❖ Disconnection
  - ❖ Bleeding
- The indication for the EVD determines the length of time it is deemed necessary. For example, children with intraventricular hemorrhage need an EVD until the CSF is clear and the protein count is less than 1 g/dL. In children with an internal ventricular shunt, CSF infection or peritonitis must be cleared before reinsertion or placement of a new shunt.[2]
- CSF specimens can be obtained with aseptic technique from an EVD (see Procedure 83).
- Child development as it relates to clinical assessment and management of an EVD, including effects of development on the child's neurologic assessment
- Principles of aseptic technique
- Appropriate pediatric dosing of analgesics and competency in procedural sedation
- Except in an emergency situation, externalization of a ventricular drain requires informed consent.

CHILD AND FAMILY ASSESSMENT

- Baseline vital signs ➥*Rationale:* Vital signs are an essential part of a complete assessment of the child.
- Baseline neurologic assessment of the child, which should include a head circumference in a child less than 2 years of age or if the cranial sutures are open ➥*Rationale:* A change in neurologic examination results may indicate increased ICP, an intracranial infection, intracranial hemorrhage, or malfunction of the EVD. If the child has signs of increased ICP, externalization becomes a medical emergency.
- Presence of meningeal signs (irritability, photophobia, headache, nuchal rigidity) or indications of increased ICP (irritability, lethargy, headache, vomiting, change in mental status) ➥*Rationale:* These signs may be used to support a diagnosis of central nervous system (CNS) infection or increased ICP from a malfunctioning EVD that causes hydrocephalus.
- Child's baseline developmental level and ability to interact ➥*Rationale:* Identifies baseline variation from the child's usual state; these factors also influence preparation of the child and interaction.
- Child's and family's understanding of the reasons for and risks and benefits of EVD procedure ➥*Rationale:* Evaluates child's and family's understanding of the procedure and provides a gauge for ongoing education.
- Current laboratory profile, including complete blood count (CBC), prothrombin time (PT), and partial thromboplastin time (PTT) ➥*Rationale:* Establishes baseline values and identifies abnormalities before procedure.
- Desire of family members to remain with the child during procedure ➥*Rationale:* Family's presence may provide support and comfort to the child during the procedure if institution-specific protocol facilitates family presence; family members should also have the choice not to remain with the child.

CHILD AND FAMILY EDUCATION

Individualized, developmentally appropriate education is provided to the family and to the child based on desire for knowledge, readiness to learn, and overall neurologic and psychosocial state.

- Provide information about CSF, including the therapeutic reasons for an external drainage system ➥*Rationale:* Providing information decreases anxiety and fear.
- Explain how the family and, if developmentally appropriate, the child can assist in ensuring proper care and safety of the drainage system ➥*Rationale:* Complications such as leakage and infection from dislodgement or disconnection can be prevented with proper care.
- Explain the importance of preventing any disconnection of the CSF drainage system or movement of child above or below the predetermined height of the system ➥*Rationale:* Moving the child above the CSF drainage

system or disconnection of the system causes rapid drainage of CSF from the ventricular system. Moving the child below the predetermined level for the drainage system prevents CSF from draining. Proper positioning of the CSF drainage system is particularly important with a system that does *not* have a valve.

- Review signs and symptoms of CNS infection, meningeal irritation, increased ICP, or any other pertinent information ➤*Rationale:* Recognition of appropriate signs and symptoms can empower the child and family and aid in diagnosis.
- Explain the importance of hourly nursing assessment of the drainage system ➤*Rationale:* Providing information decreases anxiety and fear related to frequency of assessments.
- If the family desires to stay with the child during the procedure and institution-specific protocol permits family presence, provide the family with accurate information regarding the procedure, family's role, and expectations ➤*Rationale:* Presence of family may provide support and comfort to the child, and clearly defined institution-specific protocol for family presence facilitates this; however, family members should also have the choice not to remain with the child.
- Encourage questions and answer questions as they arise ➤*Rationale:* Reinforcement of information is needed during periods of stress and is especially important if the procedure is performed emergently.

EQUIPMENT

- Intravenous (IV) pole
- CSF external ventricular drainage system
- Level (e.g., carpenter's level or laser level)
- ICP monitor (if indicated)

For Externalization of VP Shunt:

- Povidone-iodine solution or other skin antiseptic per institution-specific protocol
- Scalpel
- Suture material
- Needle holder
- Sterile scissors
- Sterile dressing kit with occlusive dressing
- Topical anesthetic
- Lidocaine 1% or 2%
- Sterile gloves
- Clean gloves
- Caps and masks
- Sterile gowns
- Personal protective equipment (eye and face protection) per institution-specific protocol

For equipment necessary for ventriculostomy and IVC placement, see Procedure 77.

Procedure for Externalized Ventricular Shunts and Drains: Catheter Management		
Steps	**Rationale**	**Considerations**
1. Ensure child and family understand procedure and questions are answered.	Evaluates and reinforces understanding of previously taught information.	Developmental level, cognitive ability, and anxiety level determine approach to and effectiveness of teaching.
2. Gather needed equipment and supplies.	Facilitates completion of task in a timely manner.	
3. Confirm that consent for procedure has been obtained.	Ensures medical-legal compliance as suggested by the Joint Commission on Accreditation of Healthcare Organizations (JCAHO).	In emergency situations, refer to institution-specific protocol or procedure for assumption of consent.
4. Wash hands.	Standard precautions; reduces transmission of microorganisms.	
5. Perform complete neurologic assessment.	Establishes a baseline for comparison with ongoing assessment.	Deterioration in the child's neurologic examination results indicates an emergent need for externalization of VP shunt or placement of an EVD.
6. Put on clean gloves.	Standard precautions.	

Procedure continues on following page

Procedure	**for Externalized Ventricular Shunts and Drains: Catheter Management**—*Continued*	
Steps	**Rationale**	**Considerations**

Externalization of a VP Shunt (steps 7 to 18; for insertion of IVC, see Procedure 77)

Steps	Rationale	Considerations
7. Apply a topical anesthetic at the approximate incision site if time allows.	Promotes child's comfort and decreases pain response.	Site of externalization varies by child. Consult with neurosurgeon or practitioner who is performing procedure to identify approximate area of externalization (i.e., the scalp, neck, upper chest wall, abdomen). Identify the child with two patient identifiers before medication administration.
8. Identify the child with appropriate patient and procedure verification process (e.g., "Time out").	Confirms correct patient, procedure, and site as recommended by JCAHO; prevents unnecessary medical procedures.	Verification process and documentation is institution specific. Use active communication techniques.
9. Ensure appropriate cardiorespiratory and hemodynamic monitoring is in place with appropriate alarm limits set and alarms activated.	Child may have decompensation during procedure.	Observe bedside monitor and obtain frequent vital signs during procedure. Emergency equipment should be readily available.
10. Assess child's pain with pain scale appropriate to child's age and developmental level. Administer pain or sedation medications as appropriate and per prescribing practitioner's order.	Externalization can be painful and may increase child's anxiety. Promotes child's comfort during procedure; facilitates completion of procedure.	See Procedure 173 for more information on age-appropriate assessment.
11. Put on personal protective equipment as appropriate; assist the practitioner who is performing the procedure with garb as necessary.	Standard precautions; protects personnel health. Hat, mask, sterile gown, and gloves may be worn by practitioner who is performing the procedure to prevent contamination of site and decrease risk of infection.	Garb required of individuals in the room during externalization varies from institution to institution; refer to institution-specific protocol.
12. Assist the practitioner who is performing the procedure with establishing a sterile field and preparing equipment.	Aseptic technique protects child from exposure to microorganisms and contamination of the surgical site, reducing likelihood of infection.	
13. Assist the practitioner who is performing procedure to prepare and drape the site.	Aseptic technique protects child from exposure to microorganisms and contamination of the surgical site, reducing likelihood of infection.	
14. Assist with local anesthetic preparation.	Local anesthetic is injected to decrease child's pain.	
15. A lateral incision is made at a point along the shunt tract as per practitioner's preference.	The surgeon determines where the shunt is exposed, depending on the etiology of the malfunction (e.g., kink in the system, broken tubing, infection, loculation, peritonitis).	
16. The shunt tubing is exposed at the incision site; the distal tubing is exposed and cut. The proximal tubing is clamped and sutured into place.	Necessary to attach distal tubing to EVD system.	If the distal tubing is removed, it is discarded in medical waste trash.

Procedure	for Externalized Ventricular Shunts and Drains: Catheter Management—*Continued*	

Steps	Rationale	Considerations
17. Prepare the EVD drainage system. Prime the system using sterile technique with sterile NS from the patient stopcock through to the drip chamber. Verify absence of leaks and that the fluid flows freely to the drainage bag. Assist practitioner to connect the proximal tubing to the EVD system.	Allows CSF to drain externally into the drainage system.	Confirm whether the VP shunt valve was removed or left intact. This affects the level at which the external drain is placed.
18. Apply a sterile occlusive dressing to the site of externalization.	Sterile occlusive dressing is necessary to prevent introduction of microorganisms.	Type of dressing may vary on basis of institution-specific protocol.

Externalized VP Shunts and IVCs (steps 19 to 31)

Steps	Rationale	Considerations
19. Position the drip chamber at the prescribed level in cm H_2O or mm Hg above the zero point with a level to ensure accuracy (Figure 80-1). *(Level VI*)*	This level determines resistance to CSF flow and therefore the amount of CSF drainage. The zero point most commonly used is the foramen of Monro. Anatomically, this is the external auditory meatus on a supine child (Figure 80-2).	If the drainage system is set at 20 cm H_2O and the ICP is less than 15 mm Hg (20 cm H_2O), no drainage occurs. However, at this level, is greater than 15 mm Hg, the system drains CSF until the desired pressure is attained.[4-7] This step is not usually necessary if the child has an externalized shunt with the valve in place; the drip chamber is leveled to the zero point.
20. Position the EVD system on an IV pole next to the head of the bed. The system must be firmly secured to the stand with the drip chamber visible at all times. *(Level VI*)*	Stabilizes the system; allows visualization of the flow chamber and the system.	This is necessary even if the child has a valve at the distal end of the EVD. Most EVD systems have a hanging cord that is looped over the IV pole to prevent the system from dropping to the floor.
21. Discard used supplies and equipment, including sharps, in appropriate receptacles.	Standard precautions; reduces the transmission of microorganisms. Protects personnel health.	
22. Remove personal protective equipment; wash hands.	Standard precautions.	

EVD Management

Steps	Rationale	Considerations
23. Assess EVD tubing at regular intervals for patency by observing for CSF oscillation in the tubing. If the fluid is not oscillating, consult with neurosurgical team. Order may be provided to briefly drop the drip chamber below the level of the foramen of Monro to assess if CSF drains into the chamber.[8] *(Level V*)*	Facilitates identification of blockage in the system; briefly lowering the drip chamber below the zero point helps to determine the patency of the drainage system.	If at any time the system appears blocked, immediately notify the neurosurgical team. If oscillation of the CSF exists, an obstruction is not likely. The CSF flow may be decreased; lowering the drip chamber may result in increased drainage of CSF. This should not be done without appropriate order from the neurosurgical team.

Procedure continues on following page

* Level V: Clinical studies in more than one or two patient populations and situations to support recommendations
Level VI: Clinical studies in a variety of patient populations and situations to support recommendations

Procedure	for **Externalized Ventricular Shunts and Drains:** **Catheter Management**—*Continued*

Steps	Rationale	Considerations

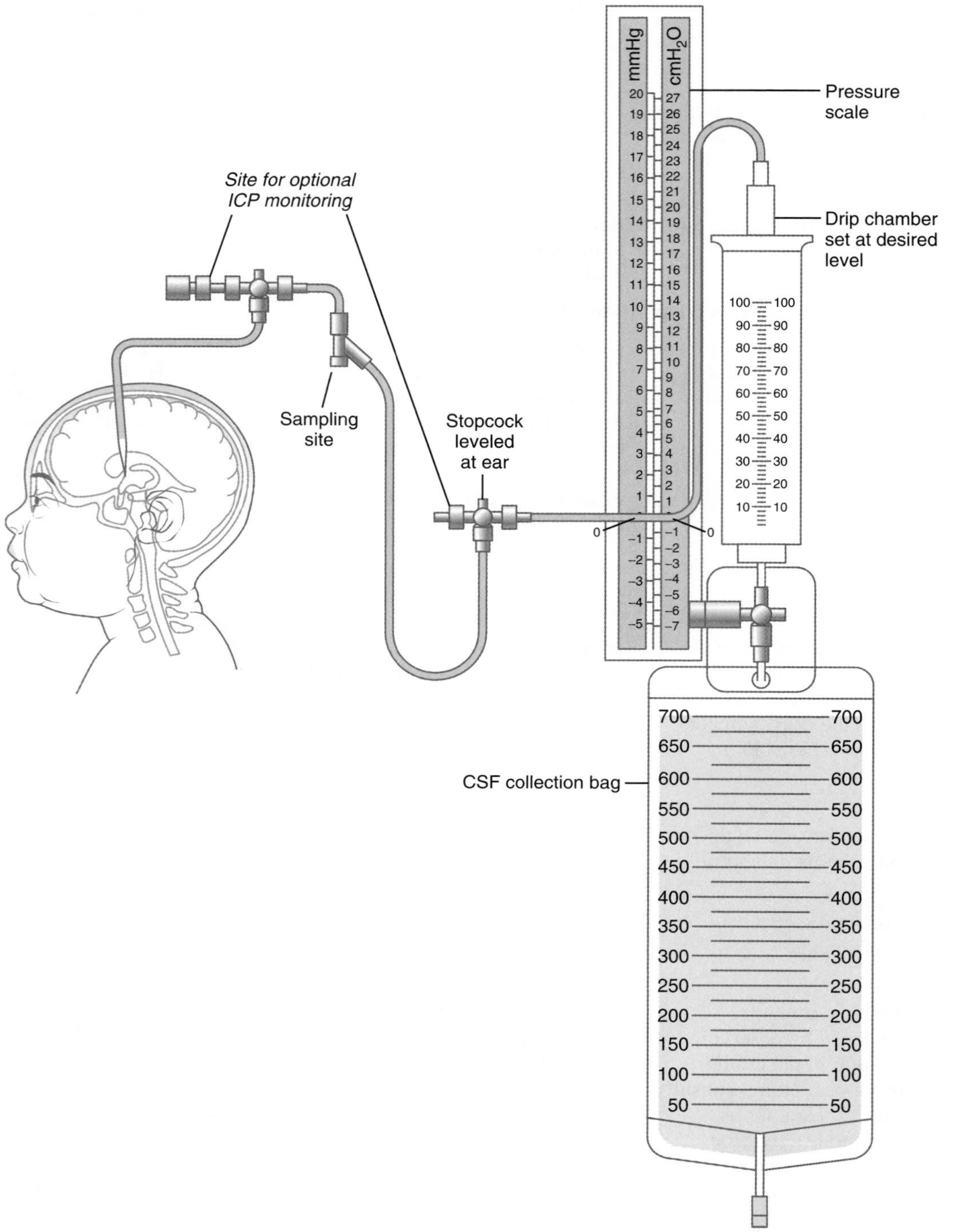

FIGURE 80-1   Example of intraventricular catheter with ICP monitoring capabilities and drainage system. Note leveling stopcock, drip chamber, pressure scale, site for attachment of ICP monitor, sampling site, and CSF collection bag.

Procedure	**for Externalized Ventricular Shunts and Drains: Catheter Management**—*Continued*	
Steps	**Rationale**	**Considerations**

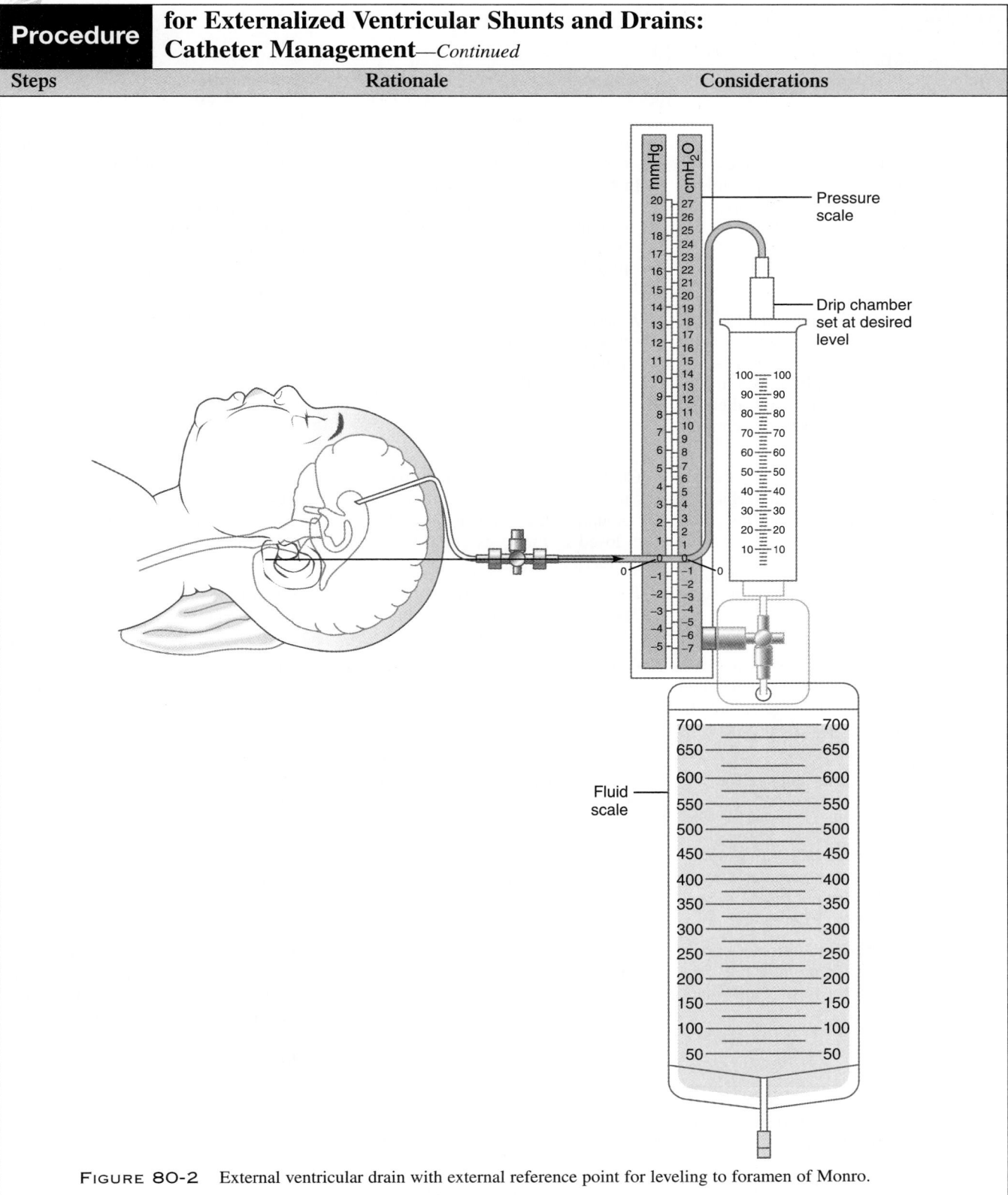

FIGURE 80-2 External ventricular drain with external reference point for leveling to foramen of Monro.

Procedure continues on following page

Procedure	for Externalized Ventricular Shunts and Drains: Catheter Management—*Continued*

Steps	Rationale	Considerations
24. Clamp the EVD if the child is moved out of bed or significantly repositioned. Unclamp immediately after repositioning or if the child's neurologic status deteriorates. *(Level V*)*	Allows movement of the child while preventing disconnections and overdrainage of CSF.[8,9] In some systems, the air filter on the drip chamber may not function when wet and CSF drainage may cease. When clamping system, prevent the filter from getting wet with CSF.	In some situations, leaving the system open may be necessary. The child must be closely monitored to prevent inadvertent disconnection or any alterations in position that may affect the CSF drainage. Confirm that the clamps are reopened after repositioning to ensure CSF drainage.
25. If the system is inadvertently disconnected, the ventricular catheter should be clamped immediately and the child placed in a supine position until the catheter is reconnected with aseptic technique. *(Level V*)*	A supine position zeroes out the ventricular pressure. If the child is supine, it is more difficult for gravity to force the flow of CSF.[4,9]	With massive hydrocephalus, some CSF leakage may occur until the system is reconnected.
26. If EVD system becomes contaminated, contact the neurosurgical team immediately. *(Level II*)*	Changing the entire system may be necessary to prevent further contamination. Maintenance of a closed system is essential to prevent infection.[9]	Maintaining a sterile drainage system is of utmost importance because the proximal catheter sits in the ventricular system of the brain.
27. See Procedure 83 for information on obtaining CSF sample.	Periodic CSF sampling may be performed to assess the status of a VP shunt infection.	Guidelines have been developed to minimize infection complications.[9]
28. Change the occlusive dressing over the EVD insertion site when soiled or loose with aseptic technique or per institution-specific protocol. *(Level II*)*	Observe the site for signs of infection whenever dressing is removed.	Scalp dressings are difficult to maintain; a full head dressing may be indicated.
29. Inspect EVD insertion site for leakage of CSF. *(Level II*)*	System malfunction may result in CSF leakage; suspect CSF leakage if the dressing is wet.	If CSF leakage is suspected, report to the neurosurgeon.
30. Change drainage bag with aseptic technique when it becomes three-fourths full or as per institution-specific protocol. *(Level VI*)*	It is recommended that the bag be changed to prevent infection and allow continued drainage.	Some institutions routinely change the bag or EVD system tubing every week.
31. Per prescribing practitioner's preference and order, monitor ICP. See Procedure 76 for further information.	Need for ICP monitoring varies based on the specific child's underlying disease process.	In EVDs without a valve, ICP monitoring with appropriately set alarm limits can serve as a disconnection notification or notification that the drip chamber has dropped below the zero point.

* Level II: Theory-based; no research data to support recommendations; recommendations from expert consensus group may exist
Level V: Clinical studies in more than one or two patient populations and situations to support recommendations
Level VI: Clinical studies in a variety of patient populations and situations to support recommendations

Expected Outcomes	Unexpected Outcomes
• Resolution of underlying condition (hydrocephalus, blood accumulation, or infection)	• Infection persists
	• Blood is not evacuated
	• The CSF does not drain
• CSF is drained appropriately	• Minimal or excessive CSF drainage due to the EVD system placed at the wrong height
	• Obstruction in the CSF drainage from tissue debris or thick CSF
	• Tear of blood vessels from overdrainage results in subdural hemorrhage
	• Collapsed ventricles
• Child is free from site infection or development of CNS infection	• Break in sterile technique results in site infection or CNS infection
• The EVD system remains intact and in place until electively removed	• Break or leakage in system
	• Inadvertent EVD removal
• Child's neurologic status remains stable throughout treatment	• Deterioration in neurologic status
• Child has acceptable level of comfort throughout procedure	• Unmanaged pain or agitation

Monitoring and Care of the Child

Activities and Interventions	Rationale	Reportable Conditions
1. Monitor child's vital signs.	Facilitates prompt identification of significant changes from baseline. Changes in blood pressure (BP) and heart rate (HR) accompanied by changes in neurologic examination results may be indicative of tentorial herniation from insufficient or excessive CSF drainage.	• Significant change from baseline • Bradycardia associated with hypertension
2. Monitor child's neurologic status.	Decrease in level of consciousness or any signs of increased ICP may indicate malfunctioning EVD system. Pallor, clamminess, headache, and lethargy may indicate overdrainage of CSF. All or most of these signs and symptoms occurring simultaneously may indicate tentorial herniation.	• Severe headache, lethargy, drowsiness, irritability • Apnea • Sluggishly reactive pupils • Pronator arm drift
3. Assess CSF color and consistency.	Change in color or consistency may indicate bleeding or infection (see Procedure 79 for more information).	• Cloudy, milky, xanthochromic CSF

4. If ICP is monitored, assess ICP waveform trends at least hourly and as needed; assess waveform for:
    Normal morphology
    Dampening of waveform
    Abnormal waveform
	Identifies abnormal waveforms. See Figures 76-1, 76-2, and 76-3 in Procedure 76 for more information and figures of abnormal wave forms.	• P2 elevations
		• A or B waveform trends
		• No numeric display on transducer-tipped catheter monitor
		• No waveform after troubleshooting

5. Prevent inadvertent dislodgement of EVD with repeated age-appropriate explanations, sedation, analgesia, and family assistance as appropriate. Encourage family to use developmentally appropriate measures to support and comfort the child.	Dislodgement of EVD may result in need for additional procedure, infection, or pneumocephaly.	• Device dislodgement • Agitation unresponsive to interventions

Documentation

- Child and family education
- Patient and procedure verification process per institution-specific protocol
- If procedure performed at bedside: date, time, type of procedure, and individual who performed the procedure
- Medications administered for procedure; child's tolerance of procedure
- Child's neurologic status before, during, and after procedure
- Presence of informed consent
- Prescribed level of the EVD system and frequent verification of accurate position
- Cerebrospinal fluid drainage amount, color, and consistency
- Regular assessment of dressing integrity
- Tubing and dressing changes
- Comfort assessment and any specific interventions provided
- Protective/restraint devices in use and related assessments per institution-specific protocol
- Unexpected outcomes and related treatment

References

1. Haines SJ: Shunt infections. In Albright AL, et al, editors: *Principles and practice of pediatric neurosurgery,* New York, 1999, Thieme Medical Publishers.
2. Kestle JRW, et al: Treatment of hydrocephalus with shunts. In Albright AL, Pollack IF, Adelson PD, editors: *Principles and practice of pediatric neurosurgery,* New York, 1999, Thieme Medical Publishers.
3. Vernon-Levett P: Intracranial dynamics. In Curley MAQ, Moloney-Harmon PA, editors: *Critical care nursing of infants and children,* ed 2, Philadelphia, 2001, Saunders.
4. Walter KA: Neurosurgical procedures. In Chen H, Sonnenday CJ, Lillemoe KD, editors: *Manual of common bedside surgical procedures,* ed 2, Philadelphia, 2000, Lippincott Williams & Wilkins.
5. Choux M, et al: *Pediatric neurosurgery,* London, 1999, Churchill Livingstone.
6. Gaskill SJ, Marlin AE: *Handbook of pediatric neurology and neurosurgery,* Boston, 1993, Little, Brown and Company.
7. Hickey JV: Intracranial hypertension: theory and management of increased intracranial pressure. In Hickey JV, editor: *The clinical practice of neurological and neurosurgical nursing,* ed 5, Philadelphia, 2003, Lippincott Williams & Wilkins.
8. Johnson E, et al: *External ventricular drains: Guidelines for nursing care.* Neuro Intensive Care Unit, Leeds,UK, 2002. http://www.neuroitu.co.uk/evd.pdf. Accessed 7/14/06.
9. Bader MK, et al: Ventriculostomies and intracranial pressure monitoring: in search of a 0% infection rate, *Heart Lung* 24(2):166-172, 1995.

Additional Readings

Andrews BT, Hammer GB: *Pediatric neurosurgical intensive care,* Rolling Meadows, IL, 1997, American Association of Neurological Association.
Barker E: *Neuroscience nursing: a spectrum of care,* Philadelphia, 2002, Mosby.
Bondurant CP, Jimenex DF: Epidemiology of cerebrospinal fluid shunt, *Pediatric Neurosurg* 23:254-259, 1995.
McLone DG, et al: *Pediatric neurosurgery: surgery of the developing nervous system,* ed 4, Philadelphia, 2001, Saunders.

Lumbar Puncture: Assist

P U R P O S E :   To assist the practitioner performing a lumbar puncture to obtain cerebrospinal fluid to support a diagnosis of central nervous system (CNS) infection, CNS malignant disease, or autoimmune disease

Michelle A. Sorscher

PREREQUISITE KNOWLEDGE

- Neuroanatomy and physiology, including the spinal cord and spinal column, of infants, children, and adolescents
- In addition to obtaining cerebrospinal fluid (CSF), a lumbar puncture (LP) may also be performed to instill medication such as chemotherapy into the central nervous system.[1-3]
- A LP is usually performed at the L3-L4 or L4-L5 interspace.
- Indications include suspected CNS infection (e.g., meningitis, encephalitis, concern for sepsis in the newborn), CNS autoimmune process, or CNS tumor.
- A LP with instillation of medication may be used in the pediatric oncology population as an adjunct to systemic chemotherapy.
- Contraindications include[1,4]:
  - ❖ Known or suspected increased intracranial pressure (ICP)
  - ❖ Noncommunicating hydrocephalus
  - ❖ Known or suspected intracranial mass of brain or spinal cord[5]
  - ❖ Known or suspected coagulopathy
  - ❖ Posterior spinal fusion in the lumbar region
- Use caution in children with suspected subarachnoid hemorrhage.
- Young children may need sedation for this procedure.
- Recommended studies[2,4]
  - ❖ Tube 1: Cultures including gram stain, bacterial, fungal, and any additional viral cultures

- ❖ Tube 2: Biochemistry profile including glucose and protein
- ❖ Tube 3: Hematology including cell count and differential
- ❖ Tube 4: Optional studies including serologies and cytologies[2]
- Complications of LP include: back pain, bleeding, CSF leak, postspinal headache, meningitis, epidural or subdural spinal hematoma, acquired epidermoid spinal cord tumor, and herniation.[1,2,4,6]
- See Procedure 79 for detailed information regarding CSF analysis.
- Computerized tomographic (CT) scan may be indicated before LP if there is a suspected mass lesion, signs of increased ICP, or intracranial bleeding.[6]
- Use of procedural sedation must be considered in children, particularly if the child cannot cooperate with proper positioning. The child must be closely monitored throughout the procedure with special attention to cardiorespiratory status during sedation and positioning. (See Procedure 177 for further information.)
- Child development as it relates to clinical assessment and LP
- Mastery of pediatric advanced life support competencies
- Competency in procedural sedation
- Informed consent is required before LP

CHILD AND FAMILY ASSESSMENT

- Child's vital signs ➤➤*Rationale:* Establishes baseline values for the child; identifies the child with increased risk for complications related to cardiorespiratory compromise.
- Baseline neurologic assessment, including mental status and sensory and motor functions; note preprocedural deficits ➤➤*Rationale:* Establishes baseline neurologic function before insertion of needle into subarachnoid space.
- Current laboratory profile, including complete blood count (CBC), prothrombin time (PT), and partial thromboplastin time (PTT) ➤➤*Rationale:* Establishes baseline values and identifies abnormalities or increased risks before procedure.
- Signs of meningeal irritation: headache, nausea/vomiting, nystagmus, nuchal rigidity, photophobia, Brudzinski's sign, fever ➤➤*Rationale:* Establishes presenting signs and symptoms before procedure.
- Child's developmental level and ability to cooperate with positioning requirements; toddlers and young children, and children with cognitive or neuromuscular disorders, may be unable to cooperate ➤➤*Rationale:* Establishes the need for sedation for the procedure. The child must remain completely still throughout the procedure.
- Status of skin at proposed LP site ➤➤*Rationale:* Identifies potential contraindications.
- Child's known allergies ➤➤*Rationale:* Identifies allergies to medications or solutions that may be used during LP.
- Previous sedation experiences of the child ➤➤*Rationale:* Identifies previous difficulties with sedation; child and family are encouraged to participate in developing plan of care.
- Child's and family's understanding of the reasons for and risks and benefits of the LP ➤➤*Rationale:* Evaluates child's and family's understanding of the procedure and provides a gauge for ongoing education.
- Desire of family members to remain with the child during procedure ➤➤*Rationale:* Family's presence may provide support and comfort to the child during the procedure if institution-specific protocol facilitates family presence; family members should also have the choice not to remain with the child.

CHILD AND FAMILY EDUCATION

Individualized, developmentally appropriate education is provided to the child and to the family based on desire for knowledge, readiness to learn, and overall neurologic and psychosocial state.

- Provide information about the procedure, including steps of the procedure and monitoring of the child ➤➤*Rationale:* Providing information may decrease anxiety and fear in both child and family.
- Explain positioning requirements for LP ➤➤*Rationale:* Providing information may decrease fear and anxiety and promote cooperation during the procedure.
- Review the pain management and sedation plan for the child, including local anesthesia, sedation, and Child Life support ➤➤*Rationale:* Providing information decreases anxiety and fear, reassures the child and family that pain will be managed appropriately, and allows child and family to verbalize concerns.
- Explain positioning required after the procedure ➤➤*Rationale:* The family's and child's knowledge of what to expect after the procedure may decrease anxiety.
- If the family desires to stay during the procedure and institution-specific protocol permits family presence, provide the family with accurate information regarding the procedure, family's role, and expectations ➤➤*Rationale:* The family is prepared for their role; clearly defined guidelines and expectations are provided.
- Encourage questions and answer questions as they arise ➤➤*Rationale:* Reinforcement of information is needed during periods of stress and is especially important if the procedure is performed emergently.

EQUIPMENT

- Sterile gloves and gowns
- Sterile drapes
- Sterile gauze pads
- Caps and masks with eye shield
- Povidone-iodine
- Alcohol pads
- Fenestrated drape
- Manometer with three-way stopcock
- Topical anesthetic, as time and situation permits
- Lidocaine 1% without epinephrine
- Syringes, 3-mL and 5-mL
- 20-gauge, 22-gauge, and 25-gauge needles
- Spinal needle, 20-gauge or 22-gauge; length appropriate for child's age
- Four numbered capped sterile specimen tubes
- Band-aid or sterile dressing supplies
- Specimen labels containing two patient identifiers
- Appropriate laboratory requisitions
- Rolls or pillows to provide support for positioning
- Bedside tables for positioning and to establish sterile field

Procedure for Lumbar Puncture: Assist

Steps	Rationale	Considerations
1. Ensure child and family understand procedure and questions are answered.	Evaluates and reinforces understanding of previously taught information.	Developmental level, cognitive ability, and anxiety level determine approach to and effectiveness of teaching.
2. Ensure presence of signed consent.	Ensures medical-legal compliance as suggested by the Joint Commission on Accreditation of Healthcare Organizations (JCAHO).	In emergency situations, refer to institution-specific protocol for assumption of consent.
3. Wash hands.	Standard precautions; reduces transmission of microorganisms.	
4. Apply topical anesthetic per prescribing practitioner's order. Draw an imaginary line between the posterior iliac crests and apply local anesthetic over the spine, 1 cm above and 1 cm below this line (see Figure 84-1).	Decreases pain and anxiety in children.	Topical anesthetic should be applied 30 to 60 minutes before procedure based on type of topical anesthetic used and manufacturer's recommendation. (Level I*) Use two patient identifiers per institution-specific protocol to identify the child before medication administration.
5. Assist practitioner gather necessary supplies and equipment for procedure.	Facilitates completion of procedure in a timely manner.	
6. Ensure appropriate cardiorespiratory monitoring is in place with appropriate alarm limits set and alarms activated.	Child may have decompensation during procedure.	Emergency equipment should be readily available. If child is receiving sedation, implement institution-specific protocol for procedural sedation.
7. Put on cap and mask; wash hands.	Standard precautions; reduces transmission of microorganisms.	Garb required for individual assisting with LP is institution specific.
8. Put on gloves and gown as required.	Decreases risk of transmission of microorganisms.	
9. Participate in identification of child with appropriate patient and procedure verification process (e.g., "Time out"). (Level II*)	Confirms correct patient, procedure, and site as recommended by JCAHO; prevents unnecessary medical procedures.	Verification process and documentation is institution specific. Use active communication techniques.
10. If prescribed, administer sedation as appropriate and per prescribing practitioner's order.	Decreases child's anxiety; facilitates positioning and child's ability to hold still.	Administration of sedation and monitoring of the child should not be the responsibility of the practitioner who is performing the procedure.
11. Assist with establishing sterile field and equipment preparation.	Maintains aseptic technique.	
12. Provide for appropriate privacy; position child in desired position depending on developmental level and ability to cooperate (see Figures 84-2 and 84-3).	Facilitates ease of needle insertion and successful puncture of the subarachnoid space. Helps to enlarge intervertebral spaces.[5] Respiratory distress is more common in side-lying position.	Both positions necessitate that the hips, knees, and neck be flexed. Privacy is an important consideration for school-aged children and adolescents.

Procedure Continues on following page

Procedure for Lumbar Puncture: Assist—*Continued*

Steps	Rationale	Considerations
Infants and small children should lie on the side in fetal position. Knees should be brought up close to the chin with neck flexed in a downward position. Sick neonates may be placed in upright position for LP.[5] Older children may be more comfortable in a sitting position lying forward with face down on a table. *(Level VI*)*		
13. Assist in identification of landmarks and anatomic site for LP.	The LP must be done below level of L3 to prevent damage to the spinal cord. Interspaces should be L3-L4 or L4-L5.[4,5]	The L3-L4 interspace is found by locating iliac crest and drawing an imaginary line from one anterior spine of ileum to the other. Intersection of this line with the spine occurs at L3-L4.[5]
14. Assist with administration of local anesthesia.	Local anesthetic decreases pain at insertion site. Systemic sedation is used based on child's age and ability to cooperate and as indicated by clinical status.	For local anesthesia, initially the skin is injected and then a deeper injection of lidocaine is administered to the interspinous ligament.
15. Once the needle is in place, instruct child to relax and breathe normally. With younger children, once needle is in place, maintain position and restrict movement. *(Level VI*)*	Increased muscle tension or intrathoracic pressure may falsely elevate CSF pressure.	Child undergoing LP may slightly straighten legs because severe leg flexion can increase intrathoracic pressure.
16. If necessary, assist in attaching manometer to the spinal needle via three-way stopcock, maintaining aseptic technique. *(Level VI*)*	Obtains CSF pressure measurement; maintains needle and field sterility. A crying uncooperative child is the most common reason for an elevated opening pressure.[5]	If performing the LP for diagnosis of infection or instillation of medications, manometer reading of CSF pressure may be omitted.
17. Assist with collection of CSF specimens.	The manometer is stabilized with one hand while the other hand turns the stopcock.	Aseptic technique must be maintained.
18. Label specimen tubes at the bedside and complete laboratory paperwork per institution-specific protocol. Label each tube with type of specimen and the order in which it was collected. *(Level II*)*	The CSF specimens must be collected in the proper sequence.	Evaluation of each numbered specimen helps differentiate between subarachnoid hemorrhage and traumatic tap. Consistent presence of red blood cells in CSF is indicative of subarachnoid hemorrhage, whereas decrease in red blood cells in consecutive samples indicates a traumatic tap.
19. Apply band-aid or dressing to site once needle is removed.	Reduces incidence rate of infection.	

* Level II: Theory-based; no research data to support recommendations; recommendations from expert consensus group may exist
 Level VI: Clinical studies in a variety of patient populations and situations to support recommendations

Procedure for Lumbar Puncture: Assist—*Continued*

Steps	Rationale	Considerations
20. Per practitioner preference or unit-specific protocol, child may be placed in supine position immediately after procedure.	Facilitates closure of dura after procedure.	Although practice may be to have the child remain supine for 1 to 4 hours after LP, a few studies in children show no decrease in the incidence rate of postdural puncture headache or other complications.[7-9] *(Level IV*)*
21. Discard used supplies and equipment, including sharps, in appropriate receptacles.	Standard precautions; reduces transmission of microorganisms. Protects personnel health.	
22. Remove personal protective equipment; wash hands.	Standard precautions.	
23. Send specimens to laboratory without delay.	Provides specimen for analysis; delay in transporting specimens to laboratory may alter results obtained.	

* Level IV: Limited clinical studies to support recommendations

Expected Outcomes	**Unexpected Outcomes**
• The LP is completed and adequate volume of CSF is obtained • The CSF specimens are placed in correct specimen tubes, labeled appropriately, and sent to the laboratory in the appropriate time frame • Child's baseline neurologic and hemodynamic status are unchanged after procedure • Child is free from complications of LP	• Cerebrospinal fluid is not obtained • Inability to complete procedure • Specimens are mislabeled • Specimens are placed in incorrect specimen tubes • Delay in sending specimens to laboratory • Herniation caused by sudden shift in intracranial contents or a change in ICP • Subdural or epidural spinal hematoma • Prolonged headache, neck stiffness, photophobia • Cranial neuropathy • Spinal abscess • Seizure • New and persistent symptoms of pain, numbness, weakness, or paralysis in lower extremities • Inability to void spontaneously

Monitoring and Care of the Child

Activities and Interventions	Rationale	Reportable Conditions
1. Monitor child's neurologic, respiratory, and cardiac status during and after procedure.	Pain or abnormal sensation radiating down one or both legs may result from spinal nerve damage or irritation and may necessitate a change in position of child or needle position. Positioning with neck flexed may impair the pediatric airway, particularly if the child is sedated.	• Respiratory depression • Motor or sensory changes • Changes in level of consciousness • Change in vital signs (VS)
2. Vital signs and neurologic assessment per institution-specific protocol.	A change in vital signs or neurologic assessment results could indicate acute hematoma formation, injury to spinal nerve, infection, or herniation.	• Bradycardia • Hypertension • Abnormal respirations • Decreased movement of lower extremities

Continued

Monitoring and Care of the Child—Cont'd

Activities and Interventions	Rationale	Reportable Conditions
3. Monitor puncture site.	Identifies complications at the site.	• Persistent bleeding at site • Persistent drainage of clear serous fluid
4. Monitor child for pain or discomfort with pain scale appropriate to child's age or developmental level. (See Procedure 173 for further information.)	Identifies traumatic complications of needle placement.	• Persistent severe back pain • Leg pain not evident before procedure

Documentation

- Child and family education
- Date and time of procedure and individual who performed the procedure
- Patient and procedure verification process per institution-specific protocol
- Medications administered for procedure and child's response; if procedural sedation is used, institution-specific documentation for procedural sedation
- Status of puncture site
- Vital signs before, during, and after procedure
- Child's neurologic status before and after the procedure
- Comfort assessment and any specific interventions provided
- Unexpected outcomes and related treatment

References
1. Berkowitz ID, et al: Meningitis, infectious encephalitis and other CNS infections. In Rogers MC, editor: *Textbook of pediatric intensive care,* ed 3, Baltimore, 1996, Williams and Wilkins.
2. Shilkofski N: Procedures. In Robertson J, Shilkofski N, editors: *The Harriet Lane handbook,* ed 17, Philadelphia, 2005, Mosby.
3. Singh NC: *Manual of pediatric critical care,* Philadelphia, 1997, Saunders.
4. Cronan KM, Wiley JF II: Lumbar puncture. In Henretig F, King C, editor: *Textbook of pediatric emergency medicine procedures,* Philadelphia, 1997, Lippincott, Williams & Wilkins.
5. Behrman RE, et al, editors: *Nelson textbook of pediatrics,* ed 17, Philadelphia, 2004, Saunders.
6. Fleisher G, Ludwig S, editors: *Pediatric emergency medicine,* ed 3, Philadelphia, 2000, Lippincott Williams & Wilkins.
7. Ebinger F, et al: Strict bed rest following lumbar puncture in children and adolescents is of no benefit, *Neurology* 62:1003-1005, 2004.
8. Janssens E, et al: Post-dural puncture headaches in children; a literature review, *Eur J Pediatr* 162:117-121, 2003.
9. Turnbull DK, Shepherd DB: Post-dural puncture headache: pathogenesis, prevention and treatment, *Br J Anaesthesia* 91(5):718-729, 2003.

Ventriculoperitoneal Shunt Tap: Assist

P U R P O S E : To assist the practitioner with performance of a ventriculoperitoneal shunt tap to identify a shunt infection, a nonfunctioning valve or shunt system, or a change in the cerebrospinal fluid flow pressure. A needle is inserted into the shunt reservoir to withdraw cerebrospinal fluid to aid in diagnosis or to decrease intracranial pressure.

Amy Carnall-Grogan

PREREQUISITE KNOWLEDGE

- Anatomy and physiology of the pediatric brain
- Hydrocephalus is an abnormal accumulation of cerebrospinal fluid (CSF) that results from an imbalance between CSF production and CSF absorption; hydrocephalus can be congenital or acquired.
- A ventriculoperitoneal shunt (VPS) is the most common type of shunt inserted for the treatment of hydrocephalus.
  - ❖ A VPS is the most common shunt inserted because the peritoneal space has a good blood supply, a large area for reabsorption, space to accommodate "extra" tubing, and decreased risk of complication associated with infection.
  - ❖ Other sites of distal shunt placement include the pleural space, right atrium, bladder, ureter, stomach, gallbladder, and fallopian tube.
- A VPS is a silastic tube that is inserted into the cerebral ventricle to divert excess CSF away from the brain to the peritoneum for reabsorption.
  - ❖ The proximal tubing is radiopaque and is usually placed in the anterior part of the lateral ventricle.
  - ❖ The proximal tubing is attached to a valve to regulate CSF drainage and allow unidirectional flow. The valve usually has a reservoir for CSF sampling and pressure assessment.
  - ❖ The distal tubing is also attached to the valve. The distal end is tunneled subcutaneously to the peritoneum or other absorptive area.

- Specific type of VPS the child has in place, if known
  - ❖ Variations in shunts may include single or double reservoir, programmable flow capability of the valve, recommended angle of penetration of the reservoir, and location of the reservoir.
- Indications for shunt tap
  - ❖ Suspected infection
  - ❖ Suspected malfunction
  - ❖ Suspected obstruction
  - ❖ To decrease intracranial pressure (ICP)
  - ❖ If immediate VPS revision is not available and the child's condition is deteriorating, tapping to remove CSF may be used temporarily to decrease ICP to less than 20 cm H_2O.
  - ❖ To assess shunt function with instillation of a contrast agent or radionuclide (i.e., shuntogram)
- Signs and symptoms of malfunctioning or infected shunt include:
  - ❖ Irritability
  - ❖ Headache
  - ❖ Lethargy
  - ❖ Emesis
  - ❖ Fever
  - ❖ Bulging fontanel in infants
  - ❖ Abdominal pain (if peritonitis is present)
  - ❖ Inflammation along shunt tract
- Shunt tap procedure should be performed with strict aseptic technique

- If a shunt tap is performed to rule out an infection, the shunt is generally tapped before the initiation of antibiotics.
- Complications of shunt tap include[1]:
  ❖ Infection (ventriculitis)
  ❖ Damage to the shunt
  ❖ Cardiorespiratory instability
  ❖ Conversion of partial shunt obstruction to complete shunt obstruction
  ❖ Bleeding
  ❖ Subdural hematoma
- Contraindications for shunt tap performance include loculated ventricles, slit-like ventricles, or small ventricles. The presence of a skin infection at the site of the reservoir is a relative contraindication.
- The opening pressure for a functioning shunt is usually not significantly higher than the valve pressure; a brisk CSF flow with a significantly higher pressure suggests a distal malfunction, whereas a slow or absent flow suggests a proximal obstruction.[2-4]
- In the presence of normal or enlarged ventricles, a spontaneous and steady flow of CSF from the proximal shunt should be expected; small ventricles may produce slow or even absent flow, which is often difficult to differentiate from shunt obstruction.[2,5]
- Child development as it relates to clinical assessment and VPS tap procedure
- Mastery of pediatric advanced life support competencies
- Informed consent is required before VPS tap procedure

CHILD AND FAMILY ASSESSMENT

- Child's baseline vital signs ➥*Rationale:* Establishes baseline values for the child; facilitates prompt recognition of change from baseline.
- Child's baseline neurologic assessment, including mental status and sensory and motor function ➥*Rationale:* Establishes baseline neurologic function before withdrawal of CSF.
- Signs of increased ICP
  ❖ Infant: Increased head circumference, full fontanel, engorged scalp veins, Macewen's sign, Cranial nerve (CN) VI palsy, irregular respirations, apnea, seizure, setting sun sign (upward gaze palsy), hyperreactive reflexes
  ❖ Older child/adolescent: Headache, nausea, vomiting, ataxia, drowsiness, blurred vision, papilledema
  ❖ Late signs: Bradycardia, hypertension, and irregular respirations (Cushing's triad) ➥*Rationale:* If the child has signs of increased ICP, this procedure becomes a medical emergency.
- Current laboratory profile including complete blood count (CBC), prothrombin time (PT), and partial thromboplastin time (PTT) ➥*Rationale:* Establishes baseline values and identifies abnormalities before procedure.
- Child's developmental level and ability to cooperate with positioning requirements ➥*Rationale:* Developmental

level affects preparation of the child and establishes whether child may need sedation for procedure.
- Child's and family's understanding of the reasons for and risks and benefits of the procedure ➥*Rationale:* Evaluates child's and family's understanding of the procedure and provides a gauge for ongoing education.
- Status of skin at proposed VPS tap site ➥*Rationale:* Identifies potential contraindications.
- Child's known allergies ➥*Rationale:* Identifies allergies to medications or solutions that may be used during shunt tap procedure.
- Desire of family members to remain with the child during procedure ➥*Rationale:* Family's presence may provide support and comfort to the child during the procedure if institution-specific protocol facilitates family presence; family members should also have the choice not to remain with the child.

CHILD AND FAMILY EDUCATION

Individualized, developmentally appropriate education is provided to the family and to the child based on desire for knowledge, readiness to learn, and overall neurologic and psychosocial state.

- Provide information about the procedure, including steps of the procedure and monitoring of the child ➥*Rationale:* Providing information may decrease anxiety and fear in both child and family.
- Explain that the child may have some discomfort when the needle punctures the skin ➥*Rationale:* Providing anticipatory information helps to decrease anxiety and promotes coping.
- Explain to the child and to the family that it is imperative that the child remain completely still during the procedure ➥*Rationale:* Any unexpected movement of the child makes CSF specimen difficult to obtain and may contaminate the procedure by disrupting the sterile field; the child and family are provided with information about expectations during the procedure.
- If the family desires to stay during the procedure and institution-specific protocol permits family presence, provide the family with accurate information regarding the procedure, family's role, and expectations ➥*Rationale:* Presence of family may provide support and comfort to the child, and clearly defined institution-specific protocol for family presence facilitates this; however, family members should also have the choice not to remain with the child.
- Encourage questions and answer questions as they arise ➥*Rationale:* Reinforcement of information is needed during periods of stress and is especially important if the procedure is performed emergently.

EQUIPMENT

- 23-gauge or 25-gauge butterfly needle
- Sterile gloves

- Clean gloves
- Syringe, 5-mL
- Sterile drapes
- Povidone-iodine solution prep sticks, pads, or other form of applicator
- Alcohol wipes

- Clippers or razor
- 4×4 gauze pads
- Specimen labels containing two patient identifiers
- Sterile specimen tubes
- Appropriate laboratory requisitions

Procedure for Ventriculoperitoneal Shunt Tap: Assist

Steps	Rationale	Considerations
1. Ensure child and family understand procedure and questions are answered.	Evaluates and reinforces understanding of previously taught information.	Developmental level, cognitive ability, and anxiety level determine approach to and effectiveness of teaching.
2. Confirm that informed consent has been obtained.	Ensures medical-legal compliance as suggested by the Joint Commission on Accreditation of Healthcare Organizations (JCAHO).	In emergency situations, refer to institution-specific protocol for assumption of consent.
3. Assist practitioner who is performing the procedure to gather equipment and supplies.	Facilitates completion of procedure in a timely manner.	
4. Ensure appropriate cardiorespiratory monitoring is in place with appropriate alarm limits set and alarms activated.	Child may decompensate during procedure.[2]	
5. Ensure emergency equipment is readily available.	Allows prompt response in case of rapid deterioration of the child's condition.	
6. Wash hands.	This is the single most important action in preventing nosocomial infections.	In a life-threatening emergency situation, immediate intervention may be necessary and may limit use of complete aseptic technique.
7. Put on clean gloves.	Standard precautions; reduces the transmission of microorganisms.	Garb required for individual assisting with shunt tap is institution specific; cap and mask may be required.
8. Participate in identifying child with appropriate patient and procedure verification process (e.g., "Time out") *(Level II*)*	Confirms correct patient, procedure, and site as recommended by JCAHO; prevents unnecessary medical procedures.	Verification process and documentation is institution specific. Use active communication techniques.
9. Assist practitioner to establish sterile field and prepare supplies.	Facilitates aseptic technique; reduces risk of infection.	
10. Position child supine with head of bed elevated 30 degrees and the child's face turned away from the side being tapped. *(Level II*)*	Provides access to the shunt bulb.	
11. Assist the practitioner to prepare and drape the area.	Facilitates aseptic technique.	

Procedure continues on following page

* Level II: Theory-based; no research data to support recommendations; recommendations from expert consensus group may exist

Procedure for Ventriculoperitoneal Shunt Tap: Assist—*Continued*

Steps	Rationale	Considerations
12. Assist child in holding the head in required position for the length of the procedure with the nondominant hand; support and comfort child throughout the procedure. *(Level II*)*	Aids the practitioner who is performing the tap by ensuring the head remains immobile during the procedure.	The child's cognitive and developmental level affects ability to cooperate with the procedure. Use developmentally appropriate techniques, such as distraction or positive reinforcement.
13. Dominant hand may be used to pass additional nonsterile supplies needed by the practitioner who is performing the procedure. *(Level II*)*	Assists the practitioner who is performing the tap to maintain sterile technique.	
14. The practitioner introduces the butterfly needle into the shunt bulb and observes for spontaneous CSF flow in the tubing.	Flow of CSF confirms placement of the needle in the shunt bulb.	
15. The practitioner attaches a stopcock with manometer to the end of the butterfly tubing and obtains an opening pressure. *(Level VI*)*	Identifies the initial ICP reading. When the outlet valve is occluded, the manometer reflects the opening pressure (ventricular pressure).[3]	
16. The practitioner allows the CSF to flow into the distal catheter.	Allows collection of CSF specimens.	No CSF flow is usually indicative of a proximal obstruction.
17. Assist practitioner to collect 2 to 3 mL of CSF in sterile specimen containers to be sent for analysis. *(Level II*)*	The CSF is sent for cell count, gram's stain, culture and sensitivity, glucose, and protein to assess for infection. Other tests are sent per the prescribing practitioner.	Send CSF specimen tubes in the numeric order indicated by the prescribing practitioner. The presence of organisms on the gram's stain confirms an infection, although absence of organism does not rule out the possibility of infection.[6]
18. The practitioner removes needle and applies gentle pressure to the scalp.	Prevents leakage of CSF.	Many manufacturers line the proximal portion of the bulb with a polymer that prevents leakage of CSF.
19. Label specimen tubes at the bedside and complete laboratory paperwork per institution-specific protocol.	Ensures specimens are labeled correctly and desired studies are requested; promotes patient safety.	
20. Ensure used supplies and equipment, including sharps, are discarded in appropriate receptacles.	Standard precautions; reduces transmission of microorganisms. Protects personnel health.	
21. Remove personal protective equipment; wash hands.	Standard precautions; reduces transmission of microorganisms.	
22. Ensure specimens are sent to laboratory without delay.	Provides specimen for analysis; delay in transporting specimens to laboratory may alter results obtained.	
23. Assess child's vital signs (VS) and neurologic status after procedure.	Assesses child's tolerance of procedure.	

* Level II: Theory-based; no research data to support recommendations; recommendations from expert consensus group may exist
  Level VI: Clinical studies in a variety of patient populations and situations to support recommendations

Expected Outcomes	Unexpected Outcomes
• CSF is obtained for analysis, including evaluation of shunt infection • Accurate ICP measurement is obtained • CSF volume is removed as a temporizing measure in the child with an occluded shunt • Child is free from complications of VPS tap • CSF specimens are placed in correct specimen tubes, labeled appropriately, and sent to the laboratory in the appropriate time frame • Child's condition remains stable throughout procedure	• Inability to obtain CSF because of occlusion of the proximal shunt • Inability to obtain ICP measurement • Inaccurate ICP measurement • Inability to remove CSF because of occlusion of the proximal shunt • Development of infection, including ventriculitis • Damage to the shunt • Cardiorespiratory instability • Conversion of partial shunt obstruction to complete shunt obstruction • Bleeding • Subdural hematoma • Specimens are mislabeled • Specimens are placed in incorrect sample tubes • Delay in sending specimens to laboratory • Decompensation of child during procedure • Deterioration of neurologic status during or after procedure

Monitoring and Care of the Child

Activities and Interventions	Rationale	Reportable Conditions
1. Monitor VS, including heart rate, blood pressure, and respiratory rate during and after procedure.	Hypotension can cause cerebral ischemia; bradycardia can result from pressure on the vagal control mechanism of the medulla.[4] If child has signs of increased ICP, vigilant monitoring is necessary to guide appropriate management.	• Bradycardia • Hypertension • Abnormal respirations • Change in level of consciousness (LOC) • Change in child's status from baseline
2. Monitor oxygen saturation.	Impaired airway clearance or decreasing respiratory rate can lead to increased O_2 requirement; hypoxia can cause cerebral ischemia.	• Pulse oximetry (SpO_2) <95% (unless child's baseline is a lower than normal SpO_2) • Headache
3. Monitor child's neurologic examination results, including LOC, during and after the procedure.	Increased ICP results in abnormal neurologic examination results. If ICP continues to rise, the child becomes lethargic, stuporous, and finally comatose.	• Changes to child's baseline neurologic examination results, including pupillary changes, focal findings • Seizures • Cushing's triad: hypertension, usually with widened pulse pressure; bradycardia; irregular respiratory pattern; this is a late response and is a compensatory mechanism to the rising ICP[5]

Documentation

- Child and family education
- Presence of informed consent
- Patient/procedure verification process per institution-specific protocol
- Date and time of procedure and individual who performed procedure
- Volume of CSF removed, appearance of CSF, and opening shunt pressure
- Child's neurologic examination results before and after procedure
- Child's tolerance of procedure
- Laboratory specimens obtained and requested studies
- Unexpected outcomes and related treatment

References

1. Duhaime A, Wiley JF: Ventricular shunt and burr hole puncture. In Henretig F, King C, editors: *Textbook of pediatric emergency medicine procedures,* Philadelphia, 1997, Lippincott, Williams & Wilkins.
2. Walter KA: Neurosurgical procedures. In Chen H, et al, editors: *Manual of common bedside surgical procedures,* ed 2, Philadelphia, 2000, Lippincott Williams & Wilkins.
3. Choux M, et al: *Pediatric neurosurgery,* London, 1999, Churchill Livingstone.
4. Gaskill SJ, Marlin AE: *Handbook of pediatric neurology and neurosurgery,* Boston, 1993, Little, Brown and Company.
5. Hickey JV: *The clinical practice of neurological and neurosurgical nursing,* ed 5, Philadelphia, 2003, Lippincott Williams & Wilkins.
6. Rogers MC, editor: *Textbook of pediatric intensive care,* ed 3, Philadelphia, 1996, William & Wilkins.

Additional Readings

Albright AL, et al, editors: *Principles and practice of pediatric neurosurgery,* New York, 1999, Thieme Medical Publishers.

Andrews BT, Hammer GB: *Pediatric neurosurgical intensive care,* Park Ridge, IL, 1997, The American Association of Neurological Surgeons.

Barker E: *Neuroscience nursing: a spectrum of care,* Philadelphia, 2002, Mosby.

McLone DG, et al: *Pediatric neurosurgery: surgery of the developing nervous system,* ed 4, Philadelphia, 2001, Saunders.

PROCEDURE 83

AP

Cerebrospinal Fluid Sampling from a Ventriculostomy/External Ventricular Drain

PURPOSE: To obtain a sterile cerebrospinal fluid (CSF) sample for testing from a closed sterile external ventricular drainage system

Delia R. Nickolaus

PREREQUISITE KNOWLEDGE

- Principles of aseptic technique
- Care of a child with a ventriculostomy or externalized ventricular shunt or drain (EVD) (See Procedures 77 and 80)
- CSF sampling may be indicated for detection of CSF infection or ventriculitis, monitoring for resolution of CSF infection, sepsis workup in the child with fever and EVD, deterioration in neurologic status, or change in appearance of CSF drainage from EVD.[1]
- Appropriate containers for specimens to be collected and minimum required volumes for those specimens
- Specimen labeling requirements
- Specimen handling requirements
- Child development as it relates to assessment of neurologic status and CSF sampling from a ventricular catheter or drain

CHILD AND FAMILY ASSESSMENT

- Child's developmental level and ability to interact ➸***Rationale:*** These factors identify baseline neurologic status and also influence preparation of the child and interaction.
- Type of drain and monitoring system in use ➸***Rationale:*** Identifies sampling port location.
- Intracranial pressure (ICP) waveform, if ICP is monitored ➸***Rationale:*** Provides a baseline assessment; facilitates identification of change in waveform after catheter manipulation.
- Child's and family's understanding of the reasons for and risks and benefits of sampling CSF ➸***Rationale:*** Evaluates child's and family's understanding of the procedure and provides a gauge for ongoing education; updates may be needed concerning the findings of previous CSF samples and the reason for subsequent analysis of CSF.
- Child's and family's understanding of the child's medical condition ➸***Rationale:*** Assesses child's and family's understanding of potential long-term consequences.
- Family's desire to be present during the procedure ➸***Rationale:*** Family may provide support and comfort during the procedure but should have the choice not to remain with the child.

CHILD AND FAMILY EDUCATION

Individualized, developmentally appropriate education is provided to the family and to the child based on desire for knowledge, readiness to learn, and overall neurologic and psychosocial state.

- Review the signs and symptoms of a CSF infection and the indications for CSF sampling. ➸***Rationale:*** Child and

AP This procedure should be performed only by physicians, advanced practice nurses, and other health care professionals (including critical care nurses) with additional knowledge, skills, and demonstrated competence per professional licensure or institutional standard.

family are assisted in understanding the reason for CSF sampling and information that will be obtained.

- Explain procedure for CSF sampling ➥*Rationale:* Child and family are assisted in understanding the method of externally draining CSF from the ventricles; providing information may decrease anxiety, especially if the child and family are reassured that the procedure is not painful.
- If ICP is monitored, explain that the pressure waveform and monitor displays are absent during CSF sampling procedure ➥*Rationale:* Reduces anxiety and fear that the child is experiencing difficulties.
- Encourage questions and answer questions as they arise ➥*Rationale:* Reinforcement of information is needed during periods of stress.

EQUIPMENT

- Sterile gloves
- Sterile syringe, 3-mL
- 22-gauge needle or needleless access device
- Sterile drape
- Mask
- Povidone-iodine antiseptic swab
- Appropriate sterile specimen containers
- Appropriate laboratory requisitions
- Specimen labels containing two patient identifiers

Procedure for CSF Sampling from a Ventriculostomy

Steps	Rationale	Considerations
1. Ensure child and family understand procedure and questions are answered.	Evaluates and reinforces understanding of previously taught information.	Developmental level, cognitive ability, and anxiety level determine approach to and effectiveness of teaching.
2. Gather needed equipment and supplies.	Facilitates completion of task in a timely manner; decreases likelihood of specimen contamination.	
3. Wash hands.	Standard precautions; reduces transmission of microorganisms.	
4. Clamp the EVD for approximately one half hour. Turn the stopcock most proximal to the child *off* to the child. If no stopcock is used, clamp the tubing between the insertion site and the sampling port. See Procedure 80 for a diagram of the sampling port. *(Level II*)*	Clamping the EVD allows CSF to accumulate in the ventricles.	Some children may not tolerate clamping of the EVD; for those children, do not clamp EVD. Unclamp immediately for any signs of increased ICP while the EVD is clamped.
5. Use two patient identifiers to verify correct child.	Promotes patient safety; ensures CSF specimen is drawn on the correct child.	
6. Using the stopcock most proximal to child, turn the stopcock off to the drainage bag and open to the child and sample port.	The stopcock *must* be turned off to the drainage system and *open* to the child to allow CSF withdrawal directly from the ventricles and not the tubing to decrease the risk of contamination.	Some EVD systems do not have a proximal stopcock; rather, they have a sampling port. For these systems, clamp the drainage tubing distal to the sampling port, between the port and the drainage collection system.
7. Put on mask; wash hands.	Decreases likelihood of contamination of closed EVD system.	
8. Place sterile drape under stopcock and sampling port closest to the child, creating a sterile field; place sterile supplies on sterile field.	Prevents contamination of the closed sterile system. Contamination of the CSF sample is least likely when obtained from sample port closest to child.	Do not obtain CSF sample from EVD drainage bag, which has the most potential to be contaminated and is not representative of the CSF in the child's ventricles.

* Level II: Theory-based; no research data to support recommendations; recommendations from expert consensus group may exist

Procedure for CSF Sampling from a Ventriculostomy—*Continued*		
Steps	**Rationale**	**Considerations**
9. Swab sample port with povidone-iodine or antiseptic per institution-specific protocol; allow to dry. *(Level II*)*	Decreases risk of contaminating the system. Swabbing before putting on gloves allows antiseptic to dry.	Chlorhexidine is not recommended for antisepsis if the possibility of contact with the meninges exists. *(Level I*)*
10. Put on gloves.	Standard precautions; decreases likelihood of EVD system contamination.	
11. If a stopcock is used, attach syringe to port and slowly and gently aspirate 2 to 3 mL of CSF over 2 to 3 minutes. If a sampling port is used, insert a 22-gauge needle or needleless access device into sampling port and gently allow 2 to 3 mL of CSF to drip freely from the needle directly into the specimen container. Alternatively, a 3-mL syringe can be attached to the needle or needleless access device and CSF can be aspirated slowly and gently over 2 to 3 minutes. *(Level II*)*	Withdrawal of CSF should be slow to prevent rapid decompression or high suction pressure, which could cause intracranial bleeding. Force should *never* be used when aspirating CSF.	CSF removal should not necessitate forceful withdrawal with the syringe. If aspiration of CSF from the system is difficult, but the system has been draining well, it may need to remain off to the drainage bag for a longer period of time. Do *not* pull hard on syringe to obtain CSF. Consult neurosurgeon if unable to obtain CSF. Needleless access device may be used if access port can be accessed with needleless access device.
12. Turn stopcock off to child while disconnecting syringe or needle.	Prevents inadvertent CSF drainage and possible introduction of air into EVD system.	
13. Place appropriate sample volume in sterile specimen containers.	Ensures accurate results are obtained.	The CSF specimens may be sent for gram stain, culture, glucose, protein, or cell count. A sample of 3 mL of CSF should be enough for these tests. Per institution-specific protocol, the CSF must be separated into individual specimen containers for the different sections of the laboratory (microbiology, etc).
14. Label specimens at the bedside and complete laboratory paperwork per institution-specific protocol.	Promotes patient safety; ensures accurate and efficient processing of specimen.	Follow institution-specific protocol for handling and labeling laboratory specimens.
15. Return all stopcocks and slide clamps to the open position to allow CSF drainage. Confirm EVD level per prescribing practitioner's order.	Reinstitutes drainage of CSF.	
16. Dispose of used supplies and equipment in appropriate receptacles.	Standard precautions; reduces transmission of microorganisms.	
17. Remove gloves, mask, and gloves; wash hands.	Standard precautions.	
18. Assess child's neurologic status after procedure.	Any change in neurologic status may indicate overdrainage of CSF or potential blood in ventricular space.	

* Level I: Manufacturer's recommendations only

Level II: Theory-based; no research data to support recommendations; recommendations from expert consensus group may exist

Expected Outcomes

- Sterile aspiration of CSF

- Child's neurologic status and ICP remain stable throughout the procedure
- The EVD continues to drain properly

Unexpected Outcomes

- Break in sterile technique during CSF aspiration
- Inability to obtain CSF from drain
- Increase in ICP after drain manipulation
- Deterioration in neurologic examination results
- Nonfunctioning EVD after CSF aspiration
- CSF leaking from around the insertion site
- Bloody CSF in previously clear CSF

Monitoring and Care of the Child

Activities and Interventions	Rationale	Reportable Conditions
1. Assess neurologic status before and after obtaining CSF; may include ICP monitoring.	Determines child's response to CSF aspiration; identifies increase in ICP.	• Deterioration in neurologic status
2. Monitor amount and type of EVD output after drain manipulation; measure and document output hourly.	Identifies change in drain output and potential complications.	• Increase in ICP after drain manipulation • The EVD no longer draining after drain manipulation • Presence of blood in previously clear CSF • CSF leaking from around the insertion site
3. Monitor temperature and vital signs.	Facilitates early detection of infection.	• Temperature greater than 38.5°C • Tachycardia • Tachypnea

Documentation

- Child and family education
- Child's tolerance of the procedure, including documentation of neurologic status before and after procedure
- Amount of CSF aspirated and studies sent
- Ease of CSF aspiration
- Procedure completed in a sterile fashion
- Appearance of CSF
- Unexpected outcomes and related treatment

Reference

1. Hader WJ, Steinbok P: The value of routine cultures of the cerebrospinal fluid in patients with external ventricular drains, *Neurosurgery* 46(5):1149-1155, 2000.

Additional Reading

Lozier AP, et al: Ventriculostomy-related infections: a critical review of the literature, *Neurosurgery* 51(1):170-182, 2002.

AP

Lumbar Puncture: Perform

P U R P O S E :   To obtain cerebrospinal fluid to support a diagnosis of central nervous system (CNS) infection, CNS malignant disease, or autoimmune disease. Lumbar puncture may also be performed to instill medication such as chemotherapy into the central nervous system.[1-3]

Michelle A. Sorscher

PREREQUISITE KNOWLEDGE

- Neuroanatomy and physiology, including the spinal cord and spinal column, of infants, children, and adolescents
- Lumbar puncture (LP) is usually performed at the L3-L4 or L4-L5 interspace.
- Principles of aseptic technique
- Indications for performing LP in infants and children[1,4]
  - ❖ Suspected meningitis
  - ❖ Diagnostic measure in children with neurologic deficits suggestive of an infectious or immunologic illness, such as Guillain-Barré syndrome, transverse myelitis, or acute disseminating encephalomyopathy
  - ❖ Administration of intrathecal medications, such as chemotherapy in children with cancer
  - ❖ Diagnostic measure to rule out CNS disease
  - ❖ Measurement of opening pressure
- Contraindications for performing an LP in infants and children[1,4,5]
  - ❖ Increased intracranial pressure (ICP) manifested clinically and radiographically

- ❖ Use caution in children with platelet dysfunction or bleeding disorder.
- ❖ Use caution in children with a known closed head injury.
- ❖ May be deferred in children with respiratory distress or hemodynamic instability until child is stabilized
- ❖ Skin infection at the proposed puncture site
- ❖ Spinal cord trauma or spinal cord compression
- ❖ Posterior spinal fusion in the lumbar region
- Complications of LP
  - ❖ Back pain
  - ❖ Bleeding
  - ❖ Spinal fluid leak
  - ❖ Postspinal headache
  - ❖ Meningitis
  - ❖ Epidural or subdural spinal hematoma
  - ❖ Acquired epidermoid spinal cord tumor
  - ❖ Herniation
- In most cases, a computed tomographic (CT) scan is performed before LP if increased ICP or space-occupying brain lesion is suspected. CT scan is recommended in any child with focal neurologic findings based on physical examination or history of focal symptoms such as seizures or papilledema.[1,4,5]
- Use of a smaller needle decreases the incidence rate of cerebrospinal fluid (CSF) leak and spinal headache. Recommended needle size guidelines are[3,4]:
  - ❖ Child <12 years: 22-gauge 1.5-inch needle
  - ❖ Child >12 years: 20-gauge or 22-gauge 3.5-inch needle

AP   This procedure should be performed only by physicians, advanced practice nurses, and other health care professionals Note: critical care nurses do not perform LPs with additional knowledge, skills, and demonstrated competence per professional licensure or institutional standard.

- Normal values[3]
  - ❖ Opening pressure, obtained with the child in the side-lying position: Older children, 5 to 20 cm H_2O; younger children, 8 to 11 cm H_2O
  - ❖ White blood cell (WBC) count: Maximum, 7 WBC/mm^3; up to 25 WBC/mm^3 in neonates and infants
  - ❖ Glucose: 40 to 80 mg/dL
  - ❖ Protein: 5 to 40 mg/dL
- Recommended studies[3,4]
  - ❖ Tube 1: Cultures including gram stain, bacterial, fungal, and any additional viral cultures
  - ❖ Tube 2: Biochemistry profile including glucose and protein
  - ❖ Tube 3: Hematology including cell count and differential
  - ❖ Tube 4: Optional studies including serologies and cytologies[5]
- See Procedure 79 for detailed information regarding CSF analysis.
- Use of procedural sedation must be considered in children, particularly if the child cannot cooperate with proper positioning. The child must be closely monitored throughout the procedure, with special attention paid to cardiorespiratory status during sedation and positioning. See Procedure 177 for further information.
- Child development as it relates to clinical assessment and LP
- Mastery of pediatric advanced life support competencies
- Competency in procedural sedation
- Informed consent is required before LP

CHILD AND FAMILY ASSESSMENT

- Child's vital signs ➤➤*Rationale:* Establishes baseline values for the child and identifies the child with increased risk for complications related to cardiorespiratory compromise.
- Baseline neurologic assessment, including mental status and sensory and motor functions; document preprocedure deficits ➤➤*Rationale:* Establishes baseline neurologic function before insertion of needle into subarachnoid space.
- Current laboratory profile, including complete blood count (CBC), prothrombin time (PT), and partial thromboplastin time (PTT) ➤➤*Rationale:* Establishes baseline values and identifies abnormalities or increased risks before procedure.
- Signs of meningeal irritation: headache, nausea or vomiting, nystagmus, nuchal rigidity, photophobia, Brudzinski's sign, and fever ➤➤*Rationale:* Establishes presenting signs and symptoms before procedure.
- Child's developmental level and ability to cooperate with positioning requirements; toddlers and young children and children with cognitive or neuromuscular disorders may be unable to cooperate ➤➤*Rationale:* Establishes the need for sedation for the procedure. The child must remain completely still throughout the procedure.
- Status of skin at proposed LP site ➤➤*Rationale:* Identifies potential contraindications.

- Child's known allergies ➤➤*Rationale:* Identifies allergies to medications or solutions that may be used during LP.
- Previous sedation experiences of the child ➤➤*Rationale:* Identifies previous difficulties with sedation; encourages child's and family's participation in developing plan of care.
- Child's and family's understanding of the reasons for and risks and benefits of the LP ➤➤*Rationale:* Evaluates child's and family's understanding of the procedure and provides a gauge for ongoing education.
- Desire of family members to remain with the child during the procedure ➤➤*Rationale:* Family's presence may provide support and comfort to the child during the procedure if institution-specific protocol facilitates family presence; family should also have the choice not to remain with the child.

CHILD AND FAMILY EDUCATION

Individualized, developmentally appropriate education is provided to the child and to the family based on desire for knowledge, readiness to learn, and overall neurologic and psychosocial state.

- Provide information about the procedure, including steps of the procedure and monitoring of the child ➤➤*Rationale:* Providing information may decrease anxiety and fear in both child and family; facilitates informed consent.
- Explain positioning requirements for LP ➤➤*Rationale:* Providing information may decrease fear and anxiety and promote cooperation during the procedure.
- Review the pain management and sedation plan for the child, including local anesthesia, sedation, and Child Life support ➤➤*Rationale:* Providing information decreases anxiety and fear and reassures the child and family that pain will be managed appropriately. Allows child and family to verbalize concerns; facilitates informed consent.
- Explain positioning necessary after the procedure ➤➤*Rationale:* Allows family and child to know what to expect after the procedure is complete; explanation may decrease anxiety.
- If family desires to stay during the procedure and institution-specific protocol permits family presence, provide the family with accurate information regarding the procedure, the family's role, and expectations ➤➤*Rationale:* Prepares the family for their role; provides clearly defined guidelines and expectations.
- Encourage questions and answer questions as they arise ➤➤*Rationale:* Reinforcement of information is needed during periods of stress and is especially important if the procedure is performed emergently.

EQUIPMENT

- Sterile gloves and gowns
- Sterile drapes
- Sterile gauze pads

- Cap and mask with eye shield
- Povidone-iodine solution
- Alcohol pads
- Fenestrated drape
- Manometer with three-way stopcock
- Topical anesthetic as time and situation permits
- Lidocaine 1% without epinephrine
- Syringes, 3-mL and 5-mL
- 20-gauge, 22-gauge, and 25-gauge needles

- Spinal needle, 20-gauge or 22-gauge, with length appropriate for child's age
- Four numbered capped sterile specimen tubes
- Band-aid or sterile dressing supplies
- Specimen labels that contain two patient identifiers
- Appropriate laboratory requisitions
- Rolls or pillows to provide support for positioning
- Bedside tables for positioning and establishing sterile field

Procedure for Lumbar Puncture: Perform

Steps	Rationale	Considerations
1. Ensure child and family understand procedure and questions are answered; obtain informed consent.	Evaluates and reinforces understanding of previously taught information. Ensures medical-legal compliance as suggested by the Joint Commission on Accreditation of Healthcare Organizations (JCAHO).	Developmental level, cognitive ability, and anxiety level determine approach to and effectiveness of teaching. In emergency situations, refer to institution-specific protocol for assumption of consent.
2. Gather needed equipment and supplies.	Facilitates completion of task in a timely manner.	
3. Wash hands.	Standard precautions; reduces transmission of microorganisms.	
4. Apply local anesthetic cream if desired and as time permits. Draw an imaginary line between the posterior iliac crests and apply local anesthetic cream to the spine 1 cm above and 1 cm below this area (Figure 84-1).[2] *(Level VI*)*	Decreases pain and anxiety levels in children.	Topical anesthetic should be applied 30 to 60 minutes before procedure based on type of topical anesthetic used and manufacturer's recommendation. *(Level I*)*
5. Ensure appropriate cardiorespiratory monitoring is in place with appropriate alarm limits set and alarms activated.	Child may clinically decompensate during procedure.	Emergency equipment should be readily available. If child receives sedation, implement institution-specific protocol for procedural sedation.
6. Provide for appropriate privacy. Position child in either sitting or lateral recumbent position with hips, knees, and neck flexed (Figures 84-2 and 84-3). *(Level II*)*	This position widens the intervertebral space and facilitates needle insertion into the subarachnoid space.[4,5] Bending the child's trunk causes the spinal cord to rise slightly, away from the site of needle insertion.[4] Privacy is an important consideration for school-aged children and adolescents.	Infants and small children should be lying on their side in fetal position. Knees should be brought up close to the chin with neck flexed in a downward position. Older children may be more comfortable in a sitting position lying forward with face down on a table. These positions can compromise the pediatric airway. Cardiorespiratory status must be frequently assessed.

Procedure continues on following page

* Level I: Manufacturer's recommendations only
  Level II: Theory-based; no research data to support recommendations; recommendations from expert consensus group may exist
  Level VI: Clinical studies in a variety of patient populations and situations to support recommendations

Procedure | **for Lumbar Puncture: Perform**—*Continued*

Steps	Rationale	Considerations

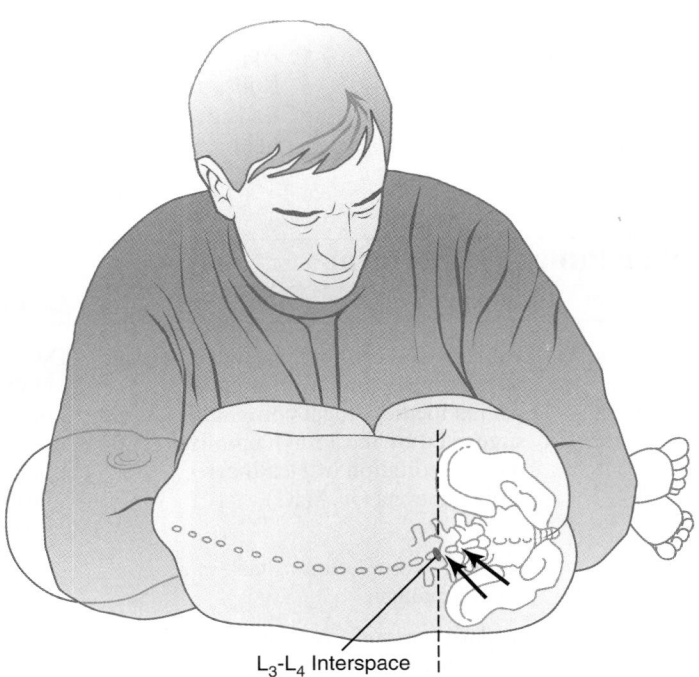

L₃-L₄ Interspace

FIGURE 84-1   Lumbar puncture landmarks. Note *landmarks* and *arrows* depicting appropriate intervertebral spaces for puncture.

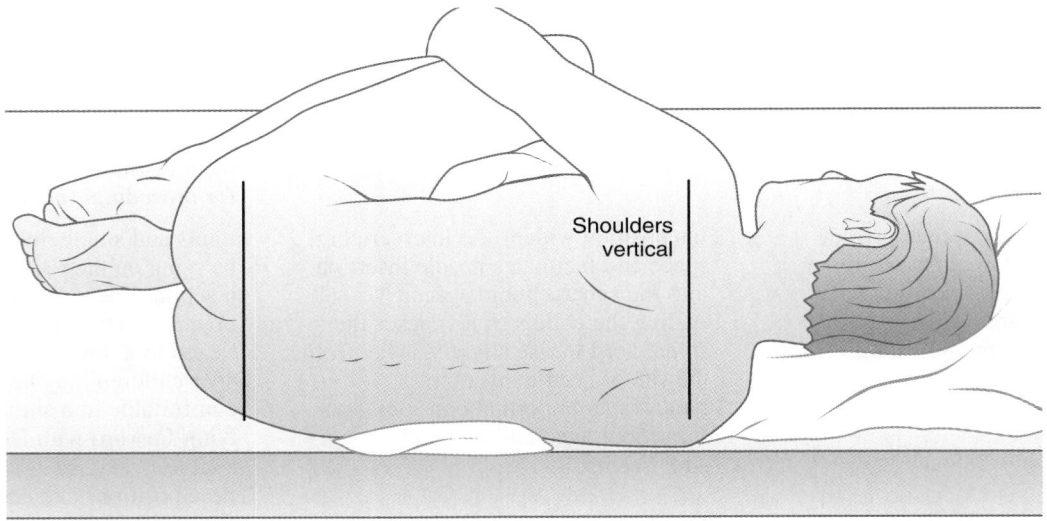

Shoulders vertical

FIGURE 84-2   Patient recumbent position. *From McGill Molson Medical Informatics Project: Lumbar puncture, Montreal, 2004, McGill University Faculty of Medicine. Text available at http://sprojects.mmi.mcgill.ca/lumbar/ introduction.htm.*

Procedure for Lumbar Puncture: Perform—*Continued*

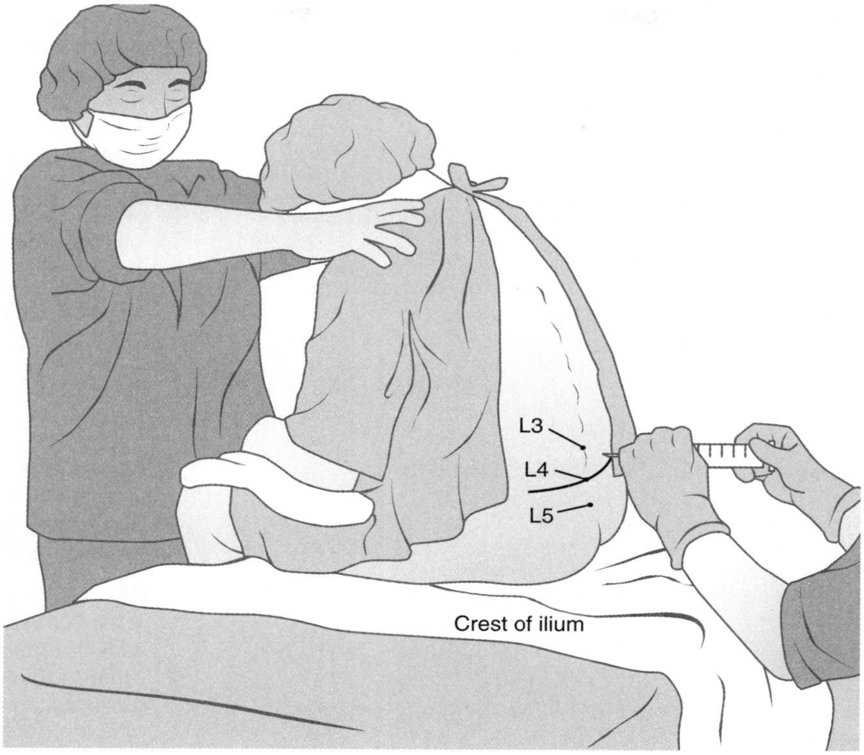

FIGURE 84-3 Patient seated position. *From McGill Molson Medical Informatics Project: Lumbar puncture, Montreal, 2004, McGill University Faculty of Medicine. Text available at http://sprojects.mmi.mcgill.ca/lumbar/introduction.htm.*

Steps	Rationale	Considerations
7. Identify child with appropriate patient and procedure verification process (e.g., "Time out"). *(Level II*)*	Confirms correct patient, procedure, and site as recommended by JCAHO; prevents unnecessary medical procedures.	Verification process and documentation are institution specific. Use active communication techniques.
8. Ensure child has received prescribed sedation, if indicated.	Decreases child's anxiety; facilitates positioning and child's ability to hold still.	Administration of sedation and monitoring of the child should *not* be the responsibility of the practitioner who performs the procedure.
9. Put on mask and cap; wash hands.	Standard precautions; reduces transmission of microorganisms.	
10. Put on sterile gown and sterile gloves.	Necessary for sterile technique; reduces transmission of microorganisms.	
11. With assistance, establish sterile field and set up sterile equipment at the bedside, including manometer, specimen tubes, lidocaine, and spinal needle.	All necessary equipment should be at bedside before the start of procedure to facilitate timely completion of procedure.	

Procedure continues on following page

* Level II: Theory-based; no research data to support recommendations; recommendations from expert consensus group may exist

AP This procedure should be performed only by physicians, advanced practice nurses, and other health care professionals (including critical care nurses) with additional knowledge, skills, and demonstrated competence per professional licensure or institutional standard.

Procedure	for Lumbar Puncture: Perform—*Continued*		
Steps	**Rationale**	**Considerations**	
12. Locate desired puncture site (intervertebral spaces L3-L4 or L4-L5; see Figure 84-1). *(Level II*)*	Most common interspace used is L4-L5, but space above or below may be used with inability to access the L4-L5 interspace.	Interspace is easily located by drawing an imaginary line between the posterior iliac crests. The intervertebral space to be punctured is at or below this line. If side-lying position is used, ensure assistant has child positioned so that hips and shoulders are perpendicular to the bed.[3,4]	
13. Cleanse skin at insertion site followed by alcohol povidone-iodine solution. Cleanse skin in a circular motion starting from the center; cleanse above and below the insertion site. *(Level II*)*	Reduces risk of transmission of microorganisms.	Cleanse skin at iliac crest if plan is to use iliac crest as a landmark during procedure.	
14. Drape area with sterile drape.	Establishes sterile field.	Drape should not obscure view of child to allow for close cardio-respiratory monitoring during procedure.[3,4]	
15. Inject lidocaine 1% with a 25-gauge needle both subcutaneously and at overlying skin. *(Level II*)*	Decreases pain from spinal needle insertion.	This step may not be necessary, especially if a topical anesthetic was used; however, one study of infant LPs performed by residents found that success rate was significantly increased with use of local anesthetic.[6]	
16. With stylet in place, slowly insert spinal needle into the L4-L5 space, angling cephalad toward the umbilicus at a 15-degree to 30-degree angle (Figure 84-4).[3-5] *(Level VI*)*	The L4-L5 intervertebal space allows entrance into the subarachnoid space below the spinal cord.	A 20-gauge or 22-gauge needle may be used depending on size of child. If bone is encountered, pull back on the spinal needle and readjust the angle. If again bone is encountered, have assistant reposition the child and flex neck and hips further. If bone is still encountered, repeat process at space immediately higher or lower.	

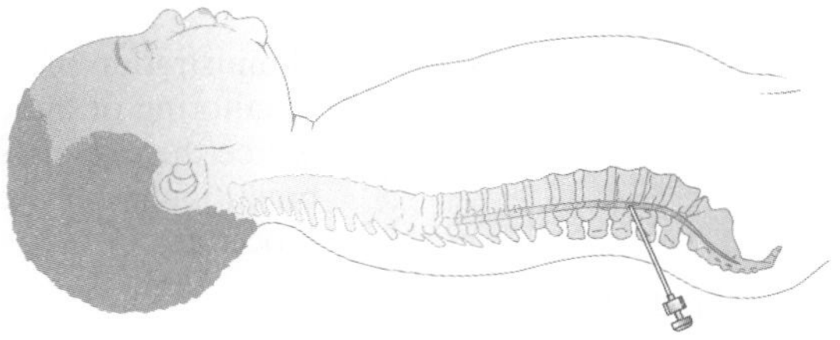

FIGURE 84-4   Note angle of needle as it enters into spinal cavity, traversing through intervertebral space.

17. Once the spinal space is accessed, withdraw stylet and check for return of CSF. If no CSF is obtained, attempt to further insert the needle and recheck for CSF. *(Level VI*)*	Needle may need to be advanced 1 to 4 cm depending on age and size of child.	Rotation of the needle 90 degrees may also facilitate CSF flow.[4] Often a "popping" sensation is felt with penetration into the spinal space; this sensation is less likely with an infant or young child.[3,4]

* Level II: Theory-based; no research data to support recommendations; recommendations from expert consensus group may exist
  Level VI: Clinical studies in a variety of patient populations and situations to support recommendations

Procedure for Lumbar Puncture: Perform—*Continued*

Steps	Rationale	Considerations
18. Attach the stopcock and manometer if an opening pressure is to be obtained. Relax child's position temporarily and measure the opening pressure. Support the needle and manometer. *(Level VI*)*	Extreme flexion can cause false elevation in CSF opening pressure. Supporting the needle throughout the procedure prevents dural tugging, which may lessen the incidence rate of postprocedure CSF leak.[4]	Opening pressure reading is not necessary in all situations. For example, if the LP is performed as part of a work up for meningitis, opening pressure measurement may not be necessary.
19. Allow approximately 1 mL of CSF to passively drain into each of four separate numbered tubes; do not aspirate CSF.	The CSF specimens must be collected in the proper sequence; adequate volume is necessary to ensure specimens can be processed.	Evaluation of each numbered specimen helps differentiate between subarachnoid hemorrhage and traumatic tap. Consistent presence of red blood cells in CSF is indicative of subarachnoid hemorrhage, whereas a decrease in red blood cells in consecutive samples indicates a traumatic tap.
20. Replace the stylet into the spinal needle before withdrawing needle. *(Level VI*)*	Facilitates needle withdrawal and reduces risk of infection.	If spinal chemotherapy has been administered, replacement of stylet is not suggested because it increases risk of chemotherapy spill.
21. Withdraw spinal needle in one fluid motion. Apply sterile gauze with direct pressure immediately.	Decreases risk of spinal fluid leak or bleeding.	
22. Per practitioner preference or unit-specific protocol, child may be placed in supine position immediately after procedure.	Facilitates closure of dura after procedure.	Although practice may be to have the child remain supine for 1 to 4 hours after LP, a few studies in children show no decrease in the incidence rate of post–dural puncture headache or other complications with this practice.[7-9] *(Level IV*)*
23. Label specimens at the bedside and complete laboratory paperwork per institution-specific protocol. *(Level II*)*	Promotes patient safety; ensures accurate and efficient processing of specimen.	Follow institution-specific protocols for handling and labeling laboratory specimens.
24. Discard used supplies and equipment, including sharps, in appropriate receptacles.	Standard precautions; reduces transmission of microorganisms. Protects personnel health.	
25. Remove personal protective equipment; wash hands.	Standard precautions.	
26. Send specimens to laboratory promptly. *(Level VI*)*	Delay in transportation of specimens to laboratory may alter results obtained.	

* Level II: Theory-based; no research data to support recommendations; recommendations from expert consensus group may exist
  Level IV: Limited clinical studies to support recommendations
  Level VI: Clinical studies in a variety of patient populations and situations to support recommendations

Expected Outcomes

- Adequate volume of CSF is obtained

- The CSF specimens are placed in correct specimen tubes, labeled appropriately, and sent to the laboratory in the appropriate time frame
- Results are available in a reasonable time

- Child's baseline neurologic and hemodynamic status is unchanged after procedure

- Child is free from complications of LP

Unexpected Outcomes

- Inability to obtain CSF
- Bloody tap that does not clear
- Inability to complete procedure
- Specimens are mislabeled
- Specimens are placed in incorrect sample tubes
- Delay in sending specimens to laboratory
- Delay in laboratory reporting
- Specimen is lost or unusable
- Herniation caused by sudden shift in intracranial contents or a change in ICP
- Subdural or epidural spinal hematoma
- Cranial neuropathy
- Seizures
- CSF leak from puncture site
- Prolonged headache, neck stiffness, or photophobia
- Bleeding
- Child is unable to void spontaneously
- New and persistent symptoms of pain, numbness, weakness, or paralysis in lower extremities
- Spinal abscess or CNS infection as a result of improper sterile technique

Monitoring and Care of the Child

Activities and Interventions	Rationale	Reportable Conditions
1. Monitor child's vital signs frequently throughout procedure.	Any change in vital signs may indicate airway compromise from positioning or from sudden change in ICP.	• Bradycardia • Hypertension • Abnormal respirations • Pulse oximetry (SpO_2) less than 95% or decreased from child's baseline value
2. Monitor child's neurologic status after LP; compare with pre-procedure assessment, particularly if child underwent sedation for procedure.	Any change in neurologic status from sudden intracranial decompression must be treated promptly.	• Deterioration in mental status • Symptoms of lower extremity weakness or numbness • Uncontrollable headache
3. Check laboratory reports for results of CSF studies, including gram stain, WBC count, red blood cell (RBC) count, glucose, and protein.	Prompt identification of abnormal results facilitates rapid treatment, which improves outcome.	• Laboratory report of lost or unusable specimens • Laboratory results not available in a reasonable time frame
4. Monitor puncture site for redness, swelling, or drainage, which could indicate infection; monitor site for hematoma.	Any change in site could indicate infection or epidural hematoma.	• CSF leak from LP site • Odor or redness at LP site • Fever
5. Monitor child for pain or discomfort with pain scale appropriate to child's age or developmental level; see Procedure 173 for further information.	Identifies traumatic complications related to needle placement.	• Persistent severe back pain or leg pain not evident before procedure • Persistent headache

Documentation

- Indication for procedure
- Informed consent
- Gauge and length of spinal needle inserted
- Patient and procedure verification process per institution-specific protocol
- Date, time, and individual performing procedure
- Amount and character of CSF collected; opening pressure, if obtained
- Laboratory studies obtained
- Vital signs before, during, and after procedure
- Medications administered for procedure and child's response; if procedural sedation is used, institution-specific documentation for procedural sedation
- Child's neurologic assessment before and after procedure
- Child's tolerance of procedure
- Status of puncture site
- Comfort assessment and any specific interventions provided
- Child and family education
- Unexpected outcomes and related treatment

References

1. Berkowitz ID, et al: Meningitis, infectious encephalitis and other CNS infections. In Rogers MC, editor: *Textbook of pediatric intensive care,* ed 3, Baltimore, 1996, Williams and Wilkins.
2. Krauss B, Brustowicz RM, editors: *Pediatric procedural sedation and analgesia,* Baltimore, 1999, Lippincott, Williams and Wilkins.
3. Shilkofski N: Procedures. In Robertson J, Shilkofski N, editors: *The Harriet Lane handbook,* ed 17, Philadelphia, 2005, Mosby.
4. Cronan KM, Wiley JF II: Lumbar puncture. In Henretig F, King C, editors: *Textbook of pediatric emergency medicine procedures,* Philadelphia, 1997, Lippincott, Williams & Wilkins.
5. Singh NC: *Manual of pediatric critical care,* Philadelphia, 1997, Saunders.
6. Baxter AL, et al: Local anesthetic and stylet styles: factors associated with resident lumbar puncture success, *Pediatrics* 117:876-881, 2006.
7. Ebinger F, et al: Strict bed rest following lumbar puncture in children and adolescents is of no benefit, *Neurology* 62:1003-1005, 2004.
8. Janssens E, et al: Post-dural puncture headaches in children: a literature review, *Eur J Pediatr* 162:117-121, 2003.
9. Turnbull DK, Shepherd DB: Post-dural puncture headache: pathogenesis, prevention and treatment, *Br J Anaesth* 91(5):718-729, 2003.

AP

Ventriculoperitoneal Shunt Tap: Perform

P U R P O S E : A ventriculoperitoneal shunt tap is performed for a suspected shunt infection, nonfunctioning valve or shunt system, or change in the cerebrospinal fluid flow pressure. A needle is inserted into the shunt reservoir to withdraw cerebrospinal fluid for evaluation or to decrease intracranial pressure.

Amy Carnall-Grogan

PREREQUISITE KNOWLEDGE

- Anatomy and physiology of the pediatric brain
- Hydrocephalus is an abnormal accumulation of cerebrospinal fluid (CSF) that results from an imbalance between CSF production and CSF absorption.
  - ✧ Hydrocephalus can be congenital or acquired.
- Most common causes of hydrocephalus in children
  - ✧ Aqueductal stenosis
  - ✧ Obstruction from brain tumor, infection, or meningeal scarring
  - ✧ Intraventricular hemorrhage
- A ventriculoperitoneal shunt (VPS) is the most common type of shunt inserted for the treatment of hydrocephalus.
  - ✧ A VPS is the most common shunt inserted because the peritoneal space has a good blood supply, a large area for reabsorption, space to accommodate "extra" tubing, and decreased risk of complication associated with infection.
  - ✧ Other sites of distal shunt placement include the pleural space, right atrium, bladder, ureter, stomach, gallbladder, and fallopian tube.

- A VPS is a silastic tube that is inserted into the cerebral ventricle to divert excess CSF away from the brain to the peritoneum for reabsorption.
  - ✧ The proximal tubing is radiopaque and is usually placed in the anterior part of the lateral ventricle.
  - ✧ The proximal tubing is attached to a valve to regulate CSF drainage and allow unidirectional flow. The valve usually has a reservoir for CSF sampling and pressure assessment.
  - ✧ The distal tubing is also attached to the valve. The distal end is tunneled subcutaneously to the peritoneum or other absorptive area.
- Specific type of VPS the child has in place, if known
  - ✧ Variations in shunts may include single or double reservoir, programmable flow capability of the valve, recommended angle of penetration of the reservoir, and location of the reservoir.
- Indications for shunt tap
  - ✧ Suspected infection
  - ✧ Suspected malfunction
  - ✧ Suspected obstruction
  - ✧ To decrease intracranial pressure (ICP)
  - ✧ If immediate VPS revision is not available and the child's condition is deteriorating, tapping to remove CSF may be used temporarily to decrease ICP to less than 20 cm H_2O.
  - ✧ To assess shunt function with instillation of a contrast agent or radionuclide (i.e., shuntogram)

- Signs and symptoms of malfunctioning or infected shunt include:
  - ❖ Irritability
  - ❖ Headache
  - ❖ Lethargy
  - ❖ Emesis
  - ❖ Fever
  - ❖ Bulging fontanel in infants
  - ❖ Abdominal pain (if peritonitis is present)
  - ❖ Inflammation along shunt tract
- A shunt tap should be performed with strict aseptic technique.
- If a shunt tap is performed to rule out an infection, tap the shunt before the initiation of antibiotics.
- Most common causative organisms are *Streptococcus epidermis* and *Staphylococcus aureus;* other organisms include gram-negative organisms.[1]
- Complications of shunt tap include[1]:
  - ❖ Infection (ventriculitis)
  - ❖ Damage to the shunt
  - ❖ Cardiorespiratory instability
  - ❖ Conversion of partial shunt obstruction to complete shunt obstruction
  - ❖ Bleeding
  - ❖ Subdural hematoma
- Contraindications for shunt tap
  - ❖ Loculated ventricles
  - ❖ Slit-like ventricles
  - ❖ Small ventricles
  - ❖ The presence of a skin infection at the site of the reservoir is a relative contraindication.
- The opening pressure for a functioning shunt is usually not significantly higher than the valve pressure; a brisk CSF flow with a significantly higher pressure suggests a distal malfunction, whereas a slow or absent flow suggests a proximal obstruction.[2-4]
- Normal opening pressure is less than 5 to 10 cm H_2O (less than the valve's preset opening pressure).
- An opening pressure of more than 20 cm H_2O indicates a shunt obstruction and necessitates immediate shunt revision.[2,3,5]
- An opening pressure of 10 to 20 cm H_2O is indeterminate.[2-4,6]
- In the presence of normal or enlarged ventricles, a spontaneous and steady flow of CSF from the proximal shunt should be expected; small ventricles may produce slow or even absent flow, which is often difficult to differentiate from shunt obstruction.[2,6]
- Computed tomographic (CT) scan results, when appropriate, should be reviewed before the shunt tap to identify the anatomy of the VPS, assess ventricular size, and identify obvious shunt problems, such as disconnection or kinking of the catheter.

- Child development as it relates to clinical assessment and VPS tap
- Mastery of pediatric advanced life support competencies
- Informed consent is required before VPS tap

CHILD AND FAMILY ASSESSMENT

- Child's baseline vital signs ➡️*Rationale:* Establishes baseline values for the child; facilitates prompt recognition of change from baseline.
- Child's baseline neurologic assessment, including mental status and sensory and motor function ➡️*Rationale:* Establishes baseline neurologic function before withdrawal of CSF.
- Signs of increased ICP
  - ❖ Infant: Increased head circumference, full fontanel, engorged scalp veins, Macewen's sign, CN VI palsy, irregular respirations, apnea, seizure, setting sun sign (upward gaze palsy), and hyperreactive reflexes
  - ❖ Older child or adolescent: Headache, nausea, vomiting, ataxia, drowsiness, blurred vision, and papilledema
  - ❖ Late signs: Bradycardia, hypertension, and irregular respirations (Cushing's triad) ➡️*Rationale:* If the child has signs of increased ICP, this procedure becomes a medical emergency.
- Current laboratory profile, including complete blood count (CBC), prothrombin time (PT), and partial thromboplastin time (PTT) ➡️*Rationale:* Establishes baseline values and identifies abnormalities before the procedure.
- Palpate the child's shunt valve to ascertain position and ability to tap before the procedure; review CT scan or shunt series if available ➡️*Rationale:* If the shunt cannot be easily palpated, the procedure may need to be performed by a neurosurgeon or with anesthesia.
- Child's developmental level and ability to cooperate with positioning requirements ➡️*Rationale:* Developmental level affects preparation of the child and establishes whether the child may need sedation for the procedure.
- Child's and family's understanding of the reasons for and risks and benefits of the procedure ➡️*Rationale:* Evaluates child's and family's understanding and provides a gauge for ongoing education.
- Status of skin at proposed VPS tap site ➡️*Rationale:* Identifies potential contraindications.
- Child's known allergies ➡️*Rationale:* Identifies allergies to medications or solutions that may be used during shunt tap.
- Desire of family members to remain with the child during the procedure ➡️*Rationale:* The family's presence may provide support and comfort to the child during the procedure if institution-specific protocol facilitates family presence; family members should also have the choice not to remain with the child.

AP This procedure should be performed only by physicians, advanced practice nurses, and other health care professionals (including critical care nurses) with additional knowledge, skills, and demonstrated competence per professional licensure or institutional standard.

CHILD AND FAMILY EDUCATION

Individualized, developmentally appropriate education is provided to the family and to the child based on desire for knowledge, readiness to learn, and overall neurologic and psychosocial state.

- When obtaining informed consent, discuss the purpose of the procedure, the possibility of alternative treatment, the potential benefits versus risks, and the expected outcomes ➤*Rationale:* Providing information regarding the risks and benefits, alternative therapies, and expected outcomes is essential in obtaining informed consent.
- Explain that the child may have some discomfort when the needle punctures the skin ➤*Rationale:* Providing anticipatory information decreases anxiety and promotes coping.
- Explain to the child and family that the child must remain completely still during the procedure ➤*Rationale:* Any unexpected movement of the child makes obtaining the CSF specimen difficult and may contaminate the procedure by disrupting the sterile field; provides the child and family with information about expectations during the procedure.
- If the family desires to stay during the procedure and institution-specific protocol permits family presence, provide the family with accurate information regarding the procedure, family's role, and expectations ➤*Rationale:* Prepares the family for their role; provides clearly defined guidelines and expectations.
- Encourage questions and answer questions as they arise ➤*Rationale:* Reinforcement of information is needed during periods of stress and is especially important if the procedure is performed emergently.

EQUIPMENT

- 23-gauge or 25-gauge butterfly needle
- Sterile gloves
- Clean gloves
- Syringe, 5-mL
- Sterile drapes
- Povidone-iodine solution preparation sticks, pads, or other form of applicator
- Alcohol wipes
- Clippers or razor
- 4×4 gauze pads
- Specimen labels that contain two patient identifiers
- Sterile specimen tubes
- Appropriate laboratory requisitions

Procedure	for Ventriculoperitoneal Shunt Tap: Perform	
Steps	**Rationale**	**Considerations**
1. Ensure child and family understand procedure and questions are answered; obtain informed consent.	Evaluates and reinforces understanding of previously taught information. Ensures medical-legal compliance as suggested by the Joint Commission on Accreditation of Healthcare Organizations (JCAHO).	Developmental level, cognitive ability, and anxiety level determine approach to and effectiveness of teaching. In emergency situations, refer to institution-specific protocol for assumption of consent.
2. Gather needed equipment and supplies.	Facilitates completion of the procedure in a timely manner.	
3. Ensure appropriate cardiorespiratory monitoring is in place with appropriate alarm limits set and alarms activated. *(Level II*)*	Children with underlying issues may decompensate rapidly during procedure.[1,5]	
4. Ensure that emergency equipment is readily available.	Allows prompt response in case of rapid deterioration of the child's condition.	
5. Wash hands. *(Level VI*)*	Correct handwashing is the single most important action in prevention of nosocomial infections.	In a life-threatening emergency situation, immediate intervention may be necessary, limiting use of complete aseptic technique.
6. Put on clean gloves.	Standard precautions; reduces the transmission of microorganisms.	

* Level II: Theory-based; no research data to support recommendations; recommendations from expert consensus group may exist
   Level VI: Clinical studies in a variety of patient populations and situations to support recommendations

Procedure for Ventriculoperitoneal Shunt Tap: Perform—*Continued*

Steps	Rationale	Considerations
7. Identify child with appropriate patient and procedure verification process (e.g., "Time out"). *(Level II*)*	Confirms correct patient, procedure, and site as recommended by JCAHO; prevents unnecessary medical procedures.	Verification process and documentation are institution specific. Use active communication techniques.
8. Position child supine with head of bed elevated 30 degrees and the face of the child turned away from side being tapped. *(Level II*)*	Provides access to the shunt bulb.	
9. Palpate scalp for shunt bulb or reservoir, which is usually in the right frontal or right occipital region within 2 cm of the scalp incision used to insert the shunt (Figure 85-1). *(Level II*)*	The shunt bulb or reservoir is the access port.	Some children may have multiple scars from other surgical procedures. Various sizes and shapes of shunt bulbs exist depending on the manufacturer.

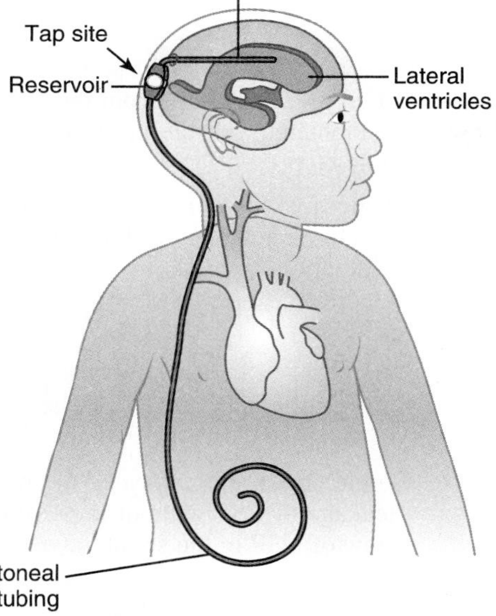

FIGURE 85-1 Ventriculoperitoneal (VP) Shunt. Note reservoir or bulb, which is used for access to CSF.

Steps	Rationale	Considerations
10. Clip or shave hair approximately 2 cm around shunt bulb. *(Level II*)*	Allows clear visualization and easier palpation of shunt bulb.	Clipping may decrease incidence rate of local skin infection.[1]
11. Wash hands.	Standard precautions; reduces the transmission of microorganisms.	Per institution-specific protocol, cap and mask may be worn for this procedure. If so, cap and mask should be put on before washing hands.
12. Establish sterile field and prepare equipment.	All necessary equipment should be at bedside before the start of procedure to facilitate completion of procedure in a timely manner.	

Procedure continues on following page

* Level II: Theory-based; no research data to support recommendations; recommendations from expert consensus group may exist

AP This procedure should be performed only by physicians, advanced practice nurses, and other health care professionals (including critical care nurses) with additional knowledge, skills, and demonstrated competence per professional licensure or institutional standard.

Procedure	for Ventriculoperitoneal Shunt Tap: Perform—*Continued*	
Steps	**Rationale**	**Considerations**
13. Put on sterile gloves. Drape the child to provide exposure to the shaved area of the scalp only.	Facilitates a sterile specimen and decreases the possibility of introduction of microorganisms into the shunt system.	Draping is sometimes omitted in an emergency situation.
14. Cleanse site with povidone-iodine solution followed by alcohol or with solution prescribed by institution-specific protocol.	Site must be sterilized to decrease risk of introduction of microorganisms into CSF.	
15. Introduce the butterfly needle into the shunt bulb at a slight oblique angle and observe for spontaneous CSF flow in the tubing. *(Level VI*)*	Flow of CSF confirms placement of the needle in the shunt bulb.	Angle used to access the shunt bulb may vary with type of shunt.
16. Attach stopcock with manometer to the end of the butterfly tubing, ensuring that the zero level on the manometer is level with the bulb and that the stopcock outlet valve is occluded; obtain opening pressure. *(Level VI*)*	Outlet valve must be occluded to obtain an accurate opening (ventricular) pressure.[5]	Stopcock is open to the patient and manometer only.
17. Turn stopcock off to patient, open to manometer and distal catheter. Allow CSF to flow into the distal catheter.	If CSF does not flow from the manometer, a distal obstruction may be present.	
18. Remove manometer and attach syringe; gently aspirate 2 to 3 mL of CSF. *(Level II*)*	Reduces volume of CSF in ventricles; obtains specimens for laboratory evaluation.	If CSF is difficult to aspirate or no CSF is obtained, suspect that the proximal end of the shunt is occluded or that the ventricles are collapsed. Aborting the procedure may be necessary.
19. Collect CSF into sterile specimen containers.	Sterile collection of CSF is essential to obtain accurate CSF analysis.	
20. Gently withdraw the needle and hold gentle pressure over the shunt bulb.	Gentle pressure is indicated to prevent leakage of CSF without impairing flow of CSF in the shunt valve.	Some manufacturers line the proximal portion of the bulb with a polymer that prevents leakage of CSF.[2,3,5]
21. Discard used supplies and equipment, including sharps, in appropriate receptacles.	Standard precautions; reduces transmission of microorganisms. Protects personnel health.	
22. Remove personal protective equipment; wash hands.	Standard precautions.	
23. Label specimens at the bedside and complete laboratory paperwork per institution-specific protocol. *(Level II*)*	Promotes patient safety; ensures accurate and efficient processing of specimen.	Follow institution-specific protocols for handling and labeling laboratory specimens.
24. Promptly send specimens to the laboratory for analysis.	The CSF is sent for cell count, Gram stain, culture and sensitivity, glucose, and protein to assess for infection. Other tests may be ordered based on the child's differential diagnosis. Delay in transportation of specimens to laboratory may alter results obtained.	The presence of organisms on the Gram stain confirms an infection, although absence of organisms does not rule out the possibility of infection.[7] See Procedure 79 for detailed information on interpretation of CSF analysis.

* Level II: Theory-based; no research data to support recommendations; recommendations from expert consensus group may exist
   Level VI: Clinical studies in a variety of patient populations and situations to support recommendations

Expected Outcomes	Unexpected Outcomes
• CSF is obtained for analysis, including evaluation of shunt infection	• Inability to obtain CSF because of occlusion of the proximal shunt
• Accurate ICP measurement is obtained	• Inability to obtain ICP measurement
	• Inaccurate ICP measurement
• CSF is removed as a temporizing measure in the child with an occluded shunt	• Inability to remove CSF because of occlusion of the proximal shunt
• Injection of contrast agents is performed if a flow study is to be obtained	• Inability to inject contrast agent
• Child's condition remains stable throughout procedure	• Decompensation during procedure
	• Deterioration of neurologic status during procedure
• Child is free from complications of VPS tap	• Development of infection, including ventriculitis
	• Damage to the shunt
	• Cardiorespiratory instability
	• Conversion of partial shunt obstruction to complete shunt obstruction
	• Bleeding
	• Subdural hematoma
• The CSF specimens are placed in correct specimen tubes, labeled appropriately, and sent to the laboratory in the appropriate time frame	• Specimens are mislabeled
	• Specimens are placed in incorrect sample tubes
	• Delay in sending specimens to laboratory

Monitoring and Care of the Child

Activities and Interventions	Rationale	Reportable Conditions
1. Monitor vital signs, including heart rate and blood pressure.	Hypotension can cause cerebral ischemia; bradycardia can result from pressure on the vagal control mechanism of the medulla. If child has signs of increased ICP, vigilant monitoring is mandatory to guide appropriate management.	• Bradycardia • Hypertension • Abnormal respirations • Change in level of consciousness (LOC) • Any change in child's status from baseline
2. Monitor oxygen saturation (SpO$_2$).	Impaired airway clearance or decreasing respiratory rate can lead to increased oxygen requirement. Hypoxia can cause cerebral ischemia.	• SpO$_2$ < 95% (unless child's baseline is a lower than normal SpO$_2$) • Headache
3. Monitor neurologic examination, including LOC during and after procedure.	Increased ICP results in an abnormal neurologic examination. If ICP continues to rise, the child becomes lethargic, stuporous, and eventually comatose.	• Changes to child's baseline neurologic examination results, including pupillary changes and focal findings • Seizures • Cushing's triad: hypertension (usually with widened pulse pressure), bradycardia and irregular respiratory pattern. Cushing's triad is a late response and is a compensatory mechanism to the rising ICP[4,6]

Documentation

- Child and family education
- Informed consent obtained
- Imaging studies obtained (e.g., CT scan)
- Patient and procedure verification process per institution-specific protocol
- Date and time of procedure and individual who performed procedure
- Volume of CSF removed and appearance of CSF
- Shunt pressure and shunt patency assessment
- Child's neurologic examination results before and after procedure
- Child's tolerance of procedure
- Plan for further assessment or definitive treatment (e.g., externalization, revision in operating room)
- Laboratory specimens and requested studies obtained
- Unexpected outcomes and related treatment

References

1. Duhaime A, Wiley JF: Ventricular shunt and burr hole puncture. In Henretig F, King C, editors: *Textbook of pediatric emergency medicine procedures,* Philadelphia, 1997, Lippincott, Williams & Wilkins.
2. Walter KA: Neurosurgical procedures. In Chen H, et al, editors: *Manual of common bedside surgical procedures,* ed 2, Philadelphia, 2000, Lippincott Williams & Wilkins.
3. Choux M, et al: *Pediatric neurosurgery,* London, 1999, Churchill Livingstone.
4. Gaskill SJ, Marlin AE: *Handbook of pediatric neurology and neurosurgery,* Boston, 1993, Little, Brown and Company.
5. Bondurant CP, Jimenex DF: Epidemiology of cerebrospinal fluid shunt, *Pediatr Neurosurg* 23:254-259, 1995.
6. Hickey JV: *The clinical practice of neurological and neurosurgical nursing,* ed 5, Philadelphia, 2003, Lippincott Williams & Wilkins.
7. Rogers MC, editor: *Textbook of pediatric intensive care,* ed 3, Philadelphia, 1996, William & Wilkins.

Additional Readings

Albright AL, editors: *Principles and practice of pediatric neurosurgery,* New York, 1999, Thieme Medical Publishers.

Andrews BT, Hammer GB: *Pediatric neurosurgical intensive care,* Park Ridge, IL, 1997, The American Association of Neurological Surgeons.

Barker E: *Neuroscience nursing: a spectrum of care,* Philadelphia, 2002, Mosby.

McLone DG, et al: *Pediatric neurosurgery: surgery of the developing nervous system,* ed 4, Philadelphia, 2001, Saunders.

PROCEDURE **86**

Cervical Traction Maintenance

P U R P O S E : To maintain reduction, alignment, and immobilization of the cervical spine with prevention or minimization of the potential complications of this therapy

Elizabeth M. Henry

PREREQUISITE KNOWLEDGE

- Anatomy and physiology of the pediatric spine and spinal cord
- Developmental differences of the pediatric spine and most common level of injury
  - ❖ Infant (0 to 2 years): Spine has tremendous mobility and elasticity as a result of underdevelopment of the neck muscles, incompletely calcified wedge-shaped vertebrae, and shallow horizontally oriented spine (facet) joints. Also, because of the large head relative to the torso, the likelihood of high cervical spine injuries (C1 to C2) is increased.
  - ❖ School-aged (2 to10 years): Muscles and ligaments strengthen, bones grow and reach a mature shape and size, and areas of cartilage and soft bone are replaced with normal calcified bone. The head is smaller in proportion to the torso. These changes shift the focus of injury from the upper cervical spine (skull to C1 to C2) to the lower cervical spine (C5 to C6).
  - ❖ Adolescents: More likely to have thoracic and lumbar injuries. Nondisplaced bony fractures are more common.
- Cervical traction may be indicated in children with injury to the cervical vertebral column, such as vertebral fracture, vertebral dislocation, or ligamentous injury.
- Cervical traction may be temporary before surgical intervention or may be longer term to align and stabilize the cervical spine and allow healing to occur.

- Specific treatment plan for cervical injury varies according to the type and level of injury and the child's clinical status and physician's preference.
- Principles of traction
- Signs and symptoms of spinal shock: hypotension, bradycardia, loss of thermoregulation, ileus, and loss of reflexes
- Signs and symptoms of overdistraction: loss of sensory or motor function
- Multisystem response to immobility and spinal cord injury
- Child development as it relates to clinical assessment and cervical traction maintenance

CHILD AND FAMILY ASSESSMENT

- Child's developmental level and ability to interact ➤*Rationale:* Both chronologic age and developmental level must be considered in the plan of care for the child. Children of different developmental levels need different management to ensure cooperation with traction and proper cervical alignment. Because of possible neuromuscular impairments or the immobility necessary for traction, the child has many self-care deficits. Older children and adolescents may struggle with this and need additional physical help or emotional support.
- Child's baseline motor and sensory function ➤*Rationale:* A thorough baseline assessment is essential for evaluation of any deterioration or improvement in motor and sensory function. A decrease in function may indicate overdistraction, which is a stretching of the spinal cord

from too much weight application, and an improvement may suggest restored neurologic function.

- Child's skin integrity ➥*Rationale:* Cervical traction impairs physical mobility, which may lead to skin breakdown. If a spinal cord injury is present, the child could have permanent immobility. Pressure ulcers can develop that are challenging to treat. Areas particularly susceptible include the sacral spine, the posterior thigh, and the heels. Children with skeletal traction in place are also at risk for disruption of any structure along the pin track (e.g., skin, facial and skull muscles, nerves, arteries or veins). The cervical traction apparatus itself can cause skin breakdown at the pin sites in skeletal traction or under the cervical halter in skin traction.
- Child's respiratory status and gas exchange[1,2] ➥*Rationale:* Impaired physical mobility and the neuromuscular dysfunction that may be associated with spinal cord injury can result in poor gas exchange, impaired secretion clearance, and pneumonia.[3] When cervical traction is used to treat posteriorly displaced odontoid fractures, a significant risk of airway obstruction from retropharyngeal swelling is seen. These children may need intubation.[1] Mortality rates from respiratory complications can be as high as 40% to 80% in the first year after injury.[3]
- Child's level of pain, using a pain scale appropriate to the child's age and developmental level (see Procedure 173 for further information) ➥*Rationale:* Severe pain and discomfort can be associated with the injury, the traction apparatus, or cervical spasms. Increased pain at the pin sites can mean a loosening of the apparatus. The effectiveness of a child's pain management regime must be continuously evaluated and revised as necessary.
- Child's cardiovascular function ➥*Rationale:* Cardiovascular responses to cervical spine injury include spinal shock, neurogenic shock, and autonomic dysfunction, all of which can make the condition of the child unstable. Monitoring the child's response to continuing immobility is critical because venous pooling, decreased venous return, and decreased cardiac output can affect cardiovascular stability. Immobility and spinal cord injury can compromise homeostasis of the sympathetic nervous system, which may also affect cardiovascular responses.
- Child's baseline musculoskeletal status ➥*Rationale:* Children with cervical traction may have musculoskeletal deformities develop. It is essential to document any joint tightness or the presence of deformities. Observe carefully for improvement or worsening during treatment.
- Child's and family's understanding of the reasons for and risks and benefits of the procedure ➥*Rationale:* Evaluates

child's and family's understanding of the procedure and provides a gauge for ongoing education.

CHILD AND FAMILY EDUCATION

- Individualized, developmentally appropriate education is provided to the family and to the child based on desire for knowledge, readiness to learn, and overall neurologic and psychosocial state.
- Review with child and family the pathology of the disease or injury that necessitates traction and the effects of spinal cord injury ➥*Rationale:* The child and family must be provided with basic information to help them understand the treatment plan.
- Discuss the principles of traction, the apparatus to be used, and the specific goals for the child ➥*Rationale:* Child and family compliance with traction is essential and can be encouraged with providing information regarding the general principles of traction.
- Ensure that the child and family understand the unique needs of the child as a result of impaired physical mobility ➥*Rationale:* Increased understanding of treatment and mobility restrictions improves compliance and collaboration.
- Positively review and reinforce strategies to maintain proper alignment of the child's spine in bed ➥*Rationale:* All involved in the child's care must understand that pillows, rolls, etc., may not be used unless proper cervical alignment necessitates that they be used in positioning the child. Research shows that instilling fear of worsening paralysis is not an effective way to ensure that the child and family do not manipulate the traction.[4]
- If halo is in place, child and family must demonstrate ability to perform pin care and maintain the halo-vest before discharge home[5] ➥*Rationale:* Ensures the family and child are prepared to manage care of the device at home; promotes patient safety.
- Encourage questions and answer questions as they arise ➥*Rationale:* Reinforcement of information is needed during periods of stress.

EQUIPMENT

- Traction apparatus (cervical tongs, halo, or cervical halter)
- Rope and pulley system
- Weights
- Appropriate bed frame for precise attachment (if indicated)

Procedure for Cervical Traction Maintenance

Steps	Rationale	Considerations
1. Ensure child and family understand procedure and questions are answered.	Evaluates and reinforces understanding of previously taught information.	Developmental level, cognitive ability, and anxiety level determine approach to and effectiveness of teaching.
2. Wash hands.	Standard precautions; reduces the transmission of microorganisms.	
3. Obtain neurovascular assessment every 1 to 2 hours for the first 12 to 24 hours after application of traction and with changes or per institution-specific protocol.[6] *(Level II*)*	It is critical to determine if the traction is impeding neurovascular function and whether child has symptoms of overdistraction.	Include assessment of skin color, temperature, capillary refill, strength of peripheral pulses, sensory status, mobility, and the presence of edema.
4. Once condition is stabilized, obtain neurovascular assessment every 4 hours with vital signs per unit-specific or institution-specific protocol.[6] *(Level II*)*	Once proper alignment is determined and the child has adequate neurovascular examination results, assessments can occur every 4 hours.	Initiate frequent assessments with any changes in the traction.
5. Maintain the traction apparatus: Each shift, assess all bolts on the equipment and tighten as necessary. Ensure the ordered amount of weight is on the traction apparatus. Ensure that the ropes run freely through the pulley system.	Provides the support necessary for proper alignment. Ropes must run freely through pulley system and weights must be suspended to ensure correct amount of traction is applied.	Ensure that the weights are suspended freely.[6]
6. For skeletal traction, assess pin sites for signs of infection. *(Level II*)*	Any break in the skin has the potential for infection.	Note any redness, tenderness, or increased drainage. The presence of some clear yellow drainage is a normal finding. This drainage can function as a lubricant for the skin.
7. Perform pin care daily per institution-specific protocol and as necessary or per prescribing practitioner's order.[7] *(Level II*)*	Decreases the possibility of infection at the pin insertion sites. Crusting is a normal protective mechanism of the skin, and crust removal could disturb healthy tissue and make it more vulnerable to infection. However, if signs of infection are present, removal of crusts may allow exudates to escape.[8]	After the first 48 to 72 hours (when drainage may be heavy), pin site care should be done daily or weekly for sites with mechanically stable bone-pin interfaces. Increase this frequency if mechanical looseness or early signs of infection are present. Chlorhexidine may be the most effective cleansing solution for pin site care. Determine whether crusting should be removed. Minimal evidence exists to indicate which pin site care regimen is most effective in reduction of infection rates. No consensus exists as to optimal frequency of pin care or whether to remove exudates and crusting. Varied opinion is seen on the appropriate method of pin site care that is optimal for these children.[7,8]

Procedure continues on following page

* Level II: Theory-based; no research data to support recommendations; recommendations from expert consensus group may exist

Procedure | for Cervical Traction Maintenance—*Continued*

Steps	Rationale	Considerations
8. For skin traction, assess the skin under traction device every shift.[9]	Early identification of any tenderness and skin breakdown under the appliance is essential to prevent further skin breakdown.	Duoderm at contact points may decrease incidence rate of skin breakdown.
9. Maintain child's position in bed.	Proper position is important to maintain the correct line of pull and prevent fracture malalignment.	Reposition the child only as permitted by the traction. Countertraction may be necessary to keep the child in correct position in the bed.
10. Perform pulmonary toilet as permitted within the limitations of the injury or the traction device.[3] *(Level VI*)*	Mobilization of secretions and clearing of the airway are critical to prevent atelectasis and pneumonia.	Provide chest physiotherapy as indicated and per prescribing practitioner's order. Consider a bed that provides kinetic therapy.[3] Encourage deep breathing and coughing with incentive spirometry and a cough-assist device. It is not recommended to position a child in cervical traction for postural drainage.
11. Maximize musculoskeletal function through active/passive range of motion exercises and the application of orthotics prescribed by therapeutic services. *(Level VI*)*	Decreases the likelihood of joint immobility and the formation of contractures.[9]	
12. Promote child's ability to maintain necessary positioning with repeated age-appropriate explanations, parental assistance, and use of services such as Child Life. Encourage family to use developmentally appropriate measures to support and comfort the child.	Maintains cervical alignment.	Child Life therapy can be extremely helpful in developing a plan with the child and family that promotes the child's ability to cope with the immobility necessary.

* Level VI: Clinical studies in a variety of patient populations and situations to support recommendations

Expected Outcomes

- Cervical alignment is maintained
- Appropriate amount of weight is applied and traction apparatus functions correctly
- Skin integrity is maintained

- Neuromuscular function remains intact
- Child is free from complications of impaired mobility

- Child has acceptable level of comfort
- Child tolerates positioning and immobility

Unexpected Outcomes

- Malalignment of cervical spine
- Malfunction of traction apparatus
- Incorrect weight applied
- Skin breakdown
- Infection at pin site
- Deterioration of motor or sensory function
- Respiratory compromise
- Hemodynamic instability
- Infection
- Inability to provide adequate nutrition
- Difficulties with bowel or bladder function
- Unmanaged pain
- Unmanaged agitation, resulting in inability to maintain proper alignment

Monitoring and Care of the Child

Activities and Interventions	Rationale	Reportable Conditions
1. Monitor vital signs per unit-specific or institution-specific protocol and as necessary.	Disturbances in the sympathetic nervous system can lead to hemodynamic instability.	• Vital signs that vary from baseline • Change in perfusion
2. Monitor oxygen saturation.	Desaturation and respiratory distress are signs of respiratory compromise, which may be related to complications of immobility or progression of injury.	• Oxygen saturation less than 95% • Increased oxygen requirement • Increased respiratory effort • Inability to manage secretions
3. Monitor intake and output closely.	Immobility and spinal cord injury can lead to urinary retention.	• Urine output consistently less than 1 mL/kg/h • Urine specific gravity more than 1.030
4. Monitor for constipation; initiate bowel regimen.	Immobility and spinal cord injury can lead to constipation. Poor gastric motility from immobility and neurogenic bowel from possible impairments in the innervations in the intestines from spinal cord injury can lead to diminished bowel emptying.	• No stool in more than 24 hours or variation from child's baseline pattern • Abdominal distension • Abdominal pain or cramps • Hard infrequent stools
5. Provide frequent neurologic assessment, including sensory and motor function.	Early recognition of change in neurologic status is essential to prevent permanent damage.	• Any deterioration in neurologic function (i.e., decrease in motor strength, loss of sensation)
6. Monitor skin for signs of impaired integrity and provide frequent skin care, including care of pin sites. Monitor pin sites for signs and symptoms of infection (see Procedures 119 and 125 for further information).	Immobility predisposes the child to skin breakdown. Frequent position changes and skin care are essential to prevent breakdown. Children with cervical traction are at increased risk of infection from prolonged immobility and the presence of a foreign body (pins) in the skin.	• Reddened skin, blisters, denuded area, drainage from wound, etc. • Purulent drainage, erythema, edema, or pain at pin sites • Pin loosening • Microbial growth from pin sites or wound, if cultured[7]
7. Monitor for signs and symptoms of respiratory infection.	Children with cervical traction need prolonged immobility; when immobility is combined with poor secretion clearance, the child may develop atelectasis and pneumonia.	• Increased airway secretions • Change in color of airway secretions • Microbial growth from airway secretions, if cultured[7] • Fever
8. Monitor for signs and symptoms of urinary tract infection or kidney stones.	Children with prolonged immobility are at risk for urinary tract infections and kidney stones.	• Cloudy urine • Foul smell to urine • Positive bacteria, nitrites, or leukoesterase in urine • Fever • Flank pain

9. Monitor for the development of deep vein thrombosis (DVT).
    Obtain clotting profile per prescribing practitioner's order.
    Establish anticoagulation therapy if indicated per prescribing practitioner's order.
    Antiembolic stockings or sequential compression devices should be applied as appropriate and per prescribing practitioner's order.[2]
	Because of prolonged immobility, children with cervical traction are at risk of DVT formation; close monitoring and care can assist in the prevention of DVT.	• Decreased perfusion (i.e., cool or cold skin) to extremity
		• Decreased peripheral pulses
		• Positive Homans' sign (with knee bent, child has calf pain with gentle dorsiflexion of ankle)

Continued

Monitoring and Care of the Child—Cont'd

Activities and Interventions	Rationale	Reportable Conditions

10. Monitor nutrition and growth.
   Assess ability to swallow before intake by mouth is allowed.[3]
   Initiate enteral or parenteral feeds as soon as appropriate per prescribing practitioner's order.
   Obtain a growth history.
   Monitor weight.
	Adequate nutrition is essential to promote healing and prevent further complications.[10]	• Inadequate caloric intake
		• Weight loss

Documentation

- Neurovascular assessment
- Weight of traction
- Vital signs
- Pin site care
- Skin assessment
- Child and family education
- Comfort assessment and interventions provided
- Unexpected outcomes and related treatment

References

1. Harrop JS, et al: Acute respiratory compromise associated with flexed cervical traction after C2 fractures, *Spine* 26(4):E50-E54, 2002.
2. Ziglar MK, Rich PB: Current concepts in evaluating cervical spine injuries, *J Trauma Nurs* 8(3):91-96, 2001.
3. Lucke KT: Pulmonary management following acute SCI, *J Neurosci Nurs* 30(2):91-104, 1998.
4. Hickey JV, Davis JM: Traction maintenance. In Lynn-McHale Wiegand DJ, Carlson K, editors: *AACN procedure manual for critical care,* ed 5, Philadelphia, 2005, Saunders.
5. The Children's Hospital of Philadelphia: Halo-vest: caring for your child. *The Children's Hospital of Philadelphia patient/family education plans,* Philadelphia, 2005, The Children's Hospital of Philadelphia.
6. The Children's Hospital of Philadelphia: Care of the patient in traction. *The Children's Hospital of Philadelphia nursing standards,* Philadelphia, 2005, The Children's Hospital of Philadelphia.
7. Holmes SB, Brown SJ: Skeletal pin site care: National Association of Orthopaedic Nurses guidelines for orthopaedic nursing: pin site care expert panel, *Orthopaedic Nurs* 24(2):99-107, 2005.
8. The Children's Hospital of Philadelphia: Orthopaedic pin care: traction and external fixators. *The Children's Hospital of Philadelphia procedure manual,* Philadelphia, 2005, The Children's Hospital of Philadelphia.
9. Fries J: Critical rehabilitation of the patient with spinal cord injury, *Crit Care Nurs Q* 28(2):179-187, 2005.
10. Harvey C: Wound healing: orthopaedic essentials, *Orthopaedic Nurs* 24(2):143-157, 2005.

Additional Readings

Brohi K, Wilson-MacDonald J: Evaluation of unstable cervical spine injury: a 6-year experience, *J Trauma Injury Infection Crit Care* 49(1):76-80, 2000.

Kyoshima K, et al: Simple cervical spine traction using a halo vest apparatus: technical note, *Surg Neurol* 59(6):518-521, 2003.

Rahimi SY, et al: Treatment of atlantoaxial instability in pediatric patients, *Neurosurg Focus* 15:1-4, 2003.

Saban KL, Ghaly RF: Spinal cervical infection: a case report and current update, *J Neurosci Nurs* 30(2):105-109,114-115, 1998.

Halo/Vest Application: Assist and Care

P U R P O S E : To provide stabilization and immobilization of the cervical spine in children with an unstable upper or lower cervical spine

Dean Barone

PREREQUISITE KNOWLEDGE

- A halo/vest is the most rigid device for external immobilization of the cervical spine[1-4] and is the only external orthosis for the cervical spine without a chin support; it thereby interferes the least with mandibular motion and eating.[5]
- The halo/vest is the orthosis of choice for an unstable upper or lower cervical spine in children.[6-9]
- There are many manufacturers of halo/vest components. The information in this procedure is based on the PMT Halo System 1200 Series (PMT Corp, Chanhassen, MN). Familiarity with the system chosen by the prescribing practitioner or institution is required.
- Anatomy and biomechanics of the cervical spine
- In-depth knowledge of manual spinal precautions, stabilization, and log roll maneuver
- Absolute contraindications for the placement of halo/vest include unstable skull fractures and open chest wounds. Other possible contraindications are at the discretion of the prescribing practitioner who applies the apparatus.
- Familiarity with the multiple treatment options available for cervical spine injuries based on type and location of injury and characteristics of the individual child, such as cervical collar or surgical intervention.
- Halo/vest packages come in multiple sizes for the halo ring and vest (Table 87-1 and Figure 87-1).
- Components of the halo/vest (Figure 87-2 and Table 87-2)
- The vest has accessibility to the anterior chest for administering chest compressions for cardiopulmonary resuscitation (CPR); see Figure 87-3.
- The halo ring is made of either steel (not compatible with magnetic resonance imaging [MRI]) or graphite (MRI

compatible). Refer to manufacturer's information for details and access points for the specific halo/vest in use.
- The halo ring is attached to the skull anteriorly with two pins and posteriorly with two pins.
- Halo rings can be used for traction before the application of the vest for reduction of the fracture. After the halo ring is in place, a rope and pulley system can be applied. Weights can be attached to the end of the rope/pulley system and serial x-rays performed to evaluate the reduction. Weight should only be applied by the prescribing practitioner because excessive traction can cause stretching and damage to the spinal cord. Once reduction is complete, the vest and struts can be applied for immobilization. See Procedure 86 for further information.
- Halo/vest is a one-time use disposable system.
- Crescent wrench and torque wrench must be kept at the child's bedside for tightening and removal of halo/vest.
- Maintenance and cleaning of the halo/vest is essential to prevent infection[8] and pin loosening.[1-4]
- Child development as it relates to clinical assessment and halo/vest application and maintenance
- Appropriate pediatric dosing of analgesics and competency in procedural sedation
- Informed consent is required before application of halo/vest.

CHILD AND FAMILY ASSESSMENT

- History of familial cervical disorders ➡*Rationale:* Family members may have experience with the application and care of halo/vest and an understanding of the pathophysiology of the disorder.

TABLE 87-1	Sizing Chart for Halo Vest and Halo Ring

Pediatric Halo Vest Sizes

Vest Size	Xyphoid Circumference	Shoulder to Xyphoid	Shoulder to Iliac	Neck Opening
PED 00	19-21 in (48-53 cm)	4 ¼ in (11 cm)	6 ¾ in (17 cm)	3 ¼ in (8 cm)
PED 0	20-21 ½ in (51-55 cm)	5 ⅛ in (13 cm)	7 ½ in (19 cm)	3 ½ in (9 cm)
PED 1	22-28 ½ in (56-72 cm)	6 ¾ in (17 cm)	9 ½ in (24 cm)	4 in (10 cm)
PED 2	22-28 ½" (56-72 cm)	7 ¼ in (18 cm)	10 ¾ in (27 cm)	4 ¼ in (11 cm)
PED 3	22-28 ½ in (56-72 cm)	8 ½ in (22 cm)	12 ¼ in (31 cm)	4 ½ in (11 cm)
PED 4	26 ½-32 ½ in (67-83 cm)	8 in (20 cm)	11 ½ in (29 cm)	4 ¾ in (12 cm)

Pediatric Halo Ring Sizes

Model	XX Small	X Small	Small	Medium	Large	X Large	XX Large
1211-1	14-17 in (36-43 cm)	16-19 in (41-49 cm)	16-21 in (41-53 cm)	21-24 in (53-61 cm)	24-26 in (61-66 cm)	26-28 in (66-71 cm)	
1201-1		14-16 in (36-41 cm)	16-19 in (41-48 cm)	19-22 in (48-56 cm)	22-24 in (56-61 cm)	24-26 in (61-66 cm)	26 in and up (66 cm and up)

Data from PMT Corp, Chanhassen, MN, 2004.

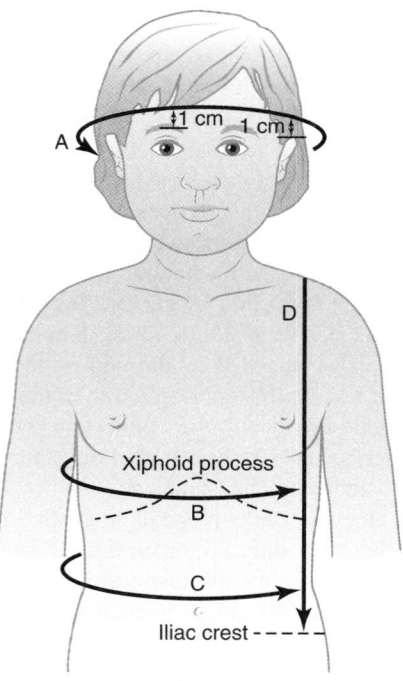

FIGURE 87-1   Measurements for Halo Vest. Measure from top of shoulder vertically down chest to line of xyphoid process. Measurement should be taken with placement of "0" of tape measure on top of shoulder and draping of tape down front of body. Reading is taken where line of tape reaches level of xyphoid. *Courtesy of PMT Corp, Chanhassen, MN, 2004.*

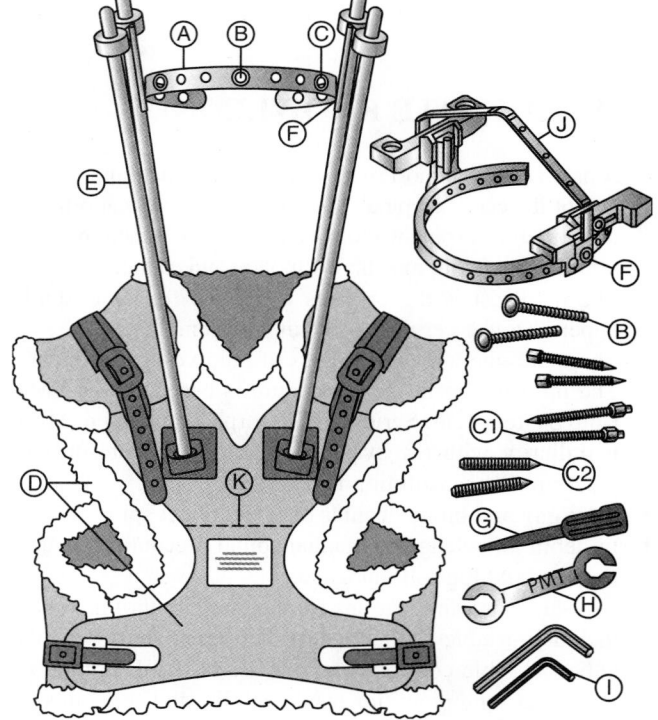

FIGURE 87-2   Parts of PMT Halo System 1200 Series. See Table 87-2 for Parts legend. *Courtesy of PMT Corp, Chanhassen, MN, 2004.*

- Child's developmental level and ability to interact ➡️*Rationale:* These factors influence preparation of the child and interaction; child may be able to understand the pathophysiology of the disorder and participate in care.
- Child's current level of consciousness and ability to cooperate ➡️*Rationale:* Child may need to be sedated for

the procedure to prevent anxiety or movement during the application process.
- Child's head circumference and torso measurements (see Figure 87-1) ➡️*Rationale:* Halo/vest comes in a variety of sizes (see Table 87-1) and must be properly fitted.

TABLE 87-2	Parts of PMT Halo System 1200 Series	
Part	**Quantity**	**Description**
A	1	**Halo ring**
B	3	**Positioning pins**
C	5	**Head pins** (standard ring) *OR*
C1	2	**Spring loaded head pins** and
C2	2	**Solid head pins** (traction ring)
D	1	**Vest with liner**
E	4	**Graphite rods**
F	2	**Head blocks**
G	1	**Small screwdriver** (standard superstructure only)
H	1	7/16-in to ½-in **Combination wrench** for locking head pins
I	2	**Allen wrenches** (1 large and 1 small)
		Note: For emergency use only. (PMT recommends torque driver for tightening head pins and superstructure.)
J	1	**Traction bail assembly** (Depending on circumstances, traction may be applied before vest application. Apply vest and put patient into traction. Traction bail assembly easily attaches to head blocks.)
K	(Feature)	**Cardiac crease**

Compare letters in Part column with labels in Figure 87-2.
Data from PMT Corp, Chanhassen, MN 2004.

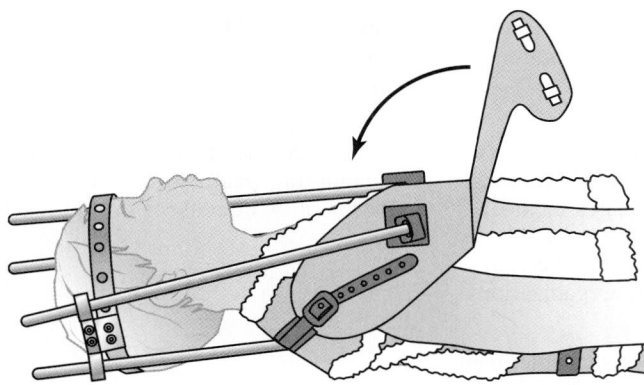

FIGURE 87-3   Performing CPR. To perform CPR, follow this procedure:
Step 1: Place child supine on posterior part of vest.
Step 2: Loosen and release side (waist) buckles.
Step 3: Anterior portion of vest is manufactured with crease in shell. Fold vest back at crease.
Step 4: With posterior portion of vest as "crash board," perform CPR as necessary.
Note: After CPR is performed on child wearing PMT Halo System, new vest must be ordered. Vest has been damaged and does not provide correct support for child. *Courtesy of PMT Corp, Chanhassen, MN, 2004.*

- Neurologic status and vital signs of the child ➻*Rationale:* Documentation of neurologic status before halo/vest application is important for baseline data and medical-legal purposes with care for a child with a cervical spine injury or disorder.
- Skin integrity of the child's torso ➻*Rationale:* Baseline data before halo/vest application.
- Child's and family's understanding of the reasons for and risks and benefits of the procedure ➻*Rationale:* Evaluates child's and family's understanding of the procedure and provides a gauge for ongoing education.
- Family's desire to be present during the procedure ➻*Rationale:* Family members may provide comfort and support to the child during the procedure but should have the choice not to remain with the child.

CHILD AND FAMILY EDUCATION

Individualized, developmentally appropriate education is provided to the family and to the child based on desire for knowledge, readiness to learn, and overall neurologic and psychosocial state.

- Inform the family, and the child as developmentally appropriate, of the reason for application of the halo/vest ➻*Rationale:* Providing information increases knowledge and may decrease the child's fear and anxiety during and after halo/vest application.
- Provide the child and family with information about the application procedure, including steps in the procedure and anticipated length of the procedure ➻*Rationale:* Because of the invasiveness of this procedure, the child and family must be educated as to what the procedure entails before the procedure.
- Explain to the child and family the importance of the child remaining still during the procedure and that medication will be used to help the child as needed ➻*Rationale:* The halo/vest is applied because of instability of the upper or lower cervical spine; if the child moves during the procedure, the child is at risk for significant neurologic injury.
- Review the plan for sedation with the family if the child is not able to cooperate with the mobility limitations during halo/vest application ➻*Rationale:* Review of the

sedation plan reassures the family that appropriate measures will be implemented to assure the child is able to be still and decreases the child's anxiety. Provides the family with the opportunity to inform the prescribing practitioner of any negative experiences the child has had with sedation in the past.

- Explain the importance of caring for the halo/vest as instructed and the potential risks that result from inadequate care of the apparatus ➤➤*Rationale:* An increased risk of infection is found in children compared with adults who wear a halo/vest.[1-4] The family is responsible for halo/vest care after discharge.
- If the child is ambulatory or is to be discharged home, explain the modifications of lifestyle, including bathing, toileting, eating, dressing, ambulation precautions, and safety precautions ➤➤*Rationale:* This information prepares the child and family for self care in the home environment.

- Encourage questions and answer questions as they arise ➤➤*Rationale:* Reinforcement of information is needed during periods of stress.

EQUIPMENT

- Halo/vest with crescent and torque wrenches
- Ruler
- Syringe, 10-mL
- 22-gauge 1.5-inch needle
- Local anesthetic
- Sterile gloves
- Clean gloves
- Alcohol swabs
- Surgical antiseptic preparation
- 4×4 pads
- Scissors and razor or surgical clippers

Procedure for Halo/Vest Application: Assist and Care

Steps	Rationale	Considerations
1. Ensure child and family understand procedure and questions are answered.	Evaluates and reinforces understanding of previously taught information.	Developmental level, cognitive ability, and anxiety level determine approach to and effectiveness of teaching.
2. Confirm that consent for the procedure has been obtained.	Ensures family understands the risks and benefits of and the alternatives to the procedure; ensures medical-legal compliance as suggested by the Joint Commission on Accreditation of Healthcare Organizations (JCAHO).	In an emergency situation, refer to institution-specific protocol for assumption of consent.
3. Gather needed equipment and supplies for halo/vest application (see Figure 87-2 and Table 87-2). *(Level I*)*	If all equipment is not available, then the procedure cannot be performed. Facilitates completion of task in a timely manner.	
4. Wash hands; put on clean gloves.	Standard precautions; reduces transmission of microorganisms.	
5. Assist with measuring head and torso as shown in Figure 87-1. *(Level I*)*	Identifies correct size of halo ring and vest.	
6. Type of halo/vest is determined by orthopedic surgeon or prescribing practitioner who applies apparatus.	Proper size and type of halo/vest is determined by child's size and injury.	The back of the halo ring can be open or closed, depending on the number of pins to be applied.[10]
7. Place all materials and instrumentation at the head of the bed; assist practitioner who applies vest to establish a sterile field and prepare equipment.	All necessary equipment should be at bedside before the start of procedure to facilitate timely completion of procedure.	The practitioner who applies the vest needs enough room to move around the child, including at the head of the bed.
8. Ensure cardiorespiratory monitoring is in place with appropriate alarm limits set and alarms activated; ensure emergency equipment and medications are readily available.	Child may clinically decompensate during the procedure, especially if sedation is given.	Refer to institution-specific protocol for monitoring requirements during procedural sedation.

* Level I: Manufacturer's recommendations only

Procedure | for Halo/Vest Application: Assist and Care—*Continued*

Steps	Rationale	Considerations
9. Identify the child with appropriate patient and procedure verification process (e.g., "Time out"). *(Level II*)*	Confirms correct patient, procedure, and site as recommended by the JCAHO; prevents unnecessary medical procedures.	Verification process and documentation is institution specific. Use active communication techniques.
10. Administer sedation and pain medication as indicated and per prescribing practitioner's order.	Prevents the child from moving; provides amnesia for duration of procedure, and reduces procedural anxiety.	Appropriate medications are selected based on child's age, weight, medical condition, and allergy profile. Administration of sedation and monitoring of the child must not be the responsibility of the practitioner who performs the procedure.
11. Assist in positioning the child supine maintaining spinal precautions; place a roll or folded towel under the child's occipital region. *(Level I*)*	Places child in appropriate position for application of the halo.	If a closed halo ring is to be used, the crown of the child's head must be off the edge of the bed and supported manually with spinal precautions to apply the ring.

Halo Ring Placement

Steps	Rationale	Considerations
12. Maintain spinal precautions as the practitioner prepares halo ring by screwing brass positioning pins into halo ring (Figure 87-4). *(Level I*)*	Positioning pins hold the halo in place during the application process.	

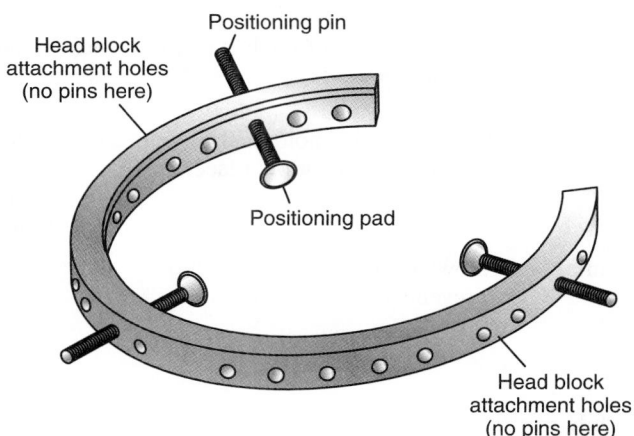

Positioning pin

Head block attachment holes (no pins here)

Positioning pad

Head block attachment holes (no pins here)

FIGURE 87-4   Brass positioning pins with white disc attached. *Courtesy of PMT Corp, Chanhassen, MN, 2004.*

Procedure continues on following page

* Level I: Manufacturer's recommendations only
  Level II: Theory-based; no research data to support recommendations; recommendations from expert consensus group may exist

Procedure	for Halo/Vest Application: Assist and Care—*Continued*	
Steps	**Rationale**	**Considerations**
13. Maintain spinal precautions while the practitioner places halo over head and aligns it with equator of the skull (Figure 87-5).	Desired location of ring.	If skull deformity is present, the placement is adjusted accordingly. Pins most commonly migrate because of poor positioning or inappropriate tightening.[11]

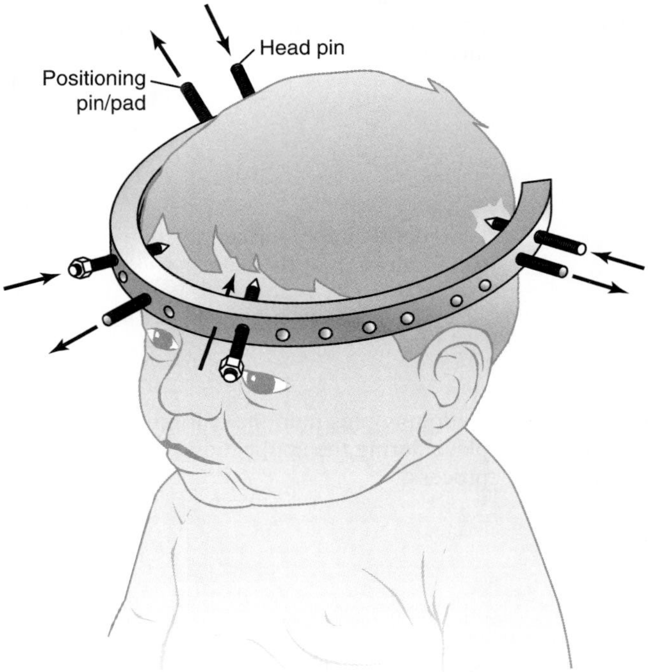

FIGURE 87-5   Placement of halo ring over equator of skull; clip or shave hair in region of permanent pin placement. *Courtesy of PMT Corp, Chanhassen, MN, 2004.*

14. Maintain spinal precautions while practitioner tightens positioning pins. *(Level I*)*	Positioning pins hold the ring in place during permanent pin placement.	Screw must be tightened such that the white disc is snug to skull and the ring is equidistant from the skull on all sides.
15. Maintain spinal precautions while practitioner identifies permanent pin site locations on equator of skull and clips or shaves hair at pin sites (see Figure 87-5).	Allows skin to be cleansed and prevents hair from entering the pin site.	Pin sites chosen must not be the sites for the head blocks.
16. Maintain spinal precautions while the practitioner cleans the skin and injects local anesthetic at the pin site locations.	Prevents infection and provides anesthesia at pin sites.	Skin antiseptic used is institution- or prescribing practitioner specific.
17. Maintain spinal precautions while practitioner screws permanent pins into designated position manually or with torque wrench.	Tightens the pins to appropriate pressure.	The torque wrench that is provided with the small end of the screw bit exposed is to be set to 2 to 4 in/lb depending on the size of the child. In children 10 months to 3 years, the pins should only be placed finger tight.[10]

* Level I: Manufacturer's recommendations only

Procedure	**for Halo/Vest Application: Assist and Care**—*Continued*	
Steps	**Rationale**	**Considerations**
18. Maintain spinal precautions while practitioner tightens lock nuts with wrench. *(Level I*)*	Prevents the screws from loosening.	Practitioner supports the halo/ring with the opposite hand to prevent torqueing the ring and placing undue pressure on the rest of the halo/ring.
19. Maintain spinal precautions while head blocks are attached (Figure 87-6) with screws and washer. The screw should be facing in toward skull with bulk of blocks above the ring. *(Level I*)*	Ensures halo ring is ready to accept the support bars after vest is attached.	Blocks are attached at the designated location.

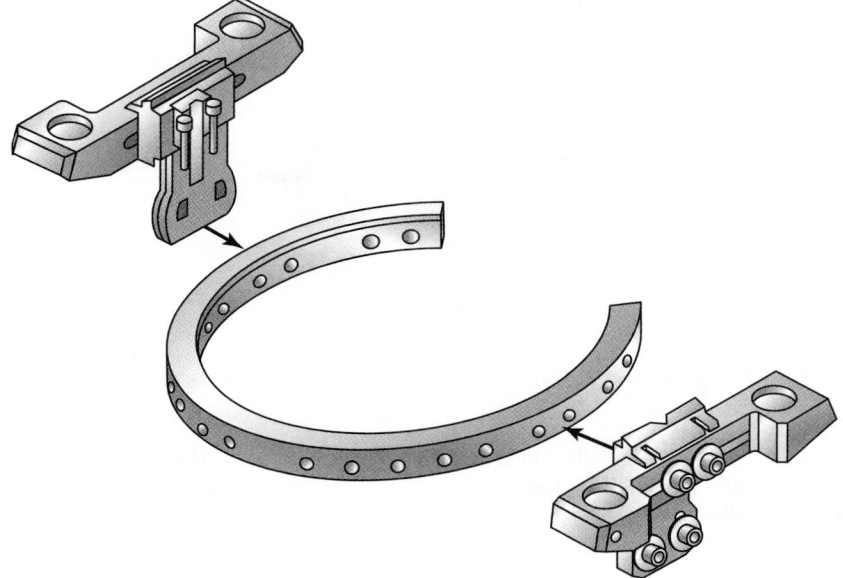

FIGURE 87-6   Attachment of head blocks. *Courtesy of PMT Corp, Chanhassen, MN, 2004.*

Vest Application

20. Maintain strict spinal precautions while practitioner assembles vest for application (Figure 87-7). *(Level VI*)*	Until the vest and rods are applied, the cervical spine is unstable and neurologic injury can occur if spinal precautions are not used.	
21. Practitioner who applies vest separates the anterior and posterior shells of the vest and removes all support rods. *(Level I*)*	Facilitates vest application.	
22. Assist with log rolling the child to the left or right; the posterior shell is placed on the bed under the child. *(Level I*)*	Places the posterior shell under child so final adjustments can be made.	Log roll precautions must be used to prevent neurologic injury.

Procedure continues on following page

* Level I: Manufacturer's recommendations only
Level VI: Clinical studies in a variety of patient populations and situations to support recommendations

Procedure | **for Halo/Vest Application: Assist and Care**—*Continued*

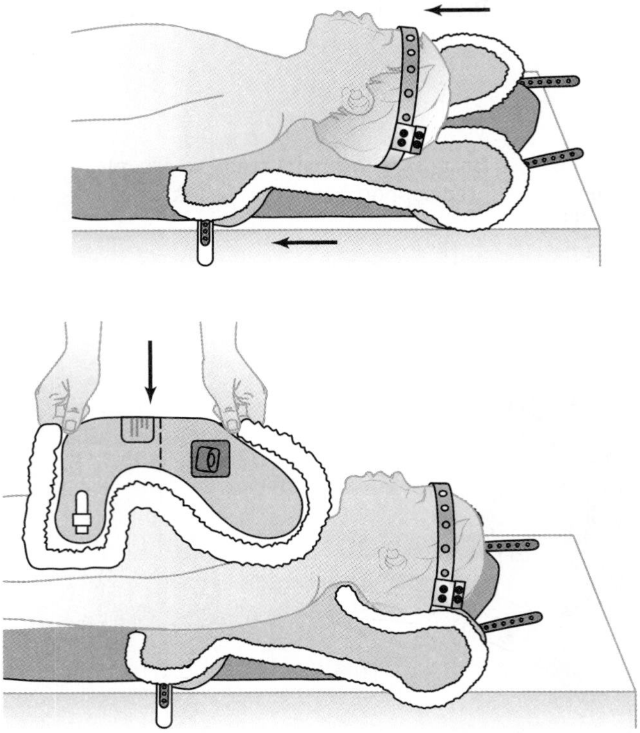

Steps	Rationale	Considerations

FIGURE 87-7   Application of vest. *Courtesy of PMT Corp, Chanhassen, MN, 2004.*

Steps	Rationale	Considerations
23. Assist with log rolling the child supine. Anterior portion of the shell is positioned on the chest of the child so that the interlocking tabs are positioned at the waist line opposite the posterior shell. *(Level I*)*	Aligns the anterior and posterior shell for tightening.	If the anterior shell is not in the right position, the posterior portion of the shell has to be adjusted.
24. Maintain spinal precautions while the practitioner who applies the vest tightens the vest and attaches the stabilization rods to the halo and vest (Figures 87-8 and 87-9). The interlocking tabs are inserted before buckling the straps. Waist straps are tightened before tightening shoulder straps. *(Level I*)*	The rods connect the halo with the vest.	Ensure that the straps are tightened equally on each side by counting the holes of the straps.
25. Maintain spinal precautions while practitioner who applies the vest verifies child is in the proper position.	Prepares the halo for final tightening.	Spinal precautions must be maintained until all adjustments to the child's position are made.
26. Maintain spinal precautions while the practitioner who applies the vest retightens the head pins and all of the screws. *(Level VI*)*	The headpins can loosen during application of vest and rods.[11]	Nut is loosened before tightening headpin and retightened after tightening head pin.
27. Discard used supplies and equipment, including sharps, in appropriate receptacles.	Standard precautions; reduces transmission of microorganisms. Protects personnel health.	

---

* Level I: Manufacturer's recommendations only
  Level VI: Clinical studies in a variety of patient populations and situations to support recommendations

Procedure   for Halo/Vest Application: Assist and Care—*Continued*

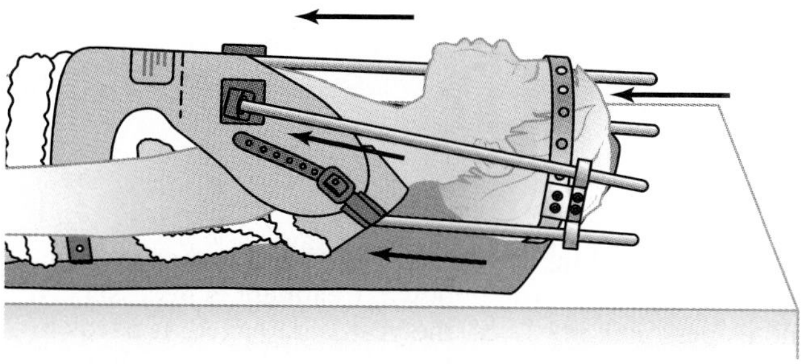

Steps	Rationale	Considerations

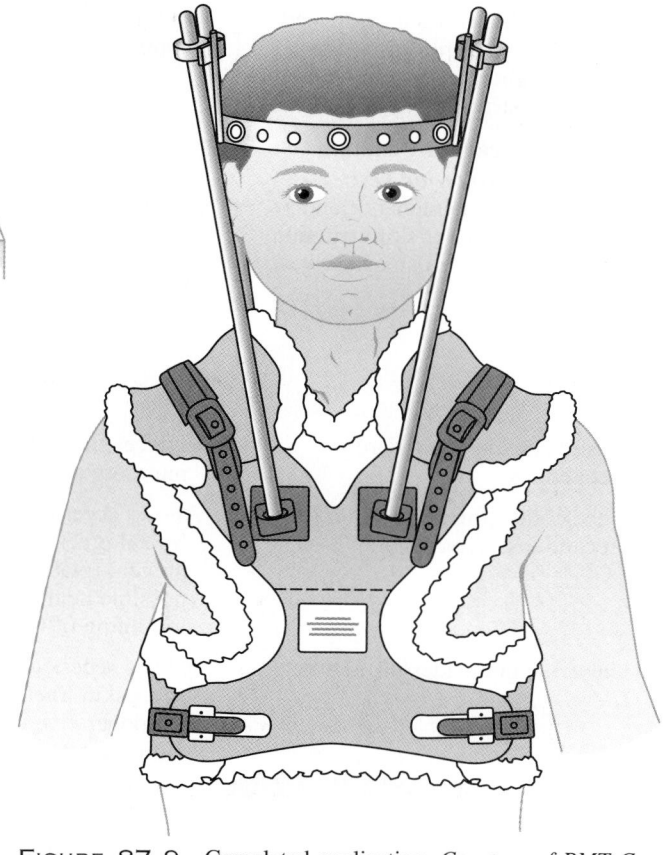

FIGURE 87-8   Application of stabilization rods. *Courtesy of PMT Corp, Chanhassen, MN, 2004.*

FIGURE 87-9   Completed application. *Courtesy of PMT Corp, Chanhassen, MN, 2004.*

Steps	Rationale	Considerations
28. Remove gloves; wash hands.	Standard precautions.	
29. Obtain cervical spine x-rays. *(Level II*)*	Medical-legal documentation of spinal alignment and adjustments to halo/vest.	Child should be appropriately sedated during x-ray in the event the halo/vest needs readjustment. After every adjustment, an x-ray should be performed. Blocks are adjusted to change the position of the cervical spine.
30. Perform neurologic examination.	Evaluates and documents child's neurologic examination after procedure.	Child should be completely awake without alteration of mental status during examination if possible; any alterations from medication or clinical condition should be noted in the medical record.

Procedure continues on following page

* Level II: Theory-based; no research data to support recommendations; recommendations from expert consensus group may exist

Procedure for Halo/Vest Application: Assist and Care—*Continued*

Steps	Rationale	Considerations
31. Ensure practitioner reevaluates and retightens all screws as indicated 24 hours after application. Ring pins are tightened first and then the rest of the structure. *(Level VI*)*	Ensures that the halo ring is tightened to torque identified during application.	
Vest Maintenance and Cleaning *To Clean Under Anterior Vest:*		
32. Provide daily maintenance and cleaning; assess for skin irritation, skin breakdown or damage to vest. *(Level I*)*	Allows evaluation of the child's skin, allows evaluation of the vest for damage, and promotes personal hygiene.	If the skin is irritated or broken down, treatment is necessary. If the vest is damaged, it needs to be replaced. Follow institution-specific protocol for individuals authorized to change the vest liner and for recommended procedure.
33. Wash hands; use standard precautions.	Reduces the transmission of microorganisms.	
34. Place child supine; maintain spinal precautions. *(Level II*)*	Allows access to the anterior chest. Spinal precautions are used to prevent rotation of the body and possible neurologic injury during loosening of the vest.	
35. Unbuckle both sides of the vest. *(Level I*)*	Allows access to the skin and sheepskin liner. If the child is uncooperative in the supine position with maintenance of spinal precautions, only unbuckle one side of the vest.	If the sheepskin does not require changing, proceed to step 37.
36. Remove the anterior vest and soiled sheepskin. *(Level I*)*	Promotes skin integrity.	The anterior sheepskin may need to be changed more often than the posterior because of soiling from eating and secretions.
37. Clean the skin with soap and water and dry with a towel. *(Level II*)*	Cleans the skin.	Do not use powders or lotions; these tend to mat the sheepskin.
38. Inspect the skin for irritation or breakdown; pay particular attention to bony prominences. *(Level II*)*	Assesses skin integrity; identifies areas of concern.	If the sheepskin is not being changed, proceed to step 40. If chest physiotherapy is prescribed, it may be performed while the anterior vest is removed.
39. Replace the sheepskin lining with a new sheepskin lining by aligning the appropriate Velcro tabs and pressing them together securely. *(Level I*)*	Secures the new liner in place.	
40. Buckle both sides of the vest. *(Level I*)*	Secures the anterior vest in place.	The vest should be able to be secured back to the original eye holes, but the need to tighten the vest to the next eye hole is not unusual as a result of weight loss. Be sure an equal number of eye holes is found on each side.

* Level I: Manufacturer's recommendations only
  Level II: Theory-based; no research data to support recommendations; recommendations from expert consensus group may exist
  Level VI: Clinical studies in a variety of patient populations and situations to support recommendations

Procedure | for Halo/Vest Application: Assist and Care—*Continued*

Steps	Rationale	Considerations
To Clean Under Posterior Vest:		
41. Be sure the vest is secure. With assistance, log roll the child to one side, maintaining spinal precautions.	Allows access to the posterior portion of the vest.	
42. Unbuckle the side of the vest facing the ceiling. *(Level I*)*	Allows access to the posterior sheepskin and child's skin.	If the sheepskin is not being changed, proceed to step 44.
43. Roll the soiled sheepskin liner toward the center of the vest. *(Level I*)*	Allows replacement of the sheepskin and cleansing and evaluation of the child's skin. Do not bunch the sheepskin too thick because the vest will be resecured before the sheepskin is completely removed.	If the sheepskin does not require changing, skip this step.
44. Clean the skin with soap and water and dry with a towel.	Daily cleansing of the skin promotes skin integrity.	Do not use powders or lotions; these tend to mat the sheepskin.
45. Inspect the skin for irritation or breakdown. *(Level II*)*	Presence of vest increases the child's risk for skin breakdown.	The most common sites for breakdown are over areas of bony prominences. If chest physiotherapy is prescribed, it may be performed while the posterior vest is removed.
46. Replace the sheepskin lining with a new sheepskin lining by aligning the appropriate Velcro tabs and pressing them together securely; unroll the new sheepskin liner to meet the edges of the soiled sheepskin liner.	Secures the liner in place on that side. Do not bunch the liner; the vest will be resecured in the next step to roll the child and complete the procedure.	If the sheepskin is not being changed, skip this step.
47. Buckle the vest. *(Level I*)*	Secures the vest and makes moving the child safe.	If the vest is unable to be secured at the eye holes previously used because of the bulk of the sheepskin, then secure it as tightly as possible and adjust the straps once the procedure is completed.
48. Repeat steps 42 to 47, but roll the soiled sheepskin liner from the midline toward the edge and unroll the new sheepskin liner from the midline toward the edge. *(Level I*)*	Completes cleaning, child's skin evaluation, and replacement of the posterior sheepskin.	
49. At the completion of the process, be sure the buckles are secure and equal amounts of eye holes are used compared with the contralateral strap.	Ensures vest is secure and provides necessary stabilization.	
50. Perform neurologic examination.	Ensures neurologic examination results are unchanged after vest manipulation.	
51. Dispose of used supplies and equipment in appropriate receptacles; wash hands.	Standard precautions; reduces transmission of microorganisms.	

* Level I: Manufacturer's recommendations only
  Level II: Theory-based; no research data to support recommendations; recommendations from expert consensus group may exist

Expected Outcomes

- Halo/vest fits properly
- Cervical spine is in anatomic position or stabilized

- Child's neurologic status is unchanged from preprocedure examination
- Child's safety is maintained

- Mobility is maintained if child's condition is neurologically intact
- Child is free from infection at the pin sites
- Skin integrity remains intact
- Child has acceptable level of comfort

Unexpected Outcomes

- Improperly fitting halo/vest
- Cervical spine not stabilized or not in anatomic position
- Neurologic injury

- Loosening of halo/vest
- Injury from fall while halo/vest is worn
- Crescent or torque wrench is not available during an emergency situation
- Inability to move because of weight and position of halo/vest
- Infection of scalp
- Skin irritation or injury from halo/vest
- Unmanaged pain
- Unmanaged anxiety

Monitoring and Care of the Child

Activities and Interventions	Rationale	Reportable Conditions
1. Assess pin sites daily for stability and signs of infection.	The risk of infection is 25% greater in children than in adults.[11] Pins may become loosened from either infection or poor care of the halo/vest.	• Loose pins • Infection: If erythema is mild or superficial with minimal drainage and pins are tight, oral antibiotic may be prescribed; if the scalp is red and swollen with large amounts of drainage or pins are loosened, the pins should be removed, intravenous (IV) antibiotics prescribed, and osteomyelitis work-up performed[11]
2. Assess halo/vest daily and as needed for loosening or damage.	Loose vest must be adjusted because it does not maintain stability of cervical spine; damaged vest must be replaced.	• Loose vest • Damage to vest
3. Assess skin integrity around and under vest daily and with vest changes.	Presence of vest increases the risk of skin irritation or breakdown.	• Skin irritation around vest edges • Skin irritation under vest • Skin breakdown
4. Assess respiratory status regularly; provide incentive spirometry or chest physiotherapy as indicated. *(Level II*)*	Application of the vest may cause a decrease in the child's vital capacity. Treatments clear the airways and enhance secretion mobilization.	• Increased pulmonary secretions • Deterioration in respiratory status
5. Monitor vital signs and neurologic evaluation results every 2 to 4 hours or as indicated.	Facilitates early recognition of deterioration in child's status.	• Unstable or deteriorating vital signs • Decrease in level of consciousness • Deterioration in sensorimotor function • Loss of sensation or function
6. Check for presence of crescent and torque wrenches at the beginning of every shift and after any transport.	Wrenches may be necessary if child must be removed emergently from halo/vest (e.g., if emergent intubation is necessary).	• Inability to locate wrenches

* Level II: Theory-based; no research data to support recommendations; recommendations from expert consensus group may exist

Monitoring and Care of the Child—Cont'd

Activities and Interventions	Rationale	Reportable Conditions
7. Keep child comfortable and support halo/vest. Provide support so child is able to be upright or semi-reclined to watch television or play games.	Child's halo/vest can loosen because of pin loosening or because the child does not protect the apparatus and bangs the halo/vest into non-moveable structures.	• Loosening of pins • Loosening or damage to halo/vest
8. Assess effectiveness of pain management strategies and provide appropriate interventions. Encourage family to assist with nonpharmacologic means to comfort and support the child.	Early identification of pain allows for immediate attention and management. Restrictions in activity and mobility may be frustrating for the child.	• Report of unresolved pain and discomfort • Changes in physiologic condition • Continued agitation despite therapy

Documentation

- Child and family education
- Child's neurologic examination results before procedure
- Presence of signed consent
- Type, model, and size of halo/vest applied
- Patient and procedure verification process per institution-specific protocol
- Time, date, and practitioner applying the halo/vest
- Medications administered for procedure and child's response; if procedural sedation is used, institution-specific documentation for procedural sedation
- X-ray obtained after procedure
- Child's neurologic examination results after procedure
- Status of pin sites; skin integrity
- Comfort assessment and any specific interventions provided
- Unexpected outcomes and related treatment

References

1. Wolf JW, Johnson RM: Cervical orthoses. In Bailey DW, Sherk HH, editors: *The cervical spine,* Philadelphia, 1983, Lippincott.
2. Callahan RA, et al: Cervical facet fusion for control of instability following laminectomy, *J Bone Joint Surg* 59:991-1002, 1997.
3. Johnson R, et al: Cervical orthosis, *Clin Orthop* 154:34-45, 1981.
4. Johnson R, et al: Immediate strength of certain cervical fusion techniques, *Orthop Trans* 4:42, 1980.
5. Prolo DJ, et al: The injured cervical spine: immediate and long-term immobilization with the halo, *JAMA* 224:591-594, 1973.
6. Pang D: Principles and pitfalls of spinal stabilization in children. In Pang D, editor: *Disorders of the paediatric spine,* New York, 1995, Raven Press.
7. Kopits SE, Steingass MH: Experience with the "halo-cast" in small children, *Surg Clin North Am* 50:935-943, 1970.
8. Baum J, et al: Comparison of halo complications in adults and children, *Spine* 14:251-252, 1989.
9. Chan RC, et al: Halo-thoracic brace immobilization in 188 patients with acute cervical spine injuries, *J Neurosurg* 58:508-515, 1983.
10. Mubarak SJ, et al: Halo immobilization for cervical spine instability in the infant. Presented at the Annual Meeting of the Pediatric Orthopedic Society of North America, 1988, Colorado Springs, CO.
11. Pang D, Sun P: Pediatric vertebral column and spinal cord injuries. In Winn HR, editor: *Youmans neurological surgery,* ed 5, Philadelphia, 2004, Saunders.

Additional Reading

Winn HR, editor: *Youmans neurological surgery,* ed 5, Philadelphia, 2004, Saunders.

AP

Cervical Collar: Placement and Management

P U R P O S E : A rigid cervical collar is placed to stabilize the cervical spine that has sustained an actual or suspected injury or to provide postoperative support. It is used to support the spine and keep it from excessive movements as the spine heals or until more definitive treatment is provided.

Dean Barone

PREREQUISITE KNOWLEDGE

- The goal of rigid cervical collar placement is maintenance of alignment of the spine in a neutral position, for prevention of new or further injury.[1]
- A rigid cervical collar alone does not provide spinal immobilization.[1] If full spinal immobilization is necessary, the child must be appropriately secured to a backboard after the collar is placed. A spine board with a head well or elevation of the child's torso with padding is recommended for maintenance of a neutral position because of the child's relatively large occiput.[1]
- A properly applied cervical collar should limit flexion and extension of the neck. A single small study of children less than 8 years old who were immobilized on a backboard with a properly fitting cervical collar in place found that all children still had some flexion of the cervical spine.[2]
- Anatomy and biomechanics of the cervical spine
- Skill in manual spinal precautions, cervical spine stabilization, and log roll maneuver

---

AP This procedure should be performed only by physicians, advanced practice nurses, and other health care professionals (including critical care nurses) with additional knowledge, skills, and demonstrated competence per professional licensure or institutional standard.

- No absolute contraindications exist for the placement of a cervical collar; however, significant neck swelling from tracheal injury or hemorrhage may limit the use of the cervical collar.[3]
- Complications of rigid cervical collar placement may include[1,4]:
  - ❖ Airway compromise (e.g., upper airway obstruction from incorrectly sized collar)
  - ❖ Increased intracranial pressure (ICP)
  - ❖ Increased aspiration risk
  - ❖ Skin ulceration
  - ❖ Increased agitation, especially in toddlers and preschoolers
- There are multiple treatment options available for cervical spine injuries based on type and location of the injury and the specific characteristics of the injured child.
- If the cervical collar is correctly fitted, the child's chin fits in the chin cup. The collar fits between the chin and the suprasternal notch and rests on the clavicles.[1,3] If the child can tuck the chin inside the collar, the collar is not fitted snugly enough.
- Components of the cervical collar
  - ❖ Cervical collars are generally made of plastic or polyurethane or both.
  - ❖ The collar may be a single unit or may have two pieces.
  - ❖ Some collar assembly may be necessary before use.

❖ In general, all models have a mechanism to allow access to the anterior neck for care of a tracheostomy or for an emergent cricoidotomy.

❖ Always refer to manufacturer's instructions for specifics of collar application and use.

• Cervical collars come in a variety of sizes and types. Single-unit collars, such as the Stifneck Pedi-Select Collar (Laerdal Medical Corp, Wappingers Falls, NY; Figure 88-1), are generally for short-term use. Two-piece collars, such as the Miami J or Miami Jr (Jerome Medical, Moorestown, NJ; Figure 88-2), have additional padding and are often used for longer periods.

• There are many manufacturers of cervical collars. Familiarity with the unit-specific or institution-specific type of collar used is necessary. The information in this procedure is based on the Miami J and Miami Jr.

• Cervical collars are a single patient use disposable system.

• Risk factors for skin breakdown under a cervical collar include presence of moisture, shock, poor nutritional status, and decreased level of consciousness.

• Child development as it relates to clinical assessment and cervical collar application

CHILD AND FAMILY ASSESSMENT

• History of familial cervical disorders ➤➤*Rationale:* Family members may have experience with the application and care of a cervical collar and an understanding of the pathophysiology of the disorder.

• Child's developmental level and ability to interact ➤➤*Rationale:* These factors influence preparation of the

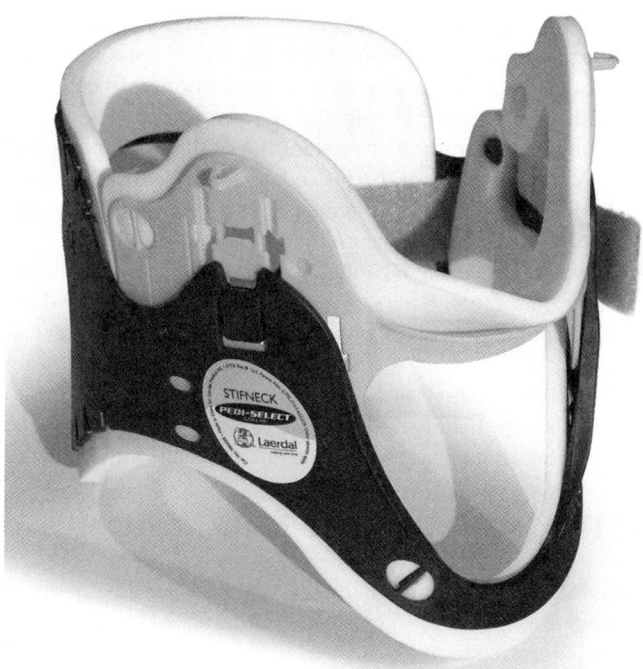

FIGURE 88-1 Stifneck® Pedi-Select™ Collar single-unit collar. *Photo courtesy of Laerdal Medical Corp, Wappingers Falls, NY, 2006. All rights reserved.*

child and interaction. Any form of restraint is particularly challenging to toddlers and preschoolers. Some children may need sedation to decrease anxiety or prevent movement during collar application.

• Size and age of child ➤➤*Rationale:* Cervical collars come in a variety of sizes and must be properly fitted.

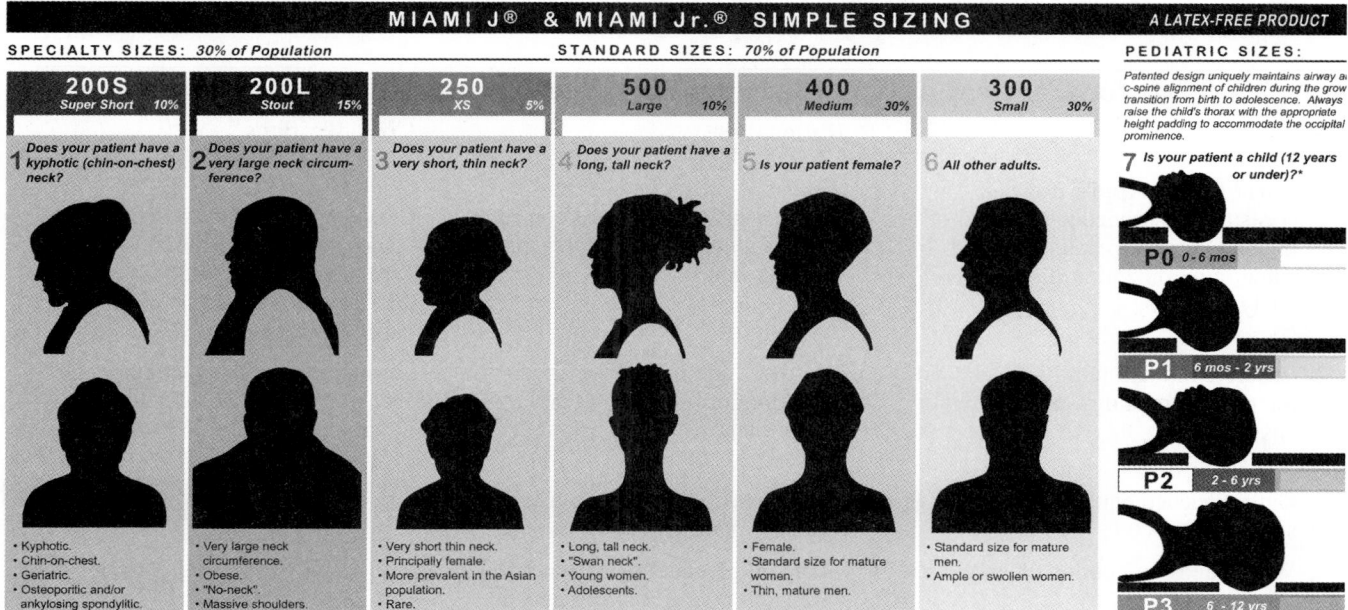

FIGURE 88-2 Sizing of Miami J® and Miami Jr.® collars. *Courtesy of Jerome Medical, Moorestown, NJ, 2006.*

- Child's neurologic status and vital signs →*Rationale:* Documentation of neurologic status is important for baseline data and medical-legal protection with care of a child with a cervical spine injury or disorder.
- Child's and family's understanding of the reasons for and risks and benefits of the procedure →*Rationale:* Evaluates child's and family's understanding of the procedure and provides a gauge for ongoing education.
- Irritation or damage to the child's skin, especially in the neck and upper torso →*Rationale:* Provides baseline data. Skin breakdown is a potential complication of cervical collar use.
- Family's desire to be present during the procedure →*Rationale:* Family may provide comfort and support to the child but should have the option not to remain with the child.

CHILD AND FAMILY EDUCATION

Individualized, developmentally appropriate education is provided to the family and to the child based on desire for knowledge, readiness to learn, and overall neurologic and psychosocial state.

- Provide information to the family and to the child about the cervical collar and the application process →*Rationale:* Providing information decreases anxiety associated with application, wearing of the cervical collar and limitations imposed by the collar.
- If developmentally appropriate, explain to the child the need to be still during the application process →*Rationale:* If the child does not remain still during the procedure, the child is at risk of neurologic injury.

- Provide information to the family and to the child about the need to wear the collar at all times, except when the collar is removed for cleaning of the skin and collar. Include information about how the cervical spine is stabilized when the collar is off. →*Rationale:* Providing this information clarifies expectations about the treatment, promotes compliance with the plan of care, and promotes the child's safety.
- If the child will be discharged with the cervical collar, educate the family, and child as appropriate, on how to care for the cervical collar →*Rationale:* Cervical collars are easily removed for personal hygiene and evaluation of skin breakdown.
- Encourage questions and answer questions as they arise →*Rationale:* Reinforcement of information is needed during periods of stress.

EQUIPMENT

Collar Application

- Sizing tape or selection chart supplied by manufacturer
- Correctly sized cervical collar
- Pad to elevate torso if needed, based on child's size
- Clean gloves

Skin Care

- Washcloths and towel
- Replacement pads
- Mild soap and water
- Small pillow or pad
- Clean gloves

Procedure	for Cervical Collar: Placement and Management	
Steps	**Rationale**	**Considerations**
Cervical Collar Application 1. Assistant positioned at the head of the bed initiates manual cervical spine immobilization if not previously initiated.	Initiates stabilization and control of the cervical spine and prevents further injury.	Child is positioned with arms at sides and head midline. Thumbs are placed on the mandible, palms are placed over ears, and fingers are placed on the occipital ridge.[1,3]
2. Ensure child and family understand the procedure and questions are answered.	Evaluates and reinforces understanding of previously taught information.	Developmental level, cognitive ability, and anxiety level determine approach to and effectiveness of teaching.
3. Gather needed equipment and supplies.	Facilitates completion of task in a timely manner.	
4. Wash hands and put on clean gloves.	Standard precautions; reduces the transmission of microorganisms.	
5. Use spinal precautions and log roll technique throughout the entire procedure. *(Level VI*)*	The child with a known or suspected cervical spine disorder or injury is at risk for serious	A minimum of two to three people is necessary for initial collar application.

* Level VI: Clinical studies in a variety of patient populations and situations to support recommendations

Procedure for Cervical Collar: Placement and Management—*Continued*

Steps	Rationale	Considerations
	neurologic injury if spinal precautions and log roll technique are not used.	
6. Position the child supine without anything under the head. *(Level I*)*	Places the child in the appropriate position for application of the collar.	If the child is less than 12 years old, place the child's torso on padding to offset the child's occipital prominence.
7. If the child is 12 years old or younger, select the appropriate collar on basis of the child's age (see Figure 88-2) or measure the child with the color-coded tape or pad supplied by the manufacturer. *(Level I*)*	Proper sizing is critical for optimal immobilization and comfort.	If the child falls between two sizes, start with the smaller size. *(Level I*)* Consider sizing children who will wear the collar in the postoperative period before surgery. *(Level I*)*
8. If the child is more than 12 years old, select the appropriate collar with the phenotype chart (see Figure 88-2) or the quick size check method (Figure 88-3). Use fingers to measure the vertical chin to shoulder distance, which should correlate with the distance from the top of the Velcro strap to the bottom edge of the plastic on the collar selected. *(Level I*)*	Proper sizing is critical for optimal immobilization and comfort.	If the child or adolescent falls between two sizes, start with the smaller size. *(Level I*)* Consider sizing children and adolescents who will wear the collar in the postoperative period before surgery. *(Level I*)*
9. Remove the selected collar from packaging and ensure padding is secure. Separate and identify anterior and posterior parts of collar.	Necessary for correct application.	Collar cannot be applied without padding in place.
10. While the assistant maintains spinal precautions, slide the posterior portion of the collar behind the child's neck. *(Level I*)*	Allows for application of the posterior portion of the cervical collar.	Be sure the collar is centered and the padding is extended beyond the plastic edges if appropriate.
11. While the assistant maintains spinal precautions, flare the edges of the anterior portion of the collar out and slide it up the chest wall and into place, "scooping" it into place snugly under the neck. Release the sides of the collar so they bend around toward the posterior portion of the collar. *(Level I*)*	Allows for application of the anterior portion of the cervical collar.	The sides should be off the trapezius muscles and the ears should be free.
12. While the assistant maintains spinal precautions, hold the collar securely and curl the ends (flaps) of the collar so they are snug against the child's neck. If the child can slip the chin inside the collar, the collar is not snug enough. *(Level I*)*	This is the final position before the Velcro straps are secured.	If the cervical collar is not snug (e.g., the collar rests on the trapezius and the ears are not free), then remove the collar while assistant maintains spinal precautions and select a new collar for application.

Procedure continues on following page

* Level I: Manufacturer's recommendations only

Procedure | **for Cervical Collar: Placement and Management**—*Continued*

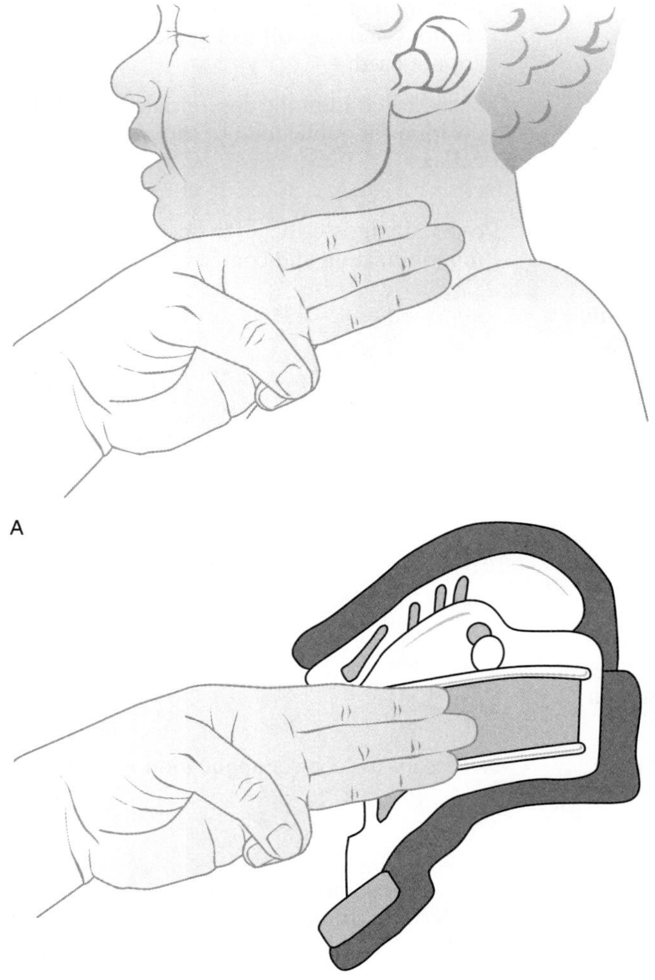

Steps	Rationale	Considerations

FIGURE 88-3 Sizing of Miami J® collar with quick size check method. *Courtesy of Jerome Medical, Moorestown, NJ, 2006.*

Steps	Rationale	Considerations
13. Apply Velcro straps one side at a time to equal lengths; ensure that no gaps are present. *(Level I*)*	If Velcro straps are not fastened equally, the collar does not provide the immobilization and comfort needed.	If the collar moves out of position or the Velcro straps are not approximated with half the surface of the Velcro, the collar needs to be replaced with a better fitting cervical collar.
14. Perform neurologic examination.	Assesses for deterioration in neurologic examination after procedure.	Child should be completely awake and mental status not altered during examination if possible; if altered mental status is present, level of consciousness should be noted.
15. Remove gloves; wash hands.	Standard precautions; reduces transmission of microorganisms.	

* Level I: Manufacturer's recommendations only

Procedure **for Cervical Collar: Placement and Management**—*Continued*

Steps	Rationale	Considerations
16. Obtain a cervical spine x-ray per prescribing practitioner's order or institution-specific protocol. *(Level II*)*	Assesses and provides documentation of alignment of the cervical spine after procedure.	If the cervical spine is not anatomically positioned, then reevaluation is necessary and consideration should be given to alternative methods of cervical immobilization.
Skin Care		
1. Ensure child and family understand procedure and questions are answered.	Evaluates and reinforces understanding of previously taught information.	Developmental level, cognitive ability, and anxiety level determine approach to and effectiveness of teaching.
2. Gather needed equipment and supplies.	Facilitates completion of task in a timely manner.	
3. Wash hands and put on clean gloves.	Standard precautions; reduces transmission of microorganisms.	
4. Use spinal precautions and log roll technique throughout the entire procedure. *(Level VI*)*	The child with a known or suspected cervical spine disorder or injury is at risk for serious neurologic injury if spinal precautions and log roll technique are not used.	A minimum of two people is necessary for skin care.
5. Position the child supine without anything under the head. Have assistant immobilize the child's cervical spine with spinal precautions. *(Level I*)*	Places the child in the appropriate position for removal of the collar with stabilization and immobilization of the cervical spine.	If the child is less than 12 years old, consider placing the child's torso on padding to offset the child's occipital prominence.
6. Open Velcro tab on left side of collar. Lift anterior portion of collar.	Necessary to visualize and clean skin.	
7. While assistant maintains spinal precautions, wash front of neck with mild soap and water and dry. Assess skin for redness, irritation, or breakdown.	Provides hygiene and facilitates assessment of skin under collar.	
8. Assess cleanliness and dryness of pads. Replace soiled or damp pads. *(Level I*)*	Soiled or damp pads increase likelihood of skin breakdown.	
9. While assistant maintains spinal precautions, reapply anterior portion of collar and refasten Velcro.	Provides support and stabilization of cervical spine.	If the child can slip the chin inside the collar, the collar is not snug enough. *(Level I*)*
10. With assistant maintaining spinal precautions, log roll the child to one side. Place a towel or small pillow under cheek. *(Level I*)*	Maintains correct alignment of cervical spine and prevents injury.	If indicated, use additional assistants to log roll child.
11. While assistant maintains spinal precautions, open Velcro tab on side of collar facing up and lift posterior portion of collar.	Necessary to visualize and clean skin.	

Procedure continues on following page

* Level I: Manufacturer's recommendations only

Level II: Theory-based; no research data to support recommendations; recommendations from expert consensus group may exist

Level VI: Clinical studies in a variety of patient populations and situations to support recommendations

AP This procedure should be performed only by physicians, advanced practice nurses, and other health care professionals (including critical care nurses) with additional knowledge, skills, and demonstrated competence per professional licensure or institutional standard.

Procedure for Cervical Collar: Placement and Management—*Continued*

Steps	Rationale	Considerations
12. While assistant maintains spinal precautions, wash back of neck with mild soap and water and dry. Assess skin for redness, irritation, or breakdown.	Provides hygiene and facilitates assessment of skin under collar.	
13. Assess cleanliness and dryness of pads. Replace soiled or damp pads. *(Level I*)*	Soiled or damp pads increase likelihood of skin breakdown.	
14. While assistant maintains spinal precautions, reapply posterior portion of collar and refasten Velcro. *(Level I*)*	Provides support and stabilization of cervical spine.	Ensure pads are not folded and extend past plastic edges of collar. *(Level I*)*
15. Reposition child supine with log roll technique or position child as desired, ensuring appropriate support and correct alignment of cervical spine. *(Level I*)*	Promotes alignment of cervical spine and skin integrity.	
16. Assess collar for appropriate fit; adjust as needed, ensuring Velcro tab length is equal on both sides of collar. *(Level I*)*	Ensures collar provides appropriate support and alignment.	If the child can slip the chin inside the collar, the collar is not snug enough. *(Level I*)*
17. Perform neurologic examination.	Assesses for deterioration in neurologic examination after manipulation of collar.	
18. Clean soiled pads per manufacturer's instructions and allow to dry completely.	Ensures replacement pads are available as needed for subsequent skin care.	
19. Discard used supplies and equipment in appropriate receptacles. Remove gloves; wash hands.	Standard precautions; reduces transmission of microorganisms.	

* Level I: Manufacturer's recommendations only

Expected Outcomes	Unexpected Outcomes
• Cervical collar is correctly sized and fitted	• Improperly placed cervical collar that allows movement of the head and neck • Collar is too large or too small and allows movement of the head and neck • Collar is too tight or too small and results in airway compromise or increased ICP
• Child's cervical spine is in anatomic position or stabilized • Child's neurologic status after collar placement is consistent with preprocedure examination results • Child's safety is maintained	• Cervical spine is unstable or in incorrect position that results in neurologic injury • Deterioration in neurologic examination after placement of collar • Injury from fall during wearing of cervical collar • Skin irritation or injury from cervical collar
• Mobility is maintained if child's condition is neurologically intact and child is able to ambulate • Skin under and around collar remains intact • Collar remains in place until discontinued by prescribing practitioner • Child has acceptable level of comfort	• Child is not able to ambulate or position self because of collar placement • Skin irritation or breakdown • Collar is removed by child or family before order for removal from prescribing practitioner • Unmanaged pain • Unmanaged anxiety

Monitoring and Care of the Child

Activities and Interventions	Rationale	Reportable Conditions
1. Assess fit of cervical collar every shift and with any manipulations of the collar.	If the collar is not fitted correctly, increased movement of the cervical spine may occur, which may result in further cervical spine injury.	• Cervical collar is not correctly sized • Cervical collar is not applied correctly
2. Monitor for complications of cervical collar placement, including upper airway obstruction from incorrectly sized collar or other respiratory complications, increased ICP, and increased aspiration risk.	Early identification of complications facilitates prompt treatment.	• Respiratory compromise • Nausea and vomiting • Increase in ICP after manipulation of cervical collar
3. Assess child's tolerance of the cervical collar; if the child removes the collar, institute spinal precautions immediately.	Removal of the cervical collar can cause the child further cervical spine injury.	• Child attempts or is able to remove collar • Increased agitation from presence of cervical collar
4. Monitor vital signs and neurologic status every 1 to 2 hours or per institution-specific protocol.	Facilitates early recognition of deterioration in child's status	• Unstable or deteriorating vital signs • Decrease in level of consciousness • Deterioration in sensorimotor function • Loss of sensation or function
5. Clean the cervical collar and replace pads as needed.	A clean cervical collar is part of the child's hygiene and prevents skin breakdown.	• Skin breakdown • Replacement pads unavailable
6. Assess skin under and around the cervical collar and provide skin care every 12 hours or per institution-specific protocol.	If the skin breaks down, the child is at risk for infection.	• Skin breakdown • Inability to provide skin care because of child's anxiety or agitation
7. Assess effectiveness of pain management strategies and provide appropriate interventions. Encourage family to assist with nonpharmacologic means to comfort and support the child.	Early identification of pain allows for immediate attention and management. Restrictions in activity and mobility may be frustrating for the child.	• Report of unresolved pain and discomfort • Changes in physiologic condition • Continued agitation despite therapy

Documentation

- Child and family education
- Child's neurologic examination results before and after placement or manipulation of cervical collar
- Type, model, and size of cervical collar applied
- Date and time collar was applied and individual who fit and applied the collar
- Medications administered for sedation or analgesia and child's response
- Interpretation of cervical spine x-ray results obtained after collar placement
- Child's tolerance of collar
- Skin assessment of area around and under collar
- Unexpected outcomes and related treatment

References

1. Trauma resuscitation and spinal immobilization. In Hazinski MF, editor: *PALS provider manual,* Dallas, 2002, American Heart Association.
2. Terloar DJ, Nypaver M: Angulation of the pediatric spine with and without cervical collar, *Pediatr Emerg Care* 13(1):5-8, 1997.
3. Emergency Nurses Association: Spinal immobilization. In Jacobs BB, Hoyt KS, editors: *Trauma nursing core course provider manual,* ed 5, Des Plaines, IL, 2000, Emergency Nurses Association.
4. Kwan I, Bunn F, Roberts I: *Spinal immobilization for trauma patients, CD002803,* 2001, updated 2003.

Additional Reading

Greenberg MS: *Handbook of neurosurgery,* ed 4, Lakeland, FL, 1997, Greenberg Graphics, Inc.

Unit **IV**
Gastrointestinal
System

SECTION THIRTEEN
**Gastrointestinal
Procedures**

PROCEDURE **89**

Abdominal Paracentesis: Assist

P U R P O S E : Abdominal paracentesis involves the percutaneous acquisition of peritoneal fluid for diagnostic evaluation or therapeutic abdominal decompression in instances in which intraabdominal pressure causes respiratory compromise from limited diaphragmatic excursion

Kelly Murawski

PREREQUISITE KNOWLEDGE

- Child development as it relates to clinical assessment and abdominal paracentesis
- Anatomy and physiology of the abdominal compartment[1,2]
- Mastery of pediatric advanced life support competencies[3]
- Conditions that may result in the development of ascites, which necessitates therapeutic or diagnostic paracentesis, include obstructive urinary tract anomalies, gastrointestinal (GI) tract perforation, congestive heart failure, portal hypertension, peritonitis, neoplasm, ventriculoperitoneal shunt obstruction, orthotopic liver transplantation, and complication of retroperitoneal or mediastinal surgery.[4-6]
- Studies such as computed tomography (CT) scan or ultrasound scan may be used to localize the fluid collection before abdominal paracentesis.[5,7]
- Rapid drainage of a large volume of peritoneal fluid may result in hypotension; albumin replacement may be initiated for volume expansion and to minimize renal or electrolyte complications.[5,7]
- Relative contraindications include prior abdominal surgery and clinical evidence of fibrinolysis and disseminated intravascular coagulopathy (DIC).[5,8] Any coagulation disorder necessitates careful planning for management.[7,9] Needle puncture for abdominal paracentesis should not be done in a cellulitic area.
- Complications of abdominal paracentesis, although rare, include introduction of contaminates into the peritoneal

space, perforation of hollow viscus, perforation of blood vessel, abdominal wall hematoma, scrotal swelling, and leakage of ascitic fluid from tap site.[8,9] Use extreme caution in children with moderate or severe coagulopathies.[8]

- Principles of aseptic technique
- Appropriate pediatric dosing of analgesics and anxiolytics and competency in procedural sedation
- Selection and use of a developmentally appropriate pain scale (see Procedure 173)
- Except in an emergency situation, informed consent is required before abdominal paracentesis.

CHILD AND FAMILY ASSESSMENT

- Child's developmental level and ability to interact ➤➤*Rationale:* These factors influence preparation of the child and interaction.
- Child's and family's understanding of the reasons for and risks and benefits of the procedure ➤➤*Rationale:* Evaluates child's and family's understanding of the procedure and provides a gauge for ongoing education; facilitates informed consent.
- Presence of abdominal abnormalities, including scars, burns, and cellulitis ➤➤*Rationale:* Abnormalities of the abdominal surface may predispose the child to complications. Previous abdominal surgery may indicate adhesions and possible fixation of intestines to the abdominal wall, which increases the risk of visceral puncture.[5,11-13]

667

- Presence of bowel or bladder distension ➧➧*Rationale:* Marked bowel distension from increased intraluminal pressure predisposes the bowel to puncture and possible leakage of bowel contents into the peritoneal cavity.[12] As with bowel distension, bladder distension may increase the risk of perforation.
- History of coagulopathy and current hematologic and coagulation study results, including prothrombin time and platelet count ➧➧*Rationale:* Presence of a coagulopathy predisposes the child to potential complications from bleeding if a blood vessel is punctured.
- History of allergies ➧➧*Rationale:* Avoids exposing the child to potential medications or material that may trigger an allergic reaction.
- Intravenous (IV) access available ➧➧*Rationale:* IV access is necessary for administration of sedation; volume resuscitation may be necessary if large volumes of fluid are removed from the abdomen.
- Current status of the child's abdomen, including bowel sounds, abdominal girth, and changes in skin characteristics ➧➧*Rationale:* Provides a baseline for comparison of abdominal status before and after the procedure.
- Child's current respiratory status, including work of breathing ➧➧*Rationale:* Provides a baseline for comparison of respiratory status before and after the procedure.
- Need for sedation and child's previous response to sedation ➧➧*Rationale:* Providing sedation to an uncooperative child reduces anxiety and facilitates a successful safe procedure minimizing complications. Issues identified during previous sedation experiences influence sedation management plan for the procedure.
- Family's desire to be present during the procedure ➧➧*Rationale:* Family may provide support and comfort measures to the child if institution-specific protocol facilitates family presence during the procedure, but family should have the choice not to remain with the child.

CHILD AND FAMILY EDUCATION

Individualized, developmentally appropriate education is provided to the family and to the child based on desire for knowledge, readiness to learn, and overall neurologic and psychosocial state.

- Provide information about abdominal paracentesis, including the reason for the procedure and the steps involved in peritoneal fluid removal ➧➧*Rationale:* Providing information decreases anxiety and fear.
- Inform the child and family of initial positioning for the procedure and whether repositioning will be necessary during the procedure ➧➧*Rationale:* Providing information decreases anxiety and fear and promotes cooperation with the procedure. The child will be positioned in a manner that facilitates fluid removal.
- Provide information about medications that will be administered for the procedure, including local anesthetics, analgesics, and anxiolytics ➧➧*Rationale:* Providing information about pain and anxiety management decreases anxiety and fear and reassures the child and family that pain will be managed.
- Provide information regarding the results of the procedure, including results of the fluid analysis ➧➧*Rationale:* Providing information decreases anxiety and fear.
- Encourage questions and answer questions as they arise ➧➧*Rationale:* Reinforcement of information is needed during periods of stress.

EQUIPMENT

- Povidone-iodine or chlorhexidine
- Sterile 4 × 4 gauze sponges
- Sterile drapes
- Sterile gloves and other protective gear, as indicated
- Lidocaine, 1%
- Syringe, 3-mL, with 25-gauge needle
- Syringes, 10-mL (2)
- 20-gauge to 22-gauge needle or over-the-needle catheter (small child)
- 16-gauge to 20-gauge needle or over-the-needle catheter (older child)
  - ❖ 15-gauge paracentesis needle (fenestrated needle with stylet) may also be used, based on practitioner's preference
- Appropriate containers for requested fluid specimens
- Appropriate laboratory requisitions
- Appropriate labels for requested specimens

Procedure for Abdominal Paracentesis: Assist

Steps	Rationale	Considerations
1. Ensure child and family understand procedure and questions are answered.	Evaluates and reinforces understanding of previously taught information.	Developmental level, cognitive ability, and anxiety level determine approach to and effectiveness of teaching.
2. Verify presence of informed consent.	Ensures medical-legal compliance as suggested by the Joint Commission on Accreditation of Healthcare Organizations (JCAHO).	For emergency situations, refer to institution-specific protocol for assumption of consent.
3. Collect all necessary equipment and supplies.	Facilitates completion of procedure without delays.	Gauge of needle or catheter is dependent on the child's size.
4. Ensure appropriate cardiopulmonary monitoring.	Critically ill children may decompensate during the procedure.	Consider the child's status when selecting the appropriate monitoring. If procedural sedation is administered, ensure availability of emergency equipment and medications.
5. Wash hands and put on personal protective equipment per institution-specific protocol.	Reduces transmission of microorganisms.	Garb for individuals in the room during the procedure varies from institution to institution; refer to institution-specific protocol.
6. Administer sedation as appropriate and per prescribing practitioner's order.	Use of sedatives may facilitate a safe successful procedure for an anxious child.	
7. Position child supine with head slightly elevated (semirecumbent position). (Level II*)	The needle is inserted in a dependent lateral position because air-filled bowel floats in ascetic fluid.[12]	Child's condition, physical examination results, or location of fluid may necessitate variation in position.
8. Identify child with appropriate patient/procedure verification process (e.g., "Time out").	Confirms correct patient, procedure, and site as recommended by JCAHO; prevents unnecessary medical procedures.	Verification process and documentation are institution specific; use active communication techniques.
9. Empty the child's bladder via catheterization or verify recent void.	Minimizes perforation of bladder and ensures bladder is located within pelvis away from site of procedure.[5,11-14] (Level II*)	
10. As indicated and per prescribing practitioner's order, place an orogastric or nasogastric tube to decompress the stomach.[2,4]	Minimizes perforation of the stomach.	
11. Assist the practitioner to establish a sterile field and prepare equipment.	Procedure is performed with aseptic technique. Ensures availability of supplies for the procedure.	
12. The practitioner cleans the abdomen with 4 × 4 pads saturated with povidone-iodine or chlorhexidine solution.	Adherence to strict aseptic technique minimizes the introduction of contaminants into the sterile peritoneal space.	

Procedure continues on following page

* Level II: Theory-based; no research data to support recommendations; recommendations from expert consensus group may exist

Procedure for Abdominal Paracentesis: Assist—*Continued*		
Steps	**Rationale**	**Considerations**
13. The abdomen is draped with sterile towels.	Creates a sterile area for the procedure.	
14. Assist the practitioner to draw up lidocaine for local anesthesia with aseptic technique maintained.	Allows the practitioner to maintain sterility for the procedure.	
15. The practitioner anesthetizes the puncture site (including skin, muscle, and peritoneum) by infiltrating the area with 1% lidocaine.	Local anesthetic minimizes pain at site of insertion during advancement of needle.[5,7,11-15]	
16. If needed, immobilize the child while the needle is inserted into the abdomen.	Immobilization assists the child to maintain position and facilitates a safe successful procedure.	
17. The practitioner inserts the needle/catheter through the skin into the peritoneal space while applying negative pressure with a syringe until fluid is obtained.	Aspiration of fluid into the syringe indicates entrance into the peritoneal space.	
18. The catheter is advanced over the needle into the peritoneum. The needle is removed.	Manipulation of the needle within the abdominal cavity may cause laceration or puncture of underlying structures.[12] Removal of the needle, with a catheter left in place, minimizes this risk while fluid is removed. *(Level II*)*	
19. Fluid is removed via aspiration into the syringe. Changing the position of the child may facilitate drainage.	Fluid flows toward dependent position.	Rapid removal of more than 15 to 20 mL of fluid/kilogram of body weight may cause hypotension from fluid shifts.[10,12]
20. Apply pressure dressing over the site after the needle or catheter is removed.	Applying pressure to site reduces the leakage of peritoneal fluid from the tap site.[11,12]	Evaluate the dressing, noting saturation with peritoneal fluid or blood. Notify the practitioner if the dressing becomes saturated.
21. Place the fluid in appropriate containers and label the containers at the bedside. Complete laboratory paperwork per institution-specific protocol. Send the peritoneal fluid for ordered studies. *(Level VI*)*	Analysis of peritoneal fluid can assist with the diagnosis of ascites, peritonitis, or hemorrhage. Culture and Gram stain identify specific pathogens.[11,12,15] *(Level VI*)* Labeling specimens at the bedside promotes patient safety and ensures accurate and efficient processing of specimen.	Fluid is typically sent for aerobic and anaerobic culture and sensitivity, Gram stain, cell count with differential, protein, glucose, LDH, pH, and amylase. Follow standard precautions in transfer of peritoneal fluid. Follow institution-specific protocol for handling and labeling laboratory specimens.
22. Discard used supplies and equipment including sharps, in appropriate receptacles.	Reduces transmission of microorganisms. Protects personnel health.	
23. Remove personal protective equipment; wash hands.	Reduces transmission of microorganisms.	

* Level II: Theory-based; no research data to support recommendations; recommendations from expert consensus group may exist
Level VI: Clinical studies in a variety of patient populations and situations to support recommendations

Expected Outcomes

- Adequate volume of peritoneal fluid is obtained percutaneously
- Peritoneal fluid is sent for ordered laboratory studies

- Child is free from complications of paracentesis

- Aseptic technique is maintained
- Child has acceptable level of comfort

Unexpected Outcomes

- Inadequate volume of fluid obtained
- Inability to obtain fluid
- Specimen tubes are labeled incorrectly
- Specimen tubes are not sent to the laboratory in required time frame, resulting in inaccurate results
- Hypotension from rapid fluid shifts
- Injury to internal structures, including perforation of blood vessel, perforation of organ, or hematoma of abdominal wall
- Infection
- Unmanaged pain or anxiety

Monitoring and Care of the Child

Activities and Interventions	Rationale	Reportable Conditions
1. Monitor cardiovascular status (heart rate, blood pressure, peripheral perfusion, and level of consciousness) every 5 to 15 minutes during the procedure and every 30 minutes for 2 hours after the procedure.[11]	Rapid removal of a large volume of fluid can cause hypotension from sudden fluid shifts.	• Hypotension
2. Monitor child's abdominal examination after procedure, including abdominal girth, pain, and bowel sounds.	Monitors for improvement in child's status after procedure or reaccumulation of fluid.	• Abdominal girth remains elevated or increases • Increasing abdominal distension
3. Evaluate child for pain or discomfort.	Presence of pain and discomfort may indicate a complication.	• Unmanaged pain
4. Assess appearance of site for leakage of fluid or development of hematoma.	Monitors for complications of the procedure.	• Hematoma • Persistent fluid leak
5. Monitor the child for complications related to the procedure.	Prompt identification of complications facilitates early intervention.	• Bleeding • Erythema, swelling around puncture site

Documentation

- Presence of informed consent
- Date and time of the procedure and individual who performed the procedure
- Medications administered for the procedure and child's response
- Paracentesis site
- Volume and appearance of fluid removed
- Laboratory studies obtained
- Child's tolerance of procedure
- Pain and anxiety assessment and specific interventions provided
- Child and family education
- Unexpected outcomes and related treatment

References

1. Sentongo T, Steinhorn D: Gastrointestinal structure and function. In Fuhrman B, Zimmerman J, editors: *Pediatric critical care,* ed 3, Philadelphia, 2006, Mosby.
2. McCance K, Huether S: *Pathophysiology: the biologic basis for disease in adults and children,* Philadelphia, 2002, Mosby.
3. Hazinski MF, et al, editors: *Pediatric advanced life support provider manual,* Dallas, 2002, American Heart Association.
4. Herzog D, et al: Ascites after orthotopic liver transplantation in children, *Pediatr Transplant* 9:74-79, 2005.
5. Lane NE, Paul RI: Paracentesis. In Henretig F, King C, editors: *Textbook of pediatric emergency medicine procedures,* Philadelphia, 1997, Lippincott, Williams & Wilkins.
6. Leibovitch I, et al: The diagnosis and management of postoperative chylous ascites, *J Urol* 167(2 Pt 1):449-457, 2002.
7. Kramer RE, et al: Large-volume paracentesis in the management of ascites in children, *J Pediatric Gastroenterol Nutrition* 33(3):245-249, 2001.
8. Kirkwood P: Paracentesis (perform). In Lynn-McHale Wiegand DJ, Carlson K, editors: *AACN procedure manual for critical care,* Philadelphia, 2005, Elsevier.
9. Hickerson S, et al: Diagnostic procedures. In Dieckmann RA, Fiser DA, Selbst SM, editors: *Pediatric emergency and critical care procedures,* ed 1, St Louis, 1997, Mosby.
10. Pache I, Bilodeau M: Severe haemorrhage following abdominal paracentesis for ascites in patients with liver disease, *Alimentary Pharmacol Therapeutics* 21(5):525-529, 2005.
11. Tuggle DW: Abdominal paracentesis. In Blummer J, editor: *A practical guide to pediatric intensive care,* ed 3, St Louis, 1990, Mosby.
12. Gunn V, Nechyba C, editors: *The Harriet Lane handbook: a manual for pediatric house officers,* ed 16, Philadelphia, 2002, Mosby.
13. Runyon BA: Paracentesis of ascitic fluid: a safe procedure, *Arch Internal Med* 146:2259-2261, 1986.
14. Dammert W: Abdominal paracentesis. In Levin DL, Morriss FC, Moore GC, editors: *A practical guide to pediatric intensive care,* ed 2, St Louis, 1984, Mosby.
15. Skale N: Peritoneal tap: paracentesis. In *Manual of pediatric nursing procedures,* Philadelphia, 1992, JB Lippincott Company.

Additional Readings

Duszak, et al: Percutaneous catheter drainage of infected intra-abdominal fluid collections; American College of Radiology, ACR appropriateness criteria, *Radiology* 215(Suppl):1067-1075, 2000.

Ergene U, et al: Current value of peritoneal tap in blunt abdominal trauma, *Eur J Emerg Med* 9:253-257, 2002.

Habeeb KS, Herrera JL: Management of ascites; paracentesis as a guide, *Postgrad Med* 101:191-200, 1997.

Balloon Gastrostomy Tube (GT) and Low-Profile GT: Removal and Reinsertion

P U R P O S E : Replacement of a dislodged balloon gastrostomy tube for prevention of narrowing of the stoma and possible surgery

Cheryl N. Bartke

PREREQUISITE KNOWLEDGE

- Child development as it relates to reinsertion of a GT
- Anatomy and physiology of the pediatric gastrointestinal (GI) tract, including structural characteristics specific to the infant and child[1,2]
- Type and size of GT the child currently uses
- Enterostomies provide access to the GI tract through the abdominal wall via tubes that extend above the skin (see Figure 96-1 in Procedure 96) or at the skin level via a low-profile device or "button" (see Figure 96-7 in Procedure 96).[3]
- A GT can be placed percutaneously or through a surgical incision.
  - ❖ A percutaneous endoscopic gastrostomy (PEG) is a tube inserted with visualization of the stomach with an endoscope and with local anesthesia. The design of the tube is such that it is held in place.[3]
  - ❖ A surgically placed tube is inserted with general anesthesia in the operating room. An incision is made in the upper left quadrant of the abdomen. The tube is secured with a purse-string suture to the stomach and abdominal wall.
- All enterostomy devices require periodic replacement because of balloon rupture, resizing, change in the type of device, and removal when the tube is no longer needed.[3,4]
- Urinary catheters can be used for short-term (temporary) GT replacement to maintain the integrity of the stoma until a proper feeding tube can be placed.[3]

- Replacement of gastrostomy-jejunostomy tubes requires added visualization and technique that can be provided with interventional radiology.

CHILD AND FAMILY ASSESSMENT

- Child's developmental level and ability to interact ➡*Rationale:* Child's developmental level influences preparation and interaction and assists in determination of the level of cooperation that the child can provide.
- Child's and family's understanding of the reasons for and risks and benefits of the procedure ➡*Rationale:* Evaluates child's and family's understanding of the procedure and provides a gauge for ongoing education.
- Signs of tube obstruction, including nausea, vomiting, and abdominal pain ➡*Rationale:* Signs and symptoms of tube displacement.
- The GT stoma condition, including redness, bleeding, skin erosion, drainage, and excess granulation tissue ➡*Rationale:* Assesses skin integrity and ability for tube reinsertion.
- Date of GT placement ➡*Rationale:* A well-established tract does not form for several weeks after placement. New GTs carry an increased risk of complications.
- Length of time the tube has been displaced ➡*Rationale:* A tube that has been out more than 4 to 6 hours often needs dilation or a smaller tube.
- Family's desire to be present during the procedure ➡*Rationale:* The family may provide support and comfort to the child but should have the choice not to remain with the child.

CHILD AND FAMILY EDUCATION

Individualized, developmentally appropriate education is provided to the family and to the child based on desire for knowledge, readiness to learn, and overall neurologic and psychosocial state.

- Explain the steps for tube removal, as indicated ➤*Rationale:* Providing information decreases anxiety and fear.
- Explain the steps involved in tube reinsertion, as indicated ➤*Rationale:* Providing information decreases anxiety and fear.
- In the case of accidental tube dislodgement, stress the importance of not pulling on the tube and provide strategies for keeping the device in place ➤*Rationale:* Avoids unnecessary pain and skin irritation.

- Encourage questions and answer questions as they arise ➤*Rationale:* Reinforcement of information is needed during periods of stress.

EQUIPMENT

- Appropriate size and type of GT and one size smaller
- Foley catheter one size smaller than GT
- Luer lock syringe of appropriate size
- Catheter-tip syringe
- Water-soluble lubricant
- Saline solution
- Tube position guard, if appropriate
- Tape or commercially available securing device
- Cotton-tipped swab

Procedure for Balloon GT and Low-Profile GT: Removal and Reinsertion

Steps	Rationale	Considerations
1. Ensure child and family understand procedure and questions are answered.	Evaluates and reinforces understanding of previously taught information.	Developmental level, cognitive ability, and anxiety level influence approach to and effectiveness of teaching. Use an interpreter if non-English speaking to ensure understanding before procedure.
2. Collect all necessary equipment and supplies.	Promotes completion of the procedure in a timely manner; may decrease child's anxiety.	Tube size and type are dependent on the original tube that was dislodged. If the tube has been placed in the past few weeks, a Foley catheter of smaller size than tube should be considered.
3. Ensure appropriate cardiopulmonary monitoring.	Some children may decompensate during the procedure.	Consider the child's status with selection of appropriate monitoring.
4. Wash hands and put on clean gloves.	Reduces the transmission of microorganisms. Protects personnel health.	
5. Position child.	Position child for comfort and visibility of the GT site.	Semi-Fowler's position with knees bent may aid in relaxing the abdominal muscles.
Device Removal		
6. Slide the external retention disc away from the exit site.	Allows for lubrication of the tube.	
7. Lubricate the tube and advance the tube slightly back and forth into the stomach.[3]	Enhances ease of removal.	A local anesthetic can be injected into the surrounding area if needed.[3]
8. If a balloon is present and inflated, withdraw the fluid from the balloon.	Prevents trauma.	
9. Firmly grasp the tube and with continuous traction, remove the tube from the stomach.	Promotes success of tube removal and reduces discomfort.	

Procedure for Balloon GT and Low-Profile GT: Removal and Reinsertion—*Continued*		
Steps	**Rationale**	**Considerations**
10. Apply a gauze dressing.	Protects the skin from gastric contents.	
Replacement		
11. Pass a lubricated cotton-tipped swab into the mucosal opening. *(Level II*)*	Assessment of the patency of the site.	Consider interventional radiology for replacement of the device if the original tube has been in for a short time period. *(Level II*)* If a tract has not been established, the GT can be misplaced into the facial planes.
12. Check GT balloon for leaks by injecting saline solution into the balloon port of the Y end of the tube with the Luer lock syringe.	Assessment of the competency of the balloon.[5] Insertion of a malfunctioning GT necessitates reinsertion.	The amount of saline solution to use is per manufacturer's recommendation. *(Level I*)*
13. Withdraw the instilled saline solution.	Returns the balloon to deflated size to facilitate insertion.	
14. Lubricate the balloon tip of the syringe with the water-soluble lubricant. *(Level II*)*	Allows for easy insertion.[5]	If resistance is met, or the tube is too big, use a Foley catheter or smaller GT.
15. Hold the tube perpendicular to the abdominal wall and aim it in the direction of the stoma tract. *(Level II*)*	Gastric tubes are replaced at a 90-degree angle.	
16. Pass the tip of the catheter into the opening of the gastrostomy site. With a steady firm pressure, push it down in the direction of the stomach. *(Level II*)*	Follow path of GT track. Sudden jerking increases the chance of abdominal wall separation.	With bleeding or a problem with reinserting the tube, stop and call prescribing practitioner.
17. Reinflate the balloon with saline solution in the amount recommended by the manufacturer. *(Level II*)*	Prevents migration of the tube.[5]	
18. Position the external retention device against the abdominal wall.	Prevents the tube from migrating.	
19. Pull gently on the tube until it meets resistance. *(Level II*)*	Ensures the tube has not migrated out of the stomach.[5]	
20. With the catheter tip syringe, gently aspirate stomach contents. *(Level II*)*	Confirms placement.	
21. Secure tube to the stomach. *(Level II*)*	Prevents further displacement of the tube.	Several commercially available products exist to assist with securing the GT. Selection is determined by availability and the child, family, and provider preference.
22. Wash hands.	Reduces transmission of microorganisms.	

* Level I: Manufacturer's recommendations only
  Level II: Theory-based; no research data to support recommendations; recommendations from expert consensus group may exist

Expected Outcomes

- The GT is removed/replaced safely and without complications

- When replaced, distal tip and balloon of the GT are located in the stomach
- When replaced, tube flushes easily and accepts enteral feedings, medications, and fluid

Unexpected Outcomes

- Bleeding
- Skin erosion
- Extreme pain
- Separation of the stomach from the abdominal wall
- Obstructed pylorus
- Aspiration
- Enlargement of stoma
- Inability to correctly position GT

- GT obstruction
- Migration of tube that causes gastric outlet obstruction

Monitoring and Care of the Child

Activities and Interventions	Rationale	Reportable Conditions
1. Monitor child's tolerance of GT removal/replacement.	Changes in child's condition may indicate complications from the removal/replacement of the GT.	• Extreme pain • Changes in vital signs
2. Monitor stoma site.	Removal/replacement of tube may cause trauma.	• Bleeding • Skin erosion • Enlargement of stoma
3. With replacement, monitor tube positioning and patency.	With replacement, the tube may be malpositioned.	• Separation of the stomach from the abdominal wall • Obstructed pylorus • Aspiration • Inability to administer feedings or medications
3. When in place, rotate the tube to ensure no added pressure against the gastric or abdominal wall.	Pressure can cause skin erosion, gastric ulceration, or migration of the internal bumper into the gastric wall (Figure 90-1).	• Inability to rotate device
4. Consider radiographic images if any concern exists regarding the location of the tube.	Provides evidence of tube location and possible complications.	• Results that indicate complications or tube dislocation
5. With accidental tube displacement, initiate strategies to prevent pulling on the device.	Prevention of displacement reduces complications.	• Inability to consistently institute strategies

Documentation

- Child's tolerance of procedure
- Size and type of tube placed/removed
- Patency of tube and ability to aspirate stomach contents (when replaced)
- Strategies to maintain correct GT placement (when replaced)
- Condition at stoma site
- Additional interventions and related outcomes
- Child and family education
- Unexpected outcomes and related treatment

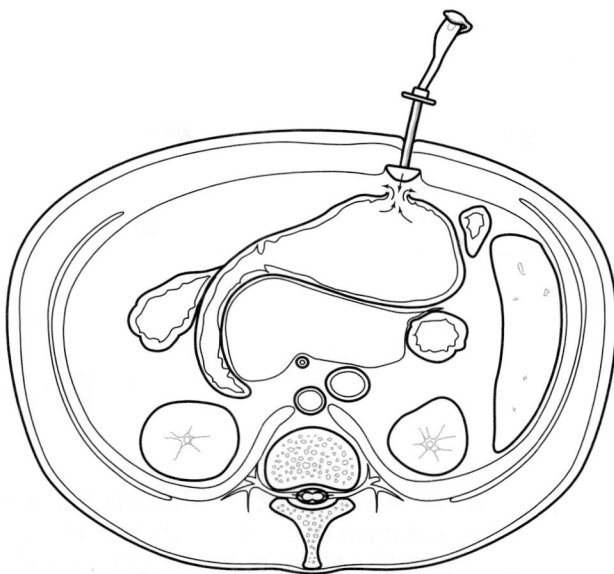

FIGURE 90-1   Migration of percutaneous endoscopic gastrostomy tube outside stomach.

References

1. Sentongo T, Steinhorn D: Gastrointestinal structure and function. In Fuhrman B, Zimmerman J, editors: *Pediatric critical care,* ed 3, Philadelphia, 2006, Mosby.
2. Thibodeau G, Patton K, editors: *Anatomy and physiology,* ed 5, Philadelphia, 2003, Mosby.
3. Rolandelli R, et al: *Clinical nutrition, enteral and tube feeding,* ed 4, Philadelphia, 2005, Elsevier.
4. Ruddy M: Procedures: replacement of gastrostomy tube. In Fleisher G, Ludwig S, Henretig F, et al, editors: *Textbook of pediatric emergency medicine,* ed 5, 2004, Philadelphia, Lippincott Williams & Wilkins.
5. Stone K, Brown P: *HEN complication chart,* Albany, NY, 2001, The Oley Foundation.

91

Bowel Irrigation

PURPOSE: Bowel irrigation is used to promote defecation in the treatment of constipation or to empty the bowel before a diagnostic or surgical procedure of the lower gastrointestinal tract

Rizalina Mauricio

PREREQUISITE KNOWLEDGE

- Child development as it relates to clinical assessment and bowel irrigation[1]
- Knowledge of gastrointestinal (GI) anatomy and physiology and anorectal function
- Bowel irrigation is intended to promote defecation and to wash out the colon and is primarily effective in cleaning the distal colon.[2]
- Bowel irrigation may be used for short-term indications, such as preparation for diagnostic or surgical procedures and treatment of constipation. Chronic indications include treatment of fecal incontinence in children with neurogenic bowel as a result of myelomeningocele and other forms of spinal dysraphism and spinal cord injury.
- Bowel irrigation stimulates peristalsis with irrigation of the colon and rectum and with distention of the rectum or colon. Other terms used for bowel irrigation include transrectal irrigation, colonic lavage, colonic irrigation, and enema.
- Rectal pulsed irrigation is a specific technique in which fluid is infused into the bowel in short pulses for approximately 30 minutes.[2]
- Substances used for bowel irrigation include tap water, sodium phosphate (e.g., Fleet, Lynchburg, Va), bisacodyl, mineral oil, and 0.9% saline solution
- When tap water is used for enemas, no significant effect on serum sodium level has been shown.[3]

- Contraindications to bowel irrigation may include recent or past bowel surgery, rectal prolapse, increased intracranial pressure, glaucoma, abnormal serum electrolytes, thrombocytopenia, neutropenia, anorectal malformations, rectal bleeding, rectal fissures, hemorrhoids, and altered renal function.
- Complications of bowel irrigation include bowel perforation, rectal prolapse, abdominal pain, cramping, and bowel rupture.[3]
- An object can only be inserted a maximum 2 cm in a preterm infant and 3 cm in a full-term infant before it hits the curvature of the bowel. A rigid object can easily perforate the bowel and cause damage if inserted too far or too forcefully.
- Whole bowel irrigation (WBI) involves the rapid administration of a large volume of an osmotically balanced solution (polyethylene glycol electrolyte solution) orally or via nasogastric tube to flush out the entire GI tract and is not the focus of this procedure. The few recommended indications for WBI include ingestion of substances not absorbed by activated charcoal (e.g., iron ingestion), ingestion of sustained-release or enteric-coated drugs, ingestion of drugs that cause concretion, and ingestion of packets of illicit drugs (body packing).[4]
- Child's usual stool pattern and date and time of last bowel movement
- The six rights of medication administration: right patient, right drug, right dose, right route, right time, and right documentation

CHILD AND FAMILY ASSESSMENT

- Family's and child's understanding of the reasons for and risks and benefits of the procedure ➻*Rationale:* Evaluates family's and child's understanding of the procedure and provides a gauge for ongoing education.
- Child's developmental level (including toilet training status) and ability to interact ➻*Rationale:* These factors influence preparation of the child and interaction. Soiling may be upsetting to children who are recently toilet trained.
- Child's known allergies ➻*Rationale:* Identifies allergies to medications or solutions that may be used during the procedure.
- Examine the perianal region and patency of anal canal ➻*Rationale:* Perianal and anorectal malformations impede administration of substances via the rectum.
- History or presence of bowel surgery, rectal prolapse, increased intracranial pressure, glaucoma, hemodynamic instability, and altered renal function ➻*Rationale:* Identifies relative contraindications to the procedure.
- Abdominal examination for distention, presence of abdominal pain, rectal hemorrhoids, rectal prolapse, and bowel sounds ➻*Rationale:* Establishes a baseline assessment for determining efficacy of the enema.
- Current laboratory profile, including complete blood count (CBC) and serum electrolytes ➻*Rationale:* Establishment of baseline values and identification of relative contraindications to the procedure.
- Previous experience with rectal medication ➻*Rationale:* Knowledge of previous experiences may help to identify successful techniques and promotion of compliance.
- Level of mobility and amount of assistance needed in positioning ➻*Rationale:* Determines the need for additional personnel and the child's ability to use a bedpan or bedside commode.
- Family's desire to remain with the child during procedure; school-aged children and adolescents should be asked their preference for family presence ➻*Rationale:* Family's presence may provide support and comfort measures to the child during the procedure, but the family should also have the choice not to remain with the child. Privacy is an important consideration for school-aged children and adolescents.

CHILD AND FAMILY EDUCATION

Individualized, developmentally appropriate education is provided to the family and to the child based on desire for knowledge, readiness to learn, and overall neurologic and psychosocial state.

- Explain the procedure to the child and family, including indications, potential side effects, anticipated length of the procedure, and attention to comfort and privacy ➻*Rationale:* Providing information decreases anxiety and fear and promotes cooperation during the procedure.
- Specifically identify the method that will be used for child to defecate (e.g., bedside commode, bedpan, diaper) ➻*Rationale:* Providing a means that is acceptable and nonthreatening to the child promotes cooperation and decreases anxiety.
- Practice deep-breathing technique with the child ➻*Rationale:* Promotes child's relaxation and comfort during the procedure.
- After the procedure, update the child and family regarding results ➻*Rationale:* Child's and family's understanding of procedure promotes involvement in plan of care.
- Encourage questions and answer questions as they arise ➻*Rationale:* Reinforcement of information is needed during periods of stress.

EQUIPMENT

- Container for water or solution with attached rectal tube (children, size 14F to 18F; infants, size 12F or infant enema syringe with bulb), if commercially prepared solution is not used
- Correct volume of lukewarm solution (0.9% saline solution, tap water, or commercially prepared enema solution)
- Water-soluble lubricant
- Bed protector
- Bedside commode chair (for children who can be transferred out of bed), bedpan, or other means to collect results
- Skin care items, such as soap, water, and towels
- Clean gloves

Procedure | for Bowel Irrigation

Steps	Rationale	Considerations
1. Ensure child and family understand procedure and questions are answered.	Evaluates and reinforces understanding of previously taught information.	Developmental level, cognitive ability, and anxiety level determine approach to and effectiveness of teaching.
2. Review prescribing practitioner's order. If medication is to be administered, ensure that the six rights of medication administration are correct; use two patient identifiers to identify the child per institution-specific protocol.	Use of the six rights of medication administration ensures the correct medication is given and avoids errors.	Ensure that the child does not have any contraindications to the medication, fluid, or method of administration. Name and medical record number or name and birth date are most commonly used for patient identification.
3. Gather needed supplies and equipment, including bedpan or commode.	Facilitates completion of procedure in a timely manner.	Amount of solution to be used and tube size are dependent on the child's size.
4. Provide for privacy.	Shows respect for child; promotes cooperation and decreases anxiety.	Privacy is an especially important consideration for school-aged children and adolescents.
5. Ensure cardiopulmonary monitoring as indicated. *(Level III*)*	Critically ill children may decompensate during the procedure.	Ensure knowledge of the child's history and current condition for providing appropriate response during an adverse reaction.
6. Wash hands and put on clean gloves.	Reduces transmission of microorganisms. Protects personnel health.	Evaluate the need for infection control measures specific to the child per institution-specific protocol.
7. Raise bed to a comfortable working height.	Promotes good body mechanics for the nurse.	
8. Place bed protector under the child and position the child on the left side or in the knee-chest position or dorsal recumbent position. *(Level IV*)*	Provides easy passage of the solution by following the natural curve of the sigmoid colon and the rectum.[5]	Consider the child's ability to tolerate the position. Ensure commode or bedpan is readily available, if indicated.
9. If required, fill the container with prescribed solution and volume; solution should be lukewarm (approximately 100°F [37.8°C]). *(Level V*)*	Solutions that are too hot or too cold can cause abdominal cramping. The volume of solution to be infused varies with solution prescribed and child's age and condition.	The standard recommended volume is 500 mL for children and 250 mL for infants. Measuring the temperature with a thermometer may be indicated. Children with spinal cord injury often have bowel dysfunction[6,7] and may need antegrade colonic irrigation (ACE) and other strategies to manage chronic evacuation disorder.[8]
10. Remove air from the solution by priming the tubing and then clamp. *(Level III*)*	Instillation of air into the GI tract can cause abdominal distention and discomfort.	Use a transparent bag and tubing so air can be seen through the irrigation set-up. If enema bottle is used, invert the bottle to expel air.

* Level III: Laboratory data; no clinical data to support recommendations
 Level IV: Limited clinical studies to support recommendations
 Level V: Clinical studies in more than one or two patient populations and situations to support recommendations

Procedure for Bowel Irrigation—*Continued*

Steps	Rationale	Considerations
11. Lubricate the tip of the rectal tube or infant enema syringe. *(Level III*)*	Facilitates insertion; promotes child's comfort.	Use water-soluble lubricant.
12. Separate the buttocks and locate the anus.	Good visibility and positioning aid in ease of procedure.	
13. Gently insert the catheter tubing or tip of commercial enema into the child's rectum to recommended depth with the tip directed towards the umbilicus (Figure 91-1). *(Level III*)*	Prevents irritation or trauma to the rectal mucosa or rectum.	Recommended depth of insertion: *Infant:* 2.5 to 3.5 cm (1 to 1.5 inches).[9] *Child:* 5 to 7.5 cm (2 to 3 inches). If pain occurs or resistance is felt, stop the procedure and confer with the prescribing practitioner.

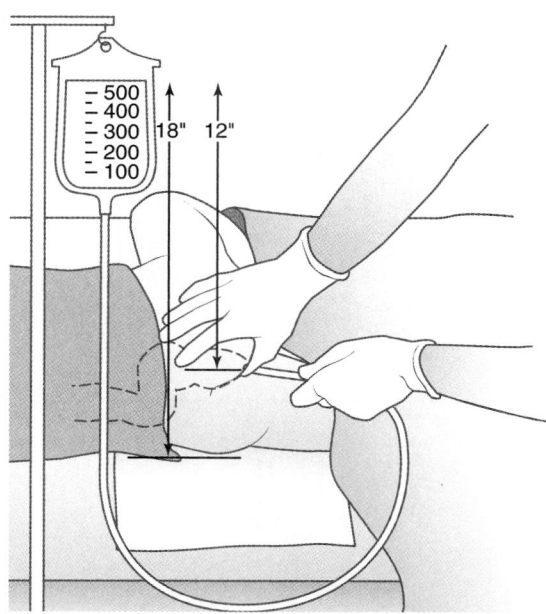

FIGURE 91-1   Bowel Irrigation. Enema is given on left side-lying position. Gently insert catheter tubing or tip of commercial enema into child's rectum to recommended depth with tip directed towards umbilicus. Bag is positioned 12 to 18 inches above rectum, depending on size of child. *Adapted from Perry A, Potter P: Clinical nursing skills and techniques, ed 5, Philadelphia, 2004, Mosby.*

Steps	Rationale	Considerations
14. Elevate the container no more than 12 to 18 inches above the rectum. *(Level III*)*	Promotes continuous slow instillation of solution, with minimization of complications.	Too rapid administration can cause painful distention of the colon and abdominal cramps. High pressure could rupture the bowel of an infant. Lower the height of the container if the child has pain or if fluid leaks around the catheter.
15. Release clamp and allow the solution to flow for 10 to 15 minutes. *(Level III*)* Hold tubing in place with one hand.	Promotes the child's comfort during infusion. Bowel contraction can cause expulsion of tube.[9]	Temporary cessation of instillation prevents abdominal cramps. For prepackaged enemas, squeeze bottle until all the solution has entered the rectum.

Procedure continues on following page

* Level III: Laboratory data; no clinical data to support recommendations

Procedure | for Bowel Irrigation—*Continued*

Steps	Rationale	Considerations
16. After instilling the solution, gently remove the rectal tubing or tip.	Prevents leakage of fluid around the tubing.	Instruct the child to take a deep breath to facilitate relaxation and fluid retention.
17. After an appropriate interval, have the child expel the solution. Transfer the child to a bedside commode or bedpan. For the child who is unable to be out of bed and cannot be lifted easily, place the bedpan by turning the child (Figure 91-2).	Longer retention of the solution promotes more effective stimulation, peristalsis, and defecation. Use of a bedpan or commode is determined by the age of the child and the child's mobility.	Holding the buttocks together may delay expelling the solution. Children with unstable conditions can be left in the dorsal recumbent position until defecation or clear bowel return is noted. Ensure catheters and tubing remain intact during transfer process. Child's face should be seen for close observation.

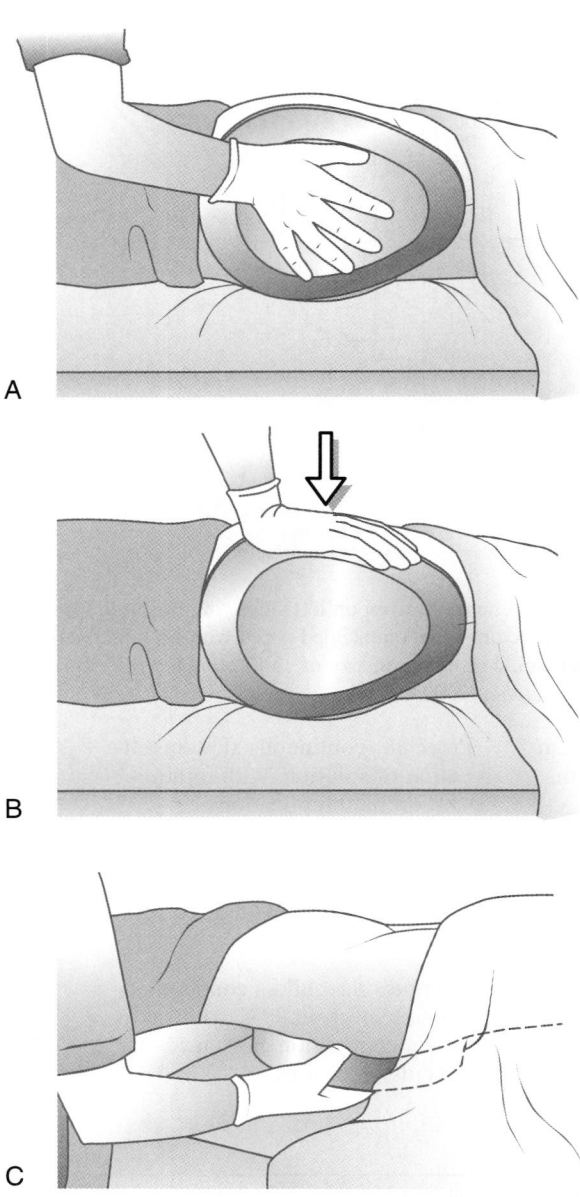

A

B

C

FIGURE 91-2   **A,** With child on left side and place bedpan firmly against buttocks. **B,** Push downward on bedpan and toward child. **C,** Roll child supine. *Adapted from Perry A, Potter P:* Clinical nursing skills and techniques, *ed 5, Philadelphia, 2004, Mosby.*

Procedure for Bowel Irrigation—*Continued*

Steps	Rationale	Considerations
18. Ensure privacy while allowing the child to expel the return solution.	Child feels more relaxed when privacy is protected.	
19. Clean the child's perianal area and assist the child to return to bed and assume a comfortable position.	Promotes comfort and prevents skin breakdown.	Limit the amount of time the child is exposed to feces; fecal contents irritate the skin.
20. Measure the amount of returned solution and the quality.	Evaluates efficacy of the procedure.	Cleansing enema should have a clear return; clear return is essential before a diagnostic procedure. If the child has a history of constipation, alternative measures can be instituted if the irrigation was not successful.
21. Dispose of used equipment and supplies in appropriate receptacles.	Reduces the transmission of microorganisms.	Follow institution-specific protocol regarding disposal of equipment for children on specific isolation precautions.
22. Remove gloves; wash hands.	Standard precautions; reduces the transmission of micro-organisms.	

Expected Outcomes

- Stool is effectively evacuated
- If the procedure is for diagnostic study preparation, the return fluid is clear
- Irrigation solution is administered and retained for desired time frame
- Irrigation tube or infant enema syringe is easily inserted into rectum
- Child is free from complications of bowel irrigation

- If medication is administered, right dose of right medication is administered to right child at right time via right route with correct documentation

- Child tolerates procedure with minimal anxiety or agitation

Unexpected Outcomes

- Stool is not completely evacuated
- Inability to obtain clear return fluid

- Child is unable to tolerate infusion of solution or retain solution because of discomfort
- Resistance to insertion of tube or syringe

- Rectal bleeding
- Electrolyte imbalance
- Abdominal pain or discomfort
- Abdominal rigidity (may indicate bowel perforation)
- Wrong dose, wrong medication, wrong route, wrong time of administration
- Medication is administered to wrong child
- Medication is not documented
- Inability to administer irrigation fluid or early termination of the procedure because of child's agitation or anxiety

Monitoring and Care of the Child

Activities and Interventions	Rationale	Reportable Conditions
1. Evaluate child's response while the rectal tube or syringe is being inserted.	Complications may arise during rectal tube insertion.	- Bleeding from the rectum - Excessive agitation or anxiety that prevents completion of procedure
2. Assess child's response during instillation of the solution.	Prompt identification of adverse effects facilitates treatment.	- Abdominal pains or cramps
3. Monitor for premature expulsion of the solution.	Desired effects of bowel irrigation may not be achieved if the solution is not retained in the rectum for the desired time.	- Solution is expelled from the rectum in less than desired time frame

Continued

Monitoring and Care of the Child—Cont'd

Activities and Interventions	Rationale	Reportable Conditions
4. Monitor rectum for skin irritation or bleeding after procedure.	Indicates altered skin integrity, which increases the risk of pain or infection; may be symptomatic of an adverse reaction to the solution.	• Perianal skin irritation or bleeding
5. Measure return volume and calculate net output.	Assesses for return of all infused fluid.	• Retention of irrigation solution
6. Monitor for indications of complications.	Early identification of complications facilitates prompt treatment.	• Signs of bowel perforation: rigid abdomen, increasing abdominal girth, hypoactive or absent bowel sounds, abdominal pain • Rectal prolapse • Significant volume of bright red blood from rectum

Documentation

- Child's response to the procedure, including changes in vital signs
- Child's abdominal examination before and after the procedure
- Type, route, and volume of fluid administered
- Color, consistency, and amount of stool and fluid returned
- Abnormal findings, such as bloody stool or presence of mucus
- Child and family education
- Unexpected outcomes and related treatment

References

1. McCance K, Huether S: *Pathophysiology: the biologic basis for disease in adults and children,* Philadelphia, 2002, Mosby.
2. Wexner SD, et al: Consensus document on bowel preparation before colonoscopy, *Gastrointest Endosc* 63(7):894-909, 2006.
3. Mattsson S, Gladh G: Tap-water enema for children with myelomeningocele and neurogenic bowel dysfunction, *Acta Paediatrica* 95:369-374, 2006.
4. Lheureux P: Position paper: whole bowel irrigation, *J Toxicol* 42(6):843-854, 2004.
5. Kayaba H, et al: Evaluation of anorectal function in patients with tethered cord syndrome: saline enema test and fecoflowmetry, *J Neurosurg (Spine)* 98:251-257, 2003.
6. De Looze D, et al: Constipation and other chronic gastrointestinal problems in patients with spinal cord injury, *Spinal Cord* 36(1):63-66, 1998.
7. Han TR, Kim JH, Kwon BS: Chronic gastrointestinal problems and bowel dysfunction in patients with spinal cord injury, *Spinal Cord* 36(7):485-490, 1998.
8. Gauderer MW, et al: Sigmoid irrigation tube for the management of chronic evacuation disorders, *J Pediatr Surg* 37(3):348-351, 2002.
9. Perry A, Potter P: *Clinical nursing skills and techniques,* ed 5, Philadelphia, 2004, Mosby.

Additional Reading

Powell M, Rigby D: Management of bowel dysfunction: evacuation difficulties, *Nurs Stand* 14(47):47-51, 2000.

Closed Surgical Drain: Care and Management

P U R P O S E : Surgical drains are placed during surgery to remove fluid or air from surgical wounds and provide adequate drainage from an operative site

Kimberly R. Bookout and Kathleen M. McLane

PREREQUISITE KNOWLEDGE

- Child development as it relates to surgical drain care and management
- Principles of aseptic technique
- Child's operative procedure, type and location of drains, and method of securing drains
- Purpose of the drain
- Penrose drains are open (static) drain systems used to drain purulent material, blood, or serum from a body cavity. Penrose drains contain latex and are usually flat rubber tubing that are sutured in place (Figure 92-1, *A).*
- Jackson-Pratt (J-P) and Hemovac (Bard Medical, Covington, Ga) drains are closed surgical drains (Figure 92-1, *B* and *C)*
  - ❖ The J-P or Hemovac drains are made of polyvinyl chloride (PVC) or silicon, which is less irritating to the body and may be less likely to cause infection.[1]
  - ❖ The J-P and Hemovac drains are threaded through the skin into the wound near the surgical site and sutured in place. The tubing is connected to a collection device that maintains a low constant suction.
  - ❖ The J-P drainage may track along the outside or within the lumen of the tubing. A gauze dressing is used to collect the drainage. The surgeon typically withdraws the drain by a few centimeters each day to allow egress of fluid and gradual healing of the wound behind the drain.
- T-tubes are silicon and are shaped like the letter T and placed into the bile duct to drain bile while the duct is

healing. T-tubes are usually left in place for 10 or more days (Figure 92-2).
- Sump suction drains are closed drains made of PVC or silicon that collect caustic drainage, such as high small bowel and pancreatic effluent.
- Type and amount of drainage expected
  - ❖ Generally, drainage is initially serosanguineous and progresses to serous or straw colored. Drainage amount is expected to decrease gradually; amount of expected drainage should be clarified with the surgical service that placed the drain.
- For closed systems, drainage is generally collected in a bulb or chamber that may be emptied without disconnection of the drain tubing from the collection device.
- The drain or collection device tubes may become clogged with clots or necrotic debris. Gentle milking or stripping of the tube may be helpful in relieving the clot.
- Procedure for drain removal (see Procedure 127)
- Procedure for dressing wounds with drains (see Procedure 128)

CHILD AND FAMILY ASSESSMENT

- Child's developmental level and ability to interact
  ➥*Rationale:* Child's developmental level influences preparation and interaction.
- Child's level of consciousness and cognitive ability
  ➥*Rationale:* These factors influence amount and type of education and interaction during the procedure.

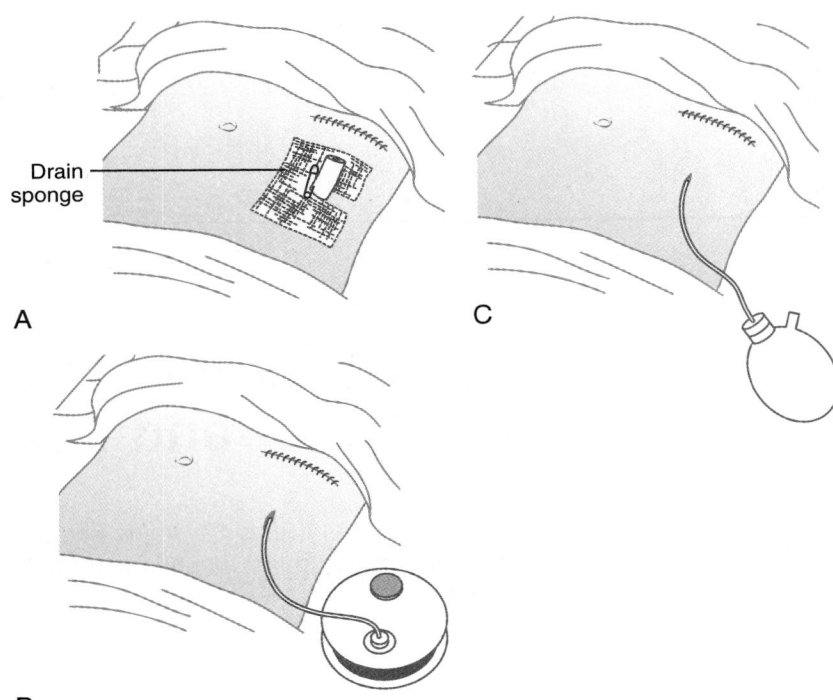

FIGURE 92-1   Drainage Systems. **A,** Penrose drain. **B,** Hemovac. **C,** Jackson-Pratt drain.

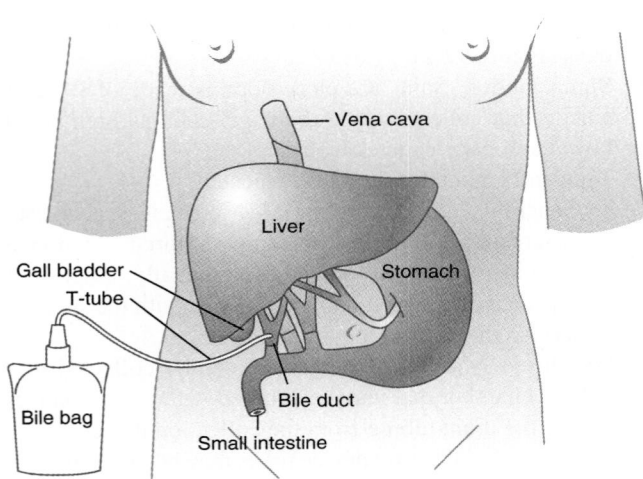

FIGURE 92-2   T-tube Drain.

- Child's known allergies ➻**Rationale:** The child may have an allergy to latex, alcohol, tape, or skin preparation products used for wound and dressing care. Penrose drains typically are made of latex.
- Child's and family's understanding of the reasons for and risks and benefits of the drain ➻**Rationale:** Evaluates child's and family's understanding of the procedure and provides a gauge for ongoing education.
- Type and appearance of drainage system and characteristics of the drainage ➻**Rationale:** Type of drain indicates

the drain characteristics with proper functioning and type of fluid expected in drain collection device.

- Observe child for signs of pain and anxiety ➻**Rationale:** Inadequate management of pain and anxiety may make future drain care more traumatic.
- Family member's desire to be present during procedure ➻**Rationale:** Family may provide comfort and support to the child during drain care but should have the choice not to remain with the child.

CHILD AND FAMILY EDUCATION

Individualized, developmentally appropriate education is provided to the family and to the child based on desire for knowledge, readiness to learn, and overall neurologic and psychosocial state.

- Provide information regarding the drain, its purpose, and expected output ➻**Rationale:** Providing information decreases anxiety and fear. Toddlers and preschoolers may be alarmed by the sight of blood or other fluids draining from the body.
- Provide information regarding local drain site care and ways in which the child or family may assist. If appropriate, demonstrate the process with a doll. Consider use of Child Life resources if available. ➻**Rationale:** Providing information decreases anxiety and fear. Medical play decreases the child's anxiety and facilitates understanding. If the child is to be discharged with the drain in place, the information initiates discharge teaching.

- Encourage questions and answer questions as they arise
  ➻*Rationale:* Reinforcement of information is needed during periods of stress.

EQUIPMENT

- Clean gloves and face shield
- 0.9% Saline solution
- Antiseptic cleanser, as indicated
- Mild soap and water
- Antibiotic ointment, as indicated
- Cotton-tipped applicators
- Gauze 4×4 or 2×2, or other appropriate dressing material
- Measuring container
- Towel or water-proof pad

If Cultures are to be Obtained:

- Appropriate sterile specimen container
- Appropriate laboratory requisitions
- Specimen labels that contain two patient identifiers

Procedure for Surgical Drains: Care and Management

Steps	Rationale	Considerations
1. Ensure child and family understand procedure and questions are answered.	Evaluates and reinforces understanding of previously taught information.	Developmental level, cognitive ability, and anxiety level determine approach to and effectiveness of teaching.
2. Position the child so that the drain is accessible and the child is comfortable. Ensure privacy.	Facilitates drain care. Respects the child's rights; drain care may necessitate exposure of the chest, abdomen, or perineum.	Privacy is an important consideration for school-aged children and adolescents.
3. Gather needed equipment and supplies.	Facilitates completion of task in a timely manner.	The type of drain determines equipment and supplies needed for drain care and management.
4. Wash hands; put on clean gloves and face shield.	Reduces transmission of microorganisms.	Contents of drain collection chamber may splash or spray when chamber is emptied. A protective gown may also be necessary.
5. If dressing is present, remove dressing, one layer at a time. Assess location and condition of exit site for redness, warmth, induration, edema, fluctuance, and rash (macular versus macular-papular). *(Level IV*)*	Removal of dressing in layers prevents inadvertent drain removal. Condition of exit site may give cues to determine infection versus normal reaction of the body to a foreign material. Condition of the skin around the drain site may indicate adequacy of absorbent dressing used.	A normal inflammatory response lasts up to 72 hours after injury. Redness at the site of approximately 0.5 to 1.0 cm is considered a normal inflammatory response.[2] *Latex/rubber drains:* Excite a profound inflammatory reaction within 24 hours that may render the drain ineffective.[2,3] *PVC drains:* Less reactive. Tubing is firm and may harden or split with prolonged use, especially when used to drain bile or caustic effluent.[2,3] *Silicon drains:* Least reactive. Very pliable and show no hardening with prolonged use.[1] A red macular rash may indicate an irritant dermatitis and necessitate additional absorption of peridrain effluent or application of a skin

Procedure continues on following page

* Level IV: Limited clinical studies to support recommendations

Procedure for Surgical Drains: Care and Management—*Continued*		
Steps	**Rationale**	**Considerations**
		barrier (petrolatum-based) or non-alcohol skin sealant. A red macular-papular rash may indicate a candidal dermatitis and necessitate antifungal cream, ointment, or powder. Increased drainage at the dressing or exit site may be an indicator of a clotted tube. Bogginess or fluctuance at the site may indicate a blockage in the tubing or a symptom of infection.[4]
6. For closed drainage systems, observe the collection chamber for drainage characteristics and ensure the chambers are compressed (J-P, Hemovac).	Drainage characteristics help to determine drain functioning and when the drain is no longer needed. Proper functioning of Hemovac and Jackson-Pratt drains requires negative pressure with flattening of the chamber.	For Hemovac drains, the springs inside the drain must be compressed to maintain suction. Jackson-Pratt drains are concave when proper suctioning is applied.

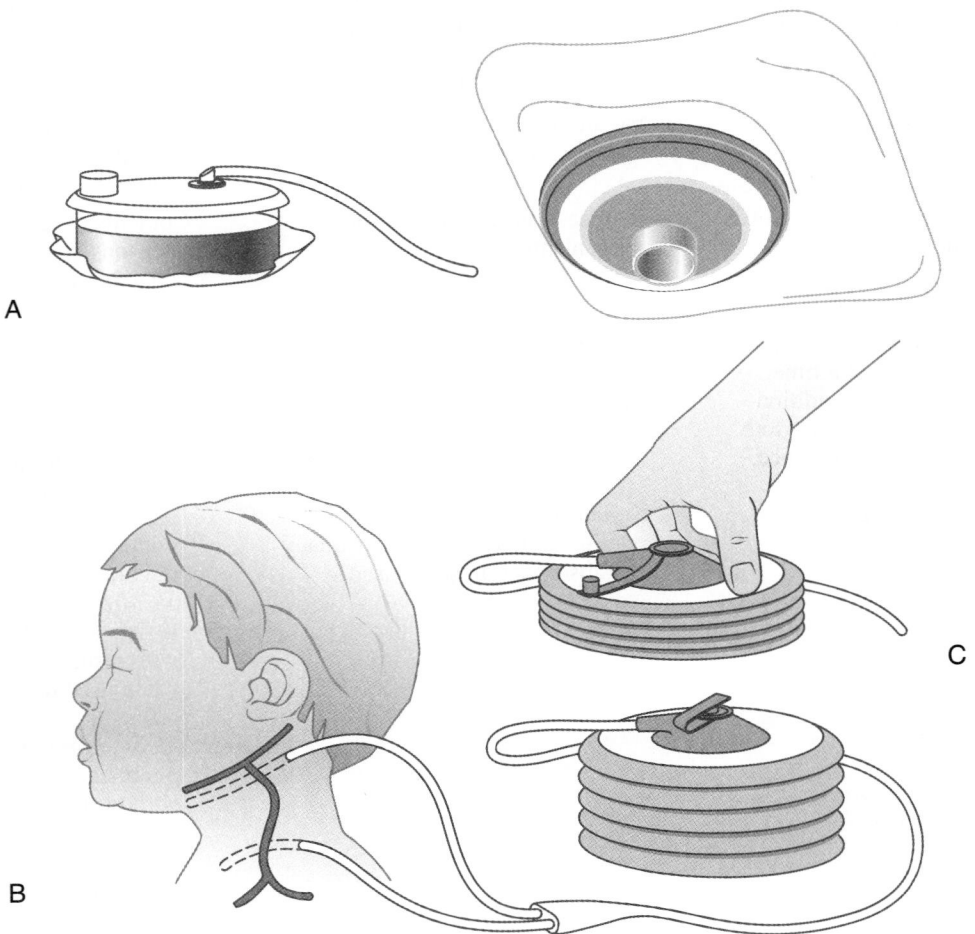

FIGURE 92-3   Hemovac Drain. **A,** Open cap on drain. **B,** Empty Hemovac drain into receptacle. **C,** Place container on flat surface. Press down until air is expelled and container is flat. Replace plug while holding container flat.

Procedure	for Surgical Drains: Care and Management—*Continued*	
Steps	**Rationale**	**Considerations**

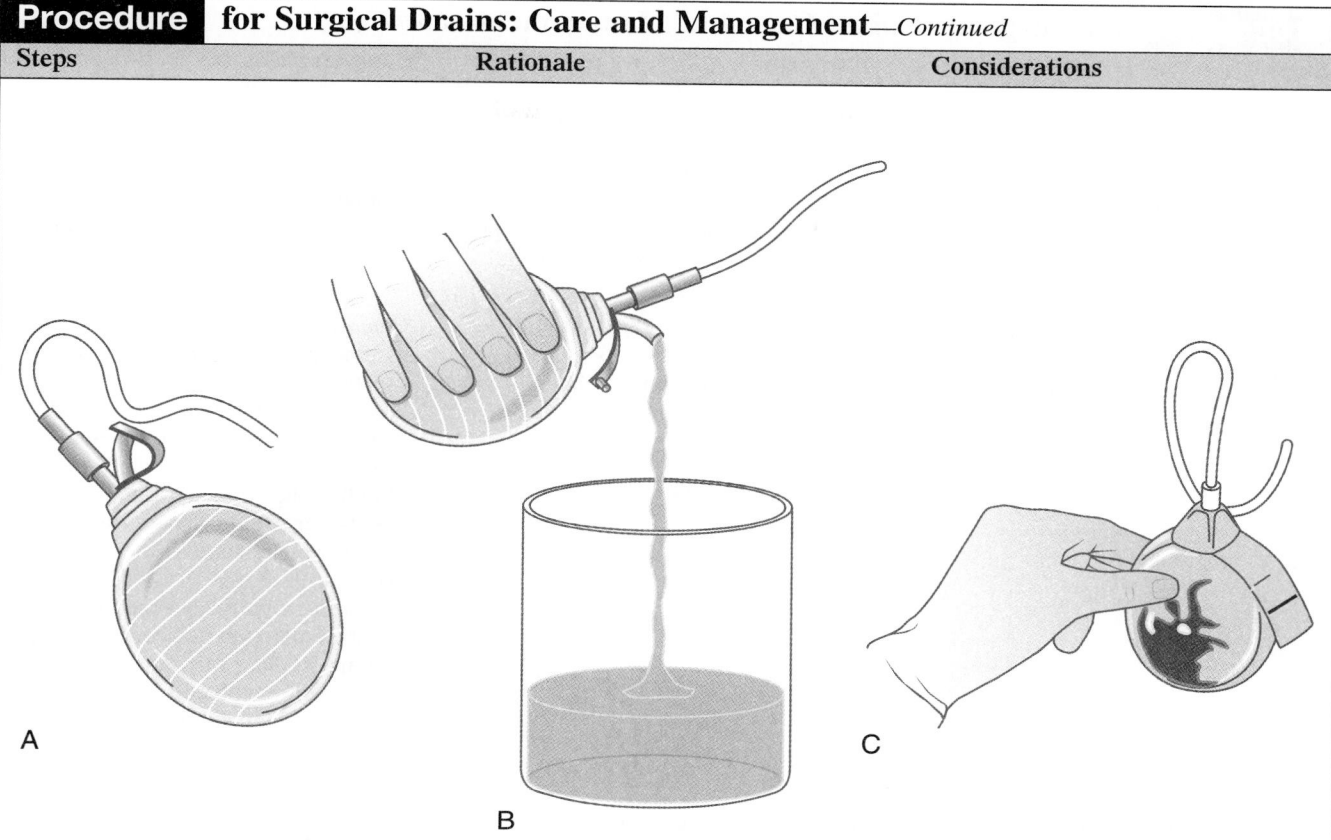

FIGURE 92-4   Jackson-Pratt Drain. **A,** J-P drain is concave when proper suctioning is applied. **B,** Empty drain into receptacle. **C,** Reestablish negative pressure by squeezing bulb and replace plug while keeping bulb compressed.

Steps	Rationale	Considerations

7. For closed drain, empty contents of collection chamber into measuring cup.
  a. Loosen any pins or clips that hold the drain system to clothing or bed linens.
  b. Open the plug on the Hemovac or J-P drain.
  c. Turn the drainage collection device upside down over the measuring cup to empty (Figures 92-3, *B,* and 92-4, *B*).
  d. The bulb of the J-P must be gently squeezed to empty. *(Level I*)*
	The drain is emptied and the output is measured and recorded to determine progression or regression of the child's condition.	Drains should be emptied per unit-specific or institution-specific protocol, typically once per shift unless otherwise indicated because of high volume of output. Drain tubing need not be disconnected from the collection device.

8. If culture of drainage or drain site is needed: a. Identify the child with two patient identifiers per institution-specific protocol.	Cultures may be obtained to identify infection. Use of two patient identifiers is recommended by the Joint Commission on Accreditation of	Refer to institution-specific protocol for appropriate patient identifiers.

Procedure continues on following page

* Level I: Manufacturer's recommendations only

Procedure for Surgical Drains: Care and Management—*Continued*

Steps	Rationale	Considerations
b. Swab insertion site or empty drainage into specimen container. c. Label specimens at the bedside and complete laboratory paperwork per institution-specific protocol.	Healthcare Organizations (JCAHO) to eliminate wrong patient/wrong procedure occurrences. Labeling of specimens at the bedside promotes patient safety and ensures accurate and efficient processing of specimens.	Follow institution-specific protocol for handling and labeling laboratory specimens.
9. If indicated, reestablish negative pressure or suction within the closed drain collection device. *(Level I*)*	Negative pressure or suction pulls the fluid into the device to promote drainage of the body cavity.	*Hemovac drain:* Place the Hemovac container on a flat firm surface. Press down on the container until all air is expelled and the container is completely flat. Replace the plug while holding the container flat. The container should remain flat when pressure is released (Figure 92-3, *C*). *J-P drain:* Gently squeeze the bulb of the collection device, expelling all air. Replace the plug while keeping the bulb compressed. The container should remain flat when pressure is released (Figure 92-4, *C*).

10. Assess tube patency of closed drain. If a tube blockage is suspected:
• Consider clearing the drainage tube by "stripping" or "milking" the tube.
    Start at the tubing exit site, pinch and roll the tubing between the thumb and forefinger. Repeat this action for the entire length of the tubing until reaching the collection device. Repeat as necessary.[4]
    or
• Grasp the tubing at the exit site with one hand to prevent dislodging the drain. Firmly pinch the tubing with the thumb and forefinger of the opposite hand. Pull the thumb and forefinger down the tubing with a firm but slow motion. Use caution not to remove drain. Repeat this as often as necessary.[4] *(Level I*)*
	Tube patency is critical to facilitate drainage of fluid or air from the body cavity.	An abrupt cessation of drainage may indicate a blockage of the tubing; therefore, patency of the tube must be established. Clots within the drain tubing are considered normal, but if clots completely obstruct the tube, they must be cleared.[4]
		If unable to clear the clot or blockage with these methods, notify the prescribing practitioner.

11. Remove soiled gloves and wash hands; put on a new pair of clean gloves.	Avoids contamination of exit site with wound drainage.	

* Level I: Manufacturer's recommendations only

Procedure	for Surgical Drains: Care and Management—*Continued*	
Steps	**Rationale**	**Considerations**
12. Cleanse skin with appropriate cleanser. *(Level IV*)*	Cleansing the skin removes old drainage or blood, which is known to harbor bacteria. Cleansing reduces the bacterial load on the skin surrounding the drain and may prevent infection at the drain site.[5-7]	Controversy exists regarding efficacy and best practice related to antiseptic cleansers.[5-9] Antiseptic skin cleansers may dry skin and cause further problems related to healing.[10] Most soap alters skin pH and remain on the skin despite rinsing with water. This elevation of pH damages the natural acid mantle and may destroy sebum, which has natural bactericidal and fungicidal properties.[10] Povidone-iodine, available in solution, cream, ointment, and scrub, has an increased bactericidal activity in lower concentrations (i.e., 1% solution). Hydrogen peroxide 3% has broad-spectrum efficacy, especially against Gram-positive bacteria. With dilution less than 3%, antibacterial activity is less effective.[5] Chlorhexidine gluconate (CHG), a commonly used surgical scrub and handwash, has been shown to be effective in the prevention of infection. CHG binds to the stratum corneum and remains active for at least 6 hours after application. It is effective against *P. aeruginosa, S. aureus,* and *E. coli.*[5-7]
13. Assess skin insertion site for stay sutures.	Identifies loosened sutures that may need to be replaced to maintain security of drain.	Notify prescribing practitioner if sutures are loose or broken.
14. Apply antibiotic ointment per prescribing practitioner's order. *(Level IV*)* • If peridrain skin is reddened, damaged, or compromised, protective skin barrier film may be applied.	May prevent infection and promote healing.	Care is often based on surgeon preference.[10] Topical application of antibiotic ointment is found to be controversial in the literature. Some clinicians use antimicrobials at the site for prophylaxis, and others leave the site open to air.[4,6,9] An alcohol-free barrier is especially helpful for broken or compromised skin. When used, ointment is applied in thin layer at the insertion site with a cotton-tipped applicator. Monitor site for reaction to ointment.

Procedure continues on following page

* Level IV: Limited clinical studies to support recommendations

Procedure for Surgical Drains: Care and Management—*Continued*

Steps	Rationale	Considerations
15. Cover with fenestrated gauze dressing or foam if indicated, for padding or absorption of drainage. *(Level IV*)*	Dressing absorbs drainage, wicking moisture away from the skin, and prevents breakdown from excess moisture or increased bacterial load.	Drain site care is carried out with aseptic or clean technique. Sterile technique is not necessary unless specifically indicated per prescribing practitioner's order or preference. Studies that evaluate the necessity of dressings at the site have shown that unless excessive drainage is found, dressings are not necessary.[9]
16. Secure dressing with tape.	Ensures dressing stays in place to absorb drainage.	Thin hydrocolloid or pectin-based wafers may be used to serve as tape anchors on compromised skin.
17. Consider use of tape to secure drain tube to skin. May also consider securing drain to child's gown below level of wound. *(Level II*)*	Avoids tension and prevents pulling or tugging on the tube. A secure drain is less likely to be removed traumatically.	Tape the drain tubing in a similar fashion as securing a urinary catheter.
18. Dispose of used supplies and equipment in appropriate receptacles.	Reduces transmission of micro-organisms.	Type and amount of drainage dictates appropriate receptacle; refer to institution-specific infection control manual.
19. Remove personal protective equipment; wash hands.	Reduces transmission of microorganisms.	

* Level II: Theory-based; no research data to support recommendations; recommendations from expert consensus group may exist
 Level IV: Limited clinical studies to support recommendations

Expected Outcomes	Unexpected Outcomes
• Surgical drain site is continuously evacuated	• Sudden increase or decrease in amount of drainage • Inability to maintain suction in drain collection chamber
• Drain site is free of infection	• Swelling or discharge at drain exit site or incision • Redness around drain exit site (>1 cm) • Presence of macular-papular rash at or surrounding drain exit site • New increased pain at exit site • Increased white blood cell count • Fever
• Drain tubing remains patent	• No drainage from drain • Increased drainage around drain exit site with no drainage in drain collection chamber
• Drain remains in place until elective removal • Child has acceptable level of comfort	• Inadvertent drain removal • Unmanaged pain or anxiety related to drain

Monitoring and Care of the Child

Activities and Interventions	Rationale	Reportable Conditions
1. Measure amount and role type of drainage each shift; compare with the previous 24-hour totals. • Weigh dressings to monitor total amount of fluid drained from the wound. More frequent measurement may be necessary for increased drainage.	Sudden increase in drainage may be indicative of serious complication. Sudden decrease in drainage may indicate a blockage or clot in the tubing or at the tip of the drain (within the surgical site). Sudden change in type of drainage (i.e., serous to bloody) necessitates further assessment per surgical team. Large volumes of wound drainage affect the child's total fluid status.	• Change in quality of drainage (especially serous drainage that becomes bloody) • Drain output of more than 15 mL/kg/shift • Drain container does not remain collapsed after emptying contents
2. Monitor insertion site for signs and symptoms of infection, indications of skin irritation, intactness of sutures and drain.	Increased redness, drainage, induration, erythema, pain, odor, or warmth may indicate infection of the soft tissue. Loosened or broken sutures put the child at risk for inadvertent drain removal.	• Erythema, induration, purulence, pain, odor, or swelling at the insertion site • Loose or broken sutures • Skin irritation • Drain tube pulled from skin/insertion site
3. Change dressing at prescribed intervals or if dressing becomes loose.	Ensures drainage is collected and measured. Ensures routine assessment of drain insertion site and surrounding skin.	• Skin irritation • Indications of infection at site
4. Evaluate effectiveness of pain management strategy with a developmentally appropriate pain assessment tool and provide appropriate interventions. • Encourage family to assist with nonpharmacologic means to comfort and support the child.	Early identification of inadequate pain control facilitates prompt treatment. Ineffective pain management may make future drain care more traumatic.	• Inadequate pain control related to drain or drain management

Documentation

- Drain type and location
- Drainage type and amount; document each drain separately
- Date and time of each dressing change
- Exit site condition
- Peridrain skin condition/tolerance of adhesive products (presence or absence of rashes, skin tears, etc.)
- Medications applied to drain exit site or peridrain skin
- Pain assessment related to drain; any specific interventions provided and effectiveness of interventions
- Child's tolerance of procedure
- Unexpected outcomes and related treatment
- Additional interventions and child's response
- Child and family education

References

1. Dingli GC: Surgical drains tutorial, October 2001.
2. Doughty D: Principles of wound healing and wound management. In Bryant RA, editor: *Acute and chronic wounds: nursing management*, St Louis, 1992, Mosby.
3. De La Pena AS, et al: General principles of surgical treatment in surgical infections. In PCS Committee on Surgical Infection: *Current concepts and management: PCS scientific publication no.3: 39-42*, Quezon City, Philippines, 1992, Philippine College of Surgeons.
4. Division of Nursing–James Cancer Hospital and Solove Research Institute: February 2003, The Ohio State University Medical Center.
5. Drousou A, et al: Antiseptics on wounds: an area of controversy, *Wounds* 15:5, 149-166, 2003.
6. White RJ, et al: Wound colonization and infection: the role of topical antimicrobials, *Br J Nurs* 10:9, 563-564, 566, 568, 2001.
7. Carson S: Chlorhexidine versus povidone-iodine for central nervous catheter site care in children, *J Ped Nurs* 19, 1, 74-80, 2004.
8. Pleat J, Duncan C: The management of surgical drains in plastic surgical units, *Nurs Res* 51:2, 73, 2002.
9. Reid R, Dumanian G: A minimalist approach to the care of the indwelling closed suction drain: a prospective analysis of local wound complications, *Ann Plast Surg* 51:6, 575-578, 2003.
10. Skewes SM: Skin care rituals that do more harm than good, *AJN* 96:10, 33-35, 1996.

Decompression Tube: Insertion and Care

P U R P O S E : A gastric decompression tube is placed for aspiration of stomach contents, gastric lavage, decompression of the gastrointestinal tract, or intestinal obstruction relief

Holly DeWald

PREREQUISITE KNOWLEDGE

- Child development as it relates to clinical assessment and gastric tube decompression
- Anatomy and physiology of the pediatric gastrointestinal (GI) tract, including structural characteristics specific to the infant and child[1]
- The primary function of a gastric decompression tube is evacuation of gas or liquid from the stomach.[2]
- A gastric decompression tube may be inserted to[2-4]:
  - ❖ Improve ventilation with minimization of gastric distension and decreased pressure on the diaphragm
  - ❖ Decrease air in the bowel
  - ❖ Minimize postoperative nausea and vomiting
  - ❖ Hasten return of bowel function after abdominal surgery
  - ❖ Decrease the risk of anastomosis leak after surgery
  - ❖ Prevent wound dehiscence
  - ❖ Decrease abdominal wound infection
  - ❖ Collect gastric contents
  - ❖ Aspirate or lavage the stomach during gastric bleeding or drug overdose
- Decompression tubes are typically large-bore plastic tubes and can be single-lumen or double-lumen tubes.[3,4]
  - ❖ Levin tubes are flexible plastic tubes with a hole at the tip and several holes along the side of the distal end of the tube (Figure 93-1). Levin tubes are not vented and may adhere to the gastric mucosa when placed to suction the tip of the tube.
  - ❖ Gastric sump tubes as more rigid plastic tubes and have two lumens the length of the tube (Figure 93-2).

- ○ The large lumen has several holes along the side of the distal end of the tube that drain air and secretions out of the stomach.

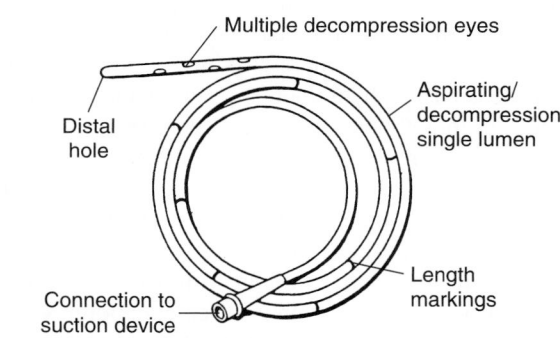

FIGURE 93-1 Nonvented single-lumen (Levin) tube.

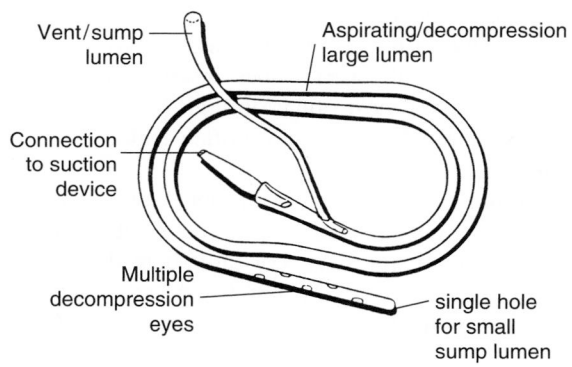

FIGURE 93-2 Vented double-lumen sump tube.

- ○ The small lumen has a single hole at the tip of the distal end of the tube; this lumen serves as an air vent that pulls air into the stomach when suction is applied, preventing the tip of the tube from adhering to the gastric mucosa.
  - ○ If fluid enters the small lumen, venting becomes ineffective; gastric reflux prevention valves are commercially available to prevent fluid from backing up into the vent lumen.
  - ❖ To be effective, the decompression tube must be large bore and made of a material that does not collapse when suction is applied. Small-bore single-lumen weighted flexible tubes used to administer feedings are not appropriate for decompression. The smallest size sump tube currently available is 8-Fr.
  - ❖ Recommended sizes for gastric decompression tubes are as follows:[4,5,6]
    - ○ Infants: <1500 g: 5-Fr
    - ○ Infants: >1500 g: 8-Fr
    - ○ Toddler: 8-Fr to 10-Fr
    - ○ Preschool-school-aged: 10-Fr to 12-Fr
    - ○ Adolescents: 12-Fr to 16-Fr
- Decompression tubes are inserted through the nostril or mouth into the stomach via the esophagus. The oral route is preferred for neonates and young infants who are obligate nose-breathers.[5] Insertion via the nasal route in infants who weigh less than 2 kg has been shown to cause decreased respiratory rate and minute ventilation, increased pulmonary vascular resistance, and increased work of breathing.[6]
- Passing of a decompression tube via the nostril is contraindicated in children with a cranial injury, including skull fracture; otorrhea or rhinorrhea, and maxillofacial injury.[7,8]
- Complications of decompression tube insertion include epistaxis, sinusitis, hydrothorax, pneumothorax including tension pneumothorax, esophageal perforation, pneumonia, transbronchial insertion into the pleura, pleural effusion, inadvertent intracranial placement, nasal septum injury, vocal cord injury, and painful swallowing.[2,7,9]
- Those patients most at risk for incorrect decompression tube placement include children with decreased level of consciousness from sedation or disease; children with an endotracheal tube or tracheostomy tube or weak cough or gag; and children who are uncooperative or agitated. In addition, operator inexperience may add risk for inadvertent tube placement.[7,9]
- A few studies in infants and children have shown that 20% to 40% of gastric tubes inserted are incorrectly placed and are most often too high (in the esophagus). Orally placed tubes are more often malpositioned than nasally placed tubes.[5,10,11]
- Abdominal radiograph is considered the most reliable method for documentation of correct position of the gastric decompression tube. For large-bore decompression tubes, studies indicate a pH of 5.5 or less obtained with a test strip with multiple colorimetric squares (pH range of 0 to 8), and observation of a grassy green, brown, or clear with shreds of off-white mucus aspirate are appropriate for confirmation of gastric placement of a decompression tube in the infant or child, including low–birth weight infants.[7,10,11]

CHILD AND FAMILY ASSESSMENT

- Child's developmental level and ability to interact ➤➤*Rationale:* Child's developmental level influences preparation and interaction and assists in determination of the level of cooperation that the child can provide.
- Child's and family's understanding of the reasons for and risks and benefits of the procedure ➤➤*Rationale:* Evaluates child's and family's understanding of the procedure and provides a gauge for ongoing education.
- History of nasal deformity, epistaxis, trauma, varices, recent esophageal or gastric surgery, esophageal malformations, or injuries ➤➤*Rationale:* These conditions can complicate or be a contraindication to tube insertion.
- With planned insertion via the nares, assess the patency of the nares ➤➤*Rationale:* A tube cannot pass through an occlusion. With the most patent nostril chosen, tube insertion is eased and tolerance of the tube may be improved.[4]
- History of ingestion of drugs or toxins ➤➤*Rationale:* Some poisons can cause esophageal perforation.
- Signs of gastric distention (e.g., vomiting, nausea, absence of or hypoactive bowel sounds) ➤➤*Rationale:* Secretions or air in the stomach increase the risk of aspiration.
- Family's desire to be present during the procedure ➤➤*Rationale:* The family may provide support and comfort to the child but should have the choice not to remain with the child.

CHILD AND FAMILY EDUCATION

Individualized, developmentally appropriate education is provided to the family and to the child based on desire for knowledge, readiness to learn, and overall neurologic and psychosocial state.

- Explain the purpose of the decompression tube and the steps involved in tube insertion ➤➤*Rationale:* Providing information decreases anxiety and fear and may promote cooperation.
- If developmentally appropriate, explain to the child how to assist in the tube insertion (e.g., swallowing during tube insertion) ➤➤*Rationale:* Elicits child's cooperation, which eases tube passage.
- Explain that tube insertion may be uncomfortable and may cause the child to gag ➤➤*Rationale:* Providing information decreases anxiety and fear.
- Encourage questions and answer questions as they arise ➤➤*Rationale:* Reinforcement of information is needed during periods of stress.

EQUIPMENT

- Appropriately sized decompression tube: Gastric sump tube or Levin tube
- Appropriately sized catheter tip syringe
- Water-soluble lubricant
- Stethoscope
- Tape or semipermeable transparent dressing to secure the tube

- Skin preparation agent
- Clean gloves
- Marker (optional)
- Gastro cult card
- Gastric pH testing equipment
- Suction source with connecting tubing

Procedure for Decompression Tube: Insertion and Care

Steps	Rationale	Considerations
1. Ensure child and family understand procedure and questions are answered.	Evaluates and reinforces understanding of previously taught information.	Developmental level, cognitive ability, and anxiety level influence approach to and effectiveness of teaching.
2. Determine method of decompression: Suction versus venting/draining.	The method of decompression determines the type of tube to use.	
3. Collect all necessary equipment and supplies.	Promotes completion of the procedure in a timely manner; may decrease child's anxiety.	Tube size is determined based on child's size.
4. Ensure appropriate cardiopulmonary monitoring.	Children may decompensate during tube insertion.	Consider the child's status in selection of appropriate cardiopulmonary monitoring.
5. Wash hands and put on clean gloves.	Reduces the transmission of microorganisms. Protects personnel health.	
6. Determine the length of tube to be inserted. Measure the tube from the tip of the child's nose to the earlobe, then from the earlobe to the xiphoid process[4,9-12] (see Figure 186-1 in Procedure 186). • Record the nearest centimeter marking on the tube or indicate location on the tube with a marker or tape. *(Level V*)*	Gives an approximation of tube length to insert. Distance from the tube entry point to the xyphoid process approximates the distance to the gastroesophageal junction. Tape or mark placed on the tube serves as a reference point if the tube becomes dislodged or is removed.	A small study done in children birth to 7 years old showed that the nose to earlobe to xiphoid process (NEX) measurement may underestimate the appropriate depth of insertion.[10] *(Level IV*)*
7. Lubricate 6 to 10 cm of the distal end of tube with water-soluble lubricant.	Lubrication facilitates passage through nares. Minimizes mucosal injury and irritation during insertion.	Use only water-soluble lubricants for tube placement. Oil-soluble lubricants cannot be absorbed by the pulmonary mucosa and may cause respiratory complications should the tube be inadvertently placed into the lungs.[3]
8. *For oral placement:* Position the end of the tube downward and insert the tube into the oral cavity over the tongue. Aim the tube	Flexing the head of an unconscious child also facilitates tube insertion. Having the child take sips of water or mimic swallowing causes the	If the child is uncooperative, use of an oral airway or bite block may prevent the child from biting the tube.

Procedure continues on following page

* Level IV: Limited clinical studies to support recommendations
Level V: Clinical studies in more than one or two patient populations and situations to support recommendations

Procedure for Decompression Tube: Insertion and Care—*Continued*

Steps	Rationale	Considerations
back and down toward the pharynx. When the tube hits the pharynx, flex the head forward (must have mobile C-spine). If appropriate, ask the child to take sips of water through a straw while the tube is advanced. *(Level IV*)* *For nasal placement:* Insert the tube into a patent nostril, aiming back and down. When the tube hits the pharynx, if the child is able and has a mobile C-spine, flex the child's head forward and have the child swallow. Advance the tube as the child swallows. *(Level IV*)*	epiglottis to close the trachea and directs the tube toward the esophagus.	If the child coughs or begins gagging, withdraw slightly, stop insertion, and allow the child to rest. Allowing the child to rest may help to decrease the risk of aspiration.
9. Continue to insert the tube until the pre-marked centimeter on the tube is reached.	Advances the tube into the stomach.	If resistance is met, rotating the tube may help placement. If unable to pass the tube after several attempts, notify the prescribing practitioner.
10. Confirm tube placement. • Aspirate and assess gastric content and test the pH per institution-specific protocol. *(Level IV*)* • Confirm placement with radiographic examination, as indicated. *(Level VI*)*	Aspirates with a pH of 5.5 or less and the appearance of grassy green, clear with white flecks, or brown indicates tube placement in the stomach.[3,4,7,8,10-12] *(Level IV*)* Radiography is considered the most reliable method of tube location confirmation.	If the pH is greater than 5.5, alternative methods to confirm placement are used. Children on H_2 blockers have a pH greater that 5.[12]
11. Secure the tube with tape or semi-permeable transparent dressing to the upper lip or cheek of the child. Avoid pressure on the rim of the nostril.	Prevents movement or inadvertent removal of tube. Pressure of the firm decompression tube on the nostril may result in skin breakdown or notching of the nostril.[3]	Avoid securing the tube to the nare. The child is at higher risk for necrotic breakdown when the tube is taped to the nare. Consider medical immobilization if the child appears to be uncooperative and presents a risk of tube dislodgement.
12. Connect the tube to suction or aspirate air with a syringe. *Double-lumen tubes:* The large lumen is connected to suction. Maintain the small lumen at a position higher than the child's stomach, which allows the vent to remain patent. *Single-lumen tubes:* Aspirate/decompress with a syringe.	Decompresses stomach; removes fluid and air. Use of intermittent suction reduces trauma to the gastric mucosa.	With a double-lumen tube, do not exceed 80 mm Hg of intermittent suction. With a single-lumen tube, do not exceed 25 mm Hg of intermittent suction.
13. Dispose of used supplies and equipment in appropriate receptacles. Remove gloves; wash hands.	Reduces transmission of microorganisms. Protects personnel health.	
14. While the decompression tube is in place, place the child in semi-Fowler's position.[7-9] *(Level V*)*	Decreases risk of aspiration of stomach contents.	Place child in semi-Fowler's position as condition permits.

* Level IV: Limited clinical studies to support recommendations
Level V: Clinical studies in more than one or two patient populations and situations to support recommendations
Level VI: Clinical studies in a variety of patient populations and situations to support recommendations

Expected Outcomes	Unexpected Outcomes
• Stomach is decompressed	• Stomach is not decompressed because of kinked, blocked, or incorrectly placed tube
• The tip of the tube is placed in the stomach	• Tracheal or bronchial intubation
	• Inadvertent pleural placement
	• Inadvertent cranial placement
	• Tube coiled in posterior pharynx or esophagus
• The tube remains patent	• Blocked tube
	• Fluid backs up into vent port of double-lumen tube, preventing effective decompression
• The tube remains in place until elective removal	• Inadvertent tube removal by child, family, or health care team
• The child's skin remains intact	• Skin irritation on face or at nares
	• Notching of the nare from pressure from tube
• The child is free from complications of decompression tube placement	• Pneumothorax from tracheal placement
	• Esophageal trauma from trauma of tube insertion
	• Bleeding from nares as result of trauma of tube insertion

Monitoring and Care of the Child

Activities and Interventions	Rationale	Reportable Conditions
1. Monitor for signs and symptoms of dehydration and electrolyte imbalances.	Gastric contents contain electrolytes and fluid essential to homeostasis.	• Dizziness, weakness, muscle cramps, concentrated urine or decreased urine output, poor skin turgor, and postural hypotension
2. Monitor intake and output. • Consider replacement fluids if ongoing output exceeds 3 to 4 mL/kg/hr.	Quantifies amount of ongoing fluid losses from the GI tract; assists in diagnosis of dehydration.	• Decreased or concentrated urine output • Increased gastric drainage • Output greater than intake
3. Maintain proper tube placement.	Proper tube placement is necessary to facilitate drainage via the decompression tube and decreases the risk of skin ulceration at the nares.	• Dislodged tube • Migrated tube • Any skin redness, breakdown, or ulceration associated with the tube
4. Assess tube position before administration of medications or irrigation solution or if the child has an episode of gagging, vomiting, or severe coughing.	Ensures tube is correctly placed before administration of fluids or medications. Tip of the tube may become displaced with episodes of gagging, vomiting, or coughing.	• Administration of medication or fluids into compartment other than stomach • Repeated episodes of retching or vomiting
5. Monitor the characteristics of the decompression tube output.	Assists with identification of tube placement and complications of tube placement.	• Significant increase or decrease in output • Output becomes bloody • Inability to irrigate tube
6. Irrigate the tube every 4 hours or per prescribing practitioner's order with 0.9% saline solution or other prescribed fluid.	Promotes patency of tube.	
7. Monitor the child for increased abdominal girth, reported feeling of fullness, or decreased gastric drainage.	May indicate that the stomach is not being decompressed.	• Increasing abdominal girth • Report of feeling distended • Significant decrease in drainage
8. If a sump tube is used, ensure the vent port remains above the level of the child's stomach. • Irrigate the vent port every 4 hours or as needed with 5 to 10 mL of air.	Fluid in the vent port decreases the effectiveness of the tube.	• Sump tube does not function effectively

Continued

Monitoring and Care of the Child—Cont'd

Activities and Interventions	Rationale	Reportable Conditions
9. Provide mouth care at least every 4 hours.	Orogastric or nasogastric tubes may cause the child to mouth breathe, drying the mouth and increasing the risk of mucosal breakdown and ulcerations. Predisposes child to sinusitis or oral infections.	• Oral ulcers • Increase in size or tenderness of the parotid glands
10. Auscultate the child's abdomen for the presence of flatus or bowel sounds.	The decompression tube may be removed once peristalsis has returned or the obstruction is relieved.	• Positive bowel sounds • Presence of flatus
11. Monitor insertion site of tube.	Frequent monitoring can prevent serious skin breakdown.	• Redness, swelling, drainage, bleeding, or skin breakdown at insertion site

Documentation

- Size and type of decompression tube
- Length of tube placed
- Location of insertion: Oral versus nare
- Amount, color, odor of gastric content obtained
- Amount of suction applied or manipulations of tube (e.g., tube is clamped)
- Intake, including amount and type of irrigation fluid and output
- Oral hygiene
- Child's tolerance of the procedure
- Difficulties encountered with tube insertion (e.g., inability to pass through right nare)
- Confirmation of tube placement and method of confirmation
- Unexpected outcomes and related treatment
- Tube insertion site assessments
- Additional interventions and related outcomes
- Child and family education

References

1. Sentongo T, Steinhorn D: Gastrointestinal structure and function. In Fuhrman B, Zimmerman J, editors: *Pediatric Crit Care,* ed 3, Philadelphia, 2006, Mosby.
2. Nelson R, et al: Prophylactic nasogastric decompression after abdominal surgery, *Cochrane Library* (1):CD004929, 2006.
3. Dulak SB: Inserting an NG tube, *RN* 69(6):24ac1-4, 2006.
4. Lockridge T, et al: Neonatal surgical emergencies: stabilization and management, *J Obstet Gynecol Neonatal Nurs* 31(3):328-339, 2002.
5. Hawes J, et al: Nasal versus oral route for placing feeding tubes in preterm or low birth weight infants, *Cochrane Database Systematic Rev* (3):CD003952, 2004.
6. Greenspan JS, et al: Neonatal gastric intubation: differential respiratory effects between nasogastric and orogastric tubes, *Pediatr Pulmonol* 8(4):254-258, 1990.
7. Metheny NA, Titler MG: Assessing placement of feeding tubes, *Am J Nurs* 101(5):36-45, 2001.
8. Hockenberry MJ, et al, editors: *Wong's nursing care of infants and children,* ed 7, St Louis, 2003, Mosby.
9. Baskin WN: Acute complications associated with bedside placement of feeding tubes, *Nutrition* 21(1):40-55, 2006.
10. Ellett ML, et al: Gastric tube placement in young children, *Clin Nurs Res* 14(3):238-252, 2005.
11. Nyqvist KH, et al: Litmus tests for verification of feeding tube location in infants: evaluation of their clinical use, *J Clin Nurs* 14:486-495, 2005.
12. Huffman S, et al: Methods to confirm feeding tube placement: application of research in practice, *Pediatr Nurs* 30(1):10-13, 2004.

Additional Readings

Bowers S: All about tubes, *Nursing* 30(12):41-48, 2000.
Koong Shiao P, Difiore TE: A survey of gastric tube practices in Level II and Level III nurseries, *Issues Comprehensive Pediatr Nurs* 19:209-220, 1996.
Lewis AM: Learning the ABCDs of pediatric assessment, *Nursing* 29(5):32H1-32H8, 1999.
Methany N: Achieving successful nasogastric tube placements in emergency situations, *Am J Crit Care* 9(5):303-306, 2000.

Esophagogastric Tamponade Tube: Care and Management

P U R P O S E : An esophagogastric tamponade tube is placed to provide temporary control of active variceal hemorrhage unresponsive to pharmacologic or endoscopic interventions

Lucy R. Paskus

PREREQUISITE KNOWLEDGE

- Child development as it relates to pediatric assessment and management of an esophagogastric tamponade tube (EGTT)
- Anatomy and physiology of the pediatric gastrointestinal (GI) tract, including structural characteristics specific to the infant and child[1]
- Mastery of pediatric advanced life support competencies[2]
- Etiology and differential diagnosis of upper GI bleeding
- Interventions available in treatment of acute variceal hemorrhage, such as vasopressin or octreotide infusion, endoscopic sclerotherapy, or endoscopic band ligation[3-5]
- Physiologic rationale for the use of an EGTT; the tube is used for tamponade of GI bleeding with a decrease in blood flow through the dilated esophageal veins.
- Purpose and location of the various balloons and ports on the EGTT[3,5]
  - ❖ The Blakemore or Sengstaken-Blakemore tube (C.R. Bard, Inc, Covington, Ga) is a latex tube with two balloons (gastric and esophageal) and a gastric aspiration port.
    - ○ Child: 12F 30-inch (76.2-cm) tube with a 4.5-inch esophageal balloon
    - ○ Intermediate: 16F 39-inch (99-cm) tube with a 6-inch esophageal balloon
    - ○ Adult: 20-F 39-inch (99-cm) tube with an 8-inch esophageal balloon
  - ❖ The Minnesota tube (C.R. Bard, Inc) is a latex tube with two balloons (gastric and esophageal) and two

aspiration ports (gastric and esophageal) this tube is available in size 18F (Figure 94-1).
- ❖ Gastric balloon: Spherical balloon that applies pressure at the esophageal-gastric junction, which decreases blood flow through the vessels that feed the varices. The gastric balloon is also used to maintain tube position.

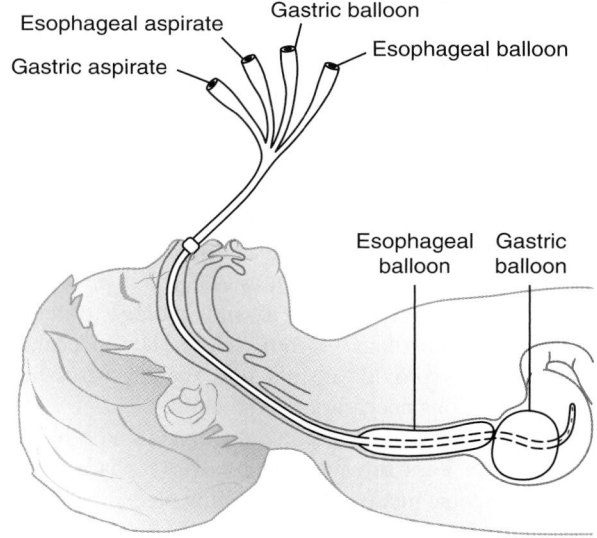

FIGURE 94-1 Minnesota tube with four lumens: esophageal balloon inflation port, esophageal aspiration port, gastric balloon inflation port, and gastric aspiration port. Note spherical gastric balloon and cylindrical esophageal balloon.

❖ Esophageal balloon: Cylindrical balloon that applies pressure directly to the varices. The esophageal balloon may not be inflated if bleeding is controlled with inflation of the gastric balloon.

❖ Gastric aspiration port: Used to remove blood and secretions from the stomach

❖ Esophageal aspiration port: Used to remove secretions from the esophagus

- The need for draining both gastric and esophageal secretions. Esophageal ports are not present on all tubes; in these cases, an additional drainage tube must be placed above the esophageal balloon.

- Risks and complications of the EGTT include atelectasis, aspiration pneumonia, airway obstruction, tube migration, esophageal ulceration or rupture, duodenal rupture, sinusitis, nasal trauma or ulceration, and lip ulceration.[3,5,6]

- Relative contraindications to use of an EGTT include recent esophageal surgery, esophageal strictures, and bleeding that has stopped.[6-8]

- Pediatric airway management[2]

- Management of the child with an endotracheal tube (see Procedure 2)

- Circulatory assessment of the child

- Selection and use of a developmentally appropriate pain scale (see Procedure 173)

- Appropriate pediatric dosing of analgesics and sedatives

- Competency in pediatric sedation

- Understand parenteral hydration and nutritional needs

CHILD AND FAMILY ASSESSMENT

- Child's developmental level and ability to interact ➤*Rationale:* These factors influence preparation of the child and interaction during the procedure.

- Family's support system and desire to be present during procedure ➤*Rationale:* This procedure is usually done emergently, and institution-specific protocol may or may not allow family presence. Family may need additional support in coping with the crisis, whether or not they choose to be present during the procedure.

- Child's medical and surgical history ➤*Rationale:* Esophageal strictures and recent esophageal surgery are relative contraindications to EGTT placement.[7,8]

- Child's known allergies, especially latex allergy or history of allergy to kiwi or bananas ➤*Rationale:* The EGTT contains latex; exposure to know allergen is prevented.

- Review of child's GI system and etiology of current variceal hemorrhage ➤*Rationale:* The information obtained may provide insight into specific assessments and precautions necessary for the child.

- Pharmacologic and endoscopic attempts to stop bleeding ➤*Rationale:* Less invasive and less risky pharmacologic and endoscopic methods of controlling bleeding should be attempted before insertion of a EGTT.[8] Re-bleeding can occur if sclerotherapy or band ligation was performed.[3]

- Child's current hemodynamic status ➤*Rationale:* Children with variceal bleeds are at high risk for volume deficits and hemodynamic instability.

- Child's current sedation level and previous sedation experiences ➤*Rationale:* Moderate sedation is necessary for successful passage of the tube and maintenance of tube placement; previous difficulties with sedation or sedation strategies that have been effective in the past are identified.

- Nutrition and fluid status ➤*Rationale:* The child will need parenteral hydration or nutrition while the EGTT is in place.

- Child's current respiratory status ➤*Rationale:* Displacement of EGTT or aspiration of upper GI contents can lead to respiratory distress.

- Family's desire to be present during the procedure ➤*Rationale:* The family may provide support and comfort to the child but should have the choice not to remain with the child.

CHILD AND FAMILY EDUCATION

Individualized, developmentally appropriate education is provided to the family and to the child based on desire for knowledge, readiness to learn, and overall neurologic and psychosocial state.

- Review the purpose of the EGTT and explain the steps involved in tube placement ➤*Rationale:* Providing information decreases anxiety and fear.

- Discuss the plan of care for the child while the tube is in place (e.g., the child will be intubated and unable to eat or drink) and the anticipated length of time tube will remain in place (typically less than 48 hours) ➤*Rationale:* Understanding of the plan of care decreases anxiety and fear.

- Discuss the importance of the tube not being dislodged ➤*Rationale:* Providing information may decrease anxiety and fear, increase compliance, and decrease the risk of complications, such as re-bleeding or esophageal rupture.

- Discuss the importance of reporting of pain, especially chest and back pain because this may be a sign of displaced balloon or esophageal rupture ➤*Rationale:* Providing information may decrease anxiety and fear and increase compliance; facilitates child's and family's participation in the plan.

- Discuss the plan for sedation and the specific goals of increasing the child's comfort level, decreasing the gag reflex, decreasing intraabdominal pressure to minimize bleeding, and maintaining the tube in proper position ➤*Rationale:* Providing information may increase compliance; knowledge that the child's anxiety will be managed may be reassuring to the child and family.

- Review the necessity of maintenance of tension on the tube to keep the gastric balloon tight against the gastroesophageal junction, which compresses fundal veins and keeps the balloon positioned properly in the esophagus ➤*Rationale:* Providing information may increase compliance and facilitate the child's and family's participation in the plan of care.

- Encourage questions and answer questions as they arise ➤*Rationale:* Reinforcement of information is needed during periods of stress, especially if the tube is placed emergently.

EQUIPMENT

- Appropriate sized EGTT (e.g., Sengstaken-Blakemore tube)
- Football helmet *or* traction set-up, to secure tube
- Catheter tipped syringe, 60-mL
- Luer lock syringe, 60 mL
- Decompression tube (e.g., Salem sump)
- Water-soluble lubricant
- Suction regulators and suction drainage containers (two)
- Pair of scissors, kept at bedside for emergent balloon decompression

- Rubber-tipped clamps (two)
- Three-way stopcock
- Pressure manometer
- Catheter adaptor to connect manometer to balloon inflation ports
- Waterproof tape (e.g., Hy-tape, Hy-tape International, Patterson, NY)
- Clean gloves
- Eye and face shield
- Gown

Procedure | for Esophagogastric Tamponade Tube: Care and Management

Steps	Rationale	Considerations
1. Ensure child and family understand procedure and questions are answered.	Evaluates and reinforces understanding of previously taught information.	Developmental level, cognitive ability, and anxiety level determine approach to and effectiveness of teaching.
2. Gather needed equipment and supplies.	Facilitates completion of the task in a timely manner.	Size of tube selected is based on child's size. 12F is the smallest tube size available.
3. Wash hands and put on clean gloves, gown, and face shield.	Reduces transmission of micro-organisms.	Gown and face shield are highly recommended because blood is likely to be splattered during this procedure.
4. Ensure child is adequately sedated and airway is protected.[5-7] *(Level IV*)*	Adequate sedation increases the child's comfort level and facilitates tube placement. Typically, children are endotracheally intubated before this procedure.[9]	A cuffed endotracheal tube is used to further decrease the risk of pulmonary aspiration.[8]
5. Assist practitioner who is placing the EGTT with gastric lavage before EGTT tube placement.[6]	Gastric lavage empties the stomach contents and decreases the risk of pulmonary aspiration while also allowing for assessment of bleeding.[8]	A large-bore gastric tube and 0.9% saline solution may be used for lavage (see Procedure 95).[8]
6. Check balloons and channels on the tube for proper functioning.[6,8,10,11] *(Level II*)*	Confirms integrity of balloons and patency of channels before tube placement.	
7. Lubricate tube with water-soluble lubricant.[5,7,9,10] *(Level II*)*	Use of lubricant may ease passage of the tube. Petroleum lubricant damages latex balloon.	Lubricate not only the tip but also along the length of the balloons.[6,10]
8. Position child in semierect position with head of bed elevated 45 degrees.[3,10,11] *(Level II*)*	Decreases risk of aspiration; child may vomit as tube is passed.	If unable to position child in semierect position, then place child in left side-lying position.[6,10]

Procedure continues on following page

* Level II: Theory-based; no research data to support recommendations; recommendations from expert consensus group may exist
Level IV: Limited clinical studies to support recommendations

Procedure for Esophagogastric Tamponade Tube: Care and Management—*Continued*

Steps	Rationale	Considerations
9. Practitioner advances the tube through the mouth or nose into the stomach to a pre-measured distance or to the 40-cm (child) or 50-cm (intermediate or adult) mark and inflate the gastric balloon with 20 to 50 mL of air.[7,10] *(Level II*)*	Initially just enough air is put in the gastric balloon to keep it positioned in the stomach until placement can be confirmed.	A gastroenterologist or other practitioner skilled in EGTT insertion should perform this procedure.[6,13] *(Level II*)*
10. A radiograph that includes the lower test and upper abdomen is obtained and interpreted.[6,8,12] *(Level II*)*	Placement of the gastric balloon in the stomach must be confirmed before full inflation of the gastric balloon.[6,12] *(Level IV*)*	Inflation of the gastric balloon in the esophagus or duodenum could cause rupture.[5,6,12] Endoscopy and ultrasound scan have also been used to verify tube placement.[6,12]
11. After correct placement of the gastric balloon is confirmed, more air is inserted in the gastric balloon and the gastric balloon is pulled up to gastroesophageal junction. One or two padded clamps are used to occlude the gastric balloon inflation port 2 to 3 cm from the end of the port.[3,6,7,10]	Full expansion of the gastric balloon allows for optimal pressure to be distributed over the gastric surface at the gastroesophageal junction. Clamping of the balloon port prevents the balloon from deflating. Avoid clamping the inflation port at the narrowest portion to prevent damage to the tube.	Total air volume varies from 50 to 200 mL, dependent on the size of the tube and child.[3,6,7,10] *(Level II*)* Air is generally recommended to inflate the balloon to prevent small particles from blocking the inflation track and because air is radiopaque.[6]
12. Mark the tube with tape or a marker at the point the tube exits the nose or mouth.[3,6] *(Level II*)*	Facilitates identification of a displaced tube.	
13. Connect the tube to traction set up or securely tape to face mask of football helmet (Figure 94-2).[6,8,14] *(Level II*)*	Tension applied to the tube compresses the fundal veins to slow bleeding.[6,14]	A 500-mL to 1000-mL intravenous fluid bag (2 to 3 lb) can be used for traction.[6,8] *(Level II*)*

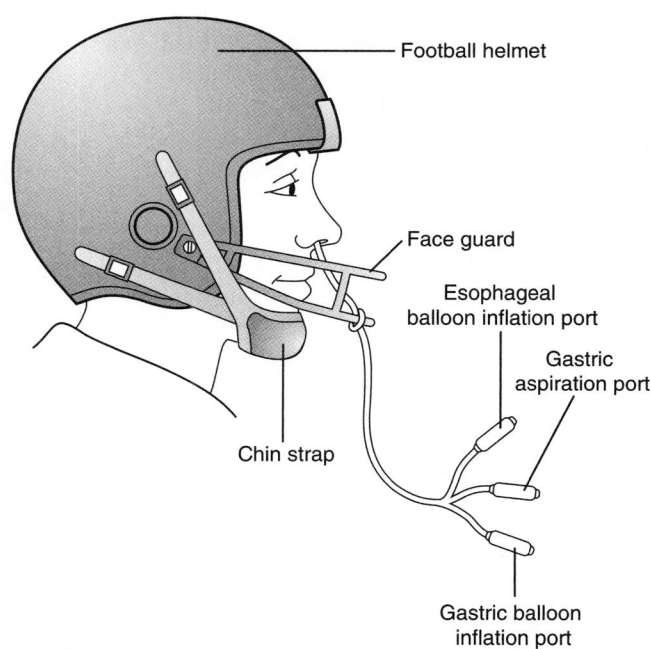

Football helmet

Face guard

Esophageal balloon inflation port

Gastric aspiration port

Chin strap

Gastric balloon inflation port

Figure 94-2   Use of football helmet to stabilize EGTT. *From Lynn-McHale Wiegand DJ, Carlson K, editors: AACN procedure manual for critical care, ed 5, St Louis, 2005, Saunders.*

Procedure	for Esophagogastric Tamponade Tube: Care and Management—*Continued*	
Steps	**Rationale**	**Considerations**
14. If bleeding continues, the prescribing practitioner may choose to inflate the esophageal balloon.[6,8] *(Level II*)* • Attach a stopcock to the catheter adapter. • Insert the catheter adapter into the esophageal balloon lumen. • Tape the catheter adapter–balloon lumen with waterproof tape. • Attach the pressure manometer to one port of the stopcock and a 60-mL Luer lock syringe to the other port of the stopcock. • With the stopcock open to the syringe and manometer, air is slowly injected until the desired pressure for the esophageal balloon is reached. The lowest pressure needed to stop bleeding is used. • The esophageal balloon port is occluded with a padded clamp, and the stopcock is turned off to the patient.	The esophageal balloon is designed to apply direct tamponade to esophageal varices.	The recommended pressure range for the esophageal balloon is 20 to 40 mm Hg. Generally, this therapy is limited to 12 to 24 hours because of the risk of pressure necrosis.[6,8,11] *(Level II*)*
15. Place the gastric aspiration port to low intermittent wall suction.[6,8,11] *(Level II*)*	Suction empties stomach contents and facilitates assessment of gastric bleeding.	Monitor volume and type of secretions.
16. Place the esophageal aspiration port to low intermittent wall suction.[6,8] *(Level II*)*	The gastric and esophageal balloons obstruct the swallowing of secretions and pooled secretions could be aspirated.[4-6,15]	If the EGTT does not have an esophageal aspiration port, a gastric tube is placed above the esophageal balloon to drain oral
17. Discard used supplies and equipment in appropriate receptacles.	Reduces transmission of micro-organisms.	
18. Remove and discard personal protective equipment; wash hands.	Reduces transmission of micro-organisms.	

* Level II: Theory-based; no research data to support recommendations; recommendations from expert consensus group may exist

Expected Outcomes	Unexpected Outcomes
• Upper GI bleeding is controlled • Improved hemodynamic stability	• Continued variceal hemorrhage • Hemodynamic instability • Shock
• Tube placed and maintained in correct position	• Respiratory distress from migration of EGTT into esophagus • Inadvertent EGTT removal
• Correct traction and balloon pressures maintained as ordered	• Balloon deflation from inflation port damage • Incorrect traction • Failure to monitor balloon pressures
• Child's nose and mouth are kept clean and free of pressure areas • Child is free from complications of EGTT placement	• Pressure areas that lead to skin breakdown • Ruptured esophagus • Pulmonary aspiration of GI contents
• Fluid and electrolyte abnormalities and anemia are identified and treated appropriately	• Unrecognized electrolyte abnormalities • Unrecognized anemia • Unrecognized dehydration
• Child demonstrates an expected level of comfort	• Uncontrolled anxiety or agitation

Monitoring and Care of the Child

Activities and Interventions	Rationale	Reportable Conditions
1. Monitor respiratory status.	Respiratory distress could indicate aspiration of GI contents or dislodgement of tube.	• Deterioration of respiratory status
2. Monitor hemodynamic status.	Continued GI bleeding or rebleeding may result in shock. Hypertension increases the risk of rebleeding.[5]	• Signs of poor peripheral perfusion: tachycardia, cool extremities, delayed capillary refill time, weak peripheral pulses • Hypertension

3. Monitor the child for proper tube position and ensure that the tube is secured:
  • To a traction system with a 500-mL to 1000-mL bag of intravenous fluid
    Or
  • To the face mask of an appropriately sized football helmet
	Proper positioning is critical for effectiveness of the tube and to decrease the risk of complications.
	Traction is necessary to avoid migration of the tube and to keep the gastric balloon snug at the gastroesophageal junction.
		• Dislodged or displaced tube
		• Inability to maintain traction

4. Ensure that the gastric balloon is securely clamped. *(Level II[*])*	Maintains balloon volume as ordered (50 to 200 mL depending on size of tube and child)[3,6] to optimize tamponade effect and to decrease risk of tube migration.	• Gastric balloon unclamped and deflated (emergent if esophageal balloon remains inflated)
5. Ensure that a pair of scissors is readily available at the bedside at all times.[3,6,7,10] *(Level II[*])*	If the child has a sudden unexplained increase in peak inspiratory pressure or acute respiratory distress, the gastric tube may have migrated into the esophagus. The balloons can be rapidly deflated with the scissors to cut the balloon ports.	• Sudden unexplained increase in peak inspiratory pressures • Acute onset of respiratory distress
6. Ensure that a second EGTT of the same size is readily available at the bedside.[6]	Allows prompt tube replacement if the tube fails or is emergently removed.	• Back-up tube of same size is not available
7. Use a manometer attached to the stopcock on the esophageal balloon port to check pressure in the esophageal balloon every 1 to 4 hours or per prescribing practitioner's order. Adjust the pressure via a syringe attached to the stopcock per prescribing practitioner's orders; typically, pressure is maintained between 30 and 40 mm Hg, depending on tube size.[3,6,10] *(Level II[*])*	Pressure must be maintained for optimal control of bleeding and decreased risk of complications (e.g., esophageal necrosis or esophageal rupture).	• Inability to maintain esophageal balloon pressure within ordered parameters
8. Every 12 hours, the esophageal balloon is completely deflated for 5 minutes (per prescribing practitioner's order) and then reinflated and the stopcock is closed to the child and the tubing clamped.[3,6,10] Refer to state Nurse Practice Act and institution-specific protocol for individuals authorized to deflate and inflate the esophageal balloon. *(Level II[*])*	Decreases the risk of esophageal necrosis. With closure of the stopcock *and* clamping of the tubing, the balloon is less likely to deflate. No randomized controlled studies show the appropriate frequency and duration of esophageal balloon deflation/reinflation.	• Inability to deflate or inflate esophageal balloon

* Level II: Theory-based; no research data to support recommendations; recommendations from expert consensus group may exist

Monitoring and Care of the Child—Cont'd

Activities and Interventions	Rationale	Reportable Conditions
9. Irrigate the gastric and esophageal aspiration ports every 4 to 6 hours or per prescribing practitioner's order.	Ensures patency and functioning of aspiration ports; prevents pooling of blood or secretions in the esophagus or stomach.	• Blockage of aspiration ports
10. Monitor gastric and esophageal drainage.	Monitors for rebleeding and volume deficits and clot formation that obstructs drainage tubes.	• Sudden increase or decrease in volume of drainage • Change in type of drainage (e.g., increased bloody drainage)
11. Monitor pain and sedation levels; administer pain and sedation medications as indicated and per prescribing practitioner's order.	Pain, especially chest pain, could be a sign of tube migration[6]; sedation is usually necessary until the tube is removed. An agitated child may bite down on and damage the tube.	• Inadequate pain management • Anxiety or agitation unresponsive to sedation • Decrease in balloon pressure after episode of agitation
12. Monitor fluid and electrolyte status.	Parenteral hydration and electrolyte replacement are necessary while EGTT is in place.	• Altered electrolyte levels • Indications of dehydration or overhydration
13. Monitor complete blood count, coagulation studies; ensure type and cross match is available.[5]	Significant or ongoing bleeding may necessitate blood product replacement.	• Expired type and cross match • Decreasing or abnormal hemoglobin and hematocrit levels • Prolonged prothrombin or partial thromboplastin time
14. Monitor for pressure areas, especially where tube exits the mouth or nose.[3,5,6,9] *(Level II*)*	A high risk for pressure sores from the tube exists because of the continuous traction necessary to maintain tube position.	• Areas of pressure or skin breakdown
15. Provide oral and nasal care every 2 to 4 hours[3,5,6,9] *(Level II*)*	Monitors for pooling of oral and esophageal secretions and for child hygiene and comfort.	• Continued pooling of oral and esophageal secretions • Mouth or nose irritation • Signs and symptoms of rebleeding[3,6,9]
16. In preparation for discontinuation of the tube, the esophageal balloon is first deflated for 12 to 24 hours and then both the esophageal and the gastric balloons are deflated and tension is released for 12 to 24 hours, before removal of the tube.[3,4,6-8,10] *(Level II*)*	The gastric balloon remains inflated initially to maintain the position of the deflated esophageal balloon and to allow one site to be assessed at a time for rebleeding. The tube is left in place even with both ports deflated so that if rebleeding does occur the balloons can simply be reinflated.[8-9]	

* Level II: Theory-based; no research data to support recommendations; recommendations from expert consensus group may exist

Documentation

- Date and time of tube insertion
- Individual who inserted tube
- Size and type of tube inserted
- Radiographic confirmation of tube placement
- Quantity of air placed in gastric balloon; quantity of air placed in esophageal balloon, if inflated
- Inflation/deflation status of gastric and esophageal balloons
- Medications administered for tube insertion
- Mechanism by which traction is applied
- Placement of decompression tube above esophageal balloon if three-port EGTT is used
- Child's tolerance of the procedure
- Periodic assessment of gastric balloon pressure (and esophageal balloon pressure if inflated)
- Volume and character of drainage from gastric and esophageal ports or gastric port and esophageal decompression tube
- Manipulations of tube (inflation, deflation, repositioning)
- Unexpected outcomes and related treatment
- Child and family education

References

1. Sentongo T, Steinhorn D: Gastrointestinal structure and function. In Fuhrman B, Zimmerman J, editors: *Pediatric critical care,* ed 3, Philadelphia, 2006, Mosby.
2. Hazinski M.F., et al: *Pediatric advanced life support provider manual,* Dallas, American Heart Association, 2002.
3. Christensen T: The treatment of esophageal varices using a Sengstaken-Blakemore tube: considerations for nursing practice, *Nurs Crit Care* 9(2):58-63, 2004.
4. Zargar SA, et al: Endoscopic ligation compared with sclerotherapy for bleeding esophageal varices in children with extrahepatic portal venous obstruction, *Hepatology* 36(3):666-672, 2002.
5. Simone S: Gastrointestinal critical care problems. In Curley MAQ, Moloney-Harmon P, editors: *Critical care nursing of infants and children,* ed 2, St. Louis, 2001, Saunders.
6. Greenwald B: The Minnesota tube: its use and care in bleeding esophageal and gastric varices, *Gastroenterol Nurs* 27(5):212-217, 2004.
7. McCormick PA, et al: How to insert a Sengstaken-Blakemore tube, *Br J Hosp Med* 43(4):274-277, 1990.
8. Pasquale MD, Cerra FB: Sengstaken-Blakemore tube placement: use of balloon tamponade to control bleeding varices, *Crit Care Clin* 8(4):743-753, 1992.
9. Chulay M, et al: *AACN handbook of critical care nursing,* New York, 1997, McGraw-Hill Medical.
10. C.R. Bard, Inc: *Blakemore esophageal nasogastric tube package insert,* Covington, GA, 1998, C.R. Bard Inc.
11. Zimmerman TA: Thinking critically about the Sengstaken-Blakemore tube, *Crit Care Nurs* 6(3):72-75, 1986.
12. Lin TC, et al: Endoscopic placement of Sengstaken-Blakemore tube, *Journal of Clinical Gastroenterology* 31(1):29-32, 2000.
13. Kelly DJ, et al: Airway obstruction due to a Sengstaken-Blakemore tube, *Anesthesia Analgesia* 85(1):219-221, 1997.
14. Noble KA: Name that tube, *Nursing* 33(3):56-62, 2003.
15. Haddock G, et al: Esophageal tamponade in the management of acute variceal hemorrhage, *Digest Dis Sci* 34(6):913-918, 1998.

Additional Reading

Sengstaken RW, Blakemore AH: Balloon tamponade for the control of hemorrhage from esophageal varices, *Ann Surg* 131(5):781-789, 1950.

PROCEDURE **95**

Gastric Lavage

P U R P O S E : Gastric lavage is a method of flushing the stomach with water or saline solution with a large-bore gastric tube for the purpose of gastrointestinal decontamination, posttoxic ingestion, gentle blood and blood clot clearing, and active rewarming and as a cooling technique

Gretchen Delametter

PREREQUISITE KNOWLEDGE

- Child development as it relates to clinical assessment and gastric lavage
- Anatomy and physiology of the pediatric gastrointestinal (GI) tract, including structural characteristics specific to the infant and child[1,2]
- The narrowness of the nasal passage, especially in infants and young children, limits the ease of insertion of a large-bore tube; therefore, gastric lavage tubes may be more easily placed orally.
- Gastric lavage is contraindicated in a child who has ingested a corrosive substance or a hydrocarbon, who has ingested a sharp object, or who has a surgical or medical condition that increases the risk for hemorrhage or GI perforation.
- A child who cannot protect the airway should undergo intubation before gastric lavage.[3]
- Complications of gastric tube insertion include epistaxis; sinusitis; hydrothorax; pneumothorax, including tension pneumothorax; esophageal perforation; pneumonia; transbronchial insertion into the pleura; pleural effusion; inadvertent intracranial placement; nasal septum injury; vocal cord injury; and painful swallowing.[4-6]
- Controversy exists regarding the efficacy of gastric lavage more than 1 to 2 hours after a toxic ingestion. Even with performance in relative proximity to the ingestion, the amount of toxin recovered is dependent on whether the substance is liquid or in pill form.[4] Gastric

lavage 1 hour after ingestion is likely most helpful for medications that are enteric-coated, long-acting, and sustained-release. Children with sluggish gastric motility may also benefit from gastric lavage after the initial postingestion period.[4,7]

- To prevent aspiration, the recommended positioning for children undergoing gastric lavage is left lateral or semi-Fowler's position.[4]
- Room temperature sterile water and saline solution are the preferred irrigants for flushing blood and blood clots; iced solutions have no proven benefit.[4,8]
- The recommended solution for gastric lavage is saline solution in children less than 5 years old. Sterile water may cause hyponatremia in the young child or infant.
- Use of activated charcoal in gastric lavage may increase the risk of aspiration.[8]
- Warmed saline solution for hypothermia is effective; however, the child with obtunded hypothermia needs airway protection before the procedure. Rapid rewarming of the extremities without simultaneous core warming measures may cause a decrease in core temperature from the influx of cool blood centrally. Extremity rewarming alone may lead to dysrhythmias, acidosis, and cardiopulmonary arrest.
- Cold gastric lavage can be combined with evaporative cooling measures to treat the child with heatstroke. Cooling measures are discontinued when the rectal temperature reaches 40°C.

CHILD AND FAMILY ASSESSMENT

- Child's developmental level and ability to interact ➥*Rationale:* Child's developmental level influences preparation and interaction and assists in determining the level of cooperation that the child can provide.
- Child's and family's understanding of the reasons for and risks and benefits of gastric lavage ➥*Rationale:* Evaluates child's and family's understanding of the procedure and provides a gauge for ongoing education.
- History of nasal deformity, epistaxis, trauma, varices, recent esophageal or gastric surgery, esophageal malformations, or injuries ➥*Rationale:* These conditions may be causative or may complicate the procedure.
- Monitor cardiorespiratory, hemodynamic, and neurologic status ➥*Rationale:* Changes in vital signs may be the first indication of child's tolerance and complications. Certain types of ingestion may cause electrocardiogram changes.[9] Passage of the gastric lavage tube may cause vagal stimulation. Changes in oxygen saturation may indicate tube dislodgement, aspiration, or intolerance of procedure. Hypothermia and heatstroke intervention may cause changes in hemodynamic status or cardiac rhythm.
- Baseline chemistry profile, hemoglobin and hematocrit, coagulation studies, liver function tests, and serum or urine drug screen, as indicated ➥*Rationale:* Provides baseline information for following trends.
- Family's desire to be present during the procedure ➥*Rationale:* The family may provide support and comfort to the child but should have the choice not to remain with the child.

CHILD AND FAMILY EDUCATION

Individualized, developmentally appropriate education is provided to the family and to the child based on desire for knowledge, readiness to learn, and overall neurologic and psychosocial state.

- Explain the purpose of the gastric lavage and the steps and rationale for the procedure ➥*Rationale:* Providing information decreases anxiety and fear and may promote cooperation.
- If developmentally appropriate, explain to the child how to assist in the tube insertion (i.e., swallowing during tube

insertion) ➥*Rationale:* Elicits child's cooperation, which eases tube passage.
- Explain that tube insertion may be uncomfortable and may cause the child to gag ➥*Rationale:* Providing information decreases anxiety and fear.
- Explain the purpose of the cardiorespiratory monitor ➥*Rationale:* Provides information regarding need for monitoring and helps to reduce anxiety regarding the monitor and alarms.
- Evaluate need for information regarding accidental ingestions, hypothermia and heatstroke, and safety in the home ➥*Rationale:* Child and family may need information regarding prevention or treatment for accidental events.
- Encourage questions and answer questions as they arise ➥*Rationale:* Reinforcement of information is needed during periods of stress.

EQUIPMENT[4,8-13]

- Clean gloves
- Eye protective wear
- Face shield
- Protective gowns
- Lavage tube (large-bore)
- Irrigating syringe, 50-mL or 60-mL
- Irrigation bowl or irrigation kit
- Water-soluble lubricant
- Lavage fluid (sterile water or saline solution)
- Disposable basin for aspirate
- Sterile container for aspirate laboratory sample, as indicated
- Suction source and tubing
- Oropharyngeal suction tip catheter
- Y connector and infusion tubing for continuous lavage with drainage container
- Stethoscope
- Emergency intubation equipment (see Procedure 15)
- Endotracheal suction equipment (see Procedure 2)
- Cardiac/respiratory monitor, including pulse oximetry and blood pressure monitor and appropriately sized cuff (if noninvasive blood pressure), as indicated
- Rectal thermometer or temperature probe for continuous monitoring if necessary
- Guaiac paper
- pH paper
- Peripheral intravenous (IV) catheter and set for insertion, as indicated

Procedure for Gastric Lavage

Steps	Rationale	Considerations
1. Ensure child and family understand procedure and questions are answered.	Evaluates and reinforces understanding of previously taught information.	Developmental level, cognitive ability, and anxiety level influence approach to and effectiveness of teaching. Use an interpreter if patients and family are non-English speaking to ensure understanding before procedure.
2. Collect all necessary equipment and supplies.	Promotes completion of the procedure in a timely manner; may decrease child's anxiety.[4,9,11]	Tube size is determined on basis of child's size.
3. Wash hands. Put on clean gloves and other protective equipment.	Reduces the transmission of microorganisms. Protects personnel health.	
4. Ensure appropriate cardiopulmonary monitoring. Complete assessment, including laboratory parameters.	Children may decompensate during tube insertion.[4,9,11,12]	Consider the child's status in selection of appropriate cardiopulmonary monitoring. Ensure laboratory parameters are stable for procedure.
5. Consider placement of a peripheral IV based on the child's condition and treatment needs.	Critically ill children may have decompensation during procedure.	
6. Determine the length of tube to be inserted. Measure the tube from the tip of the child's nose to the earlobe, then from the earlobe to the xiphoid process (see Figure 186-1 in Procedure 186). • Record the nearest centimeter marking on the tube or use a marker or tape to indicate location. *(Level V*)*	Gives an approximation of tube length to insert. Distance from the tube entry point to the xyphoid process approximates the distance to the gastroesophageal junction. Tape or mark placed on the tube serves as a reference point if the tube becomes dislodged or is removed.	Results of a small study done in children birth to 7 years old showed that the nose to earlobe to xiphoid process (NEX) measurement may underestimate the appropriate depth of insertion.[14] *(Level IV*)*
7. Lubricate 6 to 10 cm of the distal end of tube with water-soluble lubricant.	Lubrication facilitates passage through nares. Minimizes mucosal injury and irritation during insertion.	Use only water-soluble lubricants for tube placement. Oil-soluble lubricants cannot be absorbed by the pulmonary mucosa and may cause respiratory complications should the tube be inadvertently placed into the lungs.[15]
8. *For oral placement:* Position the end of the tube downward and insert the tube into the oral cavity over the tongue. Aim the tube back and down toward the pharynx. When the tube hits the pharynx, flex the head forward (must have mobile C-spine). If appropriate, ask the child to take sips of water through a straw while the tube is advanced. *(Level IV*)*	Flexing the head of an unconscious child also facilitates tube insertion. When the child takes sips of water or mimics swallowing, the epiglottis closes the trachea and directs the tube toward the esophagus.	If the child is uncooperative, use of an oral airway or bite block may prevent the child from biting the tube. If the child coughs or begins gagging, withdraw slightly, stop insertion, and allow the child to rest. Allowing the child to rest may help to decrease the risk of aspiration.

Procedure continues on following page

* Level IV: Limited clinical studies to support recommendations
Level V: Clinical studies in more than one or two patient populations and situations to support recommendations

Procedure	for Gastric Lavage—*Continued*	
Steps	Rationale	Considerations

For nasal placement:
    Insert the tube into a patent nostril, aiming back and down. When the tube hits the pharynx, if the child is able and has a mobile C-spine, flex the child's head forward and have the child swallow. Advance the tube as the child swallows. *(Level IV*)*

Steps	Rationale	Considerations
9. Continue to insert the tube until the premarked centimeter on the tube is reached.	Advances the tube into the stomach.	If resistance is met, rotation of the tube may help placement. If unable to pass the tube after several attempts, notify the prescribing practitioner.
10. Aspirate and assess gastric content and test the pH level per institution-specific protocol. *(Level IV*)* Confirm placement with radiographic examination, as indicated. *(Level VI*)*	Aspirates with a pH level of 5.5 or less and the color grassy green, clear with white flecks, or brown indicate tube placement in the stomach.[5,14-17] *(Level IV*)* Radiography is considered the most reliable method of tube location confirmation.	In addition to pH level, also consider guaiac testing to provide baseline data.[4,8,10,11] Children undergoing H_2 blocker therapy have a pH level greater that 5.[15]
11. Secure tube (Figure 95-1).	Prevention of dislodgement or displacement.	
12. Place the child in semi-Fowler's position or on left lateral side if not otherwise contraindicated.	This positioning reduces the risk of aspiration. The left lateral position maximizes the approach to the stomach and minimizes pyloric emptying.[4,9,18]	
13. Aspirate gastric contents.	Hand aspiration withdraws gastric contents.	Gastric contents should be placed in basin for overt examination.[4,8-12]

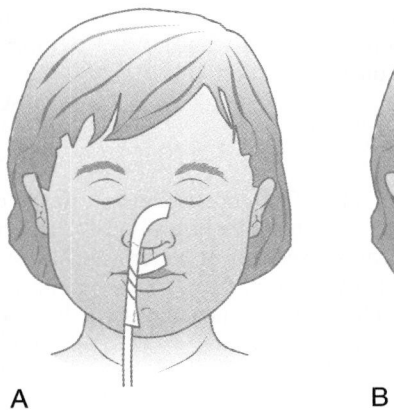
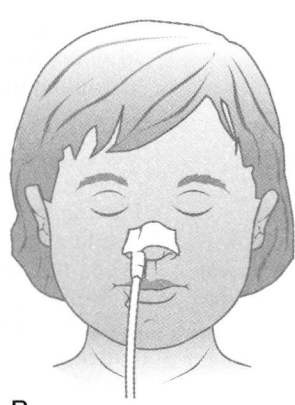

A   B

FIGURE 95-1   Securing of Nasoenteric Tube. One half of strip of tape is applied to nose. Split lower portion to tip of nose. **A,** Wrap one half of split tape around tube. **B,** In opposite direction, wrap second half of the tape around tube.

* Level IV: Limited clinical studies to support recommendations
  Level VI: Clinical studies in a variety of patient populations and situations to support recommendations

Procedure for Gastric Lavage—*Continued*

Steps	Rationale	Considerations
14. Load irrigating syringe with room temperature saline solution or water.	Room temperature fluid is effective in clearing blood and clots from the GI tract.	Cold gastric lavage may be helpful as an adjunct to other cooling measures in the treatment of heatstroke. Warmed saline solution may add in rewarming the child with hypothermia.
15. With syringe, instill solution into stomach via lavage tube.	Provides dilution to ingested toxins and rinses toxins from the GI tract (ingestion). Assists with freeing blood and clots from the GI tract (hemorrhage).	If gastric lavage is used for rewarming or cooling, the solution should have a dwell time before drainage and instillation of more fluid.
16. Aspirate gastric contents with instilled solution.	Remove unwanted fluids.	The same volume of irrigant instilled should return when syringe is aspirated.
17. Repeat steps 13 to 16 according to plan of care.	Multiple passes are often necessary to remove toxins (ingestions) and blood (hemorrhage).	For those children with GI hemorrhage, continue intermittent lavage until aspirated fluid returns to clear and is free of clots.
18. Clamp between lavage periods.	Prevents leakage of contents.	
19. Remove tube slowly, as indicated when no longer needed.	Minimizes vomiting risk.[4,11]	
20. Dispose of equipment and gastric content in appropriate receptacles.	Reduces transmission of micro organisms.	If requested, send aspirates for laboratory analysis.
21. Remove gloves, eye wear, gown, and face shield and wash hands.	Reduces transmission of microorganisms. Protects personnel health.	

Expected Outcomes

- Evacuation of gastric contents that contain ingested materials
- Evacuation of blood and clots from stomach

- The tip of the tube is correctly placed in the stomach without complications

- Prevention of absorption of ingested agents

- Rewarming measures successful
- Cooling measures successful
- The tube remains in place until elective removal

Unexpected Outcomes

- Inability to clear toxin or blood
- Trauma to upper GI tract (e.g., esophageal perforation)
- Tracheal or bronchial intubation
- Inadvertent pleural placement
- Inadvertent cranial placement
- Tube coiled in posterior pharynx or esophagus
- Hemodynamic instability
- Cardiac dysrhythmias
- Fluid and electrolyte imbalance
- Inability to stabilize core temperature

- Inadvertent tube removal by child, family, or health care team

Monitoring and Care of the Child

Activities and Interventions	Rationale	Reportable Conditions
1. Monitor cardiorespiratory status during and after procedure as plan of care dictates.	Physiologic parameters may change over time depending on absorption of ingested agent, loss of blood, and changes in temperature and hemodynamics.	• Significant changes in heart rate, respiratory rate, blood pressure, temperature, and pulse oximetry
2. Monitor neurologic status during and after procedure as plan of care dictates.	Side effects may cause changes in level of consciousness long after lavage.	• Altered level of consciousness or loss of gag reflex
3. Monitor the volume and characteristics of the lavage fluid.	Dictates the frequency and amount of gastric lavage.	• Inability to aspirate volume instilled • Continuous bloody output without resolution
4. Monitor laboratory data.	Laboratory data indicate changes in electrolytes, blood volume status, and toxin levels.	• Abnormal laboratory values

Documentation

- Tube size, confirmation of tube placement, and method of confirmation
- Lavage solution, including volume and type of fluid
- Gastric content, including description and volume of aspirate
- Laboratory data results
- Child's tolerance of the procedure
- Unexpected outcomes and related treatment
- Additional interventions and related outcomes, including medications administered
- Child and family education

References

1. Sentongo T, Steinhorn D: Gastrointestinal structure and function. In Fuhrman B, Zimmerman J, editors: *Pediatric critical care,* ed 3, Philadelphia, 2006, Mosby.
2. Thibodeau G, Patton K, editors: *Anatomy and physiology,* ed 5, Philadelphia, 2003, Mosby.
3. Mokhlesi B, et al: Adult toxicology in critical care: part I: general approaches to the intoxicated patient, *Chest* 123:577, 2003.
4. Phillips JK: Gastric lavage in hemorrhage and overdose. In Lynn-McHale Wiegand DJ, Carlson K, editors: *AACN procedure manual for critical care,* Philadelphia, 2005, Elsevier.
5. Metheny NA, Titler MG: Assessing placement of feeding tubes, *Am J Nurs* 101(5):36-45, 2001.
6. Baskin WN: Acute complications associated with bedside placement of feeding tubes, *Nutr Clin Pract* 21(1):40-55, 2006.
7. Blazys D: Use of lavage in treating overdose, *J Emerg Nurs* 26:343, 2000.
8. Bond G: The role of activated charcoal and gastric emptying in gastrointestinal decontamination: a state of the art review, *Ann Emerg Med* 39(3):273-286, 2002.
9. Tucker J: Indications for, techniques of, complications of, and efficacy of gastric lavage in the treatment of the poisoned child, *Curr Opin Pediatr* 12(2):163-165, 2000.
10. Bosse G, Barefoot J, Pfeifer M, et al: Comparison of three methods of gut decontamination in tricyclic antidepressant overdose, *J Emerg Med* 13(2):203-209, 1995.
11. Bowden V, Greenberg C: *Pediatric nursing procedures,* Baltimore, 2003, Lippincott Williams & Wilkins.
12. Shrestha M, George J, Chiu M, et al: A comparison of three gastric lavage methods using the radionuclide gastric emptying study, *J Emerg Med* 14(4):413-418, 1996.
13. Tintinalli J, Ruiz E, Krome R, editors: *Emergency medicine,* ed 4, New York, 1996, McGraw-Hill.
14. Dulak SB: Inserting an NG tube, *RN* 69(6):24,ac1-4, 2006.
15. Ellett ML, et al: Gastric tube placement in young children, *Clin Nurs Res* 14(3):238-252, 2005.
16. Nyqvist KH, et al: Litmus tests for verification of feeding tube location in infants: evaluation of their clinical use, *J Clin Nurs* 14:486-495, 2005.
17. Huffman S, et al: Methods to confirm feeding tube placement: application of research in practice, *Pediatr Nurs* 30(1):10-13, 2004.
18. Shannon M: Primary care: ingestion of toxic substances by children, *NEJM* 342:186, 2000.

Gastrostomy and Gastrostomy-Jejunostomy Tubes: Care and Management

P U R P O S E : Gastrostomy tubes and gastrostomy-jejunostomy tubes are feeding tubes placed through the abdominal wall into the stomach or jejunum to vent air and drainage and to provide medications, fluids, and nutrition. Gastrostomy and gastrostomy-jejunostomy tubes are indicated for children who cannot take adequate nutrition by mouth because of anomalies of the throat, esophagus, or bowel; respiratory distress; or severe debilitation or unconsciousness.

Shannon Stone McCord

PREREQUISITE KNOWLEDGE

- Child development as it relates to clinical assessment and care and management of the child with a gastrostomy (GT) or gastrostomy-jejunostomy (GJ) tube
- Anatomy and physiology of the pediatric gastrointestinal (GI) tract, including structural characteristics specific to the infant and child[1,2]
- GT and GJ tubes are indicated for children with GI tracts that are functional (food can be digested and absorbed) who are unable to swallow adequate oral nutrition, have gastric reflux, are at risk for aspiration, or need supplemental feeding therapy for more than 1 to 3 months.
- Enterostomies provide access to the GI tract through the abdominal wall via tubes that extend above the skin or are at the skin level via a low profile device or "button"[3]
- GT and GJ tubes can be inserted percutaneously or through a surgical incision
  - ❖ A percutaneous endoscopic gastrostomy (PEG) is a tube inserted with visualization of the stomach with an endoscope and with local anesthesia. The design of the tube is such that it is held in place (Figure 96-1).[4]
  - ❖ A surgically placed tube is inserted with general anesthesia in the operating room. An incision is made in

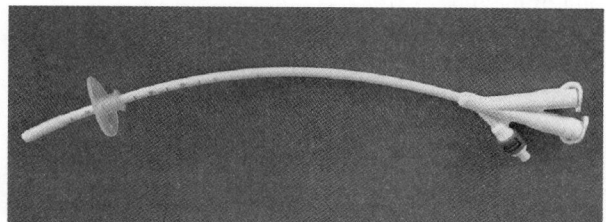

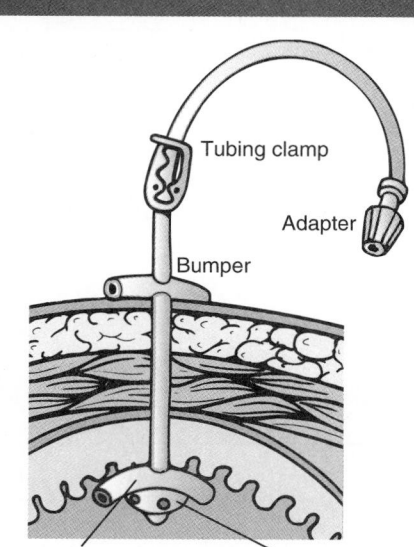

Tubing clamp

Adapter

Bumper

Internal cross bar   Mushroom catheter tip

FIGURE 96-1   Percutaneous endoscopic gastrostomy placed into stomach. *Perry A, Potter P:* Clinical nursing skills and techniques, *ed 5, Philadelphia, 2004, Mosby.*

the upper left quadrant of the abdomen. The tube is secured with a purse-string suture to the stomach and abdominal wall.

- Postoperative complications of enterostomy tube placement include site leakage, skin infection, formation of granulation tissue, discomfort, internal tube migration that causes erosions or obstructions, vomiting, and diarrhea.
- A low profile device is a skin level device with a one-way valve, an internal anchor, and external anchor, and a connecting device (Figure 96-2).[4] "Buttons" are usually substituted 4 to 8 weeks after the GT is initially placed. The appropriate decompression and feeding tube devices must be used with these tubes for adequate decompression of the stomach and reduction of bloating of the stomach and leaking and for prevention of breakage of the one-way valve. Low profile devices usually last several months and are replaced when the valve fails or the tube leaks (see Procedure 90).
- GJ tubes are indicated for children who are prone to aspiration and who have gastric motility disorders.[27]
- GJ tubes are small-bore flexible feeding tubes with a stylet threaded through the gastrostomy tube or stoma into the jejunum (Figure 96-3). The stylet is removed after placement.
- GJ tubes generally have three ports: a jejunal port for feeding, a gastric port for suction and drainage, and a balloon port for inflation and deflation of the balloon (Figure 96-4).
- GJ tubes should *not* be rotated. Rotation can cause kinking of the tube.

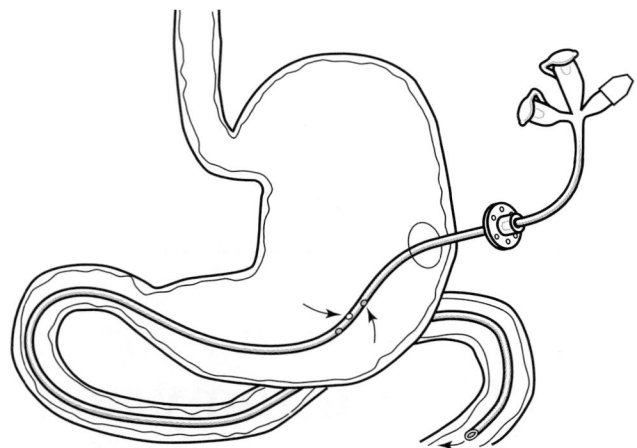

FIGURE 96-3 Gastrostomy-jejunostomy Tube Placement. Gastrostomy-jejunostomy tube placed with endoscopic insertion. GJ tubes are small-bore flexible feeding tubes threaded through gastrostomy button or stoma into jejunum. *From Rolandelli R, et al:* Clinical nutrition: enteral and tube feeding, *ed 4, Philadelphia, 2005, Elsevier.*

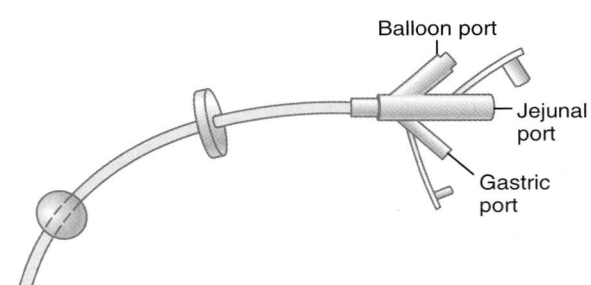

FIGURE 96-4 Gastrostomy-jejunostomy Tube. Gastrostomy-jejunostomy tubes generally have three ports: jejunal port for feeding, gastric port for suction and drainage, and balloon port for inflation and deflation of balloon.

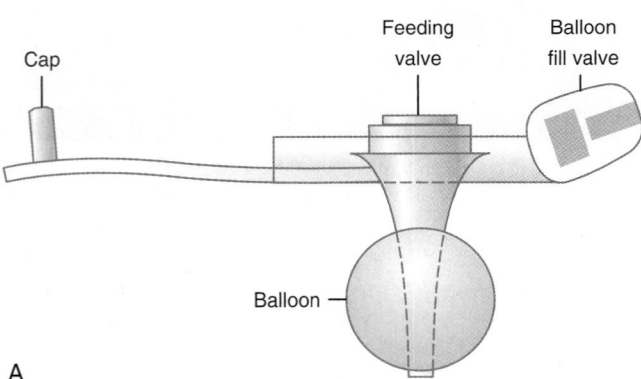

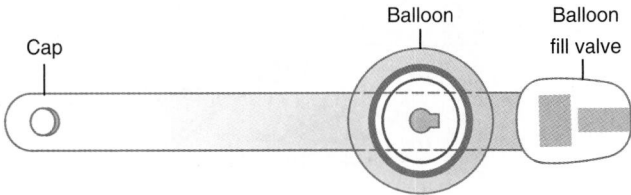

FIGURE 96-2 Gastrostomy "button" is skin level device with one-way valve, internal anchor, external anchor, and connecting device. **A,** Side view. **B,** Top view (as seen once inserted).

- Risks to GT and GJ tube placement may include hemorrhage, bowel perforation, peritonitis, wound separation, infection, and bowel obstruction from the operative procedure.
- Gastrostomy and GJ tubes can be stabilized with a tube holder or baby nipple, which assists in stabilization of the tube and prevention of dilation of the stoma.[5]
- The formation of granulation tissue is a normal occurrence around a stoma site. The tube stimulates production of epithelial tissue. The treatment for granulation tissue is chemical burn of the tissue with silver nitrate. Granulation tissue has no sensation.[6]

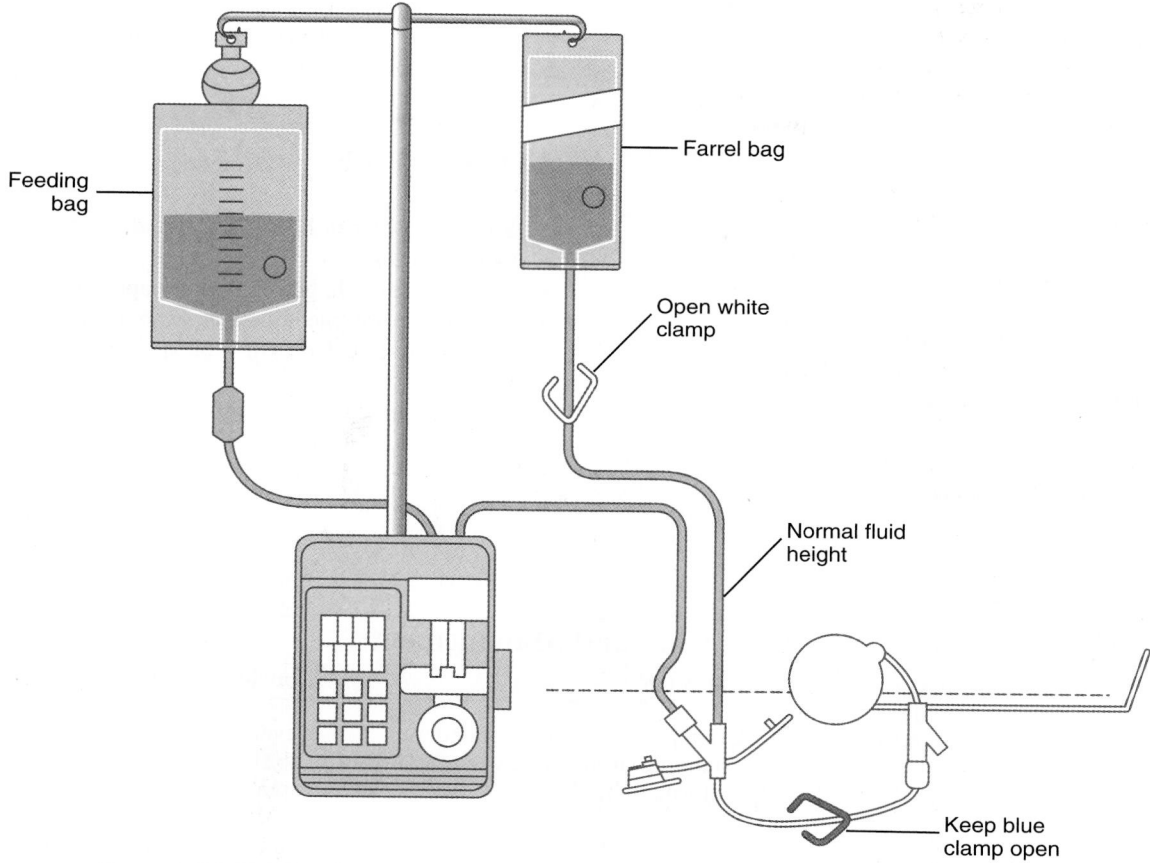

FIGURE 96-5   Farrell valve bag. Vent via Y tubing (Farrell valve) for at least 30 minutes after feedings.

- A Farrell valve bag (CORPAK MedSystems, Wheeling, IL) is used in children with poor gastric motility who are undergoing enteral feedings via a gastrostomy or GJ tube (Figure 96-5). This device decompresses the stomach and provides an outlet for gastric contents.
- Education regarding the placement of GT and GJ tubes occurs before surgery or before the procedure to prepare the child and family. Pictures of the GI anatomy or of other children with GT or GJ tubes often assist the family in understanding aspects of the tube and assists them with appropriate questions.

CHILD AND FAMILY ASSESSMENT

- Child's developmental level and ability to interact ➻**Rationale:** Child's developmental level influences preparation and interaction and assists in determining the level of cooperation that the child can provide.
- Child's and family's understanding of the reasons for and risks and benefits of the procedure ➻**Rationale:** Evaluates child's and family's understanding and provides a gauge for ongoing education.

- Tube site condition, including skin redness, rash, edema, drainage, and excess granulation tissue ➻**Rationale:** Assesses skin integrity and determines the need for topical barrier creams or medication and dressings. Scant tan or serous yellow drainage or crusting is normal.
- Signs of gastric distention (e.g., vomiting, nausea, absence of or hypoactive bowel sounds) ➻**Rationale:** Secretions or air in the stomach increase the risk of aspiration and leakage.
- Gastrointestinal symptoms, including diarrhea and vomiting ➻**Rationale:** Identification of the child's feeding tolerance.[7-9]
- Family's desire to be present during the procedure ➻**Rationale:** The family may provide support and comfort to the child but should have the choice not to remain with the child.

CHILD AND FAMILY EDUCATION

Individualized, developmentally appropriate education is provided to the family and to the child based on desire for knowledge, readiness to learn, and overall neurologic and psychosocial state.

- Provide information regarding the reason for GT or GJ tube and explain the steps involved in tube insertion ➤➤*Rationale:* Providing information decreases anxiety and fear.
- Explain the purpose of the GT and GJ tube care and the steps involved in the procedure ➤➤*Rationale:* Providing information decreases anxiety and fear and may promote cooperation.
- Explain the need for device stabilization ➤➤*Rationale:* Prevents the need for reinsertion or additional x-ray and prevention of potential leaking.
- Stress the importance of not pulling on the tube and provide strategies for keeping the device in place ➤➤*Rationale:* Avoids unnecessary pain and skin irritation.

- Encourage questions and answer questions as they arise ➤➤*Rationale:* Reinforcement of information is needed during periods of stress.

EQUIPMENT

- Soap and water or half-strength hydrogen peroxide
- Cotton swabs
- Clean wash cloth, gauze, or soft paper towel
- Skin barrier ointment, cream, swab, or wipe (optional)
- Foam fenestrated dressing or split gauze (optional for leaking)
- Clean gloves

Procedure | for GT or GJ Tubes: Care and Management

Steps	Rationale	Considerations
1. Ensure child and family understand procedure and questions are answered.	Evaluates and reinforces understanding of previously taught information.	Developmental level, cognitive ability, and anxiety level influence approach to and effectiveness of teaching. Use an interpreter if family is non-English speaking to ensure understanding before procedure.
2. Collect all necessary equipment and supplies.	Promotes completion of the procedure in a timely manner; may decrease child's anxiety.	Assessment of the tube site before the procedure helps determine the supplies needed.
3. Wash hands and put on clean gloves.	Reduces the transmission of microorganisms. Protects personnel health.	
4. Remove old dressing and tube stabilizer (if present). Check for skin redness, rash, edema, drainage, and excess granulation tissue.	Evaluates the presence of infection, leaking, cellulitis, and dermatitis.	If infection is suspected, a culture of the site may be necessary. If leaking is present, assess the tube for proper size, balloon functioning, and tube stability.
5. Clean the skin around the tube site with soap and water. *(Level VI*)* Dry the skin completely.	Cleansing of the skin helps prevent infection by removing the drainage that migrates from the gastrostomy tract. Ensuring that the skin is dry protects the skin from moisture and acidic secretions.[5,10]	Especially with new stomas (less than 6 weeks), consider cleaning with half-strength hydrogen peroxide. The effervescence of hydrogen peroxide may provide some mechanical benefit to loosening debris and blood and necrotic tissue. Hydrogen peroxide may also dry the skin. *(Level II*)*

* Level II: Theory-based; no research data to support recommendations; recommendations from expert consensus group may exist
  Level VI: Clinical studies in a variety of patient populations and situations to support recommendations

Procedure	**for GT or GJ Tubes: Care and Management**—*Continued*	
Steps	**Rationale**	**Considerations**
6. Consider application of a skin barrier cream or ointment (e.g., petrolatum, zinc-based) if the site is leaking or red. *(Level VI*)*	Protects the skin from moisture and acidic secretions.[11]	For a fungal rash, a fungal cream, ointment, or powder is used around the site.
7. Apply a foam dressing or one split gauze, if drainage is present (Figure 96-6, *A*). *(Level V*)*	A dressing wicks away drainage from the skin.[5,12]	Foam dressings are more absorbent and wick away more drainage than gauze dressings, which the keeps skin drier and less prone to dermatitis and skin breakdown. When drainage is not present, no dressing is necessary (Figure 95-6, *B*). A pouching system protects the skin from large amounts of fluid leaking and prevents further skin irritation and breakdown.[5,13]
8. Flush tubing. *GT:* Flush with 5 to 10 mL tap water after medications and with feedings. For children with fluid restriction or for infants, 1 to 5 mL is typically adequate. *GJ tubes:* Flush gastric and jejunal ports every 4 to 6 hours with 5 to 10 mL of warm tap water in children and 1 to 5 mL of water in infants. *(Level II*)*	Flushing keeps the tube patent and reduces drug/food interactions between the medications and formula.[8,14-17]	The weight of the child and other comorbidities are considered in the appropriate amount of flush volume. The volume of flush is also determined by the amount of fluid needed to clear the dead space of the tube. For a low profile device, a syringe may be used to directly inject flush into the "button."

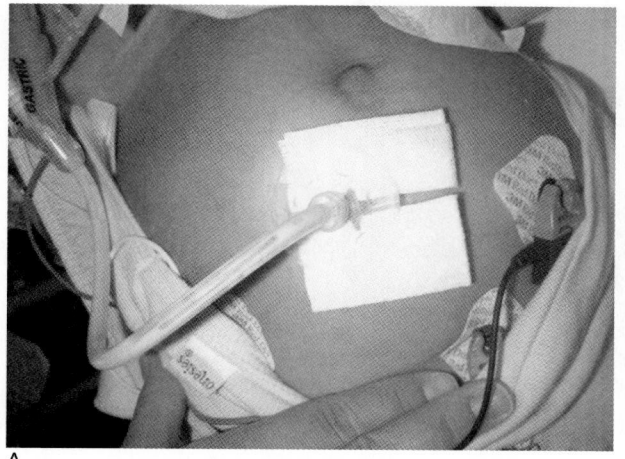
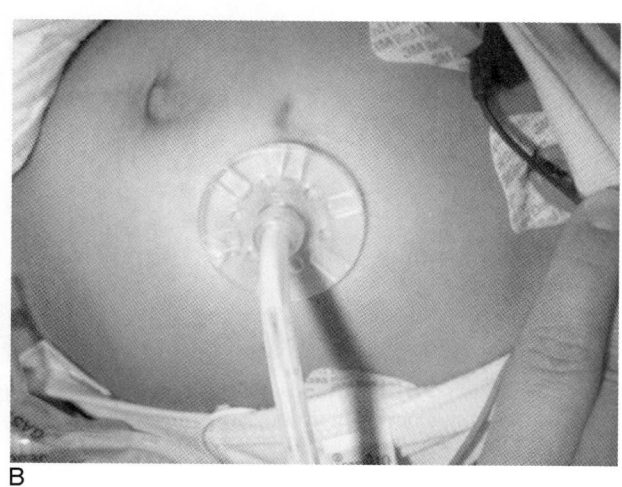

A   B

FIGURE 96-6   **A,** Gastrostomy tube with one split gauze, applied if drainage is present. **B,** Gastrostomy tube site without dressing. When drainage is not present, no dressing is necessary.

Procedure continues on following page

* Level II: Theory-based; no research data to support recommendations; recommendations from expert consensus group may exist
Level V: Clinical studies in more than one or two patient populations and situations to support recommendations
Level VI: Clinical studies in a variety of patient populations and situations to support recommendations

Procedure	for GT or GJ Tubes: Care and Management—*Continued*	
Steps	**Rationale**	**Considerations**

9. Vent tubing.
    GT: Vent via syringe or Y tubing (Farrell valve) for at least 30 minutes after feedings (Figure 96-5).
    Low profile device: Vent via appropriate decompression or feed set tube for at least 30 minutes after feedings.
    GJ: Vent via gastric port with gravity drainage. Do not use continuous or high intermittent suction. *(Level II*)*
	Gastric decompression.
	The pressure may collapse the tube or injure the stomach tissue and cause bleeding.	

Administer Feedings
10. Check placement.
    GT: Attach a syringe and withdraw gastric aspirate *or* lower syringe below stomach level and check for gastric aspirate in syringe.
    Gastric low profile device: Attach decompression tube and check for gastric aspirate.
    GJ tube: Check centimeter marking on tube. If tube has changed from the recorded measurement, contact the practitioner.
	Prevents feedings from being misplaced outside the stomach or jejunum.[7,8,14-18]	Do not discard residuals because they contain valuable electrolytes that may be refed.
		For large residuals, stop or slow feeding rate.
		Tube placement is most reliably confirmed with abdominal radiography with contrast. *(Level IV*)*
		For GJ tubes, there is no need to check gastric aspirate.

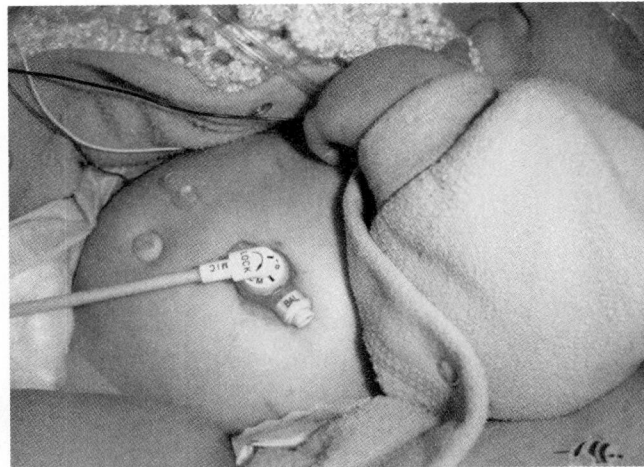

FIGURE 96-7   Gastrostomy Button. For feeding via gastrostomy button, feeding set adapter is inserted into gastrostomy port with firm twist.

* Level II: Theory-based; no research data to support recommendations; recommendations from expert consensus group may exist
Level IV: Limited clinical studies to support recommendations

Procedure for GT or GJ Tubes: Care and Management—*Continued*

Steps	Rationale	Considerations

11. Attach tubing.
    GT: Attach a tube adaptor to the end of the GT and then attach the tube feeding.
    Low profile device: Insert the feed set adaptor to the gastrostomy port with a firm twist (Figure 96-7).
	Provides connection between the feeding tubing and the tube or low profile device.
	For low profile devices, use of the specific feeding tube adaptor made by the manufacturer is especially important.
		The incorrect adaptor may break the one-way valve, necessitating a new device.[15,16]
		The Mic-Key button has one tube for feeding and venting air.
		The BARD button has two tubes: one tube for feeding and one tube for venting.

12. Infuse feedings.
 • *Intermittent feedings:*
    a. Connect feeding syringe and tubing to the feed set tubing.
    b. Instill formula slowly with gravity flow for at least 20 to 30 minutes.
    c. Flush with water or air (see step 8).
    d. Vent the GT tube of gas (see step 9).
    e. Disconnect the feeding and close the "button."
 • *Continuous feedings:*
 GT:
    a. Prime the feeding tubing with the formula.
    b. Connect to the feeding set adaptor and set feeding rate as ordered.
 • *GJ tube:*
    a. Connect the primed feeding tube set connector to the jejunal port (Figure 96-8).
    b. Set the ordered pump rate and start the pump.
    c. Flush the jejunal and gastric ports (see step 8).
	Prevents cramping, diarrhea, and vomiting.[7]
	Reduces abdominal bloating and leaking.[14-17]
	GJ feedings are always administered continuously because of the volume restrictions of the jejunum.
	Minimizes the potential for clogging the small lumen of the jejunal tube.[12,15,16-19]
		Consider raising the head of the bed to help prevent aspiration for feeding administered via gastrostomy.
		If formula appears in the gastric port, stop the feedings and notify the physician. *(Level VI*)*

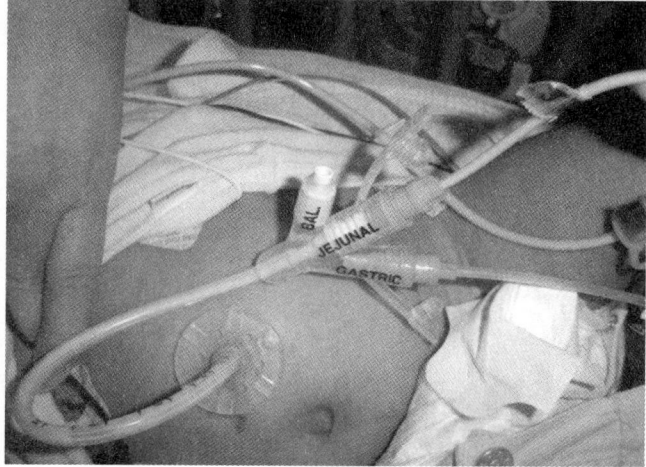

FIGURE 96-8   Feeding with gastrostomy-jejunostomy tube. Primed feeding tube set is connected to jejunal port.

Procedure continues on following page

* Level VI: Clinical studies in a variety of patient populations and situations to support recommendations

Procedure   for GT or GJ Tubes: Care and Management—*Continued*

Steps	Rationale	Considerations
13. Separate feeding set from feeding port and cleanse connection with soap and water. Disconnect.	Removes oily build-up and keeps the connection clean.[15,16]	
14. Rinse feeding sets, syringes, and tubing with warm tap water every 4 hours before refilling with formula or per policy.	Reduces bacterial contamination.[7,8,19]	Change tubing sets every 24 hours.
Administer Medication		
15. Verify placement (see step 10).	Prevents medications from being misplaced outside the stomach or jejunum.[7,8,14-18]	Use a syringe no smaller than 10 mL to avoid excess pressure and potential tube rupture.
16. Consider checking tube for patency by flushing with air or water (see step 8).	Flushing keeps the tube patent and reduces drug/food interactions between the medications and formula or milk.[8,9,14,20]	
17. Prepare medication.	Administering medications in liquid form minimizes the risk of clogging the tube.	If tablets or powders are used, they must be mixed with 10 to 20 mL of warm water to prevent the tube from clogging.
18. Connect to medication syringe. • *GT low profile device:* Connect to the medication or feeding port and push in the medication. • *GJ tubes:* Connect the medication syringe to the GT port of the tube and push in medications.	Medications can be given directly into the GI tract.	Depending on the pharmacokinetics of the medication, some medications may be given via the jejunal port.
19. Flush the tube (see step 8). *(Level IV*)*	Clears the medication from the tube, prevents drug/food interactions, and promotes tube patency.	
Tube Dislodgement and Reinsertion		
20. Cover the opening with a dry gauze dressing.	Prevents leakage and injury to stoma.	Displacement is usually the result of balloon underinflation or slipping of the tube.
21. Replace tube. *GT:* See Procedure 90. *GJ tube:* Contact the practitioner who inserted the tube and follow manufacturer's guidelines for repositioning. *(Level I*)*	Safe replacement of the tube.	Generally, replacement should occur within 4 to 6 hours because the stoma may close.

* Level I: Manufacturer's recommendations only
Level IV: Limited clinical studies to support recommendations

Expected Outcomes	Unexpected Outcomes
• Gastrostomy site remains healthy and free from complications and infection • Patent tube/device provides fluids, medications, and nutrition	• Cellulitis • Dermatitis • Leaking • Obstructive granulation tissue • Tube clogging • Tube dislodgement

Monitoring and Care of the Child

Activities and Interventions	Rationale	Reportable Conditions
1. Monitor the site for redness, rash, blisters, pain, odor, site drainage, or granulation tissue.	Determines the condition of the site and any necessary interventions.	• Cellulitis • Dermatitis • Red maculopapular rash • Bleeding; extra tissue growing around the stoma
2. Cleanse the site with soap and water and dry once to twice daily. (*Level VI**)	Cleansing and good hygiene reduce the bacterial load and reduce the chance of infection.[5,10]	• Unresolved or worsening redness, rash, swelling, pain, odor, drainage, or granulation tissue
3. Rotate GT "button" in a circle one to two times with care.	Assists with tube and track integrity.	• Clogged tube • Disruption in skin integrity
4. Monitor the GT/GJ for leakage of formula around the site.	The balloon may be leaking or may need to be reinflated, or the one valve may be broken, necessitating tube replacement.	• Leaking tube • Dilated stoma • Balloon deflated or ruptured • Improper balloon or tube placement • Tube dislodgement
5. Apply cream or ointment, as indicated. • To protect the skin, apply a barrier zinc-based or petrolatum-based cream, ointment, or nonalcohol skin preparation solution.	Barrier creams and ointments assist in protection of the skin and prevention of skin breakdown.[21]	• Unresolved or worsening redness, rash, swelling, odor, or drainage
• For fungal rash, apply antifungal powder, cream, or ointment.	Protects the skin and treats the yeast.	
6. For moderate to large drainage or leakage, consider application of a fenestrated foam dressing or ostomy pouch.	Foam dressings are more absorbable than gauze dressings and wick drainage away from the skin, thus decreasing skin irritation and a favorable environment for yeast and skin breakdown.	• Disruption in skin integrity despite treatment • Inadequate absorbency with current treatment plan
7. For granulation tissue, consider application of silver nitrate to granulation tissue twice weekly until resolved.	Provides treatment and better stabilizes the tube.[11,22]	• Unresolving or excessive granulation tissue • Burnt healthy tissue
8. Flush before and after medications and formula administration (see Procedure step 8).	Prevents clogging of the tube with formula or medication.[12,23]	• Clogged tube
9. *GT:* Check residuals every 4 hours or before feedings/medications.	Identifies the GI intolerance.[7,9]	• Residuals greater than or equal to two times the hourly rate

Documentation

- Size and type of tube placed
- Length of tube placed (GJ tube)
- Condition at tube site
- Tube patency
- Child's tolerance of procedure
- Child and family involvement in care
- Additional interventions and related outcomes
- Unexpected outcomes and related treatment
- Child and family education

References

1. Sentongo T, Steinhorn D: Gastrointestinal structure and function. In Fuhrman B, Zimmerman J, editors: *Pediatric critical care,* ed 3, Philadelphia, 2006, Mosby.
2. Thibodeau G, Patton K, editors: *Anatomy and physiology,* ed 5, Philadelphia, 2003, Mosby.
3. Rolandelli R, et al: *Clinical nutrition: enteral and tube feeding,* ed 4, Philadelphia, 2005, Elsevier.
4. Perry A, Potter P: *Clinical nursing skills and techniques,* ed 5, Philadelphia, 2004, Mosby.
5. Bryant RA: *Acute and chronic wounds: nursing management,* St. Louis, 1992, Mosby.
6. Smith P: *Care of the child with a gastrostomy tube/button, esophageal atresia,* retrieved October 25, 2006, from http://www.eatif.org/tube-button.html.
7. *American Society for Enteral and Parental Nutrition (ASPEN) guidelines,* 26(Suppl):1, 2002.
8. Eisenberg P: Enteral nutrition: indications, formulas, and delivery techniques, *Nurs Clin North Am* 24(2):1989.
9. US Department of Health and Human Services and Maternal Child Health Bureau: *Gaining and growing: assessing nutritional care of preterm infants: technical aspects of enteral feeding (tube feeding),* 2000.
10. Drousou A, et al: Antiseptics in wounds: area of controversy, *Wounds* 15(5):149-166, 2003.
11. Metry DW, Herbert AA: Topical therapies and medications in the pediatric patient, *Pediatr Clin North Am* 47(4):867-874, 2000.
12. Krasner D: *Chronic wound care: a clinical source book for healthcare professionals,* ed 3, Wayne, PA, 2001, HMP Publications, Inc.
13. Irving S, et al: Nutrition for the critically ill child: enteral and parenteral support, *AACN Clin Iss* 11(4):541-558, 2000.
14. Burd A, Burd RS: *Adv Neonatal Care* 3(4):197-205, 2003.
15. Ballard: *MIC-KEY care guide,* Draper, UT, 1999, Ballard Medical Products.
16. Ballard: *MIC transgastric jejunal feeding tube patient care guidelines,* Draper, UT, 1995, Ballard Medical Products.
17. Wong D et al: Pediatric variations of nursing interventions. In *Wong's nursing care of infants and children,* ed 7, St.Louis, 2003, Mosby.
18. Ross Medical Nutritional System: *Preventing microbial contamination of enteral formulas and delivery systems,* 1-28, 1996.
19. Centers for Disease Control and Prevention: *Enterobacter sakazakii* infections associated with the use of powdered infant formula, *MMWR Weekly* 2004.
20. Guenter P: *Administering medications via feeding tubes: what consultant pharmacists need to know,* 1999, Society of Consultant Pharmacists, Inc.
21. Metheny N, et al: Effect of feeding tube properties and three irrigants on clogging rates, *Nurs Res* 37(3):165-169, 1988.
22. Dunford C: Hypergranulation tissue: a review of the formation, causes and management of hypergranulation tissue, *J Wound Care* 8:506-507, 1999.
23. Belknap D, et al: *Am J Crit Care* 6(5):383-392, 1997.

Additional Readings

Baker S, et al: *Pediatric enteral nutrition,* New York, 1994, Chapman and Hall.

Cincinnati Children's Hospital Medical Center: *Gastrostomy-jejunostomy tube care, patient education program, parent education program II,* Cincinnati, 2003, Cincinnati Children's Hospital Medical Center.

Guenter P, et al: Enteral nutrition therapy, *Nurs Clin North Am* 32:651-668, 1997.

Guenter P, Silkroski M: *Tube feeding: clinical guidelines and nursing protocols,* Gaithersburg, MD, 2001, ASPEN.

Hagelgans NA, Janusz BH: Pediatric skin care issues for the home care nurse: part 2, *Pediatr Nurs* 20(1): 1994.

Rollins H: Hypergranulation tissue at gastrostomy sites, *J Wound Care* 9:127-129, 2000.

Rombeau JL, Rolandelli RH, editors: *Enteral and tube feeding,* ed 3, Philadelphia, 1997, Saunders.

Intraabdominal Pressure Monitoring

P U R P O S E : Pressure is monitored within the abdominal cavity to uncover intraabdominal hypertension, to quickly address abdominal compartment syndrome, and to minimize any related complications

Cynthia A. Gould

PREREQUISITE KNOWLEDGE

- Child development as it relates to clinical assessment and intraabdominal pressure (IAP) monitoring, including urinary catheterization
- Anatomy and physiology of the pediatric gastrointestinal (GI) and urinary tracts, including structural characteristics specific to the infant and child[1]
- Principles of aseptic technique
- IAP can be measured directly via a catheter inserted into the abdomen or indirectly with an indwelling catheter inserted into the bladder[2-6]
- IAP is serially measured and correlated with other assessment findings.[2,3]
- Relevant terms, as defined by The World Congress on the Abdominal Compartment Syndrome (WCACS), include[2]:
  - ❖ Intraabdominal pressure: The pressure within the abdominal cavity, measured at end expiration, expressed in millimeters of Mercury (mm Hg), with the child supine and the transducer zeroed at the midaxillary line
  - ❖ Bladder pressure obtained with continuous irrigation with a three-way indwelling bladder catheter is considered the "gold standard" for indirect continuous IAP measurement.
  - ❖ Abdominal perfusion pressure (APP): IAP – mean arterial pressure (MAP)
- IAP parameters[3]
  - ❖ Normal: 0 to 5 mm Hg
  - ❖ Mildly elevated: 10 to 20 mm Hg
- ❖ Moderately elevated: 20 to 40 mm Hg
- ❖ Severe elevation: >40 mm Hg
- ❖ Intraabdominal hypertension (IAH): An IAP of 12 mm Hg or more with use of three standardized measurements obtained 4 to 6 hours apart or an APP of 60 mm Hg or less with use of two standardized measurements obtained 1 to 6 hours apart
- ❖ Abdominal compartment syndrome (ACS): Organ system dysfunction that occurs as a result of an acute increase in IAP.[5]
  - ○ The WCACS defines ACS as an IAP of 20 mm Hg or more with or without APP of less than 50 mm Hg with use of two standardized measurements obtained 1 to 6 hours apart and single or multiple organ system failure not previously present.
  - ○ Primary ACS: Condition associated with injury or disease of the abdominopelvic region or a condition that develops after abdominal surgery.
  - ○ Secondary ACS: Conditions that do not originate from the abdomen (e.g., sepsis or capillary leak, burns) that result in the signs and symptoms seen with primary ACS.
- Abdominal decompression may be recommended when IAP reaches 25 to 30 mm Hg.[4,5]
- Parameter recommendations are based on adult data. Limited research is available regarding normal IAP in the pediatric population.
- Factors that may affect the accuracy of IAP measurements include[3]:
  - ❖ Neurogenic bladder
  - ❖ Abdominal packing

- ❖ Pelvic fracture or hematoma
- ❖ Intraperitoneal adhesions
- ❖ Head of bed elevation
- ❖ Previous abdominal or genitourinary surgery
- Common causes of IAH [2,5,6]
  - ❖ Blunt abdominal trauma with intraabdominal bleeding from splenic, hepatic, and mesenteric injury
  - ❖ Pelvic trauma
  - ❖ Bowel obstruction
  - ❖ Abdominal masses
  - ❖ Peritonitis
  - ❖ Abdominal surgery
  - ❖ Liver transplant
  - ❖ Interstitial edema as a result of massive fluid resuscitation
  - ❖ Pneumoperitoneum during laparoscopic procedures
- Pathophysiologic effects of IAH on other body systems[2,5,6]
  - ❖ Decreased cardiac output (CO) from decreased venous return
  - ❖ Impaired pulmonary function related to increased intrathoracic pressure that results in decreased lung compliance, increased airway pressures, and decreased tidal volume
  - ❖ Renal dysfunction from decreased CO that results in decreased renal plasma flow and decreased glomerular filtration rate
  - ❖ Increased intracranial pressure (ICP) from increased central venous pressures; increased ICPs have been associated with IAP of more than 25 mm Hg
  - ❖ Venous stasis in the legs
- Indications for IAP monitoring[2,3]
  - ❖ Postoperative period after abdominal surgery
  - ❖ Period after open or blunt abdominal trauma
  - ❖ Distended abdomen and clinical assessment consistent with ACS: Oliguria, hypoxia, increased peak end expiratory pressures, hypotension, change in neurologic examination results
- Indwelling urinary catheter placement in the child (see Procedure 108)
- An absolute contraindication for insertion of a urinary catheter is suspected urethral tear.
- Complications related to indwelling catheters: Bladder spasms, trauma, urethral tear or perforation, catheter encrustation, urethral strictures, catheter knotting, and urinary tract infection[7-9]
- Appropriate set up, use, and troubleshooting of hemodynamic monitoring systems (see Procedure 63)

CHILD AND FAMILY ASSESSMENT

- Child's developmental level and ability to interact ➤➤*Rationale:* Child's developmental level influences preparation and interaction; urinary catheterization is particularly threatening to preschool and school-aged children.[10]
- Child's and family's understanding of the reasons for and risks and benefits of the procedure ➤➤*Rationale:* Evaluates

child's and family's understanding of the procedure and provides a gauge for ongoing education.

- History of abdominal surgery or genitourinary tract abnormalities, including perforation ➤➤*Rationale:* These conditions may affect accuracy of IAP monitoring.
- History of blunt abdominal trauma ➤➤*Rationale:* IAH can develop after blunt abdominal trauma.
- Previous catheterizations ➤➤*Rationale:* A negative experience with catheterization may increase the child's anxiety and decrease the child's ability to cooperate with the procedure.[11,12]
- History of allergy to povidone-iodine; allergy to lidocaine if topical anesthetic is to be used for urinary catheterization ➤➤*Rationale:* Procedure may need to be modified based on allergies to these substances.
- Family's and child's concerns about the procedure, including culturally related concerns concerning urinary catheterization ➤➤*Rationale:* Parents from some cultures may fear that catheterization of the female results in loss of virginity.[10]
- Family's desire to be present during the procedure ➤➤*Rationale:* Family may provide support and comfort measures to the child but should have the choice not to remain with the child during the procedure.

CHILD AND FAMILY EDUCATION

Individualized, developmentally appropriate information is provided to the family and to the child based on desire for knowledge, readiness to learn, and overall neurologic and psychosocial state.

- Provide information regarding the procedure for IAP monitoring, including specific steps in the procedure and an explanation of the equipment ➤➤*Rationale:* Providing information may decrease fear and anxiety, foster trust, and facilitate cooperation.
- Provide information on the child's condition as it relates to IAP monitoring and identification of IAH ➤➤*Rationale:* Providing information facilitates child's and family's understanding of potential outcomes of undiagnosed IAH.
- Provide information about the risks and benefits of the procedure ➤➤*Rationale:* Supports the family's right to information concerning the procedure and encourages participation in the child's care.
- Encourage questions and answer questions as they arise ➤➤*Rationale:* Reinforcement of information is needed during periods of stress.

EQUIPMENT

If the standard two-way bladder catheter is used, refer to Procedure 108.

If a three-way bladder catheter is to be placed, refer to Procedure 107.

- Sterile urine collection system
- 10-mL to 20-mL syringe
- Sterile 0.9% saline solution
- 18-gauge needle, if sampling port on urine collection system does not have a needleless access device
- Povidone-iodine or other antiseptic per institution-specific protocol
- Short pressure tubing extension with luer lock

- Transducer set up with standard pressure tubing (or manometer if transducer unavailable)
- Three-way stopcock
- Clamp
- A preassembled IAP monitoring device, such as the AbViser AutoValve (Wolfe Tory Medical, Inc, Salt Lake City, Utah); substituted for the syringe, needle, pressure tubing, transducer, and stopcock

Procedure | for Intraabdominal Pressure Monitoring

Steps	Rationale	Considerations
1. Ensure child and family understand procedure and questions are answered.	Evaluates and reinforces understanding of previously taught information.	Developmental level, cognitive ability, and anxiety level determine approach to and effectiveness of teaching.
2. Gather needed equipment and supplies.	Facilitates completion of task in a timely manner.	Bladder catheter size is dependent on age and size of child (see Table 108-1 in Procedure 108).
3. Ensure appropriate cardiopulmonary monitoring.	Decompensation may occur during procedures in some children.	Consider child's status in selection of appropriate level of monitoring.
4. Wash hands. *(Level VI*)*	Reduces transmission of micro-organisms.	
5. With aseptic technique, assemble transducer and prime with 0.9% saline solution.	Fluid-filled system is required to transmit pressure reading and waveform to monitor display.	
6. Attach the free end of the transducer tubing to the three-way stopcock; attach the short extension tubing to the male end of the stopcock (Figure 97-1). Prime tubing and all stopcock ports with 0.9% saline solution.	Fluid-filled system is required to transmit pressure reading and waveform to monitor display.	
7. Connect the transducer system to the bedside monitor and ensure system is functioning. Select an appropriate scale (Figure 97-2).	Allows display of IAP reading and waveform.	
8. If necessary, place bladder catheter (see Procedure 108).	Bladder catheter is used to obtain indirect IAP measurement.	The smallest available three-way bladder catheter is 14F.

Intermittent IAP Measurement

NOTE: If commercial IAP measurement system is used, follow manufacturer's directions.

9. Place child in supine and flat position.[2-4] *(Level II*)*	Avoids downward pressure on bladder that results in an inaccurate reading.	If the child cannot tolerate being placed flat, document the degree of elevation of the head of the bed and obtain all IAP measurements at the same level of elevation.
10. Clamp drainage tube distal to the sampling port on urine collection system tubing.[2-4] *(Level II*)*	Ensures instilled saline solution enters the bladder to establish fluid column and obtain accurate IAP.	

Procedure continues on following page

---

* Level II: Theory-based; no research data to support recommendations; recommendations from expert consensus group may exist

Level VI: Clinical studies in a variety of patient populations and situations to support recommendations

Procedure for Intraabdominal Pressure Monitoring—*Continued*

Steps	Rationale	Considerations

Transducer
Sampling port
Bladder catheter

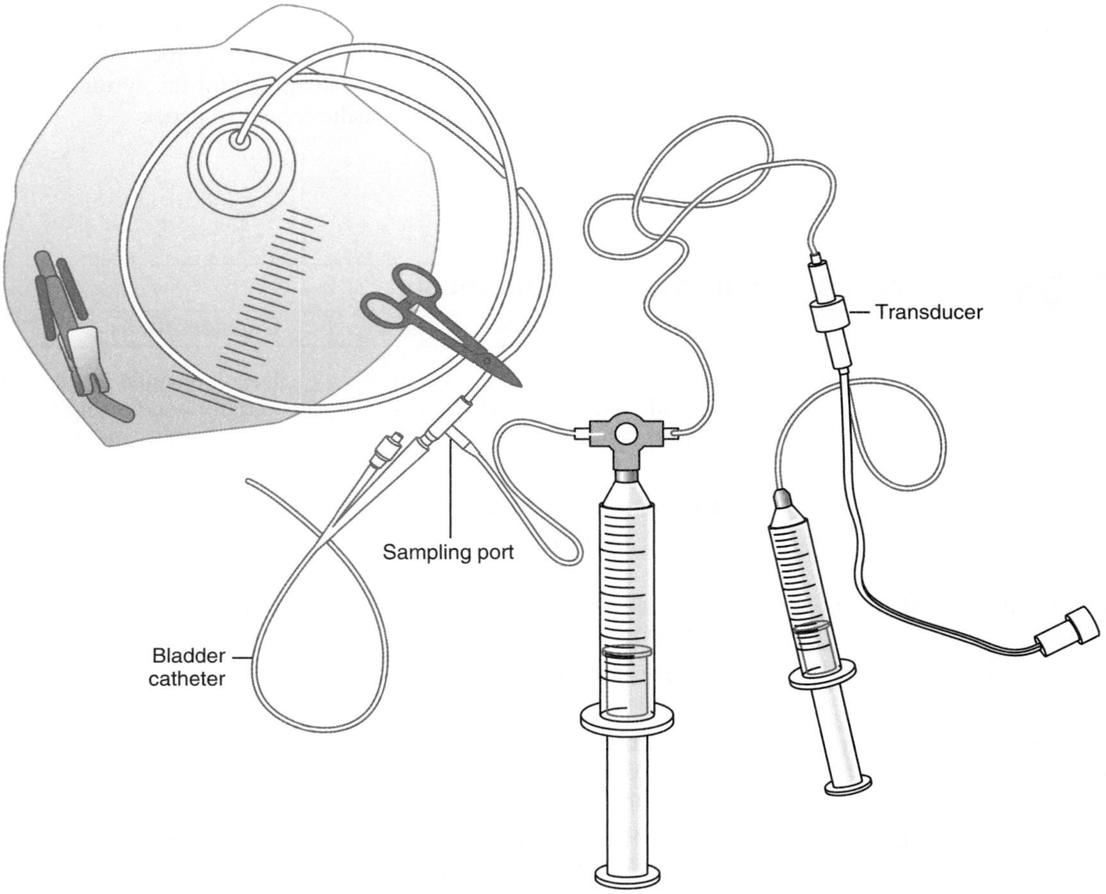

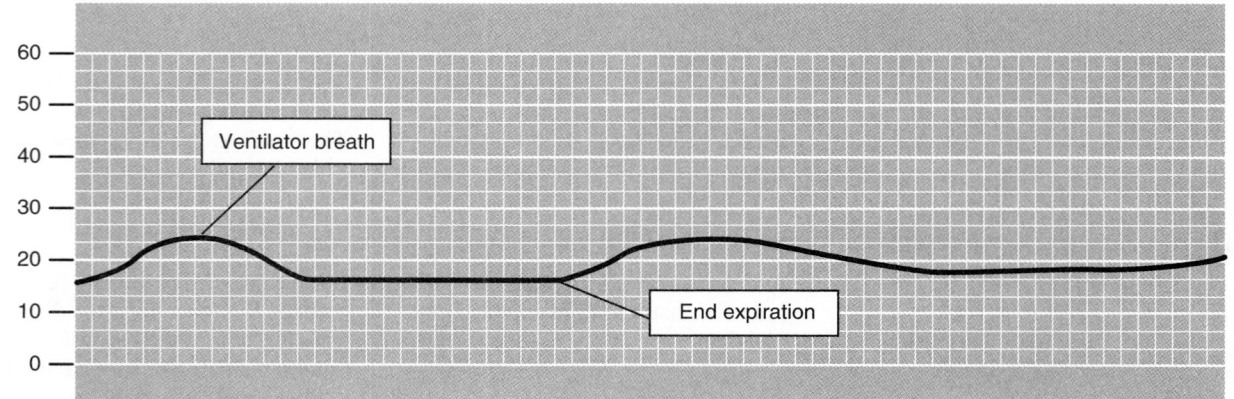

FIGURE 97-1 Set up for intermittent intraabdominal pressure monitoring.

60
50
40
30
20
10
0
Ventilator breath
End expiration

FIGURE 97-2 Intraabdominal pressure waveform. IAP read at end expiration is 16 mm Hg in this patient with mechanical ventilation.

Procedure for Intraabdominal Pressure Monitoring—*Continued*

Steps	Rationale	Considerations
11. Level transducer to midaxillary line; zero monitor and transducer.[2,3,5,13,14] *(Level II*)*	Levels transducer to the bladder and establishes atmospheric pressure as zero reference point.	See Procedure 63 for further discussion of pressure transducer systems.
12. Clean sampling port with povidone-iodine or other antiseptic per institution-specific protocol and allow to dry.	Minimizes risk of urinary tract infection.	
13. Attach extension tubing at the end of the transducer system to the sampling port on the urine collection system via the needleless access device.	Connects pressure monitoring system to the bladder catheter.	If the sampling port cannot be accessed with a needleless device, attach the 18-gauge needle to the extension tubing and insert the needle into the sampling port.
14. Attach syringe with 0.9% saline solution to the open stopcock port. Turn the stopcock so that it is open to the syringe and the bladder catheter and instill volume of saline solution specified in prescribing practitioner's order (1 mL/kg, to a maximum of 20 mL) into the bladder.[15,16] *(Level IV*)*	Establishes a fluid-filled column, required for accurate IAP measurement.	Initial studies suggest that the volume that results in the most accurate measurement of IAP in children less than 40 kg is 1 mL/kg with a maximum of 20 mL of 0.9% saline solution.[15,16]
15. Turn the stopcock open to the transducer system and the bladder catheter and off to the syringe. • Obtain the IAP reading at end expiration as a mean pressure reading. *(Level II*)*	The IAP is read as a mean pressure. Obtain the pressure reading at end expiration to eliminate the effect of transmitted intrathoracic pressure.	The waveform is relatively flat, with slight respiratory variations.[2-4] If a transducer is not available, a manometer can be used as an alternative. Connect manometer to stopcock, open stopcock to manometer and bladder catheter, and determine water level in the manometer, read as cm H_2O. The midaxillary line remains the reference point for this method.
16. After obtaining pressure reading, unclamp the drainage tubing. Ensure fluid drains out of bladder.	Unclamping drainage tubing allows urine and instilled saline solution to drain from bladder.	
17. If a needle was used to access the sampling port, remove the needle. Cap the system with a sterile cap.	Ensures patient safety; prevents needlestick injury.	
18. Discard used supplies and equipment in appropriate receptacle. Wash hands.	Reduces transmission of micro-organisms.	
19. Subtract volume of saline solution instilled in the bladder from next hour's urine output measurement to determine actual urine output.	Saline solution is allowed to passively drain into urine collection system; known volume of saline solution instilled must be subtracted from total volume in collection system to obtain actual volume of urine.	

Procedure continues on following page

Procedure continues on following page

* Level II: Theory-based; no research data to support recommendations; recommendations from expert consensus group may exist
Level IV: Limited clinical studies to support recommendations

Procedure for Intraabdominal Pressure Monitoring—*Continued*

Steps	Rationale	Considerations
Continuous IAP Measurement		
20. See previous steps 1 to 5; insert three-way bladder catheter.	Prepares system for IAP measurement.	Intermittent and continuous IAP measurement techniques result in similar measurements for 75% of patients.[13]
21. Set up the pressure transducer system to a continuous infusion of 0.9% saline solution via pressure bag or infusion pump.[13] *(Level IV*)*	Continuous infusion of fluid in to the bladder is required for accurate measurement.	Pressure bags typically deliver 3 to 4 mL/h; infusion pump can be programmed for this rate.
22. Connect the transducer system to the bedside monitor and ensure system is functioning. Select an appropriate scale.	Allows display of IAP reading and waveform.	
23. Attach the free end of the pressure transducer tubing to the irrigation port of the three-way bladder catheter.	Ensures bladder is continually filled with fluid, maintaining the fluid-filled column required for accurate pressure readings.	
24. Attach the urine collection system to the drainage arm of the catheter.	Allows continuous drainage of urine.	
25. Level the transducer at the iliac crest at the midaxillary line and zero the transducer according to manufacturer's directions.[13] *(Level IV*)*	Levels transducer to the bladder and establishes atmospheric pressure as zero reference point.	See Procedure 63 for further discussion of pressure transducer systems.
26. Observe monitor for waveform and numeric display of IAP. Set alarm limits per prescribing practitioner's order or unit-specific protocol.	Ensures system is functioning. Appropriate alarm limits facilitate early identification of elevations in IAP.	The IAP is read as a mean pressure.
27. Discard used supplies and equipment in appropriate receptacles; wash hands.	Reduces transmission of microorganisms.	

* Level IV: Limited clinical studies to support recommendations

Expected Outcomes	Unexpected Outcomes
• Accurate IAP is obtained	• IAP values are not accurate
• IAH is identified and treated	• IAH is not identified or treated
• IAP trends are monitored and support clinical decision making	• Inconsistent trends of IAP
• Accurate urine output is obtained	• Inaccurate calculation of urine output if volume of saline solution instilled is not subtracted from next hour's output
• The child is free from complications of IAP monitoring	• Bladder perforation
	• Urinary tract infection
	• Hematuria

Monitoring and Care of the Child

Activities and Interventions	Rationale	Reportable Conditions
1. Monitor child's tolerance of procedure.	Children may decompensate during the procedure.	• Any adverse change in child's status • Blood from Foley catheter • Intraabdominal pressure greater than 10 mm Hg
2. Monitor IAP at specified intervals.	Monitoring IAP trends over time promotes early identification of IAH.	• An IAP greater than 10 mm Hg or predetermined threshold • Upward trend of IAP
3. Monitor for complications of IAP measurement.	Facilitates early identification of complications and promotes prompt treatment.	• Blood in urine • Sudden cessation of urine output • Indications of urinary tract infection
4. Monitor for signs and symptoms of ACS.	IAP measurements should be correlated with clinical assessment.	• Signs and symptoms of ACS without increase in IAP measurements
5. If continuous IAP monitoring is used, subtract volume of saline solution instilled from urine output.	Volume instilled must be subtracted from urine output to obtain correct urine output volume.	• No urine output from catheter • Incorrect intake/output calculation

Documentation

- Size and type of bladder catheter placed
- Volume of saline solution instilled for measurement
- The IAP measurement obtained
- Degree of elevation of head of bed, if other than flat
- Urine output
- For continuous IAP measurement, rate of saline solution infusion and volume of urine obtained
- Child's tolerance of procedure
- Child and family education
- Additional interventions and related outcomes
- Unexpected outcomes and related treatment

References

1. Sentongo T, Steinhorn D: Gastrointestinal structure and function. In Fuhrman B, Zimmerman J, editors: *Pediatric critical care,* ed 3, Philadelphia, 2006, Mosby.
2. Sugrue M: Abdominal compartment syndrome, *Curr Opin Crit Care* 11:333-338, 2005.
3. Gallagher J: Ask the experts: monitoring intra-abdominal pressure via an indwelling urinary catheter, *Crit Care Nurs* 26(1):67-70, 2006.
4. Cuthbertson SJ: Nursing care for raised intra-abdominal pressure and abdominal decompression in the critically ill, *Intens Crit Care Nurs* 16:175-180, 2000.
5. DeCou JM, et al: Abdominal compartment syndrome in children: experience with three cases, *J Pediatr Surg* 35(6):840-842, 2000.
6. Oda J, et al: Hypertonic lactated saline resuscitation reduces the risk of abdominal compartment syndrome in severely burned patients, *J Trauma Injury Infection Crit Care* 60:64-71, 2006.
7. Bukowski TP, Freedman AL: Catheterization problems of infants, *Contemp Urol* 66-74, 1999.
8. Elizondo AP, et al: Elimination of bleeding associated with urinary catheterization in neonates, *Neonatal Network* 20:25-34, 2001.
9. Smith AB, Adams L: Insertion of indwelling urethral catheters in infants and children: a survey of current nursing practice, *Pediatr Nurs* 24:229-234, 1998.
10. Hockenberry MJ, et al, editors: *Wong's nursing care of infants and children,* ed 7, St Louis, 2003, Mosby, Inc.
11. Kleiber C, McCarthy AM: Parent behavior and child distress during urethral catheterization, *JSPN* 4:95-104, 1999.
12. Stashinko E, Goldberger J: Test or trauma? The voiding cycstourethrogram experience of young children, *Issues Comprehens Pediatr Nurs* 21:85-96, 1998.
13. Balogh Z, et al: Continuous intra-abdominal pressure measurement technique, *Am J Surg* 188:679-684, 2004.
14. Fusco MA, et al: Estimation of intra-abdominal pressure by bladder pressure measurement: validity and methodology, *J Trauma* 50:297-302, 2001.
15. Davis PJ, et al: Comparison of indirect methods of measuring intra-abdominal pressure in children, *Intens Care Med* 31(3):471-475, 2005.

16. Ejike JC, Mathur M: Optimal bladder volumes for intra-abdominal pressure measurement in small children, *Crit Care Med* 33(12 suppl):A93, 2005.

Additional Readings

Balogh Z et al: Both primary and secondary abdominal compartment syndrome can be predicted early and are harbingers of multiple organ failure, *J Trauma* 54:848-861, 2003.

Sanchez NC, et al: What is normal intra-abdominal pressure? *Am Surgeon* 67:243-248, 2001.

Walker J, Criddle LM: Pathophysiology and management of abdominal compartment syndrome, *Am J Crit Care* 12:367-371, 2003.

Ostomy Appliance: Change

P U R P O S E : An ostomy appliance provides an external pouch for collection of stool or urine through a stoma opening at the skin level

Kimberly R. Bookout and Kathleen M. McLane

PREREQUISITE KNOWLEDGE

- Child development as it relates to clinical assessment and ostomy appliance change
- Anatomy and physiology of the gastrointestinal (GI) tract[1,2]
- Understanding of the characteristics of a stoma (Figure 98-1)
  - ❖ The bowel is highly vascularized, and stomas are typically red in color.
  - ❖ The stoma has no nerve sensors for pain. The child has no pain when the stoma is touched or cleansed.
  - ❖ The stoma may be edematous after surgical creation and decreases in size during the next 6 to 8 weeks.
- Developmental differences in characteristics of the skin (e.g., premature and young infants have a less well-developed epidermal barrier, which necessitates the use of wound products that do not further damage the epidermal barrier.)[3,4]
- The goals of ostomy pouching are protection of the skin, containment of drainage, odor control, facilitation of accurate measurement of effluent, and promotion of the child's mobility.[3,5,6]
- In general, pouches are applied to stay in place for at least 24 hours.[3,5]
- Ostomies may be temporary or permanent.
- Purpose and type of stoma and expected effluent
  - ❖ Colostomy
    - ○ Ascending: Stool has higher liquid content, may contain semisolid particles.
    - ○ Transverse: Stool is thick, semisolid.

- ○ Descending/sigmoid: Stool is thicker, more formed (Figure 98-2).
- ❖ Ileostomy: Watery stools; large amount of effluent; may become slightly thicker as diet is advanced; output contains digestive enzymes and is caustic to the skin (Figure 98-3).
- ❖ Jejunostomy: Constant watery output; highly acidic effluent; high volume
- ❖ Urostomy: Urine output; constant drainage of effluent (Figure 98-4)
- ❖ Mucous fistula: Often accompanies colostomy or ileostomy; the mucous fistula may be pouched with the fecal ostomy or separated and covered with Vaseline gauze or a nonadherent gauze (Figure 98-5)
- Fecal stomas are pouched with drainable appliances with a wide opening to drain fecal matter and must be emptied when one third to one half full of stool or gas (Figure 98-6, *A*).
- Urinary stomas are pouched with appliances that have a tap and may be connected to a metered drainage bag with a connector; if not connected to a drainage bag, pouches must be emptied when one third to one half full of urine (Figure 98-6, *B*).
- Urinary stomas should have a constant output. Fecal stomas that are high in the GI tract (jejunostomy, ileostomy) also have a constant output. Fecal stomas that are lower in the GI tract generally resume the child's "normal" bowel routine and may function less frequently.
- Stomas should be beefy red as a result of the highly vascularized tissue.[7-9]
- Wound care resources available within the institution, such as wound ostomy continence nurses (WOCNs), are

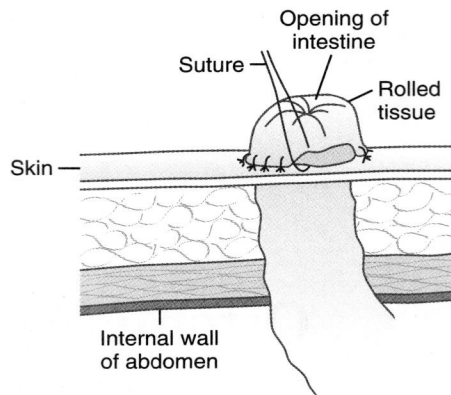

FIGURE 98-1 Creation of stoma.

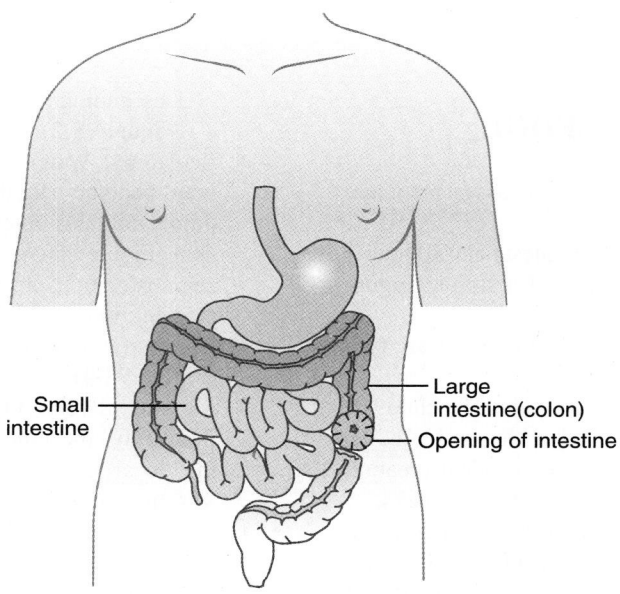

FIGURE 98-2 Colostomy.

consulted to facilitate selection of appropriate supplies and equipment.
- Ostomy pouches are disposable.
- Patching of a leaking pouch does not typically solve a leak; a leaking pouch must be changed to avoid problems with skin breakdown.
- Stomas shrink for 6 to 8 weeks after surgery. Patterns that identify the stoma opening need to be "resized" weekly to allow for shrinkage.

- Pouches may be one-piece (pouch and flange are attached) or two-piece (pouch is separate from flange or wafer).
  - ❖ One-piece pouches may be cut-to-fit and are available in premature, newborn, infant, toddler, and adult sizes (Figure 98-7).
  - ❖ Two-piece pouches are available in multiple cut-to-fit sizes. Use of precut pouches during the immediate postoperative period is not recommended because of

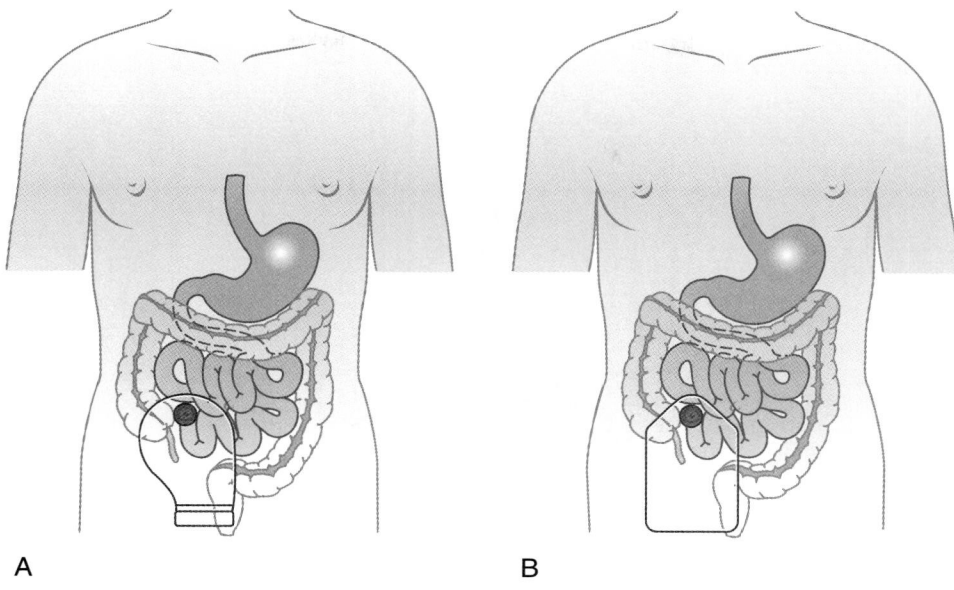

A   B

FIGURE 98-3   Ileostomy.

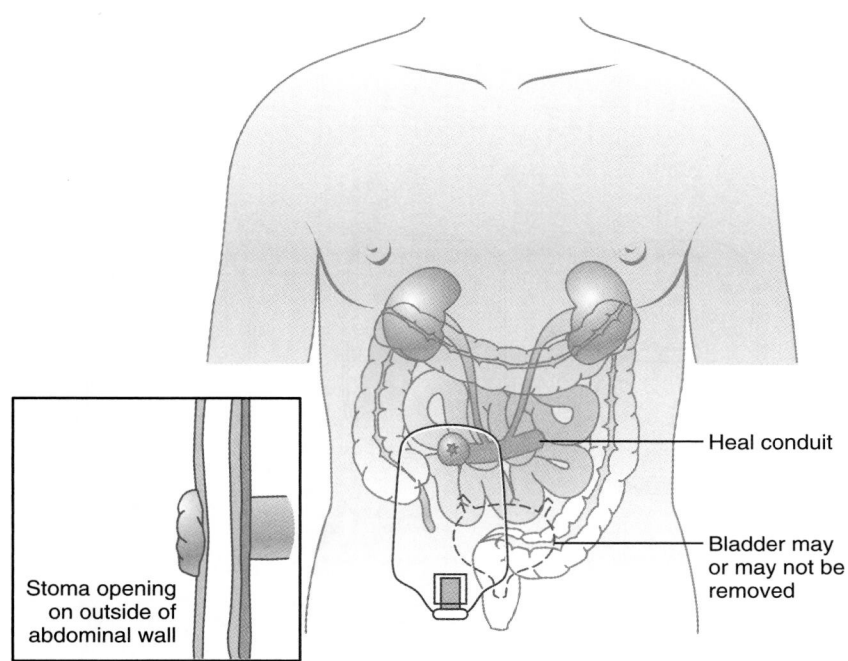

Stoma opening
on outside of
abdominal wall

Heal conduit

Bladder may
or may not be
removed

FIGURE 98-4   Urostomy.

stoma shrinkage. Two-piece pouching systems are not recommended in premature or small infants because pressure is needed to snap the two pieces together[3] (Figure 98-8).

CHILD AND FAMILY ASSESSMENT

• Child's developmental level and ability to interact ➡️*Rationale:* Determines the child's ability to understand the procedure and learn ostomy care. For the infant or toddler, parents provide all care; the school-aged child is partially involved in care; and adolescents perform all care related to the ostomy.

• Child's and family's understanding of the procedure and the ability to perform ostomy care ➡️*Rationale:* Evaluates understanding of the procedure and provides a gauge for ongoing education. Family and child may be experienced in the care of the ostomy.

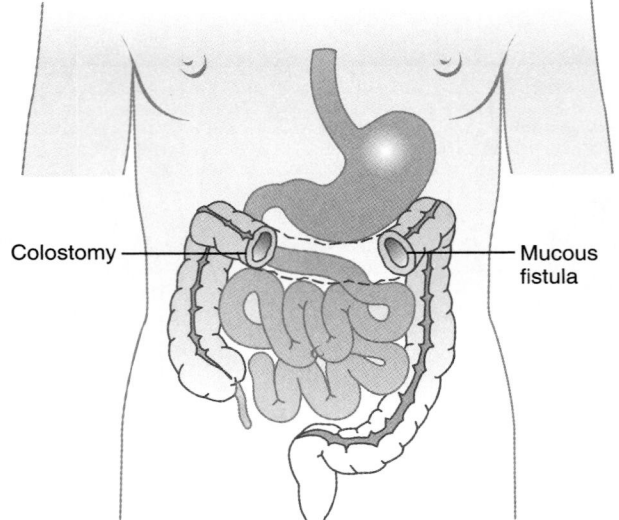

FIGURE 98-5   Mucous fistula.

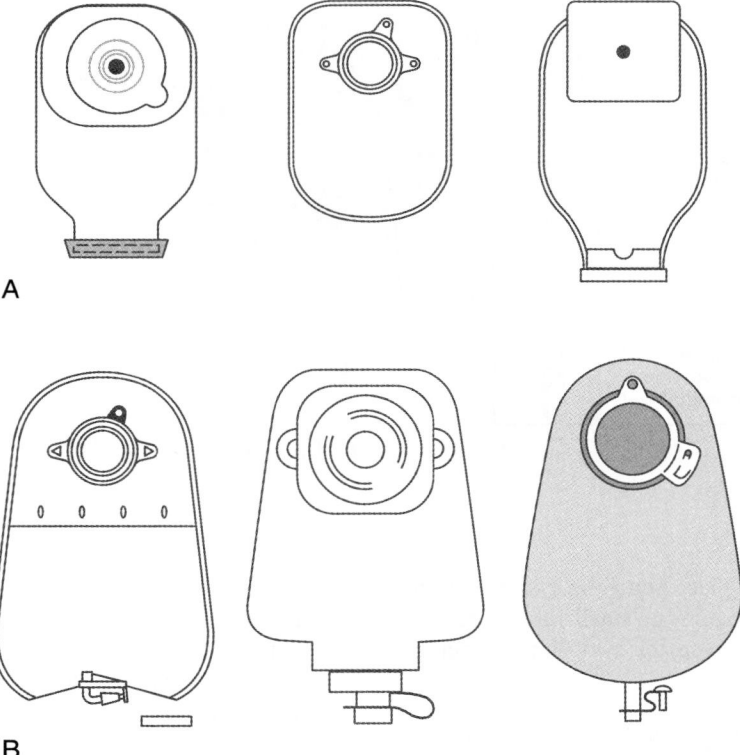

FIGURE 98-6   Ostomy Appliance Bags. **A,** Pouch for fecal stomas with wide opening for drainage. **B,** Pouch for urinary stomas with tap for liquid drainage.

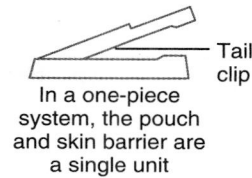
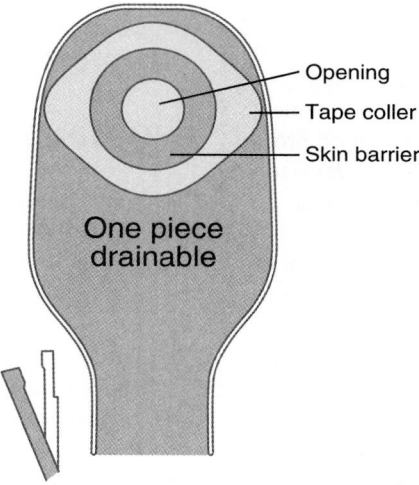

FIGURE 98-7   One-piece pouching system. The pouch and skin barrier are a single unit.

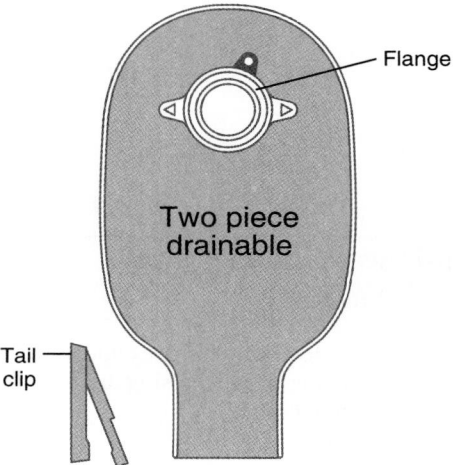

FIGURE 98-8   Two-piece pouching system. In a two-pole system, the pouch attaches to the skin barrier with flange.

- Known allergies ➼*Rationale:* The child may have an allergy to latex, tape, skin preparation products, or pouching appliances used for ostomy care.
- Type and age of fistula ➼*Rationale:* Identifies appropriate products necessary for ostomy care and pouching.
- Appearance of the stoma, surrounding skin, and stoma output ➼*Rationale:* The stoma is typically small and red in color. Stoma output varies based on specific type of stoma. Changes in stoma appearance, integrity of surrounding skin, or stoma output may indicate problems of the stoma or GI tract.
- Products currently used to pouch the ostomy ➼*Rationale:* Identifies supplies needed to pouch ostomy.

CHILD AND FAMILY EDUCATION

Individualized, developmentally appropriate education is provided to the family and to the child based on desire for knowledge, readiness to learn, and overall neurologic and psychosocial state.

- Provide information about the ostomy, including type of ostomy, expected output, and pouch selection ➡️*Rationale:* Providing information facilitates child's and family's acceptance of the stoma; the child and family are prepared to manage the stoma in the home environment.
- Provide the child and family with information on procedural steps and rationale for changing pouch ➡️*Rationale:* Providing information decreases anxiety and fear and improves compliance with procedure.
- Involve a Child Life Specialist with developmentally appropriate instruction and role playing ➡️*Rationale:* Child Life Specialists have extensive training in age-appropriate teaching techniques and the use of medical play.
- Provide handouts, brochures, or written instructions to reinforce teaching ➡️*Rationale:* Written information reinforces teaching and provides the family with a resource that can be used in the home environment.
- As part of teaching, involve the child and family in ostomy care and pouch change ➡️*Rationale:* Participating in care builds the child's and family's confidence in self care and prepares the child to return to school and other activities after hospitalization.
- Educate the family and child on the specifics of bathing, clothing, activity, diet, and routine pouch care ➡️*Rationale:* Providing information regarding daily care needs facilitates the child's and family's return to self-care.
- Encourage questions and answer questions as they arise ➡️*Rationale:* Reinforcement of information is needed during periods of stress.

EQUIPMENT

- Appropriately sized pouch/flange for fecal or urinary stoma (see Figure 129-1 in Procedure 129)
- Clean gloves
- Scissors
- Pen
- Washcloths (two) or disposable cloths and towel (one)
- Skin preparation sealant (optional)
- Adhesive remover (optional)
- Paste (optional) and syringe (for infants and toddlers)
- Pectin powder or antifungal powder (as needed)
- Skin barrier ring or strips (as needed)
- Tail closure: flexible for infant pouches; rigid for toddler, school-aged child, and adolescent pouches

Procedure   for Ostomy Appliance: Change

Steps	Rationale	Considerations
1. Ensure child and family understand procedure and questions are answered.	Evaluates and reinforces understanding of previously taught information.	Developmental level, cognitive ability, and anxiety level determine approach to and effectiveness of teaching.
2. Gather needed equipment and supplies.	Facilitates completion of procedure in a timely manner.	For preexisting ostomy, check child's stoma before pouch selection and determine type of stoma, stoma size, and child's preference for one-piece versus two-piece appliance. For children with high-output stomas (e.g., urinary, jejunal, or ileal), use of a urostomy pouch to a urinary drainage bag may be helpful.

Procedure for Ostomy Appliance: Change—*Continued*		
Steps	**Rationale**	**Considerations**
3. Wash hands; put on clean gloves.	Reduces transmission of micro-organisms. Protects personnel health.	
4. Use pattern or template to draw opening on back of barrier or wafer[7] (Figure 98-9). Date and mark the paper as "PATTERN" and indicate top and bottom for future use. *(Level I*)*	Facilitates appropriate fit of pouch around stoma. Use of the pattern ensures pouch opening is cut to appropriate size, which is especially helpful for difficult to pouch stomas.	The opening for the stoma may be placed off center to accommodate tubing, drains, incisions, umbilicus, or wounds. The pouch opening may be cut slightly larger than the stoma. Squeezing the soft retention ring (often a red rubber catheter) to elongate and fit through the opening as the pouch is applied may be necessary.

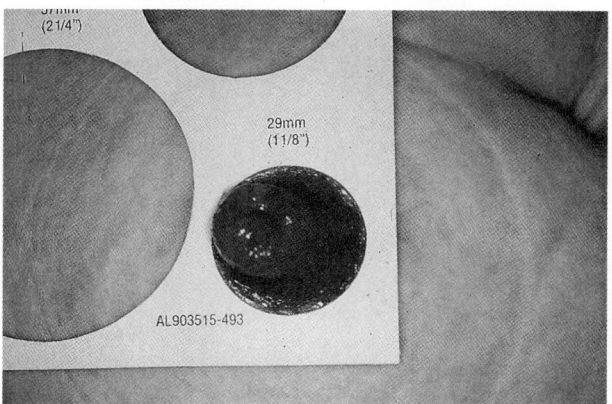

FIGURE 98-9   Measurement of ostomy.

5. For a stoma that is stabilized with a rigid retention rod, apply small amounts of paste to either side of the rod to seal and level the skin. Then, proceed with routine pouch change.	A retention device or rod needs added paste to ensure seal.	The retention rod is under the wafer, which may necessitate additional expertise with application of the appliance. Consult the WOCN if available.
6. Cut opening to fit stoma. No more than 1/8 inch of skin is exposed around stoma (Figure 98-10, *A*). *(Level II*)*	Use of a cut-to-fit appliance is recommended because the stoma has variations in size for up to 6 to 8 weeks after surgery. The barrier/wafer is designed to protect the skin from stoma effluent.	Multiple stomas may be pouched together if they are in close proximity. However, pouching of a mucous fistula is not necessary. A nonadherent gauze may be placed over the mucous fistula to protect from external trauma.

Procedure continues on following page

* Level I: Manufacturer's recommendations only
    Level II: Theory-based; no research data to support recommendations; recommendations from expert consensus group may exist

Procedure | for Ostomy Appliance: Change—*Continued*

Steps	Rationale	Considerations
7. Trim edges of barrier to accommodate additional drains, tubes, catheters, wounds, or incisions. *(Level II*)*	Trimming the edges of the barrier facilitates access to additional tubes, drains, or dressings and prevents the need to change the pouch each time a dressing change is indicated.	Petrolatum-based ointments used with adjacent wounds or incisions can seep under the barrier/wafer and cause the barrier to become loose or "float off." Consider other moist wound-healing product options as indicated.
8. For a two-piece appliance, snap pouch to flange. *(Level II*)*	Snapping the pouch to the wafer can be painful if child is in the early postoperative period because the procedure necessitates firm pressure on the abdomen.	Check the pouch and wafer for a secure attachment. If attachment is not secure, leaks may occur between the pouch and barrier/wafer.
9. Peel off paper backing (Figure 98-10, *B*).	Barrier/wafer adhesive is protected by paper backing.	Limit handling of the adhesive because this may decrease its effectiveness.
10. Apply bead of paste to cut opening (Figure 98-10, *C*). *(Level II*)*	Paste is used to augment the seal between the barrier and the skin.	Paste is applied *only* at the cut opening. Too much paste may

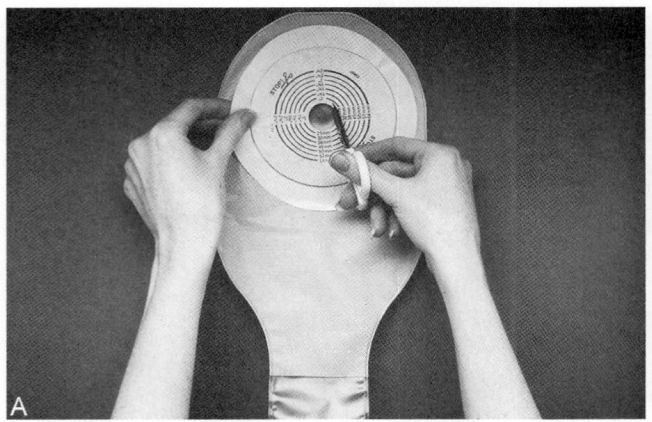
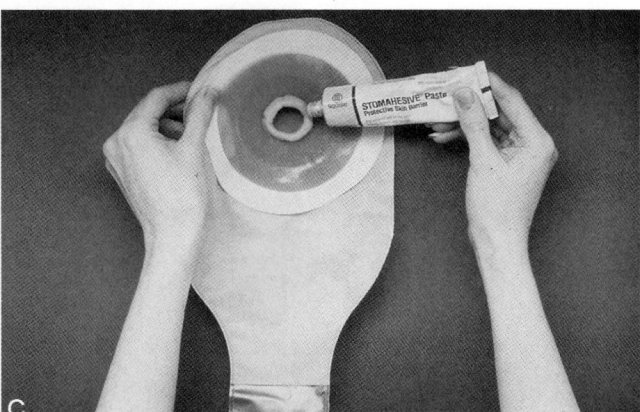
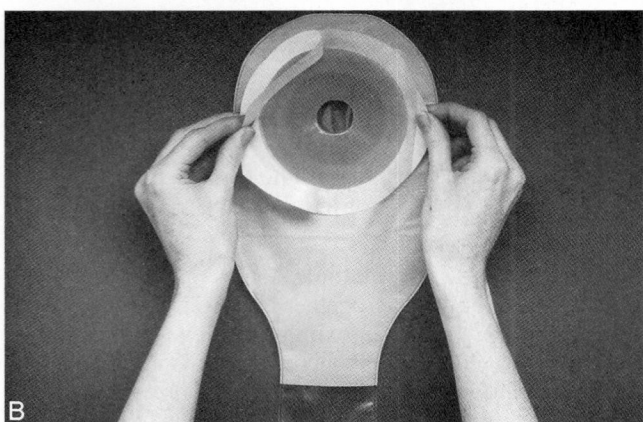

FIGURE 98-10   Attachment of ostomy pouch.

* Level II: Theory-based; no research data to support recommendations; recommendations from expert consensus group may exist

Procedure for Ostomy Appliance: Change—*Continued*		
Steps	**Rationale**	**Considerations**
	It prevents watery liquid stool from seeping under barrier/wafer and causing a leak. Application of the paste to the barrier/wafer (instead of the skin around the stoma) facilitates keeping the peristomal area clean and dry.	interfere with adhesion of barrier/wafer. Paste contains a small amount of alcohol and, if skin is irritated, may burn for a few seconds after application. With use of an infant or toddler pouch, load a 3-mL or 5-mL syringe with a small amount of paste for application. With an older child or adult pouch, apply paste directly from tube. Paste can be difficult to remove from the skin unless it has been in place 24 hours or more. Paste is not recommend for use with urinary stomas and is considered optional in colostomies that are lower in the GI tract, such as the descending or sigmoid colon. High-output stomas or those with constant output may soil paste if paste is applied to the skin versus the pouch. This paste must then be removed and more must be applied before the new pouch can be placed. Use pastes and adhesives with care in the premature infant or neonate because the skin/ostomy bond may be stronger than the bond of skin layers.[3,5]
11. Set prepared pouch/wafer aside (sticky side up). *(Level II*)*	Preparation of new pouch before removal of the old pouch allows the nurse to work without feeling rushed and facilitates keeping peristomal skin clean and dry.	High-output stomas or those with constant output may be difficult to contain during preparation of a new pouch.
12. Remove old pouch and cleanse area around the stoma. With use of adhesive remover, cleanse the skin with warm water. Limit use of soap on the skin surrounding the stoma. *(Level II*)*	If the current pouch has been in place less than 24 hours, adhesive remover may facilitate removal of paste. Adhesive remover contains alcohol, which may burn irritated skin. Residue must be removed with water. Soaps may also leave a residue that can cause dermatitis. In addition, many soaps contain moisturizers that can interfere with adhesion of the pouch to the skin.	Adhesive remover is optional and is not recommended for infants 6 months of age or younger. Water may not completely remove the residual that remains after adhesive remover use. Commercially prepared wipes are not recommended for use around ostomies because they contain lanolin, alcohol, or fragrances. The stoma may bleed during the cleansing process, which is

Procedure continues on following page

* Level II: Theory-based; no research data to support recommendations; recommendations from expert consensus group may exist

Procedure	**for Ostomy Appliance: Change**—*Continued*	
Steps	**Rationale**	**Considerations**
		considered normal. Typically, the bleeding stops without intervention. If bleeding persists, apply slight pressure and a cold water compress.
13. Pat the skin dry with a soft cloth or gauze pad. If indicated, shave or clip peristomal hair.[5,7,8,10,11] *(Level II*)*	Gentle cleansing and drying is preferred for prevention of stomal bleeding. Peristomal skin must be thoroughly dry to allow adhesion of the new pouch. Removal of peristomal hair reduces the occurrence of folliculitis and may decrease pain with pouch removal.	Rubbing of peristomal skin increases irritation. With shaving of the area, shave outward from the stoma to prevent injury to the stoma and thoroughly rinse the area with water after use of soaps or shaving cream. Refer to institution-specific protocol before shaving the area.
14. Apply skin barrier sealant to peristomal skin.[5,7,8,8,11] *(Level II*)*	Skin barriers are often used for added protection of peristomal skin, especially if the skin is thin and friable.	Skin barrier usage is optional. Some manufacturers recommend use; others do not and state that it interferes with adhesion. Non–alcohol-based skin barriers are available and are recommended for children with red broken skin and for infants. If skin is red and weepy, the addition of a pectin-based powder is helpful to control drainage from the open skin yet maintain an adequate seal of the pouch. Use powders with caution in infants and children to avoid inhalation of the powder.
15. Center the barrier/wafer over the stoma and apply (Figure 98-11). *(Level I*)*	Ensures appropriate fit of ostomy appliance.	Barrier/wafer adhesive is designed to stay in place 3 to 7 days and becomes less adherent over time and easier to remove. Cutting the opening of the barrier "off center" may be necessary to accommodate drains, tubes, or anatomic features, such as the umbilicus.
16. Ensure an adequate seal by running a finger over the pouch and around the cut opening (in the area the paste was applied). • Remove any additional paper backing from tape edges and secure to abdomen from the stoma outward.	Ensures adequate seal of the appliance to prevent leakage of effluent.	Consider use of tape to "frame" the edges of the barrier at the skin level to promote a seal.

* Level I: Manufacturer's recommendations only
  Level II: Theory-based; no research data to support recommendations; recommendations from expert consensus group may exist

Procedure	for Ostomy Appliance: Change—*Continued*	
Steps	**Rationale**	**Considerations**

17. Cover wafer with hand for 30 to 60 seconds to warm adhesive. *(Level II*)*

Holding the palm of the hand over the barrier/wafer for 30 to 60 seconds helps warm the barrier to further enhance the seal of the appliance.[3]

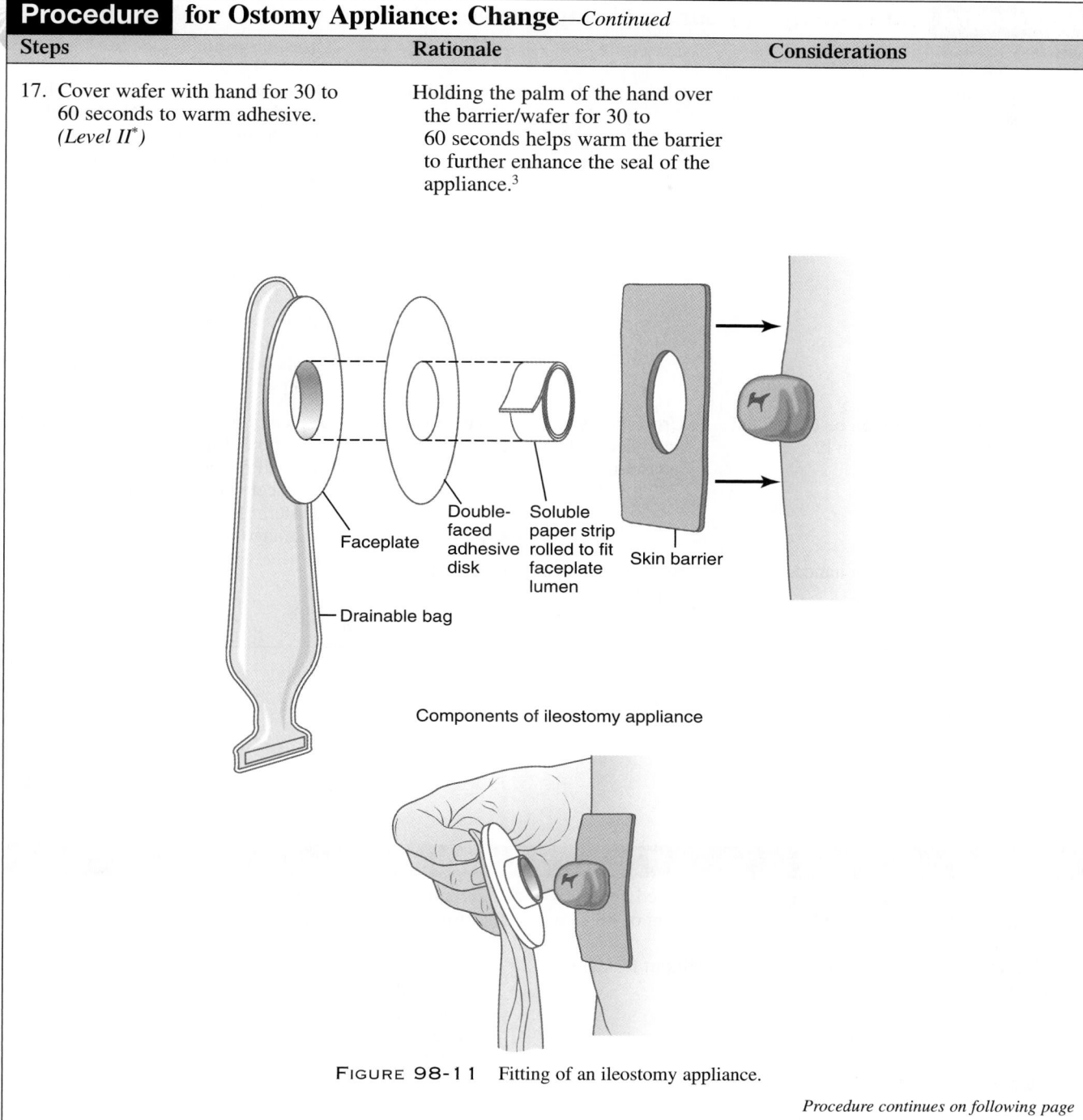

Faceplate

Double-faced adhesive disk

Soluble paper strip rolled to fit faceplate lumen

Skin barrier

Drainable bag

Components of ileostomy appliance

FIGURE 98-11   Fitting of an ileostomy appliance.

Procedure continues on following page

* Level II: Theory-based; no research data to support recommendations; recommendations from expert consensus group may exist

Procedure	for Ostomy Appliance: Change—*Continued*	
Steps	**Rationale**	**Considerations**
18. Apply tail closure or close urostomy tap.	Closes pouch to contain effluent.	*Do not* wrap the pouch around the plastic tail closures. This stretches the closure device so that subsequent pouches may not be able to hold the normal volume. With use of a flexible tail closure with infant or toddler pouches, remove the paper backing and apply to the tail of the pouch 1/2 to 1 inch from the end. Wrap the pouch end two to three times around the closure and fold the ends of the closure toward the center.
19. A urostomy may then be connected to a drainage collection bag.	Urostomy is a high-output stoma and necessitates a larger collection system.	Typically two adapters are included in a box of urostomy pouches that allow the pouch to be connected to an external drain system (leg bag or urinary drainage bag).
20. Remove gloves; wash hands.	Reduces transmission of micro-organisms. Protects personnel health.	

Expected Outcomes

- Appropriately sized ostomy appliance is placed without difficulty and remains in place for a minimum of 48 to 72 hours
- Effluent is contained within the pouch without leakage
- Peristomal skin remains intact

- Stoma remains red or pink

- Minimal amount of stomal bleeding with appliance change

Unexpected Outcomes

- Peristomal skin is exposed to effluent
- Ostomy appliance change is needed before 48 hours

- Appliance leakage
- Peristomal skin breakdown (allergic contact dermatitis, irritant dermatitis, fungal infection, folliculitis)
- Injury to peristomal skin during appliance removal
- Stomal necrosis
- Stomal retraction
- Prolapse of stoma
- Stomal bleeding that persists after appliance change

Monitoring and Care of the Child

Activities and Interventions	Rationale	Reportable Conditions
1. Empty pouch when it contains one third to one half full of stool, gas, or urine. *(Level II*)*	Prevents pouch from becoming too heavy and disrupting the seal of the pouch at the skin level.	• Change in output
2. Change pouch every 3 to 7 days or with leakage. *(Level II*)*	Pouches changed at appropriate intervals facilitate the protection of the skin by the barrier/wafer. Barrier/wafer adhesive is designed to degrade over 3 to 5 days or a 7-day period; if adhesive is allowed to remain in place for extended wear, skin breakdown is possible. Three days is considered an adequate wear time for most newborn/toddler pouches; 5 to 7 days of wear time are considered normal for adult-size pouches; in the premature and newborn population, a more realistic wear time may be only 24 to 48 hours because of the gentle adhesive used for pouching systems.	• Altered skin integrity that prevents pouch from staying well attached
3. Monitor duration of stomal bleeding with pouch changes.	Bleeding that persists beyond the pouch change may indicate the need for laboratory tests for assessment of clotting status.[7,11] Ensure adequate intervention to stop stomal bleeding.	• Persistent stomal bleeding
4. Monitor color of stoma.	A color change may indicate ischemia and necrosis of the stoma. Change is usually noticeable within 12 to 24 hours but may occur as late as 5 to 7 days after surgery.	• Change in color of stoma (stomal necrosis can occur up to 5 to 7 days after surgery)
5. Monitor output for color, amount, and consistency each time the pouch is emptied.	A change in output can be an early warning of a more severe problem. Intestinal obstruction, stenosis, food blockage, and obstruction at the exit wound are potential causes of change in output.	• Sudden increase or decrease in stoma output • Significant change in color or consistency of output
6. Monitor peristomal skin for breakdown (e.g., rash, epidermal stripping).[5-9]	Red flat rashes with partial thickness skin loss are likely the result of irritation from effluent of stoma.	• Candidal rash around the stoma • Skin breakdown around the stoma
7. When a red macular popular rash is present, apply antifungal powder.	A red macular papular rash with satellite lesions is indicative of candidiasis and must be treated with an antifungal powder.	• Rash that does not resolve
8. When drainage is present, consider application of a pectin-based powder. Apply to moist skin only and brush away excess.	A pectin-based powder is beneficial in absorbing wound drainage and may improve the wear time of the pouch. Powder is applied to the moist skin only; excess powder prevents pouch from adhering to skin.	• Drainage not controlled by pectin powder
9. If available, a WOCN is consulted to facilitate education.	WOCNs have extensive expertise and can provide validated teaching tools.	

* Level II: Theory-based; no research data to support recommendations; recommendations from expert consensus group may exist

Documentation

- Stoma size, shape, and color
- Stoma output (urine color, clarity, and quantity; fecal quantity, color, and consistency)
- Supplies used in stoma care
- Child and family response to the stoma care
- Child and family involvement in care
- Involvement of WOCN
- Additional interventions and related outcomes
- Child and family education, including any literature provided
- Unexpected outcomes and related treatment

References

1. Sentongo T, Steinhorn D: Gastrointestinal structure and function. In Fuhrman B, Zimmerman J, editors: *Pediatric critical care,* ed 3, Philadelphia, 2006, Mosby.
2. McCance K, Huether S: *Pathophysiology: the biologic basis for disease in adults and children,* Philadelphia, 2002, Mosby.
3. Rogers V: Managing preemie stomas: more than just the pouch, *J Wound Ostomy Continence* 30(2):100-110, 2003.
4. Lund C: Prevention and management of infant skin breakdown, *Nurs Clin North Am* 34(4):907-920, 1999.
5. Garvin G: Caring for children with ostomies and wounds. In Wise B, et al, editors: *Nursing care of the general pediatric surgical patient*, Gaithersberg, MD, 2000, Aspen Publications.
6. Rolstad B, Bryant R: Management of drain sites and fistulas. In Bryant R, editor: *Acute and chronic wounds: nursing management,* ed 2, Philadelphia, 2000, Mosby.
7. Hampton BG: Peristomal and stomal complications. In Hampton BG, Bryant RA, editors: *Ostomies and continent diversions: nursing management,* St Louis, 1992, Mosby.
8. McCann EM: Common ostomy problems. In Milne CT, et al, editors: *Wound, ostomy, and continence nursing secrets,* Philadelphia, 2003, Hanley & Belfus, Inc.
9. Haglegans, NA, Janusz, HB: Pediatric skin care issues for the home care nurse: part 2, *Pediatr Nurs* 20(1):69-75, 1994.
10. Harrell-Bean HA, Klell CA: Neonatal ostomies, *JOGN Nurs* 12(3 suppl):69s-73s, 1983.
11. Garvin G: Skin care considerations in the neonate for the ET nurse, *J Enterostomal Therapy* 17:225-230, 1990.

Additional Readings

Black P: Treating peristomal skin problems in the community, *Br J Community Nurs* 7(4):212,214-217, 2002.

Boarini J: Principles of stoma care for infants, *J Enterostomal Therapy* 16:21-25, 1989.

Erwin-Toth P, Doughty DB: Principles and procedures of stomal management. In Hampton BG, Bryant RA, editors. *Ostomies and continent diversions: nursing management,* St Louis, 1992, Mosby.

Hollister, Inc: *What's right for my baby?* Libertyville, IL, 2003, Hollister Inc, USA.

ConvaTec: *A parent's guide to ostomy care for infants and children,* Princeton, NJ, 2000; ConvaTec, A Bristol-Myers Squibb Company.

Percutaneous Peritoneal Lavage: Assist

P U R P O S E : A technique of abdominal cavity lavage or washing used in the diagnosis of intraperitoneal bleeding, intraabdominal hollow viscus injury, or other intraabdominal pathology[2-4]

Orlando R. Chapa

PREREQUISITE KNOWLEDGE

- Child development as it relates to clinical assessment and percutaneous peritoneal lavage (PPL)
- Anatomy and physiology of the abdominal viscera in the child
- In the young child, the bladder extends into the abdomen.[1]
- Percutaneous peritoneal lavage is used as a diagnostic tool for children who have[2-9]:
  - ❖ Hemodynamic instability and are unable to be transported for computed tomography (CT)
  - ❖ Fluid in the peritoneum (as noted on CT scan) without solid organ injury
  - ❖ Blunt abdominal injury and altered mental status or young age, which result in unreliable abdominal examination results
  - ❖ An equivocal ultrasound scan and no obvious source of bleeding
- Specifically, PPL is used to identify intraabdominal hemorrhage, visceral injury, perforation, pancreatitis, peritonitis, strangulating bowel, intestinal obstruction, and malignant cells in peritoneal washing.[2-4]
- Percutaneous peritoneal lavage may also be used as a warming technique in the child with extreme hypothermia.
- Peritoneal fluid is normally a straw-colored serous fluid.
- A laparotomy is indicated when the PPL results reflect intraabdominal pathology.
- Indications of "positive" PPL results and intraabdominal pathology include[2-7]:

- ❖ Grossly bloody fluid
- ❖ Red blood cell (RBC) count of greater than 100,000/mm^3 (the threshold may be lower in the child with a penetrating injury to the abdomen or lower chest)
- ❖ White blood cell (WBC) count of more than 500/mm^3
- ❖ Presence of bacteria, bile, stool, or amylase in the returned abdominal fluid
- Complications of PPL include bleeding of wound or omentum, wound infection, abdominal wall hematoma, small bowel or colon perforation, bladder puncture, mesenteric laceration, iliac vessel injury, ovarian laceration, and infusion of fluid into the abdominal wall or retroperitoneum; the complication rate with PPL is approximately 1%.[2-4,9-11]
- Relative contraindications to PPL include pregnancy (catheter may be inserted above the fundus), previous abdominal surgery (catheter may be inserted away from the area of abdominal scar location), pelvic fracture (catheter may be inserted in a supraumbilical location), inability to decompress stomach or bladder (catheter may be inserted in an infraumbilical location), and morbid obesity.[4,11]
- The availability of CT and ultrasound scans, including focused assessment with sonography for trauma (FAST), has significantly decreased the frequency of PPL.[2-4,9-10]
- Ultrasound scan may be used before or during the procedure to assist with catheter placement.
- A false-positive result may result from bleeding from the needle puncture site.

- Causes of false-negative PPL results include injury with minimal bleeding, retroperitoneal duodenal rupture, extraperitoneal rupture of the kidney or bladder, and viscus perforation when PPL is performed less than 3 hours from the time of injury.[3]
- Understanding of thermoregulation in the infant and child (see Procedure 187)
- Understanding of laboratory values, especially with respect to coagulation study results
- Selection and use of pediatric pain scale appropriate to child's age and developmental level (see Procedure 173)
- Informed consent is required before PPL.

CHILD AND FAMILY ASSESSMENT

- Child's developmental level and ability to interact ➛***Rationale:*** These factors influence preparation of the child and interaction.
- Child's and family's understanding of the reasons for and risks and benefits of the procedure ➛***Rationale:*** Evaluates child's and family's understanding of the procedure and provides a gauge for ongoing education.
- Medical history, including potential for pregnancy if the child is a female more than 12 years of age ➛***Rationale:*** Identifies absolute or relative contraindications to PPL.
- Baseline vital signs, cardiorespiratory status, and abdominal examination results, including abdominal girth ➛***Rationale:*** Establishes baseline parameters, which can be compared with subsequent assessments.
- Child's current level of pain and anxiety ➛***Rationale:*** Establishes a baseline; facilitates development of an appropriate pain and anxiety management plan.
- Presence of bowel or bladder distension ➛***Rationale:*** Distended viscera increase the risk of perforation during PPL.[4,5]
- Coagulation study results, including prothrombin time (PT), partial thromboplastin time (PTT), and platelet count ➛***Rationale:*** Abnormal coagulation study results increase the risk of intra-procedural and post procedural bleeding.
- Results of radiology studies ordered and performed before the procedure ➛***Rationale:*** Subsequent evaluation of free abdominal air is hampered because of pneumoperitoneum from procedure.[5]
- Family's desire to remain with the child during the procedure ➛***Rationale:*** The family's presence may provide comfort and support to the child during the procedure; family should also have the choice not to remain with the child.

CHILD AND FAMILY EDUCATION

Individualized, developmentally appropriate education is provided to the family and to the child based on desire for knowledge, readiness to learn, and overall neurologic and psychosocial state.

- Provide the family and child with information about the reasons for PPL, steps in the procedure, and pain management strategies planned ➛***Rationale:*** Providing information may decrease the child's and family's anxiety; facilitates informed consent.
- If the family desires to stay during the procedure, provide the family with accurate information regarding the procedure, the family's role, and expectations ➛***Rationale:*** Facilitates cooperation during and after the procedure; clearly defined guidelines and expectations are provided.
- Explain postprocedure care, including monitoring for fever, abdominal pain, decreased urine output, bleeding, and leakage of fluid from the wound site and the importance of the child or family reporting any of these symptoms noted ➛***Rationale:*** Ongoing assessment of unexpected outcomes; the family is involved in the child's care.
- Encourage questions and answer questions as they arise ➛***Rationale:*** Reinforcement of information is needed during periods of stress and is especially important if PPL is performed emergently.

EQUIPMENT

- Skin antisepsis
  - Sterile gloves
  - Cleansing solution: Povidone iodine, chlorhexidine, or other skin antiseptic per institution-specific protocol
  - Sterile 4×4 gauze sponges
  - Clippers or razor, if shaving is necessary
- Sterile field
  - Mask with face shield or mask and goggles
  - Sterile gowns and gloves
  - Sterile towels or fenestrated drape
  - Caps may be worn per institution-specific protocol
- PPL equipment
  - Access needle (e.g., Veress needle, angiocatheter)
  - Peritoneal catheter (e.g., peritoneal dialysis catheter)
  - Flexible guidewire
  - Intravenous (IV) tubing set without valves or volumetric device
  - Stopcock
  - Extension tubing and collection bag for effluent (empty IV bag may be used to collect effluent)
  - Syringes, 10-mL and 20-mL
  - Warmed 0.9% saline solution or Ringer's lactate solution per prescribing practitioner's order
  - Preassembled kit or gather:
    - Section 1.01 Scissors
    - Section 1.02 Needle holder
    - Section 1.03 Hemostats (2)
    - Section 1.04 Scalpel handle and no. 15 or 11 blade
  - Suture material, practitioner preference
  - Syringe, 3-mL or 5-mL, with 25-gauge needle
  - Lidocaine, 1% or 2%, with epinephrine
  - Specimen labels with two patient identifiers
  - Appropriate laboratory requisitions
  - Appropriate sterile specimen tubes

Procedure for Percutaneous Peritoneal Lavage: Assist

Steps	Rationale	Considerations
1. Ensure child and family understand procedure and questions are answered.	Evaluates and reinforces understanding of previously taught information.	Developmental level, cognitive ability, and anxiety level determine approach to and effectiveness of teaching. In an emergency situation, teaching may be deferred.
2. Confirm presence of informed consent. *(Level II[*])*	Ensures medical-legal compliance as suggested by the Joint Commission on Accreditation of Healthcare Organizations (JCAHO).	In emergency situations, refer to institution-specific protocol for assumption of consent.
3. Ensure appropriate cardiorespiratory monitoring is in place with appropriate alarm limits set and alarms activated.	Child may decompensate during the procedure.	Monitor vital signs throughout the procedure. Emergency equipment should be readily available.
4. Ensure child's stomach and bladder are decompressed; if needed, place orogastric or nasogastric decompression tube and urinary catheter.[4,11] *(Level I[*])*	Avoids bowel or bladder puncture.	A child who is toilet trained may be able to void when requested, avoiding the need to place a urinary catheter. See Procedures 93 and 108 for further information on placement of gastric decompression tube or indwelling urinary catheter.
5. Assemble necessary equipment and supplies.	Facilitates completion of procedure in a timely manner and maintenance of sterile field.	
6. Wash hands and put on personal protective equipment: sterile gown, cap, mask, eye protection.[4] *(Level II[*])*	Reduces transmission of microorganisms. Protects personnel health.	Garb required of individuals in the room during the procedure varies from institution to institution; refer to institution-specific protocol.
7. Identify child with institution-specific patient and procedure verification process (e.g., "Time out"). *(Level II[*])*	Confirms correct patient, procedure, and site as recommended by JCAHO; prevents unnecessary medical procedures.	Verification process and documentation are institution specific. Use active communication techniques.
8. Assist practitioner who performs procedure to establish sterile field and prepare equipment.	Aseptic technique protects child from exposure to microorganisms and contamination of procedure site, reducing likelihood of infection. Ensures all equipment is available and easily accessed.	
9. Assist practitioner to set up lavage equipment. Practitioner attaches IV tubing to stopcock and passes off tubing end with IV bag spike. Spike warmed fluid and prime IV set and stopcock. If fluid is to be drained into collection bag, practitioner attaches extension tubing to stopcock and collection bag.	Ensures fluid is available as soon as catheter is placed. Closed system is established. Asepsis is maintained. Warmed solution prevents hypothermia in the child.	Refer to institution-specific protocol for variations in equipment set-up. In the smaller child, syringe may be used for manual instillation and aspiration of fluid.

Procedure continues on following page

* Level I: Manufacturer's recommendations only
  Level II: Theory-based; no research data to support recommendations; recommendations from expert consensus group may exist

Procedure	for Percutaneous Peritoneal Lavage: Assist—*Continued*	
Steps	**Rationale**	**Considerations**
10. Assist with clipping or shaving of hair, if needed, and cleansing of skin. Umbilicus is cleansed last.	Provides skin antisepsis. Clipping hair rather than shaving may decrease incidence rate of skin micro-abrasions, decreasing incidence rate of local skin infection.	Shaving can cause skin micro-abrasions and increase infection risk.[12] Umbilicus is considered a "dirty area" and should be cleansed last.[12]
11. Sterile drapes are placed to isolate the intended site of catheter insertion.	Maintains asepsis; reduces transmission of microorganisms.	The periumbilical area is generally used; a supraumbilical site may be used in the younger child to avoid puncture of the bladder.[3,12] Areas with surgical scars are avoided to reduce the risk of bowel perforation caused by adhesions.[3,12] *(Level IV*)*
12. Assist with administration of local anesthetic, generally 1% or 2% lidocaine with epinephrine.	Provides pain control. Epinephrine constricts local vessels, decreasing bleeding, which reduces false-positive results.[4,5,11,13] *(Level II*)*	Maximal dose of lidocaine is 4.5 mg/kg, to a maximum of 300 mg. Maximal dose of lidocaine with epinephrine is 7 mg/kg, to a maximum of 500 mg.[13]
13. Practitioner performs initial tap with introducer needle, Veress needle, or other needle/trocar apparatus.[3,4,5,11]	Accesses peritoneal space to assess for abdominal pathology.	Veress needle is a needle with a spring-loaded obturator, used most commonly in laparoscopic procedures. Practitioner may avoid use of trochar to decrease incidence rate of false-positive results.[11]
14. Initial aspirate is drawn and sent for laboratory assessment. Label specimen tubes at the bedside and complete laboratory paperwork per institution-specific protocol.	Confirms abdominal pathology. Labeling tubes at the bedside promotes patient safety by ensuring the specimens are correctly labeled and identified.	Free return of 10 mL of blood is considered a positive result, suspicious for hemoperitoneum. Surgical intervention may be necessary.[5,6,11,14] Studies obtained may include RBC, WBC, amylase, lipase, alkaline phosphate, culture, and sensitivity.[3-5,15]
15. If the tap is dry (no fluid is obtained), insertion of the lavage catheter proceeds. A small incision in the skin through the linea alba may be made.[3,4,11]	Facilitates further assessment of peritoneal space. Use of a small incision facilitates catheter insertion.[3,4,11]	Per practitioner preference, a flexible guidewire may be passed first to facilitate placement of lavage catheter.
16. After insertion of lavage catheter, stopcock, IV tubing, and IV fluids are attached to the catheter (Figure 99-1). *(Level II*)*	Facilitates administration of fluid into peritoneal space for diagnostic or therapeutic rinse.	
17. Saline solution, 0.9 % or Ringer's lactate, 10 to 20 mL/kg to a maximum of 1 L, is quickly infused into the peritoneal space (see Figure 99-1).[3-5,11,13]	Instilled fluid "rinses" the peritoneal space.	Fluid may be instilled with gravity or with syringe. Refer to prescribing practitioner's order or institution-specific protocol for fluid used for lavage.

* Level II: Theory-based; no research data to support recommendations; recommendations from expert consensus group may exist

Level IV: Limited clinical studies to support recommendations

Procedure for Percutaneous Peritoneal Lavage: Assist—*Continued*

Steps	Rationale	Considerations

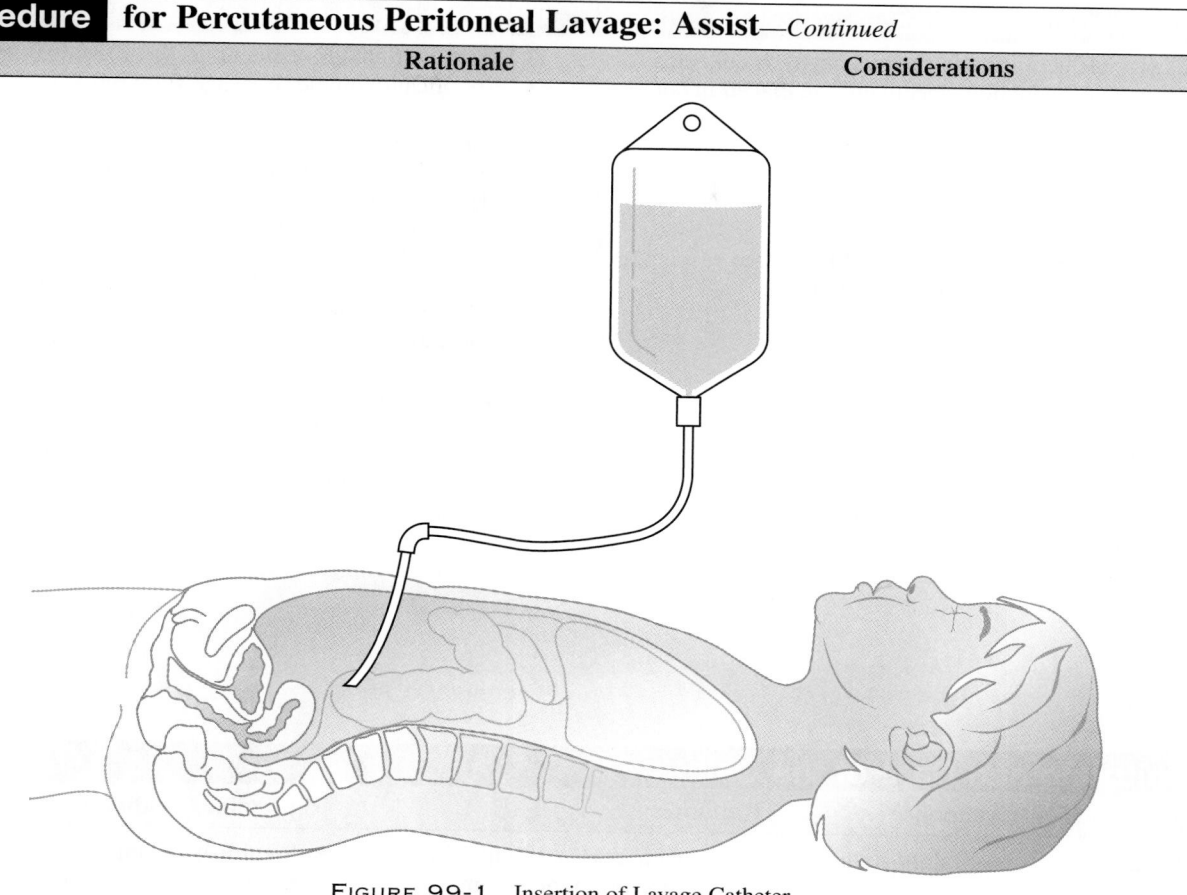

FIGURE 99-1   Insertion of Lavage Catheter.

Steps	Rationale	Considerations
18. Fluid is drained by placing the empty IV fluid bag in a dependent position, orienting the stopcock so that it is open to the collection bag and patient and placing the collection bag in a dependent position or gently aspirating with the syringe.[3-5,11] *(Level II*)*	Removes instilled fluid for assessment.	Child may be turned side to side to promote fluid distribution and drainage.[11] Send additional fluid for laboratory studies per prescribing practitioner's order.
19. Practitioner removes lavage catheter at completion of procedure. If incision was made, incision is closed with suture and a dressing is applied.[4,11]	Catheter is no longer needed; sutures close surgical wound; decreases risk of infection.	If surgery is necessary, the incision may be left open and packed with saline solution–soaked gauze. Take care not to remove packing and thus further contaminate abdominal cavity.
20. Dispose of used supplies and equipment, including sharps, in appropriate receptacles.	Standard precautions; reduces the transmission of microorganisms. Protects personnel health.	
21. Remove personal protective equipment; wash hands.	Reduces the transmission of microorganisms. Protects personnel health.	
22. If PPL results are positive, prepare the child for transport to the operating room.	Positive PPL results indicate intra-abdominal pathology that necessitates abdominal surgery.	

* Level II: Theory-based; no research data to support recommendations; recommendations from expert consensus group may exist

Expected Outcomes	Unexpected Outcomes
• Lavage effluent from peritoneal cavity is collected for diagnostic evaluation; specimens are placed in correct specimen tubes, labeled appropriately, and sent to the laboratory in the appropriate time frame • Child's cardiorespiratory status remains stable throughout PPL • Child's temperature remains stable or rises • Child is free from complications of PPL • Child has acceptable level of comfort throughout the procedure	• Inability to obtain effluent • Significant volume of lavage fluid remains in abdomen after PPL • Specimens are mislabeled, placed in incorrect tubes, or not sent to the laboratory in a timely manner • Hypotension, hypovolemia • Respiratory compromise • Hypothermia after PPL is performed • Lavage fluid is infused into abdominal wall or retroperitoneum • Laceration of catheter with loss in the peritoneal cavity • Wound infection • Laceration of major vessel • Perforation of bladder, colon, small bowel, stomach • Ovarian laceration • Unmanaged pain or agitation

Monitoring and Care of the Child

Activities and Interventions	Rationale	Reportable Conditions
1. Monitor child's respiratory status.	Increased abdominal fluid (either via lavage or ongoing hemorrhage) can impede diaphragmatic excursion, resulting in respiratory distress.	• Significant change in respiratory rate or work of breathing from baseline • Oxygen saturation less than 92% or significant change from baseline • Increased work of breathing: retractions, nasal flaring, paradoxic breathing
2. Monitor child's hemodynamic status.	Hemorrhagic shock related to abdominal bleeding or PPL-induced bleeding is a potential complication.	• Significant change from baseline heart rate (tachycardia or bradycardia) • Decreased peripheral pulses • Decreased capillary refill • Hypotension
3. Monitor child's temperature.	Identifies developing hypothermia or improvement in child's temperature if PPL was used as a rewarming therapy.	• New or persistent hypothermia
4. Monitor volume of effluent returned.	Identifies retained lavage fluid.	• Volume of retained lavage fluid
5. Monitor child's pain and/or anxiety level.	Prompt identification of pain and anxiety facilitates effective pain management.	• Unresolved pain or anxiety
6. Monitor for potential complications of PPL, including bowel or bladder perforation.	Percutaneous approach does not allow for direct visualization of visceral structures.	• Acute abdominal pain, distention, rigidity, guarding, increasing abdominal girth • Decreased bowel sounds • Blood in urine • Increased temperature
7. Monitor for signs of infection (systemic or localized).	Peritonitis from either abdominal trauma or PPL is a potential complication.	• Fever, chills • Redness, swelling at insertion site • Purulent drainage from the insertion site

Documentation

- Presence of informed consent
- Pre-procedural and postprocedural vital signs, respiratory status, and abdominal examination results, including abdominal girth
- Patient-procedure verification process per institution-specific protocol
- Decompression of stomach and bladder before PPL
- Date and time of PPL and individual who performed procedure
- Location of catheter insertion site
- Type and amount of fluid instilled
- Characteristic of effluent, including color, clarity, and particulate matter
- Medications administered and child's response
- Total lavage input minus total effluent output to determine net volume loss
- Record of specimens sent for laboratory evaluation
- Assessment of insertion site after procedure
- Child's tolerance of procedure
- Additional interventions and related outcomes
- Unexpected outcomes and related treatment
- Child and family education

References

1. McCance K, Huether S: *Pathophysiology: the biologic basis for disease in adults and children,* ed 4, Philadelphia, 2002, Mosby.
2. Davis JR, et al: Ultrasound: impact on diagnostic peritoneal lavage, abdominal computed tomography, and resident training, *Am Surg* 65:555-559, 1999.
3. Kumar A, et al: Diagnostic peritoneal lavage for assessing acute abdomen in pediatric oncology and stem cell transplantation patients, *J Pediatr Hematol Oncol* 26(12):824-826, 2004.
4. Nagy KK, et al: Experience with over 2500 diagnostic peritoneal lavages, *Injury Int J Care Injured* 31:479-482, 2000.
5. Hicks BA: Multiple trauma. In Levin DL, Morriss FC, editors: *Essentials of pediatric intensive care,* ed 2, New York, 1997, Churchill Livingstone, Inc.
6. Hazinski MF: *Manual of pediatric critical care,* St Louis, 1999, Mosby.
7. Saunders JC, et al: Percutaneous diagnostic peritoneal lavage using a Veress needle versus an open technique, *J Trauma Injury Infect Crit Care* 44(5):883-888, 1998.
8. Tyroch AH, et al: The association between Chance fractures and intra-abdominal injuries revisited: a multi-center review, *Am Surg* 71(5):434-438, 2005.
9. Dolich MO, et al: 2576 ultrasounds for blunt abdominal trauma, *J Trauma Injury Infect Crit Care* 50:108-112, 2001.
10. Ollerton JE: Prospective study to evaluate the influence of FAST on trauma patient management, *J Trauma Injury Infect Crit Care* 60(4):785-791, 2006.
11. Ruddy RM, et al: Illustrated techniques of pediatric emergency procedures. In Fleisher GR, et al, editors: *Textbook of pediatric emergency medicine,* ed 5, Philadelphia, 2006, Lippincott Williams & Wilkins.
12. Meeker MH, Rothrock JC, editors: *Alexander's care of the patient in surgery,* ed 11, St Louis, 1999, Mosby.
13. Sieberry GK, Iannone R, editors, *The Harriet Lane handbook,* ed 15, St Louis, 2000, Mosby.
14. Colony CS, Driscoll CE: Paracentesis and peritoneal lavage, *Patient Care* 29(13):137-146, 1995.
15. Simone S: Gastrointestinal critical care problems. In Curley MAQ, Moloney-Harmon PA, editors: *Critical care nursing of infants and children,* ed 2, Philadelphia, 2001, Saunders.

Additional Reading

Sweeny JF, et al: Diagnostic peritoneal lavage: volume of lavage effluent needed for accurate determination of negative lavage, *Injury* 25:659-661, 1994.

pH Monitoring Study: Care and Management

P U R P O S E : Esophageal pH monitoring provides a continuous measure of enteral pH for identification of the acid reflux associated with gastroesophageal reflux disease

Gretchen Delametter, Catherine A. Cochran, and Rémi Hueckel

PREREQUISITE KNOWLEDGE

- Child development as it relates to clinical assessment, care, and management of the child undergoing a pH monitoring study
- Anatomy and physiology of the pediatric upper gastrointestinal (GI) tract, including structural characteristics specific to the infant and child[1,2]
- Gastroesophageal reflux (GER) is the abnormal retrograde flow of acid and pepsin into the lower esophagus that is typically caused by motor dysfunction of the lower esophageal sphincter (Figure 100-1).[3,4]
- The child's current length in centimeters[5,6]
- Antireflux medication taken by the child and when last dose occurred[5,7-9]
- Symptomatology and pathophysiology of gastroesophageal reflux disease (GERD), including differences between age groups[6-8,10,11]
  - ❖ Infants often have vomiting, anorexia, dysphagia, odynophagia, arching of the back during feeds, irritability, failure to thrive, chronic respiratory disorders, recurrent stridor, chronic cough, and recurrent pneumonia.
  - ❖ Toddlers typically have intermittent vomiting.
  - ❖ Older children and adolescents usually have chronic heartburn, regurgitation and reswallowing, and abdominal pain.
- Gastroesophageal reflux disease has been associated with upper airway symptoms and apparent life-threatening events (ALTE).[8,12]
- Esophageal pH monitoring is performed with transnasal or oral placement of a microelectrode into the lower

esophagus. A device connected to the microelectrode records the pH every few seconds (Figure 100-2, *A*).[5,7,9,13]
- The distal end of the probe is placed at the level that corresponds to 87% of the distance from the nares to lower esophageal sphincter, based on the child's length. Fluoroscopic visualization may also be used for determination of the pH probe length (Figure 100-2, *B*).[10]
- Esophageal pH monitoring measures the frequency and duration of episodes of acid reflux, defined as esophageal pH of less than 4.[5-9,13]
- Esophageal pH monitoring does not detect nonacidic or postprandial reflux episodes.
- Episodes of nonacidic GER may cause complications in infants, such as ALTE, cough, or aspiration pneumonia.[6-9]
- Specially trained individuals place the esophageal pH monitoring device and connect it to the computer for periods of 8, 12, or 24 hours.[5,7-9,13]
- A variety of esophageal pH monitoring probes is available.[7,9]

CHILD AND FAMILY ASSESSMENT

- Child's developmental level and ability to interact ➤*Rationale:* Child's developmental level influences preparation and interaction and assists in determination of the level of cooperation that the child can provide.
- Child's and family's understanding of the reasons for and risks and benefits of the pH study ➤*Rationale:* Evaluates child's and family's understanding of the procedure and provides a gauge for ongoing education.
- History of signs and symptoms of GER ➤*Rationale:* Notation of child's history of signs and symptoms of

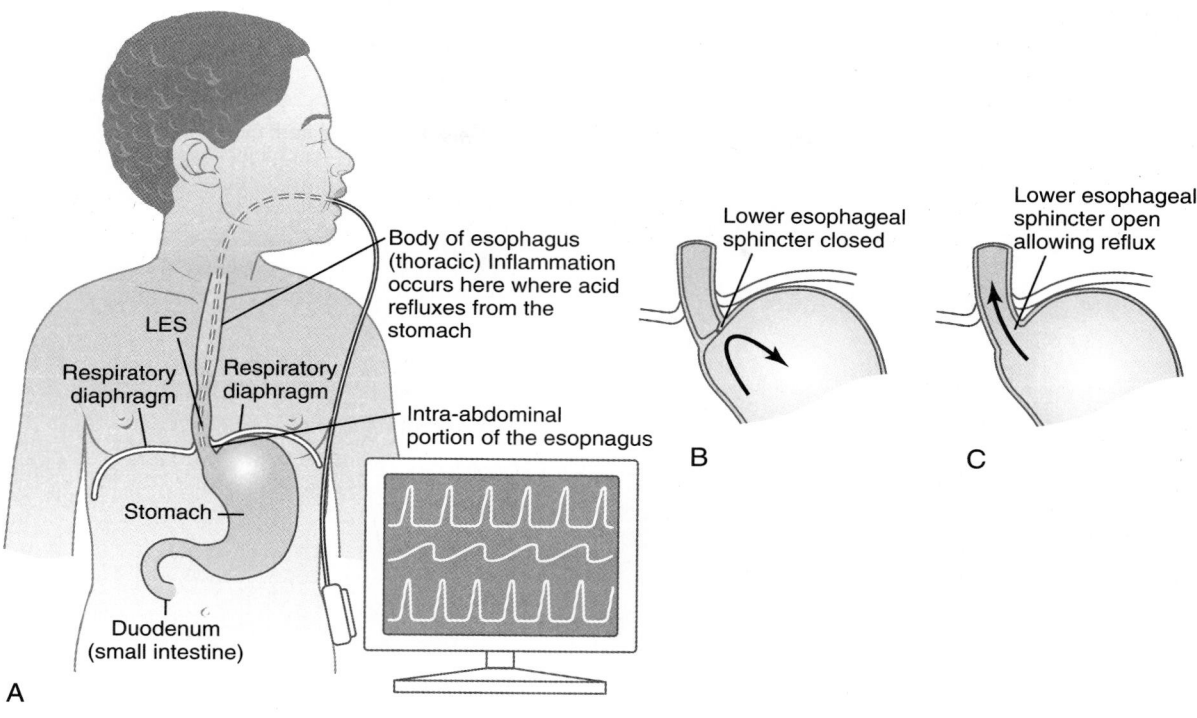

FIGURE 100-1   Gastroesophageal Reflux. **A,** Anatomy of esophagus and stomach. **B,** Lower esophageal sphincter closed. **C,** Lower esophageal sphincter open, allowing reflux.

GER assists in diagnosis and interpretation of pH study.

• Any antireflux medication the child has taken and when the last dose occurred ➧*Rationale:* Antireflux medications affect the results and interpretation of the pH monitoring study.

• Family's desire to be present during the procedure ➧*Rationale:* The family may provide support and comfort to the child but should have the choice not to remain with the child.

CHILD AND FAMILY EDUCATION

Individualized, developmentally appropriate education is provided to the family and to the child based on desire for knowledge, readiness to learn, and overall neurologic and psychosocial state.

• Explain the purpose of the pH probe study and the steps involved in tube insertion ➧*Rationale:* Providing information decreases anxiety and fear and may promote cooperation.

• Provide information regarding care and management of pH probe and the computerized recording device ➧*Rationale:* An understanding of the care and management supports a successful study.

• Ensure that child and family understand event log documentation with computerized recorder instructions ➧*Rationale:* An understanding of the care and management supports a successful study.

• Encourage questions and answer questions as they arise ➧*Rationale:* Reinforcement of information is needed during periods of stress.

EQUIPMENT

• Equipment and supplies are generally brought to the bedside by the specially trained individual who places the pH probe
• Event log or event journal
• Personal protective equipment
• Tape

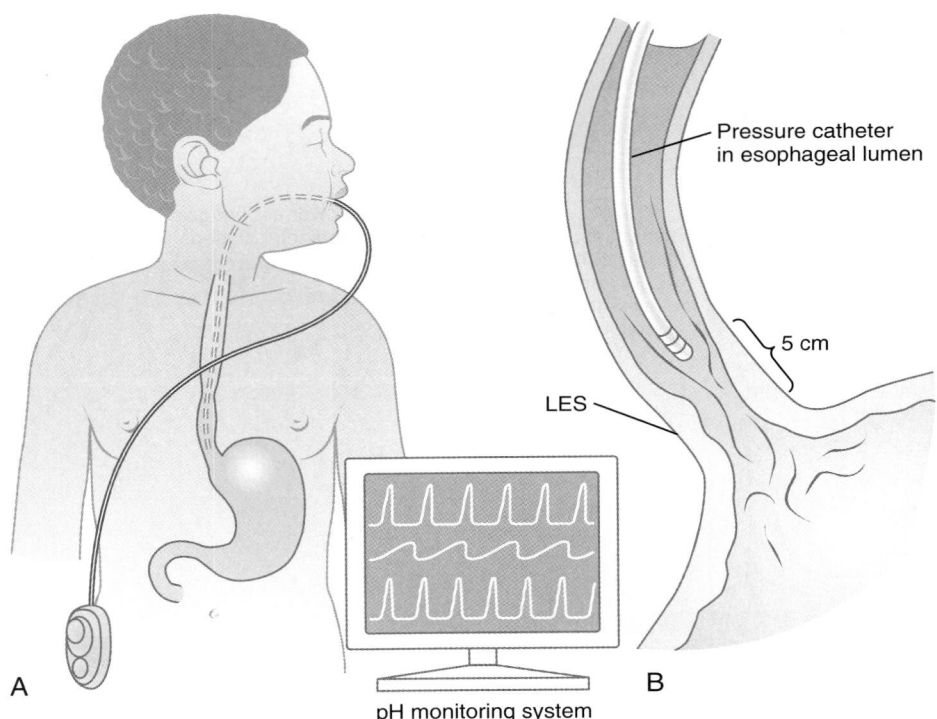

Pressure catheter
in esophageal lumen

5 cm

LES

A

B

pH monitoring system

FIGURE 1OO-2   pH Probe Study. **A,** Child during pH probe study. **B,** Placement of pH probe in esophagus.

Procedure for pH Monitoring Study: Care and Management

Steps	Rationale	Considerations
1. Review prescribing practitioner's order for esophageal pH monitor and schedule with appropriate personnel.	Preparation promotes completion of procedure in a timely manner.	
2. Ensure child and family understand procedure and questions are answered.	Evaluates and reinforces understanding of previously taught information.	Developmental level, cognitive ability, and anxiety level influence approach to and effectiveness of teaching. Use an interpreter if non-English speaking to ensure understanding before procedure.
3. Determine nothing by mouth (NPO) status and last time antireflux medication was administered.	Timing of NPO status before procedure is determined by institution-specific protocol.	Depending on the age and condition of the child, intravenous (IV) fluids may be required while child's status is NPO.
4. Collect equipment necessary to assist skilled clinician with esophageal pH probe placement.	Promotes completion of the procedure in a timely manner; may decrease child's anxiety. Assistance provides safety of the child during procedure.	
5. Wash hands. Put on clean gloves and other protective equipment.	Reduces the transmission of microorganisms. Protects personnel health.	
6. Obtain the child's length.	The child's height/length is needed for calculation of distance of probe insertion.	

Procedure	for pH Monitoring Study: Care and Management—*Continued*	
Steps	**Rationale**	**Considerations**
7. Ensure appropriate cardiopulmonary monitoring.	Children may need cardiorespiratory monitoring during the study.	Consider the child's status in selection of appropriate cardiopulmonary monitoring.
8. Assist skilled clinician with proper placement of esophageal pH probe. (*Level IV**)	Assistance may be needed to ensure proper positioning of probe, immobilization during probe placement, and safety.[7]	Parent or caregiver may provide comfort during procedure. A second assistant may be needed to help the child.
9. Assist with securing the probe in place with tape.	Taping prevents probe dislodgement.	Medical restraint devices per institution-specific protocol may be indicated during study to further prevent probe dislodgement.
10. Obtain a chest x-ray, as directed.	Typically needed to verify probe position.	
11. Reexplain to the family and child (as appropriate) the handling of the computerized event recorder while procedure is underway. (*Level I**)	Safety and care provide for uninterrupted study.[8]	Prevention of the recorder from getting wet; being exposed to x-rays, metal detectors, or strong radiation; or being dropped assists in ensuring accurate data are recorded. Do not attempt to open or service the recorder. Do not attempt to download data.
12. Use the event log to document events.	Event log provides useful information for the interpretation phase.	Computerized recorder has event button to push during events.
13. Discontinue pH probe per institutional guidelines.	Timing of probe removal with end of timed procedure.	pH probe may be done for 8, 12, or 24 hours. Removal of the probe and discontinuation of the procedure are done in the appropriate time following institution-specific protocol.
14. Wash hands. Dispose of clean gloves and other protective equipment.	Reduces the transmission of microorganisms. Protects personnel health.	

* Level I: Manufacturer's recommendations only.
  Level IV: Limited clinical studies to support recommendations

Expected Outcomes	Unexpected Outcomes
• Esophageal pH probe is in proper position • Esophageal pH probe and computerized recorder function properly during study • Interpretable results have been obtained	• Esophageal pH probe dislodgement • Computerized recorder malfunction • Missed reflux event because of pH probe buried in a musosal fold • False or negative study results caused by dietary or limited activity from intolerance of probe

Monitoring and Care of the Child

Activities and Interventions	Rationale	Reportable Conditions
1. Monitor child's tolerance during placement of the esophageal pH probe.	Changes in the child's condition may indicate complications of probe placement.	• Respiratory distress
2. Ensure event log documentation occurs and event log button is pushed when indicated.	Event log provides useful information for the interpretation phase.	• Event log button does not work on computerized recorder
3. Ensure placement of esophageal pH probe during monitoring time.	Proper probe placement throughout study ensures appropriate interpretation of results.	• Probe dislodgement

Documentation

- Time of placement of probe
- Child's tolerance of study
- Time of end of study and probe removal
- Child's tolerance of the procedure
- Additional interventions and related outcomes, including medications administered
- Child and family education
- Unexpected outcomes and related treatment

References

1. Sentongo T, Steinhorn D: Gastrointestinal structure and function. In Fuhrman B, Zimmerman J, editors: *Pediatric critical care,* ed 3, Philadelphia, 2006, Mosby.
2. McCance K, Huether S: *Pathophysiology: the biologic basis for disease in adults and children,* St Louis, 2002, Mosby Inc.
3. Biddle W: Gastroesophageal reflux disease; current treatment strategies, *Gastroenterol Nurs* 25(6):258, 2003.
4. Williams J: Gastroesophageal reflux disease: clinical manefestations, *Gastroenterol Nurs* 26(5):195-201, 2003.
5. Mahajan L, et al: Reproducibility of 24-hour intraesophageal pH monitoring in pediatric patients, *Pediatrics* 101:260-263, 1998.
6. Napierkowski J, Wong R: Extraesophageal manifestations of GERD, *Am J Med Sci* 326:285-299, 2003.
7. Richter J: Diagnostic tests for gastroesophageal reflux disease, *Am J Med Sci* 326:300-308, 2003.
8. Rudolph C, Mazur L, Lynnette J, et al: Guidelines for evaluation and treatment of gastroesphogeal reflux in infants and children: recommendations of the North American Society for Pediatric Gastroenterology and Nutrition, *JPGN* 32: S1-S31, 2001.
9. Sarani B, et al: Esophageal pH monitoring, indications, and methods, *J Clin Gastroenterol* 34:200-206, 2002.
10. Behrman R., et al: *Nelson's textbook of pediatrics,* ed 17, Philadelphia, 2004, Saunders.
11. Hassell E: Decisions in diagnosing and managing chronic gastroesophageal reflux disease in children, *J Pediatr* 146:S3-S12, 2005.
12. Rosbe KW, Kenna MA, Auerbach AD: Extraesophageal reflux in pediatric patients with upper respiratory symptoms, *Arch Otolaryngol Head Neck Surg* 129(11):1213-1220, 2003.
13. Emmerson A, et al: Assessment of three methods of pH probe positioning in preterm infants, *JPGN* 35:69-72, 2002.

Additional Reading

Sandhill Scientific, Inc: *Manufacturer's recommendations,* Highlands Ranch, CO, Sandhill Scientific, Inc.

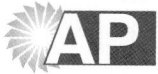

101

Abdominal Paracentesis: Perform

PURPOSE: Abdominal paracentesis involves the percutaneous acquisition of peritoneal fluid for diagnostic evaluation or therapeutic abdominal decompression in instances in which intraabdominal pressure causes respiratory compromise from limited diaphragmatic excursion

Kelly Murawski

PREREQUISITE KNOWLEDGE

- Child development as it relates to clinical assessment and abdominal paracentesis
- Anatomy and physiology of the abdominal system[1,2]
- Directly beneath the abdominal wall are the intestines and bladder.[3]
- With ascites, the bowel tends to float to the midline.[3]
- Mastery of pediatric advanced life support competencies[4]
- Conditions that may result in the development of ascites, with therapeutic or diagnostic paracentesis needed, include obstructive urinary tract anomalies, gastrointestinal (GI) tract perforation, congestive heart failure, portal hypertension, peritonitis, neoplasm, ventriculoperitoneal shunt obstruction, orthotopic liver transplantation, and complication of retroperitoneal or mediastinal surgery.[5-7]
- Studies such as computed tomographic (CT) scan or ultrasound scan may be used for localization of the fluid collection before abdominal paracentesis.[6,8]
- Rapid drainage of a large volume of peritoneal fluid may result in hypotension. Albumin replacement may be initiated for volume expansion and minimization of renal or electrolyte complications.[6,8]

- Relative contraindications include prior abdominal surgery and clinical evidence of fibrinolysis and disseminated intravascular coagulopathy.[3,6] Any coagulation disorder requires careful planning for management.[8,9] Needle puncture for abdominal paracentesis should not be performed in a cellulitic area.
- Complications of abdominal paracentesis, although rare, include introduction of contaminates into the peritoneal space, perforation of hollow viscus, perforation of blood vessel, abdominal wall hematoma, scrotal swelling, and leakage of ascitic fluid from tap site.[6,9,10] Extreme caution must be used in children with moderate or severe coagulopathies.[9]
- Principles of aseptic technique
- Appropriate pediatric dosing of analgesics and anxiolytics and competency in procedural sedation
- With use of a paracentesis kit, follow the manufacturer's instructions for performance of procedure.
- Except in an emergency situation, informed consent is required before abdominal paracentesis.

CHILD AND FAMILY ASSESSMENT

- Child's developmental level and ability to interact
  ➤➤*Rationale:* Child's developmental level influences preparation and interaction.
- Child's and family's understanding of the reasons for and risks and benefits of the abdominal paracentesis
  ➤➤*Rationale:* Evaluates child's and family's understanding

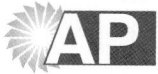

of the procedure and provides a gauge for ongoing education; facilitates informed consent.

- Presence of abdominal abnormalities, including scars, burns, and cellulitis ➤➤*Rationale:* Abnormalities of the abdominal surface may predispose the child to complications. Previous abdominal surgery may indicate adhesions and possible fixation of intestines to the abdominal wall, which increase the risk of intestinal puncture.[6,9-11]
- Presence of bowel and bladder distension ➤➤*Rationale:* Marked bowel distension from increased intraluminal pressure predisposes the bowel to puncture and possible leakage of bowel contents into the peritoneal cavity.[10] As with bowel distension, bladder distention may increase the risk of perforation.
- Child's current respiratory status, including work of breathing ➤➤*Rationale:* Identifies potential complications related to sedation administration. Provides a baseline for comparison of respiratory status before and after the procedure.
- Fluid and electrolyte status ➤➤*Rationale:* Peritoneal fluid removal may lead to shifts in serum electrolyte levels and a decrease in circulatory blood volume.
- History of coagulopathy ➤➤*Rationale:* Presence of a coagulopathy predisposes the child to potential complications from bleeding if a blood vessel is punctured.
- History of allergies ➤➤*Rationale:* Exposing the child to potential medications or material that may trigger an allergic reaction is avoided.
- Availability of intravenous (IV) access ➤➤*Rationale:* IV access is needed for administration of sedation; volume resuscitation may be necessary if large volumes of fluid are removed from the abdomen.
- Evaluate the need for sedation and the child's previous response to procedural sedation ➤➤*Rationale:* Sedation provided to an uncooperative child reduces the child's anxiety and facilitates a successful safe procedure, thereby minimizing complications. Issues identified during previous sedation experiences influence the sedation management plan for the procedure.
- Family's desire to be present during the procedure ➤➤*Rationale:* Family may provide support and comfort measures to the child if institution-specific protocol facilitates family presence during the procedure, but family should have the choice not to remain with the child.

CHILD AND FAMILY EDUCATION

Individualized, developmentally appropriate education is provided to the family and to the child based on desire for knowledge, readiness to learn, and overall neurologic and psychosocial state.

- Provide information about abdominal paracentesis, including the reason for the procedure and the steps involved in removal of peritoneal fluid ➤➤*Rationale:* Providing information decreases anxiety and fear and facilitates informed consent.
- Inform the child and family of initial positioning for the procedure and whether repositioning will be necessary during the procedure ➤➤*Rationale:* Providing information decreases anxiety and fear and promotes cooperation with the procedure. The child will be positioned in a manner that facilitates fluid removal.
- Provide information about medications that will be administered for the procedure, including local anesthetics, analgesics, and anxiolytics ➤➤*Rationale:* Providing information about pain and anxiety management decreases anxiety and fear and reassures the child and family that pain will be managed.
- Provide information regarding the results of the procedure, including results of the fluid analysis ➤➤*Rationale:* Providing information decreases anxiety and fear and includes the family in the plan of care.
- Encourage questions and answer questions as they arise ➤➤*Rationale:* Reinforcement of information is needed during periods of stress.

EQUIPMENT

- Povidone-iodine or chlorhexidine
- Sterile 4×4 gauze sponges
- Sterile drapes
- Sterile gloves and other protective gear, as indicated
- Lidocaine, 1%
- Syringe, 3-mL or 5-mL, with 25-gauge needle
- Syringes, 10-mL (two)
- 20-gauge or 22-gauge needle or over-the-needle catheter (for small child)
- 16-gauge or 20-gauge needle or over-the-needle catheter (for older child)
  - ❖ 15-gauge paracentesis needle (fenestrated needle with stylet) may also be used, based on practitioner's preference
- Appropriate containers for requested fluid specimens
- Appropriate laboratory requisitions
- Appropriate labels for requested specimens

OR

- Paracentesis kit with needle
- If gradual drainage of peritoneal fluid is desired for decompression (optional):
  - ❖ Three-way stopcock
  - ❖ IV tubing and sterile empty IV bag

Procedure for Abdominal Paracentesis: Perform

Steps	Rationale	Considerations
1. Ensure child and family understand procedure and questions are answered. Obtain informed written consent from child's legal guardian.	Evaluates and reinforces understanding of previously taught information; ensures medical-legal compliance as suggested by the Joint Commission on Accreditation of Healthcare Organizations (JCAHO). The family and child have a right to information regarding the risks and benefits of the procedure.	Developmental level, cognitive ability, and anxiety level determine approach to and effectiveness of teaching. In emergency situations, refer to institution-specific protocol for assumption of consent. Use an interpreter if patient or family is non-English speaking to ensure understanding before procedure.
2. Collect all necessary equipment and supplies.	Facilitates completion of procedure in a timely manner; eliminates stepping away from the sterile field.	Gauge of needle or catheter is dependent on the child's size. If a kit is used, only gather equipment and supplies not contained in the kit.
3. Ensure appropriate cardiopulmonary monitoring.	Critically ill children may have decompensation during the procedure.	Consider the child's status in selection of the appropriate monitoring. If procedural sedation is used, ensure the availability of emergency equipment and medications.
4. Ensure sedation is administered as indicated and per prescribing practitioner's order.	Use of sedatives may facilitate a safe successful procedure for an anxious child.	Individual who performs the procedure should not be responsible for monitoring child's cardiopulmonary status during sedation administration.
5. Wash hands.	Reduces transmission of microorganisms.	
6. Position the child supine with head slightly elevated (semirecumbent position). (Level II*)	The child's position facilitates removal of fluid.	Child's condition, physical examination results, and location of fluid may cause the child's position to vary.
7. Identify child with appropriate patient/procedure verification process (e.g., "Time out").	Confirms correct patient, procedure, and site as recommended by JCAHO; prevents unnecessary medical procedures.	Verification process and documentation are institution specific; use active communication techniques.
8. Assess and percuss abdomen to locate fluid collection and evaluate for the presence of scars or cellulitis.	Localizes fluid collection; identifies site for needle insertion. Adhesion of bowel to abdominal wall may be present beneath area of scarring, increasing the risk of intestinal perforation if percutaneous paracentesis is attempted. Avoid areas of cellulitis to minimize risk of infection.[9-12]	Ultrasound or CT scan may assist with localization of fluid pockets in the child with minimal fluid or with a history of abdominal surgeries/procedures.[6,9] (Level IV*)
9. Ensure the bladder is empty with verification of recent void or straight catheterization.	Minimizes perforation of bladder and ensures bladder is located within pelvis away from site of procedure.[6,8-12] (Level II*)	

Procedure continues on following page

---

* Level II: Theory-based; no research data to support recommendations; recommendations from expert consensus group may exist
Level IV: Limited clinical studies to support recommendations

AP This procedure should be performed only by physicians, advanced practice nurses, and other health care professionals (including critical care nurses) with additional knowledge, skills, and demonstrated competence per professional licensure or institutional standard.

Procedure for Abdominal Paracentesis: Perform—*Continued*

Steps	Rationale	Considerations
10. Identify landmarks for approach (Figure 101-1): *Midline:* Midway between the umbilicus and pubic symphysis. *Right or left lower quadrant:* Below the umbilicus, several centimeters above the inguinal ligament, in the midclavicular line.	Insertion of the needle in a dependent and lateral position minimizes the risk of entering the bowel.[9-11] Air-filled bowel floats in ascetic fluid.[10] *(Level II*)*	Site of needle entry may vary depending on location of fluid and age of child. With side-lying position, the left side is preferred.[3]

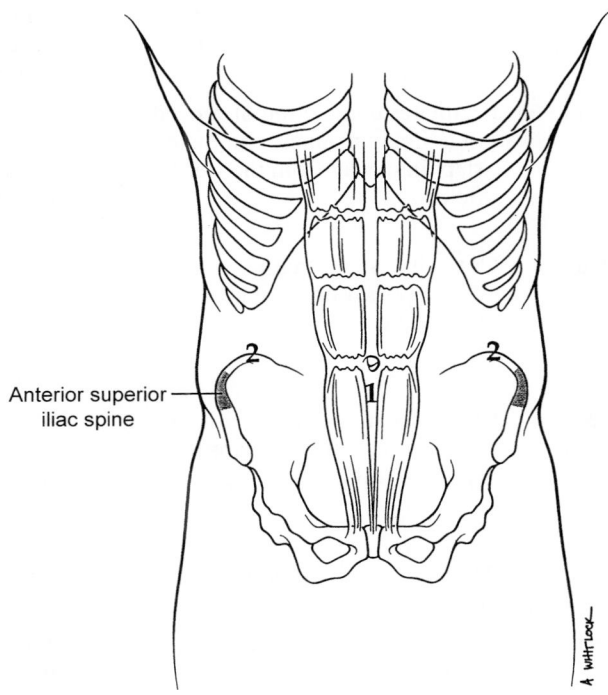

Anterior superior iliac spine

FIGURE 101-1   Landmarks for Paracentesis. *1,* Midline: Midway between umbilicus and pubic symphysis. *2,* Right or left lower quadrant: Below umbilicus, several centimeters above inguinal ligament, in midclavicular line.

Steps	Rationale	Considerations
11. Wash hands; put on sterile gloves.	Aseptic technique is used for this procedure.	Garb for individuals in the room during the procedure varies from institution to institution; refer to institution-specific protocol.
12. Clean the skin with 4×4 gauze pads saturated with an antiseptic solution.	Adherence to strict aseptic technique minimizes the introduction of contaminants into the peritoneal space.	
13. Drape the area with sterile towels or drape.	Creates a sterile area for the procedure.	
14. Anesthetize the puncture site by infiltration of the area with 1% lidocaine with the 25-gauge needle and 3-mL syringe. Include the skin, muscle wall, and peritoneum.	Local anesthetic minimizes pain at site of insertion during advancement of needle.[6,8-12]	
15. Insert the needle perpendicular to the skin while applying negative pressure to syringe with the Z-track technique; apply traction to the skin caudally while inserting the needle (Figure 101-2, *A*).	The Z-track technique reduces leakage of fluid through the puncture site by eliminating a direct track.[6,9-11]	After the needle penetrates the peritoneum and fluid is obtained, release traction of skin.

* Level II: Theory-based; no research data to support recommendations; recommendations from expert consensus group may exist

Procedure for Abdominal Paracentesis: Perform—*Continued*

Steps	Rationale	Considerations

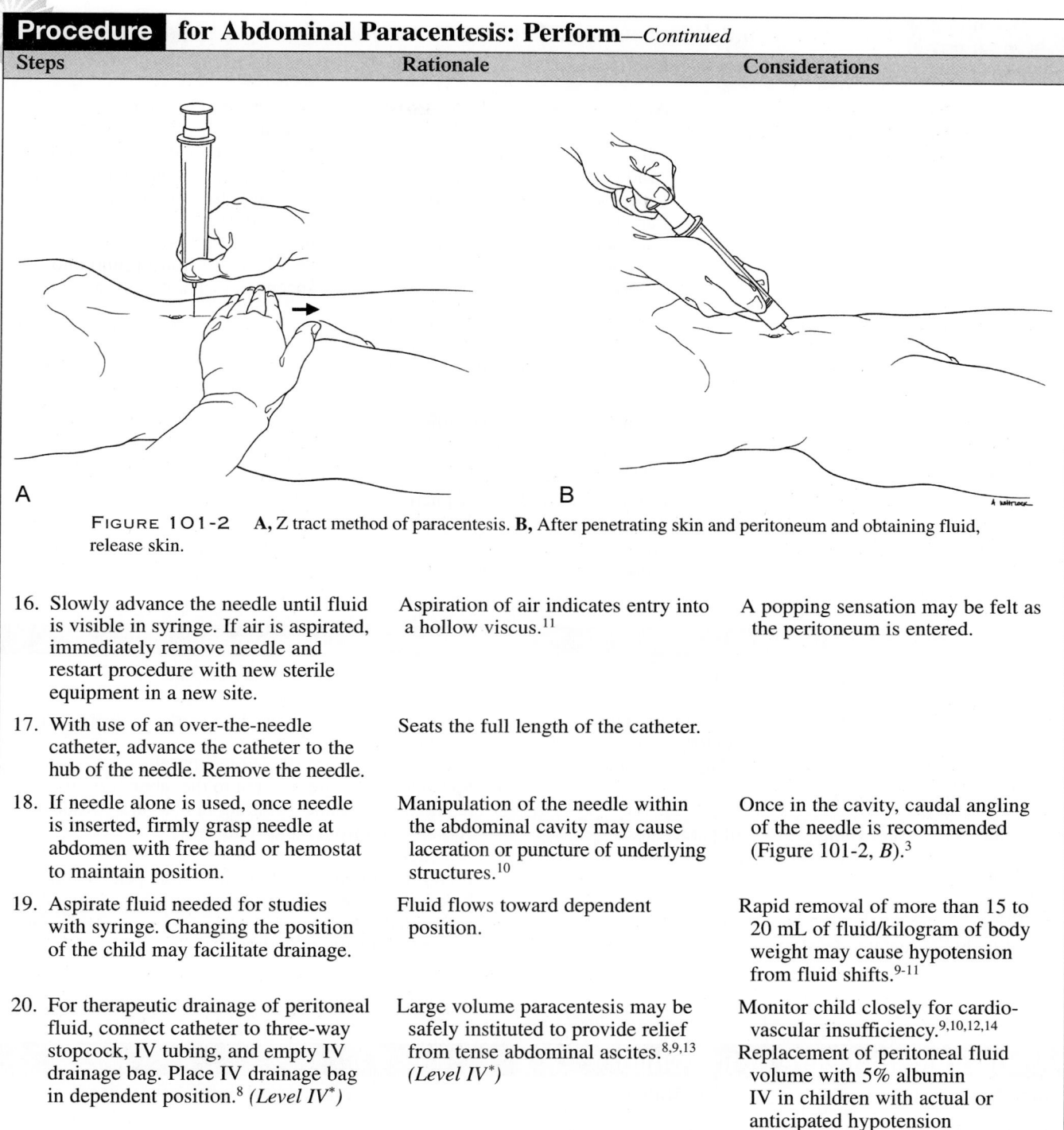

FIGURE 101-2 **A,** Z tract method of paracentesis. **B,** After penetrating skin and peritoneum and obtaining fluid, release skin.

Steps	Rationale	Considerations
16. Slowly advance the needle until fluid is visible in syringe. If air is aspirated, immediately remove needle and restart procedure with new sterile equipment in a new site.	Aspiration of air indicates entry into a hollow viscus.[11]	A popping sensation may be felt as the peritoneum is entered.
17. With use of an over-the-needle catheter, advance the catheter to the hub of the needle. Remove the needle.	Seats the full length of the catheter.	
18. If needle alone is used, once needle is inserted, firmly grasp needle at abdomen with free hand or hemostat to maintain position.	Manipulation of the needle within the abdominal cavity may cause laceration or puncture of underlying structures.[10]	Once in the cavity, caudal angling of the needle is recommended (Figure 101-2, *B*).[3]
19. Aspirate fluid needed for studies with syringe. Changing the position of the child may facilitate drainage.	Fluid flows toward dependent position.	Rapid removal of more than 15 to 20 mL of fluid/kilogram of body weight may cause hypotension from fluid shifts.[9-11]
20. For therapeutic drainage of peritoneal fluid, connect catheter to three-way stopcock, IV tubing, and empty IV drainage bag. Place IV drainage bag in dependent position.[8] *(Level IV*)*	Large volume paracentesis may be safely instituted to provide relief from tense abdominal ascites.[8,9,13] *(Level IV*)*	Monitor child closely for cardio-vascular insufficiency.[9,10,12,14] Replacement of peritoneal fluid volume with 5% albumin IV in children with actual or anticipated hypotension is effective in restoring fluid balance.[10]

Procedure continues on following page

* Level IV: Limited clinical studies to support recommendations

Procedure   for Abdominal Paracentesis: Perform—*Continued*

Steps	Rationale	Considerations
21. Place the fluid in appropriate containers and label the containers at the bedside. Complete laboratory paperwork per institution-specific protocol.	Analysis of peritoneal fluid assists with the diagnosis of ascites, peritonitis, or hemorrhage. Culture and Gram stain can identify specific pathogens.[13,14] *(Level VI*)* Labeling specimens at the bedside promotes patient safety and ensures accurate and efficient processing of specimen.	Consider sending fluid for aerobic and anaerobic culture and sensitivity, Gram stain, cell count with differential, protein, glucose, lactic dehydrogenase (LDH), pH, and amylase. *(Level VI*)* Follow standard precautions in transfer of peritoneal fluid into specimen containers.
22. After fluid is collected, remove catheter or needle and apply pressure over the site. Cover the site with a pressure dressing.	Application of pressure to the site reduces the leakage of peritoneal fluid from the tap site.[9,10]	
23. Discard used supplies and equipment, including sharps, in appropriate receptacles.	Reduces transmission of micro-organisms. Protects personnel health.	
24. Remove gloves and personal protective equipment; wash hands.	Reduces transmission of micro-organisms.	

* Level VI: Clinical studies in a variety of patient populations and situations to support recommendations

Expected Outcomes

- Adequate volume of peritoneal fluid is obtained percutaneously
- Removal of peritoneal fluid results in abdominal decompression and improved respiratory status
- Peritoneal fluid is sent for ordered laboratory studies

- Child is free from complications of paracentesis
- Aseptic technique is maintained

- Child has acceptable level of comfort

Unexpected Outcomes

- Inadequate volume of fluid obtained
- Inability to obtain fluid
- Abdominal compression and respiratory distress do not improve
- Specimen tubes are labeled incorrectly
- Specimen tubes are not sent to the laboratory in required time frame, resulting in inaccurate results
- Hypotension from rapid fluid shifts
- Infection
- Injury to internal structures, including perforation of blood vessel, perforation of organ, or hematoma of abdominal wall
- Unmanaged pain or anxiety

Monitoring and Care of the Child

Activities and Interventions	Rationale	Reportable Conditions
1. Monitor cardiovascular status (heart rate, blood pressure, peripheral perfusion, and level of consciousness) every 5 to 15 minutes during the procedure and every 30 minutes for 2 hours after the procedure.[11]	Rapid removal of a large volume of fluid can cause hypotension from sudden fluid shifts.	• Hypotension
2. Monitor child's abdominal examination results after procedure, including abdominal girth, pain, and bowel sounds.	Monitors for improvement in child's status after procedure or reaccumulation of fluid.	• Abdominal girth remains elevated or increases • Increasing abdominal distension
3. Evaluate child for pain or discomfort.	Presence of pain and discomfort may indicate a complication.	• Unmanaged pain

Monitoring and Care of the Child—Cont'd

Activities and Interventions	Rationale	Reportable Conditions
4. Assess appearance of site for leakage of fluid or development of hematoma. 5. Monitor the child for complications related to the procedure.	Monitors for complications of the procedure. Prompt identification of complications facilitates early intervention.	• Hematoma • Persistent fluid leak • Bleeding • Erythema, swelling around puncture site

Documentation

- Informed consent process
- Results of preprocedural laboratory studies
- Preprocedural and postprocedural assessment of the abdomen
- Technique used, including size and type of needle or catheter, location of puncture site, skin antisepsis, local anesthesia
- Sedation prescribed and administered
- Amount and appearance of fluid removed
- Respiratory status before, during, and after procedure
- Postprocedure site assessment
- Laboratory studies sent and results of laboratory analysis
- Child's tolerance of procedure
- Unexpected outcomes and related treatment
- Child and family education

References

1. Sentongo T, Steinhorn D: Gastrointestinal structure and function. In Fuhrman B, Zimmerman J, editors: *Pediatric critical care,* ed 3, Philadelphia, 2006, Mosby.
2. McCance K, Huether S: *Pathophysiology: the biologic basis for disease in adults and children,* Philadelphia, 2002, Mosby.
3. Kirkwood P: Paracentesis (perform). In Lynn-McHale Wiegand DJ, Carlson K, editors: *AACN procedure manual for critical care,* Philadelphia, 2005, Elsevier.
4. Hazinski MF, Zaritzky AL, Nadkarni V, et al, editors: *Pediatric advanced life support provider manual,* Dallas, 2002, American Heart Association.
5. Herzog D, et al: Ascites after orthotopic liver transplantation in children, *Pediatr Transplant* 9:74-79, 2005.
6. Lane NE, Paul RI: Paracentesis. In Henretig F, King C, editors: *Textbook of pediatric emergency medicine procedures,* Philadelphia, 1997, Lippincott, Williams & Wilkins.
7. Leibovitch I, et al: The diagnosis and management of postoperative chylous ascites, *J Urol* 167(2 Pt 1):449-457, 2002.
8. Kramer RE, et al: Large-volume paracentesis in the management of ascites in children, *J Pediatr Gastroenterol Nutr* 33(3):245-249, 2001.
9. Hickerson S, et al: Diagnostic procedures. In Dieckmann RA, et al, editors: *Pediatric emergency and critical care procedures,* ed 1, St Louis, 1997, Mosby.
10. Pache I, Bilodeau M: Severe haemorrhage following abdominal paracentesis for ascites in patients with liver disease, *Alimentary Pharmacol Therapeutics* 21(5): 525-529, 2005.
11. Tuggle DW: Abdominal paracentesis. In Blummer J, editor: *A practical guide to pediatric intensive care,* ed 3, St Louis, 1990, Mosby.
12. Gunn V, Nechyba C, editors: *The Harriet Lane handbook: a manual for pediatric house officers,* ed 16, Philadelphia, 2002, Mosby.
13. Dammert W: Abdominal paracentesis. In Levin DL, Morriss FC, Moore GC, editors: *A practical guide to pediatric intensive care,* ed 2, St Louis, 1984, Mosby.
14. Runyon BA: Paracentesis of ascitic fluid: a safe procedure, *Arch Int Med* 146:2259-2261, 1986.

Additional Readings

Duszak RL, et al: Percutaneous catheter drainage of infected intra-abdominal fluid collections; American College of Radiology, ACR appropriateness criteria, *Radiology* 215(Suppl):1067-1075, 2000.
Ergene U, et al: Current value of peritoneal tap in blunt abdominal trauma, *Eur J Emerg Med* 9:253-257, 2002.
Habeeb KS, Herrera JL: Management of ascites; paracentesis as a guide, *Postgrad Med* 101:191-200, 1997.

PROCEDURE

102

Apheresis: Assist

P U R P O S E : Apheresis is an automated procedure in which blood is withdrawn, a portion is separated and retained, and the remainder is retransfused to the child or donor. Therapeutic apheresis may be a first-line or adjunctive treatment to remove abnormal blood components. Donor apheresis is used to collect products for transfusion or transplant.

Cynthia L. Smitka and Sheryl A. Woloskie

PREREQUISITE KNOWLEDGE

- Apheresis is the separation and removal of a specified blood component through an automated process of centrifugation or filtration.
  - Whole blood is removed from a vein through a large-bore needle or one port of a double-lumen central venous catheter (CVC).
  - The blood is anticoagulated with citrate or heparin and enters the apheresis machine where it is separated into components.
  - The machine is programmed to collect one of these components and to send the remainder of the blood back to the child via a second peripheral line or port of a CVC.
  - The apheresis machine is equipped with blood filters, a warmer, and air detectors to prevent adverse events.
- Apheresis is used for a variety of diseases, which have been categorized from I to IV according to benefit versus risk and known efficacy (Table 102-1).[1]
- Decisions to treat pediatric patients with apheresis are often based on clinical data from adult studies, although presentations and therapeutic responses differ in children.[2] Nevertheless, apheresis technology has proven beneficial and sometimes life-saving in a growing number of childhood disorders.
- Plasmapheresis, or therapeutic plasma exchange (TPE), is the most frequently performed of these procedures and is used to non-selectively remove autoantibodies, para-

proteins, immunoglobulins, toxins, or drugs and to replace clotting factors.
  - In plasmapheresis, exchange or replacement fluid is determined by current and comorbid conditions. 0.9% saline solution, 5% albumin, or donor plasma may be used.
  - Typically, 1 to 1.5 total blood volumes (TBVs) are exchanged every other day for an average of five treatments, depending on response. Some conditions, such as thrombotic thrombocytopenic purpura or hemolytic uremic syndrome, warrant daily plasma exchange.
- Leukapheresis is the removal of white blood cells to reduce the circulating number in hyperleukemic states or to obtain granulocytes or mononuclear, dendritic, or hematopoetic progenitor cells for transfusion.
  - No exchange fluid is necessary, although albumin or red blood cells (RBCs) may be transfused concurrently to maintain hemodynamic stability.
  - Leukapheresis is performed once a day, until the desired response is obtained or the cell dose is collected; it is usually limited to one or two procedures.
  - Hematopoetic progenitor cell collection is a specialized form of leukapheresis that targets precursor cells for bone marrow transplant.
- Erythrocytapheresis is the removal or exchange of red blood cells for the treatment of diseases such as sickle cell anemia or polycythemia.
  - The number of RBC units needed to complete the exchange varies depending on the child's size.

| TABLE 102-1 | Guidelines for Therapeutic Hemapheresis[1] *(Level III*)* |

Disease	Procedure	Indication Category
Neurologic disorders		
Chronic inflammatory demyelinating polyradiculoneuropathy	Plasma exchange	I
Acute inflammatory demyelinating polyradiculoneuropathy (AIDP or Guillian-Barré syndrome)	Plasma exchange	I
Myasthenia gravis	Plasma exchange	I
Lambert-Eaton myasthenic syndrome	Plasma exchange	II
Multiple sclerosis and related disorders	Plasma exchange	
Acute fulminant central nervous system demyelination		II
Relapsing or progressive		III
Paraneoplastic neurologic syndromes	Plasma exchange	III
	Immunoadsorption	III
Paraproteinemic polyneuropathies	Plasma exchange	I
Demyelinating polyneuropathy IgG/IgA	Immunoadsorption	III
Polyneuropathy with IgM (with or without Waldenstrom's macroglobulinemia)	Plasma exchange	II
	Immunoadsorption	III
Cryoglobulinemia with polyneuropathy	Plasma exchange	II
Multiple myeloma with polyneuropathy	Plasma exchange	III
POEMS syndrome	Plasma exchange	III
Systemic (AL) amyloidosis	Plasma exchange	IV
Inflammatory myopathies	Plasma exchange	III
Polymyositis or dermatomyositis	Leukapheresis	IV
Inclusion-body myositis	Plasma exchange	III
	Leukapheresis	IV
Rasmussen's encephalitis	Plasma exchange	III
Stiff-person syndrome	Plasma exchange	III
Sydenham's chorea/pediatric autoimmune disorders associated with streptococcal infections (PANDAS)	Plasma exchange	II
Hematologic diseases		
ABO-incompatible hematopoietic cell transplant	Plasma exchange (recipient)	II
Erythrocytosis/polycythemia vera	Erythrocytapheresis	II
Leukocytosis and thrombocytosis	Cytapheresis	I
Thrombotic thrombocytopenic purpura	Plasma exchange	I
Posttransfusion purpura	Plasma exchange	I
Sickle cell disease	Red cell exchange	I
Myeloma/paraproteins/hyperviscosity	Plasma exchange	II
Myeloma/acute renal failure	Plasma exchange	II
Coagulation factor inhibitors	Plasma exchange	II
Aplastic anemia/pure red cell aplasia	Plasma exchange	III
Cutaneous T-cell lymphoma	Photopheresis	I
	Leukapheresis	III
Hemolytic disease of the newborn	Plasma exchange	III
Platelet alloimmunization and refractoriness	Plasma exchange	III
	Immunoadsorption	III
Malaria/babesiosis	Red cell exchange	III
Renal and metabolic diseases		
Antiglomerular basement membrane antibody disease (Goodpasture's syndrome)	Plasma exchange	I
Rapidly progressive glomerulonephritis	Plasma exchange	II
Hemolytic-uremic syndrome	Plasma exchange	III
Renal transplantation		
Rejection	Plasma exchange	IV
Presensitization	Plasma exchange	III
Recurrent focal glomerulosclerosis	Plasma exchange	III
Heart transplant rejection	Plasma exchange	III
	Photopheresis	III
Acute hepatic failure	Plasma exchange	III

* Level III: Laboratory data; no clinical data to support recommendations.

TABLE 102-1	Guidelines for Therapeutic Hemapheresis[1]—Cont'd	

Disease	Procedure	Indication Category
Familial hypercholesterolemia	Selective adsorption	I
	Plasma exchange	II
Overdose poisoning	Plasma exchange	III
Phytanic acid storage disease	Plasma exchange	I
Autoimmune and rheumatic diseases		
Cryoglobulinemia	Plasma exchange	II
Idiopathic thrombocytopenic purpura	Immunoadsorption	II
Raynaud's phenomenon	Plasma exchange	III
Vasculitis	Plasma exchange	III
Autoimmune hemolytic anemia	Plasma exchange	III
Rheumatoid arthritis	Immunoadsorption	II
	Lymphoplasmapheresis	II
	Plasma exchange	IV
Scleroderma/progressive systemic sclerosis	Plasma exchange	III
Systemic lupus erythematosus	Plasma exchange	III

From Jones HG, Bandarenko N: Management of the therapeutic apheresis patient. In McLeod BC, Price TH, Weinstein R, editors: *Apheresis: principles and practice*, ed 2, Bethesda, MD, 2003, American Association of Blood Banks.
Category I, Standard acceptable therapy; *Category II,* sufficient evidence to suggest efficacy usually as adjunctive therapy; *Category III,* inconclusive evidence of efficacy or uncertain risk:benefit ratio; *Category IV,* lack of efficacy in controlled trials.

❖ Red blood cell exchange may be performed every 4 to 6 weeks in lieu of ongoing transfusion.
- Thrombocytapheresis is the collection of platelets for transfusion or for a decrease in the number circulating in proliferative disorders.
- Specially trained health care professionals, such as blood bank personnel, perform apheresis.
- If possible, the apheresis team should be consulted before vascular access devices are placed to ensure that they are appropriate for the necessary therapy.
- Before apheresis can be performed, the child's gender, height and weight, total blood volume (TBV), and hematocrit level must be determined. These data are necessary to calculate the amount of blood to be processed and whether the blood cell separator should be primed with donor blood.
  ❖ Certain circumstances may necessitate a blood prime of the apheresis machine to maintain isovolemia during the procedure.
    ○ The extracorporeal volume (volume of blood necessary to fill the pump circuit) exceeds 10% to 15% of the child's total blood volume (usually children who weigh less than 20 kg).
    ○ Children whose conditions are unstable or severely anemic
- Blood products should be leukocyte reduced and irradiated if used for potential bone marrow transplant candidates or recipients.
- Apheresis has general risks that apply to all populations and procedures.
  ❖ Adverse effects may include:
    ○ Infection, bleeding, or thrombosis associated with line placement

    ○ Volume deficit or volume overload
    ○ Citrate toxicity with resultant hypocalcemia or allergic or vasovagal reactions
  ❖ Prescribed medications that the child is receiving may be removed during the procedure. Drugs that are highly bound to plasma proteins (e.g., antiarrhythmics, bronchodilators, anticonvulsants, and antibiotics) are effectively removed (65% to 70%) in a one TBV plasma exchange.
  ❖ Angiotensin-converting enzyme (ACE) inhibitors have been associated with severe hypotension and anaphylactoid reactions during extracorporeal therapies.[3] These drugs should be held for up to 1 week before apheresis, depending on duration of action.
- A collaborative relationship between the intensive care unit (ICU) nurse and apheresis staff is essential to ensure safe patient care.
- The child may need medications for sedation, analgesia, or reaction prevention before initiation of the procedure.
- Principles of aseptic technique
- Mastery of pediatric advanced life support competencies
- Child development as it relates to clinical assessment and apheresis
- Informed consent is required prior to apheresis

CHILD AND FAMILY ASSESSMENT

- Initial physical examination, including current height, weight, and vital signs ➤*Rationale:* Pretreatment assessment identifies comorbid conditions that may further complicate apheresis. The results provide a baseline for comparison, which allows for treatment modifications or interventions as needed. Changes in weight during or after apheresis are an indicator of fluid balance.[4,5]

- Child's and family's understanding of the reasons for and risks and benefits of the procedure ➥*Rationale:* Evaluates child's and family's understanding of the procedure and provides a gauge for ongoing education.
- Inspection of vascular access site for signs of infection or bleeding ➥*Rationale:* Catheter insertion sites provide a portal of entry for infection, with increased risk in children with immunocompromised conditions.
- Inspection of catheter patency and ease of aspiration of blood from both ports. If patency is in question, redress site or change the child's position to determine whether a thrombolytic agent needs be instilled in the CVC before apheresis ➥*Rationale:* Consistent steady blood flow is essential to apheresis. If the catheter appears to be partially or completely occluded, the occlusion must be resolved before the procedure is initiated.
- Assessment of circulation to the limb distal to the access site[4] ➥*Rationale:* The placement of a CVC may compromise blood flow in the relatively small vessels of children.
- Draw pretreatment laboratory specimens per prescribing practitioner's order, including complete blood count, electrolytes, coagulation studies, and immunoglobulins ➥*Rationale:* Some blood loss occurs with each procedure. Children whose conditions are unstable or who have low hematocrit levels may need blood prime or a transfusion during treatment. Clotting factor, platelet, and antibody levels are decreased with each apheresis procedure. Metabolism and half-life of the anticoagulants vary with each child. Clotting may be prolonged after apheresis. In addition, anticoagulants and replacement fluids can lower calcium, magnesium, and potassium levels.
- Review medication orders for indicated prophylactic medications, potential interactions, and dose scheduling that may conflict with extracorporeal therapy ➥*Rationale:* Medication may be indicated before the transfusion of blood products during apheresis. Analgesics or sedatives may be necessary to facilitate cooperation. Postponement of scheduled medications until after apheresis ensures the full dose is delivered. ACE inhibitors must be held.
- Family members desire to be present during procedure ➥*Rationale:* Family may provide support and comfort to the child but should have the choice not to remain with the child.

CHILD AND FAMILY EDUCATION

Individualized, developmentally appropriate education is provided to the family and to the child based on desire for knowledge, readiness to learn, and overall neurologic and psychosocial state.

- Explain the procedure, purpose, side effects, anticipated outcomes, and duration of the treatment. Answer any questions the child or family may have. ➥*Rationale:* Providing information decreases anxiety or fear and allows family and child participation in decision making to increase cooperation during the procedure.
- Explain the apheresis circuit and that blood will be visible in the tubing outside of the child's body ➥*Rationale:* This explanation decreases concerns that the child is losing blood. Actions can be taken to shield the child's view of the tubing to decrease anxiety.
- If appropriate, explain how the child and family can assist apheresis personnel through body positioning, operating clamps on central lines, or flushing of CVC ports ➥*Rationale:* Many children have had long-term indwelling catheters and have been assisting their caregivers in these procedures. Active involvement gives a sense of control, decreases fear, and increases cooperation.
- Explain the need for sterile technique during connection to and from the apheresis machine and during CVC dressing changes ➥*Rationale:* Aseptic technique decreases the risk of infection.
- Explain the need to limit mobility during treatment to prevent kinking of apheresis lines and disruption of blood flow ➥*Rationale:* Steady blood flow prevents interruption of the procedure and ensures quality cell collections.
- Explain the need for careful monitoring of the child's vital signs and laboratory values during the procedure ➥*Rationale:* The child and family are alerted to the need for frequent interventions, which decreases anxiety.
- In a developmentally appropriate manner, explain the importance of the child informing the nurse of any symptoms or problems during the treatment ➥*Rationale:* Symptoms can be an important sign of procedure-related complications.
- Encourage questions and answer questions as they arise ➥*Rationale:* Reinforcement of information is needed during periods of stress.

EQUIPMENT

The apheresis staff generally brings the following equipment and supplies:

- Blood cell separator machine (i.e., COBE BCT Spectra, [Gambro BCT, Lakewood, CO])
- Blood cell separator tubing set and warmer tubing
- Replacement and prime fluids as ordered
- Blood administration tubing
- Laboratory specimen tubes
- Heparinized syringes for measurement of ionized calcium level
- Activated clotting time (ACT) monitoring device if heparinization is necessary
- Admixtures of calcium gluconate or calcium chloride, as ordered
- Equipment for managing and accessing the CVC or peripheral access device
- 0.9% saline solution flush and heparin

Procedure for Apheresis: Assist

Steps	Rationale	Considerations
1. Ensure child and family understand procedure and questions are answered.	Evaluates and reinforces understanding of previously taught information.	Developmental level, cognitive ability and anxiety level will determine approach to and effectiveness of teaching.
2. Identify child using appropriate patient verification process and verify prescribing practitioner's order for treatment.	Confirms correct patient and procedure as recommended by the Joint Commission for Accreditation of Healthcare Organizations (JCAHO).	Use two patient identifiers per institution specific protocol.
3. Confirm consent for procedure and blood transfusion, if indicated.	Ensures child and family have been informed and offered the opportunity to ask questions.	
4. Administer premedication to child as ordered.	Helps prevent adverse reactions and promote relaxation, thereby improving blood flow.	
5. Withhold routine medications until after procedure.	Protein-bound drugs are effectively removed during plasmapheresis.[5]	Use of ACE inhibitors must be reported immediately to apheresis team.
6. Send laboratory specimens as ordered by apheresis team.	Current blood count, type, and screen; coagulation studies; and chemistries are essential.	Allows apheresis staff to prepare appropriate replacement and prime solutions. Use two patient identifiers when obtaining laboratory specimens.
7. Two appropriate healthcare providers independently verify correctness of blood products administered during apheresis and validate child's identity using two patient identifiers per institution-specific protocol.	Prevents blood transfusion errors.	Relatively large quantities of plasma or red blood cells are necessary for exchange procedures.
8. Provide support to child and family and apheresis personnel by continuing necessary nursing care during the procedure.	This procedure can be technically difficult in small children, necessitating the apheresis team to focus on the pump and circuit.	
9. Arrange for developmentally appropriate diversional activities during the procedure.	Lessens apprehension and fear.	Quiet activities with minimal movement of the child, such as viewing videotapes or listening to music, are most appropriate.

Expected Outcomes

- Vascular access is achieved and maintained without complication

- Procedure is completed without disruption

- Therapeutic goals (symptomatic relief, laboratory value normalization) are achieved without complication

Unexpected Outcomes

- Infection, bleeding, hematoma, thrombus or air embolism, dislodgement of catheter, poor blood flow through circuit, decreased circulation in accessed limb
- Loss of access
- Technical problems with circuit
- Child's refusal to cooperate with apheresis team
- Treatment-related complications, including fluid and electrolyte imbalance, hypotension, blood loss, excessive anticoagulation, citrate toxicity with hypocalcemia, allergic or transfusion reaction, transfusion-transmitted disease[5]

Monitoring and Care of the Child

Activities and Interventions	Rationale	Reportable Conditions
1. Perform preapheresis and ongoing assessment, including vital signs, weight, intake, and output. *(Level V*)*	Establishes baseline value before treatment is initiated and monitors for complications during treatment. Fever or chills may indicate infection or transfusion reaction. Maintenance of isovolemia is challenging in pediatric apheresis.	• Hypotension/hypertension • Tachycardia/bradycardia • Arrhythmia • Fever/hypothermia • Abnormal weight gain or loss • Edema

2. Monitor laboratory values, before, during, and after treatment, including:
    Calcium/ionized calcium
    Sodium/potassium
    Bicarbonate
    Coagulation studies
    Immunoglobulin level
    Complete blood count
    Lactic acid dehydrogenase (LDH) *(Level V*)*
	Anticoagulant citrate-dextrose binds with calcium and metabolizes to sodium and bicarbonate.
	Administration of older blood products may increase potassium levels.
	Citrate and heparin prolong clotting times.
	Fibrinogen and immunoglobulin levels drop with each successive plasmapheresis.
	Platelets and red blood cells are lost with each procedure.
	Hemolysis and platelet activation may occur in the extracorporeal circuit.
		• Hypocalcemia
		• Hypernatremia
		• Severe metabolic alkalosis (a slight metabolic alkalosis is expected after apheresis with citrate anticoagulation)
		• Hyperkalemia
		• Prolonged ACT/partial thromboplastin time (PTT) more than 4 hours after apheresis
		• Fibrinogen, immunoglobulin M (IgM), IgG, and IgA values below normal limits
		• Thrombocytopenia or anemia

3. Monitor vascular access insertion site and dressing between treatments. *(Level V*)*	Children who undergo apheresis are at risk of line sepsis from altered immunologic status. Peripheral or central venous lines necessitate extra protection and scrutiny in children.	• Inflammation, drainage, or tenderness at CVC • Bleeding • Kinking • Catheter clotting • Fever
4. Monitor neurovascular status of accessed limb between treatments.[4] *(Level V*)*	Large-bore CVC may impede blood flow, especially in the femoral vein.	• Diminished capillary refill • Diminished peripheral pulses • Pallor, mottling, or duskiness • Pain • Swelling
5. Monitor child for symptoms of complications associated with apheresis. *(Level V*)*	Complications can arise quickly during and after treatment.	• Transfusion reaction: fever, chills, hives, urticaria, swelling, wheezing, or dyspnea • Electrolyte imbalance: abdominal pain or cramping, nausea, vomiting, tachycardia, or irregular pulse • Fluid imbalance: decreased or increased urine output, diarrhea, or edema

* Level V: Clinical studies in more than one or two patient populations and situations to support recommendations

Documentation

- Child and family education
- Condition of vascular access, including patency, quality of blood flow, ease of access, and presence of bruit if arteriovenous (AV) fistula
- Date, time, and duration of treatment
- Condition of catheter insertion site, date and time of dressing change, flushing of ports, and heparinization
- Vital signs throughout apheresis
- Blood returned to the child at the completion of treatment; returning blood to the child should be done only if ordered by a prescribing practitioner and is dependent on the child's size and clinical status[5]
- Unexpected outcomes and related treatment
- Response to apheresis and progress toward goals of treatment
- Laboratory assessment results
- Fluid balance
- Daily weight

References

1. Jones HG, Bandarenko N: Management of the therapeutic apheresis patient. In McLeod BC, Price TH, Weinstein R, editors: *Apheresis: principles and practice,* ed 2, Bethesda, MD, 2003, American Association of Blood Banks.
2. Rogers RL, Cooling LW: Therapeutic apheresis in pediatric patients. In McLeod BC, Price TH, Weinstein R, editors: *Apheresis: principles and practice,* ed 2, Bethesda, MD, 2003, American Association of Blood Banks.
3. Weinstein R: Hypocalcemic toxicity and atypical reactions in therapeutic plasma exchange, *J Clin Apheresis* 16:210-211, 2001.
4. Giuliano KK: Assisting with plasmapheresis. In Lynn-McHale DJ, Carlson KK, editors: *AACN procedure manual for critical care,* ed 4, Philadelphia, 2001, Saunders.
5. Kim HC: Therapeutic pediatric apheresis, *J Clin Apheresis* 15:129-143, 2000.

Additional Readings

Adams RJ: Lessons from the Stroke Prevention Trial in sickle cell anemia (STOP) study, *J Child Neurol* 15:334-349, 2001.

Demeocq F, et al: Successful blood stem cell collection and transplant in children weighing less than 25kg, *Bone Mar Trans* 13:43-50, 1994.

Gorlin JB: Therapeutic plasma exchange and cytapheresis. In Nathan DG, Orkin SH, editors: *Hematology of infancy and childhood,* ed 5, Philadelphia, 1998, Saunders.

Kishimoto M, et al: Treatment for the decline of ionized calcium levels during peripheral blood progenitor cell harvesting, *Transf* 42:1340-1347, 2002.

Krafte-Jacobs B, et al: Catheter related thrombosis in critically ill children: comparison of catheters with and without heparin bonding, *J Pediatr* 126:50-54, 1995.

Ruggenenti P, et al: Thrombotic microangiopathy, hemolytic uremic syndrome and thrombotic thrombocytopenic purpura, *Kidney Int* 60:831-846, 2001.

Schlenke P, et al: Clinically relevant hypokalaemia, hypocalcaemia, and loss of hemoglobin and platelets during stem cell apheresis, *J Clin Apheresis* 15:230-235, 2000.

Continuous Renal Replacement Therapy

P U R P O S E : Continuous renal replacement therapy (CRRT) is a continuous extracorporeal blood purification therapy for critically ill children whose clinical state contraindicates conventional hemodialysis. Children with renal failure who have symptoms of fluid overload, electrolyte abnormalities, acid-base imbalance, sepsis, or ongoing high levels of toxic metabolites or who need excessive fluid or parenteral nutrition are candidates for CRRT therapy.

Chris Angeletti and Rhonda Gengler

PREREQUISITE KNOWLEDGE

- Anatomy and physiology of the renal system
- Indications and appropriate candidates for this therapy include children with acute renal failure related to congenital heart disease, acute tubular necrosis, hemolytic uremic syndrome, sepsis, and burns. Because CRRT is a slow continuous therapy, it is generally better tolerated by the child with a hemodynamically unstable condition than is hemodialysis.[1-4]
- Contraindications to CRRT may include coagulopathy, liver disease or active bleeding. (*Note:* these are not absolute contraindications in most institutions, especially transplant centers.)
- Understanding of the different types of CRRT[3]
  - ❖ Slow continuous ultrafiltration (SCUF): Therapy that removes fluid through ultrafiltration
  - ❖ Continuous venovenous hemofiltration (CVVH): Therapy that removes solutes through convection with a replacement solution; may also be used for fluid removal
  - ❖ Continuous venovenous hemodialysis (CVVHD): Therapy that removes solutes through diffusion with a dialysate; may also be used for fluid removal
  - ❖ Continuous venovenous hemodiafiltration (CVVHDF): Therapy that removes solutes through diffusion with a dialysate and convection with a

replacement solution; may also be used for fluid removal
- Understanding of dialysis terminology (i.e., arterial: access port from which blood is removed from the child, not really an arterial catheter; venous: access port through which blood is returned to the child)
- Specific training for initiation and maintenance of CRRT, including pump and circuit management per institution-specific protocol
- Volume of the specific filter circuit to be used
- Complications related to CRRT, including hypotension, blood loss, hyperglycemia, hypothermia, air embolus, blood leak, complications related to administration of anticoagulants, and complications related to presence of large-bore central venous catheter[3]
- Aseptic technique
- Knowledge of central venous catheters and related care (see Procedures 139, 140, and 141 for further information)
- Understanding of extracorporeal volume (ECV) and its significance in identification of children who may need a blood or albumin prime. Extracorporeal volume (amount of blood that is contained in the blood circuit outside of the child's vascular space) is 10% of the child's estimated blood volume (EBV). The EBV is calculated as dry weight in kilograms multiplied by 70 mL. This number is multiplied by 0.1 or 10%, which gives the amount of safe

ECV for a child. If ECV is more than 10%, blood or albumin may be needed to prime the circuit or transfuse on initiation of therapy.[2,4]

- Infants and small children with a large ECV are at risk for hypothermia. The addition of a blood warmer to the CRRT circuit may be necessary for this population.
- Understanding of the roles of dialysis and bedside nurse, if system is jointly managed

CHILD AND FAMILY ASSESSMENT

- Assess dialysis catheter to ensure brisk blood return and ability to flush easily ➤➤*Rationale:* Patent intravenous (IV) access is essential for good blood flow through the dialysis circuit. The best flow is achieved with a short large-diameter catheter.
- Informed consent for CRRT has been obtained by the prescribing practitioner according to institution-specific protocol ➤➤*Rationale:* Some institutions require specific consent forms for high-risk procedures such as CRRT.
- Child's developmental level and ability to interact ➤➤*Rationale:* These factors influence preparation of the child and interactions during the procedure.
- Child's fluid status, including edema, respiratory distress, hypertension, pretreatment weight, and vital signs ➤➤*Rationale:* Establishes baseline which allows assessment of effectiveness of the therapy and child's response to therapy.
- Fill volume of the arterial and venous lumens of the access catheter ➤➤*Rationale:* This information is needed to access or relock the catheter.
- Child's and family's understanding of the reasons for and risks and benefits of the procedure ➤➤*Rationale:* Evaluates child's and family's understanding of the procedure and provides a gauge for ongoing education.

CHILD AND FAMILY EDUCATION

Individualized, developmentally appropriate education is provided to the family and to the child based on desire for knowledge, readiness to learn, and overall neurologic and psychosocial state.

- Explain the child's need for CRRT to the child and family in developmentally appropriate terms. If possible, show the additional equipment that will be placed at the child's bedside. Introduce any additional staff who may now be involved in the child's care and explain their roles. ➤➤*Rationale:* Information and ongoing communication with family helps to increase comfort level, decrease anxiety, and enhance trust.
- Explain the procedure, side effects, anticipated outcomes, and duration of the treatment and the need for continuous monitoring during the procedure ➤➤*Rationale:*

Information about the procedure and aspects the nurse monitors can decrease anxiety and fear.

- Explain the CRRT circuit and that blood will be visible in the tubing outside of the child's body ➤➤*Rationale:* This explanation decreases concerns that the child is losing blood. Actions can be taken to shield the child's view of the tubing to decrease anxiety if necessary.
- Explain the need for frequent laboratory specimens ➤➤*Rationale:* This information may decrease anxiety over excessive blood loss.
- Provide the family with teaching materials; allow time for questions ➤➤*Rationale:* Information sharing helps reduce anxiety and enhance trust.
- Encourage questions and answer questions as they arise ➤➤*Rationale:* Reinforcement of information is needed during periods of stress.

EQUIPMENT

- A continuous hemofiltration pump system (i.e., Gambro Prisma [Gambro BCT, Lakewood, CO] or similar system)
- Tubing system (including hemofilter) designed for selected pump
- Additional infusion pumps, warming devices, or other disposable equipment if necessary
- One large-bore dual-lumen dialysis catheter or two single-lumen large-bore uncuffed catheters (must be in place and the placement confirmed)
- Kits or supplies for accessing or deaccessing dialysis catheter
  - ❖ Sterile syringes for withdrawal of heparin or blood, flushing lines
  - ❖ Sterile 0.9% saline solution
  - ❖ Sterile gloves
  - ❖ Antiseptic pads (70% isopropyl alcohol) or other disinfectant per institution-specific protocol
  - ❖ Sterile gauze pads
  - ❖ Mask
  - ❖ Personal protective equipment
  - ❖ Caps
  - ❖ Sterile field
  - ❖ Adhesive remover pads
- Ordered CRRT fluids, including all or some of the following:
  - ❖ Priming fluid
  - ❖ Dialysate
  - ❖ Replacement fluid
  - ❖ Anticoagulant
  - ❖ Electrolyte infusions
  - ❖ Anticoagulant antagonist
- Instrument and associated supplies for monitoring activated clotting times or other identified monitoring
- Appropriate form to document various aspects of CRRT

Procedure for Initiation of CRRT

Steps	Rationale	Considerations
1. Ensure child and family understand procedure and questions are answered.	Evaluates and reinforces understanding of previously taught information.	Developmental level, cognitive ability, and anxiety level will determine approach to and effectiveness of teaching.
2. Verify child's identity and prescribing practitioner's order for treatment.	Familiarizes the bedside nurse with indications for CRRT and expected outcomes. Ascertains correct patient and correct procedure as suggested by the Joint Commission for Accreditation of Healthcare Organizations.	Use two patient identifiers per institution specific protocol.
3. Obtain needed CRRT fluids from pharmacy and verify that they are correct with the six rights of medication administration: right patient, right drug (fluid), right dose, right time, right route, and right documentation.	The CRRT fluids are individualized to the specific patient situation. Dialysate and replacement fluids may be needed to prime the circuit. Verifying contents of fluids promotes patient safety.	These fluids are costly and often need special additional preparation by pharmacy.[3] Use of two patient identifiers promotes patient safety.
4. Place child on a bed with a scale, if available.	Changes in child's weight help determine effectiveness of therapy. Use of a bed with a built-in scale decreases the likelihood that access is inadvertently removed.	
5. Gather all necessary equipment and supplies and place at the child's bedside.	Initiation and maintenance of CRRT is complex; placement of all needed supplies nearby helps maximize nursing workflow.	
6. Allow CRRT equipment to acclimate to the child's room temperature, if required by the manufacturer. *(Level I*)*	The CRRT systems often rely on scales, which are sensitive to temperature change, to measure fluid removal/administration.	
7. Prime CRRT circuit with prescribed fluids as recommended by manufacturer. *(Level I*)*	Ensures that pump is functioning and circuit is ready for hookup as soon as central venous catheter is accessed.	
8. Pull curtain around bed or close door. Both nurse and child should wear mask and goggles.	Standard precautions; protects the child's privacy.	
9. Wash hands. Remove tape, gauze, or labels from dialysis catheter lumens. Use adhesive remover if applicable.	Standard precautions; reduces transmission of microorganisms.	
10. Prepare sterile field.	Maintains sterile environment to prevent contamination of catheter.	The catheters used for CRRT are large in diameter and have a large insertion site. Both can easily be contaminated.
11. Put on sterile gloves.	Prevents the spread of microorganisms and maintains sterility.	.
12. Using sterile technique prepare 0.9% saline solution syringes for flushing catheter (10 mL) and syringe for heparin bolus, if ordered.	Prevents the spread of microorganisms and maintains sterility.	Small flush volumes may be used if child cannot tolerate this volume.

* Level I: Manufacturer's recommendations only

Procedure for Initiation of CRRT—*Continued*

Steps	Rationale	Considerations
13. Vigorously scrub catheter arterial hub and cap connection with alcohol pads or prepare for access per institution specific protocol. *(Level IV*)*	Solution of 70% isopropyl alcohol has been shown to be effective for cleansing inanimate objects. It is rapidly bactericidal, tuberculocidal, fungicidal, and virucidal.	Alcohol should be allowed to dry thoroughly.
14. Ensure catheter is clamped.	Prevents blood loss when cap is removed.	
15. Remove cap with sterile gauze pad and discard. Attach empty syringe to hub.	Prevents the spread of micro-organisms and maintains sterility.	
16. Open the catheter clamp with a sterile gauze pad and withdraw waste equal to or greater than the filling volume of the catheter per institution-specific protocol.	Removes heparin or locking solution from lumen and assesses patency of the catheter.	If clots are noted in waste volume withdrawn, withdraw further waste volume to remove all clots
17. Clamp catheter and discard waste syringe in appropriate receptacle.	Standard precautions. Ensures anticoagulant is discarded.	
18. Attach 0.9% saline solution flush syringe.	Prepares flush.	
19. Flush lumen vigorously with 5 to 10 mL 0.9% saline solution.	Ensures patency of the catheter lumen.	Smaller flush volumes may be used if necessary.
20. Clamp catheter lumen.	Prevents inadvertent blood loss.	
21. Repeat steps 13 to 20 with the venous lumen of the catheter.	Removes heparin or locking solution from venous lumen and ensures patency of the catheter lumen.	
22. Administer heparin bolus if ordered before initiation of therapy.	Heparin is given to prevent clotting of blood when it comes in contact with CRRT tubing.[2,3]	Complete this step only if heparin is used for anticoagulation therapy. Assess activated clotting time (ACT) before administration of heparin bolus.[3] Heparin is usually ordered at 10 to 20 units/kg IV to be given if ACT is less than 150 to 165 seconds.
23. Clamp the arterial lumen clamp and remove syringe.	Clamping prevents blood loss.	
24. Attach "arterial end" or access line of the primed tubing set to arterial (red) lumen of catheter following manufacturer's recommendations.	Individual pumps have different recommendation for connecting patients.	Inflow (red) lumen is referred to as the "arterial" lumen, but it is a venous line. Outflow (blue) lumen is at times referred to as venous lumen. Lumens may be inter-changed so that blood is withdrawn from the blue lumen if patency or resistance is a problem; however, some recirculation does occur.
25. Repeat steps 23 and 24 with the venous (blue) lumen and venous or return end of the tubing set.	Required to complete circuit.	
26. Start blood pump at a low rate and gradually increase to ordered settings.	Pump set up should be done according to institution-specific protocol and manufacturer's instructions.	

Procedure continues on following page

* Level IV: Limited clinical studies to support recommendations

Procedure | **for Initiation of CRRT**—*Continued*

Steps	Rationale	Considerations
27. Secure blood lines to bed and child.	Prevents pulling of blood lines and loss of access.	
28. Discard used equipment and supplies in appropriate trash receptacles. Remove gloves and wash hands.	Standard precautions; decreases transmission of microorganisms.	

Procedure | **for Terminating Therapy and Locking Catheters**

Steps	Rationale	Considerations
1. Ensure child and family understand procedure and questions are answered.	Evaluates and reinforces understanding of previously taught information.	Developmental level, cognitive ability and anxiety level will determine approach to and effectiveness of teaching.
2. Obtain needed supplies, including prescribed locking solution for the catheter.	Ensures that all needed supplies are available and minimizes likelihood that sterile field is contaminated.	Medication used to lock catheters is child and institution specific.
3. Pull curtain around bed or close door. Both nurse and child should wear mask and goggles.	Maintains standard precautions and protects the child's privacy.	
4. Wash hands. Remove any tape, gauze, or labels from CRRT catheter lumens.	Standard precautions; reduces the spread of microorganisms.	
5. Prepare sterile field.	Maintains sterile environment to prevent contamination of catheter.	
6. Determine the need for return of blood within the circuit. Return circuit blood to child per institution specific protocol or manufacturer's instructions.	Prevents blood loss to circuit and may prevent need for further transfusion.	Returning blood to the child should be done only if ordered by a prescribing practitioner and is dependent on the child's size and clinical status.[3,4] Procedure for the terminating treatment differs with individual pumps.
7. Turn off pump. Clamp the catheter lumens and circuit tubing.	When terminating treatment, clamping the tubing prevents blood loss and contamination.	
8. Put on sterile gloves.	Reduces the spread of microorganisms.	
9. Using sterile technique prepare 0.9% saline solution syringes for flushing catheter (10 mL) and syringes for heparin or other prescribed medication to lock catheter lumens.	Reduces the spread of microorganisms and maintains sterility. The 0.9% saline solution is used to clear blood from lumens of catheters.	
10. Vigorously scrub catheter arterial (red) hub and tubing connection with alcohol pads or other antiseptic solution per institution specific protocol, then disconnect the tubing.	Reduces the spread of microorganisms.	

Procedure for **Terminating Therapy and Locking Catheters**—*Continued*

Steps	Rationale	Considerations
11. Attach 0.9% saline solution filled syringe. Open the catheter clamp with a sterile gauze pad.	Reduces the spread of micro-organisms.	
12. Aspirate slightly to ensure the absence of air in the lumen; then vigorously flush the lumen with 0.9% saline solution.	Clears catheter lumen of residual blood, decreasing the possibility of clot formation.	Smaller volumes of 0.9% saline solution may be used for small children who cannot tolerate 10 mL flushes.
13. Reclamp lumen, attach sterile cap, and flush with heparin solution (concentration per institution specific protocol) or other prescribed locking medication at the filling volume of the lumen.	Prevents clot formation when catheter is not in use.	Fill volumes of the lumens are generally marked on the catheter lumen.
14. Repeat steps 10 to 13 for the venous (blue) lumen.	Completes circuit removal and locks venous lumen.	
15. Once both lumens are capped and heparin is instilled make certain that the clamps on both lumens are engaged.	Prevents blood loss.	
16. Remove circuit from pump and discard circuit in an appropriate trash receptacle.	Standard precautions: prevents the transmission of microorganisms.	
17. Remove gloves, mask, and goggles.	No further risk of blood exposure.	
18. Apply appropriate label to catheter lumens (e.g., "Do not infuse, for dialysis only"). Label with the volume and concentration of heparin or other medication used to lock the catheter and the date, time, and initials.	Assures catheter is used only for dialysis purposes. Label serves as notification of the time and date that the catheter was flushed last and the amount and strength of heparin or other locking medication used.	Some institutions allow certain dialysis catheters to be used to draw blood or for other reasons. Refer to institution-specific protocol and Procedure 139.
19. Wash hands.	Standard precautions.	

Expected Outcomes

- Hemodynamic stability is maintained during initiation and maintenance of therapy
- Desired fluid removal is achieved
- Desired electrolyte levels are attained
- Resolution of acid-base disturbances
- The ACT or ionized calcium levels are within prescribed range during and after CRRT
- Vascular access remains patent throughout therapy

Unexpected Outcomes

- Hemodynamic instability during or after initiation of therapy
- Excessive or inadequate fluid removal
- Unstable serum electrolytes
- Acid-base disturbances are not resolved
- Uncontrolled or excessive bleeding

- Clotting of vascular access
- Inadvertent removal of vascular access

Monitoring and Care of the Child

Activities and Interventions	Rationale	Reportable Conditions
1. Monitor child's weight before start of therapy, then every 12 to 24 hours.	Weight is an indication of fluid loss or excess.	• Significant change in weight
2. Monitor intake and output hourly.	Ensures that goals of therapy with regard to fluid removal are achieved.	• Ultrafiltrate volume less than anticipated
3. Maintain sterile technique throughout treatment.	Use of sterile technique helps reduce infection risk.	• Any significant break in sterile technique during therapy
4. Monitor vital signs every 15 minutes for the first hour of therapy, then hourly. Monitor temperature hourly.	Some instability during initiation of therapy can be expected, particularly in small infants and children who need high-dose vasopressor support.[2-4]	• Changes in baseline vital signs or ongoing vital sign instability • Heat loss related to blood flow rate and volume of blood in the circuit, which may lead to hypothermia, especially in small children and infants

5. Monitor the following serum laboratory studies:
  Electrolytes, phosphorus, calcium, and magnesium every 4 to 6 hours, until condition is stable
  Serum glucose every 2 to 4 hours until stable
  Blood urea nitrogen (BUN)/ creatinine, complete blood cell count (CBC), platelets, and prothrombin time (PT)/partial thromboplastin time (PTT) daily
	Electrolyte balance is essential to maintenance of successful renal replacement therapy.
	Although balanced replacement fluids are given, electrolyte deficiency or excess can occur.[3]
		• Significant changes in serum electrolyte levels

6. Monitor clotting times.
  With heparin, monitor ACT every 30 minutes until condition is stable, then every 1 to 2 hours
  With a different method of anticoagulation therapy, refer to institution specific guidelines for monitoring
  With citrate regional anticoagulation therapy, monitor circuit and child's ionized calcium every hour until condition is stable, then every 4 to 6 hours
	Filter life and efficiency is maximized with proper anticoagulation maintenance.
	Heparin has a short half life; therefore, during initiation, clotting levels must be monitored frequently.
	Citrate lock may occur.
		• Inability to maintain clotting times within prescribed parameters
		• Inability to maintain ionized calcium levels within prescribed parameters; a rising total calcium level with a declining or sustained patient ionized calcium level is known as citrate lock[3]

7. Visually inspect ultrafiltrate hourly for changes in color.	Pink or red color in the ultrafiltrate is indicative of filter membrane rupture.	• Pink or red color in the ultrafiltrate
8. Visually inspect filter hourly for clots and air bubbles.	Large clots or air bubbles decrease effectiveness of the filter.	
9. Keep circuit tubing and access sites uncovered and within view, with attention paid to avoid bending or kinking.	Bending of the tubing or access sites can cause a pressure build up in the CRRT circuit and can potentially cause filter membrane rupture.	• A continued rise in system pressures despite correction or any kinking or bending of the tubing or access site
10. Monitor circuit, filter, and patient pressures.	Rising pressures indicate potential problems with circuit, filter, or patient access.	• Pressures outside the set range should be reported to the appropriate personnel (i.e., dialysis nurse or prescribing practitioner)
11. Monitor child for signs or symptoms of hemorrhage.	Children on CRRT with anticoagulation therapy are at high risk for bleeding from the increase in clotting times.	• Any bleeding or hemorrhage or suspicion of bleeding • Sudden changes in neurologic status

Monitoring and Care of the Child—Cont'd

Activities and Interventions	Rationale	Reportable Conditions
12. Ensure the circuit is changed per manufacturer's recommendations or institution-specific protocol. 13. Clamp inflow and outflow lines of circuit in the event of unexpected disconnection of bloodlines or system rupture.	Intermittent changes of circuit and filter are necessary to decrease infection risk and to stay within the recommended filter life. The child could have quick exsanguination from disconnect or rupture.	• A child whose condition may be too unstable to endure a circuit change • A suddenly clotted circuit • Any instances of circuit rupture/disconnect

Documentation

- Fluid balances, hourly totals, and filter pressures on CRRT flow sheet
- Time of initiation and discontinuation of therapy
- Patency of vascular access
- Child's tolerance of initiation and discontinuation of therapy
- Anticoagulation monitoring results and associated infusion adjustments
- Catheter dressing changes and condition of insertion site
- Circuit assessment
- Circuit change and reason for circuit change (e.g., routine change membrane rupture)
- Intravenous fluids and replacement fluids should be documented on Medication Adminstration Record
- Any unexpected events related to CRRT therapy and related treatment

References

1. Andreoli SP: Acute renal failure, *Curr Opin Pediatr* 14:183-188, 2002.
2. Flynn J: Choice of dialysis modality for management of pediatric acute renal failure, *Pediatr Nephrol* 17:61-69, 2002.
3. Maxvold N, Bunchman T: Renal failure and renal replacement therapy, *Crit Care Clin* 19:563-575, 2003.
4. Goldstein S: Overview of pediatric renal replacement therapy in acute renal failure, *Artific Organs* 27(9):781-785, 2003.

Additional Readings

Barenbrock M, et al: Effects of bicarbonate- and lactate-buffered replacement fluids on cardiovascular outcome in CVVH patients, *Kidney Int* 58:1751-1757, 2000.

Brophy PD, et al: AN-69 membrane reactions are pH-dependent and preventable, *Am J Kidney Dis* 38(1):173-178, 2001.

Brunet S, et al: Diffusive and convective solute clearances during continuous renal replacement therapy at various dialysate and ultrafiltration flow rates, *Am J Kidney Dis* 34(3):486-492, 1999.

Bunchman T, et al: Pediatric hemofiltration: normocarb dialysate solution with citrate anticoagulation, *Pediatr Nephrol* 17:150-154, 2002.

Chadha V, et al: Citrate clearance in children receiving continuous venovenous renal replacement therapy, *Pediatr Nephrol* 17:819-824, 2002.

Continuous Renal Replacement Therapies Web site: www.crrtonline.com; CRRT Inc.; © 2006; updated 1/21/2006; accessed 6/14/2006.

Goldstein S, et al: Outcome in children receiving continuous venovenous hemofiltration, *Pediatrics* 107(6):1309-1312, 2001.

Kornecki A, et al: Continuous renal replacement therapy for non-renal indications: experience in children, *IMAJ* 4:345-348, 2002.

Lowrie L: Renal replacement therapies in pediatric multiorgan dysfunction syndrome, *Pediatr Nephrol* 14:6-12, 2000.

Maxvold N, et al: Amino acid loss and nitrogen balance in critically ill children with acute renal failure: a prospective comparison between classic hemofiltration and hemofiltration with dialysis, *Crit Care Med* 28(4):1161-1165, 2000.

Mehta R, et al: A randomized clinical trial of continuous versus intermittent dialysis for acute renal failure, *Kidney Int* 60:1154-1163, 2001.

The Pediatric CRRT Web site: www.pcrrt.com; Dr. Tim Bunchman; ©2006; updated 3/2006; accessed 6/14/2006.

Reeves J, et al: Continuous plasma filtration in sepsis syndrome, *Crit Care Med* 27(10):2096-2104, 1999.

Symons J, et al: Continuous renal replacement therapy in children up to 10 kg, *Am J Kidney Dis* 41(5):984-989, 2003.

Williams D, et al: Acute renal failure: a pediatric experience over 20 years, *Arch Pediatr Adolesc Med* 156:893-900, 2002.

Zimmerman D, et al: Continuous veno-venous haemodialysis with a novel bicarbonate dialysis solution: prospective cross-over comparison with a lactate buffered solution, *Nephrol Dialysis Transplant* 14:2387-2391, 1999.

Hemodialysis: Assist

PURPOSE: Hemodialysis is performed for acute or chronic renal failure to restore electrolytes and acid-base balance to desired levels, manage fluid volume status, and remove toxins in cases of overdoses or ingestions that are dialyzable

Chris Breen and Kim Windt

PREREQUISITE KNOWLEDGE

- Hemodialysis is a procedure used for the treatment of acute and chronic renal failure. It removes waste products (i.e., urea) from the blood, restores normal electrolyte balance, and removes excess fluid. It can also be used to clear the body of toxins from overdoses or ingestions of toxic materials.
- Basic concepts of hemodialysis
  - ❖ Diffusion: Movement of solutes from an area of higher concentration to an area of lower concentration; diffusion in hemodialysis occurs across the semipermeable membrane that separates the blood compartment from the dialysate compartment in the artificial kidney or dialyzer
  - ❖ Osmosis: Movement of water across a membrane permeable to water; the water moves from an area of lesser solute concentration to an area of higher solute concentration between the compartments in the dialyzer
  - ❖ Ultrafiltration: The process by which plasma water is removed because of a pressure gradient between the blood and dialysate compartments in the dialyzer
- Components of the hemodialysis system
  - ❖ Dialysis machine
    - ○ Blood pump: Keeps the blood moving through the tubing and dialyzer (extracorporeal circuit).

  - ○ Dialysis machine can be programmed for specific procedure parameters.
  - ○ Dialysis machine has an air detector, blood leak detector, and other pressure monitors related to the procedure.
- ❖ Reverse osmosis (RO) machine
  - ○ Connects to a tap water faucet
  - ○ Tap water goes to the RO machine for purification. The RO machine is connected to the hemodialysis machine. The purified water comes from the RO to the hemodialysis machine and mixes with the dialysate for the procedure.
  - ○ An appropriate drain is needed for the RO and hemodialysis machine waste water.
- ❖ Dialyzer or artificial kidney: A cylinder-shaped filter with a semipermeable membrane to create two separate compartments: the blood compartment and the dialysate compartment. Diffusion and osmosis occur here.
- ❖ Dialysate: A premixed solution of water, bicarbonate, and electrolytes. The concentration of electrolytes is the same as that of normal plasma, which helps to create a concentration gradient for removal of excess electrolytes from the child's blood.
- ❖ Extracorporeal or blood circuit: Blood tubing that carries blood from the child through the dialyzer and back to the child. The blood pump controls the speed

of the blood moving through the circuit. This speed is expressed in milliliters/minute.

❖ Vascular access: To perform hemodialysis, vascular access is necessary. It can be provided in three ways: arteriovenous (AV) fistula (a surgically created anastomosis between an artery and a vein), AV graft (formed by surgical placement of a piece of synthetic material between an artery and a vein), or double-lumen catheter in a central vein (Figures 104-1 and 104-2).

○ An AV fistula or graft is used for children who undergo maintenance hemodialysis for end-stage renal disease.

○ The catheter must be of a size appropriate for the child but must also be large enough to accommodate the ordered blood pump speed.

○ In acute situations, a double-lumen catheter is the access of choice, unless a functioning AV fistula or AV graft is present.

○ A double-lumen catheter can be used immediately after placement and verification of position with chest x-ray. Common insertion sites are the femoral, internal jugular (IJ), or external jugular (EJ) veins.

○ The blood circuit starts and ends at the vascular access as the blood tubing is attached to the lumens of the catheter (Figure 104-3).

• Understanding of safe extracorporeal volume (ECV). Extracorporeal volume (amount of blood that is con-tained in the blood circuit outside of the child's vascular space) is 10% of the child's estimated blood volume (EBV). The EBV is calculated as dry weight in kilograms multiplied by 70 mL. This number is multiplied by 0.1 or 10%, which gives the amount of safe ECV for a child. If the ECV is more than 10%, blood or albumin may be needed to prime the tubing and dialyzer for the hemodialysis procedure.[1] *(Level V*)*

• Knowledge of child development as it relates to clinical assessments and hemodialysis

• Clinical findings of hypervolemia or hypovolemia in the child

• Pediatric hypertension or hypotension management

• Pediatric blood pressure assessment

• Renal physiology

• The indications for hemodialysis include:
  ❖ Primary renal disease: Renal agenesis, dysplasia, obstructive uropathies, nephrotic syndrome
  ❖ Secondary renal disease (i.e., sepsis, multiple organ failure, cancer)
  ❖ Nonrenal dialyzable toxins (i.e., lithium, ethylene glycol, salicylates, ammonia, isopropyl alcohol)

• Normal and abnormal laboratory values as it relates to renal insufficiency or disease

• Vascular accesses used for hemodialysis (AV fistula, AV graft, and central venous catheters)

---

* Level V: Clinical studies in more than one or two patient populations and situations to support recommendations

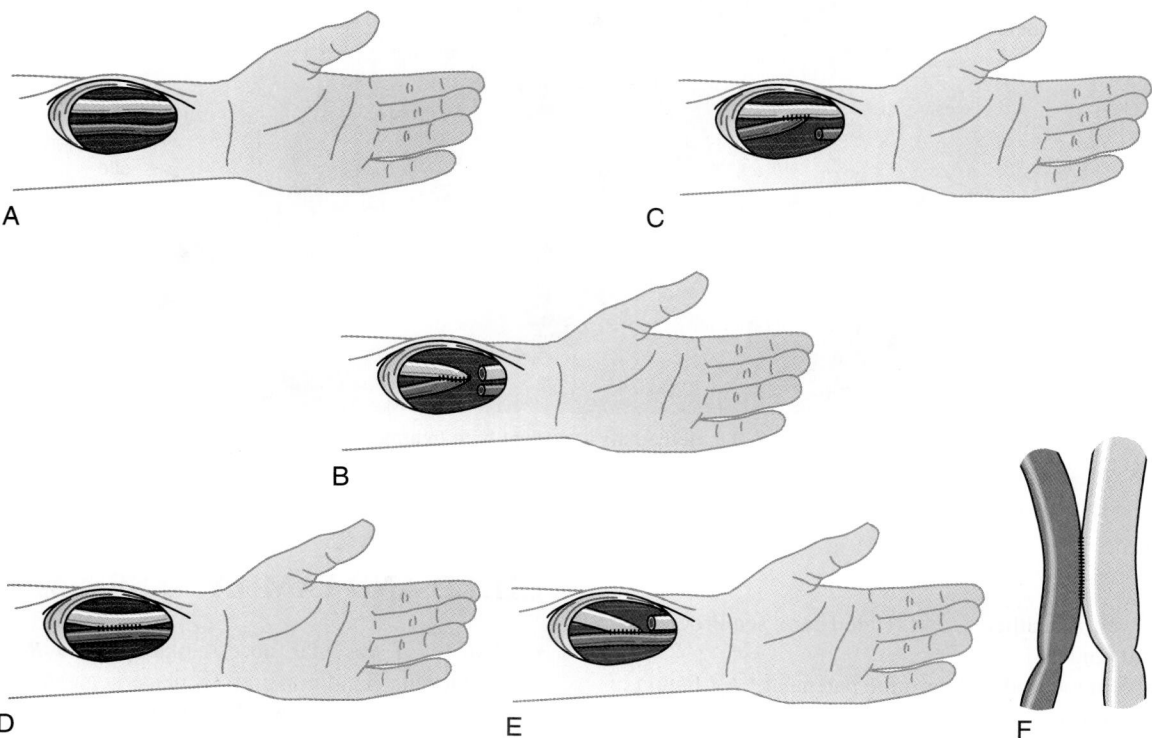

FIGURE 104-1 Examples of Various Configurations for AV Fistula Anastomoses. **A,** Normal artery-vein relationship. **B,** End-to-end anastomosis. **C,** End-vein to side-artery anastomosis. **D,** Side-to-side anastomosis. **E,** Side-vein to end-artery anastomosis. **F,** Side-to-side converted to end-to-end anastomosis. *Reprinted from American Nephrology Nurses Association:* Core curriculum for nephrology nursing, *ed 4, Pitman, NJ, 2001, ANNA.*

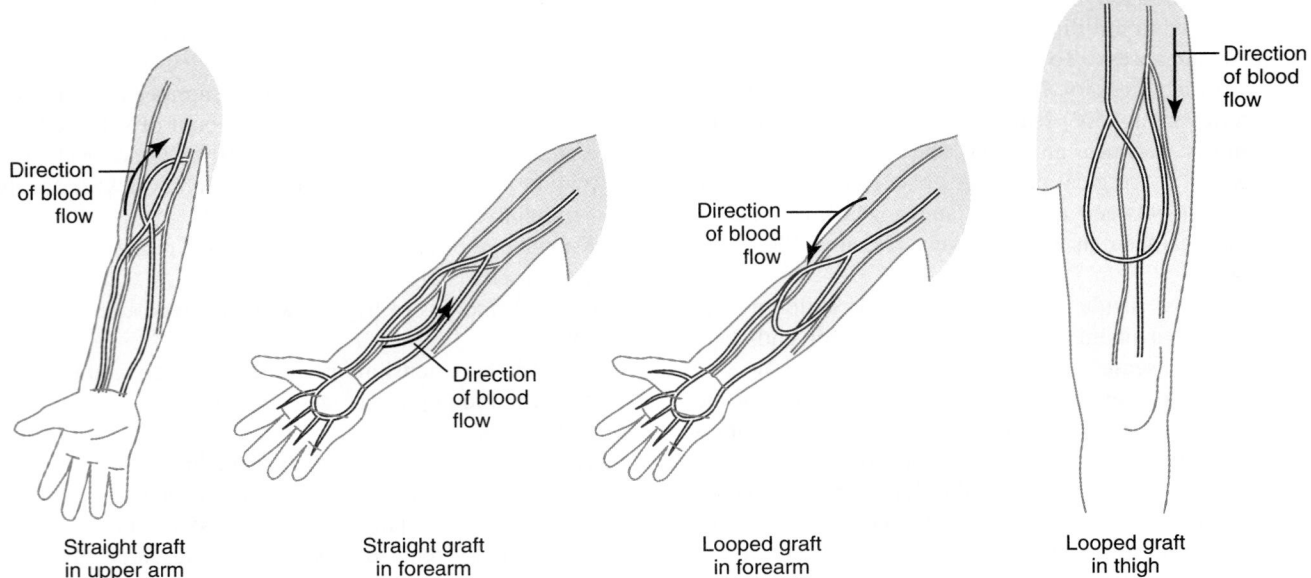

FIGURE 104-2 Frequently used AV graft configurations. *Reprinted from American Nephrology Nurses Association:* Core curriculum for nephrology nursing, *ed 4, Pitman, NJ, 2001, ANNA.*

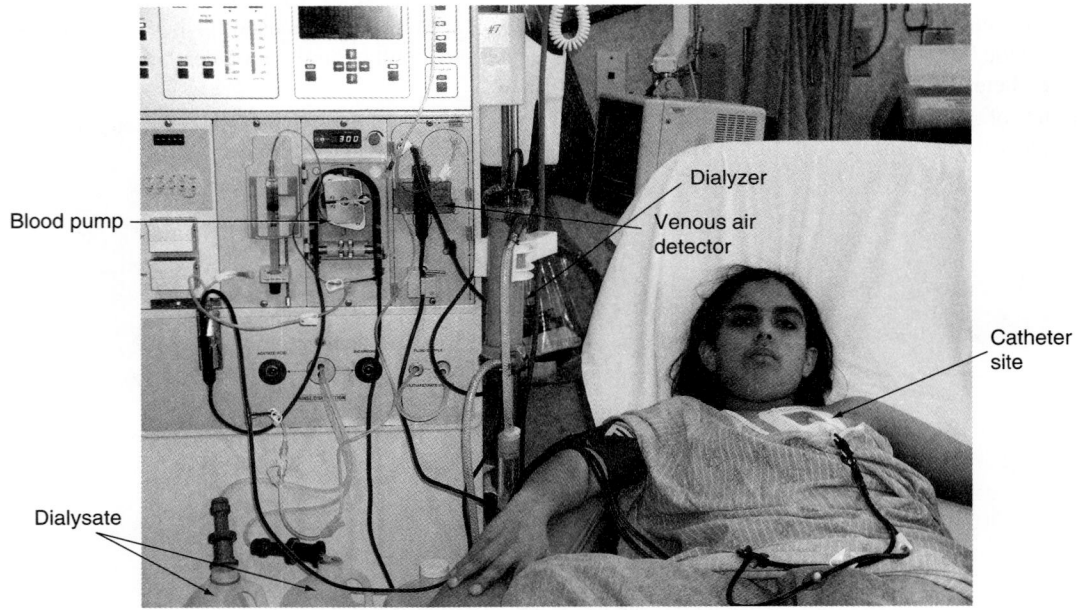

FIGURE 104-3 Hemodialysis patient with treatment in progress.

- Central venous catheters and related care; see Procedures 139, 140, and 141
- Assessment method to determine patency of AV fistula or AV graft (auscultation of the bruit with stethoscope or Doppler ultrasound scan; the thrill can be palpated)
- Principles of aseptic technique
- Mastery of pediatric advanced life support competencies
- Informed consent is required prior to hemodialysis

CHILD AND FAMILY ASSESSMENT

- History of vascular access placement ➥*Rationale:* A functioning fistula or graft in place negates the need for catheter placement. An AV fistula or AV graft in place dictates the use of the opposite extremity for blood pressure monitoring, intravenous (IV) insertion, venipuncture for laboratory specimens, and arterial line placement. Previous central venous catheter placement or a nonfunctioning AV fistula or AV graft may result in stenosis or occlusion of a central vessel.

- History of acute or chronic hemodialysis ➠*Rationale:* Previous experience with this procedure affects the level of understanding the child and family may have of the procedure.
- If child has an AV fistula or AV graft, assessment of the bruit/thrill ➠*Rationale:* Absence of the bruit/thrill indicates a clotted AV fistula or AV graft. Diminished bruit/thrill indicates decreased blood flow through the AV fistula or AV graft and can be related to decreased blood pressure.[1]
- Child's developmental level and ability to interact ➠*Rationale:* These factors influence preparation for the procedure and interactions during the procedure.[1]
- Child's level of consciousness ➠*Rationale:* Altered consciousness may affect the child's ability to give feedback concerning symptoms during the procedure.
- Child's fluid status, including edema, respiratory distress, hypertension, and predialysis weight ➠*Rationale:* Hypervolemia may occur in the presence of renal failure. Predialysis weight is compared with postdialysis weight for evaluation of fluid removal and status.
- Child's hemodynamic stability ➠*Rationale:* Cardiac instability or hypotension that necessitates vasopressors may be a contraindication for hemodialysis.
- Child's and family's understanding of the reasons for and risks and benefits of hemodialysis ➠*Rationale:* Evaluates child's and family's understanding; provides a gauge for ongoing education.
- Family's desire to be present during the procedure ➠*Rationale:* Family may provide support and comfort to the child but should have the choice not to remain with the child.

CHILD AND FAMILY EDUCATION

Individualized, developmentally appropriate education is provided to the family and to the child based on desire for knowledge, readiness to learn, and overall neurologic and psychosocial state.

Bedside Nurse:

- Explain and review the need for hemodialysis ➠*Rationale:* Providing information decreases anxiety and fear.
- If appropriate vascular access has not yet been obtained, explain and review the need for vascular access and

possible sites for catheter placement ➠*Rationale:* Promotes an understanding of the procedure.

- Explain the procedure for vascular access placement and use of sedation for the placement ➠*Rationale:* Providing information about the procedure and how the child may feel with sedation decreases anxiety and fear.
- Encourage questions and answer questions as they arise ➠*Rationale:* Reinforcement of information is needed during periods of stress.

Dialysis Nurse

- Explain the hemodialysis procedure and possible side effects (hypotension, dizziness, nausea) and treatment of symptoms ➠*Rationale:* Providing information about the procedure and treatment of adverse effects can decrease anxiety and fear.
- Encourage the child (as appropriate for age and condition) and family to notify the nurse of any symptoms experienced during the procedure ➠*Rationale:* Educates the child and family regarding the importance of reporting symptoms immediately and reinforces previously taught information.
- Explain the need for continuous monitoring during the hemodialysis procedure ➠*Rationale:* The child and family are alerted regarding the need for frequent interventions during the procedure, which decreases anxiety.
- Explain the need for laboratory specimens to check for appropriate correction of blood levels (i.e., electrolytes, ammonia) as they pertain to the indication for hemodialysis ➠*Rationale:* Alerts the child and family to the need for frequent blood specimens, which may decrease anxiety.

EQUIPMENT

- Basic monitoring equipment (blood pressure monitor, pulse oximeter, and other basic procedural equipment found within the unit)
- The dialysis nurse generally brings the following equipment and supplies:
  - Portable RO water purifying machine
  - Dialysis machine
  - Appropriately sized blood tubing and dialyzer
  - Dialysate
  - Activated clotting time (ACT) equipment

Procedure | for Hemodialysis

Steps	Rationale	Considerations
1. Ensure child and family understand procedure and questions are answered.	Evaluates and reinforces understanding of previously taught information.	Developmental level, cognitive ability and anxiety level will determine approach to and effectiveness of teaching.
2. Identify child using appropriate patient verification process and verify prescribing practitioner's order for treatment.	Confirms correct patient and procedure as recommended by the Joint Commission for Accreditation of Healthcare Organizations (JCAHO). Familiarizes the nurse with reasonable indicators for hemodialysis and expected outcomes.	Use two patient identifiers per institution-specific protocol.
3. Ensure child is located in a room with an appropriate water source and drain.	Hemodialysis equipment requires a constant water source and a drain for the waste.	
4. Assist with placement of catheter for use with hemodialysis if needed. See Procedure 140 for more information.	A properly placed catheter is essential to the hemodialysis procedure.	Preferred sites for catheter placement are femoral, right IJ, or right EJ veins. Use of the subclavian vein is not recommended because stenosis could limit future vascular access creation.[1] *(Level V*)*
5. Verify position of catheter with radiographic study.	Catheter tip should be at the level of the caval atrial junction or into the right atrium to ensure optimal blood flow.[2] *(Level II*)*	
6. Obtain preprocedure weight and vital signs.	Establishes baseline weight assessment relative to the child's dry weight and aids in fluid removal evaluation. *(Level V*)*	Dry weight is considered ideal body weight without additional fluid.
7. Assist dialysis nurse with set up and supplies as needed.	Labeling and sending blood specimens obtained by the dialysis nurse at the initiation or during the procedure may be the responsibility of the bedside nurse.	
8. Regularly assess the child in collaboration with the dialysis nurse during the procedure.	Comprehensive care of the child includes dialysis-related assessments performed by the dialysis nurse and nondialysis-related assessments performed by the bedside nurse. Communication and collaboration are essential for the continuum of care.	Assessment and observation by both the bedside nurse and the dialysis nurse in conjunction with machine and other monitoring devices is essential. Dialysis nurse performs ongoing assessment during the hemodialysis procedure, including blood pressure, fluid removal, respiratory status, deviation from baseline status, integrity of the hemodialysis circuit, and performance of the vascular access.

* Level II: Theory-based; no research data to support recommendations; recommendations from expert consensus group may exist
  Level V: Clinical studies in more than one or two patient populations and situations to support recommendations

Procedure for Hemodialysis—*Continued*

Steps	Rationale	Considerations
9. All nondialysis procedures and medications should be maintained by the bedside nurse as appropriate during hemodialysis procedure.	The dialysis nurse is responsible for the hemodialysis procedure. Some medications may be held during the hemodialysis procedure because they are removed with hemodialysis.	If the kidneys excrete medications, they could be removed with hemodialysis.[1] *(Level V*)*
10. Assist the dialysis nurse with termination of the hemodialysis procedure as needed.	Facilitates maintenance of vascular access.	Catheter lumens are instilled with high-concentration heparin at the filling volume of the lumen after the procedure. Lumens should be labeled to indicate that high-concentration heparin is instilled. Before use or flushing of the catheter, withdraw and discard heparin per institution-specific protocol.[1] *(Level II*)* Note: In many institutions, hemodialysis catheters are not accessed for purposes other than hemodialysis unless ordered by the nephrologists; refer to institution-specific protocol.
11. Obtain postprocedure weight and vital signs.	Assessment of achieved fluid removal is verified with posthemodialysis weight. New baseline status may be achieved after fluid removal or correction of electrolytes or toxin levels. (i.e., respiratory status or blood pressure). *(Level V*)*	
12. Dialysis nurse gives report to the bedside nurse at the conclusion of procedure and documents outcomes.	Summarizes interventions performed during the procedure (i.e., use of 0.9% saline solution bolus versus medication for decreased blood pressure); collaboration about expected and unexpected outcomes.	

* Level II: Theory-based; no research data to support recommendations; recommendations from expert consensus group may exist
    Level V: Clinical studies in more than one or two patient populations and situations to support recommendations

Expected Outcomes

- Vascular access is achieved and maintained without complications

- The ACT and partial thromboplastin time (PTT) are within prescribed range during and after hemodialysis procedure
- Accumulated waste products or toxins are removed

Unexpected Outcomes

- Clotting or impaired patency of the vascular access
- Decreased circulation in the vascular access extremity
- Redness, drainage, or tenderness at the catheter insertion site
- Bruit/thrill of fistula or graft diminished or absent after procedure
- Dislodgement of catheter used for hemodialysis procedure
- Postprocedure bleeding or hematoma formation at the AV fistula or AV graft needle insertion sites

- Inability to achieve goals of treatment

Continued

Expected Outcomes

- Targeted reduction of blood urea nitrogen (BUN) value
- Restoration of acid-base balance

- Desired electrolyte or toxin levels (i.e., drug levels)

- Desired fluid removal without adverse complications

Unexpected Outcomes

- Complications related to hemodialysis procedure: adverse respiratory, neurologic, cardiac, gastrointestinal, or fluid/electrolyte changes
- Technical problems with the hemodialysis machine or RO water purifying machine
- Inability to achieve targeted fluid loss

Monitoring and Care of the Child

Activities and Interventions	Rationale	Reportable Conditions
1. Perform and record preprocedure and postprocedure weights.	Predialysis weight is useful to determine the amount of fluid to be removed during the procedure. Postprocedure weight shows actual amount of fluid removed. Daily weights monitor the increase or decrease in weight and fluid status.	• Abnormal or unexpected increase or decrease in weight
2. Perform baseline and ongoing assessments, including: Vital signs Presence of edema Bulging or depressed fontanel Intake and output Neurologic status	Essential to establish baseline. Fluid restriction is indicated with acute or chronic renal failure. Although rarely seen, a rapid reduction of urea puts the child at risk for disequilibrium syndrome; this occurs with a rapid osmolar shift that can cause cerebral edema manifested by changes in neurologic examination and seizures.[3] (Level V*) Monitor for complications during and after procedure.	• Hypertension or hypotension • Fever or hypothermia • Tachycardia or bradycardia • Cardiac dysrhythmias • Tachypnea or bradypnea • Rales or change in breath sounds • Change in level of consciousness • Seizures
3. For newly placed access, monitor circulation to the extremity, including capillary refill, pulses distal to the access, color and temperature of the extremity, and sensation. (Level V*)	Large-bore access may impede blood flow.	• Diminished capillary refill • Diminished or absent pulses • Pale, mottled, or cyanotic extremity • Cool to touch • Pain • Diminished or absent sensation or movement
4. Perform catheter dressing changes per institution-specific protocol. Monitor site for redness, drainage, tenderness, or catheter dislodgement. Culture exit site as needed. Obtain blood culture for fever per institution-specific protocol.	Redness, drainage, and tenderness are symptoms of infection at the catheter exit site. Fever may be an indicator of catheter-related sepsis.[1,4] (Level II*)	• Redness, drainage, tenderness, or catheter dislodgement • Fever or chills
5. Monitor patency of AV fistula or AV graft if present. Palpate along the length of the AV fistula or graft for a thrill and auscultate for presence of bruit.	Diminished or absent bruit or thrill can indicate decreased blood flow, clotting, or stenosis of the AV fistula or AV graft. Use Doppler ultrasound scan to assess the access if unable to auscultate bruit with a stethoscope or palpate the thrill.	• Absence of bruit or thrill • Decrease in integrity of the bruit or thrill from previous assessment
6. If the child has an AV fistula or graft, post a sign over the child's bed: "No venipunctures or blood pressures in affected limb."[4] (Level V*)	Use of occluding equipment (i.e., tourniquets or blood pressure cuffs) could cause the fistula or graft to clot by constricting the blood flow through the fistula or graft.[5]	• Use of extremity with AV fistula or graft for venipuncture or blood pressure

---

* Level II: Theory-based; no research data to support recommendations; recommendations from expert consensus group may exist
Level V: Clinical studies in more than one or two patient populations and situations to support recommendations

Monitoring and Care of the Child—Cont'd

Activities and Interventions	Rationale	Reportable Conditions
7. Pharmacologic management: Monitor peak and trough drug levels (i.e., antibiotics) per prescribing practitioner's order or institution-specific protocol. Adjust medication doses as ordered by prescribing practitioner	Medications excreted by the kidneys may be removed with hemodialysis.[1] *(Level V*)*	• Medication levels out of therapeutic range
8. Monitor child's response to medications: Level of pain or sedation Blood pressure Cardiac arrhythmia Titrate medications as ordered to achieve desired effect.	Medications excreted by the kidneys may be removed with hemodialysis.[1] *(Level V*)*	• Inability to achieve expected patient response
9. Monitor laboratory results after procedure per prescribing practitioner's order or institution-specific protocol. Electrolytes, especially potassium, are not recommended to be obtained until 1 to 2 hours after procedure. *(Level V*)*	Laboratory values change with hemodialysis. A rebound increase is seen in serum potassium and lithium levels within 1 to 2 hours after hemodialysis procedure ends.[6,7] Careful consideration should be taken before replacement or correction of posthemodialysis electrolyte levels.[6]	• Levels obtained 1 to 2 hours after hemodialysis out of expected range[6]
10. Observe for signs of unexpected bleeding.	Heparin is frequently used to anticoagulate the circuit during a hemodialysis procedure unless coagulopathy is present.	• Prolonged or unexpected bleeding

* Level II: Theory-based; no research data to support recommendations; recommendations from expert consensus group may exist
  Level V: Clinical studies in more than one or two patient populations and situations to support recommendations

Documentation

Bedside Nurse
- Child and family education
- Date and time of access placement
- Type of access: AV fistula, AV graft, or catheter
- Location and integrity of access
- With catheter use for reasons other than dialysis, documentation of catheter size, length, and lumen volumes
- Vital signs throughout the procedure
- Daily, preprocedure, and postprocedure weights
- Interventions (medications, IV fluids, etc.) provided not related to hemodialysis
- Laboratory assessment data
- Unexpected outcomes and related treatment

Dialysis Nurse
- Child and family education as it relates to hemodialysis
- Date and time of hemodialysis procedure initiation and length of procedure
- Child's response to and tolerance of procedure
- Integrity of catheter, AV fistula, or AV graft: patency, quality of blood flow, and problems associated with access procedure
- Condition of catheter insertion site and any signs or symptoms of infection
- Presence and quality of bruit with AV fistula or AV graft for vascular access
- Needle size used for cannulation of AV fistula or AV graft, if applicable
- Type of hemodialysis machine used, size of tubing and dialyzer, and potassium and calcium bath/acid
- Blood pump speed with arterial and venous pressures during the procedure

Continued

Documentation—Cont'd

Bedside Nurse

Dialysis Nurse

- Vital signs during the procedure and preprocedure and postprocedure vital signs
- Net fluid removed during the procedure
- Use of a blood or albumin prime if indicated
- Medication, IV fluids, or blood products administered during the procedure related to hemodialysis
- Preprocedure and postprocedure weights
- Laboratory studies obtained before, during, or after procedure (i.e., ACT/PTT, electrolytes, blood cultures)
- Amount of heparin used during the procedure
- Unexpected outcomes related to the procedure and related treatment

References

1. American Nephrology Nurses Association: *Core curriculum for nephrology nursing,* ed 4, Pitman, NJ, 2001, ANNA.
2. NKF-K/DOQI: *Clinical practice guidelines for vascular access,* New York, 2001, National Kidney Foundation.
3. Flynn JT: Choice of dialysis modality for management of pediatric acute renal failure, *Pediatr Nephrol* 17(1):61-66, 2002.
4. Kovalik E, Schwab S: Treatment approaches for infected hemodialysis vascular catheters, *Curr Opin Nephrol Hypertension* 11(6):593-596, 2002.
5. Konner K., et al: Arteriovenous fistula, *J Am Soc Nephrol* 14(6):1669-1680, 2003.
6. Daugirdas JT, et al, editors: *Handbook of dialysis,* ed 3, Philadelphia, 2001, Lippincott Williams & Wilkins.
7. Meyer RJ, et al: Hemodialysis followed by continuous hemofiltration for treatment of lithium intoxication of children, *Am J Kidney Dis* 37(5): 2001.

Additional Readings

Beathard GA: Physical examination of the dialysis vascular access, *Semin Dialysis* 11(44):231-236, 1998.

Goldberg EA: Physical assessment of children ages 1-10, part 1 and 2, *ANNA J.* 24(2):209-230, 1997.

Schwab SJ: Vascular access for hemodialysis, *Kidney Int* 55(5):2078-2090, 1999.

Smoyer WE, et al: A practical approach to continuous hemofiltration in infants and children, *Dialysis Transplant* 24(11):633-640, 1995.

Williams DM, et al: Acute kidney failure: a pediatric experience over 20 years, *Arch Pediatr Adolesc Med* 156(9):893-900, 2002.

Peritoneal Dialysis: Catheter Exit Site Care

P U R P O S E : A peritoneal dialysis (PD) catheter is surgically placed into the abdomen and remains in place for the duration of therapy. Proper care of the catheter and exit site is essential in prevention of infection.

Patricia O'Connor

PREREQUISITE KNOWLEDGE

- Principles of aseptic technique
- Management of the PD catheter
- Appropriate preparation and pain management are essential before wound care is performed on a child.
- Frequent dressing changes during the first 2 weeks are not necessary unless dressings are wet. Recommendations are to change dressing no more often than once a week for the first 2 weeks and then two to three times per week for the following 4 weeks, or until the exit site is well healed. Infrequent dressing changes decrease the risk of contamination and local trauma to the exit site.[1-4] *(Level VI*)*
- The child may be mobilized gently on the first postinsertion day. The child should not return to school for at least 1 week.[3,5]
- The child should not engage in heavy exercise before 6 weeks after implantation.[3,5]
- No showering is allowed during the 6 weeks after implantation. Tub baths are contraindicated for the duration of PD therapy.[3,5-7]
- Exit site care for the period just after catheter insertion (minimum, first 6 weeks postimplantation) is carried out

as a sterile procedure to minimize bacterial colonization of the exit and tunnel during the early healing period.
- After the first 6 weeks, or when the incision and catheter exit site are well healed, exit site care follows strict aseptic procedure during hospitalization.
  - ❖ Home care instructions generally describe a clean technique after showering (children with PD catheters should not take tub baths), at a minimum every other day; more often with infection or crust formation at exit site. These instructions should follow outpatient dialysis center or homecare protocols.

CHILD AND FAMILY ASSESSMENT

- Child's developmental level and ability to interact ➤*Rationale:* These factors influence preparation and interaction.
- Assess for allergies, including latex, alcohol, and any skin preparation products or types of tape ➤*Rationale:* Decreases likelihood of an allergic reaction to substances used in procedure.
- Examination of PD catheter and abdominal exit site for signs and symptoms of infection, leakage, or drainage ➤*Rationale:* Catheter insertion site provides a portal of entry for infection, which could result in septicemia or peritonitis. If the exit site appears to be infected, further interventions (e.g., site change, culture, antibiotics) may be necessary.

---

* Level VI: Clinical studies in a variety of patient populations and situations to support recommendations

- Assess child's and family's understanding of the procedure and their ability and desire to perform exit site care after discharge ➻*Rationale:* Evaluates and reinforces understanding of previously taught information. Guide for further teaching.

CHILD AND FAMILY EDUCATION

Individualized, developmentally appropriate education is provided to the child and to the family based on desire for knowledge, readiness to learn, and overall neurologic and psychosocial state. Encourage questions and answer questions as they arise, and reinforce information as needed.

- Explain the procedure and reason for exit site care to the family and child at a developmentally appropriate level. Use the resources of a Child Life Specialist if available. ➻*Rationale:* Decreases child's anxiety and discomfort. If appropriate, show the procedure to be performed on a doll. Toddlers may need the parents to help alleviate anxiety. Preschoolers need simple concise explanations. School-aged children need thorough preparation for all procedures, including all the steps involved. Adolescents also need preparation and information and have a high need for privacy.
- Discuss the child's and family's role in catheter and exit site care ➻*Rationale:* Cooperation is elicited; child and family are prepared to provide exit site care in the home.
- Explain the need for strict aseptic technique in manipulation of the PD catheter to decrease the chance of peritoneal infection because pathogens can be introduced into the abdominal cavity via the catheter ➻*Rationale:* Providing information decreases anxiety and fear and promotes compliance.

EQUIPMENT

- Clean and sterile gloves (one pair each)
- Gowns and face protection as indicated
- Masks for self, child, and anyone in the room during dressing change
- Mupirocin calcium ointment if ordered or per institution-specific protocol
- Sterile applicators
- Soft absorbent gauze dressings
- Tape
- Cath-secure device if used

For Early Exit Site Care

- Mild nonirritating agent for skin cleansing
- Sterile water or saline solution for rinsing
- Sterile field

For Chronic Exit Site Catheter Care

- 2% chlorhexidine gluconate, or alternate skin antiseptic if indicated

Procedure for Peritoneal Dialysis: Catheter Exit Site Care

Steps	Rationale	Considerations
Early Exit Site Care: First 6 Weeks After Implantation Recommendations are to change dressing no more than once a week for the first 2 weeks and then two to three times per week for the following 4 weeks, or until the exit site is well healed.		
1. Ensure child and family understand procedure and questions are answered.	Evaluates and reinforces understanding of previously taught information.	Developmental level, cognitive ability and anxiety level will determine approach to and effectiveness of teaching.
2. Administer premedication to child with prescribed analgesic, if indicated, during early postimplantation period.	Decreases anxiety and increases comfort.	
3. Gather needed equipment and supplies.	Presence of all materials facilitates completion of procedure in a timely manner.	
4. Close door and turn off any portable fans.	Prevents unnecessary circulation of airborne pathogens.	
5. Place child in position of optimal comfort that allows visualization of and access to exit site. Optimize lighting in room and provide privacy.	Provides for effective exit site visualization and enhances child's ability to tolerate procedure.	Privacy is an important consideration for school-aged children and adolescents.
6. Put on surgical mask and mask child and anyone in the room during access of PD catheter.	Decreases the risk of contamination from airborne pathogens.	

Procedure for Peritoneal Dialysis: Catheter Exit Site Care—*Continued*		
Steps	**Rationale**	**Considerations**
7. Expose area.	Allows access to site for procedure.	
8. Wash hands for 3 minutes with antimicrobial soap.	Reduces risk of transmission of microorganisms.	
9. Prepare sterile field on a clean flat surface.	Peritoneal dialysis-related infections account for more than 75% of lost catheters.[8] Treatment failure in children is most often the result of recurrent catheter site infection and resultant peritonitis.[9-11]	Risk factors for early infection include: • Wound hematoma. • Sutures at exit site. • Early colonization of exit site. • Excessive catheter manipulation.
10. Determine how many and what types of dressings are necessary.	Availability of appropriate supplies facilitates procedure and decreases likelihood of sterile field contamination.	
11. Open each dressing by peeling apart the edges of package, maintaining sterility. Place dressing supplies on sterile field.	Prevents cross-contamination.[12,13]	
12. Prepare tape.	Facilitates securing dressing, when in place.	
13. Put on clean gloves and remove old dressing. *Do not* use scissors.	Avoids risk of cutting PD catheter.	
14. Examine the appearance of exit site and note the presence of any inflammation, purulent discharge, odor, or sutures. *(Level VI*)*	Purulent drainage from the exit site indicates the presence of infection. Erythema may or may not represent infection.[14,15]	Sutures are never placed at the exit site; if sutures are present, provider needs to be notified. Sutures interfere with healing and granulation at the exit site.[15,16]
15. Wash hands and put on sterile gloves.	Application of new dressing is a sterile procedure; prevents cross contamination.	
16. Place sterile drape on child's abdomen, under catheter, but away from exit site to be cleansed.		
17. Keep catheter immobilized with avoidance of excessive movement at the exit site. *(Level VI*)*	The goal is minimization of catheter manipulation and subsequent trauma. Excessive movement interferes with epithelialization and healing of the exit site.[4,17-22]	
18. A mild nonirritating agent should be used to clean the exit site, surrounding skin, and catheter. Do not disturb any scab formation.	Strong oxidizing agents, such as povidone-iodine and hydrogen peroxide, should not be used because they interfere with epithelialization over the granulation tissue beneath the scab.[1,21,23-27]	
19. Rinse exit site with sterile water or saline solution (*not* tap water) with sterile applicators.	Unless chlorinated, tap water and well water can be contaminated with *pseudomonas*.[27]	
20. Dry exit site with sterile gauze or applicators.	Facilitates dressing application.	

Procedure continues on following page

* Level VI: Clinical studies in a variety of patient populations and situations to support recommendations

Procedure for Peritoneal Dialysis: Catheter Exit Site Care—*Continued*

Steps	Rationale	Considerations
21. Mupirocin calcium ointment may be applied to the exit site after cleaning to prevent infections per prescribing practitioner's orders or institution specific protocol. *(Level VI*)*	Mupirocin has been shown to be effective in prevention of exit site infections in children who carry *Staphylococcus aureus* on their skin but is widely used for other individuals as well.[5,15,28-31]	
22. Place an absorbent sterile dressing over the exit site and tape on all four sides.	Transparent occlusive dressings are not to be used alone because drainage tends to pool at the exit site and in the sinus.[32]	
23. Immobilize the catheter.	Avoids trauma to exit site.[13,33]	
24. Discard soiled materials in an appropriate receptacle.	Standard precautions; reduces the transmission of microorganisms.	
25. Remove gloves and wash hands.	Standard precautions; reduces the transmission of microorganisms.	

Chronic Exit Site Catheter Care, for Well-healed Exit Site

No clear consensus exists as to when the child may begin to shower or change to chronic exit site care. When the exit site can be classified as good or equivocal, then showering and chronic care are recommended.[2,4,22,34]

1. Gather needed equipment and supplies.	Presence of all materials facilitates completion of procedure in a timely manner.	
2. Follow previous steps 3 to 17.		
3. If child is 2 months of age or older, cleanse exit site, surrounding skin, and PD catheter with 2% chlorhexidine gluconate. If the child is less than 2 months of age or sensitive to chlorhexidine gluconate, use povidone-iodine or consult prescribing practitioner for recommended substitution. Mupirocin calcium ointment may be applied to the exit site after cleansing to prevent infections, per prescribing practitioner orders or institution specific protocol. *(Level VI*)*	Use of 2% chlorhexidine gluconate is the preferred skin antiseptic,[16,27,35] however, it is *not* to be used in infants less than 2 months of age because of the potential for excessive skin irritation and increased drug absorption.[26]	Chlorhexidine solutions contain alcohol as a stabilizer. Alcohol can cause deterioration of polyurethane catheters (such as the Cruz catheter, PD-Midwest, LLC, New York, NY). Use povidone-iodine as alternate or consult with provider for appropriate skin antisepsis.
4. Apply an absorbent sterile dressing over the exit site and tape on all four sides.	Dressings often help to secure the catheter. Young children, because of the nature of their play and typical hygiene, should always have an exit site dressing.	To date, no studies prove that a dressing over a healthy healed exit site prevents infection; however, dressings are recommended to be worn when the exit site is likely to get dirty or wet.
5. Cover the PD catheter with the dressing. The extension set should remain on top of the dressing.	Allows access for PD. Both the catheter and the extension set should be immobilized with tape or other cath-secure device to avoid trauma to exit site or dislodgement of catheter.	

* Level VI: Clinical studies in a variety of patient populations and situations to support recommendations

Procedure for Peritoneal Dialysis: Catheter Exit Site Care—*Continued*

Steps	Rationale	Considerations
6. Discard soiled materials in an appropriate receptacle.	Standard precautions; reduces transmission of microorganisms.	
7. Remove gloves, wash hands.	Standard precautions; reduces transmission of microorganisms.	
8. Document appropriate information in the medical record.	Documents status of exit site, child's ability to tolerate procedure, and other pertinent information.	

Expected Outcomes

- Exit site heals

- Exit site and surrounding skin is free of maceration and erosion

- Exit site is free of signs of infection or compromised tissue perfusion
- The PD catheter remains intact
- Child has acceptable level of comfort
- Child and family receive appropriate education and support

Unexpected Outcomes

- Wound healing (granulation and contraction) not noticeably progressing on a weekly basis
- Cross contamination of wound
- Maceration or erosion of exit site
- Damage to exit site (hemorrhage, dehiscence) from excessive manipulation of PD catheter
- Signs of infection
- Signs of compromised tissue perfusion
- Dislodgement of PD catheter
- Unmanaged pain
- Inappropriate or incomplete education

Monitoring and Care of the Child

Activities and Interventions	Rationale	Reportable Conditions
1. Monitor child and exit site for signs and symptoms of infection or trauma. *(Level V*)*	Ongoing assessment for wound infection is essential to exit site healing and the prevention of peritonitis. The exit site must be free from infection or an inflammatory response occurs that interferes with wound healing.[23,32]	• Bleeding, inflammation, purulent drainage, or odor at exit site or on dressing • Fever • Disconnection of the extension set or any contamination of catheter • Indications that catheter has been contaminated
2. Monitor exit site dressing for intactness and catheter transfer set for kinking, loose connection, and puncture site.	Dressing must be changed if it is no longer occlusive. Kinking, loose connection, or puncture in transfer set may result in contamination of the catheter, necessitating a catheter change.	
3. Monitor effectiveness of pain management strategy.	Ineffective pain management makes future dressing changes more traumatic.	• Inadequate pain relief during dressing change

* Level V: Clinical studies in more than one or two patient populations and situations to support recommendations

Documentation

- Exit site assessment: drainage, odor, presence of inflammation or trauma (e.g., catheter has been forcibly pulled; aggressive crust removal has resulted in redness or bleeding) to the exit site
- Unexpected outcomes and treatments provided
- Description of surrounding skin, including color, moisture, and integrity
- Child and family education
- Exit site care
- Nursing interventions
- Date and time of dressing application
- Pain scores
- Child's tolerance of procedure

References

1. Nelson DB, Dilloway MA: Principles, products and practical aspects of wound care, *Crit Care Nurs Q* 25(1):33-54, 2002.
2. Prowant BF: Peritoneal dialysis. In Lancaster LE, editor: *Core curriculum for nephrology nurses,* ed 4, Pitman, NJ, 2001, American Nephrology Nurses Association, Jannetti Publications.
3. Strippoli GFM: Catheter-related interventions to prevent peritonitis in peritoneal dialysis: a systematic review of randomized, controlled trials, *J Am Soc Nephrol* 15(10):2735-2746, 2004.
4. Twardowski ZJ, Nichols K: Peritoneal dialysis access and exit site care. In Gokal R, et al, editors: *Textbook of peritoneal dialysis,* ed 2, Boston, 2000, Kluwer Academic Publishers.
5. Tacconelli E, et al: Mupirocin prophylaxis to prevent *Staphylococcus aureus* infection in patients undergoing dialysis: a meta-analysis, *Infect Dis Clin North Am* 37(12):1629-1638, 2003.
6. Holloway M: Peritoneal dialysis orders in children. In Nissenson AR, Fine RN, editors: *Dialysis therapy,* ed 3, Philadelphia, 2002, Hanley & Belfus.
7. Neu AM: Infant and neonatal peritoneal dialysis. In Nissenson AR, Fine RN, editors: *Dialysis therapy,* ed 3, Philadelphia, 2002, Hanley & Belfus.
8. Ash SR: Peritoneal access devices and placement techniques. In Nissenson AR, Fine RN, editors: *Dialysis therapy,* ed 3, Philadelphia, 2002, Hanley & Belfus.
9. Johnson RJ, Feehally J, editors: *Comprehensive clinical nephrology,* ed 2, St Louis, 2003, Mosby.
10. Vas SI: Peritonitis in peritoneal dialysis patients. In Nissenson AR, Fine RN, editors: *Dialysis therapy,* ed 3, Philadelphia, 2002, Hanley & Belfus.
11. Warady BF, et al: ISPD guidelines/recommendations: consensus guidelines for the treatment of peritonitis in pediatric patients receiving peritoneal dialysis, *Peritoneal Dialysis Int* 20(6):610-624, 2000.
12. Hayes DD: Performing peritoneal dialysis: clinical do's and don't's, *Nursing 2003* 33(3):17-18, 2003.
13. Lancaster LE, editor: *American Nephrology Nurses Association core curriculum for nephrology nursing,* Pitman, NJ, 2001, American Nephrology Nurses Association, Jannetti Publications.
14. Branom RN: Is this wound infected? *Crit Care Nurs Q* 25(1):55-62, 2002.
15. Piraino B, et al: ISPD guidelines/recommendations: peritoneal dialysis-related infections recommendations: 2005 update, *Peritoneal Dialysis Int* 25(2):107-131, 2005.
16. Shonjania K, et al: *Making health care safer: a critical analysis of patient safety practices,* Rockville, MD, 2001, Agency for Healthcare Research and Quality.
17. Brandt ML, Brewer ED: Peritoneal catheter placement in children. In Nissenson AR, Fine RN, editors: *Dialysis therapy,* ed 3, Philadelphia, 2002, Hanley & Belfus.
18. Burrows-Hudson S, Prowant BF, editors: *Nephrology nursing standards of practice and guidelines for care,* Pitman, NJ, 2005, American Nephrology Nurses Association, Jannetti Publications.
19. Daugirdas JT, et al, editors: *Handbook of dialysis,* ed 3, Philadelphia, 2001, Lippincott, Williams & Wilkins.
20. Diaz-Buxo JA: Management of peritoneal catheter malfunction, *Peritoneal Dialysis Int* 18(3):256-259, 1998.
21. Flanigan M, Gokal R: Peritoneal catheters and exit-site practices toward optimum peritoneal access: a review of current developments, *Peritoneal Dialysis Int* 25(2):132-139, 2005.
22. Twardowski ZJ: Peritoneal catheter exit-site and tunnel infections. In Nissenson AR, Fine RN, editors: *Dialysis therapy,* ed 3, Philadelphia, 2002, Hanley & Belfus.
23. Hess CT, Kirsner RS: Orchestrating wound healing: assessing and preparing the wound, *Adv Skin Wound Care* 16(5):246-257, 2003.
24. Howard R: The appropriate use of topical antimicrobials and antiseptics in children: neonatal skin care, *Pediatr Ann* 30(4):219-224, 2001.
25. Maloney J, Fisher B: Skin integrity. In Moloney-Harmon PA, Czerwinski SJ, editors: *Review of pediatric critical care,* Philadelphia, 1997, Saunders.
26. Taquino LT: Promoting wound healing in the neonatal setting: process versus protocol, *J Perinatal Neonatal Nurs* 14(1):104-118, 2003.
27. Watson AR, Gartland C: *Guidelines by an Ad Hoc European Committee for Elective Chronic Peritoneal Dialysis in Pediatric Patients,* 2001, on behalf of Paediatric Peritoneal Dialysis Working Group. Watson AR. Gartland C. European Paediatric Peritoneal Dialysis Working Group. Guidelines by an Ad Hoc European Committee for Elective Chronic Peritoneal Dialysis in Pediatric Patients. Peritoneal Dialysis International. 21(3):240-244, 2001 May-Jun.
28. Amato D, et al: Staphylococcal peritonitis in continuous ambulatory peritoneal dialysis: colonization with identical strains at exit site, nose, and hands. *Am J Kidney Dis* 37(1):43-48, 2001.
29. Bernardini J, et al: Randomized double blinded trial of antibiotic exit site cream for the prevention of exit site infection in peritoneal dialysis patients, *J Am Soc Nephrol* 16:539-545, 2005.

30. Briggs J, editor: Clinical effectiveness of different approaches to peritoneal dialysis catheter exit-site care, *Best Practice: Evidence Based Practice Information for Health Care Professionals* (8)1:1-6, 2004.

31. Lobbedez T, et al: Routine use of mupirocin at the peritoneal catheter exit site and mupirocin resistance: still low after 7 years, *Nephrol Dialysis Transplant J* 19:3140-3, 2004.

32. Clark JJ: Wound repair and factors influencing healing, *Crit Care Nurs Q* 25(1):1-12, 2002.

33. Li PK, et al: Comparison of clinical outcome and ease of handling in two double-bag systems in continuous ambulatory peritoneal dialysis: a prospective, randomized, controlled, multicenter study, *Am J Kidney Dis* 40(2):373-380, 2002.

34. National Kidney Foundation–DOQI: Clinical practice guidelines for peritoneal dialysis adequacy, 2001, National Kidney Foundation, Inc. Anonymous. II. NKF-K/DOQI Clinical Practice Guidelines for Peritoneal Dialysis Adequacy: update 2000. *Am J Kidney Dis* 37(1 Suppl 1):S65-S136, 2001 Jan.

35. Centers for Disease Control and Prevention: *Guideline for the prevention of surgical wound infections,* Rockville, MD, 1999, US Department of Health and Human Services.

Additional Readings

Chadha V, et al: Adequacy of peritoneal dialysis in pediatric patients. In Nissenson AR, Fine RN, editors: *Dialysis therapy,* ed 3, Philadelphia, 2002, Hanley & Belfus.

Curley MAQ, Moloney-Harmon PA, editors: *Critical care nursing of infants and children*, Philadelphia, 2001, Saunders.

Health Care Financing Administration: *End stage renal disease clinical performance measures project,* Baltimore, 1999, Department of Health and Human Services, Health Care Financing Administration, Office of Clinical Standards and Quality.

Jabs K, Warady BA: The impact of the dialysis outcomes quality initiative guidelines on the care of the pediatric end-stage renal disease patient, *Adv Renal Replacement Ther* 6(1):97-106, 1999.

Munford PR: Psychosocial adjustment and treatment of children and adolescents with ESRD. In Nissenson AR, Fine RN, editors: *Dialysis therapy,* ed 3, Philadelphia, 2002, Hanley & Belfus.

National Kidney Foundation-DOQI: Clinical practice guidelines for peritoneal dialysis adequacy, *Am J Kidney Dis* 30(Suppl 3): S94-99, 1997.

Piraino B: Peritoneal dialysis catheter replacement: save the patient and not the catheter, *Semin Dialysis* 1(16):72-75, 2003.

Peritoneal Dialysis: Pass Management

P U R P O S E : Dialysate fluid is instilled into and drained from the peritoneal cavity to remove fluid and toxins, regulate electrolyte levels, and manage azotemia via diffusion and osmosis

Patricia O'Connor

PREREQUISITE KNOWLEDGE

- Peritoneal dialysis (PD) involves the transport of solutes and water across a filter or semipermeable membrane (the peritoneum) that separates two-fluid filled compartments:
  - ❖ The blood in the peritoneal capillaries, which in renal failure contain excess urea, creatinine, and potassium
  - ❖ The peritoneal cavity that contains dialysis solution, which typically contains sodium, chloride, lactate, and a hyperosmolar/high concentration of glucose
- Mechanism of PD, including the principles of diffusion, osmosis, ultrafiltration, and absorption. During the course of a peritoneal dialysis dwell, these transport processes occur simultaneously.
  - ❖ Diffusion: The passive movement of *solutes* through a semipermeable membrane from an area of higher concentration to an area of lower concentration. Uremic solutes and potassium diffuse from the peritoneal capillary blood down the concentration gradient into the PD solution. Glucose, lactate, and, to a lesser extent, calcium diffuse in the opposite direction.
  - ❖ Osmosis: The passive movement of *solvent* through a semipermeable membrane from an area of higher concentration to one of lower concentration. In PD, this process is referred to as *ultrafiltration*. The relative hyperosmolarity of the PD solution leads to ultrafiltration of water and associated solutes across the membrane.

- ❖ Absorption: Constant absorption of water and solute from the peritoneal cavity both directly and indirectly into the lymphatic system
- Dialysate fluid (dialysate) is infused into the peritoneal cavity through a flexible abdominal catheter (Figures 106-1 and 106-2).
- The dwell volume that can be tolerated is related to the size of the infant or child. The larger the volume of dialysate, the more effective the removal of blood urea nitrogen (BUN), creatinine, and potassium. The most limiting factor is compromise of respiratory excursion by direct pressure on the diaphragm.
- Peritoneal dialysis involves repeated fluid exchanges or cycles; each cycle has three phases: instillation or fill, dwell, and drain.
  - ❖ During the *instillation* or *fill phase,* the dialysate is infused into the peritoneal cavity through an abdominal catheter.
  - ❖ During the *dwell phase,* the dialysate remains in the peritoneal cavity, which allows osmosis and diffusion to occur. Dwell time varies based on the child's clinical need and is ordered by the prescribing practitioner. Use of dialysate with a high concentration of glucose enhances fluid removal.
  - ❖ During the *drain phase,* the dialysate and the excess extracellular fluid, wastes, and electrolytes are drained from the peritoneal cavity via the abdominal catheter.
  - ❖ Table 106-1 is a review of types of PD.
- Peritoneal dialysis can be performed manually, with a single tubing and bag set-up (manual PD) that fills and

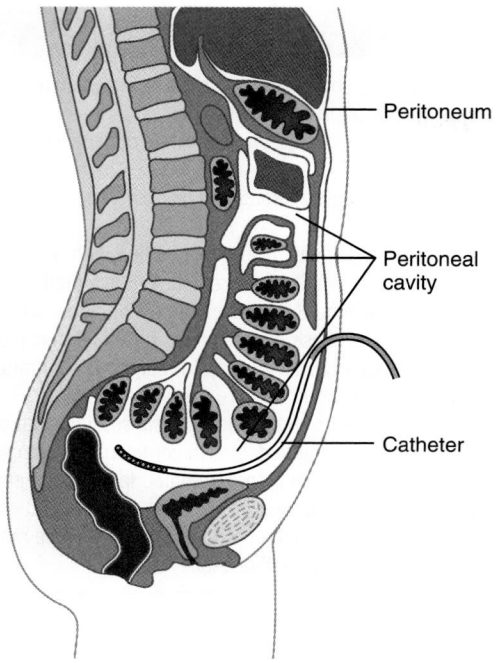

FIGURE 106-1 Placement of Peritoneal Catheter. Inside of abdomen is lined with thin membrane called peritoneum that surrounds intestines and other internal organs. In peritoneal dialysis, this cavity is filled with dialysis fluid that enters body through permanently implanted catheter. *Used with permission from the Kidney Foundation of Canada.*

drains with gravity or with a cycler machine (CCPD) that may use gravity or a pump. With a cycler machine, multiple exchanges are programmed into the machine and run automatically, most frequently during hours of sleep. Cycler machines are used in the inpatient setting and for home PD therapy (see Figure 106-3 for cycler set-up).

- Most children have a 6-inch "transfer set" or extension tubing that attaches to the PD catheter at the skin level exit site. This catheter remains in place between PD therapy and is exchanged by the prescribing practitioner in sterile conditions about every 6 months or according to institution-specific protocol or if contamination occurs. If this extension is not in place and the PD catheter becomes contaminated, surgical replacement of the PD catheter is usually necessary.
- Dialysate should be heated to approximately 37°C before instillation. Methods for heating dialysate include:
  - ❖ Automated cyclers that heat dialysate to the necessary temperature
  - ❖ Heating cabinet
  - ❖ Incubator
  - ❖ Heating pad
  - ❖ Sunshine
  - ❖ *Not recommended:* microwave, water baths

CHILD AND FAMILY ASSESSMENT

- Child's developmental level and ability to interact ➥*Rationale:* These factors influence preparation and interaction.
- Family's desire to be present during the procedure ➥*Rationale:* Family members may provide support and comfort measures to the child but should have the choice not to remain with the child. Also, knowledge of presence of family allows planning in terms of provision of protective equipment.
- Known allergies ➥*Rationale:* Decreases the possibility of allergic reaction.[1]
- Baseline vital signs, respiratory status, abdominal assessment, and pertinent laboratory results (blood glucose

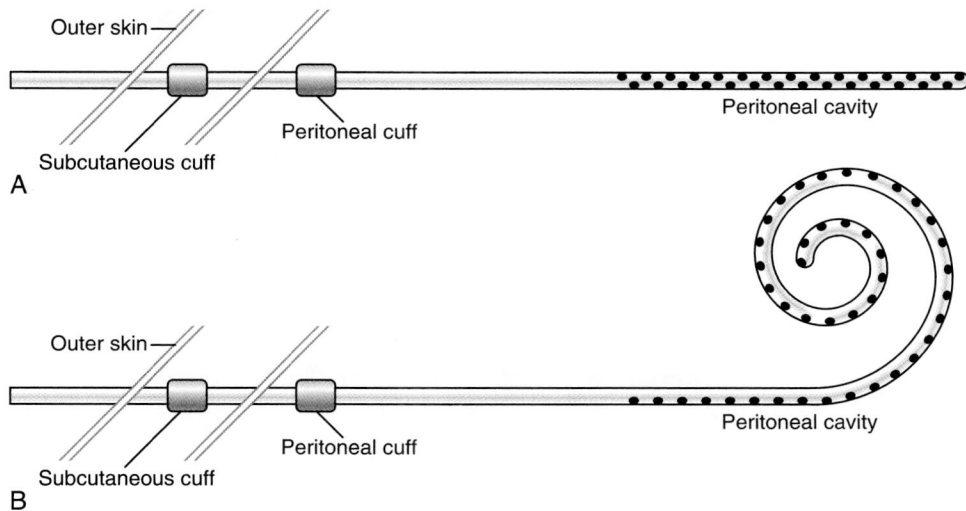

FIGURE 106-2 Types of PD Catheters. Standard catheter for PD is made of soft tubing for comfort and has Dacron cuffs that merge with patient's scar tissue to keep it in place. End of tubing that is inside abdomen has many holes to allow for free flow of dialysis solution in and out. Diagram shows two double-cuff Tenckhoff peritoneal catheters: standard (**A**) and curled (**B**). *Used with permission from National Institute of Health/National Institute of Diabetes and Digestive and Kidney Diseases (NIDDK).*

TABLE 106-1	Types of Peritoneal Dialysis
Continuous Ambulatory PD (CAPD)	Dialysis solution is constantly present in abdomen. Solution is typically changed three to five times daily. Exchanges are performed manually.
Nocturnal (or Nightly) Intermittent PD (NIPD)	At bedtime, patient hooks up to automated cycler that performs multiple exchanges through night.
Continuous Cycling PD (CCPD)	Patient carries PD solution in abdominal cavity throughout day but performs no exchanges.
Automated PD (APD)	Combines CCPD, sometimes referred to as "day dwell" or "last fill," with NIPD during sleep. In some programs, most patients with PD are treated with this method.[20]
Automated PD (APD) with daytime exchanges	For some children with CCPD, single daytime dwell does not provide adequate clearance once residual function is lost. These children need NIPD and multiple daytime exchanges. Daytime exchanges can be performed manually or by returning to cycler machine (sometimes called "PD Plus").[20]
Tidal PD (TPD)	Volume of PD solution remains in peritoneum throughout dialysis session, with only partial drain after each fill. This can be useful to deal with common APD complication of pain at end of each drain cycle. Cyclers can be programmed to tidal with each exchange or to completely drain every few cycles.[20]
Rapid Flush PD	Sometimes used to wash peritoneum when peritonitis is suspected. Multiple manual fills, each followed by immediate drains (no dwell phase).

Some information adapted from Daugirdas JT, et al, editors: *Handbook of dialysis,* ed 3, Philadelphia, 2001, Lippincott, Williams & Wilkins.

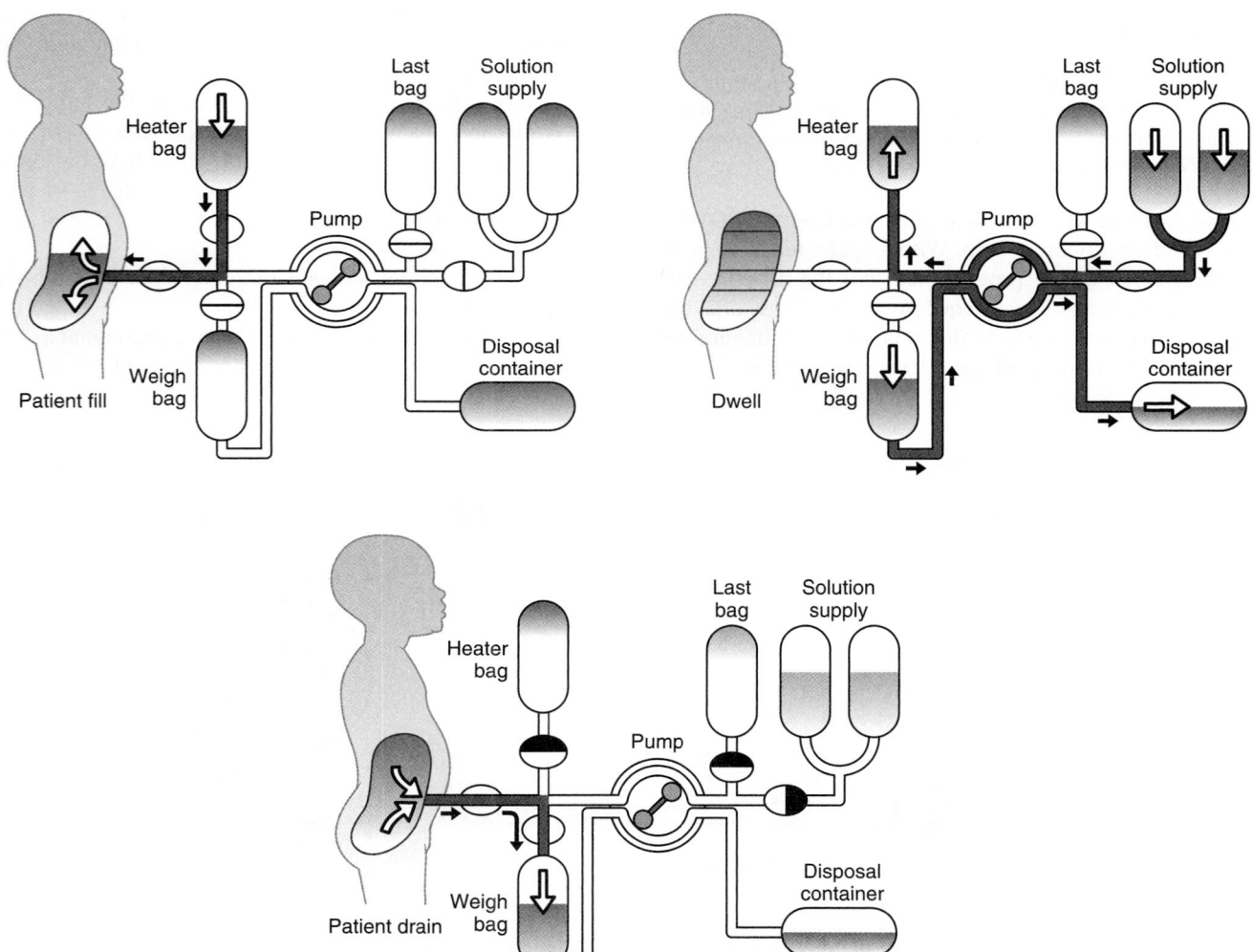

FIGURE 106-3   Peritoneal Dialysis via Cycler. Example of system used for cycler-assisted peritoneal dialysis. Solution is heated, instilled into abdomen where it dwells for prescribed length of time, and then drained. This drainage is called effluent. Cycler either works by gravity with scales to determine amount of fill and drain or by pumps that measure amount of fill and drain. Last bag of solution may have different concentration to last throughout day.

level, potassium, sodium, calcium, phosphorus, magnesium, and renal function tests) ➤➤*Rationale:* Children with renal failure often have altered baseline results, in both physical and laboratory values. Having this information before treatments are started is helpful so that interventions, including the type and amount of dialysate fluid, can be individualized.

- Volume status, as indicted by: weight, skin turgor, edema, breath sounds, intake, and output. Abdominal girth measurements may also be used to determine whether child is retaining dialysate. ➤➤*Rationale:* PD is often initiated for the control of hypervolemia. Knowledge of the child's pretreatment volume status is essential to allow for ongoing assessment and the individualization of treatment goals and interventions.

- Examination of PD catheter and abdominal exit site for signs and symptoms of infection, leakage, or drainage. Signs and symptoms of peritonitis include: cloudy effluent, abdominal pain, fever, chills, and rebound tenderness. ➤➤*Rationale:* The catheter insertion site provides a portal of entry for infection that may result in septicemia or peritonitis. If the insertion site or effluent appears to be infected, further interventions (e.g., site change, culture, antibiotics) may be necessary.

- Examination of the peritoneal catheter and tubing for kinking, puncture sites, and loose connections ➤➤*Rationale:* Adequate flow is essential for optimal treatment success. A dysfunctional catheter can alter outcomes.

- Child's and family's understanding of the reasons for and risks and benefits of the procedure ➤➤*Rationale:* Evaluates child's and family's understanding of the procedure and provides a gauge for ongoing education.

CHILD AND FAMILY EDUCATION

Individualized, developmentally appropriate education is provided to the family and to the child based on the desire for knowledge, readiness to learn, and overall neurologic and psychosocial state.

- Explain the procedure and reason for PD to family and child. If appropriate, show the procedure to be performed on a doll. Toddlers may need parents to help alleviate anxiety. Preschoolers need simple concise explanations. School-aged children need thorough preparation for all procedures, including all the steps involved. Adolescents also need preparation and information and have a high need for privacy. Use the resources of a Child Life Specialist if available. Encourage and answer questions as they arise and reinforce information as needed. ➤➤*Rationale:* Providing information decreases child's and family's anxiety and discomfort and promotes cooperation with the procedure.

- Discuss the child's and family's role in PD ➤➤*Rationale:* Child's cooperation is elicited, and child and family are prepared for PD management on discharge.

- Explain the need for strict aseptic technique during abdominal catheter access to decrease the chance of peritoneal infection ➤➤*Rationale:* Promotes child's and family's cooperation.

- Explain the three phases of PD (fill, dwell, and drain) and possible interventions associated with each phase ➤➤*Rationale:* Providing an explanation decreases the child's and family's anxiety and discomfort and promotes cooperation with the procedure.

- Explain the potential for feelings of fullness and possible shortness of breath during the dwell phase from pressure of the dialysate fluid on the diaphragm and that this may be normal for the dwell phase ➤➤*Rationale:* Providing an explanation decreases the child's and family's anxiety and fear and promotes cooperation with the procedure.

EQUIPMENT

To initiate PD:

- Masks
- Goggles
- Sterile gloves
- Sterile 4×4 gauze
- Sterile waterproof barrier
- 2% Chlorhexidine gluconate (if child is 2 months or older) or appropriate skin antiseptic
- Povidone-iodine solution, if caps not impregnated with povidone-iodine
- Tape
- Equipment for collection of cell count or culture specimens (if ordered):
  - ❖ Sterile collection container
  - ❖ Tube for cell count
  - ❖ Labels with two patient identifiers
- Method for heating dialysate
- Additional equipment for initiation of PD includes the following:
  - ❖ Manual PD:
    - ○ Sterile field
    - ○ Peritoneal dialysis tubing with drainage bag (Y-set) and dialysate solution supplied by pharmacy or multiple-spiked manifold with dialysate bags attached
  - ❖ Cycler PD:
    - ○ Cycler machine
    - ○ Appropriately sized cycler tubing or set
    - ○ Drainage bags or connection to drain directly to toilet
    - ○ Dialysate solution dispensed by pharmacy

To discontinue PD:

- Masks
- Goggles
- Sterile gloves
- Sterile 4×4 gauze pads
- Tape
- Catheter caps impregnated with povidone-iodine, or if unavailable, povidone-iodine solution, sterile container to soak cap, and sterile field

Procedure | for Peritoneal Dialysis

Steps	Rationale	Considerations
Initiation of PD		
1. Ensure child and family understand procedure and questions are answered.	Evaluates and reinforces understanding of previously taught information.	Developmental level, cognitive ability, and anxiety level will determine approach to and effectiveness of teaching.
2. Verify PD orders and patient identification using two patient identifiers.	Reduces the possibility of error.[1]	An even smaller margin of error exists in caring for infants and children.
3. Check dialysate bags for correctness of prescribed solution and additives, expiration date, clarity, and leaks.	Assesses for expiration or contamination of dialysate.	
4. Warm dialysate fluid to 37° C (98.6° F). *(Level II*)*	Fluid that is cooler than normal body temperature can cause cramping and discomfort. Fluid that is too warm can cause tissue damage.[2,3]	
5. Close door and turn off any portable fans. Put on surgical mask and mask child and anyone in the room during access of PD catheter.	Reduces transmission of microorganisms; reduces contamination from airborne pathogens.[4-8]	
6. Position child in a comfortable position, ensuring access to PD catheter.	Proper positioning ensures child's comfort, optimizes respiratory function, and facilitates optimal flow through PD catheter.	
7. Wash hands for 3 minutes with antimicrobial soap. *(Level VI*)*	Reduces transmission of microorganisms.	
8. If PD is to be performed via cycler, program machine according to prescribing practitioner's orders, following manufacturer's instructions. *(Level I*)*	Procedure for set-up varies between different manufacturers' cyclers.	Special training is needed to deliver PD via cycler. Only nurses who have completed a competency-based training program to the particular cycler to be used are qualified to do so.
9. Connect and prime tubing with dialysate, with removal of all air. Clamp tubing.	Fills tubing with dialysate. Decreases chance of introduction of air into the abdominal cavity.	Use hands-free spiking device if available. Air in the peritoneum can be painful to the child and interfere with filling.
10. If povidone-iodine impregnated cap is present, put on sterile gloves and proceed to step 17.	If impregnated caps are used, further disinfection is not required.	
11. If cap is *not* impregnated with povidone-iodine, prepare sterile field.	If caps are not povidone-iodine impregnated, further disinfection is required.	
12. Pour povidone-iodine onto sterile 4×4 gauze pads.	Povidone-iodine serves as a bacteriocidal agent.[9-13]	
13. Put on sterile gloves.	Reduces transmission of microorganisms.	
14. Saturate four 4×4 gauze pads in povidone-iodine solution and perform a 1-minute scrub of catheter-cap connection.	Reduces transmission of microorganisms.[4]	Remove any crust or drainage from around catheter-cap connection.

* Level I: Manufacturer's recommendations only
 Level II: Theory-based; no research data to support recommendations; recommendations from expert consensus group may exist
 Level VI: Clinical studies in a variety of patient populations and situations to support recommendations

Procedure for Peritoneal Dialysis—*Continued*

Steps	Rationale	Considerations
15. Wrap second povidone-iodine soaked 4×4 gauze pad around catheter-cap connection; leave in place for 3 to 5 minutes.	Provides disinfection.	
16. After 3 to 5 minutes, remove povi-done-iodine soaked 4×4 gauze pad and discard in appropriate receptacle.	Provides access to catheter-cap connection.	
17. With nondominant hand, pick up the PD catheter with a sterile 4×4 gauze pad; remove cap.	Prevents contamination.	
18. Connect catheter to dialysate tubing.	Ensures a tight connection.	
19. If cell count and culture are requested, obtain with initial drain, before first fill; or if peritoneal cavity is dry, after first fill is complete with next drain, per prescribing practitioner's orders. Collect specimen using sterile technique, with gravity drainage to a sterile collection container after wasting the first 2 to 3 mL of fluid within the catheter lumen. Label specimens at bedside.	Direct aspiration to a syringe, if the peritoneum is dry or near empty, can cause discomfort and contribute to fibrin sheath and occlusion of catheter, especially in small children with small lumen catheters.[5,14] Labeling specimens at the bedside promotes patient safety.	Capture of the first cloudy drainage for culture is important.[15] Most laboratories require 5 mL or greater for culture and an additional 5 to 7 mL for cell count; follow institution-specific laboratory guidelines.
Instillation (fill cycle): 20. With use of a cycler, unclamp catheter and tubing. Begin PD therapy per manufacturer's instructions. Continue until therapy complete, and then proceed to step 34. With performance of manual PD, use a prepared multispiked manifold from pharmacy or a Y-set with a "flush before fill" technique (Figure 106-4). Flush the Y-set with approximately 100 mL to the drainage bag, with the child's catheter closed; then open the catheter and set flow rate as prescribed. *(Level VI*)*	Spiking of dialysis bags is a high-risk procedure for contamination of the system. A multiple-bag manifold prepared by pharmacy under the hood or a "flush before fill" technique reduces the risk of contamination.[5,15-19]	Time for fill depends on the height of the dialysate bag, position of child, and patency of the catheter. Lower rates of peritonitis with this method are attributed to the initial flush clearing of any bacteria that may have been introduced during the connection procedure. Also, because the tubing and bag are disconnected between exchanges, less mechanical stress may result in fewer episodes of minor trauma and therefore fewer exit site and tunnel infections. This reduction, in turn, may reduce the peritonitis rate.[20]
21. With use of a Y-set, when inflow is complete, clamp the dialysate tubing and follow subsequent disconnect procedure (see Discontinuation of PD) after each fill. Repeat steps for the necessary number of exchanges.	The Y-set was developed to free children from remaining attached to the transfer set and empty bag between exchanges. Studies have revealed an important added benefit: significantly lower rate of peritonitis with the Y-set with a "flush before fill" technique than with a straight set (a single bag that is used to fill, then is rolled up under child's clothes, and later rolled out to drain after the desired dwell time).[18,20]	

Procedure continues on following page

* Level VI: Clinical studies in a variety of patient populations and situations to support recommendations

Procedure for Peritoneal Dialysis—*Continued*

Steps	Rationale	Considerations

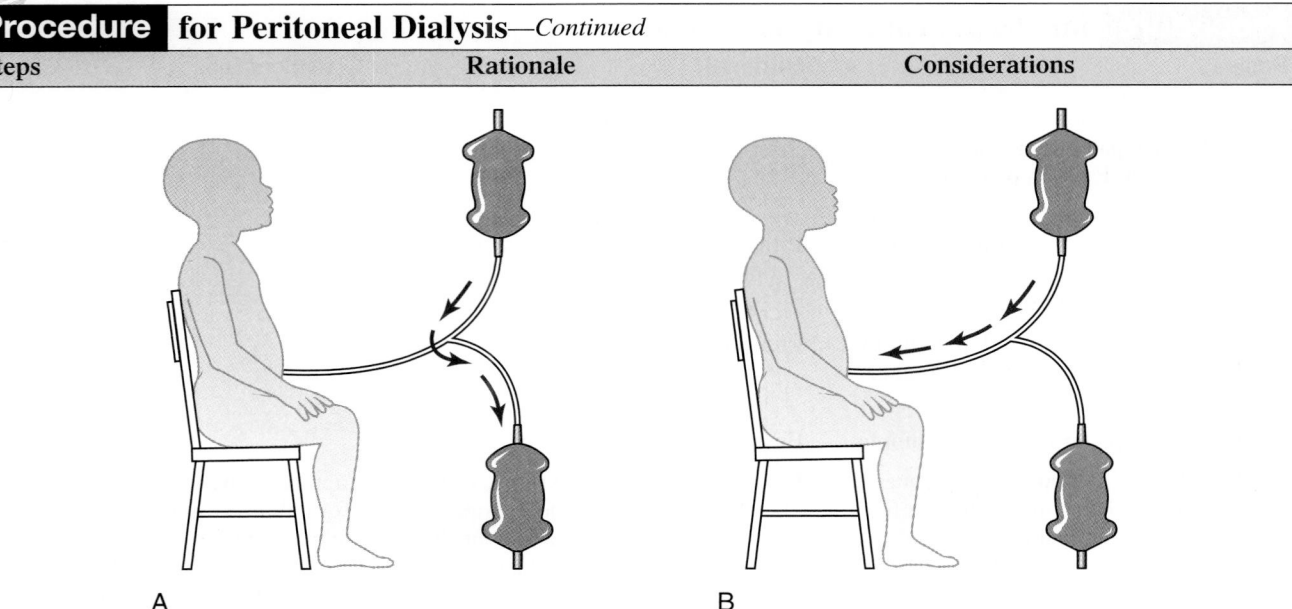

A   B

FIGURE 106-4   Manual Peritoneal Dialysis "Flush-before-fill" Strategy Used with Y Transfer Sets. **A,** Small volume of fresh dialysis solution is drained directly into drainage container (either before or just after drainage of abdomen). This acts to wash away any bacteria that may have been introduced in limb of Y leading to new bag at time of connection. **B,** Fresh solution is introduced through rinsed connector.

Dwell Cycle

Steps	Rationale	Considerations
1. Begin dwell cycle.	Exchange of substances occurs during dwell cycle.	Dwell time is determined by the number of cycles needed or prescribed in a 24-hour period. With use of a cycler, the cycles are preprogrammed. Drainage of effluent on a cycler can be to drainage bags or can be routed directly into a toilet or appropriate container.

Outflow (Drain) Cycle

Steps	Rationale	Considerations
1. With use of a manifold set-up, after the necessary dwell time, the first fill bag is reversed (placed lower than the midabdominal area of the child) and becomes the first drainage bag. The same "flush before fill" technique mentioned previously should be followed before each instillation, but the child remains connected to the manifold throughout the treatment until the necessary number of exchanges are completed. This is generally an inpatient manual PD method.	Drainage removes fluid that carries wastes removed during the dwell cycle. Use of a manifold decreases the number of times system is opened, decreasing the risk of infection.	Allow 15 to 20 minutes for outflow (drain) or as prescribed by the prescribing practitioner; record amount of effluent. With use of a cycler, the next fill occurs automatically after the drain is complete. Effluent is measured by the cycler and recorded.
2. With use of the Y-set, the same connection procedure used previously is followed: Put on surgical mask and mask child and anyone in the room during access of PD catheter. Wash hands for 3 minutes with antimicrobial soap. (*Level VI**)	Reduces transmission of microorganisms.	

* Level VI: Clinical studies in a variety of patient populations and situations to support recommendations

Procedure for Peritoneal Dialysis—*Continued*

Steps	Rationale	Considerations
3. Connect Y-set and prime tubing with dialysate, removing all air. Clamp tubing.	Prepares set for outflow cycle; if tubing is not primed dialysis will not drain out.	
4. With the nondominant hand, pick up the PD catheter with a sterile 4×4 gauze pad; remove cap.	Prevents contamination.	
5. Connect to the Y-set.	Required for fluid removal.	
6. Place drainage bag below midabdominal area.	Enhances gravity outflow.	
7. Unclamp to permit drainage from peritoneal cavity.	Opens pathway for outflow of fluid.	
8. Observe appearance of effluent.	An empiric diagnosis of peritonitis should be made if the peritoneal fluid is cloudy, the effluent white blood cell count (WBC) is greater than 100/mm^3, and at least 50% of the WBCs are polymorphonuclear leukocytes.[19,21]	Effluent may be bloody or pink tinged after catheter insertion but should become clear and colorless to light yellow after the first few exchanges and should remain odorless. Effluent may be slightly frothy because of protein content.
9. Clamp or close catheter and clamp tubing when effluent is completely drained.	Decreases leakage and contamination.	
10. Refill abdomen after use of the "flush before fill" technique again.	Begins next cycle.	
11. Repeat steps for ordered number of exchanges.	Repeated exchanges are required with PD in order to remove waste products.	

Discontinuation of PD

Steps	Rationale	Considerations
1. If child's abdomen is to be left empty, observe outflow of last PD cycle, then clamp both the catheter and the PD tubing when effluent is completely drained.	Turning child from side to side ensures the abdomen is empty of dialysate.	
2. If child's abdomen is to be left with a last fill (day dwell), instill as ordered; then clamp both the catheter and the PD tubing.	Ensures fluid will remain in abdomen.	
3. Put on surgical mask and mask child and anyone in room during de-access of PD catheter. Wash hands with antimicrobial soap.	Reduces transmission of microorganisms; reduces contamination from airborne pathogens.[22-25]	
4. With use of a povidone-iodine impregnated cap, put on sterile gloves and proceed to step 9.	If cap is impregnated, no further disinfection is required.	
5. If a povidone-iodine impregnated cap is not used, prepare sterile field.	If cap is not impregnated, further disinfection is required.	
6. Pour povidone-iodine into a sterile container containing a sterile catheter cap.	Acts as a bactericidal agent for cap.	
7. Put on sterile gloves.	Reduces risk of transmission of microorganisms.	

Procedure continues on following page

Procedure for Peritoneal Dialysis—*Continued*

Steps	Rationale	Considerations
8. Remove catheter cap from package and place on sterile field.	Reduces transmission of microorganisms.	
9. With sterile 4×4 gauze pads, disconnect the catheter from the PD tubing.	PD cycles have been completed for the day; tubing is no longer needed.	
10. Carefully connect catheter cap to catheter.	Ensures a tight connection.	
11. Securely tape catheter to abdomen. The PD catheter is covered by the dressing, but the extension set must remain on top of the dressing for access to PD. Both the catheter and the extension set are immobilized with tape or other cath-secure device.	Avoids trauma to exit site or dislodgement of catheter. Excessive movement interferes with epithelialization and healing of the exit site.[26-31]	
12. Exit site care may or may not be done at this time. If indicated, see Procedure 105.	Exit site care is performed with each dressing change and is done no more than once a week for the first 2 weeks after catheter placement, then once every 1 to 2 days, usually after showers.	If child is too young to shower, care is done with daily sponge baths; tub baths are contraindicated for the duration of PD.
13. Discard soiled materials in an appropriate receptacle.	Standard precautions; reduces transmission of microorganisms.	
14. Measure effluent.	Effluent volume indicates additional fluid removed or fluid remaining in peritoneal cavity.	Not indicated if last fill is to remain in abdomen.
15. Remove gloves and wash hands.	Standard precautions; reduces transmission of microorganisms.	
16. Calculate fluid balance.	Assesses progress of therapy.	Note that all dialysis solutions contain an overfill. For example, 2-L bag may actually contain 2050 or 2080 mL.

Expected Outcomes

- Therapeutic goals of PD are achieved

- Catheter and access site are maintained without complication

- Peritoneal dialysis access site functions properly; instillation and drainage of dialysate occurs without problems
- Respiratory status is adequate throughout treatment
- Child has acceptable level of comfort
- Child and family receive appropriate education and support

Unexpected Outcomes

- Electrolyte abnormalities remain
- Excess fluid is not removed
- Drainage or leakage from the exit site
- Introduction of pathogens into the PD catheter
- Signs and symptoms of peritonitis or bowel perforation
- Signs and symptoms of infection at the exit site
- Dislodgement of the PD catheter
- Disconnection of the extension set or tubing
- Poor dialysate flow during instillation or drainage

- Respiratory complications during procedure
- Unmanaged pain
- Inadequate preparation and support

Monitoring and Care of the Child

Activities and Interventions	Rationale	Reportable Conditions
1. Perform and record predialysis and postdialysis daily weights. *(Level VI*)*	A baseline predialysis weight is important in deciding how much fluid is to be removed and in guiding ongoing treatment.[10, 18, 20]	• Abnormal increase or decrease in weight
2. Perform baseline and ongoing assessments, including the following: vital signs, presence of edema, intake and output, and abdominal assessment. *(Level VI*)*	Establishing a baseline before therapy and monitoring throughout PD therapy for any complications are important.[10,18,20]	• Hypotension • Hypertension • Fever • Hypothermia • Crackles • Edema • Abdominal distention or tenderness • Respiratory distress
3. Monitor electrolyte levels during treatment at a frequency determined by institution-specific protocol or prescribing practitioner's orders.	Fluids and electrolytes shift during PD.[3,20]	• Abnormal laboratory values
4. Administer medications to correct ongoing metabolic abnormalities as ordered. *(Level VI*)*	The goal for the care of children with ESRD is normal growth and development.[12,32] Common medications administered to children with renal failure include: Vitamin D and calcium carbonate to prevent or treat bone disease. Erythropoietin and iron to treat anemia. Stool softeners because constipation can impair drainage of PD fluid. Phosphate binders to treat hyperphosphatemia.	• Failure to thrive • Inadequate dietary intake • Lethargy • Difficulty with medication administration
5. Monitor blood glucose at the beginning of the treatment and as indicated, or according to institution-specific protocol.	The glucose in the dialysate solution predisposes children to hyperglycemia, especially diabetics.[3,7,18,26,28,33]	• Hyperglycemia • Hypoglycemia
6. Monitor the integrity of the PD set-up. *(Level V*)*	Disconnection in the set-up provides a portal of entry for pathogens, which can lead to peritonitis.[3,15,28,33,34]	• Cloudy dialysate • Fever • Tachycardia • Purulent drainage • Pain or tenderness
7. Monitor for any difficulty filling or draining. *(Level VI*)*	Children may need repositioning, especially during sleep, to facilitate flow through the PD catheter. Catheters may become kinked or occluded. Fibrin clots can obstruct drainage; heparin may be added to the dialysate fluid to prevent or treat this. If clotting is suspected, urokinase may be used to clear the catheter.	• Inability to fill or drain • Volume of dialysate remaining in the abdomen
8. Ensure proper functioning of cycler, if cycler is used.	The nurse who performs PD must be competent to program and troubleshoot the cycler. If the equipment malfunctions, or if the child needs resuscitation, the nurse needs to know how to immediately drain the child's abdomen.	• Any problems with cycler function

* Level V: Clinical studies in more than one or two patient populations and situations to support recommendations
  Level VI: Clinical studies in a variety of patient populations and situations to support recommendations

---

Documentation

- Child and family education
- Weight before and after treatment
- Date and time of treatment initiation
- Length and parameters of treatment
- Condition of abdominal catheter and exit site at time of treatment
- Date and time of dressing application
- Amount and appearance of effluent
- Exit site care
- Child's tolerance of procedure
- Unexpected outcomes and related treatment
- Vital signs throughout the procedure
- Nursing interventions
- Intake and output
- Laboratory assessment data
- PD fluid used

References

1. Strippoli GFM, et al: Catheter-related interventions to prevent peritonitis in peritoneal dialysis: a systematic review of randomized, controlled trials, *J Am Soc Nephrol* 15(10):2735-2746, 2004.
2. Hayes DD: Performing peritoneal dialysis: clinical do's and don't's, *Nursing 2003* 33(3):17-18, 2003.
3. Lancaster LE, editor: *American Nephrology Nurses Association core curriculum for nephrology nursing,* Pitman, NJ, 2001, American Nephrology Nurses Association, Jannetti Publications.
4. Amato D, et al: Staphylococcal peritonitis in continuous ambulatory peritoneal dialysis: colonization with identical strains at exit site, nose, and hands, *Am J Kidney Dis* 37(1):43-48, 2001.
5. Ash SR: Peritoneal access devices and placement techniques. In Nissenson AR, Fine RN, editors: *Dialysis therapy,* ed 3, Philadelphia, 2002, Hanley & Belfus.
6. Bernardini J, et al: Randomized double blinded trial of antibiotic exit site cream for the prevention of exit site infection in peritoneal dialysis patients, *J Am Soc Nephrol* 16:539-545, 2005.
7. Centers for Disease Control and Prevention: *Guideline for the prevention of surgical wound infections,* Rockville, MD, 1999, US Department of Health and Human Services.
8. Clark JJ: Wound repair and factors influencing healing, *Crit Care Nurs Q* 25(1):1-12, 2002.
9. Briggs J, editor: Clinical effectiveness of different approaches to peritoneal dialysis catheter exit-site care, *Best Practice: Evidence Based Practice Information for Health Care Professionals* (8)1:1-6, 2004.
10. Hess CT, Kirsner RS: Orchestrating wound healing: assessing and preparing the wound, *Adv Skin Wound Care* 16(5):246-257, 2003.
11. Maloney J, Fisher B: Skin integrity. In Moloney-Harmon PA, Czerwinski SJ, editors: *Review of pediatric critical care,* Philadelphia, 1997, Saunders.
12. Nelson DB, Dilloway MA: Principles, products and practical aspects of wound care, *Crit Care Nurs Q* 25(1):33-54, 2002.
13. Twardowski ZJ, Nichols K: Peritoneal dialysis access and exit site care. In Gokal R, Khanna R, Krediet R, et al, editors: *Textbook of peritoneal dialysis,* ed 2, Boston, 2000, Kluwer Academic Publishers.
14. Diaz-Buxo JA: Management of peritoneal catheter malfunction, *Peritoneal Dialysis Int* 18(3):256-259, 1998.
15. Warady BF, et al: ISPD guidelines/recommendations: consensus guidelines for the treatment of peritonitis in pediatric patients receiving peritoneal dialysis, *Peritoneal Dialysis Int* 20:(6):610-624, 2000.
16. Johnson RJ, Feehally J, editors: *Comprehensive clinical nephrology,* ed 2, St Louis, 2003, Mosby.
17. Li PK, et al: Comparison of clinical outcome and ease of handling in two double-bag systems in continuous ambulatory peritoneal dialysis: a prospective, randomized, controlled, multicenter study, *Am J Kidney Dis* 40(2):373-380, 2002.
18. Prowant BF: Peritoneal dialysis. In Lancaster LE, editor: *Core curriculum for nephrology nurses,* ed 4, Pitman, NJ, 2001, American Nephrology Nurses Association, Jannetti Publications.
19. Tacconelli E, et al: Mupirocin prophylaxis to prevent Staphylococcus aureus infection in patients undergoing dialysis: a meta-analysis, *Infect Dis Clin North Am* 37(12):1629-1638, 2003.
20. Daugirdas JT, et al, editors: *Handbook of dialysis,* ed 3, Philadelphia, 2001, Lippincott, Williams & Wilkins.
21. Zabat E: When your patient needs peritoneal dialysis, *Nursing 2003* 33(8):52-54, 2003.
22. Howard R: The appropriate use of topical antimicrobials and antiseptics in children: neonatal skin care, *Pediatr Ann* 30(4):219-224, 2001.
23. Lobbedez T, et al: Routine use of mupirocin at the peritoneal catheter exit site and mupirocin resistance: still low after 7 years, *Nephrology Dialysis Transplant J* 19:3140-3143, 2004.
24. Taquino LT: Promoting wound healing in the neonatal setting: process versus protocol, *J Perinatal Neonatal Nurs* 14(1):104-118, 2003.
25. Neu AM. Infant and neonatal peritoneal dialysis. In: Nissenson AR, Fine R, eds. *Dialysis therapy,* ed 3, Philadelphia, 2002, Hanley & Belfus.
26. Brandt ML, Brewer ED: Peritoneal catheter placement in children. In Nissenson AR, Fine RN, editors: *Dialysis therapy,* ed 3, Philadelphia, 2002, Hanley & Belfus.
27. Branom RN: Is this wound infected? *Crit Care Nurs Q* 25(1):55-62, 2002.

28. Burrows-Hudson S, Prowant BF, editors: *Nephrology nursing standards of practice and guidelines for care*, Pitman, NJ, 2005, American Nephrology Nurses Association, Jannetti Publications.

29. Flanigan M, Gokal R: Peritoneal catheters and exit-site practices toward optimum peritoneal access: a review of current developments, *Peritoneal Dialysis Int* 25(2): 132-139, 2005.

30. Twardowski ZJ: Peritoneal catheter exit-site and tunnel infections. In Nissenson AR, Fine RN, editors: *Dialysis therapy*, ed 3, Philadelphia, 2002, Hanley & Belfus.

31. Vas SI: Peritonitis in peritoneal dialysis patients. In Nissenson AR, Fine RN, editors: *Dialysis therapy*, ed 3, Philadelphia, 2002, Hanley & Belfus.

32. Holloway M: Peritoneal dialysis orders in children. In Nissenson AR, Fine RN, editors: *Dialysis therapy*, ed 3, Philadelphia, 2002, Hanley & Belfus.

33. Shonjania K, et al: *Making health care safer: a critical analysis of patient safety practices*, Rockville, MD, 2001, Agency for Healthcare Research and Quality.

34. Watson AR, Gartland C: *Guidelines by an Ad Hoc European Committee for elective chronic peritoneal dialysis in pediatric patients*, 2001, on behalf of Paediatric Peritoneal dialysis Working Group. Watson AR. Gartland C. European Paediatric Peritoneal Dialysis Working Group. Guidelines by an Ad Hoc European Committee for Elective Chronic Peritoneal Dialysis in Pediatric Patients. Peritoneal Dialysis International. 21(3):240-4, 2001 May-Jun.

Additional Readings

Chadha V, et al: Adequacy of peritoneal dialysis in pediatric patients. In Nissenson AR, Fine RN, editors: *Dialysis therapy*, ed 3, Philadelphia, 2002, Hanley & Belfus.

Curley MAQ, Moloney-Harmon PA, editors: *Critical care nursing of infants and children*, Philadelphia, 2001, Saunders.

Health Care Financing Administration: *End stage renal disease clinical performance measures project*, Baltimore, 1999, Department of Health and Human Services, Health Care Financing Administration, Office of Clinical Standards and Quality.

Jabs K, Warady BA: The impact of the dialysis outcomes quality initiative guidelines on the care of the pediatric end-stage renal disease patient, *Adv Renal Replacement Ther* 6(1):97-106, 1999.

Ledermann SE, et al: Long-term outcome of peritoneal dialysis in infants, *J Pediatr* 136(1):24-29, 2000.

Munford PR: Psychosocial adjustment and treatment of children and adolescents with ESRD. In Nissenson AR, Fine RN, editors: *Dialysis therapy*, ed 3, Philadelphia, 2002, Hanley & Belfus.

National Kidney Foundation-DOQI: Clinical practice guidelines for peritoneal dialysis adequacy, *Am J Kidney Dis* 30(Suppl 3):S94-99, 1997. Anonymous. II. NKF-K/DOQI Clinical Practice Guidelines for Peritoneal Dialysis Adequacy: update 2000. *Am J Kidney Dis* 37(1 Suppl 1):S65-S136, 2001 Jan.

Nelson P, Salusky IB: Nutritional management of children on peritoneal dialysis. In Nissenson AR, Fine RN, editors: *Dialysis therapy*, ed 3, Philadelphia, 2002, Hanley & Belfus.

Piraino B: Peritoneal dialysis catheter replacement: save the patient and not the catheter, *Semin Dialysis* 1(16):72-75, 2003.

Schaefer F: Dialysis in inborn errors of metabolism. In Nissenson AR, Fine RN, editors: *Dialysis therapy*, ed 3, Philadelphia, 2002, Hanley & Belfus.

Twardowski ZJ: Tidal peritoneal dialysis. In Nissenson AR, Fine RN, editors: *Dialysis therapy*, ed 3, Philadelphia, 2002, Hanley & Belfus.

Wassner SJ: Growth in children with ESRD. In Nissenson AR, Fine RN, editors: *Dialysis therapy*, ed 3, Philadelphia, 2002, Hanley & Belfus.

Zappacosta AR: Growth in children with ESRD. In Nissenson AR, Fine RN, editors: *Dialysis therapy*, ed 3, Philadelphia, 2002, Hanley & Belfus.

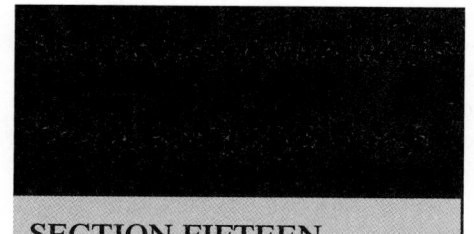

Special Renal Procedures

PROCEDURE **107**

Continuous Bladder Irrigation

P U R P O S E : Continuous bladder irrigation may be performed to prevent clots from obstructing the urinary tract in children with hemorrhagic cystitis or may be used to administer medications in conditions such as infection

Charlene Leonard and Ruth M. Lebet

PREREQUISITE KNOWLEDGE

- Anatomy and physiology of the urinary tract
- Principles of aseptic technique
- An absolute contraindication for insertion of a urinary catheter is suspected urethral tear
- Complications related to indwelling catheters, including: bladder spasms, trauma, urethral tear or perforation, catheter encrustation, urethral strictures, catheter knotting, and urinary tract infection[1-3]
- Indwelling urinary catheter insertion procedure (see Procedure 108)

CHILD AND FAMILY ASSESSMENT

- History of urogenital malformations, surgeries, or injuries, such as history of hypospadias repair **➤➤Rationale:** These conditions may complicate passage of catheter.
- Family's and child's concerns about the procedure, including culturally related concerns **➤➤Rationale:** Parents from some cultures may fear that catheterization of the female results in loss of virginity.[4]
- Level of consciousness or developmental delay **➤➤Rationale:** These conditions may hinder the ability of the child to participate in or understand the procedure. Urinary catheterization is particularly threatening to preschool and school-aged children.
- Previous catheterizations experienced by the child **➤➤Rationale:** A negative experience with catheterization

in the past may increase the child's anxiety and decrease the child's ability to cooperate during the procedure.[5,6]
- Child's and family's understanding of the reasons for and risks and benefits of the procedure **➤➤Rationale:** Evaluates child's and family's understanding of the procedure and provides a gauge for ongoing education.
- Family's desire to be present during the procedure **➤➤Rationale:** Family may provide support and comfort measures to the child but should have the choice not to remain with the child. The older school-aged child or adolescent may prefer that the family not be present.
- History of allergy to povidone-iodine; allergy to lidocaine if topical anesthetic is to be used **➤➤Rationale:** Procedure may need to be modified based on allergies to these substances.
- Appropriate size of urinary catheter for the particular child (see Procedure 108, Table 108-1) **➤➤Rationale:** The smallest three-way indwelling urinary catheter is 14F. This procedure is not recommended in children for whom this size catheter is too large.

CHILD AND FAMILY EDUCATION

Individualized, developmentally appropriate education is provided to the family and to the child based on desire for knowledge, readiness to learn, and overall neurologic and psychosocial state.

- Provide information about the indwelling catheter, including the reason for catheter insertion and continuous irrigation and an explanation of steps involved in catheter insertion ➥*Rationale:* Information allows for informed consent to the procedure.

- If developmentally appropriate, explain how the child can assist with the procedure (i.e., blowing, breathing, or other relaxation techniques as the tip of the catheter is passed through the urethral sphincter) ➥*Rationale:* Encouraging participation by the child facilitates the child's feeling of control and promotes more comfortable passage of the catheter.[4-6]
- Explain the need to avoid pulling or placing tension on the catheter once in place ➥*Rationale:* Tube removal with the balloon inflated can cause injury and pain.
- Explain the need for the child and family to notify staff of discomfort after irrigation begins ➥*Rationale:* Distended bladder or pain can indicate serious complications.

EQUIPMENT

- Appropriately sized three-way indwelling latex-free urinary catheter
- Catheter insertion tray with the following supplies (or gather supplies):
  - ❖ Sterile latex free gloves
  - ❖ Povidone-iodine solution and cotton balls or povidone-iodine applicators
  - ❖ Drape
  - ❖ Underpad
  - ❖ Forceps or tweezers
  - ❖ Specimen collection container
- Sterile lubricant, if not included in insertion tray
  - ❖ 2% lidocaine lubricant jelly in specialized applicator may be used per institution-specific protocol
- Syringe for balloon inflation (may be included in catheter insertion tray)
- Device or tape to secure catheter to child
- Hanging spring scale, if available
- Y-type bladder irrigation set; if this type of set is not available, intravenous tubing may be used
- Irrigating fluid (either sterile saline solution or medication solution as prescribed)
- If Y-type bladder irrigation set is not available, sterile urinary drainage bag
- Intravenous (IV) pole or stand

Procedure for Continuous Bladder Irrigation

Steps	Rationale	Considerations
1. Ensure child and family understand procedure and questions are answered.	Evaluates and reinforces understanding of previously taught information.	Level of consciousness and developmental delay may preclude child or family from understanding and assisting with procedure.
2. Collect all necessary supplies and equipment.	Minimizes interruption of procedure to obtain needed supplies; facilitates maintenance of sterile field during procedure.	The smallest three-way indwelling urinary catheter is 14F. Procedure is not possible or recommended in children for whom this catheter is too large.
3. Provide for child's privacy.	Procedure necessitates exposure of genitalia.	School-aged children are generally modest and removal of underwear and exposure of genitalia may cause this age group significant anxiety.[5,6]
4. Position child supine.	Facilitates placement of catheter.	Positioning female child with bent knees and legs spread apart improves visualization of anatomy.
5. Wash hands.	Reduces transmission of microorganisms; standard precautions.	
6. Open packaging, maintaining sterility.	Minimizes risk of infection; prepares equipment for use.	
7. Check irrigating solution against prescribing practitioner's order, taking allergies into consideration if the fluid contains medication.	Reduces risk of adverse reaction to irrigation solution.	Use two patient identifiers when checking solution against prescribing practitioner's order.

Procedure for Continuous Bladder Irrigation—*Continued*

Steps	Rationale	Considerations
8. Insert the spike of the tubing into the irrigation fluid and prime the tubing. When priming is complete, clamp the tubing.	Air in the tubing can cause bladder distention and discomfort.[1]	
9. Hang bag and tubing from spring scale on IV pole if spring scale is available. If not available, hang solution on the IV pole.	Spring scale allows more precise measurement of fluid instilled.	
10. Put on sterile gloves.	Aseptic technique; decreases risk of infection.	
11. Insert and secure three-way indwelling urinary catheter with sterile technique per institution-specific protocol (see Procedure 108).	Three-way catheter allows fluid to be continuously instilled into and drained from the bladder, keeping the bladder free from clots and debris.	
12. Send any specimens that have been ordered before initiating continuous bladder irrigations.	Irrigation fluid alters composition of urine.	When sending specimens, use two patient identifiers to be sure the correct specimens are sent for the correct child. Label specimens at the bedside.
13. With use of a Y-type irrigation set and a single-lumen catheter, remove sterile cap from administration set and insert the set into the catheter. With use of IV tubing and a drainage collection bag with a two-lumen catheter, attach drainage bag to one lumen of catheter and IV tubing from irrigation solution to the second lumen of catheter, maintaining sterility.	Y-type irrigation set has two arms (hence, the name "Y"). One arm attaches to the irrigation solution and the other attaches to the drainage collection bag.	
14. Open clamp to irrigation solution. Visualize drip chamber and ensure free flowing solution. Adjust flow rate of the solution to the rate ordered.	Initiates irrigation.	Flow rate is ordered based on the child's size and the goals of therapy.
15. Open clamp on drainage bag and ensure free flowing urine and irrigation solution.	Adequate drainage must be maintained to prevent bladder distention and discomfort.	
16. Instruct child and family, if appropriate, to notify staff of any discomfort.	Encourages child and family to promptly report symptoms; facilitates prompt identification of problems.	If the child has severe abdominal pain, stop the irrigation temporarily and investigate to ensure that the bladder is not distended.
17. Monitor hourly inflow of solution with spring scale if available; if not available, determine hourly inflow with graduated markings of the irrigation solution container. Monitor hourly output with drainage bag. Subtract output from inflow. Record difference as urine output.	Careful intake and output is required to ensure irrigation is occurring as ordered and child has adequate urine output.	The rate of instillation of irrigation solution is ordered by the prescribing practitioner and is dependent on the goals of therapy. An alternative method is to infuse solution with IV pump, recording hourly intake from data on pump.
18. Discard used supplies in the appropriate trash receptacle. Remove gloves and wash hands.	Standard precautions.	

Expected Outcomes

- Indwelling urinary catheter placed in child's bladder
- Irrigation solution instills freely

- Urine and irrigation solution drain freely

- Child is free from infection

Unexpected Outcomes

- Tip of catheter is placed in the urethra
- Obstruction of outflow leads to bladder distention and perforation
- Irrigation solution is absorbed systemically
- Catheter becomes obstructed; irrigation solution and urine are retained
- Secondary infection develops

Monitoring and Care of the Child

Activities and Interventions	Rationale	Reportable Conditions
1. Monitor hourly intake and output.	Discrepancy in intake and output may reflect catheter obstruction, bladder perforation, or systemic absorption of irrigation solution.[7-9]	- Fluid retained in bladder - Distended abdomen or bladder - Abdominal pain
2. Monitor color and consistency of drainage.	Changes in color or appearance may indicate bleeding, infection, or presence of mucous.[7-9]	- Cloudy fluid that was previously clear - Increase in blood or mucous in drainage
3. Monitor child's comfort related to catheter placement.	Increasing irritability may reflect developing complications.	- Removal of catheter by child
4. Assess security of catheter and integrity of surrounding skin and catheter.	An inappropriately sized catheter can lead to skin breakdown, secondary infection, or inappropriate intake and output measurement.[7-9]	- Skin breakdown at catheter site - Leakage of fluid from around the catheter

Documentation

- Child and family education
- Size of catheter placed
- Child's tolerance of procedure
- Irrigation fluid used and rate of irrigation
- Hourly intake and output and character of effluent
- Unexpected outcomes and related treatment

References

1. Bukowski TP, Freedman AL: Catheterization problems of infants, *Contemp Urology* 66-74, 1999.
2. Elizondo AP, et al: Elimination of bleeding associated with urinary catheterization in neonates, *Neonatal Network* 20:25-34, 2001.
3. Smith AB, Adams L: Insertion of indwelling urethral catheters in infants and children: a survey of current nursing practice, *Pediatr Nurs* 24:229-234, 1998.
4. Hockenberry MJ, et al, editors: Wong's nursing care of infants and children, ed 7, St. Louis, Mosby, 2003.
5. Kleiber C, McCarthy AM: Parent behavior and child distress during urethral catheterization, 4:95-104, 1999.
6. Stashinko E, Goldberger J: Test or trauma? The voiding cystourethrogram experience of young children, *Issues Comprehensive Pediatr Nurs* 21:85-96, 1998.
7. Breuninger et al. *Handbook of nursing procedures,* Springhouse, PA, 2001, Springhouse.
8. Perry AG, Potter PA: *Clinical nursing skills & techniques,* ed 4, St. Louis, 1998, Mosby.
9. Suddarth D, editor: *Lippincott manual of nursing practice,* Philadelphia, 1991, Lippincott.

Indwelling Urinary Catheter: Insertion and Removal

P U R P O S E : An indwelling urinary catheter is placed transurethrally into the bladder to allow precise monitoring of urine output

Ruth M. Lebet

PREREQUISITE KNOWLEDGE

- Anatomy and physiology of the infant's and child's urinary tract (Figure 108-1 reviews the external female genitalia)
- Principles of aseptic technique
- An absolute contraindication for insertion of a urinary catheter is suspected urethral tear.
- Indwelling urinary catheters are usually double-lumen catheters with an inflatable retention balloon that keeps the catheter in place. For premature and small infants, single-lumen feeding tubes are sometimes used.[1-3]
- Specialized indwelling urinary catheters may also be used for temperature monitoring, intra-abdominal pressure monitoring or bladder irrigation; see Procedures 97 and 107.
- Complications related to indwelling catheters: bladder spasms, trauma, urethral tear or perforation, catheter encrustation, urethral strictures, catheter knotting, and urinary tract infection[1-3]
- Child development as it relates to clinical assessment and insertion of an indwelling urinary catheter.

CHILD AND FAMILY ASSESSMENT

- Child's developmental level and ability to interact ➤*Rationale:* These factors influence preparation of the child and interaction; urinary catheterization is particularly threatening to preschool and school-aged children.
- Family's and child's concerns about the procedure, including culturally related concerns ➤*Rationale:* Parents from some cultures may fear that catheterization of the female results in loss of virginity.[4]
- Family's desire to be present during the procedure ➤*Rationale:* Family may provide support and comfort measures to the child but should have the choice not to remain with the child. The older school-aged child and adolescent may prefer that the family not be present.
- History of surgery of the genitourinary (GU) tract or urinary tract abnormalities ➤*Rationale:* These conditions may complicate passage of the catheter.
- Previous catheterizations experienced by the child ➤*Rationale:* A negative experience with catheterization in the past may increase the child's anxiety and decrease the child's ability to cooperate with the procedure.[5,6]
- History of allergy to latex or povidone-iodine; allergy to lidocaine if topical anesthetic is to be used[7] ➤*Rationale:* Procedure may need to be modified based on allergies to these substances.

CHILD AND FAMILY EDUCATION

Individualized, developmentally appropriate education is provided to the family and to the child based on desire for knowledge, readiness to learn, and overall neurologic and psychosocial state.

- Provide information about the indwelling catheter, including the reason for catheter placement, anatomy of

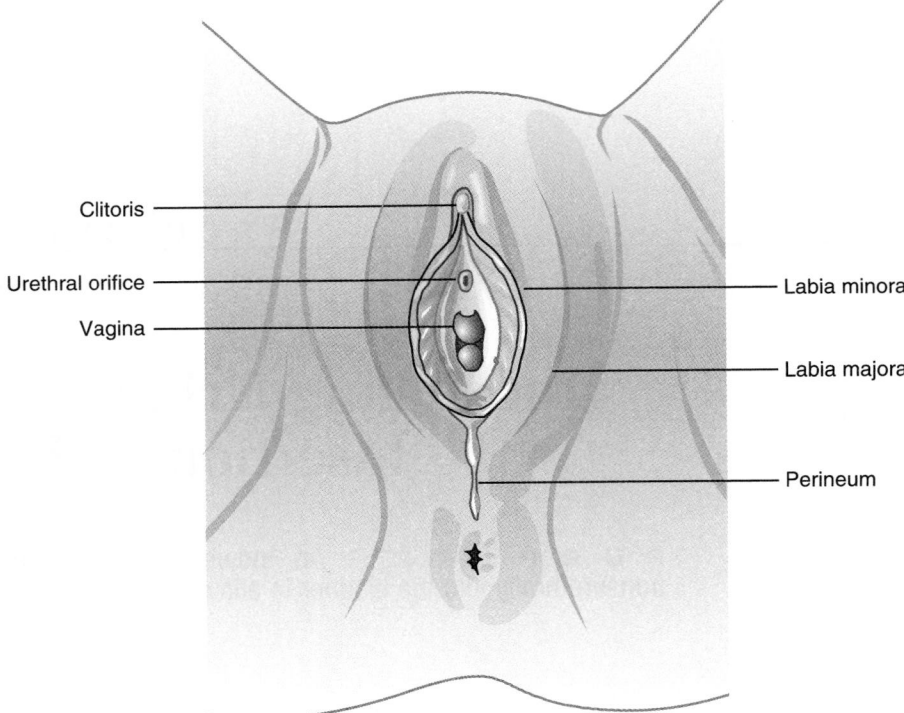

FIGURE 108-1   External female genitalia.

the GU tract, and an explanation of steps involved in catheter insertion ➻**Rationale:** Providing information decreases anxiety and fear.

- If developmentally appropriate, explain how the child can assist with the procedure (i.e., blowing, breathing, or other relaxation techniques as the tip of the catheter is passed through the urethral sphincter) ➻**Rationale:** Encouraging participation by the child facilitates the child's feeling of control and promotes more comfortable passage of the catheter.[4-6]
- Provide information about the steps involved in catheter removal before removal of the catheter ➻**Rationale:** Providing information decreases anxiety and fear, promotes cooperation with the procedure.

EQUIPMENT

Catheter Insertion

- Appropriately sized urinary catheter (Table 108-1)
- Sterile lubricant (may be included in insertion tray)
  - ❖ 2% Lidocaine lubricant jelly in specialized applicator may be used per institution-specific protocol
- Syringe for balloon inflation (may be included in catheter insertion tray)
- Sterile urine collection system
- Sterile gloves
- Tape, Foley StatLock (Venentec International, San Diego, CA), or transparent dressing to secure catheter
- Catheter insertion tray with the following supplies (or gather supplies):

TABLE 108-1	Urinary Catheter Size Selection[1-4] (Level II*)	
Age	Male Catheter Size	Female Catheter Size
Premature infant	3.5F to 5F	3.5F to 5F
Newborn	5F	5F to 6F
Infant	5F to 6F	6F to 8F
Toddler/preschooler	8F to 10F	8F to 10F
School-aged	8F to 10F	8F to 12F
Adolescent	12F	12F to 14F

*Level II: Theory-based; no research data to support recommendations; recommendations from expert consensus group may exist.

- ❖ Sterile latex-free gloves
- ❖ Povidone-iodine solution and cotton balls or povidone-iodine applicators
- ❖ Drape
- ❖ Underpad
- ❖ Forceps or tweezers
- ❖ Appropriate sterile specimen container
- ❖ Appropriate laboratory requisition(s)
- ❖ Specimen labels containing two patient identifiers

Catheter Removal

- Syringe for balloon deflation
- Clean gloves
- Alcohol pads, if StatLock has been used to secure catheter

Procedure for Indwelling Urinary Catheter: Insertion and Removal

Steps	Rationale	Considerations
Catheter Insertion		
1. Ensure child and family understand procedure and questions are answered.	Evaluates and reinforces understanding of previously taught information.	Developmental level, cognitive ability and anxiety level will determine approach to and effectiveness of teaching.
2. Collect all necessary equipment and supplies.	Preparation and presence of all materials facilitates completion of procedure in a timely manner and ability to maintain sterile field during procedure.	Catheter size is dependent on the child's size (see Table 108-1).[1,2]
3. Provide for child's privacy.	Procedure necessitates exposure of genitalia.	School-aged children are generally modest and removal of underwear and exposure of genitalia may cause this age group significant anxiety.[5,6]
4. Position child supine.	Facilitates placement of catheter.	Positioning female patients with bent knees and legs spread apart improves visualization of anatomy.
5. Wash hands.	Reduces transmission of microorganisms. Standard precautions.	
6. Open catheter insertion tray if used. Establish sterile field and place equipment and supplies so that they are easily obtained during the procedure.	Prepares equipment for use and maintains sterility.	
7. In sterile manner, place catheter onto sterile field.	Prepares equipment for use and maintains sterility.	Most manufacturers no longer recommend testing balloon on catheters with inflatable balloons because testing may result in larger French size after deflation. *(Level I*)*
8. If local anesthetic is to be used, place sterile specialized syringe with applicator containing 2% lidocaine jelly onto sterile field.	Use of local anesthetic promotes pain control and minimizes negative effects related to painful procedures.[7] *(Level IV*)*	Invasive procedures are especially traumatic for toddlers and preschool-aged children.[5,6]
9. Place sterile underpad under child's buttocks.	Provides a sterile waterproof barrier and delineates field.	
10. Put on sterile gloves.	Prevents contamination of urinary catheter with skin flora.	
11. Open lubricant jelly and squeeze onto sterile field.	Lubricant facilitates passage of the tube through the urethra.	
12. Open povidone-iodine applicators or pour povidone-iodine solution over cotton balls on field.	Facilitates application of preparation solution.	If child is allergic to povidone-iodine, mild soap and water towelettes may be used for cleansing.
13. If local anesthetic is to be used, apply cotton ball soaked with lidocaine 2% solution to area around urethral meatus for 2 minutes.[7] *(Level IV*)*	Allows local anesthetic to be absorbed, decreasing pain and discomfort with catheter placement.	Encourage family or support person to use distraction techniques with the child during the remainder of the procedure. Distraction has been shown to be effective in decreasing child's perception of pain and anxiety related to the procedure.[5,6]

Procedure continues on following page

Procedure for Indwelling Urinary Catheter: Insertion and Removal—*Continued*

Steps	Rationale	Considerations
14. Clean area around urethral meatus with cotton balls soaked in povidone-iodine solution held with tweezers or forceps. Use soap and water towelettes if child is allergic to povidone-iodine. Use a new cotton ball or towelette for each wipe. After cleansing, continue to keep non-dominant hand on area, to allow solution to dry. *(Level IV*)*	Decreases likelihood that flora on the skin is introduced to the urethra or bladder. Povidone-iodine is effective when dry.	*For females:* Separate labia with thumb and index finger of non-dominant hand and cleanse perineal area, cleaning from front to back. *For males:* Retract foreskin gently until meatus is seen in uncircumcised males. Hold penis with non-dominant hand and cleanse head of penis in a circular motion, beginning at the meatus and cleaning to the outer edge of the glans. Note: Nondominant hand is now considered contaminated.
15. If local anesthetic is to be used, instill 0.5 to 2 mL of 2% lidocaine jelly with specialized syringe applicator into the urethra and wait 2 minutes. Repeat instillation and waiting period twice more, for a total of three instillations. *(Level IV*)*	Allows lidocaine to be absorbed by local tissue, decreasing pain sensation.	Volume of lidocaine instilled increases with the age of the child.[7]
16. Holding catheter in sterile dominant hand, lubricate catheter tip with lubricating jelly. Place end of catheter in sterile specimen container.	Facilitates passage of the catheter through the urethra. Placement of end of catheter in specimen container allows culture to be obtained if needed and allows collection of urine.	
17. Insert catheter into the urethral meatus and gently advance appropriate distance for child's age. Catheter should generally be advanced at least 2 to 3 cm beyond the point at which urine flow is noted.[1-3] *(Level II*)*	Insertion length should be at least 2 cm beyond the point at which urine flow is noted in females. For males through preschool age, insert the catheter 7.5 to 10 cm past the point at which urine flow is noted. For school-aged and older male patients, insert the catheter 12.5 cm past the point at which urine flow is noted.[1,3] Insertion of the catheter only until urine flow is noted may result in a balloon placed in the distal end of the urethra because the eye hole of the catheter is at the tip of the catheter and the balloon is below the eye hole. A balloon that is inflated in the urethra may cause urethral damage.[1-3]	Recommended lengths take into consideration length of the anterior and posterior urethra and balloon.[3] *For females:* If catheter is placed in the vagina, leave catheter in place and attempt again with a new sterile catheter. This decreases the likelihood of reentering the vagina a second time. *For males:* Hold the penis at a 60-degree to 90-degree angle from the body. This straightens the urethra and allows easier insertion. Slight resistance may be noted when the catheter reaches the urethral sphincter. If the child is able to cooperate, use relaxation techniques and continue to advance the catheter. *Do not* force insertion against resistance.
18. Inflate balloon with the syringe with sterile water to the volume indicated by the manufacturer. Once the balloon is inflated, gently pull back on the catheter to ensure catheter is positioned at the bladder neck. *(Level I*)*	Retention balloon helps keep the catheter in place.	If resistance is found to inflating the balloon, do not continue to inflate. Do not use air or saline solution to inflate the balloon. Normal saline solution may evaporate and leave salt crystals, which may make balloon deflation difficult. Balloons inflated with air may float above the level of urine in the bladder.[8]

* Level I: Manufacturer's recommendations only
    Level II: Theory-based; no research data to support recommendations; recommendations from expert consensus group may exist
    Level IV: Limited clinical studies to support recommendations

Procedure	for Indwelling Urinary Catheter: Insertion and Removal—*Continued*	
Steps	**Rationale**	**Considerations**
		In uncircumcised males, return the foreskin to its original position after balloon is inflated to prevent paraphimosis.
19. In sterile fashion, attach catheter to the drainage system.	Allows collection of urine.	
20. Secure catheter to the child's thigh, allowing enough slack so that the child can move leg without pulling on the catheter.	Pulling on the catheter causes trauma to the urethra. Securing device such as StatLock or Velcro leg strap may decrease skin trauma.	If StatLock is used to secure the catheter, apply the StatLock to the catheter before applying to the skin. *(Level I*)* Avoid excessive slack, which may result in kinking of the catheter.
21. Ensure that the drainage bag is always positioned below the level of the bladder and that no dependent loops are present.	Bag positioned below the bladder prevents reflux of urine into the bladder and promotes gravity drainage. Dependent loops prevent drainage of urine.	
22. If culture or urinalysis is sent, label specimens at the bedside and complete laboratory paperwork per institution-specific protocol.	Promotes patient safety; ensures accurate and efficient processing of specimen	Follow institution specific protocol for handling and labeling lab specimens
23. Dispose of used supplies and equipment into appropriate trash container. Wash hands.	Standard precautions.	
Catheter Removal		
1. Ensure child and family understand procedure and questions are answered.	Evaluates and reinforces understanding of previously taught information.	
2. Collect all necessary equipment and supplies.	Preparation and presence of all materials facilitates completion of procedure in a timely manner.	
3. Provide for child's privacy.	Procedure necessitates exposure of genitalia.	School-aged children are generally modest and removal of underwear and exposure of genitalia may cause this age group significant anxiety.[5,6]
4. Position child supine.	Facilitates removal of catheter.	
5. Wash hands.	Reduces transmission of microorganisms. Standard precautions.	
6. Put on clean gloves.	Standard precautions.	
7. Deflate balloon with withdrawal of sterile water.	Balloon deflation prevents trauma to urethra.	If saline solution was used to inflate the balloon, salt crystals may form, which make deflation of the balloon difficult.
8. Remove catheter in a steady controlled motion.	Rapid forceful removal prevents identification of resistance to removal.	If resistance is met during catheter removal, catheter should be left in place and urologist should be consulted.

Procedure continues on following page

* Level I: Manufacturer's recommendations only

Procedure for Indwelling Urinary Catheter: Insertion and Removal—*Continued*

Steps	Rationale	Considerations
9. Gently remove material used to secure catheter.	Decreases local skin trauma.	Alcohol pad is used to remove StatLock device. (*Level I**)
10. Dispose of equipment into appropriate trash container, including gloves. Wash hands.	Standard precautions.	

* Level I: Manufacturer's recommendations only

Expected Outcomes

- Catheter and balloon are located in bladder

- Urine drains well

- Urine remains clear and without sediment
- Skin remains intact
- Child is free from complications of catheter insertion

Unexpected Outcomes

- Inflation of balloon in urethra
- Inability to advance catheter
- Inability to inflate balloon
- Urine does not drain due to occlusion of catheter with sediment
- Urine does not drain because of placement of catheter in false passage
- Sediment or cloudy urine
- Skin breakdown
- Urethral tear
- Knotting of catheter (most commonly occurs with single-lumen tubes without retention balloon)
- Bladder perforation
- Anaphylaxis
- Inability to remove catheter from the urethra

Monitoring and Care of the Child

Activities and Interventions	Rationale	Reportable Conditions
1. Monitor child's tolerance of procedure.	Changes in child's condition may indicate complications from the procedure.	- Removal of the tube by the child (note whether the balloon was inflated at the time the catheter was removed) - Symptoms of stomach or lower abdominal pain, which may indicate bladder spasms or infection
2. Monitor urine output regularly.	Decreased urine output may indicate mechanical problems with the system, such as catheter kinking, obstruction of the catheter, or dislodgement of the catheter.	- Change in character of urine, including blood, cloudy character, foul smell, or sediment - No urine drainage in 2 hours - Excessive, cloudy, or bloody drainage from the urethral meatus

Documentation

- Child and family education
- Child's response to procedure
- Size and type of catheter placed, individual placing the catheter
- Length of catheter inserted
- Unexpected outcomes and related treatment

References

1. Bukowski TP, Freedman AL: Catheterization problems of infants, *Contemp Urol* 66-74, 1999.
2. Elizondo AP, et al: Elimination of bleeding associated with urinary catheterization in neonates, *Neonatal Network* 20:25-34, 2001.
3. Smith AB, Adams L: Insertion of indwelling urethral catheters in infants and children: a survey of current nursing practice, *Pediatr Nurs* 24:229-234, 1998.
4. Hockenberry MJ, et al, editors: *Wong's nursing care of infants and children,* ed 7, St Louis, Mosby, 2003.
5. Kleiber C, McCarthy AM: Parent behavior and child distress during urethral catheterization, *JSPN* 4:95-104, 1999.
6. Stashinko E, Goldberger J: Test or trauma? The voiding cystourethrogram experience of young children, *Issues Comprehens Pediatr Nurs* 21:85-96, 1998.
7. Gerard LL, et al: Effectiveness of lidocaine lubricant for discomfort during pediatric urethral catheterization, *J Urol* 170:54-567, 2003.
8. Robinson J: Urethral catheter selection, *Nurs Stand* 15(25):39-42, 2001.

Indwelling Urinary Catheter: Irrigation

PURPOSE: Indwelling urinary catheter irrigation is performed to assess or maintain patency of the catheter, prevent blood clots from forming, flush out stagnant or infected urine, and prevent bladder distention

Suzanne Porfyris

PREREQUISITE KNOWLEDGE

- Anatomy and physiology of the urinary tract, including urethra, bladder, ureters, and kidneys
- Principles of aseptic technique specific to indwelling urinary catheters
- Principles of gravity drainage, with awareness that in caring for children with indwelling urinary catheters with drainage bags, backup of stagnant urine from the bag or bag drainage tube must be prevented by keeping the drainage bag below the level of the bladder at all times
- Force should not be used in attempting to irrigate a catheter because damage to the urethra, bladder, or ureters could occur.
- Child development as it relates to clinical assessment and indwelling urinary catheter irrigation

CHILD AND FAMILY ASSESSMENT

- History of blood, blood clots, sediment, stones, or other debris in the urine ➥*Rationale:* These conditions may complicate the catheter irrigation process by causing blockage once the irrigation procedure is completed.
- Child's developmental level and ability to interact ➥*Rationale:* These factors influence preparation for and interaction during the procedure.

- Level of consciousness and cognitive ability ➥*Rationale:* Identifies the child's ability to use a prearranged signal to indicate an inability to continue holding still during the irrigation procedure.
- Child's and family's understanding of the reasons for and risks and benefits of the procedure ➥*Rationale:* Evaluates child's and family's understanding of the procedure and provides a gauge for ongoing education.
- Family's desire to be present during the procedure ➥*Rationale:* Family may provide support and comfort measures to the child, but they should have the choice not to remain with the child.

CHILD AND FAMILY EDUCATION

Individualized, developmentally appropriate education is provided to the family and to the child based on desire for knowledge, readiness to learn, and overall neurologic and psychosocial state.

- Provide information about the catheter irrigation procedure, including the reason for the procedure and an explanation of steps involved in irrigating the catheter ➥*Rationale:* Providing information decreases anxiety and fear and may increase cooperation during the procedure.
- If developmentally appropriate, explain how child can assist with catheter irrigation procedure (i.e., holding still during the procedure) ➥*Rationale:* Contamination of the

catheter may occur if the child actively moves around during the procedure.

- Encourage questions and answer questions as they arise ➥*Rationale:* Reinforcement of information is needed during periods of stress.

EQUIPMENT

- Sterile irrigation solution prescribed
- Sterile irrigation set with 30-mL to 60-mL catheter-tip syringe or a sterile 30-mL to 60-mL catheter-tip syringe and sterile container for irrigation solution
- Sterile gloves
- Antiseptic swabs
- Sterile basin for collection of drained irrigation fluid
- Sterile cap for the drainage system tubing end
- Underpad to protect bedding
- Disposable sterile towel or drape
- Graduated container

Procedure for Indwelling Urinary Catheter: Irrigation

Steps	Rationale	Considerations
1. Ensure family and child understand procedure and questions are answered.	Prevents anxiety over the need for the procedure and promotes cooperation.	Developmental level, cognitive ability, and anxiety level determine approach to and effectiveness of teaching.
2. Collect equipment and supplies.	Preparation and presence of all materials facilitates completion of procedure without delays and decreases likelihood of contamination of catheter.	
3. Inform child and family that child will be positioned for easy access to the catheter tubing.	Allows child and family to anticipate manipulation of the catheter and facilitates coping with possible discomfort associated with movement of the catheter.	Ensuring that the catheter is anchored to the leg of the child with an appropriate device reduces the likelihood of discomfort associated with manipulation of the catheter and tubing.
4. Provide privacy and assist the child into a comfortable position.	Procedure may necessitate exposure of the child's genitalia. Child and family cooperation is increased if respect for privacy and comfort is shown.	Assistance may be needed to hold the child in a comfortable position during the procedure. The family should have the option not to hold the child.
5. Place protective underpad beneath child's buttocks.	Prevents soiling of the bed with irrigation solution and urine.	The pad also provides a clean field for placement of basin for drainage of irrigation solution.
6. Wash hands.	Standard precautions; reduces transmission of microorganisms.	
7. Open sterile irrigation set, sterile basin, and antiseptic swabs and arrange equipment.	Establishes sterile field; reduces transmission of microorganisms.	If an irrigation set is not available, create a sterile field with a sterile towel or drape and place the catheter tipped syringe, antiseptic swabs, sterile container for irrigation solution, and sterile cap for the end of the catheter tubing on the sterile field.
8. Pour sterile irrigation solution into sterile irrigation set tray or sterile container.	The bladder is considered sterile; sterile irrigant must be used.	Aseptic technique is maintained during set up of equipment.
9. Put on sterile gloves.	Maintains aseptic technique.	

Procedure continues on following page

Procedure for Indwelling Urinary Catheter: Irrigation—*Continued*

Steps	Rationale	Considerations
10. Place sterile towel or drape on surface within easy reach and place sterile basin on the sterile towel, within reach of the site of the catheter and drainage tubing connection.	Maintains aseptic technique.	
11. Cleanse connection between the indwelling catheter and the drainage tubing with antiseptic swabs. *(Level IV*)*	Contaminants on the outside of the tubing and catheter are removed, decreasing the likelihood of contamination of the catheter when disconnected for irrigation procedure.[1-4]	Cleansing should be done by scrubbing the connection for at least 20 seconds.
12. Disconnect the indwelling urinary catheter from the drainage tube, place the catheter end in the sterile basin, and place sterile cap on the drainage tubing end.	Open end of indwelling urinary catheter remains in sterile field at all times, decreasing the likelihood of contamination.	
13. Draw up 30 to 60 mL, or prescribed amount of irrigation solution if less than 30 to 60 mL, into the catheter-tip syringe. *(Level II*)*	The volume of solution in the syringe should be small enough to avoid overdistention of the bladder.[1,5,6]	The syringe size and amount of irrigation solution instilled is dependent on child's size. The volume of irrigation solution used in the syringe should be decreased if child is uncomfortable with initial volume used.
14. Slowly inject irrigation solution into indwelling urinary catheter.	Fast injection of solution may cause discomfort.[5,6]	
15. Remove the syringe from the end of the catheter and allow indwelling catheter to drain into the sterile basin.	Passive drainage of urine decreases the likelihood of trauma to the bladder.	
16. Repeat procedure until the amount of fluid ordered is instilled and returned. *(Level II*)*	Instillation of the total ordered amount of irrigation solution in increments increases patient comfort during the procedure and decreases the likelihood of trauma to the bladder from instillation of a large volume of irrigation solution.[1,5]	
17. Remove sterile cap from the end of the connection tubing and reconnect the indwelling urinary catheter to the drainage tubing.	Reestablishes drainage system.	Aseptic technique is maintained throughout the procedure.
18. Transfer solution in the sterile basin to graduated container to measure total volume returned. Determine amount of irrigation solution returned and amount of urine drained during the procedure.	Determination of whether all the irrigation solution is returned is necessary because retained irrigation solution indicates some form of blockage in the indwelling catheter or bladder.[1,5,6]	
19. Ensure child is positioned comfortably and urine is freely flowing to the collection bag.	Ensures system is intact and functioning.	
20. Discard used supplies in appropriate trash receptacle. Wash hands.	Standard precautions; reduces transmission of microorganisms.	

* Level II: Theory-based; no research data to support recommendations; recommendations from expert consensus group may exist
Level IV: Limited clinical studies to support recommendations

Expected Outcomes	Unexpected Outcomes
• Easy inflow and outflow of irrigation solution in catheter • Urine flows freely from catheter after procedure completed • Volume of irrigation solution instilled is returned • Child is free from trauma to bladder or urethra as a result of the procedure	• Irrigation solution cannot be instilled into catheter • Irrigation solution does not drain freely through the catheter • Irrigation solution is entirely retained in the bladder • Urethral or bladder trauma causes blood in the urine

Monitoring and Care of the Child

Activities and Interventions	Rationale	Reportable Conditions
1. Monitor child's tolerance of procedure.	Changes in child's condition may indicate complications from catheter irrigation.	• Pain or discomfort during the procedure
2. Monitor free flow of urine from catheter after the procedure.	Irrigation of catheter may dislodge debris, causing the catheter to clog.	• Clogged catheter that does not drain freely • Any volume of irrigation solution retained in the bladder
3. Monitor for bladder distention or palpable bladder after procedure is completed.	Bladder distention indicates a partially or completely clogged catheter.	• Distended bladder
4. Monitor characteristics of urine obtained after procedure is completed.	Abnormal characteristics of urine, such as blood, sediment, and cloudiness, may indicate trauma or infection after the procedure.	• Frank blood, sediment, or cloudy urine in drainage bag after procedure for child with no prior blood or abnormal characteristics in the urine

Documentation

- Education of child and family
- Amount of solution instilled and amount drained after procedure
- Use of aseptic technique
- Description of solution drained: color, clarity, blood, or debris visible in the irrigation solution
- Irrigation solution used
- Note of whether catheter drains urine freely after the procedure
- Child's tolerance of procedure
- Unexpected outcomes and related treatment

References

1. Gates A: The benefits of irrigation in catheter care, *Prof Nurse* 16(1):835-838, 2000.
2. Getliffe K: Care of urinary catheters, *Nurs Stand* 10(1):25-31, 1995.
3. Sobel JD, Kaye D: Urinary tract infections. In Mandell GL, Bennett JE, Dolin R, editors: *Principles and practices of infectious diseases,* ed 5, Philadelphia, 2000, Churchill Livingstone.
4. US Department of Health and Human Services: *Semiannual Report: aggregate data from the National Nosocomial Infection Surveillance System (NNIS), December,* Atlanta, 1999, Centers for Disease Control.
5. Potter A, Griffin Perry A: *Basic nursing: a critical thinking approach,* ed 4, St Louis, 1999, Mosby.
6. Wong DL: *Whaley and Wong's nursing care of infants and children,* ed 6, St Louis, 1999, Mosby.

Additional Readings

Christensen B, Kockrow E: *Adult health nursing,* St Louis, 1999, Mosby.
Kalowicz K: *Urologic nursing,* Philadelphia, 1995, Saunders.

Indwelling Urinary Catheter: Urinalysis Collection

P U R P O S E : To obtain a fresh urine specimen for measurement of the normal and abnormal physiologic constituents of urine and correlation of the results with known disease processes

Suzanne Porfyris

PREREQUISITE KNOWLEDGE

- Anatomy and physiology of the urinary tract, including urethra, bladder, ureters, and kidneys
- Principles of aseptic technique specific to indwelling urinary catheters
- Principles of gravity drainage, with understanding that indwelling urinary catheter drainage bags must be kept lower than the level of the bladder to prevent backup of stagnant urine from the bag or bag drainage tube into the bladder
- Timely processing of urine specimen once collected is necessary to prevent bacterial growth and pH changes
- Child development as it relates to clinical assessment and manipulation of an indwelling urinary catheter

CHILD AND FAMILY ASSESSMENT

- History of blood, blood clots, sediment, stones, or other debris in the urine ➡️*Rationale:* These conditions may complicate the catheter urine collection process by causing blockage of the collection needle and syringe or causing blockage once the collection procedure is completed.
- Child's developmental level and ability to interact ➡️*Rationale:* These factors influence preparation and interaction.

- Child's and family's understanding of the reasons for and risks and benefits of the procedure ➡️*Rationale:* Evaluates child's and family's understanding of the procedure and provides a gauge for ongoing education.
- Family's desire to be present during procedure ➡️*Rationale:* Family may provide support and comfort measures to the child, but they should have the choice not to remain with the child during the procedure.

CHILD AND FAMILY EDUCATION

Individualized, developmentally appropriate education is provided to the family and to the child based on desire for knowledge, readiness to learn, and overall neurologic and psychosocial state.

- Provide information about the catheter urinalysis collection procedure, including the reason for the procedure and an explanation of steps involved ➡️*Rationale:* Information decreases anxiety and fear.
- If developmentally appropriate, explain how child can assist with the collection procedure (i.e., holding still during the procedure) ➡️*Rationale:* Contamination of the specimen may occur if the child actively moves around during the procedure.
- Encourage questions and answer questions as they arise ➡️*Rationale:* Reinforcement of information is needed during periods of stress.

EQUIPMENT

- Clean specimen container
- Sterile 10-mL syringe and needleless access device or needle

- Clean gloves
- Antiseptic swabs
- Tubing clamp or rubber band
- Specimen labels containing two patient identifiers
- Appropriate laboratory requisitions

Procedure for Indwelling Urinary Catheter: Urinalysis Collection		
Steps	**Rationale**	**Considerations**
1. Ensure child and family understand procedure and questions are answered.	Evaluates and reinforces previously taught information.	Developmental level, cognitive ability and anxiety level will determine approach to and effectiveness of teaching.
2. Explain to child and family that the needleless access device or syringe and needle used to collect the specimen will not cause any discomfort for the child.	Prevents anxiety over the use of a syringe and needle and promotes cooperation.	
3. Explain why the catheter will be clamped before specimen collection.	Prevents anxiety over clamping and promotes understanding of the need to collect urine from the bladder rather than from the drainage bag.	
4. Gather all needed equipment and supplies.	Presence of needed supplies and equipment facilitates completion of procedure in a timely manner.	Refer to manufacturer's recommendations for information on devices that can be used to access the sampling port; some ports can be accessed with a needleless access device.
5. Wash hands and put on clean gloves.	Standard precautions; reduces transmission of microorganisms.	
6. Utilize two patient identifiers to verify correct child. *(Level II*)*	Promotes patient safety; ensures specimens are being obtained from the correct child.	Compare information on specimen labels with child's ID band or utilize mechanism described in institution-specific protocol.
7. Identify the sampling port in the drainage tubing. Clamp drainage tubing below the port for approximately 15 minutes. Use either a tubing clamp or a rubber band around a fold in the tubing (Figure 110-1). *(Level II*)*	Collection of fresh urine from the catheter tubing is aided by prevention of free flow of urine into the drainage bag for a short period of time.[1,2]	Clamp time necessary may be greater or less than 15 minutes, depending on the rate of urine production. Indwelling urinary catheters should not be clamped for greater than 30 minutes in most cases.
8. Once fresh urine has collected in the clamped drainage tubing, inform the child and family that the child will be positioned for easy access to the catheter tubing.	Allows child and family to anticipate manipulation of the catheter and facilitates coping with possible discomfort associated with movement of the catheter.	Ensuring that the catheter is anchored to the leg of the child with an appropriate device reduces the likelihood of discomfort associated with manipulation of the catheter and tubing.
9. Cleanse tubing entry port with antiseptic swab. *(Level VI*)*	Prevents entry of bacteria into the catheter.[1-5]	Refer to institution-specific protocol for antiseptic solution used.

Procedure continues on following page

* Level II: Theory-based; no research data to support recommendations; recommendations from expert consensus group may exist
   Level VI: Clinical studies in a variety of patient populations and situations to support recommendations

Procedure | for Indwelling Urinary Catheter: Urinalysis Collection—*Continued*

Steps	Rationale	Considerations

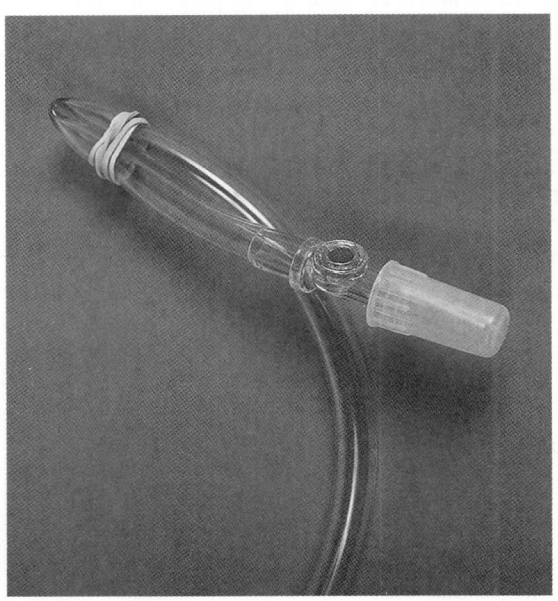

FIGURE 110-1 Method for clamping indwelling urinary catheter tubing before urinalysis collection with rubber band. Tubing is kinked and banded at least 3 cm below collection port. *From Elkin MK, et al, editors: Nursing interventions and clinical skills, ed 2, St Louis, 2000, Mosby.*

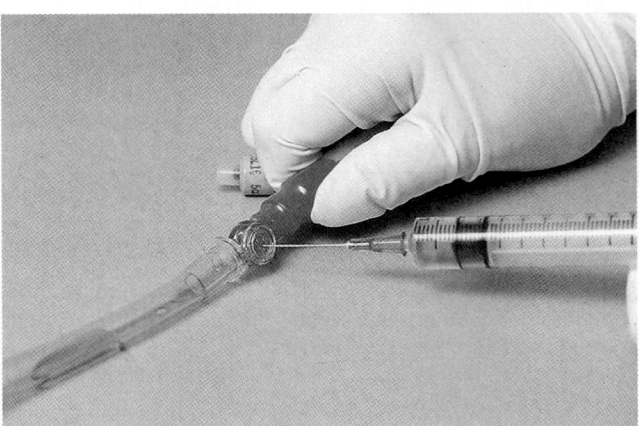

FIGURE 110-2 Withdrawal of urine from collection port of indwelling urinary catheter drainage tube, with needle and syringe inserted at 90-degree angle in sampling port. Follow manufacturer's recommendations for device used to access sampling port; some systems may be accessed with needleless cannula. *From Elkin MK, et al, editors: Nursing interventions and clinical skills, ed 2, St Louis, 2000, Mosby.*

Steps	Rationale	Considerations
10. Attach syringe to needleless access device or needle and insert device or needle at 90-degree angle into the sampling port of the drainage tubing (Figure 110-2).	Ensures entrance of needleless access device or needle into the tubing lumen.[1]	Refer to manufacturer's recommendations for information on devices that can be used to access the sampling port; some ports can be accessed with a needleless access device. If needle is used, refer to manufacturer's recommendation for gauge of needle used to access sampling port.
11. Draw 10 mL urine into syringe.	Ensures proper volume of specimen for testing without contamination.[1,4]	Volume of urine necessary for testing may vary among laboratories.
12. Transfer urine from syringe into clean container.	Urinalysis does not necessitate a sterile specimen.	
13. Do not recap needle. Dispose of uncapped needle and syringe in proper receptacle. *(Level V*)*	Reduces risk of needle stick injury.	
14. Cap specimen container securely. Label specimen(s) at the bedside and complete laboratory paperwork per institution-specific protocol *(Level II*);* send to laboratory within 30 minutes of collection.	Prevents spillage and alteration of test results from long delay between time of collection and time of processing in the laboratory.[1,4,5] Promotes patient safety; ensures accurate and efficient processing of specimen	Follow institution-specific protocol for handling and labeling lab specimens.

* Level II: Theory-based; no research data to support recommendations; recommendations from expert consensus group may exist
  Level V: Clinical studies in more than one or two patient populations and situations to support recommendations

Procedure for Indwelling Urinary Catheter: Urinalysis Collection—*Continued*

Steps	Rationale	Considerations
15. Unclamp the catheter and allow urine to flow into the drainage bag. Visually check to ensure flow of urine from the indwelling catheter. *(Level V*)*	Allows urine to drain with gravity and prevents stasis of urine in the bladder.[5]	Be sure to leave drainage bag hanging at a level below the bladder.
16. Discard supplies in appropriate trash receptacles. Remove gloves and wash hands.	Standard precautions; reduces transmission of microorganisms.	

* Level V: Clinical studies in more than one or two patient populations and situations to support recommendations

Expected Outcomes

- Fresh uncontaminated urine is provided to the laboratory for analysis

- Urine specimen is placed in correct specimen container, labeled appropriately and sent to the lab in the appropriate time frame.
- Catheter drains freely after collection procedure

Unexpected Outcomes

- Urine has bacterial overgrowth and changes in pH caused by storage at room temperature before processing in the laboratory
- Specimen is mislabeled
- Specimen is placed in incorrect container
- Delay in sending specimens to lab
- Blockage to free flow of urine from indwelling urinary catheter

Monitoring and Care of the Child

Activities and Interventions	Rationale	Reportable Conditions
1. Monitor free flow of urine from catheter after the procedure.	Clamping of the catheter or drainage tubing might cause kinking of tubing, preventing proper drainage of urine.	- Kinked catheter that does not drain freely
2. Monitor whether bladder is distended and palpable after procedure is completed.	Bladder distention indicates a partially or completely kinked or clogged catheter.	- Distended bladder - Pain

Documentation

- Child and family education
- Amount of solution drained after procedure
- Use of aseptic technique
- Description of solution drained: color, clarity, or debris visible in the solution
- Length of time catheter clamped for procedure
- Note of whether catheter drains urine freely after the procedure
- Unexpected outcomes and related treatment

References
1. Elkin MK, et al: *Nursing interventions and clinical skills,* ed 2, St Louis, 2000, Mosby.
2. Wong DL, editor: *Whaley and Wong's nursing care of infants and children,* ed 6, St Louis, 1999, Mosby.
3. Getliffe K: Care of urinary catheters, *Nurs Stand* 10(1): 25-31, 1995.
4. Potter A, Griffin Perry A, editors: *Basic nursing: a critical thinking approach,* ed 4, St Louis, 1999, Mosby.
5. Warren JW: Nosocomial urinary tract infections. In Mandell G, et al, editors: *Principals and practices of infectious diseases,* ed 5, Philadelphia, 2000, Churchill Livingstone.

Additional Reading
Christensen B, Kockrow E, editors: *Adult health nursing,* St Louis, 1999, Mosby.

Urine Culture: Indwelling Catheter or Suprapubic Tube

P U R P O S E : A sterile urine specimen is obtained from an indwelling catheter to assess for the presence of microorganisms

Susan Mills

PREREQUISITE KNOWLEDGE

- Anatomy and physiology of the urinary tract
- Principles of aseptic technique
- Types of indwelling urinary catheters and related materials
- Needle or needleless access device that may be used to access the sampling port of the urine collection system
- Signs and symptoms of a urinary tract infection
- Necessary urine volume for specimen
- Specimen container requirements
- Specimen labeling requirements
- Appropriate specimen storage, if necessary
- When a specimen is obtained from a urine collection system, careful attention to the aspiration procedure is important to keep the collection system intact.
- Strict aseptic technique is necessary in obtaining the sample to prevent sample contamination.
- Child development as it relates to clinical assessment and manipulation of an indwelling urinary catheter

CHILD AND FAMILY ASSESSMENT

- History of blood, blood clots, sediment, stones, or other debris in the urine *➥Rationale:* These conditions may complicate the catheter urine collection process by causing blockage of the collection needle and syringe or causing blockage once the collection procedure is completed.

- Child's developmental level and ability to interact *➥Rationale:* These factors influence preparation and interaction.
- Child's and family's understanding of the reasons for and risks and benefits of the procedure. *➥Rationale:* Evaluates child's and family's understanding of the procedure and provides a gauge for ongoing education.
- Child's and family's understanding of the signs and symptoms of a urinary tract infection *➥Rationale:* Educates the child and family of the signs and symptoms to be reported to allow communication of symptoms promptly. Education also helps the child and family understand the importance of obtaining a sterile specimen.

CHILD AND FAMILY EDUCATION

Individualized, developmentally appropriate education is provided to the family and to the child based on desire for knowledge, readiness to learn, and overall neurologic and psychosocial state.

- Discuss the need to collect urine from the catheter with the family and child if appropriate *➥Rationale:* Providing information decreases fear and increases understanding of the procedure.
- Explain the need to clamp the urine collection system to obtain the specimen and encourage the child and family to report any discomfort immediately *➥Rationale:* The

explanation decreases anxiety related to catheter manipulation and informs the child and family of when to notify a nurse.
- Educate the child and family about the collection procedure, including the introduction of the needle or needleless access device into the sampling port ➥*Rationale:* Education decreases anxiety related to the use of a needle.
- If developmentally appropriate, explain how the child can assist with the procedure by holding still during collection of the specimen ➥*Rationale:* Contamination of the specimen may occur if the child moves during the procedure.
- Encourage questions and answer questions as they arise ➥*Rationale:* Reinforcement of information is needed during periods of stress.

EQUIPMENT

- Antibacterial solution: 70% alcohol or per institution-specific protocol
- 3-mL syringe with a 1-inch 21-gauge needle or needleless access device
- Nonmetal clamp or rubber band
- Sterile specimen container
- Copy of prescribing practitioner's order
- Specimen labels containing two patient identifiers
- Appropriate laboratory requisitions
- Clean gloves

Procedure	for Urine Culture: Indwelling Catheter or Suprapubic Tube	
Steps	**Rationale**	**Considerations**
1. Ensure child and family understand procedure and questions are answered.	Evaluates and reinforces understanding of previously taught information.	Developmental level, cognitive ability and anxiety level influence approach to and effectiveness of teaching.
2. Collect all necessary equipment and supplies.	Presence of all of the supplies in the room eliminates delay, which can help decrease anxiety.	
3. Wash hands and put on clean gloves.	Standard precautions: reduces transmission of microorganisms.	
4. Review prescribing practitioner's order for urine culture. If urinalysis is also ordered, see Procedure 110 for further information. Identify child using two patient identifiers.	Promotes patient safety; ensures that correct tests are obtained from correct patient.	Use two patient identifiers as described in institution-specific protocol.
5. Position child for easy access to the urine collection system tubing. Provide appropriate privacy for the child.	Accessing the sampling port may necessitate some exposure of the child's perineal area.	
6. Identify the sampling port in urine collection system tubing. With the nonmetal clamp or rubber band, clamp tube below sampling port until sufficient urine collects. *(Level II*)*	Clamping tube allows fresh urine to collect in tube. A fresh sample gives the most accurate results.[1]	Do not clamp the tube for longer than 30 minutes to prevent discomfort to child and growth of organisms.[2,3] See Procedure 110 for illustration of clamping tubing.
7. Cleanse aspiration port with 70% alcohol or other antimicrobial solution per institution-specific protocol. *(Level VI*)*	Prevents microorganisms from the outside of the sampling port from entering the closed system of the indwelling catheter.[2,3]	Povidone-iodine or other antimicrobial solutions may be used.
8. Insert a sterile 1-inch 21-gauge needle or needleless access device into the cleansed sampling port. *(Level I*)*	Allows for removal of a sterile specimen.	Avoid inserting the needle into the shaft of the catheter or puncturing the catheter tubing. Refer to manufacturer's recommendations for information on devices that can be used to access the sampling port; some ports can be accessed with a needleless access device. See Procedure 110 for illustration of accessing sampling port.

Procedure continues on following page

* Level I: Manufacturer's recommendations only
  Level II: Theory-based; no research data to support recommendations; recommendations from expert consensus group may exist
  Level VI: Clinical studies in a variety of patient populations and situations to support recommendations

Procedure for Urine Culture: Indwelling Catheter or Suprapubic Tube—*Continued*

Steps	Rationale	Considerations
9. Aspirate the necessary amount of urine for specimen collection, generally 3 mL for urine culture.[1]	Proper amount of urine must be obtained for ordered tests to be run by the clinical laboratory.	
10. Remove needle or needleless access device from sampling port and transfer urine into the sterile specimen container. Cap specimen immediately.	Urine specimen remains sterile, allowing for more accurate test results.	
11. Unclamp catheter and allow urine to drain by gravity into the collection bag.	Unclamping and draining urine immediately after specimen collection reduces urinary retention, stasis, and potential for migration of microorganisms into the bladder or kidneys.[2,3]	Care must be taken after the tube is unclamped to allow urine to drain into the bag to reduce potential of infection.
12. Remove and discard gloves and supplies in appropriate trash receptacles. Wash hands.	Standard precautions: prevents transmission of microorganisms.	
13. Label specimen immediately while still at the bedside.	Allows for a "double-check" and prevents the possibility of sending the wrong specimen or mislabeling the specimen.	Labeling should always be done by the person who collected the specimen while still with the child to decrease the likelihood of an error.
14. Send specimen to the laboratory immediately.	Prevents rapid growth of microorganisms in the specimen, which results in the possibility of inaccurate results.[1]	Urine should not remain at room temperature for longer than 30 minutes. If the specimen cannot be transported immediately, it can be refrigerated for up to 4 hours.[1]

Expected Outcomes

- Sterile urine specimen is obtained without damage to the catheter

- Fresh urine is provided to the laboratory
- Catheter drains freely after collection procedure
- Urine specimen is placed in correct specimen container, labeled appropriately and sent to the lab in the appropriate time frame.

Unexpected Outcomes

- Specimen contamination
- Catheter integrity is compromised by puncture of the balloon or tubing
- Microorganisms are introduced into closed catheter system
- Delay in sending specimen results in contamination
- Urinary retention
- Specimen is mislabeled
- Specimen is placed in incorrect container
- Delay in sending specimens to lab

Monitoring and Care of the Child

Activities and Interventions	Rationale	Reportable Conditions
1. Monitor child's tolerance to catheter clamping.	Child may report or show signs of discomfort from the buildup of urine in the catheter.	• Pain or cramping
2. Monitor for free flow of urine from catheter into urine collection system after specimen collection.	If balloon or catheter is punctured, catheter may not drain properly.	• Balloon or tubing puncture
3. Monitor for signs and symptoms of urinary tract infection.	If appropriate aseptic technique is not used, child is at risk for introduction of microorganisms into the closed catheter system, which may result in urinary tract infection.	• Signs and symptoms of a urinary tract infection

Documentation

- Child and family education
- Length of time catheter clamped for procedure
- Amount of urine withdrawn for specimen
- Note of whether catheter drains urine freely after the procedure
- Unexpected outcomes and related treatment

References

1. National Committee for Clinical Laboratory Standards: Urinalysis and collection, transportation, and preservation of urine specimens; approved guidelines, ed 2, *NCCLS GP-16A2* 21(19):4-21, 1999.

2. Nettina SM, editor: *The Lippincott manual of nursing practice,* ed 7, Philadelphia, 2001, Lippincott Williams & Wilkins.

3. Potter A, Griffin Perry A, editors: *Clinical nursing skills and techniques,* ed 4, St Louis, 1998, Mosby.

Urine Culture: Intermittent Catheterization

P U R P O S E : A urinary catheter is placed into the bladder via the urethra to allow drainage of urine to obtain a sterile urine sample for analysis or culture

Kelly Pruden

PREREQUISITE KNOWLEDGE

- Anatomy and physiology of the urinary tract
- Principles of aseptic technique
- Absolute contraindications for insertion of a urinary catheter include a suspected urethral tear
- Complications related to intermittent catheterization include: urethral trauma, urethral tear, bacteriuria and urinary tract infection, creation of false passage, bladder perforation, urethritis, hematuria, and urethral stricture.[1-6]
- Transurethral catheterization provides a high degree of sensitivity in diagnosis of a urinary tract infection[7]
- Child development as it relates to clinical assessment and insertion of a urinary catheter

CHILD AND FAMILY ASSESSMENT

- Child's developmental level and ability to interact ➤*Rationale:* Information should be provided in terminology understood by both family and child.[8] Urinary catheterization is particularly threatening to preschool and school-aged children. These factors influence preparation of the child and interaction.
- Child's and family's understanding of the reasons for and risks and benefits of the procedure ➤*Rationale:* Evaluates child's and family's understanding of the procedure and provides a gauge for ongoing education.

- Family's and child's concerns about the procedure, including culturally related concerns ➤*Rationale:* Parents from some cultures may fear that catheterization of the female results in loss of virginity.[9]
- Desire of family to remain with child during the procedure ➤*Rationale:* Families may be a source of support and comfort during procedures but should have the choice not to remain with the child. School-aged children or adolescents may prefer that family does not remain.[10]
- Genitourinary (GU) abnormalities, including previous surgery of the GU system ➤*Rationale:* Passage of the urinary catheter through the urethra may be complicated by these conditions.
- History of catheterization ➤*Rationale:* A negative experience with the procedure may influence the child's coping strategies and increase anxiety level.[10,11]
- Assessment of the child's allergy history (e.g., latex, povidone-iodine, and lidocaine) ➤*Rationale:* Modification of the procedure may be necessary based on allergies to these substances.

CHILD AND FAMILY EDUCATION

Individualized, developmentally appropriate education is provided to the child and family based on desire for knowledge, readiness to learn, and overall neurologic and psychosocial state.

- Provide developmentally appropriate information regarding the procedure to the child and family; include the rationale for catheterization, anatomy of the GU system, and a description of the steps necessary for collection of specimen ➤➤*Rationale:* Providing information decreases fear and anxiety.
- If developmentally appropriate, provide information to the child regarding relaxation techniques that may be used during the procedure ➤➤*Rationale:* The use of non-pharmacologic methods to assist with relaxation during procedures may be beneficial in decreasing pain perception and diminishing distress.[10]
- Encourage questions and answer questions as they arise ➤➤*Rationale:* Reinforcement of information is needed during periods of stress.

EQUIPMENT

- Appropriately sized urinary catheter (Table 112-1)
- Sterile water-soluble lubricant (may be included in insertion tray)
  - Lidocaine lubricant may be used per institution-specific protocol
- Sterile gloves
- Catheter insertion tray with the following supplies (or gather supplies):
  - Sterile latex-free gloves of appropriate size
  - Povidone-iodine solution and sterile cotton balls or povidone-iodine applicators
  - Drape
  - Underpad or diaper
  - Forceps or tweezers
  - Sterile specimen collection container
- Light source
- Specimen labels containing two patient identifiers
- Appropriate laboratory requisitions

TABLE 112-1	Urinary Catheter Size Selection[2,5,6,12] *(Level II*)*	
Age	Male Catheter Size	Female Catheter Size
Premature infant	3.5F to 5F	3.5F to 5F
Newborn	5F	5F to 6F
Infant	5F to 6F	6F to 8F
Toddler/preschooler	8F to 10F	8F to 10F
School-aged	8F to 10F	8F to 12F
Adolescent	12F	12F to 14F

*Level II: Theory-based; no research data to support recommendations; recommendations from expert consensus group may exist.

Data from Bukowski TP, Freedman AL: Catheterization problems of infants, *Contemp Urol* 66-74, 1999; Elizondo AP, Gilbert J, Wearden ME, et al: Elimination of bleeding associated with urinary catheterization in neonates, *Neonatal Network* 20:25-34, 2001; Smith AB, Adams L: Insertion of indwelling urethral catheters in infants and children: a survey of current nursing practice, *Pediatr Nurs* 24:229-234, 1998; Hockenberry MJ, Wilson D, Winkelstein ML, et al, editors: *Wong's nursing care of infants and children,* ed 7, St Louis, Mosby, Inc.

Procedure for Urine Culture: Intermittent Catheterization

Steps	Rationale	Considerations
1. Ensure child and family understand procedure and questions are answered.	Evaluates and reinforces understanding of previously taught information.	Developmental level, cognitive ability and anxiety level determine approach to and effectiveness of teaching.
2. Collect all necessary equipment and supplies.	Preparation and presence of all equipment at hand facilitates completion of procedure without delays and ability to maintain sterile field during procedure.	Catheter size is dependent on the child's size and age (see Table 112-1). Catheter choice should be that of the smallest diameter that allows adequate drainage.[2]
3. Provide privacy for child.	Procedure necessitates exposure of genitalia.	School-aged children are generally modest and removal of underwear and exposure of genitalia may cause this age group significant anxiety.[11]
4. Utilize two patient identifiers to verify correct child. *(Level II*)*	Promotes patient safety; ensures specimens are being obtained from the correct child.	Compare information on specimen labels with child's ID band or utilize mechanism described in institution-specific protocol.
5. Place child in supine position.	Assists with the visualization of the urethral opening.	Position female children with knees flexed, feet flat on bed, and legs rotated laterally.

Procedure continues on following page

Procedure for Urine Culture: Intermittent Catheterization—*Continued*

Steps	Rationale	Considerations
6. Position light source.	Allows optimum visualization.	Light source should be in close enough proximity to allow optimum visualization while avoiding contamination of sterile field.
7. Wash hands.	Standard precautions. Reduces transmission of micro-organisms.	
8. Open catheter insertion tray while maintaining sterile technique. Establish sterile field and place supplies and equipment within easy reach.	Allows for assembling of equipment while maintaining sterile field.	
9. With sterile technique, place catheter within sterile field.	Allows for assembling of equipment while maintaining sterile field.	An extra catheter should be readily available in the event that initial catheter becomes contaminated, is malpositioned into the vagina, or is determined to be the incorrect size.
10. If local anesthetic is used, place sterile syringe containing 2% lidocaine onto sterile field.	The use of topical anesthetic supports pain control and decreases the negative effects associated with painful medical procedures.[12] *(Level IV*)*	Urethral catheterization is an invasive procedure that may cause stress and pain in the pediatric population.[11]
11. Place underpad or diaper under patient's buttocks.	Provides a waterproof barrier.	
12. Put on sterile gloves.	Standard precautions. Prevents contamination of catheter with microorganisms.	
13. Open sterile water soluble lubricant and squeeze onto sterile field.	Lubricant assists with entry of catheter into urethra.	
14. Open povidone-iodine applicators or pour povidone-iodine solution over sterile cotton balls on sterile field.	Facilitates application of solution.	Mild soap and water can be used if child has a history of allergy to povidone-iodine.
15. If topical anesthetic is used, apply cotton ball soaked with 2% lidocaine to urethral meatus for 2 minutes.[12] *(Level IV*)*	Allows for absorption of local anesthetic, thereby diminishing pain with catheterization.	The use of distraction techniques throughout the procedure may decrease fear and anxiety and diminish pain perception.[8]
16. Clean area around urethral meatus with povidone-iodine applicators or cotton balls saturated with povidone-iodine with forceps or tweezers. Use soap and water towelettes if child has an allergy to povidone-iodine. Use a clean applicator, cotton ball, or towelette with each wipe. Allow solution to dry. *(Level IV*)*	Decreases the potential for introduction of microorganisms from the skin into the urethra or bladder.	*For female child:* With nondominant hand, separate the labia with thumb and index finger. Cleanse perineal area from front to back. *For male child:* In uncircumcised male, gently retract foreskin until meatus is visualized. Holding penis with nondominant hand, cleanse head of penis in a circular motion, beginning at the meatus and cleansing toward the outer edge of the glans. *Note:* Nondominant hand is no longer considered sterile.

* Level IV: Limited clinical studies to support recommendations

Procedure for Urine Culture: Intermittent Catheterization—*Continued*

Steps	Rationale	Considerations
17. If local anesthetic is used, instill 0.5 to 2.0 mL of lidocaine into the urethra. Wait 2 minutes and repeat twice. *(Level IV*)*	Permits local tissue to absorb lidocaine, thus diminishing pain sensation.	The volume of lidocaine used is determined by the age of the child.[12]
18. Hold catheter in sterile dominant hand and lubricate tip of catheter with water-soluble lubricant. Place distal end of catheter within sterile collection container.	Lubrication facilitates the introduction and passage of catheter through the urethra.	
19. Insert catheter into the urethral meatus and gently advance appropriate distance, dependant on child's age. Advance catheter 2 to 3 cm further than the point at which urine flow is noted.[2,5,6] *(Level II*)*	Length of insertion should be at least 2 cm past the point of visualization of urine in females. In preschool-aged males, insert catheter 7.5 to 10 cm past the point of visualization of urine flow. In males of school age and older, catheter should be inserted 12.5 cm past the point of urine flow.[2,5]	*For females:* If catheter is inadvertently introduced into the vagina, do not remove the catheter. Attempt catheterization into the urethra with a second sterile catheter to prevent reentering the vagina a second time. *For males:* The penis should be held at a 60-degree to 90-degree angle, promoting straightening of the urethra, which allows for easier insertion of the catheter. When the catheter reaches the urethral sphincter, slight resistance may be noted. Use relaxation techniques and distraction while attempting to advance the catheter. Avoid forcibly advancing the catheter against resistance.
20. Collect 10 to 20 mL of urine into sterile specimen container. Allow remaining urine to drain into separate urine collection device.	Allows for sterile collection of urine for analysis.	
21. Remove catheter.	No longer required.	
22. Label specimen(s) at the bedside and complete laboratory paperwork per institution-specific protocol *(Level II*);* send to laboratory within 30 minutes of collection.	Prevents alteration of test results from long delay between time of collection and time of processing in the laboratory. Promotes patient safety; ensures accurate and efficient processing of specimen.	Follow institution-specific protocol for handling and labeling lab specimens.
23. Dispose of equipment into appropriate containers. Wash hands.	Standard precautions.	

* Level II: Theory-based; no research data to support recommendations; recommendations from expert consensus group may exist
Level IV: Limited clinical studies to support recommendations

Expected Outcomes

- Catheter is appropriately placed into the bladder
- Urine specimen is obtained in a sterile manner
- Urine drains from bladder well

- Skin remains intact
- Child is free from complications of urinary catheterization

- Urine specimen is placed in correct specimen container, labeled appropriately and sent to the lab in the appropriate time frame.

Unexpected Outcomes

- Kinking of catheter
- Urine specimen is contaminated
- Inability to advance catheter
- Urine is not obtained
- Urethral trauma
- Introduction of bacteria into the urinary tract, causing urinary tract infection
- Urethral tear
- Placement of catheter into vagina
- Bladder perforation
- Anaphylaxis
- Specimen is mislabeled
- Specimen is placed in incorrect container
- Delay in sending specimens to lab

Monitoring and Care of the Child

Activities and Interventions	Rationale	Reportable Conditions
1. Monitor child's tolerance to procedure.	A change in child's condition may indicate complications from procedure.	• Inability to pass catheter • Symptoms of lower abdominal or stomach pain that may be indicative of bladder spasms or urinary tract infection
2. Monitor characteristics of urine obtained.	Deviation from the normal characteristics may be indicative of a urinary tract infection.	• Blood in urine, foul smell, cloudy color, or presence of sediment

Documentation

- Child and family education
- Child's tolerance of procedure
- Size and type of catheter used
- Amount, color, and clarity of urine from catheterization
- Local anesthetic used
- Specimen collected
- Disposition of specimens, results, and analysis
- Unexpected outcomes and related treatment

References

1. Berkov S, Das S: Urinary tract infection and intermittent catheterization, *Infections Urol* 11:165-168, 1998.
2. Bukowski TP, Freedman AL: Catheterization problems of infants, *Contemp Urol* 66-74, 1999.
3. Cravens DD, Zweig S: Urinary catheter management, *Am Family Physician* 61:369-376, 2000.
4. Day RA, et al: A pilot study comparing two methods of intermittent catheterization: limitations and challenges, *Urol Nurs* 23:143-158, 2003.
5. Elizondo AP, et al: Elimination of bleeding associated with urinary catheterization in neonates, *Neonatal Network* 20(6):25-34, 2001.
6. Smith AB, Adams LL: Insertion of indwelling urethral catheters in infants and children: a survey of current nursing practice, *Pediatr Nurs* 24:229-234, 1998.
7. American Academy of Pediatrics: Practice parameter: the diagnosis, treatment, and evaluation of the initial urinary tract infection in febrile infants and young children, *Pediatrics* 103:843-852, 1999.
8. Burns CE, et al, editors: *Pediatric primary care: a handbook for nurse practitioners,* ed 2, Philadelphia, 2000, Saunders.
9. Hockenberry MJ, et al, editors: *Wong's nursing care of infants and children,* ed 7, St Louis, Mosby, Inc., 2003.
10. American Academy of Pediatrics: The assessment and management of acute pain in infants, children, and adolescents, *Pediatrics* 108:793-797, 2001.
11. Kleiber C, McCarthy AM: Parent behavior and child distress during urethral catheterization, *JSPN* 4:95-104, 1999.
12. Gerard LL, et al: Effectiveness of lidocaine lubricant for discomfort during pediatric urethral catheterization, *J Urol* 170:564-567, 2003.

Additional Readings

Baskin LS, Kogan BA, editors: *Handbook of pediatric urology,* ed 2, Philadelphia, 2005, Lippincott-Raven.
Kunin CM: Nosocomial urinary tract infections and the indwelling catheter, *Chest* 120:10-12, 2001.

AP

Urine Culture: Suprapubic Aspirate

P U R P O S E : A needle aspiration of the bladder is performed to obtain a sterile urine specimen for culture, gram stain, or urinalysis in children less than 2 years of age

Tresa E. Zielinski

PREREQUISITE KNOWLEDGE

- Normal abdominal anatomy and physiology
- A full bladder increases success of the procedure; the child should not have voided within 1 hour of the procedure.[1,2]
- Contraindications include genitourinary abnormalities,[3] evidence of an existing coagulopathy or thrombocytopenia, abdominal distension of unknown etiology, recent abdominal surgery, or suspicion of intestinal obstruction.[1,2]
- Informed consent is required prior to obtaining a urine culture via suprapubic aspirate.

CHILD AND FAMILY ASSESSMENT

- Child's developmental level and ability to interact ➤➤*Rationale:* These factors influence preparation of the child and interaction; suprapubic aspiration may be threatening to the toddler.
- Family's desire to be present during the procedure ➤➤*Rationale:* Family may provide support and comfort measures to the child but should have the choice not to remain with the child.
- History of surgery of the genitourinary (GU) tract or urinary tract abnormalities or history of coagulopathy, thrombocytopenia, or other bleeding disorders ➤➤*Rationale:* These conditions may complicate the procedure or be a direct contraindication to the procedure.
- History of allergy to povidone-iodine ➤➤*Rationale:* Procedure may need to be modified based on allergies to this substance.
- Child's and family's understanding of the reasons for and risks and benefits of the procedure ➤➤*Rationale:* Evaluates child's and family's understanding of the procedure and provides a gauge for ongoing evaluation.

CHILD AND FAMILY EDUCATION

Individualized, developmentally appropriate education is provided to the family and to the child based on desire for knowledge, readiness to learn, and overall neurologic and psychosocial state.

- Explain the importance of sterile specimen for culture, urinalysis, or gram stain ➤➤*Rationale:* Family should understand the reason for the invasive procedure versus noninvasive methods of urine collection.
- Provide procedure details ➤➤*Rationale:* Family should have an understanding of what to expect and have questions and fears addressed.

- Explain the expected outcomes and signs and symptoms of complications ➤➤*Rationale:* As partners in the child's care, the family should know what to watch for after the procedure in case complications arise.

EQUIPMENT

- Sterile gloves
- Povidone-iodine swabs or other skin antiseptic per institution-specific protocol
- Alcohol swabs
- 1-inch to 1.5-inch 25-gauge needle for preterm infants and a 1.5-inch 22-gauge needle for all other children
- 3-mL sterile syringe
- Sterile specimen container
- Specimen labels containing two patient identifiers
- Appropriate laboratory requisitions

Procedure	for Urine Culture: Suprapubic Aspirate	
Steps	**Rationale**	**Considerations**
1. Ensure child, as appropriate, and family understand procedure and questions are answered.	Evaluates understanding of and reinforces previously taught information; facilitates informed consent	Developmental level, cognitive ability and anxiety level will determine approach to and effectiveness of teaching.
2. Obtain informed consent.	Invasive procedures require informed consent.	Informed consent procedures and documentation are institution specific.
3. Consider use of topical analgesic, such as EMLA® (Astra-Zeneca Pharmaceuticals, Wilmington, DE), or topical anesthetic skin refrigerant.	Procedure can be painful.	If topical analgesic is used, apply according to manufacturer's recommendations and leave in place for the appropriate time before procedure. *(Level I*)*
4. Collect all supplies and recruit an assistant unless child is sedated or on a neuromuscular blocking agent.	Availability of all supplies allows completion of procedure in a timely manner.	Needle size used depends on stock supply available.
5. Conduct a final patient verification process; use two patient identifiers to identify child.	Confirms correct patient, procedure, and site, as recommended by the Joint Commission on Accreditation of Healthcare Organizations.	Active communication techniques promote patient safety.
6. Position child in frog-leg position and request that assistant immobilize the child (Figure 113-1).	Safe immobilization of child prevents motion during procedure, decreasing the likelihood of injury.	This position stabilizes the pelvis.
7. Wash hands and put on sterile gloves.	Reduces transmission of microorganisms.	
8. Cleanse skin from the urethra to the umbilicus with povidine-iodine swab or other skin antiseptic.	Removes microorganisms; prevents introduction of bacteria into the bladder.	
9. Identify the suprapubic crease, the site for puncture: draw imaginary line in the midline from umbilicus to the superior portion of the symphysis pubis. Site for puncture is 1 to 2 cm above symphysis pubis in the midline[1,2] (Figure 113-2).	Identifies puncture site.	
10. In the male, apply gentle pressure to penile shaft; apply pressure to urethral meatus in the female.[1,3]	May prevent occurrence of voiding during procedure.	

* Level I: Manufacturer's recommendations only

Procedure	**for Urine Culture: Suprapubic Aspirate**—*Continued*	
Steps	**Rationale**	**Considerations**

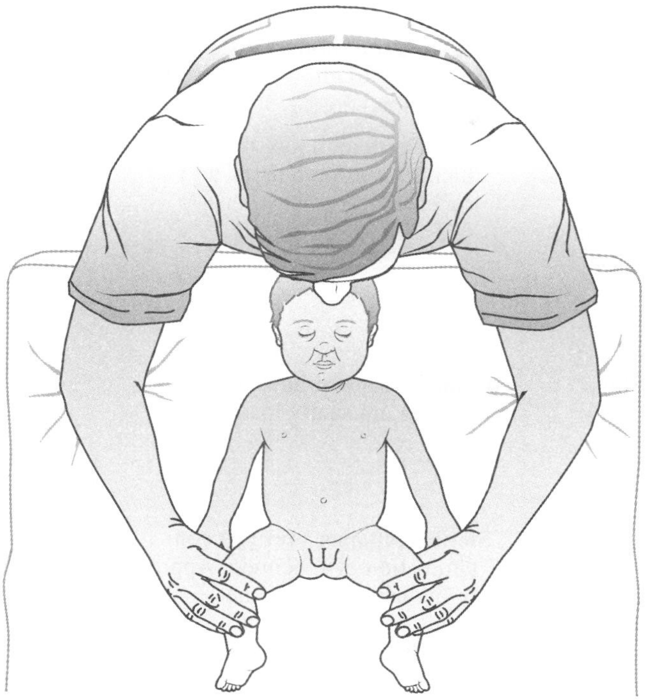

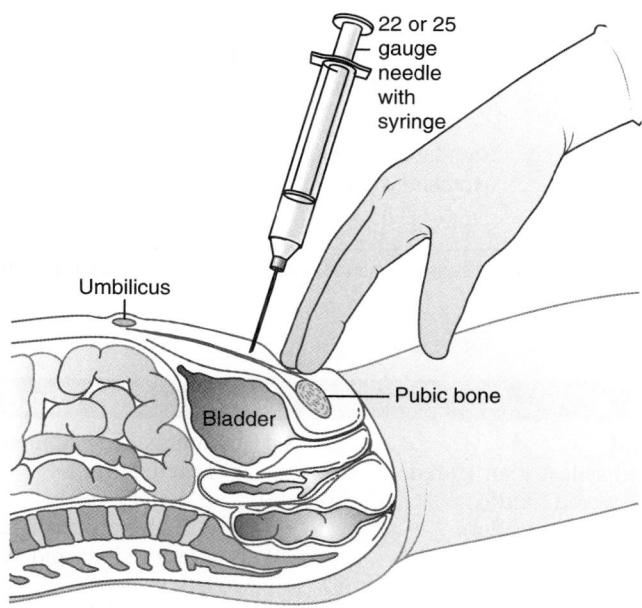

FIGURE 113-1   Child in frog-leg position, with assistant immobilizing legs.

FIGURE 113-2   Suprapubic crease is site for puncture.

Procedure continues on following page

Procedure for Urine Culture: Suprapubic Aspirate—*Continued*

Steps	Rationale	Considerations
11. After identifying suprapubic crease, insert needle perpendicular to the skin and maintain gentle suction on syringe until urine begins to flow into syringe.	With maintenance of gentle suction, the needle can be inserted the shortest distance necessary to allow urine aspiration.	Needle should not be inserted more than 2.5 cm.[3]
12. If unsuccessful, do not remove needle from below the surface of the skin. Instead, change the angle of the needle 10 to 20 degrees, aiming caudally, and reinsert as previously described. Attempt procedure at two different angles varying by 10 degrees.[1,2]	Decreases likelihood of introducing microorganisms into the bladder.	
13. If third attempt is unsuccessful, further attempts are not likely to yield urine unless done with ultrasound scan guidance or after 1 hour of hydration.[1,3]	Bladder may not have urine or may be unusually located.	
14. Place urine obtained in sterile specimen container. Label specimen(s) at the bedside and complete laboratory paperwork per institution-specific protocol *(Level II*)*; send to laboratory within 30 minutes of collection.	Sterile container prevents contamination of specimen. Appropriate label on container promotes patient safety. Promptly sending specimen to the lab prevents alteration of test results from long delay between time of collection and time of processing in the laboratory.	Follow institution-specific protocol for handling and labeling lab specimens.
15. Cleanse skin of povidone-iodine and place adhesive bandage over puncture site.	Povidone-iodine left on the skin may cause local irritation.	
16. Discard supplies in appropriate trash containers. Remove gloves; wash hands.	Standard precautions; prevents transmission of microorganisms.	

* Level II: Theory-based; no research data to support recommendations; recommendations from expert consensus group may exist

Expected Outcomes

- Sterile urine specimen obtained
- Microscopic hematuria defined as less than 10 red blood cells (RBCs) on high-powered field[1,2]
- Child is free from complications of procedure

- Urine specimen is placed in correct specimen container, labeled appropriately and sent to lab in appropriate time frame.

Unexpected Outcomes

- Contaminated specimen
- Gross hematuria

- Fecal matter aspirated; usually benign; simply observe for signs and symptoms of peritonitis[1,2]
- Anxiety
- Infection of abdominal wall around puncture site[1,2]
- Specimen is mislabeled
- Specimen is placed in incorrect container
- Delay in sending specimen to lab

Monitoring and Care of the Child

Activities and Interventions	Rationale	Reportable Conditions
1. Monitor puncture site for redness, swelling, warmth, tenderness, and drainage.	Evaluates for signs and symptoms of infection.	• Any signs or symptoms of infection
2. Monitor urine output and urine quality with urine dip for hematuria.	Microscopic hematuria is expected and should resolve within 24 hours.	• Gross hematuria

Documentation

- Patient/procedure verification process
- Date and time of procedure
- Procedure performed
- Individual who performed procedure
- Pain level and interventions
- Follow-up care necessary
- Laboratory studies obtained and results
- Unexpected outcomes and related treatment

References

1. Dieckman RA, et al, editors: *Pediatric emergency & critical care procedures,* Mosby-Year Book, Inc, 1997, St Louis.
2. Henretig FM, King C, editors: *Textbook of pediatric emergency procedures,* Baltimore, 1997, Williams & Wilkins.
3. Gunn VL, Nechyba C, editors: *The Harriet Lane handbook,* Philadelphia, 2002, Mosby.

Unit VI
Oncology/
Hematology
System

SECTION SIXTEEN
Oncology/Hematology
Procedures

P R O C E D U R E **114**

Bone Marrow Aspiration and Biopsy: Assist

P U R P O S E : To identify hematopoietic diseases, assess therapeutic response to treatment for these diseases, and detect chromosomal abnormalities

Kathryn Carnighan Kuhn

PREREQUISITE KNOWLEDGE

- Child development as it relates to clinical assessment and bone marrow aspiration
- Mastery of pediatric advanced life support competencies
- Principles of aseptic technique
- Appropriate pediatric dosing of analgesics and competency in procedural sedation
- Anatomy of the bone marrow: "after the blood itself, bone marrow is the largest and most widely distributed organ in the body" (p. 2460).[1]
  - ❖ Bone marrow is the site of hematopoiesis (the process of formation and development of blood cell lineages).
  - ❖ The marrow is composed of two parts: the hematopoietic cells and the stromal cells that support the proliferation and differentiation of these cells from stem cells.
- Diagnostic or surveillance purpose of exam
  - ❖ Hematopoietic abnormalities are more easily detected and manifest earlier in the bone marrow than in peripheral blood.
  - ❖ Flow cytometry analysis allows identification of malignant clones.
  - ❖ Cytogenetic analysis allows detection of chromosomal abnormalities associated with hematologic malignancies.
  - ❖ Chimerism studies allow evaluation of engraftment status following allogeneic transplant.
- A bone marrow aspiration provides information about cellular morphology and relative distribution of cell types,

whereas a biopsy allows the most reliable evaluation of overall bone marrow cellularity and the adequacy of bone marrow reconstitution following transplant. The bone marrow biopsy is also useful in the instance of a "dry tap" when aspirate is unable to be obtained, which occurs in approximately 4% of cases and is related to malignant cell proliferation, aplasia, or radiation fibrosis.[1]

- Assessment of lab studies, coupled with child's clinical history, must be understood so the procedure can be performed safely.
- Contraindications include certain bleeding disorders, surgery and/or trauma, and past radiation to site.
- Risks include bleeding, infection, and/or injury to the bowel.
- Informed consent is required before bone marrow aspiration and biopsy.

CHILD AND FAMILY ASSESSMENT

- Child's developmental level and ability to interact ➤➤*Rationale:* These factors influence preparation of the child and interaction.
- History and physical findings ➤➤*Rationale:* Determines if bone marrow examination is needed, risk factors and/or contraindications for procedure, and if child will tolerate prone and/or side-lying positioning during procedure.
- Review results of lab studies including platelet count and prothrombin time/partial thromboplastin time (PT/PTT) ➤➤*Rationale:* Provides baseline studies. Generally accepted

that thrombocytopenia, no matter how profound, is *not a* contraindication for bone marrow aspiration and/or biopsy.[1,2,3] The nurse, however, must be familiar with institution-specific transfusion protocol. Coagulation factor deficiencies are considered contraindications to the procedure, but may be corrected (i.e., factor products, fresh frozen plasma [FFP], vitamin K) before the procedure.[1,2,3] The procedure should be postponed if aspirin is taken within preceding 48 hours.[3]

- Degree of sedation needed based on child's age and experience with painful procedures ➨*Rationale:* Promotes comfort. All children and adolescents should receive sedation for both bone marrow aspiration and biopsy.[4,5,6] Sedation should not be administered by the same practitioner performing the bone marrow procedure to ensure patient safety and adequate pain control.
- Previous sedation experiences ➨*Rationale:* This may influence the type of sedation used.
- Child's and family's understanding of the reasons, risks, and benefits of the procedure ➨*Rationale:* Evaluates child's and family's understanding of the procedure and provides a gauge for ongoing education.
- Family's desire to be present during the procedure ➨*Rationale:* Family may provide support and comfort during the procedure, but should have the choice not to remain with the child.

CHILD AND FAMILY EDUCATION

Individualized, developmentally appropriate education is provided to the child and to the family based on desire for knowledge, readiness to learn, and overall neurologic and psychosocial state.

- Explain steps of procedure and sequence of events ➨*Rationale:* Promotes understanding and alleviates fear and anxiety. Ensures that child and family are making an informed decision.
- Reassure the family and child that pain and antianxiety medications will be given before and during the procedure ➨*Rationale:* Bone marrow aspiration and biopsy are two of the most painful procedures for children.[4,5,6] Appropriate pain management alleviates pain during the

procedure, decreases anxiety about future procedures, and creates a controlled setting in which the practitioner may safely perform the procedure. The cooperation of the child for subsequent procedures is directly influenced by the painlessness and ease of the initial procedure.[7]

- Child's and family's understanding of the reasons for and risks and benefits of the procedure ➨*Rationale:* Reinforces previous teaching and protects child and family autonomy.
- For outpatient procedures, teach family signs and symptoms of site infection and complications that warrant a return to the clinic or hospital. Teach family to keep pressure dressing intact for 12 hours, and area clean and dry for 24 hours. ➨*Rationale:* Provides family with information needed to provide safer care for the child at home.
- Encourage questions and answer questions as they arise ➨*Rationale:* Reinforcement of information is needed during periods of stress.

EQUIPMENT

- Aspiration needle (e.g., Illinois)
- Biopsy needle and stylet (e.g., Jamshidi)
- Skin antiseptic agent
- Clean gloves, protective eyewear, mask, gown
- Sterile gloves
- 1% lidocaine vial
- Sterile 0.9% saline vial
- Preservative-free heparin (1:1000) vial
- Three or four 20-mL syringes
- #11 scalpel blade
- Two 25-gauge and two 19-gauge needles
- Sterile fenestrated drape
- Sterile 2×2 and 4×4 gauze
- Preservative-free heparin tubes (quantity dependent on desired samples)
- Sterile specimen container
- Sterile labels and pen, if available
- Alcohol wipes
- Pressure dressing
- Slides (preparation and preparation material per institution-specific requirements)

Procedure	**for Bone Marrow Aspiration and Biopsy: Assist**	
Steps	Rationale	Considerations
1. Ensure child and family understand procedure and questions are answered.	Evaluates and reinforces understanding of previously taught information.	Developmental level, cognitive ability, and anxiety level will determine approach to, and effectiveness of, teaching.
2. Confirm that consent for procedure has been obtained.	Ensures medicolegal compliance as suggested by the Joint Commission on Accreditation of Healthcare Organizations (JCAHO).	

Procedure for Bone Marrow Aspiration and Biopsy: Assist—*Continued*

Steps	Rationale	Considerations
3. If required for sedation plan, ensure fasting guidelines have been implemented per institution-specific protocol. *(Level VI*)*	Prevents sedation complications related to emesis/aspiration.	NPO time is related to child's age and type of diet.
4. Gather needed equipment and supplies.	Facilitates completion of procedure in a timely manner.	Quantity of tubes required is dependent on desired samples to be obtained. Slide preparation and materials needed are per institution-specific protocols.
5. Identify the child using appropriate patient/procedure verification process (e.g., "Time out").	Confirms correct patient, procedure and site as recommended by JCAHO; prevents unnecessary medical procedures. Use of at least two patient identifiers improves the accuracy of identification.	Verification process and documentation are institution specific; use active communication techniques.
6. Wash hands.	Standard precautions; reduces transmission of microorganisms.	
7. Ensure appropriate monitoring, including pulse oximetry is in place and that the child has functioning venous access if required for sedation administration. *(Level III*)*	Continuous monitoring allows assessment of child's status while sedated. Functioning venous access may be required to administer emergency medications or sedation as needed.	Alarm limits should be individualized to the child.
8. Assist with positioning child—either side lying with knees to chest or prone with towel under hips to elevate pelvis (see Figure 117-2 in Procedure 117).	Facilitates procedure and ensures appropriate procedure site.	Side-lying or prone position based on size and clinical status of child.
9. Assist with opening supplies or bone marrow tray, establishing sterile field; place necessary syringes and aspiration/biopsy needles on a sterile tray using sterile technique.	Maintains sterility and prepares supplies.	
10. Put on eye protection, clean gown, mask, cap, and gloves.	Standard precautions; reduces transmission of microorganisms. Protects personnel from exposure to blood-borne pathogens.	Use of mask and clean gown is per institution-specific protocol for procedure.
11. Assist with preparation of heparinized syringes. Invert vial of preservative-free heparin so that practitioner may withdraw 1 to 2 mL into a 20-mL syringe(s).	Heparinized aspirate is used for flow cytometry, cytogenetics, and chimerism studies. Quantity of heparinized syringes will depend on the type of diagnostic tests performed.	
12. Discard gloves, wash hands, put on sterile gloves.	Minimizes transmission of microorganisms. Maintains sterile technique.	

Procedure continues on following page

* Level III: Laboratory data, no clinical data to support recommendations
Level VI: Clinical studies in a variety of patient populations and situations to support recommendations

Procedure for Bone Marrow Aspiration and Biopsy: Assist—*Continued*

Steps	Rationale	Considerations
13. Assist with cleansing selected procedure site with antiseptic solution.	Decreases risk of introducing infectious organisms during procedure.	
14. Assist with the administration of 1% lidocaine as needed.	Local anesthetic.	
15. Assist with processing aspirate specimen by placing drops of aspirate on slide to look for spicules.	Spicules are white-appearing fragments that contain bone marrow particles. Their presence is indicative of an adequate location within the bone marrow cavity.	Appropriate slide preparation is crucial and process varies by institution— some require providers to prepare samples, others provide lab techs. Adequate training in slide preparation is essential and beyond the scope of this procedure.
16. Assist with processing additional heparinized samples. Place aspirate in preservative-free heparin tubes or cap syringes for later disposition.	Heparinized samples are required for cytogenetic, flow cytometry, and chimerism studies.	3 to 5 mL is generally adequate for most laboratory analyses; refer to institution-specific guidelines.
17. Assist with placement of biopsy core sample in container with sterile 0.9% saline–soaked gauze.	Prevents core specimen from becoming dry and unsuitable for interpretation.	
18. Using dry sterile gauze, assist with holding pressure to site for 3 to 5 minutes, followed by the application of a sterile pressure dressing.	Minimizes risk of bleeding and hematoma.	
19. Discard used supplies and equipment in appropriate receptacle; ensure sharps are safely disposed.	Standard precautions; reduces transmission of microorganisms. Protects personnel health.	
20. Remove gloves; wash hands.	Standard precautions; reduces transmission of microorganisms.	

Expected Outcomes

- Adequate samples collected

- Procedure is completed without complications
- Respiratory status remains stable
- Sedation level is adequate during procedure
- Child demonstrates acceptable level of comfort during and after procedure

Unexpected Outcomes

- Fibrotic or hypocellular marrow prevents aspiration collection
- Inadequate biopsy core obtained
- Bleeding, infection, injury to the bowel
- Respiratory distress or failure
- Unmanaged anxiety or agitation
- Unmanaged pain

Monitoring and Care of the Child

Activities and Interventions	Rationale	Reportable Conditions
1. Provide appropriate analgesics before, during, and after the procedure; assess effectiveness of pain management strategy. Encourage the family to assist in using nonpharmacologic means to comfort and support the child.	Promotes comfort, minimizes fear, and decreases anxiety regarding future procedures. *(Level V*)*	• Unmanaged pain
2. Monitor vital signs and pulse oximetry throughout the procedure and sedation recovery phase per institution-specific protocol.	Monitors for complications of sedation.	• Changes in vital signs or oxygen saturation from baseline • Delayed recovery from sedation

* Level V: Clinical studies in more than one or two patient populations and situations to support recommendations

Monitoring and Care of the Child—Cont'd

Activities and Interventions	Rationale	Reportable Conditions
3. Assess procedure site for bleeding or hematoma. If the child is to be discharged postprocedure, review signs and symptoms of site infection, complications that warrant a return to the clinic or hospital, and dressing and site care with family before discharge.	Determines presence of procedure-related complications. Reinforces home care instructions with family.	• Bleeding, hematoma, erythema, discharge, fever

Documentation

- Consent for procedure
- Patient/procedure verification process
- Vital signs throughout procedure and recovery per institution-specific protocol
- Sedation required for procedure and response
- Preparation of child including antiseptic cleansing, positioning, and site selection
- Compliance with fasting guidelines, if appropriate
- Diagnostic and/or monitoring studies sent for laboratory analysis
- Unexpected outcomes and related treatment
- Child's tolerance of procedure including any complications
- Education of child and family, including postprocedure instructions

References

1. Ryan DH, Cohen HJ: Bone marrow aspiration and morphology. In Hoffman R, et al, editors: *Hematology basic principles and practice,* ed 3, New York, 2000, Churchill Livingstone.
2. Head DR, Pui CH: Diagnosis and classification. In Pui CH, editor: *Childhood leukemias,* Cambridge, 2000, Cambridge University Press.
3. Nguyen DT, Diamond LW: Approach to the bone marrow. *Diagnostic hematology: a pattern approach,* Oxford, UK, 2000, Butterworth Heinemann.
4. Collins JJ, Weisman SJ: Management of pain in childhood cancer. In Schechter NL, et al, editors: *Pain in infants, children, and adolescents,* ed 2, Philadelphia, 2003, Lippincott Williams & Wilkins.
5. Hertzog JH, et al: Prospective evaluation of propofol anesthesia in the pediatric intensive care unit for elective oncology procedures in ambulatory hospitalized children. *Pediatrics* 106:742-747, 2000.
6. McGrath PA: Acute pains. In McGrath PA, editor: *Pain in children: nature, assessment, and treatment.* New York, 1990, Guilford Press.
7. Miller DR: Normal blood values from birth through adolescence. In Miller DR, et al, editors. *Blood diseases of infancy and childhood,* ed 7, St. Louis, 1995, Mosby.

Additional Readings

Oakes LL, Rosenthal-Dichter C: Hematology and immunology. In Slota MC, editor: *Core curriculum for pediatric critical care nursing,* Philadelphia, 1998, Saunders.

Trewhitt KG: Bone marrow aspiration and biopsy: collection and interpretation, *Oncol Nurs Forum* 28:1409-1417, 2001.

Red Cell Exchange Transfusion: Manual and Automated

P U R P O S E : To remove abnormal red blood cells and replace them with normal red blood cells as therapy for children with intrinsic red cell defects or extracorpuscular defects thus reducing blood viscosity and vascular stasis

Lucy Thompson

PREREQUISITE KNOWLEDGE

- Child development as it relates to clinical assessment and red blood cell exchange (RBCX) transfusion
- Mastery of pediatric advanced life support competencies
- Principles of aseptic technique
- Physiologic indicators for the red cell exchange transfusion therapy: the "presence of abnormal red blood cells (RBCs) in the circulation due to intrinsic red cell defects or extracorpuscular defects."[1] Intrinsic defects of red cells result from disorders of hemoglobin, the erythrocyte membrane, and red cell enzymes.[1]
- The individual disease characteristics for which the exchange is being performed. For example, hemoglobinopathies such as methemoglobinemia, sickle cell disease, β-thalassemia syndrome, and hemoglobins with high oxygen affinity.[1,2]
- The differences between automated and rapid manual RBCX transfusions
  - ❖ *Automated red cell exchange transfusion:* the goal of pheresis is to rapidly reduce hemoglobin S (Hb S) to less than 30%, with the child's hemoglobin being transfused up to 10 gm/dL.[3]
  - ❖ *Rapid manual partial exchange transfusion:* Packed red cells are initially transfused while whole blood is removed to reduce the percentage of Hb S without further increasing the hemoglobin levels. This technique is applicable to adults and children and is based on the initial hematocrit (Hct) and body weight in kilograms.
- ❖ *Chronic transfusion:* Transfuse 5 to 10 mL/kg of packed red cells every 3 to 4 weeks to maintain a Hct of more than 30%.
- ❖ Calculation of total blood volume (TBV); accuracy of calculating TBV may be affected by health and disease states, physiologic state, and body compensation.
  - ○ TBV = 89 – 105 mL/kg in premature infants
  - ○ TBV = 82 – 86 mL/kg in term neonates
  - ○ TBV = 73 – 82 mL/kg in infants and preschool children
  - ○ TBV = 70 mL/kg in adults (75 mL/kg with chronic anemia)
  - ○ Red cell volume of child = TBV × Hct
- General goal of treatment: to establish less than 30% Hb S in the circulation with an Hb of 10 gm/dL.[3]
  - ❖ *For Hct up to 19% (Hb > 6.5 gm/dL):* Give packed cells equal to 30 mL/kg body weight while removing an equal volume of child's whole blood. Remove an additional 40 mL/kg of the child's whole blood while replacing with mL for mL equivalents of donor whole blood.[3]
  - ❖ *For Hct between 20% and 30% (Hb 6.6 to 10 gm/dL):* Exchange 10 mL/kg body weight by giving packed cells while removing whole blood, then exchange another 70 mL/kg body weight, giving donor whole

blood equivalents for child's whole blood volumes removed.[3]

❖ **For Hct greater than 30% (Hb 10 gm/dL):** Exchange whole blood removed with 0.9% saline for 10 mL/kg body weight, and then exchange subsequent child's whole blood removed with donor whole blood equivalents.[3]

- Hemodynamic effects of rapid blood loss that are dependent on the volume lost, child's size, and clinical condition.
  ❖ Hemodynamically stable children can lose up to 15% of their TBV and experience no changes in cardiac output or oxygen consumption as a result of compensation through vasoconstriction of the great veins.[1]
  ❖ Losses greater than 15% of the child's TBV result in signs and symptoms of decreased cardiac output such as decreased pulses, pallor, hypotension, tachycardia, and endocrine and metabolic compensation.
  ❖ Losses greater than 30% of the child's TBV result in circulatory shock due to hypovolemia. Signs and symptoms of hypovolemia are tachycardia, orthostatic hypotension, narrow pulse pressure, apprehension, weakness, nausea, lightheadedness, pallor, thirst, cool skin, and loss of consciousness.
- Effective hemodynamic compensation throughout the procedure is dependent on the child's pulmonary, cardiac, and renal function.
- Intravascular volume management during the procedure is directly dependent on continual evaluation of the child's clinical condition.
- Informed consent is required before red cell exchange transfusion.

For Automated Red Cell Exchange Transfusion

- Maintaining an appropriate ratio of extracorporeal volume (ECV) of the apheresis system to the child's TBV is essential in ensuring procedural hemodynamic stability.
  ❖ Volume of the circuit used in the apheresis equipment must be known in order to calculate ECV.
- The engineering of apheresis equipment is adult based; hence the performance of safe procedures in children requires modification of the equipment's procedural protocol; for example, the manual calculation of the child's total red cell replacement volume.
- Specific training for initiation and maintenance of automated red cell exchange transfusion, including pump and circuit management per institution specific protocol

CHILD AND FAMILY ASSESSMENT

- History of hematologic disorders including effectiveness of treatment modalities and regimens ➥*Rationale:* Identifies potential adverse reactions and contraindications of planned treatment.
- Child's developmental level and ability to interact ➥*Rationale:* These factors influence preparation of the child and interaction.

- Child's and family's understanding of the reasons for and risks and benefits of the procedure, as well as experience with RBCX ➥*Rationale:* Evaluates child's and family's understanding of the procedure and provides a gauge for ongoing education.
- Level of consciousness and cognitive ability ➥*Rationale:* Assesses the child's potential need for sedation and analgesia before, during, and after the procedure.
- Admission history and primary presenting problem ➥*Rationale:* Identifies possible contraindications of treatment with other presenting problems.
- Current hemodynamic status ➥*Rationale:* Determines hemodynamic status and anticipates child's needs.
- Patency of existing vascular access devices (VADs) ➥*Rationale:* Adequate vascular access is necessary to perform RBCX.
- Assess baseline vital signs including neurologic status, bedside blood glucose, color, tone, and behavior ➥*Rationale:* Establishing baseline allows prompt identification of status changes during procedure.
- Current laboratory value status ➥*Rationale:* Identifies conditions requiring treatment before, during, and following the procedure.
- Family's desire to be present during the procedure ➥*Rationale:* Family may provide support and comfort to the child, but should have the choice not to remain with the child.

CHILD AND FAMILY EDUCATION

Individualized, developmentally appropriate education is provided to the child and to the family based on desire for knowledge, readiness to learn, and overall neurologic and psychosocial state.

- Provide information describing the individual case specific reason(s) for the procedure, the processes involved in performing the procedure and the expected outcomes of the procedure ➥*Rationale:* Providing information decreases anxiety and fear; allows the child and family to construct specific questions related to the procedure, its risks and expected outcomes; and allows the child and family to express fears associated with particular aspects of the procedure.
- Provide information outlining the risks associated with the transfusion of blood products ➥*Rationale:* Providing information decreases anxiety and fear, facilitates informed decision making.
- If appropriate, explain that preparation for the procedure requires the child to undergo insertion of a VAD; provide an approximate time frame required for placement of vascular access ➥*Rationale:* The risks and time period associated with the acquisition of vascular access should be clearly understood by the child and family; may decrease family's anxiety associated with long procedure time.
- Educate the child and family about specific disease characteristics and signs and symptoms of improvement and deterioration ➥*Rationale:* An informed patient population aids in gathering accurate, precise information.

- Educate the child and family about the goals of treatment
  ➥*Rationale:* Awareness of the treatment goals will assist in alleviating child and family anxiety associated with the procedure, environment, and staff.
- Encourage questions and answer questions as they arise
  ➥*Rationale:* Reinforcement of information is needed during periods of stress.

EQUIPMENT (MANUAL RED CELL EXCHANGE TRANSFUSION)

- Blood administration set with blood infusion filter
- Blood wastage bag
- Sterile drapes and gowns
- Stopcocks
- Various size syringes
- Alcohol swabs
- Disposable surgical caps
- Surgical face masks
- Eye protection
- Two or three pairs sterile gloves
- Sterile 4×4 gauze
- Sterile 2×2 gauze
- Sterile 0.9% saline for injection
- Blood tubes for complete blood count (CBC), serum bilirubin (SBR), requested laboratory specimens

- Arterial blood gas syringes
- Labels with appropriate information
- Resuscitation cart and equipment
- Supplies to obtain vascular access or access existing vascular access
- Red blood cell exchange patient information sheet or institution specific documentation form
- Blood products per prescribing practitioner's order

ADDITIONAL EQUIPMENT (FOR AUTOMATED RED CELL EXCHANGE TRANSFUSION)

- Equipment software including instructions for setup and priming procedure
- RBCX blood tubing set
- Single-stage channel filter
- 1000-mL bag 0.9% saline—stored at room temperature
- 19-gauge needles
- Supplies for the child's VAD, or two 17-gauge Terumo® apheresis needles (Terumo Medical Corporation, Somerset, NJ)
- Relevant therapeutic apheresis documents
- Anticoagulant: ACD-A stored at room temperature

Procedure | for Manual Red Cell Exchange Transfusion

Steps	Rationale	Considerations
1. Ensure family understands procedure and questions are answered.	Evaluates and reinforces understanding of previously taught information.	Developmental level, cognitive ability and anxiety level will determine approach to and effectiveness of teaching.
2. Gather needed equipment and supplies.	Facilitates completion of procedure in a timely manner.	
3. Confirm that consent for procedure has been obtained.	Ensures medicolegal compliance as suggested by the Joint Commission on Accreditation of Healthcare Organizations (JCAHO).	
4. Calculate the volume of RBCs to be exchanged using the same formula as prescribing practitioner.	Validates calculation is correct; RBCX volumes may vary depending on the child's history and current medical status.	
5. Verify child's identity using at least two patient identifiers per institution-specific protocol.	Promotes patient safety per JCAHO recommendations; improves the accuracy of patient identification.	Refer to institution-specific protocols for patient identification.
6. Obtain requested blood studies: generally, complete blood count (CBC), type and cross-match.	CBC and platelet count results that are less than 8 hours old are preferable. Blood study results must be available before beginning the procedure.	Blood specimens may be collected the day before the scheduled procedure for outpatients. Hospital inpatients should have blood specimens processed stat. Hypokalemia and hypocalcemia detected prior to the procedure should be corrected before the procedure begins.

Procedure for Manual Red Cell Exchange Transfusion—*Continued*

Steps	Rationale	Considerations
7. The prescribing practitioner will request the desired number of RBC units to be cross-matched according to institution-specific protocol for RBCX transfusions and the desired goal Hct for the individual child. NOTE: **Only** the child's prescribing practitioner can decide the desired end Hct.	The average Hct of all replacement red cell units is: Sum of Hct in each replacement red cell unit ÷ number of red cell units.[3] The prescribing practitioner's order for the total red cell replacement volume will correspond to the total volume of cross-matched units ordered.	Prefiltered, sickle-dex–negative RBCs should be ordered.[4,5] NOTE: To perform an *even exchange,* aim for the same Hct as noted at the beginning of the RBCX. To *hypertransfuse* or increase the Hct, aim for a Hct higher than at the beginning of the RBCX. To *decrease Hct,* aim for a lower Hct than at the beginning of the RBCX.
8. Wash hands and put on personal protective equipment including eye protection as appropriate.	Standard precautions; reduces transmission of microorganisms and protects personnel from exposure to blood-borne pathogens.	
9. Ensure appropriate cardio-respiratory monitoring; infants should be placed on a heated warmer bed.	Child may demonstrate hemodynamic instability or decompensate during the procedure; consider the child's status when selecting appropriate monitoring. Infants are at risk for hypothermia.	Dysrhythmias may occur as a result of acute changes in serum electrolytes especially potassium and calcium. Intravascular volume management during the procedure is directly dependent on continuous evaluation of the child's clinical condition.
10. Ensure the child is NPO before the procedure. Evacuate gastric contents using an appropriate size gastric tube as indicated.	Potential hypoperfusion to the gut during the exchange transfusion places the child at risk of significant injury. Infants are at risk of developing necrotizing enterocolitis (NEC) during the procedure.	Orogastric and nasogastric tubes should remain to free drainage throughout the procedure.
11. Assist with insertion of vascular access lines as required; if child has VAD already present, assess patency.	Functioning vascular access is required in order to perform RBCX.	A double-lumen central venous catheter or peripheral IV and arterial line may be used to perform this procedure.
12. Two appropriate health care providers check each blood product unit for correctness and validate with prescribing practitioner's order per institution-specific protocol; revalidate patient identity with at least two patient identifiers before administration of each blood product unit.	Use of two patient identifiers improves the accuracy of patient identification. Two provider-independent verifications of correct patient, product, and volume is highly recommended. This procedure requires a prescribing practitioner's order.	
13. Set up blood warmer following manufacturer's instructions; verify appropriate functioning of alarm system. (*Level I*[*])	Ensuring all equipment is properly functioning at beginning of the procedure will decrease the likelihood of ending the procedure prematurely.	Faulty equipment that has not been repaired and/or checked by biomedical engineering poses a threat to patient safety.
14. Prepare sterile field.	Ensures that all necessary equipment is present and accessible to practitioner performing the procedure.	Readily available, well-organized equipment will aid in optimizing patient outcomes during emergency situations.
15. Place filter and disposable blood wastage bag on field using aseptic technique.	Aseptic technique should be maintained throughout the procedure to minimize the risk of infection.	

Procedure continues on following page

* Level I: Manufacturer's recommendations only

Procedure for Manual Red Cell Exchange Transfusion—*Continued*

Steps	Rationale	Considerations

16. Connect tubing in the following order:
    Blood product bag
    Infusion filter
    Blood coil or blood warmer tubing
    Attach tubing to blood product bag and flush to remove air
	Assemble the equipment in a methodic and systematic manner to ensure that all steps are complete. Ensure that all blood products are checked and filtered before administration.	Maximizing the opportunity for the donor blood to warm to 36.7° to 37° C will aid in decreasing the child's hemodynamic instability throughout the procedure.

17. Attach the following tubing in the order specified immediately before beginning exchange: **For Blood Removal** • Extension tubing from arterial line to two three-way stopcocks. • Syringe is attached to proximal three-way stopcock for blood withdrawal and sampling • Arterial line transducer and tubing is attached to distal three-way stopcock to enable intermittent blood pressure measurements. • Blood disposal bag is attached to distal three-way stopcock. **For Blood Infusion** • Extension tubing from warmer blood coil to three-way stopcock. • Extension tubing from three-way stopcock to venous access line. • Syringe is attached to three-way stopcock to enable aliquot infusion of blood to the child.	Forms a closed system, minimizing risk of infection.	Blood products also may be infused via infusion pump at a continuous rate.
18. Connect removal and infusion tubings to appropriate access lines using appropriate aseptic technique.	Establishes mechanisms for blood administration and withdrawal.	Aseptic technique in addition to minimal line interruption will significantly reduce the risk of bloodstream infections. In situations in which asepsis is interrupted, the procedure should be suspended until aseptic technique has been reestablished.
19. Practitioner performing procedure will remove first syringe of blood from child and pass it to assistant. Place in appropriate laboratory specimen tubes labeled per institution-specific protocol and "preexchange" per prescribing practitioner's order.	Blood specimens are labeled and sent stat for laboratory analysis. Follow-up and reporting of blood results is an essential part of the nursing role and responsibility throughout this procedure.	A blood glucose level must be checked with each blood sample that is obtained. Correcting blood glucose fluctuations should be a priority throughout the procedure. Children experiencing multisystem organ failure as a result of sepsis may require the collection of additional laboratory specimens.
20. Blood is drawn out of the child in aliquots specified in the	Blood is to be withdrawn only from the arterial line; administration of	Observe for arterial spasm and decreased perfusion.

Procedure for Manual Red Cell Exchange Transfusion—*Continued*

Steps	Rationale	Considerations
prescribing practitioner's order via the arterial access device, and discarded via the waste line. *(Level II*)*	blood through the arterial line could compromise perfusion to the hand.	
21. Simultaneously, warmed donor blood (packed red blood cells [PRBCs] or whole blood as specified in the prescribing practitioner's order) is drawn into a syringe in the exact same aliquot and administered to the child via the venous access device. *(Level II*)*	A slow, set rate should be used for the removal and injection of blood.	
22. Blood is exchanged slowly using a closed system and three-way stopcock until the desired amount of blood has been exchanged. All recording is done by the RN assisting with the procedure. *(Level II*)*	A closed exchange system reduces the risk of infection through minimal line interruption. The calculated total volume to be exchanged should be independently verified by two practitioners to ensure accuracy. Performing the procedure at a slow pace enables accurate assessment of the child's hemodynamic status throughout the procedure. A slow procedure is a safe procedure.	Isovolumetric exchange transfusions decrease the risk of hemodynamic instability due to the simultaneous removal and replacement of blood volume, and the minimal change in cardiac output. Donor blood should be shaken every 30 minutes during the procedure to prevent the settling of red cells.
23. Inform the prescribing practitioner at regular intervals when predetermined volumes of blood have been administered and removed from the child. Obtain laboratory specimens and administer electrolyte replacement per prescribing practitioner's order.	Child may experience an acute change in blood glucose levels and serum electrolytes, especially calcium and potassium during the procedure requiring immediate replacement. Calcium levels are particularly affected by the use of blood products containing the anticoagulant preservative citrate phosphate dextrose (CPD).	The anticoagulant preservative CPD binds with ionic calcium and magnesium to produce significant depression of these cations.[4,5] Low ionized calcium levels may produce cardiac effects such as a prolonged Q-T interval (>0.2 second).
24. On completion of the procedure, obtain and send requested specimens per prescribing practitioner's order. Blood specimens are sent stat and are labeled "postexchange."	Coagulation studies, blood counts, and electrolytes must be monitored at completion of the procedure in order to identify and correct any abnormalities and ascertain hemodynamic and clinical chemistry status.	Assessment and treatment of unstable rebounding laboratory values is a priority in the child's postexchange care.
25. Discard blood removed, tubing, and blood product bags in appropriate biohazardous waste material containers.	Standard precautions; reduces exposure of health care workers to blood. The waste red blood cells are not to be transfused back to the child.	Use standard precautions at all times.
26. Flush access lines and connect to infusions or saline or heparin lock per prescribing practitioner's order or institution-specific protocol.	Clearing blood from the access lines prevents clot formation and maintains patency of access.	
27. Remove personal protective equipment; wash hands.	Standard precautions; reduces transmission of microorganisms.	

Procedure continues on following page

* Level II: Theory based, no research data to support recommendations: recommendations from expert consensus group may exist

Procedure for Automated Red Cell Exchange Transfusion—*Continued*

Steps	Rationale	Considerations

There are a variety of apheresis systems available. Although attempting to be as generic as possible, the following equipment and procedural steps pertain in part to the COBE Spectra Version 4.7 software (Gambro BCT, Lakewood, CO).[6] This procedure should be performed only by individuals with specific training in initiation and maintenance of automated red cell exchange equipment, including pump and circuit management per institution-specific protocol.

Steps	Rationale	Considerations
28. Refer to steps 1 through 12 above.		
29. Set up and prime machine according to procedure for setup and priming for therapeutic red cell exchange as per manufacturer's guidelines. *(Level I*)*	Ensuring all equipment is properly functioning at beginning of the procedure will decrease the likelihood of ending the procedure prematurely.	Faulty equipment that has not been repaired and/or checked by biomedical engineering poses a threat to patient safety.
30. Record lot numbers and expiration dates of the blood tubing set, normal saline solution, and ACD-A on the therapeutic apheresis record.	Accurate documentation of all equipment and solutions used throughout the procedure *is* required for patient safety and any adverse procedural reaction investigations.	
31. Connect replacement solution spikes to replacement fluid (prefiltered leukocyte-poor PRBC). *(Level I*)*	Ensures aseptic technique to reduce infection risks.	
32. Enter requested patient data into machine. Data requested generally includes gender, height, weight. *(Level I*)*	This information provides important data for the automated TBV calculation used as part of the RBCX.	Intravascular volume management during the procedure is directly dependent on continuous evaluation of the child's clinical condition.
33. Confirm patient data input. *(Level I*)*	Accurate information will aid in preventing hemodynamic instability throughout the procedure.	
34. Enter child's Hct. *(Level I*)*	Ensure the use of CBC results from within the last 8 hours when possible.	
35. Enter average replacement fluid Hct. *(Level I*)*	The average Hct of all replacement red cell units is: Sum of Hct in each replacement red cell unit ÷ Number of red cell units[3]	This information may be supplied by the blood bank when units are dispensed.
36. Enter desired end Hct per prescribing practitioner's order. *(Level I*)*	Data are used by the pump.	To perform an *even exchange*, enter the same Hct as entered in step 34. To *hypertransfuse or increase the Hct*, enter a Hct higher than entered in step 34. To *decrease hematocrit*, enter a lower Hct than entered in step 34.
37. Enter desired fluid balance (generally 100%).	In isovolumetric exchange, no fluid is removed or added.	
38. If display reads "Calculate replacement fluid volume needed?" Press "No." *(Level I*)*	The prescribing practitioner's order specifies total red cell replacement volume: sum of volumes of crossmatched units ordered for the child.	
39. Enter total replacement fluid volume by adding volume of all units crossmatched.	Volume is included in prescribing practitioner's order.	

* Level I: Manufacturer's recommendations only

Procedure for Manual Red Cell Exchange Transfusion—*Continued*

Steps	Rationale	Considerations
40. The screen will display the red cell exchange results based on data entered. Approve red cell exchange results. *(Level I*)*	Carefully check all information to ensure the accuracy of the data entered.	
41. Connect child to the machine following manufacturer's instructions.	Required for initiation of RBCX.	
42. Initiate therapy per manufacturer's instructions.	Begins RBCX.	If the child will not tolerate a volume deficit equal to the tubing volume, return prime solution to the child per manufacturer's instructions.
43. Perform checks on the red cell/plasma interface every 30 minutes throughout the procedure to ensure red cells are not accumulating in the channel. *(Level I*)*	Ensures red cells are not accumulating in the channel.	
44. Obtain laboratory specimens and administer electrolyte replacement per prescribing practitioner's order.	Child may experience an acute change in blood glucose levels and serum electrolytes, especially calcium and potassium during the procedure, requiring immediate replacement. Calcium levels are particularly affected by the use of blood products containing the anticoagulant preservative CPD.	Anticoagulant preservative CPD binds with ionic calcium and magnesium to produce significant depression of these cations.[4,5] Low ionized calcium levels may produce cardiac effects such as a prolonged Q-T interval (>0.2 second).
45. Display on machine will alert when the procedure is complete. Terminate therapy per manufacturer's instructions. Do not perform rinseback.	Rinseback returns waste RBCs to child. Waste red blood cells are not to be transfused back to the child.	
46. Follow steps 24 through 27 above to complete procedure.		

* Level I: Manufacturer's recommendations only

Expected Outcomes

- Measurable improvement of underlying abnormal physiology and/or disease process
- Stable hemodynamic status

- Child remains free from transfusion-related complications

- Laboratory blood values remain within the child's normal limits
- Fluid balance neutral

- Intravascular catheters intact

Unexpected Outcomes

- Child's status is not improved after procedure

- Shock resulting from multiple factors
- Cardiac arrest
- Air or blood embolus
- Infection and sepsis related to invasive procedure
- Transfusion reaction: hives, fever, chills
- Chronic blood loss with repeated procedures
- Clinically significant hypoglycemia, hypocalcemia, hypokalemia, or hyperkalemia
- Volume overload resulting in congestive heart failure
- Insufficient blood cells resulting in anemia
- Hemorrhage as a result of coagulopathy
- Unable to access or flush catheters

Monitoring and Care of the Child

Activities and Interventions	Rationale	Reportable Conditions
1. Monitor vital signs and neurologic status every 15 minutes throughout procedure; more often if unstable. Observe the child continually.	Ensures adequate cardiac output and developmentally appropriate neurologic status.	• Changes in the child's color, behavior, and hemodynamic status should be reported *immediately* to prescribing practitioner. • Hemodynamically stable children can lose up to 15% of their TBV and experience no changes in cardiac output or oxygen consumption as a result of compensation through vasoconstriction of the great veins.[6]
2. Routine observations and monitoring of vital signs begun after completion of procedure, if observations are within normal limits.	Monitors for complications of procedure.	• Deterioration in vital signs
3. On completion of the procedure, observe child for signs of complications, including heart failure, hypocalcemia, hypoglycemia, sepsis, acidosis, shock or bleeding, and intestinal perforation due to ischemia of the bowel (decreased blood flow to intestine resulting from increased back pressure created in the portal venous system). *(Level II*)*	Replacement of partial or total blood volume is a high risk procedure requiring intensive observation, monitoring, and documentation of child's status. Monitor the child closely for the first 12 hours following the procedure to ensure hemodynamic stability.	• Indications of congestive heart failure • Hypocalcemia • Hypoglycemia • Indications of infection • Hypotension • Poor peripheral perfusion • Bleeding • Increasing abdominal girth • Fever
4. Obtain frequent blood specimens per prescribing practitioner's order during and after the procedure.	Facilitates identification of abnormalities and implementation of treatment for changes in glucose, electrolyte, and CBC values. Frequent arterial blood gas (ABG) analysis will allow for the accurate ongoing assessment of the child's acid-base balance as well as electrolyte status. The high glucose content of CPD may stimulate insulin secretion, leading to rebound hypoglycemia following the transfusion. This hypoglycemia usually occurs 30 minutes to 2 hours after the exchange has been completed.[6] CPD has approximately half the acid load of acid citrate dextrose (ACD) preservative and the pH remains the same for approximately 7 days. ACD has a pH of 6.7 after 2 to 3 days.[4,5,6]	• ALL abnormal laboratory values
5. Provide routine postphlebotomy care if peripheral veins were used or follow institution-specific protocol for care of a VAD. Observe permanent VADs and insertion sites for signs of line fractures, leakage, redness, and edema.	Promotes long-term functioning of venous access. Identifies complications such as infection, infiltration, leaking at site, and hemorrhage.	• Oozing, bleeding, redness, edema at insertion site • Line fracture • Infiltrate
6. Monitor the child closely for signs of a transfusion reaction. See Procedure 136 for further information.	Prompt identification of transfusion reaction facilitates treatment.	• Fever • Chills • Hives • Respiratory distress

* Level II: Theory based, no research data to support recommendations: recommendations from expert consensus group may exist

Documentation

- Consent for procedure
- Patient/procedure verification process
- Individuals participating in the procedure
- Child and family education
- All medications administered and the child's response to medications
- Total red cell volume exchanged, including total in and total out
- Time of commencement and completion of exchange procedure
- Frequent vitals signs, pertinent observations
- For each unit administered: blood product lot or unit number and type, individuals checking blood products, time infusion was started and completed
- Record lot numbers of all blood products as per institution-specific protocol in the appropriate section of the medical record
- For automated RBCX, documentation of equipment/solutions used during procedure is required to ensure patient safety and facilitate follow-up of any adverse reactions requiring further investigation
- Unexpected outcomes and related treatment

References

1. Kim HC: Therapeutic pediatric apheresis, *J Clin Apheresis* 15:129-157, 2000.
2. Golden P, Weinstein R: Treatment of high-risk, refractory acquired methemoglobinemia with automated red blood cell exchange. *J Clin Apheresis* 13:28-31, 1998.
3. Eckman J, Platt A: *Sickle cell information center protocols: transfusion therapy,* Atlanta, 1997, The Sickle Cell Information Center. www.scinfo.org/transfus.htm.
4. American Association of Blood Banks: *Standards for blood banks and transfusion services,* ed 22, Bethesda, MD, 2003, American Association of Blood Banks.
5. American Association of Blood Banks: *Technical manual,* ed 14, Bethesda, MD, 2002, American Association of Blood Banks.
6. Children's Hospital of Pittsburgh Institute of Transfusion Medicine Clinical Services: *Procedure for red blood cell exchange on COBE Spectra.* Pittsburgh, 2004, Children's Hospital of Pittsburgh Therapeutic Hemapheresis/Outpatient Department.

Whole Blood Exchange Transfusion

PURPOSE: Whole blood that has been resuspended to a specific hematocrit using compatible fresh frozen plasma is used to replace the neonate's own blood to treat certain disease processes

Lucy Thompson

PREREQUISITE KNOWLEDGE

- Specific physiology for which the transfusion is being instituted, e.g., nonimmune indirect hyperbilirubinemia inadequately controlled with phototherapy, multisystem organ failure, toxic substance removal, hemolytic disease of the newborn (ABO incompatibility, Rh isoimmunization)
- General principles of blood and blood component administration; refer to Procedure 132.
- Management of blood transfusion reactions; refer to Procedure 136.
- Details of the blood products to be used throughout the procedure, the appropriateness of these products (hematocrit, cytomegalovirus (CMV) status, irradiated, washed), and the total blood volume to be exchanged
  - ❖ Immunocompromised neonates should receive irradiated blood products.
  - ❖ Blood should be CMV negative.
  - ❖ Blood less than 48 hours old is preferred to avoid elevated potassium levels; if not available, red blood cells (RBCs) reconstituted with fresh frozen plasma are used. Washed blood has excess potassium removed.
- Techniques used and potential risks involved in gaining intravascular access, especially when central venous and arterial access is used; refer to Procedure 196.
- Anatomic placement of intravascular lines, in particular those inserted via the umbilicus
  - ❖ Vessels commonly used for exchange transfusion include umbilical artery and vein; umbilical vein alone; umbilical vein and peripheral arterial line; and central vein.
- Concept of isovolumetric and discontinuous techniques for exchange transfusions
  - ❖ *Isovolumetric exchange transfusion:* the simultaneous withdrawal and replacement of the same blood volume using two individual intravascular sites, one artery and one vein.[1,2] This method results in a more consistent arterial pressure.[3]
  - ❖ *Discontinuous exchange transfusion:* the withdrawal and then replacement of blood aliquots via a single catheter site, usually a vein.[1,2] This method is often referred to as the intermittent push-pull method.
- Concept of early and late whole blood exchange transfusions
  - ❖ *Early exchange transfusion:* procedure is performed in the first 9 to 12 hours of life, based on cord hemoglobin values.[1]
  - ❖ *Late exchange transfusion:* procedure is performed after 9 to 12 hours of life.[1]
- Details of the calculated blood volume to be exchanged[1]
  - ❖ Double-volume exchange transfusion removes approximately 85% to 90% of the neonate's red cells, leaving the serum bilirubin (SBR) at around 50% of the preexchange level. The SBR will rebound at approximately 4 hours postexchange transfusion to 60% of the preexchange level.[1,2] Typically used to manage neonates with severe hyperbilirubinemia or hemolytic disease.[4]

❖ Single-volume exchange transfusion removes approximately 70% to 75% of the neonate's red cells, and is most often used for the management of severe anemia in the presence of heart failure.[1,4] Single volume may also be used in the treatment of polycythemia; in this instance blood is removed and replaced with 0.9% saline

❖ Refer to Box 116-1 for formulas used to calculate exchange volumes.

- Complications of exchange transfusion
  ❖ Heart failure due to incorrectly calculated exchange volume
  ❖ Hypocalcemia due to binding of calcium by blood preservation substances
  ❖ Hyperglycemia followed by hypoglycemia related to dextrose used in blood preservation
  ❖ Sepsis
  ❖ Acidosis related to low pH of banked blood
  ❖ Shock or bleeding
  ❖ Intestinal perforation due to:
    ○ Ischemia of the bowel caused by decreased blood flow to intestine resulting from increased back-pressure created in the portal venous system when large volumes are administered via an umbilical vein
    ○ Hypotension resulting in decreased blood flow to the bowel when large volumes are removed

- Informed consent is required for exchange transfusion, unless impractical because of procedural urgency with family unavailable to provide consent.
- Mastery of neonatal advanced life support competencies
- Principles of aseptic technique

CHILD AND FAMILY ASSESSMENT

- Family's understanding of the reasons for and risks and benefits of the procedure ➡️*Rationale:* Evaluates child's and family's understanding of the procedure and provides a gauge for ongoing education.
- History of hematologic disorders including effectiveness of treatment modalities and regimens ➡️*Rationale:* Identifies potential adverse reactions/contraindications of planned treatment.

- Developmental level ➡️*Rationale:* Family's developmental level influences educational approach and procedural preparation.
- Level of consciousness ➡️*Rationale:* Determines the neonate's sedation and analgesia requirements before, during, and after the procedure; assesses neurologic status.
- Admission history and primary presenting problem ➡️*Rationale:* Identifies possible contraindications of treatment with other presenting problems.
- Obtain baseline assessment of neurologic status, abdominal girth, bedside blood glucose, color, tone, and behavior ➡️*Rationale:* Allows identification of status changes from baseline during procedure.
- Current hemodynamic status ➡️*Rationale:* Inadequate hemodynamic status may require treatment before initiating procedure.
- Details of current type and cross-match plus other pertinent laboratory values including direct Coombs', complete blood count (CBC), electrolyte, and coagulation status ➡️*Rationale:* Facilitates treatment of abnormal laboratory values before, during, and following the procedure.
- Function of gastrointestinal tract ➡️*Rationale:* Gut hypoperfusion is a significant risk factor during and after the procedure.
- Family's desire to be present during the procedure ➡️*Rationale:* Family may provide comfort and support during the procedure, but should have the option not to remain with the neonate.

CHILD AND FAMILY EDUCATION

Individualized, developmentally appropriate education is provided to the family and to the child based on desire for knowledge, readiness and ability to learn and understand new information, and overall neurologic and psychosocial state. As whole blood exchange transfusions are performed primarily on neonates, education is focused on the family.

- Provide information describing the individual case-specific reason(s) for the procedure, processes involved in performing the procedure, and the expected outcomes of the procedure ➡️*Rationale:* Providing information decreases anxiety and fear; allows the family to construct specific questions related to the procedure, its risks, and expected outcomes;

Box 116-1	**Calculation of Exchange Volume**

Single-Volume Exchange =

Term infant's blood volume (85 mL/kg) $\times \dfrac{\text{Desired Hct} - \text{observed Hct}}{\text{RBC unit Hct} - \text{observed Hct}}$

Double-Volume Exchange =

Term infant's blood volume (85 mL/kg) $\times 2 \times \dfrac{\text{Desired Hct} - \text{observed Hct}}{\text{RBC unit Hct} - \text{observed Hct}}$

For the very low–birth weight infant blood volume should be calculated as 100 mL/kg.

From: Murray NA, Roberts AG: Neonatal transfusion practice, *Arch Dis Child Fetal Neonatal Ed* 89:F101-F107, 2004; Nepean Hospital. Neonatal exchange transfusion. *Nepean hospital neonatal intensive care policy and procedure manual,* Sydney, Australia, 2000, Nepean Hospital; Royal Prince Alfred Hospital. Exchange transfusion. *Royal Prince Alfred hospital department of neonatal medicine nursing protocols,* Sydney, Australia, 1999, Royal Prince Alfred Hospital.

and allows the family to express fears associated with particular aspects of the procedure.

- Provide information outlining the risks associated with the transfusion of blood products ➻***Rationale:*** Providing information decreases anxiety and fear, facilitates informed decision making.
- If vascular access has not yet been obtained, explain that preparation for the procedure requires the neonate to undergo insertion of intravascular access devices and provide a general time frame for catheter insertion ➻***Rationale:*** The risks and time period associated with placing intravascular access should be clearly understood by the family; lengthy procedure time may increase anxiety of the family.
- Encourage questions and answer questions as they arise ➻***Rationale:*** Reinforcement of information is needed during periods of stress.

EQUIPMENT[5]

- Sterile drapes and gowns
- Exchange transfusion tray containing the following (assemble supplies if tray not available):
  - Blood waste bag
  - Stopcocks
  - Extension tubing(s)
  - Alcohol swabs
  - #11 knife blade
  - Sterile 4×4 gauze, 5 to 10
  - Sterile 2×2 gauze, 5 to 10
- Blood-warming device and associated tubing
- Blood infusion filter and tubing (refer to institution-specific protocol)
- ½-, 1-, and 2-inch adhesive tape
- Povidone-iodine solution
- 4-0 silk, two packages
- Disposable surgical caps, surgical face masks, protective eyewear
- Two or three pairs sterile gloves
- 0.9% saline for injection
- Sterile 5-, 10-, or 20-mL syringes
- Blood tubes for requested blood specimens
- Labels for requested blood specimens
- Preheated warmer bed
- Emergency cart and equipment

Procedure for Whole Blood Exchange Transfusion[2,3,5,6]

Steps	Rationale	Considerations
It is recommended that the individuals who start the procedure finish the procedure.		
1. Ensure family understands procedure and questions are answered.	Evaluates and reinforces understanding of previously taught information.	Developmental level, cognitive ability and anxiety level will determine approach to and effectiveness of teaching.
2. Independently verify the calculated total volume to be exchanged in the prescribing practitioner's order.	Ensures accuracy of volume to be administered.	Notify prescribing practitioner if there is a discrepancy in calculation.
3. Gather needed equipment and supplies	Facilitates completion of procedure in a timely manner.	
4. Confirm that consent for procedure has been obtained.	Ensures medicolegal compliance as suggested by the Joint Commission on Accreditation of Healthcare Organizations (JCAHO).	For emergency situations, the organization may have a protocol/procedure in place for assumption of consent.
5. Place neonate on heated warmer bed; maintain normothermia. Refer to Procedure 191.	Reduces incidence of cold stress.	Neonates weighing less than 2 kg, premature or very low–birth weight (VLBW) neonates are more susceptible to significant heat loss due to minimal stores of brown fat.
6. Ensure appropriate cardiorespiratory monitoring.	Neonate may demonstrate hemodynamic instability and decompensation throughout the procedure.	Dysrhythmias may occur as a result of acute changes in serum electrolytes, especially potassium and calcium.
7. Suspend enteral feeds before the procedure and evacuate the neonate's gastric contents using an appropriate size gastric tube.	Hypoperfusion to the gut during the exchange transfusion places the neonate at risk of developing necrotizing enterocolitis (NEC).	Orogastric or nasogastric tubes should remain on free drainage throughout the procedure.

Procedure	for Whole Blood Exchange Transfusion[2,3,5,6]—*Continued*		
Steps	**Rationale**	**Considerations**
8. Identify the neonate using appropriate patient/procedure verification process (e.g., two patient identifiers, "Time out").	Confirms correct patient, procedure and site as recommended by JCAHO; promotes patient safety and prevents unnecessary medical procedure.	Verification process and documentation are institution specific. Use active communication techniques.
9. Wash hands and put on personal protective equipment including gloves and eye protection as appropriate.	Standard precautions; reduces transmission of microorganisms and protects personnel from exposure to blood-borne pathogens.	
10. As required, assist with obtaining vascular access.	Adequate vascular access is required for completion of the procedure.	Refer to Procedures 195 and 196.
11. Obtain required blood products from blood bank; two individuals check blood product, patient identity and prescribing practitioner's order per institution-specific protocol.	Promotes patient safety as recommended by JCAHO; ensures right patient, right product.	Verification procedure for administration of blood products and documentation of verification procedure is institution specific.
12. Set up blood warmer following manufacturer's instructions; verify appropriate functioning of alarm system. (*Level I**)	Administration of warmed blood (36.7°–37° C) prevents cold stress; ensuring all equipment is properly functioning at commencement of the procedure will decrease the likelihood of ceasing the procedure prematurely.	Faulty equipment that has not been repaired and/or checked by biomedical engineering poses a threat to patient safety.
13. Assist with instrument tray setup and establishing sterile field.	Ensures that all equipment is present and accessible to the individual performing procedure.	Readily available, well-organized equipment will aid in optimizing patient outcomes during episodes of hemodynamic instability or emergency situations.
14. Remove disposable blood wastage bag from sterile tray using sterile gloves.	Aseptic technique should be maintained throughout the procedure to minimize the risk of infection.	
15. Connect tubing in the following order: Blood component bag Blood filter Blood tubing Blood-warmer tubing or set	Assemble the equipment in a methodic and systematic manner to ensure that all steps are complete. Ensure that all blood products are checked and filtered before administration.	Maximizing the opportunity for the reconstituted donor blood to warm to 36.7°–37° C will aid in decreasing the neonate's hemodynamic instability throughout the procedure.
16. Attach blood tubing and blood warmer tubing to blood and flush to remove air.	Prevents air embolus.	
17. Practitioner performing the procedure will attach the following tubing in order specified immediately before	Tubing will form a closed system, minimizing risk of infection.	

Procedure continues on following page

* Level I: Manufacturer's recommendations only.

Procedure for Whole Blood Exchange Transfusion[2,3,5,6]—Continued

Steps	Rationale	Considerations
beginning the exchange: Extension tubing Stopcock Second extension tubing connected to stopcock Blood waste bag		
18. Blood tubing is attached to one stopcock; tubing is flushed with blood or 0.9% saline to remove air. If discontinuous exchange is performed, single closed system is attached to vascular access catheter. If isovolumetric exchange is performed, one closed system containing blood and blood tubing is attached to umbilical vein catheter (UVC) or central venous access. Second closed system consisting of extension tubing, stopcock, and waste bag is attached to arterial access (Figure 116-1).	Establishes closed system or systems; decreases risk of bloodstream infection.	Minimal line interruption will significantly reduce the risk of blood stream infections. In situations in which asepsis is interrupted, the procedure should be suspended until aseptic technique has been reestablished.
19. Practitioner performing the procedure will remove first aliquot of blood from the neonate and hand to assistant. Place in appropriate tubes labeled with neonate's name and "preexchange" as per prescribing practitioner's order.	Establishes baseline before exchange.	Blood specimens are labeled and sent stat for laboratory analysis. A blood glucose level must be checked with each blood sample that is obtained. Correcting blood glucose fluctuations should be a priority throughout the procedure. Patients experiencing multisystem organ failure as a result of sepsis may require the collection of additional blood specimens.
20. In isovolumetric exchange, blood is removed from the neonate in appropriate aliquots via the arterial access device and discarded into the waste bag. *(Level II*)*	Arterial access facilitates removal of blood; if a single catheter is used blood may be removed via the UVC.	Aliquots of 10 to 20 mL for a term neonate or 5 to 10 mL for a severely anemic or preterm neonate are recommended.[3] Observe arterial access for arterial spasm and decreased perfusion.
21. In isovolumetric exchange, warmed donor blood is simultaneously drawn into a syringe in the *identical* aliquot and administered to the neonate via a venous access device. *(Level II*)* In discontinuous exchange via a single catheter, an aliquot is slowly removed from the neonate over approximately 90 seconds and discarded into the waste bag. An aliquot of the same volume is then drawn up into the syringe from the blood bag and administered to the neonate over approximately 90 seconds.	A *slow, set rate* for exchange cycles (blood out/blood in) of approximately 3 minutes is recommended to minimize blood pressure fluctuations.[3]	Blood may also be administered as a continuous infusion via syringe pump.
22. Blood is exchanged slowly using a closed system and 3-way stopcock until the desired amount of blood has been exchanged. All recording is	A closed exchange system reduces the risk of infection through minimal line interruption. Performing the procedure	Isovolumetric exchange transfusions decrease the risk of hemodynamic instability due to the simultaneous removal and replacement of blood

* Level II: Theory based, no research data to support recommendations: recommendations from expert consensus group may exist

Procedure	for Whole Blood Exchange Transfusion[2,3,5,6]—*Continued*	
Steps	**Rationale**	**Considerations**

Isovolumetric Exchange Setup

Discontinuous Exchange Setup

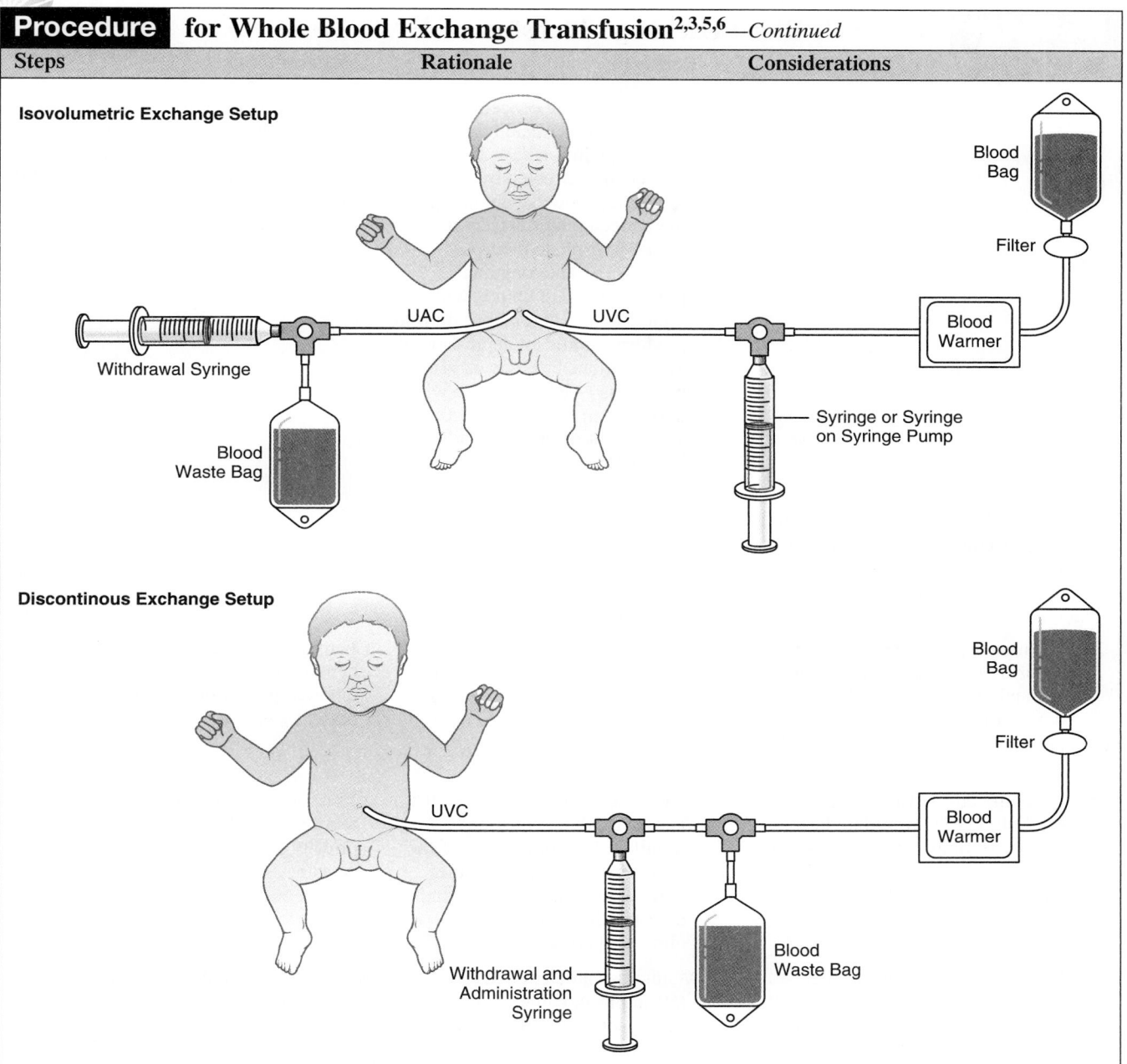

FIGURE 116-1   Examples of setups for isovolumetric and discontinuous exchange transfusions.

done by the clinician assisting with the procedure. *(Level II*)*	at a slow pace (5- to 20-mL increments) enables accurate assessment of the neonate's hemodynamic status throughout the procedure.	volume, resulting in minimal change in cardiac output. Donor blood should be shaken every 30 minutes during the procedure to prevent the settling of red cells. A typical exchange should be completed in less than 2 hours.[3]
23. Send laboratory specimens as requested throughout the procedure per prescribing practitioner's order.	Neonate may experience an acute change in blood glucose levels and serum electrolytes, especially calcium and potas-	Hypokalemia and hypocalcemia detected before the procedure should be corrected before the procedure begins.

Procedure continues on following page

* Level II: Theory based, no research data to support recommendations: recommendations from expert consensus group may exist

Procedure   for Whole Blood Exchange Transfusion[2,3,5,6]—*Continued*

Steps	Rationale	Considerations
	sium during the procedure requiring immediate replacement. Calcium levels are particularly affected by the use of blood products containing the anticoagulant preservative citrate phosphate dextrose (CPD). The anticoagulant preservative CPD binds with ionic calcium and magnesium to produce significant depression of these cations.[1,7] Frequent arterial blood gas (ABG) analysis will allow for the accurate ongoing assessment of the neonate's acid-base balance as well as electrolyte status.	Low ionized calcium levels may produce cardiac effects such as a prolonged Q-T interval (>0.2 second). Calcium gluconate may be prescribed if ionized calcium levels decrease significantly during the procedure.
24. Inform the practitioner performing the procedure when a total of 90 mL, 190 mL, 290 mL, etc, of blood has been administered and removed.	Ensures administration and removal of appropriate volumes; serves as a double check between the recorder and practitioner.	
25. Monitor the neonate continuously, ensuring close observation with each administration of blood and during the calcium infusion. Notify prescribing practitioner promptly of hemodynamic status changes.	Ensures prompt identification and treatment of hemodynamic instability.	Changes in color, behavior, and hemodynamic status should be reported *immediately* to the prescribing practitioner.
26. On completion of the procedure, send blood to appropriate labs as per prescribing practitioner's order. Blood specimens are sent stat and are labeled "postexchange."	SBR, coagulation studies, CBC, and electrolytes must be monitored at completion of the procedure in order to further correct any abnormalities and ascertain hemodynamic and clinical chemistry status.	Assessment and treatment of unstable rebounding laboratory values is a priority in the neonate's postexchange care.
27. Resume infusions to vascular catheter(s) per prescribing practitioner's order or assist with catheter removal.	Maintains catheters that will be left in place; catheters that are no longer required will be removed.	Refer to Procedure 196 for further information.
28. Discard used supplies and equipment in appropriate receptacles.	Standard precautions; reduces the transmission of microorganisms.	
29. Remove personal protective equipment; wash hands.	Standard precautions; reduces the transmission of microorganisms.	

Expected Outcomes

- Measurable improvement/correction of underlying abnormal physiology and/or disease process
- Closed system remains intact throughout procedure
- Hemodynamic status remains stable

- Laboratory blood values remain within normal limits

Unexpected Outcomes

- Laboratory values or neonate's status is not improved after procedure
- Break in system, interruption of asepsis
- Shock
- Emboli—air or blood
- Cardiac arrest
- Infection and/or sepsis related to invasive procedure
- Clinically significant hypocalcemia, hypoglycemia, hypokalemia

Expected Outcomes	Unexpected Outcomes
• Fluid balance remains neutral	• Hemorrhage—coagulopathy • Blood overload—congestive heart failure • Insufficient blood administration results in anemia
• Intravascular catheters remain intact and functional	• Catheter perforation of gut • Unable to administer or remove blood from catheters
• Gut function remains unchanged from baseline	• Signs of gut hypoperfusion • Aspiration of feeds
• Neonate remains free from transfusion related complications	• Transfusion reaction related to administration of wrong blood • Electrolyte/metabolic imbalance related to blood preservative, old blood
• Neonate demonstrates acceptable level of comfort	• Unmanaged pain

Monitoring and Care of the Child

Activities and Interventions	Rationale	Reportable Conditions
1. Monitor vital signs every 15 minutes during the procedure, or more frequently with unstable hemodynamic status.	Replacement of partial or total blood volume is a high risk procedure requiring intensive observation, monitoring, and documentation of neonate's status; prompt identification of hemodynamic instability facilitates prompt treatment.	• Hemodynamic instability
2. Monitor hourly vital signs including neurologic assessment for a minimum of 6 hours following the procedure. Routine observations begun after this time if observations are within normal limits.	Assesses for complications of procedure; ensures adequate cardiac output and developmentally appropriate neurologic status.	• Hemodynamic instability • Changes in neurologic status
3. Assess gut functioning including abdominal girth measurements every 3 to 4 hours with auscultation of bowel sounds, urinary analysis per prescribing practitioner's order, and testing of all stool samples for blood.	Assesses for signs of gut perforation and NEC resulting from a lowered gut perfusion during the procedure.	• Increased abdominal girth • Changes in abdominal perfusion, in particular redness around the umbilicus • Abnormal urinary analysis • Positive blood in stools
4. Resume feeds 12 to 24 hours following the procedure per prescribing practitioner's order.	Allows appropriate interval for identification of gut-related complications before restarting feeds; assess for rebound serum bilirubin (SBR) before restarting feeds.	• Feeding intolerance
5. Obtain frequent blood specimens per prescribing practitioner's order.	Allows identification and prompt initiation of treatment for changes in SBR, glucose, electrolyte, and CBC values. The high glucose content of CPD may stimulate insulin secretion, leading to rebound hypoglycemia following the transfusion. This hypoglycemia usually occurs 30 minutes to 2 hours after the exchange has been completed.[8] CPD has approximately half the acid load of acid citrate dextrose (ACD) preservative and the pH remains the same for approximately 7 days. ACD has a pH of 6.7 after 2 to 3 days.[7,8]	• Abnormal laboratory values

Continued

Monitoring and Care of the Child—Cont'd

Activities and Interventions	Rationale	Reportable Conditions
6. Monitor intravascular access sites and devices.	Observes for signs of infection, infiltration, hemorrhage, and leakage around intravascular access sites.	• Excessive ooze, bleeding, redness, or edema.
7. Assess effectiveness of pain management strategy and provide appropriate interventions. Encourage family to assist in using nonpharmacologic means to comfort neonate.	Early identification of pain allows for immediate attention.	• Unmanaged pain • Continued irritability, changes in physiologic condition

Documentation

- Consent for procedure
- Patient/procedure verification process
- Individuals participating in the procedure
- Vital signs, pertinent observations
- Total blood volume exchanged
- Initiation and completion times of procedure
- Time and volume of each aliquot withdrawn and administered
- Education of family
- Laboratory specimens sent and results obtained
- Medications administered and the neonate's response to these medications
- Blood product unit number and type
- Comfort assessment and any specific interventions provided
- Unexpected outcomes and related treatment

References

1. American Association of Blood Banks: *Technical manual,* ed 14, Bethesda, MD, 2003, American Association of Blood Banks.
2. Royal Prince Alfred Hospital. Exchange transfusion. *Royal Prince Alfred Hospital department of neonatal medicine nursing protocols,* Sydney, Australia, 1999, Royal Prince Alfred Hospital.
3. Kenner C, Lott JW, editors: *Comprehensive neonatal nursing: a physiologic perspective,* ed 3, Philadelphia, 2003, Saunders.
4. Murray NA, Roberts AG: Neonatal transfusion practice, *Arch Dis Child Fetal Neonatal Ed* 89:F101-F107, 2004.
5. Children's Hospital of Pittsburgh: Whole blood exchange transfusion. *Children's Hospital of Pittsburgh Patient Care Policy and Procedure Manual,* Pittsburgh, 2003, Children's Hospital of Pittsburgh.
6. Nepean Hospital. Neonatal exchange transfusion. *Nepean hospital neonatal intensive care policy and procedure manual,* Sydney, Australia, 2000, Nepean Hospital.
7. American Association of Blood Banks: *Standards for blood banks and transfusion services*, ed 22, Bethesda, MD, 2003, American Association of Blood Banks.
8. Institute of Transfusion Medicine Clinical Services. *Procedure for red blood cell exchange on COBE Spectra,* Pittsburgh, 2004, Children's Hospital of Pittsburgh Therapeutic Hemapheresis/Outpatient Department.

AP
Bone Marrow Aspiration and Biopsy: Perform

P U R P O S E : To diagnose hematopoietic diseases, assess therapeutic response to treatment for these diseases, and detect chromosomal abnormalities

Kathryn Carnighan Kuhn

PREREQUISITE KNOWLEDGE

- Child development as it relates to clinical assessment and bone marrow aspiration
- Mastery of pediatric advanced life support competencies
- Principles of aseptic technique
- Appropriate pediatric dosing of analgesics and competency in procedural sedation
- Anatomy of the bone marrow: "after the blood itself, bone marrow is the largest and most widely distributed organ in the body."[1]
  - ❖ Bone marrow is the site of hematopoiesis (the process of formation and development of blood cell lineages).
  - ❖ The marrow is composed of two parts: the hematopoietic cells and the stromal cells that support the proliferation and differentiation of these cells from stem cells.
- Diagnostic or surveillance purpose of exam
  - ❖ Hematopoietic abnormalities are more easily detected and manifest earlier in the bone marrow than in peripheral blood
  - ❖ Flow cytometry analysis allows identification of malignant clones
  - ❖ Cytogenetic analysis allows detection of chromosomal abnormalities associated with hematologic malignancies
  - ❖ Chimerism studies allow evaluation of engraftment status following allogeneic transplant
- Anatomy of the bilateral posterior superior iliac crests, anterior iliac crests, and tibia. At birth all bone cavities are filled with hematopoietic cells, but by adolescence the bulk of hematopoietic cells have been replaced by adipose tissue, and hematopoietic marrow is found only in centrally located bones such as the iliac crests, sternum, skull, clavicles, and proximal ends of the humeri and femurs.[1]
- Appropriate aspiration and biopsy site selection based on child's age and clinical history
- Clinical and technical competence performing a bone marrow aspiration and biopsy
- Hematopoietic abnormalities are more easily detected and manifest earlier in the bone marrow than in peripheral blood.
- A bone marrow aspiration provides information about cellular morphology and relative distribution of cell types, whereas a biopsy allows the most reliable evaluation of overall bone marrow cellularity and the adequacy of bone marrow reconstitution following transplant. The bone marrow biopsy is also useful in the instance of a "dry tap" when aspirate is unable to be obtained, which occurs in approximately 4% of cases and is related to

malignant cell proliferation, aplasia, or radiation fibrosis.[1] In these instances a core biopsy should be obtained for a "touch prep," which may be useful in determining morphology and cell types—qualities typically defined by the aspirate sample. If an attempt at aspiration is repeated, move to a new area of bone and use a new aspiration needle because a clot may have lodged in needle's hollow core.

- Assess laboratory studies coupled with child's clinical history to ensure procedure is performed safely
- Contraindications to bone marrow aspiration including certain bleeding disorders, surgery and/or trauma, and past radiation to site
- Risks of bone marrow aspiration are minimized with use of appropriate technique, but include bleeding, infection, and/or injury to the bowel. Sternal aspiration is associated with more serious potential complications related to proximity to the heart and major vessels.
- Specifics of individual state's nurse practice act that delineates regulations concerning performing bone marrow aspiration and/or administering sedation
- Informed consent is required before bone marrow aspiration and biopsy.

CHILD AND FAMILY ASSESSMENT

- Child's developmental level and ability to interact ➤➤*Rationale:* These factors influence preparation of the child and interaction.
- Obtain thorough history and physical ➤➤*Rationale:* Determines whether and what type of bone marrow examination is needed, risk factors and/or contraindications for procedure, and if child will tolerate prone and/or side-lying positioning during procedure.
- Obtain laboratory studies including platelet count and prothrombin time/partial thromboplastin time (PT/PTT) ➤➤*Rationale:* Provides baseline studies. It is generally accepted that thrombocytopenia, no matter how profound, is *not* a contraindication for bone marrow aspiration and/or biopsy[1,2,3]; however, practitioner must be familiar with institution-specific transfusion protocols. Coagulation factor deficiencies are considered contraindications, but may be corrected (i.e., factor products, fresh frozen plasma [FFP], vitamin K) before the procedure.[1,2,3] The procedure should be postponed if aspirin has been taken within preceding 48 hours.[3]
- Anatomy of the child considering age, medical history, and history of previous bone marrow aspirations/biopsies ➤➤*Rationale:* Determines what anatomic site would be most appropriate for procedure based on age and previous therapy. Sternal aspiration is absolutely contraindicated in children.[1,2,3] The preferred site is the posterior superior iliac crest, although the tibia can be used in children younger than 12 months.[1,2,3] Radiation fibrosis, severe osteopenia, or recent bone marrow aspirations/biopsies should be considered when selecting a procedure site.

- Degree or type of sedation needed based on child's age, experience with painful procedures, and sedation history ➤➤*Rationale:* Promotes child's comfort and decreases anxiety. All children and adolescents should receive sedation for both bone marrow aspiration and biopsy.[4,5,6] Review of previous sedation history may influence choice of sedative to be used. Sedation should not be administered by the practitioner performing the bone marrow procedure to ensure patient safety and adequate pain control. Review institution-specific protocol regarding the administration of procedural sedation before the procedure.
- Child's and family's understanding of the reasons for and risks and benefits of the procedure ➤➤*Rationale:* Evaluates child's and family's understanding of the procedure and provides a gauge for ongoing education.
- Family's desire to be present during the procedure ➤➤*Rationale:* Family may provide support and comfort during the procedure, but should have the choice not to remain with the child.

CHILD AND FAMILY EDUCATION

Individualized, developmentally appropriate education is provided to the child and family based on desire for knowledge, readiness to learn, and overall neurologic and psychosocial state.

- Explain purpose of procedure, risks (bleeding, injury to bowel, infection), and benefits. Obtain informed consent ➤➤*Rationale:* Promotes child's and family's understanding and alleviates fear and anxiety. Ensures that child and family are making an informed decision. Ensures medicolegal compliance.
- Reassure the family and child that pain and antianxiety medications will be given before and during the procedure ➤➤*Rationale:* Bone marrow aspiration and biopsy are two of the most painful procedures for children.[4,5,6] Appropriate pain management alleviates pain during the procedure, decreases anxiety about future procedures, and creates a controlled setting in which the practitioner may safely perform the procedure. The cooperation of the child during subsequent procedures is directly influenced by the painlessness and ease of the initial examination.[7]
- Assess the child's and family's understanding of the need for the procedure and the steps of the procedure itself. Review informed consent ➤➤*Rationale:* Reinforces previous teaching and protects child and family autonomy. Allows opportunity for questions to be asked and answered.
- For outpatient procedures, teach family signs and symptoms of site infection, complications that warrant a return to the clinic or hospital. Teach family to keep pressure dressing intact for 12 hours, and area clean and dry for 24 hours. ➤➤*Rationale:* Provides family with information needed to provide safe care for the child at home.
- Encourage questions and answer questions as they arise ➤➤*Rationale:* Reinforcement of information is needed during periods of stress.

EQUIPMENT

- Aspiration needle (e.g., Illinois)
- Biopsy needle and stylet (e.g., Jamshidi)
- Skin antiseptic agent
- Sterile gloves, protective eyewear, mask, and gown
- 1% lidocaine vial
- Sterile 0.9% saline vial
- Preservative-free heparin (1:1000) vial
- Three or four 20-mL syringes
- #11 scalpel blade

- Two 25-gauge and two 19-gauge needles
- Sterile fenestrated drape
- Sterile 2×2 and 4×4 gauze
- Preservative-free heparin tubes (quantity dependent on desired samples)
- Sterile specimen container
- Sterile labels and pen, if available
- Alcohol wipes
- Pressure dressing
- Slides (preparation and preparation materials per institution-specific protocol)

Procedure | for Bone Marrow Aspiration and Biopsy: Perform

Steps	Rationale	Considerations
1. Review procedure, consent, and preprocedural teaching with child and family; ensure questions have been answered.	Reinforces previous teaching and facilitates informed consent.	Developmental level, cognitive ability, and anxiety level will determine approach to and effectiveness of teaching.
2. Ensure appropriate pain and anxiety management plan.	Bone marrow aspiration and biopsy are among the most painful procedures performed in the pediatric population.[4,5,6]	Consider clinical status and developmental level of child.
3. If required for sedation plan, ensure fasting guidelines have been implemented per institution-specific protocol. *(Level VI*)*	Prevents sedation complications related to emesis/aspiration.	NPO time is related to child's age and type of diet.
4. Identify the child using appropriate patient/procedure verification process (e.g. two patient identifiers, "time out").	Confirms correct patient, procedure and site as recommended by the Joint Commission on Accreditation of Healthcare Organizations (JCAHO); prevents unnecessary medical procedures. Use of at least two patient identifiers improves the accuracy of identification.	Verification process and documentation is institution-specific; use active communication techniques.
5. Ensure appropriate monitoring is in place and that child has functioning venous access if required for sedation administration. *(Level III*)*	Continuous monitoring allows assessment of child's status while sedated. Functioning venous access may be required to administer emergency medications or sedation as needed.	Emergency equipment, including airway-management supplies, should be readily available.
6. Wash hands.	Standard precautions; reduces the transmission of microorganisms.	

Procedure continues on following page

* Level III: Laboratory data, no clinical data to support recommendations
  Level VI: Clinical studies in a variety of patient populations and situations to support recommendations

Procedure   for Bone Marrow Aspiration and Biopsy: Perform—*Continued*

Steps	Rationale	Considerations
7. Position child: either side-lying with knees to chest or prone with towel under hips to elevate pelvis. Identify bony landmarks of posterior iliac crest (Figures 117-1 and 117-2). Insertion site is the midpoint of the superior spine of the posterior iliac crest.	Facilitates procedure and ensures ability to access appropriate procedure site.	Choice of side-lying or prone position based on size and clinical status of child.

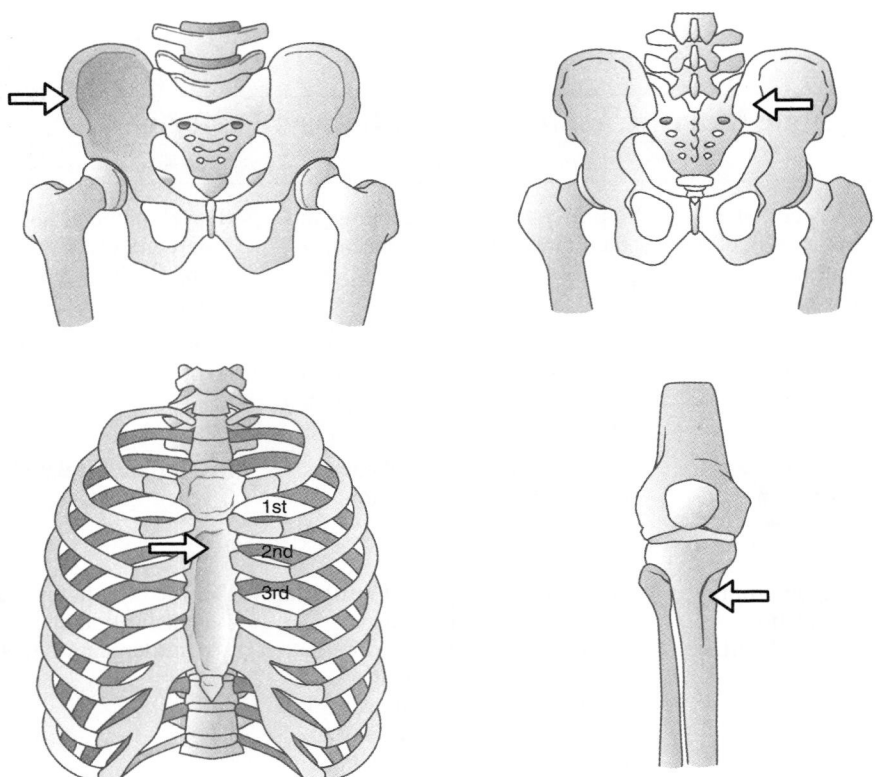

FIGURE 117-1   Common anatomic locations of bone marrow sampling. *(From Head DR, Pui CH: Diagnosis and classification. In Pui CH, editor:* Childhood leukemias, *Cambridge, 2000, Cambridge University Press, p 20.)*

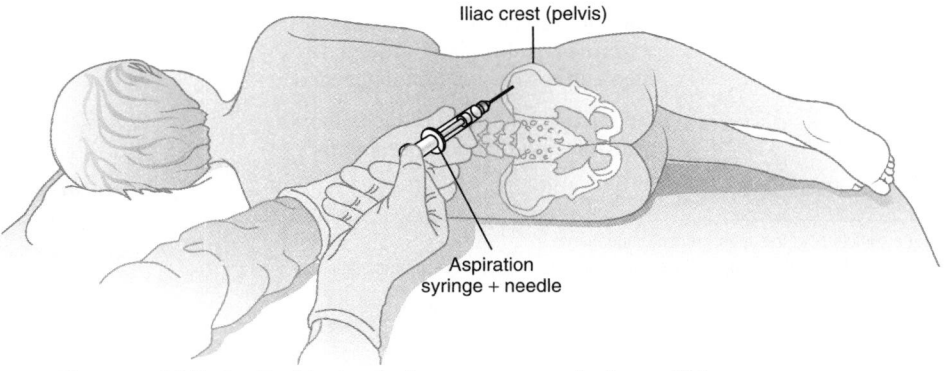

FIGURE 117-2   Positioning for bone marrow aspiration and biopsy.

Procedure for Bone Marrow Aspiration and Biopsy: Perform—*Continued*

Steps	Rationale	Considerations
8. Open supplies or bone marrow tray and place necessary syringes and aspiration/biopsy needles on sterile tray using sterile technique (Figure 117-3). Label all specimen containers and slides before beginning procedure.	Maintains sterility and prepares supplies.	Many types of aspiration/biopsy needles are available. Select based on child's size and personal preference. Familiarize yourself with the institution-specific bone marrow tray available. Know what additional supplies must be obtained before the procedure.

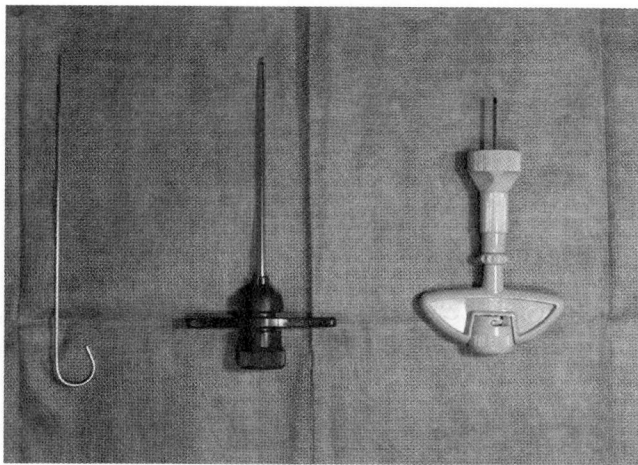

FIGURE 117-3 Bone marrow aspiration needles.

Steps	Rationale	Considerations
9. Open vial of preservative-free heparin and set aside.	Prepares supplies.	
10. Put on eye protection, clean gown, and sterile gloves. Organize sterile supplies (or contents of bone marrow tray if available). In sterile fashion, draw up 5 to 10 mL of 1% lidocaine solution into 10-mL syringe. Whenever possible, label syringe with sterile label and pen, maintaining sterile field. Test obturator of both aspiration and biopsy needles to ensure free movement within the needles. Remove sternal guard from aspiration needle.	Prepares sterile supplies and ensures proper functioning of equipment. Allows for organization of tray contents, anticipation of additional supplies needed before start of procedure, and minimization of delays. Labeling syringes prevents against incorrect medication administration, promotes patient safety	Removal of the sternal guard assumes that a sternal aspiration is *not* being performed. Sterile labels and pens are increasingly available in sterile trays, or may be obtained from the operating room. Use of non-sterile labels would break sterility and potentially contaminate the field.
11. With assistance, withdraw 1 to 2 mL of preservative-free heparin into a 20-mL syringe(s) and coat full barrel of syringe with swirling motion, pulling plunger back and forth several times. Discard heparin, leaving only 0.25 mL in syringe.	Heparinized aspirate is used for flow cytometry, cytogenetics, and chimerism studies; quantity of heparinized syringes will depend on the type of diagnostic tests being performed. Coating syringe prevents clotting. Minimal residual heparin in syringe prevents	If an assistant is not available during the procedure, plan to tape inverted vials to the edge of the procedure table so that you may withdraw the contents of the vials unassisted without breaking sterility. Take special care to avoid confusing heparinized and lidocaine syringes.

Procedure continues on following page

Procedure | for Bone Marrow Aspiration and Biopsy: Perform—*Continued*

Steps	Rationale	Considerations
	heparin from disrupting morphology.	
12. Cleanse selected procedure site with antiseptic solution.	Reduces risk of introducing infectious organisms during procedure.	
13. Using a 25-gauge needle inject 1% lidocaine into the subcutaneous tissue overlying the selected anatomic site, creating a subepidermal wheal. Massage over the site of injection to increase distribution of lidocaine.	Local anesthetic; decreases pain during procedure.	Always provide local anesthetic even when systemic sedation or analgesia is used.
14. Using a 19-gauge needle firmly inject 1% lidocaine into the periosteum, withdrawing and redirecting the needle several times.	Minimizes pain by anesthetizing highly innervated periosteum; allows assessment of the anatomy and integrity of the bone before insertion of biopsy/aspiration needles.	Needle length necessary to reach the periosteum will depend on the size of the child.
15. Using #11 surgical blade, make a small incision in the skin overlying the posterior iliac crest.	Allows for easier penetration of the aspiration needle through the skin.	May not be necessary in smaller children because skin is easily penetrated.
16. Stabilize the handle of the aspiration needle in the palm of one hand with the index finger of the same hand braced at distal end of needle. Place the thumb and second finger of the other hand on the iliac crest to guide the needle and facilitate correct positioning (Figure 117-4).	Sliding off the periosteum is a common cause of failure.[2] Careful positioning and stabilization increase chance of successful aspiration and minimize risk of injury to the child.	

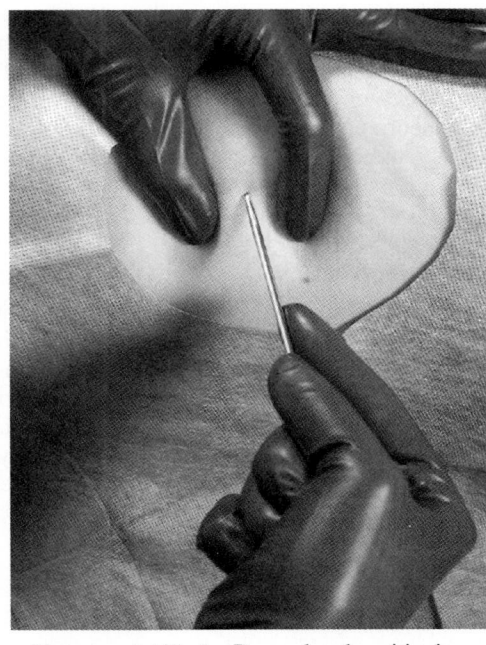

FIGURE 117-4   Proper hand positioning.

Procedure | for Bone Marrow Aspiration and Biopsy: Perform—*Continued*

Steps	Rationale	Considerations

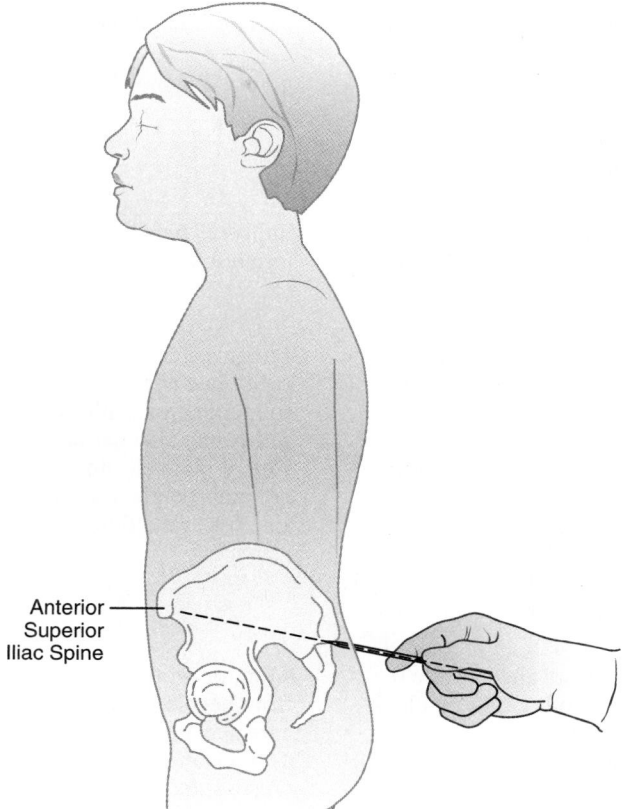

FIGURE 117-5   Needle direction.

Insert the needle into the skin through the incision, aiming toward the anterior iliac crest, and push through the tissue until reaching the periosteum. Advance through the periosteum and cortex using a twisting motion until needle is firmly in place. A "give" sensation occurs once needle passes through the cortex and into the medullary cavity (Figure 117-5).

Anterior Superior Iliac Spine

17. Remove obturator and attach nonheparinized syringe to needle hub; swiftly pull plunger back full length of syringe until 1 mL bone marrow is obtained.

Initial sample will be used to prepare direct smear, which is used for evaluation of cellular morphology; heparin can create an artifact effect that disrupts and distorts morphology. Smaller volumes of bone marrow decrease the likelihood of contamination with peripheral blood.

If aspirate not obtained, replace obturator and advance needle farther or pull out to periosteum and reposition. The aspiration step creates intense pain, so ensure adequate analgesia and sedation before withdrawing marrow.

18. Remove syringe from needle hub and promptly place a few drops of aspirate on slide to look for spicules.

Spicules are white-appearing fragments that contain bone marrow particles. Their presence is indicative of an adequate location within the bone marrow cavity.

Appropriate slide preparation is crucial, and the process varies by institution: some require practitioners to prepare samples, others provide laboratory technicians. Adequate training in slide preparation is essential and beyond the scope of this discussion; consult with institution-specific laboratory services.

Procedure continues on following page

Procedure for Bone Marrow Aspiration and Biopsy: Perform—*Continued*

Steps	Rationale	Considerations
19. Once appropriate location in marrow is confirmed by presence of spicules, attach heparinized syringe(s) and collect additional samples, rotating the needle 90 degrees with each sample obtained. Place aspirate in preservative-free heparin tubes or cap syringes for later disposition.	Rotating the needle minimizes the likelihood of a sample diluted with peripheral blood.	3 to 5 mL is generally adequate for most laboratory analyses; refer to institution-specific protocols.
20. After all aspirate specimens are obtained, withdraw needle and apply pressure to site with dry sterile gauze.	Minimizes bleeding and hematoma formation.	If attempt at aspiration is repeated, move to new area of bone and use new aspiration needle because clot may have lodged in needle's hollow core.
21. To obtain biopsy, use same hand placement to stabilize and guide needle and insert biopsy needle through established insertion site in skin moving to a new area of the periosteum. Ensure that obturator is in lock position. Aiming toward the anterior iliac crest, twist needle until it is firmly anchored in the bone; remove obturator.	Obturator should remain in place until bone is reached to avoid contamination with skin, muscle, and connective tissue. Using new area of bone eliminates possibility of hemorrhagic specimen unsuitable for evaluation.	
22. Continue to advance needle 0.5 to 1.5 cm into bone using clockwise/counterclockwise twisting motion. Replace obturator into biopsy needle to gauge size of specimen. When adequate sample obtained, remove obturator.	Obturator protruding 0.5 to 1.5 cm from needle indicates an adequate core specimen. Rotating needle as it advances cuts rather than crushes the bone.	Take care not to push core out when inserting and reinserting obturator.
23. Twist the needle 360 degrees three or four times in both directions followed by vigorous rocking from 3 to 9 o'clock and 6 to 12 o'clock several times. Before removal push the needle in 2 to 3 mm and move the needle slightly laterally.	Rocking and rotating allows core to break attachment. Advancing needle before removal pushes core into needle. Moving laterally minimizes loss of core in original needle tract.	
24. Insert stylet provided with biopsy needle into distal tip of the needle, pushing core out through the handle side. Place core in sterile 0.9% saline-soaked gauze.	Minimizes damage to the core that would be caused by forcing it through tapered distal tip. Prevents core from becoming dry and unsuitable for interpretation.	An adequate core specimen will measure at least 1 cm. If an inadequate biopsy core is obtained, i.e., too small or not at all, change location on the periosteum and reattempt collection. Depending on the size of the child, it may be possible to remain on the same iliac crest and move to a new area, or in the case of a smaller child, it may be necessary to repeat the procedure on the contralateral iliac crest. Ensure that biopsy needle hollow core is free of debris or use new biopsy needle.

Procedure for Bone Marrow Aspiration and Biopsy: Perform—*Continued*

Steps	Rationale	Considerations
25. Using dry sterile gauze, hold pressure to site for 3 to 5 minutes, followed by the application of a sterile pressure dressing.	Minimizes risk of bleeding and hematoma.	
26. Discard used supplies and equipment in appropriate container; ensure sharps are disposed of safely.	Standard precautions; reduces transmission of microorganisms. Protects personnel health.	
27. Remove protective equipment, including gloves; wash hands.	Standard precautions; reduces transmission of microorganisms.	

Expected Outcomes

- Adequate aspirate and biopsy samples collected

- Procedure is completed without complications
- Minimal pain during procedure related to use of adequate systemic analgesia and local anesthesia
- Sedation level is adequate during procedure
- Respiratory status remains stable during procedure

Unexpected Outcomes

- Unable to obtain marrow due to fibrotic or hypocellular marrow
- Inadequate core biopsy specimen obtained
- Bleeding, infection, injury to the bowel
- Unmanaged pain

- Unmanaged anxiety or agitation
- Respiratory distress or failure related to sedation/analgesia

Monitoring and Care of the Child

Activities and Interventions	Rationale	Reportable Conditions
1. Ensure adequate and appropriate analgesia before, during, and after the procedure.	Promotes comfort, minimizes fear, and decreases anxiety regarding future procedures. Postprocedural pain is generally mild and of short duration.	• Unmanaged or intractable pain
2. Monitor vital signs and pulse oximetry before, during, and after procedure.	Monitors child's response to positioning and procedure.	• Changes in vital signs or oxygen saturations from baseline • Hypoxia, bradycardia
3. Assess procedure site. If performed as an outpatient procedure, review complications with family that warrant a return to the clinic or hospital.	Determines presence of procedure related complication. Ensures family is aware of reasons to contact practitioner after discharge.	• Bleeding, hematoma, erythema, discharge, fever

Documentation

- Education of child and family including informed consent
- Patient/procedure verification process
- Compliance with fasting guidelines
- Preparation of child including sterile prep, positioning, site, and use of systemic analgesics or sedatives and local anesthetics
- Size and type of needles used
- Diagnostic and/or monitoring studies sent for laboratory analysis
- Child's tolerance of procedure
- Unexpected outcomes and related treatment
- Postprocedure instructions

References

1. Ryan DH, Cohen HJ: Bone marrow aspiration and morphology. In Hoffman R, et al, editors: *Hematology basic principles and practice,* ed 3, New York, 2000, Churchill Livingstone.
2. Head DR, Pui CH: Diagnosis and classification. In Pui CH, editor: *Childhood leukemias,* Cambridge, 2000, Cambridge University Press, p. 20.
3. Nguyen DT, Diamond LW: *Approach to the bone marrow. Diagnostic hematology: a pattern approach,* Oxford, 2000, Butterworth-Heinemann.
4. Collins JJ, Weisman SJ: Management of pain in childhood cancer. In Schechter NL, et al, editors: *Pain in infants, children, and adolescents,* ed 2, Philadelphia, 2003, Lippincott Williams & Wilkins.
5. Hertzog JH, et al: Prospective evaluation of propofol anesthesia in the pediatric intensive care unit for elective oncology procedures in ambulatory hospitalized children. *Pediatrics* 106:742-747, 2000.
6. McGrath PA: Acute pains. In McGrath PA, editor. *Pain in children: nature, assessment, and treatment,* New York, 1990, Guilford Press.
7. Miller DR: Normal blood values from birth through adolescence. In Miller DR, et al, editors: *Blood diseases of infancy and childhood,* ed 7, St. Louis, 1995, Mosby.

Additional Readings

Trewhitt KG: Bone marrow aspiration and biopsy: collection and interpretation, *Oncol Nurs Forum* 28: 1409-1417, 2001.
Weitberg AB: Study of bone marrow. In Handin RI, et al, editors: *Blood principles and practice of hematology,* Philadelphia, 1995, Lippincott.

Unit **VII**
Musculoskeletal
System

SECTION SEVENTEEN
**Musculoskeletal
Procedures**

PROCEDURE **118**

Brace and Splint Application

P U R P O S E : Braces and splints are applied for injury immobilization and minimization of complications; protection and maintenance of postoperative correction; pain relief; maintenance of proper alignment; correction of deformity; promotion of function; symptomatic relief of chronic conditions

Bridget A. Thomas

PREREQUISITE KNOWLEDGE

* Child development as it relates to clinical assessment and splinting
* Anatomy and physiology of the integumentary, musculoskeletal, neurologic, and vascular systems
* Orthoses are often used to prevent deformity, improve and stabilize gait, maintain alignment, and support the limbs, trunk, or neck. They must be fitted to avoid muscle stress, imbalance, and skin breakdown.
* Bracing or splinting is an individual treatment that may be designed by an occupational therapist, physical therapist, orthotist, or prescribing practitioner. The type of device, positioning, and length of time it is worn are determined by the prescribing practitioner and therapist. Commercial splints and braces also are available. Follow the manufacturer's guidelines for measurement when selecting pediatric sizes for commercial splints and braces.
* Complications of brace and splint application include skin breakdown, nerve compression, disuse atrophy, compartment syndrome, and vascular compromise.

CHILD AND FAMILY ASSESSMENT

* Child's developmental level and ability to interact **➧➧*Rationale:*** These factors influence preparation of the child and interaction.

* Child's and family's understanding of the reasons for and risks and benefits of the procedure **➧➧*Rationale:*** Evaluates child's and family's understanding of the procedure and provides a gauge for ongoing education.
* Integumentary, musculoskeletal, neurologic, and vascular status of the extremity or area to be splinted or braced **➧➧*Rationale:*** Provides baseline data for comparison of elements such as skin breakdown, nerve compression, disuse atrophy, compartment syndrome, and vascular compromise. Disrupted integument may increase risk of infection; altered neurovascular status due to pain or edema should improve with brace application and stability.[1,2,3]
* Child's fluid status **➧➧*Rationale:*** Presence of edema or dehydration increases likelihood of disruption of skin integrity. Edema decreases joint mobility.
* Child's pain level **➧➧*Rationale:*** Provides data for postapplication comparison; assesses the need for an intervention for comfort; effective pain control facilitates child's cooperation during and after splint application.
* Child's anxiety or irritability level **➧➧*Rationale:*** Child's inability to tolerate the procedure related to anxiety may increase pain or cause secondary injury.
* Family members desire to be present during the procedure **➧➧*Rationale:*** Family members may provide comfort and support but should have the choice not to remain with the child.

CHILD AND FAMILY EDUCATION

Individualized, developmentally appropriate education is provided to the family and to the child based on desire for knowledge, readiness to learn, and overall neurologic and psychosocial state.

- Provide information about specific splint/brace to be used, explaining the reason for application, and describing/demonstrating the procedure ➤➤*Rationale:* Decreases anxiety and fear, increases cooperation.
- If developmentally appropriate, explain any unusual sensations the child will experience during splint or brace application (e.g., warmth or cold, wetness) ➤➤*Rationale:* Providing information appropriate to the child's developmental level about sensations that will be experienced during the procedure helps the toddler, preschool, and school-aged child cope more effectively during the procedure.[3]
- Discuss wear schedule for splint or brace ➤➤*Rationale:* Prevents misuse of device, which could lead to injury.
- Review signs and symptoms of vascular compromise and skin breakdown. Encourage child and/or family to report any indications of compromise or breakdown as soon as they are identified ➤➤*Rationale:* Helps to quickly identify unintended outcomes of device application and prevent injury.

- Encourage questions and answer questions as they arise ➤➤*Rationale:* Reinforcement of information is needed during periods of stress.

EQUIPMENT

- Soft, nonrigid splints (bandaging material, blanket, cloth, cravat, foam rubber, pillow, cervical collar, clavicle strap, sling and swathe, binder)
- Hard, rigid or semirigid splints (aluminum, pliable metals, cardboard, fiberglass, wire ladder, leather, molded plastic, plaster, vacuum, wood, backboards, cervical collar, finger splint, wrist splint, knee immobilizer, ankle support, orthopedic shoe)
- Pneumatic, inflatable splints (air splint, pneumatic anti-shock garment)

Additional equipment may include:
- Measuring tape
- Padding materials
- Soft cotton roll (e.g., Webril)
- Cotton stocking material
- Tape
- Elastic bandage (e.g., ACE wrap)
- Safety pins
- Gauze bandage
- Velcro straps

Procedure for Brace and Splint Application

Steps	Rationale	Considerations
1. Ensure that child and family understand procedure and questions are answered.	Evaluates and reinforces previously taught information.	Developmental level, cognitive ability, and anxiety levels will affect approach to and effectiveness of teaching.
2. Gather necessary equipment and supplies.	Preparation and presence of all needed materials facilitates completion of procedure in a timely manner.	Splints and braces are applied with prescribing practitioners order or per unit-specific protocol.
3. Choose the appropriate-sized splint or brace. The splint may have to be improvised or altered to fit the deformity.	Improperly fitting device may cause injury.[1,2,4] *(Level II*)*	Splints may be fitted and custom made. If using prefabricated splint or brace, follow manufacturer's directions for measurement of device. The extremity should not be forced to fit the splint. *(Level I*)*
4. Obtain neurovascular and integumentary assessment before splint or brace application.	Ensures baseline assessment is obtained before apparatus is placed. Disrupted integument may increase risk of infection.	Altered neurovascular status due to pain or edema should improve with brace application and stabilization of injury.
5. Ensure zippers, knots, or attachments of the splinting device will not be directly over an injury site. Remove jewelry before applying extremity splints and cervical collars.	Foreign bodies may cause injury and skin breakdown. Rough surfaces may cause pressure injury or skin breakdown.[2,4]	

* Level I: Manufacturer's recommendations only
Level II: Theory based, no research data to support recommendations: recommendations from expert consensus group may exist

Procedure for Brace and Splint Application—*Continued*

Steps	Rationale	Considerations
6. Perform any needed assembly or preparation of splint or brace materials. Follow manufacturer's instructions for commercial products.	Facilitates prompt application of splint.	If wet plaster or fiberglass splinting materials are to be used, cool water is recommended to prepare these products. Use of very warm or hot water may cause the splint to release more heat as it hardens.[5]
7. Wash hands.	Standard precautions; reduces transmission of microorganisms.	
8. Assist child to a comfortable position that allows easy access to the extremity. Support the extremity to be splinted in anatomically correct position. *(Level IV*)*	Facilitates application; ensures proper positioning of extremity into splint or brace.[2]	Braces and splints in anatomically incorrect positions may contribute to contractures or misalignment.
9. Apply protective clothing or soft cotton roll to the area to be splinted or braced under the device. Pad bony prominences when rigid splints are used (Figure 118-1). *(Level II*)*	Protective clothing and padding help prevent disruption of skin integrity.[2]	Excessive protective clothing or padding may alter the fit or function of the device; refer to manufacturer's instructions with commercial splints or braces. For devices made by physical therapist, occupational therapist, or practitioner, follow instructions provided.

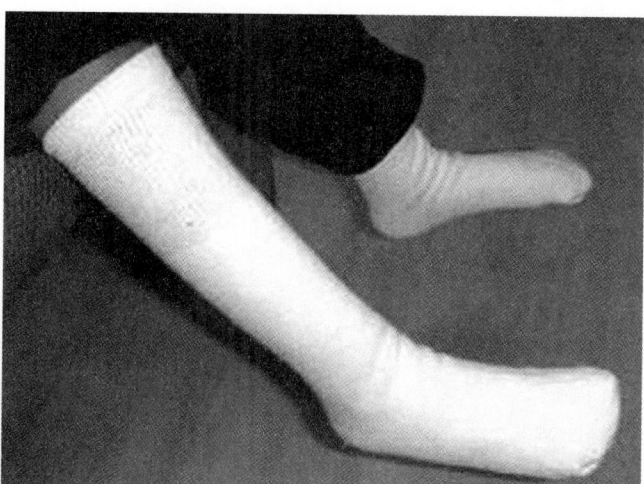

FIGURE 118-1   Application of protective clothing. (*Photo courtesy of Scheck and Siress, Inc.*)

10. Apply appropriate splint or brace (Figures 118-2 through 118-5). Secure with Velcro, tape, bandage, wet plaster or fiberglass, or safety pins. If the limb is wrapped circumferentially, the wrapping material should be expandable and nonconstricting.	Use of inappropriate device may lead to injury or compromise. Secure the splint or brace so that it does not become dislodged or loosened. Wrapping material should not cause vascular compromise.[3,4,6]	Compartment syndrome may develop in any area with vascular compromise. *(Level VI*)* Hold splint in position until material has hardened if this is required.
11. Discard used materials in appropriate receptacle; wash hands.	Standard precautions; reduces transmission of microorganisms.	

Procedure continues on p. 883

* Level II: Theory based, no research data to support recommendations: recommendations from expert consensus group may exist
Level IV: Limited clinical studies to support recommendations
Level VI: Clinical studies in a variety of patient populations and situations to support recommendations

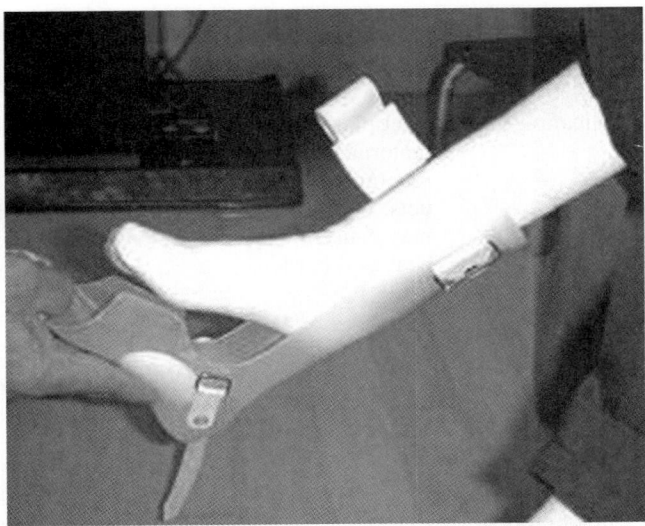

FIGURE 118-2 Leg is placed into splint. *(Photo courtesy of Scheck and Siress, Inc.)*

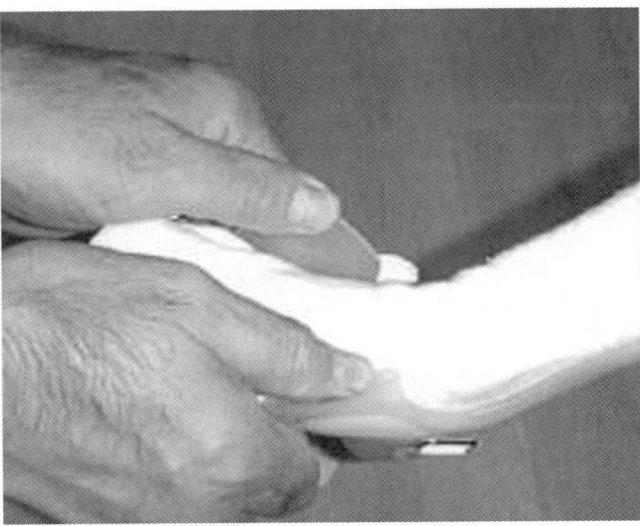

FIGURE 118-3 Leg is slid into place; fit is assessed for potential pressure points. *(Photo courtesy of Scheck and Siress, Inc.)*

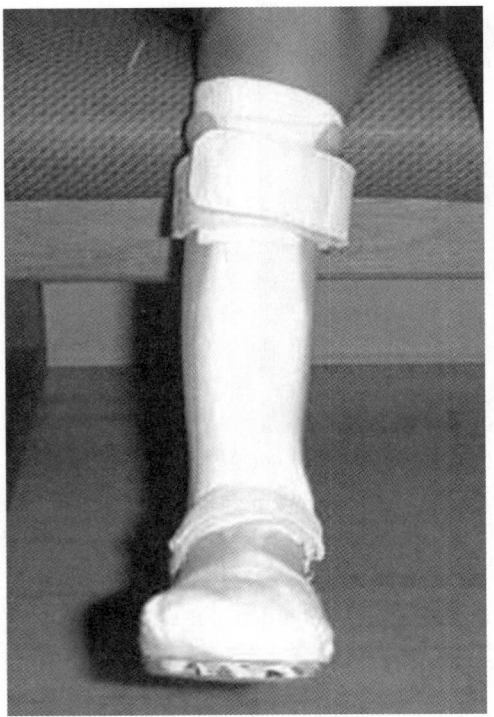

FIGURE 118-4 Splint is secured with Velcro straps. *(Photo courtesy of Scheck and Siress, Inc.)*

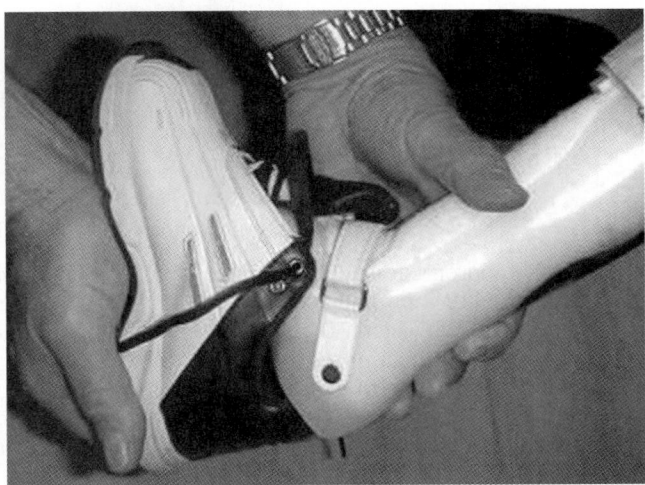

FIGURE 118-5 Shoe is applied over splint. *(Photo courtesy of Scheck and Siress, Inc.)*

Procedure   **for Brace and Splint Application**—*Continued*

Steps	Rationale	Considerations
12. Implement brace maintenance instructions, such as wear schedule, elevation, and rest periods.	Improper positioning may lead to injury or skin disruption. Elevation of extremity aids in decreasing edema. Not wearing the device for the prescribed amount of time is not therapeutic. Overwearing of the device may lead to injury or disruption in skin integrity.[2,3,4] *(Level IV*)*	
13. Evaluate neurovascular status and child's level of comfort following brace application. Loosen or remove splint and notify prescribing practitioner if there is deterioration in neurovascular status of the extremity or increasing pain.	Change in neurovascular status indicates an ill-fitting device and could result in nerve or tissue injury.[6] Identification of pain allows prompt treatment; presence of pain may indicate problems with device application.	

* Level IV: Limited clinical studies to support recommendations

---

Expected Outcomes	**Unexpected Outcomes**
• Splint or brace remains in place and fits snugly around supported area with good alignment • Splinted or braced area has good perfusion, sensation • Skin remains intact • Child demonstrates acceptable level of comfort • Brace or splint site is free from infection • Child tolerates brace or splint	• Loosely fitting device that does not provide proper support, immobility, or alignment of prescribed area • Vascular compromise, ischemia, compartment syndrome of affected extremity • Disruption of skin integrity • Unmanaged or increased pain • Infection at brace or splint site • Child is unable to tolerate wearing brace or splint

---

Monitoring and Care of the Child

Activities and Interventions	Rationale	Reportable Conditions
1. Splint or brace remains intact.	Device must fit snugly with proper alignment to be effective.	• Splint or brace falls off, is damaged, or moves out of place
2. Assess extremity for color, motion, sensation, edema, infection, and skin integrity.	Injury can result from improperly fitting device.	• Change in color, decreased pulses, decreased sensation, edema, skin breakdown, or infection
3. Monitor pain or discomfort.	Device should not cause pain.	• Pain unrelieved by removal and reapplication of device
4. Assess effectiveness of pain management strategy and provide appropriate interventions. Encourage family to assist in using nonpharmacologic means to comfort and support the child.	Allows prompt pain management.	• Ineffective pain management

Documentation

- Child and family education
- Integumentary, neurovascular, and musculoskeletal status
- Application and removal of splint or brace
- Length of time splint or brace is on
- Type and location of brace or splint
- Child's ability to tolerate brace or splint
- Unexpected outcomes and related treatment

References

1. Proehl J, editor: *Emergency nursing procedures,* ed 2, Philadelphia, 2000, Saunders.
2. Salmond S, et al, editors: NAON *core curriculum for orthopaedic nursing,* ed 3, Pittman, NJ, 1996, Janetti.
3. Hockenberry MJ, editor: *Wong's nursing care of infants and children,* ed 7, St. Louis, 2003, Mosby.
4. Pifer G: Casting and splinting: prevention of complication, *Top Emerg Med* 22(3):48-54, 2000.
5. Henretig FM, King C, editors: *Textbook of pediatric emergency procedures,* Baltimore, 1997, Williams & Wilkins.
6. Fleisher G, Ludwig S, editors: *Textbook of pediatric emergency medicine,* ed 4, Philadelphia, 2000, Lippincott Williams & Wilkins.

External Fixation Device: Pin Care

PURPOSE: To assess the fixator pin insertion sites for signs and symptoms of infection, remove exudate, and cleanse to prevent infection

Amanda Johnson

PREREQUISITE KNOWLEDGE

- Child development as it relates to clinical assessment and pin care
- Appropriate pediatric dosing of analgesics
- Anatomy and physiology of the musculoskeletal and integumentary systems
- The insertion of pins into the skin and bone can cause local infections as well as cellulitis and osteomyelitis.
- Numerous types of pins are used with external fixation devices. One does not need to know the type of pin, but instead the signs and symptoms of infection, such as erythema, warmth at site, pain at site, swelling, odor, and purulent drainage.
- Minimal evidence exists to indicate which pin site care regimen is most effective in reducing infection rates. No consensus exists as to optimal frequency of pin care or whether to remove exudates and crusting.[1] Follow institution-specific protocol when available.
- Patient safety goal: to reduce the risk of healthcare–associated infections

CHILD AND FAMILY ASSESSMENT

- Child's developmental level and ability to interact ➻*Rationale:* These factors influence preparation of the child and interaction.

- Child's and family's understanding of the reasons for pin care ➻*Rationale:* Evaluates child's and family's understanding of the procedure and provides a gauge for ongoing education.
- Musculoskeletal and integumentary status at the pin site ➻*Rationale:* Provides baseline data for identification of skin breakdown or indications of infection.
- Child's comfort level and history of pain or anxiety with previous pin care ➻*Rationale:* Identifies the need for an intervention for comfort or anxiety; promotes the child's ability to cope.

CHILD AND FAMILY EDUCATION

Individualized, developmentally appropriate education is provided to the family and the child based on desire for knowledge, readiness to learn, and overall neurologic and psychosocial state.

- Provide information regarding the reason for pin care to the family and the child (if appropriate) ➻*Rationale:* Decreases anxiety and fear.
- Explain how pin care will be performed, frequency, signs of complications, and that pin care will be continued after discharge ➻*Rationale:* Prepares the family to assume responsibility for their child's care. Knowledge will enhance compliance with home care and allow for identification of unexpected outcomes.

- Provide information to the child (as developmentally appropriate) or family about how they can assist with the procedure ➤➤*Rationale:* Allows child to participate in own care as appropriate, promoting coping and cooperation; assesses learning; allows the family to begin to practice skills they will need in the home setting.
- Encourage questions and answer questions as they arise ➤➤*Rationale:* Reinforcement of information is needed during periods of stress.

EQUIPMENT

- Sterile cotton-tipped applicators
- Clean gloves
- Sterile saline solution or other cleaning solution per institution-specific protocol
- Sterile container for cleaning solution
- Sterile 30-mL syringe
- Absorbent pads to place under site
- Gauze pads (size depends on amount of drainage)
- Tape

Procedure for External Fixation Device: Pin Care

Steps	Rationale	Considerations
1. Ensure child and family understand procedure and questions are answered.	Evaluates and reinforces understanding of previously taught information.	Developmental level, cognitive ability, and level of anxiety will determine approach to and effectiveness of teaching.
2. Gather needed equipment and supplies.	Preparation and having all materials present facilitates completion of procedure without delay.	
3. Provide for appropriate privacy; position the child to facilitate pin care.	Respects child's privacy; provides access to pin sites, facilitating completion of procedure.	Privacy is an important consideration for school-aged children and adolescents.
4. Wash hands; put on clean gloves.	Standard precautions; reduces the transmission of microorganisms.	
5. Place absorbent pad under the external fixation device.	Prevents bed from becoming saturated with saline.	
6. Pour approximately 30 mL of sterile saline or appropriate volume of cleaning solution into sterile container.	Prevents contamination of solution in multiuse container.	Hydrogen peroxide should not be used because it has been associated with pin site irritation.[2,3,4]
7. Draw sterile saline into syringe.	Syringe will be used to irrigate pin sites.	
8. Remove any gauze and tape from pin sites.	Allows visualization of the site.	If gauze is crusted to skin, moisten gauze with 0.9% saline to provide easy removal.
9. Assess skin surrounding pin site.	Ensures early identification of signs of infection.	
10. Irrigate all pin sites with sterile saline solution. *(Level II*)*	Pressure from syringe helps remove exudates and crusted areas, and cleanses the pin site thoroughly.[2,3,4]	Serous drainage may be present for the first 2 or 3 days.
11. Use dry sterile cotton-tipped applicators to wipe around each pin site. Change cotton-tipped applicator with each pin site (Figure 119-1). *(Level II*)*	Helps remove exudates and crusted areas, and dries the site completely. Changing the cotton-tipped applicator decreases cross contamination.[2,3,4,5]	A damp cotton-tipped applicator may be used if crusted areas are hard to remove.

* Level II: Theory based, no research data to support recommendations: recommendations from expert consensus group may exist

Procedure for External Fixation Device: Pin Care—*Continued*

Steps	Rationale	Considerations

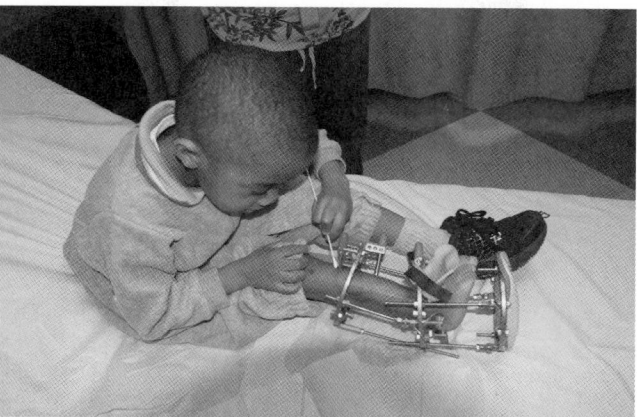

FIGURE 119-1   Pin sites are dried using sterile cotton-tipped applicators.

Steps	Rationale	Considerations
12. Cover each pin site with gauze and secure with tape. *(Level II*)*	Contains oozing. Helps prevent infection from touch and airborne contaminents.[2,3,4,5]	Do not cut gauze because threads of gauze may adhere to and infect the site. The practice of covering pin sites varies among institutions. Refer to institution-specific protocol.
13. Discard used supplies in appropriate receptacle.	Standard precautions; reduces the transmission of microorganisms.	
14. Remove gloves and wash hands.	Standard precautions; reduces the transmission of microorganisms.	

* Level II: Theory based, no research data to support recommendations: recommendations from expert consensus group may exist

Expected Outcomes

- Pin sites are free from infection
- Child is free from pain at pin sites
- Pin sites are free from irritation, bloody drainage
- Child tolerates pin care with acceptable level of comfort and minimal or no anxiety
- Child and/or family becomes competent at performing pin care

Unexpected Outcomes

- Infection at pin site (local, cellulitis, or osteomyelitis)
- Pain at pin sites
- Irritation or bleeding at pin site
- Unable to complete pin care due to child's pain or anxiety
- Family and/or child is unable to perform pin care

Monitoring and Care of the Child

Activities and Interventions	Rationale	Reportable Conditions
1. Perform pin care twice a day or more often as indicated or prescribed.	Keeps pin site clean; allows assessment of pin sites.	• Evidence of infection: redness, swelling, pain at the insertion site; discharge, pus, or odor
2. Assess pain and effectiveness of pain management strategies. Encourage family to assist in using nonpharmacologic means to comfort and support the child.	Allows early intervention for pain; promotes the use of diversional activities. Identifies the need for orthopedic consult if pins are loosened or dislodged.	• Unrelieved pain: may be associated with infection or dislodgment of pin

Documentation

- Child and family education
- Integumentary and neuromuscular status at pin sites
- Location of pin sites
- Drainage from pin sites
- Any loosening or dislodgment of pins and associated interventions
- Pain interventions and child's response
- Child's ability to tolerate the procedure
- Unexpected outcomes and related treatment

References

1. Temple J, Santy J: Pin site care for preventing infections associated with external bone fixators and pins, *Cochrane Database Syst Rev* 1:CD00455, 2004.
2. Bernardo L: Evidence-based practice for pin site care in injured children, *Orthop Nurs* 20(5):29-34, 2001.
3. Brereton V: Pin-site care and the rate of local infection, *J Wound Care* 10(1):42-44, 1998.
4. Wood M: A protocol for care of skeletal pin sites, *Nurs Times* 97(24):66-68, 2001.
5. Mckenzie L: In search of a standard for pin site care, *Orthop Nurs* 18(2):73-78, 1999.

External Fixator Lengthening Device: Adjustments

P U R P O S E : An external fixator ("exfix") placed on an extremity to correct a deformity, lengthen a limb, or stabilize a fracture is adjusted in small increments to allow gradual lengthening of the bone

Lee Brady

PREREQUISITE KNOWLEDGE

- Child development as it relates to clinical assessment and device adjustments
- Anatomy and physiology of the musculoskeletal, neurovascular, and integumentary systems
- Congenital or developmental differences specific to the child and desired correction
- Purpose of the adjustment to be performed
- Type of fixator used[1,2]
  - ❖ Circular fixators, such as the Ilizarov, encircle the fixated extremity and are attached to the bone with wires or pins.
  - ❖ Unilateral fixators are placed perpendicular to the fixated extremity and are attached to the bone with pins; refer to Figure 120-1 for an example of a unilateral fixator.
- Patient-specific information regarding adjustments provided by the prescribing practitioner: amount of lengthening (e.g., one quarter turn, 0.25 mm), frequency of the adjustments, and when the lengthening process is to begin (usually 7-10 days after the fixator has been placed)[1]
- Complications of external fixation and lengthening devices including pin site infection, osteomyelitis,

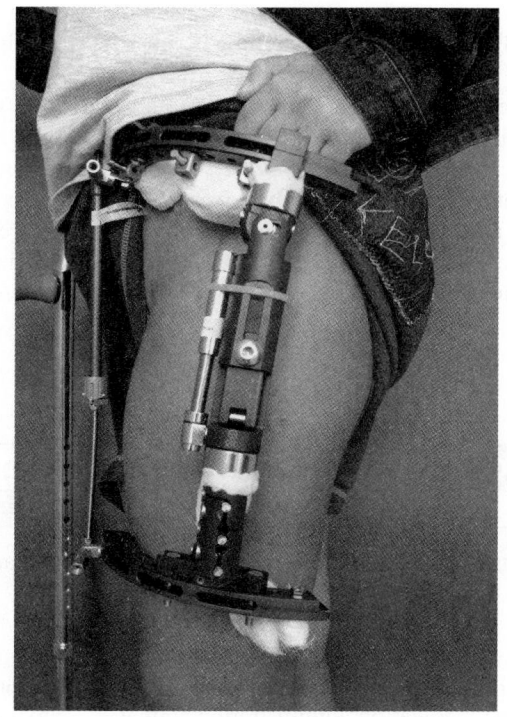

FIGURE 120-1 An example of a unilateral fixator.

contractures, nerve injury, vascular injury, refractures, and premature consolidation[1,2,3]
- Implications of incorrect manipulation or adjustment of the fixator including disruption of the bone and impaired growth of new tissue[1,2]
- Appropriate pediatric dosing of analgesics

CHILD AND FAMILY ASSESSMENT

- Child's developmental level and ability to interact ➡*Rationale:* These factors influence preparation of the child and interaction.
- Child's and family's understanding of the reasons for and risks and benefits of the procedure ➡*Rationale:* Evaluates child's and family's understanding of the procedure and provides a gauge for ongoing education.
- Child's history of limb-lengthening surgeries ➡*Rationale:* Many children have multiple limb-lengthening surgeries and may already have some familiarity with the procedure. Previous experiences may have been positive or negative and this will influence the present hospitalization. Caretakers may already be experts in their child's fixator management and should function as resources for nursing staff.
- Assess family's desire to perform the lengthening maneuvers ➡*Rationale:* Many families will be performing these adjustments independently at home and may wish to begin the lengthening maneuvers under supervision during the hospital stay. Others may require significant encouragement to participate.
- Assess child's previous reactions to any turning of the fixated extremity ➡*Rationale:* Some children react negatively to the prospect of turning because they anticipate it will be painful.
- Assess child's pain experiences and the child's and family's identification of pain management strategies that have been helpful ➡*Rationale:* Identifies pain management strategies likely to be successful; encourages child and family to participate in developing plan of care.
- Assess the musculoskeletal, neurovascular, and integumentary status of the fixated extremity ➡*Rationale:* Provides baseline data for ongoing assessment. Facilitates identification of complications such as skin breakdown.

CHILD AND FAMILY EDUCATION

Individualized, developmentally appropriate education is provided to the family and to the child based on desire for knowledge, readiness to learn, and overall neurologic and psychosocial state.

- Teaching strategies may include the use of models or dolls with fixators applied ➡*Rationale:* Allows the child to visualize the fixator, facilitating coping. This teaching strategy may be especially effective with preschool and school-aged children.
- Education may be provided preoperatively for elective limb-lengthening procedures and is generally started by a clinician from the orthopedic surgical team. This teaching is then reinforced after the surgery has been performed ➡*Rationale:* Allows learning to begin in a less stressful environment and ongoing reinforcement of learning.
- Explain that adjustments to the device are done in such small increments that the child generally does not feel discomfort as the turns are completed ➡*Rationale:* Providing information helps to reduce anxiety.
- Explain that in order to reach some of the adjustment points, the child may need to move the extremity so as to enhance visualization of the device ➡*Rationale:* Allowing the child and family rather than the staff to move the extremity may help reduce discomfort associated with movement and facilitate coping.
- Encourage questions and answer questions as they arise ➡*Rationale:* Reinforcement of information is needed during periods of stress.

EQUIPMENT

- A wrench may be necessary for certain types of fixators. These are generally metric wrenches supplied by the manufacturer of the specific device. Other fixators have preset computer-controlled units attached to the fixator.

Procedure	**for External Fixator Lengthening Device: Adjustments**	
Steps	Rationale	Considerations
1. Ensure child and family understand procedure and questions are answered.	Evaluates and reinforces previously taught information.	Developmental level, cognitive ability and anxiety level will determine approach to and effectiveness of teaching.
2. If premedication has been prescribed, time medication administration so that adjustment is performed at the time of peak effectiveness.	Promotes effective pain or anxiety management.	

Procedure **for External Fixator Lengthening Device: Adjustments**—*Continued*

Steps	Rationale	Considerations
3. Collect necessary supplies (wrenches).	Preparation and presence of all needed materials facilitates completion of procedure in a timely manner.	
4. Review medical record for specific orders for adjustment (turns, sites).	Turns must be done at the predetermined rate/site to avoid complications and optimize outcomes. Depending on the type and number of fixators, there may be different turning schedules for different sites.[2]	Orders should be written in a consistent, clear manner, such as "one quarter turn four times a day on rods 1 and 2."
5. Wash hands.	Standard precautions; reduces the transmission of microorganisms.	
6. Identify child using two patient identifiers per institution-specific protocol.	Promotes patient safety; ensures that prescribed treatment is delivered to the correct child.	
7. Identify which site(s) are to be turned.	Turns done at the wrong site may negatively affect the outcome of therapy.	Turn sites that have been manually marked by the orthopedic team may be color coded if they are to be done in groups.
8. Identify direction in which the device is to be turned.	Turns done in the wrong direction will negatively affect the outcome of therapy.	Most manufacturers place small arrows on the devices; however, some are unmarked. The orthopedic team may add larger, more easily identified arrows or other indicators of the direction of the turns (e.g., clockwise or counterclockwise).
9. Perform adjustment for each device according to the manufacturer's directions. Refer to Figure 120-2 for one example of an adjustment.	Mechanism to adjust the device varies among manufacturers.	If device has a locking mechanism, the device will need to be unlocked before making the adjustment.

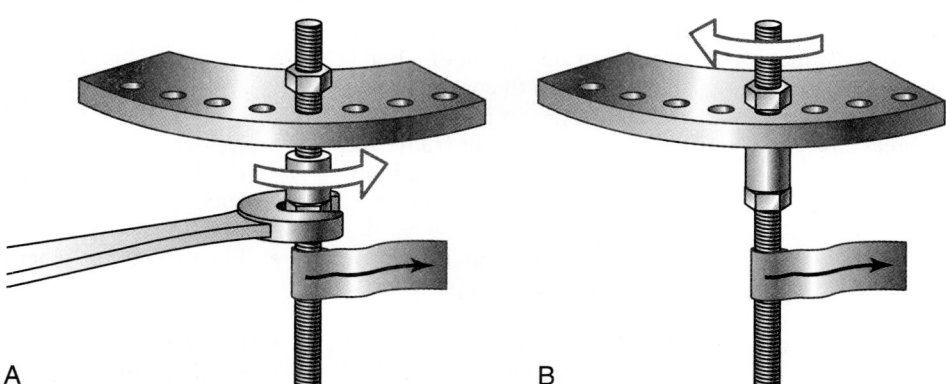

A   B

FIGURE 120-2   An Example of a Fixator Adjustment. **A,** A flag is attached to the unit to indicate the direction of the turn. **B,** The locking mechanism is relocked. *Drawing courtesy of D. Paley, MD, Rubin Institute for Advanced Orthopedics, Baltimore, MD, © 2003.*

10. If locking mechanism is present, lock the device after the adjustment according to the manufacturer's directions. Refer to Figure 120-2 for an example of a locking mechanism.	Locking the device helps prevent accidental turns, either as the child moves or if the child plays with the device. Not all devices have a locking mechanism.	

Procedure continues on following page

Procedure for External Fixator Lengthening Device: Adjustments—*Continued*

Steps	Rationale	Considerations
11. Assess skin under fixator device and assess pin or wire insertion sites.	Ensures early identification of skin breakdown or complications such as infection.	
12. Cover the device with a protective garment if child or family desires.	Many children are more comfortable with the devices out of sight. Covers may also help prevent the child from accidentally resetting the fixator or contaminating pin sites.	Stockinette or other soft cloth product may be used as a temporary cover. Many families sew their own covers, based on the dimensions of the particular device.
13. Wash hands.	Standard precautions; reduces the transmission of microorganisms.	

Expected Outcomes

- Fixator moves a small, but noticeable amount
- Child is comfortable during the adjustment

- Skin under fixator device remains intact
- Child and/or family is able to perform the adjustments correctly and to complete the adjustments at the correct intervals

Unexpected Outcomes

- Fixator will not adjust
- Child experiences unexpected discomfort
- Unmanaged pain
- Skin breakdown under fixator device
- Family is unable to perform adjustments correctly or is unable to follow the adjustment schedule

Monitoring and Care of the Child

Activities and Interventions	Rationale	Reportable Conditions
1. Monitor for pain or discomfort; assess effectiveness of pain management strategy and provide appropriate interventions. Encourage family to assist in nonpharmacologic means to comfort and support the child.	Postoperative pain is expected, but unusual pain may indicate nerve stretch.[3] Sudden onset of pain can indicate a "pop" or disruption of a bone that has begun to consolidate prematurely.[3]	• Burning, sudden pain, or numbness
2. Monitor for skin breakdown or indications of rod infection.	Breakdown may occur from excessive skin movement around pin sites or device pressure on an edematous extremity.[3]	• Evidence of skin breakdown • Evidence of infection at rod insertion sites
3. Monitor fixator settings.	Some types of fixators may move on their own and may need to be reset.	• Fixator settings other than those prescribed
4. Monitor child's compliance with the device.	Some children may try to imitate adjustment of the fixator and actually change the settings.	• Child alters fixator settings significantly
5. Assess ability to perform adjustments.	Difficulty in performing adjustments may indicate a problem with the fixator.	• Inability to perform adjustments
6. Monitor fixator to ensure it remains intact, is aligned correctly, and that rods are secure.	Device must be intact and aligned correctly to be effective.	• Fixator is damaged or moves out of place • Rods appear loose at insertion sites

---

Documentation

- Child and family education including child's or family's ability to perform adjustment
- Time, amount, and site of turns
- Musculoskeletal, neurovascular, and integumentary status of fixated extremity
- Assessment of pin or wire insertion sites and any care provided
- Child's ability to tolerate fixator adjustments and strategies used to facilitate coping
- Comfort assessment and any specific interventions provided
- Unexpected outcomes and related treatment

References

1. Chiang PP, et al: Limb lengthening: a review focused on complications for the emergency physician, *Top Emerg Med* 22(3):23–34, 2000.
2. Beeman J, Diehl B: A credentialing program for nursing staff caring for pediatric patients with an Ilizarov apparatus, *Rehab Nurs* 20(5):278–282, 1995.
3. Paley D: Problems, obstacles, and complications of limb lengthening by the Ilizarov technique, *Clin Orthop Relat Res* 250:81–104, 1990.

Additional Reading

Paley D: *Principles of deformity correction,* Berlin, Germany, 2003, Springer-Verlag.

PROCEDURE **121**

Burn Wound Care

P U R P O S E : Burn wound care is provided to all children who sustain partial and full thickness wounds to any area on their bodies to reduce the amount of bacteria present at the site, keep the wound bed moist, and remove devascularized tissue that may interfere with adequate wound healing

Laurie DeMondo Jaffe

PREREQUISITE KNOWLEDGE

- Anatomy and physiology of the skin
- Understanding of the pathophysiology of burn injuries
- Classification of burn injury and appearance[1-3]
  - ❖ Superficial burns involve the epidermis only.
    - ○ Burns are pink or red, painful, and dry.
    - ○ Burns heal in 3 to 4 days.
    - ○ Burns generally heal without scar formation or loss of pigmentation.
  - ❖ Superficial partial thickness burns involve the epidermis and some of the dermis
    - ○ Burns are pink and moist; they blister and are very painful.
    - ○ Burns usually heal in 2-3 weeks by re-epithelialization.
    - ○ Burns have minimal risk of scar formation and some pigmentation loss.
  - ❖ Deep partial thickness burns involve the epidermis and most of the dermis.
    - ○ Burns appear white, mottled pink and white, or red; the wound bed may have adherent soft eschar; they are not as painful as superficial wounds.
    - ○ Burns need at least 4 weeks to heal (healing involves the development of granulation tissue) or require surgical intervention.
    - ○ Scar formation is likely, as is pigmentation loss.
  - ❖ Full thickness burns involve the epidermis, dermis, and may involve the subcutaneous fat.
    - ○ Burns appear black, brown, white or red; the texture is leathery or waxy; thrombosed vessels are usually present; they are dry and nonpainful; the edges of the wound may be painful if not as deep.
    - ○ Burns have thick scar formation and loss of pigmentation.
    - ○ Great variability exists in healing time; surgical intervention is necessary for wound closure.
- Child development as it relates to clinical assessment and support of the child during the procedure[4-6]
- Burn wound care (BWC) can be provided in almost any setting; depending on the cleanliness of the environment, a sterile field may need to be created.
- The goals of BWC are to control the growth of microorganisms, prevent infection, prevent the wound from converting, promote healing, prevent sepsis, and minimize scarring.[1-3,7,8]
- The frequency of BWC is dictated by institution-specific protocol, types of topicals used, and the child's wound status; frequency varies from twice a day to every 72 to 96 hours.[1-3,7,8]
- Topical wound care agents and biosynthetic dressings commonly used in BWC[1-3,7-10]:
  - ❖ Topical antimicrobial agents, such as sulfadiazine, mafenide acetate and bacitracin keep the wound moist, minimize wound flora, and delay wound colonization.
  - ❖ Enzymatic topical preparations debride the wound bed by digesting necrotic tissue.

- ❖ Biologic dressings
  - ○ Homograft is skin harvested from human donors used as a temporary cover for burns.
  - ○ Skin substitutes are placed to form a protective barrier and provide a growth matrix for tissue regeneration.
  - ○ Biosynthetic dressings are temporary dressings; they consist of a biologic and a man made component.
- ❖ Synthetic dressings are temporary dressings that protect the wound and may or may not be occlusive.
  - ○ Impregnated gauze dressings are very commonly used with topical antimicrobial agents and are nonocclusive and nonadherent; they provide protection, prevent drying and keep the topical antimicrobials in place.
  - ○ Foam dressings are nonocclusive, absorb exudates, and keep the wound moist; not intended for long-term use.
  - ○ Polyurethane dressings are occlusive, maintain a moist environment, and prevent exposure to microorganisms and are generally not used on burn wounds.
- ❖ There are several silver impregnated gauze dressings that are used to keep bacteria colony counts low. They are not changed as frequently (every 3 to 7 days) as most dressings.
- ❖ Vacuum-Assisted Closure (VAC™) dressing (Kinetic Systems, Inc., San Antonio, TX) is a negative-pressure dressing that removes exudates and minimizes exposure to microorganisms; it is changed every 2 to 5 days.
- Burn wound care is painful; children need emotional, physical, and analgesic support. A multidisciplinary team is most effective in meeting the child's needs.[1-6]
- Appropriate pediatric dosing of analgesics and anxiolytics
- Aseptic technique
- Use of developmentally appropriate pain assessment scales (see Procedure 173 for more information)

CHILD AND FAMILY ASSESSMENT

- History of illnesses or drug allergies ➤*Rationale:* These conditions may impact the mode of BWC selected and the medications used.
- Child's developmental level and ability to interact ➤*Rationale:* These factors influence preparation of the child, selection of an appropriate pain scale, interaction during the procedure, and personnel who may be needed during the procedure.
- Interaction between family and child ➤*Rationale:* Identifies effective and ineffective methods used by the family to support the child.
- Depth of burns, the areas involved, and the dressing type used ➤*Rationale:* Assists in prediction of the need for and most appropriate analgesia, supplies necessary, and specifics of procedure.
- Previous pain and sedation experiences of child and family and the child's and family's identification of pain and anxiety management strategies that have been helpful in the past[5-7] ➤*Rationale:* Identifies pain management strategies likely to be successful; the child and family are encouraged to participate in development of a plan of care.
- Child's and family's understanding of the reasons for and risks and benefits of the procedure ➤*Rationale:* Evaluates child's and family's understanding of the procedure and provides a gauge for ongoing education.
- Desire of family members to be present during BWC ➤*Rationale:* Family members may provide comfort and support during the procedure, but they should have the choice not to remain with the child. Institution-specific protocol may limit family presence.

CHILD AND FAMILY EDUCATION

Individualized, developmentally appropriate education is provided to the family and to the child based on desire for knowledge, readiness to learn, and overall neurologic and psychosocial state.

- Explain the purpose and frequency of BWC ➤*Rationale:* Information decreases anxiety and fear and provides the family with information that they need to support the child.
- Explain the need for analgesia and anxiolytics and possible reactions the child may have to medications ➤*Rationale:* This information prepares the child and family for what may be experienced after wound care (e.g., increased lethargy, increased irritability, and decreased appetite).
- Explain the process of BWC and the anticipated length of the procedure ➤*Rationale:* This information prepares the child and family for the length of the procedure and allays fears that could be associated with waiting if the family is not with the child during BWC.
- Explain the need for additional support that the child may have after BWC ➤*Rationale:* The family is prepared to address the needs of the child after BWC.
- Review the pain and anxiety management plan for the child, including Child Life support, sedation, and other methods as outlined in institution-specific protocols ➤*Rationale:* Providing information decreases anxiety and fear and reassures the child and family that pain will be managed appropriately.
- Encourage questions and answer questions as they arise ➤*Rationale:* Reinforcement of information is needed during periods of stress.

EQUIPMENT

- Analgesics or anxiolytics appropriate for the child's age and weight and the specific procedure to be performed per prescribing practitioner's order (Table 121-1)
- Burn wound cleansing agents
- Burn wound topicals or antimicrobial dressings (topical wound care agents and biosynthetic dressings)
- Hydrotherapy source

- Sterile and clean gloves
- Burn wound pads or 4×4 gauze
- Sterile or nonsterile scissors
- Debridement set
- Nonadherent dressing

- Gauze rolls
- Flexible net dressing (not necessary but helpful for increased mobility)
- Personal protective equipment, including eye and face protection, mask, and gown as appropriate

TABLE 121-1	Pain Control Recommendations

Event	Pain Medication Guidelines

Background pain	All patients receive acetaminophen 15 mg/kg po every 4 hours
	Maximum dose:
	    Children <12 years, 2.6 g in 24 hours
	    Children >12 years, 4 g in 24 hours[11]
	If more background medication is necessary:
	    Children > 3 years, morphine 0.3 mg/kg po every 4 hours
	    Children < 3 years, morphine 0.1 mg/kg po every 4 hours

Immediate postoperative period (first 24 hours)	Morphine 0.3 mg/kg po and midazolam 0.5 mg/kg po every 3 to 4 hours or alternate each every 3 to 4 hours
	Morphine 0.03 mg/kg IV and midazolam 0.03 mg/kg IV every 2 to 4 hours or alternate each every 2 to 4 hours
	    Children > 5 years, morphine PCA pump
	        PCA dose, 0.05 mg/kg morphine
	        PCA lockout interval, 6 to 15 minutes
	        PCA 4-hour limit, 0.2 to 0.3 mg/kg

Dressing changes and hydrotherapy	Morphine 0.3 mg/kg po and midazolam 0.3 mg/kg po Morphine 0.03 mg/kg IV and midazolam 0.03 mg/kg IV Ketamine 0.5 to 2 mg/kg IV Propofol 0.5 to 1 mg/kg IV Nitrous oxide 50% by patient-controlled face mask
Rehabilitation therapy	Morphine 0.1 to 0.3 mg/kg po Morphine 0.03 mg/kg IV
Reconstructive surgery postoperative period	Hydrocodone 0.1 to 0.2 mg/kg po q 4 to 6 hours with: hydrocodone 5 mg/acetaminophen 500 mg Hydrocodone/acetaminophen elixir: 5 mL contains hydrocodone 2.5 mg, acetaminophen 167 mg

po, By mouth; *IV,* intravenously; *PCA,* patient controlled analgesia; *q,* every.
From Herndon DN, editor: *Total burn care,* ed 2, London, 2002, Saunders.

Procedure for Burn Wound Care

Steps	Rationale	Considerations
1. Ensure child and family understand procedure and questions are answered.	May serve to reduce child's and family's anxiety.[5-7] Evaluates and reinforces understanding of previously taught information.	Developmental level, cognitive ability, and anxiety level determine approach to and effectiveness of teaching.
2. Gather needed equipment and supplies.	Facilitates completion of task in a timely manner.	
3. Assess child's pain and anxiety level; administer premedication with analgesics and anxiolytics per prescribing practitioner's order (see Table 121-1).	Promotes child's comfort during procedure; ensures adequate pain and anxiety control; promotes compliance with future procedures.[4-6]	Child Life Specialist may be helpful in working with the child to use nonpharmacologic pain and anxiety control techniques.

Procedure continues on following page

Procedure for Burn Wound Care—*Continued*

Steps	Rationale	Considerations
4. If necessary, transport child to procedure location.	Specialized equipment necessary for BWC may require transport.	Performance of BWC in a specific location may assist the child in coping with the procedure; provision to the child of a "safe" area in which procedures are not performed may decrease anxiety.[5]
5. Ensure appropriate physiologic monitoring throughout BWC.	BWC may increase demand for oxygen delivery by 100%. Children with critical burn injuries are at risk for decompensation during wound care.[7]	At a minimum, oxygen saturation should be monitored.
6. Maintain a warm environment and minimize exposure for protection from hypothermia. Provide for appropriate privacy; position child to promote child's comfort and facilitate procedure.	Preservation of child's body temperature is important for maintenance of hemodynamic and metabolic demands. Location of burn wounds may necessitate exposure of the child; respects the child's rights.	Privacy is an important consideration for school-aged children and adolescents.
7. Wash hands; put on personal protective equipment (gloves, gown, and mask) as indicated for the specific procedure.	Standard precautions; reduces transmission of microorganisms.	All members of team present during BWC should adhere to standard precautions.
8. Remove splints if necessary; remove dressings and discard in appropriate receptacle.	Standard precautions; reduces transmission of microorganisms.	Eschar or drainage (devitalized human tissue) may be present on burn wound dressings.
9. Remove gloves; put on sterile or clean gloves per institution-specific protocol.	Burn wound precautions; contact is made with openings in the skin.	
10. Gently cleanse wounds with cleansing agent per prescribing practitioner's order or institution-specific protocol (e.g., 0.9% saline solution or bacteriostatic soap) and clean cloth or gauze pad. Use soft circular motions. *Never scrub.* (*Level II**)	Wound care that is done too aggressively may damage newly formed epithelial cells and delay wound healing.[1,2,7]	The child is not immersed in water because immersion increases potential for cross contamination of wounds and may result in lowering the patient's body temperature too rapidly. Water should flow over wounds and immediately be drained away; use shower or hydrotherapy stretcher (bed bath for child with hemodynamically unstable condition).
11. Debridement of devitalized necrotic tissue may be performed at this time if necessary; institution-specific protocol dictates who performs this procedure.	Presence of devitalized tissue at the wound site increases bacterial counts at the wound bed and places the patient at risk for development of wound infection.[1-3,7]	
12. Rinse wound beds and pat dry in preparation for dressing.	Some topical preparations may be difficult to apply if wounds are wet. (*Level I**)	
13. Put on a new pair of sterile or clean gloves.	Burn wound precautions; minimizes cross contamination.	

* Level I: Manufacturer's recommendations only
  Level II: Theory-based; no research data to support recommendations; recommendations from expert consensus group may exist

Procedure for Burn Wound Care—*Continued*

Steps	Rationale	Considerations
14. Apply topical agents or dressings per prescribing practitioner's order or institution-specific protocol.	Nonadherent dressings keep topical medications in place and protect the wound bed from dressing adherence. Dressing is dependent on the product or agent used. Refer to the manufacturer's recommendation for dressing to be used with specific agent placed on burn. *(Level I*)*	A complete history of child's allergies is necessary before application of any burn dressings or medications.
15. Wrap the affected area with gauze rolls or burn wound pads as needed. Attention to range of motion is crucial. All digits should be wrapped independently. Dressings should not be restrictive enough to inhibit movement. *(Level II*)*	Maintenance of range of motion throughout the wound healing phase is essential for good functional outcomes after wound closure.[1-3,5-7]	Appropriate pain management is crucial for compliance with rehabilitation interventions.
16. Praise the child for doing well during and after procedure.[4-6] *(Level II*)*	Positive reinforcement may result in increased compliance with future procedures.[4-6]	
17. Discard used supplies and equipment, including sharps, in appropriate receptacles.	Standard precautions; reduces transmission of microorganisms.	
18. Remove personal protective equipment; wash hands.	Standard precautions. Protects personnel health.	
19. Return child to room and family members if they were not present for dressing change. Once again, provide child with positive reinforcement.	Return to room signals end of procedure; positive reinforcement may result in increased compliance with future procedures.[4-6]	

* Level I: Manufacturer's recommendations only
  Level II: Theory-based; no research data to support recommendations; recommendations from expert consensus group may exist

Expected Outcomes

- Burn wound care is completed within shortest amount of time possible without complications
- Child's pain and anxiety related to burn wound care are effectively controlled
- Wound healing progresses with daily improvements noted

- Wound is free from infection

- Cardiorespiratory status and temperature remain stable throughout procedure

Unexpected Outcomes

- Time for completion of procedure is prolonged

- Unmanaged pain or anxiety
- Regression and inability to use coping skills
- Wound healing does not progress
- Wounds convert to deeper wounds necessitating surgical intervention
- Infection develops in wound
- Systemic infection develops
- Hypothermia related to prolonged exposure to environment and water
- Child has decompensation from stress of procedure and inadequate respiratory support

Monitoring and Care of the Child

Activities and Interventions	Rationale	Reportable Conditions
1. Obtain vital signs, including temperature, before and after procedure.	Child is at risk for development of hypothermia with prolonged exposure.	• Hypothermia or hyperthermia • Vital sign instability
2. Assess size of wound, wound color, absence or presence of drainage, extent of wound healing, and location of wound.	Monitors progress of wound healing.	• Indications that wound is not healing
3. Monitor burn wound for indications of presence of infection.	Early identification of infection facilitates prompt treatment.	• Delayed wound healing • Indications of infection at burn wound • Increased temperature • Increased white blood cell count
4. Assess child's pain and anxiety before, during, and after the procedure.	Prompt identification of pain or anxiety facilitates rapid treatment.	• Report of unresolved pain and discomfort • Continued irritability or changes in physiologic condition
5. Assess effectiveness of pain and anxiety management strategies and provide appropriate interventions. Encourage family to assist with nonpharmacologic means to comfort and support the child.	Because of painful stimuli and hypermetabolic state, child may need increased medication doses. Facilitates modifications to management strategies as indicated.	• Pain or anxiety refractory to medication administration • Inability to perform or complete the procedure because of increased pain or anxiety levels
6. Presence of bleeding through burn wound dressings.	Some types of wound beds bleed after stimulation.	• Wounds that continue to bleed despite intervention
7. Monitor perfusion to the extremity or area of the burn wound.	Compromised circulation inhibits healing of the burn wound.	• Indications of inadequate perfusion in the area of the burn wound • Indications of inadequate systemic perfusion
8. Monitor caloric and protein intake and nutritional status.	Severe burns result in increased metabolic requirements and catabolism.[1]	• Inadequate delivery of calories or protein • Child does not tolerate enteral feeds • Weight loss

Documentation

- Child and family education
- Medications administered for pain and anxiety control and effectiveness
- Location and appearance of wounds
- Specific procedures performed (e.g., sharp debridement)
- Topicals and dressings applied
- Members of team who participated in BWC
- Unexpected outcomes and related treatments

References

1. Merz J, et al: Wound care of the pediatric burn patient, *AACN Clin Iss* 14(4):429-441, 2003.
2. Honari S: Topical therapies and antimicrobials in the management of burn wounds, *Crit Care Nurs Clin North Am* 16(1):1-11, 2004.
3. Sheridan RL: Burns, *Crit Care Med* 30(11supplement):S500-514, 2002.
4. Tarnowski KJ, editor: *Behavioral aspects of pediatric burns,* New York, 1994, Plenum Press.
5. Dise-Lewis JE: A developmental perspective on psychological principles of burn care, *J Burn Care Rehabil* 22(3):255-260, 2001.
6. Smith M, et al: Unique considerations in caring for a pediatric burn patient: a developmental approach, *Crit Care Nurs Clin North Am* 16(1):99-108, 2004.
7. Herndon DN, editor: *Total burn care,* ed 2, London, 2002, Saunders.
8. Trofino RB, editor: *Nursing care of the burn injured patient,* Philadelphia, 1991, F.A. Davis Company.
9. Lukish JR, et al: The use of a bioactive skin substitute decreases length of stay for pediatric burn patients, *J Pediatr Surg* 36(8):1118-1121, 2001.
10. Heimbach DM, et al: Multicenter postapproval clinical trial of Integra dermal regeneration template for burn treatment, *J Burn Care Rehabil* 24(1):42-48, 2003.
11. Takemoto CK, et al: *Pediatric dosage handbook,* ed 12, Hudson, OH, 2005, Lexi-Comp, Inc.

Additional Readings

Bishop JF: Burn wound assessment and surgical management, *Crit Care Nurs Clin North Am* 16(1):145-177, 2004.

Deitch E, Rutan R: *The challenges of children: the first 48 hours,* Chicago, 2003, American Burn Association Education Committee.

Herdon DN, et al: Management of the pediatric patient with burns, *J Burn Care Rehabil* 14:3-8, 1993.

Owens VF, et al: Ketamine: a safe and effective agent for painful procedures in the pediatric burn patient, *J Burn Care Res* 27(2):211-217, 2006.

Donor Site Care

P U R P O S E : To keep the area of the donor site clean and moist and to promote wound healing

Laurie DeMondo Jaffe

PREREQUISITE KNOWLEDGE

- Anatomy and physiology of the skin
- Dressing preferences vary greatly on the basis of surgeon preference and institution-specific protocol.[1-3]
  - ❖ Open technique: No dressing is applied; the wound is covered with ointment; wound care may be performed several times a day.
  - ❖ Semiopen technique: The wound bed is covered with a topical antibiotic impregnated dressing or biosynthetic dressing.
  - ❖ Closed technique: An occlusive dressing is applied to the donor site and is changed depending on the product and institution-specific guidelines.
- Dressings that provide a moist healing environment, such as transparent films, hydrocolloid dressings, and calcium alginates, are associated with the shortest time to healing in split-thickness donor sites.[1-3] *(Level VI*)*
- Understanding of the pathophysiology of the surgically created donor site (DS), which is usually a superficial partial thickness site that heals with epithelialization[1,3]
- Care of this superficial site involves keeping the area clean and moist to promote the epithelialization process. Daily intervention may only include assessment for indications of wound healing, identification of infection, and dressing reinforcement.
- Exudate from the wound appears to have a role in promotion of epithelialization.[3] *(Level IV*)*

- The frequency of DS care is dictated by institution-specific protocol, type of dressings used, depth of surgical site, and needs of the individual child.[1-5]
- Superficial DS should heal within 5 to 14 days after the harvesting procedure.[1-5]
- Donor site care may be painful; children need emotional, physical, and analgesic support.[6] Consultation with Child Life Therapy and Pain Management facilitates development of a multidisciplinary plan of care.
- Child development as it relates to clinical assessment and support of the child during the procedure
- Principles of aseptic technique
- Appropriate pediatric dosing of analgesics and anxiolytics
- Use of developmentally appropriate pain assessment scales (see Procedure 173 for more information)

CHILD AND FAMILY ASSESSMENT

- History of illnesses or known allergies ➻*Rationale:* These conditions may interfere with the performance of wound care and medications used.
- Child's developmental level and ability to interact ➻*Rationale:* These factors influence preparation of the child, selection of an appropriate pain scale, interaction during the procedure, and personnel who may be necessary during the procedure.
- Interaction between family and child ➻*Rationale:* Identifies effective and ineffective methods used by the family to support the child.
- Depth of DS, the areas involved, and the dressing type used ➻*Rationale:* Assists in predicting the need for and

---

* Level IV: Limited clinical studies to support recommendations
Level VI: Clinical studies in a variety of patient populations and situations to support recommendations

the most appropriate analgesia, the supplies necessary, and the specifics of the procedure.

- Previous pain and sedation experiences of the child and family and the child's and family's identification of pain and anxiety management strategies that have been helpful in the past ➤*Rationale:* Identifies pain management strategies likely to be successful; child and family are encouraged to participate in development of plan of care.
- Child's and family's understanding of the reasons for and risks and benefits of procedure ➤*Rationale:* Evaluates child's and family's understanding of the procedure and provides a gauge for ongoing education.
- Desire of family members to be present during DS care ➤*Rationale:* Family members may provide comfort and support during the procedure, but they should have the choice not to remain with the child. Institution-specific protocol may limit family presence.

CHILD AND FAMILY EDUCATION

Individualized, developmentally appropriate education is provided to the family and to the child based on desire for knowledge, readiness to learn, and overall neurologic and psychosocial state.

- Explain the need for care and the frequency at which it will occur ➤*Rationale:* Providing information may reduce anxiety and assist the family in supporting the child.
- Explain the need for analgesia and possible reactions the child may have to specific medications ➤*Rationale:* Providing information prepares the family and child for what may be experienced after wound care (e.g., increased lethargy, increased irritability, decreased appetite).
- Discuss the properties of the dressing placed on the DS ➤*Rationale:* Providing information prepares the child and family for what may be experienced with the DS dressing. Some dressings produce a foul odor or drainage, which may cause unnecessary fear for the child and family. Knowledge of what to expect decreases anxiety.
- Explain what occurs during DS care and that the procedure may be long ➤*Rationale:* Providing information prepares the child and family for the length of procedure and

allays fears that could be associated with waiting if the family is not with the child during DS care.

- Explain the need for additional support the child may have after DS care ➤*Rationale:* The family is prepared to address the needs of the child after DS care.
- Review the pain and anxiety management plan for the child, including Child Life support, sedation, and other methods as outlined in institution-specific protocols ➤*Rationale:* Providing information decreases anxiety and fear and reassures the child and family that pain will be managed appropriately.
- Encourage questions and answer questions as they arise ➤*Rationale:* Reinforcement of information is needed during periods of stress.

EQUIPMENT

For Intact DS Dressings that Do Not Necessitate Removal:

- Donor site dressings per prescribing practitioner's order
- Sterile or clean scissors
- Analgesics or anxiolytics appropriate for child's age and weight and specific procedure to be performed per prescribing practitioner's order (see Table 121-1) in Procedure 121
- Compression bandages
- Clean gloves
- Sterile gloves

For DS that Appears Infected or Converted:

- Analgesics or anxiolytics appropriate for child's age and weight and specific procedure to be performed per prescribing practitioner's order (see Table 121-1)
- Burn wound cleansing agents per institution-specific protocol or prescribing practitioner's order
- Wound topicals per institution-specific protocol or prescribing practitioner's order
- Hydrotherapy source or 0.9% saline solution irrigation
- Sterile and clean gloves
- Burn wound pads or 4×4 gauze
- Sterile or clean scissors
- Nonadherent dressing
- Gauze rolls or compression bandages
- Stretchy dressing (not necessary but extremely helpful for increased mobility)

Procedure for Donor Site Care

Steps	Rationale	Considerations
Dressing Reinforcement		
1. Ensure child and family understand procedure and questions are answered.	May serve to reduce child's and family's anxiety. Evaluates and reinforces understanding of previously taught information.	Developmental level, cognitive ability, and anxiety level determine approach to and effectiveness of teaching.
2. Gather needed equipment and supplies.	Facilitates completion of task in a timely manner.	
3. Assess child's pain and anxiety level; administer premedication with analgesics and anxiolytics per prescribing practitioner's order (see Procedure 121, Table 121-1).	Promotes child's comfort during procedure; ensures adequate pain and anxiety control and promotes compliance with future procedures.[4-6]	Child Life Specialist may be helpful in working with the child to use nonpharmacologic pain and anxiety control techniques.
4. Wash hands; put on personal protective equipment (gloves, gown, and mask) as indicated for the specific procedure.	Standard precautions; reduces transmission of microorganisms.	
5. Provide for appropriate privacy; position child to promote child's comfort and facilitate procedure.	Location of DS may necessitate exposure of the child; respects the child's rights.	Privacy is an important consideration for school-aged children and adolescents.
6. Assess DS covering for adherence of dressing, leakage, collection of secretions, foul odor, or abnormal color.	The presence of loose dressing or leakage necessitates dressing reinforcement. *(Level I*)* The presence of foul odor, abnormal color, and collection of secretions could be signs of DS infection that need different interventions.[4]	Discuss findings with prescribing practitioner to facilitate appropriate changes to plan of care for child (e.g., removal of DS dressing and treatment of area as burn wound; see Procedure 121).
7. Cleanse DS dressing and surrounding area of all leakage.	Leakage could serve to macerate the noninjured tissue.	
8. Dry area.	Protects healthy tissue from maceration.	
9. Reinforce DS dressing at site of leak. If dressing is loose, it may need to be removed and a new DS dressing applied.	The DS dressing must be adherent without presence of leakage to provide a moist environment for epithelialization.[2-5] *(Level I*)*	
10. Wrap reinforced dressing with compression bandage.	Promotes adherence of colloidal dressing.[5] *(Level I*)*	
11. Dispose of used supplies and equipment in appropriate receptacles.	Standard precautions; reduces transmission of microorganisms.	
12. Remove personal protective equipment; wash hands.	Standard precautions.	
Care of Donor Site with Foul Drainage or Abnormal Color		
1. Reinforce education surrounding procedure and reasons for removal of the donor site dressings. Answer any questions that child or family may have.	Reinforces information regarding procedure. May serve to reduce anxiety in family or child.[6]	Child may not be able to understand teaching. Educating the family facilitates family's ability to support child.[6]
2. Gather needed equipment and supplies.	Facilitates completion of task in a timely manner.	

* Level I: Manufacturer's recommendations only

Procedure for Donor Site Care—*Continued*

Steps	Rationale	Considerations
3. Ensure appropriate cardiorespiratory monitoring throughout DS care.	Analgesic and anxiolytic medications, especially when given together, may adversely affect child's hemodynamic and respiratory status.[4]	At minimum, oxygen saturation should be monitored.
4. Assess child's pain and anxiety level; administer premedication with analgesics and anxiolytics per prescribing practitioner's order (see Table 121-1).	Promotes child's comfort during procedure; ensures adequate pain and anxiety control and promotes compliance with future procedures.[4-6]	Pain medication administered orally takes longer to reach effective levels but provides longer periods of pain relief. Intravenous (IV) pain medication acts relatively quickly but also is metabolized quickly because of child's hypermetabolic state. A combination of both is usually most effective in extensive wound care procedures.[4,5] *(Level II*)*
5. Wash hands; put on personal protective equipment (gloves, gown, and mask) as indicated for the specific procedure.	Standard precautions; reduces transmission of microorganisms.	All members of team present during wound care procedure should use appropriate standard precautions.
6. Remove DS dressings and discard in appropriate receptacles.	Standard precautions; reduces transmission of microorganisms.	
7. Remove clean gloves; put on sterile gloves.	Aseptic technique used; contact is made with openings in the skin.	
8. Gently cleanse wounds with cleansing agent per prescribing practitioner's order or institution-specific protocol (e.g., 0.9% saline solution or bacteriostatic soap) and gauze pad. Use soft circular motions. *Never scrub. (Level II*)*	Wound care that is done too aggressively may damage newly formed epithelial cells and delay wound healing.[4-6]	
9. Rinse wound beds and pat dry in preparation for new dressing.	Some topical preparations may be difficult to apply if wounds are wet.	
10. Put on a new pair of sterile gloves.	Reduces cross contamination of wound.	
11. Apply topical ointments or dressings per prescribing practitioner's order. This usually involves topical creams and nonstick dressing applied over medication.	Nonstick dressings serve to keep the topical medication in place and protect the wound bed from dressing adherence.	A complete history of child's allergies is necessary before application of any burn dressings or medications.
12. Praise child for doing well during and after procedure.	Positive reinforcement may result in increased compliance with future procedures.[6]	
13. Discard used supplies and equipment in appropriate receptacles.	Standard precautions; reduces transmission of microorganisms.	
14. Remove gloves; wash hands.	Standard precautions.	

* Level II: Theory-based; no research data to support recommendations; recommendations from expert consensus group may exist

Expected Outcomes

- Donor site heals without complications and minimal scarring

- Donor site is free from infection
- Child's pain and anxiety related to DS and care are effectively controlled

Unexpected Outcomes

- Donor site healing is delayed
- Significant scarring at DS
- Wound at DS converts to deeper wound, which results in prolonged healing times and increased risk of scarring
- Donor site becomes infected
- Unmanaged pain or anxiety

Monitoring and Care of the Child

Activities and Interventions	Rationale	Reportable Conditions
1. Monitor DS for presence of leakage so that dressing can be reinforced as needed.	Prompt assessment of leakage prevents drying out of DS bed and promotes effective wound healing.	• Excessive leakage from DS
2. Monitor for bleeding through DS dressings.	Bleeding is not uncommon in the immediate postoperative period and may necessitate dressing removal and cautery.	• Bleeding from DS
3. Monitor DS for indications of wound healing or presence of infection.	Monitors progress of wound healing. Early identification of infection facilitates prompt treatment.	• Delayed wound healing • Indications of infection at DS • Increased temperature • Increased white blood cell count
4. Assess child's pain and anxiety before, during, and after the procedure	Prompt identification of pain facilitates rapid treatment	• Report of unresolved pain and discomfort • Continued irritability or changes in physiologic condition
5. Assess effectiveness of pain and anxiety management strategies and provide appropriate interventions. Encourage family to assist with nonpharmacologic means to comfort and support the child.	Because of painful stimuli and hypermetabolic state, child may need increased medication doses. Facilitates modifications to management strategies as indicated.	• Pain or anxiety refractory to medication administration • Inability to perform or complete the procedure because of increased pain or anxiety levels
6. Monitor perfusion to the extremity or area of the DS.	Compromised circulation inhibits healing of the DS.	• Indications of inadequate perfusion in the area of the DS • Indications of inadequate systemic perfusion

Documentation

- Child and family education
- Specific procedures performed (e.g., dressing reinforced, dressing removed)
- Medications administered for pain and anxiety control and effectiveness
- Location and appearance of DS; type of dressings used in procedure
- Medications used for DS care
- Members of team involved in DS care
- Child's response to procedure
- Unexpected outcomes and related treatment

References

1. Disa J, et al: Evaluation of a combined calcium sodium alginate and bio-occlusive membrane dressing in the management of split-thickness skin graft donor sites, *Ann Plast Surg* 46(4):405-408, 2001.
2. Kilinic H, Sensoz O, Ozdemir R, et al: Which dressing for split-thickness skin graft donor sites? *Ann Plast Surg* 46(4):409-414, 2001.
3. Rakel BA, et al: Split-thickness skin graft donor site care: a quantitative synthesis of the research, *Appl Nurs Res* 11(4):174-182, 1998.
4. Herndon DN, editor: *Total burn care,* ed 2, London, 2002, Saunders.
5. Trofino RB, editor: *Nursing care of the burn injured patient,* Philadelphia, 1991, F.A. Davis Company.
6. Tarnowski KJ, editor: *Behavioral aspects of pediatric burns,* New York, 1994, Plenum Press.

Additional Readings

Deitch E, Rutan R: *The challenges of children: the first 48 hours,* Chicago, 2003, American Burn Association Education Committee.
Herdon DN, et al: Management of the pediatric patient with burns, *J Burn Care Rehabil* 14:3-8, 1993.

Skin Graft Care

PURPOSE: To deliver appropriate care to the skin graft, promote graft take and prevent graft loss

Laurie DeMondo Jaffe

PREREQUISITE KNOWLEDGE

- Skin function, anatomy, and physiology
  - ❖ The epidermis is the most external layer of the skin and is composed of epithelium that consists mainly of keratinocytes. The epidermis has no blood vessels; nutrients diffuse to the epidermis from the vascular supply of the dermis.[1]
  - ❖ The dermis is composed of two levels and consists of connective tissue, capillaries, collagen, elastic fibers, mast cells, nerve endings, and lymphatics.
- Type of skin graft applied
  - ❖ Sheet graft is a single solid sheet of material; meshed graft is a sheet with interstices or slits. Meshing allows the sheet to be expanded in size, covering a larger area, and promotes escape of fluid, such as blood or exudate, which promotes graft "take" (union of the graft with the recipient area).[1-3]
  - ❖ Split-thickness graft consists of the entire epidermis and the uppermost layer of the dermis; full-thickness graft has all of the epidermis and dermis intact. Full-thickness grafts are generally smaller in size.[1-3]
  - ❖ Autograft is skin taken from one location on the child and placed in a second location; allograft or homograft is skin taken from another individual of the same species (e.g., cadaver); xenograft is skin taken from another species (e.g., pig). Allografts and xenografts are temporary.[1-5]
  - ❖ Cultured grafts are sheets of skin grown from small sections of the child's own skin; this process takes about 16 days and the resulting graft is extremely delicate.[4,5]
- ❖ Biologic skin graft dressings, which may be used as temporary grafts[2,4]
- Mechanism of healing involved with skin grafting
  - ❖ Successful take of a graft requires the recipient wound bed to be free of necrotic tissue and infection.[1,2]
  - ❖ Graft receives nutrients from exudates for the first 24 to 48 hours; during this time, a fibrin network develops.[1-3]
  - ❖ Capillaries develop from the wound bed and move toward the graft.[3-5]
- Graft survival is promoted by[1-3]
  - ❖ Close approximation of the wound bed and graft through appropriate dressing application and prevention of hematoma or seroma formation beneath the graft
    - ○ Various types of dressings are applied, all with the goal of: providing uniform pressure across the graft, preventing adherence of the dressing, absorbing exudate, maintaining a clean environment, and immobilizing the graft.
    - ○ Closed dressings are commonly used.[6]
  - ❖ Prevention of shearing forces and tension, which cause mechanical disruption of the graft, through positioning and immobilization
  - ❖ Gentle handling of the graft
  - ❖ Prevention of infection
- Standard healing times
  - ❖ First-degree wounds heal in 5 to 7 days.
  - ❖ Second-degree wounds (partial thickness) heal in 1 to 3 weeks.
  - ❖ Third-degree wounds (full thickness) may take several months to heal without surgical intervention.

- Immobilization techniques used after skin grafting; body parts are positioned in specific ways to prevent graft loss.
  - Graft site is generally kept elevated to minimize edema[2]
- Principles of aseptic technique
- Appropriate pediatric dosing and administration of analgesics and anxiolytics and competency in procedural sedation
- Use of developmentally appropriate pain assessment scales (see Procedure 173 for further information)
- Pain management and anxiety reduction techniques effective in infants and children
- Consultation with Pain Management and Child Life Specialist should be considered to facilitate and optimize this procedure.

CHILD AND FAMILY ASSESSMENT

- History of illnesses or drug allergies ➻***Rationale:*** These factors may interfere with the performance of skin graft care and medication selection.
- Child's developmental level and ability to interact ➻***Rationale:*** These factors influence preparation of the child, selection of an appropriate pain scale, interaction during the procedure, and personnel who may be necessary during the procedure.
- Interaction between family and child ➻***Rationale:*** Identifies effective and ineffective methods used by the family to support the child.
- Type of skin graft used, area of graft, splinting methods used, and the presence of skin staples or sutures ➻***Rationale:*** Assists in predicting the need for and most appropriate analgesia, supplies necessary, and specifics of procedure.
- Previous pain and sedation experiences of child and family and the child's and family's identification of pain and anxiety management strategies that have been helpful in the past ➻***Rationale:*** Identifies pain management strategies likely to be successful; child and family are encouraged to participate in development of plan of care.
- Child's and family's understanding of the reasons for and risks and benefits of procedure ➻***Rationale:*** Evaluates child's and family's understanding of the procedure and provides a gauge for ongoing education.
- Desire of family members to be present during skin graft care ➻***Rationale:*** Family members may provide comfort and support during the procedure, but they should have the choice not to remain with the child. Institution-specific protocol may limit family presence.

CHILD AND FAMILY EDUCATION

Individualized, developmentally appropriate education is provided to the family and to the child based on desire for knowledge, readiness to learn, and overall neurologic and psychosocial state.

- Explain the need for skin graft care that is required for optimal graft adherence ➻***Rationale:*** Providing information may reduce anxiety and assist the family in supporting the child.
- Discuss the appearance of the skin graft in the immediate postoperative period ➻***Rationale:*** Child and family members may have unrealistic expectations of what the graft might look like. Preparing them for what to expect decreases the fear and dissatisfaction that they may experience on initial viewing of the skin graft.
- Explain the need for immobilization of the skin graft area ➻***Rationale:*** Prevents inappropriate handling of the graft site, which could result in graft shearing or loss; promotes of understanding of and compliance with plan of care.
- Discuss the likelihood of postoperative edema, why it may occur, and when it should resolve ➻***Rationale:*** Anxiety and fear that may be associated with seeing the child in the immediate postoperative period are reduced.
- Describe the need for additional support that the child may need after the skin graft procedure ➻***Rationale:*** The family is prepared to address the needs of the child.
- Explain that skin grafting is a mechanism of wound closure and does not serve to eliminate potential risk for scarring ➻***Rationale:*** Promotes realistic expectations on the part of the family of the results of skin grafting surgery.
- Describe the steps and process, timing, and expectations involved in skin graft care ➻***Rationale:*** Providing information may reduce anxiety and fear of the family and the child.
- Review the pain and anxiety management plan for the child, including Child Life, therapy, sedation, and other methods as outlined in institution-specific protocols ➻***Rationale:*** Providing information decreases anxiety and fear and reassures the child and family that pain will be managed appropriately.
- Encourage questions and answer questions as they arise ➻***Rationale:*** Reinforcement of information is needed during periods of stress.

EQUIPMENT

- Analgesics or anxiolytics appropriate for child's age and weight and specific procedure to be performed per prescribing practitioner's order
- Cleansing agent per prescribing practitioner's order or institution-specific protocol
- Staple or suture removal kit as indicated
- Dressings per prescribing practitioner's order
- Splinting material per prescribing practitioner's order
- Scalpel or 25-gauge or 27-gauge needle
- Clean and sterile gloves
- Burn pads or 4×4 pads for cleansing

Procedure for Skin Graft Care

Steps	Rationale	Considerations
1. Ensure child and family understand procedure and questions are answered.	May serve to reduce child's and family's anxiety.[7-9] Evaluates and reinforces understanding of previously taught information.	Developmental level, cognitive ability, and anxiety level determine approach to and effectiveness of teaching.
2. Obtain needed equipment and supplies.	Facilitates completion of task in a timely manner.	
3. Assess child's pain and anxiety level; administer premedication with analgesics and anxiolytics per prescribing practitioner's order (see Table 121-1 in Procedure 121).	Promotes child's comfort during procedure; ensures adequate pain and anxiety control and promotes compliance with future procedures.[7-9]	The removal of staples is usually frightening for the child. Medication for anxiety control may be helpful. Child Life Specialist may be helpful in working with the child to use nonpharmacologic pain and anxiety control techniques.
4. If necessary, transport child to procedure location; attach appropriate monitoring devices.	Analgesic and anxiolytic medications, especially when given together, may adversely affect child's hemodynamic and respiratory status.	Performance of graft care in a specific location may assist the child in coping with the procedure; providing the child with a "safe" area where procedures are not performed may decrease anxiety.
5. Wash hands; put on personal protective equipment (gloves, gown, and mask) as indicated for the specific procedure.	Standard precautions; reduces transmission of microorganisms.	
6. Provide for appropriate privacy; position child to promote child's comfort and facilitate procedure.	Location of graft site may necessitate exposure of the child; respects the child's rights.	Privacy is an important consideration for school-aged children and adolescents.
7. Carefully remove splints.	Prevents disruption of graft.	Timing of initial dressing change varies based on type of graft used, surgeon preference, and institution-specific protocols.[2]
First 24 to 48 Hours		
8. Assess graft site for presence of fluid accumulation under graft. Open fluid-filled blister with a 25-gauge or 27-gauge needle per institution-specific protocol.[2]	Fluid accumulation under graft could result in ineffective epithelialization and result in graft loss.[1,2,5]	Fluid tends to accumulate under sheet grafts. If a sheet graft was used, daily assessment should include assessment of fluid accumulation.[5]
Postoperative Days 3 to 5		
9. Carefully remove splints and dressings; discard dressings in appropriate containers. Cleanse splint before reapplication.	Prevents lifting of the graft off the wound bed.[1] Standard precautions; prevents cross contamination.	Care must be taken when removing dressing if dressing is adherent to skin graft site; 0.9% saline solution may be used to moisten dressing before removal.[1]
10. Remove staples or sutures per institution-specific protocol.	Graft is usually adherent enough to tolerate staple or suture removal. *(Level II*)*	Grafts may be secured with suture, staple, or tapes.[2]

* Level II: Theory-based; no reasearch data to support recommendations; recommendations from expert consensus group may exist

Procedure | for Skin Graft Care—*Continued*

Steps	Rationale	Considerations
11. Gently cleanse all graft sites that needed intervention with cleanser per prescribing practitioner's order. *(Level II*)*	Aggressive cleansing could result in graft loss.	
12. Remove gloves and put on new sterile pair.	Decreases cross contamination.	
13. Reapply dressing to skin graft per prescribing practitioner's order or institution-specific protocol.	Meshed skin grafts have openings called interstices. The interstices must remain moist for epithelialization to occur.[7] *(Level II*)*	Depending on the specific type of graft, garamycin gauze, xeroform gauze, or topical antibiotics may be prescribed.
14. Reapply splint as indicated.	Immobilization in the immediate postoperative period is necessary for graft adherence.[7,9]	Frequent assessment of splint fit is essential for proper immobilization.
15. Discard used supplies and equipment, including sharps, in appropriate receptacles.	Standard precautions; reduces transmission of microorganisms. Protects personnel health.	
16. Remove gloves and personal protective equipment; wash hands.	Standard precautions; reduces the transmission of microorganisms.	
17. Transport child back to room if necessary.	Returns child to safe location.	

* Level II: Theory-based; no research data to support recommendations; recommendations from expert consensus group may exist

Expected Outcomes

- Skin graft take of 100%
- Graft site is free from infection
- Child's pain and anxiety are effectively controlled during skin graft care
- Child and family have a realistic expectation of what the graft initially looks like and of long-term outcomes

- Child or family verbalize that skin graft procedure is intended to close the wound, not eliminate scarring

Unexpected Outcomes

- Graft sloughs and is lost
- Graft site becomes infected
- Unmanaged pain or anxiety during skin graft care

- Unrealistic expectations of initial graft appearance
- Child or family is unable to state long-term outcomes of skin grafting
- Family or child expects that no scarring is associated with the skin graft

Monitoring and Care of the Child

Activities and Interventions	Rationale	Reportable Conditions
1. Assess graft site for accumulation of fluid under graft bed; this is particularly important with the use of sheet grafts.	Fluid accumulation could result in graft loss.[1]	• Fluid accumulation under graft
2. Assess graft site for adherence of graft.	Allows early identification and prompt treatment of problems with graft.	• Graft does not appear to be adhered
3. Monitor graft site for signs of infection.	Infection may lead to loss of graft.[1]	• Redness, swelling, or purulent drainage at the graft site • Increased temperature • Increased white blood cell count
4. Assess child's pain and anxiety before, during, and after the procedure.	Prompt identification of pain or anxiety facilitates rapid treatment. Staple removal is frightening for most children; anxiety control is almost always necessary.	• Report of unresolved pain and discomfort • Continued irritability or changes in physiologic condition
5. Assess effectiveness of pain and anxiety management strategies and provide appropriate interventions. Encourage family to assist with nonpharmacologic means to comfort and support the child.	Because of painful stimuli and hypermetabolic state, child may need increased medication doses. Facilitates modifications to management strategies as indicated.	• Pain or anxiety refractory to medication administration • Inability to perform or complete the procedure because of increased pain or anxiety levels
6. Examine positioning of extremity and fit and effectiveness of splint.	Inappropriate positioning or splint application may result in graft loss.[1] Splints may become loose when postoperative edema decreases. Inappropriately fit splints may cause damage to the graft or other parts of the extremity in contact with the splint.	• Ill-fitting splints • Excessive swelling of distal extremity • Damage to the graft • Damage to surrounding skin
7. Monitor perfusion to the extremity or area where the graft is placed.	Compromised circulation inhibits take of the graft.	• Indications of inadequate perfusion in the area of the graft • Indications of inadequate systemic perfusion

Documentation

- Appearance and location of skin graft
- Dressings applied
- Members of team involved in graft care
- Necessary interventions to the skin graft site (e.g., opening fluid-filled areas, staple or suture removal)
- Medications administered for pain and anxiety control and effectiveness
- Medications administered for graft care
- Child and family education
- Child's response to the procedure
- Unexpected outcomes and related treatment

References

1. Mendez-Eastman S: Full-thickness skin grafting: a procedural review, *Plast Surg Nurs* 24(2):41-45, 2004.
2. Mendez-Eastman S: Skin grafting: preoperative, intraoperative and postoperative care, *Plast Surg Nurs* 21(1): 49-51, 2001.
3. Andreassi A, et al: Classification and pathophysiology of skin grafts, *Clin Dermatol* 23:332-337, 2005.
4. Balasubramani M, et al: Skin substitutes: a review, *Burns* 27:534-544, 2001.
5. Richters CD, et al: Immunology of skin transplantation, *Clin Dermatol* 23:338-342, 2004.
6. Moisidis E, et al: A prospective, blinded, randomized, controlled clinical trial of topical negative pressure use in skin grafting, *Plast Reconstruct Surg* 114(4):917-922, 2004.
7. Herndon DN, editor: *Total burn care,* ed 2, London, 2002, Saunders.
8. Tarnowski KJ, editor: *Behavioral aspects of pediatric burns,* New York, 1994, Plenum Press.
9. Trofino RB, editor: *Nursing care of the burn injured patient,* Philadelphia, 1991, F.A. Davis Company.

Additional Readings

Ben-Bassat H: Performance and safety of skin allografts, *Clin Dermatol* 23:365-375, 2005.

Deitch E, Rutan R: *The challenges of children: the first 48 hours,* Chicago, 2003, American Burn Association Education Committee.

Herdon DN, et al: Management of the pediatric patient with burns, *J Burn Care Rehabil* 14:3-8, 1993.

Qaryoute S, et al: Usage of autograft and allograft skin in treatment of burns in children, *Burns* 27:599-602, 2001.

Intracompartment Pressure Monitoring

P U R P O S E : To measure intracompartment pressure and identify compartment syndrome in children who are believed to have compartment syndrome but are unable to verbalize early clinical warning signs

Dawn Marie Daniels

PREREQUISITE KNOWLEDGE

- Anatomy of the involved limb, including muscle compartments of the limb (Figure 124-1)
- Two mechanisms lead to compartment syndrome: a decrease in compartment size or an increase in compartment volume. Constrictive casts or dressings can decrease the size of the compartment and place the child at risk. Etiologies that can increase the compartment volume include trauma or surgery to an extremity, fractures, massive fluid resuscitation, and intravenous infiltrations. Young children and those who are cognitively impaired are at an increased risk because of the inability to participate in the clinical examination.[1,2]
- When tissue pressure is elevated within the affected compartment, microcirculation is decreased, which can lead to nerve and tissue ischemia and possible necrosis of the tissues within the compartment, resulting in irreversible muscle or nerve damage.[2,3]
- The clinical examination is an important indicator of compartment syndrome. Signs and symptoms are often referred to as the "five P's": pain, paresthesia, pallor, pulselessness, and paralysis. Unfortunately, many of these are late signs of compartment syndrome and may be difficult to assess in a young or cognitively impaired child.[2,4]

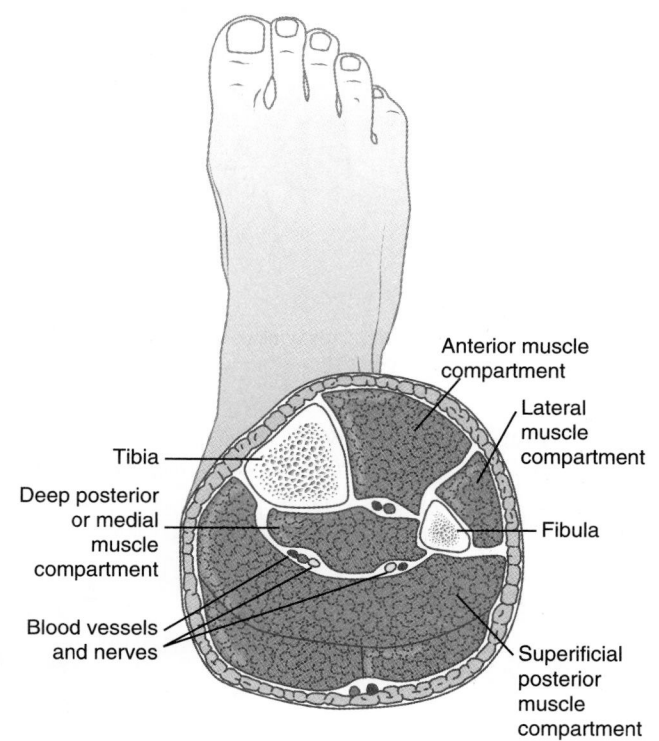

FIGURE 124-1 Muscle compartments of lower leg. *From Edwards S: Acute compartment syndrome, Emerg Nurs 12(3): 32-38, 2004.*

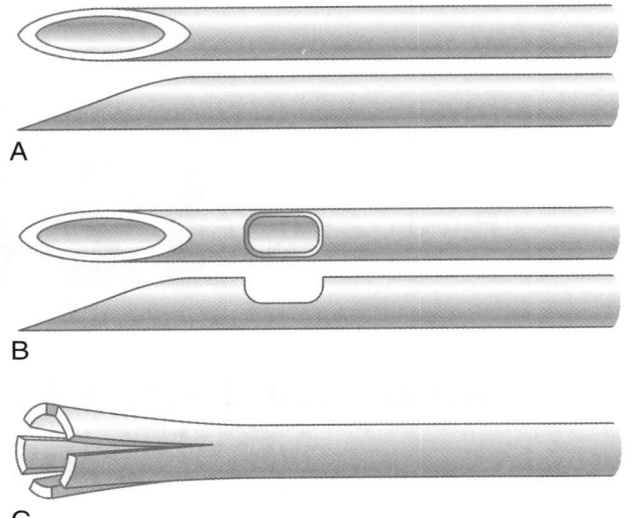

A

B

C

FIGURE 124-2 Catheters Used to Measure Compartment Pressure. **A,** Straight needle. **B,** Side-ported needle. **C,** Slit catheter. *From Boody AR, Wongworawat MD: Accuracy in the measurement of compartment pressures: a comparison of three commonly used devices,* J Bone Joint Surg *87-A(11):2415-2422, 2005.*

- Normal intracompartment pressure is 0 to 4 mm Hg. Some investigators advocate surgical intervention at 30 mm Hg, and others advocate it at 40 to 50 mm Hg; still others advocate for a fasciotomy when the compartment pressure is within 20 mm Hg of the child's diastolic pressure.[5]
- A variety of devices may be used to monitor compartment pressures:
  - ❖ Large-gauge straight needle (Figure 124-2)
  - ❖ Large-gauge side-ported needle (see Figure 124-2)
  - ❖ Slit catheter: A flexible catheter with slits cut in the end of the catheter placed into the muscle compartment through an introducer (see Figure 124-2)
  - ❖ Wick catheter: A flexible catheter with Dacron fibers at the end of the catheter that extend into the muscle tissue of the compartment, placed into the muscle compartment through an introducer (Figure 124-3)
  - ❖ Fiber optic catheter
  - ❖ Stryker Intra-Compartmental Pressure Monitor System (Stryker Instruments, Kalamazoo, Mich; Figure 124-4)
- After the needle or catheter is placed into the muscle compartment, it is attached to a monitoring system that

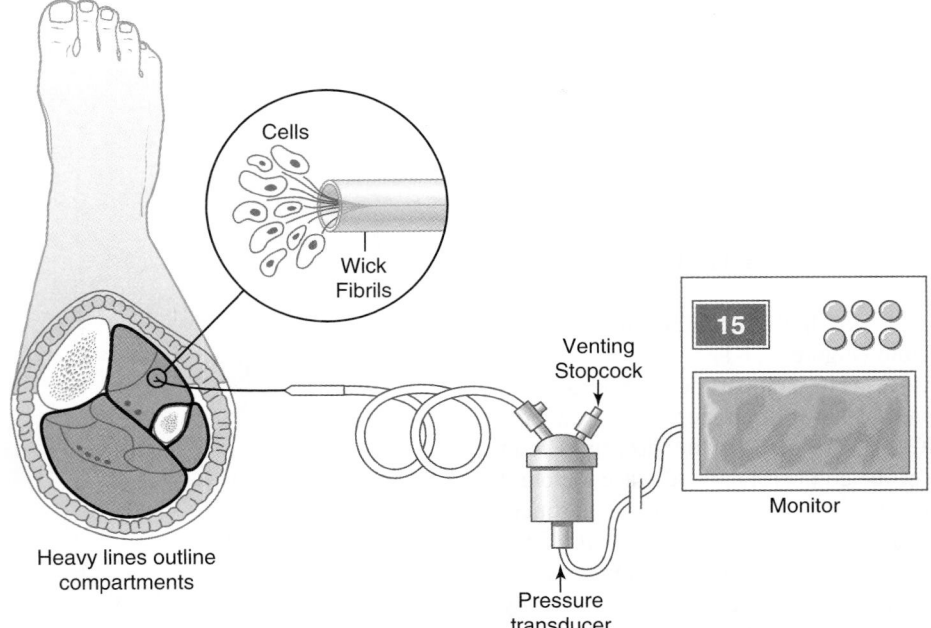

FIGURE 124-3 Wick catheter inserted into muscle compartment and attached to monitoring system. *From Pradka L: Use of the wick catheter for diagnosing and monitoring compartment syndrome,* Orthopaed Surg *4(4):17-18, 1985.*

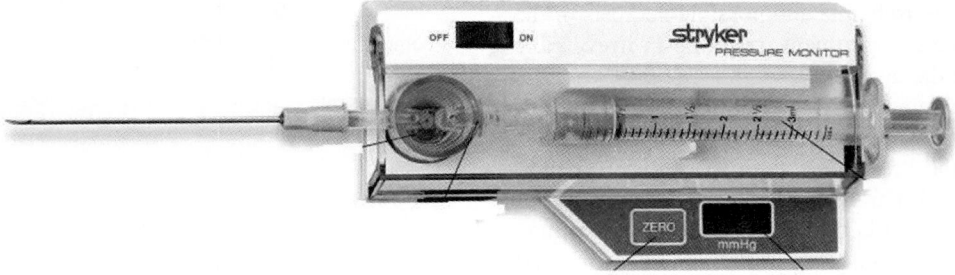

FIGURE 124-4 Handheld Stryker Intra-Compartmental Pressure Monitor System. *Courtesy of Stryker Instruments, Kalamazoo, Mich.*

consists of a transducer and bedside monitor or a machine designed specifically for monitoring compartment pressure (see Figure 124-3).

- Intracompartment pressure monitoring may be intermittent or continuous.
- Aseptic technique is essential to prevent complications.
- Child development as it relates to clinical assessment and intracompartment pressure monitoring
- Preparation of the child and adequate pain management are essential before a procedure is performed on a child.
- Selection and use of developmentally appropriate pain scale for pain assessment (see Procedure 173 for further information
- Appropriate pediatric dosing of analgesics and competency in procedural sedation
- Informed consent is generally required before invasive intracompartment pressure monitoring

CHILD AND FAMILY ASSESSMENT

- Child's developmental level and ability to interact ➥*Rationale:* These factors influence preparation of the child and interaction.
- Child's and family's understanding of the reasons for and risks and benefits of the procedure and of interventions planned if the pressure is found to be significantly elevated ➥*Rationale:* Evaluates child's and family's understanding of the procedure and provides a gauge for ongoing education.
- History of disorders or factors that increase the risk for bleeding, such as hemophilia, disseminated intravascular coagulation, anticoagulant therapy, and thrombocytopenia ➥*Rationale:* These processes both increase the risk for the development of compartment syndrome and increase the risk of complications after pressure monitoring.
- Clinical assessment of extremities bilaterally for signs and symptoms that may indicate the onset of compartment syndrome ➥*Rationale:* Clinical symptoms indicate the need for further measurements. Assessment of both the affected and the nonaffected limb assists the clinician in detection of abnormalities.
- Family's desire to be present during the procedure ➥*Rationale:* Family members may provide comfort and support to the child, but they should have the choice not to remain with the child.
- Support and comfort measures needed for the child ➥*Rationale:* Support and comfort measures must be individualized for each child; identification of techniques that have been successfully used with the child in the past promotes successful coping.
- Need for analgesia and sedation during the procedure ➥*Rationale:* The procedure is painful; each child's need for pain and sedation medication varies.
- Child's weight ➥*Rationale:* Dosing of sedatives and analgesics is based on the child's weight.

- Child's known allergies and previous experience with sedatives and analgesics ➥*Rationale:* Prevents exposure of child to medications known to produce an allergic reaction; identifies issues related to sedation or analgesia the child has had in the past.

CHILD AND FAMILY EDUCATION

Individualized, developmentally appropriate education is provided to the family and to the child based on desire for knowledge, readiness to learn, and overall neurologic and psychosocial state.

- Provide information on indications for and possible complications of invasive intracompartment pressure monitoring to the child and family ➥*Rationale:* Providing information may decrease anxiety and fear.
- Explain the procedure to the family and, if developmentally appropriate, to the child ➥*Rationale:* Providing information may decrease anxiety and fear.
- Explain planned interventions if the pressure is significantly elevated ➥*Rationale:* Information about next steps may decrease anxiety and fear.
- Explain the plan for pain management and sedation for the procedure ➥*Rationale:* Assurance to the family and child that pain and anxiety will be managed may decrease fear and anxiety.
- Explain how the family can provide support and comfort to the child. If the family chooses not to stay, explain how this support will be provided. ➥*Rationale:* Support to the child may decrease fear and anxiety and assist in the child's cooperation.
- Encourage questions and answer questions as they arise ➥*Rationale:* Reinforcement of information is needed during periods of stress.

EQUIPMENT

- Chlorhexidine, povidone-iodine, or other antiseptic solution per institution-specific protocol for skin preparation
- Local anesthetic
- Introducer needle (angiocath) 18-gauge or larger if wick or slit catheter is placed
- Catheter to be inserted: side-ported needle, slit catheter, wick catheter, or fiber optic catheter
- Pressure monitoring device: electronic handheld device, pressure transducer system, or manometer
- Three-way stopcock
- A 20-mL or 30-mL syringe
- Transducer and pressure tubing
- Sterile 0.9% saline solution: 50 mL
- Clean gloves
- Sterile gloves
- For continuous monitoring: occlusive sterile dressing and hypoallergenic tape

Procedure for Intracompartment Pressure Monitoring

Steps	Rationale	Considerations
1. Ensure child and family understand procedure and questions are answered.	Evaluates and reinforces understanding of previously taught information.	Developmental level, cognitive ability, and anxiety level determine approach to and effectiveness of teaching.
2. Gather needed equipment and supplies.	Facilitates completion of task in a timely manner.	
3. Confirm that consent for procedure has been obtained.	Ensures medical-legal compliance as suggested by the Joint Commission for Accreditation of Healthcare Organizations (JCAHO).	For emergency situations, refer to institution-specific protocol for assumption of consent.
4. Turn on monitor, select appropriate scale (30 or 60 mm Hg), and connect pressure cable.[6]	Ensures that the monitor is ready to provide an accurate pressure reading.	Several different mechanisms and monitors are available for monitoring pressure, including manometer, portable bedside electronic devices, handheld units, and cardiac monitoring systems with pressure monitoring capabilities.
5. Wash hands.	Standard precautions; reduces transmission of microorganisms.	
6. Assemble the pressure tubing, transducer, and stopcock. Maintain sterility at the end of the tubing.[6]	Prepares the monitoring system; maintenance of sterility reduces the transmission of microorganisms.	See Procedure 63 for further information. The fiber optic system does not need a fluid-filled column. The Stryker Intra-Compartment Pressure System has a built-in pressure transducer.
7. Draw up 30 mL of 0.9% saline solution; flush the transducer/pressure tubing system.[6]	Establishes a fluid-filled column; ensures that no air is in the system to interfere with pressure reading.	When flushing the system, ensure that no air bubbles are in the system.
8. Connect transducer system to pressure cable.	Allows transmission of the signal to the monitor.	
9. Wash hands and put on clean gloves.	Standard precautions; reduces the transmission of microorganisms.	
10. Identify the child with appropriate patient and procedure verification process (e.g., "Time out").	Confirms correct patient, procedure, and site as recommended by JCAHO; prevents unnecessary medical procedures.	Verification process and documentation is institution-specific. Use active communication techniques.
11. Assist the practitioner inserting monitoring device with site preparation:[6] Remove any dressings or splints. Clip hairs if appropriate. Clean site with chlorhexidine or povidone-iodine.	Facilitates visualization of the site. Reduces skin flora; decreases the potential for infection.	Refer to institution-specific protocol for antiseptic solution used for site preparation; chlorhexidine is not recommended for use in children less than 2 months of age.

Procedure for Intracompartment Pressure Monitoring—*Continued*

Steps	Rationale	Considerations
12. Remove gloves and wash hands.	Standard precautions; reduces the transmission of microorganisms.	
13. Prepare local anesthetic per prescribing practitioner's order or institution-specific protocol.	Local anesthetic assists with pain control.	Some children may need additional analgesics and sedatives. In addition, nonpharmacologic pain techniques should be used as appropriate.
14. Level the transducer with the planned insertion site and zero the monitor according to manufacturer's instructions.[6-9] *(Level IV*)*	Calibrates the machine with the insertion point to ensure accurate reading.	
15. Connect the catheter to the end of the pressure tubing. *(Level V*)*	The catheter is inserted into the compartment for a reading; special catheters are needed to ensure accuracy with the readings.[2,5-10]	Catheter may have a side port to prevent plugging of the catheter as the compartment is entered.
16. Validate that the catheter will reflect changes in pressure by first holding the catheter level with the transducer (it should read zero) and then slowly raising the catheter to eye level (it should increase to 30 to 50 mm Hg).[6] *(Level II*)*	Ensures that the system is functioning properly and is able to detect changes in pressure.	Failure to change readings when the catheter is raised could indicate air leaks or malfunctioning of the transducer system. Very slow increases in pressure when the transducer is raised could indicate the presence of air bubbles in the system.
17. Assist the practitioner with insertion of introducer and pressure monitoring catheter.	Introducer is used to facilitate insertion of the slit or wick catheter.	A handheld device may be more appropriate for single measurement readings (see Figure 124-4).
18. Read the intracompartment pressure displayed on the monitor.	Determines the pressure in the compartment.	
19. If continuous or intermittent measures are to be obtained, secure the catheter with a transparent occlusive sterile dressing and tape (Figure 124-5).	Prevents the catheter from becoming dislodged. May reduce infection. Transparent dressing facilitates visualization of the site.	

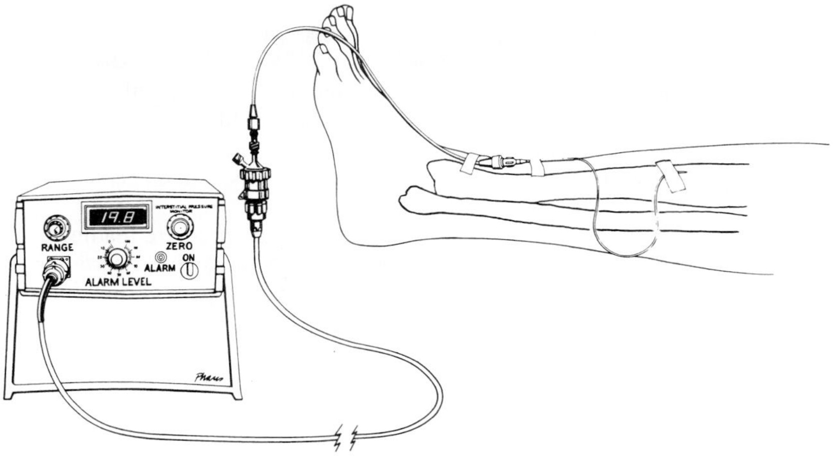

FIGURE 124-5   Catheter is secured with occlusive dressing and tape. *From Gallagher JJ: Intracompartmental pressure monitoring. In Lynn-McHale Wiegand DJ, Carlson K, editors:* AACN procedure manual for critical care, *ed 5, Philadelphia, 2005, Saunders.*

Procedure continues on following page

---

* Level II: Theory-based; no research data to support recommendations; recommendations from expert consensus group may exist
Level IV: Limited clinical studies to support recommendations
Level V: Clinical studies in more than one or two patient populations and situations to support recommendations

Procedure for Intracompartment Pressure Monitoring—*Continued*

Steps	Rationale	Considerations
20. Validate accuracy of catheter placement and system integrity by palpating the area over the catheter tip[6] (Figure 124-6).	Patient movement and palpation over the insertion site should result in changes in pressure measurements.	

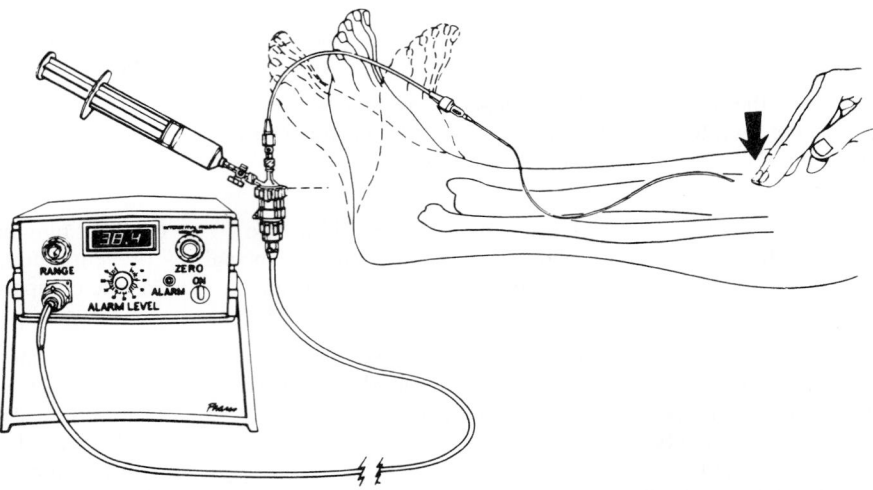

FIGURE 124-6   System's response is evaluated by palpating area over catheter tip or having child flex and extend joint distal to catheter insertion; displayed waveform and value should temporarily increase. *From Gallagher JJ: Intracompartmental pressure monitoring. In Lynn-McHale Wiegand DJ, Carlson K, editors:* AACN procedure manual for critical care, *ed 5, Philadelphia, 2005, Saunders.*

Steps	Rationale	Considerations
21. Dispose of supplies and used equipment, including sharps, in appropriate receptacles.	Standard precautions; reduces transmission of microorganisms; protects personnel health.	
22. Remove gloves; wash hands.	Standard precautions.	

Expected Outcomes

- The catheter is placed without difficulty or complications
- Compartment pressure is normal; or if compartment pressures are elevated, appropriate therapeutic interventions are initiated
- Accurate pressure readings are obtained
- Child is free from infection
- Child has acceptable level of comfort

Unexpected Outcomes

- Inability to place catheter
- Excessive bleeding at insertion site
- Nerve damage
- Muscle tissue damage
- Inaccurate pressure readings
- Infection at device insertion site
- Unmanaged pain or anxiety

Monitoring and Care of the Child

Activities and Interventions	Rationale	Reportable Conditions
1. Perform neurovascular checks of affected extremity every hour or more often as needed.	Facilitates early detection of signs and symptoms of compartment syndrome.	• New onset of pain or worsening of pain in spite of analgesics • Pain that occurs with passive flexion or extension of the affected limb • Paresthesia (burning or tingling sensation) of the affected extremity • Pallor: change in color (cyanosis, pallor, or mottling) or skin temperature of the affected extremity • Paralysis of the affected extremity • Pulses: weakening or loss of pulses in the affected extremity • Increased edema or tenseness of the extremity
2. Obtain compartment pressure measurements per prescribing practitioner's order and when increases occur.	Detects increasing pressure that could necessitate surgical intervention.	• Increasing pressures
3. Monitor insertion site for signs of infection.	Presence of the invasive catheter is a potential source of infection.	• Fever • Drainage from the insertion site • Increase in white blood cell count • Increase in skin temperature around the insertion site • Edema at the site
4. Monitor insertion site for signs of bleeding.	Bleeding may occur from the insertion site.	• Serious—sanguineous or serous sanguineous drainage from the site • Erythema at the site • Edema at the site
5. Assess child's comfort at initiation and throughout procedure; evaluate effectiveness of pain management strategy and provide appropriate interventions. Encourage family to assist with nonpharmacologic means to comfort and support the child.	Early identification of inadequate pain control facilitates prompt treatment.	• Unmanaged pain or anxiety • Continued irritability or changes in physiologic condition
6. Assist with removal of catheter when monitoring is no longer needed; cover site with dry sterile dressing.	Catheter should be removed as soon as possible to decrease risk of infection.	• Indications of infection at insertion site

Documentation

- Child and family education
- Presence of informed consent
- Institution-specific documentation of patient and procedure verification process
- Sedation and analgesia provided for the procedure and documentation of procedural sedation per institution-specific protocol
- Type of catheter inserted
- Individual who inserted the catheter
- Insertion site condition before and after catheter insertion
- Neurovascular assessments of the affected extremities
- Compartment pressure measurements
- Comfort assessment and any specific interventions provided
- Child's response to procedure
- Unexpected outcomes and related treatment

References

1. Barnes MR, et al: A technique for the long term measurement of intra-compartmental pressure in the lower leg, *J Biomed Engineer* 7:35-39, 1985.
2. Block EF, et al: Compartment syndrome in the critically injured following massive resuscitation: case reports, *J Trauma-Injury Infect Crit Care* 39(4):787-791, 1995.
3. Donahue P, Wheeler WE: A method for rapid intracompartmental pressure measurement, *West Virginia Med J* 88(5):195, 1992.
4. Hargens AR, Ballard RE: Basic principles for measurement of intramuscular pressure, *Operative Techniques Sports Med* 3(4):237-342, 1995.
5. Heppenstall RB, et al: Vascular injuries and compartment syndromes. In Bucholz RW, Heckman JD, editors: *Rockwood & Green's fractures in adults,* vol 1, ed 5, Philadelphia, 2001, Lippincott, Williams & Wilkins, pp. 319-352.
6. Gallagher JJ: Intracompartmental pressure monitoring. In Lynn-McHale Wiegand DJ, Carlson K, editors: *AACN procedure manual for critical care,* ed 5, Philadelphia, 2005, Saunders.
7. Johansen K, Watson J: Compartment syndrome: new insights, *Semin Vasc Surg* 11:294-301, 1998.
8. Russell WL, et al: Utilization and wide clinical implementation using the wick catheter for compartment pressure measurement, *Surg Gynecol Obstet* 160(3):207-210, 1985.
9. Willis RB, Rorabeck CH: Treatment of compartment syndrome in children, *Orthopaed Clin North Am* 21:401-412, 1990.
10. Wilson SC, et al: A simple method to measure compartment pressures using an intravenous catheter, *Orthopedics* 20(5):403-406, 1997.

Additional Readings

Hargens AR, Mubarak SJ: Laboratory diagnosis of compartment syndromes. In Mubarak SJ, et al, editors: *Compartment syndrome and Volkmann's contractures,* Philadelphia, 1981, Saunders, pp. 106-122.

Larson M, et al: Detecting compartmental syndrome using continuous pressure monitoring, *Focus Crit Care* 13(5):51-56, 1986.

McDermott AG, et al: Monitoring acute compartment pressures with the S.T.I.C. catheter, *Clin Orthopaed Related Res* 190:192-198, 1984.

Mubarak SJ: Etiologies of compartment syndromes. In Mubarak SJ, et al, editors: *Compartment syndrome and Volkmann's contractures,* Philadelphia; 1981, Saunders.

Musgrave, DS, Mendelson, SA: Pediatric orthopedic trauma: principles in management. *Critical Care Medicine,* 30(11 Suppl): S431-443, 2002.

Owen CA: Clinical diagnosis of acute compartment syndromes. In Mubarak SJ, et al, editors: *Compartment syndrome and Volkmann's contractures,* Philadelphia, 1981, Saunders.

Prayson, MJ, et. al: Baseline compartment pressure measurements in isolated lower extremity fractures without clinical compartment syndrome, *Trauma-Injury Infect Crit Care,* 60(5): 1037-1040, 2006.

Thompson GH, Behrens F: Fractures of the tibia and fibula. In Green NE, Swiontkowski, editors: *Skeletal trauma in children,* ed 2, Philadelphia, 1998, Saunders.

Willy C, et al: Measurement of intracompartmental pressure with use of a new electronic transducer-tipped catheter system, *J Bone Joint Surg* 81(2):158-168, 1999.

Skin Assessment Techniques

PURPOSE: To identify conditions of the skin that may be some of the first visible clues to many underlying infectious, metabolic, and neurologic disorders and to identify alterations in skin integrity that necessitate intervention

Jacqueline Simpson Dunne

PREREQUISITE KNOWLEDGE

- The skin is the body's largest organ.
- Anatomy and physiology of the skin
  - ❖ Skin consists of two layers that cover a third fatty layer. The outer layer is called the epidermis, a tough protective layer that contains melanin (protecting the skin against the rays of the sun and giving the skin color). The second layer, located under the epidermis, is the dermis and contains nerve endings, sweat glands, sebaceous glands, and hair follicles. Under these two skin layers is a fatty layer of subcutaneous tissue.
- Functions of the skin
  - ❖ The body's first line of defense against infection
  - ❖ Forms a protective barrier against germs and other organisms; keeps outside the body what belongs outside the body
  - ❖ Helps maintain a constant body temperature
- Risk factors that make newborns and children vulnerable to skin breakdown
  - ❖ The newborn infant has less well-developed adnexal structures, no protective endogenous flora, and increased susceptibility to external irritants. At birth, all the structures within the skin are present, but many of the functions of the integumentary systems are immature. The epidermis and dermis are very thin. Even the slightest friction can cause blister formation. Neonates also have less adipose tissue, which makes them more susceptible to pressure ulcers.
  - ❖ Condition of skin (dehydrated, presence of edema)

- ❖ Nutritional status
- ❖ Tissue oxygenation status
- ❖ Specific diagnosis
- ❖ Presence of graft-versus-host disease (GVHD) of the skin
- ❖ Neurologic status
- ❖ Immobility
- ❖ Presence of indwelling catheters, tubes, peripheral intravenous (IV) lines, dressings, wounds, or tissue injury
- ❖ Pharmacologic factors
- ❖ Drug-related allergies
- Age-specific diagnoses that contribute to increased risk of skin breakdown. Certain bacterial and viral diseases are specific for specific age groups. Familiarity with some of the more common diseases is important.
  - ❖ Erythema toxicum: Usual age, neonates
  - ❖ Staphylococcal scalded-skin syndrome: Usual age, infants
  - ❖ Kawasaki disease: Usual age, 6 months to 6 years
  - ❖ Measles: Usual age, infants to young adults
  - ❖ Chickenpox: Usual age, 80% at 1 to 14 years
  - ❖ Roseola: Usual age, 6 months to 3 years
  - ❖ Hand-foot-and-mouth disease: Usual age, young children
  - ❖ Enteroviral exanthems (coxsackievirus, echovirus, other enteroviruses): Usual age, young children
  - ❖ Toxic shock syndrome/Streptococcal toxin: Usual age, young children
  - ❖ Meningococcemia/Meningococcus: Usual age, less than 5 years

- ❖ Scarlet fever: Usual age, school-aged children
- ❖ Rubella: Usual age, adolescents to young adults
- Specific risk factors pertinent to the child with immunosuppression
- Knowledge of the Braden Q Scale (Table 125-1)
- Knowledge of risk factors for tissue injury and breakdown and the interventions necessary to prevent injury and breakdown (Figure 125-1)
- Anatomy and physiology of hair and nails

TABLE 125-1	Modified Braden Q Scale (for Pediatric Use) for Early Identification of Relative Risk for Pressure Ulcers				
	Intensity and Duration of Pressure				Score
Mobility The ability to change and control body position	**1. Completely immobile:** Does not make even slight changes in body or extremity position without assistance	**2. Very limited:** Makes occasional slight changes in body or extremity position but is unable to completely turn self independently	**3. Slightly limited:** Makes frequent although slight changes in body or extremity position independently	**4. No limitations:** Makes major and frequent changes in position without assistance	
Activity The degree of physical activity	**1. Bedfast:** Confined to bed	**2. Chairfast:** Ability to walk severely limited or nonexistent Cannot bear own weight or must be assisted into chair or wheelchair	**3. Walks occasionally:** Walks occasionally during day but for very short distances, with or without assistance Spends most of each shift in bed or chair	**4. All patients too young to ambulate or walks frequently:** Walks outside room at least twice a day and inside room at least once every 2 hours during waking hours	
Sensory Perception The ability to respond in a developmentally appropriate way to pressure-related discomfort	**1. Completely limited:** Unresponsive (does not moan, flinch, or grasp) to painful stimuli because of diminished level of consciousness or sedation or limited ability to feel pain over most of body surface	**2. Very limited:** Responds to only painful stimuli Cannot communicate discomfort except by moaning or restlessness or has sensory impairment that limits the ability to feel pain or discomfort over half of body	**3. Slightly limited:** Responds to verbal commands but cannot always communicate discomfort or need to be turned or has some sensory impairment that limits ability to feel pain in one or two extremities	**4. No impairment:** Responds to verbal commands Has no sensory deficit that limits ability to feel or communicate pain or discomfort	
	Tolerance of the Skin and Supporting Structure				
Moisture Degree to which skin is exposed to moisture	**1. Constantly moist:** Skin is kept moist almost constantly with perspiration, urine, drainage, etc Dampness is detected every time patient is moved or turned	**2. Very moist:** Skin is often but not always moist Linen must be changed at least every 8 hours	**3. Occasionally moist:** Skin is occasionally moist, necessitating linen change every 12 hours	**4. Rarely moist:** Skin is usually dry; routine diaper changes; linen only needs changing every 24 hours	
Friction and Shear *Friction:* Occurs when skin moves against support surfaces *Shear:* Occurs when skin and adjacent bony surface slide across one another	**1. Significant problem:** Spasticity, contracture, itching, or agitation leads to almost constant thrashing and friction	**2. Problem:** Needs moderate to maximum assistance in moving Complete lifting without sliding against sheets is impossible Frequently slides down in bed or chair, necessitating frequent repositioning with maximum assistance	**3. Potential problem:** Moves freely or needs minimal assistance During a move, skin probably slides to some extent against sheets, chair, restraints, or other devices Maintains relative good position in chair or bed most of the time but occasionally slides down	**4. No apparent problem:** Able to completely lift patient during a position change; moves in bed and chair independently and has sufficient muscle strength to lift up completely during move Maintains good position in bed or chair at all times	

Continued

TABLE 125-1	Modified Braden Q Scale (for Pediatric Use) for Early Identification of Relative Risk for Pressure Ulcers—Cont'd

	Tolerance of the Skin and Supporting Structure				Score
Nutrition *Usual* food intake pattern	**1. Very poor:** NPO or maintained on clear liquids or IV lines for more than 5 days *or* albumin less than 2.5 mg/dL *or* never eats a complete meal Rarely eats more than half of any food offered Protein intake includes only two servings of meat or dairy products per day Takes fluids poorly Does not take a liquid dietary supplement	**2. Inadequdate:** Is on liquid diet or tube feed/TPN that provides inadequate calories or minerals for age *or* albumin less than 3 mg/dL *or* rarely eats a complete meal and generally eats only about half of any food offered Protein intake includes only three servings of meat or dairy products per day Occasionally takes a dietary supplement	**3. Adequate:** Is on tube feed or TPN that provides adequate calories and minerals for age *or* eats over half of most meals Eats a total of four servings of protein (meat, dairy products) each day Occasionally refuses a meal but usually takes a supplement if offered	**4. Excellent:** Is on a normal diet that provides adequate calories for age For example: Eats/drinks most of every meal/feeding Never refuses a meal Usually eats a total of four or more servings of meat and dairy products Occasionally eats between meals Does not need supplementation	
Tissue perfusion and oxygenation	**1. Extremely compromised:** Hypotensive (MAP <50 mm Hg or <40 mm Hg in a newborn) *or* the patient does not physiologically tolerate position changes	**2. Compromised:** Normotensive; oxygen saturation may be less than 95% *or* hemoglobin may be less than 10 mg/dL *or* capillary refill may be more than 2 seconds; serum pH is less than 7.40	**3. Adequate:** Normotensive, oxygen saturation may be less than 95%; hemoglobin may be less than 10 mg/dL *or* capillary refill may be more than 2 seconds; serum pH is normal	**4. Excellent:** Normotensive, oxygen saturation more than 95%; normal hemoglobin; capillary refill less than 2 seconds	

Key for Modified Braden Q Scale Score:
Minimal score for each subscale is 1 (more risk)
Maximal score for each subscale is 4 (less risk)

Potential scores range from 7 to 28 points
The lower the score, the higher the patient's risk for pressure ulcers

Modified Braden Q Scale score of 16 or less: trigger for implementing more aggressive preventative interventions

Total Score

NPO, Nothing by mouth; *TPN*, total parenteral nutrition; *MAP* Mean Arterial Pressure.
From Quigley SM, Curley MAQ: Skin integrity in the pediatric population: preventing and managing pressure ulcers, *J Soc Pediatr Nurs* 1(1):7-18, 1996.

- Procedures for diagnostic purposes:
  - Culture of the lesion
  - Biopsy
  - Examination of specimen with wood lamp
  - Examination of specimen with potassium hydroxide (KOH) preparation
  - Tzanck smear
  - Immunoflourescence studies
  - A biopsy of the skin for diagnosis in children is rarely done.[1] These procedures, excluding culture of the lesion, are usually done by a dermatologist. In most instances, when more than a simple culture of the lesion is necessary, a dermatologic consult should be obtained.

CHILD AND FAMILY ASSESSMENT

- Child's developmental level and ability to interact ➤➤*Rationale:* These factors influence preparation of the child, interaction, and examination.
- Child's and family's understanding of the reasons for and risks and benefits of the procedure ➤➤*Rationale:* Evaluates child's and family's understanding of the procedure and provides a gauge for ongoing education.
- An accurate and detailed history ➤➤*Rationale:* A thorough and accurate history is essential to help confirm a diagnosis.
- In the newborn population, assessment for complications during pregnancy, problems during birth, appearance of child's skin at birth, history of infant being "yellow" or

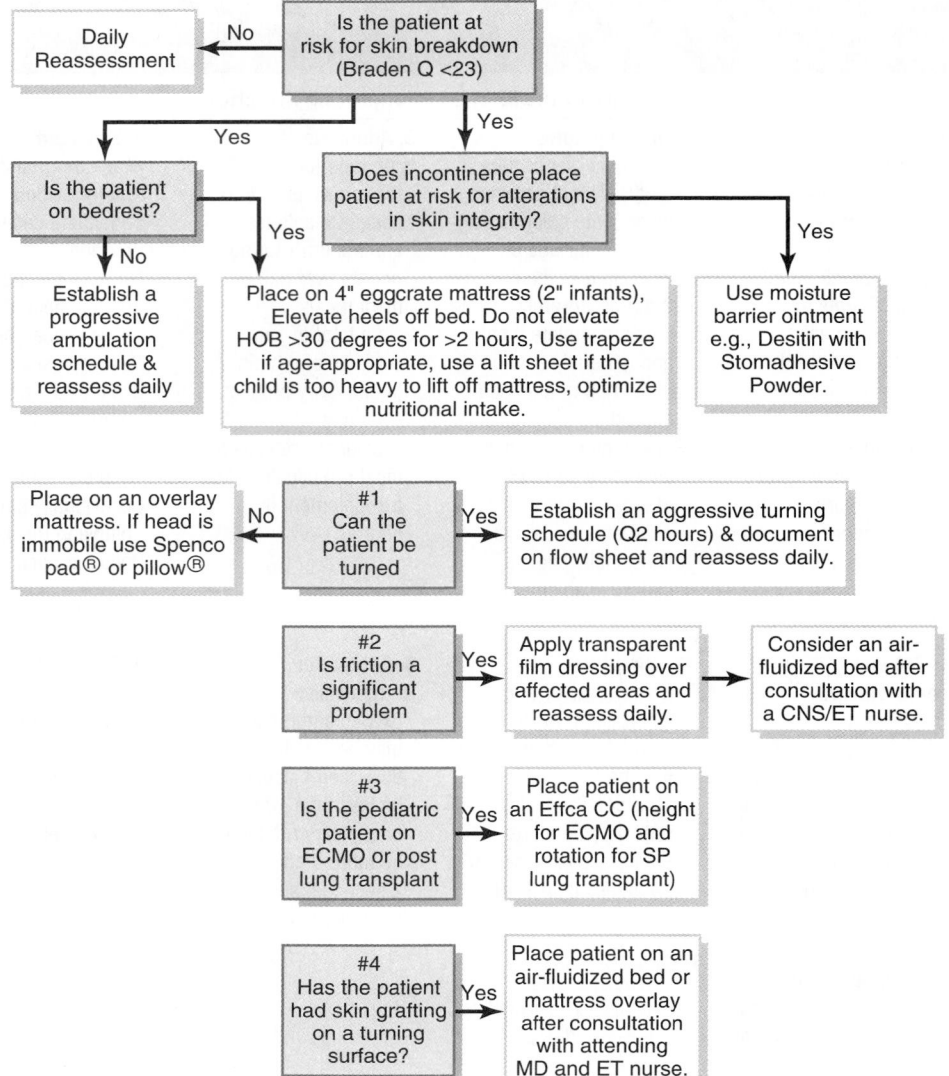

FIGURE 125-1   Skin Care Algorithm. *From Quigley S, Curley MAQ: Skin integrity in the pediatric population: preventing and managing pressure ulcers, J Soc Pediatr Nurs 1(1):7-18, 1996.*

jaundiced at birth, prematurity, and medications given at birth (e.g., antibiotics) ➤➤*Rationale:* Some disorders occur more commonly in the newborn period. Newborns are more susceptible to external irritants, have an increased relative absorption of topical agents, and differ in the ability to bind, metabolize, and excrete drugs.[2]

- Immunization status ➤➤*Rationale:* Certain communicable diseases can cause a rash in the child.
- Use of diaper creams or bathing products ➤➤*Rationale:* Certain ingredients may irritate the skin.
- Child's known allergies ➤➤*Rationale:* Seasonal or drug allergies may cause a rash.
- Signs of injury ➤➤*Rationale:* Provides a baseline for skin alterations; facilitates evaluation of ongoing status.
- Dietary history ➤➤*Rationale:* Some skin disorders can develop as a result of dietary changes or deficiencies. Poor nutritional status can lead to skin breakdown.[3]
- Family history of skin disorders ➤➤*Rationale:* Some conditions, such as psoriasis and eczema, can be genetically inherited.[2]

- Current symptoms
  - ❖ First appearance
  - ❖ Spread or change in color or appearance
  - ❖ Itching or pain
  - ❖ Treatment, including method used, length of treatment, and results
  ➤➤*Rationale:* Facilitates assessment and diagnosis
- Assessment in the pediatric oncology population
  - ❖ Recent chemotherapeutic agents the child has received
  - ❖ Bone marrow or peripheral blood stem cell transplant
  - ❖ Presence of neutropenia
  - ❖ Presence of an indwelling broviac or percutaneous catheter
  ➤➤*Rationale:* Children whose conditions or treatments cause neutropenia or who have indwelling catheters are at increased risk for infection. Children who have undergone bone marrow transplant are at risk for infection and GVHD.
- Desire of family members to be present during the procedure ➤➤*Rationale:* Family may provide comfort and

support during the procedure but should have the choice not to remain with the child.

CHILD AND FAMILY EDUCATION

Individualized, developmentally appropriate education is provided to the family and to the child based on desire for knowledge, readiness to learn, and overall neurologic and psychosocial state.

- Provide information about basic functions of the skin ➤*Rationale:* Information decreases fear and anxiety.
- Explain that a culture, with a sterile culture swab, may be needed to obtain a specimen ➤*Rationale:* Anxiety and fear about a noninvasive procedure are reduced.
- Explain that a more invasive procedure, such as a biopsy, may be needed to confirm diagnosis ➤*Rationale:* Understanding is promoted, and anxiety and fear are decreased.
- If biopsy is performed, explain the purpose of topical anesthetic cream (EMLA [Astra-Zeneca, Wilmington, DE] or ELA-Max [Ferndale Laboratories, Ferndale, MI]) and lidocaine (to reduce pain at biopsy site) ➤*Rationale:* Cooperation with procedure is promoted, and anxiety and fear are decreased.
- Provide brief explanation to the child, in a developmentally appropriate manner, of how the procedure will take place; consider use of the child's favorite doll or a book ➤*Rationale:*

Children have a fear of needles and invasive procedures. Explaining the procedure in a developmentally appropriate or age-appropriate manner to the child helps decrease anxiety, thereby increasing cooperation during the procedure.
- Educate the child and family on ways to minimize risk factors based on age, disease status, and special needs ➤*Rationale:* Particular risk factors for skin are associated with certain ages and disease processes; this information allows the family to participate in the child's care.
- Encourage questions and answer questions as they arise ➤*Rationale:* Reinforcement of information is needed during periods of stress.

EQUIPMENT

- Measuring tape
- Topical anesthetic cream (e.g., EMLA or ELA-Max)
- Transparent dressing (e.g., Op-site [Smith and Nephew, Largo, FL] or Tegaderm [3M, St. Paul, MN])
- Lidocaine, 1% to 2%
- 27-gauge or 30-gauge needle
- Sterile or clean gloves
- Sterile scissors and forceps
- Skin antiseptic, such as povidone-iodine or chlorhexadine
- Sterile culture swab
- Skin marker
- Sterile culture container

Procedure for Skin Assessment

Steps	Rationale	Considerations
1. Ensure child and family understand procedure and questions are answered.	Evaluates and reinforces understanding of previously taught information.	Developmental level, cognitive function, and anxiety level determine approach to and effectiveness of teaching.
2. Gather needed equipment and supplies.	Facilitates completion of task in a timely manner.	
3. Ensure examination area has adequate lighting and privacy and is warm.	Peripheral cyanosis may result from anxiety or a cold examination room. Examination may necessitate exposure of the genital area.	Artificial light can distort colors and mask jaundice. Privacy is an important consideration for school-aged children and adolescents.
4. Provide child with appropriate toys or books during the examination.	Encourages the child to cooperate.	"Pretend" examination on child's favorite doll or toy may alleviate the child's fears.
5. Note skin color; assess for increased pigmentation, loss of pigmentation, redness, pallor, cyanosis, or jaundice. *(Level VI*)*	Oxyhemoglobin, a bright red pigment, predominates in arteries and capillaries. Cyanosis is a result of loss of oxygen to the tissues and thereby changes to deoxyhemoglobin, which produces a darker and somewhat bluer pigment.[4] In assessment of pallor; assess surrounding	In people of color, the palms and soles may be useful areas to assess color of skin. *(Level II*)*

Procedure continues on following page

---

* Level II: Theory-based; no research data to support recommendations; recommendations from expert consensus group may exist
Level VI: Clinical studies in a variety of patient populations and situations to support recommendations

Procedure for Skin Assessment—*Continued*

Steps	Rationale	Considerations
	areas such as nailbeds, lips, and mucous membranes. Lack of oxyhemoglobin is best discerned where the horny layer of the epidermis is thinnest and causes the least scatter.	
Assessment of newborn's skin color		
6. Provide adequate lighting and warm examination room.	Facilitates good visualization; cold environment may cause changes in skin color.	Newborns may have a variety of "normal" skin changes (Box 125-1).
7. Provide pacifier if appropriate.	Sucking provides comfort for the newborn.	May not be applicable if child's respiratory status is compromised or if child has anatomic defect of the lips or palate. *(Level II*)*
8. Note color; acrocyanosis or jaundice. If jaundice is present, assess and document the distribution and degree of skin discoloration. Also, include color of sclera. *(Level VI*)*	Acrocyanosis is a purplish blue discoloration of lips, hands, and feet, and is common in newborns. Most noticeable during periods of chilling or crying. Jaundice may suggest liver disease or excessive hemolysis of red blood cells (RBCs).	Signs of jaundice warrant further work-up.
Systematic inspection of skin from head to toe, front and back		
9. Inspect for signs of breakdown.	Identifies alterations in skin integrity.	Utilize Braden Q Scale to identify children at risk for skin breakdown (see Table 125-1).
10. If breakdown is noted, assess and document location, surrounding area, and any drainage.	Establishes baseline description of altered skin integrity.	Stage pressure ulcers (Table 125-2). Box 125-2 has documentation guidelines.
11. Carefully place measuring tape alongside area of breakdown and note length and depth in terms of centimeters.	Establishes baseline size of breakdown; facilitates assessment of progression or decrease in size.	
12. If rash is noted: assess and document color and location and note raised papules and assessment of surrounding area.	In evaluation of children with a rash or lesion, a cursory examination of the skin is appropriate.[2]	Box 125-3 and Box 125-4 have descriptions of primary and secondary lesions.

13. Special considerations for newborns:
    Frequently change sites of pulse oximetry probe to prevent skin breakdown.
    Observe all IV or central line sites; use minimal amount of tape because skin is thin and prone to tears.
	The newborn has an increased susceptibility to external irritants. Small breaks in skin can serve as a portal of entry for bacteria. *(Level IV*)*	Pulse oximeter probes may cause a localized burn to newborn's affected extremity. When tape is necessary, a protective barrier should be used first, if possible. If frequent tape removal is necessary, a protective barrier (e.g., Duoderm [Convatec, Princeton, NJ]) may be used. *(Level I*)*

* Level I: Manufacturer's recommendations only
  Level II: Theory-based; no research data to support recommendations; recommendations from expert consensus group may exist
  Level IV: Limited clinical studies to support recommendations
  Level VI: Clinical studies in a variety of patient populations and situations to support recommendations

Procedure for Skin Assessment—*Continued*

Steps	Rationale	Considerations
14. Special consideration in pediatric oncology populations: Perform careful assessment and inspection of skin. The child who has undergone bone marrow transplant (BMT) or peripheral blood stem cell transplant (PBSCT) should be assessed for GVHD.	Children who undergo immuno-suppressive treatment are at risk for increased bacterial infections. A common complication in transplantation is acute GVHD, which is an immunologic response in which donor T-cells attack the "seemingly" foreign host. A macular-papular rash that begins on palms, soles, and ears then progresses to the entire body is a clinical manifestation of GVHD.[5]	Any area of skin breakdown *must* be documented. Further treatment (e.g., antibiotic therapy) may be necessary to prevent systemic infection. *(Level IV*)*
15. Special considerations for immobile or critically ill children that place them at greater risk for pressure ulcers: Inspect all areas of skin with particular attention to bony prominences, heels, elbows, sacrum, and occiput. Note location, size, depth, and color of surrounding tissue.	Children who are immobile or critically ill are at increased risk for skin breakdown from immobility, decreased sensory perception, poor nutrition, or inadequate tissue perfusion and oxygenation.[3]	Preventative measures may be indicated with this population for prevention of tissue injury. The use of gel-pads and specialty beds should be considered. Frequent repositioning, as tolerated, is a must with this population to reduce risk of tissue injury.
16. Carefully measure areas of altered skin integrity.	Establishes baseline.	
17. If discharge is present, put on clean gloves.	Standard precautions; reduces transmission of microorganisms.	Contact precautions may be required.
18. Per prescribing practitioner's order or institution-specific protocol, use sterile culture swab to collect specimen of discharge by carefully swiping area when discharge is initially noted.	Facilitates assessment of discharge for presence of organisms. *(Level IV*)*	Culture is generally obtained when presence of discharge is initially identified.
19. Palpate skin to assess temperature, texture, turgor, and edema.	Necessary for identification of abnormal findings.	
20. Inspect and palpate lesions; note location, pattern, size, shape, mobility, consistency, color, and presence of exudates.	Necessary for thorough assessment.	See Box 125-3.
21. Note whether lesion is primary or secondary.	Primary lesions arise from previously normal skin. Secondary lesions result from changes in primary lesion.[2]	See Box 125-3 and Box 125-4.
22. Note pain or discomfort related to alterations in skin integrity.	Facilitates early identification and prompt treatment of pain.	Use pain assessment tool appropriate to child's age and developmental level (see Procedure 173).
23. Discard used supplies and equipment in appropriate receptacles.	Standard precautions; reduces the transmission of microorganisms.	
24. Remove gloves; wash hands.	Standard precautions.	

* Level IV: Limited clinical studies to support recommendations

TABLE 125-2	Staging Pressure Ulcers
Stage I	Nonblanchable erythema of intact skin that does not disappear when pressure is relieved; the heralding lesion of skin ulceration. Skin discoloration, warmth, edema, induration, or hardness may also be indicators.
Stage II	A partial thickness loss of skin layers involving epidermis or dermis. The ulcer is superficial and presents clinically as an abrasion, blister, or shallow crater.
Stage III	A full thickness of skin is lost, involving exposure of subcutaneous tissues with damage or necrosis that may extend down to, but not through, underlying fascia. The ulcer presents clinically as a deep crater with or without undermining of adjacent tissue.
Stage IV	A full thickness of skin and subcutaneous tissue is lost, with extensive destruction, tissue necrosis, or damage or exposure to muscle, bone, or supporting structures. Undermining and sinus tracts may also be associated with stage IV pressure ulcers.

From National Pressure Ulcer Advisory Panel: Pressure ulcers prevalence, cost and risk assessment; consensus development conference statement, *Decubitus* 2:24-28, 1989.

Box 125-1	Normal Newborn Skin Changes

- **Cutis marmorata:** Bluish-purple mottling of trunk and extremities from vasodilation of peripheral small vessels. Usually resolves after 2 to 3 weeks.
- **Salmon patches:** Vascular "reddish" stains usually seen at nape of neck and eyelids
- **Port wine stain:** Red, flat, and unilateral. Possibility of Sturge-Weber syndrome must be ruled out.[2]
- **Hemangiomas:** Initially appear as flat red patches and darken and thicken over time
- **Mongolian spots:** Bluish-gray flat birthmarks; usually fade by 2 to 3 years of age

Adapted from: Williams J, et al L: Skin. In Rudolph A, et al, editors: *Rudolph's fundamentals of pediatrics,* ed 3, New York, 2002, McGraw-Hill.

Box 125-3	Primary Skin Lesions

- **Macule:** Flat area of circumscribed color change; nonpalpable lesion
- **Papule:** Raised, palpable, less than 0.5 cm
- **Nodule:** Papule that has enlarged in all three dimensions
- **Plaque:** Flat-topped lesion, less than 0.5 cm; lacks significant depth and height
- **Wheal:** Edematous or fluid-filled area of dermal edema
- **Vesicle:** Blister that contains clear fluid; may contain milky or purulent fluid
- **Papulosquamous:** Scaly violaceous papules or plaques
- **Eczematous:** Inflammatory lesions that ooze or are crusted or thickened

Adapted from Williams J, et al: Skin. In Rudolph A, et al, editors: *Rudolph's fundamentals of pediatrics,* ed 3, New York, 2002, McGraw-Hill.

Box 125-4	Secondary Skin Lesions

- **Erosion:** Disruption of skin lacking part or all of epidermis; usually moist and red; sometimes crusted over
- **Ulcer:** Deeper erosion; all or part of dermis is missing
- **Fissure:** Linear wedge-shaped erosion or ulcer
- **Scale:** Visible flake on skin surface
- **Crust:** Yellowish firm covering on surface of skin; may have exudates
- **Excoriation:** Scratch mark; may be linear or oval depression of skin
- **Lichenification:** Thickening of epidermis
- **Atrophy:** Area of depressed or thin skin
- **Sclerosis:** Firm smooth induration or thickening of skin

Adapted from Williams J, et al: Skin. In Rudolph A, et al, editors: *Rudolph's fundamentals of pediatrics,* ed 3, New York, 2002, McGraw-Hill.

Box 125-2	Assessment and Documentation Guidelines

- Size (record in centimeters or millimeters)
  - ❖ Height: Longest vertical
  - ❖ Width: Widest horizontal
  - ❖ Depth: Point of greatest depth
- Extent of Tissue Involvement
  - ❖ Partial thickness
  - ❖ Full thickness
  - ❖ Stage (pressure ulcers only)
- Presence of Undermining and Tracts
  - ❖ Use the face of a clock to describe location
  - ❖ Measure greatest depth
- Anatomic Location
- Type of Tissue in Wound Bed
  - ❖ Granulation
  - ❖ Muscle
  - ❖ Fibrinous
  - ❖ Eschar
  - ❖ Epithelialization
  - ❖ Bone
  - ❖ Necrotic
  - ❖ Slough
- Color (describe in percentage of wound to 100%)
  - ❖ Red/pink
  - ❖ Yellow
  - ❖ Black/brown/tan
- Exudate
  - ❖ Amount: Scant, minimal, moderate, heavy
  - ❖ Malodorous
  - ❖ Serous
  - ❖ Purulent
  - ❖ Serosanguineous
- Condition of Surrounding Skin
  - ❖ Intact
  - ❖ Denuded
  - ❖ Macerated
  - ❖ Erythema
- Wound Edges
  - ❖ Open-pink, new skin visible
  - ❖ Closed-thick and rolled

Expected Outcomes	Unexpected Outcomes
• Full assessment of skin is obtained • Skin is free of breakdown • Areas of skin breakdown are assessed, documented, and treated appropriately; areas of breakdown heal • Child has acceptable level of comfort	• Inability to obtain full assessment of skin • Areas of skin breakdown are noted • Areas of breakdown are not identified, documented, or treated appropriately and skin damage progresses • Unmanaged pain related to skin injury

Monitoring and Care of the Child

Activities and Interventions	Rationale	Reportable Conditions
1. Continually assess condition of skin and note any signs of breakdown.	Newborns, critically ill children, and children with immunosuppression are at risk for skin breakdown.	• New onset of rash, papules, or skin lesions • Any signs of injury • Worsening rash or lesions • Identified risk factors • Braden Q score of 16 or less • Need for interventions such as specialty beds
2. Implement a skin care algorithm if child is identified as having risk factors for alterations in skin integrity (see Figure 125-1).	Identification of children at risk and prompt initiation of preventative measures promote good skin integrity. Acutely ill children with a Braden Q score of 16 or less have been shown to be at risk for stage II pressure ulcers.[3] *(Level IV*)*	
3. Assess effectiveness of pain management strategy and provide appropriate interventions. Encourage family to assist with nonpharmacologic means to comfort and support the child.	Monitoring effectiveness of pain management strategies allows modification of plan as necessary.	• Unresolved pain or discomfort • Continued irritability or changes in physiologic condition

* Level IV: Limited clinical studies to support recommendations

Documentation

• Risk factors identified for altered skin integrity
• Skin assessment using documentation guidelines in Box 125-2
• Presence of pressure ulcers using pressure ulcer staging scale
• Interventions provided
• Measurement of pressure ulcer, rash, or area of breakdown, including length, depth, color, and discharge present and condition of surrounding area
• Child and family education
• Use of Braden Q Scale to assess level of risk for tissue injury and breakdown
• Unexpected outcomes and related treatment

References

1. Behrman RE, et al: Evaluation of the patient. In Behrman RE, Kliegman RM, Jenson H, editors: *Nelson's textbook of pediatrics,* ed 17, Philadelphia, 2004, Saunders, pp. 2155-2157.
2. Williams J, et al: Skin. In Rudolph A, Kamei R, Overby K, editors: *Rudolph's fundamentals of pediatrics,* ed 3, New York, 2002, McGraw Hill Medical Publishing Division, pp. 437-443.
3. Curley M, et al: Predicting pressure ulcer risk in pediatric patients: the Braden Q scale, *Nurs Res* 52(1):22-35, 2003.
4. Bickley L, Hoeckelman R: The skin. In Bickley L, Hoeckelman R, editors: *Bates' guide to physical examination and history taking,* ed 7, Philadelphia, 1999, Lippincott, pp. 145-150.
5. Cimiotti J: Peripheral blood transplantation and graft versus host disease: a case study, *J Pediatr Oncol Nurs* 20(3): 182-187, 2002.

Additional Reading

Turnbull R: Skin assessment in children: a methodical approach, *Nurs Times* 96(41):33-34, 2000.

PROCEDURE **126**

Cleansing, Irrigating, Culturing, and Dressing Wounds

P U R P O S E : To optimize wound healing; culture may be necessary to isolate and guide treatment of organisms in the wound

Patricia O'Connor

PREREQUISITE KNOWLEDGE

- An understanding of the wound-healing process
- In a child, the process of wound healing follows the same pathway as in adults but at a faster rate.
- Wounds heal by primary, secondary, or tertiary intention[1] (Figure 126-1).
  - ❖ Primary intention occurs when all layers of the wound (skin, subcutaneous tissue, and muscle) margins are well approximated. Most clean or clean/contaminated surgical wounds fall into this category. Surgical suturing of tissue layers helps to approximate the wound edges and to allow for primary intention.
  - ❖ Secondary intention occurs from ulceration and laceration in which the edges cannot be approximated, such as an evulsion or a third-degree burn. Increased inflammation and a greater chance of infection are often seen. Often excess debris, cells, and exudates must be cleaned away before healing can take place. Healing begins from the edges inward and from the bottom of the wound upward.
  - ❖ Repair by tertiary intention occurs when suturing is delayed or the wound later breaks down and is sutured or resutured when granulation is present.
- Wound assessment is the foundation for selection of the correct method to promote wound healing.
- Open wounds tend to heal more slowly and tend to be more painful for the child.
- Goals of wound care must be established so that the correct wound care products are used (Table 126-1).

- Pediatric wound care must be delivered in a developmentally appropriate manner.
- Adequate preparation and pain management are essential before wound care is performed on a child.
- Cause of the specific wound
- Wound care strategies should use moist wound-healing techniques.
- Effective and speedy healing of open wounds is promoted when the wound is kept clean and moist.[1]
- When open wounds have excessive drainage, application of absorptive dressings or more frequent dressing changes facilitates healing.[1]
- Avoid chemical or mechanical trauma in wound cleansing.[1]
- Wound infection is present if organisms are present at 10^5 colony-forming units per mL.
- Wound infection may be treated locally or systemically or with combination therapy.
- Healing may be delayed in infected wounds; sterile wound cultures isolate organisms and allow differentiation between colonization and active infection in a wound bed.[1]
- Principles of aseptic technique
- Appropriate pediatric dosing of analgesics

CHILD AND FAMILY ASSESSMENT

- Child's developmental level and ability to interact ➼*Rationale:* These factors influence preparation of the child, interaction, and selection of appropriate pain scale.
- Allergies, including latex, alcohol, tape, and skin preparation products ➼*Rationale:* These substances are found

FIRST INTENTION (Primary union)   SECOND INTENTION (Granulation)   THIRD INTENTION (Secondary suture)

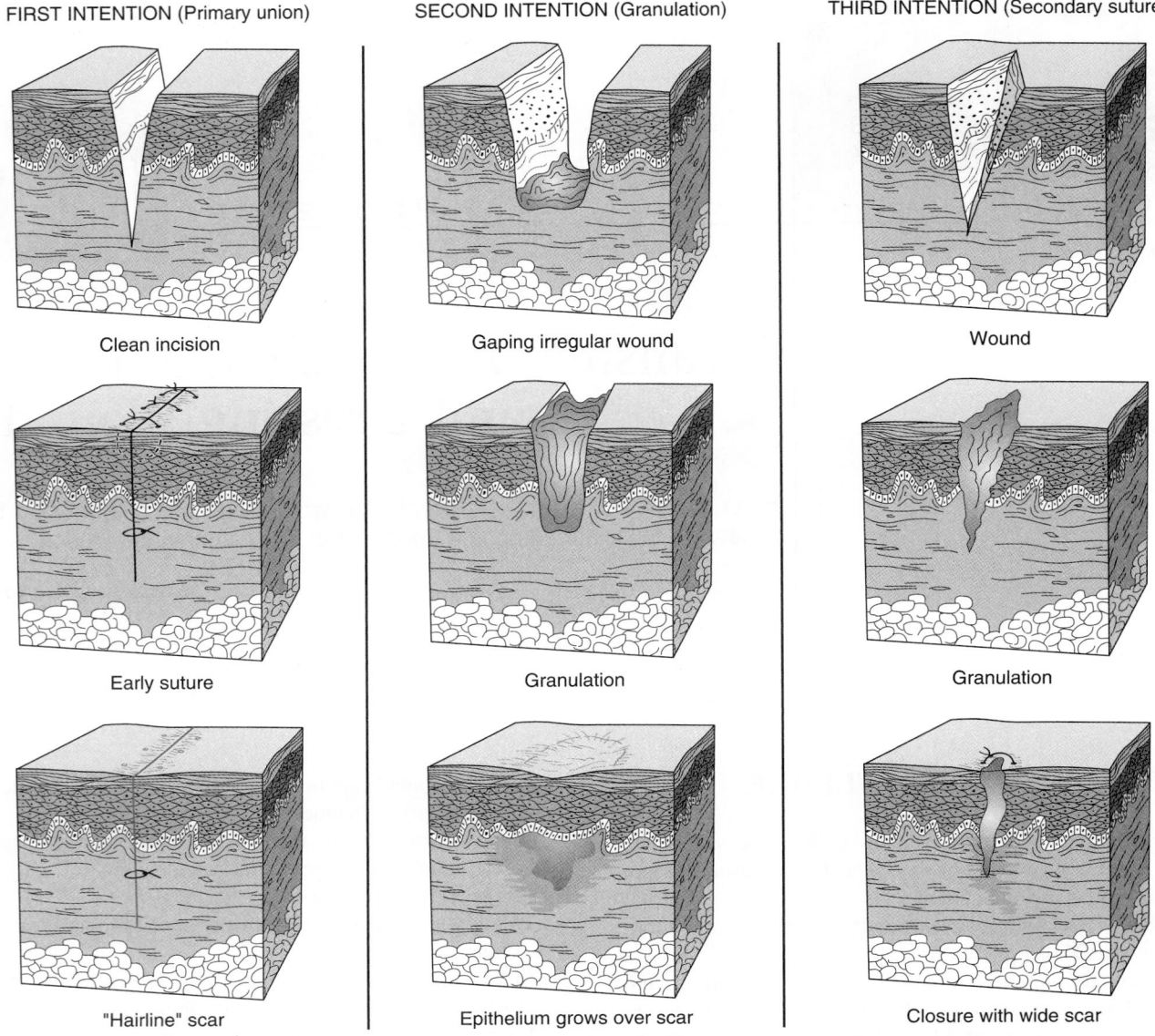

Clean incision	Gaping irregular wound	Wound
Early suture	Granulation	Granulation
"Hairline" scar	Epithelium grows over scar	Closure with wide scar

FIGURE 126-1   Wound healing by primary, secondary, and tertiary intention. *From Makic MBF: Cleansing, irrigating, culturing, and dressing an open wound. In Lynn-McHale Wiegand DJ, Carlson K, editors:* AACN procedure manual for critical care, *ed 5, Philadelphia, 2005, Saunders.*

in many products used to dress wounds; patient safety is promoted by ensuring the child is not exposed to known allergens.
• Assessment of the wound for:
  ❖ Drainage
  ❖ Foul-smelling drainage or odor
  ❖ Color of tissue bed: darkened areas, pale red, green, or yellow
  ❖ Erythema
  ❖ Change in amount or color of wound drainage
  ❖ Presence and depth of pocket or tunnel
  ➨*Rationale:* Assessment of the wound bed provides information about the healing process and assists in early identification of wound infection; true wound bed assessment cannot be completed until after the wound bed has been cleansed.

• Assessment of the child for pain, elevated temperature, and elevated white blood cell count ➨*Rationale:* The presence of these factors may indicate infection.
• Child's and family's understanding of the procedure and their ability and desire to perform wound care after discharge if indicated ➨*Rationale:* Evaluates understanding of the procedure and provides a gauge for ongoing education; wound care may need to be continued in the home after discharge.
• Family's desire to be present during the procedure ➨*Rationale:* Family may provide support, comfort, and distraction during the procedure, facilitating the child's cooperation. In general, the family should have the option not to remain during the procedure. If the child will require wound care in the home after discharge, family members need to be present during wound care to learn the care necessary.

TABLE 126-1	Types of Surgical Dressings			
Dressing Category	**Description**	**Example**	**Indication**	**Comments**
Gauze dressing sponges	Made of cotton or synthetic fabric that is absorptive and permeable to water, gas, or vapor	Topper sponges General-use gauze (2×2 or 4×4) Kerlix (Kendall, Mansfield, MA)	• Cover surgical wounds • Nonselective debridement • Keep a wound bed that needs frequent inspection moist	Can be used dry, wet-to-dry, or moist
All-absorbent combined	Cotton-filled dressing that is typically used as "over-dressing"	Surgipad (Johnson & Johnson, New Brunswick, NJ), ABD	• Cover gauze or hydrophilic dressings for added wound protection • Stabilization of dressings • Drainage absorption	May be used unaccompanied over intact surgical wounds
Hydrocolloids	Water-based nonadherent polymer-based dressing with some absorptive properties	Duoderm (ConvaTec, Princeton, NJ) Restore (Hollister, Libertyville, IL) Replicare (Smith & Nephew, Largo, FL) Confeel (Coloplast, Marietta, GA) Hydrocol (Bertek, Research Triangle Park, NC) Nu-Derm Hydrocolloid (Johnson & Johnson, New Brunswick, NJ) Sorbex (Bard, Covington, GA) Tegasorb (3M, St. Paul, MN) Ultec Pro Alginate (Kendall, Mansfield, MA)	• Used around mild to moderately draining wounds as a skin protector to preserve intact skin • Stage I to wIll pressure ulcers • Some IV infiltrates	Easy to apply Waterproof Dressing must extend 1.5 to 2 inches past wound to obtain adequate adherence Interacts with wound fluid to form a gel that some misinterpret as infection Do not use around tracheostomy stomas; gel may travel down tracheostomy tract
Hydrogel	Contains a gel composed primarily of water	Vigilon (Bard, Covington, GA) Geliperm (Fougera, Melville, NY) Curagel (Kendall, Mansfield, MA) Flexigel (Smith & Nephew, Largo, FL) Nu-Gel (Johnson & Johnson, New Brunswick, NJ) Tegagel (3M, St. Paul, MN)	• Wounds with minimal or no exudates • Dermabrasion type wounds to enhance epithelialization	Mild absorptive properties Nonadherent; requires a secondary dressing to hold it in place May be used in conjunction with topical antibiotics
Polyurethane transparent film	Transparent adhesive dressing; allows free flow of oxygen through the pores; impermeable to bacteria	Tegaderm (3M, St. Paul, MN) Op-Site (Smith-Nephew, Largo, FL)	• Secure and protect IV catheter sites • Preventative dressing on skin that is at risk for abrasion • Superficial wounds such as blisters	Lacks absorptive capabilities

Continued

TABLE 126-1	Types of Surgical Dressings—Cont'd			
Dressing Category	**Description**	**Example**	**Indication**	**Comments**
Hydrophobic occlusive	Impermeable nonadhering dressing that protects from air and moisture-borne contamination	Petroleum gauze	• Used around chest tubes and any fistula or stoma that drains digestive juices	Relatively nonabsorptive
Hydrophilic permeable	Allows drainage to penetrate dressing but remains somewhat nonadhering	Oil-based gauze Telfa pads (Kendall, Mansfield, MA)	• Oil-based gauze used on abraded and open ulcerated or granulating wounds	Telfa pads are generally reserved for simple, closed, stable wounds
Nonadhesive foam	Polyurethane foam	Biopatch (Johnson & Johnson, New Brunswick, NJ) Lyofoam (ConvaTec, Princeton, NJ) Needs a secondary dressing to hold it in place	• Ideal for use around tracheostomy sites to prevent trauma and absorb moisture	Mild absorption May be used in conjunction with topical antibiotics
Calcium alginate	Nonwoven fibers derived from seaweed Dressing forms an absorptive gel when it comes in contact with wound exudates	Sorbsan (Bertek, Research Triangle Park, NC) Kaltostat (ConvaTec, Princeton, NJ) Algisite M (Smith & Nephew, Largo, FL) Algiderm (Bard, Covington, GA) Curasorb (Kendall, Mansfield, MA) Nu-Derm Alginate (Johnson & Johnson, New Brunswick, NJ) Seasorb (Coloplast, Marietta, GA) Tegagen HI and HG (3M, St. Paul, MN)	• Used on moderate to heavily exudating wounds	Highly absorptive; absorbs 20 times its weight in exudates Requires a secondary dressing Not appropriate for use in abdominal wounds with large areas of exposed intestinal mucosa because of the potential for systematic absorption of calcium/sodium

Wound management technology is constantly progressing. This table represents a comprehensive review of dressing categories and products available at publication. Practitioners should consider the most current research, availability, and total costs.
Data compiled from:
Branom RN: Is this wound infected? *Crit Care Nurs Q* 25(1):55-62, 2002.
Hess CT: Product update 2002, *Adv Skin Wound Care* 15(6):287-295, 2002.
Hess CT, Kirsner RS: Orchestrating wound healing: assessing and preparing the wound, *Adv Skin Wound Care* 16(5):246-257, 2003.
Howard R: The appropriate use of topical antimicrobials and antiseptics in children: neonatal skin care, *Pediatr Ann* 30(4):219-224, 2001.
Maloney J, Fisher B: Skin integrity. In Moloney-Harmon P, Czerwinski SJ, editors: *Review of pediatric critical care,* Philadelphia, 1997, Saunders.
Nelson DB, Dilloway MA: Principles, products and practical aspects of wound care, *Crit Care Nurs Q* 25(1):33-54, 2002.
Nettina SM, editor: *Lippincott manual of nursing practice,* ed 7, Philadelphia, 2000, Lippincott, Williams & Wilkins.
Taquino LT: Promoting wound healing in the neonatal setting: process versus protocol, *J Perinatal Neonatal Nurs* 14(1):104-118, 2000.
Thompson J: A practical guide to wound care, *RN.* 63(1):48-53, 2000.
Wysocki AB: Evaluating and managing open skin wounds: colonization versus infection, *Adv Pract Acute Crit Care* 13(3):382-397, 2002.

CHILD AND FAMILY EDUCATION

Individualized, developmentally appropriate education is provided to the family and to the child based on desire for knowledge, readiness to learn, and overall neurologic and psychosocial state.
• Explain the procedure and reason for wound cleansing, irrigation, culture, or dressing change to the family and to the child at a developmentally appropriate level. Toddlers may need their parents to help alleviate anxiety. Preschoolers need simple concise explanations. School-aged children need thorough preparation for all procedures, including all the steps involved. Adolescents also need preparation and information and have a high need for privacy. ➤*Rationale:* Child's anxiety and discomfort is decreased, and compliance and child and family

participation are improved and promoted. The extra time taken to prepare the child or adolescent and family beforehand is well invested. If appropriate, show the procedure to be performed on a doll. Use the resources of Child Life Specialists if available.

- Explain the age-appropriate pain scale to be used to assess the child's pain (see Procedure 173) ➝*Rationale:* Ongoing assessment of the child's pain and response to pain medications are facilitated; the family and child are reassured that pain will be monitored and attended to.
- Explain the need for the child to be in a position of comfort and to be able to remain still during the procedure ➝*Rationale:* Providing information may decrease anxiety and promote cooperation with the procedure.
- Explain the procedure and reason for wound culture, as necessary ➝*Rationale:* Providing information may decrease anxiety and discomfort and promote compliance.
- If wound care is to be continued after discharge, discuss child's and family's role in wound cleansing, irrigation, culturing, or dressing management ➝*Rationale:* Wound care may need to be continued in the home. Providing information facilitates child's cooperation and prepares the child and family for wound management on discharge.

EQUIPMENT

- Clean and sterile gloves (two pairs)
- Gown and eye and face protection as indicated
- Sterile barrier or drape to establish sterile field
- Saline solution (NS), 0.9%
- Waterproof barrier
- Hypoallergenic tape
- Adhesive tape remover
- Sterile gauze (4×4)
- Abdominal (ABD) dressings for wounds with moderate to excessive drainage or as secondary dressing

- Moisture-enhancing dressing for wounds with minimal drainage
- Other type of dressing appropriate to the specific wound (see Table 126-1)

For Wound Irrigation

- Sterile 30-mL to 35-mL Luer-lock syringe and 18-gauge to 20-gauge intravenous (IV) catheter (needle removed) for irrigation, if necessary
- Irrigating solution, per prescribing practitioner's order

For Wound Culture

- Swab culture tubes
- Sterile collection container
- Two sterile serum-tipped swabs
- Specimen labels with two patient identifiers and appropriate laboratory requisitions

For Tissue Biopsy

- Scalpel
- Sterile forceps
- Sterile container
- Specimen labels with two patient identifiers and appropriate laboratory requisitions

For Needle Aspiration

- 10-mL syringe and 22-gauge needle
- Sterile container
- Specimen labels with two patient identifiers and appropriate laboratory requisitions

Additional Equipment Required May Include:

- Montgomery straps
- Skin barrier for application of Montgomery straps

Procedure for Cleansing, Irrigating, Culturing, and Dressing Wounds		
Steps	**Rationale**	**Considerations**
Preparatory Phase 1. Ensure that child and family understand procedure and questions are answered.	Evaluates and reinforces understanding of previously taught information.	Developmental level, cognitive ability, and anxiety level determine approach to and effectiveness of teaching.
2. Check prescribing practitioner's orders regarding wound care.	Facilitates preparation; ensures child receives correct treatment.	
3. Administer premedication per prescribing practitioner's order; use two patient identifiers when identifying child per institution-specific protocol.	Promotes child's comfort during procedure. Ensures medication is administered to the correct child.	Pain that is not adequately treated during a procedure increases the child's anxiety related to subsequent procedures.

Procedure continues on following page

Procedure for Cleansing, Irrigating, Culturing, and Dressing Wounds—*Continued*

Steps	Rationale	Considerations
4. Determine how many and what types of dressings are necessary; gather needed equipment and supplies.	Facilitates completion of task in a timely manner.	If dressing is changed regularly, a listing of required supplies is helpful and promotes consistency.
5. Wash hands.	Standard precautions; reduces transmission of microorganisms.	
6. Have child lie in bed or place child on treatment table in a comfortable position, ensuring wound is visible and accessible; expose dressing.	Promotes child's comfort and facilitates access to wound.	
7. Ensure adequate lighting, privacy, and appropriate room temperature.	Respects child's right to privacy. Child is at risk for hypothermia if wound dressing and irrigation necessitate exposure.	Younger smaller infants and children are at increased risk for hypothermia. Privacy is an important consideration for school-aged children and adolescents.
8. Place dressing supplies on a clean flat surface. Open each dressing by peeling apart the edges of package, maintaining sterility; leave each dressing within the open package.	Keeps supplies visible and within easy reach of practitioner. Maintains asepsis.	
9. Prepare tape.	Facilitates completion of task without interruption.	
10. Position waterproof barrier under area to be dressed to collect drainage.	Protects skin integrity and bed linen.	
11. Place disposable bag or receptacle nearby to collect soiled dressings.	Prevents spread of infectious material.	
Removing Old Dressing 12. Put on clean gloves.	Clean gloves are adequate if care is used not to touch wound.[2,3]	
13. Loosen all tape and gently pull tape ends toward the wound. Use adhesive removal pads as necessary.	Makes dressing removal less painful and less traumatizing to the skin and wound.	Adhesive removal pads should not be used on the skin of premature infants because it can cause disruption to skin surfaces.[4]
14. Remove old dressings, one layer at a time, and place in the appropriate disposal container.	Hasty removal of dressings can cause trauma to wound bed and dislodge existing drains. This process is less painful and less traumatic to the newly healing and granulating tissues.[5,6]	Adherent dressing removal may be facilitated by moistening with sterile NS or adhesive remover.
15. Assess wound bed for color, consistency, odor, and amount of drainage. *(Level VI*)*	Exudate volume that persists or is suddenly increased may indicate bacteria, local infection, or suspicion of osteomyelitis, even in the absence of the classical clinical signs of infection.[7]	The wound bed must be cleansed to obtain a complete assessment.[1]

* Level VI: Clinical studies in a variety of patient populations and situations to support recommendations

Procedure for Cleansing, Irrigating, Culturing, and Dressing Wounds—*Continued*

Steps	Rationale	Considerations
16. Remove soiled gloves and discard in appropriate receptacle; wash hands.	Standard precautions; reduces transmission of microorganisms.	
Cleansing and Irrigating Wounds		
17. Wash hands; put on personal protective equipment.	Standard precautions; reduces transmission of microorganisms.	If large amounts of drainage or potential for splashing are anticipated, gowns and eye and face protection should be used.
18. Position wound cleansing materials and soiled contamination container within easy reach.	Avoids cross-contamination; prevents awkward body position.	
19. Establish sterile field; open sterile gauze and required supplies on field with aseptic technique.	Reduces contamination.	
20. If irrigating wound, warm sterile water or NS to body temperature and place in a sterile container. (*Level VI*[*])	Use gravity to direct flow of irrigation solution away from wound bed.	
21. Put on sterile gloves.	Maintains aseptic technique.	
22. Attach 18-gauge IV catheter (needle removed) to syringe for irrigation; draw up irrigating solution into syringe.	Allows cleansing solution to be directed to desired location. Ensures wound drainage moves away from wound. Directs solution away from intact skin.[1]	Isopropyl alcohol should not be used on preterm or term infants; povidone-iodine should not be used on preterm infants or with term infants with an open wound or a wound under an occlusive dressing because of percutaneous absorption and risk for toxicity.[4,6,8]
23. With catheter kept 1 to 3 cm from wound surface, direct solution onto wound bed, irrigating from area of least to greatest contamination. Continue with irrigation until return solution is clear. (*Level IV*[*])	Enhances healing by removing excess debris.[1] A 30-mL to 35-mL syringe with an 18-gauge catheter provides approximately 8 psi, which is appropriate amount of force to remove debris without creating wound bed damage.[1,6] Irrigating with pressures more than 15 psi may cause tissue damage and reinitiation of the inflammatory process, which delays wound healing.[1,9,10]	Irrigation with a catheter may not be necessary; a slip-tip 30-mL to 35-mL syringe may be used to gently irrigate open wounds that are granulating well.[1] Increasing the size of the syringe *decreases* the psi; increasing the bore of the catheter tip or decreasing the size of the syringe *increases* the pressure.
24. When cleansing closed wound, use gauze moistened with sterile water or NS; cleanse from the top to base or center to edges; use new gauze with each area cleansed (Figure 126-2). Clean from least to greatest area of contamination.[1]	Do not use cytotoxic cleansing solution. Hydrogen peroxide destroys fibroblasts, which are the cells most closely associated with granulation and tissue healing.[11] NS irrigations have been shown to be effective in reducing bacteria count in wounds.[12]	The rule of thumb for irrigating solutions is never put anything in an open wound that you would not put in your eye.

Procedure continues on following page

[*] Level IV: Limited clinical studies to support recommendations
Level VI: Clinical studies in a variety of patient populations and situations to support recommendations

Procedure | **for Cleansing, Irrigating, Culturing, and Dressing Wounds**—*Continued*

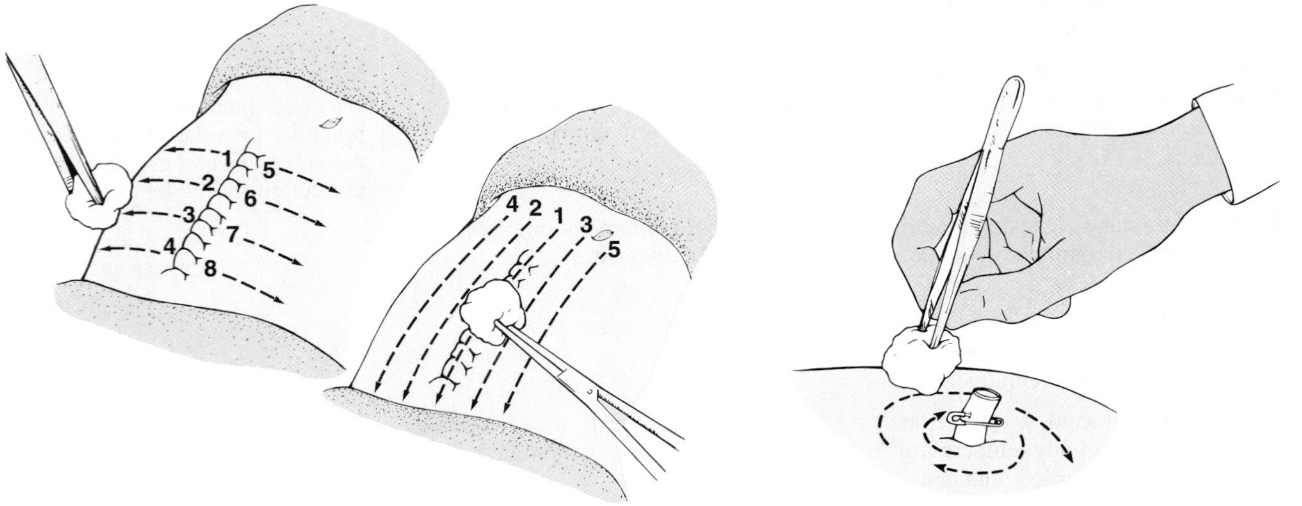

Steps	Rationale	Considerations

FIGURE 126-2   Cleaning a wound. *From: Potter PA, Perry A:* Basic nursing: essentials for practice, *ed 5, St. Louis, 2003, Mosby.*

Steps	Rationale	Considerations
	Prevents wound contamination during the cleansing process.	If cleansing around a drain, clean from the drain site outward in a circular motion (see Figure 126-2); discard gauze with each circle.
25. Dry intact skin around wound with sterile gauze.	Prevents healthy skin surrounding the wound from remaining moist, which may cause maceration.[1,2,13]	
26. Discard used supplies and equipment in appropriate receptacle.	Standard precautions; reduces transmission of microorganisms.	
27. Remove personal protective equipment; wash hands.	Standard precautions.	

Obtaining a Wound Culture (Swab or Needle Aspiration)

Steps	Rationale	Considerations
28. Gather needed equipment and supplies.	Facilitates completion of task in a timely manner.	
29. Wash hands; put on clean gloves.	Standard precautions.	
30. With aseptic technique, clean wound before obtaining culture.	Ensures debris contamination is not cultured.[14,15] Culturing the wound is a sterile procedure. Do not irrigate a wound with antiseptic solution before culturing; this may reduce the number of or kill the organisms being isolated.[16]	
31. Open sterile gloves, package containing sterile syringe and needle, and package containing sterile cotton-tipped culture swabs. Keep all packages within the sterile packages until used.	Prepares supplies needed to obtain culture.	

Procedure for Cleansing, Irrigating, Culturing, and Dressing Wounds—*Continued*

Steps	Rationale	Considerations
32. Aspirate 5 to 10 mL drainage liquid into syringe and place in sterile collection container. *(Level V*)*	Ensures adequate specimen is collected; prevents contamination.[1]	Use this method when large amounts of drainage are present or with deep wounds.[1]
33. If liquid material is unobtainable, swab desired area with cotton-tipped swab, saturating as much as possible.	Apply the moistened swab applicator to a limited cleaned area of 1 cm.[14,17] Swab center of wound rather than wound edges; prevents contamination from skin flora and wound debris.[1]	
34. Crush ampule of medium in culturette and close culturette securely; ensure culture medium surrounds swab.	Keeps specimen from drying and provides growth-supporting medium for culture.	Consult laboratory personnel for any questions regarding appropriate culture medium. If anaerobic culture is collected, tube must be kept upright to prevent carbon dioxide from escaping.[1]
35. Label specimens at the bedside and complete laboratory paperwork per institution-specific protocol.	Promotes patient safety; ensures accurate and efficient processing of specimen.	Follow institution-specific protocol for handling and labeling specimens.
36. Discard used supplies and equipment in appropriate receptacle.	Standard precautions; reduces transmission of microorganisms.	
37. Remove gloves; wash hands.	Standard precautions.	
Tissue Biopsy		
38. Obtain informed consent for procedure per institution-specific protocol.	Ensures medical-legal compliance as suggested by the Joint Commission for Accreditation of Healthcare Organizations (JCAHO).	This procedure should only be performed by practitioner with advanced training in performing this skill and in compliance with institution-specific protocol.
39. Wash hands; put on sterile gloves.	Standard precautions; procedure is sterile.	
40. Obtain a tissue sample approximately 1 to 2 cm in size in width and depth with scalpel and forceps.[1]	Ensures adequate sample is obtained.[14]	Obtain sample with care to avoid large blood loss or damage to underlying tissue.[1]
41. With sterile gauze, apply pressure to tissue sampling site.[1] *(Level IV*)*	Ensures hemostasis of area from which sample was obtained.[1,14]	
42. Place tissue sample in appropriate sterile container.	Prevents contamination of sample.	Consult laboratory for specimen handling requirements.
43. Label specimens at the bedside and complete laboratory paperwork per institution-specific protocol.	Promotes patient safety; ensures accurate and efficient processing of specimen.	Follow institution-specific protocol for handling and labeling specimens.
44. Discard used supplies and equipment, including sharps, in appropriate receptacles.	Standard precautions; reduces transmission of microorganisms; protects personnel health.	
45. Remove gloves; wash hands.	Standard precautions.	
Dressing Open Wounds		
46. Gather needed equipment and supplies.	Ensures all necessary materials are available before procedure is started.	Review prescribing practitioner's order regarding application of gauze or polyester sponges for dressing.

Procedure continues on following page

* Level IV: Limited clinical studies to support recommendations
Level V: Clinical studies in more than one or two patient populations and situations to support recommendations

Procedure for Cleansing, Irrigating, Culturing, and Dressing Wounds—*Continued*

Steps	Rationale	Considerations
47. Wash hands; put on appropriate personal protective equipment.	Standard precautions.	
48. Establish sterile field; open sterile gauze 4×4 pads and soak with NS.[1]	Dress wound with sterile procedure whether wound is sterile or clean to prevent contamination of wound with microorganisms.[18]	
49. Put on sterile gloves; wring out 4×4 pads so they are damp, not dripping.[1]	Use of moisture protects wound bed, facilitates tissue proliferation, and decreases scarring and pain.[1,13,19]	Overpacking of wound increases pressure, compromising perfusion and wound healing.[1] Dressing products that absorb drainage or provide moisture may be used for packing.[1]
50. Apply 4×4 pads over wound bed, gently packing gauze to wound edge; do not exceed wound edge. (*Level V**)	Moist dressing must stay within edges of wound bed to prevent surrounding skin maceration.	Choose size of gauze based on size of wound and anticipated drainage.[1]
51. Cover moist packing with dry 4×4 pads or ABD.[1]	Protects wound and facilitates absorption of moisture.[1]	
52. Secure dressing in place with tape or Montgomery straps.[1] *Tape:* Apply across wound dressing and 1 to 2 inches beyond dressing onto skin.	Holds dressing in place.	Hypoallergenic tape may decrease skin trauma.[1]
Montgomery straps (Figure 126-3): Apply liquid or hydrocolloid barrier to skin around wound where Montgomery straps will be placed.[1]	Provides a protective barrier; promotes adherence of Montgomery straps.[1]	
Remove paper backing from straps; apply to skin with gentle, even pressure.[1]	Attaches Montgomery straps to skin.	
With criss-cross method, lace cotton tape (twill tape, umbilical tape, tracheostomy ties) through holes in Montgomery straps.[1]	Straps secure dressing in place.[1]	
53. Discard used supplies and equipment in appropriate receptacles.	Standard precautions; reduces transmission of microorganisms.	
54. Remove personal protective equipment; wash hands.	Standard precautions.	

* Level V: Clinical studies in more than one or two patient populations and situations to support recommendations

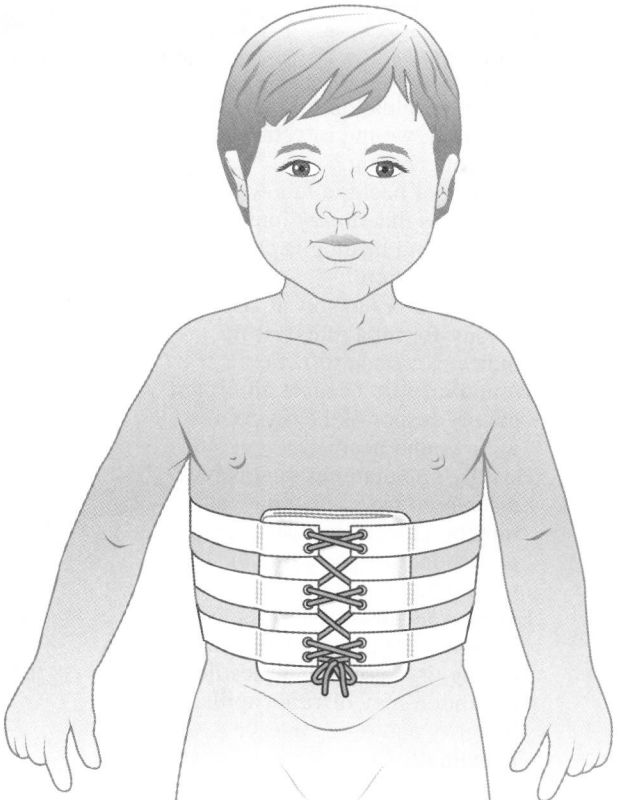

FIGURE 126-3   Montgomery strap application.

Expected Outcomes	Unexpected Outcomes
• Child has signs of wound healing	• Wound tunneling or tracking develops • Wound healing (granulation and contraction of wound) does not progress • Wound bed damage such as hemorrhage or dehiscence from excessive force used during irrigation[1]
• Child has acceptable level of comfort with dressing change	• Unmanaged pain or anxiety with dressing change
• Child and family receive appropriate education and support	• Inadequate or inappropriate education
• Causative organism of infection identified from culture specimen obtained[1]	• Inability to identify organism from culture
• Skin surrounding wound remains healthy and intact	• Skin maceration • Skin erosion
• Wound is free from infection or altered tissue perfusion[1]	• Changes in amount or character of drainage[1] • Cross-contamination of wound[1] • Compromised tissue perfusion
• Adequate biopsy specimen is obtained without complications	• Inability to obtain sufficient tissue for biopsy • Hemorrhage from tissue biopsy[1]

Monitoring and Care of the Child

Activities and Interventions	Rationale	Reportable Conditions
1. Evaluate wound bed and surrounding skin with each dressing change.[1] *(Level V*)*	Ongoing evaluation for wound infection; wound infection prevents healing.[1] Presence of bacteria in a wound in quantities that do *not* interfere with wound healing is defined as colonization.[1] Presence of organisms at 10^5 colony-forming units per mL indicates wound infection.[9,14,20] Wound infection causes an inflammatory response that interferes with wound healing.[1,19,21] Healthy granulation tissue is red; discolored tissue may indicate infection, necrotic tissue, poor perfusion, or hypoxemia of wound bed.[1]	• Increased erythema, especially extending beyond wound margin[1] • Edema • Purulent exudates • Odor to exudates • Increased pain • Fever • Darkened areas on tissue bed[1] • Pale red tissue bed[1] • Changes in amount or color of drainage[1]
2. Assess wound dressing for bleeding.[1]	Excessive stimulation of the healing wound's fragile capillary bed during tissue biopsy or needle aspiration may disrupt capillary integrity and result in excessive bleeding.[1]	• Bleeding that persists despite mild pressure to wound bed[1] • Excessive bleeding[1]
3. Monitor wound bed and edges for development of pockets or tunnels.[1]	Secondary or tertiary intention wound healing puts wounds at increased risk of development of pockets or tunnels. Pocket: A saclike small empty or hollow space in the wound bed or at the wound edge.[1] Tunnel: Completely closed passageway with open ends that permit entrance or exit to the passageway.[1]	• Presence of pocket or tunnel[1] • Depth of pocket or tunnel[1]
4. Assess child's comfort at initiation and throughout procedure; evaluate effectiveness of pain management strategy and provide appropriate interventions. Encourage family to assist with nonpharmacologic means to comfort and support the child.	Early identification of inadequate pain control facilitates prompt treatment. Ineffective pain management makes future dressing changes more traumatic.	• Inadequate pain relief before, during, or after dressing change

* Level V: Clinical studies in more than one or two patient populations and situations to support recommendations

Documentation

- Child and family education
- Premedication given, child's tolerance of procedure, and response to pain medication
- Wound assessment: Appearance of wound before and after cleansing or irrigation, drainage or odor, status of granulation or necrotic tissue, presence of pocket or tunnel[1]
- Wound size[1]
- Status of surrounding skin, including color, moisture, and integrity[1]
- Procedure performed (cleansing, irrigation, culturing) and date and time[1]
- Medications administered
- Unexpected outcomes and related treatment

References

1. Makic MBF: Cleansing, irrigating, culturing, and dressing an open wound. In Lynn-McHale Wiegand DJ, Carlson K, editors: *AACN procedure manual for critical care,* ed 5, Philadelphia, 2005, Saunders.
2. Nelson DB, Dilloway MA: Principles, products and practical aspects of wound care, *Crit Care Nurs Q* 25(1):33-54, 2002.
3. Nettina SM, editor: *Lippincott manual of nursing practice,* ed 7, Philadelphia, 2000, Lippincott, Williams & Wilkins.
4. Bowden VR, Smith-Greenberg C, editors: *Pediatric nursing procedures,* Philadelphia, 2003, Lippincott, Williams & Wilkins.
5. Ovington LG: Hanging wet-to-dry dressings out to dry, *Home Healthcare Nurs* 19(8):477-483, 2001.
6. Taquino LT: Promoting wound healing in the neonatal setting: process versus protocol, *J Perinatal Neonatal Nurs* 14(1):104-118, 2000.
7. Ovington LG: Dealing with drainage, *Home Healthcare Nurs* 20(6):368-374, 2002.
8. Howard R: The appropriate use of topical antimicrobials and antiseptics in children: neonatal skin care, *Pediatr Ann* 30(4):219-224, 2001.
9. Agency for Health Care Policy and Research: *Clinical practice guidelines: treatment of pressure ulcers,* Rockville, MD, 1994, US Department of Health and Human Services.
10. Milne C, Houle T: Current trends in wound care management, *Orthoped Nurs* 21(6):11-18, 2002.
11. Maloney J, Fisher B: Skin integrity. In Moloney-Harmon P, Czerwinski SJ, editors: *Review of pediatric critical care,* Philadelphia, 1997, Saunders.
12. Garvin G: Caring for children with ostomies and wounds. In Wise BW, McKenna C, Garvin G, et al, editors: *Nursing care of the general pediatric surgical patient,* Gaithersburg, MD, 2000 Aspen.
13. Capasso V, Munro BH: The cost and efficacy of two wound treatments, *AORN J* 77(5):984-1004, 2003.
14. Branom RN: Is this wound infected? *Crit Care Nurs Q* 25(1):55-62, 2002.
15. Thompson J: A practical guide to wound care, *RN* 63(1): 48-53, 2000.
16. Cuzzell JZ: The right way to culture a wound, *Am J Nurs* 93(5):48-50, 1993.
17. Campton-Johnston S, Wilson J: Infected wound management: advanced technologies, moisture-retentive dressings, and die-hard methods, *Crit Care Nurs Q* 24(2):64-77, 2001.
18. Centers for Disease Control and Prevention: *Guideline for the prevention of surgical wound infections,* Rockville, MD, 1999, US Department of Health and Human Services.
19. Clark JJ: Wound repair and factors influencing healing, *Crit Care Nurs Q* 25(1):1-12, 2002.
20. Wysocki AB: Evaluating and managing open skin wounds: colonization versus infection, *Adv Pract Acute Crit Care* 13(3):382-397, 2002.
21. Hess CT, Kirsner RS: Orchestrating wound healing: assessing and preparing the wound, *Adv Skin Wound Care* 16(5):246-257, 2003.

Additional Readings

Bauer J: Market choices: wound dressings, *RN* 66(10):63-64, 2003.

Briggs J, editor: Solutions, techniques and pressure for wound cleansing, *Best Pract Evidence Based Pract Info Health Care Professionals* 7(1):1-6, 2003.

Fernandez R, et al : The effectiveness of solutions, techniques and pressure in wound cleansing, *JBI Reports* 2(7):231-270, 2004.

Hess CT: Product update 2002, *Adv Skin Wound Care* 15(6): 287-295, 2002.

Leininger SM: The role of nutrition in wound healing, *Crit Care Nurs Q* 25(1):13-21, 2002.

Nichols RL: Preventing surgical site infections: a surgeon's perspective, *Emerging Infectious Dis* 7I(2):220-224, 2001.

Ovington LG: Battling bacteria in wound care, *Home Healthcare Nurs* 19(10):622-630, 2001.

Quigley SM, Curley MAQ: Skin integrity in the pediatric population: preventing and managing pressure ulcers, *J Soc Pediatr Nurs* 1(1):7-18, 1996.

Quigley SM, Whitney DE: Skin integrity. In Curley MAQ, Moloney-Harmon PA, editors: *Critical care nursing of infants and children,* ed 2, Philadelphia, 2001, Saunders.

St. Clair K, Larrabee JH: Clean versus sterile gloves: which to use for postoperative dressing changes? *Outcomes Manage* 6(1):17-21, 2002.

Valente J, et al: Wound irrigation in children: saline solution or tap water? *Ann Emerg Med* 41(15):609-616, 2003.

Wong D, et al, editors: *Nursing care of infants and children,* ed 7, St. Louis, 2003, Mosby.

Drain Removal

P U R P O S E : To safely remove wound drainage systems

Dena L. Jarog and Maureen A. Madden

PREREQUISITE KNOWLEDGE

- Purpose of the drain; drains are placed to provide an exit for blood, pus, and other fluids.
- Location of the drain, how the drain is secured, and whether the drain is still needed[1]
- The clinician who removes the drain should demonstrate competence because an improperly removed drain could result in significant injury to the tissue.[1]
- Adequate preparation and pain management are essential before drain removal from a child.
- Education and preparation for drain removal must be delivered in a developmentally appropriate manner.
- Goals of wound care must be established so that the correct wound care products are used after drain removal.[1]
- Institution-specific protocols regarding drain removal
- Principles of aseptic technique
- Appropriate pediatric dosing of analgesics

CHILD AND FAMILY ASSESSMENT

- Child's developmental level and ability to interact
  ➟*Rationale:* Determines the child's ability to understand the procedure and to learn about dressing changes and drain removal. If the family and child are not able to understand teaching, they will not be able to properly care for the wound site.
- Child's and family's understanding of the reasons for and risks and benefits of drain removal ➟*Rationale:* Evaluates child's and family's understanding of the procedure and provides a gauge for ongoing education.

- Known allergies ➟*Rationale:* The child may have an allergy to latex, alcohol, tape, or skin preparation products used for wound and dressing care.
- Assessment of wound site for signs of infection and readiness for drain removal. Signs of infection include[2]:
  - ❖ Redness
  - ❖ Swelling
  - ❖ Elevated temperature
  - ❖ Pain at the site
  - ❖ Elevated white blood cell count
  - ❖ Foul drainage from exit site
  - ❖ Pressure or tenderness at exit site
  Signs of readiness for drain removal include:
  - ❖ Volume of drainage had decreased to minimal amount
  - ❖ Consistency of drainage without evidence of infection
  ➟*Rationale:* Detection of infection at an early stage can assist with appropriate intervention; assessing readiness for removal prevents complications of premature drain removal.
- Desire of family members to be present during procedure
  ➟*Rationale:* Family may provide comfort and support to the child during drain removal but should have the choice not to remain with the child.

CHILD AND FAMILY EDUCATION

Individualized, developmentally appropriate education is provided to the family and to the child based on desire for knowledge, readiness to learn, and overall neurologic and psychosocial state.

- If appropriate, demonstrate the procedure to be performed on a doll. Use the resources of a Child Life Specialist if available. ➡*Rationale:* Medical play decreases child's anxiety and facilitates the child's understanding of the procedure.
- Prepare the child and family for drain removal by explaining the reason for removing the drain. Explain to the child the need to remain still through the procedure. ➡*Rationale:* Providing information decreases anxiety and increases cooperation. The child should remain still to decrease the possibility of tissue damage to drain site. The family can assist with this task by staying with and distracting the child. Additional personnel may be needed to assist with keeping the child still.
- Explain care for the drainage site once the drain is removed. Use of an interpreter if needed is important to give instruction and assure understanding of education.

➡*Rationale:* The family understands what to look for when changing the dressing or watching the site for any changes.
- Encourage questions and answer questions as they arise ➡*Rationale:* Reinforcement of information is needed during periods of stress.

EQUIPMENT

- Clean gloves
- Gown, eye and face protection
- Sterile gauze 4×4 pads
- Suture removal kit or sterile scissors as necessary
- Dressing kit or sterile 4×4 pads and tape
- Adhesive tape remover

Procedure   for Drain Removal

Steps	Rationale	Considerations
1. Explain procedure in a developmentally appropriate manner and provide appropriate support. Ensure child and family understand procedure and questions are answered.	Evaluates and reinforces understanding of previously taught information. The extra time taken to prepare the child or adolescent and family beforehand is well invested because cooperation is increased and anxiety is decreased.	Toddlers may need parents to help alleviate anxiety. Preschoolers need simple concise explanations. School-aged children need thorough preparation for all procedures, including all the steps involved. Adolescents also need preparation and information and have a high need for privacy.
2. Have child lie in bed or place child in a position of comfort on table in the treatment room; ensure drain is visible and easily accessible.	Facilitates drain removal.	
3. Determine how many and what types of dressings are necessary to dress wound after drain removal.	Ensures needed supplies are available; facilitates completion of task in a timely manner.	
4. Assess child's pain level with an age-appropriate scale and administer premedications per prescribing practitioner's order (see Procedure 173). Identify child with two patient identifiers per institution-specific protocol before medication administration.	Administration of medication before the procedure may help eliminate pain and anxiety for the child and increase comfort. Use of two patient identifiers promotes patient safety, ensuring the correct medication is administered to the correct child.	Pain that is not adequately treated during a procedure increases the child's anxiety related to subsequent procedures. Nonpharmacologic interventions such as imagery and distraction may help lessen anxiety and pain for the child.
5. Gather needed supplies and equipment; place dressing supplies on a clean flat surface, such as an overbed table, and in a position that facilitates good body mechanics.	Facilitates completion of task in a timely manner.	

Procedure continues on following page

Procedure for Drain Removal—*Continued*

Steps	Rationale	Considerations
6. Ensure privacy by closing curtains and doors; prevent child from becoming chilled.	Allows child to feel protected and comfortable. Infants and small children are at risk for hypothermia if large amounts of skin must be exposed.	Older children may be asked whether they are comfortable with family staying for the dressing change.
7. Wash hands.	Reduces transmission of micro-organisms.	
8. Expose dressing.	Allows visualization of drain site.	
9. Put on gown, gloves, and mask, including eye protection.	Standard precautions; maintains aseptic technique.	
10. Loosen all tape and gently pull tape ends toward the drain. Use adhesive removal pads as necessary.	Makes dressing removal less painful and less traumatizing to the skin and wound.	Adhesive removal from the skin of premature infants and children can cause disruption to skin surfaces.[2]
11. Remove old dressing from wound site, one layer at a time, and place in the appropriate disposal container. *(Level VI*)*	Hasty removal of dressings can cause trauma to wound bed and prematurely dislodge existing drains.	
12. Remove old gloves and replace with new clean gloves.	Gloves may become contaminated with exudates during dressing removal.	
13. If sutures are present, open sterile scissors or suture removal kit.	Reduces the possibility of contamination of the exposed wound site.	
14. Carefully cut any sutures.	Releases drain from tissue suture anchors.[1]	Be careful not to cut drain tubing.
15. Open sterile 4×4 pad if a suture removal kit is not used; place close to drain exit site; instruct child to take a deep breath and blow like blowing out candles or use other distraction techniques. *(Level IV*)*	Gauze catches body fluids that leak as drain is removed.[1] Distraction techniques may help the child experience less pain as the drain is removed.	
16. Smoothly and rapidly withdraw drain.[1]	Removes drain.	Do not force drain removal. If resistance to removal is found, stop and contact prescribing practitioner. Inspect drain on removal to ensure intact removal and no retained pieces remain.
17. Re-dress site with either gauze and tape or a dressing kit.[3]	Protects the open wound site from infection.	
18. Dispose of used equipment and supplies in appropriate receptacles.	Standard precautions; reduces transmission of microorganisms.	
19. Remove personal protective equipment and gloves; wash hands.	Standard precautions.	

* Level IV: Limited clinical studies to support recommendations
  Level VI: Clinical studies in a variety of patient populations and situations to support recommendations

Expected Outcomes

- Drain is removed intact and without difficulty

- Minimal drainage from drain exit site[1]
- Exit site is free of infection, inflammation, or fluid accumulation[1]
- Wound site continues to heal without complications

- Child has acceptable level of comfort

Unexpected Outcomes

- Tissue trauma beneath skin surface from resistance or difficulty in drain removal
- A portion of the drain tubing remains in the wound or in body cavity
- Inability to remove drain, requiring further intervention
- Fluid accumulation beneath skin at drain exit site[3]
- Infection or inflammation at drain exit site[1]
- Fluid accumulation at drain exit site[1,3]
- Drain exit site does not approximate, leading to improper healing that requires intervention[1]
- Unmanaged pain or anxiety

Monitoring and Care of the Child

Activities and Interventions	Rationale	Reportable Conditions
1. Assess for drainage from exit site.[1]	Drainage should be minimal and stop within 24 hours after removal. Continued drainage could indicate accumulation of fluid beneath the skin that may need evacuation.[1]	• Persistent drainage • Presence of subcutaneous fluid (seroma or hematoma) as evidenced with palpation or visualization
2. Monitor for signs and symptoms of infection.[1]	Infection must be treated immediately to assure progression of wound healing.	• Erythema, pain, swelling, increased temperature, increased white blood count, foul drainage, pressure, or tenderness at drain site[1]
3. Assess child's comfort at initiation and throughout procedure; evaluate effectiveness of pain management strategy and provide appropriate interventions. Encourage family to assist with nonpharmacologic means to comfort and support the child.	Early identification of inadequate pain control facilitates prompt treatment. Ineffective pain management makes future dressing changes more traumatic.	• Inadequate pain relief before, during, or after drain removal

Documentation

- Condition of wound at time of drain removal and dressing change
- Type of drain removed, date and time, and individual who removed drain
- Medications administered
- Comfort assessment and any specific interventions provided
- Child's tolerance of procedure
- Document drain removed intact and no evidence of retained pieces
- Amount of drainage in drain chamber before removal
- Child and family education
- Unexpected outcomes and related treatment

References

1. Makic MBF: Drain removal. In Lynn-McHale Wiegand DJ, Carlson KK, editors: *AACN procedure manual for critical care,* ed 5, Philadelphia, 2005, Saunders.
2. Bowden VR, Smith-Greenberg C, editors: *Pediatric nursing procedures,* Philadelphia, 2003, Lippincott, Williams & Wilkins.
3. Rolstad BS, et al: Principles of wound management. In Bryant RA, editor: *Acute and chronic wounds: nursing management,* St Louis, 2000, Mosby.

Additional Reading

Kane DP, Kranser D: Wound healing and wound management. In Krasner D, Kranes D, editors: *Chronic wound care: a clinical source book for healthcare professionals,* ed 2, Wayne, PA, 1997, Health Management Publications.

Dressing Wounds with Drains

PURPOSE: To promote wound healing by properly dressing a wound with a drain

Joy Hultman

PREREQUISITE KNOWLEDGE

- An understanding of the wound healing process
- Children progress through three phases of wound healing: inflammatory phase, cellular proliferation, and maturation.
- Drains are placed in wounds to provide an exit for blood, pus, and other fluids because excessive wound fluid may create pressure in the wound bed and compromise perfusion and healing.[1]
- Drains may be passive or active
  - ❖ A passive drain, such as a penrose drain, relies on gravity to remove excess fluid in or around the wound.
  - ❖ Passive drains are rarely sutured; thus, extra care must be taken when dressing a wound with this type of drain.
  - ❖ An active drain has an expandable chamber that creates a low-pressure suction to adequately remove fluid from the wound site.[2]
- Wound assessment is the foundation of selecting the correct method to enhance wound healing.
- Child's drain placement and anticipated time drain will be left in place
- Wound and drain care in children must be delivered in a developmentally appropriate manner.
- Adequate preparation and pain management are essential before wound care is performed on a child.
- Careful selection of wound care products promotes wound healing.
- Wound dressings can be designed to protect, debride, or absorb excess drainage.
- Assessment of the wound includes the quantity, color, consistency, and odor of the drainage.
- Principles of aseptic technique

CHILD AND FAMILY ASSESSMENT

- Child's developmental level and ability to interact ➤➤*Rationale:* Identifies the child's ability to understand the procedure and learn about dressing changes; guide for selection of appropriate pain scale.
- Child's and family's understanding of the reasons for and risks and benefits of the procedure ➤➤*Rationale:* Evaluates child's and family's understanding of the procedure and provides a gauge for ongoing education.
- Known allergies ➤➤*Rationale:* The child may have an allergy to latex, specific tape types, or skin preparation products used in wound care; promotes patient safety by ensuring the child is not exposed to known allergens.
- Presence of signs and symptoms of infection, including[1]:
  - ❖ Redness at wound or drainage site
  - ❖ Pain
  - ❖ Elevated temperature
  - ❖ Elevated white blood cell count
  - ❖ Change in wound color, odor, or quantity of drainage
  - ❖ Edema
  ➤➤*Rationale:* Early detection of infection allows for prompt interventions and improved patient outcomes.
- Child's pain history ➤➤*Rationale:* Previous pain experiences can help to determine what works best to alleviate the child's pain.
- Family's desire to be present during the procedure ➤➤*Rationale:* Family may provide support, comfort, and distraction during the procedure, facilitating the child's cooperation. In general, the family should have the option not to remain during the procedure. If the child will need wound care in the home after discharge, family members

must be present during wound care to learn the care necessary.

CHILD AND FAMILY EDUCATION

Individualized, developmentally appropriate education is provided to the family and to the child based on desire for knowledge, readiness to learn, and overall neurologic and psychosocial state.

- Explain the dressing type, frequency of dressing changes, and the reason as indicated to family and child. Toddlers may need family to help alleviate anxiety. Preschoolers need simple concise explanations. School-aged children need thorough preparation for all procedures, including all the steps involved. Adolescents also need preparation and information and have a strong need for privacy. ➤*Rationale:* Providing information in developmentally appropriate terms facilitates understanding. Information decreases anxiety and fear.
- If appropriate, demonstrate the procedure to be performed on a doll. Use the resources of Child Life Specialists if available. ➤*Rationale:* Providing information decreases anxiety and discomfort and encourages compliance.
- Review the child's and family's role during wound care and dressing change[1] ➤*Rationale:* Providing information decreases anxiety and promotes cooperation and prepares the child and family to provide dressing changes in the home.
- Explain the age-appropriate pain scale to be used to assess the child's pain (see Procedure 173) ➤*Rationale:* Ongoing assessment of the child's pain and response to

pain medications; the family and child are reassured that pain will be monitored and attended to.
- Explain the need for the child to be in a position of comfort and be able to remain still during the dressing change; explain how the family can assist with this task by staying with the child and providing distraction ➤*Rationale:* Providing information decreases anxiety and promotes compliance.
- Explain the need for a sterile field and how the family can assist with ensuring the child does not touch the sterile supplies ➤*Rationale:* Providing information decreases anxiety and promotes compliance.
- Encourage questions and answer questions as they arise ➤*Rationale:* Reinforcement of information is needed during periods of stress.

EQUIPMENT

- Clean gloves
- Sterile gloves
- Gowns, eye and face protection as indicated
- Wound cleansing solution per prescribing practitioner's order
- 4×4 sterile gauze pads
- 4×4 split drain dressings
- Materials to secure the dressing (hypoallergenic tape or Montgomery straps)
- Skin protection barrier if Montgomery straps are to be placed
- Sterile field barrier
- Appropriate trash receptacle

Procedure for Dressing Wounds with Drains

Steps	Rationale	Considerations
1. Review the prescribing practitioner's order for dressing change or review institution-specific protocol.	Ensures dressing is performed as specified.	
2. Review steps of the dressing change with child and family in a developmentally appropriate manner; ensure child and family understand procedure and questions are answered.	Evaluates and reinforces understanding of previously taught information.	Developmental level, cognitive ability, and anxiety level determine approach to and effectiveness of teaching.
3. Assess child's pain level with an age-appropriate scale and administer pre-medications per prescribing practitioner's order (see Procedure 173). Identify child with two patient identifiers per institution-specific protocol prior to medication administration.	Administration of medication before the procedure may help eliminate pain and anxiety for the child and increase comfort. Use of two patient identifiers for patient identification promotes patient safety.	Pain that is not adequately treated during a procedure increases the child's anxiety related to subsequent procedures. Nonpharmacologic interventions such as imagery and distraction may help lessen anxiety and pain for the child.

Procedure for Dressing Wounds with Drains—*Continued*

Steps	Rationale	Considerations
4. Determine how many and what types of dressings are necessary; gather needed equipment and supplies.	Facilitates completion of task in a timely manner.	If dressing is changed regularly, a listing of required supplies is helpful and promotes consistency.
5. Position child in a comfortable position that allows direct visualization of the wound. Respect child's modesty and prevent child from being chilled.	Facilitates complete assessment of the wound and drain site. Small children and infants are at risk for hypothermia if large areas of skin are exposed.	Privacy is an important consideration for school-aged children and adolescents.
6. Ensure privacy by closing curtains and doors.	Allows child to feel protected and comfortable.	Older children may be asked whether they are comfortable with family staying for the dressing change.
7. Wash hands.	Standard precautions; reduces transmission of microorganisms.	
8. Put on clean gloves and personal protective equipment as appropriate.	Standard precautions.	If large amounts of drainage or potential for splashing are anticipated, gowns, eye and face protection should be used.
9. Unpin drain if attached to child's gown or clothing.	Decreases the chance of accidental dislodgement of the drain.	Place the closed drain lower than the wound to prevent drainage from flowing back into the wound.[3]
10. Loosen tape by holding skin taut with one hand while peeling back the edges with the other hand and pulling the tape toward the wound. *(Level IV*)*	Decreases tension on the wound and avoids pulling the wound edges apart or traumatizing the skin.[3]	Involve a Child Life Specialist if available or another individual to help keep child distracted and still to help prevent the drain from being dislodged.
11. Remove old dressing slowly one layer at a time; dispose of in an appropriate receptacle. *(Level II*)*	Prevents accidental dislodgement of the drain.	Do not pull on the drain tubing because this can loosen stitches or dislodge drain.
12. Remove gloves and wash hands.	Standard precautions; reduces transmission of microorganisms.	
13. With aseptic technique, establish sterile field; open supplies onto sterile field.	Maintains aseptic technique.	
14. Put on sterile gloves.	Sterile procedure.	
15. Clean and irrigate wound with cleansing solution (see Procedure 126).	Facilitates removal of debris, necrotic tissue, and excess clots.[3]	Use cleansing solution per prescribing practitioner's order or institution-specific protocol.
16. Remove gloves and replace with new sterile gloves.	Cleansing solution can make gloves wet and sticky.	
17. Apply appropriate dressing on or around drain.	Helps to stabilize the drain and collect drainage.	

Procedure continues on following page

* Level II: Theory-based; no research data to support recommendations; recommendations from expert consensus group may exist
Level IV: Limited clinical studies to support recommendations

Procedure | for Dressing Wounds with Drains—*Continued*

Steps	Rationale	Considerations

Dressing a Closed Drainage System

Steps	Rationale	Considerations
18. Place single precut bifurcated 4×4 gauze pad around the drain. *(Level IV*)*	Gauze absorbs drainage to keep the skin dry and intact. Moisture can cause breakdown of healing skin.[4]	If precut bifurcated sponges are not available, one can be made by cutting gauze 4×4 pad with sterile scissors so that it has a slit in it.
19. Place another 4×4 pad on top of first 4×4 pad in the opposite direction. *(Level II*)*	Allows circumferential coverage of the drain.	
20. Loop the tubing once on top of the 4×4 pad and tape it down securely (Figure 128-1).	Decreases the length of the drain tubing and gives the drain added support.	Do not wrap gauze around the drain; may dislodge drain.

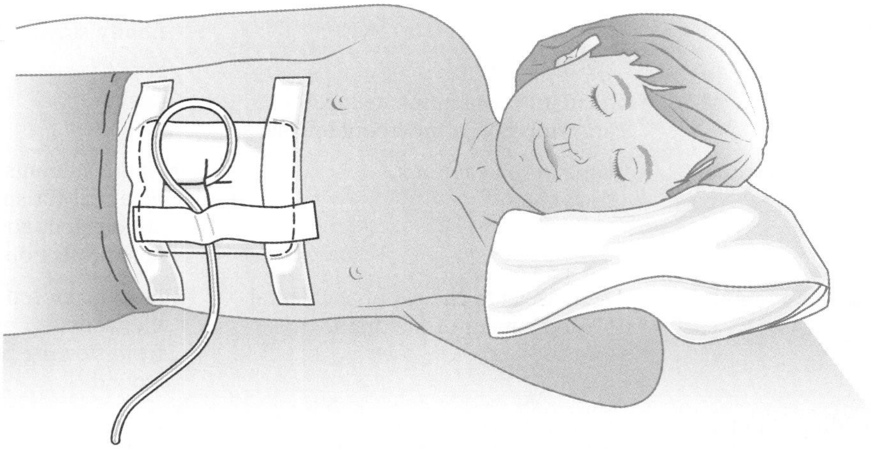

FIGURE 128-1   Loop drain tubing once on top of 4×4 pads and tape securely.

Steps	Rationale	Considerations
21. Create a tape tab on drain tubing and pin to gown or clothing.	Allows child to move around freely without dislodging the drain.	Pin the drain so that it is out of reach from small children; do not pin drain to the bed.

Dressing an Open Drainage System

Steps	Rationale	Considerations
22. Apply precut bifurcated 4×4 pad around drain.	Helps to stabilize the drain while keeping skin dry (Figure 128-2).	Assess drain site; 2×2-size gauze may be sufficient if child is small.

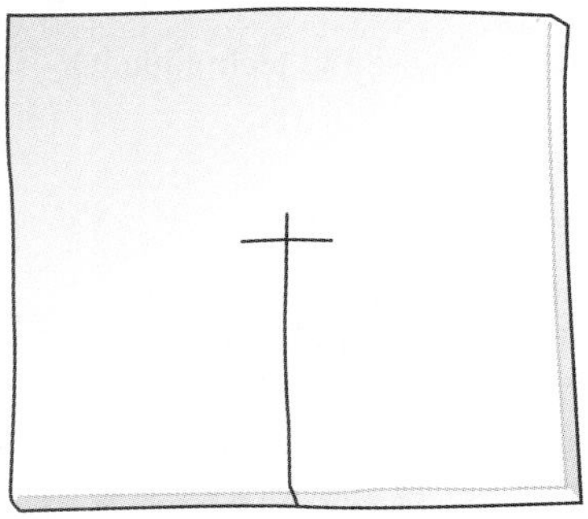

Precut sponge

FIGURE 128-2   Precut bifurcated sponge.

* Level II: Theory-based; no research data to support recommendations; recommendations from expert consensus group may exist
  Level IV: Limited clinical studies to support recommendations

Procedure for Dressing Wounds with Drains—*Continued*

Steps	Rationale	Considerations
23. Layer additional precut 4×4 pads on the drain.	Absorbs additional drainage.	Once dressed, do not layer additional gauze on site. Changing the gauze more frequently is better than keeping a substantial layer. If changing dressing frequently, consider measuring the quantity of drainage by weighing discarded dressing gauze.
24. Apply abdominal (ABD) pad or other absorptive dressing over the top of 4×4 pads.	Provides added wound protection, absorption, and stabilization of dressings.	
25. Secure dressing in place with tape or Montgomery straps.	Secures dressing.	If dressing is changed frequently, consider the use of Montgomery straps.
• Hypoallergenic tape: Apply tape across the dressing extending only about 2 inches on each side of dressing.[1]	Two inches of tape on each side should be enough to stabilize the dressing.	
• Montgomery straps (see Figure 126-3 in Procedure 126).	Montgomery straps are used when dressing a wound with a large amount of drainage and when frequent dressing changes are needed.	Use a skin sealant to adhere the straps securely to the skin without causing damage to healthy skin.
• Peel off paper back of each side of a Montgomery strap and place one on each side of the wound. *(Level I*)*	Secures Montgomery straps to the skin for repeated use.	If premade straps are not available, they can be made.
• Lace cotton twill tape through the holes in a crisscross fashion; tie in a bow. *(Level I*)*	Stabilizes dressing without using tape that can irritate healthy skin.[1]	Tie in a bow, rather than a knot so that the strings are easily removed and may be used with subsequent dressing changes.
26. Discard used supplies and equipment in appropriate receptacles.	Standard precautions; reduces transmission of microorganisms.	
27. Remove personal protective equipment; wash hands.	Standard precautions.	

* Level I: Manufacturer's recommendations only

Expected Outcomes

- Drains remain intact and patent[1]
- Wound healing progresses
- Skin around drain remains clean, dry, and intact[1]

- Drains sites show no signs of infection

- Wound drainage reduces in volume over time[1]

- Child has acceptable level of comfort during dressing change

Unexpected Outcomes

- Drains are dislodged or obstructed
- Wound does not heal
- Skin erosion or maceration around wound drain site or surrounding skin[1]
- Redness, swelling, or increased temperature of skin at drain site
- Foul-smelling wound drainage or drainage at drain site
- Change in character or volume of drainage
- Volume of wound drainage does not decrease over time or increases
- Unmanaged pain or anxiety with dressing change

Monitoring and Care of the Child

Activities and Interventions	Rationale	Reportable Conditions
1. Assess amount of wound drainage in relation to the child's overall intake and output.	Children can have a fluid and electrolyte imbalance with excessive drainage.	• Increased drainage • Tachycardia • Hypotension • Oliguria • Fever
2. Monitor for signs of infection.	Drains assist with the removal of excess fluid but can also be a portal of entry for microorganisms.[1,2,5]	• Erythema • Edema • Pain • Elevated temperature • Elevated white blood cell count • Foul-smelling drainage
3. Assess patency of drain.	Drains can easily become kinked, dislodged, or obstructed.[1,6]	• Sudden decrease or cessation of drain output • Increased drainage around drain
4. Assess child's comfort at initiation and throughout procedure; evaluate effectiveness of pain management strategy and provide appropriate interventions. Encourage family to assist with nonpharmacologic means to comfort and support the child.	Early identification of inadequate pain control facilitates prompt treatment. Ineffective pain management makes future dressing changes more traumatic.	• Inadequate pain relief before, during, or after dressing change

Documentation

- Child and family education
- Medications administered, including solutions for irrigation
- Wound assessment, including status of surrounding skin
- Description of drainage, including quantity, color, consistency, and odor
- Type of dressing applied
- Date and time of dressing change and individual who performed dressing change
- Pain levels before, during, and after procedure and response to pain medications
- Unexpected outcomes and related treatment

References

1. Makic MBF: Dressing wounds with drains. In Lynn-McHale Wiegand DJ, Carlson K, editors: *AACN procedure manual for critical care,* ed 5, Philadelphia, 2005, Saunders.
2. Noble KA: Name that tube, *Nursing* 33(3):56-62, 2003.
3. Nettina SM, editor: *The Lippincott manual of nursing practice,* ed 7, Philadelphia, 2001, Lippincott Williams & Wilkins.
4. Lampert RH, editor: *Pediatric surgery,* ed 3, Philadelphia, 2000, Saunders.
5. Wise B, editor: *Nursing care of the general pediatric surgical patient,* Gaithersburg, MD, 2002, Aspen.
6. Ovington LG: Dealing with drainage, *Home Healthcare Nurs* 20(6):368-374, 2002.

Additional Readings

Autio L, Olsen KK: The four s's of wound management: staples, sutures, steri-strips and sticky stuff, *Holistic Nurs Pract* 16(2):80-88, 2002.
Doherty GM, et al: *The Washington manual of surgery,* St Louis, 2002, Lippincott.
Taquino L: Promoting wound healing in the neonatal setting: process versus protocol, *J Perinatal Neonatal Nurs* 14(1):104-118, 2002.

Fistulas/Wounds: Care and Management

PURPOSE: A draining wound/fistula is pouched to contain wound effluent, protect the periwound/fistula skin, and obtain accurate intake and output

Vittoria Pontieri-Lewis

PREREQUISITE KNOWLEDGE

- Goals for wound/fistula pouching and effective management are achievement of[1-3]:
  - ❖ Skin protection
  - ❖ Containment of drainage
  - ❖ Odor control
  - ❖ Patient comfort
  - ❖ Accurate measurement of effluent
  - ❖ Patient mobility
  - ❖ Cost containment
- In general, wound drainage collectors or ostomy pouches should be applied to stay in place for at least 24 hours.[1,2]
- Etiology of wound (wound versus fistula):
  - ❖ Wound is defined as trauma to any of the tissues of the body, especially trauma caused by physical means and with interruption of continuity of tissue.
  - ❖ Fistula is defined as an abnormal passage from one epithelialized surface to another epithelialized surface.[3]
- Wound assessment includes the assessment of the site, drainage, and healing process.[3]
- Careful selection of wound care products is important to promote wound healing.[2]
- Developmental differences in characteristics of the skin: Premature and young infants have a less well-developed epidermal barrier, which necessitates the use of wound products that do not further damage the epidermal barrier.[1,4]
- See Procedure 126 for further details regarding wound healing.

- Institution-specific protocol for care and management of wounds and fistulas
- Wound care resources available within the institution, such as a Wound Ostomy Continence Nurse.
- Fistula/wound management in children must be delivered in a developmentally appropriate manner.
- Adequate preparation and pain management are essential before fistula/wound care is performed on a child.
- Principles of aseptic technique
- Appropriate pediatric dosing of analgesics

CHILD AND FAMILY ASSESSMENT

- Child's developmental level and ability to interact ➤➤*Rationale:* Determines the child's ability to understand the procedure and learn about dressing changes.
- Known allergies ➤➤*Rationale:* The child may have an allergy to latex, different tape types, or skin preparation products or pouching appliances used in wound care.
- Signs and symptoms of wound infection[2]: erythema; pain; elevated temperature; elevated white blood cell count (WBC); changes in color, odor, or amount of wound drainage; and pressure or tenderness at wound site ➤➤*Rationale:* Early identification of wound infection allows prompt treatment.
- Type and age of wound or fistula ➤➤*Rationale:* Identifies appropriate products necessary for wound care or pouching.
- Child's pain history ➤➤*Rationale:* Previous pain experiences can help determine most effective strategies to alleviate the child's pain.

- Child's and family's understanding of the procedure and their ability and desire to perform wound/fistula care after discharge if indicated ➤➤*Rationale:* Evaluates child's and family's understanding of the procedure and provides a gauge for ongoing education; wound/fistula care may need to be continued in the home after discharge.
- Family's desire to be present during the procedure ➤➤*Rationale:* Family may provide support, comfort, and distraction during the procedure, facilitating the child's cooperation. In general, the family should have the option not to remain during the procedure. If the child will need wound/fistula care in the home after discharge, family members must be present during wound care to learn the care necessary.

CHILD AND FAMILY EDUCATION

Individualized, developmentally appropriate education is provided to the family and to the child based on desire for knowledge, readiness to learn, and overall neurologic and psychosocial state.

- Provide child and family with information on procedural steps and rationale for changing pouch ➤➤*Rationale:* Providing information decreases anxiety and fear and improves compliance with procedure.
- If developmentally appropriate, explain how the child can assist with changing the dressing or pouch ➤➤*Rationale:* Procedure may be facilitated with child's assistance; eliciting the child's cooperation helps to prepare the child for wound management after discharge.
- Explain the age appropriate pain scale used to assess the child's pain, as indicated ➤➤*Rationale:* Facilitates ongoing assessment of the child's pain and response to pain medications.
- Explain the need for the child to be in a position of comfort and to be able to remain still during the dressing and pouching of wound/fistula ➤➤*Rationale:* Providing information may decrease anxiety and promote cooperation with the procedure.
- Explain importance of preventing child from pulling pouch ➤➤*Rationale:* Unnecessary pain is avoided, and pouch wear time is enhanced.

- If wound/fistula care is to be continued after discharge, discuss child's and family's role in wound/fistula management ➤➤*Rationale:* Wound/fistula care may need to be continued in the home; providing information facilitates child's cooperation and prepares child and family for wound/fistula management on discharge.
- Encourage questions and answer questions as they arise ➤➤*Rationale:* Reinforcement of information is needed during periods of stress.

EQUIPMENT

- Clean and sterile gloves
- Sterile field barrier
- Sterile gauze
- 0.9% saline solution (NS) for wound cleaning
- Drainage pouch or ostomy appliance (Figure 129-1)
- Skin sealant, powder, paste, and skin barrier rings or strips as appropriate
- Scissors
- Tape
- Gowns and face protection, as necessary

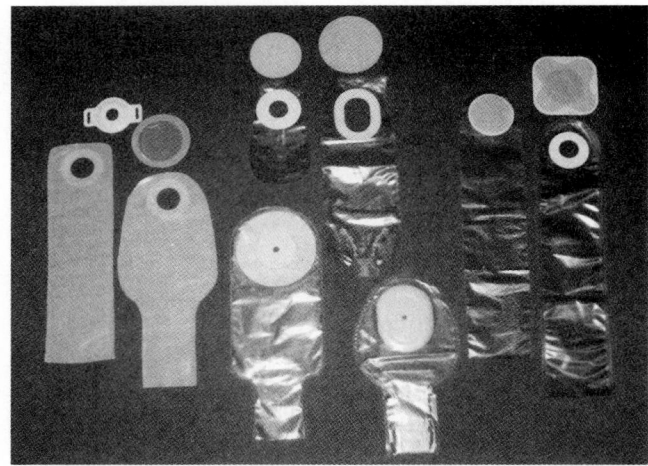

FIGURE 129-1 Examples of appliances for pouching fecal stomas. *From Rogers VE: Managing preemie stomas: more than just the pouch,* J Wound Ostomy Continence *30(2):105, 2003.*

Procedure for Fistulas/Wounds: Care and Management

Steps	Rationale	Considerations
1. Ensure child and family understand procedure and questions are answered.	Evaluates and reinforces understanding of previously taught information.	Developmental level, cognitive ability, and anxiety level determine approach to and effectiveness of teaching.
2. Administer premedication per prescribing practitioner's order; use two patient identifiers when identifying child per institution-specific protocol.	Promotes child's comfort during procedure. Ensures medication is administered to the correct child.	Pain that is not adequately treated during a procedure increases the child's anxiety related to subsequent procedures.
3. Gather needed equipment and supplies.	Facilitates completion of procedure in a timely manner.	Have all equipment ready before removal of the old pouch.
4. Have child lie in bed or place child on treatment table in a comfortable position, ensuring wound/fistula is visible and accessible; expose dressing.	Provides for effective wound/fistula visualization and enhances child's tolerance for procedure.	
5. Ensure privacy by closing curtains and doors.	Allows child to feel comfortable and protected.	Ask older child's preference in terms of parents staying for the dressing change.
6. Wash hands.	Standard precautions; reduces transmission of microorganisms.	
7. Put on clean gloves and personal protective equipment as indicated.	Standard precautions; protects personnel health.	
8. Gently remove old pouch by pushing underlying skin with fingertip and pulling pouch or dressing away from skin.[1] *(Level II*)*	Prevents tissue trauma to underlying skin.[1]	A moist cloth may be applied to loosened edges of drainage pouch to assist with removal.[1] An adhesive remover may also be used, except on infants.[1] *(Level IV*)*
9. Discard old dressing or pouch in appropriate receptacle.	Reduces risk of cross contamination.	
10. Cleanse wound and periwound/fistula skin with NS or sterile water and gently dry skin (see Procedure 126 for further details).[1,2,4] *(Level II*)*	Cleans wound bed and reduces risk of infection.	Use of soap for cleaning is not recommended because soap leaves residue that may cause chemical dermatitis or interfere with pouch adherance.[1]
11. Control wound drainage by placing gauze over wound/fistula.[1]	Protects periwound skin from effluent.	
12. Measure fistula or wound length, depth and width.[3]	Accurate wound measurements promote better pouch adherence and decrease risk of periwound/fistula skin irritation.[1-3]	
13. Trace pattern of wound/fistula onto the skin-barrier surface of pouch.[3]	The opening should fit the size of the wound/fistula to avoid periwound/fistula skin irritation from the effluent.[1,3]	
14. Cut the skin barrier pouch to the size of the pattern.[3] *(Level II*)*	Cutting correctly sized opening helps reduce risk of skin irritation and leakage.[1,2]	

Procedure continues on following page

* Level II: Theory-based; no research data to support recommendations; recommendations from expert consensus group may exist
Level IV: Limited clinical studies to support recommendations

Procedure   for Fistulas/Wounds: Care and Management—*Continued*

Steps	Rationale	Considerations
15. Run a finger around the cut edge of the barrier to smooth rough edges before applying pouch.[1]	Decreases risk of skin irritation from the barrier.	
16. If indicated, apply paste or skin barrier rings or strips around the wound or fistula or to the back of the pouch barrier. Fill in uneven skin surfaces with paste or caulking strips[1-3]; let set for 60 seconds. *(Level IV*)*	Pastes and skin barrier rings or strips help to level irregular skin surfaces and extend the duration the pouch barrier remains effective.[1-3] When used, a thin bead should be applied to the skin and then smoothed into place with a gloved finger or tongue blade. Applying paste into a small syringe may help for an easier delivery system.[1]	Pastes and skin barrier rings or strips should be used with caution in infants because some products contain alcohol. If needed, choose a paste that is alcohol free.[1,2,5] Pastes, cements, and adhesives should be used with care in the premature infant or neonate because the skin/ostomy bond may be stronger than the bond of skin layers.[1,2]
17. If indicated, apply powder to denuded or irritated periwound skin.[1-3] *(Level IV*)*	Absorbs moisture from superficial denuded skin before application of skin sealants or pouch.	Caution must be used with powders on infants and children to avoid inhalation of the powder that could result in severe respiratory symptoms. If used, protect infant's face during application. Use a minimal amount of powder; gently brush, do not blow away, excess powder. For ease of application, apply small amount on gloved finger and apply to site.[1]
18. If indicated, apply skin sealant to periwound skin.[1-3] *(Level IV*)*	Skin sealants may be used under a pouch to protect fragile skin during removal of pouch. They may help to improve pouch adherence and protect the periwound skin from effluent.	Skin sealants should be used with caution in infants and children because some products contain alcohol. If a skin sealant must be used with premature infants, use only an alcohol-free sealant and allow it to dry completely before pouch application.[1,2,4,5] Skin sealants may interfere with pouch adherence.[1]
19. Warm the pouch.[1]	Warming the pouch barrier may help to enhance pouch wear time and molding to contours of child's skin[1]; pouch may be warmed by placing between palms of hands for 1 to 2 minutes.	Do not warm pouch under lights or a microwave because this may burn the skin.[1]
20. Remove adhesive paper from drainage pouch. Center new pouch over wound/fistula; gently press in place to mold and secure pouch to child.[2,3]	Gentle even pressure over the pouch helps to increase seal and pouch wear time. Attempt to avoid wrinkles from developing on skin barrier during application. Wrinkles may cause a leak in the pouching system.	For children who are supine for significant amounts of time, consider angling the pouch to the side as opposed to toward the feet to facilitate drainage of effluent away from the wound/fistula stoma.[1] In premature and small infants, two-piece pouching systems are not recommended because pressure is required to snap the two pieces together.[1]

* Level IV: Limited clinical studies to support recommendations

Procedure for Fistulas/Wounds: Care and Management—*Continued*

Steps	Rationale	Considerations
21. Close bottom of pouch spout; if child produces large amounts of effluent, attach pouch spout to bedside drainage bag.[1]	Protects from effluent spillage and provides accurate output measurements. Attaching pouch to bedside drainage facilitates drainage of effluent.	Draining effluent away from pouch barrier may increase pouch wear time.
22. Assess for adherence of drainage pouch.	Leaking of the pouch may lead to maceration and skin breakdown to the periwound/fistula skin. If leakage occurs, pouch should be changed immediately.	
23. Discard used supplies and equipment in appropriate receptacles.	Standard precautions; reduces transmission of microorganisms.	
24. Remove personal protective equipment; wash hands.	Standard precautions.	

Expected Outcomes

- Periwound/fistula skin remains intact
- Wound drainage is effectively collected and contained
- Wound healing is enhanced by removal of effluent from wound/fistula
- Child has appropriate fluid volume status and electrolyte levels
- Child has acceptable level of comfort during dressing change

Unexpected Outcomes

- Periwound/fistula skin is irritated by leakage of wound effluent
- Wound effluent is not collected, and periwound/fistula skin becomes denuded
- Wound healing is delayed by inappropriate management of wound/fistula effluent
- Dehydration from increased effluent output that is not replaced appropriately
- Abnormal electrolyte levels from increased effluent output that is not replaced appropriately
- Unmanaged pain or anxiety with dressing change

Monitoring and Care of the Child

Activities and Interventions	Rationale	Reportable Conditions
1. Assess periwound/fistula skin.	Maintenance of intact skin is the first line of prevention against infection.	- Erythema of periwound/fistula skin - Denuded skin - Candida rash
2. Monitor amount and character of wound effluent.	Excessive wound drainage may result in fluid and electrolyte imbalances, which may necessitate fluid or electrolyte replacements.[1-3]	- Hypotension - Tachycardia - Oliguria
3. Assess for effective pouch adherence.	Leaking from the pouch may result in periwound/fistula skin denudement.[1-3]	- Leakage of effluent from around pouch
4. Monitor wound for signs of infection.	Early identification of infection promotes prompt treatment.	- Erythema - Elevated WBC count - Elevated temperature - Wound drainage changes in color, amount, and odor - Pain

Documentation

- Child and family education
- Wound/fistula effluent characteristics, including significant change in wound or effluent
- Volume of effluent
- Medications administered
- Type and size of wound pouch
- Treatment related to periwound/fistula skin care
- Intake and output
- Child's response to procedure
- Unexpected outcomes and related treatment

References

1. Rogers V: Managing preemie stomas: more than just the pouch, *J Wound Ostomy Continence* 30(2):100-110, 2003.
2. Garvin G: Caring for children with ostomies and wounds. In Wise B, et al, editors: *Nursing care of the general pediatric surgical patient,* Gaithersberg, MD, 2000, Aspen Publications.
3. Rolstad B, Bryant R: Management of drain sites and fistulas. In Bryant R, editor: *Acute and chronic wounds: nursing management,* ed 2, Philadelphia, 2000, Mosby.
4. Lund C: Prevention and management of infant skin breakdown, *Nurs Clin North Am* 34(4):907-920, 1999.
5. Irving V: Reducing the risk of epidermal stripping in the neonatal population: an evaluation of an alcohol free barrier film, *J Neonatal Nurs* 7:5-8, 2001.

Additional Reading

Hampton B, Bryant R: *Ostomies and continent diversions: nursing management,* Philadelphia, 1992, Mosby.

Vacuum-Assisted Closure (V.A.C.) System: Management of Negative Pressure Therapy

P U R P O S E : A negative-pressure wound therapy system such as the V.A.C. (Vacuum-Assisted Closure) system (Kinetic Concepts Inc. (KCI), San Antonio, TX) is used for the acceleration of wound healing through the debridement of necrotic tissue, removal of tissue edema and infectious material, and promotion of granulation tissue

Beth Broering and Andrea M. Kline

PREREQUISITE KNOWLEDGE

- Basic understanding of normal wound healing
- Wounds that heal by secondary intention need a clean moist environment to promote tissue granulation.
- Wound assessment is the foundation of selection of the correct method to enhance wound healing.
- Wounds for which negative-pressure wound therapy (NPWT) may be considered include: chronic, acute, traumatic, partial-thickness, dehisced, diabetic ulcers, pressure ulcers, flaps, and grafts.[1-5]
- The V.A.C. system is a computerized therapy unit used to apply negative pressure or suction to the wound bed by way of a foam sponge and tubing system placed in the wound and covered with an occlusive drape (Figure 130-1).[1,2,4,5]
- Negative pressure may be applied continuously or intermittently; pressures range from 50 to 125 mm Hg.[1,4]
- For NPWT to function correctly, the dressing must provide an airtight seal.[1,4,5]
- NPWT promotes wound healing by[1,2,3,5]:
  - ❖ Decreasing tissue edema with removal of interstitial fluid from the wound
  - ❖ Decreasing bacterial counts in the wound bed
  - ❖ Promoting granulation tissue formation
  - ❖ Increasing local blood flow

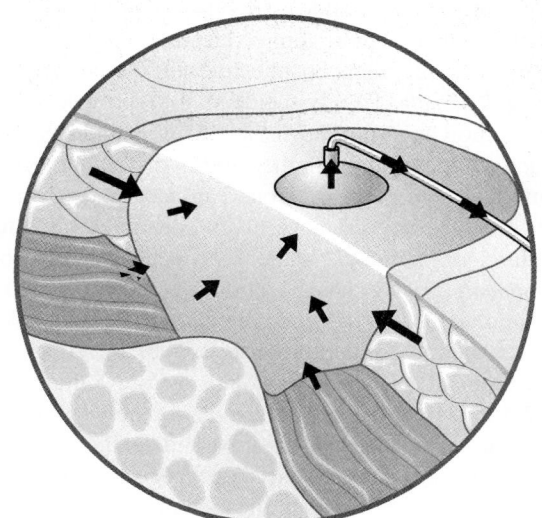

FIGURE 130-1   Vacuum-Assisted Closure Therapy Illustration. Interstitial fluid and infective material are pulled from wound bed through sponge into tubing and collected in canister. *Courtesy of KCI, San Antonio, Tx.*

- Dressing changes are generally performed every 48 to 72 hours. In one small study of children, sponge change was necessary more frequently in very young children because of an increased rate of granulation tissue formation.[2]

- Complications of NPWT include: bleeding, late wound infection, pain with sponge changes and odor.
- Contraindications for NPWT include: malignant disease in the wound, untreated osteomyelitis, nonenteric and unexplored fistula, and necrotic tissue with eschar present.[4,5]
- Debridement of nonviable tissue is necessary before use of NPWT.[1,5]
- Wound care provided to infants and children must be delivered in a developmentally appropriate manner.
- Poor nutritional status impacts the body's ability to heal.[5]
- Developmentally appropriate preparation and pain management are essential before wound care is performed on a child.
- Precautions should be taken with children with active bleeding, with difficult wound hemostasis, and on anticoagulation therapy.[5]
- Principles of aseptic technique
- Appropriate pediatric dosing of analgesics and sedatives
- Mastery of pediatric advanced life support competencies

CHILD AND FAMILY ASSESSMENT

- Child's developmental level and ability to interact ➤*Rationale:* These factors influence preparation and interaction. Child's ability to use a prearranged signal for discomfort during the procedure is identified, and selection of appropriate pain scale is guided. See Procedure 173 for further information.
- Child's and family's understanding of the reasons for and risks and benefits of the procedure ➤*Rationale:* Evaluates child's and family's understanding of the procedure and provides a gauge for ongoing education.
- Desire of family members to be present during the procedure ➤*Rationale:* Family members may provide support and comfort measures to the child but should have the choice not to remain with the child during the procedure.
- Signs and symptoms of wound infection: erythema at site, foul-smelling drainage, pain, edema, elevated temperature, or increased white blood cell (WBC) count ➤*Rationale:* Early identification of infection permits appropriate local or systemic therapies to be initiated and reduces the risk for compromise to wound healing.
- Measurement of size of wound before initiation of NPWT and at each dressing change ➤*Rationale:* Provides information about the status of wound healing.
- Child's previous pain and dressing change experiences and the child's and family's identification of pain management strategies that have been helpful in the past ➤*Rationale:* Identifies pain management strategies likely to be successful; encourages the child and family to participate in developing plan of care. The dressing change may be performed with moderate sedation to decrease anxiety.

CHILD AND FAMILY EDUCATION

Individualized, developmentally appropriate education is provided to the family and to the child based on desire for knowledge, readiness to learn, and overall neurologic and psychosocial state.

- Provide the child and family with information about the NPWT device and improved wound healing ➤*Rationale:* Providing information decreases anxiety and fear; compliance with therapy is promoted.
- Explain the procedure and the reason for changing the dressing to the family and to the child in developmentally appropriate terms ➤*Rationale:* Providing information decreases anxiety and discomfort; compliance with procedure is promoted. Toddlers need family presence to help alleviate anxiety. Preschoolers need simple concise explanations. School-aged children need thorough preparation for all procedures, including all the steps involved. Adolescents also need preparation and information and have a strong need for privacy.
- Explain the pain scale to be used to assess the child's pain ➤*Rationale:* An ongoing assessment of the child's pain and response to pain medications is facilitated.
- Explain that some discomfort may occur with dressing changes and some pressure may be associated with the NPWT. Discuss plan for analgesic therapy, and if appropriate, arrange a signal the child can use during dressing change to indicate pain. ➤*Rationale:* Anxiety is reduced, and understanding of the procedure and compliance with plan of care are promoted.
- Explain how the equipment operates and that the therapy unit should be running at all times ➤*Rationale:* Anxiety is reduced, understanding of the procedure and compliance with plan of care are promoted.
- Provide plan for dressing change therapy and expected length of therapy ➤*Rationale:* Anxiety is reduced, and understanding of the procedure and compliance with plan of care are promoted.
- Encourage questions and answer questions as they arise ➤*Rationale:* Reinforcement of information is needed during periods of stress.

EQUIPMENT

- Clean gloves
- Personal protective equipment: mask, gown, and eye protection, as indicated if splashing of body fluids or blood is anticipated
- Sterile water or 0.9% saline (NS) solution for cleansing
- The NPWT system device (e.g. Kinetic Concepts Incorporated [KCI], San Antonio, Tx, V.A.C. Therapy device; Figure 130-2)
- Sponge/foam dressing specific to the NPWT system
- System sponges are available in small, medium, and large sizes. (Table 130-1 has recommended guidelines for foam use).
  - ❖ Black (GranuFoam, KCI, San Antonio, TX) sponge is hydrophobic, is the most effective at stimulating growth of granulation tissue, and enhances exudate removal.

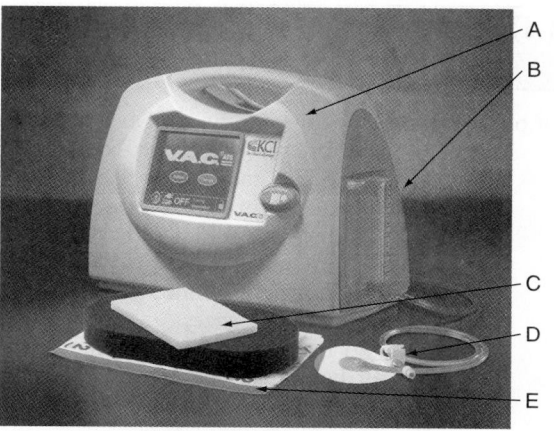

FIGURE 130-2   Vacuum-Assisted Closure System, including: **A,** therapy unit; **B,** collection canister; **C,** GranuFoam (black) hydrophobic sponge and VersaFoam (white) hydrophilic sponge; **D,** disc with suction tubing; and **E,** drape. *Courtesy of KCI, San Antonio, Tx.*

❖ White (VersaFoam, KCI, San Antonio, TX) sponge is hydrophilic and premoistened with sterile water and offers nonadherent properties. A higher minimum negative pressure (≤125 mm Hg) is required. This sponge is recommended for more controlled growth of granulation tissue or when patients cannot tolerate the pain sometimes associated with the black foam.
• The V.A.C. suction tubing (see Figure 130-2)
• The V.A.C. drainage canister (see Figure 130-2)
• Skin preparation
• Razor or scissors for shaving or trimming hair
• Scissors
• Sterile water or other solution per prescribing practitioner's order
• Optional: Liquid skin barrier or hydrocolloid wafer (i.e., Tegaderm [3M, St. Paul, MN]; Duoderm [ConvaTec, Bristol-Myers Squibb. NY, NY]) to protect fragile skin of the periwound area

TABLE 130-1	Recommended Guidelines for Foam Use		
	V.A.C. GranuFoam (Black)	V.A.C. VersaFoam (White)	Either
Deep acute wounds with moderate granulation tissue present	X		
Deep pressure ulcers	X		
Flaps	X		
Exquisitely painful wounds		X	
Superficial wounds		X	
Tunneling/sinus tracts/undermining		X	
Deep trauma wounds			X
Wounds that need controlled growth of granulation tissue			X
Diabetic ulcers			X
Dry wounds			X
Post–graft placement (including bioengineered tissues)			X
Shallow chronic ulcers			X

Used with permission of KCI, San Antonio, TX.

Procedure	**for Vacuum-Assisted Closure Wound Therapy System: Management**	
Steps	**Rationale**	**Considerations**
Initiating Therapy		
1. Review the prescribing practitioner's order for dressing change or review institution-specific protocol.	Ensures dressing is performed as specified.	
2. Ensure child and family understand procedure and questions are answered.	Evaluates and reinforces understanding of previously taught information.	Developmental level, cognitive ability, and anxiety level determine approach to and effectiveness of teaching.

Procedure continues on following page

Procedure for Vacuum-Assisted Closure Wound Therapy System: Management—*Continued*

Steps	Rationale	Considerations
3. Determine how many and what types of dressings are necessary; gather needed equipment and supplies.	Facilitates completion of procedure in a timely manner.	Sponge, tubing, and canister are all in sterile packaging. NPWT may be initiated in the operating room and performed as a sterile procedure depending on prescriber's preference for sterile versus clean dressing. Sponge size is dependent on wound size. A listing of necessary supplies is helpful and promotes consistency.
4. Ensure appropriate cardiopulmonary monitoring.	Critically ill children may decompensate during the procedure or from administration of analgesics or sedatives.	Consider the child's status and sedation/analgesia administration when selecting monitoring.
5. Wash hands.	Standard precautions; reduces transmission of microorganisms.	
6. Assess child's pain level with an age-appropriate scale; administer premedication per prescribing practitioner's order and use two patient identifiers per institution-specific protocol. *(Level II*)*	Promotes child's comfort during procedure, which may be uncomfortable.[1,2,5] Ensures medication is administered to the correct child.	Pain that is not adequately treated during a procedure increases the child's anxiety related to subsequent procedures. Ensure appropriately sized resuscitation equipment is available. Nonpharmacologic interventions such as imagery and distraction may also help lessen anxiety and pain for the child. Involve a Child Life Specialist, if available.
7. Position child in a position that is comfortable and allows for direct visualization of the wound. Respect the child's modesty, and prevent child from being chilled.	Direct visualization allows for a complete assessment of the wound and dressing site.	Smaller infants and young children are at increased risk for hypothermia.
8. Ensure child's privacy by closing curtains and doors.	Allows child to feel protected and comfortable.	Privacy is an important consideration for school-aged children and adolescents. Older children can be asked whether they prefer family members to stay or leave the room for the dressing change.
9. Wash hands.	Standard precautions; reduces transmission of microorganisms.	
10. Put on clean gloves; consider gown and eye or face shield if potential for splashing of blood and body fluids.	Standard precautions; protects personnel health.	Dressing change may be done as a clean or sterile procedure.[1,5]
11. Gently remove previous dressing by holding the skin taut with one hand and loosening the edges and peeling back the dressing towards the wound, with the other hand (if applicable).[4,5] *(Level IV*)*	Decreases tension on the wound and avoids pulling the wound edges apart and traumatizing the skin. Necessary for wound assessment.	

* Level II: Theory-based; no research data to support recommendations; recommendations from expert consensus group may exist
  Level IV: Limited clinical studies to support recommendations

Procedure for Vacuum-Assisted Closure Wound Therapy System: Management—*Continued*

Steps	Rationale	Considerations
12. Assess wound bed for color, consistency, odor, and amount of drainage.[5] *(Level VI*)*	Exudate volume that persists or is suddenly increased may indicate bacteria, local infection, or osteomyelitis, even in the absence of the classical clinical signs of infection.[3,5]	
13. Discard soiled dressing and sponge in appropriate receptacles; remove soiled gloves and wash hands.	Standard precautions; reduces transmission of microorganisms.	
14. If dressing change is done as a sterile procedure, establish sterile field on a clean surface; open sterile packages containing sponges, drape, and drainage tubing onto established field with aseptic technique. If clean technique is used, open packages, keeping contents clean.	Prepares supplies for dressing change; maintains sterility if sterile procedure used.	
15. Put on new pair of clean or sterile gloves.	Decreases contamination and reduces transmission of microorganisms.	
16. Irrigate wound with NS or alternative solution per prescribing practitioner's order.[1,3,5] *(Level VI*)*	Cleansing solution should not be cytotoxic. Hydrogen peroxide destroys fibroblasts, which are the cells most closely associated with granulation and tissue healing.[6] NS solutions facilitate removal of dead tissue and are effective in reducing bacteria count in wounds.[7]	Warm NS or irrigation solution to room or body temperature before irrigating wound.
17. Clean and dry periwound area with sterile gauze. *(Level II*)*	Prevents tissue maceration and further tissue breakdown surrounding the wound.[8]	
18. Shave or clip hair around wound border (extending approximately 3 to 5 cm outside wound margins).	Improves adherence of adhesive drape and reduces pain on removal during dressing changes.	
19. Evaluate need for application of skin preparation or hydrocolloid wafer to periwound skin and apply as needed.	Periwound skin that is fragile, excoriated, or not completely intact can be protected from further breakdown with application of a skin preparation before the drape application or the wound edges can be framed with a skin barrier product (i.e., Duoderm [Convatec, Bristol Myers Squibb, NY, NY]).[5]	Ensure that child has no allergies to skin preparation or wound dressing products before placement on skin.
20. Measure and document dimensions of wound and pathology. Select appropriate foam material.	Tracks size of wound, progress of healing, and changes in character of wound.	See Table 130-1 for foam selection recommendations.
21. Ensure adequate amount of V.A.C. foam to fill the entire wound cavity (more than one size or piece may be used).[4,5] *(Level IV*)*	Entire wound area must be covered.[1,4,5]	

Procedure continues on following page

---

* Level II: Theory-based; no research data to support recommendations; recommendations from expert consensus group may exist
  Level IV: Limited clinical studies to support recommendations
  Level VI: Clinical studies in a variety of patient populations and situations to support recommendations

Procedure | **for Vacuum-Assisted Closure Wound Therapy System: Management**—*Continued*

Steps	Rationale	Considerations
22. Cut the V.A.C. foam geometrically to fit the size and shape of the wound, including any tunneling or undermined areas (multiple pieces or sizes of sponge may be used to fill a wound bed).[4,5] *(Level IV*)*	The subatmospheric pressure of the V.A.C. system must be applied to the wound bed completely and uniformly to be most efficacious.	Cutting a template of the wound size and shape on paper and then cutting the sponge from the paper template may be helpful. When multiple pieces of sponge are used, document the number of pieces used to ensure all pieces are removed during dressing changes or discontinuation of therapy.[5]
23. Cut occlusive drape to size to cover sponge and at least 5 cm of intact skin (a larger area may be preferred depending on location of wound).[1,4,5] *(Level II*)*	An intact drape ensures that the negative pressure is achieved and maintained.	Do not discard extra drape supplies because these pieces may be used to seal small leaks in the dressing or for future dressing changes.[4] This use is dependent on the prescribing practitioner's request for sterile versus clean dressings. If preference is for sterile dressing changes, do not save for future dressing changes; discard extra pieces.
24. If exposed tendons, nerves, or blood vessels are found and polyurethane sponge is used, a protective barrier may be placed in the wound bed (e.g., Adaptic, Johnson & Johnson, New Brunswick, NJ) per prescribing practitioner's order.[5]	Protects exposed tendons, nerves, or blood vessels.	
25. Place the sponges into the wound cavity, ensuring sponges reach the edge of the wound margins, including areas of tunneling or undermining. If more than one piece of sponge is used, sponge edges must be in contact with each other.[1,4,5] *(Level II*)*	Ensures uniform application of the subatmospheric pressure. Sponges must be in contact with each other to ensure uniform and consistent subatmospheric pressure.	Extra sponge can be saved for future dressings, if dressing changes are done in clean manner. If prescribed as sterile dressing change, discard remaining pieces.
26. Place the suction tubing onto the sponges. Tubing should be positioned away from bony prominences.[1,4,5] *(Level II*)*	Prevents pressure on bony prominences and the potential for skin breakdown.	
27. Cover the foam and at least 3 to 5 cm of healthy skin with the transparent drape.[1,4,5] *(Level II*)*	Ensures an occlusive seal and permits uninterrupted suction to wound.	
28. Place a piece of sponge or other gauze padding on healthy skin under tubing and secure tubing several centimeters away from wound (Figure 130-3).[1,3-5]	Prevents pull or tension on the primary dressing and minimizes the potential for leaks.	
29. Remove drainage canister from packaging and insert canister into the V.A.C. therapy unit until it clicks into place. *(Level I*)*	Canister must be securely locked into V.A.C. therapy unit for unit to function properly.	

* Level I: Manufacturer's recommendations only
  Level II: Theory-based; no research data to support recommendations; recommendations from expert consensus group may exist
  Level IV: Limited clinical studies to support recommendations

Procedure for Vacuum-Assisted Closure Wound Therapy System: Management—*Continued*		
Steps	**Rationale**	**Considerations**

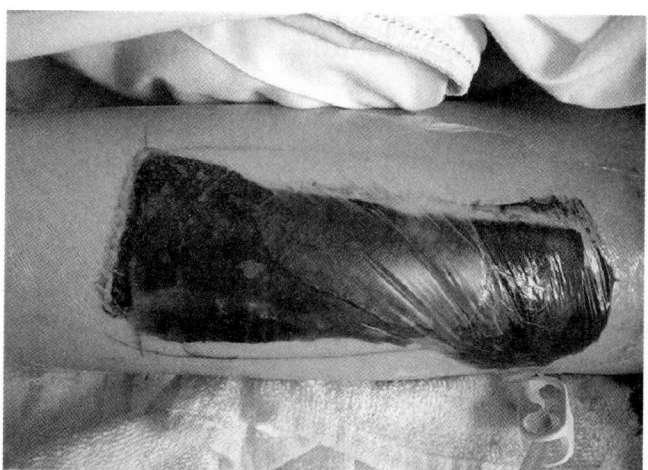

FIGURE 130-3   Wound dressed with V.A.C. system, tubing secured away from wound.

Steps	Rationale	Considerations
30. Connect tubing from dressing to tubing from suction canister. Ensure both clamps are open. *(Level I*)*	Clamps must be open for negative pressure on wound to be achieved.	
31. Turn the green-lit power button on the side of the V.A.C. therapy unit to "on."	Turns on the V.A.C. therapy unit; does *not* turn on suction.	
32. Press the "therapy on/off" button located on front of the unit and ensure that the dressing compresses. *(Level I*)*	Initiates subatmospheric pressure therapy. The default negative pressure is 125 mm Hg. Negative pressure can be adjusted lower per prescribing practitioner's order.	Negative pressure therapy should be maintained at the prescribed setting or 125 mm Hg.
33. Ensure that suction is maintained and no leaks occur. Cover leaks with excess drape or by gently pressing around wound edges and the area of the suction tubing on the sponge.[1,2,4,5] *(Level II*)*	Dressing must be completely sealed for therapy unit to function.	The most common location of air leaks is around the suction tubing at the dressing.[4,5]
34. Discard used supplies in appropriate receptacles.	Standard precautions; reduces transmission of microorganisms.	Excess sponges and drape can be saved for future dressing changes if prescribed as clean dressing change.
35. Remove gloves and personal protective equipment; wash hands.	Standard precautions; reduces transmission of microorganisms.	
Dressing Change		
36. Perform steps 1 to 10 as described previously.	The V.A.C. NPWT may be used as long as the wound is present; no time limit exists to providing therapy.	
37. Turn "therapy on/off" button located on the front of the unit to "off."	Terminates subatmospheric negative pressure.	Therapy unit may also be turned off completely, which prevents the unit from alarming.

Procedure continues on following page

* Level I: Manufacturer's recommendations only
  Level II: Theory-based; no research data to support recommendations; recommendations from expert consensus group may exist

Procedure	for Vacuum-Assisted Closure Wound Therapy System: Management—*Continued*	
Steps	**Rationale**	**Considerations**
38. Close clamps on tubing attached to dressing and tubing attached to collection canister.	Prevents spilling or splashing of wound exudate fluid.	
39. Disconnect tubing attached to dressing from tubing attached to collection canister.	Prevents pulling on suction tubing from wound site.	
40. Gently remove previous dressing by holding the skin taut with one hand and loosening the edges and peeling back the dressing towards the wound, with the other hand.[4,5] *(Level IV*)*	Decreases tension on the wound and avoids pulling the wound edges apart and traumatizing the skin; facilitates wound assessment.	
41. Assess wound bed on dressing removal for color, consistency, odor, and amount of drainage.[5] *(Level VI*)*	Exudate volume that persists or is suddenly increased may indicate bacteria, local infection, or osteomyelitis, even in the absence of the classical clinical signs of infection.[3,4]	
42. Discard soiled dressing or sponge in appropriate receptacles; remove soiled gloves and wash hands.	Standard precautions; reduces transmission of microorganisms.	
43. Perform remainder of procedure following steps 14 to 35 as described previously.	Completes dressing change.	When turning back on the therapy unit, "existing patient" should be selected on the initial screen. Assess wound and document any change in size of wound and changes in characteristics to help track wound healing, lack of healing, or presence of infection.

* Level IV: Limited clinical studies to support recommendations
  Level VI: Clinical studies in a variety of patient populations and situations to support recommendations

Expected Outcomes	**Unexpected Outcomes**
• Vacuum therapy is initiated and maintained without interruption from leaks • Wound develops healthy granulation tissue • Child tolerates therapy at the recommended suction pressure • Serosanguinous drainage from wound accumulates in canister • Skin around wound remains clean, dry, and intact • Child has acceptable level of comfort during dressing change	• Dressing seal becomes dislodged and creates leaks and loss of suction to wound • Wound becomes infected; development of granulation tissue is delayed • Excessive bleeding develops from exposed vessels or excessive growth of granulation tissue into the sponge • Suction pressure must be reduced because of unmanaged pain • Frank bloody drainage noted in tubing or canister • Interstitial fluid is not removed from wound bed • Skin erosion or maceration of skin surrounding wound • Unmanaged anxiety or pain during dressing change

Monitoring and Care of the Child

Activities and Interventions	Rationale	Reportable Conditions
1. Monitor size and characteristics of wound.	Assesses progress of wound; identifies indications of infection.	• Evidence of purulent drainage from wound; antibiotic coverage that may need to be initiated or adjusted • Evidence of necrotic tissue in wound • Evidence of exposed blood vessels, tendons, or bone
2. Monitor characteristic of drainage from wound. 3. Monitor child's tolerance of negative pressure therapy; assess effectiveness of pain management strategy and provide appropriate interventions. Encourage family to assist with nonpharmacologic means to comfort and support the child.	Promotes early identification of complications. Early identification of pain facilitates prompt treatment; additional analgesia or antianxiety medications may be necessary.	• Frank blood in canister or tubing • No drainage in canister or tubing • Continued discomfort or anxiety with therapy despite intervention • Continued irritability; changes in physiologic condition

Documentation

- Size of wound
- Medications placed in wound bed
- Color, odor, drainage, and characteristics of the wound
- Number and type of foam sponges or pieces of sponges used
- Evidence of exposed blood vessels, tendons, nerves, or bone
- Amount of suction applied to wound and whether therapy is continuous or intermittent
- Protective barriers placed under foam on skin edge (disc wafers, Duoderm®, transparent dressing)
- Protective barriers placed in the wound bed (e.g., Adaptic) and number of pieces used
- Child's response to procedure
- Unexpected outcomes and related treatment

References

1. DeFranzo AJ, et al: The use of vacuum-assisted closure therapy for the treatment of lower-extremity wounds with exposed bone, *Plast Reconstructive Surg* 108(5):1184-1191, 2001.
2. Mooney JF, et al: Treatment of soft tissue defects in pediatric patients using the V.A.C. system, *Clin Orthopaed Related Res* 376:26-31, 2000.
3. Wongworawat MD, et al: Negative pressure dressings as an alternative technique for the treatment of infected wounds, *Clin Orthoped Related Res* 1(414):45-48, 2003.
4. KCI: *V.A.C. therapy guidelines,* retrieved April 2006, from http://www.kci1.com/2-B-128_Clin_Guidelines_Blue_Book_1-05.pdf.
5. Mendez-Eastman S: Guidelines for using negative pressure wound therapy, *Adv Skin Wound Care* 14(6):314-324, 2001.
6. Centers for Disease Control and Prevention: *Guideline for the prevention of surgical wound infections,* Rockville, MD, 1999, US Department of Health and Human Services.
7. Clark JJ: Wound repair and factors influencing healing, *Crit Care Nurs Q* 25(1):1-12, 2002.
8. Nelson DB, Dilloway MA: Principles, products and practical aspects of wound care, *Crit Care Nurs Q* 25(1):33-54, 2002.

Additional Reading/Internet Learning

KCI: *KCI International On-Line Learning (Self-Paced) Course,* from http://www.KCI1.com, click education, view available online wound education courses.

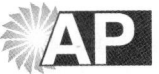

Suturing Wounds

P U R P O S E : To close minor wounds that result from tissue injuries in such a way that cosmetic and functional outcomes are maximized

Marisa Mize and Ruth M. Lebet

PREREQUISITE KNOWLEDGE

- Laceration is the most common specific injury that brings children to pediatric emergency departments; half of these lacerations occur in children less than 5 years of age.[1]
- Knowledge of the anatomy and physiology of the skin[1,2]
  - ❖ The skin is the largest organ of the body with two major layers.
    - ○ The epidermis is the outermost layer; functions are protection against infection and restriction of water loss; skin color is a function of this layer.
    - ○ The dermis is the inner layer; functions are provision of nourishment and strength. The dermis is composed of connective tissue and contains capillaries, lymphatics, and nerve endings.
  - ❖ The subcutaneous tissue is located beneath the dermis and is made of areolar and fatty connective tissue; it also contains blood vessels and nerves.
- Wound healing is a sequential process.[2]
  - ❖ When clotting systems are activated, a fibrin meshwork is produced.
  - ❖ Within this meshwork, macrophages appear that release factors that guide migration and stimulate proliferation of fibroblasts. Healthy pink friable granulation tissue appears; endothelial cells of advancing capillaries migrate to form epithelial bridges between the wound margins.
  - ❖ Epithelial bridging occurs at different rates, depending on the tissue edge location. Everted sutured skin edges epithelialize within 18 to 24 hours; approximated skin edges may take 36 hours to epithelialize, and inverted skin edges may take up to 72 hours to complete epithelialization.
- Suturing is the process of approximating body tissues and holding them together with threads. It is a mechanism of primary wound closure.[1-5]
  - ❖ The goals of suturing are to stop bleeding, to preserve function by limiting damage to nerves and blood vessels, to prevent infection and promote healing by eliminating dead space, and to restore appearance by realigning and apposing the skin edges.[1,3-5]
  - ❖ Sutures are placed to temporarily support the wound edges until skin regenerates tissue strong enough to maintain closure of the wound.[2,4]
  - ❖ Correctly sutured wounds accurately approximate deep tissue layers to each other with minimal tension on the surrounding tissues and avoid tissue ischemia and strangulation from sutures that are tied too tight.
- Common suture errors include[3-5]:
  - ❖ Sutures tied too tight: Tissue edema that occurs after suturing is not allowed. Vascular compromise of wound edges may occur and result in delayed wound healing, necrosis of wound edge, and undesirable appearance.

❖ Sutures tied too loose: Wound edges are not well approximated: may result in undesirable appearance or sutures coming undone.

❖ Overlapping or inverted (curled inward) wound edges: may delay or prevent wound healing; may cause formation of a ridge, resulting in a more obvious scar.

❖ Sutures placed too near wound edge: Sutures pull out, resulting in poor or delayed wound healing and further injury.

• Sutures are foreign bodies; use the fewest sutures needed for the shortest time period necessary and the smallest size of suture appropriate for the task.[1,2,4,5]

• Risk of infection is generally accepted to decrease with closing of clean wounds within 3 to 8 hours of injury and use of aseptic technique in all aspects of wound management. Each wound should be assessed individually to identify the most appropriate treatment plan.[2-5]

• Consultation with or referral to the appropriate service should be made for[1-4]:

❖ Wounds with damage to the blood supply, nerves, or joint

❖ Wounds with underlying fracture

❖ Wounds on the face

❖ Wounds with extensive tissue damage or infection

❖ Wounds with poor vascular supply or wounds that are difficult to completely clean

❖ Any wound believed to be beyond the practitioner's expertise

• Children are less likely than adults to have wound infections develop. However, contaminated wounds or wounds infected with saliva, feces, or purulent exudates or wounds open for a significant time (12 to 24 hours) may benefit from delayed primary closure: wound dressing for 4 or more days with suture closure on or after the fourth day to decrease risk of infection. Consultation with specialty services may be helpful with this decision.[1,4,5]

• Needles used to suture wounds

❖ Curved needles are either tapered or cutting. A curved needle with an angle of 135 degrees is generally used for skin closure.

❖ Tapered needles are used in soft tissues (intestine, blood vessels, muscles, and fascia) and produce minimal tissue damage.

❖ Reverse cutting needle is preferred for general wound repair. The cutting edge is located on the outside of the curve, which prevents suture from cutting through tissue.[1-3]

❖ Most needles are swaged (molded around) the suture material for convenience, safety, and speed in suturing.[2]

❖ Needles should always be handled with needle holders to prevent needle damage to surrounding tissue and to the practitioner.[1-3]

• Suture materials (see Table 131-1 for further information)[1-3]

❖ Suture size is indicated by "0." The smaller the number, the larger the suture; 6-0 suture is fine, and 3-0 suture is large.

❖ Absorbable sutures (natural gut, synthetic polymers) are used for layered closures. Synthetic suture is generally preferred because of increased strength and longevity and decreased infection rates.

❖ Nonabsorbable sutures are made of natural fibers (silk, cotton, linen) or synthetic fibers (nylon, polyethylene, Dacron) and are typically used for superficial lacerations.

❖ Braided or multifilament sutures may harbor infection in the small spaces between layers but are stronger than monofilament; monofilament has less of an inflammatory response and so is best suited for skin closure, but knots are less dependable.

❖ Nonabsorbable synthetic monofilament sutures (e.g., 4-0 or 5-0 nylon) are preferred for skin closure.

TABLE 131-1	Suture Selection and Removal by Anatomic Region	
Region	**Suture**	**Suture Removal**
Face	Skin: 6-0 nylon or polypropylene P3 needle	4 days
Scalp	3-0, 4-0, 5-0 Nylon or polypropylene FS-2 needle or larger	5 to 7 days
	Galea: 2-0 Vicryl, Dexon, Maxon, PDS	Absorbable
Hand	5-0 or 6-0 Nylon or polypropylene FS-2 needle	Joint, 10 to 14 days; other areas, 7 to 10 days
	No deep sutures	
Extremities	Skin: 4-0 or 5-0 nylon or polypropylene FS-2 needle	Joint, 10 to 14 days; other areas, 7 to 10 days
	Deep: 4-0 Vicryl, Dexon, Maxon, PDS	Absorbable
Trunk	Skin: 4-0 or 5-0 nylon or polypropylene FS-2 needle	7 days
	Deep: 4-0 Vicryl, Dexon, Maxon, PDS	Absorbable
Oral mucosa and tongue	5-0 to 6-0 Vicryl, Dexon, Maxon, PDS	Absorbable

Vicril (Ethicon, Inc., Somerville, NJ), Polyglactin; Dexon (United States Surgical, North Haven, CT), polyglycolic acid; Maxon (United States Surgical, North Haven, CT), glycolide trimethylene carbonate; PDS (Ethicon, Inc., Somerville, NJ), polydioxanone.

Adapted from Grisham J, Perro M: Laceration repair. In Diekmann RA, et al, editors: Illustrated textbook of pediatric emergency & critical care procedures, Philadelphia, 1996, Mosby.

AP This procedure should be performed only by physicians, advanced practice nurses, and other health care professionals (including critical care nurses) with additional knowledge, skills, and demonstrated competence per professional licensure or institutional standard.

Synthetic braided absorbable sutures provide the best closure for interrupted dermal sutures and ligation of bleeding vessels.

❖ Preferred knotting technique involves a square knot or double loop followed by a square knot.

❖ Anticipate swelling of the injured tissue; as a result, sutures tighten automatically within 12 to 24 hours. If sutures are tied too tightly, ischemia of the wound edge may occur.

❖ The more tension on a wound, the closer the stitches should be placed.

- The wound must be copiously irrigated before suturing to remove bacteria and dirt from the wound.[1-5] Saline solution 0.9% is the irrigation solution of choice. The efficacy of an irrigation system in removal of foreign material is directly related to the force of the irrigant stream and the size of the particles removed. Larger particles are more easily removed than smaller particles. High-pressure irrigation is more efficient than low-pressure irrigation.

  ❖ Irrigation with a bulb-type syringe generates relatively low pressures; irrigation with a 30-mL syringe fitted with a 19-gauge needle generates intermediate pressures.

  ❖ For wounds contaminated with bacteria or foreign material, use a 30-mL syringe fitted with either an 18-gauge angiocath or a 19-gauge needle and press down firmly on the plunger to irrigate wound.

  ❖ Splashshield devices are available to avoid splashes. The plastic shields are attached to the syringe instead of a needle and the wound is irrigated, with the shield held just above the skin surface.

  ❖ Always wear protective goggles during the irrigation process. After irrigation, the wound should be reexplored for foreign materials.

- Wounds with a glass foreign body need special attention during irrigation and exploration, before suturing. Retained glass is more likely to be present if the child has a sensation of foreign body. Wounds of the head and foot caused by glass are especially likely to have a glass foreign body. Consider an x-ray if a concern exists that glass fragments may be present in the wound.

- Sutures must be completely removed at the appropriate time to prevent tissue inflammation and possible infection or stitch marks (see Table 131-1 for recommended timing of suture removal).[1-5]

- Techniques that may minimize scar formation[1,3-5]

  ❖ Use techniques that reduce tension on the wound, such as tissue undermining.

  ❖ Evert skin edges.

  ❖ Match skin heights on each side of the wound carefully; go in and out of each wound edge with a separate pass of the needle.

  ❖ Handle tissue gently.

  ❖ Place percutaneous sutures so that depth is greater than width.

- Alternatives to suturing may be considered, if appropriate (Table 131-2).

- If suturing alternatives are used, skin surrounding the repaired wound should be cleansed of remaining blood or iodine and covered with a nonadherent dressing to protect against invading bacteria.

- Principles of aseptic technique

- Blood, wounds, and needles are frightening to most children. Ensuring anesthesia of the wound before manipulation of the wound is critical. Consider moderate anxiolytic sedation, particularly for younger children, to facilitate cooperation and decrease anxiety, especially in the case of larger wounds or wounds where a good cosmetic repair is important.[1-3] Child Life Therapists, if available, are skilled in working with the child before and during the procedure to provide support and non-pharmacologic anxiety management techniques, such as distraction.

CHILD AND FAMILY ASSESSMENT

- History of present injury, including mechanism of injury, time since injury, and environment where injury occurred ➠*Rationale:* Better understanding of the nature of injury, appropriate type of wound repair, and potential complications to wound healing.

- Child's medical history and known allergies ➠*Rationale:* Identifies factors that may predispose the child to infection or poor wound healing; identifies allergies to medications or solutions that are used in laceration repair.

- Size, location, depth, and type of wound; damage to peripheral nerve, blood supply, or motor function; presence of foreign bodies in wound ➠*Rationale:* Determines appropriate exploration, type of closure, or need for referral to consultant.

- Immunization history and tetanus status ➠*Rationale:* Identifies the child who needs tetanus prophylaxis (Table 131-3).

- Child's developmental level and ability to interact ➠*Rationale:* These factors influence preparation and interaction throughout the procedure, including selection of appropriate pain scale; assesses child's ability to cooperate during the procedure.

- Previous pain and sedation experiences of child and family and the child's and family's identification of pain and anxiety management strategies that have been helpful in the past ➠*Rationale:* Identifies pain management strategies likely to be successful or previous difficulties with sedation; encourages child's and family's participation in developing plan of care.

- Child's and family's understanding of the reasons for and risks and benefits of the procedure ➠*Rationale:* Evaluates child's and family's understanding of the procedure and provides a gauge for ongoing education.

- Family's desire to be present during procedure ➠*Rationale:* Family may provide support and comfort to the child during the procedure but should have the choice not to remain with the child.

TABLE 131-2	Alternatives to Suturing		
Method	**Recommended Uses**	**Technique**	**Comments**
Skin tape, such as Steri-Strips (3M, St. Paul, MN) Shur-strip (Derma Sciences, Inc., Princeton, NJ)	Used in place of sutures to repair simple lacerations, with easily approximated edges and not under tension or pressure Wounds closed with skin tape have significantly lower incidence rate of infection than those closed with conventional sutures *(Level IV*)*	Place skin tape after adequate hemostasis; tape does not adhere to wet skin Clean and dry skin around laceration Apply adhesive, such as tincture of benzoin, to skin surrounding wound; significantly increases sticking power of tapes Realign dermis and epithelium Place strips perpendicular to wound, leaving some space between strips Consider placing strips across ends of tape strips, parallel to wound	Do not use skin tape on infants and young children because they tend to peel off tape Tape is impractical for areas of motion, such as elbows and knees, and for areas that may become wet Parents should be instructed to leave tapes in place as long as possible Avoid pulling tape too tight, which causes wound edges to overlap and results in ridge Tapes are allowed to fall off spontaneously
Skin staples (stainless steel)	Staples can be placed more rapidly than sutures Lower infection rate and less foreign body reaction Especially useful for closing small scalp lacerations	Clean and prepare wound as for suturing Have assistant evert wound edges Place staples according to stapler manufacturer's instructions Remove staples with staple remover to ensure all of staple is removed, prevent tissue damage on removal, and maximize child's comfort	When only one or two staples are needed, placement of staples rapidly with topical anesthesia alone is less painful than first injecting with lidocaine Staples are not recommended for use on face, hands, or feet or in children who need MRI or CT studies Timing for removal is same as for sutures
Tissue adhesive or skin glue: Most commonly used adhesives are fibrin glue and octyl cyanoacrylate	Particularly useful in clean wounds less than 4 cm long and of 0.5 cm width or less	Clean wound and ensure hemostasis Hold edges of wound together with fingers or forceps; *invert* wound edges Apply drops of adhesive to wound surface with 27-gauge needle or applicator Hold wound edges together for additional 20 to 30 seconds With skin glue use, first hold wound edges together, then apply thin layer of glue Glue sets in 1 to 2 minutes	Heat production may occur during polymerization Use extreme caution near eyes because glue adheres to cornea and lids if it runs into eye Adhesive sloughs off after 7 to 10 days Do not use in wounds under significant tension Instruct family not to use ointments or lotions on wound because this dissolves glue or adhesive
Hair ties	Hair ties may be used to close small scalp lacerations that do not need subcutaneous tissue repair	Clean wound Use few strands of hair on each side of wound to tie a knot as with suture Repeat along length of incision as needed	Hair used for ties should be cut at time usually indicated for suture removal

*Level IV: Limited clinical studies to support recommendations.
MRI, Magnetic resonance imaging; *CT,* computed tomography.

Information compiled from McNamara R, Loiselle J: Laceration repair. In Henretig F, King C, editors: *Textbook of pediatric emergency medicine procedures,* Philadelphia, 1997, Lippincott, Williams & Wilkins.
Selbst SM, Attia MW: Minor trauma; lacerations. In Fleisher GR, Ludwig S, Henretig FM, editors: *Textbook of pediatric emergency medicine,* ed 5, Philadelphia, 2005, Lippincott, Williams & Wilkins.
Grisham J, Perro M: Laceration repair. In Diekmann RA, Fiser DH, Selbst SM, editors: *Illustrated textbook of pediatric emergency & critical care procedures,* Philadelphia, 1996, Mosby.

TABLE 131-3 Recommendations for Tetanus Prophylaxis		
Vaccination History	**Clean Minor Wounds**	**All Other Wounds**
Unknown or less than three doses	Td or Tdap (Tdap preferred for ages 11 to 18 years)	Td or Tdap (Tdap preferred for ages 11 to 18 years) *plus* TIG
Three or more doses and 5 or less years since last dose		
Three or more doses and 6 to 10 years since last dose		Td or Tdap (Tdap preferred for ages 11 to 18 years)
Three or more doses and more than 10 years since last dose	Td or Tdap (Tdap preferred for ages 11 to 18 years)	Td or Tdap (Tdap preferred for ages 11 to 18 years)

Td, Tetanus toxoid, reduced diphtheria toxoid; *Tdap,* tetanus toxoid, reduced diphtheria toxoid, acellular pertussis; *TIG,* tetanus immune globulin.
See http://www.cdc.gov/mmwr/preview/mmwrhtml/00041645.htm.
From Centers for Disease Control and Prevention: Emergency preparedness and response, retrieved April 28, 2006, from http://www.bt.cdc.gov/disasters/hurricanes/katrina/tetanus.asp.

CHILD AND FAMILY EDUCATION

Individualized, developmentally appropriate education is provided to the family and to the child based on desire for knowledge, readiness to learn, and overall neurologic and psychosocial state.

- Provide information about the suturing procedure, including the reason for the repair and an explanation of steps involved in suturing ➻*Rationale:* Providing information decreases anxiety and fear.
- If developmentally appropriate, explain how child can assist with suturing procedure ➻*Rationale:* Suturing is facilitated by child's cooperation.
- Explain the need for the child to be in a position of comfort and to be able to remain still during this procedure ➻*Rationale:* The family can assist with this task by staying with the child and providing distraction.
- Review the pain and anxiety management plan for the child, including local anesthesia, sedation, and Child Life support ➻*Rationale:* Providing information decreases anxiety and fear and reassures the child and family that pain will be managed appropriately.
- Explain that during the suturing the child may have a tugging sensation but should have minimal discomfort ➻*Rationale:* Providing information decreases anxiety and fear.
- If the family chooses to stay with the child during the procedure, explain that the focus should be the support of the child rather than observation of the procedure performed. Explain techniques the family can use for support and distraction. ➻*Rationale:* Defining the family's role and providing information on appropriate techniques for support of the child clearly establishes the family's role.

- Explain the need for aftercare, including pain or other medication, observation for signs and symptoms of infection, care of the wound, use of splints as needed for immobilization, follow-up necessary, how to contact practitioner, and anticipated time sutures are left in place. Written information to reinforce teaching may be helpful. ➻*Rationale:* Encourages family's participation in care and prompt intervention to treat possible infection; written information may facilitate compliance with discharge instructions.
- Encourage questions and answer questions as they arise ➻*Rationale:* Reinforcement of information is needed during periods of stress.

EQUIPMENT

- Good light source
- Local anesthetic (without epinephrine)
- Povidone-iodine
- 0.9% Saline solution (NS) for irrigation
- Eight to 10 sterile 4×4 gauze sponges
- A 30 mL to 60 mL syringe for irrigation
- Splashshield device or 18-gauge or 19-gauge needle or angiocath
- Sterile drapes, fenestrated and plain
- Clean and sterile gloves
- Mask, eye and face protection
- A 6-inch needle holder
- Suture material with appropriate needle
- Curved and straight mosquito hemostats
- Tissue scissors
- Tissue forceps
- Scalpel handle and no. 10 or 15 blade
- Skin hooks

Procedure for Suturing Wounds

Steps	Rationale	Considerations
1. Ensure child and family understand procedure and questions are answered.	Evaluates and reinforces understanding of previously taught information.	Developmental level, cognitive ability, and anxiety level determine approach to and effectiveness of teaching.
2. Gather needed equipment and supplies; recruit assistant to help child hold still.	Facilitates completion of task in a timely manner; delays in procedure may increase child's anxiety and apprehension. Most children need some assistance remaining still initially despite anesthetic administration.	In general, prepare equipment that might be frightening to the child away from the bedside.
3. Obtain informed consent. *(Level II*)*	Ensures medical-legal compliance as suggested by the Joint Commission on Accreditation of Healthcare Organizations (JCAHO).	In emergency situations, follow institution-specific protocol for assumption of consent.
4. Identify the child with appropriate patient and procedure verification process (e.g., "Time out").	Confirms correct patient, procedure, and site as recommended by JCAHO; prevents unnecessary medical procedures.	Verification process and documentation are institution specific; use active communication techniques.
5. Position child comfortably and with wound easily accessible and visible; if needed, provide temporary immobilization. Ensure adequate lighting.	Ensuring comfort of child and practitioner facilitates completion of procedure. Temporary immobilization may be necessary to prevent further injury to the child or injury to the practitioner. Adequate lighting is necessary for good visualization of the wound and repair.	
6. Wash hands and put on personal protective equipment. *(Level II*)*	Standard precautions; reduces transmission of microorganisms. Protects personnel health.	Use aseptic technique to decrease contamination of wound.
7. Clean area around wound with 1% povidone-iodine solution or other cleansing agent per institution-specific protocol. *(Level II*)*	Prepares area for administration of local anesthetic.	
8. If appropriate, apply topical solution or gel, such as LET (lidocaine, 4%; epinephrine, 0.1%; tetracaine, 0.5%) for 20 minutes before procedure. If LET is not appropriate, infiltrate perimeter of wound through subcutaneous tissue exposed by the laceration with small gauge (27-gauge or 30-gauge) 1.5-inch needle, slowly injecting local anesthetic while advancing needle; if possible, start needle advancement	Topical anesthetic avoids use of needle, which is frightening to most children. Provides for maximum comfort and facilitates cooperation during suturing; improves ability to explore wound.[1-4]	Application of LET has been shown to be effective as adequate anesthesia for small uncomplicated lacerations.[1,4-6] *(Level VI*)* In one study of children undergoing suturing of face or scalp laceration, LET gel was found to be as effective and more efficacious than LET solution.[6] *(Level IV*)* Applying pressure around the wound or immobilization of site may also decrease pain.

Procedure continues on following page

* Level II: Theory-based; no research data to support recommendations; recommendations from expert consensus group may exist
Level IV: Limited clinical studies to support recommendations
Level VI: Clinical studies in a variety of patient populations and situations to support recommendations

Procedure for Suturing Wounds—*Continued*

Steps	Rationale	Considerations
for subsequent injections by entering through previously anesthetized area (Table 131-4 has local anesthetic options). *(Level VI*)*		If wound is heavily contaminated, consider injecting anesthetic through intact skin surrounding the wound.[1,5]
9. Ensure adequate hemostasis and anesthesia.	Hemostasis is necessary to adequately visualize the wound.	
10. Examine wound thoroughly for foreign bodies, deep tissue layer damage, joint involvement, and injury to nerve, vessel, or tendon. *(Level II*)*	Prevents further damage; identifies wounds that should be referred to specialty service.[1-4]	The wound may need to be further extended, with a scalpel, to ensure adequate exploration.[2,4,5] During examination of extremity wounds, put the extremity through its full range of motion.[1,4]
11. Irrigate the wound with 200 mL to 1 L NS as appropriate to the wound, with a 20-mL to 50-mL syringe and splashguard or syringe and 18-gauge to 19-gauge needle. The tip of the needle of syringe should remain about 2 cm above the wound.[1-4] *(Level VI*)*	Removes foreign substances and reduces bacterial contamination.	Scrubbing is not routinely necessary. If wound is significantly contaminated, wound should be cleaned with a substance that is not toxic to the tissues. Consider warming irrigation fluid if the child is small or large amounts of fluid are necessary.
12. Clean wound and area around wound with 1% povidone-iodine solution or other cleansing agent per institution-specific protocol. *(Level II*)*	Cleaning wound decreases incidence rate of infection.	Do not use povidone-iodine surgical scrub, alcohol, hydrogen peroxide, or detergent scrubs that are toxic to tissues.[4,5]
13. With tissue forceps, remove particles of foreign material that remain after irrigation.[1-4] *(Level VI*)*	Avoids "tattooing" of skin; decreases risk of infection.	Extension of the wound with scalpel may be necessary to identify all foreign material in wound.[1,2,4]
14. In general, hair removal is not necessary. If necessary, remove hair near the wound.	Use of electric clippers or scissors to clip hair, rather than razors, have been associated with decreased infections.[2,4] *(Level IV*)*	Avoid removing hair over eyebrows; regrowth may be abnormal or delayed.[1,4]
15. Remove gloves; wash hands.	Standard precautions; prevents cross contamination.	
16. Prepare sterile field and place instruments on field with aseptic technique.	Prepares instruments for use and ensures needed supplies are readily available. Decreases transmission of microorganisms.	Suture and needle selected are based on location of and type of wound; appropriate suture and needle selection ensures minimal tissue trauma and appropriate support of wound edges.[1-4]
17. Drape the area with plain and fenestrated drapes as appropriate.	Creates a sterile field to reduce risk of infection.	Covering a child's face may increase the child's agitation; use of plain drapes alone may be considered.[4]
18. Reexamine the wound for devitalized tissue that necessitates removal or debridement; use sharp scissors or scalpel to remove tissue.[1,2,4]	Creates well-defined wound edges, facilitating good approximation of tissues.	Remove as little tissue as possible; excessive tissue removal may increase difficulty of wound repair.[1,2,4] Cuts made should be perpendicular and completely through the dermis.[1]

* Level II: Theory-based; no research data to support recommendations; recommendations from expert consensus group may exist
Level IV: Limited clinical studies to support recommendations
Level VI: Clinical studies in a variety of patient populations and situations to support recommendations

Procedure for Suturing Wounds—*Continued*

Steps	Rationale	Considerations
19. If needed, undermine or loosen the wound from subcutaneous fat beneath the dermis with scissors or scalpel (Figure 131-1). Distance undermined should be approximately twice the width of wound.[1,2,4,5] *(Level II*)*	Decreases tension on the surrounding skin; facilitates closure of the wound and may minimize scar formation.	Avoid undermining in contaminated wounds because this may increase risk of infection from disruption of blood supply.[1]

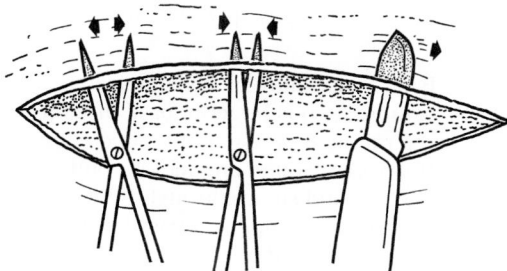

FIGURE 131-1   Techniques for Undermining Wound Edge. *From Grisham J, Perro M: Laceration repair. In Diekmann RA, editors:* Illustrated textbook of pediatric emergency & critical care procedures, *Philadelphia, 1996, Mosby.*

Steps	Rationale	Considerations
20. Simple Interrupted Suture: Pick up needle with needle holders so that it is between the jaws of and perpendicular to the needle holder, about one third the needle length from the swage end of needle.[1-4] *(Level II*)*	Facilitates stitch placement and decreases risk of needle breakage. Use of needle holders prevents injury to practitioner. Figure 131-2 is a diagram of this stitching technique.	For soft tissue repair, needle is placed in holder close to swage (thread) end. For tougher tissue, needle is placed in holder closer to point, to minimize risk of needle breaking.[1] This stitch is most commonly used for closing wounds in children. More complex wounds may necessitate a different stitching technique.[1,4,5]

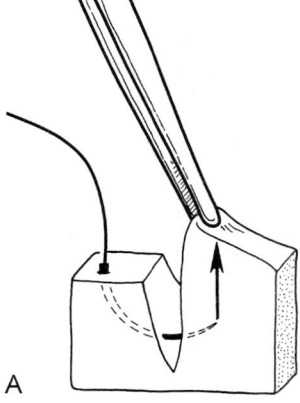
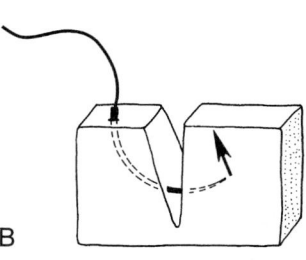

A   B

FIGURE 131-2   Technique for Simple Interrupted Stitch. *From Grisham J, Perro M: Laceration repair. In Diekmann RA, editors:* Illustrated textbook of pediatric emergency & critical care procedures, *Philadelphia, 1996, Mosby.*

Procedure continues on following page

* Level II: Theory-based; no research data to support recommendations; recommendations from expert consensus group may exist

Procedure for Suturing Wounds—*Continued*

Steps	Rationale	Considerations
21. Grasp the needle holder firmly in the dominant hand; thumb and ring finger are placed in rings with index finger on hinge of blades.[3,5] *(Level II*)*	Facilitates good control of needle and proper stitch placement with minimal manipulation.	
22. Position free end of suture away from practitioner.[2]	Ensures free end of suture is clearly visible; ensures that it does not become caught up when knot is made.	
23. While supporting wound edge opposite practitioner with tissue forceps, fingers or skin hook enter skin with needle at a 90-degree angle 2 to 5 mm from wound edge. Move the suture through the skin by rotating the wrist, following the curve of the needle.	Facilitates suture placement such that suture loop is larger at base of loop to promote eversion of wound edge. If sides of wound are uneven, pull needle and suture through first wound edge and then pass through second wound edge.[1,5] *(Level II*)*	Hand should start prone; as wrist rotates and turns supine, needle is passed toward practitioner and in the direction of the needle curve. Place sutures closer to wound edge in delicate areas where minimizing scar formation is important, such as the face.[1,4,5] *(Level II*)*
24. Grasp the needle point with tissue holders; unclamp needle holder jaws.	Stabilizes needle; maintains position in tissue.	
25. Grasp needle with needle holder; pull the desired length of suture through the wound, leaving approximately 2 cm on side of wound opposite practitioner.	Facilitates tying knot.	
26. Tie suture knot with instrument tie[1,2,4,5]: Grasp long length of suture (on side of wound closest to practitioner) with nondominant hand. Grasp needle holder in dominant hand. Loop suture twice around tip of needle holder. Grasp short (free) end of suture with needle holder and pull through loops, toward practitioner, creating a "throw." Tighten knot until skin edges just come together. Reverse process (short end of suture is now on side of wound closest to practitioner), looping suture *once* around needle holder. Repeat for a total of four or five throws. *(Level II*)*	Four or five throws are necessary to ensure security of knot and prevent unraveling. Use of more than five throws weakens suture. Figure 131-3 has a diagram of the instrument tie.	Precisely approximate wound edges without causing tissue ischemia. For each throw, hands reverse position; apply equal and opposing tension to the suture ends.
27. Cut ends of suture with scissors, holding blades perpendicular to suture and keeping knot in view between the blades; leave approximately 3-mm "ears."	Ears of knot compensate for enlarged suture loop with knot slippage and prevent knot from untying. Ensures enough suture remains to facilitate suture removal.	
28. Place knot to side of wound.[1,2,4,5] *(Level II*)*	Placement of knots to side prevents inflammation, scarring, or entrapment of sutures.[1,2,4,5]	

* Level II: Theory-based; no research data to support recommendations; recommendations from expert consensus group may exist

Procedure for Suturing Wounds—*Continued*

Steps	Rationale	Considerations

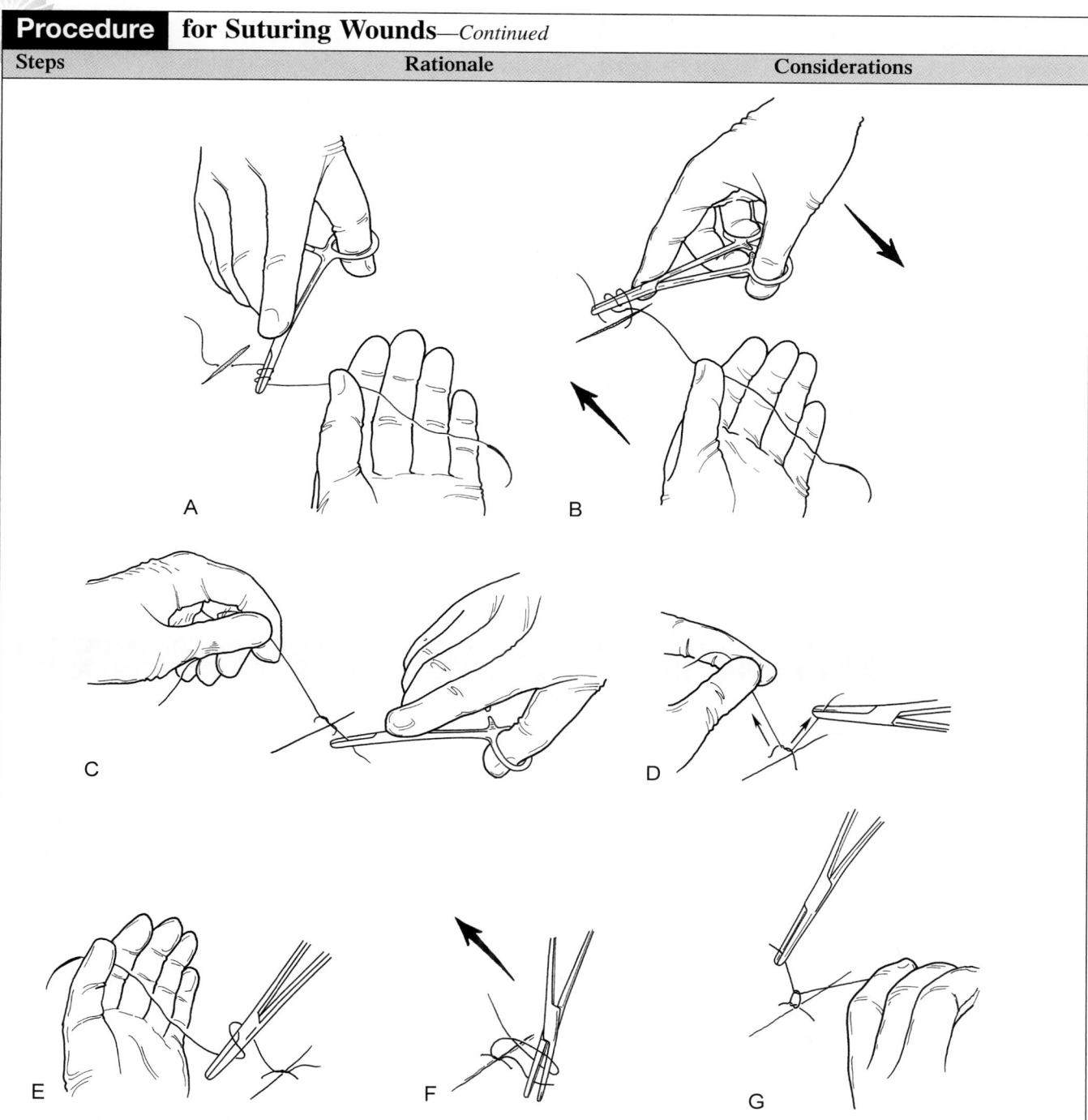

FIGURE 131-3 Instrument Tie. *From Grisham J, Perro M: Laceration repair. In Diekmann RA, editors: Illustrated textbook of pediatric emergency & critical care procedures, Philadelphia, 1996, Mosby.*

Steps	Rationale	Considerations
29. Repeat steps 20 to 28 until wound is appropriately closed, placing sutures about 2 to 5 mm apart.	Additional sutures are needed to close wound.	Sutures should be placed closer together when minimization of scar formation is important.[1,4,5] (*Level II**)

Procedure continues on following page

Procedure for Suturing Wounds—*Continued*

Steps	Rationale	Considerations
		Wounds may be closed starting at one end and moving toward the other end or by placing the first stitch in the middle of the wound and then continuing to place sutures in a bisecting fashion lateral to the midpoint.[1,3,5]
30. Remove equipment and supplies and sterile drapes.	Clears area of sharps.	
31. Clean area around wound; cover wound with nonadherent sterile dressing.	Protects wound from further injury and contamination; absorbs any secretions.	
32. Dispose of used supplies and equipment, including sharps, in appropriate receptacles.	Standard precautions; reduces transmission of microorganisms. Protects personnel health.	
33. Remove personal protective equipment; wash hands.	Standard precautions.	

TABLE 131-4   Local Anesthesia Techniques

Local Anesthetic	Dose	Administration	Indications	Contraindications
Lidocaine 1% with or without epinephrine • Onset of anesthesia, 5 to 15 minutes • Duration, 1 to 2 hours • Lidocaine with epinephrine at ratio of 1:100,000 assists with hemostasis but should only be used in areas of good perfusion	Maximum dose, 4 mg/kg or 0.5 mL/kg of plain lidocaine; 7 mg/kg or 0.7 mL/kg of lidocaine with epinephrine	Slow injection via small (27-gauge to 30-gauge) 1.5-inch needle into wound margins Reduce discomfort by slowly injecting solution while advancing needle with solution warmed to body temperature, adding sodium bicarbonate in 1:10 ratio to lidocaine to buffer pH	Commonly used for most infiltrative and regional anesthesia	Lidocaine with epinephrine is not recommended for use on digits, feet, ear, tarsal plate of eye, bridge of nose, nipple, or penis
Procaine 1% • Onset of anesthesia, 5 to 10 minutes • Duration, 60 to 90 minutes	Maximum dose, 7 to 10 mg/kg or 0.7 to 1 mL/kg	Slow injection via small (27-gauge to 30-gauge) 1.5-inch needle into wound margins Reduce discomfort by slowly injecting solution while advancing needle with solution warmed to body temperature, adding sodium bicarbonate in 1:10 ratio to buffer pH	Infiltrative and regional anesthesia	
Bupivicaine hydrochloride 0.25% • Onset of anesthesia, 10 to 20 minutes • Duration, 4 to 6 hours	Maximum dose, 2 mg/kg or 0.8 mL/kg	Slow injection via small (27-gauge to 30-gauge) 1.5-inch needle into wound margins Reduce discomfort by slowly injecting solution while advancing needle with solution warmed to body temperature, adding sodium bicarbonate in 1:10 ratio to buffer pH	Infiltrative and regional anesthesia, especially in older children and when longer anesthetic effect is desirable	

TABLE 131-4	Local Anesthesia Techniques—Cont'd			
Local Anesthetic	**Dose**	**Administration**	**Indications**	**Contraindications**
LET: Lidocaine 4%, epinephrine 0.1%, tetracaine 0.5%; available as solution or gel • Onset of anesthesia, 20 to 30 minutes • Duration, up to 1 hour	Maximum dose, 2 to 3 mL of LET	Administer within inner margins of laceration until cavity is filled. Equal amount of LET is applied with cotton ball or swab (not gauze) over wound; apply for 10 to 15 minutes	Useful for superficial injuries, particularly in young children Most effective around face	Should not be used on mucosal regions, such as mouth, or when epinephrine is contraindicated Gel may be more efficacious than solution[6] *(Level IV*)*

*Level IV: Limited clinical studies to support recommendations

Information compiled from McNamara R, Loiselle J: Laceration repair. In Henretig F, King C, editors: *Textbook of pediatric emergency medicine procedures,* Philadelphia, 1997, Lippincott, Williams & Wilkins.

Selbst SM, Attia MW: Minor trauma; lacerations. In Fleisher GR, Ludwig S, Henretig FM, editors: *Textbook of pediatric emergency medicine,* ed 5, Philadelphia, 2005, Lippincott, Williams & Wilkins.

Grisham J, Perro M: Laceration repair. In Diekmann RA, Fiser DH, Selbst SM, editors: *Illustrated textbook of pediatric emergency & critical care procedures,* Philadelphia, 1996, Mosby.

Lewis L, Stephan M: Local and regional anesthesia. In Fleisher GR, et al, editors: *Textbook of pediatric emergency medicine,* ed 5, Philadelphia, 2005, Lippincott, Williams & Wilkins.

Expected Outcomes

- Bleeding is controlled

- Function is preserved
- Wound edges remain well approximated throughout healing process
- Wound heals with minimal scarring

- Wound remains free from infection

- Pain and anxiety are well controlled

Unexpected Outcomes

- Continued bleeding from the wound site
- Hematoma formation
- Loss of function
- Wound dehiscence

- Tissue necrosis at wound edge from sutures tied too tightly
- Significant scarring
- Need for scar revision
- Local wound infection
- Sepsis
- Unmanaged pain and anxiety that result in difficulty with completion of procedure

Monitoring and Care of the Child

Activities and Interventions	Rationale	Reportable Conditions
1. Monitor for evidence of infection.[2]	Early identification of infection facilitates prompt treatment.	• Wound is red, edematous, tender, or warm or has increased drainage • Red streaks around the wound • Signs of systemic infection: fever, chills, increased white blood cell count (WBC)
2. Consider systemic antibiotics for[1,4]: Heavily contaminated wounds Animal or human bites Crush injuries Wounds longer than 5 cm Wounds repaired more than 12 hours after injury	Prevents wound infection.	• Allergies to antibiotics

Continued

Monitoring and Care of the Child—Cont'd

Activities and Interventions	Rationale	Reportable Conditions
Children at increased risk of infection because of medical condition (e.g., valvular heart disease, immunocompromise)		
3. Assess effectiveness of pain and anxiety management strategies and provide appropriate interventions. Encourage family to assist with nonpharmacologic means to comfort and support the child.	Because of painful stimuli, child may need increased medication doses. Facilitates modifications to management strategies as indicated.	• Pain and anxiety refractory to medication administration • Difficulty completing the procedure because of increased pain or anxiety levels
4. If indicated, splint wounds under tension.[2,4]	Decreases lymphatic flow, decreasing the spread of microorganisms. Provides support and limits movement in the active child, promoting wound healing.	• Sutures are pulled out • Wound edges dehisce
5. Ensure wound and dressing are kept clean and dry (child may shower but not take a bath).[2]	Promotes wound healing. Wet dressing may be a source of infection.	• Indications of wound infection
6. Change dressing after 2 days and then every day until sutures are removed. Wound edges may be cleaned with NS or half-strength peroxide, and lubricating ointment may be applied.[1,2]	Decreases risk of wound contamination and infection. Lubricating ointment prevents scab formation and may promote epithelialization.[1,4]	• Indications of wound infection • Delayed wound healing
7. If child receives moderate sedation for wound repair, ensure appropriate cardiorespiratory monitoring and availability of emergency equipment and medications per institution-specific protocol.	Facilitates identification of complications of moderate sedation and prompt treatment.	• Respiratory depression • Cardiovascular instability

Documentation

- Child and family education, including discharge instructions on care of wound, if applicable
- Time since injury
- Mechanism of injury
- Location and appearance of wound
- Patient and procedure verification process
- Individual who performed the suturing
- Date and time of wound repair
- Procedure used to clean wound
- Procedure used to close wound, including type of suture used and number of stitches placed
- Administration of tetanus toxoid, if given, and specific type
- Pain, sedation, local anesthetic medications, or antibiotics given and child's tolerance
- Dressing applied, if applicable
- Unexpected outcomes and related treatment

References

1. McNamara R, Loiselle J: Laceration repair. In Henretig F, King C, editors: *Textbook of pediatric emergency medicine procedures,* Philadelphia, 1997, Lippincott Williams & Wilkins.
2. Kirkwood P: Suturing. In Lynn-McHale Wiegand DJ, Carlson K, editors: *AACN procedure manual for critical care,* ed 5, Philadelphia, 2005, Saunders.
3. Castille K: Suturing, *Nurs Stand* 12(41):41-48, 1998.
4. Selbst SM, Attia MW: Minor trauma—lacerations. In Fleisher GR, et al, editors: *Textbook of pediatric emergency medicine,* ed 5, Philadelphia, 2005, Lippincott Williams & Wilkins.
5. Grisham J, Perro M: Laceration repair. In Diekmann RA, et al, editors: *Illustrated textbook of pediatric emergency & critical care procedures,* Philadelphia, 1996, Mosby.
6. Resch K, et al: Topical anesthesia for pediatric lacerations: a randomized trial of lidocaine-epinephrine-tetracaine solution versus gel, *Ann Emerg Med* 32(6):693-697, 1998.

Additional Readings

Barkin RM, Rosen P: Soft tissue injuries. *Emergency pediatrics: a guide to ambulatory care,* ed 6, Philadelphia, 2005, Mosby.

Buttaravoli P, Stair T: Laceration simple. *Minor emergencies: splinters to fractures,* Philadelphia, 2000, Mosby.

Kahn ANGA, et al: Cosmetic outcome of scalp wound closure with staples in the pediatric emergency department: a prospective, randomized trial, *Pediatr Emerg Care* 18(3):171-173, 2002.

PROCEDURE **132**

Blood and Blood Component Administration and Blood Pump Use

P U R P O S E : To provide blood or blood components to children in a safe and timely manner and minimize the risk of complications

Grace Macek

PREREQUISITE KNOWLEDGE

- Specific indications for the blood or blood component administration and expected outcomes
- Types of blood and blood components available for transfusion include: whole blood, red blood cells, platelets, fresh frozen plasma, cryoprecipitate, and granulocytes.[1,2]
  - ❖ *Whole blood* is used for massive hemorrhage and trauma. Whole blood contains red blood cells, white blood cells, platelets, and coagulation factors and is generally transfused over a maximum of 4 hours.
  - ❖ *Platelets* are used for active bleeding related to thrombocytopenia, platelet dysfunction, or platelet count of less than 20,000 without active bleeding present; institution-specific protocols may vary. The usual pediatric dose is 10 mL/kg infused over a maximum of 4 hours. This dose raises the platelet count by approximately 50,000 mm[3]. Peak posttransfusion concentration is achieved 45 to 60 minutes after completion of transfusion.
  - ❖ *Red blood cells* are used to improve tissue oxygenation associated with anemia. Packed red blood cells are infused at a rate of 2 to 3 mL/kg/h unless rapid replacement is necessary for blood loss or shock. The transfusion dose is 10 to 20 mL/kg over 4 hours. One mL/kg increases hemoglobin by approximately 0.5% to 0.7%.
  - ❖ *Fresh frozen plasma* is used for bleeding related to decreased coagulation factors, reversal of warfarin effects, or treatment of coagulation defects. Usual

dosage is 10 to 20 mL/kg infused over a maximum of 4 hours unless rapid replacement is necessary.
  - ❖ *Cryoprecipitate* is used for defective plasma proteins. When fresh frozen plasma is slowly thawed, the precipitate contains enriched factor VIII, von Willebrand's factor (vWF), fibrinogen, and factor XIII. Cryoprecipitate is used in children with thrombotic thrombocytopenic purpura (TTP) refractory to fresh frozen plasma and other fibrinogen deficiencies and may be infused over 5 minutes or up to 4 hours.
  - ❖ *Granulocytes* are used in children with neutropenia who have a serious infection that has not responded to antiinfective therapy.[1]
- Special preparations of blood and blood components include[1,3]:
  - ❖ *Leukocyte reduction* removes white cells from the blood and blood components to reduce the frequency of recurrent febrile nonhemolytic transfusion reactions. These reactions are typically manifested by an increase in temperature of 1°C or more as a result of antibodies against white cells or the action of cytokines generated by the transfused component or the child.[1] These reactions occur in approximately 1% of transfusions. Leukocyte reduction has also been shown to reduce the incidence rate of human leukocyte antigen (HLA) alloimmunization and the risk of cytomegalovirus (CMV) transmission.[1] Leukocyte reduction removes at least 85% of white cells but does not prevent graft versus host disease (GVHD).

❖ *CMV seronegative* blood has been tested in the blood bank and has been shown not to have antibodies to CMV. CMV can be transmitted through a blood transfusion and can be characterized by retinitis, gastroenteritis, and interstitial pneumonitis,[3] which may not be severe for the immunocompetent child but may be fatal in a seronegative immunocompromised child. CMV negative blood is indicated for individuals who are CMV seronegative and at risk for severe CMV infections, such as women who are pregnant and their fetuses, infants with low birth weight, recipients of marrow transplant and solid-organ transplant, and recipients with severe immunocompromise and HIV infection.[1,3]

❖ *Irradiated blood components* prevent proliferation of T lymphocytes, which is the immediate cause of GVHD. T lymphocytes in the transfused component engraft in the recipient and react against tissue antigens in the recipient.[1] Children at risk who should be considered to receive irradiated blood components include fetuses receiving intrauterine transfusions, immunocompromised children, children receiving a blood component from a blood relative, and recipients of bone marrow transplant.[1,3]

❖ *Washing* of blood and blood components removes unwanted plasma proteins, including antibodies. This method is indicated when these components are suspected to predispose the child to significant transfusion reactions.

• Once the integrity of the unit is disrupted, the component is only good for 4 hours at room temperature or 24 hours if the unit is kept refrigerated at a temperature of 1°C to 6°C.

• A blood warmer may be used if clinically indicated for circumstances such as exchange transfusion, massive transfusion, or children with cold-reactive antibodies. For prevention of hemolysis, warming of blood is only to be performed with a U.S. Food and Drug Administration (FDA)–cleared device and blood should not be warmed greater than 37°C.[1]

• All blood and blood components must be inspected before administration for presence of clot formation or color changes; if clot formation or color changes are present, the blood should be returned to the blood bank for further inspection to assess for possible bacterial contamination.[1,3]

• Blood for transfusion contains preservatives that may lead to electrolyte abnormalities such as hypocalcemia, hyperkalemia or hypokalemia, acidosis or alkalosis, especially when large volumes are transfused.[1]

• Units of blood can be divided into aliquots (smaller portions) for neonates and children, which allows for serial transfusions from the same unit of blood, reducing exposure to multiple donors.

• Understanding of ABO group and Rh type compatability (Table 132-1)

• Signs and symptoms of a transfusion reaction and appropriate management (see Procedure 136 for further information)

• Principles of aseptic technique

• Child development as it relates to clinical assessment and blood component administration

• Signed consent is required before initiation of transfusion

CHILD AND FAMILY ASSESSMENT

• History of previous transfusions and any suspected transfusion reaction ➥*Rationale:* Child may need pretransfusion medication to prevent febrile, nonhemolytic, or allergic reactions.

• Signs or symptoms of hemorrhage, such as external bleeding, trauma, or changes in vital signs (e.g., elevation in heart rate or change in blood pressure) ➥*Rationale:* These indications can suggest hypovolemic shock that necessitates rapid replacement of volume with packed red blood cells.

• Changes in oxygen carrying capacity as evidenced by decreased oxygen saturation with pulse oximetry, decrease in partial pressure of oxygen in arterial blood (PaO_2), respiratory changes, or decreased hemoglobin ➥*Rationale:* These indications can suggest anemia that necessitates transfusion of packed red blood cells to increase oxygen carrying capacity of hemoglobin.

• Type of vascular access available for transfusion of the prescribed blood component ➥*Rationale:* Child must have functioning and appropriate vascular access for administration of blood component.

• Child's developmental level and ability to interact ➥*Rationale:* These factors influence preparation of the

TABLE 132-1	ABO Group and Rh Type Compatibilities	
Recipient Blood Type	**Compatible Red Blood Cell**	**Compatible Plasma and Platelets**
O	O	O, A, B, AB
A	A, O	A, AB
B	B, O	B, AB
AB	AB, A, B, O	AB
Rh type	Red Blood Cell Rh type	Plasma Rh type for transfusion
Positive	Positive or negative	Positive or negative
Negative	Negative	Positive or negative

Note: Whole blood must be ABO identical with recipient.
Data from American Association of Blood Banks, America's Blood Centers, and the American Red Cross: *Circular of information for the use of human blood and blood components,* Bethesda, MD, 2002, American Association of Blood Banks.
Hockenberry MJ, et al: *Wong's nursing care of infants and children,* ed 7, Philadelphia, 2003, Mosby.

child and interaction. The sight of blood may be especially frightening for toddlers and preschool-aged children.

- Child's and family's understanding of the reasons for and risks and benefits of the procedure ➥*Rationale:* Evaluates child's and family's understanding of the procedure and provides a gauge for ongoing education.
- Family's and child's concerns about the procedure, including cultural or religious concerns ➥*Rationale:* Some cultures and religions have prohibitions or restrictions against the receipt of blood or blood components. In addition, some families have concerns about the safety of banked blood.
- Family's desire to be present during the procedure ➥*Rationale:* Family may provide support and comfort to the child during the procedure but should have the choice not to remain with the child.

CHILD AND FAMILY EDUCATION

Individualized, developmentally appropriate education is provided to the family and to the child based on desire for knowledge, readiness to learn, and overall neurologic and psychosocial state.

- Explain the reason for the administration of the blood component and the component the child will receive ➥*Rationale:* Providing information decreases fear and anxiety.

- Explain the need for consent before transfusion ➥*Rationale:* The family is informed of their rights and the benefits and risks of transfusion.
- Explain the signs and symptoms of a transfusion reaction and that the nurse should be notified immediately if any sign or symptom is seen ➥*Rationale:* The child or family may be the first to notice the signs or symptoms of transfusion reaction and can immediately notify the nurse, promoting prompt action. Encourages the child and family to be participants in the child's care.
- Encourage questions and answer questions as they arise ➥*Rationale:* Reinforcement of information is needed during periods of stress.

EQUIPMENT

- Blood or blood component as prescribed
- Blood infusion pump
- Appropriate blood or blood component transfusion administration set
- Sodium chloride solution (0.9%) for intravenous (IV) administration
- Alcohol pad
- Clean gloves
- IV connecting device
- Thermometer
- Stethoscope
- Blood pressure monitoring device or sphygmomanometer
- Blood warmer as indicated

Procedure	**for Blood and Blood Component Administration and Blood Pump Use**	
Steps	**Rationale**	**Considerations**
1. Ensure child and family understand procedure and questions are answered.	Evaluates and reinforces understanding of previously taught information.	Developmental level, cognitive ability, and anxiety level determine approach to and effectiveness of teaching.
2. Verify presence of signed consent for blood administration. *(Level II*)*	Protects the child's and family's right to be informed. Ensures medical-legal compliance as suggested by the Joint Commission on Accreditation of Healthcare Organizations (JCAHO).	In emergency situations, refer to institution-specific protocol for assumption of consent.
3. Verify the prescribing practitioner's written order for blood or blood component transfusion.[1]	Required for administration of any blood components.	The written order should include the type of blood, special preparation, quantity, and duration of transfusion.
4. Verify that a current type and screen are available at the blood bank.	Blood components must be cross matched to the child for ABO group and Rh type compatibility to decrease chance of transfusion reaction.	Type and screen can last for 24 to 72 hours depending on institution-specific protocol. If components are needed immediately, O negative blood can be given without type and screen.[2]

Procedure continues on following page

Procedure	for Blood and Blood Component Administration and Blood Pump Use—*Continued*	

Steps	Rationale	Considerations
5. Wash hands; put on clean gloves.	Standard precautions; reduces transmission of microorganisms.	
6. Assess patency of child's IV line.	If IV line is not patent, a new IV line must be placed before blood component is obtained for transfusion.	A large-bore IV line is ideal for transfusion of blood components. Use largest gauge possible.
7. Administer pretransfusion medications per prescribing practitioner's order.	Children with known sensitivities to blood may be administered premedication to prevent a transfusion reaction.	Premedication for febrile reactions can include antipyretics, antihistamines, and steroids.
8. Obtain blood or blood component from blood bank when ready to initiate transfusion.	Blood components remain in blood bank storage until needed.	Generally, if blood components cannot be immediately used after being obtained, they must be returned to the blood bank within a specified amount of time, usually 15 minutes. Per some institution-specific protocols, blood components, except platelets, may be stored in a temperature-regulated refrigerator once dispensed from the blood bank.[1]
9. Two registered nurses (RNs) independently identify the child with two patient identifiers; ensure that the medical record number and spelling of first and last names listed on the child's identification band match those listed on the blood component label and the blood component slip issued by the blood bank. *(Level II*)*	Promotes patient safety; confirms blood component issued is administered to correct child.	Two patient identifiers should be used for patient identification per institution-specific protocol; most commonly, name and birth date or name and medical record number are used.
10. Two RNs, one of whom is the transfusionist, independently verify the following[1]: *(Level II*)*	Independent verification by two individuals reduces the likelihood of error.	
a. Type of blood component to be administered listed on the blood component slip agrees with the blood component container label and the prescribing practitioner's order.[1] *(Level II*)*	Ensures child receives prescribed blood component.	
b. The ABO group and Rh type compatibility listed on the blood component slip agree with the blood component container label and are appropriate based on the child's ABO group and Rh type.[1] *(Level II*)*	Verifies child's blood type against blood component unit to assure correct ABO group and Rh type are transfused.	See Table 132-1 for appropriate ABO group and Rh typing for transfusion. Whole blood must be ABO identical with recipient.[1]
c. Unit number and expiration date and time listed on the blood component slip agree with the blood component container label.[1] *(Level II*)*	Ensures child does not receive an expired blood component.	

* Level II: Theory-based; no research data to support recommendations; recommendations from expert consensus group may exist

| Procedure | for Blood and Blood Component Administration and Blood Pump Use—*Continued* | | |

Steps	Rationale	Considerations
d. Special processing required per prescribing practitioner's order or unit-specific or institution-specific protocol is listed on the blood component slip and agrees with the blood component container label.[2] *(Level II*)*	Decreases likelihood of transfusion reactions or complications related to the transfusion.	
11. Inspect blood component for abnormal appearance, such as color changes, cloudiness, or clot formation; if abnormal appearance is present, return unit to blood bank for further inspection.[1,3] *(Level II*)*	May suggest bacterial contamination.	
12. If all information is correct, both RNs sign the transfusion record. If any errors are noted, do not hang the unit of blood. Notify the blood bank immediately.	Documents independent verification process. Unit is returned to blood bank for further investigation if errors are noted.	Delay in notifying blood bank or returning unit to blood bank may result in the unit being unusable.
13. Obtain tubing specific for blood or blood component administration; close roller clamps on tubing.	Blood and blood components must be filtered.[1,3] Closing roller clamps prevents spillage of blood.	All blood components must be transfused through blood tubing that has a 170-micron to 260-micron filter to remove clots and aggregates.[1]
14. With use of Y connector blood tubing: a. Spike a 250-mL or larger bag of 0.9% sodium chloride.	Sodium chloride (0.9%) is used to prime tubing because other IV fluids may cause precipitation when combined with blood component preservatives.[1]	
b. Open roller clamp and primes entire length of tubing with 0.9% sodium chloride.	Primes entire length of tubing and removes all air, decreasing risk of emboli.	
c. Close the roller clamp to the bag of 0.9% sodium chloride.	Stops flow of priming fluid.	
d. Spike blood component; ensure roller clamp remains closed.	Accesses the blood component for transfusion.	
15. If non-Y tubing is used to administer blood: a. Spike blood component; ensure roller clamp remains closed.	Accesses the blood component for transfusion.	
b. Open roller clamp to the blood component and carefully prime entire length of tubing, ensuring all air bubbles are removed. Close roller clamp.	Primes entire length of tubing and removes all air, decreasing risk of emboli.	

Procedure continues on following page

* Level II: Theory-based; no research data to support recommendations; recommendations from expert consensus group may exist

Procedure **for Blood and Blood Component Administration and Blood Pump Use**—*Continued*		
Steps	**Rationale**	**Considerations**
c. Turn off and disconnect IV fluids if infusing in IV line to be used for blood component administration.	Blood components cannot run simultaneously with maintenance IV fluids which may cause precipitation when combined with blood component preservatives.[1]	If child is not being fed and blood component will be administered in child's only IV access, assess whether prescribed length of transfusion will adversely affect child's blood glucose level, particularly in infants.
d. Flush line with 0.9% sodium chloride.	Sodium chloride (0.9%) is used to clear line because other IV fluids and medications, such as heparin, may cause precipitation when combined with blood component.	
16. Connect IV tubing to pump designated for blood transfusion.	Pump controls the rate of infusion to prevent fluid overload.	
17. Connect the IV tubing to the child's IV line.	Necessary to initiate transfusion.	
18. Before beginning transfusion, obtain a set of vital signs, including temperature.[1] *(Level II*)*	Baseline vital signs are compared with vital signs obtained during transfusion for prompt identification of signs and symptoms of a possible transfusion reaction.	
19. Open roller clamp to blood component.	Necessary to initiate blood component transfusion.	
20. Start pump. Unless otherwise specifically indicated by the child's clinical condition, infusions should be run slowly for the first 15 minutes (e.g., 1 mL/kg/h) and then increased to the desired rate.[1] *(Level II*)*	Acute reaction is generally seen in the first 15 minutes of the transfusion.	Infusion rate for some blood components, such as leukocytes, may be specified by institution-specific protocol.
21. After the first 15 minutes, set pump rate on basis of prescribing practitioner's order: quantity of blood to be transfused divided by ordered length of time for transfusion. Set total volume to be transfused.	Ensures blood component is administered as prescribed; prevents excess volume from being infused.	Infants and children are at risk for volume overload; monitor intake and output closely.
22. Obtain a set of vital signs 15 minutes after start of transfusion. Continue to obtain vital signs at intervals specified by institution-specific protocol until transfusion is completed.	Facilitates prompt identification of a possible transfusion reaction. Acute transfusion reactions usually occur within the first 15 minutes of infusion.[1]	No evidence is found to support a specific interval for vital signs after the first 15 minutes, and recommendations vary widely from every 15 minutes to every hour; refer to institution-specific protocol for vital sign frequency. If reaction is suspected, stop transfusion and notify prescribing practitioner. Notify blood bank and return blood component to blood bank for inspection. Refer to institution-specific protocol for management of a suspected transfusion reaction.

* Level II: Theory-based; no research data to support recommendations; recommendations from expert consensus group may exist

Procedure	for Blood and Blood Component Administration and Blood Pump Use—*Continued*	
Steps	**Rationale**	**Considerations**
		Provide appropriate supportive care to the child if a possible transfusion reaction is identified (see Procedure 136 for further information).
23. At completion of transfusion, stop pump and close roller clamps.	Discontinues the infusion.	Transfusion should be completed within 4 hours of initiation.[1] *(Level II*)*
24. Disconnect the blood infusion tubing; flush the IV with 0.9% sodium chloride.	Tubing is no longer needed; clears the IV line of blood and reduces risk of clotting the IV.	
25. Obtain posttransfusion vital signs.	Monitors for signs and symptoms of a possible transfusion reaction.	
26. Discard tubing in appropriate receptacle.	Standard precautions; reduces the transmission of microorganisms.	
27. Note volume of transfusion and duration of transfusion.	Information is necessary for accurate intake recording; facilitates evaluation of fluid balance.	Infants and children are susceptible to fluid volume overload. Maintain accurate intake and output documentation.
28. Remove gloves; wash hands.	Standard precautions; reduces transmission of microorganisms.	

* Level II: Theory-based; no research data to support recommendations; recommendations from expert consensus group may exist

Expected Outcomes	**Unexpected Outcomes**
• Child does not have transfusion reaction or disease transmission	• Transfusion reaction, including hemolytic transfusion reaction, immune-mediated platelet destruction, febrile nonhemolytic reaction, allergic or anaphylactoid reactions, or transfusion-related acute lung injury
	• Transmission of an infectious disease or CMV
	• Delayed immunologic complications including GVHD, delayed hemolytic reaction, or alloimmunization
• Child receives correctly administered prescribed blood component over prescribed time; administration is correctly documented	• Blood component is administered with IV fluids that contain dextrose or medications
	• Wrong blood component is administered
	• Blood component is not administered over the prescribed time
	• Blood component is administered to wrong child
	• Blood component administration is not documented correctly
• Restoration or maintenance of normovolemic status	• Circulatory overload from volume of blood component
• Restoration of hemostasis, correction of coagulopathies, or improvement in oxygen carrying capacity	• Coagulation profile remains altered
	• Hemostasis is not restored
	• Oxygen carrying capacity is not improved
• Electrolytes remain within normal limits	• Electrolyte abnormalities, such as hyperkalemia or hypocalcemia
• Normothermia is maintained	• Hypothermia
	• Hyperthermia related to transfusion reaction

Monitoring and Care of the Child

Activities and Interventions	Rationale	Reportable Conditions
1. Monitor child's vital signs before initiation of transfusion and throughout transfusion.	Changes in vital signs may indicate a transfusion reaction.	• Elevation of temperature more than 1°C • Elevated heart rate • Increased or decreased blood pressure • Tachypnea
2. Repeat laboratory data (hemoglobin, platelet count, coagulation factors) at completion of transfusion per prescribing practitioner's order.	Evaluates for improvement after transfusion is completed.	• No improvement in laboratory data or continued bleeding despite transfusion
3. Monitor child's respiratory and circulatory status throughout the transfusion.	Monitors for indications of fluid overload or transfusion reaction.	• Child reports dyspnea • Deterioration in vital signs
4. Monitor intake and output throughout transfusion.	Rapid administration of blood components may place child at risk for volume overload.	• Decreased urine output • Change in character of urine
5. Monitor patency of IV throughout transfusion.	Monitors for IV infiltration; prevents subcutaneous administration of blood and potential tissue injury.	• IV infiltration

Documentation

- Child and family education
- Verification of signed consent
- Independent verification by two individuals that correct blood component was administered to correct patient
- Individual administering blood component
- Vital signs before transfusion, throughout transfusion, and after transfusion
- Blood component and volume of component transfused
- Child's tolerance of transfusion
- Status of IV access before and at completion of transfusion
- Unexpected outcomes and related treatment

References

1. American Association of Blood Banks, America's Blood Centers and the American Red Cross: *Circular of information for the use of human blood and blood components,* Bethesda, MD, 2002, American Association of Blood Banks.
2. Brunetti M, Cohen J: Hematology. In Robertson J, Shilkofski N, editors: *The Harriet Lane handbook,* ed 17, St Louis, 2005, Mosby.
3. Quirolo KC: Transfusion medicine for the pediatrician, *Pediatr Clin North Am* 49(6):1211-1238, 2000.

Additional Readings

Curley MAQ, Moloney-Harmon PA, editors: *Critical care nursing of infants and children,* Philadelphia, 2001, Saunders.
Davis K, Hui CH, Quested B: Transfusing safely: a 2006 guide for nurses, *Austral Nurs J* 13:6:17-20, 2005.
Vincent JL, Piagnerelli M: Transfusion in the intensive care unit, *Crit Care Med* 34(5 supp):S96-S101, 2006.

P R O C E D U R E **133**

Blood Glucose Monitoring

P U R P O S E : To rapidly measure the blood glucose level of a child whose condition is identified as appropriate for this type of point of care testing done at the bedside

Mary Astor Gomez

PREREQUISITE KNOWLEDGE

- Point-of-care (POC) blood glucose monitoring is a measurement of glucose that can be done at any time on a portable machine and with the use of a reagent (test) strip.
  - ❖ Clinical laboratories measure serum glucose; POC devices measure glucose in a whole blood specimen and generally factor the results so that results are comparable with serum glucose test results.[1]
  - ❖ Several types of POC devices and reagent strips exist. Depending on the specific device used, blood may be applied to the reagent strip before or after it is placed in the device.
- The National Committee for Clinical Laboratory Standards currently accepts POC devices that have no more than 20% variance from the laboratory standard.[2,3]
  - ❖ A POC device operating within this acceptable range could report a blood glucose level of between 64 mg/dL and 96 mg/dL in a child with a serum glucose level of 80 mg/dL measured by the laboratory.
- Training and demonstrated competency in the specific POC device used.[4]
- Blood glucose testing may be done in children with altered mental status, seizures, unresponsiveness, insulin-dependent diabetes, non–insulin dependent diabetes, or suspected hypoglycemia or hyperglycemia or for maintenance of tight glycemic control.[5]
- Normal fasting blood glucose level in the adult is between 70 and 110 mg/dL[6]
  - ❖ Normal ranges vary by age,[7] and ranges may vary slightly between laboratories:

Preterm infant: 20 to 60 mg/dL
Newborn, <1 day: 40 to 60 mg/dL
Newborn, >1 day: 50 to 80 mg/dL
Child: 60 to 100 mg/dL
More than 16 years old: 74 to 106 mg/dL

- Normal sample levels can range from 60 to 140 mg/dL depending on physical stressors, physical activities, meals, insulin administration, and intravenous (IV) solutions.
- Hypoglycemia (<60 mg/dL) may result in confusion, anxiety, weakness, dizziness, headache, trembling, and other neurologic signs.[5] Other symptoms of hypoglycemia include decreased perfusion, diaphoresis, tachycardia, and hypotension, which are similar to signs and symptoms of hypoxemia.
- Hyperglycemia is defined as a fasting blood sugar level of more than 126 mg/dL.[6] Symptoms of high glucose levels include polyuria, polydipsia, and lethargy.[5]
- Principles of standard precautions and aseptic technique
- Abnormal glucose parameters in the infant and child and when the prescribing practitioner should be notified of abnormal results.
- POC testing is a supplement to clinical laboratory testing. Studies in critically ill adults showed significant variability between POC glucose measurements and laboratory measurements that led to clinical disagreement.[1,8]
- Child development as it relates to clinical assessment and blood glucose monitoring

CHILD AND FAMILY ASSESSMENT

- History of hypoglycemia or hyperglycemia and related symptoms[8] ➥*Rationale:* These conditions may complicate the assessment of neurologic status and may dictate the method used to obtain a blood sample.
- Child's developmental level and ability to interact ➥*Rationale:* These factors influence preparation and interaction during the procedure.
- Child's level of consciousness and cognitive ability ➥*Rationale:* A blood glucose test and follow up with clinical laboratory testing may be necessary immediately for assessment of decreased level of consciousness or diminished cognitive ability as it relates to glycemic fluctuations.
- Child's and family's understanding of the reasons for and risks and benefits of the procedure ➥*Rationale:* Evaluates child's and family's understanding of the procedure and provides a gauge for ongoing education.
- Family's desire to be present during the procedure ➥*Rationale:* Family members may provide support and comfort measures to the child but should have the option not to remain with the child. Older school-aged children and adolescents should be asked their preference concerning parental presence during the procedure.

CHILD AND FAMILY EDUCATION[5,6,9]

Individualized, developmentally appropriate education is provided to the family and to the child based on desire for knowledge, readiness to learn, and overall neurologic and psychosocial state.

- Provide information about blood glucose monitoring, including the reason for the test and an explanation of steps involved in blood glucose measurement ➥*Rationale:* Providing information decreases anxiety and fear and enhances education about glycemic monitoring.[10]
- Use developmentally appropriate strategies to prepare the child and family
  - ❖ Inform parents of infants that the test causes discomfort and that the infant will cry.
  - ❖ With toddlers, incorporate the use of play to demonstrate what occurs during the test.
  - ❖ For the preschooler, consider "acting out" the procedure with a doll to help identify the child's concerns and address worries.
  - ❖ Explain or demonstrate the procedure to the school-aged child to reduce the child's anxiety. Let the child participate with selecting the finger used, opening the alcohol wipes, reading the device, and placing the adhesive bandage.
  - ❖ Explain or demonstrate the procedure to the adolescent. Identify whether the adolescent wants a parent present during the procedure. Respect privacy issues.
  ➥*Rationale:* Use of strategies appropriate to the child's age or developmental level helps the child understand the procedure and helps the parent and child cope with discomfort.
- Explain how the child can assist with the procedure (i.e., holding still) ➥*Rationale:* The procedure is less difficult with the child's cooperation.
- Explain that during the procedure, the child may feel a small prick ➥*Rationale:* Providing information decreases anxiety and fear.
- Explain the chance of local infection at the puncture site and the necessity of notifying the health care team of signs or symptoms of local infection ➥*Rationale:* Provides information about risks; encourages the child and family to participate in care.
- Explain that after the procedure a small amount of bleeding may be seen ➥*Rationale:* Providing information decreases fear and anxiety.
- Encourage questions and answer questions as they arise ➥*Rationale:* Reinforcement of information is needed during periods of stress.

EQUIPMENT[11]

- Blood glucose monitoring device
- Reagent test strips
- Alcohol wipes
- Lancet with retractable blade
- Clean gloves
- Gauze
- Adhesive bandage

Blood Sample Obtained from IV or Arterial Access

- Syringes for waste and testing sample
- Label for waste syringe
- Saline solution (0.9%) flush
- Heparin lock solution if needed

Procedure for Blood Glucose Monitoring

Steps	Rationale	Considerations
1. Ensure child and family understand procedure and questions are answered.	Evaluates and reinforces understanding of previously taught information.	Developmental level, cognitive ability, and anxiety level determine approach to and effectiveness of teaching.
2. Gather needed equipment and supplies.	Preparation and presence of all materials facilitates completion of procedure in a timely manner. Allows reagent test strip to be at room temperature for a proper reading.	Ensure test strips are not outdated.[5] Delays in procedure may increase child's anxiety level.
3. Identify child with two patient identifiers. *(Level II*)*	Promotes patient safety; ensures specimens are obtained from the correct child.	Two patient identifiers should be used for patient identification per institution-specific protocol; most commonly name and birth date or name and medical record number are used.
4. Calibrate blood glucose monitoring device per unit and manufacturer's instructions. *(Level II*)*	Ensures accurate reading.	Ensure unit is not soiled because this may affect results. Units with color reflectance technology must be kept clean.[11]
5. As required by device and institution-specific protocol, insert child's identifying information into device.	Data from POC devices may be downloaded to the laboratory for tracking and reporting purposes; specimens are tracked with child's unique identifier.	Medical record number is most commonly used to identify specimen; refer to institution-specific protocol.
6. Ensure appropriate cardiopulmonary monitoring for critically ill children.	Critically ill children may decompensate during the procedure.	Consider child's status in selection of appropriate monitoring.
7. Wash hands; put on clean gloves.	Standard precautions; reduces transmission of microorganisms.	
8. Position child comfortably and so that site for blood specimen is well visualized and accessible.	Ensures maximal comfort of the child and successful procedure.	
9. Prepare testing site *Capillary:* a. Cleanse finger with alcohol swab; allow to dry.	Allowing the finger to dry prevents contamination from alcohol and ensures proper results.	Children with poor perfusion or cool extremities may benefit from warming the capillary site before puncturing to enhance blood flow.
b. Gently squeeze above the area on the finger that is to be punctured.	Squeezing the finger pools blood to finger tip and allows for easy blood flow to obtain an adequate sample.	Excessive squeezing of the finger can introduce interstitial fluid into the sample, which dilutes the sample.[3]
Intravenous line: a. Attach appropriately sized syringe labeled "discard" or "waste" and aspirate at least three times dead space volume of catheter and tubing.[12,13] *(Level IV*)*	Any blood drawn that is potentially contaminated with medications or fluids that alter laboratory values is discarded before obtaining blood sample.	Ideally, IV line infuses saline solution. Glucose specimens drawn from the same extremity as an infusion, even if the infusion is more distal

Procedure continues on following page

Procedure for Blood Glucose Monitoring—*Continued*		
Steps	**Rationale**	**Considerations**
	Labeling discard syringe prevents blood in discard syringe from being used for blood glucose level analysis.[13]	than the sampling site, may not provide accurate results.[13] *(Level IV*)*
Arterial line: a. Attach appropriately sized syringe labeled "discard" or "waste" and aspirate at least three times dead space volume of catheter and tubing.[12,13] *(Level IV*)*	Any blood drawn that is potentially contaminated with medications or fluids that alter laboratory values is discarded before obtaining blood sample. Labeling discard syringe prevents blood in discard syringe from being used for blood glucose level analysis.[13]	Institution-specific protocol may vary on blood draws from central venous and arterial catheters. See Procedures 138 and 141 and institution-specific protocol for additional information.
10. Obtain blood sample *Capillary:* a. Puncture side of fingertip with lancet and wipe away first drop of blood with gauze. b. Allow additional blood to flow from puncture site.	Wipe the first drop of blood with gauze to decrease the risk of contamination and dilution of the blood sample with alcohol.	Use of a lancet with retractable blade decreases the risk of needlestick injury. See Procedure 148 for further information.
Intravenous line: a. With 1 mL syringe, pull back 0.2 mL blood sample.	Small syringe decreases hemolysis.[13]	
Arterial line: a. With 1 mL syringe, pull back 0.2 mL blood sample.	Small syringe decreases hemolysis.[13]	
11. Depending on the type of device used and manufacturer's instructions, insert test strip into the designated port of the device and apply blood *or* put drop of blood on test strip and insert test strip into the designated port of the device. *(Level I*)*	Necessary for activation of test strip reagent and results reporting.	Blood should be tested immediately to avoid clotting or glycolysis, which affects accuracy of results. Be sure to have sufficient sample on test strip to obtain accurate results.
12. At indicated time, read results.	Ensures an accurate reading.	
13. With finger stick sample, place adhesive bandage on child's finger and maintain pressure until bleeding stops.	Minimizes bleeding. Offers added level of comfort, both physical and emotional, at completion of procedure.	If child is likely to put fingers in mouth, use of an adhesive bandage is discouraged to reduce the risk of choking. Apply firm pressure until the bleeding stops.
14. If IV line was accessed, flush catheter and resume fluid administration or saline or heparin lock IV catheter if appropriate.	Prevents clotting of IV line.	Institution-specific protocols may vary on blood draws from central venous catheters. Refer to institution-specific protocols for additional information.
15. If arterial line was accessed, flush arterial line with sterile technique and resume fluid infusion.	Prevents clotting of arterial line.	Follow institution-specific protocols for transduced arterial lines and methods to reduce infection and prevent dislodgement and bleeding.

* Level I: Manufacturer's recommendations only
  Level IV: Limited clinical studies to support recommendations

Procedure for Blood Glucose Monitoring—*Continued*

Steps	Rationale	Considerations
16. Dispose of used supplies and equipment, including sharps, in appropriate receptacle.	Standard precautions; reduces transmission of microorganisms. Protects personnel health.	
17. Prepare device for next use and store as indicated. *(Level II*)*	Ensures proper storage, handling, and durable life of sensitive equipment.	
18. Remove gloves; wash hands.	Standard precautions; reduces transmission of microorganisms.	
19. Contact the prescribing practitioner if results are less than 40 mg/dL or greater than 110 mg/dL or as indicated in notification orders.	Alerts prescribing practitioner to results.	If results are abnormal, consider drawing glucose level to be analyzed by laboratory.

* Level II: Theory-based; no research data to support recommendations; recommendations from expert consensus group may exist

Expected Outcomes

- Blood glucose level is determined
- Sample is obtained on correct child and correctly identified in device
- Child cooperates with procedure
- Skin at puncture site is free from infection
- Minimal bleeding from puncture site
- Access line remains in place until elective removal

Unexpected Outcomes

- Inability to obtain blood sample volume adequate for test
- Inability to determine blood glucose level
- Sample is obtained on wrong child
- Incorrect identifying information is entered into the device
- Child is uncooperative, which results in difficulty obtaining sample or inability to obtain sample
- Infection at puncture site
- Excessive bleeding from puncture site
- Dislodgement of IV or arterial line

Monitoring and Care of the Child

Activities and Interventions	Rationale	Reportable Conditions
1. Monitor child's tolerance to procedure.	Changes in child's condition may indicate complications from the procedure. Assesses for agitation and increased anxiety related to repeated finger sticks.	• Agitation that results in an inability to obtain blood sample • Dislodgement of IV or arterial line • Signs of hypoglycemia or hyperglycemia
2. Monitor factors that affect device performance.	Factors such as hematocrit, altitude, temperature, and humidity and other substances such as uric acid, glutathione, and ascorbic acid may affect device performance.[14]	• Questionable device performance
3. If samples are obtained with finger or heel stick, monitor sites for signs and symptoms of infection.	Early identification of possible infection facilitates prompt treatment.	• Signs or symptoms of local infection at puncture site
4. Monitor trends in POC testing results.	Significant change in results without correlating change in child's condition may indicate device is not functioning correctly.	• Abnormal results that do not correlate with child's clinical condition

Documentation

- Child and family education
- Blood glucose level and time obtained
- How blood sample was obtained (e.g., IV, fingerstick)
- Prescribing practitioner notified of any abnormal values and treatment prescribed
- Child's response to procedure
- Unexpected outcomes and related treatment

References

1. Kanji S, et al: Reliability of point-of-care testing for glucose measurement in critically ill adults, *Crit Care Med* 33(12):2778-2785, 2005.
2. National Committee for Clinical Laboratory Standards: *Ancillary (bedside) blood glucose testing in acute and chronic care facilities; NCCLS Guideline C30-A,* Villanova, PA, 1994, National Committee for Clinical Laboratory Standards.
3. Sirkin A, et al: Selecting an accurate point-of-care testing system: clinical and technical issues and implications neonatal blood glucose monitoring, *J Specialists Pediatr Nurs* 7(3):104-112, 2002.
4. American Diabetes Association: Bedside glucose monitoring in hospitals (position statement), *Diabetes Care* 27(Suppl 1):S104, 2004.
5. Mayfield J, Havas S: Self control: a physician's guide to blood glucose monitoring in the management of diabetes, 2004, retrieved March 22, 2005, from www.aafp.org/smbg-monograph.xml.
6. American Diabetes Association: Standards of medical care for patients with diabetes mellitus, *Diabetes Care* 25(Suppl 1):S33-49, 2002.
7. Robertson J: Blood chemistries and body fluids. In Robertson J, Shilkofski N, editors: *The Harriet Lane handbook,* ed 17, Philadelphia, 2005, Mosby.
8. Finkielman JD, et al: Agreement between bedside blood and plasma glucose measurement in the ICU setting, *Chest* 127(5):1748-1751, 2005.
9. American Diabetes Association: Self-monitoring of blood glucose (consensus statement), *Diabetes Care* 17:81-86, 1994.
10. Benjamin EM: Self monitoring of blood glucose: the basics, *Clin Diabetes* 20(1):45-47, 2002.
11. US Food and Drug Administration (FDA): Glucose meters and diabetes management, retrieved February 17, 2004, from http:/www.fda.gov/diabetes/glucose.html.
12. Himberger JR, Himberger LC: Accuracy of drawing blood through infusing intravenous lines, *Heart Lung* 30(1):66-73, 2001.
13. Frey AM: Drawing blood samples from vascular access devices: evidence-based practice, *J Infusion Nurs* 26(5):285-293, 2003.
14. Sacks DB, et al: Guidelines and recommendations for laboratory analysis in the diagnosis and management of diabetes mellitus, *Diabetes Care* 25:750-786, 2002.

Additional Readings

American Diabetes Association: Type 2 diabetes in children and adolescents, *Diabetes Care* 23(3):381-389, 2000.

American Diabetes Association: Report of the expert committee on the diagnosis and classification of diabetes mellitus (committee report). *Diabetes Care* 21(Suppl 1):S5-S19, 1998.

Expert Committee on the Diagnosis and Classification of Diabetes Mellitus: Report of the expert committee on the diagnosis and classification of diabetes mellitus, *Diabetes Care* 25(Suppl 1):S5-S20, 2002.

Vilke GM, et al: Evaluation of pediatric glucose monitoring and hypoglycemic therapy in the field, *Pediatr Emerg Care* 21(1):1-5, 2005.

Fluid Administration: Rapid Infusion

PURPOSE: To rapidly restore circulating volume to reestablish peripheral perfusion and oxygen delivery to the tissues and prevent end-organ damage in the child with hemodynamic instability from intravascular losses as a result of severe dehydration, trauma, internal hemorrhage, or septic shock

Rebecca A. Steinmann

PREREQUISITE KNOWLEDGE

- Restoration of circulating volume is critical for prevention of end-organ damage in the child with hemodynamic instability from intravascular losses. Management of severe dehydration, trauma, internal hemorrhage, and septic shock frequently necessitates rapid administration of intravenous (IV) fluids to reestablish peripheral perfusion and oxygen delivery to the tissues.

- Indicators of shock include: skin signs of decreased perfusion, delayed capillary refill, tachycardia, diminished peripheral pulses, respiratory compromise, altered mental status, decreased central venous pressure (CVP), decreased pulmonary artery occlusive pressure, and/or pulmonary capillary wedge pressure (PAOP/PCWP). Hypotension often is not apparent until approximately 20% to 25% of circulating volume is acutely lost.[1] Hypotension is a late finding, a sign that complete cardiovascular collapse is imminent.[2]

- Initial fluid resuscitation involves administration of 20 mL/kg crystalloids over 5 to 20 minutes with repeated boluses based on the child's clinical response; boluses of 5 to 10 mL/kg may be prescribed if severe myocardial dysfunction is present.[3]

- Circulating volume is age dependent. Neonates have a circulating volume of 85 to 90 mL/kg, infants 75 to 80 mL/kg, children 70 to 75 mL/kg, and adolescents 65 to 70 mL/kg.[1] Each 20-mL/kg bolus restores one fourth of the child's normal circulating volume.

- Intravenous catheters for rapid infusion should have a large bore and short diameter to facilitate the rapid infusion of fluids. Usually multiple vascular access sites are used, including peripheral, central, and intraosseous sites. In infants and young children, the small diameter of the peripheral vasculature commonly limits catheter size to 22-gauge or 24-gauge catheters.

- Iatrogenic hypothermia may result from the rapid infusion of room temperature IV fluids or refrigerated blood products. Ideally, for prevention of the metabolic and myocardial consequences of hypothermia, fluids and blood should be warmed.

  ❖ Storage of crystalloid solutions in an approved fluid warming cabinet provides ready access to warmed resuscitative fluids.

  ❖ The HotLine Blood and Fluid Warmer (Smiths Medical, Dublin, Ohio) is a method to warm fluids and blood; the device uses a tubing half-set that connects to the distal portion of any conventional IV tubing[4] (Figure 134-1).

    ○ When the HotLine is used in addition to an IV pump, the volume and rate of infusion are controlled with the IV pump.

    ○ When the HotLine is used without an IV pump and runs by gravity, the volume and rate of infusion are set with the roller clamp and drip chamber of the IV tubing.

    ○ The HotLine itself does not provide rapid fluid administration; it is a mechanism to warm fluids that can be used in conjunction with rapid fluid infusion via syringe method or pressure bag method.

- Selection of an appropriate rapid infusion strategy is based on consideration of the volume to be infused and

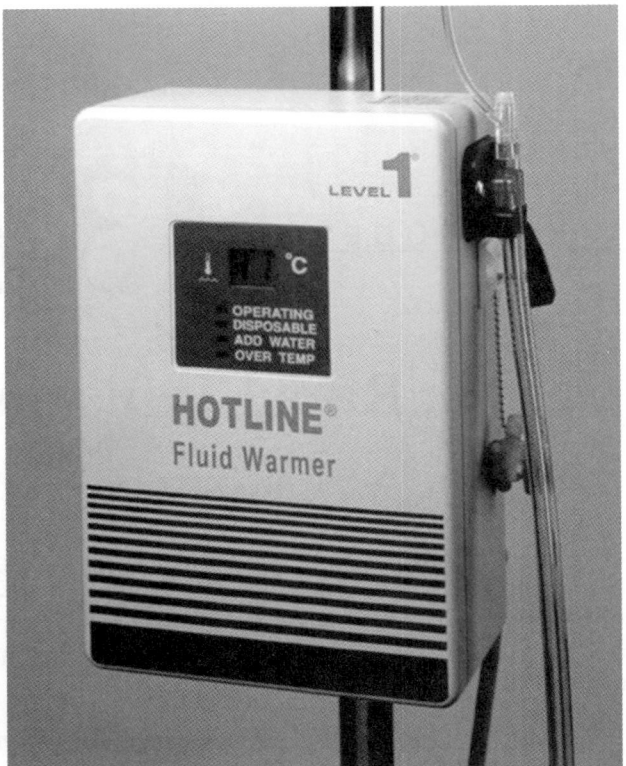

FIGURE 134-1 HOTLINE® Warming Device. *Photo courtesy of Smiths Medical ASD, Inc. Rockland, MA.*

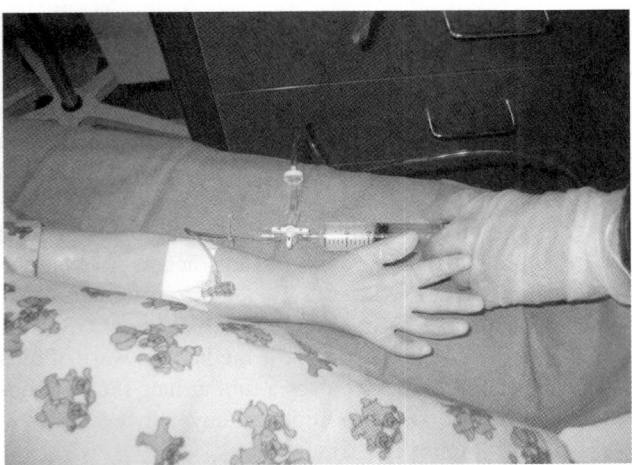

FIGURE 134-2 Three-way stopcock and syringe system for rapid fluid infusion.

the size of the catheter through which the volume will be delivered. For small-bore IV catheters (22-gauge or 24-gauge), rapid withdrawal and injection of fluids with a syringe and stopcock are efficient[3,5] (Figure 134-2). Pressure bags may be an option for children with larger catheters[6] (Figure 134-3). Pressurized rapid infusion devices, such as the Level 1 Fast Flow Fluid Warmer (Smiths Medical), may be considered for children who weigh more than 20 kg with intravenous catheter sizes of 20-gauge or larger[2,6] (Figure 134-4).

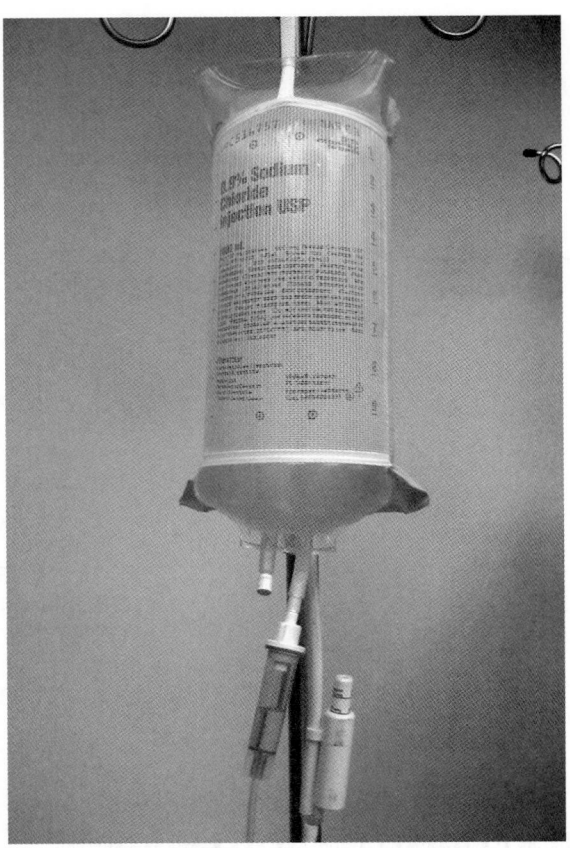

FIGURE 134-3 Pressure bag system for rapid fluid infusion.

- Indicators of volume overload: pulmonary crackles, signs of increased intracranial pressure, increased CVP, and increased PAOP/PCWP
- Ability to evaluate adequacy of fluid resuscitation based on blood gas results
- Knowledge of aseptic technique
- Mastery of pediatric advanced life support competencies
- Demonstrated competency in set up and use of the specific equipment used for rapid fluid administration and fluid warming

CHILD AND FAMILY ASSESSMENT

- Child's skin perfusion status (color, temperature, warmth), peripheral pulses, heart rate, respiratory rate, level of consciousness, blood pressure, and urinary output ➠*Rationale:* Clinical indicators of the severity of volume depletion and shock.
- Child's core temperature ➠*Rationale:* Baseline temperature determination is necessary to assess for the development of hypothermia during large volume fluid infusion.
- Child's history for precipitating events and medical history including cardiac problems ➠*Rationale:* Identifies potential cause of intravascular fluid loss and potential or actual risk of fluid overload.
- Child's hemodynamic parameters (as applicable) ➠*Rationale:* Provides baseline information regarding child's preload, afterload, and cardiac contractility.

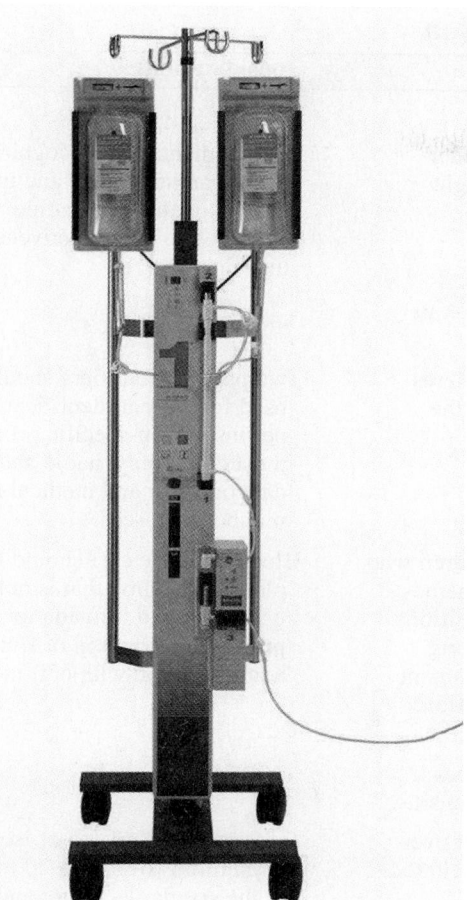

FIGURE 134-4   Level 1® Fast Flow Fluid Warmer system for rapid fluid infusion. *Photo courtesy of Smiths Medical ASD, Inc., Rockland, MA.*

- Laboratory values (blood gases, electrolytes, hemoglobin, hematocrit, and coagulation studies) ➤➤*Rationale:* Provides baseline measurements of oxygenation, identifies metabolic acidosis, presence and severity of ongoing volume loss, and presence and severity of coagulopathy, so that the necessity for intervention and the effectiveness of interventions can be determined.
- Patency and size of vascular catheters and the volume of fluid to be rapidly administered ➤➤*Rationale:* The size of the catheters and the amount of volume to be administered allow for selection of an infusion strategy that ensures the child's safety and line integrity.
- Family's understanding of the reasons for and risks and benefits of the procedure ➤➤*Rationale:* Evaluates child's and family's understanding of the procedure and provides a gauge for ongoing education.
- Family's desire to be at the child's bedside during procedure ➤➤*Rationale:* The ability to remain with the child may decrease the family's anxiety and fear. The option of being with the child during a life-threatening event reassures the family that the child is receiving optimal care, legitimizes the child's condition, and may provide some sense of comfort and control.[3] Family may provide support and comfort measures to the child but should also have the choice not to remain with the child. If the family

remains with the child, a designated health care team member should be identified to provide the family with support and updates during the procedure.[3]

CHILD AND FAMILY EDUCATION

Individualized, developmentally appropriate education is provided to the family and to the child based on desire for knowledge, readiness to learn, and overall neurologic and psychosocial state. Short simple explanations are most effective during an emergency situation.[3] Anticipate that information needs to be repeated.

- Provide information about the child's clinical status and need for fluid resuscitation and close monitoring ➤➤*Rationale:* Providing information helps the child and family understand the plan of care and decreases anxiety and fear.
- Provide information regarding the equipment to be used ➤➤*Rationale:* Providing information decreases child's and family's anxiety regarding unfamiliar equipment at the bedside.
- If family desires to stay with the child during the procedure and institution-specific protocol permits family presence, provide family with accurate information regarding procedure, family's role, and expectations ➤➤*Rationale:* The family is prepared for their role; clearly defined guidelines and expectations are provided.
- Encourage questions and answer questions as they arise ➤➤*Rationale:* Reinforcement of information is needed during periods of stress and is especially important given the emergent nature of the procedure.

EQUIPMENT

Rapid Infusion with Three-way Stopcock and Syringe
- IV fluids or blood as prescribed
- Disposable IV fluid administration set
- Three-way stopcock
- 20-mL syringe (30-mL or 60-mL syringe may also be used)
- Clean gloves

Rapid Infusion with Pressure Bag
- IV fluids or blood as prescribed
- Disposable IV fluid administration set
- Pressure bag
- Clean gloves

Rapid Infusion with Level 1 Fast Flow Fluid Warmer
- IV fluids or blood as prescribed
- Level 1 Fast Flow Fluid Warmer
- Disposable rapid infusion fluid administration set approved for use with Level 1 unit
- Distilled water for warmer
- Clean gloves

Procedure for Fluid Administration: Rapid Infusion

Steps	Rationale	Considerations
Syringe Method		
1. As time permits, ensure child and family understand procedure and questions are answered.	Evaluates and reinforces understanding of previously taught information.	Developmental level, cognitive ability, anxiety level, and urgency of the situation determine approach to and effectiveness of teaching.
2. Gather needed equipment and supplies.	Facilitates completion of task in a timely manner.	
3. Identify the child with two patient identifiers. *(Level II*)*	Promotes patient safety; ensures fluids are administered to the correct child.	Two patient identifiers should be used for patient identification per institution-specific protocol; most commonly, name and birth date or name and medical record number are used.
4. Ensure appropriate cardio-pulmonary monitoring. *(Level II*)*	Critically ill or injured children who need rapid infusion have hemo-dynamically unstable conditions. Cardiopulmonary monitoring provides continuous assessment of the child's response to fluid replacement.	Blood pressure cuff should be placed on a limb that is not being used for rapid infusion to prevent interruption of fluid administration with cuff inflation.
5. Wash hands and put on gloves.	Standard precautions; reduces transmission of microorganisms.	
6. Verify amount and type of fluid to be rapidly infused.	Ensures that the child is not over-resuscitated or underresuscitated with inappropriate fluids.	Infusion of 20 mL/kg of isotonic crystalloids over 5 to 20 minutes is the standard amount and rate of initial fluid resuscitation for a child in shock.[3]
7. Spike warmed fluid or blood with the infusion set and prime tubing. See Procedure 132 for specifics on administration of blood components.	Removes air from system, prevents air emboli.	Warmed fluid, crystalloids stored at 38°C (104°F), and IV fluid warming devices reduce the likelihood of iatrogenic hypothermia. If an IV fluid warming device is used, follow manufacturer's instructions for device use.
8. Secure the three-way stopcock to the end of the tubing and attach the 20-mL syringe (see Figure 134-2).	The three-way stopcock provides a closed system with the ability to draw measured amounts of fluid from the IV bag and manually administer measured amounts of fluid to the child while monitoring time interval.	A 20-mL syringe provides efficient delivery of fluid with the additional advantage that each syringe of fluid administered is equal to fluid resuscitation for 1 kg of the child's body weight. Larger syringes (30-mL to 60-mL) may be attached to the stopcock but generate greater resistance in withdrawing and pushing fluid and complicate the math involved in calculating the amount of fluid administered.
9. Connect system directly to the child's IV intraosseous (IO) catheter.	Prevents decreased flow rates from infusing through lengths of tubing.	Maintain aseptic technique in attaching to IV/IO catheter.

* Level II: Theory-based; no research data to support recommendations; recommendations from expert consensus group may exist

Procedure for Fluid Administration: Rapid Infusion—*Continued*

Steps	Rationale	Considerations
10. Turn stopcock off to child, open to IV bag to fill syringe.	Allows filling of syringe from IV/blood bag.	
11. Turn stopcock off to bag, open to child, and administer fluid to the child.	Manual administration of measured volume of fluid.	Allows fluid to be administered rapidly while maintaining "feel" of resistance to fluid flow.
12. Continuously monitor IV/IO site for signs of infiltration.	Extravasation may occur in delivery of fluids with pressure.	Both the anterior and posterior surfaces of extremities with IO insertions should be evaluated for signs of fluid infiltration.
13. Rapidly repeat steps 10 to 12 until initial bolus amount of fluid has been administered.	Provides desired volume to be administered in short time frame.	The full bolus should be administered over 5 to 20 minutes based on the child's clinical condition and status of IV/IO access.
14. Reassess child's skin parameters, heart rate, respiratory rate and effort, level of consciousness, and blood pressure (BP).	Evaluates child's response to initial bolus of fluid.	Additional fluid boluses may be necessary based on the child's response.
15. Dispose of used supplies and equipment in appropriate receptacles.	Standard precautions; reduces transmission of microorganisms.	
16. Remove gloves; wash hands.	Standard precautions.	
Pressure Bag Method		
1. See steps 1 to 6 listed previously in Syringe Method section.	Prepares fluid for administration.	If blood components are administered with a pressure bag, gown, eye and face protection should be worn in addition to gloves.
2. Remove the air from the IV bag with a 20-mL syringe and needle or use a needle to vent the air out of the injection port while squeezing the inverted IV bag. *(Level II*)*	Prevents an air embolism from air present in the bag (≈60 mL of air/1000 mL IV bag) being forced through the tubing under pressure.	Bags that contain blood products do not need air removal. See Procedure 132 for specifics on administration of blood components.
3. Prime the tubing with fluid.	Removes air from system.	If an IV fluid warming device is used, follow manufacturer's instructions for device use.
4. Insert the IV bag or blood bag through the lower opening of the pressure bag.	Seats fluid in pressure bag.	
5. Insert the loop at the top end of the pressure bag through the eye of the bag of fluid to be delivered.	Secures fluid bag in place within the pressure bag.	
6. Suspend the pressure bag and solution bag by the strap to the IV pole.	Prepares pressure bag system.	
7. Manually inflate pressure bag to desired pressure and begin fluid administration (see Figure 134-3).	The amount of inflation impacts the speed of fluid delivery.	Inflation should not exceed 300 mm Hg to prevent complications at the IV/IO site with crystalloid/colloid and hemolysis when red blood cells are administered.[7]

Procedure continues on following page

* Level II: Theory-based; no research data to support recommendations; recommendations from expert consensus group may exist

Procedure for Fluid Administration: Rapid Infusion—*Continued*

Steps	Rationale	Considerations
8. Continuously monitor IV/IO site for signs of infiltration.	Extravasation may occur with delivery of fluids under pressure.	Both the anterior and posterior surfaces of extremities with IO insertions should be evaluated for signs of fluid infiltration.
9. Reassess child's skin parameters, heart rate, respiratory rate and effort, level of consciousness, and BP.	Evaluates child's response to initial bolus of fluid.	Additional fluid boluses may be necessary based on the child's response.
10. Dispose of used supplies and equipment, including sharps, in appropriate receptacles.	Standard precautions; reduces the transmission of microorganisms. Protects personnel health.	
11. Remove personal protective equipment; wash hands.	Standard precautions.	

Pressure Infusion Device (Level 1 Fast Flow Fluid Warmer)

Steps	Rationale	Considerations
1. See steps 1 to 6 listed previously in Syringe Method section.	Prepares fluid for administration.	If blood components are administered under pressure, gown, eye and face protection should be worn in addition to gloves. Warmed fluids are not necessary. The Level 1 can warm fluid to 35°C to 41°C at a rate of up to 500 mL/min.[8]
2. Open Y-set administration package; ensure all connections are tight and close clamps.	Prevents accidental disconnections of tubing and spillage of fluids.	
3. Remove the air from the IV bag with a 20-mL syringe and needle or use a needle to vent the air out of the injection port while squeezing the inverted IV bag. (*Level I**)	Prevents an air embolism from air present in the bag ($\approx$60 mL of air/ 1000 mL IV bag) being forced through the tubing under pressure.	Bags that contain blood products do not need air removal. Fatal air embolism has been reported with the use of the Level 1, so care must be taken to remove all air from the IV bag.[5]
4. Spike IV fluid bag/blood and hang fluids on small hooks inside the rapid infuser pressure chamber, leaving the chamber doors open. (*Level I**)	Clearing the tubing of air before the fluid is pressurized is easier.	
5. Push the bottom end of the heat exchanger rod into the socket labeled "1." (*Level I**)	The bottom of the heat exchanger must be firmly placed or the rod does not fit into the top socket.	Firm pressure is necessary to place the tubing in the socket.
6. Insert the heat exchanger into the guide; slide the top socket labeled "2" down over the top of the rod until it clicks. (*Level I**)	Locks the heat exchanger rod into place.	
7. Insert the filter/gas vent into the holder on the lower portion of the pole assembly labeled "3" with the orange end up. (*Level I**)	Filters air and blood clots from tubing.	The vent only fits into machine one way.
8. Plug in and turn on the machine. (*Level I**)	Allows machine to begin warming up without alarming as disposable tubing is in place.	The display panel on the device should display a green "system operational" indicator light if the tubing is properly inserted.

---

* Level I: Manufacturer's recommendations only

Procedure for Fluid Administration: Rapid Infusion—*Continued*

Steps	Rationale	Considerations
9. Squeeze drip chambers so that they are half full. *(Level I*)*	Minimizes entrapment of air in the tubing. Allows visualization of the drip chamber so that flow rate can be assessed.	
10. Open the clamps on the tubing; remove the male luer cap at the end of the IV tubing and prime the line. Reclamp the tubing. *(Level I*)*	Tubing does not prime with the end cap in place.	
11. Connect infusion set directly to the child's IV/IO catheter.	Prevents decreased flow rates from infusing through additional lengths of tubing.	Maintain aseptic technique in attaching to IV/IO catheter.
12. Close the pressure chamber door and latch it. Open all the clamps on the IV tubing. *(Level I*)*	Prepares for pressurizing the chamber.	
13. Flip the toggle switch at the top of the pressure chamber to "On" (+) and begin infusion. *(Level I*)*	Pressurizes the chamber.	The pressure automatically inflates to 300 mm Hg.
14. Continuously monitor IV/IO site for signs of infiltration.	Extravasation may occur with delivery of fluids under pressure.	Both the anterior and posterior surfaces of extremities with IO insertions should be evaluated for signs of fluid infiltration.
15. At completion of infusion, reassess child's skin parameters, heart rate, respiratory rate and effort, level of consciousness, and BP.	Evaluates child's response to initial bolus of fluid.	Additional fluid boluses may be necessary based on the child's response.
16. Remove tubing from Level 1 according to manufacturer's instructions. Dispose of used supplies and equipment, including sharps, in appropriate receptacles. *(Level I*)*	Standard precautions; reduces transmission of microorganisms. Protects personnel health.	
17. Remove personal protective equipment; wash hands.	Standard precautions.	

* Level I: Manufacturer's recommendations only

Expected Outcomes

- Perfusion status is improved

- Child's core temperature remains above 36.0°C (96.8°F)

- Integrity of IV/IO sites maintained
- Child has no complications of rapid fluid administration
- System is set up and fluid administered within 20 minutes

- Prescribed type and amount of fluid is administered

Unexpected Outcomes

- Fluid overload as indicated by pulmonary crackles or signs of increased intracranial pressure
- Inability to restore normal intravascular volume despite fluid resuscitation
- Core temperature falls below 36.0°C and more aggressive rewarming interventions are necessary
- Hypothermia-induced coagulopathy develops as temperature falls below 34.5°C (94.1°F)
- Infiltration of IV/IO site
- Air embolus
- Delay in fluid administration as result of difficulties with system set up
- Incorrect type or volume of fluid is administered

Monitoring and Care of the Child

Activities and Interventions	Rationale	Reportable Conditions
1. Monitor the child's vital signs every 5 to 15 minutes until condition is stable. Assessment of vital signs may then be done every 15 to 30 minutes, until skin parameters, heart rate, and blood pressure remain stable for more than 2 hours.	Determines child's response to fluid resuscitation and the need for additional fluids.	• Persistent signs of shock despite fluid administration: poor skin perfusion, tachycardia, tachypnea, decreased level of consciousness, and hypotension
2. Assess the child's core temperature every 30 minutes at minimum.	Infants and young children have ineffective thermoregulation. The stress of shock combined with the infusion of inadequately warmed IV fluids leads to hypothermia.	• Worsening or unrelieved hypothermia
3. Assess the integrity of IV sites with each fluid bolus minimally every 15 minutes.	When fluids are infused under pressure, IV sites are at higher risk for infiltration.	• Inability to infuse prescribed fluid volume because of loss of vascular access site
4. Assess urine output every 30 to 60 minutes.	Urine output is an indication of end-organ perfusion and the adequacy of fluid resuscitation.	• Urine output: infant, <2 mL/kg/h; child, <1 to 2 mL/kg/h; adolescent, <0.5 mL/kg/h
5. Obtain blood gases and lactic acid studies per prescribing practitioner's order and monitor the results.	Serial monitoring of pH, base deficit (oxygen debt), and lactic acid provides evaluation of the adequacy of resuscitation.	• Progressive or persistent acidosis
6. Obtain hemoglobin and hematocrit studies per prescribing practitioner's order and monitor the results.	Measurements of hemoglobin and hematocrit provide data regarding ongoing blood loss.	• Abnormal hemoglobin or hematocrit results
7. Obtain coagulation studies per prescribing practitioner's order and monitor the results.	Coagulation study results determine the presence of coagulopathy and may herald the development of disseminated intravascular coagulation (DIC).	• Abnormal coagulation results
8. Obtain electrolyte studies per prescribing practitioner's order and monitor the results.	Monitoring the child's potassium level is critical because acidosis is associated with hyperkalemia; hyperchloremia may result from infusion of large volumes of sodium chloride.	• Abnormal electrolyte values

Documentation

- Child and family education
- Type and amount of fluid administered
- Site where fluid was administered
- Intake and output
- Serial evaluation of skin parameters, level of consciousness, and vital signs, including core temperature, at the completion of each fluid bolus
- Evaluation of hemodynamic parameters at the completion of each fluid bolus
- Interventions used to maintain normothermia
- IV insertions
- Serial evaluation of IV sites
- Laboratory results
- Time of reporting and name of prescribing practitioner contacted for reportable conditions
- Unexpected outcomes and related treatment

References

1. Hazinski MF: Cardiovascular disorders. In *Manual of pediatric critical care,* St Louis, 1999, Mosby.
2. Kuhn MA, Groner JI: Fluid resuscitation in the pediatric trauma patient, retrieved February 23, 2004, from http://ahc.pub.com/ahc_root_html_hot/archive/tr092001.html.
3. American Heart Association: Fluid therapy and medications for shock and cardiac arrest. In Hazinski MF, editor: *Pediatric advanced life support provider manual,* Dallas, 2002, American Heart Association.
4. *Hotline fluid warmer: instructions for use,* Rockland, MA
5. Barcelona SL, et al: A comparison of flow rates and warming capabilities of the Level I and Rapid Infusion System with various-size intravenous catheters, *Anesthesia Analgesia* 97:358-363, 2003.
6. Hawkins HS, editor: *Emergency nursing pediatric course provider manual,* ed 3, DesPlaines, IL, 2004, Emergency Nurses Association.
7. McMahon MD: Blood and fluid pressure infusers. In Proehl JA, editor: *Emergency nursing procedures,* ed 3, St Louis, 2004, Saunders.
8. McMahon MD: Blood and fluid warmers. In Proehl JA, editor: *Emergency nursing procedures,* ed 3, St Louis, 2004, Saunders.

Additional Readings

Callow C, Suddaby EC, Slota MC: Cardiovascular system. In Slota MC, editor: *AACN core curriculum for pediatric critical care nursing,* Philadelphia, 1998, Saunders.

Hawkins HS, editor: Shock. In *Emergency nursing pediatric course provider manual,* ed 3, DesPlaines, IL, 2004, Emergency Nurses Association.

Hawkins HS, editor: Medication administration. In *Emergency nursing pediatric course provider manual,* ed 3, DesPlaines, IL, 2004, Emergency Nurses Association.

Schulman CS: Massive infusion devices. In Lynn-McHale Wiegand DJ, Carlson K, editors: *AACN procedure manual for critical care,* ed 5, Philadelphia, 2005, Saunders.

Fluid Calculations: Hydration and Rehydration

P U R P O S E :   Infants and children are at high risk for alterations in fluid and electrolyte balance during times of stress and illness. Knowledge of certain fluid calculations for maintenance and restoration of fluid balance is necessary.

Cecilia Lang and Lauren Sorce

PREREQUISITE KNOWLEDGE

- Fluid and electrolyte management is an essential element of care for the infant or child who is acutely or critically ill.
- Total body fluid composition
  - ❖ Children and adults are different in makeup. Differences in the rate of metabolism and body surface area contribute to differences in fluid management. Total body water percentage for infants and children is 75% to 80%. This percentage decreases slowly with age until adulthood when it is 55% to 60% total body water.[1]
- Intracellular and extracellular fluid composition
  - ❖ Intracellular fluid (ICF) is the largest compartment of total body water (except in neonates, extracellular fluid [ECF] is more than 50% of body weight) and contains all liquid within the cell. The primary electrolytes located in the ICF are potassium and phosphate.
  - ❖ ECF is composed of interstitial fluid, plasma, and transcellular fluids, which are fluids found in the pleural, pericardial, synovial, peritoneal, and joint spaces.[2] ECF contains large volumes of sodium, chloride, and bicarbonate.
- Maintenance of fluid balance
  - ❖ Kidneys are the main system that regulate fluid balance. Imbalances in the kidney can cause disturbances in the respiratory and cardiac systems and in other body systems.

- Principle mechanisms of fluid intake and loss
  - ❖ Fluid intake is achieved mainly through the digestive system with oral intake. In the sick infant or child, fluid intake may additionally be achieved through the administration of intravenous (IV) fluids or blood products. Fluid losses can be from the gastrointestinal (GI) tract (vomiting or diarrhea), surgical wounds or drains, blood loss from trauma or surgical procedures, insensible losses from increased sweating with activity or fever; or respiratory system losses from hyperventilation.
- Fluid volume deficit
  - ❖ Fluid volume deficit is also known as dehydration. Fluid deficits represent a negative balance of total body fluid. Negative balance occurs as a result of fluid loss which may result in shifting electrolytes, third spacing of fluid and lead to ECF deficit. Recognition that fluid volume deficit in infants and children can be reflected as hypovolemia and lead to circulatory collapse if not treated promptly is important.
- Interventions to restore fluid loss
  - ❖ Once fluid volume deficit is diagnosed, identification of the source is imperative to restore fluid balance. Fluid balance can be restored with oral rehydration therapy (ORT) or IV fluid administration. If losses are the result of vomiting or diarrhea and ORT is used, adequate intake of the necessary fluids must be ensured to restore fluid balance. Blood products may be necessary to correct losses from bleeding.

- Assessment of fluid status
  - ❖ Physical assessment of the child to determine fluid balance includes evaluation of vital signs, body system assessment for signs of fluid overload or dehydration (Table 135-1 shows physical assessment findings for dehydration),[3] laboratory values such as specific gravity and electrolytes, significant body weight increases or decreases, and intake and output balance.
- Principles of aseptic technique
- Basic mathematics skills, including addition, subtraction, multiplication, division, and conversion of fractions to decimals and decimals to percentages
- Child development as it relates to clinical assessment and hydration or rehydration

CHILD AND FAMILY ASSESSMENT

- History of fluid imbalance ➠*Rationale:* Previous episodes of fluid imbalance may indicate a chronic problem or ongoing disturbances in metabolic balance.
- Child's developmental level and ability to interact ➠*Rationale:* These factors influence preparation of the child and interaction.
- Child's and family's understanding of fluid balance and the impact of common stressors ➠*Rationale:* Identification of knowledge deficits provides opportunities for education.
- Child's weight for any recent weight loss; ask the family for the child's recent weight ➠*Rationale:* Weight is the basis of fluid calculations in pediatrics and assessments of dehydration.
- History questions

- ❖ Has your child had any recent vomiting and/or diarrhea? How much and for how long?
- ❖ Has the child been urinating as usual? How many wet diapers has the child had in the last 24 hours and do they have an odor to them?
- ❖ Any recent fever? How high was the temperature and for how long was it high?
- ❖ Any recent weight gains or losses?
- ❖ What types of fluids and how much does the child drink on a daily basis?
- ❖ When your child is sick, what types of fluids do you give and how often?
- ❖ ➠*Rationale:* This information assists in assessing factors that may contribute to fluid imbalances and in identification of appropriate therapy.
- Presence and degree of dehydration (see Table 135-1) ➠*Rationale:* This knowledge directs appropriate individualized therapy.
- Signs and symptoms of fluid overload, including respiratory function, which may be impacted by significant fluid overload ➠*Rationale:* Assessment of signs and symptoms directs appropriate individualized therapy.
- Laboratory values for abnormal findings ➠*Rationale:* Identification of abnormal values direct appropriate individualized therapy.
- Abnormal findings that may be part of the child's baseline values, especially in a child who is chronically ill ➠*Rationale:* Establishes the child's usual state of health and facilitates the development of individualized therapy.
- Child's and family's understanding of the reasons for and risks and benefits of the procedure ➠*Rationale:* Evaluates child's and family's understanding of the procedure and provides a gauge for ongoing education.

TABLE 135-1	Clinical Assessment of Severity of Dehydration		
Signs and Symptoms	**Mild Dehydration**	**Moderate Dehydration**	**Severe Dehydration**
Body weight loss	3% to 5%	6% to 9%	10% or more
General appearance and condition			
Infants and young children	Alert, restless	Thirsty, restless, or lethargic; irritable to touch	Lethargic or comatose; limp, cold, sweaty, cyanotic; poor peripheral perfusion
Older children and adults	Thirsty, alert, restless	Thirsty, alert, postural hypotension	Usually conscious; apprehensive; cold, sweaty, cyanotic; wrinkled skin of fingers and toes; muscle cramps
Radial pulse	Normal rate and strength	Rapid and weak	Rapid, feeble, sometimes impalpable
Respiration	Normal	Deep, may be rapid	Deep and rapid
Anterior fontanel	Normal	Sunken	Very sunken
Systolic blood pressure	Normal	Normal or low; orthostatic hypotension	Low, may be unrecordable
Skin elasticity	Pinch retracts immediately	Pinch retracts slowly	Pinch retracts very slowly
Eyes	Normal	Sunken	Grossly sunken
Tears	Present	Reduced to absent	Absent
Mucous membranes	Moist	Dry	Very dry
Urine flow	Normal	Reduced amount and dark	Anuria/severe oliguria
Capillary refill	Normal	±2 seconds	>3 seconds
Estimated fluid deficit (mL/kg)	30 to 50	60 to 90	100 or more

From Greenbaum LA: Deficit therapy. In Berhman RE, et al, editors: *Nelson's textbook of pediatrics*, ed 17, Philadelphia, 2004, Saunders.

- Desire of family members to be present during or participate in the procedure ➻*Rationale:* Family members frequently participate in the administration of ORT and may provide support and comfort to the child during ORT, but they should have the choice not to participate.

CHILD AND FAMILY EDUCATION

Individualized, developmentally appropriate education is provided to the family and to the child based on desire for knowledge, readiness to learn, and overall neurologic and psychosocial state.

- Provide a basic understanding of fluid balance, including mechanisms for fluid losses and replacement of fluid losses with ORT or IV fluid therapy ➻*Rationale:* Providing information decreases anxiety and fear.
- Inform the family that ORT may be used for mild to moderate dehydration and that intravenous fluid (IVF) therapy is used for severe dehydration and in children who are unable to cooperate with adequate enteral intake ➻*Rationale:* Providing information decreases anxiety and fear.
- Inform the family that children have a larger amount of total body water and are more sensitive to changes in the balance of fluids than are adults. Infants and children have nearly 80% of their body composition as water, compared with almost 50% in adults. This difference, along with higher metabolic rates in children when compared with adults, makes children more susceptible to fluid imbalances. ➻*Rationale:* Provides information about risk factors for pediatric dehydration.
- Provide information to the family on signs of fluid loss in children, which may include irritability, cool or cold skin, poor skin turgor, dry mucous membranes (tongue, gums), sunken eyeballs, sunken fontanels (in infants), decreased urine output, or dark colored or malodorous urine (concentrated) ➻*Rationale:* Families who can identify problems related to fluid balance can intervene earlier and help avoid further complications.
- If the family participates in ORT to the infant or child, provide the family with guidelines on the amount of fluid to administer over a specific time period ➻*Rationale:* Facilitates appropriate therapy; involves the family in the child's care and supports the parent's role as a caregiver.
- Encourage questions and answer questions as they arise ➻*Rationale:* Reinforcement of information is needed during periods of stress.

EQUIPMENT

- Stethoscope
- Calculator
- Scale
- ORT solution (as appropriate) and means to measure and deliver fluid
- IV access
- Bag of 0.9% saline solution (NS) or lactated Ringer's (LR) IV fluid and IV tubing to maintain IV patency
- Bag of maintenance IV fluid that contains dextrose and saline per prescribing practitioner's order

Procedure for Fluid Calculations

Steps	Rationale	Considerations
Hydration		
1. Ensure child and family understand procedure and questions are answered.	Evaluates and reinforces understanding of previously taught information.	Developmental level, cognitive ability, and anxiety level determine approach to and effectiveness of teaching.
2. Obtain child's weight with scale.[2,4] *(Level II*)*	Necessary for calculation of fluid requirements.	Ask family the child's usual weight to determine fluid balance. Maintenance fluids should be calculated on basis of "dry" or baseline weight.
3. Assess child for signs and symptoms of fluid overload.	Physical assessment is a key step in the nursing process and identification of abnormal findings. IV fluid rate must be adjusted to less than maintenance in the child who is fluid overloaded.	Assess laboratory values for any abnormal findings. Assess respiratory function which may be impacted by significant fluid overload. Make note of any abnormal findings that may be part of the child's baseline, especially in chronically ill children.

* Level II: Theory-based; no research data to support recommendations; recommendations from expert consensus group may exist

Procedure for Fluid Calculations—*Continued*

Steps	Rationale	Considerations
4. Perform calculation for maintenance fluid requirements with formula from Table 135-2.[4] *(Level II*)*	Ensures correct calculations based on standardized formula. The goal of maintenance fluid administration is prevention of dehydration, electrolyte imbalances, ketoacidosis, and protein degradation.[4]	Example, for a 12-kg child: 1000 mL for the first 10 kg and 50 mL/kg for the additional 2 kg to be given in 24 h = 1000 mL + (50 mL × 2 kg) = 1000 mL + 100 mL = 1100 mL total for 24 h
5. For IV hydration, calculate the hourly IV rate with division of total intake by 24 hours.	Determines hourly rate for administration of IV fluids continuously over 24 hours.	Example: 1100 mL/24 h = 45.8 or 46 mL/h. Maintenance IV fluid is generally composed of dextrose, saline, and potassium.
6. Calculate intake for 24 hours, including total of all enteral, IV, and colloid products.[2,4,5] *(Level II*)*	Accurate documentation and calculation of intake are integral in assessing whether the child is receiving maintenance fluid requirements.	Ask child and family whether any enteral intake was not accounted for in documentation. Ask the family and child to keep track of fluid/food intake and notify nurse of any intake.
7. Calculate output for 24 hours, including all urine, stool, emesis, and drainage collected.	Accurate documentation and calculation of output are essential in assessing if the child is maintaining fluid balance.	Provide child and family with a collection container for any urine or stool and ask them to save specimen so it can be measured and recorded. Ask the family of diapered children to save diapers for measurement and documentation.
8. Calculate child's urine output for 24 hours as mL/kg/h. Divide total urine output by weight in kg then divide by 24 h. Example: 600 mL/10 kg/24 h = 2.5 mL/kg/h.	Total urine output is indicative of fluid volume status. A well-hydrated child should void at least 0.5 to 1.0 mL/kg/h.[2,4] *(Level II*)*	Inaccuracies may result if the calculation includes measurements of diapers that contain urine and stool or if urine or diaper is discarded before evaluation and documentation.

Rehydration

1. Ensure child and family understand procedure and questions are answered.	Evaluates and reinforces understanding of previously taught information.	Developmental level, cognitive ability, and anxiety level determine approach to and effectiveness of teaching.

Procedure continues on following page

* Level II: Theory-based; no research data to support recommendations; recommendations from expert consensus group may exist

TABLE 135-2	Calculation of Maintenance Fluid Requirements	
Body Weight (kg)	**Fluid Requirements for 24 h**	**Hourly Fluid Requirements***
<10	100 mL/kg	4 mL/kg/h
10 to 20	1000 mL + 50 mL/kg for each kg above 10 kg	40 mL/h + 2 mL/kg/h for each kg above 10 kg
>20	1500 mL + 20 mL/kg for each kg above 20 kg	60 mL/h + 1 mL/kg/h for each kg above 20 kg

* Intravenous fluids may also be calculated for an hourly infusion rate with this calculation.
Adapted from Greenbaum LA: Maintenance and replacement therapy. In Berhman RE, et al, editors: *Nelson's textbook of pediatrics,* ed 17, Philadelphia, 2004, Saunders.
Roberts K: Fluid and electrolyte regulation. In Curley M, Moloney-Harmon P, editors: *Critical care nursing of infants and children,* ed 2, Philadelphia, 2001, Saunders.

Procedure   for Fluid Calculations—*Continued*

Steps	Rationale	Considerations
2. With previous steps 2 to 4, calculate the child's baseline fluid requirements.	Evaluation of baseline needs is crucial to delivery of appropriate rehydration therapy.	Note any abnormal physical findings or laboratory values.
3. Calculate the fluid deficit or degree of dehydration.[2-4,6] *(Level II*)*	This classification is useful in management of dehydration. Mild dehydration is 3% to 5% weight loss, moderate dehydration is 6% to 9% weight loss, and severe dehydration is more than 10% weight loss (see Table 135-1).[4]	This calculation should be used in conjunction with clinical assessment of the child to direct treatment.
a. Divide current weight by healthy baseline weight to obtain percentage of weight loss. *(Level II*)*	Percentage of weight loss is used in determining appropriate therapy.	Example: 12-kg child at baseline; admission weight, 10.8 kg: 10.8 ÷ 12 = 0.9 or 90% of usual weight. On occasion, a healthy baseline weight is not available. In these cases, physical examination findings are needed for determination of degree of dehydration (see Table 135-1).[3,6]
b. Subtract the previous percentage from 100%.	Determines percentage of weight loss.	Example: 100% − 90% = 10% weight loss.
c. Each 1% of weight loss corresponds to 10 mL/kg estimated deficit to be replaced.[2,5]	Calculates volume of fluid replacement necessary.	Example: 10% loss in 12-kg child = 10 (% weight loss) × 10 (mL for each percent loss) × 12 kg = 1200 mL fluid deficit to be replaced
4. Mild dehydration may be treated with ORT with delivery of 50 mL/kg of oral rehydration solution given over 4 hours.[4,6] *(Level IV*)*	The child with mild fluid losses may have effective rehydration with oral solutions either by mouth or through an enteral tube. The ORT should be done only with glucose-containing and electrolyte-containing fluids such as Pedialyte or Infalyte because hyponatremia can occur with a large consumption of low-electrolyte or electrolyte-free fluids.[4]	Evaluate the child's ability to tolerate oral/enteral intake; initially small volumes should be given frequently. Amount and rate are increased or decreased based on the clinical appearance of the child and symptoms of diarrhea or emesis.
5. Moderate dehydration may be treated with ORT with 100 mL/kg of oral rehydration solution given over 4 hours.[4,6] *(Level IV*)*	The child with moderate fluid losses may have effective rehydration with oral glucose and electrolyte solutions either by mouth or through an enteral tube.	Evaluate the child's ability to tolerate oral/enteral intake. Amount and rate are increased or decreased on basis of the clinical appearance of the child and symptoms of diarrhea or emesis.
6. When a child has signs of significant fluid volume deficits evidenced by shock, rapid administration of 20 mL/kg fluid bolus with isotonic fluids (NS or LR) is necessary.[2,6,7] Additional boluses may be indicated based on the child's response to the bolus. *(Level II*)*	Fluid boluses given through rapid administration of fluid assist in restoration of the ICF and ECF.[2,6,7]	Initial fluid boluses should be given with large-bore IV access. If IV access cannot be obtained, an intraosseous line may be necessary. The child should never be given a bolus with dextrose because this creates a large dextrose load and potentially leads to an osmotic diuresis.

* Level II: Theory-based; no research data to support recommendations; recommendations from expert consensus group may exist
  Level IV: Limited clinical studies to support recommendations

Procedure for Fluid Calculations—*Continued*		
Steps	**Rationale**	**Considerations**
		Reassessment after each fluid bolus is necessary because additional boluses may be indicated with continued evidence of shock. Assessment for signs and symptoms of fluid overload, such as respiratory distress or auscultation of rales, is important after fluid boluses because some children may not tolerate the excess fluid load.[7] *(Level II*)*
7. After the initial fluid resuscitation bolus, initiate replacement of fluid loss volume over 24 to 72 hours depending on the degree of dehydration.	Fluid resuscitation that occurs too quickly can precipitate seizure activity.[2,5]	Replacement fluids usually contain both dextrose and a percentage of 0.9% saline (example: D5 1/2 NS). Potassium may be added once urine output is adequate. An accurate time check of how long the replacement fluids have been running is imperative to avoid overrehydration or underrehydration rates. Monitoring of electrolytes and renal function is important to assess child's tolerance to fluid therapies.
a. Calculate maintenance IVF rate with steps 2 to 4 in previous Hydration section.	Maintenance fluid must be provided in addition to replacement to prevent further dehydration.	Example: 12-kg child needs 46 mL/h of maintenance IVF.
b. Calculate fluid deficit with steps 3a through c in Rehydration section.	Identifies volume of fluid replacement needed.	Example: 12-kg child with 10% fluid deficit needs 1200 mL replaced.
c. For fluid replacement over a total of 24 hours, half of the total deficit is infused over the first 8 hours. Divide the calculated fluid deficit by 2 to determine the amount to be infused over the first 8 hours. Divide this number by 8 to determine the hourly replacement fluid rate.	Administration of half the deficit over 8 hours helps to prevent potential complications of rapid rehydration.	Example: 1200 ÷ 2 = 600 mL ÷ 8 hr = 75 mL/hr. In hypernatremic dehydration, fluid replacement may be administered over a longer time period to prevent rapid changes in serum sodium.[3] *(Level II*)*
d. Add the hourly IV hydration rate calculated previously to the hourly rate for the first 8 hours of fluid replacement rate calculated in step 7c to obtain the total IV infusion rate for the first 8 hours.[3,6] *(Level II*)*	Maintenance fluids must be given in addition to replacement fluids to prevent further dehydration.	Example: hydration rate 46 mL/hr + replacement rate 75 mL/hr = 121 mL/hr for the first 8 hours.
e. After the 8-hour infusion is completed, calculate the remaining fluid deficit to infuse over the next 16 hours in addition to the hydration fluid rate.[6]	Prevents potential complications of rapid rehydration.	Example: 600 mL/16 hr = 37.5 mL/h replacement rate. Add the hydration rate: 46 mL/hr + replacement rate 37.5 mL/hr = 83.5 mL/hr for the next 16 hours.
8. Once the fluid deficit has been replaced over 24 hours, continue hydration fluid rate.	Fluid deficit has been replaced; additional fluid is no longer necessary.	Example: 46 mL/h.

Procedure continues on following page

* Level II: Theory-based; no research data to support recommendations; recommendations from expert consensus group may exist

Procedure for Fluid Calculations—*Continued*

Steps	Rationale	Considerations
9. Measure, record, and calculate all intake and output.	Accurate measurement, documentation, and calculation of intake and output are integral in assessing child's fluid balance.	Review any additional intake or output with the family and document.
10. Any ongoing excessive losses (enteral tube, stool, drains, etc) may be replaced with IV fluid depending on the clinical condition of the child. The selection of IV fluid is dependent on the composition of the drainage. The ratio of fluid replacement to drainage may vary.[3,6] *(Level II*)*	If ongoing losses are not replaced, output exceeds intake and the child becomes dehydrated.	Documentation and communication to the prescribing practitioner of any significant ongoing losses, such as those from drains, excessive sweat, or respiratory secretions, are important. Ongoing losses are replaced gradually to prevent neurologic complications that may occur with rapid administration of fluids.

* Level II: Theory-based; no research data to support recommendations; recommendations from expert consensus group may exist

Expected Outcomes

- Child's fluid status is in balance with no symptoms of volume deficit or excess
- Intake and output are measured, documented, and calculated accurately
- Maintenance fluids are correctly calculated based on child's weight
- Fluid deficits are correctly calculated and replacement fluids are administered slowly over an appropriate period of time
- Child tolerates administration of fluid bolus if needed
- When ORT is implemented, family understands the basics of ORT

Unexpected Outcomes

- Child is in a state of fluid imbalance with symptoms of excess or deficit
- Incorrect measurement, documentation, or calculation of intake and output
- Child's daily requirements are incorrectly calculated, resulting in underadministration or overadministration of maintenance fluids
- Degree of dehydration incorrectly calculated, resulting in overrehydration or underrehydration
- Fluid deficit replacements are administered too quickly, resulting in neurologic changes or deficits
- Child does not tolerate fluid bolus, which necessitates treatment of volume overload
- Family does not understand the basics of ORT and chooses the wrong rehydration solutions

Monitoring and Care of the Child

Activities and Interventions	Rationale	Reportable Conditions
1. Perform serial physical assessments during administration of hydration or rehydration.	Identifies any abnormalities or physical symptoms of volume overload or dehydration.	• Abnormally high heart rate for age or low blood pressure for age • Weak pulses, poor perfusion, or significant decrease in urine output (e.g., no urine output for 2 hours)
2. Measure, document, and calculate intake and output.	Correct measurement, documentation and calculation of intake and output are integral to complete assessment of fluid status.	• Significant discrepancies between intake and output totals
3. Verify prescribed IV rate is appropriate.	Verifies accurate calculation of maintenance fluid requirement.	• Incorrect IV rate calculation

Monitoring and Care of the Child—Cont'd

Activities and Interventions	Rationale	Reportable Conditions
4. Monitor child's response to fluid boluses and assess need for further boluses.	Monitors child's response to treatment and identifies need for further intervention.	• Assessment and vital signs indicate need for further fluid boluses • Assessment and vital signs indicate child did not tolerate fluid bolus
5. Monitor child's response to administration of replacement fluids; obtain weight as part of the assessment.	Monitors child's response to treatment. Increase in weight indicates replacement of fluid losses.	• No improvement in assessment or vital signs after administration of replacement fluids • No increase in weight after administration of replacement fluids
6. Monitor status of IV access throughout IV fluid bolus and replacement administration. 7. Obtain laboratory studies per prescribing practitioner's order and monitor results.	Facilitates prompt recognition of IV infiltration and prevents significant tissue injury. Assesses response to therapy; identifies abnormalities that need further treatment.	• IV infiltration that results in compromise of circulation to the involved extremity • Abnormal laboratory values • Inability to obtain ordered laboratory studies

Documentation

- Child's weight on presentation and after rehydration
- Initial physical assessment and physical assessment after fluid administration
- Intake and output, including type and volume of fluids administered
- Assessment of IV access before and after fluid bolus administration
- Child's response to fluid bolus administration
- Laboratory studies obtained and results
- Child and family education
- Unexpected outcomes and related treatment

References

1. Bowden VR, Greenberg CS: Principles of fluid and nutritional management. *Pediatric nursing procedures,* Philadelphia, 2003, Lippincott, Williams & Wilkins.
2. Roberts K: Fluid and electrolyte regulation. In Curley M, Moloney-Harmon P, editors: *Critical care nursing of infants and children,* ed 2, Philadelphia, 2001, Saunders.
3. Greenbaum LA: Deficity therapy. In Berhman RE, et al, editors: *Nelson's textbook of pediatrics,* ed 17, Philadelphia, 2004, Saunders.
4. Greenbaum LA: Maintenance and replacement therapy. In Berhman RE, Kliegman RM, Jonson HB, editors: *Nelson's textbook of pediatrics,* ed 17, Philadelphia, 2004, Saunders.
5. Roberts KB: Fluid and electrolytes: parenteral fluid therapy, *Pediatr Rev* 22:380-387, 2001.
6. Stone B: Fluids and electrolytes. In Robertson J, Shilkofski N, editors: *The Harriet Lane handbook,* ed 17, Philadelphia, 2005, Mosby.
7. Fluid therapy and medications for shock and cardiac arrest. In Hazinski MF, editor: *PALS provider manual,* Dallas, 2002, American Heart Association.

Additional Readings

D'Angio B: Fluid and electrolyte balance in the pediatric patient, *J Intravenous Nurs* 21:153-159, 1998.

Spandorfer PR, et al: Oral versus intravenous rehydration of moderately dehydrated children: a randomized, controlled trial, *Pediatrics* 115(2):295-301, 2005.

Transfusion Reaction: Management

PURPOSE: To promptly recognize and address blood transfusion reactions to reduce potential morbidity and mortality. Appropriate treatment necessitates identification of the type of reaction that has occurred.

Joyce Weishaar

PREREQUISITE KNOWLEDGE

- Blood transfusion reactions can be acute hemolytic, febrile nonhemolytic, or anaphylactic.[1-8]
  - *Acute hemolytic reactions* are typically associated with ABO incompatibility and can cause significant morbidity and mortality. Fever is the most common symptom, accompanied by chills, rigor, lumbar pain, nausea and vomiting, hematuria, chest pain, and anxiety. A severe reaction can lead to shock, acute tubular necrosis, and disseminated intravascular coagulation (DIC). Blood transfusions are typically started at a slow rate to limit the amount of cells infused in case of an acute hemolytic reaction. The rate can be increased after 15 minutes.
  - *Febrile nonhemolytic reactions* are typically caused by antileukocyte antibodies. More recent evidence points to the mediation of bioreactive substances created by leukocytes during blood storage. These reactions are rarely serious and tend to occur in children who have had multiple transfusions. Fever and chills are the most common symptoms of a reaction and can occur during or a few hours after a transfusion. Blood may be given through a leukocyte filter or be leukocyte reduced in the blood bank to prevent febrile nonhemolytic reactions.
  - *Anaphylactic reactions* are rare and can be life threatening. They occur in children with immunoglobulin A (IgA) deficiency with development of IgA antibodies.

Severe gastrointestinal symptoms and shock can occur after infusion of only a few milliliters of blood. Transient hypertension is followed by severe hypotension. Chills and flushing may also be present, but fever is not usually a symptom. The use of washed red cells is a preventive measure for anaphylactic reactions.
  - *Urticarial or allergic reactions* are rarely serious and are characterized by hives. The transfusion may not need termination, but antihistamines may be given.
- The leading cause of transfusion-related deaths in the United States is transfusion error; the second leading cause is bacterial sepsis from contaminated blood components.[6]
  - Platelets are the most likely blood component to have bacterial contamination; risk of infection from platelets is three times higher than that of other blood components.[1,6]
- All transfusion-related adverse events must be reported to the blood bank. Deaths that occur as a result of a complication of a blood transfusion must be reported to the US Food and Drug Administration (FDA) Center for Biologics Evaluation and Research.[1]
- While not a transfusion reaction, transfusion-related acute lung injury (TRALI) is an immunologic complication of blood component administration.[1,6] Symptoms are similar to those of acute respiratory distress syndrome and generally occur within six hours of transfusion. TRALI is not common in children.
- Mastery of pediatric advanced life support techniques

CHILD AND FAMILY ASSESSMENT

- Child's history of previous transfusions and any reactions that have occurred. If a history of transfusion reaction is found, identify the medications routinely given for prevention. ➤➤*Rationale:* Previous transfusions may predispose the child to transfusion reactions. The child may need pretransfusion medications to prevent a reaction.
- Child's developmental level and ability to interact ➤➤*Rationale:* These factors influence interaction and child's reaction to the event.
- Physical assessment of the child ➤➤*Rationale:* An ongoing assessment of the child is necessary after the transfusion is discontinued to evaluate for further symptoms or the need for intervention.
- Child's and family's understanding of the reasons for and risks and benefits of the procedure ➤➤*Rationale:* Evaluates child's and family's understanding of the transfusion reaction and provides a gauge for ongoing education.

CHILD AND FAMILY EDUCATION

Individualized, developmentally appropriate education is provided to the family and to the child based on desire for knowledge, readiness to learn, and overall neurologic and psychosocial state.

- Explain to child and family that the symptoms the child has may be from a reaction to the transfusion. Assure the child and family that medications will be given to allevi-

ate the symptoms. ➤➤*Rationale:* Providing information and assurance that medications will be provided may decrease anxiety and fear of both child and family.
- Explain that blood samples and a urine sample will be sent to the laboratory for analysis to confirm the occurrence of a reaction ➤➤*Rationale:* Providing information reduces fear and anxiety.
- Explain to child and family any change in treatment necessary as a result of the transfusion reaction ➤➤*Rationale:* Providing information decreases anxiety and fear.
- Encourage questions and answer questions as they arise ➤➤*Rationale:* Reinforcement of information is needed during periods of stress.

EQUIPMENT

- Institution-specific transfusion reaction form
- Bag of 0.9% saline solution (NS) and intravenous (IV) tubing to maintain IV patency
- Appropriate biohazard container to send blood component and tubing to the blood bank and specimens to the appropriate laboratory
- Appropriate equipment to draw blood and obtain a urine sample
- Two specimen tubes for laboratory: one plain tube and one ethylenediamine tetraacetic acid (EDTA) tube
- Appropriate specimen container for urine specimen
- Specimen labels that contain two patient identifiers; specific labels may be necessary per institution-specific protocols
- Clean gloves

Procedure | for Transfusion Reaction: Management

Steps	Rationale	Considerations
1. Wash hands; put on clean gloves.	Standard precautions; reduces the transmission of microorganisms.	
2. If a transfusion reaction is suspected, stop the transfusion; remove and save blood bag and tubing.	Quick recognition and discontinuation of blood may limit the amount of cells transfused and reduce adverse events from the transfusion.	If urticaria and itching are the only symptoms, the transfusion can possibly continue. Slow or temporarily stop the transfusion and notify the prescribing practitioner.[2]
3. Hang NS with fresh tubing and connect to child's IV access.[1] (Level II*)	IV access must be maintained for emergency medications and infusion of fluid boluses.	Fresh tubing must be used so that any cells left in the infusion tubing are not administered to the child.[1]
4. Immediately notify prescribing practitioner of the transfusion reaction. (Level II*)	The prescribing practitioner assesses the child and orders further intervention as necessary.	Acute hemolytic transfusion reactions and severe anaphylactic reactions need immediate intervention to maintain child's hemodynamic stability.[3,5]

Procedure continues on following page

* Level II: Theory-based; no research data to support recommendations; recommendations from expert consensus group may exist

Procedure for Transfusion Reaction: Management—*Continued*

Steps	Rationale	Considerations
5. Assess the child's vital signs, respiratory condition, and urine output.	Early recognition of the signs and symptoms of shock or respiratory distress facilitates early intervention.	Acute hemolytic transfusion reactions can lead to acute tubular necrosis and DIC.[8]
6. Compare the blood component container, blood band tag, and child's identification band to check for clerical errors. *(Level II*)*	Verifies the correct identity of the child and the blood products; reconfirms the ABO type of both. Clerical errors account for most acute hemolytic transfusion reactions.[1,5,6]	Transfusion of ABO incompatible red blood cells is the most dangerous and most preventable of immediate reactions.[5]
7. Provide the child and family with information about the possible transfusion reaction; reassure the child and family that appropriate interventions are being implemented.	Prompt action and reassurance decrease anxiety. Most reactions are not life threatening.	Acute hemolytic reactions cause extreme anxiety and a sense of impending doom in patients.
8. Draw blood from child and fill plain and EDTA vials according to institution-specific protocol. Label specimens at the bedside and place in appropriate containers for transport to the blood bank. *(Level II*)*	The clotted sample is used for recross matching with the donor blood; the EDTA sample is used for a direct Coombs' test (DCT) and an estimation of free plasma hemoglobin.[2] Labeling of specimens at the bedside promotes patient safety. *(Level II*)*	If free plasma hemoglobin is not detected and DCT results are negative, then acute hemolytic reaction is unlikely.[2] Drawing the sample from a site other than the access used for the blood transfusion is preferred.[1] *(Level II*)*
9. Complete appropriate blood bank transfusion reaction form and other institution-specific paperwork as required.	Blood bank transfusion reaction form must be initiated and sent with the samples and donor blood to the blood bank.	The transfusion reaction form is reviewed by the blood bank medical director.
10. Place donor blood and tubing in biohazard container. Send to blood bank for evaluation, along with blood specimens drawn from the child.[1] *(Level II*)*	Blood, blood container, and tubing are evaluated by blood bank as part of the investigation.	
11. Obtain urine specimen. Label specimen at the bedside and place in appropriate container; send to the laboratory.[1,2] *(Level II*)*	Fresh urine is examined for hemoglobin, an important sign of acute hemolytic transfusion reaction.[2]	Blood may be evident in the first voided sample after the event.
12. Provide supportive care as prescribed for acute hemolytic reactions[7]: Fluid boluses may be ordered. Low-dose dopamine and diuretics may be used to maintain urine output. Blood products may be needed to support clotting if DIC is present.	Management is directed toward treatment and prevention of shock, acute tubular necrosis, and DIC.	Rapid response may be necessary to maintain stability of child.
13. Provide supportive care as prescribed for febrile nonhemolytic reactions:[2,7]	Treatment is directed toward alleviation of symptoms.	If bacterial contamination is suspected, blood cultures may be sent.

* Level II: Theory-based; no research data to support recommendations; recommendations from expert consensus group may exist

Procedure **for Transfusion Reaction: Management**—*Continued*

Steps	Rationale	Considerations
Antipyretics may be prescribed for fever. If reaction is moderate to severe, antihistamines or hydrocortisone may be prescribed.		
14. Provide supportive care as ordered for anaphylactic reactions:[3,7] IV epinephrine may be necessary for poor tissue perfusion. Fluid resuscitation may be necessary for shock. Steroids may be ordered for alleviation of symptoms.	Treatment is directed toward treatment of shock and alleviation of symptoms.	Rapid response may be necessary to maintain stability of child.
15. Provide supportive care as ordered for urticaria and allergic reactions.[3,5] Antihistamines may be ordered for reduction in symptoms.	Alleviates symptoms.	Transfusion may be restarted at a lower rate of infusion after treatment with antihistamines.
16. Discard used supplies and equipment, including sharps, in appropriate receptacles.	Standard precautions; reduces transmission of microorganisms. Protects personnel health.	
17. Remove gloves; wash hands.	Standard precautions.	

Expected Outcomes

- Symptoms of transfusion reaction are promptly identified
- Symptoms of transfusion reaction subside
- Child has no adverse sequelae as a result of the reaction

Unexpected Outcomes

- Delay in recognition of symptoms of transfusion reaction
- Symptoms do not improve or symptoms progress
- Symptoms of shock, including DIC
- Renal failure from acute tubular necrosis

Monitoring and Care of the Child

Activities and Interventions	Rationale	Reportable Conditions
1. Closely monitor vital signs; obtain full assessment of child, including assessment of perfusion and respiratory assessment.	Signs and symptoms of shock may occur as a result of acute hemolytic or severe anaphylactic transfusion reaction.	• Persistent signs of shock: poor skin perfusion, mottling, cool extremities, tachycardia, tachypnea, decreased level of consciousness, hypotension • Respiratory distress
2. Monitor urine output.	Decreased urine output can be a sign of acute tubular necrosis, a result of an acute hemolytic transfusion reaction.	• Urine output of less than 1 mL/kg/h • Blood in urine
3. Reassure child if further transfusion is necessary.	Reassurance decreases anxiety from fear of reoccurrence of reaction.	• If transfusion is in progress, severe anxiety and a sense of impending doom (in the older child or adolescent) can be a sign of a hemolytic transfusion reaction
4. Monitor child's response to therapy for the transfusion reaction.	Monitors for appropriate response to therapy.	• No improvement in child's condition after administration of prescribed therapy

Documentation

- Detailed documentation of child's symptoms
- Notification of prescribing practitioner
- Discontinuation of the transfusion and initiation of NS infusion to keep IV line patent
- Child and family education related to transfusion reaction
- Therapy initiated for transfusion reaction management
- Required blood work; donor blood and tubing sent to the blood bank
- Urine specimen sent to the laboratory
- Completion of the blood bank transfusion reaction form
- Unexpected outcomes and related treatment

References

1. American Association of Blood Banks, America's Blood Centers and the American Red Cross: *Circular of information for the use of human blood and blood components,* Bethesda, MD, 2002, American Association of Blood Banks.
2. Bansal D: Transfusion reactions, *Indian J Pediatr* 68: 133-139, 2001.
3. Brinker D, Moloney-Harmon PA: Hematologic critical care problems. In Curley MAQ, Moloney-Harmon PA, editors: *Critical care nursing of infants and children,* ed 2, Philadelphia, 2001, Saunders.
4. Bryan S: Hemolytic transfusion reaction: safeguards for practice, *J Perianesth Nurs* 17:399-403, 2002.
5. Logue G: Adverse reactions to blood transfusions. In Rakel R, Bope E, editors: *Conn's current therapy 2004,* ed 56, Philadelphia, 2004, Elsevier.
6. Quirolo KC: Transfusion medicine for the pediatrician, *Pediatr Clin North Am* 49(6):1211-1238, 2000.
7. Szymanski IO: Transfusion therapy in general practice. In Noble J, et al, editors: *Textbook of primary care medicine,* ed 3, St. Louis, 2001, Mosby.
8. Wu YY, Snyder EL: Transfusion reactions. In Hoffman R, et al, editors: *Hematology: basic principles and practice,* ed 3, New York, 2000, Churchill Livingstone, Inc.

Additional Reading

Domen RE: Allergic transfusion reactions: an evaluation of 273 consecutive reactions, *Arch Pathol Lab Med* 127:316-320, 2003.

PROCEDURE **137**

Arterial Catheter: Insertion Assist and Management

P U R P O S E : Arterial pressure lines are used to continuously monitor blood pressure, titrate vasoactive agents, and facilitate blood sampling or other laboratory specimens in children with severe cardiorespiratory disease

Marisa Mize

PREREQUISITE KNOWLEDGE

- Anatomy and physiology of the vascular system and its adjacent structures
- Principles of hemodynamic monitoring
- Principles of aseptic technique
- Principles of pressure transducer systems: refer to Procedure 63 for information on this topic.
    - ❖ Conditions or needs that warrant the use of arterial pressure monitoring include the following:
        - ○ Hypertension, hypotension, or labile blood pressure[1]
        - ○ Use of vasoactive agents such as vasopressors, vasodilators, or cardioactive drugs[1]
        - ○ Monitoring for effect of transient or intermittent dysrhythmias on blood pressure[1]
        - ○ Need to obtain frequent arterial blood gases for ventilation management or other laboratory studies without pain or discomfort to child[1]
    - ❖ Potential complications of invasive arterial monitoring

CHILD AND FAMILY ASSESSMENT

- Child's developmental level ➥*Rationale:* These factors influence preparation and interaction.
- Family's desire to be present during procedure ➥*Rationale:* Family may provide support and comfort measures to their child but should have the choice not to remain with the child.
- History of diabetes, hypertension, arterial vasospasm, thrombosis, embolism, heparin-induced thrombocytopenia (HIT) or heparin sensitivity, or allergy ➥*Rationale:* Presence of these conditions can cause complications in the extremity. If known heparin sensitivity, allergy or history of HIT, avoid use of heparin in line.
- Recent history, evaluating for prolonged bleeding or abnormal bruising. Assess the child for signs of oral, gastric, or rectal bleeding, hematomas, petechiae or oozing of blood from puncture sites. Refer to recent coagulation and platelet counts, if available ➥*Rationale:* Insertion of arterial line may be contraindicated in children with coagulopathy. Administration of blood products such as fresh frozen plasma, cryoprecipitate, or platelets may be indicated before insertion.
- Specific neurovascular and peripheral vascular assessment of the extremity to be used for arterial cannulation, including color, temperature, presence and fullness of pulses, capillary refill, and motor and sensory function (as compared with opposite extremity). *Note*: A modified Allen test is performed before cannulation of a radial or ulnar artery. Refer to Procedure 151 for information on performing an Allen test ➥*Rationale:* This test identifies any circulatory or neurovascular impairment before cannulation to avoid potential complications.

CHILD AND FAMILY EDUCATION

Individualized, developmentally appropriate education is provided to the family and to the child based on desire for knowledge, readiness to learn, and overall neurologic and psychosocial state.

- Provide information about the arterial line, including insertion procedure, use of monitor alarms, need for immobility of the extremity, and expected time catheter will be in place ➥*Rationale:* Providing information decreases anxiety and fear.
- Educate the family on procedure and possible complications as well as the actions taken to prevent complications ➥*Rationale:* The family is provided with information about and indications for procedures performed on their child, allowing informed consent.
- Explain to the family and child (if appropriate) that medications will be used to keep the child comfortable during the procedure, which may include local anesthetics, anxiolytics, and/or pain medications ➥*Rationale:* Providing information decreases anxiety and fear.
- If developmentally appropriate, explain how child can participate in the insertion of the arterial line (keeping extremity immobile) ➥*Rationale:* Providing information decreases anxiety and fear, and promotes compliance.
- Explain that the extremity must remain immobile during catheter insertion and while the catheter remains in place ➥*Rationale:* Providing information decreases anxiety and fear, and promotes compliance.
- Explain the need for the family and/or child to report any warmth, redness, pain, or wet sensation at insertion site at any time ➥*Rationale:* These sensations may indicate infection, bleeding, or disconnection of tubing.

- Encourage questions and answer questions as they arise ➥*Rationale:* Reinforcing information is needed during periods of stress.

EQUIPMENT

- If radial artery is used, appropriate-sized armboard, tape, and small roll for below wrist
- If femoral artery is used, towel or blanket to place below hips
- 2% chlorhexidine, 10% povidone-iodine or 70% alcohol based on institution-specific protocol for site preparation
- Sterile towels, sterile gloves, mask, surgical hat, sterile gown, and eye protection
- Sterile gauze pads
- Tape
- 1% lidocaine solution without epinephrine
- Appropriate-sized safety cannula over needle or procedure tray with appropriate-sized catheter over guidewire
- Syringes
- Hemodynamic monitoring system: pressure device, flush bag or syringe and syringe pump, pressurized tubing, transducer, monitor cable, and monitor
- 0.9% saline solution with heparin 1 to 3 units/mL per institution-specific protocol; papaverine, if ordered
- Suture (3.0 or 4.0 silk, needle driver may be required) or other securement device such as StatLock
- Scalpel handle and blade (if using sutures for securement)
- Additional equipment needed may include:
  - ❖ Armboard
  - ❖ Transparent or semipermeable dressing
  - ❖ Bath towel

Procedure | for Arterial Catheter: Insertion Assist and Management

Steps	Rationale	Considerations
1. Ensure that child and family understand procedure and questions are answered.	Evaluates and reinforces understanding of previously taught information.	Developmental level, cognitive ability and anxiety level will determine approach to and effectiveness of teaching.
2. Wash hands.	Standard precautions; reduces transmission of microorganisms.	
3. Assemble all equipment.	Having all materials present facilitates completion of procedure without delays.	
4. A modified Allen test should be preformed if catheter is to be inserted in the radial or ulnar artery. The posterior tibial and dorsalis pedis arteries should be	Assesses adequacy of collateral blood flow of extremity to be cannulated.	If a vascular prosthesis (e.g., hemodialysis fistula) is present in an extremity, do not place arterial catheter in that extremity.

Procedure for Arterial Catheter: Insertion Assist and Management—*Continued*		
Steps	**Rationale**	**Considerations**
assessed using a similar technique to evaluate collateral blood flow in the lower extremity, if either of these sites is to be used.[2] *(Level II*)*		
5. Obtain premixed infusion solution from pharmacy or prepare the infusion solution using aseptic technique. Heparin (1 to 3 units/mL) or papaverine (60 mg/500mL) may be added to the infusate if their use is not contraindicated.[3, 5] *(Level IV*)*	Heparinized saline flush improves the length of time catheters remain patent (up to 72 hours).[3] *(Level V*)* Standardized solutions prepared in the hospital pharmacy promote patient safety. Dextrose supports the growth of microorganisms. Use of dextrose solutions has been associated with infection.[3] *(Level VI*)*	Bag or syringe should be free from air. Follow institution-specific protocol in determining the amount of heparin added per milliliter of flush solution (usually 1-3 units/mL). No fluids other than 0.25%, 0.45%, or 0.9% sodium chloride solution may be infused through an arterial line. Heparin may prevent clot formation and papaverine may prevent arterial spasm. Use of heparin is contraindicated in children with HIT or heparin allergy.[3] Papaverine is contraindicated in neonates and children with increased intracranial pressure because it causes cerebral blood vessels to dilate, potentially aggravating intracranial hypertension or intracranial bleed.

6. Prepare the arterial line tubing set:
   Check and secure all luer-lok tubing connections.
   Connect the prepared arterial line tubing setup to the flush solution.
   Prime the line slowly, eliminating all bubbles from system.
	Removal of air from solution bag or syringe decreases risk of infusing air into the child's arterial system. This is especially critical in mixed-lesion cardiac patients.
	Air bubbles can be avoided by moving fluid through the tubing slowly and steadily. Air bubbles may cause errors in blood pressure readings.[4] *(Level V*)*
		Consider using a closed tubing system with an in-line blood discard reservoir, which may reduce the risk of hospital-acquired anemia.

7. Attach the tubing and transducer apparatus to the monitor.	Necessary for pressure readings and waveform to be displayed on the monitor.	Tubing that is wide bore, high pressure, and short (no more than 48 inches), with minimal use of stopcocks is optimal for reducing distortion of the signal to the monitor.[4] *(Level VI*)*
Assisting with Insertion 1. Unless situation is emergent, ensure that informed consent has been obtained.	Informed consent is required for all invasive procedures.	Informed consent documentation is institution specific.
2. Wash hands, put on gloves and eye protection.	Reduces transmission of microorganisms. Standard precautions are implemented because blood spray is possible.	

Procedure continues on following page

---

* Level II: Theory based, no research data to support recommendations: recommendations from expert consensus group may exist
Level IV: Limited clinical studies to support recommendations
Level V: Clinical studies in more than one or two patient populations and situations to support recommendations
Level VI: Clinical studies in a variety of patient populations and situations to support recommendations

Procedure for Arterial Catheter: Insertion Assist and Management—*Continued*

Steps	Rationale	Considerations
3. Ensure hemodynamic monitoring system is prepared and easily accessible.	Allows rapid display of waveform and activation of monitoring and disconnect alarms, which promotes patient safety.	
4. Conduct final patient verification process (e.g., timeout).	Confirms correct patient, procedure, and site, as recommended by the Joint Commission on Accreditation of Healthcare Organizations (JCAHO).	Use active communication techniques.
5. Ensure appropriate cardio-respiratory monitoring.	Sedation or anxiolytic medication, which can cause respiratory depression or hypotension, may be needed to promote successful completion of procedure.	Ensure that the alarms are activated with appropriate settings and are sufficiently audible.
6. Place child's extremity in the appropriate position with adequate lighting of insertion site.	Prepares site for cannulation, allows adequate visualization, and facilitates accurate insertion.	A soft cotton or gauze roll may be placed under the wrist and the hand may be placed on an armboard to facilitate proper positioning for radial artery cannulation. A towel roll may be placed under the hip to facilitate positioning for femoral artery cannulation.
7. Immobilize extremity during catheter insertion.	Facilitates insertion; may prevent needle from lacerating vessel wall during insertion.	Sedation may be required. Institution- or unit-specific policy for procedural sedation should be implemented as appropriate. A second person may be needed to help the child tolerate the procedure.
8. Assist with catheter placement.	Providing supplies and equipment as needed facilitates successful catheter placement.	
9. When catheter is positioned, connect flush system tubing with luer connection to arterial catheter.	Luer connection provides secure attachment, decreasing likelihood of inadvertent disconnection. Fluid-filled system is required for signal to be transmitted to monitor via transducer.	T-connector with luer connection may be used to decrease tension on catheter because pediatric arterial cannulas are often short. Catheter must be held in place until secured.
10. Observe waveform; refer to Figure 137-1 for components of the arterial waveform.	Ensures arterial tracing.	
11. Assist with securing catheter in place. Catheter may be sutured in place at the discretion of the individual placing the catheter.	Short catheters are at risk of becoming dislodged until secured.	Sutureless (e.g., StatLock) secure-ment devices can be advantageous over suture in preventing catheter-related bloodstream infections.[2] *(Level IV*)*
12. When the catheter is secured, apply a sterile gauze, transparent, or semipermeable dressing.[2]	Provides sterile environment; reduces infection.	Refer to institution-specific protocol for dressing the arterial line.
13. Apply armboard, if necessary, for medical immobilization.	Ensures correct position of extremity for optimal waveform.	Child's developmental level and ability to cooperate should be considered when using medical immobilization.

* Level IV: Limited clinical studies to support recommendations

Procedure for Arterial Catheter: Insertion Assist and Management—*Continued*

Steps	Rationale	Considerations

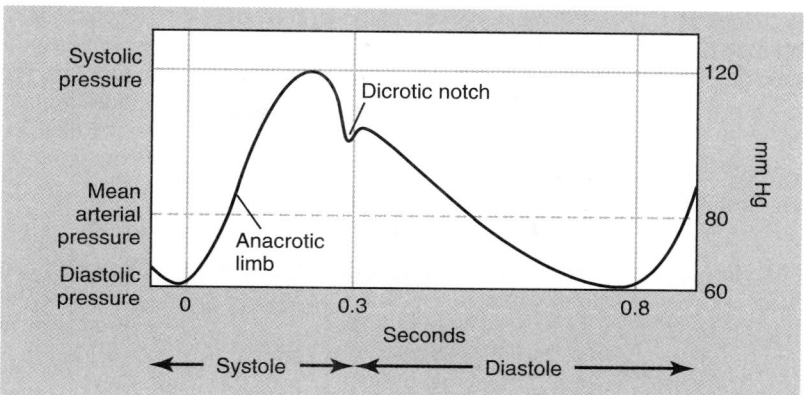

FIGURE 137-1   Components of the Arterial Waveform.

Steps	Rationale	Considerations
14. Level and zero the transducer at the phlebostatic axis (Figure 137-2).	Ensures accurate pressure readings.	Location of transducer may vary from institution to institution. Refer to institution-specific protocol.

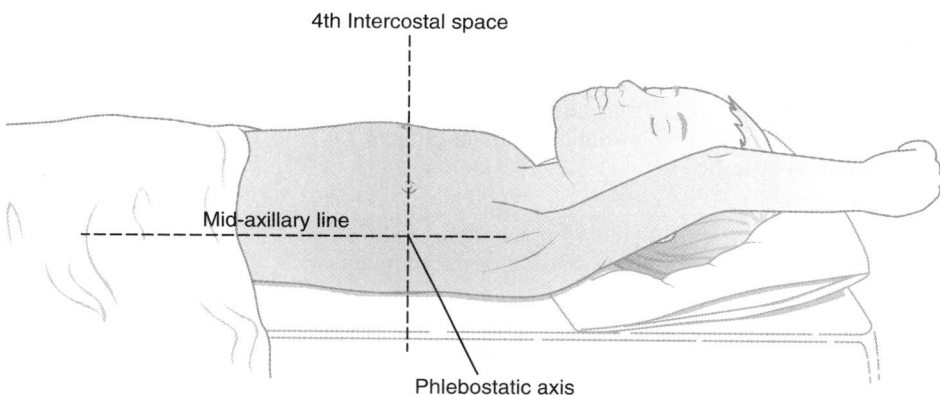

FIGURE 137-2   Locating the phlebostatic axis, which approximates the location of the right atrium. For a child in the supine position, locate the intersection of two imaginary lines, one drawn from the fourth intercostal space at the sternum toward the axilla and one drawn horizontally down the anterior axillary line. For a child in the lateral position, locate the intersection of two imaginary lines, one drawn horizontally down the sternum and one drawn vertically down the fourth intercostal space.

Steps	Rationale	Considerations
15. Set alarm parameters based on child's current blood pressure or notification parameters.	Appropriately set alarms to allow detection of inadvertent disconnection, pulseless electrical activity, significant changes in vital signs, catheter malfunction, or inadvertent catheter removal.	Ensure that the alarms are activated with appropriate settings and are sufficiently audible.
16. Evaluate extremity distal to insertion site.	Ensure adequate circulation distal to catheter placement.	
17. Discard used equipment and supplies in appropriate container: wash hands.	Standard precautions.	Ensure that all sharps are disposed of in appropriate container.

Procedure for Arterial Line Dressing Change

Steps	Rationale	Considerations
1. Frequency of dressing change is determined by dressing material used and institution-specific protocol.	Prevents infection at insertion site.	Replace the dressing if the catheter is replaced; routinely per institution-specific protocol; when the dressing becomes damp, loosened, or soiled; or if visualization of the site is required.[3]
2. Wash hands and put on clean gloves.	Reduces transmission of micro-organisms; standard precautions.	
3. Carefully remove old dressings.	Prevents inadvertent dislodgement of catheter.	A second person may be needed to help the child tolerate the procedure and to immobilize the child.
4. Observe for signs of infection, leaking at the site, presence of hematoma, kinks in catheter at exit site.	Allows identification and appropriate management of potential complications.	
5. Clean site using 2% chlorhexidine, 10% povidone-iodine, or 70% alcohol per institution-specific protocol and considering age of child.[2] Using friction, scrub site back and forth. Allow solution to dry. (*Level V**)	Reduces cutaneous colonization of microorganisms at the insertion site. Antimicrobial solutions must air-dry for maximum effectiveness.	Do not remove chlorhexidine or povidone-iodine solution from skin.[2] No guidelines have been established for use of 2% chlorhexidine in children less than 2 months of age.[2]
6. Replace transparent dressing over site, or alternate dressing recommended per institution-specific protocol.	Transparent dressing allows for visual assessment of site.	
7. Discard used supplies and equipment appropriately. Wash hands.	Standard precautions; reduces transmission of microorganisms.	

* Level V: Clinical studies in more than one or two patient populations and situations to support recommendations

Procedure for Removal of an Arterial Catheter

Steps	Rationale	Considerations
1. Check child's most recent platelet count.	Hemostasis may be difficult to achieve in the child with a low platelet count.	
2. Collect all necessary equipment and supplies.	Preparation and having all materials present facilitates completion of procedure in a timely manner.	A second person may be needed to help the child tolerate the procedure.
3. Explain procedure to child and family, including how child can assist in the procedure if appropriate, and need to hold pressure for at least 5 minutes.	Decreases anxiety and promotes cooperation.	Explanation should be tailored to the child's developmental level.
4. Wash hands and put on clean gloves and eye protection.	Standard precautions; reduces transmission of microorganisms.	If appropriate, refer to institution-specific protocol regarding removal of arterial catheters that have been sutured in or from sites other than radial artery.

Procedure | for Removal of an Arterial Catheter—*Continued*

Steps	Rationale	Considerations
5. Turn off continuous infusion and monitoring alarms.	Prevents false alarms.	Once the alarm has been deactivated, remain in the room until the catheter has been removed.
6. Carefully remove dressing.	Allows visualization of site before catheter removal.	
7. Remove sutures or other securement device.	Required for catheter removal.	Suture removal may be very threatening for some children. Encourage family support during this process.
8. Cover the site with a sterile gauze pad and briskly withdraw the catheter.	Prevents splashing of blood.	
9. Immediately apply firm pressure with sterile gauze over the insertion site.	Prevents bleeding and hematoma formation.	
10. Continue to apply pressure for at least 5 minutes for radial or ulnar artery.	Achieves hemostasis.	Duration of application of direct pressure is often increased before hemostasis is achieved in children receiving systemic heparin or thrombolytics, or those with catheters in large arteries (i.e., femoral).[3]
11. When hemostasis has been achieved, apply a pressure dressing to the site. Do not apply tape completely around the extremity.	Pressure dressing helps prevent rebleeding.	Tape that completely encircles the extremity and is applied tightly may cause ischemia of extremity.
12. Discard used supplies and equipment appropriately. Wash hands.	Standard precautions.	Ensure sharps are disposed of in an appropriate container.
13. Monitor site.	Evaluates for ongoing bleeding and vascular compromise.	Validates adequate peripheral circulation and neurovascular integrity. Changes in pulse, color, temperature, or capillary refill may indicate ischemia, arterial spasm, or neurovascular compromise.

Expected Outcomes

- Minimal discomfort at catheter insertion site
- Hemoglobin and hematocrit levels remain stable
- Adequate perfusion to the extremity where the catheter is placed

- Insertion site remains free from infection

- Adequate sensory/motor function of the extremity
- System remains secure and catheter remains in place until electively removed
- Able to withdraw blood from the catheter without difficulty

Unexpected Outcomes

- Pain or discomfort at catheter insertion site
- Decreased hemoglobin and hematocrit
- Impaired peripheral tissue perfusion of the extremity in which the catheter is located; edema, coolness, pain, paleness, or slow capillary refill of fingers or toes of cannulated extremity
- Signs of infection at the insertion site, including redness, warmth, edema, drainage
- Fever or increased white blood cell count
- Impaired sensory or motor function of the extremity
- Catheter disconnection with significant blood loss
- Inadvertent catheter removal
- Unable to draw blood from catheter

Monitoring and Care of the Child

Activities and Interventions	Rationale	Reportable Conditions
1. Monitor the extremity where the catheter is inserted on an hourly basis for indications of adequate perfusion distal to the catheter insertion site and appropriate neurovascular function.	Complications of arterial cannulation may include ischemia, arterial spasm, or neurovascular compromise.[3]	• Decreased or absent pulses • Pain or alteration in sensation of the extremity • Decreased motor function of the extremity • Change in warmth or color of the extremity or prolonged capillary refill time • Blanching of the extremity when catheter is flushed
2. Ensure monitor alarm limits are set appropriately, functioning properly, and audible at all times.	Promotes patient safety by providing notification of system disconnect, inadvertent catheter removal, changes in vital signs, and other potentially hazardous situations.	
3. Monitor waveform continuously for under- or overdamping (Figure 137-3).	An optimally damped system is necessary in order to display an adequate waveform with accurate blood pressure readings.[3] Overdamping should be assessed immediately to ensure waveform accuracy and to prevent clotting of the catheter.	Overdamped or underdamped waveform that cannot be corrected with trouble shooting maneuvers (Table 137-1)

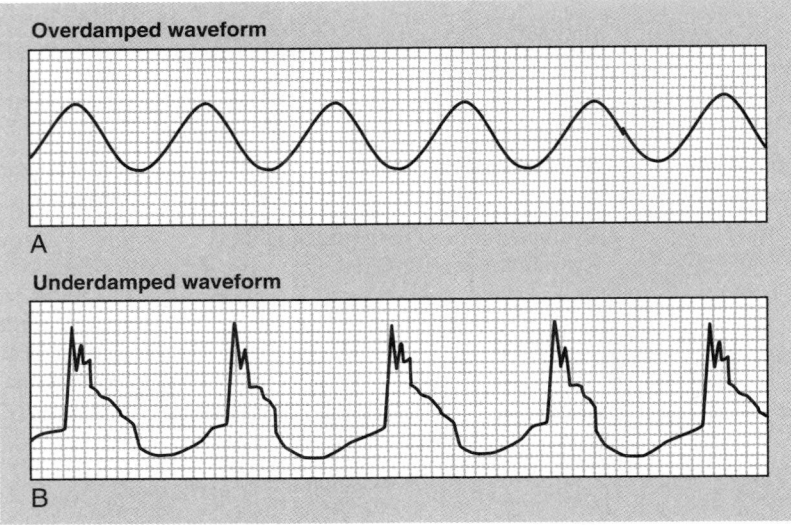

FIGURE 137-3   Over- and Underdamped Waveforms. **A,** Overdamped waveform shows the anacrotic limb (systolic upstroke) is blurred, the dicrotic notch is diminished or absent, and the wave peak is broad and flat. **B,** Underdamped waveform shows the anacrotic limb (systolic upstroke) is rapid and steep and the peak of the waveform is sharp and narrow.

Activities and Interventions	Rationale	Reportable Conditions

4. Check arterial line flush system regularly for the following:
   Fluid present in flush bag or syringe.
   Syringe pump or pressure bag is correctly functioning.
   System is free from air bubbles.
   System is intact with no loose connections.
   Catheter and system are free from kinks.
	Maintains catheter patency and ensures accurate pressure readings.	• Loss of excessive amounts of blood due to system disconnection
		• Kinked catheter with altered waveform

Monitoring and Care of the Child—Cont'd

Activities and Interventions	Rationale	Reportable Conditions
5. If using a pressure bag system, ensure inflation to 300 mm Hg.	Necessary for proper function of flush device to prevent backflow of blood into catheter and tubing.	
6. Change the pressure tubing, flush bag, and transducer per institution-specific protocol and if new catheter is inserted.	Frequent changing of the flush bag or syringe and system may cause contamination and increase risk of infection.[3]	
7. Perform a dynamic response test per institution or unit policy; most commonly done when the system is opened to air or when the accuracy of the reading is in question.	Tests the system to determines if the monitoring system is adequately reproducing the child's arterial pressure.[4] In the child it is not recommended to use continuous flow (fast flush) devices to flush catheter because of risk of delivering large volumes at high pressure. In addition, flow generated by continuous flow devices can cause arterial retrograde flow, which may cause central nervous system (CNS) embolization or acute increase in intracranial pressure (ICP).	
8. Zero the transducer per institution-specific protocol. This is most commonly done at setup, if the transducer and monitoring cable are disconnected, when the transducer is re-leveled and when values obtained do not fit clinical picture. Follow manufacturer's recommendations.	Ensures accuracy of the hemodynamic monitoring system by establishing atmospheric pressure and hydrostatic pressure reference points and eliminating zero drift of the monitoring system.[4] *(Level V*)*	
9. Level the transducer to the phlebostatic axis or the catheter tip, per institution-specific protocol.	The phlebostatic axis most accurately reflects central arterial pressure. Placing the air-fluid interface at the level of the catheter tip monitors the pressure in the specific arterial bed where the catheter tip sits. *(Level VI*)*	
10. Observe insertion site for signs of infection.	Infected catheters must be removed as soon as possible to prevent bacteremia. The tip can be sent for culture.	• Purulent drainage, tenderness or pain at insertion site, elevated temperature, or elevated white blood cells
11. Obtain an arterial waveform strip to place in the child's medical record at the start of the shift, whenever there is a change in the waveform, or per institution-specific protocol.	Printed waveform allows assessment and documentation of the adequacy of the waveform, degree of damping, or respiratory variation.[3]	
12. Monitor blood volume withdrawn from the catheter on a daily basis. Check hemoglobin or hematocrit if there is a significant blood loss through the catheter (e.g., through inadvertent disconnection).	Infants and children have smaller circulating blood volumes. Frequent blood sampling from the catheter or blood lost through inadvertent disconnection may result in clinically significant anemia.	• Decrease in hemoglobin or hematocrit

* Level V: Clinical studies in more than one or two patient populations and situations to support recommendations
  Level VI: Clinical studies in a variety of patient populations and situations to support recommendations

TABLE 137-1	Troubleshooting Waveforms			
Waveform	**Wave Description**	**Related Patient Conditions**	**Effect on Pressure Reading**	**Troubleshooting Steps**
Optimal	All components of wave clearly visible			
Overdamped waveform	Systolic upstroke is blurred Dicrotic notch diminished or absent Wave peak is broad and flat Waveform does not fall to baseline	Aortic stenosis Vasodilatation Sepsis Shock Hypovolemia	False low systolic reading False high diastolic reading	• Check the child and obtain a noninvasive blood pressure reading; severe or sudden hypotension may cause the waveform to appear overdamped • Check perfusion to the extremity where the line is located. • Attempt to aspirate and withdraw clots or air bubbles. Clots and air bubbles should be discarded, not reinfused. Using the fast-flush device or flushing with a syringe before attempting aspiration may force a clot at the catheter tip into the arterial circulation • Check for blood in the catheter • Check for air bubbles in the system • Ensure the system is set up with short, rigid tubing (48 inches is recommended) • Check that all connections are secure • Check that there are no cracks in stopcocks or tubing • If using a pressure bag, check that it is inflated to 300 mm Hg • If using a syringe pump, check that the pump is on and functioning • Check for kinks in the tubing or catheter site • Perform a fast-flush test
Underdamped waveform	Systolic upstroke is rapid and steep Peak of waveform is sharp and narrow	Hypertension Vasoconstriction Aortic regurgitation Hyperdynamic state (e.g., fever)	False high systolic reading False low diastolic reading	• Remove air bubbles • Ensure the system is set up with rigid tubing • Consider using larger-bore tubing • Consider using a damping device

Data from Shaffer R: Arterial catheter insertion (assist), care and removal. In Lynn-McHale DJ, Carlson K , editors: *AACN procedure manual for critical care,* ed 4, Philadelphia, 2001, Saunders, pp. 367-378; and McGhee B, Bridges ME: Monitoring arterial blood pressure: what you may not know, *Crit Care Nurse* 22(2): 60-79, 2002.

Documentation

- Child and family education
- Peripheral vascular and neurovascular assessment of the extremity where the catheter is inserted before and after the procedure, and with routine assessments
- Date and time of catheter insertion; size, type, and location of catheter placed
- Condition of dressing and insertion site with dressing changes and routine observations
- Child's response to insertion procedure
- Intake of flush solution (e.g., 3mL/hr)
- Type of flush solution used
- Characteristics of the waveform
- Removal of arterial catheter
- Unexpected outcomes and related treatment

References

1. Bowdle TA: Complications of invasive monitoring, *Anesthesiol Clin North America* 20(3):571-588, 2002.
2. O'Grady NP, et al: Guidelines for the prevention of intravascular catheter related infections, *MMWR Morbid Mortal Wkly Rep* 51(No.RR-10):1-29, 2002.
3. Shaffer R: Arterial catheter insertion (assist), care and removal. In Lynn-McHale DJ, Carlson K, editors: *AACN procedure manual for critical care,* ed 4, Philadelphia, 2001, Saunders, pp. 367-378.
4. McGhee B, Bridges ME: Monitoring arterial blood pressure: what you may not know. *Crit Care Nurse* 22(2):60-79, 2002.
5. Taketomo CK, et al: *Lexi-Comp's pediatric dosage handbook,* ed 10, Hudson, OH, 2003, Lexi-Comp, Inc., p. 862.

Additional Reading

Levin DL, Morriss, FC: Arterial catheters. In Levin DL, Morriss FC, editors: *Essentials of pediatric intensive care,* ed 2, St. Louis, 1997, Churchill Livingstone, p. 818.

Arterial Catheter: Blood Sampling

P U R P O S E :   To obtain blood specimens for arterial blood gas (ABG) and laboratory analysis

Beth Broering

PREREQUISITE KNOWLEDGE

- Child development as it relates to clinical assessment and blood sampling
- Aseptic technique
- Standard precautions
- General care of the site and maintenance of the arterial pressure monitoring system. Refer to Procedure 137 as well as institution-specific protocol.
- Order of draw, if several specimens of various types are being obtained (e.g., chemistry, hematology, and coagulation studies)
- Appropriate containers for specimens to be collected and minimum required blood volumes for those specimens
- Specimen labeling requirements
- Specimen handling requirements
- Neurovascular assessment of the extremities
- Damped waveform observed before or after blood sample is obtained may indicate occlusion or kinking of the catheter.
- Blood should be easily aspirated from the catheter with only gentle traction on the syringe plunger. If blood does not flow easily into the syringe, the catheter may be occluded, kinked, or in spasm.
- Arterial line tubing and monitoring systems may be "open" or "closed." Open systems use a stopcock system to withdraw blood for specimens. Closed systems contain a reservoir in the arterial line tubing that is filled with blood before obtaining specimens, clearing the line of contaminants. After specimens are obtained, the blood in the reservoir is reinfused. Benefits of closed systems are proposed to be[1]: *(Level II*)*

  ❖ Decreases potential for line contamination
  ❖ Decreases nosocomial anemia
  ❖ Minimizes blood exposure of staff, in keeping with requirements of the Occupational Safety and Health Administration

- Terminology

  ❖ Clearing the line: withdrawing a specified blood volume from the line before obtaining the actual blood sample; this is done to obtain a sample free of heparin and saline.[1]
  ❖ Discard volume: the initial blood volume obtained to clear the line; usually calculated based on the volume of the stopcock, T-connector, or pressure tubing and IV catheter.[1]
  ❖ Dead space: the volume required to fill the stopcock, T-connector or pressure tubing and IV catheter. Recommendations for discard volume to be obtained are usually between three and six times the dead space.[1,2,3] *(Level IV*)*

CHILD AND FAMILY ASSESSMENT

- Child's developmental level and ability to interact
  ➡**Rationale:** These factors influence preparation of the child and interaction.

---

* Level II: Theory based, no research data to support recommendations: recommendations from expert consensus group may exist
  Level IV: Limited clinical studies to support recommendations

1034

- Level of consciousness and cognitive ability ➧*Rationale:* Affects child's ability to participate in care.
- Child's and family's understanding of the reasons for and risks and benefits of the procedure ➧*Rationale:* Evaluates child's and family's understanding of the procedure and provides a gauge for ongoing education.
- Arterial waveform for appropriate tracing ➧*Rationale:* A waveform with a damped appearance may indicate problems with the catheter, which may cause difficulty in obtaining specimens.
- Family's desire to be present during the procedure ➧*Rationale:* Family may provide support and comfort measures to the child, but should have the choice not to remain with the child during the procedure.

CHILD AND FAMILY EDUCATION

Individualized, developmentally appropriate education is provided to the family and to the child based on desire for knowledge, readiness to learn, and overall neurologic and psychosocial state.

- Explain the purpose of drawing blood to child and family ➧*Rationale:* Reduces anxiety and facilitates an understanding of the plan of care; this is especially important if frequent samples are being obtained.
- Explain the procedure to the child and to the family; if developmentally appropriate, explain to the child that only a small amount of blood is being removed ➧*Rationale:* Reduces anxiety and fear; some children are very fearful of the sight of blood and see it as an indication that they have been hurt.

- Explain that the procedure should not cause discomfort ➧*Rationale:* Reduces anxiety and fear.
- Explain that the pressure waveform and monitor displays will be absent during blood sampling procedure ➧*Rationale:* Reduces anxiety and fear that the child is experiencing difficulties.
- Encourage questions and answer questions as they arise ➧*Rationale:* Reinforcement of information is needed during periods of stress.

EQUIPMENT

- Two or three syringes of size required to obtain discard volume and required specimens. This will vary based on size of the child, type of specimen(s) required, and minimum blood volume required for the specimen.
- Label for discard syringe
- Gloves (clean or sterile, based on institution-specific protocol)
- Alcohol wipes or other antiseptic wipes per institution-specific protocol
- 2×2 gauze sponges
- ABG syringe (when indicated)
- Vacutainer (optional)
- Luer-Lok needle or needleless access device, per institution-specific protocol
- Appropriate specimen tubes
- Appropriate laboratory requisitions
- Specimen labels containing two patient identifiers
- Container with ice, if required, for handling of specimen

Procedure for Arterial Catheter: Blood Sampling		
Steps	Rationale	Considerations
1. Ensure child and family understand procedure and questions are answered.	Evaluates and reinforces understanding of previously taught information.	Developmental level, cognitive ability, and anxiety level will determine approach to and effectiveness of teaching.
2. Gather needed equipment and supplies.	Facilitates efficient completion of procedure.	Blood specimen tubes needed depend on specimens ordered.
3. Use two patient identifiers to verify correct patient.	Promotes patient safety; ensures blood specimens are being drawn on the correct patient.	
4. Expose and position the extremity in which arterial line is inserted. Expose stopcock or transducer.	Allows easy access to site and prepares site for blood withdrawal.	
5. Silence the monitor alarms.	Prevents unnecessary alarm activation during sampling procedure.	
6. Wash hands and put on gloves.	Standard precautions; reduces risk of exposure to and transmission of microorganisms.	

Procedure continues on following page

Procedure for Arterial Catheter: Blood Sampling—*Continued*

Steps	Rationale	Considerations
Stopcock Method		
7. Identify stopcock to be used for drawing specimen. If more that one stopcock is available, the stopcock closest to the child should be used.	Minimizes amount of discard that will be required.	Number of stopcocks in the system is institution-specific protocol.
8. Label the syringe to be used for drawing discard.	Prevents blood in discard syringe from being sent to the lab for analysis.[2]	
9. Clean specimen port site or needleless access site with alcohol wipe or antiseptic swab.	Reduces transmission of micro-organisms.	Refer to institution-specific protocol for antiseptic solution used for cleaning port or needleless access site.
10. Turn stopcock so that "off" arm is toward the child ("off to the child" position) and if necessary, remove occlusive cap (Figure 138-1).	Closes port oriented toward child; prevents backflow of blood from arterial line when sampling port is opened.	Arterial waveform will be lost. Needleless access caps should not be removed.

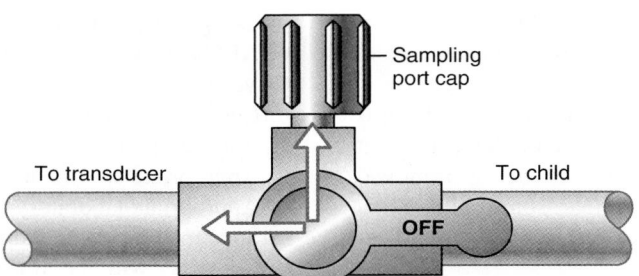

FIGURE 138-1   Stopcock in "off to child" position; ports to sampling port and transducer are open.

Steps	Rationale	Considerations
11. Attach labeled discard syringe to the stopcock or syringe with needleless access device into needleless access site.	Discard volume required will depend on the type of monitoring system, size, and length of tubing.	Dead space volume must be accurately determined to ensure samples are free of contaminants (heparin or crystalloids). Recommended discard volume is at least three times the dead space volume; two times the dead space volume for ABGs; six times the dead space volume for coagulation studies.[1-4] *(Level IV*)*
12. Rotate the stopcock so that "off" arm of the stopcock is toward the transducer ("off to the transducer" position) (Figure 138-2).	Allows withdrawal of the discard volume by opening the sampling and patient ports.	

* Level IV: Limited clinical studies to support recommendations

Procedure for Arterial Catheter: Blood Sampling—*Continued*

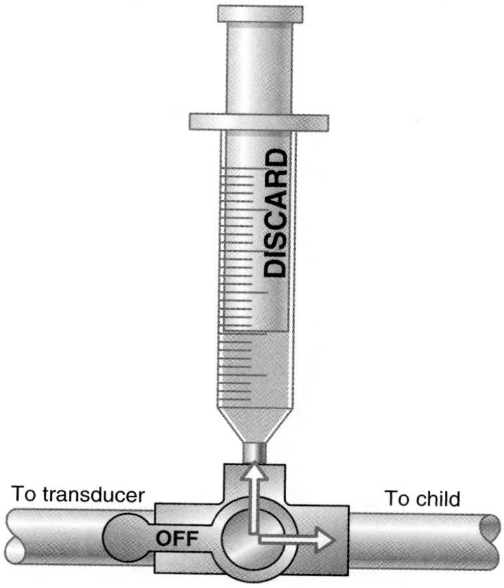

Steps	Rationale	Considerations

FIGURE 138-2   Stopcock in "off to transducer" position; ports to sampling syringe and child are open.

Steps	Rationale	Considerations
13. Slowly pull back appropriate amount of discard volume from the tubing/catheter into the syringe. *(Level V*)*	Ensures accurate blood sample free of contaminates such as heparin or crystalloids.	Do not allow blood to contaminate the transducer. If a Vacutainer is used, seat the discard collection tube to activate.
14. If a needleless access site is used, remove the syringe with discard volume. If a syringe is directly attached to the stopcock, rotate the stopcock so that the "off" arm of the stopcock is off to the syringe, child, and transducer.	Prevents excess blood withdrawal and contamination of the transducer. Prevents backflow of blood from arterial line when stopcock port is opened.	Remove the syringe with the discard volume and place to the side. Care must be taken to prevent mistaking the discard specimen from the actual specimens to be sent to the lab; this is prevented by labeling the discard syringe.[2]
15. Attach the ABG syringe or an appropriately sized syringe for the amount of blood to be sampled via the needleless access port directly to the stopcock or attach a collection tube to the Vacutainer.	Syringe or Vacutainer must be securely attached to prevent leakage of blood from stopcock and tubing.	If appropriate, discard excess heparin from ABG syringe before attaching to the stopcock port. Determine the minimum amount of blood required for laboratory analysis before sampling.
16. If needed, rotate the stopcock to the "open to the child" position; slowly withdraw the desired amount of blood.	Stopcock must be open to the child for specimen collection.	Do not pull on the syringe plunger if resistance is felt.
17. Rotate the stopcock to the "off to the syringe" position and remove the syringe (Figure 138-3).	Ensuring stopcock is turned "off to the syringe" prevents inadvertent blood loss from the system.	

Procedure continues on following page

* Level V: Clinical studies in more than one or two patient populations and situations to support recommendations

Procedure **for Arterial Catheter: Blood Sampling**—*Continued*

Steps	Rationale	Considerations

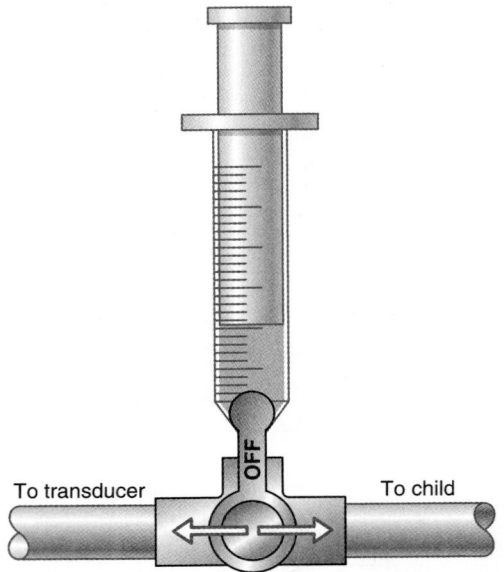

FIGURE 138-3   Stopcock in "off to syringe" position; ports to child and transducer are open.

Steps	Rationale	Considerations
18. Place blood in appropriate specimen tubes.	Required for transport of specimen to lab.	Specimen collection tubes are determined by the institution.
19. It is not recommended to reinfuse discard volume to the child.[1,2] If discard is to be returned to the child, replace syringe with discard onto stopcock. Rotate the stopcock to the "off to the transducer" position; slowly reinfuse the blood in the syringe and then rotate the stopcock to "off to the syringe" position.	Reinfusion of discard reduces the blood loss that occurs when multiple specimens are obtained over several hours or days.	Reinfuse the discard volume if this is consistent with institution-specific protocol. Concerns with reinfusing discard volume include possible contamination of the discard syringe, clots in the discard volume, and exposure of the clinician to blood.[1,2] If discard volume is reinfused, monitor site for mottling or blanching distal to the arterial line. Assess ease of reinfusion; do not force.
20. Manually flush the arterial line at the stopcock with a syringe, or at the transducer with the fast-flush device, using quick bursts.	Clears line of residual blood; prevents clot formation.	If heparin is used in the flush use only the amount of flush necessary to clear line to avoid complications associated with heparin use.
21. If occlusive cap was removed, recap the port with a sterile cap and ensure the stopcock is in the "off to the syringe" position.	Minimizes risk of contamination of system and ensures resumption of accurate monitoring.	
22. Ensure that all caps and connections are secure.	Prevents blood loss or introducing air into system.	
23. Observe for return of waveform.	Enables resumption of accurate arterial monitoring.	Notify prescribing practitioner if waveform is damped or if arterial pressures are higher or lower than expected.

Procedure for Arterial Catheter: Blood Sampling—*Continued*

Steps	Rationale	Considerations
24. Reactivate monitor alarms.	Provides for notification when arterial pressures are at an unacceptable level.	Alarm ranges are set per institution-specific protocol or child's status.
25. Label specimens at the bedside and complete laboratory paper work per institution-specific protocol.	Promotes patient safety; ensures accurate and efficient processing of specimen.	Expel any air bubbles from the ABG syringe. Place ABG syringe on ice if required by institution-specific protocol. Follow institution-specific protocol for handling and labeling lab specimens.
26. Dispose of used supplies and equipment in appropriate receptacle; ensure sharps are disposed of correctly. Wash hands.	Standard precautions; prevents transmission of microorganisms. Protects personnel health.	

Closed Blood Conservation System Method

Steps	Rationale	Considerations
27. Follow steps 1 through 6 above.	Prepare for blood sampling.	Advantages of closed blood conservation systems are reported to be as follows: allows return of discard volume while maintaining a closed system; decreases clinician exposure to blood; prevents confusion of discard syringe and specimen syringe; decreases nosocomial anemia.[1]
28. Unlock the system reservoir; refer to system manufacturer's instructions.	Allows blood conservation reservoir to fill with line clearance volume.	Mechanism that allows blood to be withdrawn into the blood conservation reservoir varies among manufacturers.
29. Slowly aspirate the required dead space volume into the blood conservation reservoir.	Ensures that specimen will not be contaminated with heparin or crystalloid.	Slowly aspirate the required dead space volume into the blood conservation reservoir.
30. Activate manufacturer's mechanism to ensure dead space volume remains in reservoir.	Prevents dead space volume from being aspirated when specimen is withdrawn.	Mechanism varies among manufacturers; frequently a stopcock is closed.
31. Clean sampling port with alcohol or other antiseptic solution per institution-specific protocol.	Prevents contamination of system and minimizes risk of nosocomial infection.	Follow institution-specific protocol for cleaning sampling ports.
32. Access sampling port with a needleless access device or needle attached to a syringe per manufacturer's recommendations; a Vacutainer also may be attached.	Accesses line to obtain specimen.	Needleless systems are preferred because they decrease the likelihood of needlestick injury. Size of syringe determined by blood volume required for requested samples.
33. Withdraw the amount of blood needed for sample.	Obtains requested specimens.	
34. Remove syringe from sampling port and place blood in appropriate specimen tubes.	Ensures accurate specimens and laboratory data.	Follow institution-specific protocol for specimen handling.

Procedure continues on following page

Procedure | for Arterial Catheter: Blood Sampling—*Continued*

Steps	Rationale	Considerations
35. Unlock reservoir and slowly return dead space volume to child; ensure all blood is returned.	Returning the volume of blood contaminated with flush or heparin solution back to the child minimizes-nosocomial anemia.	Follow manufacturer's recommendations for reinfusion of blood.
36. Close or lock reservoir according to manufacturer's recommendations.	Prevents reservoir from being inadvertently activated.	
37. Flush line with a syringe or by using fast-flush device until line is cleared of blood.	Clears line of residual blood; prevents clot formation.	
38. Ensure that all caps and connections are secure.	Prevents contamination of line or blood loss.	
39. Observe for return of waveform.	Enables resumption of accurate pressure monitoring.	Notify prescribing practitioner if waveform is damped or if arterial pressures are higher or lower than expected.
40. Reactivate monitor alarms.	Provides for notification when arterial pressures are at an unacceptable level.	Alarm ranges are set per institution-specific protocol or child's status.
41. Label specimens at the bedside and complete laboratory paperwork per institution-specific protocol.	Promotes patient safety; ensures accurate and efficient processing of specimen.	Expel any air bubbles from ABG syringe. Place ABG syringe on ice if required by institutional protocol. Follow institution-specific protocol for handling and labeling lab specimens.
42. Dispose of used supplies and equipment in appropriate receptacle; ensure sharps are disposed of correctly. Wash hands.	Standard precautions; reduces transmission of microorganisms. Protects personnel health.	

Expected Outcomes

- Adequate blood specimen obtained with minimal blood loss
- Arterial pressure monitoring is resumed without complications

- Distal extremity remains warm and pink with evidence of adequate perfusion
- Specimens are placed in correct sample tubes, labeled appropriately, and sent to the lab in the appropriate time frame

Unexpected Outcomes

- Inadequate, diluted, or hemolyzed blood specimen
- Excessive blood volume removed
- Waveform is damped or lost
- Bleeding from connections or ports
- Arterial pressures become unreliable after sampling due to contamination of transducer
- Arterial spasm
- Extremity becomes cool or mottled or demonstrates other signs or poor perfusion
- Specimens are mislabeled, placed in incorrect sample tubes, or not sent to lab in a timely fashion

Monitoring and Care of the Child

Activities and Interventions	Rationale	Reportable Conditions
1. Monitor child's response to procedure.	Allows for early identification of complications.	• Excessive pain or tingling in extremity in which catheter is located
2. Monitor ease of blood withdrawal and ability to flush catheter.	Identifies potential complications of the catheter such as kinking, occlusion, arterial spasm.	• Difficulty flushing catheter • Unable to withdraw blood • Significant blanching of site/extremity with flushing
3. Compare arterial waveform before and after blood draw.	Ensures accurate monitoring, identification of arterial spasm.	• Loss of arterial waveform
4. Attempt to group blood draws together.	Reduces the number of times the system is entered, minimizing the risk for infection or nosocomial anemia.	• Abnormal lab results
5. Monitor volume of blood drawn on a daily basis and for the duration of hospitalization.	Heightens staff's awareness of blood loss due to phlebotomy, which may decrease overall blood loss.[1,2] *(Level IV*)*	• Volume of blood withdrawn exceeds predetermined threshold
6. Monitor results of specimens obtained.	Monitors child's status; facilitates identification of possible errors in obtaining specimens (e.g., inadequate discard volume drawn results in erroneous results).	• Abnormal lab values

*Level IV: Limited clinical studies to support recommendations

Documentation

- Time of blood sampling and specimens obtained
- Amount of blood withdrawn, along with running total for hospitalization
- Color, temperature, and capillary refill of extremity after specimens obtained
- Waveform assessment after procedure completed
- Monitor alarms turned on, set appropriately, and functional
- Child's tolerance of procedure
- Results of tests
- Child and family education
- Unexpected outcomes and related treatment

References

1. Dech ZF, Szaflarski NL: Nursing strategies to minimize blood loss associated with phlebotomy, *AACN Clinical Issues* 7(2):277-287, 1996.
2. Frey AM: Drawing blood samples from vascular access devices: evidence-based practice, *J Infus Nurs* 26(5):285-293, 2003.
3. Yucha CB, DeAngelo E: The minimum discard volume: accurate analysis of peripheral hematocrit, *J IV Nurs* 19(3):141-144, 1996.
4. Shaffer RB: Blood sampling from arterial pressure lines. In Lynn-McHale DJ, Carlson K, editors: *AACN procedure manual for critical care,* ed 4, Philadelphia, 2001, Saunders, pp. 379-384.

Additional Reading

Farjo L: Blood collection from peripherally inserted central venous catheters: an institution's effort to evaluate and update its current policy, *J Infus Nurs* 26(6):374-379, 2003.

Central Venous Catheters for Hemodialysis or Hemofiltration: Blood Sampling

P U R P O S E : To obtain blood specimens for monitoring fluid and electrolyte status, hematologic stability and other ordered indices in children with known or impending renal failure either directly from the catheter or through the dialysis circuit when renal replacement therapy is in progress

Cathy Haut

PREREQUISITE KNOWLEDGE

- Child development as it relates to clinical assessment and blood drawing
- Principles of aseptic technique
- Standard precautions
- Order of draw, if several specimens are being obtained; refer to institution-specific protocol
- Appropriate containers for specimens to be collected and minimum required blood volumes for those specimens
- Specimen labeling requirements
- Specimen handling requirements
- In many institutions renal replacement therapy catheters are not accessed for purposes other than continuous renal replacement therapies (CRRT) unless ordered by a nephrologist. A prescribing practitioner's order may be necessary for the bedside nurse to obtain blood specimens directly from these catheters; refer to institution-specific protocol.
  - ❖ Catheter lumens must be labeled to indicate whether the catheter may be used for blood drawing.
- Catheter size and number of lumens as well as filling volume of lumens should be noted before accessing the catheter.
- CRRT catheter lumens are instilled with high-concentration heparin or tissue plasminogen activator (tPA) at the filling volume of the lumen when not in use ("locked").

Lumens should be labeled to indicate that high-concentrate heparin is instilled. Before use or flushing of the catheter, withdraw and discard heparin or tPA per institution-specific protocol. *(Level II*)*

- Catheter size and number of lumens is dependent on child's weight and purpose of catheter; generally, most catheters used for CRRT have two same-size lumens, ranging from size 5 Fr to 12.5 Fr.
- Hemodialysis or hemofiltration catheters are generally placed in the femoral vein, internal jugular vein or external jugular vein.[1,2,3]
- Anatomic location of catheter placement may affect the ease of blood drawing; catheters placed in femoral veins can become kinked more easily due to child's position.
- The volume of blood needed to clear the catheter (discard volume) is at least two to three times the catheter's dead space volume (volume between the blood-drawing port and tip of catheter).
- Hemodialysis or hemofiltration should not be interrupted for blood drawing. Blood-drawing ports located in the CRRT circuit should be used in this situation. When blood is drawn from the circuit, no discard volume is drawn.

---

* Level II: Theory based, no research data to support recommendations: recommendations from expert consensus group may exist

- It is preferable to obtain blood specimens for coagulation studies directly from a vein or artery or from another peripherally or centrally placed catheter *not* containing heparin or anticoagulation substances.[1,3]
- When drawing blood from multilumen catheters, it is imperative to clamp or turn off infusions entering other lumens of the catheter while obtaining blood specimen to prevent contamination of specimen with fluids infusing in other lumens.
- Stopcocks should not be attached to the lumen of a catheter.

CHILD AND FAMILY ASSESSMENT

- Child's developmental level and ability to interact ➧*Rationale:* These factors influence preparation of the child and interaction.
- Child's and family's understanding of the reasons for and risks and benefits of the procedure ➧*Rationale:* Evaluates child's and family's understanding of the procedure and need for frequent blood sampling; provides a gauge for ongoing education.
- Child's anxiety related to the sight of blood ➧*Rationale:* Facilitates developmentally appropriate preparation of the child; some children are very fearful of the sight of blood and see it as an indication that they have been hurt.
- Family's desire to be present during procedure ➧*Rationale:* Family may provide support and comfort measures to the child but should have the choice not to remain with the child.

CHILD AND FAMILY EDUCATION

Individualized, developmentally appropriate education is provided to the family and to the child based on desire for knowledge, readiness to learn, and overall neurologic and psychosocial state.

- Provide information about the rationale for blood sampling in developmentally appropriate terminology for child and family ➧*Rationale:* Providing information decreases anxiety and fear.
- Assure child and family that privacy will be protected during procedure ➧*Rationale:* Accessing femoral catheters may require exposure of the groin; providing privacy demonstrates respect and will decrease anxiety during procedure.
- Acknowledge that child and family will be able to view blood in syringe/containers; if developmentally appropriate, explain to the child that only a small amount of blood is being removed ➧*Rationale:* Reduces anxiety and fear; child and/or family may have negative reaction to the sight of blood.
- Explain how family can assist to comfort and provide support or distraction for child during blood drawing if necessary ➧*Rationale:* Promotes family participation in care; may decrease anxiety and fear.
- Encourage child to lie still during procedure. Explain positioning (extending leg, turning head) if necessary ➧*Rationale:* Promotes cooperation and facilitates completion of blood drawing.
- Encourage questions and answer questions as they arise ➧*Rationale:* Reinforcement of information is needed during periods of stress.

EQUIPMENT

- Sterile or clean gloves: refer to institution-specific protocol
  - ❖ Sterile gloves are generally used when accessing catheter.
  - ❖ Clean gloves are generally used when accessing CRRT circuit.
- Appropriate-sized syringes to remove discard volume and obtain requested specimens
- Needle or needleless access device for CRRT circuit port if specimen is obtained from circuit
- Sterile occlusive cap for catheter lumen if lumen is locked
- Solution used to lock catheter at completion of procedure, generally heparin or tPA; refer to prescribing practitioner's order
- Plastic tubing clamps, if clamps are not present on catheter
- 10-mL syringe containing 10 mL of sterile 0.9% saline
- Appropriate containers for requested blood specimens
- Appropriate laboratory requisitions
- Appropriate labels for requested specimens
- Antimicrobial disinfectant solution for cleaning port such as chlorhexidine or alcohol

Procedure	for Central Venous Catheters for Hemodialysis and Hemofiltration: Blood Sampling

Steps	Rationale	Considerations
1. Ensure child and family understand procedure and that questions are answered.	Evaluates and reinforces understanding of previously taught information.	Developmental level, cognitive ability, and anxiety level will determine approach to and effectiveness of teaching.
2. Utilize two patient identifiers to verify correct patient.	Promotes patient safety; ensures blood specimens are being drawn on the correct child.	
3. Gather necessary equipment and supplies.	Facilitates completion of procedure in a timely manner.	
4. Provide for appropriate privacy; position child to facilitate blood drawing.	Ensures appropriate privacy; facilitates obtaining specimen.	Privacy is an important consideration for school-aged children and adolescents.
5. Wash hands, put on sterile gloves.	Catheter lumen must be kept sterile while disconnecting cap or infusions.	
6. Stop infusions and clamp all lumens of catheter for 2 to 3 minutes before blood collection.[4] *(Level VI*)*	Contamination of specimen can occur if fluids are aspirated from other catheter lumens while specimen is drawn.	If triple-lumen catheter is used, one lumen is designated for blood drawing.
7. Clean junction of catheter lumen/ occlusive cap or infusion line with antimicrobial disinfectant solution.	Removes contaminants; decreases transmission of microorganisms.	Refer to institution-specific protocol for appropriate antimicrobial disinfectant solution.
8. Remove occlusive cap or disconnect infusion line from identified blood draw lumen.	Care should be taken to avoid contamination of tubing connections.	Central catheters pose high risk of blood infection.[4,5,6]
9. Attach appropriately sized syringe labeled "discard" and aspirate at least three times the catheter's dead space volume. In older children and adolescents, 5 to 10 mL is recommended discard volume.[4,7,8] *(Level IV*)*	Any blood drawn potentially contaminated with medications or fluids that will alter laboratory values is discarded before obtaining blood sample. Heparin or tPA used to lock catheters must be withdrawn and discarded before blood draw. Prevents blood in discard syringe from being sent to the lab for analysis.	Small-volume syringe exerts least amount of pressure on line when drawing blood; excessive pressure can damage catheter.[1] Infants and young children or children who require frequent blood drawing may be candidates for discard return; however, heparin and tPA are never returned to the child. If unable to draw blood from catheters locked with tPA or high concentration of heparin, do not flush catheter. Notify prescribing practitioner.
10. Attach new syringe and withdraw blood volume required for specimens.	Obtains blood for testing.	Blood volume is determined by ordered specimens.
11. Remove syringe containing specimen and flush catheter with 0.9% saline using volume adequate to clear lumen.	Prevents clotting and occlusion of catheter lumen.	Discard volume with heparin or tPA is not reinfused. Reinfusing any discard is not generally recommended; concerns with

* Level IV: Limited clinical studies to support recommendations
  Level VI: Clinical studies in a variety of patient populations and situations to support recommendations

Procedure	for Central Venous Catheters for Hemodialysis and Hemofiltration: Blood Sampling—*Continued*		
Steps	**Rationale**	**Considerations**
		reinfusing discard volume include possible contamination of the discard syringe, clots in the discard volume, and exposure of the clinician to blood.[7,8]
12. If catheter is to be locked, instill appropriate volume of heparin or tPA per prescribing practitioner's order; clamp catheter. (*Level VI**)	Maintains patency; prevents clotting of catheter lumen.	Ordered volume is usually filling volume of the catheter lumen plus 0.1 mL; refer to institution-specific protocols.
13. If occlusive cap is removed, recap the lumen with a sterile cap; otherwise reconnect tubing and resume infusion.	Reestablishes closed system.	
14. Place blood in appropriate specimen tubes.	Ensures sample is provided to laboratory for analysis.	Tubes used depend on specimen requested and laboratory guidelines.
15. Label specimens at the bedside and complete laboratory paperwork per institution-specific protocol.	Promotes patient safety; ensures accurate and efficient processing of specimen.	Follow institution-specific protocol for handling and labeling lab specimens.
16. Dispose of supplies and used equipment appropriately; remove gloves and wash hands.	Standard precautions; decreases the transmission of microorganisms.	
Drawing Blood via CRRT Circuit		
17. Complete steps 1 through 5 listed above.		
18. Identify sampling port to be used for requested specimen (generally the prefilter port).	Pre- and postfilter ports are available. Prefilter port is best indicator of child's status.	Most systems identify blood-drawing ports of circuit; refer to manufacturer's instructions.
19. Cleanse port with antimicrobial solution.	Prevents contamination of system.	
20. Insert 5- to 10-mL syringe with needle or needleless access device attached.	Size of syringe prevents negative pressure in tubing and system.	Size of needle used to puncture diaphragm or ability to use needleless access device varies among manufacturers; refers to manufacturer's instructions.
21. Draw needed amount of blood from port.	Type of specimen requested determines blood volume needed.	
22. Withdraw syringe from port.		
23. Place blood in appropriate specimen tubes.	Ensures sample is provided to laboratory for analysis.	Tubes used depend on specimen requested and laboratory guidelines.
24. Label specimens at the bedside and complete laboratory paperwork per institution-specific protocol.	Promotes patient safety; ensures accurate and efficient processing of specimen.	Follow institution-specific protocol for handling and labeling lab specimens.
25. Dispose of supplies and used equipment appropriately; remove gloves and wash hands.	Standard precautions; decreases the transmission of microorganisms.	

* Level VI: Clinical studies in a variety of patient populations and situations to support recommendations

Expected Outcomes	Unexpected Outcomes
• Blood specimen is obtained without contamination	• Lab results indicate contaminated specimen
	• Inability to obtain blood from catheter
• Sterility of catheter is maintained	• Contamination of catheter ports
• Child remains hemodynamically stable	• Excessive blood volume removed
	• Blood loss from catheter lumens or ports
• Catheter lumens remain patent	• Inability to flush catheter or obtain blood after blood has been drawn from catheter
• Catheter-locking solution remains in catheter lumens or is removed and discarded	• Child receives bolus of high-concentration heparin or tPA
• Specimens are placed in correct sample tubes, labeled appropriately, and sent to the lab in the appropriate time frame	• Specimens are mislabeled, placed in incorrect sample tubes, or not sent to lab in a timely fashion

Monitoring and Care of the Child

Activities and Interventions	Rationale	Reportable Conditions
1. Child's hemodynamic response to procedure.	Changes in heart rate or blood pressure may indicate hypovolemia if excessive blood is removed.	• Bradycardia, tachycardia, with hypertension
2. Monitor ability to obtain blood from catheter.	Assesses catheter functioning.	• Inability to draw blood from catheter; lumen may need to be cleared with antithrombolytic agent [4]
3. Attempt to group blood draws together.	Reduces the number of times the system is entered, minimizing the risk for infection or nosocomial anemia.	• Abnormal lab results
4. Monitor volume of blood drawn on a daily basis and for the duration of hospitalization.	Heightens staff's awareness of blood loss due to phlebotomy, which may decrease overall blood loss.[8,9] *(Level IV*)*	• Excessive blood volume removed; exceeds predetermined threshold
5. Monitor results of specimens obtained.	Monitors child's status; facilitates identification of possible errors in obtaining specimens (e.g., inadequate discard volume drawn results in erroneous results).	• Abnormal lab values

* Level IV: Limited clinical studies to support recommendations

Documentation

• Child and family education
• Child's response to procedure
• Unexpected outcomes and related treatment
• Time of blood sampling and specimens obtained
• Amount of blood withdrawn, along with running total for hospitalization
• Ease of obtaining blood from catheter
• Results of tests

References

1. Kaplow R, Barry, R: Continuous renal replacement therapies, *Am J Nurs* 102(11):26-33, 2002.
2. Guilano K: Continuous renal replacement therapies. In Lynn-McHale DJ, Carlson K, editors: *AACN procedure manual for critical care,* ed 4, Philadelphia, 2001, Saunders, pp. 717-732.
3. Meyer M: Renal replacement therapies, *Crit Care Clin* 16(1):29-54, 2000.
4. Himberger JR, Himberger LC: Accuracy of drawing blood through infusing intravenous lines, *Heart Lung* 30(1):66-73, 2001.
5. Masoorli S, Angeles T: Getting a line on central venous access devices, *Nursing 2002* 32(4):36-43, 2002.
6. Schmid MW: Risks and complications of peripherally and centrally inserted intravenous catheters, *Crit Care Clin* 12(2):165-173, 2000.
7. Dech ZF, Szaflarski NL: Nursing strategies to minimize blood loss associated with phlebotomy, *AACN Clin Issues* 7(2):277-287, 1996.
8. Frey AM: Drawing blood samples from vascular access devices: evidence-based practice, *J Infus Nurs* 26(5):285-293, 2003.

Central Venous Non-tunneled Catheter: Insertion Assist

P U R P O S E :   To facilitate insertion of short-term to intermediate central vascular access for administration of fluids and medications, laboratory sampling, or monitoring central venous pressure

Kelly A. Lankin

PREREQUISITE KNOWLEDGE

- Child development as it relates to clinical assessment and central venous catheter (CVC) insertion
- Mastery of pediatric advanced life support competencies
- Principles of aseptic technique
- Appropriate pediatric dosing of analgesics and competency in procedural sedation
- Indications for non-tunneled central venous access[1-5]
  - ❖ Central venous pressure measurement
  - ❖ Delivery of drugs to the central circulation, including chemotherapy
  - ❖ Rapid infusion of large volumes of fluids or blood products
  - ❖ Administration of high-concentration parenteral alimentation
  - ❖ Administration of medications that cannot infuse peripherally
  - ❖ Dialysis procedures (plasmapheresis, hemofiltration, hemodialysis)
  - ❖ Exchange transfusions
  - ❖ Provision of access in children lacking peripheral sites who require intravenous therapies
- Site options for non-tunneled CVCs include femoral, subclavian, internal and external jugular veins
  - ❖ **Internal jugular vein**
    - ○ Place the child supine, in the Trendelenburg position, approximately 20 to 30 degrees with a neck roll to hyperextend the neck. Turn the child's head opposite the side to be cannulated.
    - ○ Complications during CVC insertion using this site include pneumothorax, arterial cannulation (carotid), bleeding, infection, dysrhythmias, venous air embolism, pericardial tamponade, cerebral spinal fluid tap, chylothorax.
    - ○ A relative contraindication for this site is a coagulopathy; insertion by ultrasound is recommended.[1-5]
  - ❖ **External jugular vein**
    - ○ Place child supine, in the Trendelenburg position, approximately 20 to 30 degrees with a neck roll to hyperextend the neck. Position the child's head opposite the side to be cannulated.
    - ○ Complications during CVC insertion using this site include bleeding from site, difficulty visualizing vein for venipuncture, venous air embolism; complications with this site are low.[1-5]
  - ❖ **Subclavian vein**
    - ○ Place child in the supine position, arms by sides, in the Trendelenburg position 20 to 30 degrees with the child's head midline or slightly positioned toward the opposite side of the side to be cannulated.
    - ○ Complications during CVC insertion using this site include arterial puncture, dysrhythmias, venous air embolism, thrombosis, nerve injury, pericardial tamponade, bleeding, hemothorax, and pneumothorax.

○ Contraindications include coagulopathy, severe lung disease that cannot tolerate a pneumothorax; pneumothorax accounts for 25% to 50% of all complications with the subclavian site.[1-5]

❖ **Femoral vein**
  ○ Place the child supine, with hips abducted (rotated out), and externally rotate the thigh slightly. A roll may need to be placed underneath the hip that is to be cannulated to expose the area more appropriately.
  ○ Complications during CVC insertion using this site include arterial cannulation, retroperitoneal bleeding, accessing the bladder, thrombosis, infection, nerve damage.
  ○ This site is recommended for short-term use due to the higher risk of infection than other sites.[1-5]
  ○ Catheter sizes available: 1 Fr to 14 Fr, with one to three lumens. Catheters vary in length; length is not generally adjustable by cutting the internal tip, so length selected is based on child's size and location of insertion site. It is important to be familiar with the institution's stock of catheter brands and sizes.[4]

• Most short-term catheters, generally left in place for up to 3 weeks, are constructed of polyurethane.
• When a non-tunneled catheter is inserted and passed into the atriocaval junction dysrhythmias, such as premature ventricular contractions (PVCs), may occur during guidewire insertion. This is an indication that the guidewire is too far into the right atrium. If PVCs persist after the catheter is in place, it is possible that the catheter is in too far; catheter position must be confirmed by x-ray.
• Ideally the tip of the CVC is placed at the atriocaval junction. In this position, there is little motion of the catheter, which allows more accurate CVP measurements, less chance of blood clot formation due to the rapid flow of blood through this junction, and less chance of cardiac perforation because the catheter is not located too deeply in the right atrium.
• Except in an emergency situation, informed consent is required before placement of a central venous non-tunneled catheter.

CHILD AND FAMILY ASSESSMENT

• Child's developmental level and ability to interact ➤➤***Rationale:*** These factors influence preparation of the child and interaction; sedation and analgesics most likely will be needed; therefore it is important to determine baseline interaction/awareness.
• Child's and family's understanding of the reasons for and risks and benefits of the procedure ➤➤***Rationale:*** Evaluates child's and family's understanding of the procedure and provides a gauge for ongoing education; facilitates informed consent.
• Family's and child's history of prolonged bleeding or abnormal bruising. Assess child for signs of gastric, oral,

or rectal bleeding; hematomas; petechiae; or bleeding from puncture sites. Review recent complete blood count (CBC) and coagulation profile, if available ➤➤***Rationale:*** Assesses risk for bleeding potential during catheter placement.
• Previous or present CVCs, pacemakers, etc. ➤➤***Rationale:*** May affect insertion procedure and ease of insertion into venous system.
• Allergies to medications or substances, including dressing materials ➤➤***Rationale:*** Child will be receiving sedation, analgesics, and skin antiseptics.
• Child's hemodynamic status and vital signs ➤➤***Rationale:*** Sedation and analgesics can cause hypotension and may worsen already compromised hemodynamic status.
• History of previous response to anesthesia or procedural sedation ➤➤***Rationale:*** May influence type of sedation used for procedure to safely achieve desired results.
• Child's respiratory status ➤➤***Rationale:*** Certain positioning, sedation, and analgesics can cause respiratory distress or worsen already compromised respiratory status.
• Family's need for chaplain or social work services to provide support ➤➤***Rationale:*** Helps the family meet emotional and spiritual needs, especially during emergency CVC placement.
• Family's desire to be present during the procedure ➤➤***Rationale:*** Family members may provide comfort and support, but should have the choice not to remain with the child. In some situations, if family presence will not be permitted, allows explanation of reasons for this and promotes cooperation.

CHILD AND FAMILY EDUCATION

Individualized, developmentally appropriate education is provided to the family and to the child based on desire for knowledge, readiness to learn, and overall neurologic and psychosocial state.

• Provide information on the child's medical condition, purpose, and rationale for CVC placement ➤➤***Rationale:*** Providing pertinent information helps decrease the child and family's anxiety levels and offers reassurance during an extremely stressful period.
• Provide the family and child with information about the procedure, including analgesia and sedation that will be given, the sterile field, and positioning of the child ➤➤***Rationale:*** Providing pertinent information increases knowledge and decreases fear and anxiety related to the procedure.
• If the family is asked to leave the room during the procedure, reassure the child and family that the bedside nurse will be present to comfort the child and that the family will be notified as soon as they are able to return to the bedside. If institution-specific protocol permits family presence, provide family with accurate information regarding procedure, family's role and expectations of family ➤➤***Rationale:*** Helps to alleviate family's anxiety. If family stays at the bedside, information prepares the

family for their role; provides clearly defined guidelines and expectations.

- Educate the family and/or child about medications that will be administered for the procedure, including local anesthetics ➻*Rationale:* Knowing that anticipated pain and/or anxiety/agitation will be preemptively treated will decrease fear and anxiety of the child and family.
- Educate the family and/or child about what the line will look like and how it will be used ➻*Rationale:* Decreases parental and child anxiety and fear.
- Use interpretation services if the child or family's preferred language is not English ➻*Rationale:* Decreases barriers to communication.
- Encourage questions and answer questions as they arise ➻*Rationale:* Reinforcement of information is needed during periods of stress. This is especially important if the procedure is emergent.

EQUIPMENT

- Masks, sterile gowns, hats, sterile gloves in the appropriate sizes, protective eyewear
- Skin antiseptic solutions: chlorhexidine or 10% povidone-iodine
- Sterile towels and sterile drape
- Vascular access tray
- Appropriate size and type central line for age/route/purpose
- Local anesthetic, i.e., 1% lidocaine without epinephrine
- Sedation and/or analgesic medications as ordered
- Syringes and safety needles or needleless access device
- Saline or heparinized saline to prime and flush the line after insertion, per institution-specific protocol
- Suture material or securement device
- Sterile transparent water vapor–permeable plastic dressing or gauze and tape
- Equipment for measuring central venous pressure (CVP); refer to Procedure 142
- Cardiorespiratory monitor with pulse oximeter
- Emergency equipment

Procedure for Central Venous Non-tunneled Catheter: Insertion Assist

Steps	Rationale	Considerations
1. Ensure child and family understand procedure and questions are answered.	Evaluates and reinforces understanding of previously taught information.	Developmental level, cognitive ability, and anxiety level will determine approach to and effectiveness of teaching.
2. Gather needed equipment and supplies; bring to the bedside; assist with setting up equipment.	Facilitates completion of task in a timely manner; decreases time child is sedated and that family is out of the room.	Obtain the requested catheter in advance if it is not readily available on the unit.
3. Confirm that consent for procedure has been obtained.	Ensures medicolegal compliance as suggested by the Joint Commission on Accreditation of Healthcare Organizations (JCAHO).	For emergency situations, the organization may have a protocol or procedure in place for assumption of consent.
4. Provide for appropriate privacy.	Respects child's privacy.	Privacy is an important consideration for school-aged children and adolescents.
5. Wash hands.	Reduces the transmission of microorganisms.	
6. Identify child using appropriate patient/procedure verification process (e.g., "Time out").	Confirms correct patient, procedure and site as recommended by JCAHO; prevents unnecessary medical procedures.	Verification process and documentation are institution-specific; use active communication techniques.
7. Ensure that child is placed on a cardiorespiratory monitor and pulse oximeter.	Allows continuous monitoring during procedure for heart rate, respiratory rate, blood pressure, and oxygen saturations.	Ensure alarms are activated with appropriate settings and are sufficiently audible. Pay close attention to PVCs that may occur during the threading of the catheter—an indication that the line has passed through the atriocaval junction and into the right atrium.

Procedure **for Central Venous Non-tunneled Catheter: Insertion Assist**—*Continued*

Steps	Rationale	Considerations
8. Administer sedation and analgesia as ordered.	Child must remain still during the procedure and pain/anxiety must be alleviated. It is important to administer sedation and analgesics before positioning and preparation to alleviate anxiety.	Supplemental oxygen may need to be administered if child is not intubated.
9. Place child in the appropriate position based on the site chosen for cannulation.	Place child supine in the Trendelenburg position, with arms at the sides, for subclavian and jugular approaches to help prevent air embolism and to distend the central veins. Place child supine with the hips abducted and the thighs externally rotated (frog-legged) for the femoral approach; a roll may need to be placed under the hip on the side of cannulation.	Consult with the practitioner inserting the CVC before the procedure to discuss preferred positioning.
10. Assist the practitioner inserting the CVC to put on sterile gown/gloves, mask, cap, protective eyewear. NOTE: Everyone entering the room at this point must wear a mask.	Establishes aseptic environment; decreases transmission of microorganisms.	Once the practitioner is garbed, he or she will need assistance with opening sterile packaging and gathering other equipment required during the procedure.
11. Assist with establishing sterile field.	Establishes aseptic environment.	
12. Provide appropriate antiseptic solution to clean insertion site.	Chlorhexidine or 10% povidone-iodine; chlorhexidine is not recommended for infants less than 2 months of age. *(Level V*)*	Antiseptic solution used is based on institution-specific protocol.
13. Provide saline and/or heparinized saline to prime and flush catheter after insertion. *(Level IV*)*	Heparin is used to prevent catheter from clotting.	Catheter is flushed before and after insertion.
14. Provide sterile towels and drapes to be placed around insertion site.	Create sterile field around cannulation site.	Be sure to cover child's mouth and nose, if not intubated, with a mask or loosely applied sterile towel.
15. Open sterile packaged central venous catheter kit.	Prevents practitioner inserting catheter from contaminating gloves when removing catheter from packaging.	
16. Assist practitioner with drawing up local anesthetic.	Used for topical anesthetic in conjunction with systemic sedation and analgesia.	Local anesthetic is found in some CVC kits, depending on brand; syringe and needle may need to be provided.

Procedure continues on following page

* Level IV: Limited clinical studies to support recommendations
  Level V: Clinical studies in more than one or two patient populations and situations to support recommendations

Procedure for Central Venous Non-tunneled Catheter: Insertion Assist—*Continued*

Steps	Rationale	Considerations
17. Notify the practitioner of any dysrhythmias such as PVCs seen during introducer, guidewire, or catheter insertion.	Instrumentation may stimulate the sinoatrial (SA) node while in the right atrium, resulting in ectopic beats, including PVCs; notification alerts the practitioner to adjust placement.	Central lines are measured before insertion to verify depth of insertion and ensure that the tip is in the atriocaval junction.
18. Once the catheter is inserted, attach a CVP measurement system to display waveform and measurement if desired.	Appropriately placed central catheter will display a typical CVP wave form. See Figure 142-1 in Procedure 142 waveform assessment will also identify venous or arterial placement for an example of a typical CVP waveform.	If arterial cannulation is suspected, a blood gas can be obtained to assess for arterial placement.
19. Provide suture materials or other securement device, such as a StatLock.	Catheters are secured in place to help prevent dislodgment.	Some catheter kits have securement materials; this should be determined before starting procedure so that appropriate device or material is readily available
20. Assist with occlusive dressing application—use gauze under transparent, water vapor—permeable plastic dressing[4] or gauze and tape. *(Level VI*)*	Prevents infection; helps prevent dislodgement.	Dressing should be changed per institution-specific protocol and when it becomes nonocclusive.
21. Ensure portable chest x-ray is obtained to confirm CVC placement.	CVC placements are confirmed by chest x-ray or fluoroscopic study.	Subclavian lines have the possibility of angling up toward the head instead of toward the heart; if line is positioned toward the head, it should not be used for hypertonic or caustic solutions. Notify the practitioner immediately. Short femoral central lines may not require x-ray confirmation; refer to institution-specific protocol.
22. Once placement has been confirmed, infuse fluids through the lumen(s) as ordered or heparin lock lumen(s) not being used. *(Level IV*)*	Decreases the chance of thrombus formation.	Additional methods used to confirm placement include: CVP waveform analysis Intravenous dye contrast study Sonography
23. Remove any excess prep solution and blood from the child.	Povidone-iodine may cause skin breakdown and should be removed from the area outside the dressing; infants are most at risk.	
24. Alert family that procedure is completed; update the family about child's condition.	The family is generally anxious about success of procedure, child's condition.	Ensure that the prescribing practitioner talks with the family to provide an update about the procedure.
25. Dispose of supplies and used equipment appropriately; ensure sharps have been disposed of appropriately.	Standard precautions; reduces transmission of microorganisms; protects personnel health.	
26. Remove protective equipment; wash hands.	Standard precautions; reduces transmission of microorganisms.	

* Level IV: Limited clinical studies to support recommendations
  Level VI: Clinical studies in a variety of patient populations and situations to support recommendations

Expected Outcomes

- Child remains hemodynamically stable during CVC placement
- Respiratory status remains stable
- All CVC lumens have a blood return and flush without difficulty
- CVC tip is located at the atriocaval junction

- CVC is placed without complications

- Child remains free from infection

- Sedation level is adequate during catheter placement
- Child demonstrates acceptable level of comfort

Unexpected Outcomes

- Unstable vital signs

- Respiratory distress or failure
- Unable to flush lumens or obtain blood return

- CVC tip is not located centrally or is advanced into the atrium or ventricle
- Severe dysrhythmias with placement of long catheter
- Pneumothorax, hemothorax, chylothorax (jugular and subclavian sites)
- Arterial puncture (jugular, femoral, and subclavian sites)
- Nerve injury (subclavian, femoral, internal jugular sites)
- Retroperitoneal bleeding (femoral site)
- Cerebral spinal tap (internal jugular site)
- Bleeding (all sites)
- Venous air embolism (all sites)
- Thrombosis (all sites)
- Pericardial tamponade (all sites)
- Infection (all sites) possibly related to poor aseptic technique during insertion
- Unmanaged anxiety or agitation
- Unmanaged pain

Monitoring and Care of the Child

Activities and Interventions	Rationale	Reportable Conditions
1. Monitor vital signs and cardio-respiratory status throughout procedure.	Allows early identification of complications from procedure or sedation.	• Significant change in vital signs • Indications of airway compromise
2. Ensure dressing remains intact and occlusive; dressing changes per institution-specific protocol.	Decreases incidence of infection.	• Redness, drainage, swelling, warmth at insertion site
3. Assess all lumens for blood return, especially distal lumen if short catheter is used, and that all lumens flush without difficulty.	Distal lumen is the tip of the catheter and must always have a blood return—if the catheter is short, and the femoral site is used, the tip of the catheter could puncture the inferior vena cava and fluids could be infused into the peritoneal cavity.	• Lumens do not flush • Unable to obtain blood return
4. Monitor cardiac rhythm for ectopy.	May indicate catheter tip is located past the atriocaval junction or has migrated.	• Arrhythmias, such as persistent PVCs or ventricular tachycardia
5. Monitor site for bleeding, edema and leakage.	Edema may indicate hematoma or catheter displacement; bleeding (if significant) may need to be addressed by practitioner.	• Persistent bleeding from the catheter insertion site
6. Monitor child's tolerance of having CVC in place; evaluate pain and anxiety after insertion and provide appropriate interventions. Encourage family to assist in using nonpharmacologic means to support and comfort the child.	Early identification of pain, anxiety, or discomfort allows immediate attention.	• Unmanaged pain, anxiety, or agitation

Documentation

- Size, length, type, location of catheter, and individual placing catheter
- Presence of blood return, ability to flush catheter
- Tip location and means of verification
- Respiratory and hemodynamic status during procedure
- Medications given during procedure
- Vital signs throughout procedure and recovery, per institution-specific protocol
- Presence of ectopy
- Child and family education
- Site assessment including dressing status, bleeding from site, indications of infection
- Child's tolerance of the procedure
- Length of catheter on removal
- Unexpected outcomes and related treatment

References

1. Fiser DH, Graham J, Green JW et al. Pediatric vascular access and centeses. In Fuhrman BP, Zimmerman JJ, editors: *Pediatric critical care,* ed 3, St. Louis, 2006, Mosby, pp. 151-182.
2. Hocking G: Central venous access and monitoring, *Update in Anaesthesia* 12(13):1, 2000. http://www.nda.ox.ac.uk/wfsa/html/u12/u1213_05.htm. Accessed 6/19/2006.
3. Senett MG: Central venous catheters. In Irwin RS, Rippe JM, editors: *Intensive care medicine,* ed 5, Philadelphia, 2003, Lippincott Williams & Wilkins, pp. 17-32.
4. Hijazi OM, et al: Vascular catheters. In Levin DL, Morriss FC, editors: *Essentials of pediatric intensive care,* ed 2, New York, 1997, Churchill Livingstone, pp. 1189-1233.
5. Dolinski SY, Grohan L, Butterworth J. Procedures in the intensive care unit. In Murray MJ, et al, editors: *Critical care medicine, perioperative management,* ed 2, Philadelphia, 2002, Lippincott Williams & Wilkins, pp. 102-121.

Additional Readings

Chaiyakunapruk N, et al: Vascular catheter site care: the clinical and economic benefits of chlorhexidine gluconate compared with povidone iodine, *CID* 37(6):764-761, 2003.

Hazinski MF: *Manual of pediatric critical care,* St. Louis, 1999, Mosby.

Jacobs BR: Central venous catheter occlusion and thrombosis, *Crit Care Clin* 19:489-514, 2003.

Mooney G, Comerford D: What you need to know about central venous lines, *Nurs Times* 99(10):28-29, 2003.

Moureau N: Using alteplase to clear occlusion, *Nursing* 32(1):73, 2002.

O'Grady NP, et al: Guidelines for the prevention of intravascular catheter-related infections, *MMWR Morb Mortal Wkly Rep* 51(RR-10):1-29, 2002.

Penne K: Using evidence in central catheter care, *Semin Oncol Nurs* 18(1):66-70, 2002.

Puls L, et al: Confirmatory chest radiographs after central line placement; are they warranted? *South Med J* 96(11):1138-1141, 2003.

Simcock L: Central venous catheters; some common clinical questions, *Nurs Times* 97(19):34-36, 2001.

Simcock L: Complications of CVCs and their nursing management, *Nurs Times* 97(19):36-38, 2001.

Central Venous Non-tunneled Catheter: Care and Management

P U R P O S E : To ensure functioning of the catheter, reduce incidence of catheter-related bloodstream infections, and prevent or identify complications related to the catheter

Lara G. Smith

PREREQUISITE KNOWLEDGE

- Child development as it relates to clinical assessment and management and monitoring of a central venous catheter (CVC)
- Principles of aseptic technique
- Standard precautions
- Vascular anatomy and physiology
- Rationale for the placement of a CVC
- Maintenance of central venous pressure (CVP) monitoring system, if CVP is being monitored. Refer to Procedure 142 for further discussion of this topic.
- Complications associated with central venous access, appropriate prevention strategies, and appropriate management of complications
- Order of draw, if blood samples are being obtained

CHILD AND FAMILY ASSESSMENT

- Child's developmental level and ability to interact ➻*Rationale:* These factors influence preparation of the child and interaction; also determine safety measures necessary to maintain CVC.
- History of previous CVC ➻*Rationale:* Previous experience with CVC will ease anxiety related to care and management.
- Child's and family's understanding of the reasons for and risks and benefits of the CVC as well as routine care that

will be provided ➻*Rationale:* Evaluates child's and family's understanding of the procedure and provides a gauge for ongoing education.
- Child's and family's fears and concerns related to the CVC ➻*Rationale:* Identification of concerns and fears facilitates development of an individualized teaching plan.
- Family's desire to be present during procedures such as blood drawing and dressing changes ➻*Rationale:* Family members may provide comfort and support during the procedure, but should have the choice not to remain with the child.

CHILD AND FAMILY EDUCATION

Individualized, developmentally appropriate education is provided to the family and to the child based on desire for knowledge, readiness to learn, and overall neurologic and psychosocial state.

- Provide information about the CVC and reasons for placement ➻*Rationale:* Providing information can help decrease anxiety and fear.
- Explain the necessity of notifying the nurse when child is moving or needs to be moved ➻*Rationale:* Nursing assistance with movement can decrease the likelihood of inadvertent removal or tubing disconnection from the CVC.

- If developmentally appropriate, explain to the child reasons not to touch/pull on CVC or the tubing connected to it ➔*Rationale:* Decreases the likelihood of accidental removal or tubing disconnection.
- Review routine management and care of the CVC such as dressing changes, blood drawing, CVP monitoring ➔*Rationale:* Providing information can help decrease anxiety and fear and promotes cooperation.
- Explain the potential need for devices such as limb holders, elbow restraints or ACE wraps to keep the child from interfering with the CVC and ensure the safety of the child and the device ➔*Rationale:* Providing information can help decrease anxiety and fear and promotes cooperation.
- Encourage questions and answer questions as they arise ➔*Rationale:* Reinforcement of information is needed during periods of stress.

EQUIPMENT

- Blood sampling
  - ❖ Two or three syringes of size required to obtain discard volume and ordered specimens; this will vary based on size of the child, type of specimen(s) required, and minimum blood volume required for the specimen.

- ❖ Label for discard syringe
- ❖ Appropriate specimen tubes
- ❖ Appropriate laboratory requisitions
- ❖ Specimen labels containing two patient identifiers
- ❖ Needles or needleless access device
- ❖ Clean gloves
- ❖ Sterile 4×4 gauze
- ❖ Alcohol wipes or 10% povidone-iodine wipes per institution-specific protocol
- **Dressing change** (Note: supplies listed may come prepared in a dressing change kit)
  - ❖ Clean gloves
  - ❖ Mask
  - ❖ 2% chlorhexidine or 10% povidone-iodine per institution-specific protocol
  - ❖ Sterile 2×2 gauze
  - ❖ Tape
  - ❖ Transparent dressing
  - ❖ Sterile gloves
- Removal
  - ❖ Clean gloves
  - ❖ Sterile 4×4 gauze
  - ❖ Sterile 2×2 gauze
  - ❖ Tape or coverlet
  - ❖ Sterile scissors if CVC is sutured in place

Procedure for Central Venous Non-tunneled Catheter: Care and Management

Steps	Rationale	Considerations
Blood Sampling		
1. Ensure the child and family understand procedure and questions are answered.	Evaluates and reinforces understanding of previously taught information.	Developmental level, cognitive ability, and anxiety level will determine approach to and effectiveness of teaching.
2. Gather needed supplies and equipment.	Facilitates completion of procedure in a timely manner.	Supplies necessary may vary based on institution specifics such as type of blood draw system used; refer to institution-specific protocol.
3. Wash hands.	Standard precautions; reduces transmission of microorganisms.	
4. Use two patient identifiers to verify correct child.	Promotes patient safety; ensures blood specimens are being drawn on the correct child.	
5. If CVP is being monitored, silence the monitor alarms.	Prevents unnecessary alarm activation during sampling procedure.	
6. Put on clean gloves.	Standard precautions; reduces transmission of microorganisms.	
7. Place sterile 4×4 under stopcock or sampling port from which blood is being drawn.	Provides a clean work surface.	

Procedure	**for Central Venous Non-tunneled Catheter: Care and Management**—*Continued*	
Steps	**Rationale**	**Considerations**
8. If the CVC has more than one lumen, stop infusions running through all lumens.[1,2] *(Level II*)*	Ensures accurate lab results; prevents contamination of blood sample with fluids infusing in other lumens.	Stability of child dictates the safety of pausing infusions. If child is receiving medications for inotropic support via one of the catheter lumens, do not stop infusion. If a high-concentration dextrose solution is being infused, flush the line with normal saline before withdrawing blood.
9. Label the syringe to be used for drawing discard.	Prevents blood in discard syringe from being sent to the lab for analysis.[3]	
10. Clean specimen port site or needleless access site with alcohol wipe or antiseptic swab.[4] Remove occlusive cap from stopcock if appropriate.	Reduces transmission of microorganisms.	Refer to institution-specific protocol for antiseptic solution used for cleaning port or needleless access site.
11. Attach labeled discard syringe to stopcock closest to child or access sampling port with needleless access device. Turn stopcock open to child and catheter, off to infusion and aspirate two to six times the volume of the catheter and tubing before stopcock or sampling port (dead space).[1,3] *(Level IV*)*	Ensures fluid and medication are cleared from line, prevents contamination of sample for lab.	Dead space volume must be accurately determined to ensure samples are free of contaminants (heparin or crystalloids).
12. Remove discard syringe. Attach syringe for laboratory specimens and withdraw amount of blood required for sample.	Obtains laboratory samples.	If drawing more than one lab including a prothrombin time/ partial thromboplastin time (PT/PTT), draw the PT/PTT last to attempt to ensure heparin from transducer system flush fluid is removed from line. Some recommend never drawing coagulation studies from a heparinized Hickman catheter, though non-tunneled catheters are not specifically discussed.[3] *(Level V*)*
13. Place blood in appropriate specimen tubes.	Required for specimen processing.	Specimen collection tubes are determined by the institution
14. It is not recommended to reinfuse discard volume to the child.[3] If discard is to be returned to the child, replace syringe with discard; turn the stopcock off to the fluid, open to the child and catheter; slowly reinfuse the blood in the syringe, and then turn the stopcock to off to the syringe.	Reinfusion of discard reduces the blood loss that occurs when multiple specimens are obtained over several hours or days. Infants and smaller children with frequent blood draws cannot tolerate losing 2 to 5 mL of blood with each specimen sampling due to less circulating blood volume (approximately 75-85 mL/kg of circulating blood volume).	Reinfuse the discard volume if this is consistent with institution-specific protocol. Concerns with reinfusing discard volume include possible contamination of the discard syringe, clots in the discard volume, and exposure of the clini cian to blood.[3]
15. When blood draw is complete, flush line with saline to clear line and stopcock or sampling port of blood.	Prevents line from clotting and decreases infection risk from blood sitting in the port.[4]	

Procedure continues on following page

* Level II: Theory based, no research data to support recommendations: recommendations from expert consensus group may exist
Level IV: Limited clinical studies to support recommendations
Level V: Clinical studies in more than one or two patient populations and situations to support recommendations

Procedure for Central Venous Non-tunneled Catheter: Care and Management—*Continued*

Steps	Rationale	Considerations
16. If occlusive cap was removed, recap the port with a sterile cap and ensure the stopcock is in the "off to the syringe" position.	Minimizes risk of contamination of system and ensures resumption of accurate monitoring.	
17. Resume fluid infusion.	Maintains catheter patency.	
18. Reactivate monitor alarms if appropriate.	Provides for notification when central venous pressures are at an unacceptable level.	Alarm ranges are set per institution-specific protocol and child's status.
19. Label specimens at the bedside and complete laboratory paperwork per institution-specific protocol.	Promotes patient safety; ensures accurate and efficient processing of specimen.	Follow institution-specific protocol for handling and labeling specimens.
20. Dispose of used supplies and equipment in appropriate receptacle; ensure sharps are disposed of correctly. Wash hands.	Standard precautions; prevents transmission of microorganisms. Protects personnel health.	
Dressing Change		
1. Ensure child and family understand the procedure and questions are answered.	Evaluates and reinforces understanding of previously taught information.	Developmental level, cognitive ability, and anxiety level will determine approach to and effectiveness of teaching.
2. Gather needed supplies and equipment. If required, enlist an assistant to help with positioning child.	Facilitates completion of procedure in a timely manner.	Supplies necessary will vary based on the size of the child, and institution-specific dressing change protocol. Active infants and young children may require an assistant to position the child and keep the child's hands away from the catheter insertion site.
3. Wash hands.	Standard precautions; reduces transmission of microorganisms.	
4. Provide for appropriate privacy and position the child to facilitate access to the catheter insertion site.	Respects child's privacy; femoral lines and some chest lines require exposing the groin or chest.	Privacy is an important consideration for school-aged children and adolescents.
5. Put on clean gloves and mask.	Standard precautions; reduces transmission of microorganisms.	
6. Prepare sterile field with supplies.	Decreases length of time site is undressed.	
7. Remove old dressing.	Must be removed to clean site and place new dressing.	
8. Put on sterile gloves.[4,5] *(Level V*)*	Reduces transmission of microorganisms, reduces incidence of intravascular catheter-related bloodstream infections (CRBSI).	
9. Assess catheter site for signs of infection, infiltration.[6] *(Level IV*)*	Identifies CVC-related complications.	Signs of infection include redness, swelling, drainage, warmth, odor at the insertion site.

* Level IV: Limited clinical studies to support recommendations
  Level V: Clinical studies in more than one or two patient populations and situations to support recommendations

Procedure | **for Central Venous Non-tunneled Catheter: Care and Management**—*Continued*

Steps	Rationale	Considerations
10. Ensure sutures or line securement device is intact.	Ensures line securely in place.	Sutureless securement devices may be advantageous over suture in preventing CRBSI.[4] *(Level IV*)*
11. Clean dried blood and/or secretions with sterile gauze and 0.9% saline. *(Level II*)*	Decreases infection risk.	
12. Clean site with 2% chlorhexidine, tincture of iodine, or 70% alcohol per institution-specific protocol, scrubbing area, then allow to air-dry completely.[4] *(Level V*)*	Decreases infection risk and ensures adherence of new dressing.	At the time of publication of Centers for Disease Control and Prevention (CDC) recommendations to prevent CRBSI, the only concentration of chlorhexidine available was 2%, which caused significant dermatitis in low birth weight neonates. A 1% concentration is now available. A concentration of 0.5% was not shown to be better than povidone-iodine.[4] Do not use topical antibiotic ointment or creams at insertion sites because of their potential to promote fungal infections and antimicrobial resistance.[4] *(Level V*)*
13. Apply new dressing, either sterile gauze and tape or transparent dressing.[7] *(Level V*)*	Protects catheter and site. Transparent dressings allow for visualization of insertion site.	Studies showed no significant difference in infection occurrence between tape and gauze or transparent dressing. Tape and gauze are recommended if the site is oozing or bleeding or if child is diaphoretic. Tape and gauze dressings should be changed twice a week or when soiled or nonocclusive. Transparent dressings should be changed weekly or when soiled or nonocclusive.[4] *(Level V*)*
14. Dispose of supplies and used equipment appropriately.	Standard precautions; reduces the transmission of microorganisms.	
15. Remove mask and gloves; wash hands.	Standard precautions; reduces the transmission of microorganisms.	
Catheter Removal		
1. Ensure child and family understand reasons for the removal of the CVC.	Evaluates and reinforces understanding of previously taught information.	Developmental level, cognitive ability, and anxiety level will determine approach to and effectiveness of teaching.
2. Collect all necessary supplies and equipment.	Facilitates completion of procedure in a timely manner.	
3. Turn off infusions or move the infusions to alternate catheters.	CVC is capped or clamped off for removal.	Ensure any fluids that are being moved to a peripheral line have a glucose concentration appropriate for the line (i.e., 12.5% dextrose).
4. Wash hands.	Standard precautions: reduces transmission of microorganisms.	

Procedure continues on following page

---

*   Level II: Theory based, no research data to support recommendations: recommendations from expert consensus group may exist
    Level IV: Limited clinical studies to support recommendations
    Level V: Clinical studies in more than one or two patient populations and situations to support recommendations

Procedure for Central Venous Non-tunneled Catheter: Care and Management—*Continued*

Steps	Rationale	Considerations
5. Provide for appropriate privacy and position the child to facilitate access to the catheter insertion site.	Respects child's privacy; femoral lines and some chest lines require exposing the groin or chest.	Privacy is an important consideration for school-aged children and adolescents.
6. Put on clean or sterile gloves, and personal protective equipment per institution-specific protocol.	Standard precautions.	
7. Remove dressing.	Facilitates removing catheter.	
8. Remove sutures or securement device.	Must be removed in order to remove CVC.	
9. Place sterile gauze in hand to hold pressure over site during and after removal.	Prepares for line removal.	
10. Remove CVC in a smooth, steady movement and place sterile gauze over the site simultaneously; hold pressure for at least 5 minutes.	Stops bleeding, prevents hematoma formation; decreases risk of introduction of air embolus.	If resistance is felt during removal, do not forcibly remove catheter; notify prescribing practitioner.
11. Apply an airtight dressing to site for 24 hours, and encourage child to lie flat for 30 minutes after CVC removal.[8] *(Level IV*)*	Prevents air being sucked into the tract before it seals.	If the CVC has been in more than two weeks, consider placing petrolatum gauze over the site to help seal tract.
12. Dispose of supplies and used equipment appropriately.	Standard precautions; reduces transmission of microorganisms.	
13. Remove personal protective equipment; wash hands.	Standard precautions; reduces transmission of microorganisms.	

* Level IV: Limited clinical studies to support recommendations

Expected Outcomes

- CVC remains in place for desired length of therapy
- CVC is functional with appropriate CVP tracing, brisk blood return; flushes without difficulty

- Child is free from CVC complications

- CVC dressing remains intact and is changed at appropriate intervals; no indications of skin breakdown

- CVC removal is planned and completed without incident
- Administration sets are replaced at appropriate intervals

- Specimens obtained are placed in correct sample tubes, labeled appropriately, and sent to the lab in the appropriate time frame
- Child demonstrates acceptable level of comfort

Unexpected Outcomes

- Unplanned CVC removal
- Unable to flush CVC
- Unable to obtain blood return
- CVP waveform is damped or is not dynamic
- Unable to infuse fluids
- Localized site infection or CRBSI
- Air embolus
- Dislodgement of thrombus or fibrin sheath[9]
- Hemorrhage or bruising
- Extravasation of infusion fluids
- Pneumothorax, hemothorax, chylothorax
- Perforation or fracture of CVC
- Superior vena cava (SVC) syndrome
- Skin irritation or breakdown
- Dressing is not intact
- Dressing changes are not completed at appropriate intervals
- Catheter fracture and embolism during removal[9]
- Administration sets are not replaced at the appropriate interval
- Specimens are mislabeled, placed in incorrect sample tubes, or not sent to lab in a timely fashion

- Unmanaged pain related to CVC

Monitoring and Care of the Child

Activities and Interventions	Rationale	Reportable Conditions
1. Monitor the CVC for functionality; ease of infusion, blood return, appropriate CVP waveform.	Inability to flush or draw blood may indicate clotted catheter.	• Difficulty infusing fluids or drawing blood • CVP waveform that is damped or is not dynamic
2. Monitor site for signs and symptoms of infection.	Intervention will be required for cellulitis or bloodstream infection.	• Erythema, swelling, purulent drainage, warmth at insertion site; bruising at insertion site • Fever, increased white blood cell count
3. Monitor skin integrity at insertion site.	Monitors for local skin irritation or breakdown caused by antiseptic solutions or dressing materials.	• Skin irritation or breakdown
4. Monitor integrity of CVC dressing and securement device.	Replace dressings that are not secure to promote infection-free site.	• Grossly soiled dressing • Dressing loose for significant period of time • Sutures not intact
5. Monitor for signs of CVC-related complications.	Early identification allows prompt treatment of complications.	• Pulsatile blood flow in catheter • Swelling of head and/or neck • Swelling of extremities by insertion site, color changes, temperature changes • Dyspnea, cyanosis, hypotension, dizziness, tachycardia, weak pulse, anxiety, confusion, decreased level of consciousness • Dysrhythmias
6. Replace administration sets and occlusive caps at appropriate intervals. Recommendations for tubing and cap replacement is every 72 hours; replace tubing for blood and blood products, lipid emulsions every 24 hours, propofol infusions every 6 to 12 hours. Change needleless components of system when administration set is changed.[4]	Studies indicate that following these recommendations decreases the incidence of CRBSI. *(Level VI[*])*	• Unable to remove administration set from catheter hub

7. When accessing the catheter:
  Wipe access port with antiseptic (70% alcohol or povidone-iodine).
  Use a sterile device to access the port.
  Cap all stopcocks when not in use.
	Studies indicate that following these recommendations decreases the incidence of CRBSI.[4] *(Level VI[*])*	• Deviation from these recommendations

8. Monitor volume of blood drawn on a daily basis and for the duration of hospitalization.	Heightens staff's awareness of blood loss due to phlebotomy, which may decrease overall blood loss.[3] *(Level IV[*])*	• Significant blood volume removal, as defined by institution-specific protocol

* Level IV: Limited clinical studies to support recommendations
  Level VI: Clinical studies in a variety of patient populations and situations to support recommendations

Documentation

- Education of child and family
- Insertion site status, including skin and dressing integrity
- CVP waveform assessment, if CVP is monitored
- Dressing changes
- Tubing and fluid changes
- Time of blood sampling, specimens obtained, results of studies
- Amount of blood withdrawn, along with running total for hospitalization
- Removal of catheter
- Comfort assessment and any specific interventions provided
- Unexpected outcomes and related treatment

References

1. Arrow International. Central venous catheter nursing care guidelines. Update 12/01. www.arrowintl.com/products/critical_care/literature.asp. Accessed 5/14/06.
2. Hadaway L: Can I stop a drug infusion to draw blood? *Nursing* 33(5):14, 2003.
3. Frey AM: Drawing blood samples from vascular access devices: evidence-based practice, *J Infus Nurs* 26(5):285-293, 2003.
4. Centers for Disease Control and Prevention: Guidelines for the prevention of intravascular catheter related infections, *MMWR Morbid Mortal Wkly Rep* 51(No.RR-10):1-29, 2002.
5. Hadaway L: Infusing without infecting, *Nursing* 33(10):58-63, 2003.
6. Hadaway L: IV infiltration: not just a peripheral problem, *Nursing* 32(8):36-42, 2002.
7. Gilles D, et al: Central venous catheter dressings: a systematic review, *J Adv Nurs* 44(6):623-632, 2003.
8. Drewett S: Central venous catheter removal: procedures and rationale, *Br J Nurs* 9(22):2304-2315, 2000.
9. Knutstad K, et al: Radiologic diagnosis and management of complications related to central venous access, *Acta Radiol* 44(5):508-516, 2003.

Additional Readings

Casado-Flores J, et al: Complications of central venous catheterization in critically ill children, *Pediatr Crit Care Med* 2(1):57-62, 2001.

Chaiyakunapruk N, et al: Vascular catheter site care: the clinical and economic benefits of chlorhexidine gluconate compared with povidone iodine, *CID* 37(6):764-771, 2003.

McConnell EA: Changing a central venous catheter dressing, *Nursing* 30(4):24, 2000.

Mooney G, Comerford D: What you need to know about central venous lines, *Nurs Times* 99(10):28-29, 2003.

Moureau N: Using alteplase to clear occlusions, *Nursing* 32(1):73, 2002.

O'Grady NP, et al: Guidelines for the prevention of intravascular catheter-related infections, *MMWR Morb Mortal Wkly Rep* 51(RR-10):1-29, 2002.

Penne K: Using evidence in central catheter care, *Semin Oncol Nurs* 18(1):66-70, 2002

Puls L, et al: Confirmatory chest radiographs after central line placement: are they warranted? *South Med J* 96(11):1138-41, 2003.

Simcock L: Central venous catheters: some common clinical questions, *Nurs Times* 97(19):34-36, 2001.

Simcock L: Complications of CVCs and their nursing management, *Nurs Times* 97(19):36-38, 2001.

Central Venous Non-tunneled Catheter: Central Venous Pressure Monitoring

PURPOSE: To evaluate intravascular blood volume, or preload; estimate circulatory function, in particular cardiac function and blood volume

Kelly A. Lankin

PREREQUISITE KNOWLEDGE

- Child development as it relates to clinical assessment and central venous pressure (CVP) measurement
- Indications for CVP monitoring include hypovolemic shock, sepsis, cardiogenic shock (postcardiac surgery), hypotension, and in children receiving continuous infusions of inotropes.
- Familiarity with catheter and transducer devices; refer to Procedure 63
- Principles of hemodynamic monitoring
- Anatomy and physiology of the central vascular system
- CVP directly correlates with right atrial pressure (RAP), which reflects right ventricular end-diastolic pressure (RVEDP), as well as left ventricular function in individuals without cardiopulmonary disease.[1,2,3]
- In order to obtain accurate readings, the tip of the CVC should be located at the caval-atrial junction[1]
- Normal CVP: 4 to 8 mm Hg[1,2,3,4,5]
  - ❖ Trends are more important than actual values.
  - ❖ Treatment should not be based on CVP readings alone but accompanied by clinical assessment.
- Optimize bedside pressure monitoring system[1,3,4]: *(Level VI*)*
  - ❖ Use high-pressure tubing between transducer and child that does not exceed 36 to 48 inches in length.

- ❖ Use transparent stopcocks with luer-lok connections to maintain system integrity and permit evaluation for air bubbles.
- ❖ Remove all air bubbles in transducer system—air can alter pressure readings.
- ❖ Minimize the potential for clot formation by infusing a heparinized solution continuously (1-3 units of heparin/mL of solution).
- ❖ Zero the transducer once per shift or per institution-specific protocol.
- ❖ Use disposable transducers, which offer advantages in both low compliance and excellent time-temperature stability.
- CVP waveform components (Figure 142-1)
  - ❖ *a*-wave: atrial contraction
  - ❖ *c*-wave: closing and bulging of the tricuspid valve at the onset of ventricular systole
  - ❖ *v*-wave: passive venous filling of the right atrium during ventricular systole
  - ❖ *x*-wave: descent that represents atrial relaxation
  - ❖ *y*-wave: descent that represents rapid atrial emptying after opening of the tricuspid valve
- Conditions that cause elevated CVP measurements: tension pneumothorax, heart failure (right or left ventricle), pericardial tamponade, pulmonary stenosis, pulmonary hypertension, volume overload
- Conditions that cause decreased CVP measurements: hypovolemia, sepsis (distribution of fluid) and dehydration
- Dysrhythmias will cause abnormalities in the CVP waveform (i.e., heart block will cause pauses in the CVP

---

* Level VI: Clinical studies in a variety of patient populations and situations to support recommendations

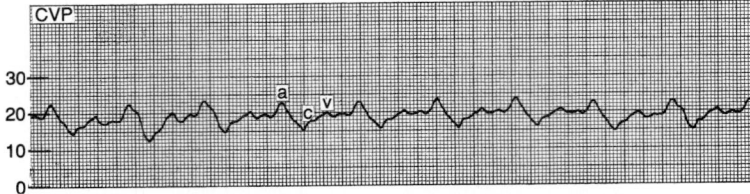

FIGURE 142-1   Components of the central venous pressure waveform. *From Arnone R: Central venous/right atrial pressure monitoring. In Lynn-McHale DJ, Carlson KK, editors:* AACN procedure manual for critical care, *ed 4, Philadelphia, 2001, Saunders, p. 412.*

waveform, tachycardic dysrhythmias will cause rapid waveform tracing).
- Positive-pressure ventilation and positive end-expiratory pressure (PEEP) can increase CVP values if intrathoracic pressure increases or can decrease CVP measurements if venous return is impeded, making interpretation of the child's volume and cardiac status difficult.[1,2,4,6,7]
- Potential complications of CVP monitoring
- Principles of aseptic technique

CHILD AND FAMILY ASSESSMENT

- Child's developmental level and ability to interact ➤➤*Rationale:* These factors influence preparation of the child and interaction.
- Patency of the central venous catheter (CVC) by checking distal port for blood return and ease of flushing—also verify that there are no visible kinks in the catheter or transducer tubing ➤➤*Rationale:* Patent CVC is necessary for accurate CVP measurements.
- Placement of tip of CVC via chest x-ray; consult prescribing practitioner ➤➤*Rationale:* Correct placement of the CVC is essential in order to obtain accurate CVP measurements. If the catheter is not in optimal position for accurate reading, value may be monitored for 'trends.'
- Child's and family's understanding of the reasons for and risks and benefits of monitoring CVP measurements ➤➤*Rationale:* Providing information decreases fear and anxiety.
- Child's hemodynamic status, including vital signs and electrocardiogram (ECG) tracing ➤➤*Rationale:* Cardiac arrhythmias or hypotension will alter the CVP waveform tracing.
- Child's hydration status ➤➤*Rationale:* CVP is a measure of intravascular volume.

CHILD AND FAMILY EDUCATION

Individualized, developmentally appropriate education is provided to the family and to the child based on desire for knowledge, readiness to learn, and overall neurologic and psychosocial state.

- Explain the procedure of attaching a transducer system to the CVC ➤➤*Rationale:* Prepares family and child for this procedure.
- Explain the meaning of CVP measurements and how these numbers, coupled with the child's assessment, may affect treatment (i.e., fluid may need to be given if CVP is low and child is hypotensive) ➤➤*Rationale:* Educates family and child on reasons for CVP measurement.
- Explain to the family and child that there will be no pain involved with this procedure ➤➤*Rationale:* Alleviates child and family anxiety related to pain.
- Explain that the waveform and readings will be monitored and that the equipment may periodically alarm; in many cases alarm activations are related to manipulation of the catheter or transducer. Assure the family and child that staff will respond to and evaluate alarms ➤➤*Rationale:* Decreases family's and child's anxiety related to monitor alarms.
- If the child does not have a CVC and one needs to be placed for CVP measurements, explain the procedure (refer to Procedure 140) ➤➤*Rationale:* Providing information decreases anxiety and fear.
- Use an interpreter if the child and/or family has limited English proficiency ➤➤*Rationale:* Decreases barriers to communication.
- Encourage questions and answer questions as they arise ➤➤*Rationale:* Reinforcement of information is needed during periods of stress.

EQUIPMENT

- Transducer kit with pressure tubing
- Pressure bag or syringe pump
- Stopcock, if not in transducer kit
- Bag or syringe of 0.9% saline with heparin 1 to 3 units/mL per institution-specific protocol or fluids to infuse through transducer system per prescribing practitioner's order
- Cardiorespiratory monitor
- Cable to connect transducer to monitor
- Sterile gloves
- Mask
- Sterile 2×2s or 4×4s
- Alcohol swabs or antiseptic wipes

Procedure	for Central Venous Non-tunneled Catheter: Central Venous Pressure Monitoring		
Steps	**Rationale**	**Considerations**	
1. Ensure family and child understand procedure and questions are answered.	Evaluates and reinforces understanding of previously taught information.	Developmental level, cognitive ability, and anxiety level will determine approach to and effectiveness of teaching.	
2. Gather needed equipment and supplies.	Facilitates completion of task in a timely manner.	Disposable transducer systems decrease the incidence of catheter–related bloodstream infections (CRBSI).[8] *(Level IV*)*	
3. Wash hands.	Standard precautions; reduces the transmission of microorganisms.		
4. Turn monitor on, if necessary, and program the monitor to read CVP measurements and display waveform.	Ensures monitor is functioning and will display CVP waveform and reading after the transducer system is assembled and attached.	Monitoring systems vary widely; refer to manufacturer's instructions for CVP monitoring setup.	
5. Assemble transducer system as required; ensure all luer connections are secure. Connect flush solution to transducer system.	Ensures a closed system; prevents introduction of microorganisms and blood loss through loose connections.	Closed, continuous flush systems decrease the incidence of CRBSI.[8] *(Level IV*)*	
6. Flush tubing with heparinized saline or prescribed fluid, eliminating all air bubbles from the system.	Transducer systems must be flushed with fluid to establish an uninterrupted fluid column; otherwise CVP measurements will be inaccurate.	If the system contains a fast-flush valve or other activation device, it must be used when flushing the tubing. A syringe may be used to flush the system; fluids do not typically flow through transducer systems with attached pressure tubing by gravity. Premixed solutions or solutions prepared in the pharmacy are preferred because they promote patient safety. *(Level IV*)*	
7. Put on mask and sterile gloves.	Manipulation of CVC using sterile technique decreases the incidence of CRBSI.[8] *(Level VI*)*	Sterile glove package can be opened and used as a sterile field; place gauze and alcohol pads onto the internal packaging. Everyone in the room will need to put on a mask, including family members, while accessing the CVC. This practice may vary; refer to institution-specific protocol.	
8. Place sterile gauze under CVC port; clean CVC port with alcohol wipe or antiseptic swab.	Reduces transmission of microorganisms.		
9. Using aseptic technique, attach the transducer system to the CVC.	Use of aseptic technique reduces the transmission of microorganisms.	Pressure tubing can be used between the transducer and the CVC, which range from 6 inches to 36 inches. *(Level IV*)*	

Procedure continues on following page

* Level IV: Limited clinical studies to support recommendations
Level VI: Clinical studies in a variety of patient populations and situations to support recommendations

Procedure	**for Central Venous Non-tunneled Catheter: Central Venous Pressure Monitoring**—*Continued*	
Steps	**Rationale**	**Considerations**
10. When using a multilumen catheter, transduce the distal port of the CVC.[9] *(Level VI*)*	The distal port of the CVC is the tip of the catheter and will give the most accurate readings for CVP measurements.[9]	Accurate CVP monitoring from the distal port requires patency of the distal port. If distal port does not have blood return, investigate the possibility of thrombus, catheter up against the vessel wall, kinks in catheter.[9]
11. Limit the number of stopcocks to three between the transducer and the child. *(Level IV*)*	Added stopcocks, like pressure tubing, will alter pressure measurements.	Stopcocks must be capped when not in use to decrease incidence of CRBSI.[8] *(Level IV*)*
12. Attach appropriate cable from the transducer to the monitor.	A connection between the transducer and the monitor must be established in order to display CVP measurements and waveforms.	Refer to manufacturer's instructions.
13. Level the transducer at the phlebostatic axis. *(Level VI*)*	Ensures accurate pressure readings; eliminates the effects of atmospheric and hydrostatic pressure.[1]	Refer to Procedure 137 for a diagram of phlebostatic axis location.
14. Zero the transducer: turn stopcock off to the child, open to the transducer and stopcock port.	Ensures accurate CVP measurements.	Follow institution specific protocol and procedure.
15. Remove the cap from the stopcock port to open the transducer to air (atmospheric pressure).	Transducer is zeroed while open to air.	Be sure to have the stopcock off to the child while open to air to prevent backflow of blood into the tubing.
16. Press zero button on the monitor and wait for confirmation that zero procedure is complete.	Zeros the transducer.	Follow manufacturer's instructions for zeroing procedure.
17. Turn stopcock off to the stopcock port and open to the transducer and child. Replace sterile cap.	Closes the system to allow CVP measurement; replace sterile cap to decrease the incidence of infection.	Stopcocks must be capped when not in use to decrease incidence of vascular CRBSI.[8] *(Level IV*)*
18. To obtain a reading, turn all stopcocks off to infusing fluids, leaving open one fluid path from the transducer to the child. *(Level V*)*	If fluids are infusing through the transducer, especially at rate of >30 mL/hr, the reading may not be accurate.[4]	Intermittent CVP readings are most accurate. There are too many variables to monitor CVP continuously (child's position, position of the transducer in relationship to the phlebostatic reference point, infusing fluids).
19. With the transducer at the phlebostatic axis obtain the CVP measurement, paying close attention to the waveform. *(Level VI*)*	The CVP waveform should be detectable—a damped waveform may indicate that the reading is not accurate.	Child's position can also affect readings; if waveform is damped or values are not following trends, then reposition the child and repeat the CVP reading. Transducer positioned above phlebostatic axis will give falsely low readings; transducer positioned below phlebostatic axis will give falsely high readings.[1]

* Level IV: Limited clinical studies to support recommendations
Level V: Clinical studies in more than one or two patient populations and situations to support recommendations
Level VI: Clinical studies in a variety of patient populations and situations to support recommendations

Procedure	for Central Venous Non-tunneled Catheter: Central Venous Pressure Monitoring—*Continued*	
Steps	**Rationale**	**Considerations**
20. After a measurement is obtained and waveform analyzed, open stopcocks to infusing fluids.	Maintains catheter patency; allows fluid administration.	
21. Set alarm parameters based on child's current CVP or notification parameters.	Appropriately set alarms to allow detection of inadvertent disconnection, significant changes in CVP, catheter malfunction, or inadvertent catheter removal.	Ensure that alarms are activated with appropriate settings and are sufficiently audible.
22. Dispose of supplies and used equipment appropriately; remove gloves and wash hands.	Standard precautions; reduces transmission of microorganisms.	

Expected Outcomes

- Dynamic CVP waveform
- Accurate pressure readings are obtained

- Distal port of CVC has brisk blood return and flushes easily
- Catheter remains in place until electively removed

- Child remains free from CRBSI
- Improvements in child's assessment after interventions guided by CVP measurements

Unexpected Outcomes

- Damped or absent CVP waveform
- Inaccurate readings are obtained related to incorrect transducer system setup, transducer not located at the phlebostatic axis, zero drift of transducer due to incorrect frequency of transducer zero, transducer not attached to distal port of multilumen catheter
- Unable to obtain blood return from distal port
- Distal port does not flush
- Inadvertent catheter removal
- Migration of catheter tip
- Indications of CRBSI
- No improvement with interventions guided by CVP measurement

Monitoring and Care of the Child

Activities and Interventions	Rationale	Reportable Conditions
1. Monitor CVP measurements and trends as prescribed; monitor CVP waveform for changes that correlate with child's clinical state.	CVP readings are used in conjunction with the child's assessment to provide necessary interventions.	• CVP readings outside notification parameters • Significant changes in CVP waveform • Damped CVP waveform despite repositioning child and flushing catheter
2. Monitor CVC site: intact, without drainage or bleeding, with occlusive dressing intact.	Monitor for indications of complications; minimize risk of CRBSI.	• Catheter inadvertently removed • Excessive bleeding from insertion site • Drainage from insertion site • Indications of infection at insertion site
3. Monitor CVC patency.	Nonpatent lines will not produce accurate CVP readings or pressure waveforms.	• Unable to flush CVC or obtain blood return

Continued

Monitoring and Care of the Child—Cont'd

Activities and Interventions	Rationale	Reportable Conditions
4. Ensure transducer system remains intact, with all connections secure, stopcock ports capped. Change flush solution and tubing every 72 to 96 hours or per institution-specific protocol. *(Level IV*)*	Decreases incidence of CRBSI; Centers for Disease Control and Prevention recommendations for CVC flush and tubing change frequency is every 96 hours.[8]	• Indications of CRBSI including fever, hemodynamic instability, positive blood cultures from CVC
5. Zero the transducer every shift and after disconnecting the pressure cable (i.e., after transducer is changed or if disconnected for transport) or any time that there is a discrepancy in trends or readings. *(Level VI*)* Level the transducer to the phlebostatic axis with changes in child's position.	Maintains accurate CVP measurements; because treatment is based on clinical changes and CVP readings, it is imperative that the readings obtained are accurate.	• Discrepancy between current and previous CVP readings despite releveling and rezeroing transducer

* Level IV: Limited clinical studies to support recommendations
  Level VI: Clinical studies in a variety of patient populations and situations to support recommendations

Documentation

- Child and family education
- CVP waveform analysis
- CVP readings
- Zeroing and leveling procedure
- CVC site inspection
- Fluid and tubing changes
- CVC patency, including blood return, ease of flushing, no kinks in catheter or tubing
- Type of CVC in place
- Unexpected outcomes and related treatment

References

1. Craig, J, et al. In Curley MAQ, Moloney-Harmon PA, editors: *Critical care nursing of infants and children,* ed 2, Philadelphia, 2001, Saunders, pp 131-231.
2. Fiser DH, et al: Pediatric vascular access and centeses. In Fuhrman BP, Zimmerman JJ, editors: *Pediatric critical care,* ed 3, St. Louis, 2006, Mosby, pp. 151-182.
3. Hazinski MF: *Manual of pediatric critical care,* St. Louis, 1999, Mosby.
4. Hocking G: Central venous access and monitoring, *Pract Proced* 12(Article 13), 2000.
5. Hijazi, OM, et al: Vascular catheters. In Levin DL, Morriss FC, editors: *Essentials of pediatric intensive care,* ed 2, New York, 1997, Churchill Livingstone, pp. 1189-1233.
6. Senett MG. Central venous catheters. In Irwin RS, Rippe JM, editors: *Intensive care medicine,* ed 5, Philadelphia, 2003, Lippincott Williams & Wilkins, pp. 17-32.
7. Dolinski SY, et al: Procedures in the intensive care unit. In Murray MJ, et al, editors: *Critical care medicine, perioperative management,* ed 2, Philadelphia, 2002, Lippincott Williams & Wilkins, pp. 102-121.
8. O'Grady NP, et al: Guidelines for the prevention of intravascular catheter related infections, *MMWR Morbid Mortal Wkly Rep* 51(No.RR-10):1-29, 2002.
9. Scott SS, et al: Influence of port site on central venous pressure measurement from triple-lumen catheters in critically ill adults, *Am J Crit Care* (17)1:60-63, 1998.

Central Venous Tunneled Catheter: Care and Management

P U R P O S E : To ensure functioning of the catheter, reduce incidence of catheter-related bloodstream infections, and prevent or identify complications related to the catheter

Marvin Siegel

PREREQUISITE KNOWLEDGE

- Indications for placement of a central venous tunneled catheter include:
  - To provide long-term infusion therapy when peripheral access is unavailable
  - To provide vesicant or hyperosmolar infusions
  - To provide multiple or complex infusion therapies
- Child development as it relates to clinical assessment and care and management of central venous tunneled catheters
- Fill volume of each lumen of the catheter
- Anatomy and physiology of the central venous system
- Complications associated with central venous access, appropriate prevention strategies, and appropriate management of complications
- Care of surgical sites
- Aseptic technique
- Standard precautions
- Centers for Disease Control and Prevention (CDC) guidelines for the prevention of catheter–related bloodstream infections (CRBSI)
- Infusion Nurses Society (INS) Standards of Practice regarding care of central venous access devices (CVADs)
- Specific state nurse practice act as it relates to care and maintenance of central venous catheters (CVCs)
- Institution-specific protocols regarding tunneled CVCs

CHILD AND FAMILY ASSESSMENT

- Child's developmental level and ability to interact **➤Rationale:** These factors influence preparation of the child's and interaction.
- Child's and family's understanding of the reasons for and risks and benefits of central venous tunneled catheter placement and management **➤Rationale:** Evaluates child's and family's understanding of the procedure and ongoing care that will be required; provides a gauge for ongoing education.
- During the initial visit identify any educational, cultural, or physical barriers to learning and performing care of the catheter **➤Rationale:** Facilitates development of an individualized educational plan, which promotes success.
- Child's and family's fears and concerns related to the central venous tunneled catheter **➤Rationale:** Identification of concerns and fears facilitates development of an individualized teaching plan.

CHILD AND FAMILY EDUCATION

Individualized, developmentally appropriate education is provided to the family and to the child based on desire for knowledge, readiness to learn, and overall neurologic and psychosocial state.

- Educate the family, and child as appropriate, about routine postoperative care of insertion site, signs and symptoms of infection, inflammation, and catheter occlusion ➥*Rationale:* Provides family with information needed to care for the child with a tunneled CVC at home; decreases anxiety and fear.
- Teach the family, and child as appropriate, the saline flush-administer medication-saline flush-heparin flush (SASH) procedure to maintain catheter patency ➥*Rationale:* Prepares the family to safely provide care for the child at home when administering medications through the CVC.
- Provide written educational material to the child and family on care and management of the tunneled catheter and the insertion site ➥*Rationale:* Providing written material permits the child or family to refer to a source of information that reinforces teaching done by the nurse. Having educational materials to refer to can help reduce anxiety and fear associated with family's responsibility for performing tasks related to CVC care.
- Have the family, and child if appropriate, give a repeat demonstration of any tasks that they are instructed to perform independently, such as routine catheter flushes ➥*Rationale:* In order to appropriately document a child and family member as being independent in performing a task, they must be observed carrying it out as instructed.
- Encourage questions and answer questions as they arise ➥*Rationale:* Reinforcement of information is needed during periods of stress.

EQUIPMENT

- Gloves, sterile and clean
- Face mask
- If available, dressing change tray containing (or gather supplies as needed):
  - ❖ Alcohol swabs or prep pads
  - ❖ Antimicrobial solution applicator/swab
  - ❖ Sterile barrier
  - ❖ Skin protectant pad/swab
- Transparent semipermeable membrane dressing
- Adhesive tape
- Extension tubing set, if required
- Needleless occlusive injection cap
- Flush solution

Procedure	for Central Venous Tunneled Catheter: Care and Management	
Steps	**Rationale**	**Considerations**
Dressing Change 1. Ensure child and family understand procedure and questions are answered.	Evaluates and reinforces understanding of previously taught information.	Developmental level, cognitive ability, and anxiety level will determine approach to and effectiveness of teaching.
2. Gather needed equipment and supplies.	Facilitates completion of task in a timely manner.	
3. Wash hands with antiseptic-containing soap or with a waterless alcohol-based product.[1,2] *(Level VI*)*	Standard precautions; reduces transmission of microorganisms.	The use of gloves does not negate the need for proper hand hygiene.
4. Position child with head turned away from insertion site.	Prevents site contamination by airborne pathogens.	Consider placing face mask on child if he or she has difficulty with this position.
5. Put on face mask.	Prevents site contamination by airborne pathogens.	
6. Put on clean gloves and remove old dressing.	Decreases risk of exposure to blood-borne pathogens.	
7. Assess insertion site for signs or symptoms of infection, inflammation, or irritation.	Entire site should be visualized and any signs of potential problem should be addressed.	If any drainage is noted the prescribing practitioner must be notified. Consider obtaining a culture of the drainage.
8. Wash hands and put on sterile gloves.[2,3,4] *(Level VI*)*	INS and CDC standards to reduce incidence of CRBSI.	If sterile gloves become contaminated they must be immediately changed for a new pair of sterile gloves.

* Level VI: Clinical studies in a variety of patient populations and situations to support recommendations

Procedure for Central Venous Tunneled Catheter: Care and Management—*Continued*

Steps	Rationale	Considerations
9. Open sterile barrier and establish sterile field for supplies.	Procedure now is considered sterile as are supplies.	Consider the need for an assistant to help, especially with an infant or young child.
10. Cleanse catheter-skin junction with alcohol pad/swab if povidone-iodine will be used.	Removes skin surface contaminants. Chlorhexadine contains alcohol; this step is not required if chlorhexadine is used.	Use friction while cleansing site in a circular motion from the center outward. Allow to air-dry.
11. Scrub the insertion site with 2% chlorhexidine and allow to air-dry.[2,5] *(Level VI*)*	Fast-acting, broad-spectrum persistent antiseptic that reduces the number of microorganism on the skin.	Not required to use a circular motion, can rub across the site as needed. Allow to air-dry for at least 30 seconds before applying new dressing. Povidone-iodine is recommended for infants less than 2 months old, and may require up to 2 minutes to air-dry.[2,4]
12. Apply transparent gauze dressing per institution-specific protocol; transparent semipermeable dressing or gauze and tape dressing.	There has been no demonstrated difference in the risk of catheter-related bloodstream infections using transparent or gauze dressings.[2,4] Occlusive dressing reduces the incidence of intra-vascular catheter–related infections. *(Level VI*)*	Replace gauze dressing every 48 hours and semipermeable dressing every 7 days.[6,7,8] If the integrity of the dressing is compromised it should be changed. Do not apply topical antibiotic ointments to insertion sites because of their potential to promote antimicrobial resistance and fungal growth. The exception to this is dialysis catheters.[7,8] *(Level VI*)* Skin protectant may be used before applying dressing, based on the child's specific need.
13. Label dressing with date, time, and clinician's name.	Allows monitoring of interval when dressing is due to be changed.	Secure perimeter of dressing with adhesive tape if needed. Dressing should remain completely occlusive.
14. Attach add-on devices (such as extension tubing) as required; ensure all devices are compatible.[2,4] *(Level IV*)*	Reduces leaks or breaks in the system to minimize CRBSI.	Change add-ons at regularly scheduled intervals per institution-specific protocol and manufacturer's recommendations.
15. Secure all connections and initiate therapy.	Maintains closed sterile system to minimize incidence of CRBSI.	Use only luer-lok products unless not available; do not use adhesive tape to secure connections.
16. Dispose of all used supplies and equipment in appropriate receptacle.	Standard precautions; reduces transmission of microorganisms.	
17. Remove gloves; wash hands.	Standard precautions; reduces transmission of microorganisms.	
Flushing Catheter 18. Ensure child and family understand procedure and questions are answered.	Evaluates and reinforces under-standing of previously taught information.	Developmental level, cognitive ability, and anxiety level will determine approach to and effectiveness of teaching.

Procedure continues on following page

* Level IV: Limited clinical studies to support recommendations
Level VI: Clinical studies in a variety of patient populations and situations to support recommendations

Procedure for Central Venous Tunneled Catheter: Care and Management—*Continued*

Steps	Rationale	Considerations
19. Gather needed equipment and supplies.	Facilitates completion of task in a timely manner.	
20. Wash hands; put on clean gloves.	Standard precautions; reduces transmission of microorganisms.	
21. Clean occlusive cap with alcohol swab for 30 seconds.	Reduces transmission of micro-organisms.	Apply friction when cleaning cap.
22. Attach syringe with appropriate volume of flush solution.	Prepares flush solution for admini-stration.	Refer to prescribing practitioner's order or institution specific proto-col for flush solution, volume, and frequency of flush. Flush solutions routinely used include heparin 10 units/ mL, heparin 100 units/mL, or 0.9% saline. Volume of flush used varies based on child's weight, volume of catheter lumen, and child's fluid status. Frequency of flush varies based on required frequency of catheter use and type of catheter.
23. Open clamp, if present.	Clamped catheter cannot be flushed.	
24. Flush using gentle pulsatile technique. *(Level II[*])*	Pulsatile technique has been shown to be effective in maintaining patency of catheter.	Many manufacturers recommend using 10-mL or larger syringes for flushing, but size used may depend on size of catheter lumen. NEVER force flush against resis-tance, no matter what size syringe is used.
25. Use positive pressure technique at completion of flush using one of two methods: • Close the catheter clamp while infusing the last 0.5 mL of flush solution; remove syringe. • At completion of flush admini-stration, apply pressure to the flush syringe plunger while closing the catheter clamp; remove syringe. *(Level II[*])*	Positive pressure technique prevents backflow of blood into the catheter lumen at the completion of the flush, decreasing the risk of clot formation.	If positive pressure cap in place, such as CLC 2000, remove syringe after flushing, then clamp CVC. If a catheter with internal valve (e.g., Groshong) is in place, clamping is not required to prevent backflow of blood.
26. Discard used supplies and equip-ment in appropriate receptacle; remove gloves and wash hands.	Standard precautions; reduces transmission of microorganisms.	

* Level II: Theory based, no research data to support recommendations: recommendations from expert consensus group may exist

Expected Outcomes

- Catheter and insertion site are infection free
- Dressing changes performed at appropriate intervals
- Catheter remains in place until electively removed
- Catheter flushes without difficulty
- Catheter is free from breaks or damage
- Child tolerates therapy as ordered

Unexpected Outcomes

- Child develops a catheter-related infection
- Dressing changes are not performed at appropriate intervals
- Inadvertent catheter removal
- Unable to flush catheter
- Catheter fracture or disruption
- Therapy is interrupted due to adverse reactions

Monitoring and Care of the Child

Activities and Interventions	Rationale	Reportable Conditions
1. Ensure radiographic confirmation of catheter tip placement.	Tip placement must be confirmed before infusion is begun to a central vein; USFDA also requires periodic reassessment of catheter replacement.	• Tip placement not within the vena caval/right atrial junction • Radiographic confirmation has not been obtained
2. Perform dressing change and site observation at regularly scheduled intervals: gauze dressing changes every 48 hours and/or if not intact; transparent dressing changes every 7 days and/or if not intact.	Dressing change at appropriate intervals decreases the incidence of CRBSI. Visual inspection and palpation of site alerts nurse of developing problem such as infiltration, infection, catheter displacement, or fracture.	• Swelling at or above the site • Redness at the site • Discharge at the site • Fluid leakage around insertion site
3. Perform cap and tubing changes at appropriate intervals: CDC recommendations for cap and tubing changes are no more frequently than every 72 hours or per manufacturer's recommendations.[2,4] *(Level III*)*	Decreases incidence of CRBSI.	• Unable to remove and replace cap and/or tubing
4. If catheter is accessed intermittently, flush catheter using heparinized saline per prescribing practitioner's order or institution-specific protocol.	Maintains catheter patency.	• Unable to flush catheter • Lack of blood return from catheter
5. Assess alterations in flow rate not corrected by change in child's position; examine catheter to ensure no mechanical problems, such as kinking of the catheter, exist.	May be indicative of the primary stages of an obstruction.	• Decreased flow rate with no improvement in flow rate with position change and no mechanical obstructions noted

* Level III: Laboratory data, no clinical data to support recommendations

Documentation

- Date of catheter insertion
- Size, type, and length of catheter
- Volume(s) of catheter lumen(s)
- Radiographic confirmation of tip location
- Type of dressing used
- Appearance of insertion site
- Medications administered via catheter, presence of blood return and ease of flushing
- Child and family education
- Unexpected outcomes and related treatment

References

1. Larson EL, et al: APIC guideline for handwashing and hand antisepsis in health care settings, *Am J Infect Control* 23:251-269, 1995.
2. Guidelines for the Prevention of Intravascular Catheter-Related Infections: Centers for Disease Control and Prevention. *MMWR Morbid Mortal Wkly Rep* 51(RR10);18:III, 2002.
3. Infusion Nurses Society: Standard S54. In *Infusion nursing standards of practice,* Cambridge, MA, 2000, Infusion Nurses Society, Inc.
4. Guidelines for the Prevention of Intravascular Catheter-Related Infections: Centers for Disease Control and Prevention. *MMWR Morbid Mortal Wkly Rep* 51(RR10);18:IV, 2002.
5. Maki DG, et al: Prospective randomized trial of povidone-iodine, alcohol, and chlorhexidine for prevention of infection associated with central venous and arterial catheters, *Lancet* 338:339-343, 1991.
6. Infusion Nurses Society: *Policies and procedures for infusion nursing,* ed 2, Norwood, MA, 2002, Infusion Nurses Society.
7. Clemence MA, et al: Central venous catheter practices: results of a survey, *Am J Infect Control* 23(1):5, 1995.
8. Zakrzewska-Bode A, et al: Mupirocin resistance in coagulase-negative staphylococci, after topical prophylaxis for the reduction of central venous catheters, *Hosp Infect* 31:189-193, 1995.

Additional Reading

Weinstein SM: *Plumer's principles and practice of intravenous therapy,* ed 7, Philadelphia, 2001, Lippincott Williams & Wilkins.

Central Venous Tunneled Catheter: Permanent Catheter Repair (Broviac® or Other Brand)

P U R P O S E :   To repair holes or fractures of the lumen(s) of a central venous tunneled catheter that may occur during use

Anne Marie Frey

PREREQUISITE KNOWLEDGE

- Anatomy and physiology of the central venous system
- Principles of aseptic technique
- Child development as it relates to clinical assessment and repair of a central venous tunneled catheter
- A tunneled central venous catheter (CVC) is a long-term silicone catheter that is tunneled under the skin during placement by a surgeon or interventional radiologist. A tissue fixation cuff on the catheter helps the catheter adhere to tissue in the tunnel, preventing the outward migration of the catheter and the inward invasion of bacteria.
- Because of the small lumen size of these catheters, holes or fractures of the lumen(s) may occur during the course of use.
- A permanent repair kit, sized specifically to fit each size catheter, is available from the corresponding manufacturer.
- Tunneled catheters are usually inserted for intermittent or continuous treatments that will take months to years, such as chemotherapy, total parenteral nutrition (TPN) in children with bowel disease, and neonates requiring months of care in the neonatal intensive care unit (NICU).
- The most common placement site is the jugular or subclavian vein; the catheter is then tunneled to a distant exit site, usually in midchest area. The tunneled catheter is initially sutured, with the transparent dressing and sutures keeping the catheter in place until the tissue fixation cuff, located in a subcutaneous tunnel under the skin, takes hold.
- Tunneled CVCs may have more than one lumen.
- Although tunneled CVCs in children are often referred to as Broviac catheters, Broviac is one brand of catheter (others, such as Cook, also manufacture pediatric tunneled CVCs).
- Repair kits are sized specifically for one size and brand of tunneled catheter and are not interchangeable: the repair kit *must* match the specific catheter.
- Tunneled catheter repair is a sterile procedure.
- Tunneled catheter repairs are considered a permanent repair of the line and can be completed multiple times on a single catheter if needed.
- Tunneled catheter repair is contraindicated if less than 5 cm of undamaged catheter remains external to the skin exit site.
- Repair of the adapter leg of multilumen catheters is contraindicated if the undamaged portion of adapter leg remaining proximal to the bifurcation or trifurcation is less than 2.5 cm.[1]
- Repaired tunneled catheters may be used for infusion after 4 hours, although in some cases it is necessary to flush the repaired segment gently to avoid blood backup into the lumen and subsequent occlusion by clot before the 4-hour mark.

- The repair joint will not achieve full mechanical strength for 48 hours.[1]

CHILD AND FAMILY ASSESSMENT

- History of multiple repairs, catheter dislodgment ➜*Rationale:* These conditions may indicate a need for reinforcement of catheter care and securement with staff or family, or positioning of exit site in a different location, out of child's reach.
- Type and size of catheter ➜*Rationale:* Repair kits are sized specifically for one size and brand of tunneled catheter and are not interchangeable: the repair kit *must* match the specific catheter.
- Child's and family's understanding of the reasons for and risks and benefits of the procedure ➜*Rationale:* Evaluates child's and family's understanding of the procedure and provides a gauge for ongoing education.
- Child's developmental level and ability to interact ➜*Rationale:* These factors influence preparation and interaction.
- Level of consciousness and cognitive ability ➜*Rationale:* Determines if child can hold still or will need distraction or positioning for comfort-type of restraint during the procedure.
- Patency of the catheter; when catheter was last flushed or used ➜*Rationale:* A break or fracture often leads to blood backflow and concomitant occlusion of tunneled catheter, which might require instillation of a fibrinolytic agent.
- Family's desire to be present during procedure ➜*Rationale:* Family may provide support and comfort to their child but should have the choice not to remain with the child.

CHILD AND FAMILY EDUCATION

Individualized, developmentally appropriate education is provided to the family and to the child based on desire for knowledge, readiness to learn, and overall neurologic and psychosocial state.

- Provide information about the tunneled catheter repair, including the reason for the repair and an explanation of steps involved in the repair procedure ➜*Rationale:* Providing information decreases anxiety and fear.
- If developmentally appropriate, explain how child can assist with the repair (i.e., hold still, don't touch anything on the "towel"; child can help make the tongue blade "bridge," etc.) ➜*Rationale:* Repair requires fine motor skills in a small area and child must hold still in order to not contaminate the site or pull apart the repair. Engaging the child in the process promotes cooperation.
- Explain the need to prevent tension on the tunneled catheter for 48 hours. ➜*Rationale:* Tunneled catheter repair would have to be repeated with risk of infection or bleeding if repair is pulled apart before achieving full mechanical strength.
- Encourage questions and answer questions as they arise ➜*Rationale:* Reinforcement of information is needed during periods of stress.

EQUIPMENT

- Sterile silicone catheter repair kit in appropriate size and lumen configuration
  - ❖ Usual contents of kit
    - ○ Silicone external replacement catheter segment
    - ○ Silicone splice sleeve and splice connector (mounted on replacement segment)
    - ○ Medical adhesive, 3-mL syringe, and 18-gauge blunt-tipped needle packed in sterile repair kit or in nonsterile envelope outside kit package
- Sterile drapes (2)
- Catheter clamp without teeth or padded hemostats (1)
- Sterile gloves (powder free) (2 pairs)
- Alcohol swabs (3 or 4)
- 4×4 sterile gauze sponges (4)
- Sterile suture removal kit (1)
- Tongue blade (1)
- Mask (1)
- 10-mL syringe (1)
- Prefilled heparin flush solution in syringe, with appropriate strength of heparin (1)
- 10-mL vial of 0.9% saline solution for flushing air out of repair segment (1)
- Tape, nonsterile latex-free (1 roll)
- Sterile suture material (3.0 nylon preferable for repair of 2.7 Fr and 4.2 Fr Broviac catheters) (1)
- Needleless end cap (1)
- Safety needle, 21- or 18-gauge (1 or 2)

Note: If repairing the main body of a multilumen catheter, the following supplies must equal the number of lumens: syringes (10 mL), needleless caps, safety needles, and heparin flushes.

Procedure for Central Venous Tunneled Catheter: Permanent Catheter Repair

Steps	Rationale	Considerations
1. Ensure child and family understand procedure and questions are answered.	Evaluates and reinforces understanding of previously taught information.	Developmental level, cognitive ability, and anxiety level will determine approach to and effectiveness of teaching.
2. Determine catheter size and brand.	Repair kit size depends on CVC size and brand.	Catheter size is written on external portion of catheter or may be available from family or medical record.
3. Gather needed equipment and supplies.	Facilitates completion of procedure in a timely manner.	
4. Put on mask; wash hands.	Prevents contamination with airborne organisms; proper hand hygiene is the first step in decreasing catheter-related bloodstream infections (CRBSIs).	Either a waterless alcohol-based product or an antibacterial soap and water can achieve the desired results.[2]
5. Prepare a sterile field on a clean work surface.	Tunneled catheter repair is a sterile procedure.	
6. Put on sterile powder-free gloves.[2] *(Level VI*)*	Standard as recommended by the Centers for Disease Control and Prevention (CDC) and the Infusion Nurses Society (INS) to prevent CRBSIs.[2,3]	Glove powder may prevent adhesion of adhesive.
7. Place the following supplies onto the sterile field: • Sterile drape • Alcohol swabs • Contents of suture removal kit • Sterile 4×4s • Needleless cap • Contents of sterile repair kit • 10-mL syringe/needle • Sterile suture material, if indicated for size of catheter	Ensures required supplies are available during procedure.	Use nylon suture for securing the repair of small-gauge catheters as indicated by manufacturer.[1] *(Level I*)*
8. While assistant holds vial of saline, withdraw saline flush into 10-mL syringe(s) and place onto sterile field.	Tunneled catheter repair is a sterile procedure.	Flush solutions may be in sterile package. If so, drop flush syringes onto sterile field.
9. Attach needleless cap to hub of repair segment and flush air out of repair segment with saline. Clamp segment and remove saline syringe.	Prevents flushing of air into child's circulatory system if blood return cannot be obtained after catheter repair.	
10. Prepare adhesive syringe in the following manner: • Remove cap from glue vial. • Flip cap over and use point in cap to pierce end of glue tube. • Apply blunt needle to 3-mL syringe provided in kit. • Remove plunger. • Squeeze adhesive into barrel of syringe (Figure 144-1).	Adhesive is sterile.	If Cook TPN catheter repair performed, assistant must squeeze glue into syringe because tube of glue is not sterile.[4]

Procedure continues on following page

* Level I: Manufacturer's recommendations only
Level VI: Clinical studies in a variety of patient populations and situations to support recommendations

Procedure | **for Central Venous Tunneled Catheter: Permanent Catheter Repair**—*Continued*

Steps	Rationale	Considerations

• Replace plunger, pushing adhesive and air out of syringe barrel to tip of blunt needle.

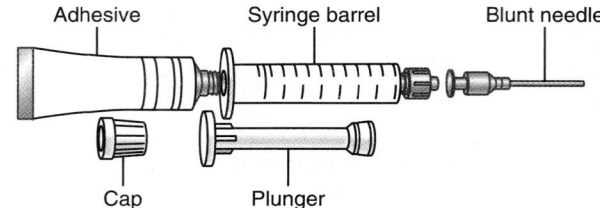

FIGURE 144-1   Prepare adhesive syringe:
• Apply blunt needle to 3-mL syringe provided in kit
• Squeeze adhesive into barrel of syringe
• Replace plunger, pushing adhesive and air out of syringe barrel to tip of blunt needle
(*From Bard, Inc.* Repair kits for Hickman, Leonard, and Broviac central venous catheters: instructions for use, *Salt Lake City, July 1997, Bard Access Systems.*)

Steps	Rationale	Considerations
11. Remove sterile gloves.	Sterile gloves not needed to position child.	
12. Place catheter clamp proximal to the damage.	Prevents blood loss or air intake when damaged portion cut off.	Clamp must be toothless, or padded if teeth present, to avoid more damage to catheter.
13. Place the child supine.	Allows a flat work surface so sterile drapes will stay in place.	Infants, toddlers, and some older children may require assistance to remain immobile during the procedure. A second person may be needed to help the child remain still.
14. Put on sterile gloves.	Standard as recommended by the CDC and the INS to prevent CRBSIs.	If powdered gloves are used, wipe powder from gloves with alcohol and sterile gauze.[1]
15. Clean damaged portion of catheter. • Hold the catheter proximal to the damaged area with an alcohol swab or sterile gauze. • Using another alcohol swab, clean the catheter 2 inches on either side of the damaged site. • Allow catheter to dry completely.	Alcohol is a disinfectant that works immediately and dries quickly.	Be sure not to place too much tension on the catheter.
16. Holding catheter with alcohol swab or with sterile gauze, slide sterile drape underneath catheter. Place portion of catheter to be removed onto sterile gauze on sterile field.	Sterile procedure.	
17. Using sterile scissors cut the damaged catheter on a 90-degree angle immediately proximal to the damaged area. Remove damaged portion with sterile gauze away from sterile field. Ensure that cut portion remains sterile.	Allows easy fit of repair segment; an angled cut would not allow secure repair.	Note: On 6.6 Fr Broviac, if white inner lumen retracts into the outer lumen, cut both lumens until flush. *(Level I*)*

---

* Level I: Manufacturer's recommendations only

Procedure for Central Venous Tunneled Catheter: Permanent Catheter Repair—*Continued*		
Steps	**Rationale**	**Considerations**
18. Insert splice connector into cut end of catheter to join with replacement catheter segment, matching up corresponding lumens if dual lumen.	Repairs catheter.	Note: 5.0 Fr Cook TPN dual-lumen catheters have equal inner lumen sizes.
19. Inject small amount of adhesive around connection of new and old segments; push new segment tightly into old catheter segment (Figure 144-2).	Joins catheter segments.	For the 2.7 and 4.2 Fr Broviac catheters, tie two clamping surgical knots on patient side of repair joint each approximately 2.5 and 5 mm from center, without occluding the catheter (Figure 144-3). *(Level I*)*

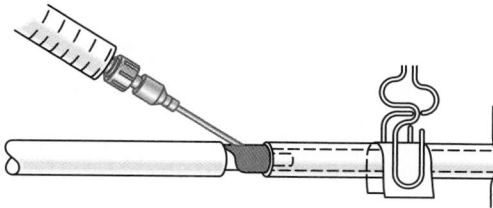

FIGURE 144-2 Perform repair by inserting splice connector into cut end of catheter to join with replacement catheter segment, matching up corresponding lumens if dual lumen. Inject small amount of adhesive around connection of new and old segments. *From Bard, Inc.* Repair kits for Hickman, Leonard, and Broviac central venous catheters: instructions for use, *Salt Lake City, July 1997, Bard Access Systems.*

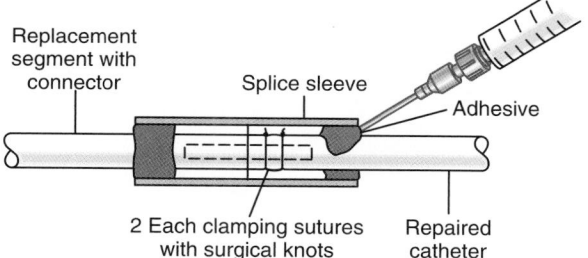

FIGURE 144-3 For the 2.7 and 4.2 Fr Broviac catheters, tie two clamping surgical knots on patient side of repair joint, each approximately 2.5 and 5 mm from center, without occluding the catheter. *From Bard, Inc.* Repair kits for Hickman, Leonard, and Broviac central venous catheters: instructions for use, *Salt Lake City, July 1997, Bard Access Systems.*

20. Position splice sleeve over repaired segment and inject the medical adhesive under both ends of the splice sleeve to completely fill the sleeve (Figure 144-4).	Reinforces repair site.	
21. Roll the splice sleeve between gloved fingers to extrude excess adhesive and wipe it away using sterile 4×4.	Removes excessive adhesive.	
22. Check patency of lumen(s).	Assesses for catheter function and/or need to use fibrinolytic agent.	At this time, a sterile field is no longer needed; mask and gloves can be removed.

Procedure continues on following page

* Level I: Manufacturer's recommendations only

Procedure **for Central Venous Tunneled Catheter: Permanent Catheter Repair**—*Continued*

Steps	Rationale	Considerations

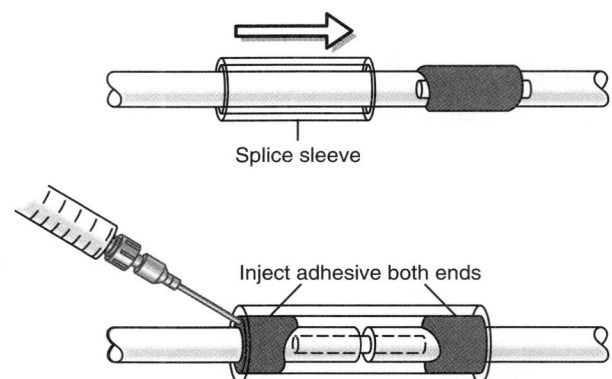

FIGURE 144-4 Push new segment tightly into old catheter segment. Position splice sleeve over repaired segment and inject the medical adhesive under both ends of the splice sleeve to completely fill the sleeve. *From Bard, Inc.* Repair kits for Hickman, Leonard, and Broviac central venous catheters: instructions for use, *Salt Lake City, July 1997, Bard Access Systems.*

- Attach saline syringe to needleless cap, and release clamp.
- Check for blood return, then flush the catheter with saline; clamp catheter and remove the syringe.
- Clean needleless cap with alcohol pad.
- Attach heparin syringe to needleless cap, open clamp on catheter, and flush with heparin.
- Close clamp, then remove the syringe.

Steps	Rationale	Considerations
23. Place the repaired joint of catheter lengthwise along the surface of a tongue blade padded with gauze and tape in place (Figure 144-5).	Forms a bridge to support the repair until full mechanical strength is achieved.	The splint may be removed after 48 hours because the glue reaches its full strength at 48 hours *(Level I*)*
24. Resume infusion at the time recommended by manufacturer.	Allows sufficient time for mechanical strength to be achieved, ensuring the repair will be successful.	Catheter may be used 4 hours after repair. If catheter is needed before 4 hours, consult with prescribing practitioner.
25. Dispose of used equipment and supplies in an appropriate receptacle; wash hands.	Standard precautions; reduces the transmission of microorganisms.	

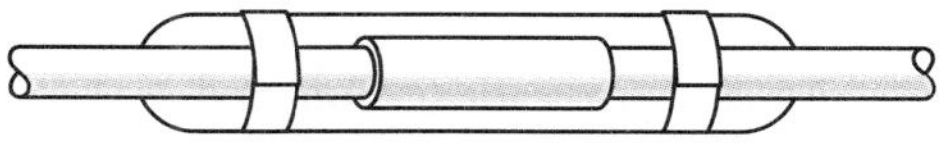

FIGURE 144-5 Place the repaired joint of catheter lengthwise along the surface of a tongue blade padded with gauze, and tape in place. *From Bard, Inc.* Repair kits for Hickman, Leonard, and Broviac central venous catheters: instructions for use, *Salt Lake City, July 1997, Bard Access Systems.*

* Level I: Manufacturer's recommendations only

Expected Outcomes

- Catheter repair is permanent
- Catheter functions after repair
- Child tolerates procedure

- Child remains free from complications of procedure

Unexpected Outcomes

- Repair leaks or comes apart
- Unable to flush catheter or obtain a blood return
- Unable to complete procedure due to child's agitation or activity level
- Air embolus
- Blood embolus
- Signs of CRBSI

Monitoring and Care of the Child

Activities and Interventions	Rationale	Reportable Conditions
1. Monitor child's tolerance to tunneled catheter repair.	Changes in child's condition may indicate complications from catheter repair.	• Agitation resulting in an inability to repair the catheter.
2. Monitor integrity of catheter after repair.	Assesses success of repair; identifies continued problems.	• Repair pulls apart or leaks
3. Monitor catheter function after repair.	Assesses need for further interventions, including administration of fibrinolytics.	• Inability to flush and/or withdraw blood from catheter
4. Assess dressing technique and manipulation of catheter by the child.	Assesses for situations that may lead to further catheter damage and identifies opportunities for reinforcement of education.	• Identification of issues that may require change in catheter exit site to protect catheter

Documentation

- Child and family education
- Catheter function after repair
- Clinician performing the repair
- Size and type of repair done
- Child's response to repair
- Medications administered
- Unexpected outcomes and related treatment

References

1. Bard, Inc: *Repair kits for Hickman, Leonard, and Broviac central venous catheters: instructions for use,* Salt Lake City, July 1997, Bard Access Systems.
2. Centers for Disease Control and Prevention: Guidelines for the prevention of intravascular catheter related infections, *MMWR Morbid Mortal Wkly Rep* 51(No.RR-10):1-29, 2002.
3. Infusion Nurses Society: *Infusion nursing standards of practice 2000,* Cambridge, MA, 2000, Infusion Nurses Society.
4. Cook Critical Care: *Cook TPN multilumen catheter repair sets: suggested instructions for use,* Bloomington, IL, 1999, Cook Critical Care.

Additional Readings

Bard, Inc. *Hickman, Leonard, and Broviac central venous catheters: long-term instructions for use,* Salt Lake City, March 1999, Bard Access Systems.
Hankins J, et al: *Infusion nurses society infusion therapy in clinical practice,* ed 2, Philadelphia, 2001, Saunders.
Weinstein S: *Plumer's principles and practice of intravenous therapy,* ed 7, Philadelphia, 2001, Lippincott Williams & Wilkins.

Intraosseous Needle: Care and Management

P U R P O S E :   An intraosseous needle is placed in the child with decompensated shock or cardiac arrest when vascular access is rapidly required and cannot be obtained through conventional means

Harriet S. Hawkins

PREREQUISITE KNOWLEDGE

- Anatomy and physiology of long bones and the bone marrow system
- A functioning intraosseous (IO) needle should stand firmly upright in the bone and should not show any indication of soft tissue swelling during flushing (Figure 145-1).
- IO needles may be used to administer resuscitation drugs, fluids, and blood products.
- It may be possible to obtain blood specimens for laboratory analysis via the IO needle.

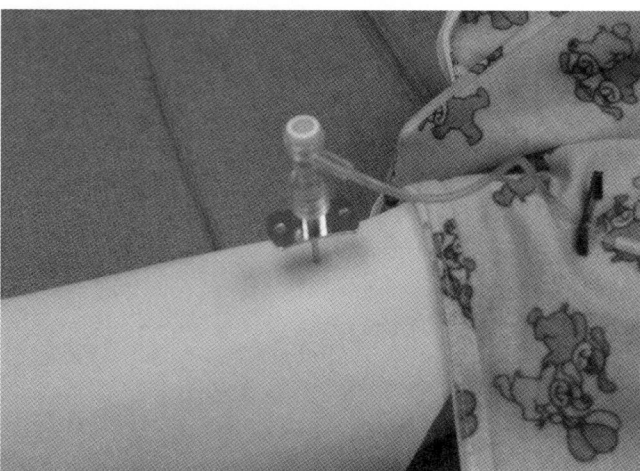

FIGURE 145-1   Intraosseous needle in proximal tibia.

- Infiltrated IO infusions can cause compartment syndrome: a limb-threatening condition observed when perfusion pressure falls below tissue pressure in a closed anatomic space
  - ❖ Changes in perfusion distal to the IO needle may indicate compartment syndrome.
- An IO infiltrate may present as edema of the posterior surface of the extremity in which the IO needle is placed.
- Extravasation of caustic medications can destroy surrounding tissue and muscle.
- All IO lines must be maintained with either a pressure bag and intravenous tubing or an intravenous pump (preferred) because gravity flow via the IO line is generally unacceptably slow.
- After resuscitation, the IO line may stay in place for up to 4 hours *(Level IV*)* during further stabilization or while awaiting placement of conventional means of vascular access.[1,2]
- Complications of IO placement[3]
  - ❖ Fracture of the bone
  - ❖ Compartment syndrome
  - ❖ Local tissue damage
  - ❖ Osteomyelitis
- Principles of aseptic technique
- Child development as it relates to clinical assessment and IO needle placement
- Refer to Procedure 154 for further information on IO needle placement.

---

* Level IV: Limited clinical studies to support recommendations

CHILD AND FAMILY ASSESSMENT

- Child's level of consciousness **➤➤*Rationale:*** If the neurologic status of the child is improving with resuscitative efforts, there may be more spontaneous movement, necessitating medical immobilization to prevent the inadvertent dislodgement of the IO needle.
- Presence of trauma in the lower extremities **➤➤*Rationale:*** Placement of an IO needle is contraindicated in a fractured extremity.
- Status of extremity in which IO needle is placed **➤➤*Rationale:*** Extravasation of medications and fluids can cause complications, the most significant of which is compartment syndrome.
- Family's understanding of recent events related to the resuscitation **➤➤*Rationale:*** After a resuscitative event, the family will have many questions and concerns and may require repeated explanations by health care providers.
- Family's desire to be present during the procedure **➤➤*Rationale:*** Having the option of being with the child during a life-threatening event reassures family that their child is receiving optimal care, legitimizes child's condition, and may provide some sense of comfort and control, but family should also have the choice not to remain with the child.[3]

CHILD AND FAMILY EDUCATION

Individualized, developmentally appropriate education is provided to the family and to the child based on desire for knowledge, readiness to learn, and overall neurologic and psychosocial state. IO needles are placed during resuscitative events; simple explanations are most effective during an emergency situation. The family may or may not have been present during the insertion, making it important for them to understand the rationale for this procedure. Anticipate that information will need to be repeated.

- Explain the rationale for IO needle placement **➤➤*Rationale:*** Education decreases fears and anxiety.
- Inform the family that the child was not in pain when the IO needle was placed **➤➤*Rationale:*** Family members need to know that their child is receiving compassionate care.
- Explain that after the IO needle has been placed, there is no pain from having the needle in the bone **➤➤*Rationale:*** Because of the way the needle looks, family members may think that there is constant pain.
- Explain that the IO needle will be removed as soon as possible, depending on child's status and ability to obtain additional means of vascular access **➤➤*Rationale:*** Family members may be less anxious if they know the IO needle will not remain in place for an extended time.
- Explain that complications from IO infusions are rare and that there should be no negative long-term effects from having the needle in the bone **➤➤*Rationale:*** The family may have concerns about the effect of this needle in their child's bone in the future.
- Explain steps in removal procedure immediately before needle removal **➤➤*Rationale:*** Preparation and explanation facilitate coping.
- Encourage questions and answer questions as they arise **➤➤*Rationale:*** Reinforcement of information is needed during periods of stress. This is especially important given the emergent nature of the procedure.

EQUIPMENT

- Tape (½-inch waterproof)
- Gauze pads
- T-connector
- Small paper or plastic cup (to be used as a "house" over the IO needle) if appropriate
- Intravenous tubing for infusion pump or intravenous tubing and pressure bag
- Measuring tape
- Clean gloves
- Adhesive bandage

Procedure	for Intraosseous Needle: Care and Management	
Steps	Rationale	Considerations
1. Ensure family understands procedure, the need to continue the IO needle on a temporary basis, and questions are answered.	Evaluates and reinforces understanding of previously taught information.	Cognitive ability and anxiety level will determine approach to and effectiveness of teaching.
2. Wash hands; put on clean gloves. (*Level VI**)	Standard precautions; reduces transmission of microorganisms.	
3. Assess security of the IO needle, making sure that the tape is secure and the dressing is dry.	During a resuscitative event, the dressing or tape may have become moist or loose.	

Procedure continues on following page

* Level VI: Clinical studies in a variety of patient populations and situations to support recommendations

Procedure for Intraosseous Needle: Care and Management—*Continued*

Steps	Rationale	Considerations
4. If retaping is necessary, gather needed equipment and supplies.	Facilitates completion of task in a timely manner.	
5. Gently remove the tape and dressing, using an assistant as necessary to help stabilize the needle and extremity.	Manipulation of the needle will cause leaking at the site and may cause dislodgement of the needle.	
6. Assess the needle insertion site and note any leaking of fluid or swelling at the site.	Continuous leaking or swelling at the insertion site may indicate extravasation of fluids.	Immediately notify the prescribing practitioner of unexpected findings.
7. Measure the circumference of the leg just distal to the insertion site. Note the condition of the skin posterior to the needle. *(Level II*)*	Establishes a baseline; if extravasation of fluid occurs, the circumference of the leg will increase and the skin will become tense and swollen, initially posterior to the needle.	
8. Clean gently around insertion site if there is any dried blood on the skin. *(Level VI*)*	Removes bacterial growth medium; decreases potential for infection.	During resuscitation, this step may have been omitted due to the need to emergently use the IO access.
9. If no leaking noted and insertion site appears intact with good color and perfusion at site, replace tape and dressing.	Blanching of the skin at insertion site may indicate extravasation of medications or fluids.	Immediately notify the prescribing practitioner of unexpected findings.

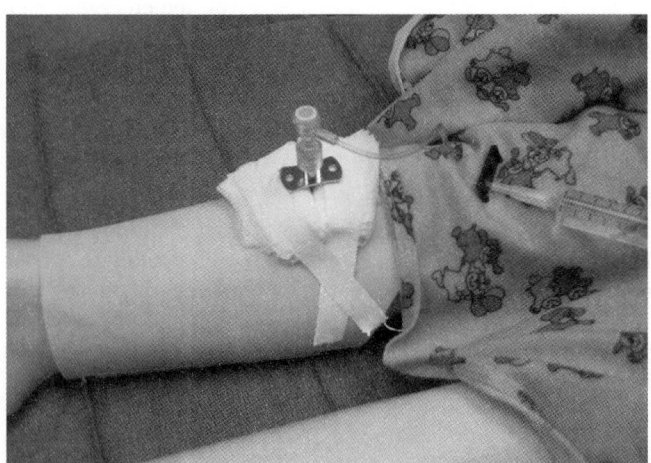

FIGURE 145-2   Folded gauze pads placed next to intraosseous needle and taped for support.

Steps	Rationale	Considerations
10. Support sides of the IO needle with folded gauze pads of appropriate size, usually 2- or 4-inch pads (Figure 145-2). *(Level II*)*	The hub of the IO needle is typically not flush with the skin, due to variety in needle length and extremity size.	
11. Tape gauze pads to extremity; do not place tape circumferentially around the leg (see Figure 145-2). *(Level II*)*	Provides support to the needle to help prevent dislodgement; circumferential taping restricts flow to the extremity.	
12. If a screw-type needle is present, cover the incision with sterile gauze pads and tape in place.	Decreases potential for infection.	

* Level II: Theory based, no research data to support recommendations: recommendations from expert consensus group may exist
  Level VI: Clinical studies in a variety of patient populations and situations to support recommendations

Procedure for **Intraosseous Needle: Care and Management**—*Continued*		
Steps	**Rationale**	**Considerations**
13. Place a paper or plastic cup over the IO needle and tape to the leg (Figure 145-3).	Protects the needle to prevent dislodgement.	Cut a slit up the side of the cup and a hole in the top of the cup to allow the T-connector to be accessible; avoid sharp edges, which may injure the skin. Monitor the skin under the cup on a regular basis.

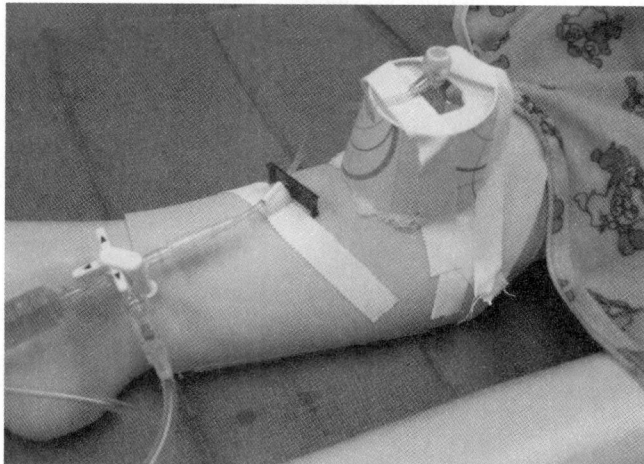

FIGURE 145-3   Paper cup "house" taped over intraosseous needle with T-connector readily accessible.

14. Tape the T-connector attached to the hub of the IO needle to the leg using a "goalpost" form (Figure 145-4).	Secures tubing and allows tension on the tape rather than the tubing if the tubing is pulled or stretched.	

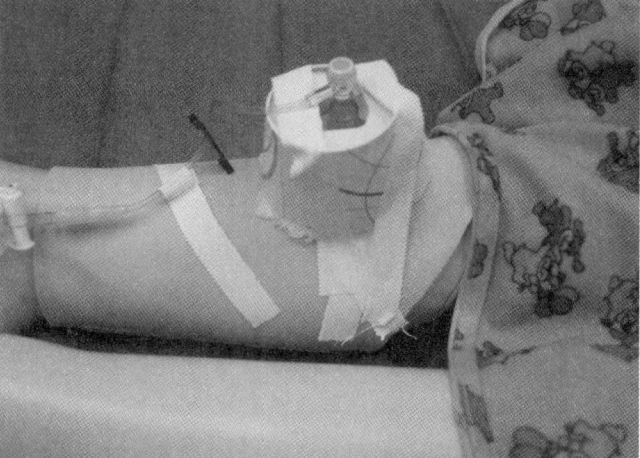

FIGURE 145-4   T-connector taped using a goalpost format to allow tension on the tape rather than the tubing.

15. For infants, consider taping the leg to an armboard to limit movement; medical immobilization may be necessary to prevent dislodgement of the needle in the child.	With improvement in status the infant or child may begin to move around and may dislodge the needle.	Do not place tape for the armboard tightly around the leg because this will contribute to swelling and prevent good assessment of perfusion.

Procedure continues on following page

Procedure for Intraosseous Needle: Care and Management—*Continued*

Steps	Rationale	Considerations
16. Attach infusion tubing from prescribed fluids to IO needle.	Continuous fluid infusion is necessary to prevent clotting of the needle.	Infusion may be via manual flushing, pressure bag and intravenous tubing system, or intravenous pump.
17. Dispose of supplies and used equipment appropriately.	Standard precautions; reduces transmission of microorganisms.	
18. Remove gloves; wash hands. *(Level VI*)*	Standard precautions; reduces transmission of microorganisms.	

Intraosseous Needle Removal

Steps	Rationale	Considerations
1. Ensure child and family understand procedure and questions are answered.	Evaluates and reinforces understanding of previously taught information.	Developmental level, cognitive ability, and anxiety level will determine approach to and effectiveness of teaching.
2. Wash hands; put on clean gloves. *(Level VI*)*	Standard precautions; reduces transmission of microorganisms.	
3. Stop continuous infusion and remove tubing.	Prevents fluid spills or spray when IO needle is removed.	
4. Gently remove the tape and dressings around the IO needle.	Allows visualization of site for needle removal.	If child is awake, have family present if possible, to provide distraction and comfort.
5. With conventional IO needle, twist gently and pull the needle out rapidly; with screw-type needle, gently but rapidly unscrew the needle. *(Level I*)*	Gently dislodging and removing the needle rapidly decreases pain.	There is brief pain on needle removal.
6. Hold gentle pressure on the insertion site until bleeding stops.	Prevents blood loss and hematoma formation at the insertion site.	Bleeding is usually minimal.
7. Cover site with small dressing or bandage.	Contains any ongoing oozing or bleeding.	Monitor insertion site for bleeding. Many children are comforted by the application of a bandage.
8. Dispose of supplies and used equipment appropriately.	Standard precautions; reduces transmission of microorganisms.	
9. Remove gloves; wash hands. *(Level I*)*	Standard precautions; reduces transmission of microorganisms.	

* Level I: Manufacturer's recommendations only
  Level VI: Clinical studies in a variety of patient populations and situations to support recommendations

Expected Outcomes

- IO line remains functional with no extravasation of medications or fluids

- IO needle remains in place until conventional access is obtained (goal is no longer than 4 hours) and IO needle is electively removed
- At termination of therapy IO needle is removed without difficulty
- Extremity where IO needle was placed remains free from complications

- Child demonstrates acceptable level of comfort during and after IO needle removal

Unexpected Outcomes[1,3,4,5]

- Leaking of medications or fluids necessitating removal of IO needle and replacement in another bone
- Occlusion of IO needle necessitating removal and replacement in another bone
- Extravasation of medications or fluids into surrounding skin
- IO needle is inadvertently removed

- Unable to remove IO needle

- Infection
- Compartment syndrome
- Osteomyelitis
- Unmanaged pain during or after IO needle removal

Monitoring and Care of the Child

Activities and Interventions	Rationale	Reportable Conditions
1. Monitor insertion site for leaking, blanching.[4] Frequency of evaluation depends on the amount of medications and fluids being given. The more the line is being used, the more frequent the evaluations need to be.	Increased leakage of fluids or obvious local infiltration at the insertion site indicates the need to change the IO needle to another site.	• Increased or continued leakage of fluids from insertion site • Any signs of local infiltration
2. Monitor for increased circumference of extremity and/or tenseness of skin posterior to IO needle.	Increased circumference indicates extravasation of medications or fluids, which can lead to compartment syndrome.	• Increase in circumference of extremity just distal to needle placement • Increased tenseness of skin posterior to needle
3. Monitor perfusion distal to IO needle.	Indications of decreased perfusion such as poor pulses, pale or mottled skin color, cool temperature, and prolonged capillary refill may indicate compartment syndrome.	• Decreased pulses, pale or mottled, cool skin, delay in capillary refill
4. Monitor the ease with which the IO needle flushes.	Assess for increased resistance when flushing the IO needle. If the needle no longer flushes at all, it may be occluded and will need to be removed.	• Increased resistance to flushing • Unable to flush IO needle
5. Monitor comfort level; encourage family to assist in using nonpharmacologic means to comfort and support the child if appropriate.	Increasing pain may indicate developing compartment syndrome.	• Increasing pain at insertion site or surrounding area

Documentation

- Location, size, and type of IO needle placed
- Date and time of placement and clinician placing IO needle
- Assessment of IO needle insertion site
- Leakage of fluids at insertion site, or lack thereof
- Perfusion distal to the IO needle
- Circumference of extremity distal to IO needle insertion site
- Ability to flush needle and ease of flushing
- Condition of leg posterior to needle
- Fluids, medications, and blood products administered via the IO needle
- Removal of IO needle
- Child and family education
- Comfort assessment and any specific interventions provided
- Unexpected outcomes and related treatment

References

1. Gluckman W, Forti RJ: Intraosseous cannulation. Retrieved March 3, 2004, from www.emedicine.com/ped/topic2557.htm.
2. Vascular access. In Hawkins HS, editor: *Emergency nursing pediatric course provider manual,* ed 3, Des Plaines, IL, 2004, Emergency Nurses Association, pp. 93-94.
3. Vascular access. In Hazinski MF, editor: *Pediatric advanced life support provider manual,* Dallas, 2000, American Heart Association, pp. 93-94.
4. Simmons CM, et al: Intraosseous extravasation complication reports, *Ann Emerg Med* 23:363-366, 1994.
5. Ribeiro JA, et al: Compartment syndrome of the lower extremity after intraosseous infusion of fluid: a report of two cases, *J Bone Joint Surg* 75A(3):430-443, 1993.

Additional Readings

Fiorito BA, et al: Intraosseous access in the setting of pediatric critical care transport, *Pediatr Crit Care Med* 6(1):50, 2005.
Vidal R, et al: Compartment syndrome following intraosseous infusion, *Pediatrics* 91:1201-1202, 1993.

Peripheral Intravenous Line: Insertion

P U R P O S E : Intravenous catheters less than 3 inches long are inserted in an extremity for the administration of solutions and/or medications or for use during certain diagnostic procedures

Marvin Siegel

PREREQUISITE KNOWLEDGE

- Anatomy of the peripheral vascular system and structure of blood vessels
- Infection control principles and site preparation required before catheter placement
- The preferred site for placement is in the most distal aspect of the selected extremity.
- Child assessment and site selection as appropriate to therapy needs
- Correct procedure for placement of catheter as recommended by manufacturer
- Correct activation of safety features of catheter as recommended by manufacturer
- Standards of care for peripheral intravenous (PIV) lines as published by the Infusion Nurses Society
- Intravenous fluids and medications appropriate to be administered via peripheral vein
- Indications that the catheter has been placed into the vessel
- Indications of infiltration or phlebitis
- Child development as it relates to clinical assessment and PIV line insertion, including distraction and other pain reduction measures suitable to age and developmental level of child
- Principles of aseptic technique

CHILD AND FAMILY ASSESSMENT

- Child's developmental level and ability to interact ➥*Rationale:* These factors influence preparation of the child and interaction.

- Child's and family's understanding of the reasons for and risks and benefits of PIV placement ➥*Rationale:* Evaluates child's and family's understanding of the procedure and provides a gauge for ongoing education.
- Before placement of PIV review the child's past and current medical history ➥*Rationale:* Medical history can reveal potential areas of complication for infusion therapy, such as hypertension, diabetes, coagulation disorders, etc. All of these can result in changes to the vascular system.
- Review child's medication profile ➥*Rationale:* Medications can cause changes to a child's electrolyte balance that can result in vascular changes.
- Perform a clinical assessment of the child including but not limited to vital signs, hydration status, skin turgor, potential vascular access sites ➥*Rationale:* Identifies potential barriers to the placement of a PIV catheter.
- Assess child's and family's previous experience with and potential benefits of using topical anesthetic cream against urgency of PIV placement ➥*Rationale:* Some children may tolerate the procedure better with the use of topical anesthetic cream.
- Family's desire to be present during the procedure ➥*Rationale:* Family may provide comfort and support to the child during PIV placement, but should have the option not to remain with the child.

CHILD AND FAMILY EDUCATION

Individualized, developmentally appropriate education is provided to the family and to the child based on desire for knowledge, readiness to learn, and overall neurologic and psychosocial state.

- Provide information to the child and/or family regarding the procedure and the plan of treatment ➤*Rationale:* Providing information reduces anxiety and fear.
- Provide information on the therapy, its duration and goals; review potential side effects ➤*Rationale:* Educates the child and family about the plan of care; provides an opportunity for the family and child to ask questions.
- If available, provide the family and child with educational materials about PIVs ➤*Rationale:* Providing written material permits the family to refer to a source of information that reinforces verbal teaching. Having educational materials to refer to can help to reduce anxiety and fear.
- Teach the child and family indications of complications with the PIV, such as swelling, pain, bleeding at the insertion site ➤*Rationale:* Informs the child and family of reasons to notify the health care team, allowing prompt assessment and intervention; encourages active participation in care by the family and child.

- Encourage questions and answer questions as they arise ➤*Rationale:* Reinforcement of information is needed during periods of stress.

EQUIPMENT

- Appropriate-sized intravenous catheter(s)
- Clean gloves
- Gauze pad
- Alcohol prep pad
- Antimicrobial skin pad/swab
- Single-use tourniquet, latex-free
- Transparent semipermeable membrane dressing
- Extension tubing with luer-lok
- Needleless cap
- Adhesive tape
- 0.9% saline flush solution or heparinized saline flush, 10 units/mL, per institution-specific protocol
- Sharps container
- Anesthetic agent: topical cream or other per child or family request

Procedure for Peripheral Intravenous Line: Insertion

Steps	Rationale	Considerations
1. Ensure child and family understand procedure and questions are answered.	Evaluates and reinforces understanding of previously taught information.	Developmental level, cognitive ability, and anxiety level will determine approach to and effectiveness of teaching.
2. Complete vascular assessment and site selection.[1,2]	Appropriate site must be identified before catheter placement.	Avoid areas of flexion, such as the wrist or bend at the antecubital space, which can lead to mechanical phlebitis. Avoid feet after walking age and in children older than 10 years. Refer to Figure 146-1 for PIV sites used in children.
3. Gather needed equipment and supplies.	Facilitates completion of task in a timely manner. Delays in performing procedure can increase the child's anxiety.	Have available appropriate-sized catheter for child's size and therapy. Ensure that sharps container is placed nearby to facilitate needle discard immediately after use.
4. Wash hands.[3] *(Level VI*)*	Proper hand hygiene is the first step in decreasing catheter-related bloodstream infections (CRBSI).	Either a waterless, alcohol-based product[4] or an antibacterial soap and water[5] can achieve the desired results.
5. Identify the child using two patient identifiers per institution-specific protocol.	Ensures the procedure is being done for the correct child; promotes patient safety as recommended by the Joint Commission on Accreditation of Healthcare Organizations (JCAHO).	

* Level VI: Clinical studies in a variety of patient populations and situations to support recommendations

Procedure   **for Peripheral Intravenous Line: Insertion**—*Continued*

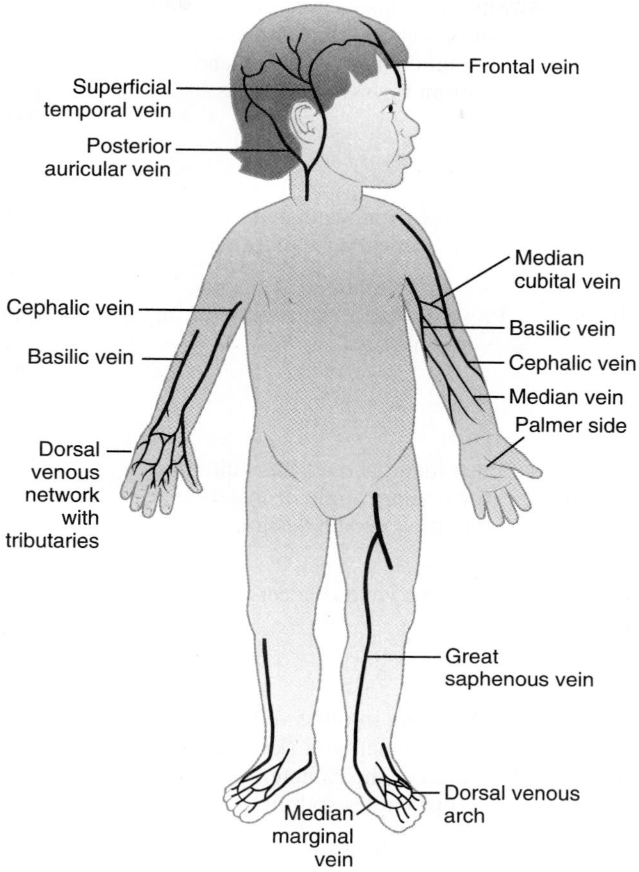

Steps	Rationale	Considerations

FIGURE 146-1   Suggested sites for venous access in children.

Labels in figure:
- Frontal vein
- Superficial temporal vein
- Posterior auricular vein
- Median cubital vein
- Cephalic vein
- Basilic vein
- Basilic vein
- Cephalic vein
- Median vein
- Palmer side
- Dorsal venous network with tributaries
- Great saphenous vein
- Median marginal vein
- Dorsal venous arch

Steps	Rationale	Considerations
6. If topical anesthetic is to be used, apply for appropriate period and in a manner as recommended by manufacturer. *(Level I*)*	Topical anesthetic must be applied for a specific time period in order to be effective.	
7. Wash hands and identify the child using two patient identifiers per institution-specific protocols.	When a period has occurred between interventions, child must be identified again to ensure patient safety.	
8. Place child in comfortable position. Use sucrose drops for infants,[6] distraction techniques, or pharmaceutical pain reduction for children as developmentally appropriate.	Lessens chance of child moving during insertion procedure, which might lead to venous perforation. Sucrose has been shown to reduce pain of needlestick procedure in infants. *(Level IV*)*	Use positioning for comfort techniques to restrain child, which promotes child's coping while still maintaining safety and immobilization.
9. Put on clean gloves.[3] *(Level VI*)*	Protects individual inserting catheter from blood exposure.	Wear gloves that fit well for best tactile sense in placing IV.

Procedure continues on following page

* Level I: Manufacturer's recommendations only
Level IV: Limited clinical studies to support recommendations
Level VI: Clinical studies in a variety of patient populations and situations to support recommendations

Procedure **for Peripheral Intravenous Line: Insertion**—*Continued*

Steps	Rationale	Considerations
10. Cleanse skin with antiseptic; 2% aqueous chlorhexidine gluconate or other antiseptic per institution-specific protocol. *(Level VI*)*	Skin antisepsis decreases the risk of infection by removing potential contaminants. Use back and forth motion for skin antisepsis.	70% isopropyl alcohol, 2% aqueous chlorhexidine gluconate,[3] or povidone-iodine solution is preferred as a skin antiseptic Note: Alcohol or povidone-iodine is recommended in infants less than 2 months old.[3]
11. Apply tourniquet.	Promotes venous distention, which assists in catheter placement.	To prevent the spread of nosocomial infections, tourniquets should be single-patient use.
12. Use nondominant hand to stabilize the selected vein.	Prevents vein from rolling during venipuncture.	Apply traction to the side of insertion site with the nondominant hand; do not put the hand on the area cleaned with antiseptic solution.
13. Penetrate the skin at a 10- to 30-degree angle with the bevel end up; follow brand specific manufacturer's recommendations. *(Level I*)*	Each manufacturer has guidelines for optimal angle of insertion based on needle design.	The deeper the vein the greater the angle of approach.
14. Observe for positive blood return in catheter or flashback chamber, depending on manufacturer's guidelines for use. *(Level I*)*	Confirms venous access.	Lower the angle of the catheter to prevent posterior wall puncture as soon as blood return is observed.
15. Advance the catheter into the vein.	Advancing into the vein until hub is in contact with skin seats the length of the catheter in the vein and promotes stability.	At least three quarters of catheter should be in skin to prevent easy dislodgement.
16. Release tourniquet.	No longer needed.	Tourniquet left on after catheter is in place can result in trauma to tissue or vein.
17. Remove stylet activating safety feature per manufacturer's guidelines. *(Level I*)*	Safety features may vary by device.	Prevents needlestick injury. Press fingers of nondominant hand over vein path to prevent backflow of blood until add-on device attached.
18. Attach add-on luer-lok tubing such as extension set or injection cap per institution-specific protocol.	Extension set tubing prevents direct manipulation of hub, which can result in phlebitis, and stabilizes catheter.	For continuous infusions a direct connection to extension tubing is appropriate. For intermittent infusions attach a needleless cap to extension tubing.
19. Cover site with a sterile transparent dressing.	Provides barrier site protection while allowing visual inspection without changing dressing.	Materials used should allow visual inspection of site and do not interfere with or impede circulation.
20. Stabilize catheter per institution-specific protocol; insertion site should be clearly visible.	Protects catheter from being dislodged.	Location of catheter and child's level of activity will direct appropriate stabilization such as use of armboard or protective cover. Stabilization should not interfere with delivery of therapy. Do not place tape directly at skin/hub junction; secure add-on devices instead.

* Level I: Manufacturer's recommendations only
Level VI: Clinical studies in a variety of patient populations and situations to support recommendations

Procedure for Peripheral Intravenous Line: Insertion—*Continued*

Steps	Rationale	Considerations
21. Secure all connections and initiate therapy as prescribed.	Ensures closed system; prevents blood loss or clotting of catheter due to backup of blood into catheter.	
22. Discard used supplies and equipment in appropriate container.	Standard precautions; reduces transmission of microorganisms.	Ensure all sharps are disposed of appropriately.
23. Remove gloves; wash hands.	Standard precautions; reduces transmission of microorganisms.	

Expected Outcomes

- Catheter is placed within the vein

- Full length of catheter is advanced into the vein

- Prescribed therapy is appropriate for peripheral intravenous line
- Therapy is tolerated and completed

- Child demonstrates acceptable level of comfort

Unexpected Outcomes

- Catheter stylet perforates the vein through one or more walls
- Catheter is placed into an artery
- Catheter is placed within the vein but cannot be advanced
- Medication or intravenous fluid is the cause of a chemical phlebitis
- Therapy is not completed as prescribed due to adverse reactions or inadvertent catheter removal
- Unmanaged pain or agitation during or after catheter placement

Monitoring and Care of the Child

Activities and Interventions	Rationale	Reportable Conditions
1. If family desires to be present for procedure and as appropriate, facilitate family participation in positioning for comfort.	Family may provide comfort to child during procedure.	• Unmanaged pain or agitation during or after catheter placement
2. Visualize and inspect insertion site and extremity where catheter is placed frequently per institution-specific protocol.	Allows early identification of complications of therapy; PIV catheters are changed at the first sign of a complication.	• Swelling at, above, or below the insertion site • Redness at the insertion site • Discharge at the insertion site • Fluid leakage around insertion site • Pain at insertion site • Change in color or temperature in extremity where catheter is placed
3. Change site if complication occurs.[3] *(Level IV*)*	Limits injury related to complications; Centers for Disease Control guidelines for prevention of CRBSI recommends leaving peripheral venous catheters in place until therapy is completed unless a complication develops.[3]	• Family or child refuses to allow catheter removal and replacement • Complications such as phlebitis, occlusion, infiltration
4. Ensure all fluids and medications administered via the catheter are appropriate for peripheral vein administration.	Prevents damage to vessel or surrounding tissue.	• Prescribed fluids or medications inappropriate for peripheral vein administration

* Level IV: Limited clinical studies to support recommendations

Continued

Monitoring and Care of the Child—Cont'd

Activities and Interventions	Rationale	Reportable Conditions
5. Inspect dressing regularly to ensure it is dry, clean, and intact. Change dressing immediately if integrity has been compromised.	Reduces risk of CRBSI; promotes security and stability of catheter.	• Inadvertent catheter removal
6. Monitor child to assess tolerance to catheter; provide medical immobilization to protect catheter if indicated.	Active and inquisitive children may play with catheter or tubing and dislodge catheter or disconnect tubing if site is not properly protected.	• Dislodgment or removal of catheter by child

Documentation

- Therapy prescribed requiring catheter placement
- Topical anesthetic used before catheter placement
- Type, length, gauge, and site of the vascular access device[7]
- Individual placing catheter
- Number of attempts made to cannulate vein
- Regular assessment of insertion site and extremity
- Comfort assessment and any specific interventions provided
- Child and family education
- Unexpected outcomes and related treatment

References

1. Hankins J, et al: *Infusion Nurses Society infusion therapy in clinical practice,* ed 2, Philadelphia, 2001, Saunders.
2. Weinstein SM: *Plumer's principles and practice of intravenous therapy,* ed 7, Philadelphia, 2001, Lippincott Williams & Wilkins, pp. 234-237.
3. O'Grady NP, Alexander M, Dellinger EP et al: Guidelines for the prevention of intravascular catheter-related infections. *MMWR Morbid Mortal Wkly Rep* 51(RR-10):1-29, 2002.
4. Pittet D, et al: Effectiveness of a hospital-wide program to improve compliance with hand hygiene, *Lancet* 356:1307-1309, 2000.
5. Larson EL, et al: APIC guideline for handwashing and hand antisepsis in health care settings, *Am J Infect Control* 23:251-256, 1995.
6. Greenberg C: Practice applications of research: a sugar-coated pacifier reduces procedural pain in newborns, *Pediatr Nurs* 28(3):271-277, 2002.
7. Infusion Nurses Society: Standard 21. In *Infusion nursing standards of practice,* Cambridge, MA, 2000, Infusion Nurses Society.

Peripherally Inserted Central Venous Catheter: Care, Management, and Removal

P U R P O S E : To facilitate administration of infusion therapy for more than 5 days, vesicant or hyperosmolar infusions, infusions in children with limited peripheral access, and multiple or complex infusion therapies

Nancy L. Moureau

PREREQUISITE KNOWLEDGE

- Anatomy of the peripheral and central vascular system and structure of blood vessels
- Principles of aseptic technique
- Indications of infiltration or phlebitis of the peripherally inserted central venous catheter (PICC)
- Rationale for the placement of a PICC
- Complications associated with PICCs, appropriate prevention strategies, and appropriate management of complications
- Location of catheter tip
- Total length of catheter and length of catheter remaining outside the insertion site
- Size, number of lumens, and type of PICC placed
- Manufacturer's recommendations for size of syringe to be used for flushing PICC
- Manufacturer's recommendations regarding use of PICC for obtaining lab specimens
- Child development as it relates to clinical assessment and management of a PICC
- State nurse practice act as it relates to care and maintenance of central venous catheters (CVC)
- Organization-specific policies and procedures regarding PICCs
- PICC care in children includes dressing changes, flushing, monitoring for complications, and removal.

CHILD AND FAMILY ASSESSMENT

- Child's developmental level and ability to interact ➤*Rationale:* These factors influence preparation of the child and interaction.
- Assess insertion site routinely for indications of infiltration or infection per institution-specific protocol ➤*Rationale:* Regular assessment facilitates early identification of complications.
- Child's and family's understanding of the reasons for and risks and benefits of the procedure ➤*Rationale:* Evaluates child's and family's understanding of the procedure and provides a gauge for ongoing education.
- Child's and family's fears and concerns related to the PICC ➤*Rationale:* Identifies concerns and fears; facilitates development of an individualized teaching plan.
- Assess the child and family for educational, cultural, or physical barriers to learning and performing care of the catheter, such as literacy, physical limitations, cultural norms ➤*Rationale:* Identifies barriers to learning that may be present.
- Family's desire to be present during procedures such as PICC removal or dressing change ➤*Rationale:* Family may provide support and comfort to the child but should have the choice not to remain with the child.

CHILD AND FAMILY EDUCATION

Individualized, developmentally appropriate education is provided to the family and to the child based on desire for knowledge, readiness to learn, and overall neurologic and psychosocial state

- Provide or reinforce information about the reasons for the PICC, anticipated duration of therapy, and goals of therapy ➤➤*Rationale:* Providing information can help decrease anxiety and fear; involves the family and child in the plan of care.
- Teach the family and child signs and symptoms of complications of a PICC including infection, inflammation, and catheter occlusion ➤➤*Rationale:* Informs the child and family of reasons to notify the health care team, allowing prompt assessment and intervention; encourages active participation in care by the family and child.
- Explain steps in procedure before performing, such as dressing change or PICC removal ➤➤*Rationale:* Providing information decreases anxiety and fear, and promotes the child's coping.
- If the child is to be discharged with the PICC in place, teach the family or child as appropriate to perform dressing changes, flushing of PICC, routine care, methods to prevent complications such as catheter dislodgement, breakage, and infection ➤➤*Rationale:* Prepares the family to safely provide care for the child at home when the child is discharged with a PICC.
- If available, provide written educational material to the child and family on care and management of the PICC and the insertion site if the child is being transferred or discharged with PICC in place ➤➤*Rationale:* Providing written material permits the family to refer to a source of information that reinforces verbal teaching. Having educational materials to refer to can help to reduce anxiety and fear.
- Have the family, and child if appropriate, give a repeat demonstration of any tasks that they will be required to perform at home such as routine catheter flushes

➤➤*Rationale:* In order to appropriately document a child or family member as being independent in performing a task, the person must be observed carrying it out as instructed.
- Encourage questions and answer questions as they arise ➤➤*Rationale:* Reinforcement of information is needed during periods of stress.

EQUIPMENT

Dressing Change

- Clean gloves
- Dressing change kit with the following supplies, or gather these supplies:
  - ❖ Gloves, sterile and clean
  - ❖ Adhesive remover pads
  - ❖ Alcohol prep pads
  - ❖ Antimicrobial skin prep
  - ❖ Sterile barrier or dressing kit with sterile over wrap
- Transparent semipermeable membrane dressing
- Tape, sterile tape strips, or securement device
- Extension tubing set, if required
- Needleless injection cap, if required

Flushing PICC

- Needleless access device
- Flushing solution in syringe per institution-specific protocol; 0.9% saline or heparinized saline, concentration per institution-specific protocol
- Alcohol swab or other antiseptic swab per institution-specific protocol

PICC Removal

- Alcohol swabs
- Disposable single-use tourniquet
- Clean gloves
- Antimicrobial ointment
- Dry sterile gauze
- Transparent dressing

Procedure	for Peripherally Inserted Central Venous Catheter (PICC): Care, Management, and Removal		
Steps	Rationale	Considerations	
Dressing Change 1. Ensure child and family understand procedure and questions are answered.	Evaluates and reinforces understanding of previously taught information.	Developmental level, cognitive ability, and anxiety level will determine approach to and effectiveness of teaching.	
2. Gather needed supplies and equipment.	Facilitates completion of task in a timely manner.	Anticipation creates fear and anxiety in children. Do not allow child to anticipate the procedure longer than 2 minutes per year of age.	

Procedure	for Peripherally Inserted Central Venous Catheter (PICC): Care, Management, and Removal—*Continued*	
Steps	**Rationale**	**Considerations**
3. Consider enlisting an assistant to help immobilize the child during the dressing change.	Young active children may move during the dressing change, contaminating the sterile field or causing the PICC to be dislodged.	
4. Wash hands. *(Level VI*)*	Standard precautions; reduces the transmission of microorganisms.	
5. Put on clean gloves and remove old dressing. If needed, use adhesive remover pads to release adhesives.	Allows visualization and inspection of site.	Refer to institution-specific protocol for frequency of dressing change. Remove transparent dressing by pulling parallel to skin.
6. Assess insertion site for signs or symptoms of infection, inflammation, or irritation.	Entire site is now visible and any signs of problem or potential problem can be identified.	If any drainage or sign of infection/complication is noted, the prescribing practitioner must be notified.
7. Remove gloves; wash hands.	Replace contaminated gloves.	Hands are to be washed after each glove removal.
8. Establish sterile field for supplies.	Aseptic technique decreases the incidence of catheter-related bloodstream infections (CRBSI).	Implement principles of sterility with supplies in center of field, prepping supplies discarded after use and gloves changed with any contamination.
9. Put on sterile gloves *(Level VI*)*	Recommendations of the Infusion Nurses Society (INS) and Centers for Disease Control and Prevention (CDC) for the prevention of CRBSI.[1,2]	
10. Apply antiseptic solution such as 2 % chlorhexidine; rub across the site with back and forth friction for at least 30 seconds. Allow to completely air-dry.[3] *(Level VI*)*	Fast-acting, broad-spectrum and persistent antiseptic that reduces the number of microorganisms on the skin.	Chlorhexidine is not recommended for use in infants less than 2 months old; povidone-iodine is recommended.
11. Apply sterile site dressing per institution-specific protocol. Use securement devices as applicable (e.g., StatLock)[4]	Sterile occlusive dressing decreases the risk of catheter-related infections. Securement devices reduce complications such as accidental dislodgement.	Do not apply topical antibiotic ointments to insertions sites because of their potential to promote antimicrobial resistance and fungal growth.[2] *(Level VI*)* Skin preparations for added protection and adherence can be applied to the outer dressing edges before applying dressing.
12. Label dressing with date, time, and initials of individual performing the dressing change.	Allows monitoring of interval when dressing is due to be changed.	
13. Attach add-on devices such as caps and extension tubing as required.	Replace devices at interval outlined in institution-specific protocol or manufacturer's guidelines to prevent CRBSI.	Attach device using aseptic technique. Devices should have a luer-lok connection. Prime extension set at same time as main administration set.

Procedure continues on following page

* Level VI: Clinical studies in a variety of patient populations and situations to support recommendations

Procedure	**for Peripherally Inserted Central Venous Catheter (PICC):** **Care, Management, and Removal**—*Continued*		

Steps	Rationale	Considerations
14. Secure all connections and initiate therapy.	Maintains closed sterile system.	Use only luer-lok products unless not available by manufacturer; do not use adhesive tape to secure connections.[5]
15. Dispose of used supplies and equipment appropriately.	Standard precautions; reduces transmission of microorganisms.	
16. Remove gloves; wash hands.	Standard precautions; reduces transmission of microorganisms.	
Flushing Catheter		
1. Ensure child and family understand procedure and questions are answered.	Evaluates and reinforces understanding of previously taught information.	Developmental level, cognitive ability, and anxiety level will determine approach to and effectiveness of teaching.
2. Gather needed supplies and equipment.	Facilitates completion of task in a timely manner.	Institution-specific protocol will indicate if heparin is used with a particular PICC line.[5] Heparin will not damage a catheter, but may not be indicated if closed-ended, valved catheters are used.
3. Wash hands. *(Level VI*)*	Standard precautions; reduces transmission of microorganisms.	
4. Prepare flush solution in syringes per institution-specific protocol or prescribing practitioner's order.	Flushing catheter reduces complications from blood cell and medication buildup within the catheter.	Flush solution must be in a form that can be administered through a PICC. Aseptic technique must be used to prevent contamination of intravenous solutions.
5. Swab access port with alcohol prep pad. *(Level VI*)*	Reduces incidence of CRBSI.[2] *(Level VI*)*	Reducing bacterial counts before to access will prevent contamination.
6. Access port for lumen and flush with push-pause, push-pause action; repeat for each lumen of catheter.	Technique creates turbulence, which is most effective in cleaning out catheter.	Never forcefully flush against resistance. Syringes 5 mL or smaller can create enough pressure to rupture a catheter when a partial or complete occlusion is present.
7. If positive pressure end cap is not in use, use positive pressure technique at end of flush: initiate a final push; then clamp catheter while pushing down on the syringe plunger; remove syringe after clamp is closed.	Positive pressure technique reduces blood reflux at the terminal end of the catheter.	Positive pressure technique is not necessary with some valved catheters or with positive pressure end caps.
8. Dispose of supplies and used equipment appropriately.	Standard precautions; reduces transmission of microorganisms.	Ensure used syringes and needles are placed into sharps disposal containers.
9. Wash hands.	Standard precautions.	

* Level VI: Clinical studies in a variety of patient populations and situations to support recommendations

Procedure	for Peripherally Inserted Central Venous Catheter (PICC): Care, Management, and Removal—*Continued*	
Steps	**Rationale**	**Considerations**

PICC Removal

Steps	Rationale	Considerations
1. Ensure child and family understand procedure and questions are answered.	Evaluates and reinforces understanding of previously taught information.	Developmental level, cognitive ability, and anxiety level will determine approach to and effectiveness of teaching.
2. Determine length of catheter at time of insertion.	Length at insertion will be compared with length at removal, to ensure catheter did not break during removal.	
3. Gather needed supplies and equipment.	Facilitates completion of task in a timely manner.	Anticipation creates fear and anxiety in children.
4. Consider enlisting an assistant to help immobilize the child during catheter removal.	Young active children may move during removal, causing the PICC to be fractured.	
5. Wash hands.	Standard precautions.	
6. Place child in supine position with arm at 45-degree extension from body. Instruct child in Valsalva maneuver if developmentally appropriate.	Positioning will reduce the risk of air emboli occurrence and ease removal. Valsalva maneuver will further reduce risk of air being drawn into the vascular system. Arm extension will allow the catheter to be removed without obstruction.	Occasional resistance to removal occurs.
7. Put on clean gloves and remove dressing, using alcohol pads as needed to release adhesive on StatLock.	Standard precautions; decreases exposure to blood-borne pathogens.	
8. Assess insertion site for signs or symptoms of infection, inflammation, irritation.	Allows identification of complications.	If drainage is noted, consult with the prescribing practitioner about obtaining a culture.
9. Grasp catheter with gloved hand around hub and catheter body. Remove with slow, even pull, moving up the catheter as line is pulled out of insertion site.[6]	Removing the PICC by grasping the catheter and not just the hub will reduce the risk of breakage. A tourniquet should be available in the event the catheter breaks for application on the arm above the breakage site.	Catheter breakage can occur if too much stress is placed on the catheter. Do not stretch the PICC or pull against resistance.[7]
10. If child is able to cooperate, have child perform the Valsalva maneuver before removal of last portion of the catheter. If child is unable to perform Valsalva, remove catheter on expiration.	Reduces risk of air entering the vascular system on removal of the PICC.	Child can also hum to create the same effect as the Valsalva maneuver.
11. Notify the prescribing practitioner if PICC resists removal.[8,9]	The prescribing practitioner is responsible for ordering referral to radiology or other measures for catheter removal.	Referral to radiology may be necessary to determine cause of inability to remove the catheter.

Procedure continues on following page

Procedure	**for Peripherally Inserted Central Venous Catheter (PICC): Care, Management and Removal**—*Continued*

Steps	Rationale	Considerations
12. Once catheter is removed, immediately apply antimicrobial ointment, dry sterile gauze, and transparent dressing with pressure to the site. Change dressing daily until the site has epithelialized.	Standard of practice per the Infusion Nurses Society.[3] Ointment on the insertion site prevents air from entering the vascular system.	Instruct the child and/or family in dressing change and site assessment if appropriate (i.e., child going home shortly after PICC removal).
13. Measure the length of catheter removed and compare with the insertion length. Notify the prescribing practitioner of any discrepancy.	Measurement verifies that entire catheter was removed and no complication occurred with removal.	
14. Dispose of supplies and used equipment appropriately.	Standard precautions; reduces transmission of microorganisms.	
15. Remove gloves; wash hands.	Standard precautions.	

Expected Outcomes

- PICC insertion site is free from infection

- Dressing is changed at appropriate intervals consistent with institution-specific protocol
- PICC functions without complications until therapy is completed
- PICC remains in place until electively removed

- Tip of PICC remains in the vena cava throughout therapy

- PICC is removed easily, without complications

Unexpected Outcomes

- Catheter-related signs of infection such as redness, drainage, pain
- Dressing is not changed at recommended intervals or is left in place when soiled, wet, or loose
- Therapy is interrupted due to adverse reactions

- PICC is inadvertently removed by child, family, or health care team
- Tip of PICC is displaced more than 2 cm during therapy; line is no longer central
- PICC line resists removal or breaks during removal

Monitoring and Care of the Child

Activities and Interventions	Rationale	Reportable Conditions
1. Ensure radiographic confirmation that PICC tip is located in the vena cava before initiating therapy; follow x-ray to monitor location of catheter tip.	Ensures catheter tip is located in a central vein before initiation of therapy and remains in appropriate location.	• Tip placement not within the vena cava • Any movement of the PICC more than 1 to 2 cm in or out of the insertion site • Indications that the PICC has moved from a central location
2. Inspect the insertion site regularly; monitor status of sutures, if present and length of catheter outside of insertion site.	Monitors for security of sutures; indications of infection, infiltration, or inflammation; possible movement of catheter tip if length of catheter outside of insertion site is increased.	• Loose sutures or inflammation or drainage at suture sites • Increase in length of catheter outside of insertion site • Redness, swelling, drainage, pain at insertion site
3. Maintain an occlusive dressing at the insertion site; gauze dressing is preferred if the site is bleeding or oozing. (*Level IV**)	Decreases the incidence of CRBSI.	• Bleeding or oozing at the insertion site

* Level IV: Limited clinical studies to support recommendations

Monitoring and Care of the Child—Cont'd

Activities and Interventions	Rationale	Reportable Conditions
4. Replace gauze dressing every 48 hours and semipermeable dressing every 7 days or when dressing is soiled, wet, or nonocclusive.[2] *(Level IV*)*	Decreases the incidence of CRBSI.	• Blood at or near the PICC insertion site • Leaking at insertion site
5. Monitor ease of flushing and ability to obtain a blood return; if gravity infusion is used, monitor for decreased flow rate not improved with position change.	Difficulty flushing or lack of blood return may be indicative of the primary stages of an obstruction.	• Unable to flush catheter • Unable to obtain blood return when previously present • If gravity administration used, unable to infuse fluids via gravity
6. Monitor neurovascular status of extremity where PICC is inserted.	Change in neurovascular status may indicate complications related to PICC location.	• Increasing size of extremity • Cool extremity • Pain in extremity

* Level IV: Limited clinical studies to support recommendations

Documentation

- Date, time, size, type, and total length of catheter at time of insertion; length of catheter outside the insertion site
- Date of dressing change and type of dressing used
- Appearance of insertion site; status of sutures if present
- Neurovascular assessment of extremity where PICC is placed
- Date and time of PICC removal, individual removing the PICC, length of PICC removed, and comparison with insertion length
- Condition of PICC at removal
- Child and family education
- Unexpected outcomes and related treatment

References

1. Infusion Nurses Society: Standard S54. In *Infusion nursing standards of practice 2000,* Cambridge, MA, 2000, Infusion Nurses Society.
2. Centers for Disease Control and Prevention: Guidelines for the prevention of intravascular catheter related infections, *MMWR Morbid Mortal Wkly Rep* 51(No.RR-10):1-29, 2002.
3. Maki DG, et al: Prospective randomized controlled trial of povidone iodine, alcohol and chlorhexidine for prevention of infection associated with central venous and arterial catheters, *Lancet* 338:339-343, 1991.
4. Yamamoto IJ, et al: Sutureless securement device reduces complications of peripherally inserted central venous catheters, *J Vasc Interv Radiol* 13(1):77-81, 2002.
5. Thacker D: Effect of heparinized saline versus normal saline on maintaining patency of a peripherally inserted central catheter, *JVAD* 2(2):16-18, 1997.
6. Masoorli S: Removing a PICC? Proceed with caution (peripherally inserted central catheter), *Nursing* 28(3):56-57, 1998.
7. Chow LM, et al: Peripherally inserted central catheter (PICC) fracture and embolization in the pediatric population, *J Pediatr* 142920:141-144, 2003.
8. Miall LS, et al: Peripherally inserted central catheters in children with cystic fibrosis: eight cases of difficult removal, *J Infus Nurs* 24(5):297-300, 2001.
9. Wall JL, et al: Peripherally inserted central catheters: resistance to removal: a rare complication, *J Intraven Nurs* 18(5):251-254, 1995.

Additional Readings

Frey AM: PICC complications in neonates and children, *JVAD* 4(2):2-11, 1999.

Infusion Nurses Society: *Policies and procedures for infusion nursing,* ed 2, Norwood, MA, 2002, Infusion Nurses Society.

Macklin D: How to manage PICCs, *Am J Nurs* 97(9):26-32, 1997.

Weinstein SM: *Plumer's Principles and practice of intravenous therapy,* ed 7, Philadelphia, 2001, Lippincott Williams & Wilkins.

Skin Puncture for Collection of Blood Samples: Fingerstick and Heelstick

P U R P O S E : To quickly obtain capillary blood samples by heelstick or fingerstick in emergent or routine situations

Margaret Grover

PREREQUISITE KNOWLEDGE

- Anatomy of primary arterial and venous blood supplies to digits and heels
- Principles of aseptic technique
- Only lab values requiring small sample sizes can be obtained via this method; consult institution-specific laboratory manual for specimens appropriate for this collection method.
- Calcaneal puncture during heelstick may result in calcified nodules of the heel, necrotizing chondritis, or osteomyelitis.[1]
- Poor peripheral perfusion, local infection, and edema are absolute contraindications to performing fingersticks or heelsticks.
- Complications of fingerstick or heelstick
- Appropriate containers for specimens to be collected and minimum required blood volumes for requested specimens
- Specimen labeling requirements
- Specimen handling requirements
- Child's developmental level as it relates to clinical assessment and capillary blood sampling
- Pain reduction measures suitable to age and developmental level of child
- The Occupational Safety and Health Administration (OSHA) and Centers for Disease Control and Prevention (CDC) recommend the use of a lancet with a retractable blade to decrease the incidence of needlestick injury and exposure to blood-borne pathogens.

CHILD AND FAMILY ASSESSMENT

- Child's developmental level and ability to interact ⇥*Rationale:* These factors influence preparation of the child and interaction.
- History of previous similar procedures ⇥*Rationale:* Past experiences influence current experiences; identifies children who may have a negative reaction to the procedure.
- Child's and family's understanding of the reasons for and risks and benefits of obtaining capillary blood sample ⇥*Rationale:* Evaluates child's and family's understanding of the procedure and provides a gauge for ongoing education.
- Family/child interaction and family's desire to be present during the procedure ⇥*Rationale:* Family should be encouraged to stay in the room if they are able to provide comfort and support to the child,[2] but should have the choice not to remain.
- Child's ability to be cooperative during the procedure ⇥*Rationale:* Additional staff may be necessary to minimize risk to child and staff during the procedure.

CHILD AND FAMILY EDUCATION

Individualized, developmentally appropriate education is provided to the family and to the child based on desire for knowledge, readiness to learn, and overall neurologic and psychosocial state.

- Explain procedure to the child and family before assembling supplies and equipment needed to perform the procedure ➤➤*Rationale:* Taking time to allay child and family concerns will not eliminate the pain of the procedure, but it will make the procedure less traumatic; seeing equipment for blood drawing in the room may increase child's anxiety level.
- Explain need to obtain laboratory studies ➤➤*Rationale:* Helping the child and family understand the value of procedures can help reduce anxiety and fear.[2]
- Explain how family can be of assistance/support to the child ➤➤*Rationale:* Children have reported feeling more safe and less scared when family members are present during invasive procedures.[2]
- Encourage questions and answer questions as they arise ➤➤*Rationale:* Reinforcement of information is needed during periods of stress.

EQUIPMENT

- Clean gloves
- Hot pack
- Alcohol swab(s)
- Sterile petroleum jelly (if desired)
- Appropriately sized lancet device with retractable blade
- 2×2 gauze
- Laboratory specimen collection tubes
- Appropriate laboratory requisitions
- Specimen labels containing two patient identifiers
- Adhesive bandage, latex-free
- Sucrose solution for pain reduction in infants
- Comfort/distraction box or small portable toys for distraction in children

Procedure	**for Skin Puncture for Collection of Blood Samples: Fingerstick and Heelstick**	
Steps	**Rationale**	**Considerations**
1. Ensure child and family understand procedure and questions are answered.	Evaluates and reinforces understanding of previously taught information.	Developmental level, cognitive ability, and anxiety level will determine approach to and effectiveness of teaching.
2. Identify child using two patient identifiers per institution-specific protocol.	Eliminates wrong patient/wrong procedure occurrences.	Patient safety requirement of the Joint Commission on Accreditation of Healthcare Organizations (JCAHO).
3. Verify prescribing practitioner's order.	Ensures that the correct specimens will be obtained.	
4. Gather and prepare needed supplies and equipment.	Prevents delays and unnecessary anticipation/anxiety on the part of the child.	
5. Wash hands.	Standard precautions; reduces the transmission of microorganisms.	
6. Select appropriate site. If possible, allow child to participate in selection of site ("Which finger would you like me to use?")	Selection of best site is crucial to successful outcome; child's participation facilitates child's coping.	Heelsticks are used for infants younger than 1 year, and fingersticks are used for children older than 1 year of age.
7. Apply hot pack to area selected for 3 to 5 minutes *(Level VI*)*	Improves blood flow to the skin surface promoting free flow of blood, which decreases hemolysis of sample.	
8. Put on clean gloves.	Standard precautions; minimizes provider's exposure to blood-borne pathogens.	
9. Cleanse area with alcohol swab using a back and forth rubbing motion; replace swab as needed until the alcohol swab is clean when removed from the skin. Allow alcohol to dry completely before performing procedure. *(Level VI*)*	Appropriate cleansing of the site will reduce chances of infection. Alcohol on the skin may lead to falsely high blood glucose values.[1]	Use new alcohol swab as needed if skin is soiled.

Procedure continues on following page

* Level VI: Clinical studies in a variety of patient populations and situations to support recommendations

Procedure	**for Skin Puncture for Collection of Blood Samples: Fingerstick and Heelstick**—*Continued*	

Steps	Rationale	Considerations
10. Immobilize child as appropriate. Use sucrose drops for infants[3] or distraction techniques for children for pain reduction as developmentally appropriate.	An assistant may be necessary to immobilize a strong, uncooperative child.	It is best to have someone other than a family member immobilize the child for the procedure. Family members should be encouraged to offer the child support during the procedure and comfort once the procedure is completed. Avoid offering bottle or juices during procedure because choking may occur.
11. Hold the leg or arm in a dependent position.	Increases blood flow to the skin surface at the selected site, promoting free flow of blood.	
12. For a heelstick, hold the heel at a 90-degree angle using one hand. For a fingerstick, hold the distal phalanx of the digit using one hand.	Increases blood flow to the skin surface and provides stability of the extremity or digit during the procedure.	
13. Using the lancet, puncture the skin on the most medial or lateral portion of the heel or on the fatpad of the distal fingertip (halfway between the center of the fingertip and the edge of the nail) (Figure 148-1). *(Level V*)*	Use of these areas results in best blood flow; calcaneal puncture may result in calcified nodules of the heel, necrotizing chondritis, or osteomyelitis.[1]	National Committee for Clinical Laboratory Standards recommends a penetration depth of no more than 2 mm for heelsticks in infants; select lancet with appropriate-sized blade. Avoid previous puncture sites. Avoid using the fingertips of the child's dominant hand if possible. Avoid heelstick in children who are walking when possible. Avoid using the curve of the heel.

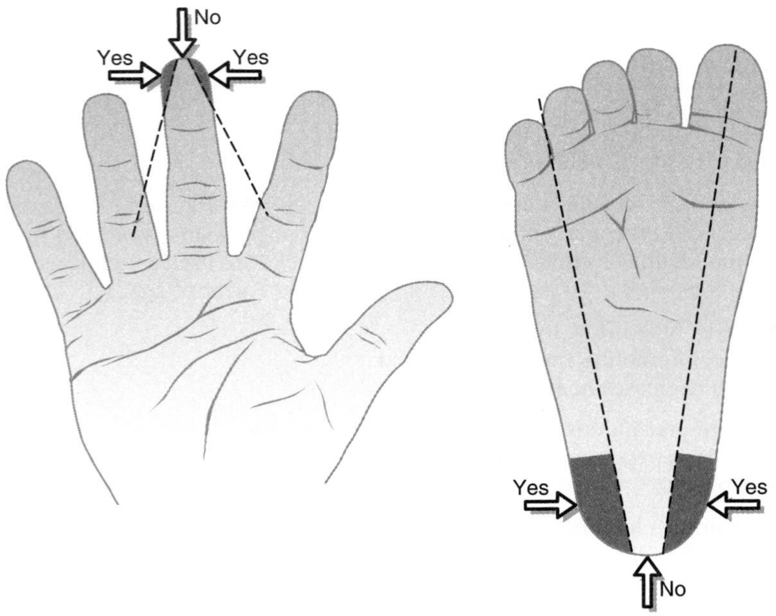

FIGURE 148-1   Recommended sites for fingerstick and heelstick.

* Level V: Clinical studies in more than one or two patient populations and situations to support recommendations

Procedure	for Skin Puncture for Collection of Blood Samples: Fingerstick and Heelstick—*Continued*	

Steps	Rationale	Considerations
14. Wipe away the first drop(s) of blood using the 2×2 gauze pad; if desired, apply a thin layer of sterile petroleum jelly to the puncture site. (*Level II**)	Petroleum jelly facilitates beading of the blood and thereby prevents excessive smearing, which will facilitate collection of the needed specimen(s).	
15. Obtain the blood sample from the puncture site using a scraping motion with the detachable capillary collector piece of the appropriate collection tube.	Sample collection is facilitated by efficient collecting of blood from puncture site.	Pediatric collection tubes contain a capillary collector piece to facilitate collection of fingerstick or heelstick samples. Avoid "milking" the heel or digit because this may increase clotting and cause hemolysis of cells which may result in falsely high potassium and bilirubin levels.[1]
16. When sample has been collected, apply pressure to the puncture site with the 2×2 gauze pad for 1 to 3 minutes.	Facilitates clotting.	A cooperative child may be helpful in holding gauze in place and applying direct pressure; family may be included in this step as well.
17. Remove the capillary collection piece of the collection tube and cap the specimen.	Ensures specimen is not lost. Minimizes staff exposure to blood-borne pathogens.	
18. Label specimens at the bedside and complete laboratory paperwork per institution-specific protocol.	Promotes patient safety; ensures accurate and efficient processing of specimen.	Follow institution specific protocols for handling and labeling lab specimens.
19. Discard lancet in sharps container at child's bedside; discard used supplies and equipment appropriately.	Standard precautions; reduces exposure to blood-borne pathogens.	
20. Apply adhesive bandage to site once hemostasis is achieved.	Protects site; if repeated capillary samples are being obtained, identifies previously used sites.	Many children find adhesive bandages comforting.
21. Remove gloves; wash hands.	Standard precautions; reduces transmission of microorganisms.	

* Level II: Theory-based, no research data to support recommendations: recommendations from expert consensus group may exist

Expected Outcomes

- Requested laboratory studies are obtained

- Sample collected is able to be analyzed
- Child and family tolerates procedure with minimum distress
- Child remains free from localized infection, bacteremia, osteomyelitis

- Calcaneal puncture is avoided

- Specimens are placed in correct sample tubes, labeled appropriately, and sent to the lab in the appropriate time frame
- Child demonstrates acceptable level of comfort after procedure is completed

Unexpected Outcomes

- Inadequate volume of blood collected for needed laboratory studies
- Hemolyzed sample resulting in erroneous results
- Child or family is traumatized by procedure

- Localized infection at puncture site
- Bacteremia
- Osteomyelitis
- Calcified nodules of the heel resulting from calcaneal puncture
- Specimens are mislabeled, placed in incorrect sample tubes, or not sent to lab in a timely fashion

- Unmanaged pain

Monitoring and Care of the Child

Activities and Interventions	Rationale	Reportable Conditions
1. Assess puncture site for active bleeding.	Bleeding may continue if inadequate pressure is applied, particularly in active children.	• Bleeding that persists after a full 5 minutes of direct pressure
2. Assess previously used puncture sites for signs of infection.	Early identification of complications facilitates prompt treatment.	• Signs of infections including redness, swelling, warmth, drainage or pain at puncture site
3. Assess effectiveness of pain management strategy and provide appropriate interventions; encourage family to assist in using nonpharmacologic means to comfort and support the child.	Use of appropriate pain management techniques facilitates the child's coping and promotes cooperation with subsequent procedures.	• Continued irritability, changes in physiologic condition • Reports of unresolved discomfort

Documentation

- Type of procedure performed, i.e., heelstick or fingerstick
- Site of procedure
- Name and credentials of person performing procedure
- Child's tolerance of procedure
- Laboratory specimens sent
- Comfort assessment and any specific interventions provided
- Child and family education
- Unexpected outcomes and related treatment

References
1. Duffy S, Steele D: Heel sticks. In Henretig FM, King C, editors: *Textbook of pediatric emergency procedures,* Baltimore, 1997, Williams & Wilkins.
2. Eichhorn DJ, et al: Family presence during invasive procedures and resuscitation, *AJN* 101:5, 2001.
3. Greenberg C: Practice applications of research: a sugar-coated pacifier reduces procedural pain in newborns, *Pediatr Nurs* 28(3):271-277, 2002.

Additional Readings
Hazinski MF: *Manual of pediatric critical care,* Philadelphia, 1998, Mosby.
Roberts J, Hedges JR: *Clinical procedures in emergency medicine,* ed 4, Philadelphia, 2003, Saunders.

Totally Implantable Central Venous Port: Accessing, Management, and De-accessing

PURPOSE: To provide repeated or prolonged access to the vascular system

Dana Etzel-Hardman

PREREQUISITE KNOWLEDGE

- Child development as it relates to clinical assessment and care of a totally implanted central venous port
- Anatomy and physiology of the cardiovascular system
- Principles of intravenous therapy
- Principles of aseptic technique
- Standard precautions
- A totally implantable central venous port otherwise known as a "port" is an internalized central venous catheter. The procedure is usually performed in the operating room or interventional radiology suite.[1] Refer to Figure 149-1 for a diagram of port placement.
  - ❖ A small reservoir made of titanium or plastic is placed subcutaneously.
  - ❖ A venous catheter is inserted and advanced into a central vein, usually through the subclavian vein but other veins also may be used.
  - ❖ The catheter is tunneled under the skin and connected to the reservoir.
- The side of the reservoir facing the skin has a self-sealing thick silicone rubber membrane, called the septum, accessed via a special noncoring needle that allows repeated use of the port without leaking.
- Before first use of the port, radiographic confirmation by chest x-ray of catheter tip placement in the superior vena cava or atrial-caval junction is required.

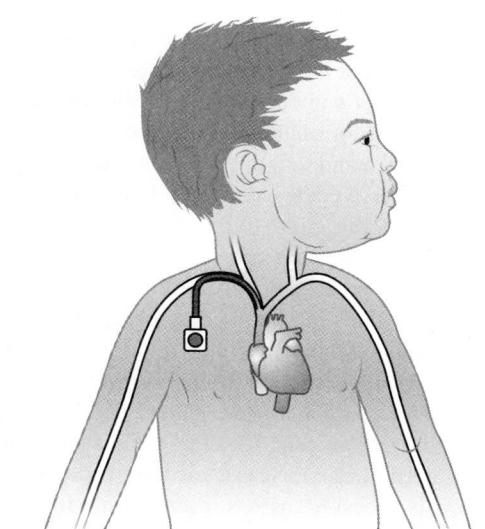

FIGURE 149-1 Totally implanted central venous access device.

- Noncoring needles (e.g., Huber) are the only acceptable needles for port access; other types of needles will cause the septum to leak.
- An infusion pump is generally recommended for infusions; situations such as administration of chemotherapeutic agents known to be vesicants, a pump may not be used.

- The subcutaneous port is generally accessed and flushed using heparin (100 units/mL, volume based on size of child) at least once every 30 days if not in use, or per manufacturer's instructions; some closed-ended (Groshong) catheters do not require a heparin flush.
- Port septum has a usual life expectancy of 1000 to 2500 punctures.
- Complications associated with ports include catheter disconnection, fragmentation, fracture, or shearing with possible embolization of the catheter; catheter rupture; erosion of port/catheter through skin and/or blood vessel; implant rejection; nerve damage.[2]
- Because there is no external catheter present, the port is easier to care for and more accepted by active pediatric or adolescent patients. When de-accessed, there is no visible indication of the port, allowing the child to feel more "normal."
- Exercise care when changing dressing to avoid dislodging the noncoring needle.
- Comparing all types of central venous access, ports have the lowest risk for catheter-related bloodstream infections (CRBSI).[3] *(Level VI*)*
- Informed consent is required before placement of a totally implanted central venous port.

CHILD AND FAMILY ASSESSMENT

- Child's developmental level and ability to interact ➥*Rationale:* These factors influence preparation of the child and interaction.
- Child's and family's understanding of the reasons for and risks and benefits of the procedure ➥*Rationale:* Evaluates child's and family's understanding of the procedure and provides a gauge for ongoing education.
- Type of port, size and length of needle used to access the port ➥*Rationale:* Needle size and length are individualized to the specific child; type of port affects solution used for flushing the catheter.
- If port has been previously accessed, have family provide insight on the child's reaction to and tolerance of accessing and de-accessing of the port, as well as any unique interventions required such as specific positioning of the child or stabilization of the port ➥*Rationale:* Allows development of an individualized plan of care; increases child's ability to cope with the procedure and increases success of accessing port.
- When port is accessed, assess insertion site routinely for indications of infiltration or infection per institution-specific protocol ➥*Rationale:* Regular assessment facilitates early identification of complications.
- Child's and family's current skills related to management of the port ➥*Rationale:* Ports are placed for long-term access; the child and family are usually responsible for managing the port in the home. The family may have routines established around accessing or managing the port, such as using topical anesthetic cream before port access or specific type of needle used to access the port.

- Family's desire to be present during procedures such as accessing, de-accessing, or dressing change ➥*Rationale:* Family may provide comfort and support to the child during the procedure, but should have the option not to remain with the child.

CHILD AND FAMILY EDUCATION

Individualized, developmentally appropriate education is provided to the family and to the child based on desire for knowledge, readiness to learn, and overall neurologic and psychosocial state.

- Teach the family and child techniques to manage pain related to accessing the port ➥*Rationale:* Use of topical anesthetics and techniques such as distraction may help the child cope with discomfort associated with repeated accessing of port.
- If port is newly placed, provide information about care and management of the port, including routine flushing of catheter ➥*Rationale:* Providing information decreases anxiety and fear of unknown. The family, and child as appropriate, will generally be involved in the care and maintenance of the port when the child is out of the hospital.
- Teach family, and child as appropriate, aseptic technique for accessing and de-accessing port, and any time the device is used ➥*Rationale:* Appropriate care of the catheter is considered to be of primary importance and is believed to play a critical role in decreasing the risk of CRBSI.[3] *(Level VI*)*
- Teach the family, and child as appropriate, the correct needles used for port access ➥*Rationale:* Specially designed noncoring needles are used to access an implanted port to prevent leaking through the septum. Use of a coring needle may require the port to be replaced.
- Teach the family and child signs and symptoms of complications related to port including infection, infiltration, and catheter occlusion ➥*Rationale:* Informs the child and family of reasons to notify the health care team, allowing prompt assessment and intervention; encourages active participation in care by the family and child.
- Explain steps in procedure before performing, such as dressing change or accessing or de-accessing port ➥*Rationale:* Providing information decreases anxiety and fear, and promotes the child's coping.
- If available, provide written educational material to the child and family on care and management of the port ➥*Rationale:* Providing written material permits the family to refer to a source of information that reinforces verbal teaching. Having educational materials to refer to can help to reduce anxiety and fear.
- Have the family, and child if appropriate, give a repeat demonstration of any tasks that they will be required to perform at home such as routine catheter flushes ➥*Rationale:* In order to appropriately document a child or family member as being independent in performing a task, the person must be observed carrying it out as instructed.

---

* Level VI: Clinical studies in a variety of patient populations and situations to support recommendations

- Encourage questions and answer questions as they arise
  ➥*Rationale:* Reinforcement of information is needed during periods of stress.

EQUIPMENT

For Port Access

- Central line dressing tray with the following supplies, or gather these supplies:
  ❖ Sterile overwrap
  ❖ 2×2 gauze
  ❖ Sterile strips
  ❖ Sterile protective barrier
  ❖ Non-latex sterile gloves
  ❖ Skin protectant
  ❖ Alcohol prep sticks or swabs
  ❖ Cleansing agents, 2% chlorhexidine or 10% povidone-iodine per institution-specific protocol

- Transparent semipermeable membrane dressing
- Masks for all individuals in the room
- Additional pair of sterile gloves
- 0.9% saline for flush
- Syringes
- Appropriate-sized noncoring needle (needle with safety mechanism, if available)
- Heparin 100 units/mL or 10 units/mL per institution-specific protocol
- Topical anesthetic cream if desired

For De-accessing Port

- Alcohol swabs
- 0.9% saline in 10-mL or larger syringe
- Clean non-latex gloves
- Heparin 100 units/mL or per institution-specific protocol
- Adhesive bandage

Procedure	for Totally Implantable Central Venous Port: Accessing, Management, and De-accessing	
Steps	**Rationale**	**Considerations**
Accessing Port		
1. Ensure child and family understand procedure and questions are answered.	Evaluates and reinforces understanding of previously taught information.	Developmental level, cognitive ability, and anxiety level will determine approach to and effectiveness of teaching.
2. Wash hands; apply topical local anesthetic to port site for appropriate time interval before accessing port per prescribing practitioner's order and as recommended by manufacturer. *(Level I*)*	Placement of needle is painful; some children tolerate the procedure more easily if topical anesthetic is used.	Other options for pain management include application of ice or a cold pack for a few minutes before accessing port.
3. Gather needed equipment and supplies included appropriate-sized noncoring needle.	Facilitates completion of task in a timely manner.	Noncoring needle sizes available for use in children include 22 or 20 gauge, ¾, 1, or 1½ inches long. The smallest gauge appropriate for therapy prescribed should be used to access the implanted port. Use shortest length that will access port.
4. Provide for appropriate privacy.	Accessing port generally requires exposure of the chest.	Privacy is an important consideration for school-aged children and adolescents.
5. Wash hands.[1,3,4] *(Level VI*)*	Standard precautions; reduces the transmission of microorganisms.	Thorough handwashing is the most important and basic technique in preventing and controlling infection.
6. Prepare sterile field using aseptic technique. Place additional supplies onto field in a sterile manner.	Having all supplies available and within easy reach during accessing of port helps to maintain sterile field.	
7. Consider enlisting an assistant to help immobilize the child during port access.	Young active children may move during the procedure, contaminating the sterile field.	

Procedure continues on following page

Procedure	**for Totally Implantable Central Venous Port: Accessing, Management, and De-accessing**—*Continued*	
Steps	**Rationale**	**Considerations**
8. Put on sterile gloves.[3,4,5] *(Level VI*)*	Aseptic technique; decreases the incidence of CRBSI.	
9. With help of assistant, draw up appropriate volume of 0.9% saline into 10-mL or larger syringe in a sterile manner.	Larger sized syringe decreases pressure when catheter is flushed; high pressures may damage catheter or blood vessels.	
10. Attach 0.9% saline syringe to non-coring needle extension tubing; prime needle.	Removes air from needle and tubing, reducing risk of air embolus.	
11. Leave syringe attached and clamp tubing. If drawing blood, do not prime needle set; attach empty syringe.	Prepares needle set to access port.	
12. Prepare cleansing agent, syringes, and dressing on sterile field. Remove gloves.	Prepares all supplies for port access; child's chest will need to be palpated to locate port and gloves will no longer be sterile.	
13. Place child supine; if child is unable to hold still during procedure use assistant to immobilize child.	Location of port requires palpation and examination in a supine position.	Occasionally a child will require a position other than supine to access port; encourage family to provide information on how port is most easily accessed.
14. If present, wipe off topical anesthetic agent.	Allows visualization of and access to site.	
15. Inspect port site for redness, swelling, or other signs of infection or infiltration.	Allows identification of problems before port is accessed.	These signs are not always indicative of infection.
16. Palpate over child's chest to locate the edges of the port housing.	Identifies area to be cleaned before port insertion.	
17. Put mask on self and child; everyone in room during procedure should mask.	Masks prevent contamination of site and sterile field with airborne organisms.	With young children, make sure the child sees your face before putting on mask.
18. Wash hands.	Standard precautions.	
19. Put on sterile gloves.[3,4,5] *(Level VI*)*	Aseptic technique is required during port access to decrease the risk of CRBSI.	
20. Use alcohol swabs to cleanse port access site, using a back and forth, scrubbing motion.[3,4,5] *(Level VI*)*	Removes skin oils and cells; reduces microbe count on skin.	
21. Disinfect site with 2% chlorhexidine; allow to air-dry.[3,4,5] *(Level VI*)*	Fast-acting, broad-spectrum and persistent antiseptic that reduces the number of microorganisms on the skin.	Chlorhexidine is not recommended for use in infants less than 2 months old; povidone-iodine is recommended for this group.[3,4]
22. Place sterile towel below port site.	Provides sterile work area.	

* Level VI: Clinical studies in a variety of patient populations and situations to support recommendations

Procedure	for Totally Implantable Central Venous Port: Accessing, Management, and De-accessing—*Continued*		
Steps	**Rationale**	**Considerations**
23. Stabilize port housing using thumb and index finger of nondominant hand.	Stabilizing port provides clear target area for needle insertion.	
24. Insert the noncoring needle through skin at a right angle to port septum and push down firmly until needle penetrates port septum and contacts rigid back of port.[1] (Figure 149-2).	Ensures proper placement of needle into port.	Do not tilt or rock the needle once the septum is punctured; it may cause damage to the septum.

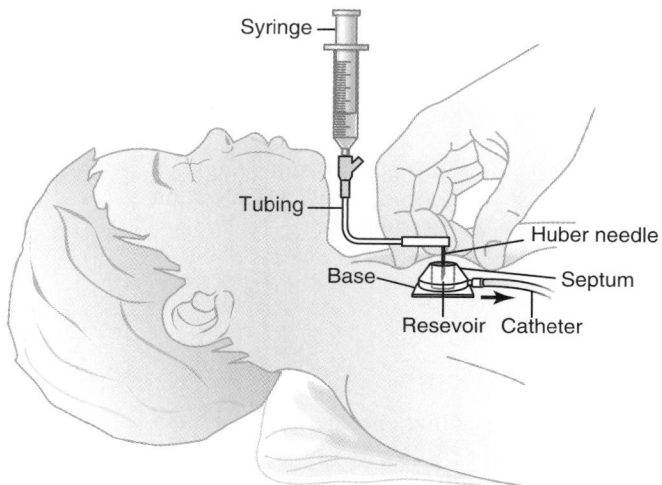

Figure 149-2   Accessing a port using a noncoring needle. Note the 90-degree angle in the needle.

25. Flush port with 20 mL of 0.9% saline if child is more than 10 kg; if less than 10 kg use 1mL/kg for flush. Apply gentle negative pressure to assess blood return.[5] *(Level II*)*	Ensures patency of port and catheter.	Do not irrigate forcefully if resistance is felt; forceful irrigation may dislodge a clot, causing it to enter the vascular system. Refer to institution-specific protocol for volume of flush used.
26. If port is to be locked, flush port with appropriate volume of heparinized saline per institution-specific protocol; 100 units/mL is concentration generally used. Flush port using a push-pause, push-pause technique.[6]	Use of heparin prevents clot formation. Push-pause, push-pause technique creates turbulence that is most effective in cleaning out catheter.	Suggested volumes for heparinized saline based on frequency of flush; refer to institution-specific protocol. **More than 10 kg** Monthly: 3 mL heparin 100 units/mL Daily: 3 mL heparin 100 units/mL More than twice daily: 3 mL heparin 10 units/mL **4 to 10 kg** Monthly:1.5 mL heparin 100 units/mL Daily:1.5 mL heparin 100 units/mL More than twice daily: 1.5 mL heparin 10 units/mL

Procedure continues on following page

Procedure	for Totally Implantable Central Venous Port: Accessing, Management, and De-accessing—*Continued*	
Steps	**Rationale**	**Considerations**
		Less than 4 kg Monthly:1 mL heparin 100 units/mL Daily:1 mL heparin 100 units/mL More than twice daily:1 mL heparin 10 units/mL
27. If positive pressure end cap is not in use, use positive pressure technique at end of flush: initiate a final push; then clamp the catheter while pushing down on the syringe plunger; remove syringe after clamp is closed. *(Level II*)*	Positive pressure technique reduces blood reflux at the terminal end of the catheter.	Positive pressure technique is not necessary with some valved catheters or with positive pressure end caps.
28. If fluid is to be administered, secure noncoring needle and dress site. • Support wings of needle with gauze, ensuring there is equal pressure above and below the length of needle and hub. • Do not cover needle insertion site with gauze. • Stabilize needle with sterile strips placed under wings of needle, adhesive side up; crisscross over the needle and secure to skin. • Apply semipermeable transparent dressing.	Prevents needle from being dislodged; allows visualization of insertion site. Stabilizes needle. Transparent dressings allow continuous inspection of the site and assist in stabilizing and securing the needle.	Port dressings and needles are changed every 7 days unless the dressing becomes damp, loosened, or soiled.
29. Attach IV tubing and begin infusion.	Initiates fluid administration.	
30. Label dressing with date, time, and initials of person performing the dressing change.	Indicates time next dressing change is due.	
31. Dispose of supplies and used equipment appropriately.	Standard precautions; reduces transmission of microorganisms.	
32. Remove gloves and mask; wash hands.	Standard precautions.	
De-accessing Port 1. Ensure that child and family understand procedure and questions are answered.	Evaluates and reinforces understanding of previously taught information.	Developmental level, cognitive ability, and anxiety level will determine approach to and effectiveness of teaching.
2. Wash hands.[3,4,5,7] *(Level VI*)*	Standard precautions.	
3. Gather needed equipment and supplies.	Facilitates completion of task in a timely manner.	
4. Provide for appropriate privacy.	De-accessing port generally requires exposure of the chest.	Privacy is an important consideration for school-aged children and adolescents.

* Level II: Theory-based, no research data to support recommendations: recommendations from expert consensus group may exist
  Level VI: Clinical studies in a variety of patient populations and situations to support recommendations

Procedure	for Totally Implantable Central Venous Port: Accessing, Management, and De-accessing—*Continued*	
Steps	**Rationale**	**Considerations**
5. Prepare 10-mL syringes with appropriate volume of 0.9% saline and heparinized saline per prescribing practitioner's order or institution-specific protocol.	Syringes smaller than 10 mL generate high pressures during flushing, which could damage catheter.	The smaller the syringe, the higher the pressure transmitted during flushing. If smaller syringe must be used because of small volume medication, NEVER force plunger against resistance.
6. Place child supine; if child unable to hold still during procedure use assistant to immobilize child.	A young child may resist procedure or pull at needle.	
7. Loosen transparent dressing.	Facilitates removal of dressing.	Adhesive remover may be used to facilitate dressing removal.
8. Put on clean gloves.	Standard precautions; minimizes exposure to blood-borne pathogens.	
9. If fluid is infusing, stop infusion; disconnect IV tubing.	No longer required; removing tubing allows access to cap for flushing.	
10. Cleanse port end cap with alcohol swab using scrubbing action.[3,4,5,7] (*Level VI**)	Removes microorganisms; decreases incidence of CRBSI.	Clean end cap (injection site) first; continue to clean around sides of cap, cleansing the whole device.
11. Clamp tubing.	Prevents backflow of blood.	Not necessary if positive pressure end cap is used.
12. Attach syringe with 0.9% saline; open clamp and flush using a push-pause, push-pause technique.	Clears any fluid or medication remaining in the port reservoir and catheter.	
13. Clamp tubing; remove saline flush syringe.	Prevents backflow of blood.	Clamping is not necessary if positive pressure end cap is used.
14. Attach heparinized saline syringe; unclamp and flush port.	Heparinization of port helps to prevent fibrin sheath and clot formation.	
15. Stabilize port using thumb and forefinger of nondominant hand; use positive pressure technique at end of flush: continue to infuse last 0.5 mL of flush while removing needle, pulling the needle straight up and out.	Positive pressure technique reduces blood reflux at the terminal end of the catheter, preventing clotting.	Noncoring needles with safety mechanism to prevent needlestick injuries are now available; follow manufacturer's instructions to activate safety mechanism while removing needle.
16. Inspect the site for signs of skin breakdown, infiltration or infection.	Allows identification of complications and prompt intervention.	Report indications of breakdown, infiltration, and infection to prescribing practitioner.
17. Apply adhesive bandage or coverlet dressing over puncture site.	Reduces risk of infection until puncture site healed.	
18. Dispose of supplies and used equipment appropriately; ensure needle is placed in sharps container.	Standard precautions; reduces transmission of microorganisms; protects staff from needlestick injuries.	
19. Remove gloves; wash hands.	Standard precautions.	

* Level VI: Clinical studies in a variety of patient populations and situations to support recommendations

Expected Outcomes

- Port is completely placed under the skin
- Child is free from indications of infection

- Catheter tip is centrally placed as confirmed by radiologic studies
- Child is free from catheter-related complications

- Needle is correctly placed into chamber of port

- Noncoring needle is used to access port

- Port functions without difficulty

- Port needle stays in place until electively removed or changed

Unexpected Outcomes

- Port erodes through skin
- Indications of infection at catheter site
- Indications of CRBSI including hypotension, poor perfusion, change in level of consciousness
- Catheter tip is not centrally located

- Catheter disconnection
- Catheter fragmentation
- Catheter embolus
- Catheter rupture
- Cardiac dysrhythmia
- Cardiac puncture
- Cardiac tamponade
- Needle is not placed into port and fluid or medication infiltrates into subcutaneous tissue or lung
- Coring needle is used to access port, disrupting septum, causing leaking of fluid and blood into subcutaneous tissue, and requiring port removal and replacement
- Fibrin sheath formation around catheter tip prevents blood sampling or fluid/medication administration
- Catheter occlusion due to precipitated medications
- Dislodgement of needle

Monitoring and Care of the Child

Activities and Interventions	Rationale	Reportable Conditions
1. Ensure radiographic confirmation that port tip is located in the vena cava or at the atrial-caval junction before initiating therapy; follow x-ray to monitor location of catheter tip.	Ensures catheter tip is located in a central vein before initiating therapy and remains in appropriate location.	• Tip placement not within the vena cava
2. Monitor port function and site for signs of infection or infiltration.	Facilitates early identification of complications and prompt treatment.	• Unable to infuse fluid or flush port • Lack of blood return • Pain at port site • Swelling at port site
3. When accessing port, note any difficulties inserting needle.	Port may flip so that metal or plastic back of reservoir is oriented toward the skin.	• Unable to access port; resistance is felt when attempting to insert needle
4. Monitor child for signs and symptoms of sepsis.	CRBSIs are a significant complication; early identification allows prompt intervention.	• Fever • Indications of poor perfusion such as increased capillary refill time, cool extremities, change in level of consciousness, weakening peripheral pulses • Increased work of breathing
5. If port is accessed, change needle and dressing every 7 days; change end cap when needle is changed.	Decreases incidence of CRBSI; allows close inspection of insertion site.	• Indications of skin breakdown under dressing
6. If continuous fluid infusion is in place, change tubing and solution every 72 hours.[3,4,5,7] *(Level IV*)*	CDC recommendations to decrease incidence of CRBSI.	• Unable to remove tubing set from needle, requiring replacement of needle before 7 days

* Level IV: Limited clinical studies to support recommendation

Documentation

- Radiologic findings documenting placement of catheter tip
- Date of dressing change and type of dressing used
- Date and time port accessed, size of noncoring needle used, presence of blood return, ease of flushing
- Assessment of needle insertion site
- Solution used to lock port
- Child and family education
- Unexpected outcomes and related treatment

References

1. Masoorli S, Angeles T: Getting a line on CVAD, *Nursing* 32(4):36-43, 2002.
2. Hadaway L: IV infiltration: not just a peripheral problem, *Nursing* 32(8):36-42, 2002.
3. Centers for Disease Control and Prevention: Guidelines for the prevention of intravascular catheter related infections, *MMWR Morbid Mortal Wkly Rep* 51(No.RR-10):1-29, 2002.
4. Hadaway L: Infusing without infecting, *Nursing* 33(10):58-63, 2003.
5. Infusion Nurses Society: Infusion nursing standards of practice, *J Intraven Nurs* 23(6S):S1-85, 2000.
6. Hadaway L: Catheter connection . . . stop start method of flushing catheters, *J Vasc Access* 7(3):57, 2002.
7. Hadaway L: What you can do to decrease catheter related infections, *Nursing* 32:36-43, 2002.

Additional Readings

Alexander H: Insertion technique for long-term venous access catheters: percutaneous vein cannulation. In Alexander H, editor: *Vascular access in the cancer patient: devices, insertion techniques, maintenance, and prevention and management of complications,* Philadelphia, 1994, Lippincott.
Hadaway L: Hub disinfection and its impact on catheter-related infections, *J Vasc Access* 6(2):33-36, 2001.
Halfman M, Reiner S, editors: *Quick guide to central venous access,* Ontario, Canada, 2002, Edwards Life Sciences.
Hankins J, et al, editors: *Infusion therapy in clinical practice,* ed 2, Philadelphia, 2001, Saunders.
Kowalski C, et al: Migration of central venous catheters: implications for initial catheter tip positioning, *J Vasc Interv Radiol* 8:443-447, 1997.
Simpson KR, et al: Interventional radiological placement of chest wall ports: results and complication in 161 consecutive placements, *J Vasc Interv Radiol* 8:189-195, 1997.
Venous access.com 2002 Home page. Central line catheter care: Tunneled, PICC, PASV, and Groshong catheters. Accessed November, 2003, from www.venousaccess.com.

Venipuncture for Blood Sampling

P U R P O S E : To obtain blood specimens for laboratory analysis; results are used to support clinical decision making

Margaret Grover

PREREQUISITE KNOWLEDGE

- Anatomy of venous vascular system; refer to Procedure 146, Figure 146-1 for location of access sites commonly used in children
- Standard precautions
- Principles of aseptic technique
- Order of draw, if several specimens of various types are being obtained (e.g., chemistry, hematology, and coagulation studies)
- Appropriate containers for specimens to be collected and minimum required blood volumes for those specimens
- Specimen labeling requirements
- Specimen handling requirements
- Injury, infection, renal grafts/fistulas compromise vasculature in extremities
- Child development as it relates to clinical assessment and performing venipuncture, including distraction and other pain reduction measures suitable to child's age and developmental level
- Although venipuncture is frequently performed in children, it remains one of the more challenging procedures performed in pediatrics.

CHILD AND FAMILY ASSESSMENT

- Child's developmental level and ability to interact ➟*Rationale:* These factors influence preparation of the child and interaction.
- Child's and family's understanding of the reasons for and risks and benefits of the procedure ➟*Rationale:* Evaluates

child's and family's understanding of the procedure and provides a gauge for ongoing education.
- History of similar procedures and child's ability to tolerate procedure as well as coping strategies that were effective, including previous experience with and potential benefits of using topical anesthetic cream against urgency of obtaining blood sample. ➟*Rationale:* Past experiences influence current experiences.
- History of injury, infection, renal grafts/fistulas in any extremity ➟*Rationale:* These factors compromise vasculature in the affected extremity; venipuncture should not be performed in affected extremity.
- Child's hydration and perfusion status ➟*Rationale:* It is more difficult to perform successful venipuncture in a dehydrated or poorly perfused child.
- Family's desire to be present during the procedure ➟*Rationale:* Family should be encouraged to stay in the room to provide comfort and support to the child, but should have the choice not to remain.
- Child's ability to cooperate during the procedure ➟*Rationale:* Additional staff may be necessary to minimize risk to child and staff during the procedure

CHILD AND FAMILY EDUCATION

Individualized, developmentally appropriate education is provided to the family and to the child based on desire for knowledge, readiness to learn, and overall neurologic and psychosocial state.

- Explain procedure to child and family before preparing bedside to perform the procedure ➟*Rationale:* Taking time, when possible, to allay child and family concerns will not eliminate the pain of venipuncture, but it will make the procedure less traumatic.

- Explain need to obtain laboratory studies ➥*Rationale:* Helping child and families understand the value of procedures can help reduce anxiety and fear.
- Explain how family can assist and support the child ➥*Rationale:* Children have reported feeling more safe and less scared when family members are present during invasive procedures.[1]
- Encourage questions and answer questions as they arise ➥*Rationale:* Reinforcement of information is needed during periods of stress.

EQUIPMENT

- Clean gloves
- Hot pack (optional)
- Alcohol swabs
- Appropriately sized butterfly needle set
- Povidone-iodine or chlorhexidine applicator if blood culture ordered
- Needleless blood-drawing setup to obtain specimen(s)
- Appropriately sized syringe(s) for needed blood sample(s)
- Single-use disposable tourniquet, latex-free
- 2×2 gauze
- Adhesive bandage or pressure dressing, latex-free
- Needleless blood transfer system (to transfer blood from syringe[s] to specimen tubes)
- Appropriate specimen tubes
- Appropriate laboratory requisitions
- Specimen labels containing two patient identifiers
- Anesthetic agent: topical cream or other per family request and as clinical situation permits

Procedure | for Venipuncture for Blood Sampling

Steps	Rationale	Considerations
1. Ensure child and family understand procedure and questions are answered.	Evaluates and reinforces understanding of previously taught information.	Developmental level, cognitive ability and anxiety level will determine approach to and effectiveness of teaching.
2. Identify child using two patient identifiers per institution-specific protocol.	Eliminates wrong patient/wrong procedure occurrences.	Patient safety requirement of the Joint Commission on Accreditation of Healthcare Organizations (JCAHO)
3. Verify prescribing practitioner's order.	Ensures that the correct specimens will be obtained.	Identify minimum amount of blood required for requested specimens; drawing minimum required blood volume decreases the incidence of iatrogenic anemia.
4. Gather and assemble needed supplies and equipment.	Prevents delays and unnecessary anticipation on the part of the child.	Identify special handling requirements for lab specimens before obtaining specimens (e.g., specimen must be placed on ice).
5. Ensure good lighting.	Facilitates visualization of venipuncture site.	For infants and young children, may use transilluminator to locate veins.
6. Wash hands; identify site.	Selection of best vein for the procedure is crucial to successful outcome.	Avoid using veins that are heavily scarred or sclerosed due to numerous previous venipuncture attempts. Do not use veins that are compromised. When possible, avoid preferred intravenous access sites. Do not use veins that are proximal to running intravenous fluids. Begin by using distal sites, moving more proximally with subsequent attempts.

Procedure continues on following page

Procedure for Venipuncture for Blood Sampling—*Continued*

Steps	Rationale	Considerations
7. If topical anesthetic was used, ensure it was applied for an appropriate time period and per manufacturer's recommendations. Remove topical anesthetic.	Topical anesthetic must be applied for a specific time period in order to be effective. Topical anesthetic must be removed prior to venipuncture in order to visualize site.	
8. Immobilize child as appropriate; consider enlisting an assistant to help with procedure.	Additional health care staff may be necessary to immobilize a strong or uncooperative child.	It is best to have someone other than a family member immobilize the child for the procedure. Family members should be encouraged to offer the child support during the procedure and comfort once the procedure is completed. Avoid offering bottle or juice during procedure, because choking may occur.
9. Put on clean gloves.	Standard precautions; reduces the transmission of microorganisms.	
10. Apply tourniquet approximately 2 to 4 inches proximal to vein.	Applying the tourniquet proximal to the vein will block venous return and distend the vein, making it more prominent.[2]	The tourniquet should not be left in place for longer than 3 to 5 minutes because this will result in a more fragile vein. The tourniquet must not be so tight as to occlude arterial flow. If needed, apply hot pack to site for 5 to 10 minutes before attempting venipuncture. To prevent the tourniquet from pinching the skin or pulling the hair, place a 4×4 gauze over the area where the tourniquet will be applied.
11. Cleanse venipuncture site with alcohol swab using a back and forth or rubbing motion until the alcohol swab is clean; replace swab as needed. If obtaining a blood culture, cleanse the site with povidone-iodine or chlorhexadine.[3] *(Level VI*)*	Appropriate cleansing of the site will decrease incidence of infection. Appropriate preparation of the site before obtaining a blood culture will minimize the risk of blood culture contaminants.	
12. Perform the venipuncture while applying slight traction to the skin and vein to better secure and visualize the vein. *(Level II*)*	Serves to stabilize and straighten the vein, allowing for easier penetration without going through the vein.[4]	
13. Insert the tip of the needle with the bevel facing upward just distal to the exact site selected for vein penetration holding the needle at a 15- to 30-degree angle.	Allows for controlled entry into the vein once the skin has been pierced.[2]	Child may move slightly, even when well immobilized, in response to the initial puncture with the needle. Entering the skin distal to the vein prevents unanticipated vein puncture, which may result in inadequate blood specimen retrieval and a large hematoma.

* Level II: Theory-based, no research data to support recommendations: recommendations from expert consensus group may exist
Level VI: Clinical studies in a variety of patient populations and situations to support recommendations

Procedure for Venipuncture for Blood Sampling—*Continued*

Steps	Rationale	Considerations
13. Enter the vein slowly. Entry into the vein is verified by the flashback of blood into the closed blood obtaining system.	Allows for controlled entry into the vein to avoid through-and-through penetration of the vein and extravasation of blood into surrounding tissues.	A slight popping sensation may be appreciated as the needle enters the vein.
14. Withdraw blood volume needed for ordered laboratory studies; consider removing the tourniquet prior to obtaining blood sample (this may only be feasible in older children and adolescents). *(Level II*)*	Specific volumes are required in order to run requested studies. Tourniquet removal is recommended to prevent hemoconcentration.[5]	If unable to easily obtain blood sample with the tourniquet off, replace the tourniquet and obtain the blood sample.
15. If not previously removed, remove the tourniquet.	Venous distention no longer required; decreases hematoma formation.	
16. Remove the needle while activating the safety lock system and dispose of needle in sharps container at bedside.	Reduces incidence of needlestick injuries.	
17. Place 2×2 gauze over puncture site and apply direct pressure for 1 to 3 minutes.	Direct pressure minimizes oozing from the site and will minimize hematoma formation by facilitating clot formation.	A cooperative child may be helpful in holding gauze in place and applying direct pressure; family may be included in this step as well.
18. Transfer blood to appropriate laboratory specimen tubes.	Specimens must be placed in correct tubes to ensure accurate results are obtained.	Order of draw specified by institution-specific laboratory should be followed to ensure specimens obtained are able to be processed and yield accurate results.
19. Label specimens at the bedside and complete laboratory paperwork per institution-specific protocol.	Promotes patient safety; ensures accurate and efficient processing of specimen.	Follow institution-specific protocols for handling and labeling lab specimens.
20. Discard used supplies in appropriate receptacle.	Standard precautions; reduces transmission of microorganisms.	
21. Apply adhesive bandage to site once hemostasis is achieved.	Decreases incidence of infection until puncture site is healed.	
22. Remove gloves; wash hands.	Standard precautions; reduces transmission of microorganisms.	

* Level II: Theory-based, no research data to support recommendations: recommendations from expert consensus group may exist

Expected Outcomes

- Venipuncture is successfully performed with one attempt

- Child and family tolerate procedure with minimum distress
- Desired laboratory specimens and accurate results are obtained

- Experience of procedure builds child/family trust in the role of the health care staff member performing the procedure
- Child remains free from complications of venipuncture

Unexpected Outcomes

- More than one attempt is required to obtain ordered laboratory studies
- Child or family is traumatized by procedure

- Inadequate blood volume is obtained; specimens cannot be processed
- Specimen is contaminated by intravenous fluids infused at another site in the extremity
- Specimen is hemolyzed
- Child or family develops mistrust of health care staff member performing the procedure

- Significant hematoma at puncture site
- Localized infection at puncture site
- Bacteremia
- Osteomyelitis

Monitoring and Care of the Child

Activities and Interventions	Rationale	Reportable Conditions
1. Assess puncture site for active bleeding.	Following puncture of the vein, bleeding may occur if inadequate pressure is applied, particularly in active children. Inadvertent arterial puncture may have occurred.	• Active bleeding that persists after 3 to 5 minutes
2. Assess perfusion distal to puncture site.	Inadvertent arterial puncture may have occurred, affecting perfusion to extremity distal to puncture site.	• Decreased or absent perfusion distal to puncture site

Documentation

- Gauge and type of needle used to perform venipuncture
- Number of attempts, location(s), name, and credentials of person performing any attempts
- Site of venipuncture
- Name and credentials of person performing procedure
- Child's tolerance of procedure
- Laboratory studies sent
- Unexpected outcomes and related treatment
- Child and family education

References

1. Eichhorn DJ, et al: Family presence during invasive procedures and resuscitation, *AJN* 101:5, 2001.
2. Smith-Temple J, Young-Johnson J: Venipuncture for blood specimen. In Smith-Temple J, Young-Johnson J: *Nurses' guide to clinical procedures,* Baltimore, 2002, Lippincott Williams & Wilkins.
3. O'Grady, NP, et al: Centers for Disease Control and Prevention: Guidelines for the prevention of intravascular catheter related infections, *MMWR Morbid Mortal Wkly Rep* 51(No.RR-10):1-29, 2002.
4. Duffy S, Steele D: Venipuncture. In Henretig FM, King C, editors: *Textbook of pediatric emergency procedures,* Baltimore, 1997, Williams & Wilkins.
5. Clinical and Laboratory Standards Institute: Procedure for the collection of diagnostic blood specimens by venipuncture; approved standard, ed 5, Wayne, PA, 2003, Clinical and Laboratory Standards Institute.

Additional Reading
Roberts J, Hedges JR: *Clinical procedures in emergency medicine,* ed 4, Philadelphia, 2003, Saunders.

AP
Arterial Catheter Insertion: Perform

P U R P O S E : An indwelling arterial catheter is inserted to allow continuous observation of systemic blood pressure and facilitate blood sampling for laboratory studies including arterial blood gases without pain or discomfort to the child[1]

Eileen Briening

PREREQUISITE KNOWLEDGE

- Anatomy of vascular system and appropriate sites for arterial catheter insertion
  - ❖ Radial artery is the preferred site; consider ulnar, femoral, dorsalis pedis, axillary, or posterior tibial artery.[2]
    - ○ Radial artery is easily accessible, collateral circulation is usually adequate, and risk of nerve injury is low. Ulnar artery is also easy to access.[2]
  - ❖ Avoid the brachial artery because the risk of thrombosis is high due to poor collateral circulation.[3]
  - ❖ Axillary artery is difficult to access but may be palpable when other pulses are difficult to palpate; risk of ischemia is low; increased risk of nerve injury and cerebral embolization.[4,5]
  - ❖ Femoral artery is easily accessible; easily palpable when other pulses are difficult to palpate; increased risk of arterial transection, bleeding, and nerve injury.[2]
  - ❖ Dorsalis pedis artery is easily accessible; collateral circulation is adequate, risk of nerve damage is low; anatomic position is variable and may be absent in up to 12% of population.[4]
- Principles of hemodynamic monitoring

- Indications for insertion of arterial catheter include:
  - ❖ Hypertension, hypotension, or labile blood pressure[2]
  - ❖ Use of vasoactive agents such as vasopressors, vasodilators, or cardioactive drugs[2]
  - ❖ Monitoring effect of transient or intermittent dysrhythmias on blood pressure[2]
  - ❖ Frequent sampling of arterial blood gases for oxygenation and ventilation management or other laboratory studies without pain or discomfort to child[2]
- Complications of invasive arterial monitoring
  - ❖ Local and systemic infection, pain and swelling, hematoma, pseudoaneurysm, thrombus formation, embolization, arteriovenous fistulas, limb ischemia, and accidental disconnection within the system with exsanguination[2,3]
  - ❖ Complications of radial artery cannulation: cerebral embolization, peripheral neuropathy
  - ❖ Complications of femoral artery cannulation: retroperitoneal hemorrhage, bowel perforation, arteriovenous fistula
  - ❖ Complications of axillary artery cannulation: cerebral embolization, injury to brachial plexus
  - ❖ Complications of brachial artery cannulation: median nerve injury and cerebral embolization[2]
- Assessment of collateral flow through the ulnar artery using the modified Allen test for radial artery cannulation[3,6] (Figures 151-1 to 151-3)
- Child development as it relates to clinical assessment and arterial catheter insertion
- Principles of aseptic technique

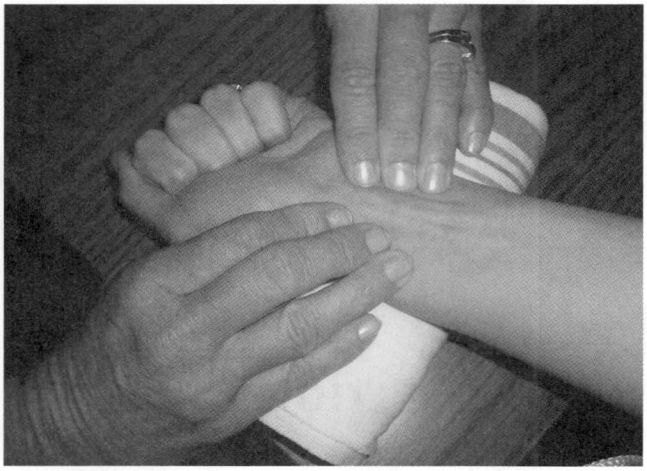

FIGURE 151-1 Performing the modified Allen test, step one: elevate the hand above the heart; compress the radial and ulnar arteries while passively opening and closing the hand.

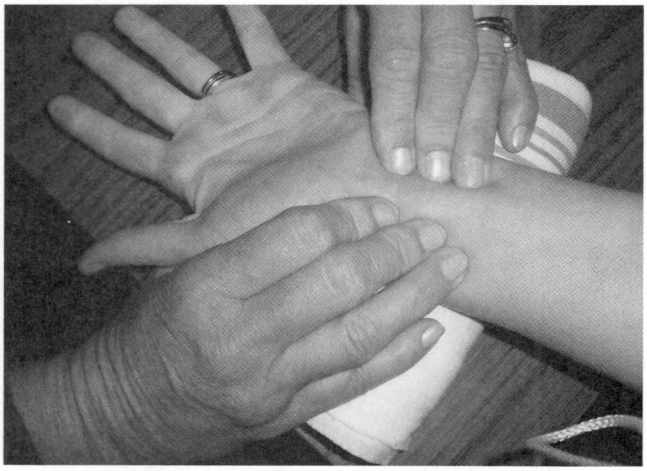

FIGURE 151-2 Performing the modified Allen test, step two: when the hand appears pale, release ulnar compression while continuing to compress the radial artery.

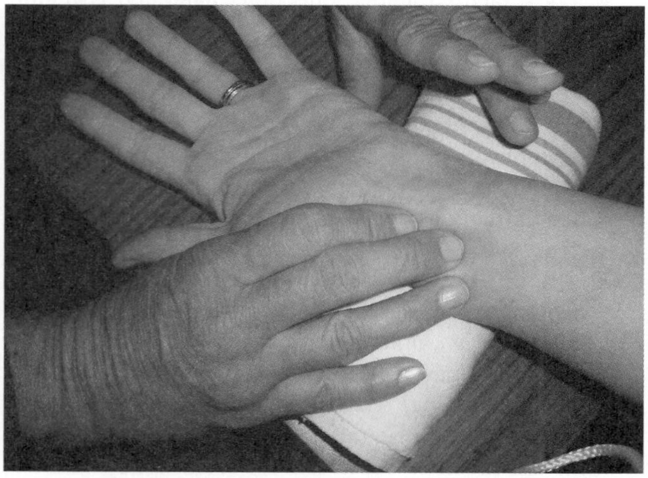

FIGURE 151-3 Performing the modified Allen test, step three: flushing of hand (return of color) indicates adequate collateral flow from ulnar artery.

- Appropriate pediatric dosing of analgesics and anxiolytics and competency in procedural sedation

CHILD AND FAMILY ASSESSMENT

- Family's or child's history of prolonged bleeding or abnormal bruising. Assess child for signs of oral, gastric, or rectal bleeding; hematomas; petechiae; or oozing of blood from puncture sites. Refer to recent coagulation studies and platelet count, if available **»Rationale:** Insertion of arterial line may be contraindicated in children with coagulopathy.[5] Blood product such as fresh frozen plasma, cryoprecipitate, or platelets may be indicated before insertion.
- Assess child for skin infection or skin breakdown at potential insertion site[7] **»Rationale:** Skin that is not intact increases risk of systemic infection.
- If radial or ulnar artery is used, perform the modified Allen test before catheter insertion **»Rationale:** Assesses for adequate collateral blood flow through ulnar artery.[3,6]
- Child's developmental level and ability to interact **»Rationale:** These factors influence preparation of the child and interaction.
- Child's and family's understanding of the reasons for and risks and benefits of procedure **»Rationale:** Evaluates child's and family's understanding of the procedure and provides a gauge for ongoing education.
- Family's desire to be present during the procedure **»Rationale:** Family may provide comfort and support to the child but should have the choice not to remain with the child.

CHILD AND FAMILY EDUCATION

Individualized, developmentally appropriate education is provided to the family and to the child based on desire for knowledge, readiness to learn, and overall neurologic and psychosocial state.

- Educate family and child as appropriate on procedure and possible complications as well as actions taken to prevent complications **»Rationale:** Family is entitled to information, indications, and rationale of procedures performed on their child; providing information allows informed participation in the decision-making process.
- Explain arterial line monitor device **»Rationale:** Providing information about monitor and alarms reduces anxiety and fear.
- Explain to the family and child as appropriate that medications will be used to keep the child comfortable, which include local anesthetic agents, anxiolytics, and/or systemic analgesics **»Rationale:** Decreases family's and child's anxiety and fear related to unmanaged pain.
- Encourage questions and answer questions as they arise **»Rationale:** Reinforcement of information is needed during periods of stress.

EQUIPMENT

- If radial artery is used, appropriate-sized armboard, tape, and small roll to use under the wrist
- If femoral artery is used, towel or blanket to place under hips
- 2% chlorhexidine, 10% povidone-iodine, or 70% alcohol[3]
- Sterile towels, gloves, and gown
- Mask
- Protective eyewear
- Surgical cap
- 1% lidocaine without epinephrine
- T-connector primed with 0.9% saline solution[1]
- Appropriate-sized safety cannula over needle or procedure tray with catheter over guidewire, sterile gauze sponges, and syringes
- 3.0 or 4.0 silk suture and needle driver or other securement device such as StatLock
- Scalpel handle and scalpel blade
- Transparent or semipermeable dressing
- Monitoring setup, including pressure transducer, transducer cable, monitor with pressure module, appropriate fluid for infusion; refer to Procedure 137.

Procedure for Arterial Catheter Insertion: Perform

Steps	Rationale	Considerations
1. Ensure child and family understand procedure and questions are answered.	Evaluates and reinforces understanding of previously taught information.	Developmental level, cognitive ability, and anxiety level will determine approach to and effectiveness of teaching.
2. Gather needed equipment and supplies.	Facilitates completion of task in a timely manner.	
3. Wash hands.	Standard precautions; reduces transmission of microorganisms.	
4. Conduct final patient verification process (e.g., "Time out") per institution-specific protocol.	Confirms correct patient, procedure and site; prevents unnecessary medical procedures.	Use active communication techniques.
5. Ensure appropriate cardio-respiratory monitoring.	Medication for pain, sedation or anxiolytic medication may be needed to facilitate successful completion of procedure.	Ensure that the alarms are activated with appropriate settings and are sufficiently audible.
6. Perform modified Allen test if radial artery or ulnar artery will be used. *(Level II*)* If dorsalis pedis artery is used, check the sufficiency of collateral circulation by compressing the dorsalis pedis and posterior tibial arteries until the great toe blanches; release posterior tibial artery and observe time of color return to the great toe. The time should be less than 10 seconds.	Assesses collateral circulation to hand or foot, ensuring placement of catheter will not compromise perfusion to extremity.[4,7]	
7. Ensure sedation, anxiolytics, or pain medication has been administered as appropriate.	Promotes comfort and safety of child during procedure; facilitates successful completion of procedure.	If procedural sedation is used, sedation should be administered by someone other than the practitioner placing the arterial catheter.

Procedure continues on following page

* Level II: Theory-based, no research data to support recommendations: recommendations from expert consensus group may exist

Procedure | for Arterial Catheter Insertion: Perform—*Continued*

Steps	Rationale	Considerations
8. If radial artery site is selected, use an armboard to immobilize forearm, wrist, and hand. Dorsiflex hand at wrist 45 to 60 degrees using a small roll under the wrist. Using tape, moderately abduct the thumb.[3]	Brings the radial artery to the skin surface and keeps the artery parallel to the long surface of the forearm, facilitating insertion.[3]	The piece of tape abducting the thumb may be removed after the catheter is inserted.
If femoral artery site is selected, form 90-degree angle between the lower extremities by placing them in a frog-leg position[3]; place a towel or blanket under the hips.	Allows the femoral vessels to align along a line from the umbilicus to the knee, facilitating insertion.[3]	
If axillary artery site is selected, abduct the upper arm between 90 and 135 degrees from the body and rotate arm palm up and place under child's head.[2,3]	Exposes the axillary artery.[2]	
9. Put on eyewear, cap, mask, sterile gown, and sterile gloves.	Provides maximal barrier to microorganisms.[5]	
10. Prepare site using 2% chlorhexidine, 10% povidone-iodine, or 70% alcohol. Using friction, scrub site back and forth; allow solution to air-dry.[8] *(Level VI*)*	Reduces cutaneous colonization of microorganisms at the insertion site.[4,5]	Do not remove chlorhexidine or povidone-iodine solution from skin.[4,8] 2% chlorhexidine is not currently recommended for children less than 2 months of age.[4]
11. Using a 25-gauge needle, infiltrate 0.5 mL of lidocaine into each side of artery.[2]	Minimizes discomfort; may reduce vasospasm.[2] *(Level II*)*	
12. Radial artery • Palpate pulse; puncture the skin at about a 30-degree angle, directing the safety catheter or needle toward the underlying artery.	If less acute angle is used, needle may lie on top of artery. If more acute angle is used, needle may pass through artery.	
• Advance the catheter (needle) slowly, watching for flashback. When blood return is noted, advance the catheter (needle) about 1 to 2 cm into the lumen of the artery.	Slowly advancing catheter allows adequate time to observe flashback.	
• At this point, lower the catheter (needle) so that it is in line with the vessel and flat to the skin. If a catheter is used, advance slowly to the hub.	Facilitates threading catheter into artery.	
• Activate safety feature to remove inner stylet. The presence of pulsatile blood confirms placement.	Prevents needlestick injury. If vein has been cannulated, blood flow will not be pulsatile.	Guidewire should pass through lumen of needle with ease. If resistance if met, withdraw guidewire and verify there is pulsatile blood flow. Needle may need to be repositioned or reinserted.[2]

* Level II: Theory-based, no research data to support recommendations: recommendations from expert consensus group may exist
  Level VI: Clinical studies in a variety of patient populations and situations to support recommendations

Procedure for Arterial Catheter Insertion: Perform—*Continued*

Steps	Rationale	Considerations
• If catheter over guidewire is used, pulsatile blood flow should be seen from hub of needle. The guidewire is inserted into lumen of needle.	Guidewire is placed into artery to maintain placement and allow catheter to be threaded over guidewire into artery.	
• Remove needle while holding guidewire in place; advance catheter over the guidewire. Insert catheter to hub and remove guidewire.[2,3]	Guidewire facilitates placement of catheter into artery.	
13. Femoral artery		
• Palpate pulse. Hold needle with syringe attached at a 45-degree angle, bevel up, below inguinal crease and just a few centimeters distal from inguinal ligament.	Landmarks facilitate locating femoral artery.	Seldinger technique.[2]
• Enter through skin, then advance needle into femoral artery. When blood is obtained, remove syringe and bring needle down against skin.	Flattening needle facilitates threading guidewire.	
• Pass guidewire through lumen of needle and advance into artery; withdraw needle while holding guidewire in place.	Guidewire is placed into artery to maintain placement and allow catheter to be threaded over guidewire into artery.	When passing dilator or catheter over guidewire, use free hand to pull skin taut below insertion site to aid passage.
• Using a scalpel, make a small incision at the insertion site.	Incision opens skin to allow dilator and catheter to be threaded into artery	
• Pass dilator over the guidewire into the artery; guidewire remains in place.	Dilates vessel, facilitates insertion of catheter into the artery.	
• Remove dilator, stabilizing guidewire.	Removes dilator to allow passage of catheter.	
• Thread catheter over guidewire and advance into artery.	Use of guidewire facilitates passage of catheter into artery.	
• Remove guidewire.	Guidewire is no longer needed once catheter is advanced into artery.	
14. Axillary artery		
• Palpate the axillary artery at the lower border of the pectoralis major muscle.		
• Fix the artery against the shaft of humerus.	Stabilizes artery, facilitates insertion of needle into artery.	
• Use the Seldinger technique as outlined in femoral artery insertion.[2]		
15. Dorsalis pedis		
• Position the foot in plantar flexion.	Positioning facilitates access to artery.	Dorsalis pedis has systolic blood pressures 5 to 20 mm Hg greater than radial artery. Mean artery pressures are about the same.[2]
• Follow technique outlined for radial artery insertion. Puncture skin where the artery is best palpated.[2]		

Procedure continues on following page

Procedure | for Arterial Catheter Insertion: Perform—*Continued*

Steps	Rationale	Considerations
16. Attach catheter to transducer/flush system; observe for presence of arterial waveform, ease of aspiration, and flushing of catheter.	Arterial waveform, brisk blood return, and ability to flush catheter easily confirm appropriate arterial cannulation.	Waveform indicating venous cannulation requires replacement of catheter.
17. Secure with suture, StatLock, and/or transparent or semipermeable dressing.	Suture or other securement device (i.e., StatLock) reduces risk of accidental dislodgment. Sterile dressing decreases risk of contamination of insertion site and assists with security of catheter.	Sutureless securement devices may be advantageous over suture in preventing catheter related bloodstream infections.[8] *(Level IV*)*
18. Dress site using gauze or transparent dressing per institution-specific protocol. *(Level IV*)*	Provides sterile environment; reduces infection.	
19. Dispose of used supplies and equipment in appropriate receptacle; ensure sharps are disposed of appropriately.	Standard precautions; reduces transmission of microorganisms; prevents needlestick injury.	
20. Remove personal protective equipment; wash hands.	Standard precautions.	

* Level IV: Limited clinical studies to support recommendations

Expected Outcomes	Unexpected Outcomes
• Arterial waveform observed on monitor with good dynamics and appropriate blood pressure readings • Blood is aspirated from catheter easily	• Damped waveform • Vasospasm of artery • No blood return from catheter • Formation of thrombi
• Child remains free from intravascular catheter–related infection • Child remains free from complications of arterial catheter insertion	• Local infection at insertion site • Systemic infection related to arterial line • Bleeding from insertion site • Hematoma at insertion site • Limb ischemia • Nerve injury • Injury to artery
• Catheter provides information allowing identification of alterations in hemodynamic stability and facilitates treatment	• Inaccurate pressure measurements or poor waveform
• Child demonstrates acceptable level of comfort throughout procedure	• Unmanaged pain or anxiety during procedure

Monitoring and Care of the Child

Activities and Interventions	Rationale	Reportable Conditions
1. Observe site for signs of bleeding.[1]	Bleeding may occur due to coagulopathy.	• Excessive bleeding or hematoma
2. Observe site and area distal to site for signs of compromised circulation.[1]	Circulation distal to insertion site may be compromised by catheter.	• Changes in perfusion, blanching, decreased capillary refill, or swelling of extremity distal to catheter insertion site
3. Observe insertion site for signs of local infection.[1]	Poor aseptic technique at time of insertion or during dressing changes increases risk of infection.[2]	• Inflammation or purulent discharge at site
4. Assess effectiveness of pain and anxiety management strategy; provide appropriate interventions.	Early identification of pain or anxiety issues allows prompt treatment and facilitates completion of procedure.	• Increased pain or agitation impeding completion of procedure

Documentation

- Procedure, risks/benefits, and indications explained to family and child (as appropriate)
- Date and time of procedure, and individual performing procedure
- Skin preparation, insertion site, and use of local anesthesia
- Size and type of catheter and technique used
- Local anesthetic agent, sedation, and/or pain medication used
- Condition of child at completion of procedure
- Unexpected outcomes and related treatment

References

1. Becker DE: Arterial catheter insertion (perform). In Lynn-McHale DJ, Carlson KK, editors: *AACN procedure manual for critical care,* ed 4, Philadelphia, 2001, Saunders, pp. 361-365.
2. Bowdle TA: Complications of invasive monitoring, *Anesthesiol Clin North America,* 20(3): 571-588, 2002.
3. Garland JS, et al: The 2002 hospital infection control practices advisory committee centers for disease control and prevention guideline for prevention of intravascular device-related infection, *Pediatrics* 10(5):1009-1013, 2002.
4. Lodato RF: Arterial pressure monitoring. In Tobin MJ, editor: *Principles and practice of intensive care monitoring,* New York, 1998, McGraw-Hill, pp. 733-756.
5. Pinsky MR: Hemodynamic monitoring in the intensive care unit, *Clin Chest Med* 24(4):549-560, 2003.
6. Kahler AC, Mirza F: Alternative arterial catheterization site using the ulnar artery in critically ill pediatric patients, *Pediatr Crit Care Med* 3(4):370-374, 2002.
7. Steinhart CM: Arterial catheterization. In Dieckmann RA, et al, editors: *Pediatric emergency and critical care procedures,* St. Louis, 1997, Mosby, pp. 213-219.
8. O'Grady NP, et al: Guidelines for the prevention of intravascular catheter related infections, *MMWR Morbid Mortal Wkly Rep* 51(No.RR-10):1-29, 2002.

Additional Readings

Levin PD, et al: Use of ultrasound guidance in the insertion of radial artery catheters, *Crit Care Med* 31(2):481-484, 2003.
McGee B, Bridges ME: Monitoring arterial blood pressure: what you may not know, *Crit Care Nurse* 22(2):60-78, 2002.
Rhee KH, Berg RA: Antegrade cannulation of radial artery in infants and children, *Chest* 107(1):182-184, 1995.

AP
Arterial Puncture: Perform

P U R P O S E : To obtain a blood sample for arterial blood gas analysis or to obtain a blood sample for laboratory analysis in a child with poor vascular access

Andrea M. Kline

PREREQUISITE KNOWLEDGE

- Anatomy of vascular system and appropriate sites for arterial puncture in the child (Figure 152-1)
  - ❖ **Radial artery** is the preferred site in the child; consider ulnar, femoral, dorsalis pedis, axillary, or posterior tibial arteries.[1,2]
    - ○ Radial artery is easily accessible, superficial; collateral circulation is usually adequate and risk of nerve injury is low.[1,2,3]
    - ○ Ulnar artery is easily accessed, but there is a risk of ischemia if ulnar collateral circulation is insufficient.
  - ❖ Avoid the **brachial artery** because the risk of thrombosis is high due to poor collateral circulation.[4]
  - ❖ **Ulnar artery,** the larger terminal branch artery of the brachial artery commences in the midline of the forearm opposite the neck of the radius. It continues on the medial side of the forearm, lying on the radial side of the ulnar nerve to continue across the palm as a superficial palmar arterial arch. The ulnar nerve provides blood supply to the medial muscles in the forearm and hand and to the ulnar nerve and is easily accessible.[3]
  - ❖ **Axillary artery** is difficult to access but may be palpable when other pulses are difficult to palpate; risk of

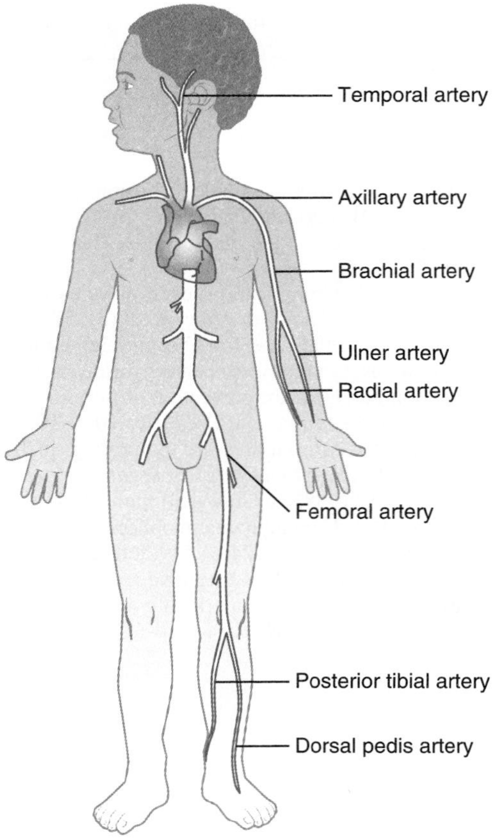

FIGURE 152-1   Arterial Sites. *From Levin DL, Morriss FC, editors:* Essentials of pediatric intensive care, *ed 2, New York, 1997, Churchill Livingstone, p. 1218.*

AP   This procedure should be performed only by physicians, advanced-practice nurses, and other health care professionals (including critical care nurses) with additional knowledge, skills, and demonstrated competence per professional licensure or institutional standard.

ischemia is low; increased risk of nerve injury and cerebral embolization.[5,6]

* **Femoral artery** is easily accessible and easily palpable when other pulses are difficult to palpate and may be more easily accessible during active cardiac arrest; increased risk of arterial transection, bleeding and nerve injury.[1]
* **Dorsalis pedis artery** is easily accessible; collateral circulation is adequate, risk of nerve damage is low; anatomic position is variable and may be absent in up to 12% of population.[5]

- Indications for arterial puncture include assessing respiratory function, obtaining laboratory samples.
- Complications of arterial puncture can include pain, swelling, hematoma, thrombus formation, thrombophlebitis, local or systemic infection, or ischemia if collateral circulation is insufficient.[1,3,4]
  * Bleeding complications may occur if child is coagulopathic or on anticoagulation therapy.[2]
- Relative complications to arterial puncture include:
  * Unpalpable artery
  * Known or suspected arterial disease at the site/distal to the site, such as aneurysm, infection, inflammation, or hematoma.
  * Previous vascular surgery involving the vessel
- Assessment of collateral flow through the ulnar artery using the modified Allen test for radial artery cannulation[1,3] (Refer to Procedure 151 for a description of the modified Allen test)
- Order of draw, if several specimens of various types are being obtained (e.g., chemistry, hematology and coagulation studies)
- Appropriate containers for specimens to be collected and minimum required blood volumes for those specimens
- Specimen labeling requirements
- Specimen handling requirements
- Principles of aseptic technique

CHILD AND FAMILY ASSESSMENT

- Family history or patient history of prolonged bleeding or abnormal bruising. Assess child for signs of oral, gastric or rectal bleeding, hematomas, petechiae, or oozing of blood from puncture sites. Refer to recent coagulation studies and platelet count, if available ➡*Rationale:* Arterial puncture may be contraindicated in children with coagulopathy.[6]
- Presence of skin infection or skin breakdown at potential site[7] ➡*Rationale:* Skin that is not intact increases risk of systemic infection.
- If radial or ulnar artery is used, perform the modified Allen test ➡*Rationale:* Assesses for adequate collateral blood flow through ulnar artery.[3,4]

- Child's developmental level and ability to interact ➡*Rationale:* These factors influence preparation of the child and interaction.
- Child's and family's understanding of the reasons for and risks and benefits of the procedure ➡*Rationale:* Evaluates child's and family's understanding of the procedure and provides a gauge for ongoing education.
- Family's desire to be present during the procedure ➡*Rationale:* Family may provide comfort and support to the child but should have the choice not to remain with the child.

CHILD AND FAMILY EDUCATION

Individualized, developmentally appropriate education is provided to the family and to the child based on desire for knowledge, readiness to learn, and overall neurologic and psychosocial state.

- Provide information about arterial puncture, including potential complications and an explanation of steps involved in obtaining blood sample ➡*Rationale:* Providing information decreases anxiety and fear.
- If developmentally appropriate, explain how child can facilitate arterial puncture (i.e. holding extremity still) ➡*Rationale:* Puncture is more easily accomplished with child's cooperation.
- Explain that the puncture may be uncomfortable; consider local or systemic pain relief ➡*Rationale:* Providing information and addressing pain management decreases anxiety and fear.
- Encourage questions and answer questions as they arise ➡*Rationale:* Reinforcement of information is needed during periods of stress.

EQUIPMENT

- Syringe(s) for collecting sample; syringe size and type will vary based on type of specimen(s) required and minimum blood volume required for the specimen
- Appropriate-sized needle or butterfly needle for child's size: suggested sizes are 25 gauge for infant, 23 gauge for toddler/school-aged child, 22 gauge for older child
- Gauze pads
- 2% chlorhexidine, 10% povidone-iodine, or 70% alcohol[4]
- Sterile gloves
- Protective eyewear (optional)
- Adhesive bandage
- Appropriate specimen tubes
- Appropriate laboratory requisitions
- Specimen labels containing two patient identifiers
- Container with ice, if required for handling of specimen

Procedure for Arterial Puncture

Steps	Rationale	Considerations
1. Ensure child and family understand procedure and questions are answered.	Evaluates and reinforces understanding of previously taught information.	Developmental level, cognitive ability, and anxiety level will determine approach to and effectiveness of teaching.
2. Gather needed equipment and supplies.	Facilitates efficient completion of procedure.	Needle size is dependent on child's size; blood specimen tubes needed are dependent on specimens ordered.
3. Wash hands. *(Level VI*)*	Standard precautions; reduces transmission of microorganisms.	
4. Identify child using two patient identifiers.	Ensures correct patient and procedure; prevents unnecessary medical procedures.	
5. Ensure appropriate cardiopulmonary monitoring.	Critically ill children may decompensate during the procedure.	Consider the child's status when selecting appropriate monitoring. Ensure that alarms are activated with appropriate settings and are sufficiently audible.
6. Perform modified Allen test if radial artery or ulnar artery will be used. *(Level II*)*	Assesses collateral circulation to hand.[2,5,8]	Select an alternate arterial site if Allen test is negative (circulation does not return after ulnar release).
7. Prepare site using 2% chlorhexidine, 10% povidone-iodine, or 70% alcohol. Using friction, scrub site using a back and forth motion.[9] *(Level V*)*	Reduces cutaneous colonization of microorganisms at the insertion site.[5,6]	Do not remove chlorhexidine or povidone-iodine solution from skin.[5,9] 2% chlorhexidine is not recommended for use in children less than 2 months of age.[5]
8. Consider use of local anesthetic agent.	Decreases discomfort associated with the procedure.	Assess allergies if anesthetic agent is to be used.
9. Put on sterile gloves.	Provides maximal barrier to microorganisms.[6]	
10. If **radial artery** is used, dorsiflex hand at wrist 45 to 60 degrees (Figure 152-2).	Brings the radial artery to the skin surface and keeps the artery parallel to the long surface of the forearm.[4]	

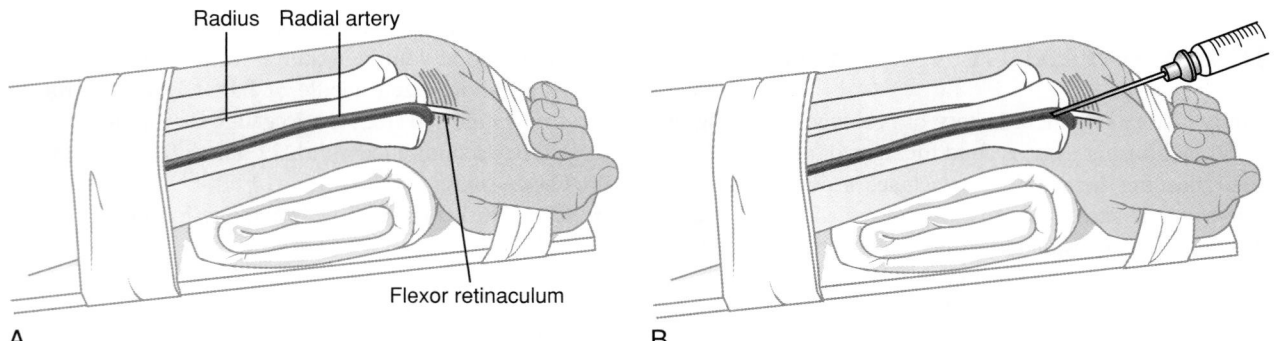

Radius   Radial artery

Flexor retinaculum

A

B

FIGURE 152-2   Radial Artery. **A,** Anatomy and **B,** cannulation. *Reproduced with permission, Pediatric Advanced Life Support, Copyright © 1997, American Heart Association, Dallas, TX. pp. 5-14*

* Level II: Theory-based, no research data to support recommendations; recommendations from expert consensus group may exist
Level V: Clinical studies in more than one or two patient populations and situations to support recommendations
Level VI: Clinical studies in a variety of patient populations and situations to support recommendations

Procedure for Arterial Puncture—*Continued*

Steps	Rationale	Considerations
If **ulnar artery** is used, palpate at wrist and identify point of maximal pulsation. Percutaneously puncture vessel at angle of 30 to 45 degrees to the horizontal.[4]		
If **femoral artery** is used, form 90-degree angle between the lower extremities by placing them in a frog-leg position[4]; place a towel or blanket under the hips.	This position allows the femoral vessels to align along a line from the umbilicus to the knee.[4]	
If **axillary artery** is used, abduct the upper arm between 90 and 135 degrees from the body and rotate arm palm up and place under the child's head.[2,4] *(Level II*)*	Exposes the axillary artery.[2]	
11. Palpate and immobilize the artery with two or three fingers of the nondominant hand while holding the needle/syringe or butterfly needle over the insertion site with the other hand. *(Level II*)*	Decreases the chance of vessel rolling; increases accuracy of puncture.	
12. Puncture the skin and arterial wall in one slow gradual motion, following the path of the artery.	A slow, gradual thrust will promote arterial entry without passing directly through the posterior wall of the vessel.	
13. Watch for backflow of blood in the syringe/tubing.	Pulsation of blood into the syringe verifies arterial puncture.	
14. Obtain blood volume required for specimen(s).	Collects sample for analysis.	If possible, avoid aspirating the blood, because this can cause hemolysis of the specimen.
15. If blood is not obtained on first attempt, withdraw the needle to just below the skin surface and advance needle at same angle but at 1 mm to either side of previous attempt.	Prevents necessity of another puncture while changing the angle to better locate the vessel.	
16. After collecting blood sample, withdraw needle; hold firm pressure with gauze over site for at least 5 minutes.	Helps achieve hemostasis, minimizes blood loss. If child is receiving an anticoagulant, hold pressure for 10 to 15 minutes.	Lack of pressure over site can lead to hematoma or unnecessary bleeding; hematomas can cause circulatory impairment and discomfort and predispose child to infection.
17. When hemostasis has been achieved, place adhesive bandage over site.	Facilitates wound healing.	

Procedure continues on following page

* Level II: Theory-based, no research data to support recommendations; recommendations from expert consensus group may exist

Procedure | for Arterial Puncture—*Continued*

Steps	Rationale	Considerations
18. Label specimens at the bedside and complete laboratory paperwork per institution-specific protocol.	Promotes patient safety; ensures accurate and efficient processing of specimen.	Expel any air bubbles from the arterial blood gas (ABG) syringe; place ABG syringe on ice if required by institution-specific protocol. Follow institution-specific protocol for handling and labeling lab specimens.
19. Dispose of used supplies and equipment in appropriate receptacle; ensure sharps are disposed of correctly.	Standard precautions; prevents transmission of microorganisms and protects personnel health.	
20. Remove protective equipment and wash hands. *(Level VI**)*	Standard precautions; reduces transmission of microorganisms.	

* Level VI: Clinical studies in a variety of patient populations and situations to support recommendations

Expected Outcomes

- Adequate volume of free-flowing blood obtained for analysis

- Viable specimens appropriate for analysis are obtained

- Specimens are placed in correct sample tubes, labeled appropriately and sent to the lab in the appropriate time frame
- Child remains free from complications of arterial puncture

Unexpected Outcomes

- Inadequate blood volume obtained or unable to obtain blood for analysis
- Bleeding from site, hematoma
- Specimens are clotted, hemolyzed, or otherwise not viable for analysis
- Specimens are mislabeled, placed in incorrect sample tubes, or not sent to lab in a timely fashion

- Bleeding from site
- Hematoma formation
- Local or systemic infection
- Circulatory impairment of the extremity distal to puncture site

Monitoring and Care of the Child

Activities and Interventions	Rationale	Reportable Conditions
1. Assess extremity distal to puncture 15 minutes after puncture performed.	Monitors for complications of arterial puncture; early identification of complications facilitates prompt treatment.	• Large hematoma • Decreased perfusion distal to puncture site • Swelling, discoloration, pain, numbness, or tingling in affected extremity
2. Monitor for bleeding at puncture site; recheck site 15 minutes after puncture performed.	Assesses for ongoing bleeding, need for additional pressure at site.	• Inability to achieve hemostasis
3. Review results of specimens obtained.	Monitors child's status; facilitates identification of possible errors in obtaining specimens.	• Abnormal lab values

Documentation

- Child's tolerance of procedure
- Child and family education
- Location of site of arterial puncture
- Date and time of puncture and specimens obtained
- Color, temperature, and capillary refill of extremity after specimens obtained
- Results of laboratory studies obtained
- Amount of blood withdrawn, along with running total for hospitalization
- Unexpected outcomes and related treatment

References

1. Bowdle TA: Complications of invasive monitoring, *Anesthesiol Clin North America* (3):571-588, 2002.
2. Springhouse Publishing Corporation. *Procedures for nurse practitioners,* Springhouse, PA, 2001, Springhouse Corporation, pp. 6-10.
3. Kahler AC, Mirza F: Alternative arterial catheterization site using the ulnar artery in critically ill pediatric patients, *Pediatr Crit Care Med* 3(4):370-374, 2002.
4. Garland JS, et al: The 2002 hospital infection control practices advisory committee centers for disease control and prevention guideline for prevention of intravascular device-related infection, *Pediatrics* 10(5):1009-1013, 2002.
5. Lodato RF: Arterial pressure monitoring. In Tobin MJ, editor: *Principles and practice of intensive care monitoring,* New York, 1998, McGraw-Hill.
6. Pinsky MR: Hemodynamic monitoring in the intensive care unit, *Clin Chest Med* 24(4):549-560, 2003.
7. Steinhart CM: Arterial catheterization. In Dieckmann RA, et al, editors: *Pediatric emergency and critical care procedures,* St. Louis, 1997, Mosby.
8. Ruengsakulrach P, et al: Preoperative assessment of hand circulation by means of Doppler ultrasonography and the modified Allen test, *J Thorac Cardiovasc Surg* 121(3):526-531, 2001.
9. O'Grady, et al: Centers for Disease Control and Prevention. Guidelines for the prevention of intravascular catheter related infections, *MMWR Morbid Mortal Wkly Rep* 51(No.RR-10):1-29, 2002.

Additional Readings

Franklin CM: The technique of dorsalis pedis cannulation: an overlooked option when the radial artery cannot be used, *J Crit Illn* 10(7):493-498, 1995.

Ino T, et al: Secondary arteriovenous fistula after a single arterial puncture, *Pediatr Int* 43(2):179-180, 2001.

Tran NQ, et al: A randomized controlled trial of the effectiveness of topical amethocaine in reducing pain during arterial puncture, *Chest* 122(4):1357-1360, 2002.

AP
Central Venous Non-tunneled Catheter Insertion: Perform

PURPOSE: Non-tunneled central venous catheters are placed for hemodynamic monitoring and to administer total parenteral nutrition, intravenous fluids, vasoactive medications and other drugs, blood, and blood products

Marcella L. Donkin

PREREQUISITE KNOWLEDGE

- Anatomy and physiology of the cardiovascular system with particular emphasis on the internal jugular vein, subclavian vein, femoral vein, and adjacent structures
- Indications for non-tunneled central venous access[1-5]
  - ❖ Central venous pressure measurement
  - ❖ Delivery of drugs to the central circulation, including chemotherapy
  - ❖ Rapid infusion of large volumes of fluids, blood, or blood products
  - ❖ Administration of high-concentration parenteral alimentation
  - ❖ Administration of medications that cannot infuse peripherally
  - ❖ Dialysis procedures (plasmapheresis, hemofiltration, hemodialysis)
  - ❖ Exchange transfusions
  - ❖ Provide access in children lacking peripheral sites who require intravenous therapies
- Factors that may increase the risk of complications related to non-tunneled central venous catheter (CVC) placement: thrombocytopenia, abnormal vascular anatomy, inexperience with non-tunneled CVC insertion, high-pressure mechanical ventilation, presence of shock, obesity, sepsis[3-5]
- Contraindications for non-tunneled CVC placement[2]
  - ❖ Congenital or acquired vascular abnormality
  - ❖ Femoral vein: vascular disease in the involved extremity, abdominal trauma
  - ❖ Relative contraindications: injury or infection of the skin over the puncture site, hypercoagulable state
- Complications of CVC placement: arterial puncture; hematoma; pneumothorax; thrombosis; infection; hemothorax; catheter embolism; vessel laceration; air embolism; dysrhythmia; pericardial effusion; cardiac tamponade; extravasation injury[3-5]
- Non-tunneled CVCs account for the majority of intravascular catheter–related bloodstream infections (CRBSI).[6]
- Principles of aseptic technique
- Appropriate pediatric dosing of analgesics and competency in procedural sedation
- Mastery of pediatric advanced life support competencies
- Child development as it relates to clinical assessment and non-tunneled CVC placement
- Except in an emergent situation, informed consent is required before placement of a central venous non-tunneled catheter.

CHILD AND FAMILY ASSESSMENT

- Child's developmental level ➠*Rationale:* Developmental level will determine ability of child to cooperate if

---

AP This procedure should be performed only by physicians, advanced practice nurses, and other health care professionals (including critical care nurses) with additional knowledge, skills, and demonstrated competence per professional licensure or institutional standard.

conscious during procedure and ability to comprehend the explanation regarding the procedure.

- Child's level of consciousness ➤➤*Rationale:* Sedation may be required in the alert or agitated child in order to place the catheter safely.
- History of central venous catheterization; difficulties or complications with catheter placement ➤➤*Rationale:* These factors may increase the difficulty of catheter insertion and may influence site selection.[3,4]
- Family's and child's (as appropriate) understanding of the reasons for and risks and benefits of procedure ➤➤*Rationale:* Evaluates child's and family's understanding of the procedure and ability to provide informed consent; provides a gauge for ongoing education.
- Family's desire to be present during the procedure ➤➤*Rationale:* Families may provide comfort and support, but should have the choice not to remain with the child. In some situations, if family presence will not be permitted, allows explanation of reasons for this and promotes cooperation.

CHILD AND FAMILY EDUCATION

Individualized, developmentally appropriate education is provided to the family and to the child based on desire for knowledge, readiness to learn, and overall neurologic and psychosocial state.

- Provide information on the child's medical condition, purpose, and rationale for CVC placement ➤➤*Rationale:* Providing information helps decrease the child's and family's anxiety levels and offers reassurance during an extremely stressful period.

- Provide the family and child with information about decrease the procedure, including analgesia and sedation that will be given, steps taken to prevent infection ➤➤*Rationale:* Providing information decreases fear and anxiety.
- If the family is asked to leave the room during the procedure, reassure the child and family that the bedside nurse will be present to comfort the child and that the family will be notified as soon as they are able to return to the bedside ➤➤*Rationale:* Helps decrease family's anxiety.
- Educate the family and/or child about medications that will be administered for the procedure, including local anesthetics ➤➤*Rationale:* Knowing that anticipated pain and/or anxiety/agitation will be preemptively treated will decrease fear and anxiety of the child and family.
- Encourage questions and answer questions as they arise ➤➤*Rationale:* Reinforcement of information is needed during periods of stress. This is especially important if the procedure must be performed emergently.

EQUIPMENT

- Sterile gloves
- Sterile gown
- Sterile towels
- Large sterile drape
- Mask
- Hat
- Central venous catheter kit with appropriate size and type of catheter
- Needle and suture or securement device (i.e., StatLock)
- Sterile dressing
- Heparinized saline flush

Procedure	for Central Venous Non-tunneled Catheter Insertion: Perform	
Steps	**Rationale**	**Considerations**
1. Ensure child and family understand procedure and questions are answered; obtain informed consent.	Evaluates and reinforces understanding of previously taught information; ensures medicolegal compliance as suggested by the Joint Commission on Accreditation of Healthcare Organizations (JCAHO).	Developmental level, cognitive ability, and anxiety level will determine approach to and effectiveness of teaching. In emergency situations, follow institution-specific protocol for assumption of consent.
2. Measure child for catheter placement; choose catheter size, type, and site.	Appropriate-sized catheter will facilitate correct placement. *Internal jugular:* the right side of the neck is preferred because the dome of the right lung and pleura is lower than the left, thus reducing the risk of pneumothorax.[1,2] *Subclavian:* catheter does not limit	Choose multilumen catheter if multiple infusions are part of treatment plan or anticipated to be required; choose single-lumen catheter if minimal number of infusions or compatible infusions ordered. Fewer lumens equals less infection risk.[6] *(Level IV*)*

Procedure continues on following page

* Level IV: Limited clinical studies to support recommendations

Procedure for Central Venous Non-tunneled Catheter Insertion: Perform—*Continued*

Steps	Rationale	Considerations
	child's movement. With the exception of tracheal secretions, this site is away from body fluids that could increase risk of infection.[2,5] *Femoral:* Cardiopulmonary resuscitation (CPR) not interrupted for line placement, easier to obtain hemostasis if artery is punctured, no risk of pneumothorax or hemothorax, easily identifiable landmarks.[2,5]	
3. Gather needed equipment and supplies.	Eliminates need for stepping away from sterile field and decreases time to complete procedure.	Catheter size and length must be appropriate for child's size and cannulation site selected.
4. Ensure appropriate cardio-pulmonary monitoring.	Allows continuous monitoring of cardiopulmonary status, alerting practitioner to changes in status during procedure.	Ensure that the alarms are activated with appropriate settings and are sufficiently audible.
5. Identify child using appropriate patient/procedure verification process (e.g., "Time out").	Confirms correct patient, procedure, and site as recommended by JCAHO; prevents unnecessary medical procedures.	Verification process and documentation are institution specific; use active communication techniques.
6. Ensure analgesics and sedation are administered as indicated and per prescribing practitioner's order.	Decreases anxiety, discomfort, and movement during catheter placement.	History of child's sedation experience and method used is helpful; consider cardiac depressant effects of some sedatives when selecting agents. Individual performing the procedure should not be responsible for monitoring child's cardiopulmonary status during sedation administration.
7. Put on mask and hat. *(Level IV*)*	Use of maximal sterile barrier precautions decreases CRBSI.	
8. Wash hands. *(Level VI*)*	Standard precautions; reduces transmission of microorganisms.	
9. Position child appropriately based on catheter insertion site selected. *Internal jugular:* Place child in Trendelenburg position. Lower child's head and turn to side opposite insertion site. Extend the neck and head by placing a towel under the shoulder on the side of the insertion site if no cervical spine injury is present.	Appropriate positioning increases ability to identify landmarks and likelihood of cannulation of correct vessel.	Some children may not tolerate certain positions due to compromised cardiopulmonary function.
Subclavian: Place shoulder roll under shoulder and parallel to spine and hyperextend neck if no cervical spine injury is present. Turn head in opposite direction of cannulation site. Place child in Trendelenburg position.	Catheter insertion site should be positioned below heart to avoid air embolism during insertion.	

* Level IV: Limited clinical studies to support recommendations
  Level VI: Clinical studies in a variety of patient populations and situations to support recommendations

Procedure for Central Venous Non-tunneled Catheter Insertion: Perform—*Continued*		
Steps	**Rationale**	**Considerations**
Femoral: Place roll under groin site to be cannulated; externally rotate hip. *(Level II*)*		
10. Wash hands. *(Level VI*)*	Reduces transmission of micro-organisms.	
11. Put on sterile gown and gloves.[6] *(Level V*)*	Use of maximal sterile barrier precautions decreases CRBSI.	
12. Open sterile CVC kit. Prep and drape area to be cannulated in sterile fashion. Use back and forth scrubbing motion with 2% chlorhexidine for children more than 2 months old or povidone-iodine solution for infants less than 2 months old; allow antiseptic solution to dry completely.[6] *(Level V*)*	Use of maximal sterile barrier precautions decreases CRBSI.	Assess contents of catheter kit to ensure that all required supplies and equipment are present for catheterization.
13. Administer local anesthetic to site.	Decreases discomfort during catheter insertion.	Calculate maximum dose of lidocaine to prevent administration of excess. Maximum recommended dose is 4.5 mg/kg in a 2-hour interval; 1% lidocaine contains 10 mg/mL.[7]
14. Flush needle and catheter with sterile saline or heparinized saline. *(Level I*)*	Ensures that catheter is patent and intact and minimizes risk of air embolus.	
15. Insert needle at appropriate site while gently aspirating with syringe. **Internal jugular** *Anterior route:* Insert needle at the midpoint of the anterior border of the sternocleidomastoid muscle, aiming toward the ipsilateral nipple at a 30-degree angle posteriorly[1,2] (Figure 153-1). *Central route:* Insert needle at the apex of the triangle formed by the sternoclavicular heads of the sternocleidomastoid muscle and the clavicle at a 30- to 45-degree angle, aiming toward the ipsilateral nipple[1,2] (Figure 153-2).	If needle is in vessel, backflash of blood will appear in syringe when aspirated. When accessing the internal jugular using the central route, blood should appear in syringe before the needle has been advanced more than 2 cm.[2]	

Procedure continues on following page

* Level I: Manufacturer's recommendations only
Level II: Theory-based, no research data to support recommendations; recommendations from expert consensus group may exist
Level V: Clinical studies in more than one or two patient populations and situations to support recommendations
Level VI: Clinical studies in a variety of patient populations and situations to support recommendations

AP This procedure should be performed only by physicians, advanced practice nurses, and other health care professionals (including critical care nurses) with additional knowledge, skills, and demonstrated competence per professional licensure or institutional standard.

Procedure | **for Central Venous Non-tunneled Catheter Insertion: Perform**—*Continued*

Steps	Rationale	Considerations

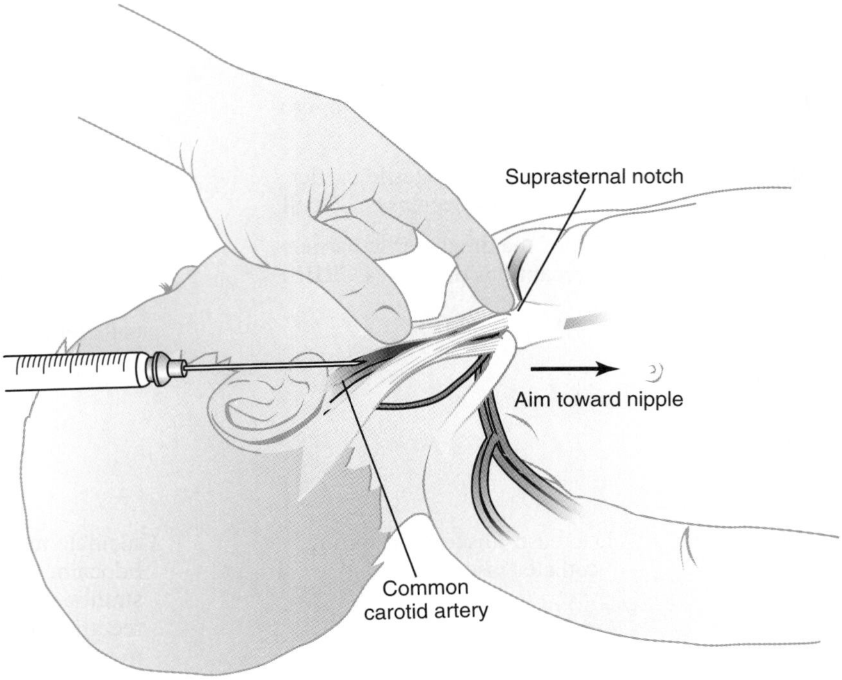

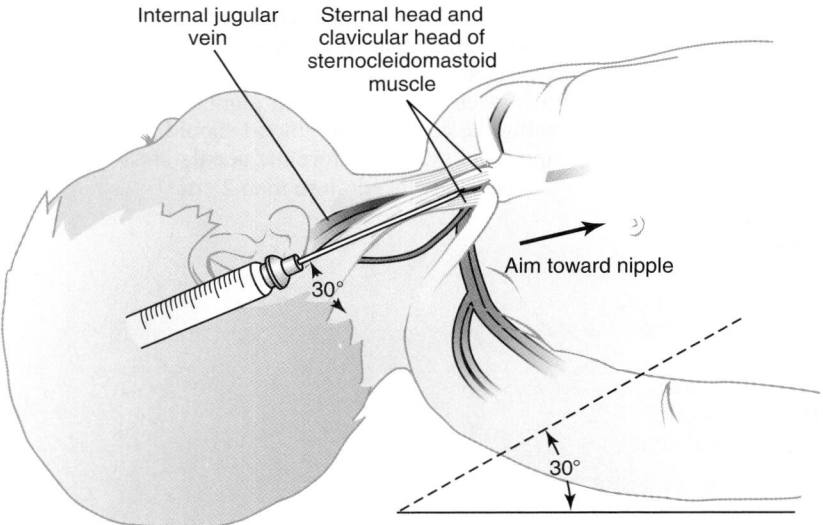

FIGURE 153-1   Internal jugular vein line placement, anterior route.

FIGURE 153-2   Internal jugular vein line placement, central route.

Procedure | for Central Venous Non-tunneled Catheter Insertion: Perform—*Continued*

Steps	Rationale	Considerations

Posterior route: Aiming toward the suprasternal notch, insert needle under the posterior border of the sternocleidomastoid muscle one third of the muscle's length from the clavicular insertion[1,2] (Figure 153-3).

Subclavian: Insert needle just under the clavicle at the junction of the middle and medial thirds of the clavicle in the direction of the suprasternal notch.[1,2] The needle should be parallel to the frontal plane, directed medially and slightly cephalad, beneath the clavicle toward the posterior aspect of the sternal end of the clavicle[1,3] (Figure 153-4).

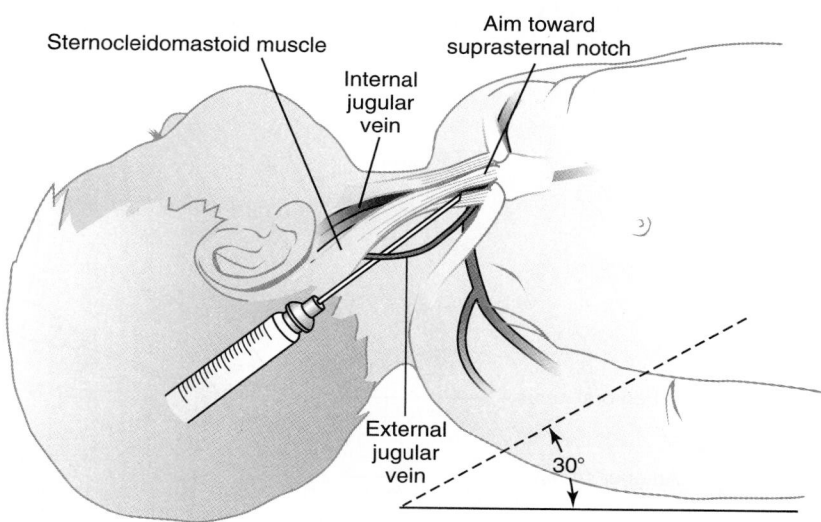

FIGURE 153-3   Internal jugular vein line placement, posterior route.

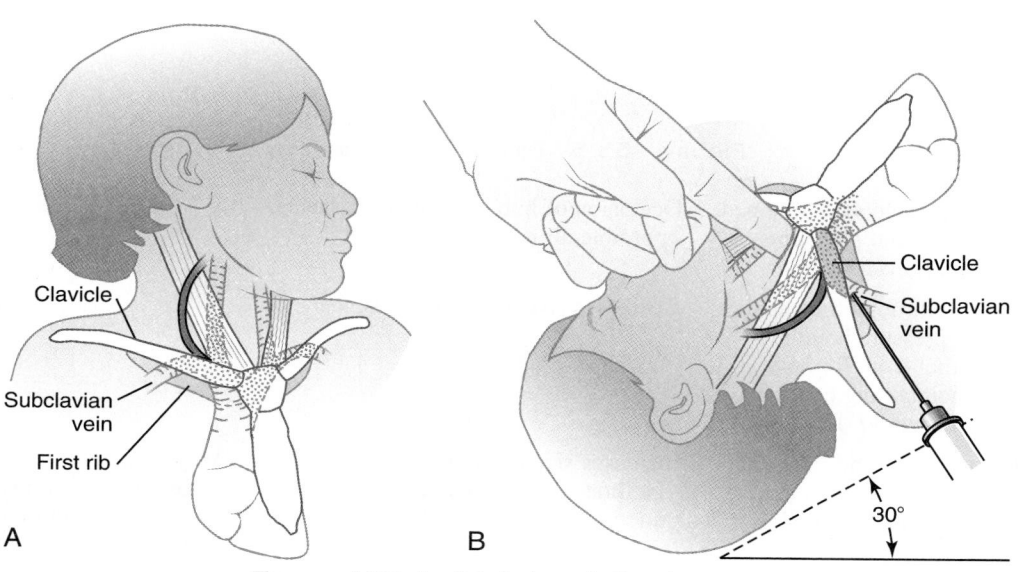

FIGURE 153-4   Subclavian vein line placement.

Procedure continues on following page

Procedure | **for Central Venous Non-tunneled Catheter Insertion: Perform**—*Continued*

Steps	Rationale	Considerations

Femoral: insert needle one finger's width below the inguinal ligament, just medial to the femoral artery. Direct the needle toward the umbilicus at a 45-degree angle[1] (Figure 153-5). *(Level VI*)*

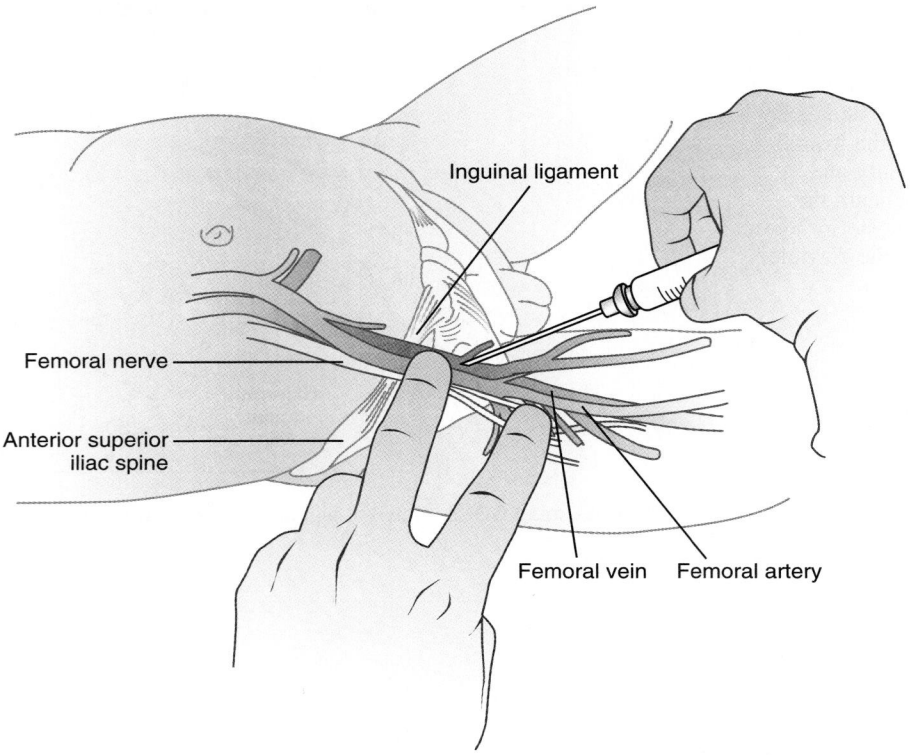

Inguinal ligament

Femoral nerve

Anterior superior iliac spine

Femoral vein   Femoral artery

FIGURE 153-5   Femoral vein line placement.

16. When backflash of blood is obtained, disconnect syringe and place finger over needle hub. *(Level VI*)*

Occlusion of hub with finger prevents possible air embolism.

17. Insert guidewire through the needle during positive pressure breath or spontaneous exhalation. Remove needle while maintaining control of guidewire.[1] *(Level VI*)*

Decreases risk of air embolus.

18. Pass dilator over wire and into vein; remove dilator while maintaining control of guidewire. *(Level VI*)*

Increases size of insertion point and facilitates ease of catheter introduction.

May be helpful to hold dilator close to insertion site, advancing with a twisting motion over guidewire to facilitate insertion. Small skin nick at site of insertion with scalpel blade directed away from wire may be necessary.

19. Pass catheter over wire. Advance catheter to predetermined surface

Advancing catheter to predetermined surface landmark increases likelihood

Do not advance catheter until guidewire is visualized through

* Level VI: Clinical studies in a variety of patient populations and situations to support recommendations

Procedure for Central Venous Non-tunneled Catheter Insertion: Perform—*Continued*

Steps	Rationale	Considerations
landmark while maintaining control of guidewire. Remove guidewire. *(Level VI*)*	of correct catheter placement. Guidewire must be removed to prevent embolus of wire and occlusion of catheter. Monitor for arrhythmias as guidewire and/or catheter are advanced.	hub and control of guidewire is obtained.
20. Assess blood return of all ports of catheter by aspirating with syringe from each port. If no blood return is present, catheter should be withdrawn slightly and aspiration should be repeated. If blood return is still not evident, catheter is in the incorrect position and should be removed. *(Level VI*)*	If catheter is in the improper position, extravasation of fluids could cause an effusion or other complications.	
21. If appropriate blood return is present and catheter is easily flushed, suture catheter in place or use securement device; apply appropriate sterile dressing. *(Level V*)*	Suture or other securement device, such as a StatLock, reduces risk of accidental dislodgement. Sterile dressing decreases risk of contamination of insertion site and assists with security of catheter.[4-6]	Sutureless securement devices may be advantageous over suture in preventing CRBSI.[6]
22. Dispose of used supplies and equipment, including sharps, in appropriate receptacles.	Standard precautions; decreases transmission of microorganisms; protects personnel health.	
23. Remove sterile garb; wash hands.	Standard precautions; reduces transmission of microorganisms.	
24. Obtain chest x-ray. *(Level VI*)*	Assesses catheter tip position and presence or absence of pneumothorax or hemothorax.[1,2]	

* Level V: Clinical studies in more than one or two patient populations and situations to support recommendations
Level VI: Clinical studies in a variety of patient populations and situations to support recommendations

Expected Outcomes	Unexpected Outcomes
• Catheter tip is located at the superior vena cava/right atrial junction or at the inferior vena cava/right atrial junction • CVC flushes easily and has brisk venous blood return • CVC is placed without complications • Child remains hemodynamically stable during CVC placement • Child demonstrates acceptable level of pain control and sedation	• CVC is not positioned centrally or is advanced into the atrium or ventricle • Dysrhythmias related to incorrect CVC position • Unable to flush CVC • Unable to obtain blood return • Blood return is bright red and pulsatile • Complications such as hemothorax, pneumothorax, bleeding, venous thrombosis, arterial puncture, heart perforation, broken catheter, air embolism, infection, dysrhythmias, nerve injury, retroperitoneal bleeding, spinal tap • Unstable vital signs • Hemodynamically significant dysrhythmia • Respiratory distress or failure related to sedation or positioning • Unmanaged anxiety or agitation • Unmanaged pain

AP This procedure should be performed only by physicians, advanced practice nurses, and other health care professionals (including critical care nurses) with additional knowledge, skills, and demonstrated competence per professional licensure or institutional standard.

Monitoring and Care of the Child

Activities and Interventions	Rationale	Reportable Conditions
1. Assess all lumens for blood return, especially distal lumen if short catheter is used, and that all lumens flush without difficulty.	Distal lumen is the tip of the catheter and must always have a blood return—if the catheter is short, and the femoral site is used, the tip of the catheter could puncture the inferior vena cava and fluids could be infused into the peritoneal cavity.	• Lumens do not flush • Unable to obtain blood return
2. Observe site for signs of bleeding.	Bleeding may occur due to coagulopathy or vessel laceration.	• Excessive bleeding or hematoma
3. Monitor for unstable vital signs and dysrhythmias throughout procedure; individual assisting with procedure and providing sedation provides this information.	Individual performing the procedure is focused on the procedure; individual providing sedation monitors cardiopulmonary status.	• Hemodynamic instability • Respiratory distress or failure • Hemodynamically significant arrhythmias
4. Monitor for indications of complications; assess cardiac, respiratory, and neurologic status at completion of procedure and compare with baseline.	Prompt identification of complications allows rapid treatment.	• Changes in vital signs indicating complications such as pneumothorax, cardiac tamponade, hematoma formation, retroperitoneal bleeding, improper catheter placement, extravasation
5. Assess position of CVC tip on chest x-ray.	Documents correct position of CVC tip.	• Catheter is not centrally located or is located in the atrium or ventricle
6. Assess effectiveness of pain and anxiety management strategy; provide appropriate interventions.	Early identification of pain or anxiety issues allows prompt treatment and facilitates completion of procedure.	• Increased pain or agitation impeding completion of procedure

Documentation

• Catheter size, length, site
• Date and time catheter placed; individual placing catheter
• Indications for procedure
• Description of procedure including number of attempts
• Sedation/analgesics used and effectiveness
• Location of catheter tip as documented by x-ray
• Child and family education
• Unexpected outcomes and related treatment

References

1. Vascular access. In Hazinski MF, editor: *Pediatric advanced life support provider manual,* Dallas, 2000, American Heart Association, pp. 93-94.
2. Fuhrman BP, Zimmerman JJ, editors: *Pediatric critical care,* ed 3, St. Louis, 2006, Mosby.
3. McGee DC, Gould MK: Preventing complications of central venous catheterization, *N Engl J Med* 348(12):1123-1133, 2003.
4. Polderman KH, Girbes AJ: Central venous catheter use. Part 1: mechanical complications, *Intens Care Med* 28:1-17, 2002.
5. Polderman KH, Girbes AJ: Central venous catheter use. Part 2: infections complications. *Intens Care Med* 28:18-28, 2002.
6. O'Grady NP, et al: Guidelines for the prevention of intravascular catheter related infections, *MMWR Morbid Mortal Wkly Rep* 51(No.RR-10):1-29, 2002.
7. Taketomo CK, et al, editors: *Lexi-Comp pediatric dosage handbook,* ed 11, Hudson, OH, 2004, Lexi-Comp, Inc.

AP
Intraosseous Needle Placement: Perform

P U R P O S E : To obtain rapid vascular access in arrest or decompensated shock state when vascular access cannot be obtained through conventional means

Harriet S. Hawkins

PREREQUISITE KNOWLEDGE

- Anatomy and physiology of the circulatory system
- Anatomy and physiology of long bones and the bone marrow system
- Child development as it relates to clinical assessment and intraosseous (IO) needle placement
- An intraosseous (IO) needle can be rapidly inserted and can be used for the administration of all resuscitation medications and fluids.[1-3]
- An intact bone is necessary for insertion of an IO needle.
- Absolute contraindications for insertion of an IO needle include recent fracture of the selected bone or a history of osteogenesis imperfecta.[3]
  - ❖ Cellulitis, infection, or burns at the site are relative contraindications.
  - ❖ Known injury to the inferior vena cava is also a relative contraindication because the infused fluid must be able to drain into the central circulation.
- IO needles are available in a variety of sizes from 12 to 18 gauge; larger-gauge needles are needed in older children.
- Several types of bone marrow needles are available; needles specifically designed for IO infusion and bone marrow aspiration needles are most commonly used.[3]

AP This procedure should be performed only by physicians, advanced-practice nurses, and other health care professionals (including critical care nurses) with additional knowledge, skills, and demonstrated competence per professional licensure or institutional standard.

- The proximal tibia is the preferred site of insertion.
  - ❖ Alternate sites include the distal anteromedial surface of the tibia, the distal femur, the iliac crest, and sternum.
- The long bone selected for IO placement must be supported on a firm or semi-firm surface (book, chart, tightly rolled towel or blanket) to prevent fractures from occurring during insertion.
- Laboratory studies (with the exception of coagulation studies) may be drawn from the IO needle at the time of insertion.[4] All tubes and requisitions must be labeled as bone marrow.
- Mastery of pediatric advanced life support competencies
- Principles of aseptic technique

CHILD AND FAMILY ASSESSMENT

- History of osteogenesis imperfecta ➤*Rationale:* This condition is a contraindication to IO placement.
- History of recent fracture injury, cellulitis or burn ➤*Rationale:* These conditions are relative contraindications to placement of an IO needle in the affected extremity.
- Child's developmental level and ability to interact ➤*Rationale:* These factors influence preparation of the child and interaction; if child is somewhat interactive, sedation may be required.
- Family's and child's (as appropriate) understanding of the reasons for and risks and benefits of procedure ➤*Rationale:* Evaluates family's and child's understanding of the procedure and provides a gauge for ongoing education.

- Family's desire to be present during the procedure ➻**Rationale:** Having the option of being with the child during a life-threatening event reassures family that their child is receiving optimal care, legitimizes child's condition, and may provide some sense of comfort and control, but family should also have the choice not to remain with the child.[3]

CHILD AND FAMILY EDUCATION

Individualized, developmentally appropriate education is provided to the family and to the child. IO needles are placed as part of resuscitation in either decompensated shock or arrest states. If the family is present, they will be understandably distraught, and every attempt should be made to facilitate their understanding of all procedures. If they are not present in the room for procedures, they should be kept informed as to what is being done and what to expect when they do see their child. Education is provided to the family based on an assessment of the family's readiness to learn; short, simple explanations are most effective during an emergency situation. Anticipate that information will need to be repeated.[3]

- Explain the reason for the IO needle placement (difficulty in obtaining vascular access via the conventional intravenous route) ➻**Rationale:** Providing information decreases anxiety and fear.
- Explain that the IO needle is easily placed and rapidly provides a route to administer medications, blood products, and fluids ➻**Rationale:** Providing information in the critical situation decreases anxiety and assures the family that the medical team is taking all appropriate actions to care for the child.

- Inform the family that the child was not in pain when the IO needle was placed ➻**Rationale:** Providing information decreases anxiety and fear. Family members should know that their child is receiving compassionate care.
- Explain that after the IO needle is in place the needle does not cause any pain ➻**Rationale:** The appearance of an IO needle can be frightening, and providing additional information will help decrease the family's fears.
- Explain that the IO needle will be removed as soon as possible after the resuscitative event ➻**Rationale:** Providing information helps reduce the family's fears and anxiety.
- Encourage questions and answer questions as they arise. ➻**Rationale:** Reinforcement of information is needed during periods of stress. This is especially important given the emergent nature of the procedure.

EQUIPMENT

- Antiseptic solution for cleaning the skin; chlorhexidine or povidone-iodine
- Appropriate needle for child's age and size
  - ❖ 18 gauge for infants and toddlers
  - ❖ 15 to 16 gauge for young children
  - ❖ 12 gauge for older children
- Sterile gloves
- Flush solution: 0.9% saline or lactated Ringer's
- Syringe: 5 or 10 mL
- Tape: ½ inch waterproof
- Gauze: 2 inch and 4 inch
- T-connector
- Intravenous tubing for infusion pump or intravenous tubing and pressure bag

Procedure	for Intraosseous Needle Placement	
Steps	**Rationale**	**Considerations**
1. Ensure child and family understand procedure and questions are answered.	Assesses family's understanding of the procedure.	In critical situations, family may not be available; procedure should not be delayed.
2. Gather needed equipment and supplies.	Preparation and having all materials present facilitates completion of procedure in a timely manner.	Needle size selected depends on the child's size; if the size initially chosen bends during the insertion attempt, the next larger size should be used.
3. Wash hands. (*Level VI**)	Standard precautions; reduces the transmission of microorganisms.	
4. Locate site for needle placement.	Ensures that appropriate location is used; if there is a break in the integrity of the bone, the fluids administered will leak out and will not be delivered to the central circulation. (*Level IV**)	IO insertion is contraindicated in a child with osteogenesis imperfecta. Needle cannot be placed in a recently fractured bone or in a bone that has recently had another IO needle. Burns or cellulitis in the extremity are also relative contraindications.

* Level IV: Limited clinical studies to support recommendations
  Level VI: Clinical studies in a variety of patient populations and situations to support recommendations

Procedure for Intraosseous Needle Placement—*Continued*

Steps	Rationale	Considerations
5. Ensure appropriate cardiopulmonary monitoring.	Facilitates early identification of decompensation during the procedure.	
6. Position the child to facilitate access to the bone to be used. If using a long bone (distal femur, proximal tibia, or distal tibia) place something firm under the bone, below the insertion site (Figure 154-1). *(Level II*)*	Proper positioning is of the utmost importance during the procedure in order to facilitate rapid needle placement and to prevent fractures.	Rapid insertion of the needle is facilitated by positioning the bone so that the flat surface to be entered is horizontal.
7. Wash hands and put on sterile gloves. *(Level VI*)*	Reduces transmission of microorganisms.	Sterile gloves should be worn as the needle may be touched during the insertion.
8. Clean site with antiseptic solution.	Reduces incidence of infection.	Institution-specific protocol may direct choice of antiseptic solution used.
9. Palpate bone to determine the exact insertion site, taking care to avoid the epiphyseal plate.	Damage of the epiphyseal plate before puberty can result in bone growth abnormalities. *(Level IV*)*	The preferred site is the proximal tibia on the tibial plateau 2 cm below and medial to the tibial tuberosity (Figure 154-2). *(Level II*)* Alternative sites include the distal tibia, 1 to 2 cm superior to the medial malleolus, and the lower third of the femur, approximately 3 cm above the lateral femoral epicondyles (Figure 154-3).
10. Check the needle to ensure that the stylet is completely engaged in the needle. If using a 12-gauge screw needle, ensure that the removable handle engages and disengages easily. *(Level I*)*	Insertion is facilitated by the use of properly functioning equipment.	Needles may become disengaged during the packaging and shipping process.
11. Insert the needle.	Gentle pressure is necessary to advance the needle through the bone without causing damage to the bone.	
Standard IO Needle		
a. Insert the needle through the skin and begin entering the bone using a gentle but firm twisting motion, back and forth. Start with gentle pressure to "seat" the needle on the surface of the bone.	Pressing too hard during the initial stages of insertion may cause the needle to slip off of the bone.	

Procedure continues on following page

* Level I: Manufacturer's recommendations only
 Level II: Theory-based, no research data to support recommendations: recommendations from expert consensus group may exist
 Level IV: Limited clinical studies to support recommendations
 Level VI: Clinical studies in a variety of patient populations and situations to support recommendations

Procedure for Intraosseous Needle Placement—*Continued*

Steps	Rationale	Considerations

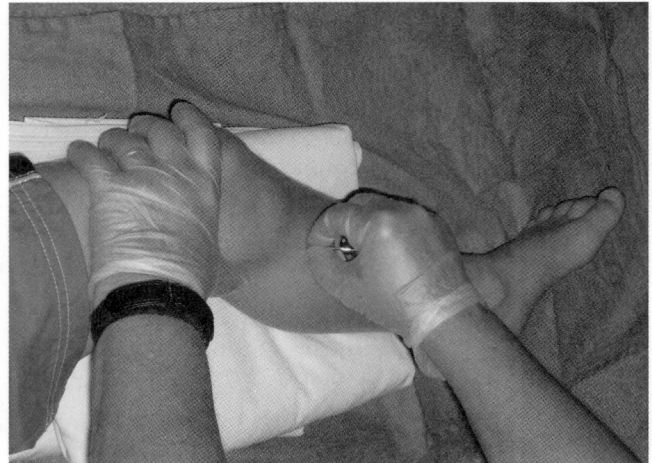

FIGURE 154-1   Insertion of intraosseous needle with leg supported on rolled sheet.

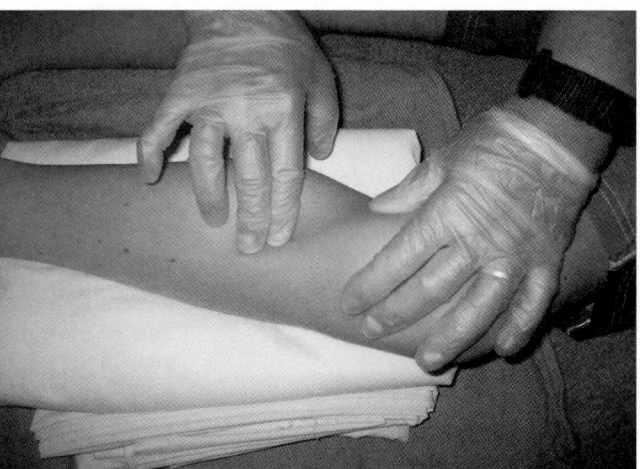

FIGURE 154-2   Proximal tibia intraosseous insertion site.

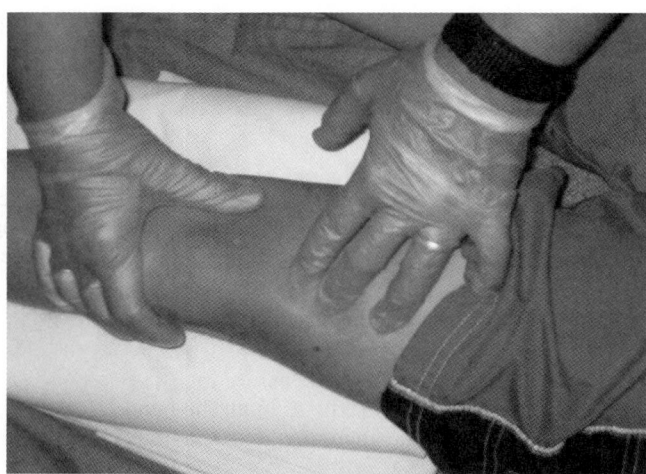

FIGURE 154-3   Distal femur intraosseouss insertion site.

Steps	Rationale	Considerations
b. As the needle enters the bone, the gentle pressure may be increased. Using twisting motion, twist the needle back and forth while applying gentle pressure until penetration through the cortex is noted.	As the needle bores through the bone, resistance will be felt and greater pressure may be required.	When the needle passes through the cortex and into the marrow cavity, the resistance will decrease, and often a "pop" is felt.
c. Remove stylet and attach a 5-mL syringe.	Stylet must be removed in order to infuse fluids or medications.	Hold the IO needle firmly in place to avoid dislodging the needle while the stylet is withdrawn.

Procedure for Intraosseous Needle Placement—*Continued*

Steps	Rationale	Considerations
Gauge Screw–Type Needle		
a. Use the scalpel enclosed in package to cut through the skin to the surface of the bone. *(Level I*)*	This needle does not have a stylet and is shorter, requiring it to be placed directly on the bone through an incision in the skin.	
b. Using a continuous rotating motion and gentle pressure, screw the needle into the bone until a lack of resistance is felt. *(Level I*)*	This screw-type needle must be inserted using a continuous clockwise motion.	The bones of older children are more dense and it is therefore more difficult to bore through the bone.
c. Remove insertion handle from needle and attach a 5-mL syringe. *(Level I*)*	Handle must be removed in order to use the needle.	Knowledge of how the particular IO needle and stylet fit together will prevent inadvertent removal or dislodging of the needle during this part of the procedure.
12. Using a 5-mL syringe, attempt to gently aspirate bone marrow.	Aspiration of bone marrow confirms placement; the marrow may be sent for laboratory testing.	Although the needle may be properly placed, bone marrow may not always be aspirated.
13. If marrow is obtained, place in appropriate tubes for laboratory testing; label appropriately.	Emergent laboratory testing may be obtained via the IO route (electrolytes, type and cross, drug screening, mixed venous gas).[4] *(Level IV*)*	Mark all tubes and requisitions "bone marrow."
14. If marrow is not obtained but the IO needle stands firmly in the bone, proper placement is assumed and the needle may be flushed.	Marrow is not always initially aspirated from appropriately placed IO needles.	
15. Remove syringe and attach a T-connector with injection port to the IO needle.	Repeated attachment of syringes directly to the IO needle may result in slight dislodgement of the needle and leaking of medications and fluids from the insertion site.	Allows delivery of fluids via manual push with a syringe, without constant manipulation of the actual needle; also allows delivery of medications directly to the IO needle.
16. Attach a 5- or 10-mL syringe to the T-connector and flush the IO needle.	Appropriately placed needle should flush relatively easily without increased resistance or obvious soft tissue swelling at the insertion site.	A very slight leakage of fluid may occur at the insertion site during initial flushing. This should be minimal. If increased or continuous, an alternate IO site should be obtained.
17. After confirmation of appropriate placement of the IO needle, resuscitation medications, blood products and fluids may be administered. *(Level IV*)*	IO needles are placed when vascular access is emergently needed and should be used immediately after insertion.	

Procedure continues on following page

* Level I: Manufacturer's recommendations only
Level IV: Limited clinical studies to support recommendations

AP This procedure should be performed only by physicians, advanced practice nurses, and other health care professionals (including critical care nurses) with additional knowledge, skills, and demonstrated competence per professional licensure or institutional standard.

Procedure for Intraosseous Needle Placement—*Continued*

Steps	Rationale	Considerations
18. Secure the needle with tape and gauze dressings.	Supporting the needle with gauze and tape will help prevent dislodgment.	Do not put tight tape circumferentially around the leg. If infiltration occurs, such tape could cause compartment syndrome.
19. Throughout resuscitation, maintain patency of the IO needle by continually infusing fluids. *(Level II*)*	Continuous infusion will help maintain patency of the line.	Appropriate methods include manual flushing, use of a pressure bag, and intravenous tubing or an intravenous pump with tubing.
20. Dispose of used supplies and equipment appropriately; stylet or scalpel should be placed in sharps container.	Standard precautions; reduces transmission of microorganisms and protects health care personnel.	
21. Remove gloves; wash hands.	Standard precautions.	
22. As soon as feasible, attempt vascular access via another means and remove the IO needle.	IO needle should be removed as soon as conventional vascular access can be obtained (preferably within 4 hours).[1,2,5] *(Level II*)*	

* Level II: Theory-based, no research data to support recommendations: recommendations from expert consensus group may exist
   Level IV: Limited clinical studies to support recommendations

Expected Outcomes

- IO needle functions properly and allows the delivery of resuscitation medications and fluids

- IO needle is placed without complications

- Child remains free from infection

Unexpected Outcomes

- IO needle becomes dislodged
- IO needle becomes occluded and will not flush
- Extravasation of fluid into surrounding tissues
- Fracture of bone during insertion attempt
- Needle breaks during insertion attempt
- Injury to individual placing needle
- Localized infection at insertion site
- Osteomyelitis

Monitoring and Care of the Child

Activities and Interventions	Rationale	Reportable Conditions
1. Monitor insertion site for leakage of fluids from site, infiltration of fluids, swelling on the posterior surface of extremity.	Early identification of nonfunctioning IO needle allows prompt treatment and identifies need for another location for access.	• Increased leakage of fluids from insertion site (may signal the need to change the IO needle to another site) • Obvious local infiltration of fluids or dependent edema
2. Monitor perfusion of the extremity distal to IO needle.	Allows prompt identification of complications.	• Any change in perfusion distal to the IO needle

Documentation

- Exact site of IO needle placement
- Condition of site, including evidence of leakage
- Time IO needle placed
- Size and type of IO needle used, number and location of placement attempts
- Name and title of person placing the needle
- Ability to flush needle
- Perfusion distal to the IO needle insertion site
- Child's tolerance of procedure
- Child and family education
- Unexpected outcomes and related treatment

References

1. Ellemunter H, et al: Intraosseous lines in preterm and full term neonates, *Arch Dis Child* 80(1);F74-F75, 1999.
2. Vascular access. In Hawkins HS, editor: *Emergency nursing pediatric course provider manual,* ed 3, Des Plaines, IL, 2004, Emergency Nurses Association, pp. 93-94.
3. Vascular access. In Hazinski MF, editor: *Pediatric advanced life support provider manual,* Dallas, 2002, American Heart Association, pp. 152-172.
4. Johnson L, et al: Use of intraosseous blood to assess blood chemistries and hemoglobin during cardiopulmonary resuscitation with drug infusions, *Crit Care Med* 27(6): 1147-1152, 1999.
5. Vidal R, et al: Compartment syndrome following intraosseous infusion, *Pediatrics* 91:1201-1202, 1993

Additional Readings

Claudet I, et al: Long term effects on tibial growth after intraosseous infusion: a prospective, radiographic analysis, *Pediatr Emerg Care* 19(6):397-401, 2003.

Fiorito BA, et al: Intraosseous access in the setting of pediatric critical care transport, *Pediatr Crit Care Med* 6(1):50, 2005.

Jun H, et al: Comparison of new screw-tipped intraosseous needle versus a standard bone marrow aspiration needle for infusion, *Am J Emerg Med* 18(2):135-139, 2000.

AP

Peripherally Inserted Central Catheter (PICC) Insertion: Perform

P U R P O S E : To insert a catheter into the peripheral veins of the upper or lower extremities of suitable length to be advanced into the superior or inferior vena cava allowing infusion of intravenous medications, parenteral nutrition, or fluids to the central circulation.[1-3] Several methods for PICC insertion are used for children, including peel-away sheath and modified Seldinger technique (MST). Peel-away sheath technique is described here.

Nancy L. Moureau

PREREQUISITE KNOWLEDGE

- Intravenous (IV) medication administration
- Anatomy of the peripheral and central vascular system and structure of blood vessels
- Principles of aseptic technique
- PICC management, including flushing, securement, and aseptic technique
- Concepts related to vascular access and central vascular catheters
- Complications of PICC insertion: bleeding, venous thrombosis, arterial puncture, heart perforation, broken catheter with embolization, air embolism, infection, dysrhythmia, catheter occlusion, phlebitis, pneumothorax[4-11]
- Competency in PICC insertion verified via completion of class/clinical learning; refer to institution- and state-specific guidelines regarding qualifications of individuals authorized to perform PICC insertion

- Child development as it relates to clinical assessment and PICC insertion
- Appropriate pediatric dosing of analgesics and competency in procedural sedation
- Informed consent is required before placing a PICC

CHILD AND FAMILY ASSESSMENT

- Child's developmental level and ability to interact ➻*Rationale:* These factors influence preparation of the child and child's ability to cooperate during the procedure.
- Age, walking status, prescribed IV fluids and medications, availability of sites ➻*Rationale:* Vein selection is based on these factors as well as previous peripheral IV history.
- Expected duration of treatment, type of treatment ➻*Rationale:* Vascular access device selection determination is based on how long the device is needed and what infusate is ordered.
- History of chronic illness and effects of illness or treatment on veins ➻*Rationale:* Previous treatment with chemotherapeutic agents, steroids, or other vesicant or irritating medications can alter the integrity of the available vasculature.
- History of failed vascular access ➻*Rationale:* Knowledge of problems with previous insertions can help to increase the success of future insertions.

- Knowledge of allergies and sensitivities ➺*Rationale:* Medication history with allergies and sensitivities is necessary to avoid complications related to the procedure.
- Child's and family's understanding of the reasons for and risks and benefits of the procedure ➺*Rationale:* Evaluates child's and family's understanding of the procedure and provides a gauge for ongoing education.
- Family members desire to be present during the procedure ➺*Rationale:* Family members may provide comfort and support to the child but should have the choice not to remain with the child.

CHILD AND FAMILY EDUCATION

Individualized, developmentally appropriate education is provided to the family and to the child based on desire for knowledge, readiness to learn, and overall neurologic and psychosocial state.

- Explain the need for vascular access, risks and benefits of the procedure, options available, and the assessment for the PICC ➺*Rationale:* Facilitates informed consent; information provided in a calm clear manner will reduce anxiety. Patient/family involvement in decision making increases the feeling of control thus reducing anxiety. Family involvement with decisions may also reduce liability.
- Provide information about the insertion steps and process, timing and expectations ➺*Rationale:* Providing information about the insertion procedure will reduce anxiety and fear by the family and the child.
- Provide information about the pain and anxiety management plan for the child including Child Life, sedation, and other methods as outlined in institution-specific protocols ➺*Rationale:* Providing information decreases anxiety and fear.
- Explain the possible complications with a PICC, including breakage, infection, dislodgement, clotting, or malpositioning ➺*Rationale:* Understanding of the possible complications facilitates informed consent and may prevent occurrence.
- Describe care and maintenance of the PICC and management in the hospital and home as applicable ➺*Rationale:* Promotes realistic understanding of care measures necessary for intermediate term vascular access and should be included as a component of education and a part of informed consent.
- Encourage questions and answer questions as they arise ➺*Rationale:* Reinforcement of information is needed during periods of stress.

EQUIPMENT

- PICC kit may include:
  - ❖ 5-mL syringe
  - ❖ Scissors
  - ❖ Forceps
  - ❖ Introducer
- Appropriately sized PICC with safety insertion device
  - ❖ Sizes available include 1.1 to 5 Fr for use in neonates to adolescents
- Tourniquet (latex-free)
- Personal protective equipment including mask, eye shield, cap, sterile gown, and sterile gloves
- Sterile drapes (full body drapes if using ultrasound)
- 2% chlorhexidine prepping agent (infants and children ≥ 2 months) or alcohol and 10% povidone-iodine (infants < 2 months) for site preparation
- Sterile and clean tape measure
- Securement device or tape (latex-free)
- Gauze 4×4, 2×2
- Flushing solution(s)
- Agents for local anesthesia, may include buffered lidocaine in tuberculin syringe, topical anesthetic cream

Procedure for Peripherally Inserted Central Catheter Insertion: Perform

Steps	Rationale	Considerations
1. Receive order for PICC insertion from prescribing practitioner.	Prescribing practitioner's order is required for insertion of PICC. The prescribing practitioner directs care.	Physician, nurse, family, and other medical personnel work as a team to administer care.
2. Review chart, medications, and history.	Identifies child-specific risk factors.	Complications may be more likely to develop if certain risk factors are present in child's history.
3. Ensure child and family understand procedure and questions are answered; confirm that informed consent has been obtained.	Ensures medicolegal compliance as suggested by the Joint Commission on Accreditation of Healthcare Organizations (JCAHO).	Refer to institution-specific protocols for obtaining and documenting informed consent.

Procedure continues on following page

Procedure	for Peripherally Inserted Central Catheter Insertion: Perform—*Continued*	
Steps	**Rationale**	**Considerations**
4. Assess child's age, developmental stage, and requirement for Child Life and/or sedation.	Trauma to the child is reduced with appropriate sedation or when Child Life assistance is provided.	Use of Child Life personnel can assist the child in managing a potentially long and possibly painful procedure. Children younger than the age of 6 years may need sedation. If sedation is used, ensure fasting guidelines are implemented per institution-specific protocol.
5. Wash hands. *(Level VI*)*	Standard precautions; reduces the transmission of microorganisms.	Performed prior to the procedure and whenever gloves are removed.
6. Assess child's veins for suitability and size of catheter most appropriate for the vein chosen; assess effect of selected site on child's comfort and activity.[10] *(Level IV*)*	Promotes successful PICC insertion.	Veins of the upper or lower extremities can be considered. Scalp veins are sometimes used in the infant. Consider the child's comfort and coping mechanisms and provide choices whenever possible, based on age and developmental level.
7. If using topical anesthetic, apply cream to site(s) identified for PICC insertion and leave in place for appropriate time interval. *(Level I*)*	Allows time for maximum numbing effect of topical agent.	Topical numbing cream must remain in place for 30 minutes to 4 hours for best anesthetic effect depending on the agent and instructions for use; refer to product insert. EMLA cream has been shown to cause vasoconstriction, which may complicate PICC insertion.
8. Gather needed supplies and equipment.	Facilitates completion of procedure in a timely manner. Have all supplies ready prior to talking with the child. Speed and organization are important to reduce the time frame and thus reduce the child's fear and anxiety.	Anxiety of a child increases with delays.
9. If child is to receive sedation, ensure appropriate monitoring is in place, emergency equipment is available, and fasting guidelines have been implemented. *(Level II*)*	Monitoring facilitates early identification of complications related to sedation; availability of emergency equipment allows prompt initiation of treatment.	Refer to institution-specific protocols related to procedural sedation.
10. Position child comfortably but securely. Using clean tape measure, measure child in centimeters for proper catheter tip placement. *For superior vena cava:* with arm extended at 45 degrees, measure from selected vein insertion site to the head of the clavicle on the right side. Add 1 to 3 cm depending on size of child	Positioning facilitates PICC insertion. Measurement determines the correct length of catheter to be inserted for proper terminal tip location in the vena cava.	Superior or inferior vena cava terminal tip is the only acceptable terminal location.[8] *(Level IV*)*

*Level I: Manufacturer's recommendations only
Level II: Theory-based, no research data to support recommendations; recommendations from expert consensus group may exist
Level IV: Limited clinical studies to support recommendations
Level VI: Clinical studies in a variety of patient populations and situations to support recommendations

Procedure for Peripherally Inserted Central Catheter Insertion: Perform—*Continued*		
Steps	**Rationale**	**Considerations**
(approximately 0 to 6 years). Older children measure from insertion site to mid section on the clavicle, then down to the third intercostal space to the right of the sternum. *For inferior vena cava:* Measure from selected vein insertion site, up the leg to groin, groin to umbilicus, umbilicus to 2 cm (two fingers) below xyphoid process.		
11. Identify child using appropriate patient/procedure verification process (e.g., "Time out")	Confirms correct patient, procedure and site as recommended by JCAHO; prevents unnecessary medical procedures.	Verification process and documentation is institution specific. Use active communication techniques.
12. Have RN/MD administer procedural sedation, if applicable. Administer local anesthetic agents as applicable to the age and activity of the child. *(Level II*)*	An RN or MD, in addition to the person performing the procedure, is required to be present if procedural sedation is used.	Refer to institution-specific protocol for procedural sedation.
13. Wash hands. Put on personal protective equipment including mask, eye shield, hat, sterile gloves, and sterile gown.[12] *(Level VI*)*	Standard precautions; reduces the transmission of microorganisms. Protects personnel from blood exposure.	Handwashing and maximum sterile barriers are used based on Centers for Disease Control recommendations.[12] Put on sterile gown before gloves, keeping cuffs over fingers; then apply gloves on top of cuffs. Use of sterile gown requires an assistant to tie the neck and reach for the front ties to complete securement in the back. It is impossible for the inserter to maintain sterility while tying own gown.
14. Establish sterile field away from possible contamination by child. Prepare the catheter and all materials in a sterile fashion before moving toward the child. Second or third assistant may be necessary to preserve sterility of the field and limit the movement of child during procedure.	Consideration for sterile field setup is necessary to maintain a strict sterile field with a child. Movement of the extremity reduces the potential for successful insertion.	Do not allow child to touch or affect the sterile field in any way that results in contamination.
15. Place sterile drape under extremity selected and prep insertion site with chlorhexidine. Use a back and forth friction scrub in a large prep area at least halfway up the extremity and halfway down, scrubbing for at least 30 seconds.[12] *(Level VI*)*	Reduces bacterial colonization and risk of contamination.	Chlorhexidine with alcohol provides a broad-spectrum kill with significant residual activity. 10% povidone-iodine is used for infants <2 months.

Procedure continues on following page

* Level II: Theory-based, no research data to support recommendations; recommendations from expert consensus group may exist
Level VI: Clinical studies in a variety of patient populations and situations to support recommendations

Procedure for Peripherally Inserted Central Catheter Insertion: Perform—*Continued*

Steps	Rationale	Considerations
16. Apply fenestrated drape over extremity; extra drapes can cover hand or foot and extend field. Always overlap drapes. Use maximum sterile drapes at all times. Use full body drapes with ultrasound guidance.	Sterile covering over extremity facilitates sterile technique during catheter insertion.	Smaller drapes can be used for smaller children. For children less than 6 years, may use fenestrated oval eye drape with smaller hole; drop eye drape into the sterile field during preparation.
17. Change gloves after prep and drape. Wash hands after each glove change. Always have extra sterile gloves available. If glove change is needed, pull cuffs down over fingers as gloves are removed; put on new sterile gloves.	Contamination is common when prepping; changing gloves ensures sterility.	
18. Prepare flushes; prefill extension sets and catheter with flow-through guidewires or catheter without guidewire. Attach syringe with flush to T-connector as appropriate for catheter. Flush with at least 1 mL of fluid.	Prevents air embolus.	Certain PICC brands may work better for the pediatric and neonatal population. Catheter preparation should be in keeping with manufacturer's recommendations for that product.
19. Measure catheter with sterile tape measure, or look at catheter markings; take care to move catheter with forceps. Apply previous measurement of child, adding on the amount to stay out of skin. Move guidewire back past trim point. Cut catheter, as needed, below guidewire, with straight cut, following manufacturer's recommendations for trimming, as needed. If no trimming is required, confirm the amount to be left out and coiled under the dressing. *(Level I*)*	Confirms proper length of catheter for insertion into the superior or inferior vena cava. Guidewire stabilizes catheter during insertion.	Refer to manufacturer's instructions for trimming catheter. NEVER CUT THE GUIDEWIRE. Bend wire 90 degrees at hub. Some catheters are manufactured so that tip is not to be cut; instead, length is adjusted externally after tip location verified (e.g., Groshong PICC). It is not recommended to trim dual lumens with staggered tips.
20. Position catheter near extremity on your dominant side; keep to center of field and away from field edges.	Facilitates maintaining sterility of catheter.	Products vary; follow manufacturer's guidelines for catheter preparation.
21. Have assistant apply tourniquet above vein selected, or apply tourniquet and change gloves. Do not apply tourniquet until needed to dilate veins.	Tourniquet allows dilation of blood vessels for easier access.	For infants may use rubber band or other forms of pressure to assist in vein dilation; ensure child does not have a latex allergy.
22. Hold introducer device with pads of fingers. A new introducer should be used for each cannulation attempt. Remove cover.	Introducer is placed to facilitate catheter insertion.	Insertion devices vary with age and size. Follow manufacturer's guidelines for insertion techniques specific to the products.
23. Approach vein below the best spot of the vein. Using a very low angle go through the skin, then into vein. When flashback is seen, drop angle of introducer, keeping point of needle up; advance a little farther into vein. *(Level II*)*	Low angle of insertion is less likely to rupture the vessel with greater chance of success.	Low and slow is a good rule for insertion of IV devices in children.

* Level I: Manufacturer's recommendations only
Level II: Theory-based, no research data to support recommendations: recommendations from expert consensus group may exist

Procedure for Peripherally Inserted Central Catheter Insertion: Perform—*Continued*		
Steps	**Rationale**	**Considerations**
24. Push off cannula into vein, holding stylet in place. Thread cannula into vein. Hold the introducer in place.	Slow, two-hand approach makes for greater success with threading of the peel-away cannula sheath into the vein. Do not retract the needle, only thread the cannula first; then pull the needle/activate the safety device.	Larger access devices require greater skill with insertion into the small veins of a child.
25. Apply digital pressure to the vein above cannula.	Control of bleeding can be achieved with digital pressure, protecting the child from complications.	
26. Remove stylet by activating safety mechanism.	Needle is no longer needed after vein access and cannula threading are complete.	Clinician safety is of vital importance. Safety devices should be properly used in all insertion procedures.
27. Use forceps to pick up catheter. Confirm blood return through cannula, then thread catheter through cannula, slowly advancing 1 inch (2.5 cm) at a time.	Greater tactile sensitivity is achieved with catheter threading by means of forceps. Forceps make handling of very small catheters easier.	If forceps are not available sterile talc free gloved fingers are acceptable.
28. After advancing 4 to 6 inches (10 to 15 cm) catheter has been advanced past the valves. Check blood return and flush catheter if applicable. Gently remove the cannula introducer, holding the catheter with the forceps. Pull back introducer on the catheter. Bend wings of peel-away introducer up, down, and then peel away. *(Level I*)*	Advancing catheter the first 10 to 15 cm can be problematic at times. The introducer can be left in place for the entire threading time if there are any threading difficulties, reason to leave the introducer or concerns over child's state of dehydration.	Valves can cause difficulties in advancing catheter in older children and children with cystic fibrosis.
29. Position child's chin toward insertion site, extending arm 45 to 90 degrees from body.	Advancement into the superior vena cava (SVC) is promoted with the head turn, which results in a change in the angle of the jugular vein.	
30. Continue to thread catheter slowly. If difficulty threading, check for blood return, pull back a little, flush, advance again. Continue to check for blood return intermittently and alternately flushing.	Slow threading reduces incidence of malpositioning and allows blood flow to advance the catheter to the right location.	Malpositioning can sometimes be avoided with certain adjustments to the procedure and slow threading.
31. Remove guidewire as appropriate, using Valsalva maneuver as developmentally appropriate whenever opening catheter system. For flow-through guidewires, which can be flushed with heparin, x-ray may be taken with guidewire in place; then removed when placement is confirmed.	Guidewire is removed to allow complete flushing and confirmation of blood return.	Guidewire may be left in place for x-ray as needed for better visualization.

Procedure continues on following page

* Level I: Manufacturer's recommendations only

Procedure | for Peripherally Inserted Central Catheter Insertion: Perform—*Continued*

Steps	Rationale	Considerations
32. Complete catheter insertion to predetermined marking. Secure based on manufacturer's recommendations.	Securement of catheter without excess length reduces complications. Use of definite method of securement and securement devices reduces complications.	Accidental dislodgement is a common problem with children and can be avoided with specific securement devices.
33. Apply preprimed extension set, cap, and sterile pressure dressing.	Extension sets added to the hub reduce manipulation of the catheter.	Pressure dressings are applied for the first 24 hours to prevent bleeding.
34. Discard used supplies and equipment in appropriate receptacle.	Standard precautions; reduces transmission of microorganisms; protects personnel health.	
35. Remove personal protective equipment; wash hands.	Standard precautions.	Biohazardous waste must be handled and disposed of in proper manner.
36. Obtain chest x-ray; confirm catheter tip location. *(Level IV*)*	Confirms correct placement of catheter tip in SVC at or near the right atrial junction. No central venous catheter may be allowed to dwell within the right atrium or in any location within the heart. Serious complications such as cardiac tamponade and pleural effusion have resulted from improper positioning.	If guidewire was left in place for confirmation of placement, remove guidewire. Serious complications are avoided with catheter placement in the SVC. Periodic checks are needed to ensure continued correct positioning. Policies are necessary to establish reporting of malpositioned catheter tips and confirmation of subsequent adjustment of position.

* Level IV: Limited clinical studies to support recommendations

Expected Outcomes

- Insertion of PICC catheter tip into the superior or inferior vena cava
- PICC is confirmed by radiology study as suitable for use
- Trauma of procedure is minimized
- PICC has blood return and is easily flushed

- PICC is placed without complications

Unexpected Outcomes

- Unable to insert PICC or catheter tip malpositioned
- Malposition of catheter tip identified by x-ray requiring radiology intervention
- Local hematoma, nerve damage, upset child, upset family
- PICC is clotted/unable to aspirate blood
- PICC is kinked
- PICC is malpositioned
- PICC does not flush
- Bleeding
- Venous thrombosis
- Arterial puncture
- Respiratory depression (sedation)
- Heart perforation
- Broken catheter
- Air embolism
- Infection
- Dysrhythmia

Monitoring and Care of the Child

Activities and Interventions	Rationale	Reportable Conditions
1. Monitor child's tolerance of procedure throughout PICC insertion.	Allows early identification of need for change in pain and sedation management plan. Evaluates effectiveness of Child Life interaction.	• Unable to complete procedure because child is overly anxious, agitated, or unable to remain still
2. Monitor vital signs throughout procedure and recovery period if child receives sedation, per institution-specific protocol.	Allows prompt identification of complications related to sedation.	• Respiratory distress or failure • Hypotension • Bradycardia • Dysrhythmias
3. Monitor insertion site following the insertion.	Identifies possible arterial insertion or nerve injury.	• Pain, excess bleeding, numbness to extremity
4. Monitor dressing for presence of blood or drainage and intactness.	Excess bleeding is not normal; may indicate vascular injury.	• Bleeding that saturates the dressing • Contamination, signs of infection or drainage around insertion site
5. Monitor catheter length outside the insertion site.	Identifies catheter dislodgment.	• Catheter tip moved out of confirmed location may only be used for isotonic or nonirritating solutions • Requires corrective action
6. Monitor for presence of pain or vibration in neck indicating catheter malpositioning or dislodgement.	Catheter may become malpositioned in jugular vein; possible malpositioning must be confirmed by x-ray.	• Pain or vibration in neck

Documentation

- Length of catheter inserted, amount of catheter in and amount out of insertion site
- Approximate blood loss, difficulties with insertion
- Extremity circumference
- Insertion site (right or left) and location, vein specific
- Brand and size of catheter
- Number of attempts
- Medications administered
- Child and family education
- X-ray confirmation of tip location in the vena cava
- Presence of blood return, ability to flush catheter
- Unexpected outcomes and related treatment

References

1. BeVier PA, Rice CE: Initiating a pediatric peripherally inserted central catheter and midline catheter program, *J Intrav Nurs* 17:201, 1994.
2. Chathas MK, Paton JB: Meeting the special nutritional needs of sick infants with a percutaneous central venous catheter quality assurance program, *J Perinat Neonatal Nurs* 10(4):72-87, 1997.
3. Chung DH, Ziegler MM: Central venous catheter access, *Nutrition* 14(1):119-123, 1998.
4. Camara D: Minimizing risks associated with peripherally inserted central catheters in the NICU, *Am J Matern Child Nurs* 26(1):17-20, 2001.
5. Duntley E, et al: Vascular erosion by central venous catheters, *Chest* 101(6):1633-1638, 1992.
6. Garland JS, et al: Comparison of 10% povidone-iodine and 0.5% chlorhexidine gluconate for the prevention of peripheral intravenous catheter colonization in neonates: a prospective trial, *Pediatr Infect Dis J* 14(6):510-516, 1995.
7. Goutail-Flaud ME, et al: Central venous catheter-related complications in newborns and infants: a 587 case survey, *J Pediatr Surg* 26(6):645-650, 1991.
8. Racadio JM, et al: Pediatric peripherally inserted central catheters: complication rates related to catheter tip location, *Pediatrics* 7(2):E28-31, 2001.

AP This procedure should be performed only by physicians, advanced practice nurses, and other health care professionals (including critical care nurses) with additional knowledge, skills, and demonstrated competence per professional licensure or institutional standard (training usually obtained in an 8 hour Basic PICC class).

9. Frey AM: PICC complications in neonates and children, *JVAD* 4(2):2-11, 1999.
10. Chow LM, et al: Peripherally inserted central catheter (PICC) fracture and embolization in the pediatric population, *J Pediatr* 142:141-144, 2003.
11. Schwengel DA, et al: Peripherally inserted central catheters: a randomized, controlled, prospective trial in pediatric surgical patients, *Anesth Analg* 99:1038-1043, 2004.
12. Centers for Disease Control and Prevention. Guidelines for the prevention of intravascular catheter related infections, *MMWR Morbid Mortal Wkly Rep* 51(No.RR-10):1-29, 2002.

Additional Readings

Frey AM: Pediatric peripherally inserted central catheter program report: a summary of 4,496 catheter days, *J Intrav Nurs* 18(6):280-291, 1995.

Fry C, Aholt D: Local anesthesia prior to the insertion of peripherally inserted central catheters, *J Infus Nurs* 24(6):404-408, 2001.

Hruszkewycz V, et al: Complications associated with central venous catheters inserted in critically ill neonates, *Infect Control Hosp Epidemiol* 12(9):544-548, 1991.

Mupanemunda RH, MacKanjee HR: A life-threatening complication of percutaneous central venous catheters in neonates, *Am J Dis Child* 146:1414-1415, 1992.

Nour S, et al: Intra-abdominal extravasation complicating parenteral nutrition in infants, *Arch Dis Child* 72(3):207-208, 1995.

Puntis JW, et al: Staff training. A key factor in reducing intravascular catheter sepsis, *Arch Dis Child* 66(3):335-337, 1991.

Seguin JH: Right-sided hydrothorax and central venous catheters in extremely low birthweight infants, *Am J Perinatol* 9(3):1`i4-1'iR, 1992.

Trotter CW: Percutaneous central venous catheter-related sepsis in the neonate. An analysis of the literature from 1990 to 1994, *Neonatal Netw* 1996; 15(3).

P R O C E D U R E **156**

Aerosolized Medication: Metered-Dose Inhaler

P U R P O S E : A metered-dose inhaler (MDI) is used to administer medication for the treatment of asthma and other reactive airway diseases. The MDI delivers a high concentration of medication to the airways with few systemic side effects.

Phyllis Slutsky and Joel M. Brown II

PREREQUISITE KNOWLEDGE

- The six rights of medication administration: right patient, right route, right drug, right dose, right time, and right documentation
- Anatomy and physiology of the upper and lower respiratory tract
- Knowledge of medication to be delivered including desired response, side effects, and contraindications
- Knowledge of equipment assembly including use of the spacer with mouthpiece or mask attachment
- Spacer use is recommended with the MDI in children less than 12 years of age or older children unable to coordinate voluntary breath with activating the inhaler.
- Working knowledge of the parts of the ventilator circuit and dead space volumes of the circuit, when an MDI is used in a ventilator circuit.

CHILD AND FAMILY ASSESSMENT

- The child's medical history, including any medication allergies or adverse responses to medication ➻*Rationale:* Determines known contraindications to medication administration.
- For the child receiving ipratropium bromide, assess for peanut allergy ➻*Rationale:* The ipratropium MDI uses soya lecithin, from a legume related to peanuts, as a suspending agent. Individuals with a soy or peanut allergy

who received ipratropium experienced anaphylactic reactions.

CHILD AND FAMILY EDUCATION

Individualized, developmentally appropriate education is provided to the family and to the child based on desire for knowledge, readiness to learn, preferred language, and overall psychosocial state.

- Review the purpose of the medication, dosing frequency, equipment assembly and use, MDI administration techniques (proper breathing, etc.), cleaning equipment, and treatment response for home use. ➻*Rationale:* Child and family must have this information in order to continue therapy correctly and safely at home.
- Return demonstration of MDI medication administration with a placebo should be observed ➻*Rationale:* Ensures safe use of MDI at home.
- Encourage questions and answer questions as they arise ➻*Rationale:* Reinforcement of information is needed during periods of stress.

EQUIPMENT

- MDI
- Spacer with mouthpiece or mask attachment (mask sizes available: infant, small child, medium child, and adult)
- Stethoscope

Procedure for MDI Medication Administration

Steps	Rationale	Considerations

MDI Medication Administration for the Child with a Natural Airway
Use of an MDI with Spacer[1-4]

Steps	Rationale	Considerations
1. Explain to child and family the purpose and procedure for medication delivery. *(Level VI*)*	Proper explanation aids in child and family's cooperation and decreases anxiety related to the procedure.	Child's developmental level and family's reading level or preferred language barriers may influence comprehension.
2. Ensure the six rights of medication administration are correct. *(Level VI*)*	Facilitates correct medication administration and avoids errors.	Two identifiers should be used for patient identification per institution-specific protocol; most commonly name and birth date or name and medical record number are used.
3. Gather medication and needed supplies.	Preparation prevents delay, which may reduce the child's anxiety.	Depending on the age of the child a mouthpiece or mask with spacer may be used.
4. Assist child to comfortable sitting or semi-Fowler's position as tolerated.	Improves delivery of the medication to the lower airways.	
5. Wash hands before assembling equipment.	Standard precautions; decreases the transmission of microorganisms.	
6. Shake the MDI unit vigorously for 3 seconds.	Ensures the medication in the canister is mixed equally with the MDI propellant before aerosolizing.	
7. Insert the MDI into the spacer and attach the mouthpiece or mask. *(Level IV*)*	Use of a spacer increases the likelihood that the full dose of medication will be delivered to the airways.	Use of an MDI with a spacer is the recommended method of administration for children and adults.[1]
8. Instruct the child to exhale completely.	Increases medication delivery.	
9. Actuate the MDI (press down on the canister) once and advise the child to breathe in slowly and deeply.	Fills spacer chamber with medication and delivers dose.	
10. **For use with a mouthpiece** (Figure 156-1): Instruct the child to seal lips around the mouthpiece and take in a slow, deep breath.	Taking slow, deep breaths activates release of the medication from the spacer unit. A tight seal ensures that no medication escapes from the unit.	If a whistling sound is heard while the child is inhaling the medication, instruct the child to breathe slower.

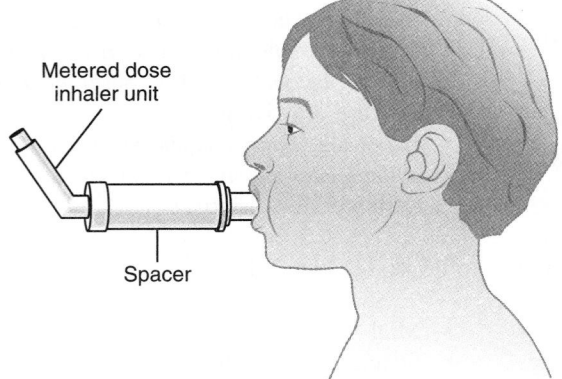

Metered dose inhaler unit

Spacer

FIGURE 156-1   Use of MDI with spacer and mouthpiece. *Extracted with permission from Living with Asthma, 2003 edition, a booklet published by Children's Hospital and Regional Medical Center, Seattle, WA.*

* Level IV: Limited clinical studies to support recommendations
Level VI: Clinical studies in a variety of patient populations and situations to support recommendations

Procedure for MDI Medication Administration—*Continued*

Steps	Rationale	Considerations

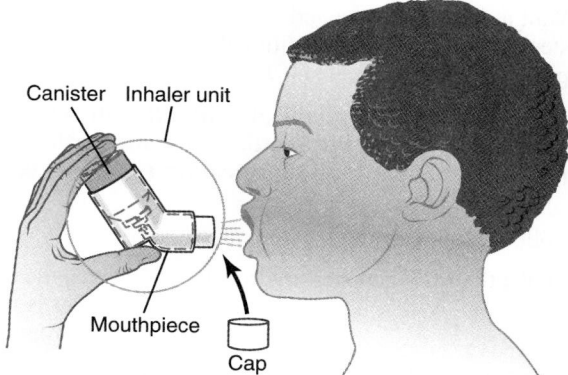

Masks are used for children who are developmentally unable to follow directions or keep the mouthpiece in the mouth.

For use with a mask (Figure 156-2):
Instruct the parent to hold the mask over the nose and mouth, making a tight seal. Hold the mask in place for at least six breaths.

The spacer unit has a vent to allow for normal breathing during medication administration.

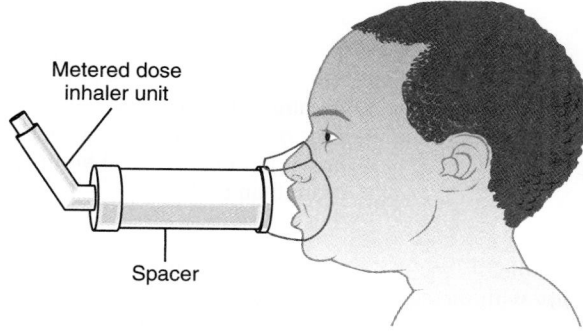

Metered dose inhaler unit

Spacer

FIGURE 156-2 Use of MDI with spacer and face mask. (*Extracted with permission from Living with Asthma, 2003 edition, a booklet published by Children's Hospital and Regional Medical Center, Seattle, WA.*)

Canister Inhaler unit

Mouthpiece

Cap

FIGURE 156-3 Use of MDI without a spacer.

11. Instruct the child to hold the breath while you count to 10. Then have the child release the breath and breathe normally. *(Level V*)*

Prolonged inspiration allows for optimal deposition of medication.

12. Wait at least 1 minute and repeat steps 8 through 11 for each additional prescribed puff. *(Level IV*)*

The medication needs a minimum of 1 minute to clear the respiratory tract.

Use of an MDI without Spacer
13. Follow steps 1 through 5 above.

Spacers are recommended for adolescents and adults to promote maximum medication deposition; however, there are adherence issues with older children in using spacers.[5]

14. Place medication canister in the mouthpiece and remove the cap (Figure 156-3).

Assembles equipment for correct delivery of medication.

15. Shake the MDI unit vigorously for 3 seconds.

Ensures the medication in the canister is mixed equally with the MDI propellant before aerosolizing.

16. Instruct the child to exhale completely.

Increases medication delivery.

17. Instruct the child to open the mouth and hold the inhaler with the mouthpiece just outside the mouth and pointing toward the back of the mouth.

Decreases amount of medication deposited on the lips, tongue, and teeth.

This positioning directs the aerosol away from the lips, tongue, teeth, and directs the medication to the back of the throat.[1,4]

Procedure continues on following page

* Level IV: Limited clinical studies to support recommendations
Level V: Clinical studies in more than one or two patient populations and situations to support recommendations

Procedure for MDI Medication Administration—*Continued*

Steps	Rationale	Considerations
18. Actuate the canister and instruct the child to take a single slow deep breath.	Administers medication dose.	
19. Instruct the child to hold the breath in as long as possible.	Breath holding will give the medication time to deposit in airways.	The goal is to have the child hold the breath for a count of 10.
20. Instruct the child to release the breath and breathe normally.		
21. Wait at least 1 minute and repeat steps 6 through 11 for additional prescribed puffs. *(Level IV*)*		
Use of an MDI with Mechanical Ventilation or Artificial Airway[6-12] **Delivery of MDI using the ventilator circuit (patients with tidal volumes greater than 500 mL and inspiratory times of 1 second or greater).**		Pressure-controlled and volume-controlled breaths are acceptable,[12] providing that the tidal volume is more than a 5L.
22. Follow steps 1 through 5 above.		
23. Shake the MDI canister vigorously.	Ensures the medication in the canister is mixed equally with the MDI propellant.	Review manufacturer's recommendations for amount of time canister should be shaken.
24. Insert the MDI into a cylindrical chamber-spacer located in the inspiratory limb just below the Y-adapter (Figure 156-4). *(Level IV*)*	Both in vitro and in vivo studies have shown that combination of an MDI and a chamber device results in four to six times greater deposition of aerosol than MDI actuation into a connector attached directly to the endotracheal tube or an in-line device that lacks a chamber.[3]	It is preferable to synchronize bronchodilator treatment with routine suction and care to decrease disconnections of the ventilator.[8]
25. Ensure that the ventilator breath is synchronized with the child's inspiratory effort.	Maximizes medication delivery.	If the child is not in synchronization with the ventilator, consider making adjustments to the ventilator settings or delivering the medication using a manual ventilation device (see step 30).
26. Actuate the MDI to correspond with the onset of inspiration by the child.[7]	Ensures maximum medication delivery into the airways.	

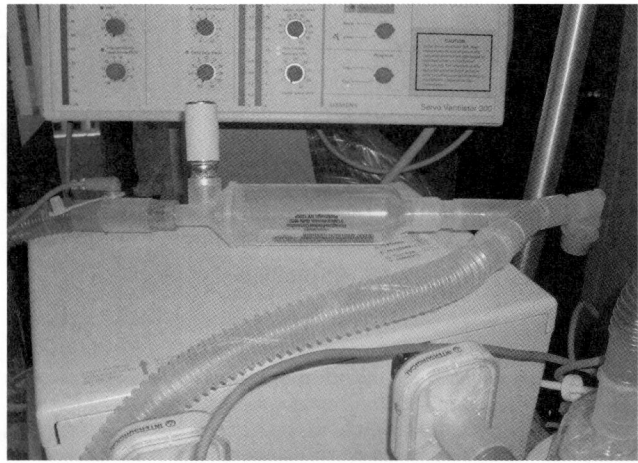

FIGURE 156-4   Placement of MDI and spacer in a ventilator circuit.

Procedure for MDI Medication Administration—*Continued*

Steps	Rationale	Considerations
27. Allow passive exhalation.	Allows appropriate gas exchange.	
28. Allow an additional five or six breaths.	Ensures that all of the medication has been delivered.	
29. Repeat actuation at 20 to 30 second intervals until the prescribed dose is delivered.	Allows the MDI to recharge to ensure consistent delivery of medication.	
Delivery of MDI using a manual resuscitation device.		
30. Shake the MDI canister vigorously.	Ensures the medication in the canister is mixed equally with the MDI propellant.	
31. Insert the MDI into a cylindrical chamber-spacer located in-line with the manual ventilation device. (*Level IV**)	Both in vitro and in vivo studies have shown that combination of an MDI and a chamber device results in four to six times greater deposition of aerosol than MDI actuation into a connector attached directly to the endotracheal tube or an in-line device that lacks a chamber.	It is preferable to synchronize bronchodilator treatment with routine suction and care to decrease disconnections to the ventilator.[8]
32. Connect the manual ventilation device and the cylindrical chamber-spacer to the artificial airway.	Assembles equipment for correct delivery of medication.	
33. Manually ventilate the child at the same rate and approximate volume or pressure delivered by the ventilator.	Ensures the child receives adequate ventilation during the procedure.	
34. Actuate the MDI to correspond with inspiration via the manual resuscitation device.[10]	Inspiration delivered should be 0.5 second or greater.	
35. Give an additional five or six manual breaths.	Ensures that all of the medication has been delivered.	
36. Repeat actuation at 20 to 30 second intervals until the prescribed dose is delivered.	Allows the MDI to recharge to ensure consistent delivery of medication.	

* Level IV: Limited clinical studies to support recommendations

Expected Outcomes	Unexpected Outcomes
• Child tolerates the medication prescribed without significant changes in vital signs • Child's breathing pattern and gas exchange improve	• Child experiences unanticipated dysrhythmias • Child exhibits no improvement in breathing pattern or gas exchange

Monitoring and Care of the Child

Activities and Interventions	Rationale	Reportable Conditions
1. Assess child's lung sounds, respiratory rate and effort, oxygen saturation values, and peak flowmeter readings as appropriate.	Compare baseline with posttreatment assessment to evaluate medication efficacy.	• No improvement from baseline or deterioration (may necessitate change in medication dosing)
2. Monitor electrocardiogram for heart rate and rhythm.	Tachycardia and other cardiac arrhythmias are side effects of bronchodilators.	• Significant increase in heart rate or any cardiac dysrhythmias

Documentation

- Name of medication administered, dose, time of administration, and child's response
- Respiratory assessment before and after MDI administration
- For mechanically ventilated children who receive medication dose via manual ventilation device, tolerance to being disconnected from the ventilator
- Child and family education
- Any anaphylactic reaction, and treatment of the reaction
- Unexpected outcomes and related treatment

References

1. Dhand R, Tobin MJ: Inhaled bronchodilator therapy in mechanically ventilated patients, *Am J Respir Crit Care Med* 156(1):3-10, 1997.
2. Guidelines for the Diagnosis and Management of Asthma Based on the Expert Panel Report 2: U.S. Department of Health and Human Services National Institutes of Health (1997), National Institutes of Health NHLBI, NIH Publication No. 97-4053.
3. Holt T: Ventilation for life: aerosol therapy during mechanical ventilation, *Am Assoc Respir Care Times,* July:18-24, 2000.
4. Scarfone, et al: Demonstrated use of metered-dose inhalers and peak flow meters by children and adolescents with acute asthma exacerbations, *Arch Pediatr Adolesc Med* 156:378-382, 2002.
5. Wong DL, et al: *Nursing care of infants and children,* ed 7, St. Louis, 2002, Mosby.
6. Asthma management in educational settings: taking asthma medications (2001). Retrieved February 2004 from www.cshcn. org/resources/AMES.htm, Children's Hospital and Regional Medical Center, Seattle, WA, AMES education project.
7. Dhand R: Basic techniques for aerosol delivery during mechanical ventilation, *Respir Care* 49(6):611-622, 2004.
8. Marik P, et al: A comparison of bronchodilator therapy delivered by nebulization and metered-dose inhaler in mechanically ventilated patients, *Chest* 115(6):1653-1657, 1999.
9. Nurses: partners in asthma care (1995, revised 1998), NIH Pub no. 95-3308, Bethesda, MD. Retrieved February 2004 from www.nhlbi.nih.gov/health/prof/lung/asthma/nurs.
10. Rubin BK, Fink JB: Aerosol therapy for children, *Respir Care Clin N Am* 7(2):175-213, 2001.
11. Piccuito, C et al: Albuterol delivery via tracheostomy tube, *Respir Care* 50(8): 1071-1076, 2005.
12. Hess, D et al: In vitro evaluation of aerosol bronchodilator delivery during mechanical ventilation: pressure-control vs. volume control ventilation, *Intensive Care Med* 29: 1145-1150, 2003.

Additional Reading

Guidelines for the diagnosis and management of asthma-update on selected topics, expert panel (2002) National Institutes of Health: NHLBI report retrieved February 2004 from www.nhlbi.nih.gov/suidelines/asthma/index.html.

Aerosolized Medication: Nebulized Medication

PURPOSE: Nebulization adds medication to inspired air by mixing particles of various sizes and using a delivery system that produces a jet of air to deliver the medication to the lungs

Cecilia Lang

PREREQUISITE KNOWLEDGE

- The six rights of medication administration: right patient, right route, right drug, right dose, right time, and right documentation
- Anatomy and physiology of the lungs and upper airways
- Indications for delivery of aerosols including airway inflammation, rhinitis, sputum collection, anesthesia, and antibiotic administration
- Common medications nebulized include saline, bronchodilators, steroids, and antibiotics
- Knowledge of medications to be administered including desired response, side effects, and contraindications
- Equipment assembly and use based on manufacturer recommendations and delivery device used
    - ❖ In-hospital use of equipment should be for single patient use only and disposable equipment should be changed at minimum once a week[1-4] *(Level V*)*
- Working knowledge of the parts of the ventilator circuit and dead space volumes of the circuit, when a nebulizer is used in a ventilator circuit
- Child development as it relates to clinical assessment and nebulized medication administration

CHILD AND FAMILY ASSESSMENT

- Baseline vital signs, respiratory assessment (including lung sounds and respiratory effort), and when indicated, peak flowmeter readings ➤*Rationale:* Provides baseline data to compare findings after treatment to monitor efficacy of medication delivery.[5]
- Determine appropriate delivery device based on assessment of child's age and ability to follow instructions, and presence of natural or artificial airway (e.g., endotracheal or tracheostomy tube) ➤*Rationale:* Selection of appropriate device is essential in providing effective delivery of medication to lungs. Artificial airways will require use of special equipment and procedures depending on various factors (tube size, ventilator, ventilator circuit, etc.).[1,5]
- Review medication order and compare with child's identifying information for six rights: patient, route, drug, dose, time, and documentation ➤*Rationale:* Reduces chance of drug administration error.
- Child's medical history, including allergies, known hypersensitivity to medication and other medications currently in use ➤*Rationale:* Influences how certain drugs will interact and which drugs are most appropriate for particular child's use.
- Child's and family's understanding of the reasons for and risks and benefits of nebulized medication administration ➤*Rationale:* Evaluates child's and family's understanding of the procedure and provides a gauge for ongoing education.

---

* Level V: Clinical studies in more than one or two patient populations and situations to support recommendations

- Child's or family's willingness to administer medication ➨*Rationale:* Provides opportunity for teaching and reinforcement of previous knowledge; assesses family's ability to continue care in the home.
- Child's developmental level and ability to interact ➨*Rationale:* These factors influence preparation of the child and interactions; assesses child's ability to follow directions for handheld versus mask delivery device.

CHILD AND FAMILY EDUCATION

Individualized, developmentally appropriate education is provided to the family and to the child based on desire for knowledge, readiness to learn, and overall neurologic and psychosocial state.

- Provide information on need for medication, dosing frequency, equipment assembly, troubleshooting, and methods of evaluating treatment response for home use of nebulizer therapy as appropriate ➨*Rationale:* Providing information decreases fear and anxiety; promotes safe and appropriate use of therapy in the home; provides child and family with symptoms to monitor for and to report to practitioner.
- Provide information related to side effects, administration techniques, and selection of appropriate delivery device based on age and cooperation of child (mask versus handheld for children less than 8 years)[1] ➨*Rationale:* Mask delivery indicated for a child if unable to follow instructions necessary for effective delivery of medication via handheld mouthpiece route.
- If child will receive nebulized medication at home, provide information on proper cleaning of equipment after treatment is complete: disassemble all parts of nebulizer and rinse each part in sterile water; shake off excess water, and allow to air-dry (hot soapy tap water for home use). Store in clean bag until next use.[1-4,6] Once a week (at home) nebulizer parts should be cleaned by soaking parts in a 1:1 solution of vinegar and water for at least 20 minutes or may soak overnight, then rinse with water and allow to dry.[1,3] *(Level V*)* ➨*Rationale:* Proper cleaning after each use decreases spread of and development of microorganisms. Sterile water has been recommended for in-hospital use for infection control related to respiratory disease transmission.[1,2,4] Tap water for home use is recommended, but may vary based on child's underlying health history (e.g., immunosuppressed, history of cystic fibrosis).
- Provide information on the importance of compliance with medication regimen for effective treatment[5] ➨*Rationale:* Providing information promotes compliance with therapy.
- Encourage questions and answer questions as they arise ➨*Rationale:* Reinforcement of information is needed during periods of stress.

EQUIPMENT

- Medication and diluent if needed (saline)
- Nebulizer with gas source (compressed oxygen or air) and reservoir for medication
- Flowmeter (for use in hospital)
- Connection tubing
- Mask or mouthpiece
- Stethoscope

---

* Level V: Clinical studies in more than one or two patient populations and situations to support recommendations

Procedure	**for Aerosolized Medication: Nebulized Medication**	
Steps	**Rationale**	**Considerations**
1. Ensure child and family understand procedure, including the purpose and procedure for medication delivery, and that questions are answered. *(Level VI*)*	Evaluates and reinforces understanding of previously taught information.	Developmental level, cognitive ability, and anxiety level will determine approach to and effectiveness of teaching.
2. Ensure the six rights of medication administration are correct. *(Level VI*)*	Facilitates correct medication administration and avoids errors.	Two identifiers should be used for patient identification per institution-specific protocol; most commonly name and birth date or name and medical record number are used.
3. Gather medication and needed supplies.	Prevents delay in medication delivery, which may decrease child's anxiety.	Supplies vary depending on device used (home machine versus hospital device), airway status (natural versus artificial airway) and child's age or developmental level.

* Level VI: Clinical studies in a variety of patient populations and situations to support recommendations

Procedure for Aerosolized Medication: Nebulized Medication—*Continued*

Steps	Rationale	Considerations
4. Wash hands.	Standard precautions; reduces the transmission of microorganisms.	
5. Assemble nebulizer equipment according to manufacturer's recommendations. *(Level I*)*	Facilitates effective delivery of medication.	Assembly may vary slightly by manufacturer model.
6. Assist child to comfortable sitting or semi-Fowler's position as tolerated by the child.	Promotes optimal lung expansion and maximal distribution of aerosolized particles to lung fields.[7,8]	Family may hold child upright in lap for optimal positioning as indicated.
7. Add prescribed medication and diluent if needed to the medication chamber of nebulizer.	Some medications are unit dosed and prediluted, whereas others may require diluent such as saline to ensure optimal drug delivery (check required fill volume for device used).[3]	If nebulized medication is delivered through a ventilator circuit, medication chamber is placed in-line in the inspiratory limb of the ventilator circuit.
8. Turn wall flowmeter to 6 to 8 L/minute or turn air compressor (for home use) on and ensure that a fine mist forms at mouthpiece or mask end of tubing.	Ensures that equipment is functioning properly.[5]	Gas source used and flow rate are determined by institution-specific protocol. Medication chamber must be upright in order for medication to be aerosolized.
9. If mouthpiece is used, instruct child to hold it with lips, using gentle pressure to form a seal around tip of mouthpiece. For face mask use, mask should be tight fitting and child should be instructed to breathe through open mouth. *(Level IV*)*	Correct fit with a tight seal around mouthpiece or face mask decreases loss of medication to air, ensuring delivery of prescribed dose. Inhaling through the mouth increases amount of medication delivered to lungs.	Infants and young children may be unable to breathe solely through their mouth. Blow-by treatments with a flexible tube may be used for infants who do not tolerate the mask on their face. However, with blow-by it is impossible to quantify the amount of medication delivered.[9] Allowing child to play with mask and equipment prior to use may decrease anxiety and promote cooperation.
10. Instruct older children to take slow, deep breaths through the mouth during treatment with occasional inspiratory holds for 10 seconds as tolerated.[1,3,9,10] *(Level V*)*	Increases optimal delivery of medication to lungs.	Medication deposition to lungs will vary in young children depending on their respiratory rate and depth of breathing during treatment.
11. Monitor child's heart rate periodically during treatment and discontinue treatment if significant rise in heart rate occurs. If child is on cardiac monitor, monitor for cardiac dysrhythmias.[1,3,5,7]	Tachycardia is a side effect of bronchodilators; it can lead to hemodynamic instability in small infants and children with cardiac disease.	Side effects usually subside shortly after treatment.
12. When the majority of medication dose is delivered, sputtering will occur in medication chamber. Tap sides of chamber to drop medication to the bottom of the chamber. *(Level IV*)*	Releases droplets of medication that may adhere to sides of medication chamber, increasing the volume of medication delivered.[1,3,5,6]	

Procedure continues on following page

* Level I: Manufacturer's recommendations only
  Level IV: Limited clinical studies to support recommendations
  Level V: Clinical studies in more than one or two patient populations and situations to support recommendations

Procedure for Aerosolized Medication: Nebulized Medication—*Continued*

Steps	Rationale	Considerations
13. Length of nebulization time should be 10 to 15 minutes on average. After sputtering occurs, continue treatment for 1 minute.[3] *(Level V*)*	Child/caregiver knowledge of length of treatment helps to increase compliance with treatment and identify when equipment may be malfunctioning.	Some medications such as antibiotics will have longer nebulization time due to the viscosity of liquid. Play or distraction during procedure may help child tolerate length of treatment.
14. When treatment is complete, turn off compressor or flowmeter and assess child's response to treatment (heart rate, respiratory rate, lung sounds, oxygen saturation values, and peak flow readings).[1,3,5]	Compare assessment findings with baseline assessment to evaluate treatment effectiveness.	For young children, it may be necessary to wait several minutes after treatment to compare heart rate and respiratory rate for accurate data because the treatment may have agitated the child.
15. Disassemble all parts of nebulizer and rinse each part in sterile water; shake off excess water and allow to air-dry.[1,2,4] Store in clean bag until next use. *(Level V*)*	Proper cleaning after each use decreases transmission and development of microorganisms.	Additional research is warranted to determine the most appropriate method for cleaning equipment. Refer to institution-specific protocol for cleaning recommendations.
16. Dispose of used supplies and equipment in appropriate receptacle.	Standard precautions; reduces transmission of microorganisms.	
17. Wash hands.	Standard precautions.	

* Level V: Clinical studies in more than one or two patient populations and situations to support recommendations

Expected Outcomes	Unexpected Outcomes
• Right medication and dose are administered to right child at right time via right route and is correctly documented	• Incorrect medication or dose administered • Medication administered via incorrect route • Medication administered at incorrect time or dose is missed • Medication is not delivered to correct child • Medication dose is not documented or is documented incorrectly
• Child's breathing pattern and gas exchange improve	• Child exhibits no improvement in breathing pattern or gas exchange
• Child tolerates treatment without significant change in vital signs	• Child experiences significant increase in heart rate or cardiac dysrhythmias
• Family or child demonstrates procedure for administering nebulized medication and verbalizes possible complications that could occur with machine (no mist or shorter nebulization time) as well as demonstrates proper cleaning of equipment	• Family or child is unable to demonstrate procedure for administering nebulized medication and cleaning of equipment
• Family or child verbalizes indications for medication, side effects, and frequency of administration	• Family or child is unable to verbalize indications for use of medication, side effects, and frequency of administration

Monitoring and Care of the Child

Activities and Interventions	Rationale	Reportable Conditions
1. Lung sounds, respiratory rate and effort, oxygen saturation values, peak flowmeter readings (for bronchodilator treatments).	Compares baseline with posttreatment assessment to evaluate efficacy of treatment.	• No improvement from baseline (may require change in dose or medication)
2. Oxygen saturation values, heart rate, and cardiac rhythm.	Tachycardia and cardiac dysrhythmias are side effects of many bronchodilator medications.	• Significant increase in heart rate or failure of heart rate to return to baseline after treatment
3. Child's tolerance of medication delivery.	Certain drugs or nebulized saline can cause bronchospasm in some children.[3]	• Any cardiac rhythm changes • Excessive coughing • Difficulty breathing • Stridor • Signs of increasing respiratory distress

Documentation

- Date and time medication administered
- Individual administering medication
- Child's response to treatment, including vital signs and lung assessment
- Child's tolerance or intolerance of medication delivery
- Child and family education
- Unexpected outcomes and related treatment

References

1. AARC Clinical Practice Guideline: Selection of an aerosol delivery device for neonatal and pediatric patients, *Respir Care* 40(12):1325-1335, 1995.
2. AARC Clinical Practice Guideline. Delivery of aerosols to the upper airway, *Respir Care* 39(8):803-807, 1994.
3. British Thoracic Society Nebulizer Project. Nebulizer therapy: guidelines [Electronic version]. *Thorax* 52 (Suppl 2):S1-S103, 1997.
4. Centers for Disease Control and Prevention: Guidelines for prevention of nosocomial pneumonia, *MMRW Morbid Mortal Wkly Re*p 46(RR-1):55, 1997.
5. Scanlan CL, et al, editors: *Egan's fundamentals of respiratory care,* ed 6, St. Louis, 1995, Mosby.
6. AARC Clinical Practice Guideline: Bland aerosol administration: 2003 revision and update. *Respir Care* 48(5): 529-533, 2003.
7. Earl B, Robbins P: Hand-held nebulizer therapy, *J Pediatr Nurs* 5(6):408-409, 1990.
8. Jacobs L: Nebulizers for children, *Advance for Nurses* 5(24):22, 2003.
9. Lee TM: Delivery devices for inhaled medications. In Grammer LC, Greenberger PA, editors: *Patterson's allergic diseases,* Philadelphia, 2002, Lippincott Williams & Wilkins.
10. Munzenberger P: Pharmacist consult: using nebulizers correctly, *Nursing* 25(4):22-25, 1995.

Continuous Intravenous Medication Infusion

P U R P O S E : To administer intravenous medications that must be delivered in large volumes or when constant plasma drug concentrations are required

Lorri Nielsen

PREREQUISITE KNOWLEDGE

- The six rights of medication administration: right patient, right route, right drug, right dose, right time, and right documentation
- Basic mathematics skills including addition, subtraction, multiplication, division; converting fractions to ratios, fractions to decimals, and decimals to percents
- Pharmaceutical math requires the nurse to know the three main systems of measurement (metric, apothecary, and household) and how to convert within these systems of measurement
- The ability to perform mathematical calculations to correctly administer medications and intravenous solutions to children
- Calculation errors with pediatric infusions can be fatal because the therapeutic range for neonates and children is very small.
- Body weight and body surface area are the most commonly used methods for determining pediatric drug dosing.
- Commonly encountered continuous infusion flow rates in pediatrics are expressed in terms of an infusion over a set time period including milliliters/hour (mL/hr), milligrams/minute (mg/min), milligrams/hour (mg/hr), micrograms/kilogram/hour (mcg/kg/hr) or micrograms/kilogram/minute (mcg/kg/min).
- When calculating flow rate (mL/hr) for medications the following must be known: the concentration of the infu-

sion, weight expressed in kilograms, the dosage to be given (i.e., mcg/kg/min, units/hour, mg/min, etc.) and that time is constant (60 minutes/hr).
- Properties of drug to be infused (mechanism of action, absorption, metabolism, excretion rate, route, and side effects).
- Infusion pumps are necessary when delivering continuous infusions to children; it is the nurse's responsibility to determine which solution set to use to deliver the required flow rate.
- Certain medications may require specialized tubing and/or filters

CHILD AND FAMILY ASSESSMENT

- History of allergies to medications, foods, or environmental allergens ➤➤*Rationale:* Knowing allergy history lessens the possibility of an allergic reaction to the medication.
- History of any kidney or liver disorders ➤➤*Rationale:* These conditions alter the metabolism and excretion of drugs.
- Age of the infant or child ➤➤*Rationale:* Neonates differ from children in their metabolism, absorption, distribution and excretion of medications.
- Fluid and electrolyte status ➤➤*Rationale:* Changes in the fluid and electrolyte status can alter the effects of certain medications.

- Height and weight ➥*Rationale:* Medication dosing is based on weight and/or body surface area.
- Child's and family's understanding of the reasons for and risks and benefits of continuous medication infusion ➥*Rationale:* Evaluates child's and family's understanding of the procedure and provides a gauge for ongoing education.

CHILD AND FAMILY EDUCATION

Individualized, developmentally appropriate education is provided to the family and to the child based on desire for knowledge, readiness to learn, and overall neurologic and psychosocial state.

- Inform the family of the name of the medication, its desired effects, and any possible side effects ➥*Rationale:* Providing information decreases anxiety; some medications may need to be discontinued due to lack of efficaciousness or unwanted side effects.

- If developmentally appropriate, explain to the child what sensations, if any, may be experienced during the infusion of the medication ➥*Rationale:* Providing information decreases fear and anxiety.
- Encourage questions and answer questions as they arise ➥*Rationale:* Reinforcement of information is needed during periods of stress.

EQUIPMENT

- Calculator
- Pen and paper
- Medication order
- Current pharmaceutical reference
- Medication to be administered
- Diluent, if required
- Appropriate intravenous tubing
- Infusion pump
- Alcohol wipes
- Possibly a stopcock, filter, and/or extension

Procedure for Continuous Intravenous Medication Infusion

Steps	Rationale	Considerations
1. Ensure child and family understand procedure and questions are answered.	Evaluates and reinforces understanding of previously taught information.	Developmental level, cognitive ability, and anxiety level will determine approach to and effectiveness of teaching.
2. To calculate drug dosages, convert the child's weight in pounds to kilograms (kg).	Kilograms are used to determine drug dosages because the metric system allows for more precise measurements.	The formula to convert weight in pounds to weight in kilograms is: Weight in pounds ÷ 2.2 = weight in kg.
3. When a drug is ordered in square meters, calculate the body surface area (BSA).	BSA is one of the most accurate methods for determining drug dosing in pediatrics.	To calculate BSA from a nomogram: • Find the child's height (in cm) in the height column. • Find the child's weight (in kg) in the weight column. • Using a ruler or straight edge, draw a straight line between these two values. • In the BSA column, note where the line intersects. This value represents the BSA in square meters.[1] See Figure 158-1 for an example of a nomogram.

Procedure continues on following page

Procedure   for Continuous Intravenous Medication Infusion—*Continued*

Steps	Rationale	Considerations

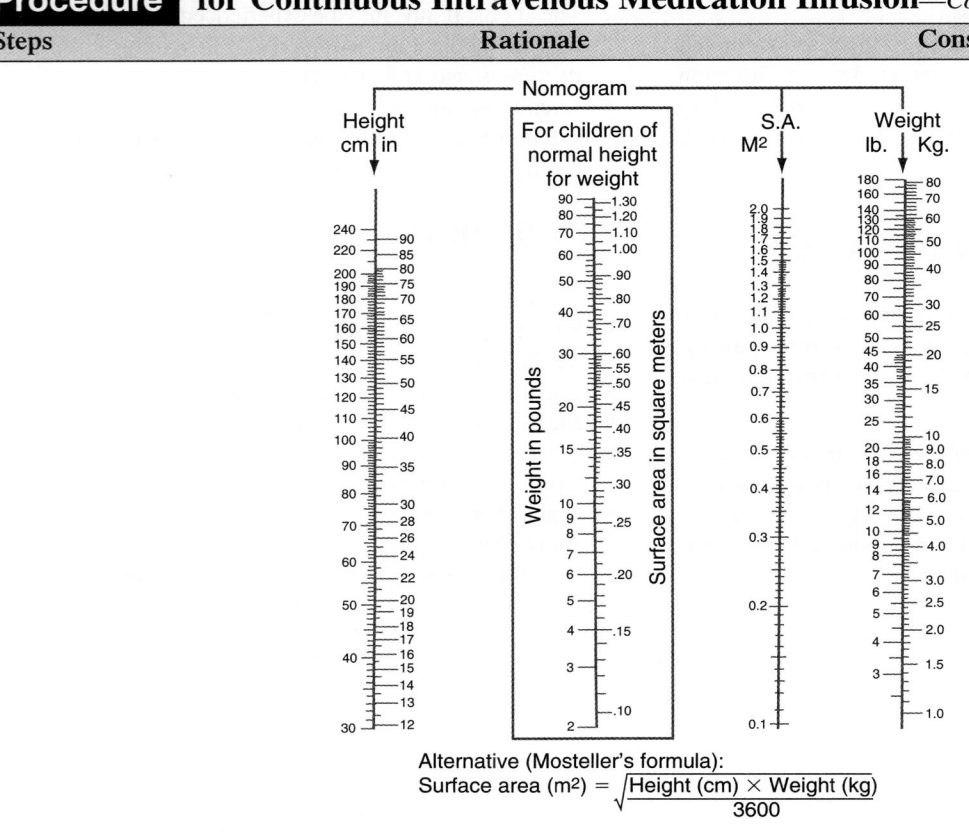

Alternative (Mosteller's formula):

$$\text{Surface area (m}^2) = \sqrt{\frac{\text{Height (cm)} \times \text{Weight (kg)}}{3600}}$$

FIGURE 158-1   The West nomogram for body surface area (BSA). *From: Berman RE, et al:* Nelson textbook of pediatrics, ed 17, Philadelphia, *2004, Saunders.*

4. Determine if the drug dose is within the recommended range based on body weight or BSA.

Accuracy when determining drug dosing is essential because the effects of medications given intravenously (IV) can be immediate and overdoses can be fatal.[1]

For example: a medication order reads cyclosporine 200 mg IV over 6 hours; the child weighs 20 kg.
Look up the recommended range for cyclosporine (5 mg/kg/day).
Calculate the recommended dose by multiplying the child's weight by the recommended dose (20 kg × 5 mg = 100 mg of cyclosporine/day).
The ordered dose is outside the recommended dosage range and must be clarified with the prescribing practitioner.

5. To calculate drug dosage using the ratio-proportion method, start with the drug information, the ratio of the **strength of the drug (H)** and the **volume of the drug (V)**. Place this information to the **left** of the equals sign. Next, set up a ratio for the dose desire, which is the relationship of the **dose ordered (D)** and the **amount to be given (G)**.

This method of determining drug dosing is very effective if the nurse remembers that a ratio is a comparison between two related items and a proportion is the equality of the two ratios.[1]

For example: a medication order reads cyclosporine 100 mg IV over 6 hours. The concentration of the drug is 50 mg/1mL. What is the volume that must be given to deliver 100 mg?

Procedure for Continuous Intravenous Medication Infusion—*Continued*

Steps	Rationale	Considerations
Place this information to the **right** of the equals sign.[1] This proportion is expressed as: H (mg)/V (mL) = D (mg)/G (mL) so that **H × G = V × D** Identify the unknown variable (either D or G) with an X.		The ratio-proportion would be set up as follows: 50 (mg)/1 (mL) = 100 (mg)/**X** (mL) so that 50 × **X** = 1 × 100 50**X** = 100 **X** = 2 mL of cyclosporine
6. Once the unknown variable has been calculated, determine if the answer calculated is correct by multiplying the product of the means (V & D) by the product of the extremes (H & G).	For a calculation to be correct, the product of the means (V & D) must equal the product of the extremes (H & G).	Using the above cyclosporine example, multiply the products of the means by the product of the extremes, which would result in the following equation: 1(mL) × 100 (mg) = 100 50 (mg) × 2 (mL) = 100 Because 100 = 100, the calculation is correct.
7. To calculate drug dosage using the formula method, the terminology remains the same; however, the formula is as follows: $$G(mL) = \frac{D\ (mg) \times V\ (mL)}{H\ (mg)}$$	The formula method, like the ratio-proportion method, is an effective method for determining drug dosing.	Using the above cyclosporine example, the equation for the formula method would look like this: $$X(mL) = \frac{100\ (mg) \times 1\ (mL)}{50\ (mg)}$$ $$X(mL) = \frac{100\ ml}{50}$$ The answer remains 2 mL of cyclosporine.
8. Use the following steps to calculate flow rates for continuous intravenous medication infusions: • Step 1: Use the ratio-proportion or formula method to determine the concentration of medication in 1 mL of fluid.	This step will be required in a formula used to determine IV flow rates.	For example: If starting a dopamine drip with a concentration of 200 mg of dopamine in 250 mL of D5W determine the amount of drug in 1 mL using the following formula: **Ratio-proportion method:** $$\frac{H\ (mg)}{V\ (mL)} = \frac{D\ (mg)}{G\ (mL)}$$ $$\frac{200\ (mg)}{250\ (mL)} = \frac{X\ (mg)}{1\ (mL)}$$ 200 mg = 250 mL X X = 0.8 mg/mL
• Step 2: If the dose ordered and the amount of medication in 1 mL are not in like amounts, convert these values to like amounts (i.e., if **mcg**/kg/min is dose ordered and the strength of the drug is in **mg**, convert mg to mcg).	To calculate flow rates, the doses must be in like amounts.	In the above example to convert 0.8 mg to mcg, multiply the number of mg by 1000 (move the decimal three places to the right). The final answer is: There are 800 mcg of dopamine in 1 mL of fluid.
• Step 3: If the infusion rate is based on body weight, determine the child's weight in kilograms.	This step is required in a formula used to determine the flow rate if the rate is based on body weight.	

Procedure continues on following page

Procedure for Continuous Intravenous Medication Infusion—*Continued*

Steps	Rationale	Considerations
• Step 4: Use the following formula to determine the flow rate ordered as a "unit"/kg/min: Dose in 1mL ÷ weight ÷ 60 (min/hr) = Amount of drug in 1 mL of fluid; then set up ratio proportion formula to determine the infusion rate.	This formula is used to determine the flow rate of medication expressed as a unit/kg/min.	Using the above dopamine example, in a 10-kg child if the desired dose is to infuse dopamine at 5 mcg/kg/min: 800 (mcg/mL) ÷ 10 (kg) ÷ 60 (min/hr) = 1.33 mcg/kg/min in 1 mL of fluid. Using ratio proportion to determine rate, $$H \times G = V \times D$$ $$1.33 \text{ mcg/kg/min} \times X = 1\text{mL} \times 5\text{mcg/kg/min}$$ $$X = \frac{1\text{mL} \times 5 \text{ mcg/kg/min}}{1.33 \text{ mcg /kg/min}}$$ $$X = 3.75 \text{ mL/min}$$
9. If a dose is ordered in a unit per kg of body weight per **hour**, use the above formula but omit the 60 (min/hr).	Because the dose ordered is expressed in terms of a unit/kg/**hr**, there is no need to multiply by 60 minutes.	The infusion will run at 3.75 mL/hr An example would be a morphine order to be infused at 50 mcg/kg/**hr**.
10. If a dose is ordered in a unit per minute, use the above formula but omit the **weight**.	Because the dose ordered is not based on body weight, there is no need to multiply by the weight in kilograms.	An example is amiodarone ordered at 0.5 mg/min.
11. A second nurse or clinical pharmacist independently performs the calculation.	Ensures that the dose and rate of the infusion are calculated correctly.	Independent verification requires that the second individual perform all calculations before comparing the results with the initial calculations.
12. Review the prescribing practitioner's order.	Ensures safe medication deliveryand minimizes the risk of medication errors.	Clarify any questions with prescribing practitioner.
13. Review information about the drug to be administered.	Knowing information such as thepurpose, action, peak onset, dosage, side effects, contraindications, and nursing implications minimizes incorrect medication delivery.	
14. Assess appropriate lab values.	Alteration in kidney and hepatic function can alter the metabolism and excretion of certain drugs.	This step is important with medications that depend on a balanced milieu (i.e., digoxin and potassium).
15. Review the child's allergy history.	Minimizes the risk of allergic reaction to medications.	
16. Assess for any potential drug-drug interaction.	Decreases the risk of interactions between different medications.	Especially important when giving medications metabolized via the cytochrome P450 pathway.
17. Ensure the six rights of medication administration are correct. *(Level VI*)*	Facilitates correct medication administration and avoids errors.	Two identifiers should be used for patient identification per institution-specific protocol; most commonly name and birth date or name and medical record number are used.

* Level VI: Clinical studies in a variety of patient populations and situations to support recommendations

Procedure for Continuous Intravenous Medication Infusion—*Continued*

Steps	Rationale	Considerations
18. Collect all necessary supplies and equipment.	Adequate preparation allows for initiation of the infusion in a timely manner.	
19. Wash hands.	Standard precautions; reduces the transmission of microorganisms.	
20. Assess the IV line for patency.	Ensures adequate delivery of the drug into the vascular system; prevents injury.	Some medications, such as those with a high osmolality, must be given via a central vein.
21. If required, reconstitute and/or dilute the medication.	Some medications come in a powdered form that requires reconstitution. Dilution of medications is often required before continuous infusion.	Use a current formulary or package insert to determine the amount and type of diluent to use and maximal concentration of the drug. Centrally infused and peripherally infused drugs may have different concentration requirements.
22. Inspect the solution for precipitates and for an expiration date.	If precipitates are present or if the medication is expired, discard the medication.	
23. Choose the correct tubing for the solution or medication being administered.	Certain medications may require specialized tubing (i.e., non–polyvinyl-chloride tubing must be used when administering nitroprusside).	
24. Prime the tubing according to the manufacturer's recommendations.	Prevents the administration of air into the vascular system.	Inspect the tubing for air, and remove any remaining air bubbles.
25. If indicated for medication to be administered via continuous infusion, ensure appropriate monitoring is in place.	Some medications administered via continuous infusion may affect heart rate or blood pressure.	
26. Wipe the injection port or stopcock with alcohol.	Aseptic technique minimizes the risk of infection.	
27. Connect the tubing to the IV access port or stopcock.	Allows for the administration of the medication into the vascular system.	
28. Administer the medication via an infusion pump according to manufacturer's instructions.	Continuous infusions must be administered via an infusion pump to ensure accurate delivery.	
29. Set the pump to infuse the medication at the correct rate and total volume to be infused.	Ensures the correct rate of medication administration.	Consider having a second nurse independently verify settings on the infusion pump.
30. Dispose of used supplies and equipment in appropriate receptacle.	Standard precautions; reduces the transmission of microorganisms.	Ensure that sharps are disposed of properly.
31. Wash hands.	Standard precautions.	

Expected Outcomes

- The medication infuses at the correct dose and the correct rate
- Right medication is administered to right child via right route and is correctly documented

- Therapeutic serum drug level is maintained

- Child remains free from local intravenous complications[1]

- Child remains free from systemic complications of intravenous therapy[1]

Unexpected Outcomes

- Miscalculation of intended drug dose or infusion rate

- Medication is not administered to the right child
- Medication is not administered via the right route
- Medication is not correctly documented
- Alteration in serum levels of medications related to alterations in metabolism and excretion
- Infiltration
- Phlebitis
- Thrombosis
- Ecchymosis or hematoma
- Sepsis
- Air embolism
- Allergic reactions
- Drug-drug interactions

Monitoring and Care of the Child

Activities and Interventions	Rationale	Reportable Conditions
1. Child's response to the medication.	Allows for the continuation of medications that are efficacious and the discontinuation of those that are not.	• Allergic reaction • Side effects of medications • Anaphylactic reaction to medication

Documentation

- Pertinent physical exam findings and changes during the course of treatment
- Name of the medication, concentration, dosage, time infusion started, rate, site of infusion, and total volume infused
- Child's response to medication
- Patency of vascular access device
- Significant laboratory values
- Child and family education
- Unexpected outcomes and related treatment

Reference

1. Hankins J, et al: *Infusion therapy in clinical practice,* ed 2, St. Louis, 2001, Saunders.

Additional Readings

Chernecky M: *Real world nursing survival guide: IV therapy,* St. Louis, 2004, Saunders.

Cieplinski-Robertson JA, et al: Administration of IV medications via soluset, *Pediatr Nurs* 29(4):283-286, 319, 2003.

Colby N, Kelly LE: Teaching medication calculation for conceptual understanding, *J Nurs Edu* 42(10):468-471, 2003.

Puryear L: Pharmacology math website, accessed October, 2005, from www.accd.edu/sac/nursing/math/default.html.

Taketomo CK, et al, editors: *Pediatric dosage handbook,* ed 12, Hudson, OH, 2005, Lexi-Comp, Inc.

Intradermal Injection

PURPOSE: To administer a very small amount of medication under the skin into the dermal layer

Kelly S. Finkbeiner

PREREQUISITE KNOWLEDGE

- The six rights of medication administration: right patient, right route, right drug, right dose, right time, and right documentation
- Intradermal injections are primarily used to perform desensitization or diagnostic skin testing; there is little absorption in the dermal layer and the injections usually produce only a localized reaction.[1-3]
- Anatomy and physiology of intradermal injection sites
- Concepts and principles of administering intradermal injections including aseptic technique
- Understanding of appropriate needle size, syringe size, and fluid amount to be administered intradermally
- Indications and contraindications to specific intradermal injections
- Patient safety, privacy, education, and comfort considerations when administering intradermal injections
- Ability to determine a positive from negative tuberculosis or allergy skin test
- Child development as it relates to clinical assessment and intradermal injection

CHILD AND FAMILY ASSESSMENT

- History of food, medication, or environmental allergies and the type of allergic reaction produced ➻*Rationale:* Many allergies may predispose a child to be allergic to the medication being administered. More caution must be taken when giving a child intradermal allergy skin testing if the child has had an anaphylactic reaction in the past. Personnel and equipment for treatment of an anaphylactic reaction must be available at the time of allergy testing.
- Medication that the child has taken in the past week ➻*Rationale:* Some medications can affect skin test result.[2]
- Child's developmental level and family's preferred learning method ➻*Rationale:* This will help the clinician educate using developmentally appropriate terms and appropriate teaching techniques.
- Child's and family's previous experience with intradermal injections ➻*Rationale:* This can affect how the child and family react to the procedure, and the clinician can address any issues. It also informs the clinician of any complications from previous intradermal injections or complications.
- Skin condition ➻*Rationale:* Identifies the most appropriate area for intradermal injection. It is important not to give intradermal injection where the child has skin breakdown as a result of an increased risk of infection or in an area with heavy hair or skin pigmentation because testing results may be difficult to assess.
- Child's ability to cooperate with the procedure and the family's desire to be present during or assist with the procedure ➻*Rationale:* This will determine if more assistance is required to prevent the child from being injured by unexpected movement during the procedure. Family members may provide comfort and support during the procedure but should have the choice not to remain with the child.
- Child's and family's understanding of the reasons for and risks and benefits of the procedure ➻*Rationale:* Evaluates child's and family's understanding of the procedure and provides a gauge for ongoing education.

CHILD AND FAMILY EDUCATION

Individualized, developmentally appropriate education is provided to the family and to the child based on desire for knowledge, readiness to learn, and overall neurologic and psychosocial state.

- Provide the family and child with appropriate verbal and written information about the medication including the purpose, why this route is preferred, possible side effects from the medication, and the intradermal injection ➤*Rationale:* It is important to give verbal and written information whenever possible because this reinforces the teaching and gives the family a resource.
- Inform the family of their exact role during the procedure. If family member has elected to participate, demonstrate the appropriate way to hold the child. ➤*Rationale:* Providing information will decrease their anxiety about their role in the procedure. It will prevent injury to the child and the caregiver. Family members should have the option not to participate in the procedure.

- If appropriate, educate the child about the procedure. Use developmentally appropriate words and avoid using words that may be viewed by the child as threatening ➤*Rationale:* Providing information decreases the child's anxiety and may increase cooperation during the procedure.
- Encourage questions and answer questions as they arise ➤*Rationale:* Reinforcement of information is needed during periods of stress.

EQUIPMENT

- Medication to be administered
- Eutectic mixture of local anesthetics (EMLA), Ela-max, or vapor coolant spray as prescribed or per institution-specific protocol
- Tuberculin syringe
- 25 to 27 gauge, ¼- to ⅝-inch needle
- Alcohol wipes
- Clean gloves
- Cotton ball or gauze pad
- Adhesive bandage
- Distraction equipment (books, toys, and bubbles)

Procedure for Intradermal Injection

Steps	Rationale	Considerations
1. Ensure child and family understand procedure and their role and questions are answered. Obtain consent when appropriate. *(Level VI*)*	Assesses and reinforces understanding of information and allows for any further questions or concerns.	Developmental level, cognitive ability, and anxiety level will determine approach to and effectiveness of teaching. Appropriate consent should be obtained for immunizations per institution-specific protocol.
2. Ensure that the six rights of medication administration are correct. *(Level VI*)*	Ensures correct medication administration and avoids errors.[1,3-6]	Two patient identifiers should be used for patient identification per institution-specific protocol; most commonly name and birth date or name and medical record number are used.
3. Wash hands.	Standard precautions; reduces the transmission of microorganisms.	
4. Select appropriate injection site: anterior aspects of the forearm, intrascapular area, anterior abdominal wall, or the inner aspect of the thigh. *(Level II*)*	Ensures injecting into the dermis.[1,3-6]	The forearm is the most commonly used site because of accessibility, decreased pain, less hair, and minimal pigmentation.[1] Other areas may be required for more extensive allergy testing.
5. Apply local anesthesia as appropriate per prescribing practitioner's order and manufacturer's instructions. *(Level IV*)*	Decreases pain at injection site.[7]	EMLA cream should be applied at least 30 minutes before injection. EMLA cream effectively decreases pain associated with skin testing and does not affect the potential indurations needed to determine if a test is positive.[7]

* Level II: Theory-based, no research data to support recommendations; recommendations from expert consensus group may exist
   Level IV: Limited clinical studies to support recommendations
   Level VI: Clinical studies in a variety of patient populations and situations to support recommendations

Procedure for Intradermal Injection—*Continued*

Steps	Rationale	Considerations
6. Gather needed equipment and supplies.	Prevents delays in performing the procedure that can increase child's anxiety level.	
7. Prepare and draw up the exact amount of medication required.	Required for medication administration.	When giving several intradermal injections mix and draw up all doses and properly label each syringe.[1]
8. Attach appropriate-sized needle to the syringe (25-27 gauge, ¼- to ⅝-inch needle). *(Level II*)*	Ensures medication is injected into the dermis with the least pain to the child.[1,3-6]	If the medication leaks onto the needle it should be wiped off with sterile gauze to prevent irritation from tracking medication through the dermis.[3,5] Changing a needle after drawing from a rubber membrane will decrease pain because the membrane dulls the needle, making it more difficult to penetrate the skin.
9. Position the child and begin to perform distraction measures. *(Level IV*)*	Proper positioning ensures child's comfort and allows the clinician to stabilize the area to ensure injection into the dermal layer. Distraction may help alleviate the child's anxiety and discomfort associated with the injection.[2,8]	It may help to stabilize the child's arm on a table or hard surface. Some distraction techniques involve books, bubbles, and toys.
10. Put on clean gloves.	Standard precautions; reduces transmission of microorganisms.	
11. Using friction, clean area with alcohol. *(Level II*)*	Alcohol is a skin disinfectant.	Clean a circular area approximately 5 to 8 cm.[1,6]
12. Allow skin to dry.	Decreases pain from introducing alcohol into the skin.[1,6]	
13. Pull skin taut with thumb and index finger.	Allows easy insertion of needle under the skin.[1,2,5,7]	
14. Insert needle bevel up at a 15-degree angle (Figure 159-1). *(Level IV*)*	Ensures that the needle is inserted into the dermal layer of the skin.[1,2,5,7]	Stop advancing the needle when the bevel is no longer in view.[1]

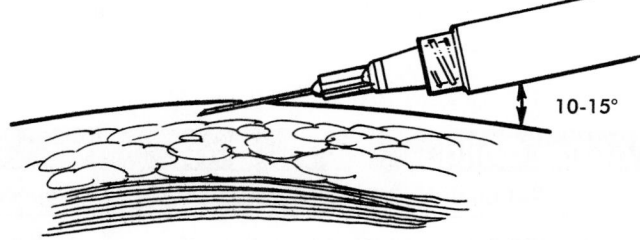

10-15°

FIGURE 159-1   Intradermal Injection sites. *From Wong DL, Hess C, editors:* Wong & Whaley's clinical manual of pediatric nursing, *ed 5, St. Louis, 2000, Mosby.*

Procedure continues on following page

* Level II: Theory-based, no research data to support recommendations; recommendations from expert consensus group may exist
Level IV: Limited clinical studies to support recommendations

Procedure | for Intradermal Injection—*Continued*

Steps	Rationale	Considerations
15. Inject medication slowly to produce a bleb or wheal.	Indicates the medication was properly injected into the dermis.[4,6]	If no bleb or wheal is noted remove needle and start again 2 inches from original site.[1]
16. Remove needle quickly and smoothly.	Decreases pain and prevents injury to the skin.[1,6]	When performing timed allergy testing be sure to note the time of the injection.
17. Apply light pressure at the injection site.	Prevents leakage of medication into the surrounding tissue.	Do not massage site because this may irritate the tissue and affect the test results.[1,6]
18. Assess injection site for complications and apply an adhesive bandage.	Allows identification of and interventions for any minor complications.	If applying multiple injections it is important to circle the site and label it to prevent confusion.[1] Tuberculosis skin test injection sites must be reassessed in 48 to 72 hours. An induration of greater than 5 mm requires further assessment to determine it is a positive skin test. Allergy skin test must be reassessed 15 to 20 minutes after application. Allergy tests are considered positive if the induration is greater than 5 mm.[9]
19. Praise child for positive behavior.	Provides a sense of accomplishment.	
20. Dispose of supplies and used equipment, including sharps appropriately.	Standard precautions; reduces transmission of microorganisms; protects personnel health.	
21. Remove gloves; wash hands.	Standard precautions.	

Expected Outcomes

- Medication produces a small bleb or wheal

- Medication produces an appropriate response and the child has no adverse reaction

Unexpected Outcomes

- Medication is administered too deep into the dermis or subcutaneous tissue; bleb or wheal is not produced
- Child has an allergic reaction to the medication
- Child has a systemic reaction to the medication
- Infection, bleeding, bruising, skin tear, or intense pain

Monitoring and Care of the Child

Activities and Interventions	Rationale	Reportable Conditions
1. Monitor injection site for response to medication or complications.	Facilitates prompt intervention for minor complications.[4]	- Positive skin test - Profuse bleeding - Indications of infection
2. Monitor for allergic reaction to the medication.	Child may develop an allergic reaction shortly after administration of the medication.	- Rash - Difficulty breathing - Seizures - Anaphylaxis
3. Assess for pain; give analgesics as indicated or prescribed.	Early identification of pain allows prompt treatment.	- Report of unresolved pain or discomfort - Continued irritability

Documentation

- Consent if obtained
- Child and family education
- Name of medication administered, dose, injection site, time of administration, and child's response
- Results of skin test
- Unexpected outcomes and related treatment

References

1. Grindel CG, et al: *Nursing procedures,* ed 3, Philadelphia, 2000, Springhouse.
2. Hill SL, Krouse JH: The effects of montelukast on intradermal wheal and flare, *Otolaryngol Head Neck Surg* 129(3):199-203, 2002.
3. Wong DL, Hess C, editors: *Wong & Whaley's clinical manual of pediatric nursing,* ed 5, St. Louis, 2000, Mosby.
4. Gilsenan I: A practical guide to giving injections, *Nurs Times* 96(33):43-44, 2000.
5. Hockenberry MJ, et al, editors: *Wong's nursing care of infants and children,* ed 7, St. Louis, 2003, Mosby.
6. McConnel EA: Do's & don'ts to administering intradermal injections, *Nursing* 30(3):17, 2000.
7. Sicherer SH, Eggleston PA: EMLA cream for pain reduction in diagnostic allergy skin testing: effects on wheal and flare responses, *Ann Allergy Asthma Immunol* 78(1):64-68, 1997.
8. Dahlquist LM, et al: Distraction for children of different ages who undergo repeated needle sticks, *J Pediatr Oncol* 19(1):22-34, 2002.
9. Burns CE, et al: *Pediatric primary care: handbook for nurse practitioners,* ed 2, Philadelphia, 2000, Saunders.

Intramuscular Injection

PURPOSE: To administer medication safely into the muscle below the subcutaneous layer

Kelly S. Finkbeiner

PREREQUISITE KNOWLEDGE

- The six rights of medication administration: right patient, right route, right drug, right dose, right time, and right documentation
- Anatomy and physiology of intramuscular (IM) injection sites
- Concepts and principles of administering IM injections, including aseptic technique
- Many medications must be injected intramuscularly to maximize the medication's therapeutic effect and minimize local reaction and injury.[1]
- The IM route is preferred for larger volumes because of the rapid absorption and low pain sensing nerves in the muscle.[2]
- Understanding of appropriate needle size, syringe size, and fluid volume per muscle size
- Indications and contraindications to specific IM injections
- Patient safety, privacy, education, and comfort considerations when administering IM injections
- Child development as it relates to clinical assessment and IM injection

CHILD AND FAMILY ASSESSMENT

- History of food, medication, or environmental allergies and the reaction produced ➤➤*Rationale:* Food allergies may predispose a child to be allergic to the medication being administered. Some immunizations contain eggs, shellfish, or other food products that can cause a child with a food allergy to have a reaction.

- Developmental level of the child's and the family's preferred learning method ➤➤*Rationale:* Facilitates education using developmentally appropriate terms and teaching techniques.
- Child's and family's experience with IM injections ➤➤*Rationale:* The child's and family's previous experience can affect how they react to this procedure, and the clinician can address any issues. It also informs the clinician of any complications from previous IM injections.
- Muscle mass and skin condition ➤➤*Rationale:* Determines the most appropriate area for IM injection. It is important not to give IM injections where a child has skin breakdown because of the increased risk of infection.
- Child's ability to cooperate with the procedure and the family's desire to be present during or assist with the procedure ➤➤*Rationale:* This will determine if more assistance is required to prevent the child from being injured by unexpected movement during the procedure. Family members may provide comfort and support during the procedure but should have the option not to remain with the child.
- Child's and family's understanding of the reasons for and risks and benefits of the procedure ➤➤*Rationale:* Evaluates child's and family's understanding of the procedure and provides a gauge for ongoing education.

CHILD AND FAMILY EDUCATION

Individualized, developmentally appropriate education is provided to the family and to the child based on desire for knowledge, readiness to learn, and overall neurologic and psychosocial state.

- Provide the family and child with appropriate verbal and written information about the medication including the purpose, why this route is preferred, possible side effects from the medication, and the IM injection ➥*Rationale:* Verbal and written information reinforces teaching and gives the family a resource.
- Inform the family of their exact role during the procedure. If family member has elected to participate, demonstrate the appropriate way to hold the child. ➥*Rationale:* Providing family with information will decrease their anxiety about their role in the procedure. It will prevent injury to the child and the caregiver. Family members should have the option not to participate in the procedure.
- If appropriate, educate the child about the procedure and why it is necessary. Use developmentally appropriate words and avoid using words that may be viewed by the child as threatening ➥*Rationale:* Decreases the child's anxiety and increase the child's cooperation during the procedure.
- Provide family and child with self-management techniques, for example, acetaminophen for fever and cool compresses for pain. Inform them when and how to notify a clinician about a problem ➥*Rationale:* Providing

information empowers the family and child to manage any minor effects from the IM injection and when/how to notify a medical professional if a problem arises.
- Encourage questions and answer questions as they arise ➥*Rationale:* Reinforcement of information is needed during periods of stress.

EQUIPMENT

- Medication to be administered
- Eutectic mixture of local anesthetics (EMLA), Ela-max, or vapor coolant spray as ordered or per institution-specific protocol
- Syringe
- Two needles, one filter needle, or small-gauge needle and one needle (21-25 gauge, ⅝-1½ inches) to administer the medication
- Alcohol wipes
- Clean gloves
- Cotton ball or gauze
- Adhesive bandage
- Distraction equipment (books, toys, and bubbles)

Procedure for Intramuscular Injection		
Steps	**Rationale**	**Considerations**
1. Ensure child and family understand procedure and questions are answered. Obtain consent when appropriate. *(Level VI*)*	Evaluates and reinforces understanding of previously taught information and encourages further questions or concerns.	Developmental level, cognitive ability, and anxiety level will determine approach to and effectiveness of teaching. Parental consent should be obtained for immunizations per institution-specific protocol.
2. Ensure that the six rights of medication administration are correct. *(Level VI*)*	Ensures correct medication is administered and avoids errors.[1-5]	Two patient identifiers should be used for patient identification per institution-specific protocol; most commonly name and birth date or name and medical record number are used.
3. Wash hands.	Standard precautions; reduces the transmission of microorganisms.	
4. Provide for appropriate privacy.	Some injection sites require exposure of the buttocks.	Privacy is an important consideration for school-aged children and adolescents.
5. Select appropriate injection site based on child's age, muscle mass, medication volume and viscosity. (Refer to Figures 160-1 through 160-4 and Table 160-1 for injection sites). *(Level VI*)*	It is important to select the most appropriate site that can safely accommodate the volume and viscosity of fluid being administered without causing injury to the child.[1-3,5,6]	The injection site selected affects how much fluid can be given and how quickly the medication will be absorbed.[1-3,5,6] Damage or scar tissue, poor muscle mass or tone, and accessibility may be contraindications to using a particular site[2] (Table 160-1).

Procedure continues on p. 1186

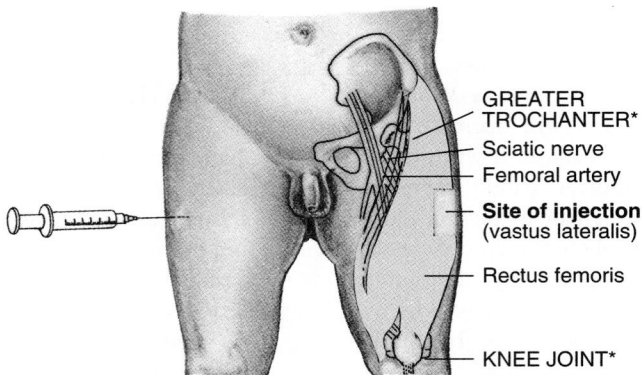

FIGURE 160-1   Vastus lateralis injection site. *(From Hockenberry MJ, et al, editors:* Nursing care of infants and children, *ed 7, St. Louis, 2003, Mosby.)*

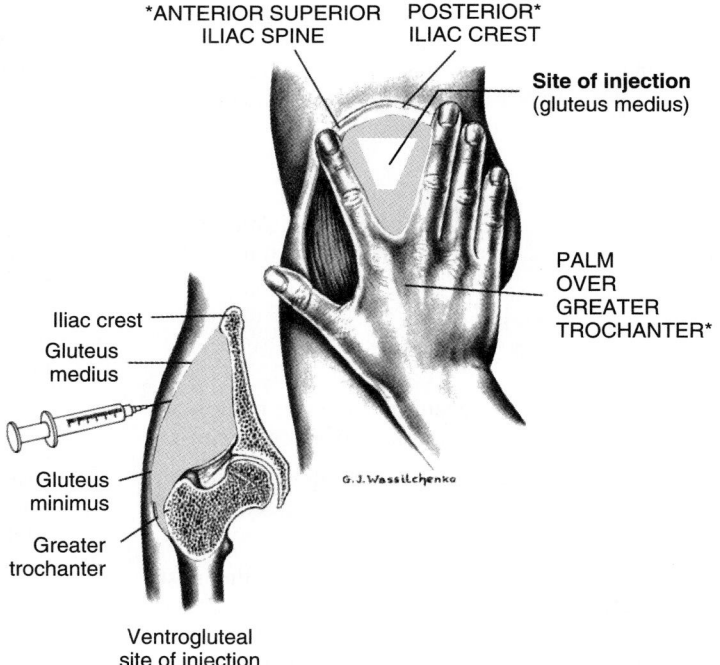

FIGURE 160-2   Ventrogluteal injection site. (Location indicated by asterisks.) *From Hockenberry MJ, et al, editors:* Nursing care of infants and children, *ed 7, St. Louis, 2003, Mosby.*

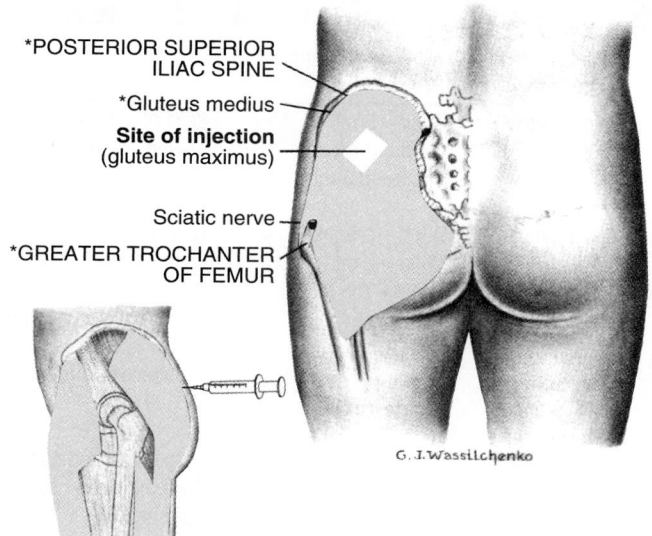

FIGURE 160-3 Dorsogluteal injection site. *From Hockenberry MJ, et al, editors:* Nursing care of infants and children, *ed 7, St. Louis, 2003, Mosby.*

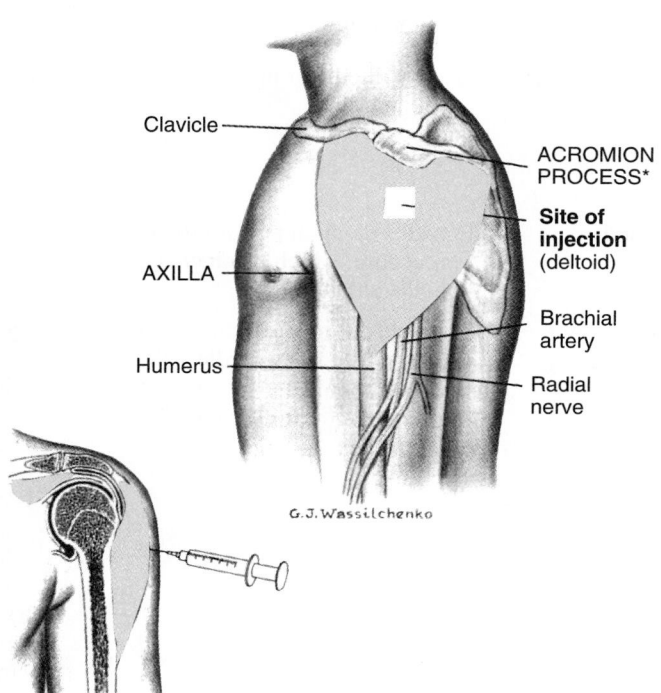

FIGURE 160-4 Deltoid injection site. (Locations indicated by asterisks.) *From Hockenberry MJ, et al, editors:* Nursing care of infants and children, *ed 7, St. Louis, 2003, Mosby.*

TABLE 160-1	Guidelines for Intramuscular Site Selection[1,2,4,5,7,10]				
Injection Site	**Patient Age**	**Needle Size**	**Maximum Fluid Volume**	**Advantages**	**Disadvantages**
Vastus lateralis	All ages	22-25 gauge ⅝-1 inch	Adult—5 mL Child—2 mL Infant—0.5 mL	Ease of access, no major blood vessels	Risk of sciatic nerve damage More painful than other sites
Ventrogluteal	All ages	22-25 gauge ½-1 inch	Adult—2.5 mL Child—2 mL Infant—0.5 mL	Low risk of complications Thin layer of subcutaneous tissue	Health care professionals less familiar with this site
Deltoid	More than 18 months	22-25 gauge ½-1 inch	All—1 mL	Faster absorption than other sites Less pain and reaction	Small muscle mass Small margin of safety with possible damage to radial and axillary nerves Low injection volume
Dorsogluteal	More than 3 years	20-25 gauge 1½ inches	Adult—5 mL Child—2 mL	Large muscle mass The child does not see the needle	Major nerves within the muscle Slow uptake of medication and thick adipose tissue Contraindicated in children who have not been walking for a year

Procedure for Intramuscular Injection—*Continued*

Steps	Rationale	Considerations
6. Apply local anesthesia as appropriate per manufacturer's instruction.	Decreases pain at injection site.[1,5]	EMLA cream should be applied at least 30 minutes prior to injection. Refer to institution-specific protocols for administration of local anesthetics.
7. Gather needed equipment and supplies.	Prevents delay in performing the procedure, which can increase child's anxiety level.	
8. Mix and draw up the exact amount of medication using a filter needle. (*Level VI**)	Required for medication administration; the filter needle will prevent drawing glass, rubber, or large particles into the syringe.[1,4]	Syringe size should be the smallest that will accommodate the volume being administered. Do not draw up an air bubble because it can decrease the accuracy of medication dose.[7] If a filter needle is unavailable, use a small-gauge needle and do not draw up all of the medication in the vial. Excess medication should be expelled from the syringe before injection.[2,7,8]
9. Attach appropriate-sized needle to the syringe. Refer to Table 160-1 for needle size and injection sites that are appropriate for child based on age.	Prevents tracking of the medication through the subcutaneous tissue.[1,5,7]	If medication leaks onto the needle, a sterile gauze should be used to wipe it off; this will prevent tracking medication through the tissue.[1,4,5]

* Level VI: Clinical studies in a variety of patient populations and situations to support recommendations

Procedure for Intramuscular Injection—*Continued*		
Steps	**Rationale**	**Considerations**
10. Position child and perform distraction measures. *(Level IV**)*	Proper positioning ensures child's comfort and allows the clinician to properly identify the site. Distraction may help alleviate the child's anxiety and discomfort associated with the injection.[9]	It is important to position the child to relax the muscle. Internally rotating the femur will relax the gluteal muscle. For the vastus lateralis site the child can sit on an adult's lap. The ventrogluteal site can be used with the child sitting, standing, lying supine or side lying.[1,7] Some distraction techniques involve books, bubbles, and toys.[9]
11. Put on clean gloves.	Standard precautions; reduces the transmission of microorganisms.	
12. Using friction, clean area with alcohol. *(Level II**)*	Alcohol is a skin antiseptic; decreases the risk of infection.[2]	Clean a circular area approximately 5 to 8 cm.[7]
13. Allow skin to dry.	Decreases pain from introducing alcohol into the subcutaneous tissue.[1,5]	
14. Pull skin laterally at injection site for Z-track technique or stretch skin. *(Level VI**)*	Increases the likelihood of administering the medication into the muscle. The Z-track method should be used on medications that are irritating to the tissue.[1,2,7]	When giving dextrose or diphtheria and tetanus toxoid, the Z-track method should always be used.[1] Initial research on applying manual pressure before injection has been shown to decrease pain in a small population of patients.[8]
15. Insert needle with a steady, smooth motion at a 90-degree angle to the skin. *(Level II**)*	Causes less displacement and shearing of the tissue, which decreases pain.[1,7]	If bone is hit, pull the needle back a small distance and wait 1 or 2 seconds and then inject the medication.[3]
16. Pull back on the plunger. *(Level VI**)*	Prevents injection of medication into a vein or artery.[1]	Pull back for 5 to 10 seconds to ensure that the needle is not in a low-flow blood vessel. If blood is noted in the syringe withdraw the needle, apply pressure at the site, and start again with a new needle, syringe, and injection site.[3,4,7]
17. Inject medication slowly at a rate of 1 mL per 10 seconds. *(Level II**)*	Allows muscle to stretch and accommodate the volume with less leaking into subcutaneous tissue.	
18. Remove needle and syringe quickly and smoothly. For retractable safety needle follow manufacturer's instructions. *(Level II**)*	Decreases pain and prevents injury to the tissue.	Some authors recommend waiting 5 to 10 seconds before removing the needle and syringe to allow the medication to diffuse into the surrounding muscle.[4,7]
19. Apply pressure at the injection site. *(Level II**)*	Prevents leakage of medication into the surrounding subcutaneous tissue.[1,5]	Do not massage the site. Use gauze, not an alcohol wipe, to prevent skin irritation.

Procedure continues on following pages

* Level II: Theory based, no research data to support recommendations: recommendations from expert consensus group may exist
Level IV: Limited clinical studies to support recommendations
Level VI: Clinical studies in a variety of patient populations and situations to support recommendations

Procedure for Intramuscular Injection—*Continued*

Steps	Rationale	Considerations
20. Assess injection site for complications and apply adhesive bandage.	Facilitates identification of and interventions for minor complications.	Notify the prescribing practitioner in the event of an injury. If applicable, reassess injection site in 2 to 4 hours for complications.
21. Praise child for positive behavior.	Provides a sense of accomplishment for the child.	Allow the child to express feelings after procedure is complete.[1]
22. Dispose of used supplies and equipment, including sharps, in appropriate receptacle.	Standard precautions; reduces transmission of microorganisms, protects personnel health.	
23. Remove gloves; wash hands.	Standard precautions.	

Expected Outcomes

- Right dose of right medication is administered to right child at right time via right route and is correctly documented
- Medication is administered into the muscle, with little discomfort to the child
- Medication is appropriately absorbed and the child has no adverse reaction to the medication

- Child demonstrates acceptable level of comfort after injection

Unexpected Outcomes

- Wrong dose, wrong medication, dose administered to wrong child, wrong time, wrong route of administration
- Medication is not documented
- Medication is administered into the subcutaneous tissue
- Local or systemic reaction to the medication
- Hematoma or abscess
- Infection
- Fibrosis of the muscle
- Glass particles injected into the muscle as a result of not using a filter needle
- Tissue damage due to movement of child during injection
- Nerve damage causing pain or paralysis
- Bone damage
- Contractures, palsy, peripheral nerve injury
- Neuropathy, bleeding, or bruising
- Persistent nodules
- Arterial puncture
- Permanent damage to sciatic nerve resulting in paralysis, fibrosis, or abscess
- Tissue necrosis and gangrene[1,2,5]
- Unmanaged pain

Monitoring and Care of the Child

Activities and Interventions	Rationale	Reportable Conditions
1. Monitor injection site.	Facilitates identification of and interventions for complications.[2]	<ul><li>Profuse bleeding</li><li>Loss of function at injection site</li></ul>
2. Monitor for allergic reactions to the medication.	Child may develop an allergic reaction shortly after administration of the medication.	<ul><li>Rash</li><li>Difficulty breathing</li><li>Seizures</li></ul>
3. Assess pain and give analgesics as prescribed or per institution-specific protocol; encourage family to use nonpharmacologic means to comfort and support the child.	Early identification of pain associated with the injection facilitates prompt treatment.	<ul><li>Report of unresolved pain or discomfort</li><li>Continued irritability</li></ul>

Documentation

- Consent as indicated
- Name of medication administered, dose, injection site, time of administration, individual administering medication, and child's response
- Child and family education
- Comfort assessment and any specific interventions provided
- Unexpected outcomes and related treatment

References

1. Hockenberry MJ, et al, editors: *Nursing care of the infant and child,* ed 7, St. Louis, 2003, Mosby.
2. Rodger MA, King L: Drawing up and administering IM injections: a review of literature, *J Adv Nurs* 31(3):574-582, 2000.
3. Gilsenan I: A practical guide to giving injections, *Nurs Times* 96(33):43-44, 2000.
4. Nicoll LH, Hesby A: IM injection: an integrative research review and guideline for evidence-based practice, *Appl Nurs Res* 16(2):149-162, 2002.
5. Wong DL, Hess C, editors: *Wong & Whaley's clinical manual of pediatric nursing,* ed 5, St. Louis, 2000, Mosby.
6. Diggle L, Deeks J: Effects of needle length on incidence of local reaction to routine immunization in infants aged 4 months: randomized controlled trial, *BMJ* 321(7266): 931-933, 2000.
7. Beyea SC, Nicoll LH: Administering IM injections the right way, *Am J Nurs* 96(1):34-35, 1996.
8. Chung JWY, et al: An experimental study on the use of manual pressure to reduce pain in IM injections, *J Clin Nurs* 11:457-461, 2002.
9. Dahlquist LM, et al: Distraction for children of different ages who undergo repeated needle sticks, *J Pediatr Oncol* 19(1):22-34, 2002.
10. Beyea SC, Nicoll LH: Administration of medications via the IM route: an integrative review of the literature and research-based protocol for the procedure, *Appl Nurs Res* 8(1):23-33, 1995.

Additional Readings

Taketomo CK, et al, editors: *Pediatric dosage handbook,* ed 12, Hudson, OH, 2005, Lexi-Comp, Inc.

Wexler DL, editor: *Needle tips and the hepatitis B coalition news.* 2004;14(1). St. Paul, MN: Immunization Action Coalition.

Intranasal Medication

PURPOSE: To administer medications via the nasal mucosa. Administration may be in the form of drops, sprays, ointments, jellies, or lotions.

Cecilia Lang

PREREQUISITE KNOWLEDGE

- The six rights of medication administration: right patient, right route, right drug, right dose, right time, and right documentation
- Anatomy and physiology of nasal passage and upper airway, including the location of sinus cavities
- Medications available as intranasal preparations include decongestants, antibiotics, anesthetics, pain medications, immunizations
- Indications for intranasal medication administration: nasal congestion; sinus problems; sedation; to anesthetize the nares for procedures
- Pharmacokinetics of intranasal medications because they can enter systemic circulation through nasal mucosa or the gastrointestinal tract if swallowed. Due to entry through nasal mucosa, drug does not pass through liver for breakdown and a larger percentage of medication reaches both desired and toxic sites of action (dosage for intranasal use may be less than or greater than other routes depending on the drug)[1]
- Contraindications to nasal medications including allergy and maxillofacial trauma
- Child development as it relates to clinical assessment and intranasal medication administration

CHILD AND FAMILY ASSESSMENT

- Age of child related to positioning needed for administration ➤➤*Rationale:* Infants and younger children may need assistance with positioning to ensure proper administration.

- Child's ability to lie supine and/or extend head if needed for administration ➤➤*Rationale:* Administration of drops requires head to be extended.[2] Positioning the child in a hyperextended position will prevent the strangling sensation caused by the medication entering the throat. Previous assessment of child's mobility ensures correct delivery method of medication as ordered.
- Condition of child's nasal passages (patency, mucosal breakdown, irritation, or drainage) ➤➤*Rationale:* Findings provide baseline to monitor effectiveness of medication. Excessive drainage or occluded nasal patency may interfere with effective medication absorption.
- Child's medical history of allergies and possible contraindications ➤➤*Rationale:* The child may have known contraindications for medication administration or substances used to administer medications, such as latex.
- Family's desire to be present during the procedure ➤➤*Rationale:* Family may provide support and comfort to their child, but should have the choice not to remain with the child.
- Family's ability to assist the child in cooperating with the procedure ➤➤*Rationale:* Family anxiety can decrease with participation. Additionally, intranasal medication may be continued following hospital discharge, and the nurse can ensure the family's ability to administer the medication.
- Age, height, and weight ➤➤*Rationale:* Medication dosing may be based on age, weight, and/or body surface area.
- Child's and family's understanding of the reasons for and risks and benefits of intranasal medication ➤➤*Rationale:* Evaluates child's and family's understanding of the procedure and provides a gauge for ongoing education.

CHILD AND FAMILY EDUCATION

Individualized, developmentally appropriate education is provided to the family and to the child based on desire for knowledge, readiness to learn, and overall neurologic and psychosocial state.

- Provide information to the family including indications for use, dose frequency, side effects, administration techniques, and sensations the child may experience during and after administration such as burning or stinging of nasal mucosa, itching or choking sensation if medication trickles down back of throat[3] ➥**Rationale:** Education decreases anxiety related to medication administration. Education related to use and administration will be needed for home administration.
- If appropriate, educate the child about the procedure. Use developmentally appropriate words, and avoid using words that may be viewed by the child as threatening ➥**Rationale:** Decreases the child's anxiety and may increase cooperation during the procedure.
- Encourage questions and answer questions as they arise ➥**Rationale:** Reinforcement of information is needed during periods of stress.

EQUIPMENT

- Prepared medication with administration device (dropper, spray, or syringe)
- Clean gloves
- Tissues
- Emesis basin
- Pillow (optional)
- Washcloth (optional)
- Suctioning equipment as needed

Procedure for Intranasal Medication

Steps	Rationale	Considerations
1. Ensure child and family understand procedure and questions are answered. *(Level VI*)*	Evaluates and reinforces understanding of previously taught information.	Developmental level, cognitive ability, and anxiety level will determine approach to and effectiveness of teaching.
2. Ensure the six rights of medication administration are correct. *(Level VI*)*	Ensures correct medication administration and avoids errors.	Two identifiers should be used for patient identification per institution-specific protocol; most commonly name and birth date or name and medical record number are used.
3. Gather needed equipment and supplies.	Prevents delay of medication administration, which can increase the child's anxiety level.	Supplies may vary based on child's age.
4. Wash hands; put on clean gloves.	Standard precautions; reduces transmission of microorganisms.	
5. Have child blow nose to clear passageway. For infants and toddlers, use bulb syringe to clear nares as indicated.[3]	Clearing nasal passage of secretions/mucus provides more effective medication delivery and absorption.	Infants and young children (<3 years of age) may require suctioning to adequately clear nasal passages. Ensure there are no contraindications to blowing nose such as increased intracranial pressure or maxillofacial trauma.
6. For nasal drops, shake container and draw up amount needed into dropper or pipette. *(Level I*)*	Ensures fine particles are mixed before administration.	

Procedure continues on following page

* Level I: Manufacturer's recommendations only
Level VI: Clinical studies in a variety of patient populations and situations to support recommendations

Procedure	**for Intranasal Medication**—*Continued*	
Steps	**Rationale**	**Considerations**

7. Place pillow under neck and shoulders and assist the child to tilt head over back edge of pillow.
 	
   For ordinary congestion, position the child semi-reclining with the head tilted toward the affected side.[4]
 	
   For ethmoid or sphenoid sinuses tilt head straight back.
 	
   For frontal or maxillary sinuses tilt head back and turn toward affected side (Figure 161-1).[3]
(Level II)*
	Correct positioning ensures medication is delivered to appropriate site of action. Hyperextension will help decrease the strangling sensation that the child may experience when the medication enters the throat.	Infants and children may need to be restrained to assume needed position. A position in which the head can be extended is optimal.[4]
		All paranasal sinuses are not developed at birth. Maxillary and ethmoid sinuses are present at birth, but not completely functional until late childhood to early adolescence.[5] Frontal and sphenoid sinuses are not functionally significant until early school age.[5] Although there are different stages of sinus development in children, younger children can suffer from sinus infections and discomfort.

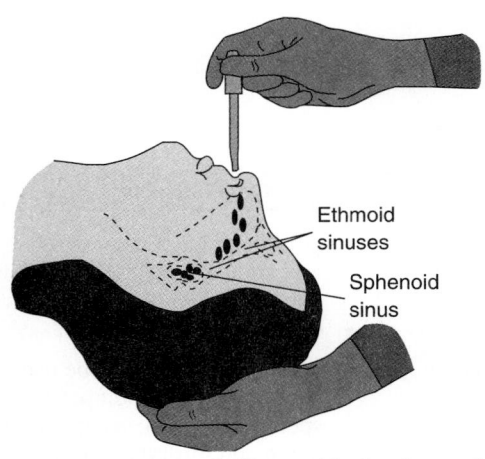
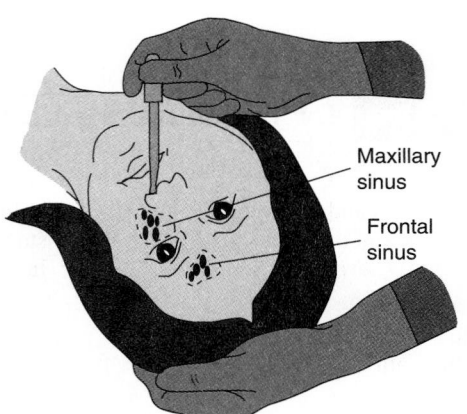

FIGURE 161-1   Patient positioning for nasal drops to sinus cavities. *From Perry AG, Potter PA, editors:* Clinical nursing skills and techniques, *ed 5, St. Louis, 2002, Mosby.*

8. Hold dropper ½ inch above nares and instill prescribed number of drops one side at a time or to affected side.[3] *(Level IV*)*	Keeping dropper above nares prevents contamination of dropper from nasal mucosa.[6]	In infants due to the small nares size, it may be necessary to place dropper ⅓ inch into nares.[4]
9. Instruct child to keep head tilted back for 3 to 5 minutes.	Aids in optimal absorption of medication and prevents leakage of medication from nares.	Hold infant or small child in position as long as tolerated.
10. Offer child a tissue to blot runny nose or wipe child's nares of any drainage; instruct child not to blow nose for several minutes. *(Level II*)*	Ensures maximum absorption of medication.	Instruct family not to blow child's nose for several minutes.
11. Keep emesis basin near the child and instruct him or her to expectorate any medication that drains into posterior pharynx or mouth. *(Level II*)*	Decreases amount of medication inadvertently delivered to the gastrointestinal tract.	Infants and young children may cough and gag during administration.

* Level II: Theory-based, no research data to support recommendations: recommendations from expert consensus group may exist
   Level IV: Limited clinical studies to support recommendations

Procedure for Intranasal Medication—*Continued*

Steps	Rationale	Considerations
12. For jelly or topical administration, place medication into nostril and instruct child to sniff into back of the nose.[1]	Ensures absorption of the medication.	Infants and young children may be unable to receive maximum benefits from this form of delivery; consider alternate routes.
13. Praise child and caregiver for positive behaviors.	Provides positive reinforcement.	
14. For nasal spray administration: follow steps 1 through 5 as above.	Preparation for both methods is the same.	
15. Shake bottle or canister as needed. *(Level I*)*	Some materials may be activated by shaking the bottle or canister.	
16. Hold head upright and press one finger against side of nose to close one nostril. *(Level II*)*	Aids in maximum inhalation of medication delivered to nostril.[7]	Infants should not have nares occluded for long because they are obligate nose breathers until 6 months of age.
17. Using right hand to hold bottle, insert tip of bottle into left nostril and squeeze bottle while inhaling. *(Level II*)*	Holding bottle in opposite hand aids in directing spray away from nasal septum and decreases irritation.[8]	For infants and young children, try to direct spray away from center of nose and spray either directly up and back, or toward outside of the nose.
18. Instruct child to try and hold breath for a few seconds and then exhale through mouth.[7] *(Level II*)*	Aids in delivery and absorption of medication.	Demonstrate to young children and have them practice before medication administration.
19. Repeat steps 15 through 18 with other hand and nostril.	Medication is delivered to both nostrils.	
20. Instruct child not to blow nose and to avoid sneezing immediately after medication administration. *(Level II*)*	Aids in effective delivery and absorption of medication.	
21. Rinse canister tip with hot water before replacing cap. *(Level IV*)*	Decreases contamination of tip with nasal flora, reducing the spread of microorganisms.	If using a canister for repeated use of saline sprays, the canister should be discarded and replaced on a regular basis to decrease the risk of contamination and infection.[6]
22. Discard used supplies and equipment in appropriate container.	Standard precautions; reduces transmission of microorganisms.	
23. Remove gloves; wash hands.	Standard precautions; reduces transmission of microorganisms.	Wash infant or child's hands if they were touching nares during or after procedure.

* Level I: Manufacturer's recommendations only
Level II: Theory-based, no research data to support recommendations: recommendations from expert consensus group may exist
Level IV: Limited clinical studies to support recommendations

Expected Outcomes

- Right dose of right medication is administered to right child at right time via right route and correctly documented

- Child is able to breathe easier through nose
- Nasal mucosa has decreased tenderness, swelling, and drainage
- Child experiences decreased sinus pain

- Child/family understands use of medication and side effects

- Child/family able to self-administer medication

Unexpected Outcomes

- Wrong dose, wrong medication, wrong route, wrong time of administration
- Medication is not documented
- Medication is administered to wrong child
- Child is unable to breathe easier through nose
- Nasal mucosa remains dry, swollen, irritated, and tender
- Child experiences nasal bleeding or complains of sinus pressure or headache
- Child/family does not understand use of medication and side effects. Child complains of stomach pain or gastrointestinal upset secondary to accidental swallowing of medication
- Child/family unable to demonstrate self-administration of medication

Monitoring and Care of the Child

Activities and Interventions	Rationale	Reportable Conditions
1. Monitor child for signs of respiratory distress (especially infants) during and immediately after administration.	Occlusion of nares or agitation in a distressed infant or child may increase an already existing respiratory compromise.	• Worsening signs of respiratory distress as evidenced by increased respiratory rate, heart rate, work of breathing, or decreased oxygen saturation value
2. Observe child for signs of side effects within 30 minutes after administration.	Systemic reactions may occur as the drug is absorbed through nasal mucosa.	• Signs of adverse drug reaction • Anaphylaxis
3. Monitor child for signs of improvement in nasal congestion and sinus pain.	Denotes efficacy of medication use.	• No improvement in symptoms
4. Monitor child for signs of nasal pain or nasal bleeding during medication use.	Improper administration or individual sensitivities may lead to these adverse reactions.	• Nasal bleeding necessitates the stoppage of medication for several days

Documentation

- Name of medication administered, dose, time of administration, individual administering medication, and child's response
- Child and family education
- Unexpected outcomes and related treatment

References

1. Gray MA: Intranasal administration of medications, *Orthop Nurs* 11(6):46-47, 1992.
2. McConnell EA: Clinical do's and don'ts: how to instill nose drops, *Nursing* 23(7):18, 1993.
3. Perry AG, Potter PA, editors: *Clinical nursing skills and techniques*, ed 5, St. Louis, 2002, Mosby.
4. Using drops and sprays, *RN*:64(1):Office nurse, 5-6, 2001.
5. Herendeen NE, Szilagy PG: Infections of the upper respiratory tract. In Behrman RE, et al, editors: *Nelson textbook of pediatrics*, ed 16, Philadelphia, 2004, Saunders, p. 1264.
6. Brook I: Bacterial contamination of saline nasal spray/drop solution in patients with respiratory tract infection, *Am J Infect Contr* 30(4):246-247, 2002.
7. Information from your family doctor. Nasal sprays: how to use them correctly, *Am Fam Phys* 62(12):2695-2696, 2000.
8. Practice pointers, *Nurse Pract* 23(12):86, 1998.

Intravenous Medication: Drip Method

PURPOSE: To deliver intravenous medications at a prescribed rate via gravity flow

Elizabeth M. Preze

PREREQUISITE KNOWLEDGE

- The six rights of medication administration: right patient, right route, right drug, right time, and right documentation.
- Ability to perform basic mathematics operations including addition, subtraction, multiplication, division, converting fractions to decimals
- Intravenous (IV) tubing drip factor, which is determined by the brand and type of IV tubing
- Properties of drug to be infused (mechanism of action, absorption, metabolism, excretion rate, route and side effects)
- Certain medications may require specialized tubing and/or filters.
- Principles of aseptic technique
- Child development as it relates to clinical assessment and IV medication administration

CHILD AND FAMILY ASSESSMENT

- History of allergies to medications, foods, or environmental allergens ➤*Rationale:* Knowing allergy history lessens the possibility of an allergic reaction to the medication or to substances used in medication administration, such as latex.
- History of any kidney or liver disorders ➤*Rationale:* These conditions alter the metabolism and excretion of drugs.
- Age of the infant or child ➤*Rationale:* Neonates differ from children in their metabolism, absorption, distribution, and excretion of medications.

- Fluid and electrolyte status ➤*Rationale:* Changes in the fluid and electrolyte status can alter the effects of certain medications.
- Height and weight ➤*Rationale:* Medication dosing is based on weight and/or body surface area.
- History of previous experience with receiving IV medications/fluids ➤*Rationale:* Family and child may already have knowledge or misconceptions of the process; this can help identify areas for further education.
- Type of IV access and patency of device ➤*Rationale:* Patent IV access is required for IV medication administration.
- Child's developmental level and ability to interact ➤*Rationale:* These factors influence preparation of the child and interaction.
- Child's and family's understanding of the reasons for and risks and benefits of the procedure ➤*Rationale:* Evaluates child's and family's understanding of the procedure and provides a gauge for ongoing education.
- Family members desire to be present during the procedure ➤*Rationale:* Family may provide comfort and support during the procedure but should have the choice not to remain with the child.

CHILD AND FAMILY EDUCATION

Individualized, developmentally appropriate education is provided to the family and to the child based on desire for knowledge, readiness to learn, and overall neurologic and psychosocial state.

- Provide information on the rationale for IV medications/fluids, and the importance of regulating IV flow rate to deliver fluids as ordered ➤➤*Rationale:* Providing information decreases anxiety and fear.

- Inform the family of the name of the medication, its desired effects, and any possible side effects ➤➤*Rationale:* Providing information decreases anxiety; some medications may need to be discontinued due to lack of efficacy or unwanted side effects.
- Provide information on nothing by mouth (NPO) status if IV fluids will be primary source of hydration ➤➤*Rationale:* Providing information may increase compliance with NPO status.
- Encourage questions and answer questions as they arise ➤➤*Rationale:* Reinforcement of information is needed during periods of stress.

EQUIPMENT

- Watch with second hand or timing device that measures seconds
- Calculator
- IV tubing with flow rate adjustment mechanism
- Volume control device (optional)
- IV solution or medication
- Labels to label and date IV fluid/medication
- Alcohol wipes
- Clean gloves

Procedure for Intravenous Medication: Drip Method

Steps	Rationale	Considerations
1. Ensure child and family understand procedure and questions are answered.	Evaluates and reinforces understanding of previously taught information.	Developmental level, cognitive ability, and anxiety level will determine approach to and effectiveness of teaching.
2. Ensure the six rights of medication administration. *(Level VI*)*	Lessens the chance of incorrect drug administration.	Two identifiers should be used for patient identification per institution-specific protocol; most commonly name and birth date or name and medical record number are used. Check child's weight in kilograms to determine if volume/dose prescribed/infused is correct.
3. Determine volume of medication to be administered and duration of infusion.	This information is needed to calculate flow rate.	
4. Determine drop factor of the IV tubing being used.	Drop factor is needed to determine drops (gtt)/mL.	Each brand of tubing has a specific drop factor, printed on product packaging. Macrodrip infusion set drop factor is typically 10 to 15 gtt/mL. Microdrip infusion set drop factor is typically 60 gtt/mL. Microdrip tubing with volume control device delivers fluid at rates less than 100 mL/hr. Macro drip tubing delivers fluid at rates greater than 100 mL/hr.

* Level VI: Clinical studies in a variety of patient populations and situations to support recommendations

Procedure for Intravenous Medication: Drip Method—*Continued*

Steps	Rationale	Considerations
5. Calculate the flow rate in gtt/min using the following formula[1]: $$\frac{\text{Volume to be administered in mL}}{\text{Administration time in min}}$$ $\times$ Drip factor in gtt/ml $$= \frac{\text{Number of gtt}}{\text{Minute}}$$	Once the volume to be administered, duration of infusion and the drop factor of the IV tubing is known, a formula can be applied to determine the correct flow rate in drops per minute.	Example: 200 mg of meropenem, total volume 10 mL, is to be administered over 30 minutes, using macrodrip tubing, which has a drip factor of 15 gtt/mL $$\frac{10 \text{ mL}}{30 \text{ min}} \times \frac{15 \text{ gtt}}{\text{mL}} = \frac{5 \text{ gtt}}{\text{min}}$$ 200 mg of meropenem, total volume 10 mL, is to be administered over 30 minutes, using microdrip tubing, which has a drip factor of 60 gtt/mL. $$\frac{10 \text{ mL}}{30 \text{ min}} \times \frac{60 \text{ gtt}}{\text{mL}} = \frac{20 \text{ gtt}}{\text{min}}$$
6. Gather needed equipment and supplies, including appropriate IV tubing (microdrip versus macrodrip).	Use of correct tubing ensures accurate delivery of IV medication.	Macrodrip tubing is used for delivery of higher infusion rates and volumes; microdrip tubing is used for delivery of slower rates and lower volumes.
7. Wash hands.	Standard precautions; reduces transmission of microorganisms.	
8. Put on clean gloves.	Standard precautions.	If the child has a latex allergy, be sure to use latex-free gloves.
9. Assess the IV line for patency.	Ensures delivery of medication into the vascular system.	Flush the child's IV catheter with 0.9% saline to determine patency before starting IV medication. Some medications, such as those with a high osmolality, may need to be given via a central vein.
10. Remove IV tubing and IV bag from packaging.	Required for setup of infusion.	
11. If tubing and fluid are to be set up, remove plastic covering on IV bag, clamp the IV tubing using roller clamp, and remove spike on IV tubing.	Prevents flow of fluid until system is set up.	Maintain sterility of IV tubing and IV bag.
12. Insert spike of IV tubing into IV bag.	Establishes fluid pathway.	
13. Hang IV bag from the IV pole at a level higher than the level of the child's IV. *(Level VI*)*	Required for gravity to assist with the flow of IV fluid.	
14. If microdrip tubing with volume control device is used, inject medication into volume control chamber.	Places medication in system.	

Procedure continues on following page

* Level VI: Clinical studies in a variety of patient populations and situations to support recommendations

Procedure for Intravenous Medication: Drip Method—*Continued*

Steps	Rationale	Considerations
15. Label tubing per institution-specific protocol.	Identifies presence of medication in tubing; identifies when tubing should be changed.	Frequency of tubing change is determined by institution-specific protocol and specific medication being administered.
16. Squeeze drip chamber to fill half full with IV fluid.	Prevents air from entering tubing during priming; if drip chamber is overfilled, drops will not be visible.	
17. Slowly open roller clamp on IV tubing and allow IV fluids to flow through tubing, clearing air bubbles during prime. *(Level I*)*	Slow flow through tubing decreases turbulence and clears air more effectively.	Gently tap on ports of IV tubing during priming to discourage air trapping. Assess for air bubbles in tubing before infusing fluids.
18. Reclamp roller clamp on IV tubing once IV fluid reaches the end of the tubing and IV tubing is completely primed.	Prevents continued flow of fluids.	
19. Check IV tubing closely for air bubbles and repeat steps 17 and 18 as necessary to remove air.	Prevents air embolus.	Avoid excess priming, which results in loss of medication.
20. Using aseptic technique, attach tubing to child's IV access. *(Level VI*)*	Necessary for administration of medication.	Refer to institution-specific protocol for means of attaching tubing (e.g., use of needleless access device).
21. Slowly release the roller clamp on IV tubing and count the drops for 1 minute. Adjust the roller clamp to increase or decrease the number of drops/minute until the desired number of drops/minute is reached.	Allows adjustment of flow rate until desired rate is achieved.	
22. Remove gloves; wash hands.	Standard precautions; reduces transmission of microorganisms.	
23. Monitor flow rate and volume administered throughout infusion.	Ensures medication is delivered over correct time frame.	
24. When medication infusion is complete, close roller clamp on tubing.	Stops flow of fluid.	
25. Remove empty medication bag and attach fluid for flush to tubing or, if volume control device is used, drop appropriate volume of flush solution into volume control chamber.[2] *(Level IV*)*	Clears medication from tubing, ensuring entire dose is administered.	Volume of fluid to be used for flush is determined by volume of tubing; a recent study done in the pediatric population demonstrated that a flush of two times the tubing volume was required to deliver more than 95% of a medication dose given via volume control device.[2] *(Level IV*)* Fluid and medication compatibility as well as institution-specific protocol determine fluid used for flush.

* Level I: Manufacturer's recommendations only
　Level IV: Limited clinical studies to support recommendations
　Level VI: Clinical studies in a variety of patient populations and situations to support recommendations

Procedure for Intravenous Medication: Drip Method—*Continued*

Steps	Rationale	Considerations
26. Slowly release the roller clamp on IV tubing and count the drops for 1 minute. Adjust the roller clamp to increase or decrease the number of drops/minute until the desired number of drops/minute is reached.	Allows adjustment of flow rate until desired rate is achieved.	
27. When flush has infused, close roller clamp.	Stops flow of fluid.	
28. Wash hands; put on clean gloves. *(Level VI*)*	Standard precautions; reduces transmission of microorganisms.	
29. If appropriate, disconnect tubing from child's IV access using aseptic technique; if tubing is to be used again, cap tubing end with a sterile cap.	Decreases incidence of infection.	
30. As appropriate to specific situation, saline or heparin lock IV access or resume IV fluid administration.	Ensures continued patency of IV access.	Refer to institution-specific protocol for maintenance of IV access.
31. Dispose of supplies and used equipment in appropriately.	Standard precautions; reduces transmission of microorganisms.	
32. Remove gloves; wash hands.	Standard precautions.	

* Level VI: Clinical studies in a variety of patient populations and situations to support recommendations

Expected Outcomes

- Right dose of right medication is administered to right child at right time via right route and correctly documented
- Medication is delivered over correct time period
- Child is free from complications of medication administration
- Child demonstrates acceptable level of comfort

Unexpected Outcomes

- Wrong dose, wrong medication, wrong route, wrong time of administration
- Medication is administered to wrong child
- Medication is not documented
- Medication infuses too quickly or too slowly
- Medication does not infuse
- Medication leaking at insertion site
- IV infiltration
- Pain related to medication administration

Monitoring and Care of the Child

Activities and Interventions	Rationale	Reportable Conditions
1. Monitor IV site for signs of infiltration: swelling, pain, inflammation, or erythema at site.	Close observation of IV site allows prompt identification of IV infiltration.	• IV infiltration • Pain at site
2. Observe child for signs of over-hydration or dehydration.	IV fluid may be infusing at the incorrect rate.	• Shortness of breath, tachycardia, restlessness, confusion, respiratory distress, and adventitious lung sound (crackles or rhonchi)
3. Monitor rate of medication infusion.	Ensures medication is administered at the correct rate.	• Medication not infusing or infused at the wrong rate
4. If child has not received medication before, observe child for indications of allergic reaction.	Close observation allows prompt identification of allergic reaction to new medications.	• Rash, hives, respiratory distress, edema, or any indications of allergic reaction

Documentation

- Appearance of IV site before and after medication infusion
- Volume of medication infused and rate of infusion
- Name of medication administered, dose, time of administration, individual administering medication, and child's response
- Child and family education
- Unexpected outcomes and related treatment

References

1. Pelletier G: Intravenous therapy calculations. In Hankins J, et al, editors: *Infusion therapy in clinical practice*, ed 2, Philadelphia, 2001, Saunders, pp. 362-374.

2. Ford N, et al: Administration of IV medications via soluset, *Pediatr Nurs* 29(4):283-286, 2003.

Intravenous Medication: Heparin Lock Method

P U R P O S E : To deliver intravenous medications via intravenous injection devices used for intermittent access

Lorri Nielsen

PREREQUISITE KNOWLEDGE

- The six rights of medication administration: right patient, right route, right drug, right dose, right time, and right documentation
- Knowledge of the different types of intravenous (IV) vascular devices
- Concepts and principles of administering IV medications including aseptic technique
- Awareness that different IV vascular devices may require different concentrations of heparin lock to ensure patency.
  - ❖ Studies in neonates, infants, and children have shown no significant difference in peripheral IV catheter longevity between those flushed with heparin 10 units/mL and those flushed with 0.9% saline.[1,2] *(Level V*)*
- Understanding of heparin's mechanism of action and side effects
- Knowledge of the signs and symptoms of heparin-induced thrombocytopenia (HIT)
- Child development as it relates to clinical assessment and medication administration via heparin lock

CHILD AND FAMILY ASSESSMENT

- Status of the vascular and hematologic systems ➤➤*Rationale:* Abnormalities of the vascular or hematologic system may predispose the child to thrombosis of the vascular device.
- History of bleeding tendencies or HIT ➤➤*Rationale:* Increases the risk of hemorrhagic or thromboembolic events.
- Current lab values ➤➤*Rationale:* Abnormal clotting factors or platelet count may place the child at an increased risk of hemorrhagic complications; severe thrombocytopenia is a contraindication to heparin lock therapy.
- History of food, medication, or environmental allergies and the reaction produced ➤➤*Rationale:* Allergies may predispose the child to be allergic to the medication being administered or to substances used in medication administration, such as latex.
- Child's age ➤➤*Rationale:* Neonates require preservative-free heparin.
- Child's developmental level and ability to interact ➤➤*Rationale:* These factors influence preparation of the child and interaction.
- Child's and family's understanding of the reasons for and risks and benefits of the procedure ➤➤*Rationale:* Evaluates child's and family's understanding of the procedure and provides a gauge for ongoing education.
- Family's desire to be present during the procedure ➤➤*Rationale:* Family may provide support and comfort to the child during the procedure but should have the option not to remain with the child.

** Level V: Clinical studies in more than one or two patient populations and situations to support recommendations

CHILD AND FAMILY EDUCATION

Individualized, developmentally appropriate education is provided to the family and to the child based on desire for knowledge, readiness to learn, and overall neurologic and psychosocial state.

- Provide the family and child with appropriate verbal and written information about the medication to be administered, including the purpose, why this route is preferred, possible side effects from the medication ➸***Rationale:*** Verbal and written information reinforces teaching and gives the family a resource.
- Provide information to the child and to the family (if developmentally appropriate) regarding the need for heparin flush and any potential side effects ➸***Rationale:*** Providing information decreases anxiety and fear.
- If appropriate, educate the child about the procedure, and why it is necessary. Use developmentally appropriate words, and avoid using words that may be viewed by the child as threatening ➸***Rationale:*** This will decrease the child's anxiety and increase the child's cooperation during the procedure.
- If developmentally appropriate, ask the child to remain still during the instillation of medication and heparin to prevent dislodgment of the vascular device ➸***Rationale:*** The vascular device may need to be replaced if it becomes dislodged during the procedure.
- Encourage questions and answer questions as they arise ➸***Rationale:*** Reinforcement of information is needed during periods of stress.

EQUIPMENT

- Heparin solution
- Medication to be administered
- 0.9% saline flush
- Alcohol swab
- Clean gloves

Procedure for Intravenous Medication: Heparin Lock Method

Steps	Rationale	Considerations
1. Ensure child and family understand procedure and questions are answered.	Evaluates and reinforces understanding of previously taught information.	Developmental level, cognitive ability, and anxiety levels will determine approach to and effectiveness of teaching.
2. Review the prescribing practitioner's order; ensure that the six rights of medication administration are correct. *(Level VI*)*	Ensures correct medication is administered and avoids errors.	Two identifiers should be used for patient identification per institution-specific protocol; most commonly name and birth date or name and medical record number are used.
3. Assess for potential drug interactions.	Decreases the risk of interactions between heparin and other medications.	Platelet inhibitors (e.g., aspirin and ibuprofen) should be used cautiously in children receiving heparin.
4. Gather needed equipment and supplies.	Facilitates completion of task in a timely manner.	
5. Wash hands.[3]	Standard precautions; reduces the transmission of microorganisms.	
6. Put on clean gloves.	Standard precautions.	
7. Clean cap or stopcock with alcohol swab for 30 seconds using friction.[3] *(Level VI*)*	Decreases risk of infection.	
8. Attach a flush syringe of 0.9% saline and gently flush to assess the IV line for patency.	Ensures delivery of the medication into the vascular system.	Determine patency before starting IV medication infusion. Some medications, such as those with a high osmolality, may need to be given via a central vein.

* Level VI: Clinical studies in a variety of patient populations and situations to support recommendations

Procedure	for Intravenous Medication: Heparin Lock Method—*Continued*	
Steps	**Rationale**	**Considerations**
9. Prepare medication for administration. After cleaning cap or stopcock with alcohol swab for 30 seconds, use aseptic technique and attach IV tubing to child's IV access.[3] *(Level VI*)*	Necessary for administration of medication.	Refer to institution-specific protocol for means of attaching tubing (e.g., use of needleless access device).
10. Administer medication.	Delivers medication to child per prescribing practitioner's order.	Medication may be administered via infusion pump, syringe pump, or gravity flow.
11. After initiating medication infusion remove gloves; wash hands.	Standard precautions; reduces transmission of microorganisms.	
12. When medication has been administered, turn off infusion device or stop gravity flow.	Stops flow of fluid.	
13. Wash hands; put on clean gloves.	Standard precautions.	
14. Disconnect IV tubing from IV access.	Allows access to IV catheter for flush and instillation of heparin.	
15. Clean cap or stopcock with alcohol swab for 30 seconds using friction.[3] *(Level VI*)*	Decreases the risk of infection.	
16. Attach syringe containing 0.9% saline and inject with enough volume to clear the device using pulsatile technique. *(Level IV*)*	Prevents clotting of the vascular device due to precipitation of heparin with incompatible medications. Pulsatile technique has been shown to be effective in maintaining patency of catheter.	Use the port closest to the child to prevent volume overload and excessive exposure to heparin.
17. Attach syringe and inject heparin solution per institution-specific protocol or prescribing practitioner's order. *(Level V*)*	Prevents clotting of the vascular access device.[4,5]	Heparin is available in 10 units/mL and 100 units/mL. Neonates should receive preservative (benzyl alcohol) free heparin to prevent the occurrence of gasping syndrome.[6] Concentration and volume of heparin used will vary based on size and type of catheter and frequency of device use.
18. Use positive pressure technique at completion of flush with one of two methods: *(Level IV*)* • Close the catheter clamp while infusing the last 0.5 mL of flush solution; remove syringe. • At completion of flush administration, apply pressure to the flush syringe plunger while closing the catheter clamp; remove syringe.	Positive pressure technique prevents backflow of blood into the catheter lumen at the completion of the flush, decreasing the risk of clot formation.	

Procedure continues on following page

Procedure continues on following page

* Level IV: Limited clinical studies to support recommendations
Level V: Clinical studies in more than one or two patient populations and situations to support recommendations
Level VI: Clinical studies in a variety of patient populations and situations to support recommendations

Procedure for Intravenous Medication: Heparin Lock Method—*Continued*

Steps	Rationale	Considerations
19. Dispose of used supplies and equipment in appropriate receptacle.	Standard precautions; reduces transmission of microorganisms.	
20. Remove gloves; wash hands.	Standard precautions.	
21. Repeat procedure each time device is used or per prescribing practitioner's order.	Maintains patency of vascular access device.	

Expected Outcomes

- Right dose of right medication is administered to right child at right time via right route and correctly documented

- Vascular access device remains patent
- Child is free from complications related to heparin administration

- Child demonstrates acceptable level of comfort

Unexpected Outcomes

- Wrong dose, wrong medication, wrong route, wrong time of administration
- Medication is administered to wrong child
- Medication is not documented
- Clotting or infiltration of vascular access device
- Development of complications (bleeding, gasping syndrome, or heparin-induced thrombocytopenia)
- Gasping syndrome
- Pain related to heparin administration or IV infiltrate

Monitoring and Care of the Child

Activities and Interventions	Rationale	Reportable Conditions
1. Monitor the IV access device for patency.	If access is not patent, new access will be required.	• Clotting of the vascular access device
2. Monitor IV site for signs of infiltration: swelling, pain, inflammation, or erythema at site.	Close observation of IV site allows prompt identification of IV infiltration.	• IV infiltration • Pain at site
3. Monitor for side effects of heparin.	Early identification of complications allows prompt treatment.	• Bleeding, bruising • Abnormal coagulation studies, decreased platelet count
4. If child has not received medication before, observe child for indications of allergic reaction.	Close observation allows prompt identification of allergic reaction to new medications.	• Rash, hives, respiratory distress, edema, or any indications of allergic reaction

Documentation

- Appearance of vascular access site
- Patency of vascular access device
- Signs or symptoms of bleeding
- Significant changes in laboratory values
- Family and child education
- Date, time, child's response, and dose of medication administered
- Concentration, volume, and time of heparin solution administered
- Unexpected outcomes and related treatment

References

1. Hanrahan KS, et al: Saline for peripheral intravenous locks in neonates: evaluating a change in practice, *Neonatal Netw* 19(2):19-24, 2000.
2. LeDuc K: Efficacy of normal saline solution versus heparin solution for maintaining patency of peripheral intravenous catheters in children, *J Emerg Nurs* 23(4):306-309, 1997.
3. Centers for Disease Control and Prevention: Guidelines for the prevention of intravascular catheter related infections, *MMWR Morbid Mortal Wkly Rep* 51(No.RR-10):1-29, 2002.
4. De Neef M, et al: The efficacy of heparinization in prolonging patency of arterial and central venous catheters in children: a randomized double-blind trial, *Pediatr Hematol Oncol* 19(8):553-560, 2002.
5. Rabe C, et al: Keeping central lines open: a prospective comparison of heparin, vitamin C and sodium chloride sealing solutions in medical patients, *Intens Care Med* 28(8):1172-1176, 2002.
6. Menon PA, et al: Benzyl alcohol toxicity in a neonatal intensive care unit, *Am J Perinatol* 1:288-292, 1984.

Additional Reading

Schmugge M, et al: Heparin-induced thrombocytopenia-associated thrombosis in pediatric intensive care patients, *Pediatrics* 109(1):1-4, 2002.

Intravenous Medication: Syringe Pump Method

P U R P O S E : To deliver intravenous (IV) medications when a small volume of medication is to be delivered over a prescribed amount of time

Elizabeth M. Preze

PREREQUISITE KNOWLEDGE

- The six rights of medication administration: right patient, right route, right drug, right time, and right documentation
- The ability to perform mathematical calculations (addition, subtraction, multiplication, division and converting fractions to decimals) used in administering medications to children
- Concepts and principles of administering medications on a syringe pump, including aseptic technique
- Ability to identify and calculate appropriate final concentration of IV medication for administration via syringe pump
  - ❖ Appropriate final concentration for an IV medication administered in a peripheral vein may be less than an IV medication administered in a central vein.
- Ability to program, load, and troubleshoot specific syringe pump being used to deliver the IV medication
- Patient safety, privacy, education, and comfort considerations when administering syringe pump medications
- Child development as it relates to clinical assessment and IV medication administration via syringe pump

CHILD AND FAMILY ASSESSMENT

- History of previous experience of having received an IV medication delivered on syringe pump ➼*Rationale:* Identifying any previous experiences may help to assess

child's and family's understanding or misconceptions, and identify areas for further education.
- History of allergies to medications, foods, or environmental allergens ➼*Rationale:* Knowing allergy history lessens the possibility of an allergic reaction to the medication or substances used in administration of medication.
- History of any kidney or liver disorders ➼*Rationale:* These conditions alter the metabolism and excretion of drugs.
- Age of the infant or child ➼*Rationale:* Neonates differ from children in their metabolism, absorption, distribution and excretion of medications.
- Fluid and electrolyte status ➼*Rationale:* Changes in the fluid and electrolyte status can alter the effects of certain medications.
- Height and weight ➼*Rationale:* Medication dosing is based on weight and/or body surface area.
- Child's and family's understanding of the reasons for and risks and benefits of medication infusion via syringe pump ➼*Rationale:* Evaluates child's and family's understanding of the procedure and provides a gauge for ongoing education.

CHILD AND FAMILY EDUCATION

Individualized, developmentally appropriate education is provided to the family and to the child based on desire for knowledge, readiness to learn, and overall neurologic and psychosocial state.

- Provide family and child, as developmentally appropriate, with rationale for the use of a syringe pump as well as IV medication being delivered ➤➤*Rationale:* Knowledge will help decrease fear and anxiety associated with new procedures and equipment.
- Provide family and child, as developmentally appropriate, with the purpose and potential side effects of medication being administered with the syringe pump ➤➤*Rationale:* Knowledge of the medication's purpose and potential side effects can help to identify potential adverse reactions early and facilitate appropriate interventions.
- Provide family and child with information about alarms and sounds produced by the pump, as well as staff response to these alerts ➤➤*Rationale:* Providing information about various alarms and alerts reduces child's or

family's anxiety related to unknown alarms and encourages child and family to notify staff when an alarm or alert occurs; reassurance that staff are attentive to alarms decreases anxiety.
- Encourage questions and answer questions as they arise ➤➤*Rationale:* Reinforcement of information is needed during periods of stress.

EQUIPMENT

- Syringe pump
- Appropriate IV tubing
- IV medication drawn up into syringe
- Alcohol wipes
- Flushes compatible with IV medication
- Clean gloves

Procedure for Intravenous Medication: Syringe Pump Method

Steps	Rationale	Considerations
1. Ensure child and family understand procedure and questions are answered.	Evaluates and reinforces understanding of previously taught information.	Developmental level, cognitive ability, and anxiety level will determine approach to and effectiveness of teaching.
2. Obtain IV medication drawn up into syringe compatible with syringe pump. (*Level I**)	Syringe pumps are programmed to work with specific brands of syringes.	Some syringe pumps can be programmed for different brands of syringes; when programming the pump, select the correct brand of syringe to ensure accurate delivery of medication.
3. Ensure the six rights of medication administration. (*Level VI**)	Lessens the chance of incorrect drug administration.	Two identifiers should be used for patient identification per institution-specific protocol; most commonly name and birth date or name and medical record number are used.
4. Assess for any potential drug interactions.	Decreases the risk of interactions between different medications and harm to the child.	Especially important when giving medications metabolized via the cytochrome P450 pathway.
5. Review child's allergy and medication history.	Promotes patient safety by avoiding inappropriate medication administration.	
6. Gather needed equipment and supplies.	Facilitates completion of task in a timely manner.	
7. Wash hands and put on clean gloves. (*Level VI**)	Standard precautions; reduces the transmission of microorganisms.	

Procedure continues on following page

Procedure for Intravenous Medication: Syringe Pump Method—*Continued*

Steps	Rationale	Considerations
8. Using aseptic technique, flush catheter to assess the patency of the IV.	Ensures that the IV medication will be delivered intravascularly.	
9. Attach medication syringe to tubing appropriate for syringe pump. *(Level I*)*	Tubing designed to fit the syringe is used to deliver the IV medication.	60-inch high-flow tubing holds 2.4 mL of fluid; 60-inch micro-volume tubing holds 0.5 mL of fluid. Refer to manufacturer's specifications. If different tubing is used, determine the volume of tubing before using with syringe pump to ensure accuracy of medication delivery.
10. Prime the tubing by applying pressure to the syringe plunger.	Prevents air embolus.	Ensure the tubing is primed with medication and is free of air.
11. Insert the syringe into the syringe pump according to manufacturer's directions.	Syringe must be seated in pump mechanism in order for medication to be delivered.	Be sure that the syringe is securely placed in the syringe pump.
12. Clean IV access port, cap, or stopcock with alcohol swab for 30 seconds using friction.[1] *(Level VI*)*	Decreases risk of infection.	Refer to institution-specific protocol for antiseptic solution used to clean IV access ports before access.
13. Using aseptic technique, connect the syringe pump tubing to the child's IV access.	Required in order to administer medication to the child.	
14. Program the syringe pump to deliver the medication at the prescribed rate; refer to manufacturer's instructions.	Ensures proper delivery of medication.	Refer to institution-specific protocol for independent verification of pump settings required if high-alert medication is being administered.
15. Start the pump and ensure medication is infusing.	Required for medication delivery.	
16. Discard used supplies and equipment in appropriate receptacle.	Standard precautions: reduces transmission of microorganisms.	
17. Remove gloves; wash hands.	Standard precautions.	
18. When medication infusion is complete, remove medication syringe from tubing and attach flush syringe with an appropriate amount of flush using aseptic technique; continue delivering medication at same rate until flush is administered.[2] *(Level V*)*	Ensures child receives the entire dose of medication at the prescribed rate.	Volume of fluid to be used for flush is determined by volume of tubing; a recent study done in the pediatric population demonstrated that a flush of two times the tubing volume was required to deliver more than 95% of a medication dose given via volume control device.[2] *(Level IV*)* Fluid and medication compatibility as well as institution-specific protocol determine fluid used for flush.

* Level I: Manufacturer's recommendations only
  Level IV: Limited clinical studies to support recommendations
  Level V: Clinical studies in more than one or two patient populations and situations to support recommendations
  Level VI: Clinical studies in a variety of patient populations and situations to support recommendations

Procedure for Intravenous Medication: Syringe Pump Method—*Continued*

Steps	Rationale	Considerations
19. When syringe pump indicates flush has been delivered, wash hands; put on clean gloves. *(Level VI*)*	Standard precautions; reduces transmission of microorganisms.	
20. Disconnect syringe pump tubing from IV line; if IV access is used intermittently, saline or heparin lock per institution-specific protocol. Refer to Procedure 163 for specific details.	Ensures continued patency of the child's IV access.	Studies in neonates, infants, and children have shown no significant difference in peripheral IV catheter longevity between those flushed with heparin 10 units/mL and those flushed with 0.9% saline.[3,4] *(Level V*)*
21. Discard used supplies and equipment in appropriate receptacle.	Standard precautions.	
22. Remove gloves; wash hands.	Standard precautions.	

* Level V: Clinical studies in more than one or two patient populations and situations to support recommendations
Level VI: Clinical studies in a variety of patient populations and situations to support recommendations

Expected Outcomes

- Right dose of right medication is administered to right child at right time via right route and correctly documented
- IV medication is delivered at desired rate
- Child is free from complications of medication administration
- Child demonstrates acceptable level of comfort

Unexpected Outcomes

- Wrong dose, wrong medication, wrong route, wrong time of administration
- Medication is administered to wrong child
- Medication is not documented
- Pump is not programmed correctly
- Syringe pump malfunction
- Medication leaking at insertion site
- IV infiltration
- Pain related to medication administration or IV infiltrate

Monitoring and Care of the Child

Activities and Interventions	Rationale	Reportable Conditions
1. Monitor syringe pump to ensure that the medication is infusing at the programmed rate.	Closely monitoring the syringe pump will allow for the detection of a malfunction of the syringe pump.	• Syringe pump malfunctions and does not deliver medication at rate programmed
2. Monitor IV site for complications related to IV medication administration; redness, swelling, pain, leaking of fluid at site.	Allows early identification of infiltration and prompt intervention, decreasing the risk of further sequelae at the site.	• IV infiltration • Extravasation of medication
3. Monitor child for adverse reaction to the medication being delivered.	Allows early identification and prompt intervention.	• Adverse drug reaction

Documentation

- Name of medication administered, dose, volume, time of administration, individual administering medication and child's response
- Appearance of the IV site before and after medication administration
- Comfort assessment and any specific interventions provided
- Child and family education
- Unexpected outcomes and related treatment

References

1. Centers for Disease Control and Prevention: Guidelines for the prevention of intravascular catheter related infections, *MMWR Morbid Moral Wkly Rep* 51(No.RR-10):1-29, 2002.
2. Ford N, et al: Administration of IV medications via soluset, *Pediatr Nurs* 29(4):283-286, 2003.
3. Hanrahan KS, et al: Saline for peripheral intravenous locks in neonates: evaluating a change in practice, *Neonatal Netw* 19(2):19-24, 2000.
4. LeDuc K: Efficacy of normal saline solution versus heparin solution for maintaining patency of peripheral intravenous catheters in children, *J Emerg Nurs* 23(4):306-309, 1997.

Additional Readings

Pelletier G: Intravenous therapy calculations. In: Hankins J, et al (eds): *Infusion therapy in clinical practice*, ed. 2, Philadelphia, 2001, Saunders, pp. 362-374.
Speakman E: Fluid, electrolyte and acid-base balances. In Potter PA, Perry AG, editors: *Fundamentals of nursing*, ed 5, St. Louis, 2001, Mosby, pp. 1229-1233.

Ophthalmic Medication

P U R P O S E : To safely administer an eye medication required to treat an infection or to provide lubrication[1]

Barbara A. Weintraub

PREREQUISITE KNOWLEDGE

- The six rights of medication administration: right patient, right drug, right dose, right route, right time, and right documentation
- Anatomy and physiology of the eye
- Concepts and principles of administering ophthalmic medications
- Signs and symptoms of various ophthalmic pathologies
- Indications and contraindications for specific ophthalmic medications
- Side effects of ophthalmic medications
  - ❖ Children are at greater risk for systemic side effects because dosing is not weight adjusted[2]
  - ❖ Side effects of antibiotic eye drops may include ocular irritation, contact dermatitis, hypersensitivity reactions, epithelial keratopathy, anaphylaxis[2]
  - ❖ Side effects of antiallergy eye drops may include ocular irritation, itching, taste alteration, eyelid edema, dry eye, dry mouth, dizziness, headache, cardiac arrhythmia[2]
  - ❖ Side effects of dilating and antiglaucoma medications may include tachycardia, bronchospasm, bradycardia, arrhythmias, somnolence.[2]
- Patient safety, privacy, education, and comfort considerations when administering ophthalmic medications
- Child development as it relates to clinical assessment and ophthalmic medication administration

CHILD AND FAMILY ASSESSMENT

- Presence of any exudates on the eyelids or eyelashes
  ➤*Rationale:* Exudates should be gently wiped away before administration of medication to prevent contamination of the eye itself.
- Appearance of the eye including erythema, swelling, or presence of foreign bodies ➤*Rationale:* The presence of these conditions may indicate the need to withhold the medication.
- Developmental level of the child and ability to interact ➤*Rationale:* These factors influence preparation of the child and interaction.
- History of previous experience of having received an eye medication ➤*Rationale:* Identifying any previous experiences may help assess child's and family's understanding or misconceptions, and identify areas for further education.
- History of allergies to medications, foods, or environmental allergens ➤*Rationale:* Knowing allergy history lessens the possibility of an allergic reaction to the medication and identifies need to avoid latex products or other substances.
- Child's and family's understanding of the reasons for and risks and benefits of eye medication administration ➤*Rationale:* Evaluates child's and family's understanding of the procedure and provides a gauge for ongoing education.
- Family's desire to be present during procedure ➤*Rationale:* Family may provide support and comfort measures to their child but should have the option not to remain with the child.
- Family's ability to assist the child in cooperating with the procedure ➤*Rationale:* Family anxiety can decrease with participation in the procedure. Additionally, eye medication may need to be continued following discharge from

the hospital, and the family's ability to correctly administer the medication must be assessed.

CHILD AND FAMILY EDUCATION

Individualized, developmentally appropriate education is provided to the family and to the child based on desire for knowledge, readiness to learn, and overall neurologic and psychosocial state.

- Provide information regarding the purpose of the medication and its expected outcome ➤*Rationale:* Providing information decreases anxiety and fear.
- Provide explanation regarding anticipated sensations or tastes associated with medication administration ➤*Rationale:* Providing information decreases anxiety and fear.

- Provide explanation to the child and to the family regarding the step-by-step procedure ➤*Rationale:* Providing information decreases anxiety and fear.
- If developmentally appropriate, explain how child can help assist with instillation of eye drops (e.g., playing a game like "peek-a-boo" or "open your eyes when I count to three") ➤*Rationale:* Medication instillation will be enhanced with cooperation of the child.
- Encourage questions and answer questions as they arise ➤*Rationale:* Reinforcement of information is needed during periods of stress.

EQUIPMENT

- Medication to be administered
- Clean gloves
- Sterile gauze

Procedure | for Ophthalmic Medication

Steps	Rationale	Considerations
1. Ensure child and family understand procedure and questions are answered.	Evaluates and reinforces understanding of previously taught information.	Developmental level, cognitive ability, and anxiety level will determine approach to and effectiveness of teaching.
2. Ensure child and family understand expected tastes and sensations during medication administration. Ensure the child and family understand why the ophthalmic route is the preferred route of administration.	Children can experience anxiety related to manipulation of eyes. Some eye medications can cause pain on instillation, or produce unpleasant tastes on drainage through the tear ducts into the nasopharynx.	Developmental level can influence understanding.
3. Gather needed equipment and supplies.	Facilitates completion of task in a timely manner.	
4. Wash hands.	Standard precautions; reduces transmission of microorganisms.	
5. Ensure that the six rights of medication administration are correct.	Lessens the chance of incorrect medication administration; eye and ear medications may be easily confused.	Two patient identifiers should be used for patient identification per institution-specific protocol; most commonly name and birth date or name and medical record number are utilized.
6. Ensure appropriate cardiorespiratory monitoring of child as appropriate for specific medication. *(Level II*)*	Some eye medications can cause a systemic reaction, such as decrease in heart rate or blood pressure if the eye drops drain down the nasolacrimal duct and are absorbed into the systemic circulation via the nasal mucosa.[2,3]	

* Level II: Theory-based, no research data to support recommendations: recommendations from expert consensus group may exist

Procedure | for Ophthalmic Medication—*Continued*

Steps	Rationale	Considerations
7. Put on clean gloves.	Standard precautions; reduces transmission of microorganisms.	
8. Assist child to a supine position.	Provides optimal access to conjunctival sac.	Infants, toddlers, and some older children may require assistance to remain immobile during the procedure. A second person may be needed to assist in immobilizing the child.
9. If crusts or drainage is present, gently cleanse from inner canthus to outer canthus.	Prevents microorganisms from entering lacrimal ducts or contaminating other eye.	
10. If child is able to cooperate, ask him or her to look at the ceiling.	Eye movement retracts sensitive cornea up and away from conjunctival sac and reduces stimulation of blink reflex.	Coach child in game of "peek-a-boo" or "opening eyes on count of three".
11. Expose lower conjunctival sac by placing the thumb or fingers of nondominant hand on the child's cheekbone, and rest the dominant hand on the child's forehead. Gently pull down with the nondominant hand (Figure 165-1). *(Level II*)*	Placement of the hands in this manner minimizes the possibility of touching the cornea, avoids putting pressure on the eyeball, and prevents the child from blinking or squinting.	
12. Approach the eye from medial side.	Decreases blink reflex.	
13. Hold medication 1 to 2 cm above the eye.	Helps prevent accidental contact of eyedropper with eye structure, reducing risk of injury to eye and transmission of infection to dropper.	

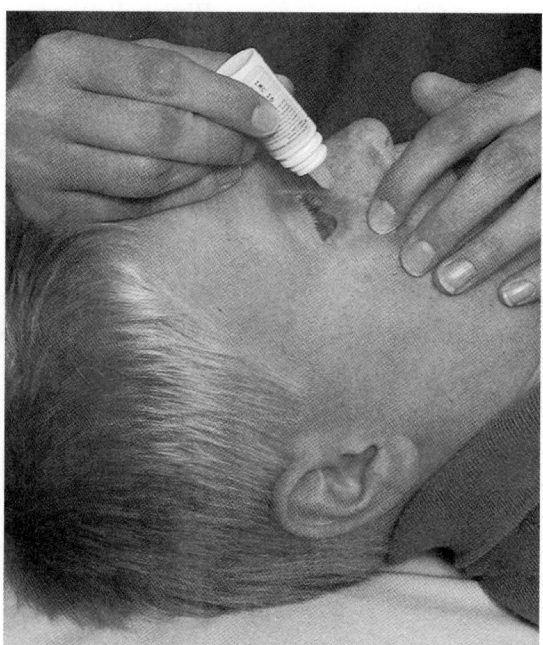

FIGURE 165-1   Administering eye drops. *Hockenberry MJ, et al:* Whaley & Wong's nursing care of infants and children, *ed 7, St. Louis, 2003, Mosby.*

Procedure continues on following page

* Level II: Theory-based, no research data to support recommendations: recommendations from expert consensus group may exist

Procedure for Ophthalmic Medication—*Continued*

Steps	Rationale	Considerations
14. Instill prescribed number of drops into exposed conjunctival sac.	The conjunctival sac normally holds 1 or 2 drops. Instillation into conjunctival sac provides even distribution across the eye.	If the child clenches the eyes tightly, instill the drops into the medial corner of the closed eye. The medication will pool in this area, and will flow onto the conjunctiva when the eye is opened.[2] *(Level IV*)*
15. Apply pressure to the nasolacrimal duct for at least 30 seconds.[3,4] *(Level III*)*	Prevents medication from draining through duct to nasal mucosa, thus preventing possible systemic absorption.	For medications with significant effect if absorbed systemically, applying pressure for up to 3 minutes is recommended.[3]
16. For ophthalmic ointment, squeeze 2 cm of ointment into the conjunctival sac, from inner canthus to outer canthus.	Avoids damaging sensitive cornea.	
17. Have the child gently close eye.	Closing the eye spreads the medication over the entire eye.	
18. Discard used supplies and equipment in appropriate receptacle.	Standard precautions; reduces transmission of microorganisms.	
19. Remove gloves; wash hands.	Standard precautions.	

* Level III: Laboratory data, no clinical data to support recommendations
Level IV: Limited clinical studies to support recommendations

Expected Outcomes

- Right dose of right medication is administered to right child at right time via right route and correctly documented

- Medication delivered to lower conjunctival sac
- Medication effects limited to eye only
- Eye remains free from injury

Unexpected Outcomes

- Medication is administered to wrong child
- Wrong dose, wrong medication, wrong route, wrong time of administration
- Medication is not documented
- Medication delivered outside conjunctival sac
- Medication produces systemic effects
- Injury to eye during medication administration due to child's agitation

Monitoring and Care of the Child

Activities and Interventions	Rationale	Reportable Conditions
1. Monitor child for systemic effects of medication.	Some eye medications can cause a systemic reaction, such as decrease in heart rate or blood pressure if the eye drops drain down the nasolacrimal duct and are absorbed into the systemic circulation.[2,3]	• Change in vital signs or level of consciousness • Bradycardia • Dysrhythmias
2. Monitor child for adverse reaction to the medication being delivered.	Allows early identification and prompt intervention.	• Adverse drug reaction • Allergic response to medication • Unable to administer medication because of extreme anxiety
3. Monitor child's tolerance of the procedure; use developmental strategies to help child tolerate procedure. If available, consider including Child Life Therapist.	Children may be very anxious during manipulation of the eyes and have difficulty tolerating the procedure.	

Documentation

- Initial assessment of eye
- Name of medication administered, eye(s) dosed, dosage, time of administration, individual administering medication, and child's response
- Child and family education
- Unexpected outcomes and related treatment

References

1. Kozier B, et al: Integral components of client care: medications. In *Fundamentals of nursing: concepts, process and practice*, ed 7, New Jersey: Upper Saddle River, 2004, Prentice-Hall
2. Wallace DK, Steinkuller PG: Ocular medications in children, *Clin Pediatr* 37(11):645-652, 1998.
3. Levy Y, Zadok D: Systemic side effects of ophthalmic drops, *Clin Pediatr* 43(1):99-101, 2004.
4. Taketomo CK, et al, editors: *Pediatric dosage handbook,* ed 12, Hudson, OH, 2005, Lexi-Comp, Inc.

Additional Reading

Wong DL, et al: *Whaley & Wong's nursing care of infants and children,* ed 6, St. Louis, 1999, Mosby.

Oral Medication

PURPOSE: To deliver medications to alert, awake children with the ability to swallow

Sarah A. Martin

PREREQUISITE KNOWLEDGE

- Medications for oral use are supplied as suspensions, tablets, gelcaps or capsules.
- The six rights of medication administration: right patient, right drug, right dose, right route, right time, and right documentation
- Anatomy and physiology of the gastrointestinal tract
- Knowledge of the medication to be administered including desired purpose, dose, side effects, and administration techniques
- The ability to perform mathematical calculations to correctly administer medications to children
- Child development as it relates to clinical assessment and oral medication administration
- Indications and contraindications for specific oral medications (nonintact gag reflex, inability to swallow)
- Patient education, comfort, safety, and privacy when administering oral medications

CHILD AND FAMILY ASSESSMENT

- Child's developmental level and ability to interact **➤➤Rationale:** These factors influence preparation of the child and interaction.
- Child's and family's understanding of the reasons for and risks and benefits of oral medication administration **➤➤Rationale:** Evaluates child's and family's understanding of the procedure and provides a gauge for ongoing education.
- History of previous experience with receiving oral medication **➤➤Rationale:** Noting any previous experiences

may help to identify successful techniques and promote compliance.

- Child's medical history, including current medications and known contraindications to prescribed medication **➤➤Rationale:** Ensures safe and proper medication administration.
- History of allergies to medications, foods, or environmental allergens **➤➤Rationale:** Knowing allergy history lessens the possibility of an allergic reaction to the medication or substances used in medication administration such as latex.
- History of any kidney or liver disorders **➤➤Rationale:** These conditions alter the metabolism and excretion of drugs.
- Height and weight **➤➤Rationale:** Medication dosing is based on weight and/or body surface area.
- Family's desire to be present during procedure **➤➤Rationale:** Family may provide support and comfort measures to their child but should have the option not to remain with the child.

CHILD AND FAMILY EDUCATION

Individualized, developmentally appropriate education is provided to the family and to the child based on desire for knowledge, readiness to learn, and overall neurologic and psychosocial state.

- Provide information regarding the purpose, dose, dosing frequency, side effects, and administration techniques of the oral medication **➤➤Rationale:** Ensures safe and proper medication administration.
- Provide explanation regarding anticipated sensations or tastes associated with medication administration

➵*Rationale:* Providing information decreases anxiety and fear.

- Provide explanation to the child and family regarding the step-by-step procedure ➵*Rationale:* Providing information decreases anxiety and fear; initiates teaching if medication is to be continued in the home.
- Encourage questions and answer questions as they arise ➵*Rationale:* Reinforcement of information is needed during periods of stress.

EQUIPMENT

- Medication to be administered
- Oral medication syringe or medicine cup
- Fluid or soft foods for mixing medications
- Nipple (optional for infants)
- Spoon (optional if mixing medications with soft foods)
- Clean gloves

Procedure for Oral Medication Administration

Steps	Rationale	Considerations
1. Ensure child and family understand procedure and questions are answered.	Evaluates and reinforces understanding of previously taught information.	Developmental level, cognitive ability, and anxiety level will determine approach to and effectiveness of teaching.
2. Ensure the six rights of medication administration. *(Level VI*)*	Lessens the chance of incorrect drug administration.	Two identifiers should be used for patient identification per institution-specific protocol; most commonly, name and birth date or name and medical record number are used. Liquid preparations are usually easiest to administer to infants. Toddlers and preschoolers may be able to take chewable tablets or eat crushed pills placed in food (e.g., pudding or applesauce).
3. Gather needed equipment and supplies.	Prevents delay in medication administration, which may decrease the child's anxiety.	For infants and young children a syringe may be needed to accurately draw up liquid medications. Oral medication syringes should be used to avoid inadvertent intravenous administration of enteral medications. Measuring doses in teaspoons or droppers has been shown to be unreliable.[1] *(Level VI*)*
4. Wash hands and put on clean gloves.	Standard precautions; reduces transmission of microorganisms.	
5. Prepare the medication for administration. Verify with the child or caregiver that the child can take the dispensed preparation (e.g., tablets can be swallowed).	Medications to be administered should be drawn up in a measuring device to insure dosing accuracy. The Medibottle (Medicine Bottle Company, Inc., Yorba Linda, CA) (Figure 166-1) has been shown to be more effective in delivering medication to infants than oral syringes.[2] *(Level IV*)*	Crush tablets as needed for mixing in small amount of sterile water, alternate beverage, or soft food for administration. Verify compatibility with liquid or solid being used. Avoid mixing medications in essential foods because the infant may refuse these foods in the future.[3] Sustained release and enteric-coated tablets should not be crushed.

Procedure continues on following page

---

* Level IV: Limited clinical studies to support recommendations
  Level VI: Clinical studies in a variety of patient populations and situations to support recommendations

Procedure	for Oral Medication Administration—*Continued*

Steps	Rationale	Considerations

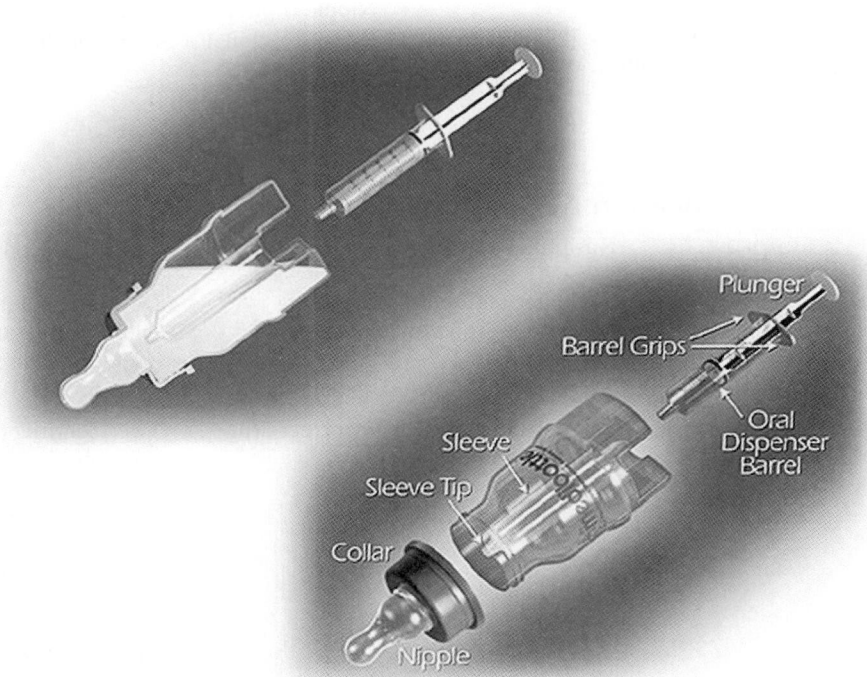

FIGURE 166-1   Medibottle. *From Medicine Bottle Company, Inc. website: www.medibottle.com/works.html Accessed 6/6/06.*

Steps	Rationale	Considerations
6. Demonstrate for the family measuring the medication if home use is anticipated.	Decreases dosing errors at home.	
7. Administer medication by age or developmentally appropriate method.[1,3,4] **Infant:** Place in a semi-reclining position. Administer the medication in increments of 0.5 to 1 mL. Place the syringe in the infant's mouth along the tongue directed toward the cheek. Allow the infant to swallow all medication before administering additional medication	Promotes effective medication administration. Allowing infant to swallow in between dispensed increments will decrease the chance of aspiration.	Infant: May use syringe, nipple measuring spoon, or medibottle.[2]

Procedure for Oral Medication Administration—*Continued*

Steps	Rationale	Considerations
increments. A nipple may also be placed in the infant's mouth and medication administered in a compatible fluid. Allow the infant to suck until all of the medication is out of the nipple. Follow the medication with 2.5 to 5 mL of water placed in the nipple. **Toddler:** Offer medication in either a cup or spoon. May need to use syringe or measuring spoon as with the infant. Some toddlers find it novel to drink out of a medication cup or cup with a sticker on it. **School age:** Offer liquid medication in a syringe or cup, or offer solid preparations. The older school-aged child may be able to swallow pills. **Adolescent:** Offer medication in a medication cup.		
8. Offer older child a "chaser" after the child swallows the medication.	Drinking a tasteful beverage immediately following the medication administration may promote cooperation with future medication doses.	Informing the older child the medication may taste unpleasant may gain the child's cooperation.
9. Praise child for cooperating.	Acknowledges child's positive behavior; promotes cooperation with future medication doses.	
10. If child refuses to take the medication, enlist parental help or consider alternate method for administration.	Forcing child to take oral medication may result in vomiting or other adverse events.	The crying child may aspirate medication, particularly when lying down.
11. If child vomits within 30 minutes of the medication being administered, confer with the practitioner prescribing medication to determine if the dose should be repeated.	Identifies medications that should be repeated.	Repeat dosing should be considered on an individual basis because the margin of safety with drugs is variable.
12. Discard used supplies and equipment in appropriate receptacle.	Standard precautions; reduces transmission of microorganisms.	
13. Remove gloves; wash hands.	Standard precautions.	

Expected Outcomes

- Right dose of right medication is administered to right child at right time via right route and correctly documented

- Child is able to swallow the medication
- Medication dose is absorbed from the GI tract
- Child/family understands the purpose and side effects of the medication
- Child/family is able to self-administer medication

Unexpected Outcomes

- Wrong dose, wrong medication, wrong route, wrong time of administration
- Medication is administered to wrong child
- Medication is not documented
- Child is unable to swallow the medication
- Child vomits the medication after administration
- Child/family does not understand the purpose and is unable to list side effects of the medication
- Child/family is unable to self-administer medication

Monitoring and Care of the Child

Activities and Interventions	Rationale	Reportable Conditions
1. Monitor child for adverse reaction to the medication being delivered according to pharmacokinetics and pharmacodynamics.	Allows early identification and prompt intervention for adverse reactions.	• Adverse drug reaction • Allergic response to medication
2. Monitor child's tolerance of the procedure; use developmental strategies to help child tolerate procedure. If available, consider consulting a Child Life Therapist.	Children may be very anxious about taking medication.	• Unable to administer medication because of extreme anxiety

Documentation

- Name of medication administered, dose, time of administration, individual administering medication, and child's response
- Child and family education
- Unexpected outcomes and related treatment

References

1. Algren C, Arnow D: Pediatric variations of nursing interventions. In Wong DL, Hockenberry M, editors: *Wong's nursing care of infants and children,* ed 7, St. Louis, 2003, Mosby, pp. 1101-1170.
2. Kraus DM, et al: Effectiveness and infant acceptance of the Rx medibottle versus the oral syringe, *Pharmacotherapy* 21(4):416-423, 2001.
3. Hockenberry MJ: *Wong's clinical manual of pediatric nursing,* St. Louis, 2004, Mosby.
4. McKenry LM, Salerno E: *Mosby's pharmacology in nursing,* ed 21, St. Louis, 2000, Mosby.

Additional Reference

Taketomo CK, et al, editors: *Pediatric dosage handbook,* ed 12, Hudson, OH, 2005, Lexi-Comp, Inc.

Otic Medication

P U R P O S E : To administer medication into the ear canal in order to provide local therapy to reduce inflammation, destroy infective organisms in the external ear canal, relieve pain, or clean the canal[1]

Barbara A. Weintraub

PREREQUISITE KNOWLEDGE

* The six rights of medication administration: right patient, right drug, right dose, right route, right time, and right documentation
* Anatomy of the ear
* Signs and symptoms indicating tympanic membrane rupture
* Concepts and principles of administering otic medications
* Indications and contraindications for specific otic medications
* Child development as it relates to clinical assessment and otic medication administration
* Patient education, comfort, safety, and privacy when administering otic medications.

CHILD AND FAMILY ASSESSMENT

* Appearance of the external ear structures, including erythema, abrasions, or discharge ➤*Rationale:* The presence of these conditions may indicate the need to withhold the medication.
* Family's desire to be present during procedure ➤*Rationale:* Family may provide support and comfort measures to the child, but should have the option not to remain with the child.
* Child's developmental level and ability to interact ➤*Rationale:* These factors influence preparation of the child and interaction.
* Family's ability to assist the child in cooperating with the procedure ➤*Rationale:* Family anxiety can decrease with

participation in the procedure. Additionally, the medication may need to be continued following discharge from the hospital, and the family's ability to correctly administer the medication must be assessed.

* History of previous experience of receiving an otic medication ➤*Rationale:* Identifying any previous experiences may help to assess child's and family's understanding or misconceptions, and identify areas for further education.
* History of allergies to medications, foods, or environmental allergens ➤*Rationale:* Knowing allergy history lessens the possibility of an allergic reaction to the medication or substances such as latex which may be used during the procedure.
* Child's and family's understanding of the reasons for and risks and benefits of otic medication administration ➤*Rationale:* Evaluates child's and family's understanding of the procedure and provides a gauge for ongoing education.

CHILD AND FAMILY EDUCATION

Individualized, developmentally appropriate education is provided to the family and to the child based on desire for knowledge, readiness to learn, and overall neurologic and psychosocial state.

* Provide information regarding the reasons for medication administration and expected outcome ➤*Rationale:* Providing information decreases anxiety and fear.
* Provide explanation to the child and family regarding the step-by-step procedure ➤*Rationale:* Providing information decreases anxiety and fear and promotes compliance

- Provide explanation regarding anticipated sensations associated with medication administration ➥*Rationale:* Providing information decreases anxiety and fear.
- If developmentally appropriate, explain how the child can help assist with instillation of ear drops (hold very still and sing the child's favorite song) ➥*Rationale:* Medication instillation will be enhanced with cooperation of the child.
- Encourage questions and answer questions as they arise ➥*Rationale:* Reinforcement of information is needed during periods of stress.

EQUIPMENT

- Medication as prescribed
- Clean gloves
- Cotton fluff (optional)
- Cotton-tipped applicators

Procedure | for Otic Medication

Steps	Rationale	Considerations
1. Ensure child and family understand procedure, including expected sensations during the procedure, and questions are answered.	Evaluates and reinforces understanding of previously taught information.	Developmental level, cognitive ability, and anxiety level will determine approach to and effectiveness of teaching.
2. Ensure the six rights of medication administration. *(Level VI*)*	Lessens the chance of incorrect drug administration; eye and ear medications may be easily confused.	Two identifiers should be used for patient identification per institution-specific protocol; most commonly, name and birth date or name and medical record number are used. Ensure the child does not have any contraindications to the medication or to the administration route.
3. Gather needed equipment and supplies.	Facilitates completion of task in a timely manner.	
4. Allow medication to come to room temperature.	Instilling cold ear drops may result in vertigo or nausea.[1]	
5. Wash hands and put on clean gloves if ear drainage is present.	Standard precautions; reduces transmission of microorganisms.	
6. Assist child into a side-lying position, with the ear to receive medication in the uppermost position.	Provides optimal access to ear for instillation of medication.	
7. Clean pinna and meatus of ear canal with cotton-tipped applicators.	Removes external discharge before medication instillation, preventing its introduction into the ear canal.	
8. Straighten ear canal. *(Level V*)*	Straightening of ear canal provides direct access to deeper external ear structures.	Children 3 years or older: pull earlobe up and back. Children less than 3 years: pull earlobe down and back.
9. Instill the correct number of drops along the side of the ear canal.	Prevents drops from escaping and allows even distribution of the medication.	

* Level V: Clinical studies in more than one or two patient populations and situations to support recommendations
  Level VI: Clinical studies in a variety of patient populations and situations to support recommendations

Procedure for Otic Medication—*Continued*

Steps	Rationale	Considerations
10. Gently press on the tragus several times. *(Level IV*)*	Assists the flow of medication into the ear canal.	
11. If desired or prescribed, insert a small piece of cotton fluff loosely into the meatus of the auditory canal for 15 minutes; do not pack tightly.	May prevent medication from draining from ear.	May vary based on medication administered or prescribing practitioner's preference.
12. Keep child in a side-lying position for at least 5 minutes.	Prevents medication from flowing out of the ear.	
13. Discard used supplies and equipment in appropriate receptacle.	Standard precautions; reduces transmission of microorganisms.	
14. Remove gloves; wash hands.	Standard precautions.	

* Level IV: Limited clinical studies to support recommendations

Expected Outcomes

- Right dose of right medication is administered to right child at right time via right route and correctly documented

- Medication is delivered to ear canal
- Goal of treatment is achieved (e.g., analgesia, decreased cerumen, resolution of infection)

Unexpected Outcomes

- Medication is administered to wrong child
- Wrong dose, wrong medication, wrong route, wrong time of administration
- Medication is not documented
- Medication is delivered outside ear canal
- No therapeutic benefit seen
- Ruptured tympanic membrane

Monitoring and Care of the Child

Activities and Interventions	Rationale	Reportable Conditions
1. Monitor child for adverse reaction to the medication being delivered.	Allows early identification and prompt intervention.	• Adverse drug reaction • Allergic response to medication
2. Monitor child's tolerance of the procedure; use developmental strategies to help child tolerate procedure. If available, consider consulting child life therapist.	Children may be very anxious during manipulation of the ears and have difficulty tolerating the procedure.	• Unable to administer medication due to extreme anxiety
3. Monitor child for anticipated effect of medication, if applicable (i.e., local analgesia).	Lack of anticipated response may indicate need to repeat medication.	• Sudden increase in pain may indicate tympanic membrane rupture

Documentation

- Initial assessment of ear canal and drainage
- Name of medication administered, ear(s) dosed, dose, time of administration, individual administering medication, and child's response
- Child and family education
- Unexpected outcomes and related treatment

Reference

1.   Kozier B, et al: Integral components of client care: medications. In *Fundamentals of nursing: concepts, process and practice*, ed 7, New Jersey: Upper Saddle River, 2004, Prentice-Hall.

Additional Readings

Taketomo CK, et al, editors: *Pediatric dosage handbook,* ed 12, Hudson, OH, 2005, Lexi-Comp, Inc.

Wong DL, et al editors: *Whaley & Wong's nursing care of infants and children,* ed 6, St. Louis, 1999, Mosby.

PROCEDURE **168**

Rectal Medication

P U R P O S E : To provide an alternative method of medication administration when oral or parenteral administration is contraindicated

Roni L. Zarge

PREREQUISITE KNOWLEDGE

- Medications for pain control, fever management, antiepileptic, evacuant or antiemetic therapy may be administered rectally, and come in a variety of formulations: suppositories, solutions, and creams.
- The six rights of medication administration: right patient, right drug, right dose, right route, right time, and right documentation
- Anatomy and physiology of the anorectal area
- Concepts and principles of administering rectal medications
- Indications and contraindications for specific rectal medications
- Contraindications to rectal medication therapy: thrombocytopenia, neutropenia, anorectal malformations, diarrhea, rectal bleeding, rectal fissures, hemorrhoids, anal area irritation, or recent anorectal surgery
- Do not divide suppository doses by cutting them, because of the possibility that all the medication may be in one area of the suppository. If the desired dose does not come prepackaged, contact the pharmacist for alternative medications.
- If the child is constipated or the rectum is full of stool, absorption of the medication may be impaired. Administration of an evacuant may be advised before administration of the desired medication.
- Child development as it relates to clinical assessment and rectal medication administration

- Patient safety, privacy, education and comfort considerations when administering rectal medications

CHILD AND FAMILY ASSESSMENT

- Child's developmental level and ability to interact ➤➤*Rationale:* These factors influence preparation of the child and interaction.
- Patency of anal canal ➤➤*Rationale:* Anorectal malformations will impede administration of medications via the rectum.
- Integrity of anal canal/rectum ➤➤*Rationale:* Identifies contraindications to administration of rectal medications.
- History of allergies to medications or environmental allergens ➤➤*Rationale:* Knowing allergy history lessens the possibility of an allergic reaction to the medication or substances used in medication administration, such as latex.
- Presence of constipation or a full rectum ➤➤*Rationale:* If the medication is surrounded by stool, it will not be absorbed efficiently.
- History of any kidney or liver disorders ➤➤*Rationale:* These conditions alter the metabolism and excretion of drugs.
- Height and weight ➤➤*Rationale:* Medication dosing is generally based on weight and/or body surface area.
- Child's and family's understanding of the reasons for and risks and benefits of rectal medication administration

1225

➤➤*Rationale:* Evaluates child's and family's understanding of the procedure and provides a gauge for ongoing education.
- Previous experience of receiving rectal medication ➤➤*Rationale:* Identifying previous experiences may help to identify successful techniques and promote compliance.
- Family's desire to be present during the procedure ➤➤*Rationale:* Family may provide support and comfort measures to their child but should have the option not to remain with the child.

CHILD AND FAMILY EDUCATION

Individualized, developmentally appropriate education is provided to the family and to the child based on desire for knowledge, readiness to learn, and overall neurologic and psychosocial state.

- Provide information about the purpose of the medication, why it must be given rectally, dosing frequency, and its expected outcome ➤➤*Rationale:* Providing information about why the procedure is necessary will decrease fear and anxiety and may promote cooperation.

- Provide information about how the medication will be administered, including attention to comfort and privacy ➤➤*Rationale:* Providing assurance of comfort and privacy will help obtain cooperation and ensure proper administration of the medication.
- Explain the need for proper positioning for rectal medication administration as well as the need to keep the buttocks held or tapered together for 5 to 10 minutes after medication administration ➤➤*Rationale:* Proper positioning during and after administration ensures maximum medication absorption.
- Encourage questions and answer questions as they arise ➤➤*Rationale:* Reinforcement of information is needed during periods of stress.

EQUIPMENT

- Medication to be administered
- Clean gloves
- Water-soluble lubricant
- Tissue or wipes

Procedure for Rectal Medication

Steps	Rationale	Considerations
1. Ensure child and family understand preprocedural teaching and questions are answered.	Evaluates and reinforces understanding of previously taught information.[1-3]	Developmental level, cognitive ability, and anxiety level will determine approach to and effectiveness of teaching.
2. Ensure child and family understand why the rectal route is the preferred route of administration. *(Level VI*)*	Evaluates and reinforces understanding of previously taught information.[1-3]	Acknowledges the possible discomfort and embarrassment that may occur during the procedure.
3. Ensure the six rights of medication administration are correct.[1,2,4-6] *(Level VI*)*	Knowing the six rights of medication administration ensures giving the correct medication and avoids errors.	Ensure the child does not have any contraindications to the medication or the way it will be administered.
4. Gather needed equipment and supplies.	Facilitates completion of procedure in a timely manner.	Equipment and supplies may vary depending on the form of medication being administered (e.g., enema bag and IV pole are needed for enema administration).
5. Provide for appropriate privacy.	Demonstrates respect for the child; decreases anxiety.	Privacy is an important consideration for school-aged children and adolescents.
6. Wash hands; put on clean gloves.	Standard precautions; reduces transmission of microorganisms.	

* Level VI: Clinical studies in a variety of patient populations and situations to support recommendations

Procedure for Rectal Medication—*Continued*

Steps	Rationale	Considerations
7. Place child on left side with left leg straight or slightly bent, and right knee bent upward (Sims' position). *(Level II*)*	Placing the child on the left lateral side facilitates rectal administration.[1,4,5]	It may be difficult to keep a child in the same position for an extended period. Child's caregiver may assist in this process using distraction techniques.
8. If administering a suppository, remove the foil wrapper. If administering a solution via an enema, remove the cap on the enema tubing or applicator tip. If administering medication via a syringe, remove cap of syringe.	Prepares medication for administration.	Follow administration directions provided by pharmacy/pharmacy reference to ensure proper administration of medication and avoid errors.
9. Coat the end of the suppository, end of enema tubing, tip of applicator or syringe with a water-soluble lubricant. *(Level IV*)*	Lubricant promotes ease of insertion of the suppository or enema applicator and comfort.[3,7]	Some enemas may come with a pre-lubricated tip.
10. Gently insert lubricated suppository, enema tubing, applicator tip, or syringe into the rectum, beyond the internal anal sphincter; approximately 2 to 3 inches. (Figures 168-1 and 168-2). *(Level II*)*	Total surface area for drug absorption in the rectum occurs above the anus.[1,4,5,7,8]	Not inserting a suppository past the internal anal sphincter may cause discomfort to the child. Not inserting a solution past the internal anal sphincter may cause premature evacuation of the medication and a less than desirable effect.

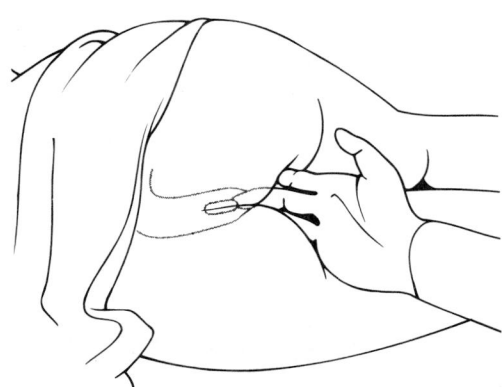

FIGURE 168-1 Insertion of a suppository. Gently insert lubricated suppository past the anal sphincter to ensure maximum absorption. *From Clark JB, et al:* Pharmacologic basis of nursing practice, *ed 6, St. Louis, 2000, Mosby.*

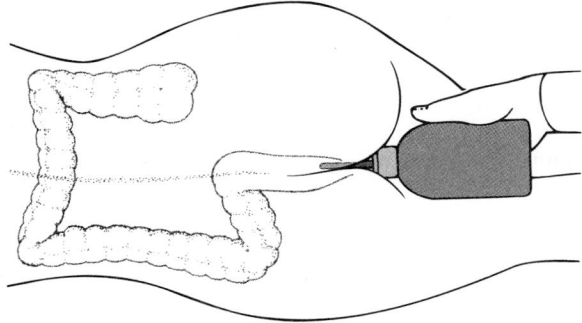

FIGURE 168-2 Insertion of an enema. Gently inset applicator tip and squeeze bottle to propel medication into the child's rectum. *From Clark JB, et al:* Pharmacologic basis of nursing practice, *ed 6, St. Louis, 2000, Mosby.*

Procedure continues on following pages

---

* Level II: Theory-based, no research data to support recommendations: recommendations from expert consensus group may exist
Level IV: Limited clinical studies to support recommendations

Procedure for Rectal Medication—*Continued*

Steps	Rationale	Considerations
11. Keep finger inserted into rectum for 3 seconds to ensure the medication has gone past the internal anal sphincter. If delivering an enema, squeeze the bottle to propel medication into the child's rectum (see Figure 168-2). *(Level II*)*	Waiting 3 seconds ensures adequate absorption of the medication.[1,4,5,7,8]	
12. Keep the child in side-lying position for 10 to 15 minutes. The buttocks should be held together for 10 to 15 minutes. *(Level II*)*	Promotes maximum amount of medication absorption. Keeping the buttocks together relieves pressure on the anal sphincter, facilitating retention and absorption of the medication.[1,4,5]	Depending on the age and cognitive level of the child, gaining cooperation of the child to maintain appropriate position and keep the buttocks held together will be variable.
13. Instruct the child to avoid having a bowel movement for as long as possible; 30 minutes is ideal. *(Level VI*)*	Retaining the medication for as long as possible allows for maximum absorption of the medication.[1,7]	Premature evacuation of the medication results in a less than desirable effect.
14. Wipe the perianal area with a tissue or wipe if any excess lubricant or medication leaked from rectum.	Increases child's comfort.	
15. Discard used supplies and equipment in appropriate receptacle.	Standard precautions; reduces transmission of microorganisms.	
16. Remove gloves; wash hands.	Standard precautions; reduces transmission of microorganisms.	

* Level II: Theory-based, no research data to support recommendations: recommendations from expert consensus group may exist
Level VI: Clinical studies in a variety of patient populations and situations to support recommendations

Expected Outcomes	Unexpected Outcomes
• Right dose of right medication is administered to right child at right time via right route and correctly documented	• Wrong dose, wrong medication, wrong route, wrong time of administration
	• Medication is administered to wrong child
	• Medication is not documented
• Medication dose is absorbed from the rectum and desired results are achieved	• Medication is not absorbed
• Medication is retained for 30 minutes	• Too rapid absorption of medication
• Medication is easily inserted into rectum	• Premature evacuation of medication
	• Resistance to the administration of the medication
	• Perianal skin irritation
• Child tolerates procedure with minimal anxiety or agitation	• Unable to administer medication because of child's agitation or anxiety

Monitoring and Care of the Child

Activities and Interventions	Rationale	Reportable Conditions
1. Monitor child's response to the medication.	Adverse changes to the child's condition following administration of a medication may be a result of a reaction to the medication.	• Adverse reaction following administration • Desired response is not obtained
2. Monitor rectum for skin irritation or bleeding after medication administration.	Indicates altered skin integrity, which increases the risk of pain and/or infection; may be symptomatic of an adverse reaction to the medication.	• Perianal skin irritation or bleeding
3. Monitor for premature expulsion of the medication.	Desired effects of the medication may not be achieved if the medication is not retained in the rectum.	• Dose is expelled from the rectum in less than 30 minutes
4. Monitor child's tolerance of the procedure; use developmental strategies to help child tolerate procedure. If available, consider consulting a Child Life Therapist.	Child may be very anxious about rectal medication administration.	• Unable to administer medication due to extreme anxiety or agitation

Documentation

- Name of medication administered, dose, time of administration, individual administering medication, effect of medication, and child's response to administration
- Child and family education
- Unexpected outcomes and related treatment

References

1. Clark JB, et al: *Pharmacologic basis of nursing practice*, ed 6, St. Louis, 2000, Mosby.
2. Henry C: The advantages of using suppositories, *Nurs Times* 95(17):50-51, 1999.
3. Shende A: Disorders of the white blood cells. In Lanzkowsky P, ed: *Manual of pediatric hematology and oncology*, ed 4, San Diego, 2005, Elsevier.
4. Craven RF, Hirnle CJ, editors: *Fundamentals of nursing: human health and function*, ed 4, Philadelphia, 2003, Lippincott Williams & Wilkins.
5. Moppett S, Parker M: Practical procedures for nurses: insertion of a suppository, *Nurs Times* 95(23):2p, 1999.
6. Russic M, Brill CK: Partnering with pharmacy for positive patient outcomes, *Semin Nurse Manag* 10(1):55-60, 2002.
7. McKenry LM, Salerno E, editors: *Mosby's pharmacology in nursing*, ed 21, St. Louis, 2003, Mosby.
8. Pasero C, McCaffery M: Opioids by the rectal route, *Am J Nurs* 99(11):20-22, 1999.

Additional Readings

Fitzgerald BJ, et al: Treatment of out-of-hospital status epilepticus with diazepam rectal gel, *Seizure* 12(1):52-55, 2003.

Scolnik D, et al: Comparison of oral versus normal and high-dose rectal acetaminophen in the treatment of febrile children, *Pediatrics* 110(3):553-556, 2002.

Sterrick M, Foley J: Educating lay careers of people with learning disability in epilepsy awareness and in the use of rectal diazepam: a suggested teaching protocol for use by healthcare personnel, *Health Bull* 57(3):198-204, 1999.

Taketomo CK, et al, editors: *Pediatric dosage handbook,* ed 12, Hudson, OH, 2005 Lexi-Comp, Inc.

Subcutaneous Injection

PURPOSE: To administer medication into the subcutaneous tissue

Kelly S. Finkbeiner

PREREQUISITE KNOWLEDGE

- The six rights of medication administration: right patient, right route, right drug, right dose, right time, and right documentation
- Indications for subcutaneous injection: this route is used when small volumes of medication need to be absorbed at a slow, steady rate and is commonly used for insulin, anticoagulation therapy, allergy desensitization, and immunizations.[1-4]
- Anatomy and physiology of subcutaneous injection sites
- Concepts and procedures of administering subcutaneous injections, including aseptic technique
- Understanding of appropriate needle size, syringe size, and fluid volume for subcutaneous tissue injection
- Indications and contraindications to specific subcutaneous injections
- Patient safety, privacy, education, and comfort considerations when administering subcutaneous injections
- Child development as it relates to clinical assessment and subcutaneous injection

CHILD AND FAMILY ASSESSMENT

- History of food, medication, or environmental allergons ➤*Rationale:* Many allergies may predispose a child to be allergic to the medication being administered. Some immunizations contain eggs, shellfish, or other food products that can cause a child with a food allergy to have a reaction.
- Developmental level of child; family's preferred learning method ➤*Rationale:* Helps the clinician educate using developmentally appropriate terms and teaching techniques.
- Child's and family's previous experience with subcutaneous injections ➤*Rationale:* This can affect how the child and family react to subcutaneous injection; it also identifies any complications from previous subcutaneous injections.
- Subcutaneous tissue and skin condition ➤*Rationale:* Determines the most appropriate area for subcutaneous injection. It is important not to give subcutaneous injections where a child has skin breakdown because of the increased risk of infection.
- Child's ability to cooperate with the procedure and the family's desire to be present during, or assist with, the procedure ➤*Rationale:* This will determine if more assistance is required to prevent the child from being injured by unexpected movement during the procedure. Family members may provide comfort and support during the procedure but should have the option not to remain with the child.
- Child's and family's understanding of the reasons for and risks and benefits of the procedure ➤*Rationale:* Evaluates child's and family's understanding of the procedure and provides a gauge for ongoing education.

CHILD AND FAMILY EDUCATION

Individualized, developmentally appropriate education is provided to the family and to the child based on desire for knowledge, readiness to learn, and overall neurologic and psychosocial state.

- Provide the family and child with appropriate verbal and written information about the medication including the purpose, why this route is preferred, possible side effects from the medication, and the subcutaneous injection ➟*Rationale:* Verbal and written information reinforces teaching and gives the family a resource.
- Inform the family of their exact role during the procedure. If family member has elected to participate, demonstrate the appropriate way for them to hold their child ➟*Rationale:* Providing family with information will decrease their anxiety about their role in the procedure. It will prevent injury to the child and the family. Family members should have the option not to participate in the procedure.
- If the family or child is going to be administering the subcutaneous injection, begin teaching as early as possible[5] ➟*Rationale:* This allows the family and the child time to learn self-administration.
- If appropriate, educate the child about the procedure. Use developmentally appropriate words and avoid using words that may be viewed by the child as threatening ➟*Rationale:* Decreases the child's anxiety and increases the child's cooperation during the procedure.
- Provide family and child with self-management techniques, for example: acetaminophen for fever, and cool compresses for pain. Provide information on when to notify a clinician about a problem and how to do this ➟*Rationale:* Empowers the family and child to handle minor effects from the subcutaneous injection and when/how to notify the medical team if a problem arises.
- Encourage questions and answer questions as they arise ➟*Rationale:* Reinforcement of information is needed during periods of stress.

EQUIPMENT

- Medication to be administered
- Eutectic mixture of local anesthetics (EMLA), Ela-max, or vapor coolant spray as prescribed or per institution-specific protocol
- 3-mL or smaller syringe
- 25- to 30-gauge, ⅜ to ⅝-inch needle
- Alcohol wipes
- Clean gloves
- Cotton ball or gauze pad
- Adhesive bandage
- Distraction equipment (book, toys, and bubbles)

Procedure for Subcutaneous Injection

Steps	Rationale	Considerations
1. Ensure child and family understand procedure and their role and questions are answered. Obtain consent when appropriate. *(Level VI*)*	Evaluates and reinforces understanding of previously taught information and encourages further questions or concerns.	Developmental level, cognitive ability, and anxiety level will determine approach to and effectiveness of teaching. Parental consent should be obtained for immunizations per institution-specific protocol.
2. Ensure the six rights of medication administration are correct.[1,2,6-8] *(Level VI*)*	Ensures correct medication is administered and avoids errors.	Two identifiers should be used for patient identification per institution-specific protocol; most commonly, name and birth date or name and medical record number are used.
3. Wash hands.	Standard precautions; reduces transmission of microorganisms.	
4. Provide for appropriate privacy.	Some injection sites require exposure of the abdomen or thighs.	Privacy is an important consideration for school-aged children and adolescents.
5. Select appropriate injection site based on child's subcutaneous tissue mass, medication volume, previous subcutaneous injection sites, and needed absorption rate. Most common subcutaneous sites are the center third of lateral aspect of upper arm, the abdomen, center third of anterior thigh.[4,8,9] *(Level VI*)*	Select the most appropriate site that can safely accommodate the fluid volume being administered without causing injury to the child. Maximum fluid volume is 1 mL.[1,2,6,7,9]	Rotating sites will prevent tissue damage and may increase absorption. The abdomen has the most rapid absorption followed by the arms, thighs, and buttocks.[4,7] Due to the different absorption rates it is important for diabetic patients to rotate sites in the same area.[4] The

Procedure continues on following page

* Level VI: Clinical studies in a variety of patient populations and situations to support recommendations

Procedure for Subcutaneous Injection—*Continued*

Steps	Rationale	Considerations
		5-centimeter radius around the umbilicus should be avoided because of the umbilical vein.[4] Damage or scar tissue, poor subcutaneous tissue mass, and accessibility may be contraindications to a particular site. It is important to inject heparin or enoxaparin (Lovenox) into the lower abdomen because it has greater surface area and is not involved in a lot of muscle activity, which will reduce bruising. If bruising does occur there is a larger surface area to absorb the bruising.[2,5]
6. Apply local anesthesia as appropriate per manufacturer's instruction.	Decreases pain at injection site.[3,4]	EMLA cream should be applied at least 30 minutes before injection. Refer to institution-specific protocols for administration of local anesthetics.
7. Gather needed equipment and supplies.	Prevents delay in performing the procedure, which can increase the child's anxiety level.	
8. Mix and draw up the exact amount of medication. Use a filter needle when drawing from glass ampules and mixing powder medication.[2] *(Level VI*)*	Necessary for administering the medication. Using a filter needle will prevent drawing glass or large particles into the syringe.[3,4]	If mixing two medications they should be drawn up in the same order every time to prevent mistakes. Due to the small dosing of many subcutaneous injections and the importance of accuracy, it may be important to have another clinician check the dosage of medication; refer to institution specific protocol.[7]
9. Attach appropriate-sized needle to the syringe; 25 to 30 gauge $3/8$ to $5/8$ inch. *(Level VI*)*	Ensures medication reaches the subcutaneous tissue.[1,2,3,6,7,9]	If medication leaks onto the needle, sterile gauze should be used to wipe off the medication; this will prevent tracking the medication through the tissue.[3,4] Changing the needle after drawing up from a rubber stopper will decrease pain because the rubber stopper dulls the needle, making it more difficult to penetrate the skin.[3] When using an insulin syringe the needle is not changed.
10. Position child and begin to perform any distraction measures. *(Level IV*)*	Proper positioning ensures child's safety and comfort. Distraction may help alleviate child's anxiety and discomfort associated with the injection.[8]	Some distraction techniques include books, bubbles, or toys.
11. Put on clean gloves.	Standard precautions; reduces transmission of microorganisms.	

* Level IV: Limited clinical studies to support recommendations
  Level VI: Clinical studies in a variety of patient populations and situations to support recommendations

Procedure for Subcutaneous Injection—*Continued*

Steps	Rationale	Considerations
12. Clean area with alcohol. *(Level III*)*	Decreases risk of infection.[4,5]	Clean a circular area approximately 5 to 8 cm.[2,5,9]
13. Allow skin to dry.	Decreases pain from introduction of alcohol into the subcutaneous tissue.[3,4]	
14. Pinch tissue with thumb and index finger. *(Level VI*)*	Isolates the subcutaneous tissue and prevents injecting into the muscle.[9]	Give the injection at 90-degree angle if 2 inches of skin are grasped.[7]
15. Insert needle with a steady, smooth motion at a 45- to 90-degree angle (Figure 169-1). *(Level VI*)*	Causes less displacement and shearing of the tissue, which decreases pain.[3]	A 45-degree angle is used with children who have little subcutaneous tissue. Heparin must be given at a 90-degree angle.[5]

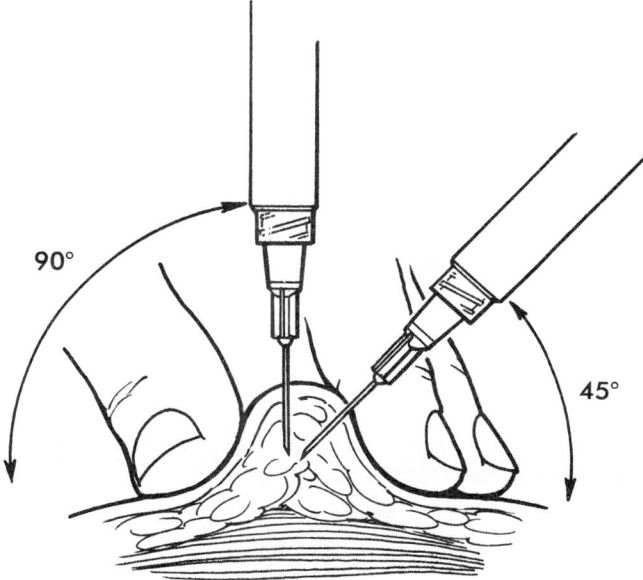

90° 45°

FIGURE 169-1 Subcutaneous injection angles. *From Wong DL, Hess C:* Wong & Whaley's clinical manual of pediatric nursing, *ed 5, St. Louis, 2000, Mosby.*

16. Pull back on plunger, except when injecting heparin or insulin. *(Level V*)*	Assesses for blood return and prevents injection of medication into a vein or artery.	Although controversial, many authors feel that if the right needle length is used, assessing for blood return is unnecessary. This is not recommended for heparin due to the risk of hematoma and is not necessary for insulin.[2-4,5,7] If blood is noted in the syringe, withdraw the needle, apply pressure at site, and start again with a new syringe and injection site.[2]
17. Inject medication slowly at a rate of 1 mL per 10 seconds. *(Level II*)*	Allows medication to be absorbed into the subcutaneous tissue.	

Procedure continues on following page

* Level II: Theory-based, no research data to support recommendations: recommendations from expert consensus group may exist
Level III: Laboratory data, no clinical data to support recommendations
Level V: Clinical studies in more than one or two patient populations and situations to support recommendations
Level VI: Clinical studies in a variety of patient populations and situations to support recommendations

Procedure for Subcutaneous Injection—*Continued*

Steps	Rationale	Considerations
18. Remove needle quickly and smoothly.	Decreases pain and prevents injury to the tissue.	
19. Apply pressure at the injection site. *(Level II*)*	Prevents leakage of the medication into the surrounding subcutaneous tissue.	Do not massage site; this can affect absorption and cause bruising.[3] Use gauze, not an alcohol wipe, to prevent irritation.[3,4]
20. Assess injection site for complications and apply an adhesive bandage. *(Level II*)*	Allows the clinician to provide interventions for any minor complications.	In the event of an injury, the prescribing practitioner should be notified. If applicable, reassess injection site in 2 to 4 hours for any complications.
21. Praise child for positive behavior.	Provides a sense of accomplishment for the child.	
22. Dispose of used supplies and equipment, including sharps, in appropriate receptacle.	Standard precautions; reduces transmission of microorganisms, protects personnel health.	
23. Remove gloves; wash hands.	Standard precautions.	

* Level II: Theory-based, no research data to support recommendations: recommendations from expert consensus group may exist

Expected Outcomes

- Right dose of right medication is administered to right child at right time via right route and correctly documented

- Medication is administered into the subcutaneous tissue with little discomfort

- The medication is appropriately absorbed and the child has no adverse reaction to the medications
- The child is free from complications of subcutaneous injection

Unexpected Outcomes

- Medication is not documented
- Medication is administered to wrong child
- Wrong dose, wrong medication, wrong route of administration, wrong time
- Severe pain with injection
- Medication is administered intradermally or intramuscularly
- Medication causes damage to the tissue
- Child has local or systemic reaction to the medication
- Infection
- Tissue damage due to child's movement
- Bleeding
- Glass particles administered into subcutaneous tissue
- Abscess
- Hematoma
- Bruising
- Tissue necrosis, gangrene
- Persistent nodule
- Lipodystrophy[1,2,3]

Monitoring and Care of the Child

Activities and Interventions	Rationale	Reportable Conditions
1. Monitor injection site for complications.	Facilitates identification of and interventions for complications.	• Profuse bleeding • Loss of function at injection site • Signs and symptoms of infection[4,9]
2. Assess for allergic reactions to the medication.	Child may develop an allergic reaction shortly after administration of the medication.	• Rash • Difficulty breathing • Seizures
3. Assess pain and give analgesics as prescribed or per institution-specific protocol; encourage family to use nonpharmacologic means to comfort and support the child.	Early identification of pain facilitates prompt treatment.	• Report of unresolved pain at the injection site • Continued irritability

Documentation

- Child and family education
- Consent if obtained
- Name of medication administered, dose, injection site, time of administration, individual administering the medication, and child's response
- Comfort assessment and any specific interventions provided
- Unexpected outcomes and related treatment

References

1. Gilsenan I: A practical guide to giving injections, *Nurs Times* 96(33):43-44, 2000.
2. Grindel CG, et al: *Nursing procedures,* ed 3, Springhouse, PA, 2000, Springhouse.
3. Hockenberry MJ, et al, editors: *Nursing care of the infant and child,* ed 7, St. Louis, 2003, Mosby.
4. Wong DL, Hess C, editors: *Wong & Whaley's clinical manual of pediatric nursing,* ed 5, St. Louis, 2000, Mosby.
5. McConnel EA: Do's & don'ts: administering subcutaneous heparin, *Nursing* 30(6):17, 2000.
6. Caffrey RM: Are all syringes created equal? How to choose and use today's insulin syringes. *Am J Nurs* 103(6):46-49, 2003.
7. Dunlap MM: Pediatric medication administration...other routes, *Growing Up With Us* 9(1):2002.
8. Dahlquist LM, et al: Distraction for children of different ages who undergo repeated needle sticks, *J Pediatr Oncol* 19(1):22-34, 2002.
9. Pope BB: How to administer subcutaneous and intramuscular injections, *Nursing* 32(1):50-51, 2002.

Additional Readings

Gehling E. Injecting insulin 101, *Diabetes Self Manage* 17(5):7-14, 2000.
Resource guide 2003: Insulin delivery, *Diabetes Forecast* 56(1):59-61, 2003.
Taketomo CK, et al, editors: *Pediatric Dosage Handbook,* ed 12, Hudson, OH, 2005: Lexi-Comp, Inc.

PROCEDURE **170**

Bispectral Index Monitoring

PURPOSE: To provide an objective measure to assess the child's level of consciousness to achieve the optimal level of sedation in the critical care environment using stand-alone monitoring

Larissa Hutchins

PREREQUISITE KNOWLEDGE

- Bispectral index (BIS) monitoring technology is available in two formats. This procedure is written for use with the stand-alone monitoring system. Integrated BIS monitoring systems are available for use with several patient-monitoring systems. Refer to specific user's manual from the manufacturer of the patient monitoring system for specifics on use of the BIS integrated system.
- The BIS monitor is an objective tool to assist the clinician in measuring the hypnotic effects of sedatives on the brain and optimize titration of sedatives administered.
- The BIS value is a continuous measure that assesses the child's level of consciousness by processing electroencephalographic (EEG) data obtained using a sensor placed on the child's forehead.
- In adults, a BIS value of 100 represents a fully awake patient. A BIS value less than 60 represents a low probability of explicit recall and that the patient is unresponsive to verbal stimulus. A BIS value of zero indicates the absence of electrical brain activity.[1]
- BIS technology is valuable to the clinician in preventing oversedation or undersedation when moderate to deep sedation is desired during mechanical ventilation. It can be used to assess level of consciousness when a child is receiving neuromuscular blockade, and assist in achieving burst suppression during pentobarbital coma.[2] It has been used in adults to assess level of consciousness

during procedures to decrease the probability of recall and anxiety. The BIS monitor has also been used to assess the neurologic status of critically ill adults who have not received sedation.[3]
- BIS monitoring is used in conjunction with ongoing clinician assessment of the child's comfort. BIS values have been shown to correlate with increasing depth of sedation and consciousness using subjective sedation assessment scales in pediatric[1,4-6] and in adult studies.[7-11] BIS values in children older than 1 year receiving general anesthesia have been shown to correlate with those obtained in adult studies.[12]
- BIS monitoring is intended for use in children older than 1 year of age. Results in children less than 1 year old should be interpreted with caution.
- BIS values should not independently be used for sedation management.
- Child development as it relates to BIS monitoring and clinical assessment
- Appropriate pediatric dosing of sedative medications

CHILD AND FAMILY ASSESSMENT

- Child's developmental level and ability to interact **➤➤Rationale:** These factors influence preparation of the child, interaction and selection of medications used for sedation.
- Child's and family's understanding of the reasons for and risks and benefits of BIS monitoring **➤➤Rationale:** Evaluates

child's and family's understanding of the procedure and provides a gauge for ongoing education.

- Child's allergies ➤➤***Rationale:*** Assesses for allergies to sensor components; sensor contains adhesive and conduction gel.
- Integrity of the skin over the child's forehead ➤➤***Rationale:*** Establishes baseline skin condition in the area where the sensor will be placed.

CHILD AND FAMILY EDUCATION

Individualized, developmentally appropriate education is provided to the family and to the child based on desire for knowledge, readiness to learn, and overall neurologic and psychosocial state.

- Provide information to the family, and child as appropriate, about the equipment or bedside monitor and the purpose of the BIS monitor; explain that BIS monitoring is used to assess level of consciousness and provide objective information about an individual child's response to sedative drugs to help achieve an optimal level of sedation ➤➤***Rationale:*** Decreases family anxiety related to presence of unfamiliar equipment.
- Explain that BIS values are used in conjunction with the clinical assessment performed by the care providers at the bedside to provide an objective assessment of the child's level of consciousness ➤➤***Rationale:*** Assures family that clinical assessment is an important component of sedation management. BIS values should not independently be used for sedation management.
- Provide family with information that the BIS values displayed may be affected by factors such as natural sleep-wake cycles, artifact, stimulation, movement, and hypothermia ➤➤***Rationale:*** Decreases family anxiety related to fluctuation in BIS values.
- Encourage questions and answer questions as they arise ➤➤***Rationale:*** Reinforcement of information is needed during periods of stress.

EQUIPMENT

- A-2000 BIS XP monitoring system (Figure 170-1)
- BIS patient interface cable (PIC) (see Figure 170-1)
- BIS pediatric sensor (Figure 170-2)
- Alcohol pad
- Gauze pad

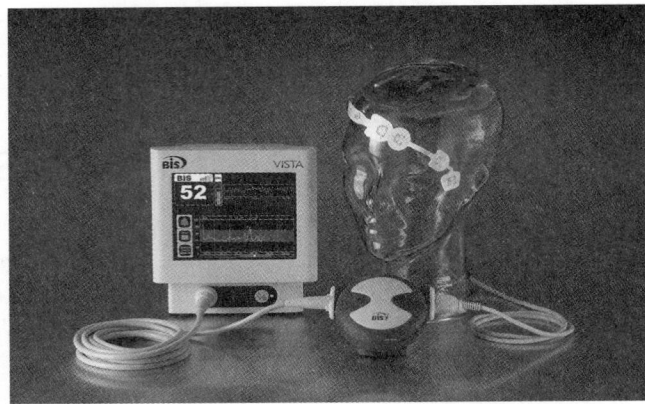

FIGURE 170-1   BIS VISTA monitoring system with BIS pediatric sensor and patient interface cable. *Photo courtesy of Aspect Medical Systems, Inc., Newton, MA, 2005.*

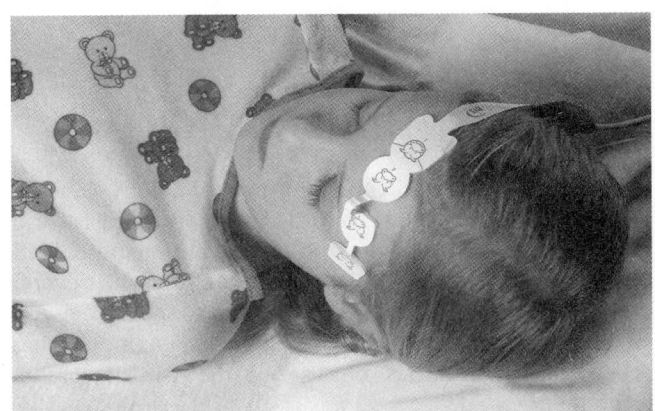

FIGURE 170-2   Pediatric BIS probe placement. *Photo courtesy of Aspect Medical Systems, Inc., Newton, MA, 2005.*

Procedure for Bispectral Index (BIS) Monitoring

Steps	Rationale	Considerations
1. Ensure child and family understand procedure and questions are answered.	Evaluates and reinforces understanding of previously taught information.	Developmental level, cognitive ability, and anxiety level will determine approach to and effectiveness of teaching.
2. Gather needed equipment and supplies.	Facilitates completion of task in a timely manner.	BIS monitoring is intended for use in children older than 1 year of age. Results in children less than 1 year old should be interpreted with caution. *(Level IV*)*

* Level IV: Limited clinical studies to support recommendations

Procedure for Bispectral Index (BIS) Monitoring—*Continued*

Steps	Rationale	Considerations
3. Connect the power cable to the back of the monitor. Ensure that the cord is fully connected to the power receptacle. Plug into AC power source. *(Level I*)*	Establishes power supply for monitor.	
4. Connect digital signal converter and patient interface cable to monitor (see Figure 170-1). *(Level I*)*	Required to connect sensor to monitor.	
5. With ballpoint pen write date and time of application of sensor. *(Level I*)*	Disposable sensor needs to be replaced every 24 hours to ensure good signal quality and to check the child's skin integrity.	
6. Wash hands.	Standard precautions; reduces transmission of microorganisms.	
7. Wipe skin with alcohol and dry with gauze pad. *(Level I*)*	Removes oil and debris for improved adherence of sensor.	
8. Apply sensor to forehead at an angle. Refer to manufacturer's instructions for positioning circles 1 through 4. Position circle 1 at center of forehead, approximately 1½ inches above bridge of nose. Apply circle 4 directly above and adjacent to the eyebrow, circle 3 on temple, between corner of eye and hairline, and circle 2 as directed. *(Level I*)*	Circles are applied across one hemisphere to obtain appropriate data.	
9. Press edges of sensor to ensure adhesion; then apply firm pressure to all 4 electrode circles for 5 seconds to ensure proper contact. *(Level I*)*	Electrode circles contain a gel. Pressing edges of sensor before applying pressure to electrode circles improves adhesion.	
10. Insert BIS extend sensor tab into the patient interface cable. *(Level I*)*	Required for transmission of signal from sensor to monitor.	
11. Turn on the power switch.	Required to initiate monitoring.	
12. Self-test is initiated; ensure that test is successful.	Ensures monitor is functioning correctly.	
13. Monitor checks sensor impedance of each electrode circle. *(Level I*)*	Sensor impedance indicates acceptable signal reception from the child to the sensor. Pass indicates impedance is good. HIGH indicates that the electrodes need to be reprepped. NOISE indicates the presence of a large external stimulus, or if there is pressure on the electrode during the check. LDOFF indicates that the electrode needs reprepping because it was lifted off.	To initiate a manual impedance check at any time during monitoring, highlight sensor check on the setup menu and press select. The impedance values will appear above each electrode on the screen.

Procedure continues on following page

* Level I: Manufacturer's recommendations only

Procedure for Bispectral Index (BIS) Monitoring—*Continued*

Steps	Rationale	Considerations
14. Identify BIS value displayed in the BIS numeric region in solid characters. *(Level I*)*	BIS calculates a value between 0 and 100 that provides a direct measure of the child's hypnotic state or level of consciousness. 0 indicates isoelectric EEG or absence of brain activity. 40 indicates deep level of sedation. <60 indicates moderate level of sedation, low probability of explicit recall, and that the child is unresponsive to verbal stimulus. 100 indicates the child is fully awake. *(Level IV*)*	The BIS value is calculated as a rolling average using a window of artifact-free time that is updated with new EEG information every second. Smoothing rate is the value averaged over a period of 30 seconds when the extend sensor is used. Smoothing rate of 30 is used in the ICU setting because it provides less variability and sensitivity to artifact. A smoothing rate of 15 seconds is used when a rapid change of the child's hypnotic state is expected such as during induction or awakening.
15. Identify battery icon on monitor screen.	The monitor automatically switches to battery backup if the power is interrupted. The battery symbol will appear in the BIS numeric region. The battery will provide 20 minutes of operation and is recharged in 4 hours when the power is on.	
16. Adjust high and low alarm limits through the setup screen if necessary. *(Level I*)*	When a high or low alarm is reached, an audible alarm sounds and the BIS value alternates between a solid and an outlined character. Press alarm silence key on the front of the monitor to stop the alarm.	When the extend sensor is in use, the alarm will silence for 120 seconds and then reactivate if the condition continues.
17. Identify the BIS values plotted over 1 hour on the BIS trend window. You may review up to 11 hours by pressing review keys and use the left arrow to scroll back in time and the right arrow to scroll forward. Secondary trend lines such as EEG, suppression ratio (SR) or signal quality index (SQI) may be added through the advanced setup menu. Highlight advanced setup and press the select key.	Allows trending of BIS values over time.	Extended memory is stored up to 23 days and can be accessed only by Aspect personnel. The secondary variable option is used for trending the EEG, SR, or SQI in addition to the BIS trend.
18. Identify SQI, located in the signal status region.	The SQI indicates the quality of the EEG signal obtained over the last 60 seconds. The bar should extend to the far right. As the SQI decreases, the BIS numeric display will change to an outlined number and will prompt a sensor-patient connection check.	
19. Identify the electromyograph (EMG) indicator located in the signal status region; the bar should be to the left side of the display.	EMG indicates muscle activity or other high-frequency artifacts. If the EMG is increased, the BIS value is less reliable.	The EMG may extend to the right when sedation is lightening, when the child is moving, experiencing seizures, is in pain, or when the neuromuscular blockade is wearing off. *(Level V*)*

* Level I: Manufacturer's recommendations only
Level IV: Limited clinical studies to support recommendations
Level V: Clinical studies in more than one or two patient populations and situations to support recommendations

Procedure for Bispectral Index (BIS) Monitoring—*Continued*

Steps	Rationale	Considerations
20. Identify the EEG waveform display.	Displays EEG activity obtained via sensor.	
21. Identify the SR value.	The SR indicates the percentage of time over the last 63 seconds that the EEG signal is suppressed.	The SR is useful in titration of pentobarbital infusions to achieve burst suppression for children in pentobarbital coma. *(Level IV*)*
22. Access setup menu to review and change monitoring options. Press menu/exit soft key on the monitor. *(Level I*)*	To review data, press right or left arrow. Press the up and down arrows to move from one menu item to the next item.	
23. To mark an event, highlight the event item on the setup menu, press select. The event is marked with an arrow on the trend display. The monitor will return to the main screen. *(Level I*)*	"Event" is used to mark an event on the trend screen display.	
24. Dispose of used supplies and equipment in appropriate receptacle; wash hands.	Standard precautions; reduces transmission of microorganisms.	

* Level I: Manufacturer's recommendations only
  Level IV: Limited clinical studies to support recommendations

Expected Outcomes

- Reliable BIS values are obtained and optimal level of sedation is provided to the child

- Child experiences no complications of undersedation

- Child experiences no complications of oversedation

Unexpected Outcomes

- Unreliable BIS value obtained because of artifact related to muscle activity, poor sensor placement or adherence, or interference
- Recall of stressful events or procedures
- Increased anxiety
- Prolonged time on mechanical ventilation resulting in increased length of stay
- Complications related to oversedation
- Increased charges related to excessive use of sedative drugs

Monitoring and Care of the Child

Activities and Interventions	Rationale	Reportable Conditions
1. Monitor child's sedation and anxiety levels.	Clinical assessment of child's sedation status is mandatory.	• Indications of over- or undersedation
2. Monitor child for complications of sedation.	Prompt identification of complications allows immediate intervention.	• Hypotension • Decreased respiratory rate • Paradoxical reaction to sedation medication
3. Monitor BIS value with vital signs and before and after stimulation.	A higher BIS value may be noted poststimulation, and a rapid return to baseline is normal. A BIS value that remains higher than expected after stimulation may indicate the need for analgesia.	• Failure of BIS to return to baseline when stimulus is removed

Continued

Monitoring and Care of the Child—Cont'd

Activities and Interventions	Rationale	Reportable Conditions
4. Monitor for changes in BIS value.	Child may require titration of sedation medications.	• High BIS score despite increased doses of sedation medications • Lower than clinically expected BIS value • Change in BIS value independent of titration of sedation medications
5. Monitor condition of skin under electrode placement.	Assess for skin irritation with daily sensor changes.	• Alterations in skin integrity • Report changes in skin integrity to Aspect Medical Systems, Inc.

Documentation

- BIS values with vital sign documentation
- BIS values before and after administration of sedation medications and procedures
- Clinical assessment of sedation and specific interventions provided
- Skin condition before sensor application and after sensor removal
- Child and family education
- Unexpected outcomes and related treatment

References

1. Berkenbosch JW, et al: The correlation of the bispectral index monitor with clinical sedation scores during mechanical ventilation in the pediatric intensive care unit, *Anesth Analg* 94:506-511, 2002.
2. Riker RR, et al: Comparing the bispectral index and suppression ratio with burst suppression of the electroencephalogram during pentobarbital infusions in adult intensive care patients, *Pharmacotherapy* 23(9):1087-1093, 2003.
3. Gilbert TT, et al: Use of bispectral electroencephalogram monitoring to assess neurologic status of unsedated, critically ill patients, *Crit Care Med* 29:1996-2000, 2001.
4. McDermott NB, et al: Validation of the bispectral index monitor during conscious and deep sedation in children, *Anesth Analg* 97:39-43, 2003.
5. Azzam MA, et al: Comparison of the bispectral index (BIS) with the comfort score to assess sedation in the pediatric intensive care unit, *Crit Care Med* 28(Suppl 12):544, 2000.
6. Crain N, et al: Assessing sedation in the pediatric intensive care unit by using BIS and comfort scale, *Pediatr Crit Care Med* 3(1):11-14, 2002
7. Simmons L, et al: Assessing sedation during intensive care unit mechanical ventilation with the bispectral index and the sedation-agitation scale, *Crit Care Med* 27(8):1499-1504, 1999.
8. Trilsch A, et al: Bispectral index (BIS) correlates with Ramsay sedation scores in neurosurgical ICU patients, *Anesthesiology* 91(3A):A295, 1999.
9. Takeda T, et al: Usefulness of the bispectral index (BIS) for mechanically ventilated patients in intensive care unit, *Crit Care Med* 28(Suppl 12):114, 2000.
10. Riker RR, et al: Validating the sedation-agitation scale with the bispectral index and visual analog scale in adult ICU patients after cardiac surgery, *Intensive Care Med* 27(5):853-858, 2001.
11. Ely EW, et al: Validating the bispectral EEG for ventilated ICU patients, *Am Respir Crit Care Med* 163(5):A899, 2001.
12. Denman WT, et al: Pediatric evaluation of the bispectral index monitor and correlation of BIS with end-tidal sevoflurane concentration in infants and children, *Anesth Analg* 90:872-877, 2000.

Additional Readings

Aspect Medical Systems, Inc. BIS by Aspect. *BIS Inservice Video*, Newton, MA: Aspect Medical Systems, Inc., 2003
Aspect Medical Systems, Inc. *Technology overview: Bispectral Index*. Newton, MA: Aspect Medical Systems, Inc., 1997.
McGaffigan P: Advancing sedation assessment to promote patient comfort, *Crit Care Nurse* 22(Suppl):29-38, 2002.
Olson D, et al: Potential benefits of bispectral index monitoring in critical care: a case study, *Crit Care Nurse* 23:45-51, 2003.

Epidural Catheter: Care and Management

P U R P O S E :   An epidural catheter is placed to provide pain relief to the abdomen, thorax, and lower extremities by injecting medications into the epidural space, decreasing the possibility of the side effects associated with systemic opioid administration

Linda L. Oakes

PREREQUISITE KNOWLEDGE

- Anatomy of the central nervous system, specifically, the location of the epidural space as a potential space between the dura mater and the vertebral canal (Figure 171-1).
- The epidural space is a potential space filled with vasculature, fat, and a network of nerve extensions. No free-flowing fluid is in the epidural space; a true space is created when fluid or air is injected into it.
- Diffusion of opioids through the dura into the cerebrospinal fluid (CSF) and then into the spinal cord directly to the analgesic action site (receptors in the dorsal horn of the spinal cord) leads to direct analgesia, eliminating many of the systemic side effects of opioids with minimal effect on motor or sympathetic function.[1]
- Indications for epidural analgesia include:
  - ❖ Postoperative pain management following thoracic, major abdominal or lower-limb surgeries. Studies in adults demonstrate superior analgesia and attenuate postoperative morbidity such as improving postoperative pulmonary function. However, there are no such studies in children.[2]
  - ❖ Oncologic pain below the T4 dermatome (nipple line) when systemic routes of analgesia are no longer an option because of unmanageable and intolerable side effects at the anticipated doses required for adequate analgesia (i.e., sedation/respiratory depression).

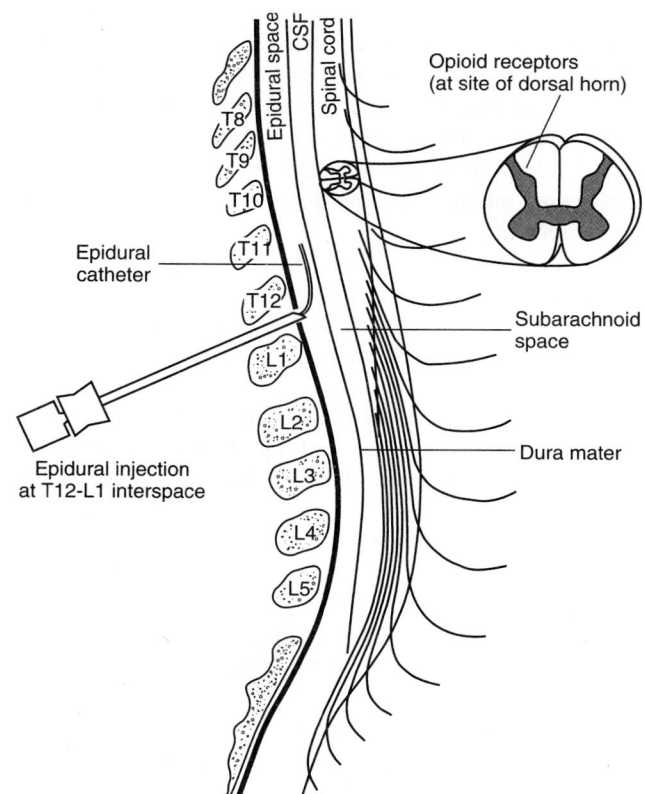

FIGURE 171-1 Anatomy of the epidural space. *From McCaffery M, Pasero C, editors:* Pain: clinical manual, *ed 2, St Louis, 1999, Mosby.*

❖ Elective amputation of a lower limb to prevent or reduce the severity of phantom pain.[2-4]
- Vigilance is required to identify signs and provide immediate management for the following rare, serious complications:
  ❖ Infection of the site and epidural space including an epidural abscess
  ❖ Bleeding into the epidural space including an epidural hematoma
  ❖ Side effects of local anesthetics such as motor blockade, cardiovascular collapse, and apnea
  ❖ Side effects of opioids such as excessive sedation, respiratory depression, and apnea
- Placement of the epidural catheter and ongoing medical direction is to be done by those trained and skilled in anesthesiology. Clinical support systems are to be available around the clock to assess for the need to titrate the infusions and to assess for and manage complications.
- Most state boards for nursing and institutions require nursing management by registered nurses who have demonstrated evidence of competency in care of patients with epidurals on an annual basis. Professional nursing organizations have endorsed the role of the RN if ongoing competency has been determined.[5] RNs must be aware of and adhere to any restrictions in their state/institution regarding administration of epidural boluses or the maintenance of epidural infusions.
- Two types of medications are often used either as a bolus or continuous infusion: opioids and local anesthetics. When given in combination, a synergistic effect provides effective analgesia at lower doses than would be possible with either type of medication alone.[2] Lower doses of either type of medication reduce the incidence and severity of side effects. Doses of medications given in the epidural space to produce analgesia are lower than the systemic requirement but higher than the intrathecal requirement.[6]
  ❖ Local anesthetics: bupivacaine or levo-bupivacaine, usually in a solution with a concentration of 0.1% (1 mg/mL) to 0.125% (1.25 mg/mL). Such dilute concentrations provide analgesia with less risk of motor blockade.
    ○ The maximal recommended loading dose as a bolus is 2.5 mg/kg (1 mL/kg of the 0.25% solution) with a maximum of 20 mL for catheters placed at the caudal level. The dose should be decreased appropriately for catheters placed at thoracic and lumbar levels.
    ○ For continuous infusions, the usual maximum dose of bupivacaine or levo-bupivacaine is 0.4 mg/kg/hr.
  ❖ Opioids: fentanyl, morphine, hydromorphone (Dilaudid)
    ○ The usual concentration for fentanyl is 2 to 5 mcg/mL; for morphine, 2 to 30 mcg/mL; for hydromorphone, 10 mcg/mL.
    ○ The maximum initial dose as a bolus of fentanyl is 1 mcg/kg/bolus; for morphine, 0.05 mg/kg/bolus.

    ○ The maximum hourly rate of a continuous infusion for fentanyl is 1 mcg/kg/hr; for morphine 8 to 12 mcg/kg/hr; for hydromorphone, 2 to 3 mcg/kg/hr.
- Continuous infusions facilitate prompt adjustment of the dose based on the child's response and avoid peaks and troughs associated with bolus doses only. Fentanyl is more lipid soluble than morphine and is readily taken up into the systemic circulation, reducing the duration of action. Effective analgesia using fentanyl will best be provided by a continuous infusion.
- Epidural catheters inserted percutaneously can be maintained with minimal risk of infection up to 3 to 5 days.[2]
- Informed consent is required before placement of an epidural catheter.
- Standard precautions and sterile technique are to be maintained during catheter manipulation.
- Child development as it relates to clinical assessment and epidural catheter management
- Mastery of pediatric advanced life support competencies
- Appropriate pediatric dosing of analgesics and sedatives and competency in procedural sedation

CHILD AND FAMILY ASSESSMENT

- The overall physical status of the child weighing risk versus benefit of placement of the epidural catheter ➥*Rationale:* The type, site of surgery, severity of postoperative pain anticipated over the next 3 to 5 days should be considered to determine the potential benefit of providing epidural analgesia.
- The presence of contraindications including but not limited to coagulopathies,[7] anatomic deformities/fractures of the spine, local infections near the site of the potential placement of the catheter or fever (systemic infection) and unstable cardiovascular status ➥*Rationale:* The presence of these clinical findings increases the risk for:
  ❖ Epidural hematoma: usually the platelet count should be greater than 70,000 mm[3] and the partial thromboplastin time (PTT) and prothrombin time (PT) within the range of normal control for the child to be eligible for placement of an epidural[1]
  ❖ Failure of catheter insertion or flow of the epidural medication
  ❖ Seeding of bacteria into the epidural space leading to epidural abscess[7]
  ❖ Further compromise of cardiovascular status
- Child's developmental level and ability to interact ➥*Rationale:* These factors influence preparation of the child and interaction.
- Child's and family's understanding of the reasons for and risks and benefits of the procedure ➥*Rationale:* Evaluates child's and family's understanding of the procedure and provides a gauge for ongoing education.
- Family's desire to be present during catheter insertion ➥*Rationale:* Family may provide support and comfort measures to their child but should have the choice not to remain with the child.

CHILD AND FAMILY EDUCATION

Individualized, developmentally appropriate education is provided to the family and to the child based on desire for knowledge, readiness to learn, and overall neurologic and psychosocial state.

- Provide information about epidural analgesia including the purpose of providing this method of pain control, the necessary safety measures to minimize the associated risks, and sensations which might be experienced such as a decreased ability to sense touch or move a lower limb ➤➤*Rationale:* Providing information decreases family's and child's anxiety and increases cooperation.
- Provide information that epidural analgesia can provide optimal relief of pain and can improve postoperative outcomes, particularly if it is used in combination with a postoperative rehabilitation program that emphasizes early mobilization, oral nutrition, and early return to normal activities[8,9] ➤➤*Rationale:* Providing the child and family with information about benefits and goals of epidural therapy facilitates compliance with the treatment plan.
- If developmentally appropriate and the insertion will be completed while the child is awake, explain how the child can assist with the insertion to improve correct catheter placement ➤➤*Rationale:* Providing information increases the child's ability to cooperate and decreases anxiety.
- Methods that will be used to assess pain using age-appropriate valid pain scales. See Procedure 173 for further information ➤➤*Rationale:* Reassuring the family that pain will be regularly assessed in an appropriate manner decreases anxiety and increases cooperation.
- Explain actions of the child and family that will assist in maintaining the integrity of the system, specifically to prevent tension on the tubing ➤➤*Rationale:* Providing the family and child with this information will reduce the incidence of catheter displacement or separation of the catheter from the infusion system. Percutaneously placed catheters are inserted through a needle, and then an adapter is applied to connect the catheter to the infusion tubing (Figure 171-2). Tension to the system can separate the adapter from the catheter.
- Encourage questions and answer questions as they arise ➤➤*Rationale:* Reinforcement of information is needed during periods of stress.

EQUIPMENT

- Continuous epidural anesthesia tray and catheter
- Skin preparation agent per institution-specific protocol
- Sterile gloves
- Infusion pump and compatible infusion tubing specific for epidural infusion
- Transparent dressing
- Tape
- Medications ordered by the anesthesiologist: a prepared loading dose and reservoir for continuous infusion (bag, syringe, or cassette as required by the infusion pump)
- One vial epinephrine (1:1,000)
- Oxygen saturation monitor
- Emergency cart with naloxone, ephedrine, 0.9% saline
- Suction equipment
- Oxygen

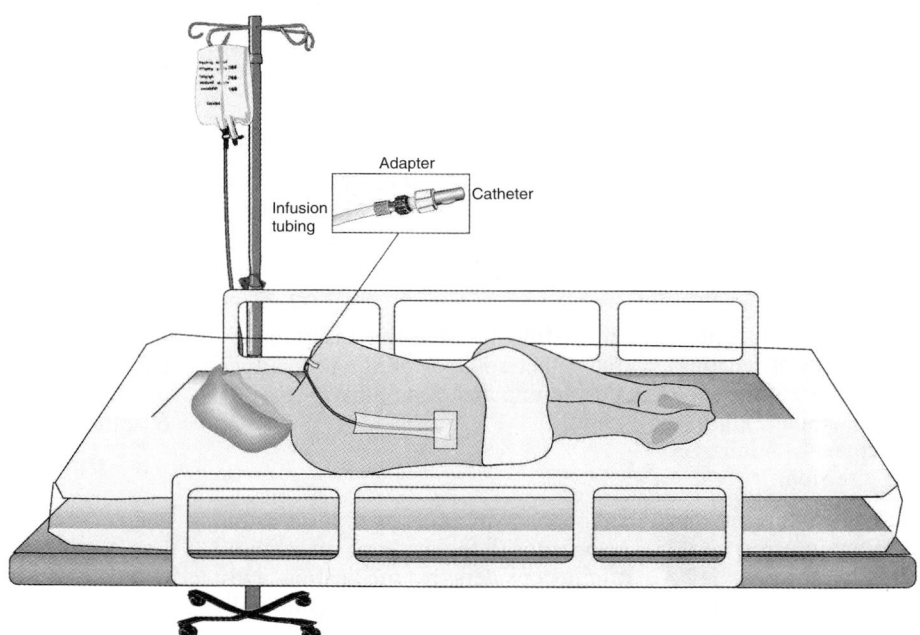

FIGURE 171-2 Placement of epidural catheter and the epidural infusion system. *Drawing courtesy of Biomedical Communications, St. Jude Children's Research Hospital, Memphis, TN, 2005.*

Procedure for Epidural Catheter: Care and Management

Steps	Rationale	Considerations
Assisting with Insertion		
1. Ensure child and family understand procedure and questions are answered.	Evaluates and reinforces understanding of previously taught information.	Developmental level, cognitive ability, and anxiety level will determine approach to and effectiveness of teaching.
2. Confirm that consent for procedure has been obtained.	Ensures medicolegal compliance as suggested by the Joint Commission on Accreditation of Healthcare Organizations (JCAHO).	
3. Apply local anesthetic cream to the anticipated insertion site as prescribed and according to manufacturer's recommendations.[10]	Reduces the pain of needle insertion for subcutaneous local anesthetic infiltration before placing the epidural needle.	Children have an intense fear of needle-related pain.
4. Gather needed equipment and supplies including local anesthetic for subcutaneous infiltration.	Facilitates completion of task in a timely manner; local anesthetic reduces the pain related to the insertion of the epidural needle.	Children have an intense fear of needle-related pain.
5. Identify child using appropriate patient/procedure verification process (e.g., "Time out").	Confirms correct patient, procedure and site as recommended by JCAHO; prevents unnecessary medical procedures.[11]	Two patient identifiers are generally used; in the inpatient setting, name and medical record number are most often used. Verification process and documentation is institution specific; use active communication techniques.
6. Wash hands.	Standard precautions; reduces the transmission of microorganisms.	Epidural infection may result in epidural abscess.
7. Ensure child has cardiopulmonary monitoring with alarms appropriately set and a patent IV.	The respiratory and cardiovascular systems of children may decompensate during the procedure. Oxygen, airway support, IV fluid boluses, and other medications may need to be administered urgently.	Consider child's status when selecting the appropriate monitoring. All emergency equipment must to be of the appropriate size for the child.
8. Compare all medications for bolus or infusion purposes to ensure consistency with prescribing practitioner's orders. Medications, their concentrations, and initial pump settings should be independently verified by another licensed staff member. Ensure all medications and solutions are preservative free. *(Level II*)*	Preservatives may cause damage to the spinal cord; only preservative-free medications and 0.9% saline should be administered via the epidural route. Assume that all multiple-dose vials contain preservatives and do not administer epidurally.	Dose is dependent on the child's age, size, underlying medical condition, and the margin of safety for that specific child.
9. Consult with the individual inserting the catheter about benefits of sedating child during the procedure if the child is not under general anesthesia at the time of placement to minimize movement during insertion.	Successful and event-free insertion of the catheter is increased with optimal positioning and immobility of the child.[2]	The child's ability to cooperate and remain immobile during the insertion is related to age and overall condition.
10. Prime infusion tubing from reservoir to the distal end of the infusion tubing. Ensure placement of an antisiphon valve or mechanism to prevent free-flow within the infusion system.	Although small amounts of air are not dangerous in the epidural space, the pump considers this medication, and therefore there is a risk the child will be undermedicated. In the event the pump malfunctions, valves or	

* Level II: Theory-based, no research data to support recommendations: recommendations from expert consensus group may exist

Procedure for Epidural Catheter: Care and Management—*Continued*

Steps	Rationale	Considerations
	mechanisms must be in place to prevent free-flow of the infusion into the child.[11]	
11. Assist the anesthesia practitioner inserting the catheter in positioning, prepping, and draping child. Support child during the remainder of the insertion.	Generally speaking, the catheter tip should be placed as close as possible to the spinal nerves carrying the pain impulses from the surgical area. Although most catheters are placed in the lumbar region, placement in the thoracic or caudal regions can provide effective analgesia and minimal risk to damaging the spinal cord and its surrounding anatomy.[2] Sitting or side-lying with the back arched out toward the anesthesia practitioner helps to spread the vertebrae apart.	The caudal approach is often used in children because it is simple, easy to perform, and with less risk of injury to the spinal column because its distal tip does not reach the caudal area. However, clinicians are concerned about its anatomic closeness to the diaper area in non–toilet trained children, thus increasing the risk of infection. Because of a more challenging placement in younger children, thoracic placement is generally reserved for older children having upper abdominal and thoracic procedures. The child's anatomy may require a variation in the flexing of the back. Family presence may be very supportive.
12. Observe child while the anesthesia practitioner confirms catheter placement by injecting a test dose to rule out intravascular placement of the catheter tip.[2] If heart rate (HR) does not increase, the needle is considered to be in the epidural space rather than a vascular space. The catheter is then threaded through the needle.[12]	Doses of local anesthetics for epidural administration are generally higher than those intended for intravascular administration. The test dose of the local anesthetic usually contains epinephrine. If child's HR increases by 20% within 30 to 60 seconds after the test dose, the catheter must be repositioned. The only absolute way to confirm placement in the epidural space is to inject contrast dye.	As in adults, signs of intravascular administration of local anesthetics include tinnitus, metallic taste, circumoral numbness, cardiovascular collapse, blurred vision, light-headedness, and seizures. Preverbal children may not be able to report subjective signs. Therefore, clinicians must depend on objective signs such as HR and blood pressure (BP).
13. Assess BP, HR, oxygen saturation (SpO_2), respiratory rate (RR), and signs of sensory or motor blockade every 3 to 5 minutes for the first 30 minutes. If boluses are given at any other time during the infusion, these parameters must be reassessed as above. If any signs of the catheter tip suggest that is in the intrathecal space, discontinue the infusion and reposition the catheter immediately.	Dosages of opioids and local anesthetics for epidural administration are approximately 10 times greater than the dosages intended for the intrathecal route.[10] If a dosage amount intended for the epidural space is given into the intrathecal space, the child may report a progressive loss of feeling and motor ability in the legs, trunk, and chest. If catheter is not repositioned, the following will occur: • Blockade of the cardiac sympathetic system leading to vasodilation and hypotension, reflex tachycardia. • Followed by bradycardia, and increasing respiratory depression. • Respiratory and cardiac arrest.	Preverbal children may not be able to report subjective signs. Therefore, clinicians must depend on objective signs such as HR and BP. Age-appropriate explanations must be given. Even if the goal of therapy is blocking the sensory nerves, this sensation may be frightening to children. If motor weakness also occurs, the child may experience feeling their legs as "heavy."
14. Connect and start the infusion as prescribed. Boldly label the pump and tubing as "epidural." The use of	Labels will decrease the risk of clinicians titrating the infusion with the wrong pump. No medications other	The usual maximum rate for epidural infusions is 14 to 16 mL/hr. Occasionally higher rates

Procedure continues on following page

Procedure for Epidural Catheter: Care and Management—*Continued*

Steps	Rationale	Considerations
indwelling filters depends on institution-specific protocol.	than those ordered by the pain management practitioner (anesthesiologist, certified registered nurse anesthetist (CRNA), pain service nurse practitioner (NP) are to be infused in the epidural catheter.	may be acceptable, not to exceed 20 mL/hr. Refer to state-specific nurse practice acts and institution-specific protocols for information on practi-tioners permitted to order epidural medications.
15. Do not insert any stopcocks within tubing system. Avoid tubing with injection ports; if such tubing is used, tape over every injection port and boldly label as "epidural," indicating the infusion is going into the epidural space.[2]	Prevention of accidental administration of nonepidural medications into the epidural infusion system is required to prevent toxicity to the central nervous system or inappropriate dosages being administered to the child.	
16. Secure catheter with a transparent dressing at the insertion site and apply tape along the entire length of catheter from the insertion site to the shoulder. Tape adapter securely to the shoulder to prevent tension and accidental disconnection of the catheter from the infusion system (see Figure 171-2). Protect dressing from contamination by urine or stool.	Transparent dressings facilitate observation of the catheter insertion site to determine early signs of leakage, infection, or displacement.[2] Percutaneously placed catheters are inserted through a needle. The needle is removed, leaving the catheter in place; an adapter is applied to connect the catheter to the infusion tubing. Because the adapter is not fused to the catheter, it can be easily separated from infusion system at the adapter site.	Age-appropriate explanations must be given to the child to explain mobility while in the bed, during ambulation, or while being held by a family member. Although being held is beneficial to the child, the integrity of the infusion system must be protected.
17. Discard used supplies and equipment, including sharps, in appropriate receptacle.	Standard precautions; reduces transmission of microorganisms. Protects personnel health.	
18. Remove gloves; wash hands.	Standard precautions; reduces transmission of microorganisms.	
Epidural Catheter Removal		
1. Ensure child and family understand procedure and questions are answered.	Evaluates and reinforces understanding of previously taught information.	Developmental level, cognitive ability and anxiety level will determine approach to and effectiveness of teaching.
2. Gather needed supplies and equipment.	Facilitates completion of procedure in a timely manner.	
3. Discontinue catheter per institution-specific protocol and as authorized by the state nurse practice act.[12]	Removing percutaneous epidural catheters is within the scope of practice for RNs in most states.[12]	Consult specific state nurse practice act and institution-specific protocol.
4. Wash hands; put on clean gloves.	Standard precautions; reduces transmission of microorganisms.	
5. Position child in sitting or side-lying position with the back arched.	Removal is facilitated when the child assumes a position similar to that of catheter placement.	
6. Remove all tape and dressing materials gently from the skin.	Required for removal of catheter.	Use adhesive remover to decrease the trauma of tape removal from the skin.
7. Apply gentle traction on the catheter to remove the catheter.	Because the catheter is not sutured in, it should slide out with application of gentle traction.	Excessive force should not be needed.

Procedure for Epidural Catheter: Care and Management—*Continued*

Steps	Rationale	Considerations
8. If resistance is felt, reposition child; retry removal. If still unable to remove the catheter contact the anesthesia/pain service.	The catheter should come out easily and painlessly.	Do not use force to remove the catheter.
9. Inspect catheter tip for the presence of a black or blue mark.	Indicates tip of the catheter was removed intact.	If no black or blue mark is seen on the tip of the catheter, it indicates the tip remains within epidural tract and will have to be surgically removed.
10. Cover insertion site with an adhesive bandage.	Decreases incidence of infection.	
11. Discard used supplies and equipment in appropriate receptacle.	Standard precautions; reduces transmission of microorganisms.	
12. Waste any remaining medication per institution-specific protocol.	Ensures appropriate management of controlled substances.	
13. Remove gloves; wash hands.	Standard precautions.	
14. Ensure that adequate analgesia will be provided by another route of delivery.	Ensures adequate pain control continues.	Refer to an equianalgesic chart in determining the appropriate dosages.

Expected Outcomes

- Pain at a level acceptable to the child or for preverbal children, less than 5/10 points (defined as controlled)
- Integrity and sterility of the epidural system is protected
- Cardiovascular status is stable
- Respiratory status is stable
- Neurologic status is stable (easily aroused and level of consciousness (LOC) is at baseline)
- Skin remains intact over bony prominences
- Aspirated epidural fluid is clear and volume is less than 1 mL
- Child is free from epidural infection or hematoma
- Catheter tip intact at removal

Unexpected Outcomes

- Pain is not controlled (an unacceptable level to the child and/or interferes with movement, cough, treatment, play, or sleep)
- The infusion system is inadvertently disconnected and sterility is not maintained
- Hypotension/cardiovascular collapse
- Respiratory depression or apnea
- Excessive sedation, irritability, seizures, motor blockade
- Skin breakdown present
- Aspirated epidural fluid is bloody (indicating possible intravascular placement) or volume is greater than 1 mL (indicating possible intrathecal placement)
- Epidural abscess or hematoma
- Catheter tip left in the epidural space as a foreign body

Monitoring and Care of the Child

Activities and Interventions	Rationale	Reportable Conditions
1. Assess pain intensity, location and quality at least every 4 hours while awake. Optimally, establish with child the trigger point (the number on the pain scale) the child considers comfortable as well as promotes activities for recovery. For further details about pain assessment, see Procedure 173. *(Level II*)*	Even though weight is generally used to predict analgesic effect, the starting doses for treatment are merely an estimate. When a starting dose is given, it is titrated according to the child's response.[10] Inadequate pain relief is addressed with gradual escalation of the epidural analgesic infusion until adequate analgesia is achieved or intolerable and unmanageable adverse effects occur.	- Inadequate pain control - Inability of the child to participate in recovery activities due to pain - Catheter is displaced from the insertion site

* Level II: Theory-based, no research data to support recommendations: recommendations from expert consensus group may exist

Continued

Monitoring and Care of the Child—Cont'd

Activities and Interventions	Rationale	Reportable Conditions
2. If the pain level requires adjustment of the epidural anticipate direction to: • Increase the infusion rate by 10% to 25%. Changes in pump settings should be independently verified by another licensed staff member. • Administer an epidural bolus of local anesthetic and/or opioid and increase the infusion by 10% to 25%. Give a bolus using the clinician-administered mechanism available on most infusion pumps. Most institutions require anesthesia staff[12] to give any boluses via syringe; syringe used should have a volume of 5 mL or greater. Refer to state nurse practice act and institution-specific protocols for individuals authorized to bolus the epidural catheter via infusion pump or syringe. *(Level II*)*	If the infusion rate is increased without a bolus, it may take 3 to 4 hours for a new steady state to be reached and relief of severe pain.[3] Administration of a bolus of a volume of 1 to 2 hours of the existing infusion over 20 to 30 minutes followed by increasing the infusion by 15% to 25% is recommended for severe pain.[3] Most pumps will have a mechanism to program a bolus which is useful to avoid potential error and time involved in syringe preparation. To prevent excessive pressure on the epidural space, small syringes are to be avoided.[12] Because of the catheter's narrow lumen, resistance is expected. If strong resistance is met, reposition the child to flex the spine; if still not able to give the bolus, stop and notify the practitioner managing the epidural catheter.	• Catheter occlusion
3. Assess BP, HR, and LOC at least every 4 hours while child is awake.[12] Increase frequency of assessment based on child's response to the infusion. If reportable conditions occur, stop the infusion, and: • For hypotension, prepare to infuse fluid boluses and/or ephedrine doses per pain management or anesthesia practitioner. • For neurologic changes, prepare to administer oxygen support, support ventilation, and administer naloxone per pain management or anesthesia practitioner.	The infusion is titrated to effect as well as side effects and adverse reactions. In rare instances, the tip of the catheter can migrate into a blood vessel or the intrathecal space at any time during epidural analgesia therapy despite correct catheter placement initially. Early signs of epidural catheter migration during continuous infusion are likely to be subtle but more pronounced if boluses are given.[5] When a bolus is given, follow the details in Procedure step 13 to rule out that the catheter tip is in the intrathecal space before medication administration.[7]	• Hypotension • Unexplained persistent tachycardia • Bradycardia or other dysrhythmias • Confusion, behavioral changes, excessive sedation • Persistent nausea or vomiting • Seizures • Other neurologic changes • Itching not controlled by prescribed antipruritics
4. Monitor RR and SpO$_2$ at least every 2 hours.[13] When excessive sedation is detected, epidural opioid doses must be decreased. *(Level II*)* • Consult the anesthesia or pain service before administering sedatives, opioids, or hypnotics ordered by another prescribing practitioner. • For children less than 6 months of age, an apnea/bradycardia monitor is recommended to be used as well.[12] *(Level II*)*	Monitoring of sedation level and respiratory status is critical to preventing significant opioid-induced respiratory depression.[7] Respiratory depression may be best prevented by noting any sedative effects from the infusion. Using lipophilic opioids such as fentanyl lessens the risk due to less rostral spread toward the respiratory center in the brainstem.[2,12] A nonsteroidal antiinflammatory drug (NSAID) that provides analgesia	• Change in respiratory pattern (i.e., depth, rate) • SpO$_2$ less than 90% • Change in ability to arouse the child • If any of the above occurs, discontinue the infusion, provide oxygen, and assist with ventilation. • Consider administration of opioid antagonists such as naloxone.

* Level II: Theory-based, no research data to support recommendations: recommendations from expert consensus group may exist

Monitoring and Care of the Child—Cont'd

Activities and Interventions	Rationale	Reportable Conditions
	without the sedative effects of opioids may be useful. Infants less than 6 months of age are at higher risk of respiratory depression. There is neither consensus nor conclusive evidence regarding which forms of electronic monitoring are most useful. If oximetry or apnea alarms are used, they must be connected to central monitors to provide audible alarms when clinicians are not at the bedside. Electronic monitoring is not a substitute for clinical assessment.	
5. Assess child's lower extremity motor function for signs of motor blockade at least every 4 hours[12] to confirm that the child can: • Wiggle the toes and lift the legs off the bed or bend the knees and lift the buttocks off the bed. Explain that any decrease in motor function will improve when the local anesthetic dose is reduced. Consider positioning the child with the side of the body that is feeling numb as the nondependent side.	The goal of administering local anesthetics is to reduce the sensation of pain without affecting the motor nerves. By using a low concentration of local anesthetic, the sensory pain fibers are blocked and motor fibers should remain intact. Decreased ability to move legs or hips may indicate the need to decrease the dose of the local anesthetic. Numbness, "heaviness," and motor weakness may be quite distressing and frightening to children. Reduction in the concentration of local anesthetic or removing all local anesthetics from the infusion may be required to improve motor function.	• Unresolved motor function deficits after the local anesthetic dose is reduced or eliminated from the infusion, which could indicate hematoma or abscess. See item 6 below for details • If the motor blockade continues to rise above the T2 level as assessed by visual disturbances or sensory disturbances in upper extremities, breathing difficulties may occur. • Numbness and tingling in areas distant to the site of injury or surgery
6. Assess for signs and symptoms of epidural abscess or hematoma: • Localized back pain • Localized tenderness • Radicular pain • Paraplegia • Sensory loss • Urinary and fecal retention • Incontinence • Defect on myelography • Localized lesion on MRI • Fever (abscess only)[2]	Child's recovery without neurologic injury depends on early recognition and aggressive treatment of epidural hematoma or abscess.	• Continued motor weakness or onset of severe back pain must be reported urgently because of the need to assess for an epidural hematoma or abscess that, if left untreated, could lead to compression, ischemia, and permanent neurologic damage. • Be prepared to transport for immediate radiologic investigation (MRI) and surgical decompression or evacuation
7. Minimize disconnections of the epidural system to only when the reservoir needs to be changed, during administration of the boluses of analgesics, or when otherwise requested by the anesthesia or pain management practitioner.	Minimizing system disconnections will decrease the risk of infection. Use only non-neurotoxic agents such as povidone-iodine to clean any ports or connecting points; if alcohol is used it could then be introduced into the infusion system and it is known to be neurotoxic.[14,10]	• Inadvertent disconnection of the epidural system
8. Assess and document integrity of the epidural dressing and the full length of the infusion system every 4 hours while child is awake. Inspect the connection of the catheter adapter to the catheter to ensure stability. Remind the child to not tug on the catheter. Reinforce any loose edges of the dressing, using care to not dislodge	A collection of fluid may be seen at the insertion site. In most cases, this is fluid from backflow out along the tract made by the insertion needle, which is larger than the epidural catheter. Usually this does not require any special treatment. Inadequate pain relief may be a result of a number of factors, including incorrect pump programming, discon-	• Concern that the epidural catheter tip is no longer in the epidural space • Obvious catheter displacement • Loose dressing • The proximal end of the catheter is no longer connected to the infu-on system at the adapter site

Continued

Monitoring and Care of the Child—Cont'd

Activities and Interventions	Rationale	Reportable Conditions

the catheter until the anesthesiologist changes the dressing.

If the proximal end of the catheter is no longer connected to the infusion system at the adapter site, do not reconnect; maintain sterility as much as possible by wrapping both ends in sterile gauze or cap tubing when possible.[6] *(Level II*)*

nection of the catheter from the infusion pump tubing, an empty reservoir, or catheter displacement.

The practice of reconnecting a catheter to the adapter is controversial, and clinicians should refer to institution-specific protocol and their state nurse practice act.

If reconnection is to be done[6]:
  Use sterile technique.
  Clean the catheter with alcohol and then allow the alcohol to dry.
  Cut the end of the epidural catheter with sterile scissors.
  Apply new epidural adapter.
  Reconnect and resume the infusion.
These steps should be performed only after consultation with the anesthesia or pain service prescribing practitioner.

9. Assess for side effects of opioids such as pruritus or urinary retention. Generally, children will have an indwelling urinary catheter. Assess for signs of bladder distention.

Itching as a side effect of the opioid occurs more frequently via epidural catheters compared to IV administration. If fentanyl is infused at a rate of more than 1 mcg/kg/hr it often leads to unacceptable pruritus.[2] Antihistamines or the titration of an infusion of naloxone typically at doses of 0.25 to 1 mcg/kg/hr may be used.[2] Clinicians should consider that antihistamines also can produce sedation.

Because analgesics are delivered close to the micturition center of the spinal cord, the detrusor muscle may be relaxed. Opioids may induce increased sphincter tone.[7] The central effects of opioids and sensory blockade of the anesthetics can interfere with perception of bladder fullness and the child's attention to bladder distention.

- Intolerable pruritus
- Bladder distention
- Excessive sedation from antihistamines

10. Promote activity as per prescribing practitioner's orders. Ambulation is to be done with the assistance of hospital staff. Observe for orthostatic hypotension before ambulation. Assess ability to bear weight before ambulation. Because motor impairment may lead to a risk of injury, instruct the family to have the child remain in bed until further assessment if motor impairment is identified.

Children need close supervision of ambulation for potential weakness and disconnection of the epidural system. Local anesthetics may interfere with motor function, and the child may be at risk for falls. Reducing or removing the local anesthetic from the epidural analgesic solution may be necessary to decrease motor blockade. Children may not bathe or shower until the epidural catheter is removed.

- Motor function impairment

11. Notify anesthesia or pain management team of any signs of infection, leakage, or catheter occlusion or displacement. Do

Changing dressing will increase the risk of catheter dislodgement because the very small lumen prevents effective suturing of the catheter to the skin

- Unexplained fever greater than 38° C
- Signs of infection, leakage of clear or bloody fluid

---

* Level II: Theory-based, no research data to support recommendations: recommendations from expert consensus group may exist

Monitoring and Care of the Child—Cont'd

Activities and Interventions	Rationale	Reportable Conditions
not flush the epidural catheter unless specifically directed by the anesthesia or pain management team. Only the anesthesia or pain management team should determine the need to change the dressing or to remove the catheter.	without obstructing flow. If entire catheter is displaced, retain the catheter for the anesthesia/pain management team to ensure entire catheter including the tip has been removed.	• Failure to infuse due to occlusion • Dressing loose • Catheter displacement
12. Assess child's skin integrity, specifically over the sacral and other pressure points. Assist in repositioning every 2 hours while awake.	Children are at increased risk for skin breakdown because of decreased sensation and decreased urge to reposition themselves.	• Skin redness over pressure points or skin breakdown
13. Reassess medications infusing at least once a shift including the concentration and pump settings as compared with the prescribing practitioner's orders. If the child has another infusion of bupivacaine, such as through a catheter into a wound or nerve sheath, the total dose of both infusions is not to exceed the 0.4 mg/kg/hr limit. For infants less than 2 months of age, the dose is reduced to 0.2 mg/kg/hr.[2,15] *(Level II[*])*	Strict attention to drug concentration and infusion rates to avoid toxic doses of medications is necessary. The absolute opioid dose is unimportant as long as the balance between pain relief and adverse effects is favorable. The goal of titration is to use the lowest dose possible to provide satisfactory pain relief with the fewest adverse effects. However, the usual maximum dose of bupivacaine is 0.4 mg/kg/hr. Higher doses may be tolerated but increase the risk of neurologic side effects.[15]	• Any medication or dose/concentration variance
14. To check placement of catheter using sterile technique[1]: • Carefully disconnect the infusion tubing and maintain sterility. • Connect an empty syringe to the epidural catheter. • Gently aspirate. • Inspect for fluid. • If blood is seen, reconnect the tubing but do not restart the infusion. • If clear fluid of more than 1 mL is obtained, reconnect the tubing to the catheter but do not restart the infusion. *(Level II[*])*	Refer to state nurse practice act or institution-specific protocol to determine individuals authorized to perform this procedure. Blood in the fluid indicates the tip of the catheter is intravascular. Clear fluid in a volume greater than 1 mL indicates that the tip of the catheter may be in the intrathecal space.	• Blood in the aspirated fluid • More than 1 mL of aspirated fluid • Catheter occlusion as indicated by inability to aspirate fluid
15. Consider the combination of continuous controlled infusion via the epidural catheter infusion and patient-administered boluses using a pump to deliver patient-controlled epidural analgesia (PCEA). Provide half of the maximum dose of bupivacaine as a continuous infusion while making the other half available as boluses with a lockout of 15 minutes for a maximum of 2 boluses per hour. Refer to Procedure 174 for more details.	PCEA permits the child to treat increased pain by self-administering doses of analgesics. This option should be considered in pediatric postoperative pain management for the older child.[16,2] Time needed for a bolus dose to take effect is longer with epidural compared with IV PCA. Thus the lockout period is longer, usually 15 to 30 minutes.[2]	

*[*] Level II: Theory-based, no research data to support recommendations: recommendations from expert consensus group may exist

Documentation

- Child and family education
- Vital signs and SpO_2
- Pain intensity (score), location, and quality
- Medications given during insertion
- Condition of dressing and insertion site
- Medications/infusion, pump settings
- Adjunctive medications for pain, nausea, pruritus
- Response to medications administered
- Level of consciousness/arousability
- Ease in removing catheter, the presence of the catheter tip on removal, condition of the insertion site
- Child's lower extremity motor function and dermatome level of sensation
- Unexpected outcomes and related treatment

References

1. Oakes LO: Caring practices: providing comfort. In Curley MAQ, Moloney-Harmon PA, editors: *Critical care nursing of infants and children,* ed 2, Philadelphia, 2001, Saunders, pp. 568-570.
2. Desparmet JF, et al: Central blocks in children and adolescents. In Schechter NL, et al, editors: *Pain in infants, children, and adolescents,* ed 2, Philadelphia, 2003, Lippincott Williams & Wilkins, pp. 339-359.
3. Fainsinger RL, et al: Amputation and the prevention of phantom pain, *J Pain Symptom Manage* 20:308-312, 2000.
4. Swope EM: Benefits of proper pain management. In St. Marie B, editor: *American Society of Pain Management Nurses: core curriculum for pain management nursing,* Philadelphia, 2002, Saunders, pp. 55-66.
5. American Nurses Association: *Role of the registered nurse in the management of analgesia by catheter technique (epidural, intrathecal, intrapleural, or peripheral nerve catheters),* Silver Spring, MD, 1991, American Nurses Association.
6. Yaster M, et al: Epidural analgesia. In Yaster M, et al, editors: *Pediatric pain management and sedation handbook,* St Louis, 1997, Mosby, pp. 114-136.
7. Slowikowski RD, Flaherty SA: Epidural analgesia for postoperative orthopaedic pain, *Orthop Nurs* 19(1):23-31, 2000.
8. Berde CB, Solodiuk J: Multidisciplinary programs for management of acute and chronic pain in children. In Schechter NL, et al, editors: *Pain in infants, children, and adolescents,* ed 2, Philadelphia, 2003, Lippincott Williams & Wilkins, pp. 477-479.
9. Wong CM, et al: The pain (and stress) in infants in a neonatal intensive care unit. In Schechter NL, et al, editors: *Pain in infants, children, and adolescents,* ed 2, Philadelphia, 2003, Lippincott Williams & Wilkins, p. 686.
10. Pasero C: *Epidural analgesia for acute pain management: self-directed learning program,* Lenexa, KS, 2005, American Society for Pain Management Nursing. www.aspmn.org, accessed 5/19/06.
11. Joint Commission Resources. Special Report: 2003 JCAHO national patient safety goals: practical strategies and helpful solutions for meeting these goals. Accessed from www.jcrinc.com/subscribers/patientsafety.asp?durki=7916&site=22&return=154, accessed 11/3/05.
12. Pasero C, et al: Opioid analgesics. In McCaffery M, Pasero C, editors: *Pain: clinical manual,* ed 2, St Louis, 1999, Mosby, pp.161-299.
13. American Pain Society: *Principles of analgesic use in treatment of acute pain and cancer pain,* ed 5, Glenview, IL, 2003, American Pain Society, pp. 24-26.
14. Paice JA, et al: Catheter port cleansing techniques and the entry of povidone-iodine into the epidural space, *Oncol Nurs Forum* 26:603, 1999.
15. Macfadyen AJ, Buckmaster MA: Pain management in the pediatric intensive care unit, *Crit Care Clin* 15:185-197, 1999.
16. Birmingham PK, Wheeler M, et al: Patient-controlled epidural analgesia in children: can they do it? *Pediatr Anesth* 96:686, 2003.

Additional Readings

Block BM, et al: Efficacy of postoperative epidural analgesia: a meta-analysis, *JAMA* 290:245, 2003.

Muir MR, et al: Monitoring practices following epidural analgesics for pain management: a follow-up survey, *J Pain Symptom Manage* 14:3-44, 1997.

Locally Administered Anesthetic Infusions

PURPOSE: To provide pain relief by placing a catheter directly into an operative site or along a nerve sheath and then connecting it to a spring-loaded device or pump to deliver a local anesthetic continuously and/or by bolus

Linda L. Oakes

PREREQUISITE KNOWLEDGE

- Local anesthetics (LAs) used in locally administered anesthetic infusions (LAAIs)
    - ❖ Bupivacaine, lidocaine, mepivacaine, and ropivacaine; bupivacaine (0.25%-0.5%; 2.5-5 mg/mL) is used most frequently with a maximum dose of 0.4 mg/kg/hr
    - ❖ Therapeutic intent: reduce pain transmitted by the peripheral nerves to the spinal cord, thus allowing for lighter general anesthesia as well as reduced dosages of systemic analgesics and their related side effects
    - ❖ Side effects of LAs: twitching, lightheadedness, perioral tingling, tinnitus, visual disturbances, motor blockade, seizures, cardiovascular collapse, and apnea (if used near the thoracic area)
- Capabilities of the specific spring-loaded device (SLD) or pump regarding
    - ❖ The volume it will deliver in mL/hr
    - ❖ The volume in mL per bolus
    - ❖ For SLDs that have a bolus mechanism: how to provide a bolus, the time needed to refill the bolus reservoir, and the maximum volume the SLD can deliver per hour. This calculation is needed to determine the maximum dose of LA per hour to ensure toxic doses are avoided.
- Percutaneous placement of the catheter is performed during the surgical procedure. Ongoing medical direction is done by surgical staff trained in placement of such catheters and LAAI. If an epidural infusion with an LA is also in place, collaboration with anesthesia or pain serv-ice staff is required to assure that the total LA dose given by the epidural and LAAI is not above the dose at risk for LA toxicity.
    - ❖ Optimal pain control can improve postoperative outcomes, particularly if it is used in combination with a postoperative rehabilitation program that emphasizes early mobilization, oral nutrition, and early return to normal activities.[1,2]
- To ensure safety, only physicians and nurses competent in managing LAAI in children including the assessment for side effect and complications should offer this method of pain control.[2]
- Monitoring and care are to be provided by RNs who have demonstrated knowledge and skills in the care of children with LAAI; professional nursing organizations have endorsed the role of the RN in the care of these children and support competency recommendations.[3]
- Standard precautions and aseptic technique are maintained during manipulation of the infusion system and medication.
- Child development as it relates to clinical assessment and LAAI

CHILD AND FAMILY ASSESSMENT

- The appropriateness of using LAAI for a specific child including any known allergies to LA ➥*Rationale:* Postoperative pain management has been demonstrated to be effective for postorthopedic surgical procedures involving upper or lower limbs.[2] Earlier discharge to the outpatient setting including the use of the LAAI at home after any motor blockade has been partially recovered has been demonstrated for adults but not for children.[1,2] Therefore, the use of LAAI should be restricted to inpatient use in children for close monitoring for side effects.[2]

- Ability to comprehend the appropriate use of the bolus mechanism of LAAI. Generally this applies to children older than 5 years of age who are not too ill or physically impaired to appropriately activate a bolus ➤➤*Rationale:* Although exceptions occur for children who become more familiar with medical technology due to chronic illnesses, the cognitive ability to understand the relationship between cause and effect and thus how and when to push a bolus button does not develop until 5 years of age.[1,4,5] However, the recommended lower age limit for children continues to fall as considerations are made for allowing proxies (nurses or family members) to initiate a PCA bolus for children too young or ill to self-boost.
- Child's developmental level and ability to interact ➤➤*Rationale:* These factors influence preparation of the child and interaction.
- Child's and family's understanding of the reasons for and risks and benefits of the procedure ➤➤*Rationale:* Evaluates child's and family's understanding of the procedure and provides a gauge for ongoing education.

CHILD AND FAMILY EDUCATION

Individualized, developmentally appropriate education is provided to the family and to the child based on desire for knowledge, readiness to learn, and overall neurologic and psychosocial state.

- Provide information about the LAAI including the purpose, expected effects, and sensations that might be experienced such as the decreased ability to feel touch or move the limb ➤➤*Rationale:* Providing information decreases anxiety and increases cooperation. Child and family need to understand reducing pain is necessary to positively affect recovery of illness or injury.
- If developmentally appropriate in children who are alert, explain to the child how to bolus with the LAAI.

Otherwise, consider proxy bolusing by a designated family member ➤➤*Rationale:* Allows the child to participate in own care and have some control over pain management; facilitates early intervention for increasing pain. Level of consciousness, developmental and cognitive level influence preparation and interaction.

- Explain the need to assist in maintaining the integrity of the system, specifically to prevent tension on the tubing system ➤➤*Rationale:* Reduces the incidence of catheter displacement.
- Educate the child and family to notify the nurse or other clinical staff when the child is experiencing pain. Appropriate pain assessment methods are used to determine the effectiveness of the LAAI. See Procedure 173 for further information ➤➤*Rationale:* If prescribed intervention is not effective, alternative pain management interventions should be implemented.
- Explain to the child and family that the goal of the LAAI is pain relief, not elimination of all pain ➤➤*Rationale:* Establishes realistic expectations related to the prescribed therapy.
- Teach the child and family nonpharmacologic methods of reducing pain that complement but do not replace pharmacologic methods such as relaxation breathing ➤➤*Rationale:* All children should learn some simple, versatile, and age-appropriate methods for pain relief during painful attacks other than relying exclusively on medications.[6]
- Encourage questions and answer questions as they arise ➤➤*Rationale:* Reinforcement of information is needed during periods of stress.

EQUIPMENT

- LAAI catheter (surgical preference)
- Skin preparation agent per institution-specific protocol
- Sterile gloves
- SLD or infusion pump and compatible infusion tubing
- LA prescribed by the surgeon
- Sterile syringe to fill the SLD with the LA
- Transparent tape

Procedure | for Locally Administered Anesthetic Infusions

Steps	Rationale	Considerations
1. Ensure child and family understand procedure and questions are answered.	Evaluates and reinforces understanding of previously taught information.	Developmental level, cognitive ability, and anxiety level will determine approach to and effectiveness of teaching.
2. Gather needed supplies and equipment.	Facilitates completion of task in a timely manner.	
3. Identify the child using two patient identifiers; name and medical record	Adherence of the National Patient Safety Goals endorsed by the Joint	Two identifiers should be used for patient identification per

Procedure for **Locally Administered Anesthetic Infusions**—*Continued*		
Steps	**Rationale**	**Considerations**
number are most often used in the inpatient setting.	Commission on Accreditation of Healthcare Organizations (JCAHO);[7] ensures right patient receives right medication.	institution-specific protocol; most commonly, name and birth date or name and medical record number are used. Children may not be able to verbalize their identities.
4. Wash hands with antimicrobial soap and dry well, or use an alcohol-based hand-hygiene product.	Standard precautions; reduces transmission of microorganisms, which is of concern with the use of invasive catheters.	
5. Ensure an IV is in place and emergency equipment is immediately available.	Adverse reactions or toxicity to the LA may develop and affect the hemodynamic status of the child.	All emergency equipment needs to be of the appropriate size for the child. Emergency drug dosages should be determined in advance.
6. Prepare the SLD or pump per prescribing practitioner's order and manufacturer's instructions, ensuring that dose available agrees with prescribing practitioner's order. Prime infusion tubing between the SLD or pump and the catheter. *(Level I*)*	Although studies have shown that complications from LAAI are extremely rare, safety is dependent on ensuring that the concentration of the LA in the SLD or pump is as per prescribing practitioner's order and will not administer a toxic dose.[2]	For infants, the spreading of the LA from the site of injection can be considerable in distance along the perineural tract.[2] Also the structures of the nerve sheaths make the absorption of the LA more rapid for infants. Maximal "safe doses" of many LAs have not been established for all LA agents.[2]
7. Boldly label the SLD or pump as "local anesthetic pump."	Labels will decrease the risk of clinicians titrating infusions with the wrong pump.	
8. Assist the surgeon in positioning, prepping, and draping the child. After the catheter is placed, secure the distal end with dressing per surgeon preference or institution-specific protocol.	The catheter tip should be placed as close as possible to the peripheral nerves carrying the pain impulse to the spinal cord.	
9. Connect the infusion tubing to the catheter and start the infusion. If the child is awake and able to comprehend the bolus technique, explain how to self-administer a bolus dose.	Self-bolusing permits the child to treat increased pain in a timely manner. Bolusing is encouraged when the child is in pain or about to begin a potentially painful action such as getting out of bed.	Age-appropriate explanations must be given. If the child cannot understand how to self-bolus, consider family members as proxy bolusers. Refer to Procedure 174 for further information on selection of family members to provide proxy boluses.
10. For children who cannot self-bolus but family proxy bolusing is not advisable, collaborate with the prescribing practitioner to consider nurse controlled analgesia (NCA).	NCA appears to be safe and convenient for providing boluses in a timely manner for children with PCA pumps.[8] NCA allows the nurse to medicate the child as soon as it is determined that the child is in pain, avoiding the time-consuming process of obtaining medications from the narcotic supply for intermittent administration.	Availability of NCA is determined by institution-specific protocol. It may also be limited to hospital units in which the nurse/patient ratio provides the time to be nearby to press the bolus button when the child is in pain.
11. Dispose of used supplies and equipment in appropriate receptacle; wash hands.	Standard precautions; reduces transmission of microorganisms.	

* Level I: Manufacturer's recommendations only

Expected Outcomes

- An acceptable level of pain as per child (defined as controlled) or less than 5/10 point scale if the child cannot self-report
- Integrity and sterility of the LAAI system is maintained

- Skin remains intact over bony prominences or edges of casting

Unexpected Outcomes

- Pain is not controlled (an unacceptable level to the child and/or interferes with movement, cough, treatment, play, or sleep)
- The LAAI system is inadvertently disconnected and sterility is not maintained
- Skin breakdown is present

Monitoring and Care of the Child

Activities and Interventions	Rationale	Reportable Conditions
1. Assess pain intensity, location, and quality every hour until pain is controlled and then at least every 4 hours while child is awake. Examine surgical dressing to ensure catheter placement. Optimally establish with the child the trigger point (the number on the pain scale the patient considers comfortable as well as promotes activities for recovery). For further details about pain assessment refer to Procedure 173. *(Level II*)*	Inadequate pain control may occur if the catheter has been dislodged. Inadequate pain control is addressed by either increasing the concentration of the LA in the LAAI (up to the toxic dose) or by administering analgesics by another route (PO, IV, IV, PCA).	• Inadequate pain control • Change in severity, location or characteristics of the pain • Inability of child to participate in recovery activities due to pain • Catheter displacement from the insertion site
2. Monitor vital signs, SpO$_2$ and cardiac rhythm per general postoperative guidelines.[2] Also assess the affected limb for hemodynamic status.	Children at risk for compartment syndrome require specific monitoring of the hemodynamic status of the relevant limb.[2] The LA may mask any pain related to the lack of perfusion to the area and prevent self-report of discomfort.	• Clinically significant changes in vital signs, SpO$_2$, and cardiac rhythm • Changes in the temperature, color, capillary refill of the affected limb

3. Assess the LAAI device every 4 hours to ensure:
  • Medication is infusing at correct rate.
  • No leakage at the site.
  • No signs of infection.
    Do not flush infusion system unless specifically directed by surgeon.
	For SLD, 2 to 4 hours are necessary to note the volume on the syringe has diminished appropriately. For electronic pumps, alarms will indicate failure to infuse.	• Failure to infuse
		• Leakage
		• Signs of infection at the catheter insertion site
		• Unexplained fever greater than 38°C

4. Assess motor function of the affected extremity every 4 hours while child is awake. If child complains of excessive numbness, consider the need to decrease the percentage of LA in the SLD or pump. Explain that lowering the percentage of LA will decrease numbness.	The goal of administered LA is to reduce the sensation of pain without affecting the motor nerves. By using a low concentration of LA, the sensory pain fibers are blocked and the motor fibers should remain intact. Decreased ability to move the extremity may indicate the need to decrease the dose of the LA. Numbness, "heaviness," and motor weakness may be quite distressing to the child.[2]	• Unresolved excessive numbness or motor block, especially after the LA concentration has been reduced.
5. Assess for side effects of LA. For side effects, discontinue the infusion immediately but do not	There are fewer side effects when dosages of the LA are less than the known toxic dose. The side effects	• Twitching • Light-headedness • Perioral tingling

* Level II: Theory-based, no research data to support recommendations: recommendations from expert consensus group may exist

Monitoring and Care of the Child—Cont'd

Activities and Interventions	Rationale	Reportable Conditions
disconnect until after notifying the prescribing practitioner.	may diminish with lower concentrations of LA administered by the LAAI.	• Tinnitus • Visual disturbances • Seizures • Unresolved inability to complete physical activities considering overall physical condition
6. Promote activity of the child as medically indicated. Ambulation is to be done with assistance of staff following assessment of ability to bear weight.	LA may interfere with motor function and the child may be at risk for falls. Reducing the percentage of LA may be necessary to decrease motor blockade.	
7. Using sterile technique, refill the LAAI device according to specific manufacturer's directions.	Ensure LA is the correct percentage according to prescribing practitioner's order.	
8. Assess child's skin integrity over the pressure points of the affected limb. Assist in repositioning every 2 hours while awake.	The use of LAs increases risk for skin breakdown because of decreased sensation and decreased urge to reposition often.	• Skin breakdown
9. Remove catheter as per prescribing practitioner's order and institution-specific protocol.	Institution-specific protocol will direct the role of the RN in the removal of LAAI catheters. The catheter should come out easily and painlessly.	• Difficulty removing the LAAI catheter
10. Waste any medication per institution-specific protocol. Ensure that pain will be controlled by another method.	Refer to analgesic guidelines in determining the appropriate dosages of analgesics given by another route or method.	• Unmanaged pain after catheter removal

Documentation

- Education of the child and family, specifically any teaching related to the proxy bolusing for the child
- Medications, concentration, SLD rate or pump settings, volume per hour (include in intake and output determinations)
- Pain intensity (score), location, and quality
- Side effects of medications
- Condition of dressing and insertion site, noting any signs of infection
- Adjunctive medications given for pain or side effects
- Motor and sensory function of affected limb
- Unexpected outcomes and related treatment

References

1. American Nurses Association: Role of the registered nurse in the management of analgesia by catheter technique (epidural, intrathecal, intrapleural, or peripheral nerve catheters), Silver Spring, MD, 1991, American Nurses Association.
2. Lehr VT, BeVier P: Patient-controlled analgesia for the pediatric patient, *Orthopaedic Nursing* 22:298-306, 2003.
3. Barber FA, Herbert MA: The effectiveness of an anesthetic continuous-infusion device on postoperative pain control, *Arthroscopy* 18:76-81, 2002.
4. Joint Commission Resources: Special report: 2003 JCAHO national patient safety goals: practical strategies and helpful solutions for meeting these goals. Accessed from www.jcrinc.com/subscribers/patientsafety.asp?durki=7916&site=22&return=154, 2003, accessed 11/3/05.
5. Berde CB, Solodiuk J: Multidisciplinary programs for management of acute and chronic pain in children. In Schechter NL, et al, editors: *Pain in infants, children, and adolescents,* ed 2, Philadelphia, 2003, Lippincott Williams & Wilkins, pp. 477-479.
6. McGrath PA, Hillier LM: Modifying the psychologic factors that intensify children's pain and prolong disability. In Schechter NL, et al, editors: *Pain in infants, children, and adolescents,* ed 2, Philadelphia, 2003, Lippincott Williams & Wilkins, pp. 85-102.
7. Rothley BB, Therrien SR: Acute pain management. In St. Marie B, editor: *American Society of Pain Management Nurses: core curriculum for pain management nursing,* Philadelphia, 2002, Saunders, pp. 239-271.
8. Dalens B: Peripheral nerve blockade in the management of postoperative pain in children. In Schechter NL, et al, editors: *Pain in infants, children, and adolescents,* ed 2, Philadelphia, 2003, Lippincott Williams & Wilkins, pp. 363-393.

Pain Assessment Scales

P U R P O S E : To use a valid, reliable measurement scale to guide pain clinical management toward meeting desired physiologic and psychologic patient outcomes. Developmentally appropriate pain scales, including CRIES, Attia, FLACC, N-PASS, and Wong-Baker FACES Pain Rating Scale, will be described.

Helen Turner and Debbie Brinker

PREREQUISITE KNOWLEDGE

- Anatomy and physiology of the peripheral nervous system, the autonomic and skeletal motor systems, and the central nervous system
- Pain assessment and management is a continuous and ongoing process that should result in satisfactory pain reduction.
- Pain is multidimensional and includes sensory, affective, cognitive, behavioral, sociocultural and physiologic dimensions.[1]
- Responses to pain must be assessed according to appropriate cognitive and developmental levels.
- There is a relationship between pain, distress, and anxiety.
- The nature of pain is subjective and individual.
- Pain can exist with no obvious cause.
- Analgesics should *not* be held until diagnosis is made, e.g., the child with abdominal pain.
- There can be up to a 30% positive placebo effect with administration of pain medications.[2,3]
- There is a tendency of caregivers (professional and family) to underreport pain.
- Factors influencing pain assessment include the following: pain history, current pain, developmental level, coping strategies used, and cultural background.
- Physiologic measures such as heart rate, blood pressure, respiratory rate, transcutaneous O_2, palmar sweating, vagal tone, and endorphin concentration provide information about general distress levels, but they are not specific indicators of children's pain.

- Pain assessment is not equivalent to sedation assessment; refer to Procedure 176 for discussion of sedation assessment scales including the Modified Motor Activity Assessment Scale and Comfort Scale.
- Both pain and sedation assessments are necessary, and accomplished together guide optimal management to prevent physiologic pain and anxiety, inefficient ventilation, hypoxia, agitation, self-harm, and awareness of the potentially very frightening environment.

CHILD AND FAMILY ASSESSMENT

- Developmental level of child and ability to interact ➤➤*Rationale:* Child's developmental level and ability to interact influence preparation, pain scale selection, and responses to pain.
- Previous pain experiences of child and family ➤➤*Rationale:* Previous pain and pain treatment experience of child and family influences response, behaviors, and expectations in current situation.
- Factors that may alter a child's ability to mount a pain response such as immobilization, neurologic deficit, and medications affecting heart rate and blood pressure ➤➤*Rationale:* Many factors can mask a child's usual physiologic response to pain.
- Child's and family's understanding of the reasons for and benefits of regular pain assessment ➤➤*Rationale:* Evaluates child's and family's understanding of the importance of pain assessment and provides a gauge for ongoing education.

CHILD AND FAMILY EDUCATION

Individualized, developmentally appropriate education is provided to the child and to the family based on desire for knowledge, readiness to learn, and overall neurologic and psychosocial state.

- Explain that consistent and accurate assessment of pain is necessary to appropriately treat the child's pain ➥*Rationale:* Providing information decreases anxiety and promotes compliance with regular assessments.
- Provide information regarding the physiologic and psychologic effect of undertreated pain ➥*Rationale:* Providing information decreases fear, anxiety, and resistance to treatment.
- Collaborate with family to learn and identify child's pain cues/behaviors; select and explain use of appropriate pain scale ➥*Rationale:* Involving the family decreases their sense of helplessness in the high-technology environment of an acute or intensive care unit. Family best understands behavioral/communication cues that the child exhibits when in distress or discomfort. Teaching family

and child (as appropriate) how the pain scale is used facilitates accurate assessment.

- Encourage questions and answer questions as they arise ➥*Rationale:* Reinforcement of information is needed during periods of stress.

EQUIPMENT

- Developmentally appropriate pain scale such as:
  - ❖ CRIES (neonatal)[4] (Figure 173-1)
  - ❖ Attia (neonate up to 1 year)[5] (Figure 173-2)
  - ❖ FLACC (2 months to 7 years of age)[6] (Figure 173-3)
  - ❖ FACES Pain Rating Scale (3 years of age and older)[8] (Figure 173-4)
  - ❖ N-PASS (infants of all gestational ages)[7] (Figure 173-5)
  - ❖ Other number scales in the school-aged or older age-group
- Stethoscope
- Cardiorespiratory monitoring
- Oxygen saturation (SpO_2) monitoring

Criteria	0	1	2
Crying	No	High pitched	Inconsolable
Requires O_2 for saturation >95%	No	<30%	>30%
Increased vital signs	HR and BP less than or equal to preop	Increase in HR or BP <20% of preop	Increase in HR or BP >20% of preop
Expression	None	Grimace	Grimace/grunt
Sleepless	No	Wakes at frequent intervals	Constantly awake

Coding Tips for Using CRIES

Crying	The characteristic cry of pain is *high pitched*.
	If no cry or cry that is not high pitched, score 0.
	If cry high pitched but baby is easily consoled, score 1.
	If cry is high pitched and baby is inconsolable, score 2.
Requires O_2 for sats >95%	Looks for *changes* in oxygenation. Babies experiencing pain manifest decreases in oxygenation as measured by transcutaneous monitoring or pulse oximetry.
	If no O_2 is required, score 0. If <30% O_2 is required, score 1.
	If >30% O_2 is required, score 2. (Consider other causes of changes in oxygenation such as atelectasis, pneumothorax, oversedation.)
Increased vital signs	Note: measure BP last because this may wake child, causing difficulty with other assessments. Use baseline preoperative parameters from a nonstressed period.
	Multiply baseline HR × 0.2; then add this to baseline HR to determine the HR, which is 20% over baseline. Do likewise for BP. Use mean BP.
	If HR and BP are both unchanged or less than baseline, score 0.
	If HR or BP is increased but increase is <20% of baseline, score 1.
	If either one is increased >20% over baseline, score 2.
Expression	The facial expression most often associated with pain is a grimace. This may be characterized by brow lowering, eyes squeezed shut, deepening of the nasolabial furrow, open lips and mouth.
	If no grimace present, score 0. If grimace alone present, score 1.
	If grimace and noncry vocalization grunt present, score 2.
Sleepless	This parameter is scored based on the infant's state during the hour preceding this recorded score.
	If he or she is continuously asleep, score 0.
	If awakened at frequent intervals, score 1. If awake constantly, score 2.

FIGURE 173–1 CRIES neonatal postoperative pain measurement scale. (From Krechel SW, Bildner J: CRIES: a new neonatal postoperative pain measurement score: initial testing of validity and reliability, *Pediatr Anesth* 5:53-61, 1995. Developed at the University of Missouri–Columbia.

INDICATORS	SCORE			TIME								
	0	1	2									
Sleeps during preceding hour	Longer naps >10 min	Short naps between 5-10 min	None									
Facial expression of pain	Calm, relaxed	Less marked, intermittent	Marked constant									
Quality of cry	No cry	Modulated: can be distracted by normal sound	Screaming, painful, high pitched									
Spontaneous motor activity	Normal	Moderate agitation	Thrashing around, incessant agitation									
Spontaneous excitability and responsiveness to ambient stimulation	Quiet	Excessive reactivity (to any stimulation)	Tremulous, clonic mvmts. Moro reflexes									
Constant, excessive flexion of finger & toes	Absent	Less marked, intermittent	Very pronounced, marked & constant									
Sucking	Strong, rhythmic with pacifying effect	Intermittent (3-4) and stops with crying	Absent or disorganized sucking									
Global evaluation of tone	Normal for age	Moderate hypertonicity	Strong hypertonicity									
Consolability	Calm before 1 min	Quiet after 1 min of effort	None after 2 min									
Sociability (eye contact) response to smile or voice, real interest in face	Easy and prolonged	Difficult to obtain	Absent									
TOTAL												

Range of total score: 0-20   Pain: Score ≥5

FIGURE 173–2   Attia behavioral pain scale. (From Barrier G, et al: Measurement of post-operative pain and narcotic administration in infants using a new clinical scoring system, *Intensive Care Med* 15[Suppl 1]:S37-S39, 1989.)

Category	Scoring		
	1	2	3
Face	No particular expression or smile	Occasional grimace or frown, withdrawn, disinterested	Frequent to constant quivering chin, clenched jaw
Legs	Normal position or relaxed	Uneasy, restless, tense	Kicking, or legs drawn up
Activity	Lying quietly, normal position, moves easily	Squirming, shifting back and forth, tense	Arched, rigid or jerking
Cry	No cry (awake or asleep)	Moans or whimpers; occasional complaint	Crying steadily, screams or sobs, frequent complaints
Consolability	Content, relaxed	Reassured by occasional touching, hugging or being talked to, distractible	Difficult to console or comfort

FIGURE 173–3   FLACC pain scale. (From Merkel SI, et al: The FLACC: a behavioral scale for scoring postoperative pain in young children, *Pediatr Nurs* 23:293-29, 1997. University of Michigan Medical Center. Copyright 1997 by Jannetti Co.)

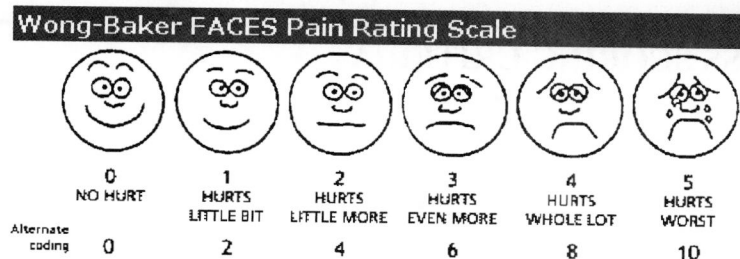

Wong-Baker FACES Pain Rating Scale

0 NO HURT	1 HURTS LITTLE BIT	2 HURTS LITTLE MORE	3 HURTS EVEN MORE	4 HURTS WHOLE LOT	5 HURTS WORST

Alternate coding   0   2   4   6   8   10

Brief word instructions: Point to each face using the words to describe the pain intensity. Ask the child to choose face that best describes own pain and record the appropriate number.

Original instructions: Explain to the person that each face is for a person who feels happy because he has no pain (hurt) or sad because he has some or a lot of pain. **Face 0** is very happy because he doesn't hurt at all. **Face 1** hurts just a little bit. **Face 2** hurts a little more. **Face 3** hurts even more. **Face 4** hurts a whole lot. **Face 5** hurts as much as you can imagine, although you don't have to be crying to feel this bad. Ask the person to choose the face that best desribes how he is feeling.

FIGURE 173–4   Wong-Baker FACES Pain Rating Scale. (From: Hockenberry MJ, et al, editors: *Wong's essentials of pediatric nursing,* ed 7, St. Louis, 2005, Mosby, p. 1259. Used with permission. Copyright, Mosby.)

N-PASS:
Neonatal Pain, Agitation, & Sedation Scale

Pat Hummel MA, RNC, NNP, PNP, APN/CNP & Mary Puchalski MS, RNC, APN/CNS

Assessment Criteria	Sedation		Normal	Pain / Agitation	
	-2	-1	0	1	2
Crying Irritability	No cry with painful stimuli	Moans or cries minimally with painful stimuli	Appropriate crying Not irritable	Irritable or crying at intervals Consolable	High-pitched or silent-continuous cry Inconsolable
Behavior State	No arousal to any stimuli No spontaneous movement	Arouses minimally to stimuli Little spontaneous movement	Appropriate for gestational age	Restless, squirming Awakens frequently	Arching, kicking Constantly awake or Arouses minimally / no movement (not sedated)
Facial Expression	Mouth is lax No expression	Minimal expression with stimuli	Relaxed Appropriate	Any pain expression intermittent	Any pain expression continual
Extremities Tone	No grasp reflex Flaccid tone	Weak grasp reflex ↓ muscle tone	Relaxed hands and feet Normal tone	Intermittent clenched toes, fists or finger splay Body is not tense	Continual clenched toes, fists, or finger splay Body is tense
Vital Signs HR, RR, BP, SpO_2	No variability with stimuli Hypoventilation or apnea	< 10% variability from baseline with stimuli	Within baseline or normal for gestational age	10-20% from baseline SpO_2 76-85% with stimulation – quick recovery	> 20% from baseline $SpO_2 \leq 75\%$ with stimulation – slow recovery Out of sync with vent

This tool is currently undergoing testing for validity and reliability, and the authors cannot accept responsibility for errors or omision or for any consequences resulting from the application or interpretation of this material

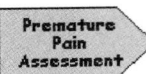

Premature Pain Assessment
+3 if < 28 weeks gestation / corrected age.
+2 if 28 - 31 weeks gestation / corrected age.
+1 if 32 - 35 weeks gestation / corrected age.

N-PASS SCORING CRITERIA

Crying/Irritability

−2 → No response to painful stimuli, e.g.:
- No cry with needle sticks
- No reaction to ETT or nares suctioning
- No response to care giving

−1 → Moans, sighs, or cries (audible or silent) minimally to painful stimuli, e.g. needle sticks, ETT or nares suctioning, care giving

0 → Not irritable—appropriate crying
- Cries briefly with normal stimuli
- Easily consoled
- Normal for gestational age

+1 → Infant is irritable/crying at intervals—but can be consoled
- If intubated – intermittent silent cry

+2 → Any of the following:
- Cry is high-pitched
- Infant cries inconsolably
- If intubated—silent continuous cry

FIGURE 173–5 N-PASS: (Neonatal Pain, Agitation and Sedation Scale). (From N-PASS: Neonatal Pain, Agitation and Sedation Scale, copyright 2004, www.n-pass.com. Used with permission.)

Behavior/State

−2 → Does not arouse or react to any stimuli
  • Eyes continually shut or open
  • No spontaneous movement

−1 → Little spontaneous movement, arouses briefly and/or minimally to any stimuli
  • Opens eyes briefly
  • Reacts to suctioning
  • Withdraws to pain

 0 → Behavior and state are gestational age appropriate

+1 → Any of the following:
  • Restless, squirming
  • Awakens frequently/easily with minimal or no stimuli

+2 → Any of the following:
  • Kicking
  • Arching
  • Constantly awake
  • No movement or minimal arousal with stimulation (inappropriate for gestational age or clinical situation, i.e., post-operative)

Facial Expression

−2 → Any of the following:
  • Mouth is lax
  • Drooling
  • No facial expression at rest or with stimuli

−1 → Minimal facial expression with stimuli

 0 → Face is relaxed at rest but not lax – normal expression with stimuli

+1 → Any pain face expression observed intermittently

+2 → Any pain face expression is continual

Extremities/Tone

−2 → Any of the following:
  • No palmar or planter grasp can be elicited
  • Flaccid tone

−1 → Any of the following:
  • Weak palmar or planter grasp can be elicited
  • Decreased tone

 0 → Relaxed hands and feet—normal palmar or sole grasp elicited—appropriate tone for gestational age

+1 → Intermittent (<30 seconds duration) observation of toes and/or hands as clenched or fingers splayed
  • Body is *not* tense

+2 → Any of the following:
  • Frequent (≥30 seconds duration) observation of toes and/or hands as clenched, or fingers splayed
  • Body is tense/stiff

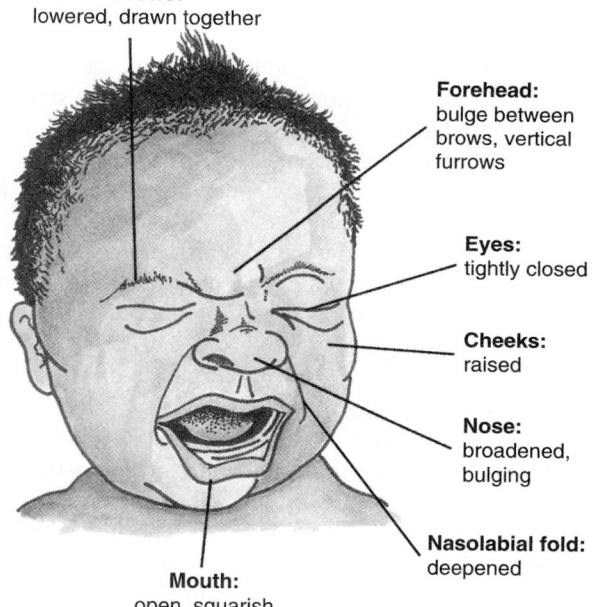

Brows: lowered, drawn together
Forehead: bulge between brows, vertical furrows
Eyes: tightly closed
Cheeks: raised
Nose: broadened, bulging
Nasolabial fold: deepened
Mouth: open, squarish

FIGURE 173–5, CONT'D   N-PASS.

Continued

Vital Signs: HR, BP, RR, & O₂ Saturations

−2 → Any of the following:
- No variability in vital signs with stimuli
- Hypoventilation
- Apnea
- Ventilated infant – no spontaneous respiratory effort

−1 → Vital signs show little variability with stimuli – less than 10% from baseline

 0 → Vital signs and/or oxygen saturations are within normal limits with normal variability – or normal for gestational age

+1 → Any of the following:
- HR, RR, and/or BP are 10-20% above baseline
- With care/stimuli infant desaturates minimally to moderately (SpO_2 76-85%) and recovers quickly (within 2 minutes)

+2 → Any of the following:
- HR, RR, and/or BP are > 20% above baseline
- With care/stimuli infant desaturates severely (SpO_2 < 75%) and recovers slowly (> 2 minutes)
- Infant is out of syynchrony with the ventilator -fighting the ventilator

Assessment of Sedation

- Sedation is scored in addition to pain for each behavioral and physiological criteria to assess the infant's response to stimuli
- Sedation does not need to be assessed/scored with every pain assessment/score
- Sedation is scored from 0 → −2 for each behavioral and physiological criteria, then summed and noted as a negative score (0 → −10)
  - A score of 0 is given if the infant's response to stimuli is normal for their gestational age
- Desired levels of sedation vary according to the situation
  - "Deep sedation" → score of −10 to −5 as goal
  - "Light sedation" → score of −5 to −2 as goal
- Deep sedation is not recommended unless an infant is receiving ventilatory support, related to the high potential for apnea and hypoventilation
- A negative score without the administration of opioids/ sedatives may indicate:
  - The premature infant's response to prolonged or persistent pain/stress
  - Neurologic depression, sepsis, or other pathology

Assessment of Pain/Agitation

- Pain assessment is the fifth vital sign – assessment for pain should be included in every vital sign assessment
- Pain is scored from 0 → +2 for each behavioral and physiological criteria, then summed
  - Points are added to the premature infant's pain score based on their gestational age to compensate for their limited ability to behaviorally or physiologically communicate pain
  - Total pain score is documented as a positive number (0 → +10)
- Treatment/interventions are indicated for scores > 3
  - Interventions for known pain/painful stimuli are indicated before the score reaches 3
- The goal of pain treatment/intervention is a score ≤ 3
- More frequent pain assessment indications:
  - Indwelling tubes or lines which may cause pain, especially with movement (e.g. chest tubes) → at least every 2-4 hours
  - Receiving analgesics and/or sedatives → at least every 2-4 hours
  - 30-60 minutes after an analgesic is given for pain behaviors to assess response to medication
  - Post-operative → at least every 2 hours for 24-48 hours, then every 4 hours until off medications

Pavulon/Paralysis

- It is impossible to behaviorally evaluate a paralyzed infant for pain
- Increases in heart rate and blood pressure may be the only indicator of a need for more analgesia
- Analgesics should be administered continuously by drip or around-the-clock dosing
- Higher, more frequent doses may be required if the infant is post-op, has a chest tube, or other pathology (such as NEC) that would normally cause pain
- Opioid doses should be increased by 10% every 3-5 days as tolerance will occur without symptoms of inadequate pain relief

FIGURE 173-5, CONT'D   N-PASS.

Procedure for Pain Assessment

Steps	Rationale	Considerations
1. Select and obtain developmentally appropriate pain scale. *(Level VI*)*	Pain scale selected must be appropriate for child's cognitive and developmental levels.	Not all pain scales are appropriate for ventilated and paralyzed infants and children.
2. Ensure child and family understand the pain assessment tool selected and questions are answered.	Evaluates and reinforces understanding of previously taught information.	Developmental level, cognitive ability, and anxiety level will determine approach to and effectiveness of teaching.
3. Quietly observe child.	Allows observation of behaviors without additional stimulation; agitation may be observed.	Multiple causes for agitation include hypoxia, emotional distress, environmental factors, drug reactions, or pain; cause must be treated.
4. Note physiologic indicators such as heart rate, blood pressure, respiratory rate, and effort before disturbing the child.	These indicators are nonspecific, but may be indicative of pain.	
5. Ask family what they believe is the child's level of pain or discomfort.	Parents know their child best and may be able to interpret behavior cues indicative of pain.	Agitation may be interpreted as pain.
6. If using observational scales, use scale as directed and determine pain score.	Pain assessment is valid only when scale is used correctly (refer to Figures 173-1 through 173-5 for descriptions of individual pain scales).	
7. If using self-report scale, tell child what you are doing and then use scale as directed to determine pain score.	Involve child when developmentally appropriate because pain is individual. Pain assessment is valid only when scale is used correctly.	Assessment can be reliable only when a child is physically and developmentally able to use the self-report scale.
8. Assess child during activities such as coughing and repositioning and compare with scores obtained when child is quiet.	Child's pain rating/assessment may vary with activity, and should guide pain management.	
9. Reassess after each pain management intervention.	Reassessment will identify effectiveness of current pain management and guide further pain management.	

* Level VI: Clinical studies in a variety of patient populations and situations to support recommendations

Expected Outcomes

- Appropriate pain scale is selected for child, resulting in accurate pain assessment
- Pain scale is less than 4/10, or value mutually decided on by child (as developmentally appropriate), family, and staff
- Child is free from side effects of pain medication

Unexpected Outcomes

- Inappropriate pain scale is selected for child, resulting in inaccurate pain assessment and untreated pain
- Inadequate pain management as indicated by pain scale value equal to or greater than 5/10 or higher than value mutually decided on by child (as developmentally appropriate), family, and staff
- Unacceptable side effects of pain medication such as nausea, vomiting, constipation, itching, sleepiness
- Over- or under-sedation

Monitoring and Care of the Child

Activities and Interventions	Rationale	Reportable Conditions
1. Monitor scores obtained using tool selected; ensure tool is appropriate for child's developmental level and physical condition.	Determines that assessment is accurate; assesses effectiveness of pain management techniques.	• Pain score equal to or greater than 5/10 or higher than value mutually decided on by child (as developmentally appropriate), family, and staff
2. Monitor cardiorespiratory status and SpO$_2$.	Alerts care providers to potential respiratory compromise or need for increase in analgesia.	• SpO$_2$ saturations less than 94% (without other physiologic cause) • Hypotension (without other physiologic cause) • Tachycardia and hypertension may be indicators for inadequately treated pain
3. Monitor for withdrawal behaviors that may include irritability, tremors, hyperactivity, seizures, insomnia, abdominal cramping, nausea, vomiting, diarrhea, sweating, fever, chills, nasal congestion, rhinitis, tachypnea, tachycardia.	The potential for withdrawal exists after 5 to 10 days of regular opioid and/or benzodiazepine administration.	• Any of the noted behaviors (without other physiologic cause)

Documentation

- Child and family education
- Pain scale used for pain assessment
- Pain assessment including pain rating using developmentally appropriate scale, documented at minimum of every 2 to 4 hours; hourly if procedures are being performed; after changes to therapy and each intervention
- Vital signs and SpO$_2$
- Pharmacologic and nonpharmacologic interventions provided in response to increased pain score
- Unexpected outcomes and related treatments

References

1. Broome ME, Huth MM: Nursing management of the child in pain. In Schechter NL, et al, editors: *Pain in infants, children, and adolescents*, ed 2, Philadelphia, 2003, Lippincott Williams & Wilkins, pp. 417-433.
2. Evans FJ: The placebo response in pain reduction. In Bonica, JJ: *Advances in neurology, vol 4*, New York, 1974, Raven Press, pp. 289-296.
3. Goodwin JS, et al, editors: Knowledge and use of placebos by house officers and nurses, *Ann Intern Med* 91:106-110, 1979
4. Krechel SW, Bildner J: CRIES: a new neonatal postoperative pain measurement score: initial testing of validity and reliability, *Pediatr Anesth* 5:53-61, 1995.
5. Barrier G, et al: Measurement of post-operative pain and narcotic administration in infants using a new clinical scoring system, *Intensive Care Med* 15(Suppl 1):S37-S39, 1989.
6. Merkel SI, et al: The FLACC: a behavioral scale for scoring postoperative pain in young children, *Pediatr Nurs* 23:293-297, 1997.
7. Hummel P, Puchalski M: The reality of neonatal pain, *Adv Neonatal Care* 2(5):233-24, 2002.
8. Wong DL, Baker C: Pain in children: comparison of assessment scales, *Pediatr Nurs* 14(1):9-17, 1988.

Additional Readings

Martin GT: Pain management for children. In James SR, et al, editors: *Nursing care of children principles and practice*, ed 2, Philadelphia, 2002, Saunders, pp. 419-438.
Oakes LL: Caring practices: providing comfort. In Curley MAQ, Moloney-Harmon PA, editors: *Critical care nursing of infants and children*, ed 2, Philadelphia, 2000, Saunders, pp. 547-576.
Wong DL, Hockenberry MJ: Family-centered care of the child during illness and hospitalization. In Hockenberry MJ, et al, editors: *Wong's nursing care of infants and children*, ed 7, St. Louis, 2003, Mosby, pp. 1046-1057.

Patient Controlled Analgesia

P U R P O S E : To deliver analgesics via a programmable infusion pump that allows the child to self-administer small amounts of opioids (boluses) based on the intensity of the pain and desire for pain relief

Linda L. Oakes

PREREQUISITE KNOWLEDGE

- An understanding of the method and the specific operations of the programmable patient controlled analgesia (PCA) pump including the rationale for specific dosages for boluses and the "lockout" time (the time set between consecutive PCA doses to prevent overdosing by excessive bolusing).
- The pharmacologic principles of administering opioids including morphine, hydromorphone, and fentanyl. Morphine is the initial choice for most children.[1] However, for children with renal dysfunction, morphine should be used with caution because of its potential accumulation and its active metabolites.[2] Fentanyl or hydromorphone is preferred over morphine in these children because of the shorter half-life and less potential for accumulation of metabolites.[2] Meperidine is not recommended because of the risk of the accumulation of its metabolite, normeperidine, which can cause central nervous system toxicity (dysphoria, agitation, and seizures) especially with children who have renal dysfunction.
- Table 174-1 provides general guidelines for initiating intravenous (IV) PCA for opioid naïve children (children who have had minimal exposure to opioids).
- The starting PCA doses need to be considered as an estimate of a child's opioid requirement. Higher starting doses will be necessary for children with chronic pain such as cancer who are often opioid tolerant. To a great extent, the success of IV PCA depends on prescribing bolus doses that can be self-administered frequently

TABLE 174-1	General Guidelines for Initiating IV PCA for Opioid Naïve Children		
Drug	Loading Dose	Continuous Infusion Dose	Bolus Dose/ Frequency
Morphine	20 mcg/kg	0 to 30 mcg/kg/hr	10-30 mcg/kg every 15-30 min
Hydromorphone	10 mcg/kg	0 to 6 mcg/kg/hr	2-6 mcg/kg every 15-30 min
Fentanyl	1 mcg/kg	0 to 1 mcg/kg/hr	0.5-1 mcg/kg every 10-15 min

enough for children to manage their pain effectively. Infants younger than 6 months tend to have a longer elimination half-life and a lower clearance rate of opioids. The duration of action of morphine is highly variable among infants in this age-group. By 6 months of age, infants require dosages nearing that of a child. For infants less than 6 months of age, use only one third to one half the starting doses listed in Table 174-1.[3-7]

- Adjunctive pain medications, such as acetaminophen and nonsteroidal antiinflammatory drugs (NSAIDs), may be used in conjunction with PCA.
- Ongoing medical direction is provided by prescribing practitioners skilled in the principles of pain management. Clinical support systems must be available around the clock to assess the need for titration of the PCA settings.
- To ensure safety, only physicians and nurses competent in managing PCAs in children, including the assessment

for side effects and complications, should offer this method of pain control.[1,2,5]

- Use of PCA can improve postoperative outcomes, particularly if used in combination with a postoperative rehabilitation program that emphasizes early mobilization, nutrition, and early return to normal activities.[1,2,4]
- Standard precautions and aseptic technique must be maintained during manipulation of the infusion system and medication.
- Child development as it relates to clinical assessment and the use of PCA
- Mastery of pediatric advanced life support competencies
- Appropriate pediatric dosing of analgesics (opioid and nonopioid)

CHILD AND FAMILY ASSESSMENT

- Appropriateness of using a PCA considering the child's:
  - Physical condition or medical interventions associated with moderate to severe pain requiring frequent administration of analgesics such as major surgery, burns, sickle cell crises, trauma, cancer, and mechanical ventilation (with sedatives) ➡*Rationale:* The use of frequent dosages of opioids is relevant for conditions resulting in severe nociceptive pain as well as pain that is continuous.
  - Ability to comprehend the appropriate use of the bolus button and motivation to do so when anticipating or having pain. Generally this applies to children older than 5 years of age who are not too ill or physically impaired such that they cannot push a button ➡*Rationale:* Although exceptions occur for children who become more familiar with medical technology due to chronic illnesses, the cognitive ability to understand the relationship between cause and effect and thus how and when to push a bolus button does not develop until 5 years of age.[1,2,8] However, the recommended lower age limit for children continues to fall as considerations are made for allowing proxies (nurses or family members) to initiate a PCA bolus for children too young or ill to self-bolus.
- The overall physical status of the child including:
  - Renal or hepatic dysfunction that may affect the clearance of the opioid thus requiring a lower dosage per hour
  - Preexisting conditions increasing the risk of respiratory depression such as sleep apnea, obesity, asthma, and upper airway obstructions, scoliosis, cystic fibrosis
  - Known allergies or previous reactions to a specific medication
  - History of substance abuse (should not be a contraindication for use of a PCA)
  - Physical ability and strength sufficient to activate a bolus dose ➡*Rationale:* These factors affect selection, dosing, monitoring, and prescribing of PCA.

- Current use of opioids for pain relief. Children with preexisting conditions (e.g., cancer) may require a higher dose of opioids via oral, IV, or transdermal routes to achieve the same effect as those who are opioid naïve ➡*Rationale:* The tolerance to an opioid (decrease in a drug's effect over time) or the need to increase the dose to achieve the same effect may be especially pertinent to those children in which the cause of pain is becoming more severe such as tumor increasing in size or causing nerve compression.
- Child's and family's understanding of the reasons for and risks and benefits of using a PCA versus other options for pain management such as short-acting IV or oral medications including controlled-release opioids ➡*Rationale:* Evaluates child's and family's understanding of PCA and provides a gauge for ongoing education.
- If proxy PCA is to be used, assess family member carefully in terms of family member's ability to follow instructions and desire to participate in bolusing the child.[1,2] ➡*Rationale:* Family member providing proxy boluses must be able to understand technique and have a desire to be responsible for their child's pain control; family should have the option to decline.

CHILD AND FAMILY EDUCATION

Individualized, developmentally appropriate education is provided to the family and to the child based on desire for knowledge, readiness to learn, and overall neurologic and psychosocial state.

- Provide information about PCA including the reason for providing this method of pain control, how to use the pump, expected outcomes, the pump's safety features to minimize the associated risks (when should the bolus button be pushed and by whom). Specifically, if the child is in pain but has not used the bolus button frequently, more explanation is needed, or the child is poorly suited to have a PCA ➡*Rationale:* Providing information decreases anxiety and increases cooperation. Children and families need to understand that pain management is necessary to positively effect recovery of illness or injury.
- If developmentally appropriate, explain how the child can bolus when in pain or in anticipation of a painful event (i.e., getting out of bed) ➡*Rationale:* Level of consciousness and developmental and cognitive level influence preparation and interaction. Maximizing the benefits of PCA involves teaching children expectations about certain recovery activities and the need to tell clinicians when these activities are too painful to perform. Necessary adjustments of the PCA settings should be made so that these important activities can be performed with minimal discomfort.
- Describe methods that will be used to assess pain using age-appropriate valid pain scales. Refer to Procedure 173 for further information ➡*Rationale:* Reassuring the

family that pain will be regularly assessed in an appropriate manner decreases anxiety and increases cooperation.

- Explain to the child and family that the goal of PCA is pain relief, not elimination of all pain ➤➤*Rationale:* Establishes realistic expectations related to the prescribed therapy.
- Explain nonpharmacologic methods of reducing pain that complement but do not replace pharmacologic methods, such as relaxation breathing ➤➤*Rationale:* All children should learn some simple, versatile, and age-appropriate methods for pain relief during painful attacks rather than relying exclusively on medications.[9]
- Encourage questions and answer questions as they arise ➤➤*Rationale:* Reinforcement of information is needed during periods of stress.
- If proxy PCA is to be used, educate the family member who will be responsible when to bolus (only when the child is awake and behavior or words tell you he or she is hurting); consider the need to bolus before diaper changes if the perianal area is excoriated ➤➤*Rationale:* Education is required to ensure safety of proxy PCA.
- If proxy PCA is to be used, educate the family member who will be responsible when *not* to bolus (while the child is sleeping, if the child is "just fussy," difficulty in waking the child, abnormal breathing is present) ➤➤*Rationale:* Education is required to ensure safety of proxy PCA.

EQUIPMENT

- Programmable PCA pump with bolus button
- Tubing with antisiphon valve specific to the PCA pump used
- Opioids ordered by the prescribing practitioner provided via a reservoir (syringe, cassette, or bag) compatible with the PCA pump
- Patient monitoring equipment per institution-specific protocol

Procedure | for Patient Controlled Analgesia

Steps	Rationale	Considerations
1. Ensure child and family understand procedure and questions are answered.	Evaluates and reinforces understanding of previously taught information.	Developmental level, cognitive ability, and anxiety level will determine approach to and effectiveness of teaching.
2. Gather needed supplies and equipment.	Facilitates completion of task in a timely manner.	
3. Identify child using two patient identifiers; name and medical record number are most often used in the inpatient setting. *(Level II*)*	Adherence to the National Patient Safety Goals endorsed by the Joint Commission on Accreditation of Healthcare Organizations (JCAHO);[10] ensures right patient receives right medication.	Two identifiers should be used for patient identification per institution-specific protocol; most commonly name and birth date or name and medical record number are used. Children may not be able to verbalize their identities.
4. Wash hands with antimicrobial soap and dry well, or use an alcohol-based handwashing product.	Standard precautions; reduces the transmission of microorganisms, which is of concern regarding intravascular catheters.	
5. Ensure appropriate cardiopulmonary monitoring, an emergency cart with naloxone, oxygen, and suction equipment are immediately available. Refer to institution-specific protocol. *(Level II*)*	Opioid pain medications affect the respiratory and cardiovascular systems of children; children may suddenly decompensate.	Consider the child's status and institution-specific protocol when selecting the appropriate monitoring. All emergency equipment must be of appropriate size for the child. Emergency drug dosages should be predetermined based on weight of the child.
6. Ensure child has a patent intravenous (IV) line. If IV must be started, apply local anesthetic cream to the site per prescribing practitioner's order and	IV is required to deliver IV PCA. Local anesthetic cream reduces the pain of needle insertion of subcutaneous local anesthetic	Children have an intense fear of needle-related pain; their ability to remain immobile during the insertion is related to age and overall condition.

Procedure continues on following page

* Level II: Theory based, no research data to support recommendations: recommendations from expert consensus group may exist

Procedure for Patient Controlled Analgesia—*Continued*

Steps	Rationale	Considerations
manufacturer's recommendations[5] before insertion.	infiltration before placing the IV needle.	
7. Program the PCA pump per prescribing practitioner's orders.	The choice of opioid depends on availability, experience of prescribing practitioner, and individual child's history of effectiveness or side effects. Some pumps provide a "lock level" to set such that the non-clinician is unable to change the settings without access to a code entered into the pump.	The same principles for use of the PCA in adults apply to children. The safety and efficacy of PCA for pediatric patients have been established. The use of protocols and standardized order sets that are developed specifically for pediatric patients is encouraged.[2]
8. Review pump settings and the medication itself and compare this with prescribing practitioner's order. A verification process including medication concentration, bolus dose (mcg or mg), and the lockout interval between boluses, the infusion rate (mcg or mg per hour) are to be independently verified by another licensed staff member. Some PCA pumps may also be programmed to limit the amount of medication given within a 4-hour period, called a 4-hour lockout.[2] (*Level II**)	Provides a mechanism such that the child self-administers boluses and builds in safety because this allows the child to determine when more medication is needed. If the child is too sleepy to bolus, this may indicate an excessive level of the analgesic. It is unlikely that children who are sedated are able to press the bolus button for additional medication. Also a PCA provides a "lockout interval" that prevents excessive bolus doses within a specified period. The lockout interval is usually set at 5- to 20-minute intervals. Smaller boluses at shorter delay intervals are best for opioid naïve children to prevent excessive sedation at peaks and for breakthrough pain at troughs.[5] Larger bolus doses at lockout intervals of 15 to 30 minutes may be required for opioid tolerant children.	The principles for adults regarding starting doses and further titration of the amount of medication apply also to children. Pediatric patients are at higher risk for adverse drug events than adults because of[2]: • Need for careful calculation of individualized doses based on age, body weight, and clinical condition. • The unique and rapidly changing pharmacokinetic parameters exhibited by infants and children at various ages and states of development. • A deficit of Food and Drug Administration (FDA)— published information regarding the dosing, pharmacokinetics, efficacy, safety, and clinical use of drugs in the pediatric population.
9. Consider the need to include a continuous infusion with bolus doses. If used in opioid naïve children, the continuous infusion dose should be less than half of dose that is projected to be needed per hour.[5] (*Level II**)	Although adult literature on pain does not support the use of a continuous infusion, most experts feel it improves satisfaction and can be done safely.[5,7] This is particularly useful at night and often provides more restful sleep by preventing the child from awakening in pain.	Children who have continuous infusions have higher ratings of satisfaction than children who do not.[5] However, providing infusions does increase the risk of sedation, thus requiring more frequent reassessments for mental status changes and respiratory effects.[1,8]
10. Prime infusion tubing from the reservoir to the distal end of infusion tubing. Ensure placement of an antisiphon valve or mechanism to prevent free flow within the infusion system.	Tubing must be primed to prevent air embolus In the event the pump malfunctions, antisiphon valves or other mechanisms must be in place to	

* Level II: Theory-based, no research data to support recommendations: recommendations from expert consensus group may exist

Procedure for Patient Controlled Analgesia—*Continued*

Steps	Rationale	Considerations
	prevent free flow of the infusion into the child.[10]	
11. Connect and start the PCA pump. Administer a loading dose if ordered by the prescribing practitioner.	A loading dose provides quicker relief of pain by shortening the time in establishing an adequate analgesic level.	
12. Ensure bolus button is within easy reach of child and explain reasons to press the bolus button.	Ensures child is able to push bolus dose button as needed. Explanation reinforces previously taught information.	Bolusing is encouraged when the child is in pain or about to begin a potentially painful action such as getting out of bed. Explanations must be appropriate to child's developmental level.
13. If child cannot self-bolus, consider possible benefit of family members' bolusing for their child ("proxy bolus"); obtain prescribing practitioner order for a family member to bolus. *(Level II*)*	Proxy bolusing is not recommended for pain from sources that are likely to resolve quickly (i.e., postoperative). However, many institutions allow proxy bolusing for children less than 5 years or if too ill to self-bolus.[7] This practice is controversial because it removes the inherent safety factor that the child must be alert and awake enough to push his or her own button.[1,2,4,11] In these instances it is likely the parent becomes medically sophisticated and able to successfully learn appropriate times to bolus for the child.[3] Evaluate child for risk factors including airway narrowing, respiratory disease, or motor impairment, and avoid proxy boluses unless very close monitoring can be provided.	Allowing a parent to bolus for the child provides some control and participation in the child's care. Parents may know best the cues their child is in pain. Careful selection of proxies and specific teaching cannot be overemphasized. A retrospective study of both parent and nurse proxy bolusing for children indicated the occurrence of opioid-related side effects may be similar to settings in which only patients pump the bolus button. Even in this institution with long-established pain services and routine use of electronic monitoring, respiratory depression for both the self-bolusing children and proxy-bolused children occurred, requiring treatment with naloxone.[11]
14. For children who cannot self-bolus and yet proxy bolusing is not advisable, collaborate with the prescribing practitioner to consider nurse controlled analgesia (NCA).	NCA appears to be safe and convenient for providing boluses in a timely manner.[1] NCA allows nurse to medicate child as soon as it is assessed that child is in pain, avoiding the time-consuming process of obtaining opioids from the narcotic box for intermittent administration.	Nurses must be cautioned not to press the PCA button for a sleeping child. NCA may be limited to hospital units in which the nurse/patient ratio provides the time to be nearby to press the bolus button when the child is in pain.

Procedure continues on following page

* Level II: Theory-based, no research data to support recommendations: recommendations from expert consensus group may exist

Procedure for Patient Controlled Analgesia—*Continued*

Steps	Rationale	Considerations
15. Review medication administration record (MAR) to determine if any other medications with known risk of sedative effects are being given and adjust the dosages of both medications as indicated.	Children with preexisting renal, hepatic, and respiratory impairment are at higher risk for respiratory depression, requiring more frequent reassessment intervals.	
16. Dispose of used supplies and equipment in appropriate receptacle.	Standard precautions; reduces the transmission of microorganisms.	

Expected Outcomes

- An acceptable level of pain as per child (defined as controlled) or less than 5 on a 10-point scale if the child cannot self-report
- Child uses PCA effectively

- Stable respiratory status
- Stable neurologic status; easily aroused
- Stable cardiovascular status
- Child is free from signs of opioid withdrawal

Unexpected Outcomes

- Pain is not controlled (an unacceptable level to the child and/or interferes with movement, cough, treatment, play, or sleep)
- Child is unable to understand PCA use or does not push bolus dose button, resulting in inadequate pain control
- Respiratory depression or apnea
- Excessive sedation
- Hypotension or bradycardia
- Signs of opioid withdrawal

Monitoring and Care of the Child

Activities and Interventions	Rationale	Reportable Conditions
1. Assess pain intensity, location, and quality every hour until pain is controlled and then at least every 4 hours while awake. Optimally establish with the child the trigger point (the number on the pain scale the child considers comfortable as well as promotes activities for recovery). Refer to Procedure 173 for further details. (*Level II**)	Even though weight is generally used to predict analgesic effect, the starting doses for treatment are merely an estimate. Initial pump settings must be adjusted according to child's response.[5] Inadequate pain relief is addressed with gradual escalation of the PCA dosages until adequate analgesia is achieved or intolerable and unmanageable adverse effects occur.	- Inadequate pain control - Changes in severity, location, or characteristics of the pain - Inability of the child to participate in recovery activities due to pain
2. Assess the child's level of consciousness (LOC) every 1 to 2 hours during the first 12 to 24 hours of starting the PCA, then at least every 4 hours while child is awake. Describe the LOC in terms of a sedation scale. Increase the frequency of reassessment based	Traditionally, the RR has been used as an indicator of opioid overdose. However, a decrease in the RR is now recognized as a late sign. The best indicator of early respiratory depression is unexpected sedation. Sedation is most likely due to the	- Confusion - Behavioral changes - Unexpected change in LOC - Excessive sedation - Change in the ability to arouse the child - Other neurologic changes

* Level II: Theory based, no research data to support recommendations: recommendations from expert consensus group may exist

Monitoring and Care of the Child—Cont'd

Activities and Interventions	Rationale	Reportable Conditions
on the child's response to the PCA setting. Eliminate any nonessential CNS depressant medications.	opioid if the PCA has just been started or if recent increase in dose.	
If analgesia is satisfactory, reduce the opioid dose by 25%.	Sedation scales that can be used to monitor child's LOC in terms of levels include the following[6]:	See Procedure 176 for additional information on assessment scales.
If reportable conditions occur[6]:	S = Sleep, easy to arouse	
• Stop the infusion. *(Levels III and IV*)*	1 = Awake and alert	
• Summon help; contact the medical team	2 = Slightly drowsy, easily aroused	
• Gently stimulate the child. *(Levels III and IV*)*	3 = Frequently drowsy, but arousable, drifts off to	
• Assess the need to start oxygen by mask at a rate of at least 6 L/min. *(Level IV*)*	4 = Somnolent, minimal or sleep during conversation no response to physical stimulation	
• Assess the need to provide bag-mask ventilation. *(Level IV*)*	Although not necessarily contraindicated with opioids, concurrent use of hypnotics, antihistamines, muscle relaxants and anxiolytics can produce sedation and respiratory depression requiring increased monitoring of LOC.[2]	
• Assess the need to call the resuscitation (code) team. *(Level IV*)*		
• If no improvement, prepare naloxone by diluting 0.1 mg in 10 mL of saline to produce a 10 mcg/mL solution; give 0.5 mL (5 mcg) every 2 minutes until child is responsive. Prepare to repeat dose within 30 minutes because the half-life of some opioids is longer than that of naloxone. *(Level IV*)*	Naloxone given to those receiving opioids for more than 1 week may lead to sudden opioid withdrawal. This can be avoided by using only small doses and titrating until the appropriate LOC is achieved.	
• Do not leave the child until the LOC has returned to baseline. *(Level IV*)* Exception: *Terminally ill children in whom sedation is an acceptable side effect.*		
• When the LOC and respiratory rate are acceptable, resume the PCA with a 50% reduction in the opioid dose.		
• Consider adding or increasing a nonopioid analgesic such as ketorolac for additional pain relief.	NSAIDs may be useful adjuvants to improve analgesia without risk of additive sedation.[2]	
3. Monitor child with pulse oximetry continuously. Assess respiratory rate (RR) and document oxygen saturation (SpO$_2$) at least every 2 hours.	All opioid naïve children are at some risk for respiratory depression when first starting PCA. Clinically significant opioid-induced respiratory depression	• Changes in respiratory pattern (i.e., depth, rate) • SpO$_2$ less than 90% • If any of these occur, stop the infusion, provide

---

* Level III: Laboratory data, no clinical data to support recommendations
  Level IV: Limited clinical studies to support recommendations

Continued

Monitoring and Care of the Child—Cont'd

Activities and Interventions	Rationale	Reportable Conditions
Consider stopping or decreasing the dose for children with sustained SpO$_2$ less than 93% especially if arousing the child is difficult.[2]	can be prevented by careful opioid titration and close monitoring for sedation. Infants less than 2 months of age should be in a monitored setting.[3] Electronic monitoring is not a substitute for frequent clinical assessments. Nursing observation is the best method for monitoring the respiratory status. No consensus or conclusive evidence exists regarding which forms of electronic monitoring are most useful. If oximetry or apnea alarms are used, they must be connected to central monitors to provide audible alarms when clinicians are not at the bedside.	oxygen, and assist with ventilation • Consider administration of opioid antagonists such as naloxone
4. Monitor for side effects of opioids; if the pain score is satisfactory reduce dose by 25% and/or: • For hypotension, consider the need for a fluid bolus. • For nausea, consider IV antiemetics including the antiserotonin drugs such as ondansetron at doses of 0.15 mg/kg with a maximum dose of 8 mg every 6 to 8 hours[2] or changing to another opioid.[2] • For constipation; a stool softener combined with a mild peristaltic stimulant should be given as soon as condition permits such as docusate sodium/senna 187 mg (Senokot-S) 10 to 20 mg/kg/dose at bedtime.[6]	Because of great interindividual variability, different opioids can produce side effects of different intensities for individual children. Changing to another opioid should be considered primarily when side effects are intolerable. Opioids cause arterial and venous vasodilation by having a direct effect on vascular smooth muscle as well as the release of histamine resulting in vasodilation and pruritus. Fentanyl is the least likely opioid for these effects. Clinicians should take into account that antihistamines and antiemetics, with the exception of the antiserotonin drugs, can also lead to excessive sedation. Opioids cause nausea by stimulation of the chemoreceptor trigger zone in the medulla. These effects are enhanced by vestibular stimulation (movement). Constipation occurs because opioids can delay gastric emptying, slow bowel motility, and decrease peristalsis. Ileus rarely occurs. All opioids are capable of causing constriction of the sphincter of Oddi and the biliary tract.[5]	• Unexplained hypotension • Intolerable nausea or vomiting unresponsive to antiemetics • Unrelieved constipation • Intolerable pruritus unresponsive to antihistamines • Bladder distention • Excessive sedation from antihistamines
• For pruritus, consider antihistamines or changing to another opioid; if unrelieved by antihistamines or changing to another opioid, consider adding a continuous infusion of naloxone typically at starting doses of 0.25 mcg/kg/hr titrating up to 1 mcg/kg/hr as needed to control pruritus.[2] • For urinary retention, consider the need for Foley catheter.	NSAIDs may be useful adjuvants to improve analgesia without risk of additive sedation.	

Monitoring and Care of the Child—Cont'd

Activities and Interventions	Rationale	Reportable Conditions
5. At least every 4 hours, assess the number of boluses the child has self-administered and the level of pain intensity. If the child has uncontrolled pain and has bolused at maximum rate: • Consider obtaining an order to administer a clinician bolus via the PCA pump per institution-specific protocol. • Consider obtaining an order to increase the infusion by 25%. • Over the next 12 to 24 hours, if child has bolused more than once per hour as an average, consider increasing continuous infusion rate such that the child's overall opioid requirement per hour can be achieved with the continuous infusion plus one bolus. *(Level II*)*	The absolute opioid dose is unimportant as long as the balance between pain relief and adverse effects is favorable. The goal of titration is to use the lowest dose to provide satisfactory pain relief with the fewest adverse effects. Ideally, the PCA infusion dose will necessitate bolusing only for expected levels of increased pain (such as on activity) as well as reasonable durations of sleep and awakening without pain. One method of determining the effectiveness of the PCA settings is to look at the number of boluses during the previous 4 to 24 hours. Bolusing more than twice per hour may indicate inadequate continuous infusion rates and/or bolus doses. If the pain level is minimal or none with few boluses, then the continuous infusion is too high.	• Excessive boluses/attempts ratio • Unrelieved pain
6. For any concerns regarding pump failure, stop the pump, obtain a new one, label the malfunctioning pump with as much information about the event as possible as well as "do not use." Send pump for evaluation per institution-specific protocol. Complete appropriate report for incidents involving a medical device.	Maintaining safety of the child is of highest importance.	• Child and/or pump-related incidents of clinical significance
7. Promote activity of the child as medically indicated. Postural hypotension may occur when sitting or standing.	Ambulation must be done initially with supervision of hospital staff.	• Unresolved inability to complete physical activities considering overall physical condition • Any medication dose/concentration variance
8. Change infusion tubing and medication reservoir when empty or per institution-specific protocol regarding IV fluid administration. When a reservoir is changed, two licensed clinicians independently verify concentration of the new infusion and recheck all pump settings to ensure accuracy. *(Level II*)*	Minimize disconnection of infusion system to only when necessary to decrease the risk of infection. Many institutions report changing only when the reservoir is empty or no less frequent than 7 days of use. The highest risk of programming errors is not recognizing a new concentration of the medication Under- or overdosing the child will occur if the reservoir and the pump program do not match.	
9. When source of pain is diminishing, decrease or stop the infusion but continue to provide adequate bolus doses. For those who have used opioids for fewer than 5 days, decrease the	Evaluate children individually and taper doses based on their pain scores and ability to perform recovery activities rather than a preconceived notion of when the PCA should be discontinued.	• Inadequate pain control • Signs of opioid withdrawal including[12] neuroexcitablity (high-pitched cry, irritability, increased wakefulness, tremors, increased muscle tone, seizures),

* Level II: Theory based, no research data to support recommendations: recommendations from expert consensus group may exist

Continued

Monitoring and Care of the Child—Cont'd

Activities and Interventions	Rationale	Reportable Conditions
opioid dose 20% to 30% every 1 to 2 days. However, for those who have been on opioids for more than 5 to 7 days, begin a slower wean by calculating the total amount of opioid used the past 24 hours. Then one of the following approaches may be useful[12,13]: • Reduce PCA dose by 20% on first day; then wean subsequent doses by 10% per day as tolerated. • Convert amount of opioid to intermittent IV doses given every 2 to 4 hours. • Determine equivalent dose of methadone every 6 hours orally according to suggested dosing recommendations. *(Level II*)*	Duration of weaning is dependent on the individual child's response. The longer children have been receiving opioids, the longer it will take to wean them without withdrawal symptoms. Children given doses of opioids for as little as 5 to 7 days may show signs of withdrawal if opioids are ceased abruptly.[7]	gastrointestinal dysfunction (poor feeding, uncoordinated and constant sucking, vomiting, and diarrhea), and autonomic dysfunction (sweating, nasal stuffiness, fever, and mottling).
10. Discontinue infusion per prescribing practitioner's order. Waste remaining medication as per institution-specific protocol. Ensure that pain will be controlled by another method.	Refer to an equianalgesic chart in determining the appropriate dosages of opioids given by another route or method.	

* Level II: Theory based, no research data to support recommendations: recommendations from expert consensus group may exist

Documentation

- Child and family education including teaching related to a family member bolusing for the child
- Medication, concentration, pump settings including continuous rate, bolus doses, and lockout interval (initial settings, ongoing reassessment, and with any change in the pump settings)
- Individuals independently verifying pump settings and medication administered
- Pain intensity (score), location, and quality
- Vital signs and SpO_2
- LOC/arousability/sedation score
- Side effects of medications and effectiveness of related treatments
- Boluses given/attempts to bolus
- Adjunctive medications given for pain or side effects
- Condition of the IV
- Nonpharmacologic methods used for pain management and their effectiveness
- Unexpected outcomes and related treatment

References

1. Berde CB, Solodiuk J: Multidisciplinary programs for management of acute and chronic pain in children. In Schechter NL, et al, editors: *Pain in infants, children, and adolescents,* ed 2, Philadelphia, 2003, Lippincott Williams & Wilkins, pp. 477-479.
2. Lehr VT, BeVier P: Patient-controlled analgesia for the pediatric patient, *Orthop Nurs* 22:298-305, 2003.
3. Di Maggio TJ: Pediatric pain management. Acute pain management. In St. Marie B, editor: *American Pain Society of Pain Management Nurses: core curriculum for pain management nursing,* Philadelphia, 2002, Saunders, pp. 367-387.
4. Grandinetti CA, Buck M: Patient-controlled analgesia: guidelines for use in children, *Pediatr Pharm* 6(11):1-4, 2000.
5. Pasero C, et al: Opioid analgesics. In McCaffery M, Pasero C, editors: *Pain: clinical manual,* ed 2, St Louis, Mosby, pp.161-299.
6. Pasero C: *Intravenous patient-controlled analgesia for acute pain management: self-directed learning program,* Pensacola, FL, 2003, American Society of Pain Management Nurses. www.aspmn.com.
7. Yaster M, et al: Opioid agonists and antagonists. In Schechter NL, et al, editors: *Pain in infants, children, and adolescents,* ed 2, Philadelphia, 2003, Lippincott Williams & Wilkins, pp. 205-207.

8. Rothley BB, Therrien SR: Acute pain management. In St. Marie B, editor: *American Pain Society of Pain Management Nurses: core curriculum for pain management nursing,* Philadelphia, 2002, Saunders, pp. 239-271.

9. McGrath PA, Hillier LM: Modifying the psychologic factors that intensify children's pain and prolong disability. In Schechter NL, et al, editors: *Pain in infants, children, and adolescents,* ed 2, Philadelphia, 2003, Lippincott Williams & Wilkins, pp. 85-102.

10. Joint Commission Resources: Special Report: 2003 JCAHO National Patient Safety Goals: practical strategies and helpful solutions for meeting these goals. www.jcrinc.com/subscribers/patientsafety.asp?durki=7916&site=22&return=154, accessed 11/3/2005, 2003.

11. Monitto CL, et al: The safety and efficacy of parent/nurse-controlled analgesia in patients less than six years of age, *Anesth Analg* 91:573-579, 2000.

12. Oakes LO: Assessment and management of pain in the critically ill pediatric patient, *Crit Care Nurs Clin North Am* 13:282-295, 2001.

13. Anghelescu D, Oakes L: Working toward better cancer pain management for children, *Cancer Pract* 10;S52-S57, 2002.

Additional Readings

American Pain Society: Principles of analgesic use in treatment of acute pain and cancer pain, ed 5, Glenview, IL, 2003, *American Pain Society:* 24-26

Oakes LO: Caring practices: providing comfort. In Curley MAQ, Moloney-Harmon PA, editors: *Critical care nursing of infants and children,* ed 2, Philadelphia, 2001, Saunders.

Tobias J: Pain management for the critically ill child in the pediatric intensive care unit. In Schechter NL, et al, editors: *Pain in infants, children, and adolescents,* ed 2, Philadelphia, 2003, Lippincott Williams & Wilkins, pp. 807-840.

Peripheral Nerve Stimulator

P U R P O S E : A peripheral nerve stimulator is used in association with the administration of neuromuscular blocking agents to obtain an objective measurement of the depth of neuromuscular blockade with assessment of nerve impulse transmission

Karen C. Bowe and Dana Garver

PREREQUISITE KNOWLEDGE

- Peripheral nerve stimulators (PNSs) are used to monitor and document the presence and degree of neuromuscular blockade when neuromuscular blocking agents (NMBAs) are given to block skeletal muscle activity.[1,2]
- An NMBA is used in the intensive care unit to produce muscle relaxation and flaccid paralysis by pharmacologic blockade at the neuromuscular junction.[1] Indications for NMBA include:
  - ❖ To optimize ventilator support
  - ❖ To decrease the child's respiratory effort
  - ❖ To decrease high peak pressures during ventilation
  - ❖ To improve severe hypoxemia
  - ❖ To decrease oxygen consumption
  - ❖ As adjunctive medication in the treatment of increased intracranial pressure
  - ❖ As an aid in recovery phase after specific surgical procedures
- NMBAs have NO sedative or analgesic properties; therefore, a combination of sedatives and analgesics should always be administered *before* the administration of an NMBA and during continuous infusion of an NMBA. This minimizes the child's awareness of paralysis and decreases exposure to noxious stimuli. In addition, sedatives and analgesics should always be given *prophylactically* to produce a relaxed unconscious child who has minimal periods of awareness and pain during paralysis.

- Monitoring of neuromuscular function and blockade with a PNS utilizing the Train-of-Four (TOF) method of stimulation is most commonly used in intensive care settings. A series of small electrical stimuli (four) delivered by the PNS produces a muscle twitch that corresponds to the percentage of nerve receptor sites occupied by NMBAs. In the absence of significant neuromuscular blockade (NMB), four muscle twitches occur. The four twitches indicate that 75% or less of receptors are blocked. Three twitches correspond to 80% blockade, and one to two twitches correlate with 85% to 90% blockade. Zero twitches indicate that 100% of the receptors are blocked, a results that exceeds the desired level of blockade (Table 175-1).
- Studies identify a TOF count of 1/4 to 2/4 as indicative of adequate block without undue risk of toxicity.[3]
- The stimulating current is measured in milliamps (mA). The usual range to elicit a muscle twitch response is 20 to 50 mA, although an increase in the current to the maximum setting of 80 mA may be necessary. Some PNSs are digital or have dialed numbers that range from 1 to 10, representing the mA range of 20 to 80. With these instruments, the usual setting is 2 to 5.
- Familiarity with the specific PNS unit used to assess NMB: some models require quality control tests prior to use to prevent errors in assessment related to malfunctioning equipment.
- Proximal and distal electrodes are placed on the child to use the PNS. Electrodes are placed:
  - ❖ Along the ulnar nerve (Figure 175-1)

TABLE 175-1	Correlation of Twitches Elicited by Train-of-Four Stimulation and Percentage of Blocked Nerve Receptors[2,3,5]

TOF (No. of Twitches) Percentage of Receptors Blocked

0/4, 100%
1/4, 90%
2/4, 85%
3/4, 80%
4/4, 75% or less

Information compiled from Martin L, Bratton S, O'Rourke P: Clinical uses and controversies of neuromuscular blocking agents in infants and children, *Crit Care Med* 27(7):1358-1366, 1999.

McManus M: Neuromuscular blockers in surgery and intensive care, part 2, *Am J Health-System Pharmacy* 58(24):2381-2399, 2001.

Arbour R: Continuous nervous system monitoring, EEG, the bispectral index, and neuromuscular transmission, *AACN Clin Iss Adv Pract Crit Care* 14(2):185-207, 2003.

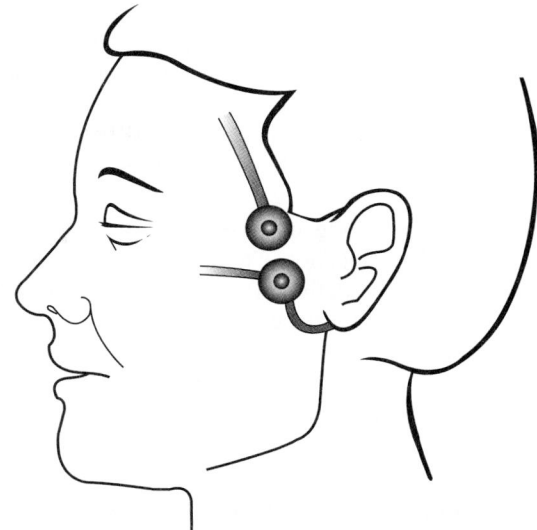

FIGURE 175-2 Placement of electrodes along facial nerve. *From Whetstone Foster JG: Peripheral nerve stimulators. In Lynn-McHale Wiegand DJ, Carlson K, editors:* AACN procedure manual for critical care, *ed 5, Philadelphia, 2005, Saunders, p. 840.*

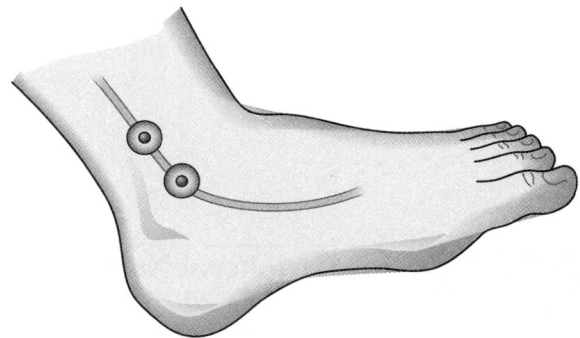

FIGURE 175-3 Placement of electrodes on foot. *From Whetstone Foster JG: Peripheral nerve stimulators. In Lynn-McHale Wiegand DJ, Carlson K, editors:* AACN procedure manual for critical care, *ed 5, Philadelphia, 2005, Saunders, p. 841.*

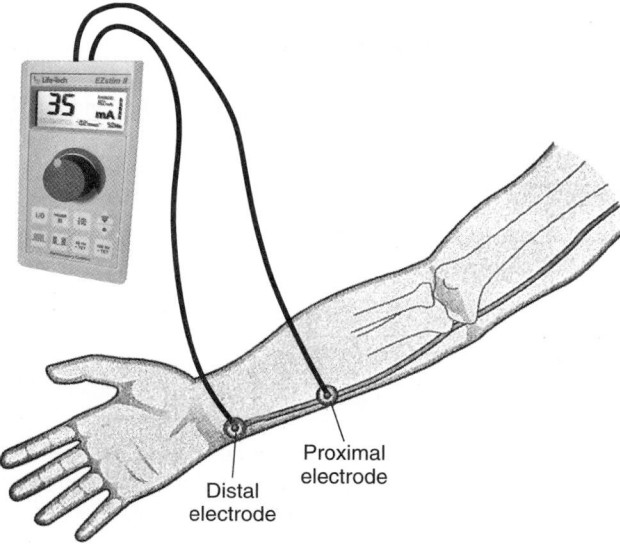

FIGURE 175-1 Placement of electrodes along ulnar nerve. *From Whetstone Foster JG: Peripheral nerve stimulators. In Lynn-McHale Wiegand DJ, Carlson K, editors:* AACN procedure manual for critical care, *ed 5, Philadelphia, 2005, Saunders, p. 839.*

❖ Along the facial nerve (Figure 175-2)
❖ Along the posterior tibial nerve (Figure 175-3)
• Use of NMBAs may result in complications that affect multiple body systems. The relative risk increases with acuity and prolonged use of NMBAs. Always evaluate response to stimulation in the context of clinical assessment findings and whether clinical goals have been met.
• Titration of medication according to clinical assessment and TOF responses provides a basis for decision making in determining the level of adequate blockade without saturation of the receptor sites. Overdose of an NMBA or accumulation of the drug can cause serious complications, including prolonged weakness or paralysis. PNS monitoring during NMBA administration results in decreased medication utilization.

• Anatomy and physiology of the neuromuscular junction
• Child development as it relates to clinical assessment, NMBA, and use of PNS
• Mastery of pediatric advanced life support competencies
• Appropriate pediatric dosing of sedatives, analgesics, and NMBA

CHILD AND FAMILY ASSESSMENT

• Selection of ideal placement of electrodes; consider arterial and venous catheters, dressings, wounds, edema, or diaphoresis ➤➤*Rationale:* Appropriate placement and adequate electrode contact improve conduction of the stimulating current.
• Child's and family's understanding of the reasons for and risks and benefits of the procedure ➤➤*Rationale:* Evaluates the child's and family's understanding of the procedure and provides a gauge for ongoing education.

- If possible, apply the electrodes and determine adequacy of the selected location and a baseline response before initiation of the NMBA ➥*Rationale:* Improves reliability of interpretation of the TOF response.
- Child's and family's previous experience with sedatives, analgesics, or NMBA ➥*Rationale:* Identifies any previous experiences and may help to assess child's and family's understanding or misconceptions and identify areas for further education. Children may have paradoxic reactions to some sedatives. Promotes selection of appropriate medications for the child.
- Allergies to sedatives, NMBA, analgesics, electrode gel, or tape ➥*Rationale:* Promotes patient safety; prevents exposure to medications or substances to which the child has a known allergy.

CHILD AND FAMILY EDUCATION

Individualized, developmentally appropriate education is provided to the family and to the child based on desire for knowledge, readiness to learn, and overall neurologic and psychosocial state.

- Provide information to the family about NMBA, clinical effect, and the reason for TOF monitoring (for example, to assess the effect of the medication and adjust the dose accordingly) ➥*Rationale:* Providing information decreases anxiety and fear.
- Show and describe the function of the equipment ➥*Rationale:* Providing information decreases anxiety and fear; ability to see and touch the equipment is helpful to visual learners.
- Describe the sensation of the stimulus as a slight stinging sensation ➥*Rationale:* Identification of a known or previously experienced sensation may be effective in decreasing anxiety associated with the procedure.
- Encourage questions and answer questions as they arise ➥*Rationale:* Reinforcement of information is needed during periods of stress.

EQUIPMENT

- Peripheral nerve stimulator
- Alcohol pads or other cleaning agent per institution-specific protocol
- Two gelled electrode pads (type used for electrocardiographic monitoring)
- Two lead wires packaged with the PNS to connect PNS to electrodes

Procedure | for Peripheral Nerve Stimulator

Steps	Rationale	Considerations
1. Ensure family (and child as appropriate) understands procedure and questions are answered.	Evaluates and reinforces understanding of previously taught information.	Developmental level, cognitive ability, and anxiety level determine approach to and effectiveness of teaching.
2. Gather needed equipment and supplies.	Facilitates completion of task in a timely manner.	
3. Identify child with two patient identifiers.	Confirms correct patient and procedure as recommended by the Joint Commission on Accreditation of Healthcare Organizations (JCAHO).	Refer to institution-specific protocol; name and medical record number are the most frequently used patient identifiers in the inpatient setting.
Testing the Ulnar Nerve 4. Wash hands.	Standard precautions; reduces the transmission of microorganisms.	
5. Locate the ulnar nerve.	The ulnar nerve is commonly used because it is superficial and easy to locate. *(Level VI*)*	The ulnar nerve is the site that is least likely to have artifact in testing for NMB.
6. Place the arm in an extended relaxed position with the palm up (see Figure 175-1).	Exposes the ulnar nerve.	

* Level VI: Clinical studies in a variety of patient populations and situations to support recommendations

Procedure	**for Peripheral Nerve Stimulator**—*Continued*	
Steps	**Rationale**	**Considerations**
7. Clean area selected for electrode placement with alcohol and allow to dry or prepare area according to manufacturer's instructions. *(Level I*)*	Cleaning and drying the skin before electrode application may improve adherence of the electrode, resulting in improved assessment.	
8. Apply gel electrodes over the ulnar nerve (see Figure 175-1). The distal electrode should be placed at the proximal flexor crease in a straight line from the base of the fifth digit. The proximal lead should be placed 1 to 2 cm along the same plane.	Accurate electrode placement facilitates stimulation of the ulnar nerve. Direct stimulation of the ulnar nerve results in flexion-adduction of the thumb.	Inaccurate placement of electrodes may cause stimulation of the muscle, resulting in flexion of the fingers. Flexion of the fingers is not an appropriate assessment of level of neuromuscular blockade.
9. Attach lead wires, matching red and black leads to receptacles of the PNS. Attach leads to electrodes.	Correct connection of the positive and negative wires allows for conduction of electrical current.	The red electrode should be placed proximally and the black electrode should be placed distally.[1]
10. Turn on PNS and select a low mA on the dial; press the TOF key.	The TOF delivers a series of four stimuli at 2 Hz each every 0.5 seconds.	When rechecking for flexion-adduction of the thumb, wait 10 to 15 seconds to allow for repolarization of the nerve.[2]
11. Observe thumb and count the number of twitches.	Number of twitches elicited is used to determine degree of NMB.	Only count the flexion-adduction of the thumb. Do not count any finger movement because it is considered artifact.
12. Depress standby button after stimulation of the nerve.	The PNS automatically delivers a series of stimuli every 10 seconds until the standby button is pressed.	
13. Turn PNS off; detach lead wires from electrodes.	Procedure has been completed.	
14. Wash hands.	Standard precautions; reduces transmission of microorganisms.	
Testing the Facial Nerve		
15. Locate the facial nerve.	Alternative spots can be used for testing when invasive lines or edema interfere with the testing of the ulnar nerve.	The orbicularis oculi has an onset and recovery time similar to the diaphragm.[2]
16. Place gel electrode on the face next to the outer canthus of the eye. Place the second electrode 2 cm below and parallel to the tragus of the ear (see Figure 175-2).	Direct stimulation of the facial nerve evokes frontalis and orbiculis oculi muscle contraction.	Facial nerve stimulation is prone to muscle artifact because of the number of small facial muscles.
17. Attach lead wires, matching red and black leads to receptacles of the PNS. Attach leads to electrodes.	Correct connection of the positive and negative wires allows for conduction of electrical current.	The red electrode should be placed proximally and the black electrode should be placed distally.[1]
18. Turn on the PNS and select a low mA on the dial and press the TOF button.	The TOF delivers a series of four stimuli at 2 Hz each every 0.5 seconds.	
19. Observe muscle twitching above the eyebrow towards the forehead; count the number of twitches.	Number of twitches elicited is used to determine degree of NMB.	

Procedure continues on following page

* Level I: Manufacturer's recommendations only

Procedure for Peripheral Nerve Stimulator—*Continued*

Steps	Rationale	Considerations
20. Depress standby button after stimulation of the nerve.	The PNS automatically delivers a series of stimuli every 10 seconds until the standby button is pressed.	
21. Turn PNS off; detach lead wires from electrodes.	Procedure has been completed.	
22. Wash hands.	Standard precautions.	
Testing the Posterior Tibial Nerve		
23. Locate posterior tibial nerve.	Determines site for electrode placement.	
24. Place one electrode approximately 2 cm posterior to the medial malleolus; second electrode is placed 2 cm directly above the first electrode (see Figure 175-3).	Accurate electrode placement facilitates stimulation of the nerve.	
25. Attach lead wires, matching red and black leads to receptacles of the PNS. Attach leads to electrodes.	Correct connection of the positive and negative wires allows for conduction of electrical current.	The red electrode should be placed proximally and the black electrode should be placed distally.[1]
26. Turn on the PNS; select a low mA on the dial and press the TOF button.	The TOF delivers a series of four stimuli at 2 Hz each every 0.5 seconds.	
27. Observe plantar flexion of the great toe and count the number of twitches.	Number of twitches elicited is used to determine degree of NMB.	
28. Depress the standby button after stimulation of the nerve.	The PNS automatically delivers a series of stimuli every 10 seconds until the standby button is pressed.	
29. Turn PNS off; detach lead wires from electrodes.	Procedure has been completed.	
30. Wash hands.	Standard precautions.	
Determining the Supramaximal Stimulation (SMS)		
31. Starting at a low current, depress TOF button and observe the number of twitches. Increase mA by 1 after each TOF series until four twitches are observed. Once four twitches are observed, continue to increase the mA by 1 until no increase is seen in the magnitude of the response. *(Level V*)*	Determination of the SMS serves as a baseline for monitoring of neuromuscular blockade. The SMS is the starting point for peripheral nerve stimulation assessment.[4]	The SMS must be determined before the administration of NMBA.
Monitoring NMB		
32. After administration of analgesia or sedation, administer NMBA bolus and start continuous infusion of NMBA.	Frequent monitoring allows for the lowest dose of NMBA to be administered.[4]	The PNS should be used in conjunction with a clinical assessment to monitor NMB.
33. Continue to monitor every 30 to 60 minutes until desired level of clinical NMB is achieved.	Desired number of twitches is 1/4 to 2/4 or according to prescribing practitioner's order.	

* Level V: Clinical studies in more than one or two patient populations and situations to support recommendations

Procedure	for Peripheral Nerve Stimulator—*Continued*	
Steps	**Rationale**	**Considerations**
34. Once desired level of NMB is achieved, continue to monitor every 4 hours or per institution-specific or unit-specific protocol.	Ongoing monitoring facilitates titration of NMBA to maintain desired degree of NMB.	
35. If 3/4 or 4/4 twitches are present, increase continuous NMBA infusion per prescribing practitioner's order or institution-specific or unit-specific protocol.	Optimizes degree of NMB.	Continually monitor level of sedation in addition to level of NMB. *(Level VI*)*
Troubleshooting		
36. If TOF = 0/4 twitches: Attempt repositioning or placement of new electrodes.	Dry electrodes can decrease conduction.	When 0/4 twitches are noted, determination of either a complete neuromuscular block or a malfunctioning TOF system is necessary.
Ensure proper placement of red (proximal) and black (distal) electrodes.	Malpositioned electrodes elicit a false reading.	
Verify lead wires are properly connected to the PNS.	Incomplete connection alters current conduction.	
Ensure sufficient time for the nerve to repolarize.	Always allow 10 to 15 seconds for the nerve to repolarize between stimulation.[4]	
Retest with another site.	Nerve desensitization may occur.	Rotation of sites on a regular basis may decrease incidence rate of nerve desensitization.
Increase the stimulation by 1 mA on the PNS. If an increase in mA does not produce a response, the NMB continuous infusion must be decreased per prescribing practitioner's order or institution-specific or unit-specific protocol.	A TOF of 0/4 could ultimately be from excessive neuromuscular blockade.[5]	

* Level VI: Clinical studies in a variety of patient populations and situations to support recommendations

Expected Outcomes

- The NMBA is titrated on basis of the TOF and clinical assessment; therefore, the least amount of NMB is administered[3,4]
- Minimal discomfort is experienced as result of the combined used of analgesia, sedation, while the child is receiving NMBA
- Skin at site of PNS electrodes remains intact
- The appropriate nerve is stimulated during PNS monitoring
- Return of 4/4 twitches occurs within 2 hours of discontinuing the NMBA continuous infusion

Unexpected Outcomes

- Clinical assessment is not used in combination with TOF
- Titration does not occur
- An increased amount of discomfort is experienced during the testing of the PNS
- The child has unrecognized pain or anxiety
- Skin irritation is noted at the site of PNS electrodes
- Failure to stimulate nerve
- Muscle artifact is noted during PNS stimulation
- The return of 4/4 twitches does not occur within 2 hours of discontinuing the NMBA continuous infusion

Monitoring and Care of the Child

Activities and Interventions	Rationale	Reportable Conditions
1. Select a site for electrode placement that is easily accessible and has the least amount of edema, invasive lines, dressings, or wounds.	An easily accessible site facilitates stimulation of the nerve. Edema and anasarca inhibit the transmission of electrical current and may result in a false reading.	• Inability to place electrodes in desired location because of invasive lines, dressings, wounds, or increased edema
2. Monitor skin at the site of electrode placement.	Risk of skin irritation from electrode gel or delivery of current.	• Skin irritation
3. Monitor child's level of NMB every 4 hours as long as TOF is maintained within parameters listed in prescribing practitioner's orders.	Frequent monitoring is necessary while the child is receiving a continuous infusion of a NMBA.	• Results not within ordered parameters
4. Do not perform "Single Twitch," "Tetany," or "Double Burst" on the PNS.	These methods for monitoring are used only in the operating room and are uncomfortable for the child.	• Inadvertent use of listed methods
5. Assess effectiveness of pain management and sedation strategies and provide appropriate interventions. Encourage family to assist with nonpharmacologic means to comfort and support the child.	Early identification of pain or agitation allows for immediate intervention.	• Increase in Comfort score or increase in other mechanisms used to assess pain and anxiety or agitation

Documentation

- Family and child education
- The time, SMS, mA, and nerve tested
- Number of twitches elicited in response to TOF recorded as 0/4, 1/4, 2/4, 3/4, or 4/4
- Any action taken on basis of the TOF
- The drugs, dose, and site of administration of NMBA
- Sedatives and analgesics administered concomitantly with NMBA
- Unexpected outcomes and related treatment

References

1. Arbour R: Mastering neuromuscular blockade, *Dimens Crit Care Nurs* 19(5):4-20, 2000.
2. Martin L, et al: Clinical uses and controversies of neuromuscular blocking agents in infants and children, *Crit Care Med* 27(7):1358-1366, 1999.
3. McManus M: Neuromuscular blockers in surgery and intensive care, part 2, *Am J Health-System Pharmacy* 58(24):2381-2399, 2001.
4. Foster J, et al: National practice with assessment and monitoring of neuromuscular blockade, *Crit Care Nurs Q* 25(2):27-40, 2002.
5. Arbour R: Continuous nervous system monitoring, EEG, the bispectral index, and neuromuscular transmission, *AACN Clin Iss Adv Pract Crit Care* 14(2):185-207, 2003.

Additional Readings

Loyola R, Dreher M: Management of pharmacologically induced neuromuscular blockade using peripheral nerve stimulation, *Dimens Crit Care Nurs* 22(4):157-164, 2003.

Murray M, et al: Clinical practice guidelines for sustained neuromuscular blockade in the adult critically ill patient, *Crit Care Med* 30(1):142-156, 2002.

Vernon D, Witte M: Effects of neuromuscular blockade on oxygen consumption and energy expenditure in sedated mechanically ventilated children, *Crit Care Med* 28(5):1569-1571, 2000.

Sedation Assessment Scales

P U R P O S E : To use a valid reliable assessment tool to guide clinical management to meet the desired physiologic and psychologic patient outcomes. The COMFORT and Modified Motor Activity Assessment Scales are described.

Maria Teresa Zapata and Mary Frances D. Pate

PREREQUISITE KNOWLEDGE

- Anatomy and physiology of peripheral nervous system, the autonomic and skeletal motor systems, and the central nervous system
- Sedation and comfort assessments are essential and, if accomplished together, guide optimal management to prevent: physiologic effects of untreated pain and anxiety, inefficient ventilation, hypoxia, agitation, self-harm (self-extubation, removal of lines, and lack of cooperation with medical treatments), and awareness of the potentially frightening environment.
- Sedation scales provide a systematic approach to detect undersedation (agitation, hypertension, tachycardia, respiratory distress, and self-harm) and oversedation (more difficult to assess because of a more insidious onset caused by drug accumulation and difficulty in differentiation from the severity of the underlying illness).
- Oversedation can lead to respiratory depression, problems in weaning from ventilator, hemodynamic instability, gastrointestinal stasis, muscle wasting, and decreased ability to communicate. Additional risks may include renal or hepatic failure from impaired excretion of the accumulated metabolites of sedatives, especially with prolonged use.
- Cultural variations, individual behavioral manifestations, and environmental factors play a role in sedation and comfort assessment and management.
- Self-report pain and sedation assessment scoring are not feasible in children who are preverbal or unable to communicate because of level of consciousness, mechanical ventilation, or chemical relaxation.
- Observational scales are used to guide sedation management; specifically providing a level of medication to promote sleep and reduce anxiety, while allowing caregivers to arouse the child for assessment and ongoing medical interventions.
- Standardized sedation tools assist with consistent assessment and documentation of levels of sedation and communication within the team of caregivers when the tool is used correctly and consistently by all caregivers who assess the child; education on how to use the tool is necessary.
- Validity and reliability testing of the COMFORT Scale has been performed in children.[1-7]
- Validity and reliability testing of the Motor Activity Assessment Scale (MAAS) for adult ventilated patients has been performed.[3,8] Results of validity and reliability testing of a modified scale for use in the pediatric population (MMAAS) have not been reported of the scale in its current form. The State Behavioral Scale incorporates components of the MAAS scale, and has been studied in the infants and young children on mechanical ventilation.[9]
- Child development as it relates to sedation assessment
- Appropriate pediatric dosing of sedatives and anxiolytics

CHILD AND FAMILY ASSESSMENT

- Presedation assessment of vital signs, including temperature, airway assessment, oxygen saturation (SpO2), weight, mental status, allergies, and oral intake ➤*Rationale:* These factors affect appropriate drug selection and dosing or may be affected by administration of sedation; these factors facilitate ongoing assessment of effectiveness of sedation plan.

- Child's usual coping methods ➤➤*Rationale:* Children with temperaments that are less adaptable are more reactive to painful stimuli.[10]
- Age and developmental level ➤➤*Rationale:* Older children's perception of pain has been shown to be less than that of younger children with the same diagnostic procedure.[10]
- Level of consciousness and cognitive ability ➤➤*Rationale:* Baseline assessment data are useful for comparison during sedation.
- Child's and family's previous experience with sedatives ➤➤*Rationale:* Identification of any previous experiences may help to assess child's and family's understanding or misconceptions and identify areas for further education. Children may have paradoxic reactions to some sedatives; selection of appropriate medications for the child is promoted.
- Family's desire to be present during procedure ➤➤*Rationale:* Family presence decreases child's anxiety and increases sense of security.
- Dose, route, and frequency of medications the child is receiving that may contribute to sedation ➤➤*Rationale:* Medications the child is receiving for purposes other than sedation may also cause sedation as a side effect.

CHILD AND FAMILY EDUCATION

Individualized developmentally appropriate education is provided to the family and to the child based on desire for knowledge, readiness to learn, and overall neurologic and psychosocial state.

- Provide information about the importance of sedation and comfort assessment in guiding medication administration to optimize sedation ➤➤*Rationale:* Providing information decreases anxiety and fear.
- Explain how the family can assist with sedation (i.e., identification of behaviors that show the child's distress) ➤➤*Rationale:* Families best understand behavioral and communication cues that child exhibits when in distress or discomfort.
- Encourage questions and answer questions as they arise ➤➤*Rationale:* Reinforcement of information is needed during periods of stress.

EQUIPMENT

- Sedation scale appropriate for the individual child
- Stethoscope
- Cardiorespiratory monitoring
- Oxygen saturation monitoring
- Timer or clock/watch with second hand (COMFORT Scale)

Procedure for Sedation Assessment

Steps	Rationale	Considerations
COMFORT Scale 1. Ensure instructions for administration of the tool are understood.[3] *(Level III*)*	If the scoring tool is not used appropriately, results are not valid.	The COMFORT Scale is intended for use in children requiring mechanical ventilation. One study supports the use of the scale to assess post-operative pain in infants.[6]
2. Identify individual child's baseline levels for heart rate (HR) and mean arterial blood pressure (MAP).	Child's current HR and MAP are compared with baseline levels during assessment period.	
3. Observe the child for 2 minutes from a location where the child's entire body and face and the monitor can be seen and score the parameters listed subsequently.[4] *(Level IV*)*	Allows observation of all items in the scale.	Most extreme (distressed) behavior observed is scored.[4]
4. Assess and score: **Alertness.** 1 Deeply asleep. 2 Lightly asleep. 3 Drowsy. 4 Fully awake and alert. 5 Hyper alert.	Rates the child's response to ambient stimulation in the environment.[4]	No stimulus is introduced by the observer. Children with neurologic deficits may have baseline alteration in alertness.

The COMFORT scale from Ambuel B, et al: Assessing stress in pediatric intensive care environments: the COMFORT scale, *J Pediatr Psychol* 17(1): 95–109, 1992. Used with permission.

* Level III: Laboratory data; no clinical data to support recommendations
  Level IV: Limited clinical studies to support recommendations

Procedure for Sedation Assessment—*Continued*

Steps	Rationale	Considerations
5. Assess and score: **Calmness/ Agitation.** 1 Calm. 2 Slightly anxious. 3 Anxious. 4 Very anxious. 5 Panicky.	Rates the child's level of emotional arousal/anxiety.[4] Agitation is behavioral communication, a sign that "something is wrong."	Causes for agitation include hypoxia, emotional distress, environmental factors, drug reactions, and pain.
6. Assess and score: **Respiratory Response.** 1 No coughing and no spontaneous respiration. 2 Spontaneous respiration with little or no response to ventilation. 3 Active breathing against ventilator or regular coughing. 4 Fighting ventilator, coughing, or choking.	Rates the child's oral and respiratory response to endotracheal tube and mechanical ventilation.[4] Synchrony with ventilator is optimal; "fighting" ventilator can be life threatening.	Consider level of ventilator support required (conventional versus oscillatory ventilation).
7. Assess and score: **Physical Movement.** 1 No movement. 2 Occasional slight movement. 3 Vigorous movement limited to extremities. 4 Vigorous movement including torso and head.	Rates frequency and intensity of physical movement.[4] Excessive movement may be evidence of agitation and can lead to injury and dislodgement of tubes; no movement can be a sign of oversedation.	Children with neuromuscular deficits or neuromuscular blockade may have altered physical movement at baseline.
8. Assess and score: **MAP Compared with Baseline.** Observe MAP five to six times during 2-minute observation period. 1 MAP below baseline. 2 MAP consistently at baseline. 3 Infrequent elevations of MAP of 15% or more (one to three during observation period). 4 Frequent elevation of MAP of 15% or more (more than three during observation period). 5 Sustained elevation of MAP of 15% or more.	Rates frequency of change from baseline.[4] Blood pressure is most often elevated in response to pain or anxiety.	Blood pressure changes can reflect changes in hemodynamic status. Preterm and newborn infants can respond with either elevated or decreased MAP.[11] Blood pressure can return to normal because of the body's inability to sustain response to stress. If the child does not have an arterial line, one MAP measurement is obtained. A few studies have identified that this parameter can be eliminated without affecting the validity of the assessment.[2,6] *(Level IV*)*
9. Assess and score: **Heart Rate Compared with Baseline.** Observe HR five to six times during 2-minute observation period. 1 Heart rate below baseline. 2 Heart rate consistently at baseline. 3 Infrequent elevations of 15% or more above baseline during observation period (one to three). 4 Frequent elevations of 15% or more above baseline during observation period (more than three). 5 Sustained elevation of 15% or more.	Rates frequency of change from baseline.[4] Heart rate is most often elevated in response to pain or anxiety.	Changes in heart rate can reflect changes in hemodynamic status. Preterm infants can respond to stress with decreased heart rate. A few studies have identified that this parameter can be eliminated without affecting the validity of the assessment.[2,6] *(Level IV*)*

Procedure continues on following page

* Level IV: Limited clinical studies to support recommendations

Procedure **for Sedation Assessment**—*Continued*

Steps	Rationale	Considerations

10. Assess and score: **Muscle Tone.**
  1 Muscles totally relaxed; no muscle tone.
  2 Reduced muscle tone.
  3 Normal muscle tone.
  4 Increased muscle tone and flexion of fingers and toes.
  5 Extreme muscle rigidity and flexion of fingers and toes.
	Assessed in comparison with a child who is awake and alert; based on child's response to rapid and slow flexion of an extremity without invasive lines.[4]
	No muscle tone can be an indication of oversedation or muscle wasting; increased muscle tone can be an indication of pain and anxiety.
		Children with neuromuscular deficits or those receiving neuromuscular blocking agents (NMBAs) have baseline alterations in muscle tone.

11. Assess and score: **Facial Tension.**
  1 Facial muscles totally relaxed.
  2 Facial muscle tone normal; no facial muscle tension evident.
  3 Tension evident in some facial muscles.
  4 Tension evident throughout facial muscles.
  5 Facial muscles contorted and grimacing.
	Assesses tone and tension of facial muscles in comparison with a child who is awake and alert.[4]
	Facial grimace is an indication of pain or distress, especially in infants.
		Children with neuromuscular deficits or those receiving NMBAs have baseline alterations in muscle tone.

12. Add the score for each dimension to obtain total score. (*Level IV**)	Optimal range is 17 to 26.[1]	A few studies have identified that HR and MAP can be eliminated without affecting the validity of the assessment. Exclusion of these parameters has been suggested because they can be affected by other factors.[4,10]
Modified Motor Activity Assessment Scale (MMAAS)[9]		
13. Ensure instructions for administration of the tool are understood.[3] (*Level III**)	If the scoring tool is not used appropriately, results are not valid.	The MMAAS is intended for use in children with normal neurologic responses who are not receiving neuromuscular blocking agents; criteria may necessitate motor movement.[10]
14. Observe the child and assign a rating from the options listed subsequently. (*Level IV**)	Careful observation of behavior determines score assigned.	No validated optimal score exists; values should be individualized to the child and the child's phase of illness.
15. Score: **−3, Unresponsive.**	May be indicative of oversedation or induction/acute phase of sedation.	Vital signs, Spo$_2$, and ETco$_2$ should be used to guide sedation management. Sedation should be titrated to meet goals. Consider drug holiday if ventilation has been prolonged or if large doses administered.

The Modified Motor Activity Assessment Scale (MMIS) from Devin JW, et al: Motor activity assessment scale: a valid and reliable scale for use with mechanically ventilated patients in an adult surgical intensive care unit, *Crit Care Med* 27(7): 1271-1275, 1999. Used with permission.

* Level III: Laboratory data; no clinical data to support recommendations
  Level IV: Limited clinical studies to support recommendations

Procedure for Sedation Assessment—*Continued*

Steps	Rationale	Considerations
16. Score: **−2, Responsive only to noxious stimuli.**	Indicative of induction/acute phase of sedation.[5]	Vital signs, SpO_2 and $ETCO_2$ should be used to guide sedation management. Sedation should be titrated to meet goals.
17. Score: **−1, Responsive to touch.**	Indicative of stabilization phase of sedation.[5]	Continue physiologic monitoring as child's condition stabilizes. Sedation goals should be met by providing minimal effective dose.
18. Score: **0, Calm and cooperative.**	Indicative of stabilization phase of sedation.[5]	Continue physiologic monitoring as child's condition stabilizes. Sedation goals should be met by providing minimal effective dose.
19. Score: **+1, Restless and cooperative.**	May indicate inadequate sedation or unrelated causes of agitation.	Assess for adequate sedation and analgesia. Encourage parental support. Child may be attempting to communicate by behavioral means. Reduce environmental stimuli. Attempt comfort measures (e.g., swaddling, repositioning, therapeutic massage).
20. Score: **+2, Agitated.**	May indicate inadequate sedation or unrelated causes of agitation.	Assess for hypoxia, inadequate ventilation, and drug withdrawal. Consider sedation weaning schedule. Provide for patient safety.
21. Score: **+3, Dangerously agitated, uncooperative.**	May indicate inadequate sedation or unrelated causes of agitation.	Assess for hypoxia, inadequate ventilation, and drug withdrawal. Consider sedation weaning schedule. Provide for patient safety.

Expected Outcomes

- Appropriate sedation scale is selected and used correctly

- Child has appropriate level of sedation that results in minimal anxiety or agitation and security and stability of invasive lines, artificial airway, etc

- Child is free from complications of sedation

Unexpected Outcomes

- Inappropriate sedation scale is selected or scale is not used appropriately, with results that are not valid
- Oversedation
- Undersedation
- Inadequate sedation, paradoxic response
- Inadvertent removal of artificial airway, invasive lines, drains, etc
- Apnea
- Hypotension
- Stridor, laryngospasm, bronchospasm
- Nausea/vomiting
- Hypotension, arrhythmias
- Emergence reactions
- Aspiration
- Increased duration of mechanical ventilation

Monitoring and Care of the Child

Activities and Interventions	Rationale	Reportable Conditions
1. Monitor child's tolerance to sedation.	Changes in child's condition may indicate complications related to sedation.	• Apnea • Hypotension • Arrhythmias • Paradoxic agitation
2. Obtain sedation score at appropriate intervals per institution-specific protocol, generally every 2 to 4 hours; trend sedation score over time.	Allows assessment of level of sedation and effectiveness and appropriateness of sedation plan; facilitates prompt intervention for undersedation or oversedation.	• Significant change in score that indicates need to reevaluate current sedation plan
3. Assess effectiveness of nonpharma-cologic interventions for agitation and anxiety; encourage family to assist with nonpharmacologic means to comfort and support the child.	Facilitates identification of non-pharmacologic means effective in managing agitation or anxiety. Family presence and interaction provides comfort and support to the child.	• Agitation or anxiety unresponsive to pharmacologic and non-pharmacologic interventions
4. Monitor for causes of agitation other than anxiety or inadequate sedation.	Physiologic factors and environ-mental stressors may cause the child to be agitated.	• Hypoxia • Inadequate ventilation • Inadequate pain control • Indications of drug withdrawal • Mental status changes

Documentation

- Presedation assessment
- Sedation scale used
- Sedation score obtained
- Interventions resulting from sedation assessment
- Sedation, analgesia, and NMBA administered (drug, dose, time, route, and child's response)
- Child and family education
- Unexpected outcomes and related treatment

References

1. Marx CM, et al: Optimal sedation of mechanically ventilated pediatric critical care patients, *Crit Care Med* 22:163-170, 1994.
2. Carnevale F, Razack S: An item analysis of the COMFORT scale in a pediatric intensive care unit, *Pediatr Crit Care Med* 3(2):177-180, 2002.
3. DeJonghe B, et al: Using and understanding sedation scoring systems: a systematic review, *Intens Care Med* 26:275-285, 2000.
4. Ambuel B, et al: Assessing distress in pediatric intensive care environments: the COMFORT scale, *J Pediatr Psychol* 17(1):95-109, 1992.
5. Brinker D: Sedation and comfort issues in the ventilated infant and child, *Crit Care Nurs Clin North Am* 16(3):365-377, 2004.
6. van Dijk M, et al: The reliability and validity of the COM-FORT scale as a postoperative pain instrument in 0 to 3-year-old infants, *Pain* 84(2-3):367-377, 2000.
7. Crain N, et al:: Assessing sedation in the pediatric intensive care unit by using the BIS and the COMFORT scale, *Pediatr Crit Care Med* 3(1):11-14, 2002.
8. Devlin JW, et al: Motor activity assessment scale: a valid and reliable scale for use with mechanically ventilated patients in an adult surgical intensive care unit, *Crit Care Med* 27(7):1271-1275, 1999.
9. Curley, MAQ, et al: State behavioral scale: A sedation assessment instrument for infants and young children sup-ported on mechanical ventilation. *Pediatr Crit Care Med* 7(2):107-114, 2006.
10. Finley GA, Schechter NL: Sedation. In Schechter NL, Berde CB, Yaster M, editors: *Pain in infants, children, and adoles-cents,* ed 2, Philadelphia, 2003, Lippincott, Williams & Wilkins.
11. Oakes LL: Caring practices: providing comfort. In Curley MAQ, Moloney-Harmon PA, editors: *Critical care nursing of infants and children,* ed 2, Philadelphia, 2001, Saunders.

Additional Readings

Hogg LH, et al: Interrater reliability of 2 sedation scales in a medical intensive care unit: a preliminary report, *Am J Crit Care* 10(2):79-83, 2001.
Wielenga JM, et al: COMFORT scale: a reliable and valid method to measure the amount of stress of ventilated preterm infants, *Neonatal Network* 23(2):39-44, 2004.

AP
Sedation for Procedures

PURPOSE: To provide safe and effective control of pain, anxiety, and motion during a procedure, allowing performance of a necessary procedure while assuring an appropriate degree of memory loss or decreased awareness

Catherine Brailer, Pamela Meadors Fox, and Cynthia Keel

PREREQUISITE KNOWLEDGE

- Individuals who provide moderate or deep sedation or anesthesia must have at a minimum competency-based education, training, and experience in the following[1-3]:
  - Evaluation of children before moderate or deep sedation and anesthesia
  - Performance of moderate or deep sedation and anesthesia, including rescue of children in a deeper-than-desired level of sedation and analgesia
- Competency-based education and training in[1-6]:
  - Advanced airway skills and airway management techniques (e.g., BLS/PALS/ACLS)
  - Pharmacology of drugs used in sedation
  - Appropriate pediatric dosing of analgesic and sedation medications
  - Recognition of dysrhythmias
- Anatomy and physiology of the pediatric airway
- Sedation is a continuum; prediction of how an individual receiving sedation will respond is not always possible.[1-6]
- The four levels of sedation and anesthesia[1,2,4,5]:
  - **Minimal sedation (anxiolysis):** A drug-induced state during which the child responds normally to verbal commands. Although cognitive function and coordi-

nation may be impaired, ventilatory and cardiovascular functions are unaffected.
  - **Moderate sedation/analgesia:** A drug-induced depression of consciousness during which the child responds purposefully to verbal commands, either alone or accompanied by light tactile stimulation. No interventions are necessary to maintain a patent airway, and spontaneous ventilation is adequate. Cardiovascular function is usually maintained.
  - **Deep sedation/analgesia:** A drug-induced depression of consciousness during which the child cannot be easily aroused but responds purposefully after repeated or painful stimulation. The ability to independently maintain ventilatory function may be impaired. The child may need assistance in maintaining a patent airway, and spontaneous ventilation may be inadequate. Cardiovascular function is usually maintained.
  - **Anesthesia:** Consists of general anesthesia and spinal or major regional anesthesia. It does not include local anesthesia. General anesthesia is a drug-induced loss of consciousness during which the child is not arousable, even with painful stimulation. The ability to independently maintain ventilatory function is often impaired. The child often needs assistance in maintaining a patent airway, and positive-pressure ventilation may be necessary because of depressed spontaneous ventilation or drug-induced depression of neuromuscular function. Cardiovascular function may be impaired.

- Ability to continuously monitor oxygenation, ventilation, and circulation during procedures that may affect the child's physiologic status[2-6]
- Ability to identify, recognize, and manage complications and risks associated with sedation including: hypoventilation, apnea, airway obstruction, cardiopulmonary impairment, vomiting, seizures, and anaphylaxis[2,4,5]
- Child development as it relates to clinical assessment and sedation administration
  - ❖ Children less that 6 years of age or children with developmental delay may need a deeper level of sedation to obtain cooperation.[1]
- Sufficient numbers of qualified staff must be available to evaluate the child, perform the procedure, and monitor and recover the child.[2,3,7]
  - ❖ Moderate sedation
    - ○ Individual with advanced life support skills is immediately available (less than 5 minutes away)
    - ○ Individual who monitors the child may assist the practitioner during the procedure and sedation for a task of short duration
  - ❖ Deep sedation
    - ○ Individual with advanced life support skills must be located within the procedure room
    - ○ Individual who monitors the child during the procedure and sedation should have no other responsibilities
- Informed consent is required before the administration of sedation for procedures.[2-5,7]

CHILD AND FAMILY ASSESSMENT

- History of cardiac or respiratory anomalies, medications, allergies, last oral intake and time, procedures or surgeries, and response to anesthesia or medications. Conditions that place the child at particular risk include: any previous problems with anesthesia or sedation medications; stridor, snoring, or sleep apnea; chromosomal abnormality; asthma; and gastroesophageal reflux.[2,3,5-7] ➠*Rationale:* These conditions may complicate the child's response to sedation and increase risk.
- Thorough physical assessment completed before sedation. Examination findings that place the child at additional risk include: obesity, short neck, limited neck extension, neck mass, dysmorphic facial feature, trauma to neck, tracheal deviation, small mouth opening, high arched palate, macroglossia, tonsillar hypertrophy, trismus, micrognathia, retrognathia, and malocclusion.[2,3,5-7] ➠*Rationale:* These conditions may complicate the child's response to sedation and increase risk.
- History of current and recent illnesses (e.g., asthma exacerbation, upper respiratory tract infection, significant nasal congestion, or need for positive pressure ventilation)[2,3,5-7] ➠*Rationale:* These conditions may increase risk of sedation.
- Child's and family's understanding of the reasons for and risks and benefits of sedation ➠*Rationale:* Evaluates child's and family's understanding of the procedure and provides a gauge for ongoing education.

- Child's developmental level and ability to interact ➠*Rationale:* These factors influence preparation and interaction and development of sedation plan.
- Desire of family members to be present during the procedure ➠*Rationale:* Family members may provide comfort and support during the procedure but should have the choice not to remain with the child. In some situations, if family presence is not permitted, identifying the family's wishes facilitates an explanation of reasons family presence is not allowed which may promote family's cooperation.

CHILD AND FAMILY EDUCATION

Individualized, developmentally appropriate education is provided to the family and to the child based on desire for knowledge, readiness to learn, and overall neurologic and psychosocial state.

- Provide information about sedation including the reasons for sedation and an explanation of steps involved in sedation ➠*Rationale:* Providing information decreases anxiety and fear.
- Ensure that risks and benefits of sedation are discussed by the person who administers the sedation[2,3,5,6] ➠*Rationale:* Providing information decreases anxiety and fear and facilitates provision of informed consent by the family.
- If developmentally appropriate, explain how the child can help during the sedation ➠*Rationale:* If the child is cooperative, many procedures can be performed in a primary sedative state, thus decreasing the risk of cardiopulmonary depression.
- Encourage questions and answer questions as they arise ➠*Rationale:* Reinforcement of information is needed during periods of stress.

EQUIPMENT

- Appropriately sized positive pressure oxygen delivery system (bag and mask)
- Oxygen source
- Nonrebreather mask and nasal cannula
- Intravenous catheters
- Airways: Oral and endotracheal, age-appropriate and size-appropriate
- Suction set-up and catheters
- Continuous cardiopulmonary monitoring system
- Pulse oximetry
- $ETCO_2$ monitor is strongly recommended for moderate and deep sedation[1,3]
- Isotonic fluids
- Syringes for medications
- Stethoscope
- Appropriately sized blood pressure cuff
- Resuscitation drugs
- Reversal agents

Procedure for Sedation for Procedures

Steps	Rationale	Considerations
1. Ensure child and family understand procedure and questions are answered.	Evaluates and reinforces understanding of previously taught information.	Developmental level, cognitive ability, and anxiety level determine approach to and effectiveness of teaching.
2. Obtain informed consent. *(Level II[*])*	Child and family must be informed about risks and benefits and consent to the proposed sedation plan.[2,3] Ensures medical-legal compliance as suggested by the Joint Commission on Accreditation of Healthcare Organizations (JCAHO).[7]	In emergency situations, follow institution-specific protocol or procedure for assumption of consent.
3. Collect all necessary equipment and supplies including emergency equipment. *(Level II[*])*	Facilitates completion of procedure in a timely manner.	Blood pressure cuff, airway, and suction equipment are dependent on the child's size.
4. Ensure airway assessment and risk assessment have been completed and risk factors identified.[1-3,5,8] *(Level II[*])*	Preprocedure evaluation decreases likelihood of adverse outcomes.	Most institutions use Mallampati's classification of airway and American Society of Anesthesiologist (ASA) classification for risk assessment; both of these are assigned by physicians or advanced care practitioners.[1-3,5,8]
5. Place child on continuous cardiopulmonary monitors and pulse oximetry; ensure airway equipment, including oxygen, is available and functioning.[1-3,5,8] *(Level VI[*])*	Provides continuous monitoring of the child during the procedure for prompt identification of complications. Critically ill children may decompensate during the procedure.	Consider the child's status in selection of appropriate monitoring.
6. Ensure pre-sedation assessment has been completed, including allergy history.[1-3,5,8] *(Level II[*])*	Appropriate preprocedure evaluation (history, physical examination) increases the likelihood of satisfactory sedation and decreases the likelihood of adverse outcomes for moderate and deep sedation.[2] Clinicians who administer sedation or analgesia should be familiar with sedation-oriented aspects of the child's medical history and how these might alter the child's response to sedation or analgesia.	Review presedation assessment to identify: abnormalities of the major organ systems; previous adverse experience with sedation or analgesia and regional and general anesthesia; drug allergies, current medications, and potential drug interactions; time and nature of last oral intake; and history of tobacco, alcohol, or substance use or abuse.[1-3,5,8]
7. Verify nothing by mouth (NPO) status. *(Level II[*])*	Children who undergo elective sedation or analgesia should be on NPO status for a period of time to allow for gastric emptying before procedure to decrease likelihood of aspiration.[2,3,5,8]	Oral intake allowances before procedure[3]: Clear liquids, 2 hours Breast milk, 4 hours Infant formula, 6 hours Nonhuman milk, 6 hours Light meal, 6 hours

Procedure continues on following page

* Level II: Theory-based; no research data to support recommendations; recommendations from expert consensus group may exist
  Level VI: Clinical studies in a variety of patient populations and situations to support recommendations

Procedure   for Sedation for Procedures—*Continued*

Steps	Rationale	Considerations
8. Identify child with appropriate patient and procedure verification process (e.g., "Time out").	Confirms correct patient, procedure, and site as recommended by JCAHO; prevents unnecessary medical procedures.[7]	Verification process and documentation is institution specific; use active communication techniques.
9. Obtain presedation vital signs, pulse oximetry, weight, and mental status assessment.[1-3] *(Level II[*])*	Provides baseline for comparison during procedure. Calculation of medications and fluid management in children is based on weight.	Monitoring with ET_{CO_2} is strongly recommended, especially during deep sedation.[1,3] Vital signs vary with age. Mental status scoring system used varies by institution.
10. Consider intravenous (IV) catheter placement for minimal sedation or anxiolysis; obtain IV access for moderate or deep sedation.[2,3,5] *(Level II[*])*	Placement of IV line is determined on basis of sedation plan and institution-specific protocol. The IV administration of sedative and analgesic medications increases the likelihood of satisfactory sedation for both moderate and deep sedation. It also decreases the likelihood of adverse outcomes.	If IV line is not placed before sedation, skilled personnel must be readily available to obtain vascular access.

11. Develop sedation plan on basis of[3-5,8]:
    Desired level of immobility for the procedure.
    Anticipated pain associated with procedure.
    Anticipated duration of the procedure.
    Risk factors identified for the individual child.
	Knowledge of these factors allows selection of appropriate drugs, doses, route, and individual to administer sedation.	

12. Administer sedation; refer to institution-specific protocol for verification of drugs, doses before sedation administration. Table 177-1 shows sedative and adjunctive medications commonly used for children.	Necessary to achieve desired level of sedation for procedure.	Sedation is generally administered in incremental doses, titrating total dose on basis of individual child's response; incremental doses may improve comfort and decrease risk.[3] *(Level II[*])* If reversal agents exist for medications administered, they should be available at bedside.
13. Provide supplemental oxygen during procedure.[3,8]	Improves clinical efficacy and reduces adverse outcomes.	Cardiac or respiratory anomalies or illnesses.
14. Monitor and document oxygenation, ventilation, and circulation every 5 minutes during procedure.[1-5,8] *(Level IV[*])*	Critically ill children may decompensate during procedure.	Child's head position should be regularly checked to assess airway patency.[2] Consider child's status in selection of appropriate monitoring.
15. Monitor child's degree of sedation and level of consciousness with scoring system before, during, and after procedure; titrate medications to achieve desired level of sedation.[1-3] *(Level II[*])*	Assures appropriate level of sedation or analgesia.	Sedation and level of consciousness scoring system varies by institution; refer to institution-specific protocol.

* Level II: Theory-based; no research data to support recommendations; recommendations from expert consensus group may exist
  Level IV: Limited clinical studies to support recommendations

Procedure for Sedation for Procedures—*Continued*

Steps	Rationale	Considerations
16. After sedation, monitor heart rate, blood pressure, respiratory rate, and oxygen saturation; document every 15 minutes or more often as necessary until institution-specific protocol.[1-3] *(Level II*)*	Close monitoring reduces adverse outcomes. Decreased procedural stimulation, delayed drug absorption after non-IV administration, and slow drug elimination may contribute to residual sedation and cardiopulmonary depression during the recovery period.	Children should be monitored in an appropriately staffed and equipped area until they are near the baseline level of consciousness. Monitoring should be continued until discharge criteria are met; refer to institution-specific protocol. If reversal agents are given during procedure, monitoring must be extended by 2 hours.
17. Assess child to ensure institution-specific protocol are met.[2-6] *(Level II*)*	Ensures patient safety and return to baseline before discharge.	Refer to institution-specific discharge criteria.
18. If appropriate, review discharge instructions with child and family.[2,3,6,7] *(Level II*)*	Evaluates and reinforces understanding of previously taught information.	Discharge instructions should include but are not limited to: • Information about expected behavior after sedation • Instructions for eating • Warning signs of complications • Special instructions in case of emergency • A telephone number to contact the medical service responsible for the child's care that is available 24 hours per day

* Level II: Theory-based; no research data to support recommendations; recommendations from expert consensus group may exist

TABLE 177-1	Medications Commonly Used for Sedation or Analgesia in the Child

Medication	Dose	Onset of Action	Duration of Action	Common Side Effects
Barbiturates				
Pentobarbitol	IV: 1-2 mg/kg; may repeat up to 6 mg/kg; not to exceed 50 mg/min IM: 2-6 mg/kg (not to exceed 100 mg) PO: 2-3 mg/kg	IV: 1-5 min IM: 5-15 min PO: 15-60 min	IV: 15-60 min IM: 2-4 h PO: 2-4 h	Apnea Hypoventilation Hypotension Hallucinations Ataxia
Thiopental	PR: 25 mg/kg	5-15 min	60-90 min	
Benzodiazepines				
Midazolam	IV: 0.05-0.1 mg/kg; titrate to effect (may repeat up to total dose of 0.4 mg/kg or 10 mg) IM: 0.05-0.15 mg/kg IN: 0.2-0.3 mg/kg PR: 0.5-0.75 mg/kg PO: 0.25-0.75 mg/kg; maximal single dose, 20 mg	IV: 1-2 min IM: 5-15 min PR: 5-10 min PO: 10 min	IV: 30-60 min IM: 30-60 min PR: 30-60 min PO: 1-2 h	Respiratory depression Ataxia Paradoxic excitation Hypotension Myoclonic seizure-like activity in neonates

Continued

TABLE 177-1	Medications Commonly Used for Sedation or Analgesia in the Child—Cont'd			
Medication	**Dose**	**Onset of Action**	**Duration of Action**	**Common Side Effects**
Lorazepam	IM/IV: 0.05-0.1 mg/kg; maximal single dose, 4 mg PO: 0.05-0.1 mg/kg; maximal single dose, 2 mg	IV: 3-5 min IM: 10-20 min PO: 60 min	IV: 2-6 h IM: 2-6 h PO: 2-8 h	Respiratory depression Ataxia Hypotension Paradoxic excitation
Diazepam	IV: 0.1-0.2 mg/kg (maximal single dose, 10 mg) IM: Not recommended PO: 0.1-0.3 mg/kg PR: 0.2-0.3 mg/kg; not recommend because of erratic absorption	IV: 2-3 min PO: 60 min (peak) PR: 5-15 min	IV: 30-90 min PR: 2-4 h	Respiratory depression Ataxia Paradoxic excitation Hypotension
Opioid Analgesics				
Fentanyl	IV: 0.25-3 mcg/kg (slowly titrate) PO: Fentanyl oralet 0.0005-0.0015 mg/kg ≥2y and ≥10 kg	IV: 2-3 min PO: 15-30 min	IV: 20-60 min PO: 2-3 h	Respiratory depression Bradycardia Nausea Pruritus Chest wall and glottic rigidity Hypotension
Morphine	IV: 0.05-0.1 mg/kg	5-10 min	2-4 h	Respiratory depression Bradycardia Nausea Pruritus Hypotension
Other				
Ketamine, dissociative analgesic/anesthetic **May produce state of general anesthesia**	IV: 0.5-2 mg/kg (slowly titrate every 3-5 min) IM: 1-4 mg/kg; consider combining with atropine 0.01-0.02 mg/kg and low dose benzodiazepine	IV: 1-2 min IM: 3-10 min	IV: 15-60 min IM: 3-10 min	Respiratory depression Apnea Laryngospasm/coughing Stimulation of salivary/tracheobronchial secretions Mild-moderate increase in BP Nystagmus Elevated ICP Emergence phenomena
Propofol **May produce state of general anesthesia**	IV: 0.5-1 mg/kg; may repeat in 0.5 mg/kg boluses or titrate as continuous infusion of 25-200 mg/kg/min	1-2 min	3-5 min	Pain with injection Respiratory depression Apnea Hypotension Metabolic acidosis
Etomidate, hypnotic agent; not recommended by US FDA for children <10 y	IV: 0.1-0.2 mg/kg	5-30 sec	5-15 min	Respiratory depression Myoclonus Adrenocortical dysfunction
Chloral hydrate, hypnotic	PO/PR: 25-100 mg/kg; maximal dose, 2 g or 100 mg/kg, whichever is less	15-30 min	2-3 h	Respiratory depression Airway obstruction Agitation Ataxia Vomiting
Reversal Agents				
Flumazenil, reversal for benzodiazepines	IV: 0.01-0.02 mg/kg; repeat every 1-2 min up to maximal dose of 1 mg	1-3 min	60 min	May induce seizures Monitor for recurrence of respiratory depression

TABLE 177-1	Medications Commonly Used for Sedation or Analgesia in the Child—Cont'd			
Medication	**Dose**	**Onset of Action**	**Duration of Action**	**Common Side Effects**
Naloxone, reversal for opioids	IV/IM/ETT: 1-10 mcg/kg for respiratory depression caused by opioids complete reversal 0.1 mg/kg; may repeat every 1-2 min	1-5 minutes	20-60 minutes	Monitor for recurrence of respiratory depression because naloxone has shorter half-life than opioids

FDA, Food and Drug Administration; *IM,* intramuscular; *PO,* orally; *PR,* per rectum; *IN,* intranasal; *BP,* blood pressure; *ICP,* intracranial pressure; *ETT,* endotracheal tube.

Data compiled from Cote C, et al: Adverse sedation events in pediatrics: analysis of medications used for sedation, *Pediatrics* 196(4):633-644, 2000.

Hazinski MF, editor: *Pediatric advanced life support provider manual,* Dallas, 2002, American Heart Association.

Kaplan RF, et al: Pediatric sedation for diagnostic and therapeutic procedures outside the operating room. In Cote CJ, et al, editors: *A practice of anesthesia for infants and children,* Philadelphia, 2001, Saunders.

Krauss B, Green SM: Sedation and analgesia for procedures in children, *N Engl J Med* 343(13):938-944, 2000.

Expected Outcomes

- Appropriate level of sedation or analgesia is achieved and procedure is performed safely

- Return to baseline vital signs and presedation level of consciousness within expected recovery period
- Child is free from side effects of medications administered
- Child is free from complications of sedation

- Child has acceptable level of comfort

Unexpected Outcomes

- Inability to achieve desired level of sedation, which leads to patient distress
- Oversedation that progresses to anesthesia
- Delayed return to baseline vital signs and level of consciousness
- Adverse drug reaction
- Respiratory compromise
- Apnea
- Aspiration
- Arrhythmia
- Hypotension
- Death
- Unmanaged pain
- Unmanaged anxiety

Monitoring and Care of the Child

Activities and Interventions	Rationale	Reportable Conditions
1. Monitor child's tolerance to sedation.	Changes in child's condition may indicate complications from sedation.	• Adverse drug reactions • Change in mental status • Paradoxic reaction to sedation medications
2. Monitor airway and cardiovascular status throughout procedure and recovery period.	Analgesics and sedatives administered together may increase likelihood of hypoxemia or ventilatory depression.[3] *(Level IV*)*	• Change in vital signs or pulse oximetry • Change in child's oxygenation, ventilation, or circulation
3. Monitor child's level of sedation throughout procedure.	Ensures desired level of sedation is achieved and maintained without oversedation or undersedation.	• Inability to achieve desired level of sedation • Level of sedation progresses to anesthesia
4. Assess effectiveness of pain management strategy during and after procedure; during recovery, encourage family to assist with nonpharmacologic means to comfort and support the child.	Many procedures are painful; early identification of pain allows prompt treatment.	• Unresolved pain and discomfort • Pain greater than anticipated from procedure

* Level IV: Limited clinical studies to support recommendations

Documentation

- Education of child and family, including documentation that discharge instructions were received and understood by a responsible person
- Informed consent
- Presedation assessment, including risk factors identified
- Child's fasting status
- Vital signs, sedation and level of consciousness score, and child's response to sedation before, during, and after procedure
- Medications administered: drug, dose, route, site, and time
- Individual who administered sedation
- Achievement of discharge criteria
- Comfort assessment and specific interventions provided
- Unexpected outcomes and related treatment

References

1. American Academy of Pediatrics Committee on Drugs: Guidelines for monitoring and management of pediatric patients during and after sedation for diagnostic and therapeutic procedures: addendum, *Pediatrics* 110(4):836-838, 2002.
2. American Academy of Pediatrics: Guidelines for monitoring and management of pediatric patients during and after sedation for diagnostic and therapeutic procedures, *Pediatrics* 89(6):1110-1115, 1992.
3. American Society of Anesthesiologists: Practice guidelines for sedation and analgesia by non-anesthesiologists, *Anesthesiology* 96(4):1004-1017, 2002.
4. Cote C: Sedation for the pediatric patient, *Pediatr Clin North Am* 41(1):31-58, 1994.
5. Kaplan RF, et al: Pediatric sedation for diagnostic and therapeutic procedures outside the operating room. In Cote CJ, et al, editors: *A practice of anesthesia for infants and children,* Philadelphia, 2001, Saunders.
6. Krauss B, Green SM: Sedation and analgesia for procedures in children, *N Engl J Med* 343(13):938-944, 2000.
7. Joint Commission on Accreditation of Healthcare Organizations: *Hospital accreditation standards,* Chicago, 2004, JCAHO.
8. Hazinski MF, editor: *Pediatric advanced life support provider manual,* Dallas, 2002, American Heart Association.

Additional Readings

Cote C, et al: Adverse sedation events in pediatrics: analysis of medications used for sedation, *Pediatrics* 196(4):633-644, 2000.

Kaplan R, Yang C: Sedation and analgesia in pediatric patients for procedures outside the operating room, *Anesthesiol Clin North Am* 20(1):184-194, 2002.

Polaner D: Sedation-analgesia in the pediatric intensive care unit, *Pediatr Clin North Am* 48(3):695-711, 2001.

Breast Milk: Administration, Collection, and Storage

P U R P O S E : Collection and storage of expressed human milk for administration in the hospital setting

Jamie A. Tumulty

PREREQUISITE KNOWLEDGE

- Breast-feeding is a natural feeding method and is endorsed by the American Academy of Pediatrics (AAP).[1] Breast milk has many benefits to the infant, including improved absorption of nutrients, enhanced gastric emptying, enhanced neurocognitive development, and improved immunity.[1] Mothers who breast-feed also benefit with improved iron status and reduction in risk of both breast and ovarian cancer.[1]

- Although breast-feeding may not be possible for all hospitalized infants, administration of expressed breast milk should be considered.

- A breast pump is used to express or draw out breast milk. Single or double pumps can be used to express breast milk (Figure 178-1).

- Single pumps pump only one breast at a time and are available for manual use and for use with a battery or electricity. Simultaneous double pumps, often referred to as hospital-grade pumps, pump both breasts at the same time, thus reducing pumping time in half over single pumping. In addition, simultaneous double pumping is often preferred because it is thought to increase the hormone responsible for milk production and may help maintain milk supply over a longer period of time.[2]

- Fresh milk may be stored at room temperature for less than or equal to 4 hours, refrigerated at 4°C for less than or equal to 48 hours, or frozen at −20°C for 3 to 12 months. Thawed or fortified milk may be stored at room temperature for less than or equal to 4 hours or refrigerated at 4°C for less than or equal to 24 hours. Thawed milk should not be refrozen.[3-6]

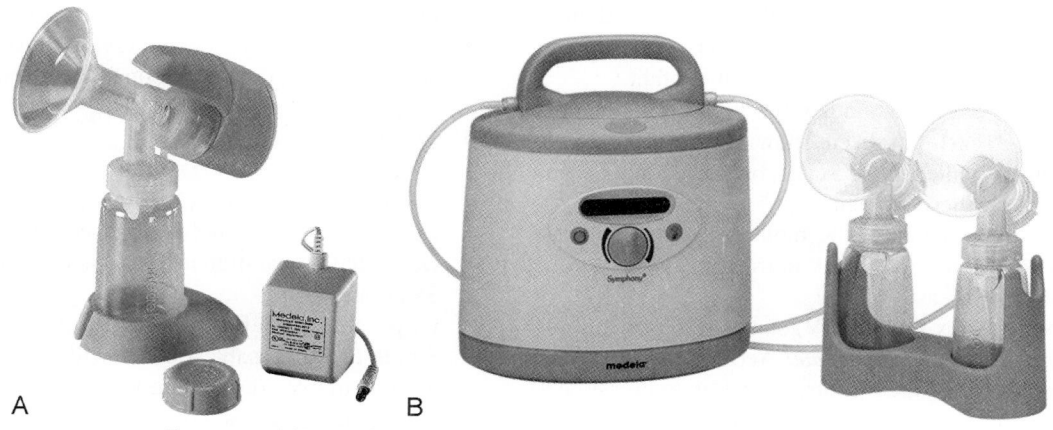

FIGURE 178-1   **A,** Single breast pump. **B,** Double breast pump.

- Do not use a microwave to warm breast milk. This process may inactivate essential nutrients and may result in nonuniform heating with the potential to cause 'hot spots,' which could cause thermal injury to the infant's oral mucosa.[1,3,4,6]
- Many drugs are secreted into breast milk and thus could be transmitted to the recipient infant.[7] Drugs such as sulfonamides, ergotamine, bromocriptine, cabergoline, pseudoephedrine, estrogens, progestins, acebutolol, meperidine, fluxetine, lithium, angiotensin-converting enzyme inhibitors, alcohol, amphetamines, marijuana, cocaine, iodine, caffeine, and anticancer agents are not recommended for breast-feeding mothers.[8]

CHILD AND FAMILY ASSESSMENT

- Family's understanding of the reasons for and benefits of breast-feeding and steps necessary to provide the infant with breast milk ➤➤*Rationale:* Evaluates understanding of procedure and provides a gauge for ongoing education.
- Breast-feeding history ➤➤*Rationale:* Feeding history is important in developing the infant's nutrition plan.
- History of lip or palate deformity, tracheoesophageal fistula, neurologic impairment, trisomy 21, or prematurity ➤➤*Rationale:* These conditions may necessitate special feeding techniques (for example, Habermann's nipple), and benefit may be derived from an oral motor therapy consult.
- History of gastroesophageal reflux disease (GERD) ➤➤*Rationale:* The condition may preclude oral infant feedings if severe or necessitate additional precautions (e.g., infant positioning, thickening agents or motility agents).
- History of galactosemia ➤➤*Rationale:* Galactosemia is a glycogen storage disease that necessitates a galactose-free diet and therefore is a contraindication for breast-feeding.
- Gastrostomy tube ➤➤*Rationale:* Although presence of a gastrostomy tube does not preclude oral infant feeding, assessment of rationale for placement of gastrostomy is necessary to determine appropriate route of feeding.
- Function of gastrointestinal (GI) tract ➤➤*Rationale:* A functional GI tract is necessary to administer enteral feedings.
- Respiratory status of infant ➤➤*Rationale:* Severe respiratory compromise or impending failure may limit the infant's ability to tolerate enteral feeding.
- Medication profile of the mother (or breast milk donor) including over-the-counter drugs, illicit drugs, and alcohol use ➤➤*Rationale:* Some medications are secreted into breast milk and may be transmitted to the infant.[7]
- The HIV status of the mother (or breast milk donor) ➤➤*Rationale:* HIV-1 has been shown to be transmitted in breast milk. In the United States, breast-feeding is contraindicated for these women.[9]
- The tuberculosis status of the mother (or breastfeeding donor) ➤➤*Rationale:* Active or untreated TB is a contraindication of breastfeeding.[1]
- The herpes simplex virus (HSV) status of the mother (or breastfeeding donor) ➤➤*Rationale:* Active herpes simplex lesions on the breast are a contraindication to breastfeeding. If only one breast is affected, the other breast can be used.[9]

CHILD AND FAMILY EDUCATION

Individualized, developmentally appropriate education is provided to the family based on desire for knowledge, readiness to learn, and overall neurologic and psychosocial state.

- Explain the health benefits of breast-feeding for infants and mothers ➤➤*Rationale:* Understanding the benefits of breast milk may encourage mothers for whom exclusive feeding at the breast is not feasible to consider feeding expressed milk.
- Explain importance of good hygiene ➤➤*Rationale:* Good hand-washing and sanitizing the breast pump before use minimizes the risk of contamination.
- Explain that cleaning the breast before pumping is not necessary ➤➤*Rationale:* Unwarranted cleaning may cause skin breakdown, which provides a potential infection site.[4]
- Explain the need for expressing milk or breast-feeding at least six times per day; with an additional three to four times per day for mothers of premature infants ➤➤*Rationale:* Adequate stimulation of the breast is essential to produce an abundant milk supply.[4] Mothers of preterm infants may need to express milk more often because the weak suck of a preterm infant compared with a full-term infant may not be sufficient to empty the breast.
- Explain proper collection technique (use of single-use solid lid containers; no nipples; one expression per container; label with name, medical identification number, date and time expressed, additives, date and time thawed)[4,6] ➤➤*Rationale:* Minimizes the risk of contamination.
- Explain the importance of proper breast milk storage ➤➤*Rationale:* Proper storage preserves the beneficial breast milk constituents and minimizes the risk of contamination.[6]
- Encourage and answer questions as they arise ➤➤*Rationale:* Reinforcement of information is needed during periods of stress.

EQUIPMENT

- Hospital-grade electric breast pump or personal collection kit
- Privacy screen, if dedicated lactation room is not available
- Disposable storage containers with solid lids (glass, polypropylene, or polycarbonate containers are preferred over bags)
- Clean gloves
- Labels
- Dedicated refrigerator (2°C to 4°C; 35°F to 40°F)
- Dedicated non–self-defrosting freezer (–4°C; –20°F)
- Dedicated preparation area with sink and soap
- Sanitizing agent
- Disposable basin for thawing frozen milk
- Single-use disposable bottles with age-appropriate disposable nipples (premature versus full-term)
- Additional feeding supplies as needed (i.e., syringe, feeding bag, feeding tube, syringe pump)

Procedure   for Breast Milk: Administration, Collection, and Storage

Steps	Rationale	Considerations
1. Identify mothers who are interested in providing breast milk for their infants as early as possible.	Adequate stimulation of the breast is essential to produce an abundant milk supply.[4]	
2. Consider contacting a Lactation Consultant, especially for inexperienced mothers. *(Level VI*)*	Lactation services may increase breast-feeding participation.[4]	
3. Locate and gather breast milk collection supplies.	Preparation and presence of all materials facilitate completion of procedure in a timely manner.	
4. Instruct the mother to clean the breast pump before milk expression.[3,4] *(Level III*)*	Sanitizing the breast pump before use minimizes the risk of contamination.	
5. Instruct the mother on the use of the pump. Encourage her to pump each breast for an additional 2 minutes after milk flow has ceased. *(Level VI*)*	Ensures that the breast is fully emptied.[4]	A variety of hospital-grade pumps are available. Refer to appropriate manufacturer instructions for use and care. (Figure 178-2).[4]

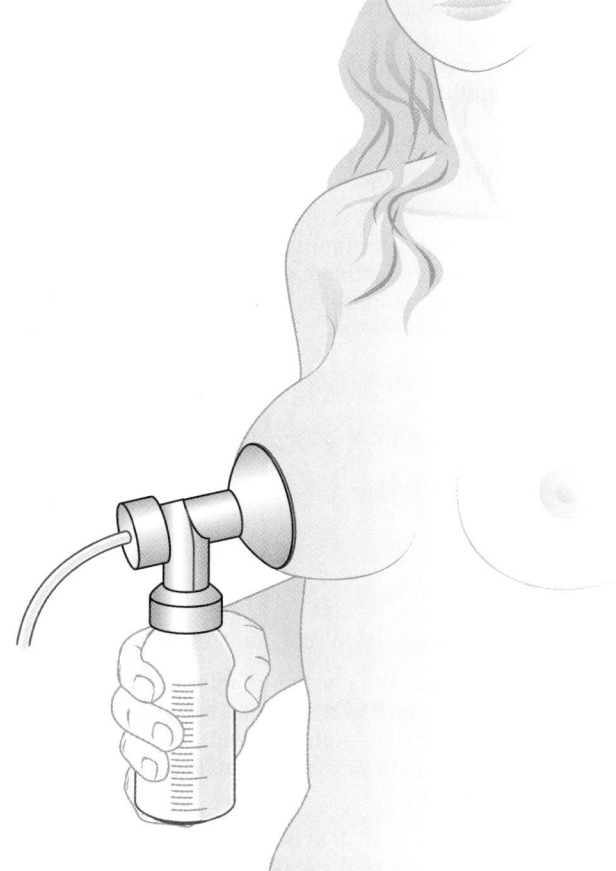

FIGURE 178-2   Use of single breast pump.

Procedure continues on following page

---

* Level III: Laboratory data; no clinical data to support recommendations
Level VI: Clinical studies in a variety of patient populations and situations to support recommendations

Procedure | for Breast Milk: Administration, Collection, and Storage—*Continued*

Steps	Rationale	Considerations
6. Instruct the mother to place expressed milk in storage container with solid lid and label with child's name, identification number, and date and time of collection.[4]	A solid lid (as opposed to a nipple) minimizes the chance of contamination.[3,6]	
7. Use fresh breast milk within 4 hours of expression. Otherwise, refrigerate or freeze breast milk.[4,6]	Bacterial growth is not increased by storing milk at room temperature for 4 hours.[3]	Refrigerated breast milk should be maintained at 4°C and used within 48 hours. If breast milk is not planned to be used within 48 hours, freeze at −20°C for up to 12 months until ready to use.[4] *(Level III*)*
8. When using of frozen breast milk, thaw by: Washing hands. Removing from freezer only the amount of breast milk needed. Labeling the date and time removed from freezer. Placing in refrigerator, in a basin of tepid water, or under tepid running water. *(Level III*)*	Loss of vitamins and cellular components is slowed by cooling breast milk quickly after expression.[6] Washing hands minimizes contamination.[4] Removal of only what is needed minimizes the potential of waste of unused thawed breast milk.[4] Labeling the date and time removed from freezer prevents multiple freeze thaw cycles and serves as the start of the 24 hours that thawed breast milk may be stored in the refrigerator.	Do not immerse lid of container under water because it increases risk of contamination. Do not use hot water (potential to cause thermal injury to infant).
9. Determine the route of breast milk administration and collect appropriate feeding supplies.	Preparation and presence of all materials facilitate completion of procedure in a timely manner.	Oral feedings require a disposable bottle and an age-appropriate nipple (premature infants may need special nipples). Bolus enteral tube feedings require a disposable syringe and feeding tubing or a feeding bag and tubing. Continuous tube feedings require a disposable syringe and tubing or bag and syringe pump.
10. Warm breast milk in basin of warm water (17°C to 22°C). *(Level III*)*		Do not microwave.
11. Wash hands, put on gloves.	Minimizes risk of contamination.	
12. Supplement and fortify breast milk as indicated.	Premature infants and infants with failure to thrive may need supplemental nutrients and additional calories for catch-up growth.[3,10]	Unfortified breast milk does not contain adequate calcium and protein to fulfill growth requirements for premature infants.[3,10]
13. Measure volume of feed to be administered. If the infant is continuously tube fed, do not exceed a volume of more than 4 hours worth of feeding. *(Level III*)*	Bacterial growth is not increased by storing milk at room temperature for 4 hours.[3,6]	

* Level III: Laboratory data; no clinical data to support recommendations

Procedure for Breast Milk: Administration, Collection, and Storage—*Continued*		
Steps	**Rationale**	**Considerations**
14. Return unused portion of breast milk to refrigerator. Discard if not used within 24 hours. *(Level III*)*	Loss of vitamins and cellular components is slowed by cooling breast milk quickly after expression.[3,6]	
15. Remove gloves and wash hands.	Reduces transmission of infection. Protects personnel health.	

* Level III: Laboratory data; no clinical data to support recommendations

Expected Outcomes

- Mother is able to express an adequate supply of milk
- Infant receives adequate nutrition and attains growth targets without complications

Unexpected Outcomes

- Inadequate milk supply
- Growth failure
- Abdominal distention
- Emesis
- Aspiration, cyanosis, or apnea
- Heme-positive diarrhea

Monitoring and Care of the Child

Activities and Interventions	**Rationale**	**Reportable Conditions**
1. Monitor infant for signs and symptoms of distress with feeding.	Feeds should be discontinued if distress is life threatening.	- Gagging, choking, cyanosis, or apnea
2. Monitor infant for feeding tolerance.	Feeding intolerance may indicate undiagnosed GI pathology.	- Abdominal distention, emesis, profuse or bloody diarrhea, or temperature instability
3. Monitor growth parameters with a growth chart.	Growth measures indicate adequacy of feeding.	- Growth velocity less than expected for age

Documentation

- Date, time, volume, and route of feed
- Any fortification of breast milk
- Infant's tolerance of feed
- Additional interventions necessary
- Unexpected outcomes and related treatment
- Daily temperatures of storage refrigerator and freezer
- Family education, specifically education provided to the mother on expressing breast milk

References

1. American Academy of Pediatrics: Breastfeeding and the use of human milk, *Pediatrics* 100(6):1035-1039, 1997.
2. Flora B: Breastpumps 101, retrieved November 11, 2005, from http://www.breastfeed-essentials.com/pumps101.html.
3. Landers S: Maximizing the benefits of human milk feeding for the preterm infant, *Pediatr Ann* 32(5):298-306, 2003.
4. Sapsford A, Lessen R: Expressed human milk. In Robbins S, Beker L, editors: *Infant feedings: guidelines for preparation of formula and breast milk in health care facilities,* 2004, Chicago, American Dietetic Association.
5. Tully M: Cost of establishing and operating a human milk bank, *J Hum Lact* 16(1):57-59, 2000.
6. Tully M: Recommendations for handling of mother's own milk, *J Hum Lact* 16(2):149-151, 2000.
7. Nice F, Snyder J, Kotansky B: Breastfeeding and over-the-counter medications, *J Hum Lact* 16(4):319-330, 2000.
8. Hale T: Medications in breastfeeding mothers of preterm infants, *Pediatr Ann* 32(5):337-47, 2003.
9. American Academy of Pediatrics: Human milk, breast feeding, and transmission of human immunodeficiency Virus Type 1 in the United States, *Pediatrics* 112(5):1196-1205, 2003.
10. Diehl-Jones WL, Fraser Askin D: Nutritional modulation of neonatal outcomes, *AACN Clin Iss* 15(1):83-96, 2004.

Additional Readings

Kleinman R: *Pediatric nutrition handbook,* ed 5, 2004, Chicago, American Academy of Pediatrics.
Morton J, editor: Breastfeeding the premature infant, *Pediatr Ann* 32(5), 2003.

Enteral Nutrition: Administration

P U R P O S E : Administration of enteral nutrition through a feeding tube supplies nutrients to the child who is unable to safely consume adequate oral nutrition

Dyana Burns Conway

PREREQUISITE KNOWLEDGE

- The principles and processes of gastrointestinal (GI) digestion and absorption
- Child development as it relates to clinical assessment and implications for delivery of enteral nutrition
- Selection of the enteral access route depends on the type and anticipated duration of nutrient delivery.
- GI congenital anomalies, severe ischemic injury, necrotizing enterocolitis, hemodynamic instability with high vasopressor support, severe acute pancreatitis, GI obstruction or bleeding, and trauma or surgery to the bowel may lead the practitioner to limit enteral feedings.[1-3] If enteral feeding is initiated, the feeding is started at a low rate to provide trophic feeds and advanced slowly with assessment for feeding intolerance.
- Enteral nutrition can be delivered through orogastric, nasogastric, transpyloric gastrostomy and jejunostomy tubes (see Procedures 182 and 184).
- Transpyloric feeding tubes are recommended for children with aspiration risk, intolerance to gastric feeds, and malabsorption problems.[1,4]
- Choice of appropriate feeding solutions and of method of administration is decided by the multidisciplinary team on the basis of sound pathophysiologic considerations of the GI[1,2] (see Procedure 180).
- Enteral nutrition has trophic effects on the GI mucosa, nourishing the enterocytes and thus maintaining the absorptive and immunologic structures of the bowel.[1]
- Knowledge and understanding of insertion and confirmation of orogastric/nasogastric tube, and transpyloric feeding tube placement (Procedures 182 and 184).

- Medication and enteral formulas may interact, reducing the effectiveness of the medication or causing enteral feeding side effects. For example, the administration of phenytoin necessitates that tube feedings are stopped for 1 hour before and a minimum of 1 hour after dose.[2]

CHILD AND FAMILY ASSESSMENT

- Child's developmental level and ability to interact ➤*Rationale:* Influences preparation and interaction.
- Child's and family's understanding of the reasons for and risks and benefits of enteral nutrition administration via feeding tube ➤*Rationale:* Evaluation of child's and family's understanding of the procedure and provides a gauge for ongoing education.
- History of cardiac, hepatic, renal, or pulmonary disease ➤*Rationale:* Chronic illness may dictate dietary restrictions in type and volume of enteral nutrition administration.
- Current anthropometric measurements including admission weight, length or height, head circumference, body mass index (>2 yrs old), skin folds if available, and plots of these values on appropriate age and gender growth charts ➤*Rationale:* The measurement and evaluation of growth parameters are part of the foundation of the nutritional assessment. Obtaining admission measurements is necessary as a baseline to determine effectiveness of enteral nutrition after initiation and advancement.
- History of conditions that impact GI malabsorption (e.g., cystic fibrosis, pancreatic insufficiency, short gut syndrome, intractable diarrhea, Crohn's disease, celiac

disease, and hepatobiliary disorders), metabolic rate and fluid status (e.g., cardiac, hepatic, renal, or pulmonary disease), food allergy, and enteropathy (e.g., autoimmune or HIV associated)[5] **>>Rationale:** These conditions influence the child's nutrition plan.

- Medications that the child is prescribed **>>Rationale:** Note potential food and drug interactions and collaborate with the prescribing practitioner.
- Gastrointestinal tract function including bowel sounds (present and normoactive), abdominal examination results (soft and nondistended), and function (flatus or stool present) **>>Rationale:** Assessment of GI function indicates the ability of the GI tract to tolerate enteral feeding.
- Fluid balance assessment **>>Rationale:** Fluid balance assessment is a key element in determining enteral nutrition requirements.
- Proper insertion and confirmation of orogastric or nasogastric tube placement or transpyloric feeding tube placement **>>Rationale:** Correct placement of feeding tube provides necessary nutrition and decreases the risk of complications.
- Assessment that the child and family understand the need for enteral nutrition **>>Rationale:** Understanding of previously taught information is assured.

CHILD AND FAMILY EDUCATION

Individualized, developmentally appropriate education is provided to the family and to the child based on desire for knowledge, readiness to learn, and overall neurologic and psychosocial state.

- Explain procedure for enteral nutrition administration to both the child and family. Discuss treatment regimen and possible length of therapy. **>>Rationale:** Providing information decreases anxiety and fear.
- For older children, teach reporting of signs and symptoms of nausea, abdominal fullness, and abdominal cramping **>>Rationale:** Early detection of feeding intolerance decreases the child's discomfort.
- Encourage and answer questions as they arise **>>Rationale:** Reinforcement of information is needed during periods of stress.

EQUIPMENT

- Prescribed enteral formula
- Enteral feeding bag or 60-mL syringe with administration set
- Enteral feeding pump as indicated
- A 20-mL or 30-mL syringe, to check tube placement
- White tape or sticker label

Procedure | for Enteral Nutrition: Administration

Steps	Rationale	Considerations
1. Ensure that child and family understand pre-procedural teaching.	Evaluates and reinforces understanding of previously taught information.	Developmental level, cognitive ability, and anxiety level determine approach to and effectiveness of teaching.
2. Gather all necessary equipment and supplies.	Preparation and presence of all materials facilitates completion of procedure in a timely manner.	
3. Verify prescribing practitioner's order for enteral feedings. *(Level VI*)*	Decreases the risk of error.	Order should include type of formula, volume to be delivered, and rate or length of infusion.
4. Wash hands and put on clean gloves.	Reduces transmission of microorganisms. Protects personnel health.	
5. Check placement of feeding tube. *(Level VI*)*	Prevents delivery of feeding into the esophagus or lungs.[1-3, 6-9]	Obtaining an abnormal x-ray is the recommended method for determination of tube placement.[10] Although not 100% reliable, pH testing appears to be the most accurate nonradiologic alternative for determination of tube location.[3,10,11]

Procedure continues on following page

* Level VI: Clinical studies in a variety of patient populations and situations to support recommendations

Procedure	**for Enteral Nutrition: Administration**—*Continued*	
Steps	**Rationale**	**Considerations**
		If child must be supine, monitor for aspiration closely. Use of a transpyloric feeding tube is highly recommended.
6. For gastric feedings, head of bed is elevated at least 30 to 45 degrees. *(Level V*)*	Decreases the risk of pulmonary aspiration of gastric contents.[2,5,7,8]	Especially important for children with gastroesophageal reflux disease (GERD) and other children at risk for aspiration.
7. Close clamp on the enteral feeding bag and pour up to 4 hours of room-temperature formula (or breast milk) into the bag. *(Level V*)*	Hang no more than 4 hours worth of feeding to prevent bacterial overgrowth in the formula.[1,2,8]	
8. Hang bag on intravenous (IV) pole and prime tubing, purging the system of air. Load administration set into enteral feeding pump. *(Level II*)*	Priming of tubing before administration purges the system of air.	
9. Check for gastric residuals before starting feeding. Attach a syringe to the orogastric or nasogastric feeding tube and aspirate gastric contents if possible. *(Level V*)*	Determines the stomach's readiness for feeding.[2,5,8,9]	An increase in gastric residual volume may occur because of formula intolerance or delayed gastric emptying. Assessment of feeding residuals is difficult with transpyloric or jejunostomy tubes.
10. Perform pH and guaiac test on gastric residual. If guaiac results are negative, return the gastric aspirate to stomach with the same syringe. *(Level V*)*	Gastric aspirate contains enzymes and secretions essential for digestion of nutrients.	
11. Flush feeding tube with water. *(Level V*)*	Prevents clogging of tube.[1,2,8,12]	Exact volume of water depends on the size and volume of feeding tube, the child's age and size, and the child's fluid requirements or restrictions. May flush with a higher volume if child needs additional free water. For children who require fluid restriction, consider reducing water volume to no more than 5 to 10 mL.
12. Connect feeding bag set to distal end of feeding tube. *(Level II*)*	Initiates administration of feeding.	
13. Remove gloves and wash hands.	Reduces transmission of microorganisms. Protects personnel health.	
14. Begin infusion. *Continuous feeding via feeding pump:* Set prescribed infusion flow rate for continuous feeding and start infusion.	Administers feeding.	Give infants a pacifier to satisfy oral needs.

* Level II: Theory-based; no research data to support recommendations; recommendations from expert consensus group may exist
  Level V: Clinical studies in more than one or two patient populations and situations to support recommendations

Procedure for Enteral Nutrition: Administration—*Continued*

Steps	Rationale	Considerations
Bolus feeding via syringe method: Remove the plunger from a 30-mL or 60-mL syringe. Attach syringe to the distal end of the feeding tube. Pour the enteral formula into the syringe and administer slowly by gravity. *(Level V*)*		A feeding bag may also be used for bolus feedings depending on the volume of feeding administered.
15. Label enteral feeding bag and administration set with date, time hung, type of formula, and amount of formula. Change bag and administration set every 24 hours. *(Level VI*)*	Changing bag and administration set every 24 hours prevents bacterial overgrowth in set.[2]	
16. If indicated, administer water boluses as prescribed. *(Level VI*)*	Enteral formulas do not contain sufficient water to meet fluid requirements for older children. High osmolality formulas could lead to dehydration.[2,9]	To provide additional free water, the formula can be diluted with the necessary water and the infusion rate increased depending on the volume tolerated by the child.
17. To administer medications, stop feeding infusion and flush tube with water. Administer the medication, then flush with water and resume feeding. *(Level V*)*	Prevents clogging of tube.[2,12] Reduces mixing of drug and nutrient.	Determine drug-nutrient incompatibilities before administration of the medication. The flush volume depends on the size and volume of the tubing, the fluid requirements or restrictions of the child, and the age and size of the child.
18. Declogging the tube: Attach a 20-mL or 30-mL syringe to the end of the tube and attempt to aspirate fluid. Fill the syringe with 5 mL of warm water or carbonated beverage (ginger ale or cola) and attempt to instill with manual pressure and a back-and-forth motion with the plunger. Clamp the tube for 5 to 10 minutes. Aspirate or flush the tube. *(Level V*)*	Flushing frequently with water maintains a patent feeding tube.[12]	If declogging method fails, notify the prescribing practitioner and replace the tube.

* Level V: Clinical studies in more than one or two patient populations and situations to support recommendations
Level VI: Clinical studies in a variety of patient populations and situations to support recommendations

Expected Outcomes	Unexpected Outcomes
• Maintain growth velocity for age and gender • Provide nutrients safely and without complications • Maintain fluid balance	• Failure to attain growth targets • Infection • Pulmonary aspiration • Hyperglycemia/hypoglycemia • Drug and nutrient interactions • Dehydration • Vomiting • Diarrhea

Monitoring and Care of the Child

Activities and Interventions	Rationale	Reportable Conditions
1. Weigh and measure child routinely; compare with baseline measurements. Document measurements on appropriate growth chart.	Evaluates response to enteral feeding. Growth measures reflect nutrition adequacy.	• Significant changes in growth velocity • Growth measures plotted at less than 5th percentile or more than 95th percentile
2. Monitor fluid intake and output, including urine output, emesis, and stools.	Evaluates for dehydration or fluid overload. Diarrhea can occur as a response to intolerance to enteral formula, lactose intolerance, prolonged use of antibiotics, or bacterial contamination of formulas.	• Dry mucous membranes • Poor skin turgor • Fluid imbalance • Vomiting • Oliguria • Diarrhea
3. Monitor laboratory values (electrolytes, liver function tests, serum proteins, hemoglobin, hematocrit), including daily monitoring of serum glucose levels as indicated.	Metabolic complications, such as electrolyte imbalances, dehydration, overhydration, hypoglycemia, or anemia, can occur with artificial modes of providing nutrition.[6,13,14] Infants are especially vulnerable to hypoglycemic or hyperglycemic conditions.	• Electrolyte imbalance • Elevated liver function test (LFT) results • Decreased total protein, albumin, and prealbumin levels • Increased transferrin level • Decreased hemoglobin and hematocrit levels • Glucose level of more than 120 mg/L or less than 60 mg/L (or as indicated)[15]
4. Monitor for proper tube placement with radiographic confirmation before usage.	Prevents delivery of feeding into the esophagus or lungs.	• Improper tube placement
5. Auscultate bowel sounds every 4 hours.	Evaluation of GI motility and function helps predict the ability for the child to absorb and tolerate enteral feedings.	• Decreased or absent bowel sounds
6. Aspirate gastric residuals before every feeding or at least every 4 hours	Large residuals indicate decreased gastric motility or emptying. Continuation of feeds with large residuals increases the risk of vomiting and pulmonary aspiration.[16]	• Notify practitioner if residual is greater than the amount delivered in previous 2 hours for continuous feed or greater than one half the volume delivered for intermittent or bolus feed[16]
7. Measure abdominal girth at baseline as indicated.	Increasing abdominal girth may indicate intolerance to enteral feeding and decreased GI function.	• Abdominal girth increased more than 10% from baseline
8. Monitor indices of oxygenation and ventilation.	Aspiration is a risk whenever artificial enteral feedings are administered.	• Changes in work of breathing • Alterations in arterial blood gases, oxygenation saturation, or end tidal carbon dioxide ($ETCO_2$)
9. Assess patency of feeding tube every feeding or at least every 8 hours.	Clogged feeding tubes prevent the administration of enteral feeding.	• Inability to aspirate or flush feeding tube
10. Perform mouth care every 2 hours and as needed.	Decreases bacterial flora in the oral cavity and prevents drying and cracking of oral mucosa.	• Mouth lesions or breakdown

Documentation

- Fluid balance (weight, intake and output, emesis, stools)
- Growth measures
- If continuous feeding, rate of infusion
- If bolus feeding, total volume delivered and time delivered
- Indications of feeding intolerance (abdominal girth, residual volumes)
- Size and type of tube used for feeding
- Confirmation of tube placement, method used, and date and time of initiation
- Type and strength of enteral nutrition
- Mouth care completed and oral cavity condition
- Comfort assessment and any specific interventions provided
- Additional interventions necessary
- Child and family education
- Unexpected outcomes and related treatment

References

1. Grant MC, Martin S: Delivery of enteral nutrition, *AACN Clin Iss* 11(4):507-516, 2000.
2. Lynn-McHale DJ, Carlson KK: *AACN procedure manual for critical care,* ed 4, Philadelphia, 2001, Saunders.
3. Metheny, NA, Stewart BJ: Testing feeding tube placement during continuous tube feedings, *Appl Nurs Res* 15(4):254-258, 2002.
4. Bowers S: All about tubes: your guide to enteral feeding devices, *Nursing* 30(12):41-48, 2000.
5. Davies AR, et al: Randomized comparison of nasojejunal and nasogastric feeding in critically ill patients, *Crit Care Med* 30(3):586-590, 2002.
6. Colagiovanni L: Nutrition: taking the tube...nasogastric tube-feeding...methods to test tube position, *Nurs Times* 95(21):63-64,67,71, 1999.
7. Ellett MLC, Beckstrand J: Examination of gavage tube placement in children, *J Soc Pediatr Nurs* 4(2):51-60, 1999.
8. Fellows LS, et al: Evidence-based practice for enteral feedings: aspiration prevention strategies, bedside detection, and practice change, *Med Surg Nurs* 9(1):27-31, 2000.
9. Irving SY, et al: Nutrition for the critically ill child: enteral and parenteral support, *AACN Clin Iss* 11(4):541-558, 2000.
10. AACN: Practice alert: verification of feeding tube placement, *AACN News* 22(5).
11. Metheny N, Meert K: Monitoring feeding tube placement, *Nutr Clin Pract* 19(5):487-495, 2004.
12. Lord LM: Restoring and maintaining patency of enteral feeding tubes, *Nutr Clin Pract* 18(5):422-426, 2003.
13. Bettler J, Roberts KE: Nutrition assessment of the critically ill child, *AACN Clin Iss* 11(4):498-506, 2000.
14. Nevin-Folino NL: *Pediatric manual of clinical dietetics,* ed 2, 2003, Pediatric Nutrition Practice Group, Chicago, American Dietetic Association.
15. Syrinivasan V, et al: Association of timing, duration, and intensity of hyperglycemia with intensive care unit mortality in critically ill children, *Pediatr Crit Care Med* 5:329-336, 2004.
16. McClave SA, Snider HL: Clinical use of gastric residual volumes as a monitor for patients on enteral tube feeding, *JPEN* 26(6 Suppl):S43-50, 2002.

Additional Readings

Burd RS, Lentz CW: The limitations of using gastric residual volumes to monitor enteral feedings: a mathematical model, *Nutr Clin Pract* 16(6):349-354, 2001.

Hildebrandt LA, et al: Comparison of post-pyloric vs. gastric enteral formula administration, *Topics Clin Nutr* 17(3):44-51, 2002.

Neumann DA, DeLegge MH: Gastric versus small-bowel tube feeding in the intensive care unit: a prospective comparison of efficacy, *Crit Care Med* 30(7):1436-1438, 2002.

Enteral Nutrition: Selection of Formulas and Fortification

P U R P O S E : To describe the selection of commercially available formulas and formula fortification on the basis of the nutritional needs of the infant and child

Jamie A. Tumulty

PREREQUISITE KNOWLEDGE

- The principles and processes of gastrointestinal (GI) digestion and absorption
- For infants, breast milk is preferred when available. The benefits of breast milk include improved absorption of nutrients, enhanced gastric emptying, enhanced neurocognitive development, and improved immunity.[1,2] A lower incidence rate of food allergy is also seen with breast milk-fed infants.[3] Benefits for the mother include improved iron status and reduction in risk of both breast and ovarian cancer.[1,2] Breastmilk feeding is endorsed by the American Academy of Pediatrics (AAP).[1,3]
- Age-appropriate and size-appropriate maintenance fluid calculation (Table 180-1)
- General nutritional requirements for infants and children based on age, size, and condition (Figure 180-1)
- Gastrointestinal congenital anomalies, severe ischemic injury, necrotizing enterocolitis, hemodynamic instability with high vasopressor support, severe acute pancreatitis, GI obstruction or bleeding, and surgery or trauma to the bowel may lead the practitioner to limit enteral feedings.[4-6] If enteral feeding is initiated, the feeding is started at a low rate to provide trophic feeds and advanced slowly with assessment for feeding intolerance.
- Formulas are configured to support various health conditions, including prematurity, renal disease, and malabsorption (Tables 180-2 and 180-3).
- Premature infants have special dietary considerations because of the immature GI tract. Medium chain triglycerides (MCTs) are necessary because of decreased fat absorption.[7] Infants who are premature and small for gestational age (SGA) also have reduced iron stores.[2,7] Premature infants also benefit from formulas with lower renal solute load (reduced osmolality), increased protein, and increased calcium and phosphorous. In addition, premature infants who weigh less than 1800 g should not be fed soy-based formulas because of concerns regarding weight gain, bone mineralization, and aluminum toxicity (Table 180-4).[7]
- Infants and children with congestive heart failure or renal failure may benefit from fluid restriction. A more calorically dense formula may be desired (i.e., 24 to 30 kcal/oz). Close monitoring of these children is necessary because this formula causes an increase in renal solute load (increased osmolality) and a potential for dehydration.
- A special low-sodium and phosphorous formula may be helpful for infants and children with renal disease. Soy formulas should be avoided in this population. Peptide-based formulas are favored over amino acid formulas because they have lower osmolality.[7]

TABLE 180-1	Daily Fluid Requirement for Children
Weight (kg)	**Fluid**
1-10 kg	100 mL/kg
11-20 kg	1000 mL + 50 mL/kg for each kg over 10 kg
>20 kg	1500 mL + 20 mL/kg for each kg over 20 kg

Example: A 15-kg child needs 1250 mL/d or 52 mL/h of continuous infusion.

Age (years)	RDA (kcal / kg /day)	REE (kcal / kg /day)	PRO* (gm / kg / day)
.5 - 1.0	90 - 108	55	2 - 2.5
1 - 3	85 - 102	50	1.2 - 3.0
4 - 6	70 - 90	45	1.1 - 3.0
7 - 10	60 - 70	40	1.0 - 3.0
11 - 13	45 - 55	30	1.0 - 2.5
15 - 18	36 - 45	27	0.8 - 1.2

Several methods can be used to estimate energy needs. Caloric requirements are commonly estimated by:

1. RDA (Recommended Dietary Allowance). **The upper end of caloric range** assumes age-appropriate activity. Many acutely or chronically ill children require fewer calories because of their relatively low activity levels. **The lower end of the caloric range** is the REE plus stress/activity adjustments for acutely ill children. Children with very low activity levels or with very high levels of stress may have calorie needs outside of these ranges.

2. **REE** (Resting Energy Expenditure) plus the addition of a stress factor to adjust for critical illness. REE is typically multiplied by a factor of 1.5 to 1.6 for the moderately stressed critically ill child.

Stress Factors in Critically Ill Children	
Condition	**Stress Factor**
Sepsis, trauma	1.5
Ventilated, sedated patient	1.2 or 1.3
Burns	2.0

Reference: Verger J, Schears G. Nutrition Support. In Curley MAQ, Moloney-Harmon PA. *Critical Care Nursing of Infants and Children*, ed 2, Philadelphia: Saunders, 2001.

3. **TEE** (Total Energy Expenditure) is REE plus the addition of factors to adjust for acute and critical illness, activity, and growth. TEE (kcal/kg/day) = REE (kcal/kg/day) + REE (kcal/kg/day) x [Factors i.e., Maintenance + Injury + Activity]

Factors:
Maintenance	= 0.2
Activity	= 0.1 - 0.25
Fever	= 0.13 per degree Celsius > 38
Multiple injuries	= 0.4
Burns	= 0.5-1
Growth	= 0.5

TEE Calculation Example for a 3-Year-Old Child
REE + REE x (factors i.e., Maintenance + Activity + Growth)
= 50 kcal/kg/day + 50 kcal/kg/day x (0.2 + 0.1 + 0.5)
= 50 kcal/kg/day + 50 kcal/kg/day x (0.8)
= 50 kcal/kg/day + 40 kcal/kg/day
= 90 kcal/kg/day

*Stress and injury can increase energy (calories and protein) needs by 30 – 50% depending on the intensity of the insult or injury.

(Reference: Gunn VL, Nechyba C. *The Harriet Lane Handbook*, ed 6, Philadelphia: Mosby, 2002.)

FIGURE 180-1 Daily Energy Requirements for Children. *From Verger J, Schears G: Nutrition support. In Curley MAQ, Moloney-Harmon PA, editors:* Critical care nursing of infants and children, *ed 2, Philadelphia, 2001, Saunders. Gunn VL, Nechyba C:* The Harriet Lane handbook, *ed 6, Philadelphia, 2002, Mosby.*

TABLE 180-2	Formula Characteristics and Related Conditions			
Lactose-Free	Soy-Based	Peptide-Based	Amino Acid–Based	Isotonic
Premature infants **Bowel resection** **Inflammation** Lactase is diminished with these conditions; therefore, lactose-containing formulas should be avoided.	**Milk allergy:** Soy-based formulas do not contain milk protein. **Galactosemia:** An enzyme deficiency that prevents metabolism of galactose, which may result in mental retardation, hepatic disease, renal Fanconi's syndrome, and cataracts. Galactose-containing foods including milk-based formulas are be avoided.[8] **Strict vegetarian diet:** Soy-based formulas are derived from plants. *Avoid* in infants less than 1800 g: Because these products can cause aluminum toxicity, delayed weight gain, and bone mineralization.	**Renal disease:** Metabolized whole protein increases BUN. Peptide-based formulas contain short chain peptides which are more easily absorbed. Children with renal disease need careful attention to electrolytes and may need low potassium and calcium supplements. **Short bowel syndrome:** Peptides are better tolerated than intact proteins. Peptide-based formulas have lower osmolality than amino acid-based.	**Food allergy:** Peptides are smaller molecules and less allergenic than whole protein. Free amino acids are nonimmunogenic. **Enteropathy** (i.e., autoimmune or HIV associated) **Malabsorption problems** (i.e., cystic fibrosis, pancreatic insufficiency, short gut syndrome, intractable diarrhea, Crohn's disease, and hepatobiliary disorders)	**Delayed gastric emptying:** High-osmolar formula inhibits gastric emptying. **Dumping syndrome:** Caused by rapid gastric emptying of carbohydrates, which results in hyperglycemia and diarrhea. Decreased incidence rate with isotonic feedings. **Osmotic diarrhea:** Hyperosmolar formulas contribute to loose stools in some infants and children.

BUN, Blood urea nitrogen; *CF,* cystic fibrosis.
From Chang T, Kleinman R: Standard and specialized formulas. In Walker WA, Watkin JB, Dugga C, editors: *Nutrition in pediatrics,* ed 3, London, 2003, BC Decker.
Irving S, Derengowski S, Hicks F, et al: Nutrition for the critically ill child: enteral and parenteral support, *AACN Clin Iss* 11(4):541-58, 2000.
Kleinman R: *Pediatric nutrition handbook,* ed 5, 2005, Chicago, American Academy of Pediatrics.

TABLE 180-3	Indication for Selected Adult Formulas
Condition	Formulas
Caloric density, high nitrogen	Nutrient 1.5, Nutrient 2.0, Boost High Protein, Boost Plus, Ensure High Protein, Ensure Plus, Ensure Plus HN, Impact 1.5, Isosource 1.5, Isosource HN, Levity Plus, Nova Source 2.0, Rebalance HN, Resource Plus, Resource 2.0, Subdue Plus Ultra cal HN Plus
Chronic liver disease	HepaticAid
Crohn's disease	Modulen IBD
Fat malabsorption	Portagen, Lipisorb
Hyperglycemia	Glytrol, Resource Diabetic, Glucerna
Hemodialysis/renal disease	Magnacal, Nepro, NutriRenal, NovaSource Renal, RenalCal
Immune support	Advera, Immun-Aid
Pulmonary disease	NovaSource Pulmonary, NutriVent, PulmoCare, Respalor, Oxcepa
Wound healing	Crucial, Replete, Traumacal

Kleinman, R.: *Pediatric nutrition handbook,* ed 5, 2004, Chicago, American Academy of Pediatrics.

- Children with chylothorax may benefit from low-fat or fat-free formula. Long chain fatty acids from digestion are absorbed through the lymph system, whereas medium and short chain fatty acids are absorbed directly into the bloodstream.[8,9]
- Children with hemodynamic instability may not be candidates for total enteral nutrition but rather may benefit from trophic feeds supplemented with parenteral nutrition.
- Conditions that increase metabolic needs (such as burns and fever) impact nutritional needs and often necessitate an increase in caloric intake to meet the child's energy needs. Formulas with a higher caloric density can help to meet these needs.
- Children need close monitoring of growth parameters (weight, length/height, and head circumference), and the use of appropriate growth charts is recommended.
- Normal values for serum electrolytes (sodium, potassium, calcium, phosphate, magnesium, blood urea nitrogen, creatinine, and glucose); liver function tests (transaminases, alkaline phosphate, and bilirubin); serum proteins (total protein, albumin, prealbumin, and transferrin); and hemoglobin and hematocrit

CHILD AND FAMILY ASSESSMENT

- Child's developmental level and ability to interact **➻Rationale:** Influences preparation and interaction.
- Child's and family's understanding of the reasons for formula selection **➻Rationale:** Evaluates family's understanding of formula selection and provides a gauge for ongoing education.
- Historic growth data; birth weight, length, and head circumference are especially important for infants **➻Rationale:** Comparing growth parameters with normal values guides nutritional requirements (such as additional calories for catch-up growth, limiting of calories for obesity).
- Function of GI tract **➻Rationale:** A functional GI tract is necessary for enteral feeding.
- Feeding and formula history **➻Rationale:** Important considerations in determination of route and type of feeding.
- History of conditions that lead to GI malabsorption (i.e., cystic fibrosis, pancreatic insufficiency, short gut syndrome, intractable diarrhea, Crohn's disease, celiac disease, and hepatobiliary disorders), food allergy, or enteropathy (autoimmune or HIV associated)[7] **➻Rationale:** These conditions often necessitate a special formula choice, including peptide-based or amino acid–based formulas (see Tables 180-2 and 180-3).
- History of galactosemia **➻Rationale:** Galactosemia is an inborn error of metabolism in which defective enzyme activity prevents normal carbohydrate metabolism. Cow's milk formula is contraindicated in infants and children with this condition.[7]
- Family atopic history **➻Rationale:** This history may be used to identify children at risk of development of food allergy.[3]
- History of angioedema, urticaria, wheezing, rhinitis, vomiting, eczema, pulmonary hemosiderosis, malabsorption with vilous atrophy, enterocolitis, esophagitis, or colic[3] **➻Rationale:** These conditions may indicate undiagnosed food allergy and necessitate further investigation before formula selection.
- History of vomiting, wheezing, esophagitis, or failure to thrive **➻Rationale:** These conditions may indicate gastroesophageal reflux disease (GERD), which may necessitate specialized formula with added rice (AR) starch.[7]
- History of renal disease **➻Rationale:** Renal disease may necessitate an alternative formula choice low in sodium and phosphorous.
- Cultural or religious dietary restrictions **➻Rationale:** Individualized nutritional plans consider the child's cultural and religious preferences. Strict vegetarians may need soy-based formula.[7]
- History of developmental delay or mental retardation **➻Rationale:** These children are at risk of developing obesity and osteopenia related to low resting energy expenditure and may need decreased caloric intake.
- Conditions that necessitate fluid restriction, such as renal failure and congestive heart failure **➻Rationale:** A calorically dense formula (24 to 30 kcal/oz) may be desired for these children.
- Presence of chylothorax **➻Rationale:** Children with chylothorax need low-fat or fat-free formula until its resolution.[8,9]
- Hypermetabolic state (fever or burns) **➻Rationale:** Infants and children in a hypermetabolic state need increased calories/protein for healing.[8]

CHILD AND FAMILY EDUCATION

Individualized, developmentally appropriate education is provided to the family based on desire for knowledge, readiness to learn, and overall neurologic and psychosocial state.

- If applicable, explain the health benefits of breast milk and breast-feeding for infants and mothers **➻Rationale:** Understanding the benefits of breast-feeding may encourage mothers to consider initiating and continuing with breast-feeding.
- Explain any special dietary needs of the child (based on assessment), the importance of any fortifiers added to breast milk or formula, and instructions on preparing feeding **➻Rationale:** Knowledge decreases fear and anxiety and may increase compliance of prescribed feeding regimen.
- Explain feeding route and schedule **➻Rationale:** May increase compliance of prescribed feeding regimen.
- Encourage questions and answer questions as they arise **➻Rationale:** Reinforcement of information is needed during periods of stress.

EQUIPMENT

- Sanitizing agent
- Clean gloves
- Selected formula
- Selected fortifiers
- Volume measuring device
- Powder measuring device (scale preferred over "scoop" method)
- Disposable storage containers with solid lids (glass, polypropylene, or polycarbonate containers are preferred)
- Labels
- Single-use disposable bottles with age-appropriate disposable nipples (premature versus full-term)
- Disposable syringe and feeding tubing or feeding bag (for children who are tube fed)
- Dedicated refrigerator (2°C to 4°C; 35 °F to 40°F)

Procedure   Enteral Nutrition: Selection of Formulas and Fortification

Steps	Rationale	Considerations
1. Assess nutritional needs including nutrition status and anthropometric measurements, clinical and fluid status, medical history, metabolic laboratory values, and allergies.[4] *(Level VI*)*	Formula selection, fortification, and initiation and advancement of enteral feeds is based on needs of infant or child.	
2. Estimate fluid, caloric and protein requirements based on weight and age of the child (see Figure 180-1). • Estimate resting energy (caloric) needs. • Increase resting energy requirements depending on stress level of the child.	Determination of the child's fluid, caloric and protein needs help to develop an individualized plan of care. Resting energy requirements vary by age and condition. After establishing the child's baseline requirements, addition or subtraction of calories is necessary based on the child's condition.	Although standard recommendations are available for healthy children (e.g., World Health Organization, Schofield's equation, Centers for Disease Control recommendations), indirect calorimetry is a more precise alternative for prediction of a sick child's energy requirements.[4,8] Stress and injury may increase energy requirements, necessitating a 30% increase for mild to moderate stress, a 50% increase for severe stress, and an increase of 100% for burns.[4] *(Level VI*)* A decrease in requirements by up to 30% is considered if the child is pharmacologically sedated and receiving muscle relaxants.[4] *(Level V*)*
3. For the infant, determine whether breast milk is to be used. Infants who exclusively receive breast milk need a multivitamin supplement (e.g., Poly-vi-sol (Bristol-Myers/Squib) which contains vitamin D, calcium, iron, fluoride, and other vitamins). *(Level IV*)*	Breast milk as a nutritive choice is endorsed by AAP.[1,3,8] Vitamin D is needed to prevent rickets; human milk does not contain the amount in fortified commercial formula.[2]	
4. Choose age-specific enteral formula based on clinical assessment of needs (Tables 180-4 to 180-8).	Commercially available formulas are designed to meet caloric, osmolar, and nutrient needs of children according to age.	In the hospital setting, ready-to-feed formula is preferred, followed by concentrate.[10] Premature infants may need additional supplements and increased calories for catch-up growth. Many premature infant formulas or Lipil formulas contain a blend of docosahexanoic (DHA) and arachidonic (ARA) fatty acids, which are long chain polyunsaturated fatty acids important in brain and retinal development.[2,7] *(Level IV*)*

* Level IV: Limited clinical studies to support recommendations
  Level V: Clinical studies in more than one or two patient populations and situations to support recommendations
  Level VI: Clinical studies in a variety of patient populations and situations to support recommendations

Procedure	**Enteral Nutrition: Selection of Formulas and Fortification**—*Continued*	
Steps	**Rationale**	**Considerations**
5. Determine whether nutrient supplements are needed to meet nutritional goals.	Caloric modifiers are available to increase protein, carbohydrates, and fat calories (Table 180-9). *(Level V*)*	
6. Gather necessary equipment and supplies in designated formula preparation area.		
7. Sanitize work surface, wash hands, and put on gloves.	Minimizes contamination and eliminates the need for terminal sterilization, which may inactivate nutrients.[10]	
8. If supplements are added, determine amount of supplement to be added per unit volume of formula by weighing powder.	Weight is a more accurate measure of powder than volume.	Stock amounts (greater than the requirement of one feed) may be prepared and stored at 4°C for up to 24 hours.[10]
9. Label prepared formula with child's name, identification number, location, base formula plus additives, caloric density per volume, volume prepared, expiration date and time, route of administration with frequency or rate, "for enteral use only," "refrigerate until used," and "shake well."[10]		

* Level V: Clinical studies in more than one or two patient populations and situations to support recommendations

TABLE 180-4	**Selected Preterm Infant Formulas (Milk-Based)**

		Composition			
Formula	**Ingredients**	**Protein (g/100 kcal)**	**Carbohydrate (g/100 kcal)**	**Fat (g/100 kcal)**	**Calories (kcal/oz)**
Enfamil Premature Lipil*	DHA, ARA, iron	3	11	5.1	20
(20 and 24 cals/oz)		3	11	5.1	24
EnfaCare Lipil*	DHA, ARA, iron	2.8	10.4	5.3	22
Neosure Advance†	DHA, ARA, iron	2.6	10.3	5.5	22
Similac Special Care Advance†	DHA, ARA, available with and	2.71	10.6	5.43	20
(20 and 24 cals/oz)	without iron	2.71	10.6	5.43	24
Similac Natural Care Advance†	DHA, ARA, low iron, HMF	2.71	10.6	5.43	24
Similac 60:40†	No DHA, ARA, low iron, low phosphorus	2.22	10.2	5.59	20

DHA, Docosahexanoic fatty acids; *ARA,* arachidonic fatty acids; *HMF,* human milk fortifier.
Data from Kleinman, R: *Pediatric nutrition handbook,* ed 5, 2004, Chicago, American Academy of Pediatrics.
*Mead Johnson Nutritionals, Evansville, IN.
†Ross Products Division, Abbott Laboratories, Columbus, OH.

TABLE 180-5	Selected Full-Term Infant Formulas				
		Composition			
Formula	Ingredients	Protein (g/100 kcal)	Carbohydrate (g/100 kcal)	Fat (g/100 kcal)	Calories (kcal/oz)
Milk-Based					
Carnation Good Start	Available with and without iron				
Enfamil*	Available with and without iron	2.1	10.9	5.3	20
Enfamil AR Lipil*	Iron, DHA, ARA	2.5	11	5.1	20
Enfamil Lipil*	Available with and without iron, DHA, ARA	2.1	10.9	5.3	20
Similac† (20 and 24 cals/oz)	Available with and without iron	2.07	10.8	5.40	20
		2.73	10.5	5.3	24
Similac Advance†	Available with and without iron, DHA, ARA	2.07	10.8	5.40	20
Lactose-Free					
Enfamil Lactofree Lipil*	Iron, DHA, ARA	2.1	10.9	5.3	20
Similac Lactose Free†	Iron, DHA, ARA	2.14	10.7	5.40	20
Soy-Based					
Enfamil Prosobee*	Iron	2.5	10.6	5.3	20
Enfamil Prosobee Lipil*	Iron, DHA, ARA	2.5	10.6	5.3	20
Similac Isomil†	Iron	2.45	10.3	5.46	20
Similac Isomil Advance†	Iron, DHA, ARA	2.45	10.3	5.46	20
Similac Isomil DF†	Iron, fiber	2.66	10.1	5.46	20
Peptide-Based					
Enfamil Nutramigen Lipil*	Iron	2.8	10.3	5.3	20
Enfamil Pregestimil* (20 and 24 cals/oz)	Iron, MCT	2.8	10.2	5.6	20
		2.8	10.2	5.6	24
Similac Alimentum†	Iron	2.75	10.2	5.54	20
Similac Alimentum Advance†	Iron, MCT, DHA, ARA	2.75	10.2	5.54	20
Amino Acid–Based					
EleCare†	Iron	3.01§	10.7	4.76	20
Neocate‡	Iron	3.1§	11.7	4.5	20

DHA, Docosahexanoic fatty acids; *ARA,* arachidonic fatty acids; *MCT,* medium chain triglycerides: *AR,* added rice; *DF,* diarrhea formula.

Data from Kleinman R: *Pediatric nutrition handbook,* ed 5, 2004, Chicago, American Academy of Pediatrics.

*Mead Johnson Nutritionals, Evansville, IN.

†Ross Products Division, Abbott Laboratories, Columbus, OH.

‡Scientific Hospital Supplies North America, Gaithersburg, MD.

§Peptide and amino acid formulas do not contain whole protein. Values given represent protein equivalents.

TABLE 180-6	Selected Infant/Toddler Formulas (9 to 24 Months)				
		Composition			
Formula	Ingredients	Protein (g/100 kcal)	Carbohydrate (g/100 kcal)	Fat (g/100 kcal)	Calories (kcal/oz)
Milk-Based					
Enfamil Next Step Lipil*	Iron, DHA, ARA	2.6	10.5	5.3	20
Soy-Based					
Enfamil Next Step Prosobee Lipil*	Iron, DHA, ARA	3.3	11.8	4.4	20
Similac Isomil 2+†	Iron, low osmolality	2.45	10.3	5.46	20

DHA, Docosahexanoic fatty acids; *ARA,* arachidonic fatty acids.

Data from Kleinman R: *Pediatric nutrition handbook,* ed 5, 2004, Chicago, American Academy of Pediatrics.

*Mead Johnson Nutritionals, Evansville, IN.

†Ross Products Division, Abbott Laboratories, Columbus, OH.

TABLE 180-7	Selected Pediatric Formulas (1 to 10 Years)

| Formula | Ingredients | Composition | | | |
		Protein (g/100 kcal)	Carbohydrate (g/100 kcal)	Fat (g/100 kcal)	Calories (kcal/oz)
Milk-Based					
Enfamil Kindercal*	Lactose-free, gluten-free, kosher, fiber	2.83	12.7	4.15	31.8
Enfamil Kindercal TF (tube feeding)*	Lactose-free, gluten-free, kosher, fiber	2.83	12.7	4.15	31.8
Nutren Junior[†]	Lactose-free, gluten-free, kosher, fiber	3	11	4.96	30
Pediasure[‡] (flavored)	Lactose-free, gluten-free, kosher	3	11	4.98	30
Peptide-Based					
Peptamin Junior[†]	Lactose-free, gluten-free, kosher	3[¶]	13.76	3.84 + MCT	30
Peptide One +[§]	Lactose-free, gluten-free, kosher	3.1[¶]	10.6	5 + MCT	30
Amino Acid–Based					
Neocate Junior[§]	Lactose-free, gluten-free, kosher	3[¶]	10.4	5	30
Neocate One +[§]	Lactose-free, gluten-free, kosher	3[¶]	14.6	3.5	30
Pediatric EO28[§] (flavored)	Lactose-free, gluten-free, kosher	3[¶]	14.6	3.5	30
Vivonex Pediatric[∥]	Lactose-free, gluten-free, kosher, + MCT	3[¶]	15.75	2.94	24

MCT, Medium chain triglyceride; *TF,* tube feeding.
Data from Kleinman R: *Pediatric nutrition handbook,* ed 5, 2004, Chicago, American Academy of Pediatrics.
*Mead Johnson Nutritionals, Evansville, IN.
[†]Nestle Clinical Nutrition, Deerfield, IL.
[‡]Ross Products Division, Abbott Laboratories, Columbus, OH.
[§]Scientific Hospital Suppllies North America, Gaithersburg, MD.
[||]Novartis Nutrition Corp., Minneapolis, MN.
[¶]Peptide and amino acid formulas do not contain whole protein. Values given represent protein equivalents.

TABLE 180-8	Selected Adolescent Formulas

| Formula | Uses | Composition | | | |
		Protein (g/100 kcal)	Carbohydrate (g/100 kcal)	Fat (g/100 kcal)	Calories (kcal/oz)
Milk-Based					
Boost*	Oral supplement	41.5	17.1	1.7	30.3
Ensure[†]	Oral supplement or tube feeding	3.75	16.7	2.5	31.8
Impact[‡]	Glutamine for wound healing	5.6	13	2.8	30
Jevity[†]	Tube feeding with fiber	4.18	14.62	3.29	31.8
Nutren 1.0[§]	Tube feeding with fiber	4	12.7	3.8	30
Ultracal*	Oral supplement or tube feeding with fiber	4.25	13.4	3.7	31.8
Soy-Based					
Isosource[§]		3.58	14.16	3.25	36
Peptide-Based					
Criticare HN*	Malabsorption, short bowel syndrome	3.58[||]	21	0.5	31.8
Peptamen[‡]	Malabsorption	4[||]	12.7	3.9 + MCT	30
Subdue*	Malabsorption	5[||]	13	3.4 + MCT	30
Amino Acid-Based					
Intensical*		6.2[||]	11.5	3.23	39
Nestle f.a.a[§]	Oral or tube feeding, malabsorption, food allergy	5[||]	17.6	1.12 + MCT	30
Tolerex[‡]	Chylothorax	2.1[||]	23	0.15	30
Vivonex[‡] (can be flavored)	Malabsorption, severe food allergy	4.5[||]	19	0.67	30

MCT, Medium chain triglycerides; *faa,* free amino acids.
Data from Kleinman R: *Pediatric nutrition handbook,* ed 5, 2004, Chicago, American Academy of Pediatrics.
*Mead Johnson Nutritionals, Evansville, IN.
[†]Ross Products Division, Abbott Laboratories, Columbus, OH.
[‡]Novartis Nutrition Corp., Minneapolis, MN.
[§]Nestle Clinical Nutrition, Deerfield, IL.
[||]Peptide and amino acid formulas do not contain whole protein. Values given represent protein equivalents.

TABLE 180-9	Composition of Selected Nutritional Supplements (Modifiers)				
		Composition			
Formula	Ingredients	Protein (g)	Carbohydrate (g)	Fat (g)	Calories (kcal)
Multicomponent					
Duocal (per 100 g)†	Corn, coconut, and MCT oils; hydrolyzed corn starch; vegetable oil	0	73	22	492
Human Milk Fortifier (four packets in 100 mL)	Enfamil brand‡	1.1	<0.4	1	15
	Similac brand†	1.0	1.8	0.36	14
Protein					
Casec (per 15 mL)‡	Calcium caseinate, soy lecithin	4			17
Promod (15 mL)§	Whey lecithin	3			17
Carbohydrate					
Polycose Liquid (per mL)§	Glucose polymers		0.5		2
Polycose Powder (100 g)§	Glucose polymers		94		380
Fat					
Corn Oil (per mL)	Corn oil				8
MCT Oil (per mL)‡	MCT			0.9	7.7
Microlipid (per mL)‡	Safflower oil emulsion			0.5	4.5
Safflower Oil (per mL)	Safflower oil				8

MCT, Medium chain triglycerides.

Data from Kleinman R: *Pediatric nutrition handbook,* ed 5, 2004, Chicago, American Academy of Pediatrics.

*Nestle Clinical Nutrition, Deerfield, IL.

†Scientific Hospital Suppllies North America, Gaithersburg, MD.

‡Mead Johnson Nutritionals, Evansville, IN.

§Ross Products Division, Abbott Laboratories, Columbus, OH.

Expected Outcomes	Unexpected Outcomes
• Maintenance of growth velocity appropriate for age and gender • Infant receives adequate nutrition safely and without complications	• Failure to meet growth targets • Abdominal distention • Emesis • Heme-positive diarrhea • Infection • Pulmonary aspiration

Monitoring and Care of the Child

Activities and Interventions	Rationale	Reportable Conditions
1. Weigh and measure child routinely; compare with baseline measurements. Document measurements on appropriate growth chart.	Evaluates response to enteral feeding. Growth measures reflect nutrition adequacy.	• Significant changes in growth velocity • Growth measures plotted at less than 5th percentile or more than 95th percentile
2. Monitor for feeding tolerance.	Feeding intolerance may indicate undiagnosed GI pathology or food allergy.	• Abdominal distention, emesis, profuse or bloody diarrhea, temperature instability, or residual feed greater than twice the prescribed feeding volume[4,&box;]
3. Monitor electrolytes, glucose, and metabolic laboratory values. 4. Monitor for signs and symptoms of infection.	Determines the efficacy of nutritional therapy[4,9] Infection is a stress that may increase energy requirements.	• Electrolyte derangements; including elevated liver function tests, decreased prealbumin and total protein, increased transferrin, decreased hemoglobin and hematocrit, glucose levels >120 mg/dl, and <60 mg/dl hypophosphakonia, hypomagnesemia, hypokalemia

Documentation

- Formula selection and fortification
- Date, time, volume, and route of feed
- Child's tolerance of feed
- Child's allergies
- Additional interventions necessary
- Child and family education
- Unexpected outcomes and related treatment

References

1. American Academy of Pediatrics: Breastfeeding and the use of human milk, *Pediatrics* 100(6):1035-1039, 1997.
2. Diehl-Jones WL, Fraser Askin D: Nutritional modulation of neonatal outcomes, *AACN Clin Iss* 15(1):83-96, 2004.
3. American Academy of Pediatrics Committee on Nutrition: Hypoallergenic infant formulas, *Pediatrics* 106(2):346-9, 2000.
4. Irving S, et al: Nutrition for the critically ill child: enteral and parenteral support, *AACN Clin Iss* 11(4):541-58, 2000.
5. Metheny NA, Stewart BJ: Testing feeding tube placement during continuous tube feedings, *Appl Nurs Res* 15(4):254-258, 2002.
6. Grant MC, Martin S: Delivery of enteral nutrition, *AACN Clin Iss* 11(4):507-516, 2000.
7. Chang T, Kleinman R: Standard and specialized formulas. In Walker WA, et al, editors: *Nutrition in pediatrics,* ed 3, London, 2003, BC Decker.
8. Kleinman R: *Pediatric nutrition handbook,* ed 5, 2005, Chicago, American Academy of Pediatrics.
9. Suddaby EC, Schiller S: Management of chylothorax in children, *Pediatr Nurs* 30(4):290-295, 2004.
10. Teske S, Robbins S: Formula preparation and handling. In Robbins S, Beker L, editors: *Infant feedings: guidelines for preparation of formula and breast milk in health care facilities,* 2004, Chicago, American Dietetic Association.

Additional Readings

Carver JD: Advances in nutritional modifications of infant formulas, *Am J Clin Nutr* 77(6):1550S-1554S, 2003.

Fulhan J, Collier S: Update on pediatric nutrition: breastfeeding, infant nutrition, and growth, *Curr Opin Pediatr* 15:323-332, 2003.

Sentongo T, Mascarenhas MR: Newer components of enteral formulas, *Pediatr Clin North Am* 49(1):113-125, 2002.

Serrano AS, Mannick EE: Enteral nutrition, *Peds Rev* 24(12): 417-423, 2003.

Growth Assessment: Obtaining Anthropometric Measurements

P U R P O S E : To describe the methods of obtaining and evaluating weight, length or height, and head circumference

Jamie A. Tumulty

PREREQUISITE KNOWLEDGE

- Standard growth measurements include weight, height or length, and head circumference.
- Weight is the most frequently measured parameter and is a screening tool for detection of abnormalities of growth and assessment of adequacy of nutritional interventions. Weight measurement is necessary to calculate body surface area (BSA). In addition, weight is the basis of dosing for most pediatric medications.
- Infants are weighed on a pan scale (accurate to 0.01 kg) with a tray large enough to adequately support an infant or young child who weighs up to 20 kg or 40 lb (Figure 181-1).
- Older children who can stand are weighed on a stand-up scale (Figure 181-2), whereas children (>2 years of age) who are mechanically ventilated and are bedridden need sling scales or special scale beds for weight measurement
- Measuring length and height are screening tools to detect abnormalities in linear growth and are necessary for calculating BSA and body mass index (BMI). BSA and BMI are used in determination of the dosage of several medications, including chemotherapy.[1,2] *(Level VI*)*
- A length board is necessary for measurement of infant length and provides the most reliable measurement of length in infants.[1,3] A length board is a measuring board with fixed headboard and adjustable footboard (Figure 181-3).

- Children require a stadiometer for measuring height and standing scales for measuring weight (Figure 181-4).[2,4]
- Head circumference is measured with a nonstretchable tape measure (Figure 181-5).
- All infants and children require the use of appropriate reference growth charts to evaluate growth measurements.
- Measurement accuracy is essential for correct plotting on age-specific and gender-specific growth curves.[1] In the United States, the Centers for Disease Control and Prevention (CDC) 2000 growth charts are recommended

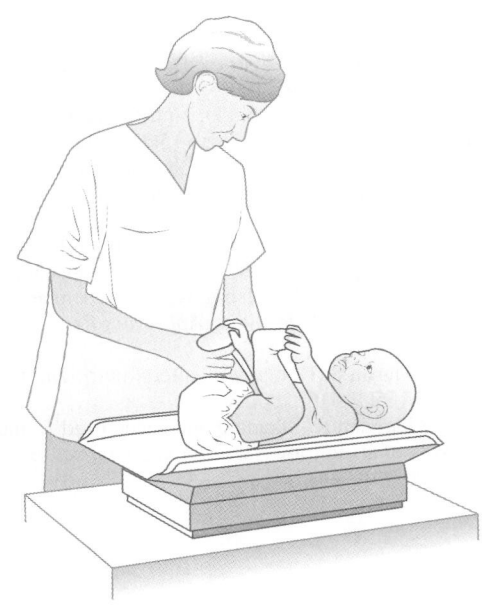

FIGURE 181-1 Infant weight with pan scale.

* Level VI: Clinical studies in a variety of patient populations and situations to support recommendations

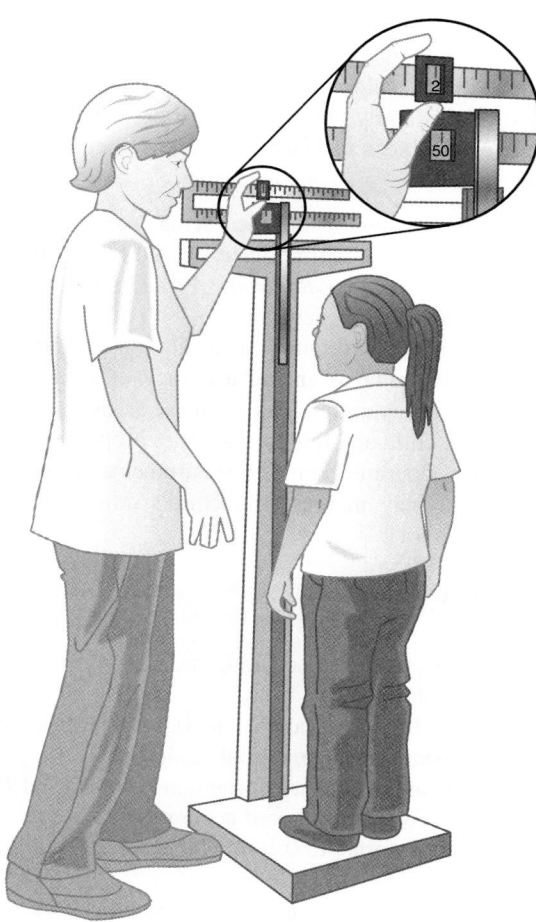

FIGURE 181-2 Child weight with stand-up scale.

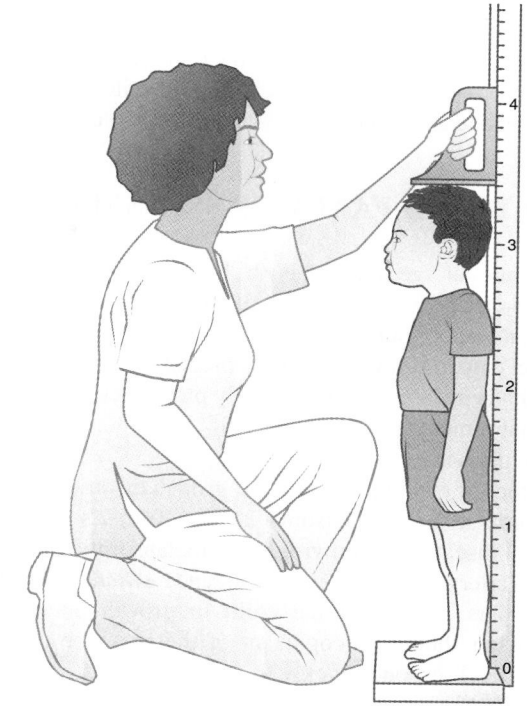

FIGURE 181-4 Child height with stadiometer.

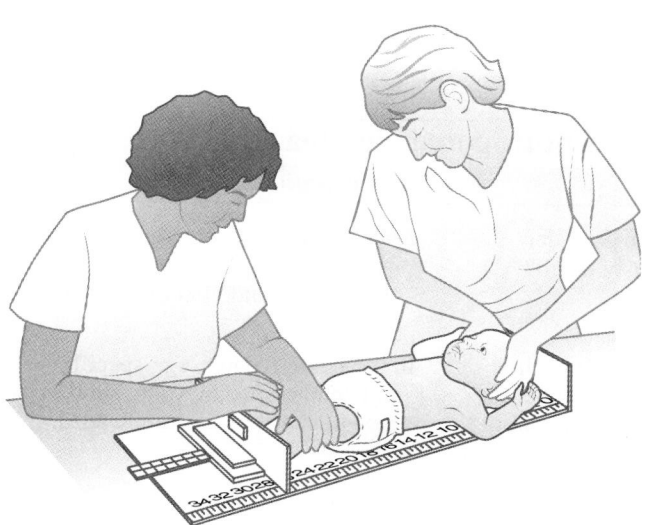

FIGURE 181-3 Infant length with length board.

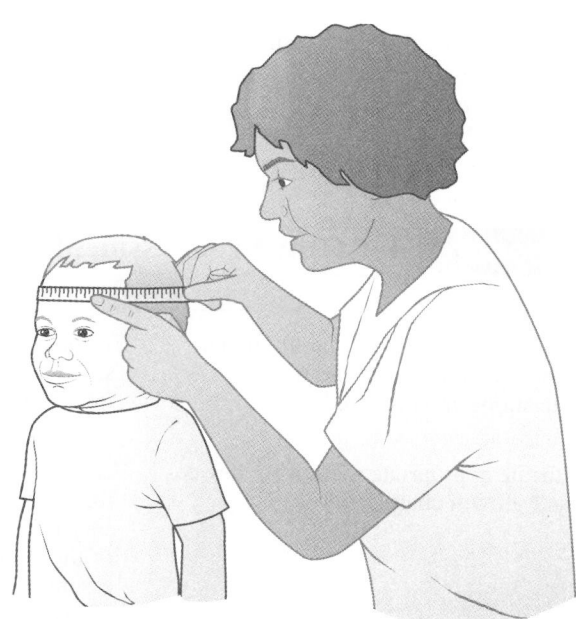

FIGURE 181-5 Infant head circumference.

over previous National Center for Health Statistics (NCHS) growth charts. The sample used to support the development of the 2000 growth charts included a larger number of diverse infants and children.[5] Age-specific and gender-specific growth charts are available at www.cdc.gov/growthcharts. In addition, there are specific growth charts for some conditions such as prematurity and Trisomy 21.

• The following guidelines are suggested for determining significant weight loss: greater than 2% in 1 week, greater than 5% in 1 month, greater than 7.5% in 3 months, and greater than 10% in 6 months.[6] With use of a growth chart, growth parameters less than the 5th percentile (underweight) and greater than the 95th percentile (overweight) necessitate attention.

CHILD AND FAMILY ASSESSMENT

- Gestational age, date of birth, birth weight, length, and head circumference (especially important for infants)[1] **→Rationale:** Foundation for evaluation of growth. An exact date of birth allows more precise calculation of age, which is necesssary to accurately plot the anthropometric measurements on age-specific and gender-specific growth charts.
- History of endocrine disorders; growth disorders; genetic disorders, such as Trisomy 21 and Turner's syndrome; renal disease; hypothyroidism; malabsorption disease; food allergy; and feeding intolerance **→Rationale:** These disorders predispose the child to growth delays. The clinician should be cognizant of the presence of a disorder and respond quickly to any deviation from normal growth.
- History of hydrocephalus or intraventricular hemorrhage **→Rationale:** These conditions may predispose an infant to abnormally large head circumference. The clinician should be cognizant of the presence of a disorder and respond quickly to any deviation from normal growth in these infants.
- History of familial short stature[1,2] **→Rationale:** Short stature in a child may be a normal finding if both parents are short.

CHILD AND FAMILY EDUCATION

Individualized, developmentally appropriate education is provided to the family and to the child based on desire for knowledge, readiness to learn, and overall neurologic and psychosocial state.

- Explain the procedure for measuring weight, length or height, and head circumference, including the purpose, steps, and rationale **→Rationale:** Providing information decreases fear and anxiety.
- Instruct the child and family regarding the importance of removing clothing to ensure accuracy of measurement **→Rationale:** Preparation may decrease anxiety.
- Instruct the child and family regarding proper posture for obtaining accurate height measurements **→Rationale:** Preparation may increase the child's compliance with proper technique.

EQUIPMENT

- Infant scale capable of accurate measurement to 0.01 kg (in good calibration)[1,2]
- Adult or child scale accurate to 0.1 kg (various types available: beam-balance, digital readout)[1,2]
- Measuring table or board for infants, with fixed headboard and movable footboard accurate to 0.1 cm[1-3]
- Stadiometer accurate to 0.1 cm (for child and adolescent measurement)[1,2]
- Narrow nonstretchable tape measure accurate to 0.1 cm[1,2]
- Appropriate age-specific, gender-specific, and disease-specific growth charts[1,2,5]
- Privacy curtain or private room

Procedure for Growth Assessment: Obtaining Anthropometric Measurements

Steps	Rationale	Considerations
1. Ensure that child and family understand the procedure and that questions are answered.	Evaluates and reinforces understanding of previously taught information.	Developmental level, cognitive ability, and anxiety level determine approach to and effectiveness of teaching.
2. Locate appropriate measuring devices and growth charts. (*Level VI**)	Facilitates completion of task in a timely manner. Equipment necessary is based on age and mobility of the child. Growth charts are essential for accurate evaluation of growth measures.	In the United States, age-specific and gender-specific CDC 2000 growth charts are recommended.
3. Assist the child in removal of shoes and clothes. Provide privacy for the child to disrobe.	Removal of shoes and clothes ensures that weight and stature measurements are not falsely elevated but reflect the true weight and stature of the child.	The American Academy of Pediatrics (AAP) recommends nude weights and should be weighed without diapers.[1,2]

* Level VI: Clinical studies in a variety of patient populations and situations to support recommendations

Procedure for Growth Assessment: Obtaining Anthropometric Measurements—*Continued*

Steps	Rationale	Considerations
Measuring Weight		
4. Obtain the appropriate scale for age and condition of the child.	Scale choice is based on the size of the child and the child's ability to stand.	Children less than 2 years of age need flat pan scale (see Figure 181-1). Bedridden children more than 2 years of age need sling scale or special scale. A standing scale is used for children able to stand (see Figure 181-2).
5. Zero the scale before measurement so the scale registers zero before the child is placed or steps on the scale.	Zeroing the scale ensures that the weight obtained reflects the true weight of the child.	If a hospital gown is worn, the weight of the gown should be subtracted from the child's weight.[1]
6. Assist the infant or child to age-appropriate scale.		
7. Record weight to nearest 0.01 kg for infants and nearest 0.1 kg for children.	Accuracy of measurement is important in interpretation of the data.	
8. Plot weight measurements on age-specific and gender-specific growth charts, including weight for age, weight for height, and BMI.	Plotting of weight measurements allows a deviation from normal or easy visualization of a change in growth velocity.[1]	Special growth charts are necessary for certain infant or child populations, including infants who are preterm and very low birth weight and children with other conditions (such as Trisomy 21).[1,5]
Measuring Linear Growth		
4. For recumbent length, obtain a length board (see Figure 180-3). a. Person one holds the crown of the head against the fixed head board with the external auditory meatus aligned with the lower edge of the orbit, perpendicular to the measuring board.[1,3] b. Person two holds the ankles of the infant or child and slides the footboard up until the heels are firmly positioned against it. The knees are then pressed down so that the dorsal surface touches the measuring board.[1,3] c. Record length to the nearest 0.1 cm.	A length board is used for infants or children with conditions that preclude standing erect.[1] Children with developmental disabilities, musculoskeletal disorders, or medical conditions that render them unconscious may need recumbent length measurements. Two-person length board measurement of recumbent length in infants is more accurate than alternative tape measure lengths.[1,3] *(Level VI*)* Gently pressing the knees down reflects full leg extension for a more accurate length measurement.	This method of measurement requires two people.
5. Obtain a stadiometer to measure standing height. a. Have the child stand erect, with feet flat on the floor, looking straight ahead, with heels, buttocks, shoulders, and head against the measuring board. Instruct child to "make yourself as tall as possible with your heels on the ground"[1] (see Figure 181-4).	Stadiometers are used for children more than 2 years old who are able to stand. Measure the child erect to determine stature (or height). To obtain an accurate height measurement, the child must stand straight and tall.	

Procedure continues on following page

* Level VI: Clinical studies in a variety of patient populations and situations to support recommendations

Procedure | **for Growth Assessment: Obtaining Anthropometric Measurements**—*Continued*

Steps	Rationale	Considerations
b. Lower the horizontal rule of the stadiometer firmly onto the crown of the child's head so that it is a right angle with the vertical rule.[1] c. Record stature measurement to the nearest 0.1 cm.		
6. Plot length measurements on age-specific and gender-specific growth charts including length for age, weight for height, and BMI.	Plotting of measurements tracks growth over time. A deviation from normal or easy visualization of a change in growth velocity can be easily visualized.[1]	Special growth charts are necessary for certain infant or child populations, including infants who are preterm and very low birth weight and those children with other conditions (such as Down syndrome).[1,5]
Head Circumference 4. Obtain a nonstretchable tape measure to measure head circumference.	Nonstretchable tape measures add accuracy to the measurement. This technique is used to routinely measure the maximal head circumference in children less than 2 years of age.	
5. Position one end of nonstretchable tape measure on the forehead above the supraorbital ridges (see Figure 185-5).		
6. Circle the tape measure above the infant's ears and around the head so that it passes over the occiput and returns to the forehead above the supraorbital ridge.[1]		
7. Pull tape measure taut; record measurement to the nearest 0.1 cm.[1]		
8. Plot head circumference measurements on age-specific and gender-specific growth charts.	Plotting of measurements tracks growth over time. A deviation from normal or a change in growth velocity can be easily visualized.[1]	
Body Mass Index 9. Formula: BMI = (weight in kg)/ (height in m).[1] • The CDC BMI charts are available for gender and ages 2 to 20 years.	Measure of weight relative to height. Used as an indicator of degree of obesity for children greater than 2 years of age. *(Level VI*)*	Underweight: BMI for age or weight for length less than 5th percentile. Risk of overweight: BMI for age or weight for length from 85th to 95th percentile. Overweight: BMI for age or weight for length more than 95th percentile.
Percent Ideal Body Weight (IBW) 10. Formula: IBW = (actual weight)/ (IBW at 50% for age) × 100.	The IBW is the recommended weight range for height. Calculation is used to determine acute and chronic nutritional status as compared with the standard. *(Level V*)*	

* Level V: Clinical studies in more than one or two patient populations and situations to support recommendations
Level VI: Clinical studies in a variety of patient populations and situations to support recommendations

Expected Outcomes	Unexpected Outcomes
• Accurate measurement of growth trajectory	• Poor measurement technique that leads to inaccuracies in growth measures

Monitoring and Care of the Child

Activities and Interventions	Rationale	Reportable Conditions
1. Monitor abnormal variations in growth measures.	May indicate pathology or inaccuracy of measurement.	• A growth parameter less than 5th or more than 95th percentile • "Rapid decline" in growth curve from previous measurements

Documentation

- Weight, stature, head circumference, and method of measurement
- Plot of percentiles of weight, stature, and head circumference for age
- Calculation of BMI for children greater than 2 years of age
- Any abnormal findings or variations in growth velocity
- Additional interventions necessary during measurements
- Child's response to measurements
- Unexpected outcomes and related treatment
- Child and family education

References

1. Kleinman R, editor: *Pediatric nutrition handbook,* ed 5, 2004, Chicago, American Academy of Pediatrics.
2. Zemel B, et al: Evaluation of methodology for nutritional assessment in children: anthropometry, body composition, and energy expenditure, *Ann Rev Nutr* 17:211-35, 1997.
3. Corkins M, et al: Accuracy of infant admission lengths, *Pediatrics* 109(6):1108-11, 2002.
4. Lab 3-2: Taking growth measurements, from http://www.humankinetics.com/lifeSpanMotorDevelopment/OSL/PICS/lab0302.pdf.
5. Ogden C, et al: Centers for Disease Control and Prevention 2000 growth charts for the United States: improvements to the 1977 National Center for Health Statistics version, *Pediatrics* 109(1):45-60, 2002.
6. Nevin-Folino NL, editor: *Pediatric manual of clinical dietetics,* ed 2, 2003, Chicago, American Dietetic Association.
7. Seidel H, et al, editors: *Mosby's guide to physical examination,* ed 4, Philadelphia, 1999, Mosby.

Orogastric/Nasogastric Tube: Insertion and Removal

P U R P O S E : An orogastric (OG)/nasogastric (NG) tube is inserted into the stomach for gastric air decompression, removal of gastric contents, supply of fluid and nutrients, and medication administration

Dyana Burns Conway

PREREQUISITE KNOWLEDGE

- Anatomy and physiology of the upper and lower gastrointestinal (GI) tract
- A functioning GI tract is necessary for digestion and absorption of enteral nutrition.
- The size of the child and the purpose of the tube influence the type and size of the tube chosen. A small-bore feeding tube is used to provide enteral nutrition; a small-bore Salem sump or Levin tube is used for gastric decompression; and a large-bore Salem sump tube or lavage tube (i.e., Ewald) is used for gastric lavage.
- A OG/NG tube is contraindicated with suspected basilar skull fracture or maxillofacial trauma because of the risk for inadvertent tube placement into the brain via the cribriform plate or ethmoid bone.
- An abdominal x-ray is the only reliable method of confirmation of enteral tube placement.[1,2] Although results are not 100% reliable, good evidence suggests that pH testing of GI secretions is the most accurate nonradiologic method for determination of enteral tube location (Figure 182-1).[2-6]
- Gastric aspirate has a pH of 5 or less and is usually grassy green or clear and colorless, with off-white to tan mucus shreds.[2-6] An aspirate from a small tube placed in the intestine often has a pH of 6 or greater, is usually bile

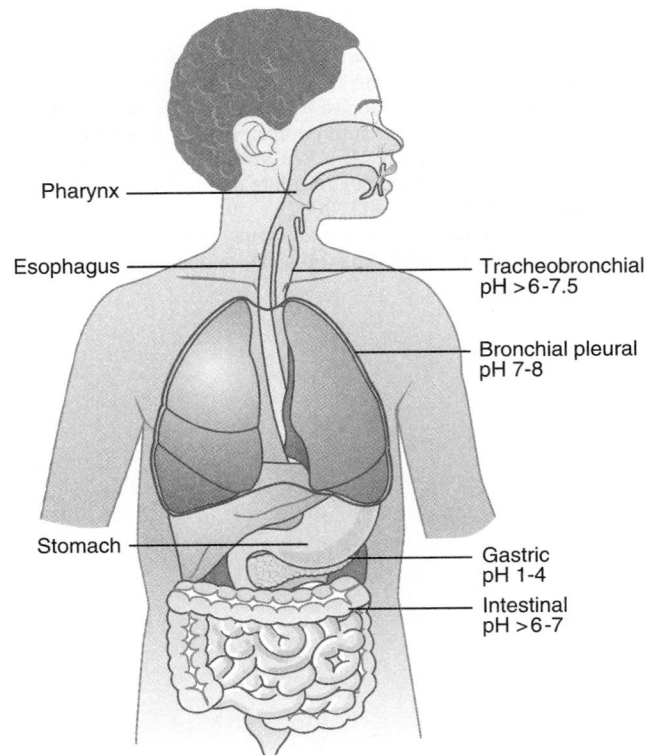

Pharynx

Esophagus

Tracheobronchial
pH >6-7.5

Bronchial pleural
pH 7-8

Stomach

Gastric
pH 1-4

Intestinal
pH >6-7

FIGURE 182-1 Normal pH readings for aspirates. Values are approximate.

stained, and ranges in color from light to golden yellow or brownish green. In addition, the aspirate is usually thicker and more translucent than fluid from a tube with a tip located in the stomach.[2] An aspirate from a tube inadvertently positioned in the tracheobronchial tree has the appearance of fluid from the tracheobronchial tree, whereas an aspirate from the pleural space is usually watery and straw colored. Both locations produce a pH of 6 or greater.[1-5]

CHILD AND FAMILY ASSESSMENT

- Child's developmental level and ability to interact ➻*Rationale:* Influences preparation and interaction.
- Child's and family's understanding of the reasons for and risks and benefits of OG/NG tube insertion ➻*Rationale:* Evaluates child's and family's understanding of the procedure and provides a gauge for ongoing education.
- Desire of family members to be present during the procedure ➻*Rationale:* The presence of family may provide comfort and support; although family members should have the choice not to remain with the child.
- History of nasal or palate deformity, gastric fundoplication, gastric or esophageal surgery, or esophageal and pyloric malformations or injuries ➻*Rationale:* These conditions may complicate the passage of an OG/NG tube.
- Level of consciousness and cognitive ability ➻*Rationale:* Determine if a prearranged signal that the child uses to indicate gagging during tube passage is appropriate.
- Status of upper respiratory tract ➻*Rationale:* Excessive upper airway secretions interfere with the child's ability to tolerate passage of the tube.
- Patency of the nares ➻*Rationale:* A tube cannot pass through an occlusion.
- Function of GI tract ➻*Rationale:* A functional GI tract is necessary for administration of enteral feedings.

CHILD AND FAMILY EDUCATION

Individualized, developmentally appropriate education is provided to the family and to the child based on desire for knowledge, readiness to learn, and overall neurologic and psychosocial state.

- Provide information about the OG/NG tube, including the reason for insertion and an explanation of steps involved in tube insertion ➻*Rationale:* Knowledge decreases anxiety and fear.
- Discuss appropriate expected outcomes of the procedure ➻*Rationale:* Allows the family and medical team to formulate similar goals and expectations.
- Explain how the older child can assist with passage of the tube by swallowing during tube insertion ➻*Rationale:* The tube passes easily with the child's cooperation.
- Explain that the child may gag during tube insertion ➻*Rationale:* Providing information decreases anxiety and fear.
- Explain the need to prevent tension on the feeding tube once in place ➻*Rationale:* Tube reinsertion may be necessary if the tube is displaced or removed.
- Encourage questions and answer questions as they arise ➻*Rationale:* Reinforcement of information is needed during periods of stress.

EQUIPMENT

- Levin tube or Salem sump (infant, 6F to 10F; child, 8F to 14F)[7,8]
- Feeding tube (infant, 5F to 10F; child, 10F to 14F)[7,8]
- Tape or semipermeable transparent dressing to secure tube
- Skin preparation agent
- Clean gloves
- Water-soluble lubricant
- Appropriately sized syringe
- Stethoscope
- Marker (optional)
- Bedside suction equipment, as indicated

Procedure for Orogastric/Nasogastric Tube: Insertion		
Steps	**Rationale**	**Considerations**
1. Ensure child and family understand procedure and questions are answered.	Evaluates and reinforces understanding of previously taught information.	Developmental level, cognitive ability, and anxiety level determine the approach to and effectiveness of teaching.
2. Collect all necessary equipment and supplies.	Preparation and presence of all materials facilitate completion of procedure without delays.	Tube selection is dependent on size of the child and intended use of tube (i.e., air decompression, gastric feeding).
3. Have suction available, if indicated.	Suction is readily available for removal of emesis.	

Procedure continues on following page

Procedure for Orogastric/Nasogastric Tube: Insertion—*Continued*

Steps	Rationale	Considerations
4. Ensure appropriate cardiopulmonary monitoring.	Children who are critically ill may have decompensation during the insertion.	Consider the child's status in selection of appropriate monitoring.
5. Wash hands and put on clean gloves.	Reduces transmission of microorganisms. Protects personnel health.	
6. Position the child in the supine position. Head of bed may be flat or elevated 30 to 45 degrees as condition permits. *(Level II*)*	Elevation of head of bed 30 to 45 degrees decreases risk of aspiration.[7]	Infants, toddlers, and some older children depending on cognitive ability may need assistance to remain immobile during the procedure. A second person may be needed to help with the procedure. Parental presence may be supportive.
7. Estimate depth of tube insertion by measuring tube from the tip of nose to the earlobe, then from the earlobe to the tip of the xiphoid process. Mark this point with a marker or small piece of tape (Figure 182-2). *(Level IV*)*	Length approximates the distance to the gastroesophageal junction.[9]	

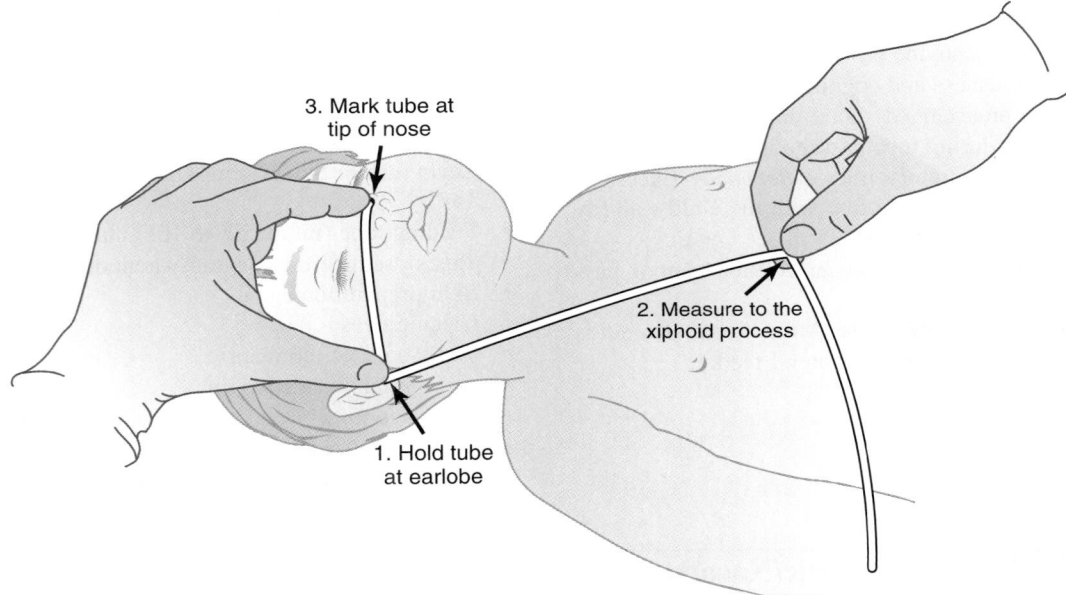

3. Mark tube at tip of nose

2. Measure to the xiphoid process

1. Hold tube at earlobe

FIGURE 182-2   Measurement of length of gastric tubes.

Steps	Rationale	Considerations
8. Lubricate the distal tip of tube with water-soluble lubricant. *(Level I*)*	Lubrication facilitates passage through nares.	Some manufacturers make self-lubricating tubes. If tube is self lubricating, dip tip of tube in water before insertion.
9. Gently but steadily thread the tube through either the mouth or one of the nares (aiming posterior and parallel to nasal septum) to the previously identified mark (Figure 182-3). *(Level IV*)*	Allows for ease in following the normal anatomy.[7,8,10]	

* Level I: Manufacturer's recommendations only
   Level II: Theory-based; no research data to support recommendations; recommendations from expert consensus group may exist
   Level IV: Limited clinical studies to support recommendations

Procedure **for Orogastric/Nasogastric Tube: Insertion**—*Continued*

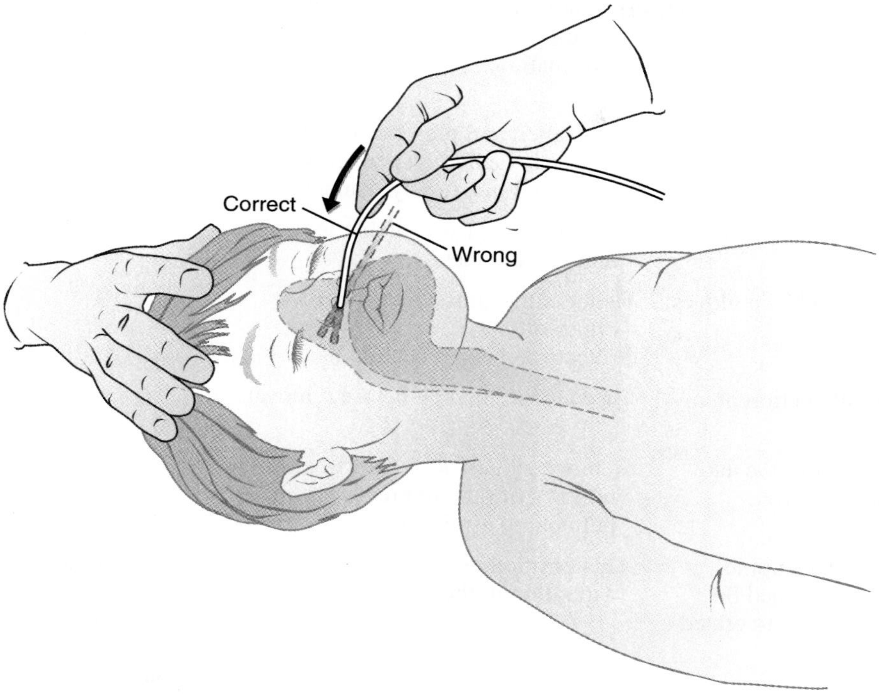

Steps	Rationale	Considerations

FIGURE 182-3   Insertion of nasogastric tube.

Steps	Rationale	Considerations
10. If the child is cooperative, ask the child to continuously swallow sips of water during insertion of tube. Infants may be offered a pacifier. *(Level IV*)*	Swallowing assists passage of the tube into the esophagus instead of the trachea.[9] Sucking on a pacifier promotes passage of the tube into the esophagus.	Difficult passage, choking, coughing, cyanosis, and decreased oxygen saturations are indications of possible tracheal intubation. Remove tube and reattempt placement at a different angle.
11. Obtain an abdominal x-ray for visual confirmation of correct tube placement.[1,2] Although not a substitute, aspiration of stomach contents with a syringe and testing of the pH is also used routinely to confirm tube location.[1,2,6] *(Level IV*)*	Radiography is the most reliable method of determining tube placement. pH testing appears to be the most accurate nonradiologic alternative for determination of tube location.	Other than radiography, most methods of confirming tube placement have a wide error margin. Do not rely on the auscultation method to confirm tube placement.[1,2]
12. Apply skin preparation to face where tube will be secured and allow to dry.	Prepares surface of skin to help adherence of tape. Provides a protective barrier for the skin.	
13. Stabilize the tube by taping securely above the upper lip or cheek. Avoid taping the tube to the nare (see Figure 95-1 in Procedure 95).	Tube is more secure when taped to a nonmobile area; taping prevents tube from migrating into wrong position.	
14. Remove gloves and wash hands.	Reduces transmission of infection. Protects personnel health.	
15. Record length of the tube at the mark located at the mouth or nostril.	Monitoring of placement after the tube is first positioned ensures correct placement.	Recheck this measurement each shift and before each usage.

Procedure continues on following page

* Level IV: Limited clinical studies to support recommendations

Procedure for Orogastric/Nasogastric Tube: Removal

Steps	Rationale	Considerations
1. Ensure child and family understand preprocedural teaching.	Evaluates and reinforces understanding of previously taught information.	Developmental level, cognitive ability and anxiety level determine the approach to and effetiveness of teaching.
2. Collect all necessary equipment and supplies.	Preparation and presence of all materials facilitate completion of procedure in a timely manner.	
3. Have suction available if indicated.	Suction is readily available for removal of emesis.	
4. Wash hands and put on clean gloves.	Reduces transmission of microorganisms. Protects personnel health.	
5. If applicable, turn off suction or continuous feeding.	Discontinue therapy before removal.	
6. Attach syringe to end of tube and remove all air and fluid from stomach.	Remove all gastric contents before removal of tube to prevent pulmonary aspiration.	
7. Position the child in the supine position. Elevate head of bed 30 to 45 degrees or higher, if tolerated by the child. *(Level II*)*	This position decreases the risk of aspiration in the event of emesis.	Infants, toddlers, and some older children depending on cognitive ability may need assistance to remain immobile during the procedure. A second person may be needed to help with the procedure. Parental presence may be supportive.
8. Gently remove tape from under the lip or cheek.	Careful removal of tape prevents any skin breakdown.	Consider use of skin adhesive remover to assist in the removal of tape.
9. Pull tube out of mouth or nose in a steady motion.	Quick and steady removal decreases the amount of discomfort to the child.	
10. Dispose of tube in appropriate receptacle and wash hands.	Reduces transmission of microorganisms.	

* Level II: Theory-based; no research data to support recommendations; recommendations from expert consensus group may exist

Expected Outcomes	Unexpected Outcomes
• Distal tip of tube is located in the stomach	• Tracheal/bronchial intubation as indicated by choking, coughing, cyanosis, or decreased oxygen saturations • Tube coiled in posterior pharynx or esophagus
• Tube patency • Uncomplicated tube placement and use	• Clogged or kinked tube • Esophageal tear from trauma of tube passing • Skin irritation at nares • Pneumothorax from inadvertent pleural placement • Aspiration of stomach contents despite appropriate placement

Monitoring and Care of the Child

Activities and Interventions	Rationale	Reportable Conditions
1. Monitor child's tolerance to OG/NG tube placement.	Changes in child's condition may indicate complications from tube placement.	• Agitation that results in an inability to place the tube
2. Monitor for correct position when tube is used intermittently to administer feeding, medications, and fluid.	Incorrect position before administration of contents through the tube can cause pulmonary aspiration or other complications.	• Change in respiratory or cardiovascular status during placement • Indication of tube outside the stomach • Removal of tube by the child
3. Check tube patency every 2 hours or as indicated.	Frequent monitoring of patency assures continuation of therapy and minimal interruptions.	• Clogged or kinked tube
4. If tube is used for gastric decompression, monitor output (color, amount, type, pH, guaiac) every 4 hours and as needed.	Excessive volume loss can cause the child to become hypovolemic or can cause electrolyte imbalances.	• Increased output or sudden change in output; positive guaiac or output has frank blood, "coffee-ground," black, or brown color • Abnormal pH • Ulceration, drainage, or foul odor
5. Assess nasal and oral cavity and provide oral care every 4 hours and as needed.	OG/NG tubes may cause the child to mouth breathe, drying the mouth and increasing the risk of mucosal breakdown and ulcerations. Predisposes child to sinusitis or oral infections.	
6. Monitor insertion site of tube.	Frequent monitoring can prevent serious skin breakdown.	• Redness, swelling, drainage, bleeding, or skin breakdown at insertion site
7. Monitor child's vital signs per unit standards. Perform respiratory and GI assessments every 2 hours and as needed.	Frequent monitoring of changes in vital signs and respiratory or GI assessment provide early detection of complications.	• Continued choking, coughing, cyanosis, or decreased oxygen saturations • Increased abdominal distention or abdominal girth or change in bowel sounds

Documentation

- Response to insertion (or removal)
- Size, type, and length of tube placed
- Tube site assessments
- Oral care
- If applicable, amount of type of irrigation fluid
- If present, appearance and volume of gastric secretions
- Additional interventions necessary during insertion
- Child and family education
- Unexpected outcomes and related treatment

References

1. National Guideline Clearinghouse: Access for administration of nutrition support, *JPEN J Parenter Enteral Nutr* 26(1 Suppl):33SA-41SA, 2002. Text available at http://www.guideline.gov/summary/summary.aspx?ss= 15&doc_id=3630&nbr=2856.
2. AACN: Practice alert: verification of feeding tube placement, *AACN News* 22(5).
3. Metheny N, Titler M: Assessing placement of feeding tubes, *AJN* 101(5):36-45, 2001.
4. Westhus N: Methods to test feeding tube placement in children, *MCN Am J Matern Child Nurs* 29(5):282-287, 2004.
5. Huffman S, Jarczyk K, Bayne A, et al: Methods to confirm feeding tube placement: application of research in practice, *Pediatr Nurs* 30(1):10-13, 2004.
6. Metheny N, Meert K: Monitoring feeding tube placement, *Nutrition Clin Pract* 19(5):487-495, 2004.
7. Henretig FM, King C: *Textbook of pediatric emergency procedures,* ed 4, 1999, Philadelphia, Lippincott Williams & Wilkins.
8. Hockenberry MJ: *Wong's, clinical manual of pediatric nursing,* ed 6, St. Louis, 2003, Mosby.
9. Grant MC, Martin S: Delivery of enteral nutrition, *AACN Clin Issues* 11(4):507-516, 2000.
10. Lynn-McHale DJ, Carlson KK: *AACN Procedure Manual for Critical Care,* ed 4, Philadelphia, 2001, Saunders.

Additional Readings

Ellett ML, Maahs J, Forsee S: Prevalence of feeding tube placement errors & associated risk factors in children, *MCN Am J Matern Child Nurs* 23(5):234-239, 1998.

Klasner AE, Luke DA, Scalzo AJ: Pediatric orogastric and nasogastric tubes: a new formula evaluated, *Ann Emerg Med* 39(3):268-72, 2002.

Parenteral Nutrition: Administration

P U R P O S E : Administration of parenteral nutrition (PN) is intended to safely provide nutritional support to children who are unable to receive adequate enteral nutrition

Sharon Y. Irving

PREREQUISITE KNOWLEDGE

- Pediatric fluid, electrolyte and caloric requirements (Table 183-1; see Table 180-1)
- Children who cannot fully meet fluid, electrolyte, and nutritional requirements through the oral or enteral route for nutrition are prescribed parenteral nutrition (PN) as sole or adjunct therapy to meet nutritional requirements.
- PN is indicated when the child's gastrointestinal (GI) function is inadequate to support nutritional needs or when enteral feeding is contraindicated, such as with GI obstruction, bleeding, or hemodynamic instability with high vasopressor support.[1,2]
- Relative contraindications for PN include inadequate intravenous (IV) access, short duration of therapy (usually less than 5 days), unstable fluid and electrolyte status, and death that is imminent from underlying disease state or child's condition.[3,4]
- PN consists of a complex hyperosmolar formulation of dextrose, amino acids, electrolytes, minerals, vitamins, and trace elements. The composition of these components makes it suitable to meet the child's nutritional needs.
- Central access is usually preferred over peripheral access for long-term delivery of maximum fluid and nutrient requirements. Peripheral PN, however, has less complications associated with its administration.[5]
- Peripheral PN has a final dextrose concentration of 12.5% or less and is intended to supplement dietary intake.

TABLE 183-1	Daily Electrolyte Requirements for Children	
Electrolyte	**Maintenance Requirement**
Sodium	2 to 4 mEq/kg/d
Potassium	2 to 4 mEq/kg/d
Magnesium	0.25 to 1.0 mEq/kg/d
Calcium	0.5 to 3 mEq/kg/d
Phosphorus	0.5 to 2 mmol/kg/d

From Kleinman R: *Pediatric nutrition handbook*, ed 5, 2004, Chicago, American Academy of Pediatrics.

- Centrally delivered PN therapy is intended to provide the child's total nutritional needs with dextrose concentrations 15% or greater.
- Lipid solutions (i.e., intralipids) provide fats and essential fatty acids. Lipid solutions may be infused separately or as an admixture (three-in-one solution with lipid emulsion mixed with amino acid–glucose solution and administered through a single line).[5] When administered from a separate bottle, intralipids are "piggy-backed" into the PN infusion distal to the PN in-line filter, close to the child's IV site. A separate infusion pump is necessary.
- Intralipid solution is available in 10% and 20% concentrations. The 20% solution is the infusion of choice because of the increased caloric density (2 kcal/mL). Use of a filter with lipid solutions is not necessary unless the lipids are delivered in an admixture or a combined PN intralipid solution. In this case, a 1.2-micron filter is appropriate.

- Cycling of PN may be preferred. Physiologically, cycled PN allows enzymes and hormones to regulate similar to conventional eating and fasting patterns.[1,5,6] Cycled PN is typically infused over 10 to 16 hours per day. To decrease the prescribed delivery time, the cycled time is compressed by 2 to 4 hours daily until the infusion goal is met. An indication for cycled PN is to optimize normalcy for children on long-term therapy. Cycled PN may also be prescribed to foster the child's appetite.[1]
- Knowledge of institution-specific protocol policy regarding PN handling and administration
- Knowledge of operation of electronic infusion device suitable for PN delivery

CHILD AND FAMILY ASSESSMENT

- Child's developmental level and ability to interact ➥*Rationale:* Influences preparation and interaction.
- Child's and family's understanding of the reasons for and risks and benefits of administering parenteral nutrition ➥*Rationale:* Evaluates child's and family's understanding of the procedure and provides a gauge for ongoing education.
- Family's desire and ability to be involved with child's care ➥*Rationale:* The family can provide support to the child and maintain some control in the care of the child.
- Child's underlying diagnosis and indication for therapy ➥*Rationale:* Direction for central versus peripheral administration is provided.
- Laboratory findings, including electrolytes (baseline sodium, potassium, calcium, phosphate, magnesium, blood urea nitrogen, creatinine, and glucose), liver function tests (transaminases, alkaline phosphate, and bilirubin), serum proteins (total protein, albumin, prealbumin, and transferring), and hemoglobin (Hgb) and hematocrit (Hct) ➥*Rationale:* Baseline laboratory values provide data for selection and formulation of type and amount of formula and the need for electrolyte supplementation. Depressed baseline protein levels indicate malnourishment. Hgb and Hct values screen for anemia and iron status.
- Child's preillness nutritional status ➥*Rationale:* Identifies risk factors and challenges associated with meeting the child's nutritional needs.[3,6,7]
- Current anthropometric measurements, including admission weight, length or height, head circumference, body mass index, skin folds if available, and plots of these values on appropriate age and gender growth charts ➥*Rationale:* The measurement and evaluation of growth parameters are part of the foundation of the nutritional assessment. Admission measurements are necessary to determine effectiveness of enteral nutrition after initiation and advancement.
- Use and function of the GI tract, including ability and tolerance of oral or tube feeding ➥*Rationale:* PN may be used to provide partial or full nutritional support.[2,5,7]
- Child's IV access ➥*Rationale:* Access (either central or peripheral) determines the concentration of nutrients that can be supplied.

CHILD AND FAMILY EDUCATION

Individualized, developmentally appropriate education is provided to the family and to the child based on desire for knowledge, readiness to learn, and overall neurologic and psychosocial state.

- Explain the procedure for administering PN, including the purpose, steps, and rationale ➥*Rationale:* Providing information decreases fear and anxiety.
- Discuss appropriate expected outcomes for the administration of PN ➥*Rationale:* The family and health care team can formulate similar goals and expectations.
- Provide developmentally appropriate information to child and family regarding PN therapy ➥*Rationale:* If the child is able to understand the importance of therapy, external complications may be decreased (e.g., child can help "protect" IV access, child will not play with the tubing or infusion device, etc). Appropriate education can minimize or avoid contradiction or omission of information.[3]
- Explain the nursing care involved with PN administration, including handling the solution and tubing, care of the insertion site, and insertion site dressing changes ➥*Rationale:* Family and child are educated "standard" care during PN administrator, particularly the factors associated with care of the insertion site.[6]
- Encourage questions and answer questions as they arise ➥*Rationale:* Reinforcement of information is needed during periods of stress.

EQUIPMENT

- Prescribing practitioner's order for PN solution
- Prescribed PN solution
- Electronic infusion device suitable for continuous PN infusion
- Appropriate IV administration set for infusion device
- In-line 0.22-micron IV filter, compatible with IV administration set[6]
- Clean gloves
- Alcohol pads or swabs
- Povidone-iodine pads or swabs (see institution policy)
- Needleless injection cannula and appropriately sized syringe
- Normal saline solution flush

Procedure for Parenteral Nutrition: Administration

Steps	Rationale	Considerations
1. Verify prescribing practitioner's order for PN.	Minimizes risk of error.	
2. Compare the order with the pharmacy label affixed to PN container on arrival to the nursing unit. Check for expiration date and time of solution.[2,6] *(Level VI*)*	Reduces error in administration.	The PN order includes dextrose, protein, and additive concentrations of the solution the PN order also includes rate of infusion and length of time for infusion. Return solution to pharmacy if discrepancies exist.
3. Compare child's name and identifying number with label on the PN solution container.	Assures PN is administered to the correct child.	
4. Gather and assemble all equipment and supplies, including the IV tubing and connectors necessary for administration of PN; secure a clean clutter free area to assemble tubing.	Connection of the tubing before spike into PN container minimizes transmission of bacteria by decreasing the contact sites once the fluid has been accessed.	After assembly, ensure that all open ports are clamped or closed.
5. Wash hands and put on clean gloves.	Reduces transmission of microorganisms. Decreases exposure to blood and body fluids.	
6. Access the PN solution with the assembled IV tubing with in-line filter and slowly prime the tubing. *(Level V*)*	Systematic approach to administration of PN reduces risk of error and infection. Slow priming of tubing allows visualization of solution for particulate matter and leaks in the tubing.	Ensure removal of all air and inspect solution for precipitation. *NOTE:* Some infusion devices do not allow the tubing to be primed before insertion into the device.
7. Clamp child's access port.	Reduces possibility of air embolism.[1]	
8. Following institutional policies, cleanse the catheter port. • For separate administration of lipids, follow procedure for both access ports. *(Level IV*)*	Minimizes bacteria at catheter insertion site.[1,6]	
9. Attach primed tubing to electronic infusion pump. Set administration rate for PN as prescribed. *(Level II*)*	An infusion pump is essential to ensure the solution is delivered with accuracy and allows for close monitoring of hourly administration.[1,5,6]	
10. Attach primed IV line to the child's access site. Ensure no air is found at connection site. Set prescribed rate of infusion and other parameters on infusion pump. *(Level I*)*	This completes the priming process and the solution is ready for infusion.	All connections should be luer-lock connections to ensure prevention of accidental disconnections. Minimizing the risk of disconnection is essential for patient safety.
11. Recheck PN orders for infusion rate of PN solution and ensure infusion device is set at the prescribed rate. Open all clamps and start infusion pump.	Open clamps before starting pump to prevent pressure build-up and "bolus" infusion to child on pump start-up. Consistent infusion rate minimizes metabolic complications associated with PN (Table 183-2).	

Procedure continues on following page

* Level I: Manufacturer's recommendations only
Level II: Theory-based; no research data to support recommendations; recommendations from expert consensus group may exist
Level IV: Limited clinical studies to support recommendations
Level V: Clinical studies in more than one or two patient populations and situations to support recommendations
Level VI: Clinical studies in a variety of patient populations and situations to support recommendations

Procedure for **Parenteral Nutrition: Administration**—*Continued*

Steps	Rationale	Considerations
12. Ensure PN bag and tubing are labeled according to institution-specific protocol for date, time, and other information, as required.	Confirmation of prescribed PN solution to the correct child at the prescribed rate of infusion.	
13. If lipid solution is ordered, prime and administer. Follow steps 1 to 12. • Remove cap and spike with administration set.	A separate administration set and priming is necessary for administration of lipid solutions.	
14. For cycled PN:		
a. To begin cycled infusion, rate is increased every 15 minutes for an hour until at prescribed hourly rate. *(Level V*)*	Graduated increase in starting cycled PN prevents hyperglycemia.[1,5,6,8]	For children with hepatic dysfunction, cycled PN may allow for excess glycogen to clear during off hours.[1]
b. Check bedside glucose 1 to 2 hours into infusion when at goal rate.	Blood glucose levels can be labile when changes are made in the administration of high concentrations of dextrose.	
c. During the last hour of infusion, the rate is decreased every 15 minutes for 1 hour until off.	Graduated decrease in stopping cycled PN prevents hypoglycemia.[1,5,6]	Notify prescribing practitioner if glucose level is more than 120 mg/dL.
d. Check bedside glucose 1 hour after PN is discontinued.	Blood glucose levels can be labile when changes are made in the administration of high concentrations of dextrose.	Notify prescribing practitioner if glucose level is less than 60 mg/dL.
e. At the end of PN infusion, turn off infusion pump and disconnect PN tubing from catheter. Flush catheter with normal saline solution or heparin per institution-specific protocol.		

* Level V: Clinical studies in more than one or two patient populations and situations to support recommendations

TABLE 183-2	Complications Associated With Parenteral Nutrition		
Complication	**Sign**	**Cause**	**Intervention**
Catheter Associated			
Insertion	Pneumothorax	Pleural puncture	Special attention to insertion technique
	Hemothorax	Trauma to vessels	
	Brachial plexus injury	Nerve damage	
	Air embolism	Air into vasculature	
	Dysrhythmia	Catheter tip irritating cardiac muscle	
Thrombus formation	Intraluminal blood clot	Venous status	Special attention to catheter selection for site and duration of therapy
	Solution precipitate	Sluggish venous flow	
	Inability to flush catheter/occlusion	Precipitates in PN solution	Heparin in PN solution
		Thrombus formation	
Phlebitis	Infiltration into surrounding tissues	Extravasation of solution	Monitor site for signs of extravasation (i.e., redness, edema, pain at catheter site)
			Infuse intralipid solution to reduce osmolarity

TABLE 183-2	Complications Associated With Parenteral Nutrition—Cont'd		
Complication	**Sign**	**Cause**	**Intervention**
Infection			
Local or insertion site	Edema or erythema at insertion site	Frequent manipulation of catheter Frequent manipulation of occlusive dressing Unsecured occlusive dressing	Minimize handling of catheter Sterile technique for dressing change (follow institution protocol)
Bloodstream	Change in child's vital signs (i.e., fever, tachycardia, tachypnea, or hypotension) Change in laboratory values (i.e., leukocytosis, bandemia, thrombocytopenia) Positive blood culture and gram stain results	Migration of bacteria or micro-organisms into catheter along subcutaneous tract or into catheter lumen Seeding from another infection source Contamination of PN solution	Hand sanitization before handling catheter, IV tubing, or PN solution Minimize manipulation of catheter and insertion site dressing Meticulous technique with dressing changes, solution changes (in accordance with institutional protocol) Dedicate line (if possible) solely to infusion of PN
Metabolic			
Hydration abnormality	Fluid overload or dehydration Increase or decrease in laboratory values (i.e., BUN, creatinine, Hct, serum sodium, and osmolality) Change in urine output	Inadequate fluid calculation or infusion Unaccounted fluid losses Renal insufficiency Cardiac insufficiency	Close attention to fluid balance Frequent evaluation of child's status (i.e., fever, significant change in urine output, onset or cessation of diarrhea)
Hyperglycemia	Increased blood glucose Increased urine output	Increased glucose in PN Metabolic stress Concurrent corticosteroid administration Rapid administration of PN Insufficient insulin response	Decrease in dextrose concentration in PN Slow PN infusion rate Initiate low-dose continuous insulin infusion
Hypoglycemia	Decreased blood glucose Diaphoresis Pallor Lethargy	Low dextrose concentration in PN solution Insulin infusion Undiagnosed endocrine disorder Severe sepsis Acute discontinuation of PN	Increase dextrose concentration in PN solution Stop or decrease insulin infusion Treat sepsis Taper PN rate to off Do not abruptly stop PN
Electrolyte imbalance	Abnormal electrolyte values	Electrolyte requirements change with illness and hydration status	Frequent monitoring of blood chemistries with necessary adjustments
Hyperammonemia	Change in mental status or lethargy Asterixis (a flapping movement or tremor of the hands)	Increased protein intake Hepatic insufficiency	Decrease protein intake
Azotemia	Increased BUN Mild dehydration Increased urine specific gravity	Increased protein to nonprotein (carbohydrates and fat) caloric intake	Decrease percentage of amino acid added to PN Change the solution amino acid to Nephramine
Fatty acid deficiency	Dry flaky skin despite adequate fluid intake Thrombocytopenia	Inadequate lipid intake with PN solution	Provide lipids at least two times per week Give oral fats if tolerated Provide topical fats daily for absorption
Hyperlipidemia	Increased serum triglyceride Cloudy blood specimen	Increased intralipid administration Familial hyperlipidemia Renal insufficiency	Check triglyceride levels 4 hours after initiation of lipid administration and daily until stable Stop infusion if level ≥400 mg/dL (or per institution protocol)

BUN, Blood urea nitrogen; *Hct,* hematocrit.

Worthington P, Reyen L: Administration and management of parenteral nutrition. In Worthington PH, editor: *Practical aspects of nutritional support: an advanced practice guide,* Philadelphia, 2004, Saunders.

Donahue M: Parenteral nutrition. In McHale DJ, Carlson KK, editors: *AACN procedure manual for critical care,* ed 4, Philadelphia, 2001, Saunders.

Irving SY, et al: Nutrition for the critically ill child: enteral and parenteral support, *AACN Clin Issues* 11(4):541-58, 2000.

Expected Outcomes

- Maintain growth velocity appropriate for age and gender
- Balanced fluid status
- Metabolic markers (chemistry panel, metabolic panel, complete blood cell count, and lipid levels) within normal limits for the child
- Catheter and catheter site is free of infection

Unexpected Outcomes

- Failure to meet growth targets
- Fluid overload or dehydration
- Metabolic derangements

- Infection at catheter site or systemic infection

Monitoring and Care of the Child

Activities and Interventions	Rationale	Reportable Conditions
1. Weigh and measure child routinely; compare results with baseline measurements. Document measurements on appropriate growth chart.	Evaluates response to enteral feeding. Growth measures reflect nutrition adequacy.	• Significant changes in growth velocity • Growth measures plotted at less than 5th percentile or more than 95th percentile
2. Triglyceride level 4 hours after intralipid infusion initiated. If level is 400 mg/dL or more, stop infusion and recheck every 4 hours until level is 200 mg/dL or less (or acceptable level for the child)	Hyperlipidemia usually occurs within 4 hours of initiation of the infusion.[2]	
3. Laboratory values (chemistry/metabolic panel) every 12 hours for initial 24 to 48 hours of infusion and then at prescribed frequency.	Monitoring of laboratory values ensures adequate fluid, electrolyte, and nutrition needs (see Figure 180-1, Table 180-1, and Table 183-1).	• Electrolyte imbalance • Elevated liver function test (LFT) results • Decreased total protein, albumin, and prealbumin levels • Increased transferrin value • Decreased Hgb and Hct values • Glucose level of more than 120 mg/L or less than 60 mg/L (or as indicated)[8] • Dehydration • Fluid overload
4. Complete blood count every 24 hours for first 48 hours, then twice each week, or as prescribed.	Acute changes may be the first sign of infection.	• More than 10% variation from child's baseline values
5. Monitor and record vital signs and fluid status at prescribed intervals.	Subnormal or elevated temperature and changes from normal range of vital sign parameters may be indicators of infection or child's intolerance of PN.	• Acute changes or significant trend changes from child's baseline status
6. Catheter insertion site.	Site edema, erythema, or tenderness may be precursor to systemic infection. Leakage from the site may be indicative of a crack or tear in the catheter.	• Erythema • Tenderness • Edema • Any type of drainage from the site

Documentation

- Date and time of initiation of PN
- Baseline and routinely measured laboratory values
- Assessment of catheter insertion site
- Growth parameters
- Vital signs and physical assessment findings
- Additional interventions necessary
- Child and family education
- Unexpected outcomes and related treatment

References

1. Donahue M: Parenteral nutrition. In McHale DJ, Carlson KK, editors: *AACN procedure manual for critical care,* ed 4, Philadelphia, 2001, Saunders.
2. Worthington P, Gilbert KA, Wagner BA: Parenteral nutrition for the acutely ill, *AACN Clin Issues* 11(4): 559-579, 2000.
3. American Society for Parenteral and Enteral Nutrition, Board of Directors: Guidelines for the use of parenteral and enteral nutrition in adult and pediatric patients, *JPEN* 26(suppl):1SA-138SA, 2000
4. University of South Carolina School of Medicine: Section 14: adult parenteral nutrition, from http://www.med.sc.edu:1060/nutrition/nm.htm. Retrieved October 10, 2006.
5. Irving SY, et al: Nutrition for the critically ill child: enteral and parenteral support, *AACN Clin Issues* 11(4):541-558, 2000.
6. Worthington P, Reyen L: Administration and management of parenteral nutrition. In Worthington PH, editor: *Practical aspects of nutritional support: an advanced practice guide,* Philadelphia, 2004, Saunders.
7. McGinnis C: Parenteral nutrition focus: nutrition assessment and formula composition, *J Infus Nurs* 25:54-64, 2002.
8. Syrinivasan V, Spinella P, Drott H, et al: Association of timing, duration, and intensity of hyperglycemia with intensive care unit mortality in critically ill children, *Pediatr Crit Care Med* 5:329-336, 2004.

Additional Readings

American Society for Parenteral and Enteral Nutrition: Standard of practice for nutrition support nurses, from http://www.nutritioncare.org/profdev/standardsnurse/htm. Retrieved October 10, 2006.

Deshpande KS: Total parenteral nutrition and infections associated with use of central venous catheters, *Am J Crit Care* 12:326-327,380, 2003.

Lyman B: Metabolic complications associated with parenteral nutrition, *J Infus Nurs* 25:36-44, 2002.

Transpyloric Feeding Tube: Insertion

P U R P O S E : A transpyloric feeding tube is inserted into the gastrointestinal (GI) tract and advanced past the pylorus in the child who is at risk for aspiration and in situations in which gastric feedings are not preferred. The transpyloric tube is used for administration of nutrients, fluid, and medications.

Ruth M. Lebet and Judy Trivits Verger

PREREQUISITE KNOWLEDGE

- Child development as it relates to clinical assessment and procedure
- Anatomy and physiology of the upper and lower GI tract
- A functioning GI tract is necessary for digestion and absorption of enteral nutrition.
- Tubes specifically designed for transpyloric placement are typically small bore and are packaged with guidewires already in the lumen to assist with passage of the tube.
- Small-bore feeding tubes are not designed for drainage of GI contents.
- Absolute contraindications for insertion of a nasoenteric feeding tube are basilar skull fracture, mechanical bowel obstruction, and esophageal varices. Recent esophageal or gastric anastomoses are relative contraindications.

CHILD AND FAMILY ASSESSMENT

- Child's developmental level and ability to interact ➙*Rationale:* Influences preparation and interaction.
- Child's and family's understanding of the reasons for and risks and benefits of administering parenteral nutrition ➙*Rationale:* Evaluates child's and family's understanding of procedure and provides a gauge for ongoing education.
- History of nasal or palate deformity, gastric fundoplication, gastric or esophageal surgery, and esophageal and pyloric malformations or injuries ➙*Rationale:* These conditions may complicate the passage of a feeding tube.
- Level of consciousness and cognitive ability ➙*Rationale:* Determine the need for and ability to prearrange a signal that the child will use to indicate gagging during tube passage.
- Status of upper respiratory tract ➙*Rationale:* Excessive upper airway secretions interfere with the child's ability to tolerate passage of the tube.
- Patency of the nares ➙*Rationale:* A tube cannot pass through an occlusion.
- Function of GI tract ➙*Rationale:* A functional gut is needed to administer enteral feedings.
- Desire of family members to be present during procedure ➙*Rationale:* Family members may provide support and comfort measures to the child but should have the choice not to remain with the child.

CHILD AND FAMILY EDUCATION

Individualized, developmentally appropriate education is provided to the child and to the family based on desire for knowledge, readiness to learn, and overall psychosocial state.

- Provide information about the transpyloric feeding tube, including the reason for the feeding tube and an explanation of steps involved in tube insertion ➙*Rationale:* Providing information decreases anxiety and fear.
- If developmentally appropriate, explain how the child can assist with passage of the tube (i.e., swallowing small

sips of water during tube insertion) ➥*Rationale:* Tube passes more easily with the child's cooperation.

- Explain that the child may gag during tube insertion ➥*Rationale:* Providing information decreases anxiety and fear.
- Explain the need to prevent tension on the feeding tube once it is in place ➥*Rationale:* Tube reinsertion and an additional x-ray may be necessary if the tube is displaced or removed.

EQUIPMENT

- Weighted or nonweighted soft flexible feeding tube with stylet designed for transpyloric placement (size guide-

lines: ≤10 kg, 5F or 6F; >10 kg, 8F; a 10F tube may be used in adolescents)[1-4]
- Saline solution–filled syringe (to flush tube with guidewire in place before procedure)
- Skin preparation agent
- Tape or semipermeable transparent dressing to secure tube
- Clean gloves
- Water-soluble lubricant (if tube is not prelubricated)
- Appropriately sized syringe
- Stethoscope
- Pacifier for infants
- Marker (optional)

Procedure for Transpyloric Feeding Tube: Insertion

Steps	Rationale	Considerations
1. Ensure that child and family understand preprocedural teaching.	Evaluates and reinforces understanding of previously taught information.	Developmental level influences understanding.
2. Collect all necessary equipment and supplies.	Preparation and presence of all materials facilitate completion of procedure in a timely manner.	Tube size is dependent on the child's size.
3. Ensure appropriate cardiopulmonary monitoring if indicated.	Some children may decompensate during the procedure.	Children who are critically ill may need more intensive monitoring.
4. Administer prokinetic agent (i.e., erythromycin or metoclopramide) as per institution-specific protocol. *(Level IV*)*	These agents may promote movement of the tube across the pylorus.[2,4-7]	Dose is dependent on weight of child and allergy history.
5. Wash hands.	Reduces transmission of microorganisms.	
6. Put on clean gloves.	Protects personnel health.	
7. Decompress stomach and consider removal of previously placed tube.	Passing a small-bore tube may be difficult with an oral or nasal gastric tube already in place.	Gastric tube may still be necessary for gastric decompression and may necessitate reinsertion after placement of a transpyloric tube.
8. Measure the tube from the tip of nose to the earlobe and then from the earlobe to the xiphoid process. Mark this distance on the tube (gastric mark). Measure the tube from the gastric mark to the left midaxillary line (pyloric mark). Mark this distance on the tube (Figure 184-1). *(Level IV*)*	To ensure accuracy of tube placement. Distance from the tube entry point to the xiphoid process approximates distance to the gastroesophageal junction. Distance from the gastric point to the left midaxillary line approximates the distance to the pylorus.[5]	Nearest centimeter mark can also be used to estimate length of tube placement.
9. Position the child in the right lateral recumbent position. Head of bed may be flat or elevated 30 to 45 degrees as condition permits. *(Level II*)*	Placing the child's right side down ensures that the pylorus is the lowest point within the stomach and may facilitate movement of the tube across the pylorus.[2-4,6,7]	The child may be supine for insertion of the tube to the gastric mark but should be turned right side down for passage past the pylorus. Infants, toddlers, and some older children may need assistance to

Procedure continues on following page

Procedure for Transpyloric Feeding Tube: Insertion—*Continued*

Steps	Rationale	Considerations

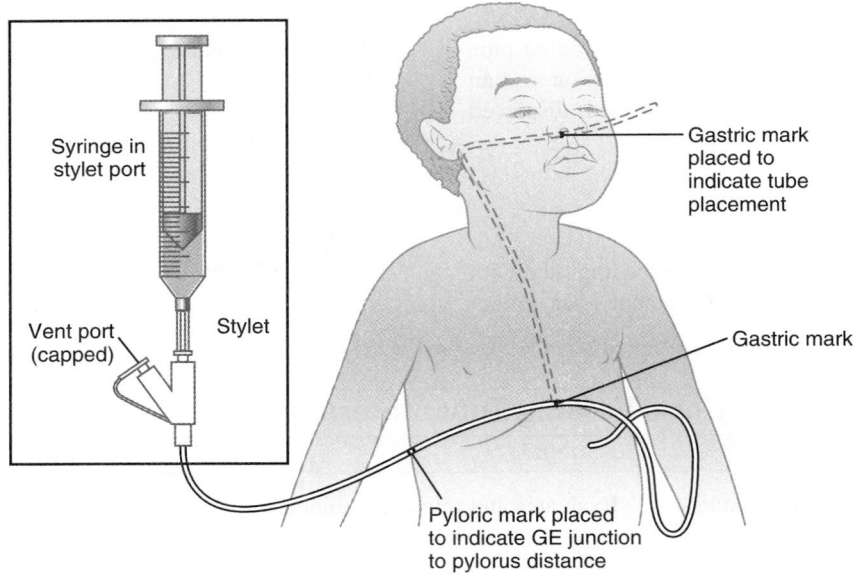

FIGURE 184-1   Gastric mark identifies estimated length needed for nasogastric (NG) placement. Spacing between gastric and pyloric marks equals distance from xiphoid process to right lateral costal margin, approximating estimated distance from gastroesophageal (GE) junction to pylorus. *From Harrison AM, et al: Nonradiographic assessment of enteral feeding tube position,* Crit Care Med *25:2055, 1997.*

Steps	Rationale	Considerations
		remain immobile during the procedure. A second person may be needed to help the child.
10. Flush tube with approximately 5 mL of water. Remove stylet before flushing tube if necessary. *(Level I*)*	Confirms patency and function of tube and facilitates removal of stylet after tube placed.	Volume of the flush used is based on assessment of the child, length and diameter of tube, manufacturer's recommendations, and institution-specific protocol.
11. If stylet was removed, reinsert and ensure that the guidewire is screwed in tightly.	Firmly secured guidewire assists with appropriate insertion.	If the tube has a secondary port, ensure that it is closed.
12. Ensure distal tip of the tube is lubricated. *(Level I*)*	Lubrication facilitates passage through nares.	If tube is self lubricating, dip the tip of tube in water. If tube does not have self lubrication, a water-soluble lubricant can be applied to the tube tip.
13. Gently but steadily thread the tube through nare (aiming posterior and parallel to nasal septum) to previously identified gastric mark. *(Level IV*)*	Allows for ease in following the normal anatomy.[3,5,7] Transpyloric tubes are typically inserted via the nares.	The child's anatomy may necessitate a variation in the angle of insertion. Assessment of the child's developmental level determines whether a second person is needed to help the child tolerate the procedure. Parental presence may be supportive.

* Level I: Manufacturer's recommendations only
  Level IV: Limited clinical studies to support recommendations

Procedure for Transpyloric Feeding Tube: Insertion—*Continued*

Steps	Rationale	Considerations
		Difficult passage, choking, coughing, cyanosis, and decreased oxygen saturations are indications of possible tracheal intubation. Remove tube and reattempt placement.
14. If the child is able to cooperate, ask the child to continuously swallow sips of water. *(Level IV*)*	Swallowing assists passage of the tube into the esophagus instead of the trachea.	Infants may be offered a pacifier.
15. Confirm stomach placement with auscultation or aspiration of stomach contents. *(Level IV*)*	Insufflation of air heard over the left side of the abdomen is typically used to confirm gastric placement.[1-8]	Smaller amounts of air are recommended for infants and young children.
16. Steadily advance and twist the tube toward the pylorus to the previously identified pyloric mark. *(Level IV*)*	Twisting the tube in a clockwise direction during advancement may help the tube move through the pylorus.[4,6]	Do not force the tube at any time. If resistance is felt, pull back to the gastric mark and reattempt passage through the pylorus.
17. Attach a syringe with 10 mL of air to the distal end of the tube.	Necessary for air insufflation.	
18. Quickly advance the tube approximately 5 cm simultaneously injecting 5 to 10 mL of air into the tube while auscultating over the right side of the abdomen. *(Level IV*)*	Advancing the tube the additional length ensures transpyloric placement.[3,5] Injecting air while inserting the tube may promote movement of the tube tip further into the small bowel.[3,4,7] If the tube has passed the pylorus, air is best auscultated over the right side of the abdomen.	Requires a second person. One person injects air and auscultates while the second advances the tube. Sounds of air injected in the small bowel sound higher pitched than air injected in the stomach (Figure 184-2).[2-6]

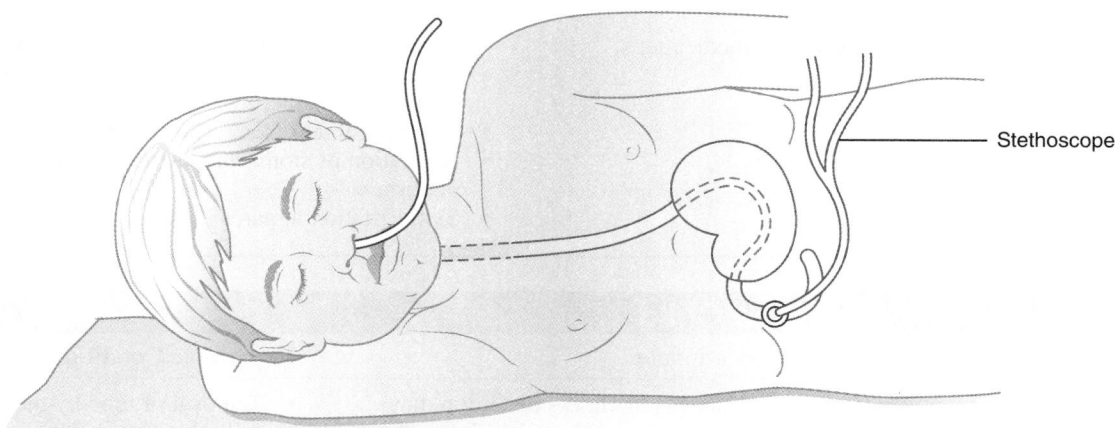

Stethoscope

FIGURE 184-2   When tube has passed through pylorus, insufflated air can be clearly auscultated over right upper quadrant. *From Ugo PJ, et al: Bedside postpyloric placement of weighted feeding tubes,* Nutrition Clin Pract *7:285, 1992.*

19. Confirm tube placement with inability to aspirate injected air. Tube placement may also be confirmed with ability to aspirate clear yellow bile. *(Level I*)*	The small bowel should not contain large amounts of air. Aspirates with pH of 7 or more and bilirubin of 5 mg/dL or more have been shown to be indicators of transpyloric placement.[3,6,8]	If a large amount of air can be aspirated, pull tube back to gastric mark and reattempt transpyloric insertion.

Procedure continues on following page

* Level I: Manufacturer's recommendations only
 Level IV: Limited clinical studies to support recommendations

Procedure for Transpyloric Feeding Tube: Insertion—*Continued*

Steps	Rationale	Considerations
20. When postpyloric placement has been confirmed, mark the tube at the nare.	Allows caregivers to identify whether the tube has been displaced.	
21. Apply skin preparation to face where tube will be secured and allow to dry.	Prepares surface of skin to help adherence of tape. Provides a protective barrier for the skin.	
22. Tape tube securely above the upper lip or cheek. Avoid taping the tube to the nare (see Figure 95-1).	Tube is more secure when taped to a nonmobile area; taping prevents tube from migrating into wrong position.	Consider medical restraint devices to maintain patency and position of tube as indicated by the needs of the child and institutional protocol.
23. Remove gloves and wash hands.	Reduces transmission of infection. Protects personnel health.	
24. Leave guidewire in place and obtain abdominal x-ray to verify placement. *(Level VI*)*	Abdominal x-ray verification is the safest way to ensure correct placement. Leaving the guidewire in allows the nurse to reposition tube if necessary.[3-5]	Never reinsert guidewire into the tube once it has been removed from the tube. *(Level I*)*
25. When placement is verified, hold tube at nares; remove and dispose of guidewire.	Guidewire removal is necessary to allow enteral feeding.	

* Level I: Manufacturer's recommendations only
  Level VI: Clinical studies in a variety of patient populations and situations to support recommendations

Expected Outcomes | Unexpected Outcomes

Expected Outcomes	Unexpected Outcomes
• Distal tip of tube is located in small bowel	• Tracheal or bronchial intubation as indicated by choking, coughing, cyanosis, and decreased oxygen saturations
• Patent tube accepts enteral feedings, medications, and fluid	• Pneumothorax from inadvertent pleural placement • Tube coiled in posterior pharynx, esophagus, or stomach • Esophageal tear from trauma of tube passing • Aspiration of stomach contents despite appropriate placement
• Skin integrity is maintained	• Skin irritation at nares

Monitoring and Care of the Child

Activities and Interventions	Rationale	Reportable Conditions
1. Monitor child's tolerance to feeding tube placement.	Changes in child's condition may indicate complications from tube placement.	• Removal of tube by the child • Agitation that results in an inability to place the tube • Persistent vomiting during placement attempts • Continued choking, coughing, cyanosis, and decreased oxygen saturations • Ulceration, drainage, or foul odor
2. Assess nasal and oral cavity and provide oral care every 4 hours and as needed.	Feeding tubes may cause the patient to mouth breathe, drying the mouth and increasing the risk of mucosal breakdown and ulcerations. Presence of the tube predisposes child to sinusitis or oral infections.	

Monitoring and Care of the Child—Cont'd

Activities and Interventions	Rationale	Reportable Conditions
3. Monitor insertion site of tube.	Frequent monitoring can prevent serious skin breakdown.	• Redness, swelling, drainage, bleeding, or skin breakdown at insertion site
4. Monitor child's vital signs per unit standards. Perform respiratory and gastrointestinal assessments every 2 hours and as needed.	Frequent monitoring for change in vital signs and respiratory or gastrointestinal assessment provide early detection of complications.	• Continued choking, coughing, cyanosis, and decreased oxygen saturations • Increased abdominal distention or abdominal girth; change in bowel sounds

Documentation

- Response to insertion
- Size, type, and length of tube placed
- Tube site assessments
- X-ray interpretation
- Oral care
- Additional interventions necessary during insertion
- Child's response to insertion
- Unexpected outcomes and related treatment
- Child and family education

References

1. Harrison AM, et al: Nonradiographic assessment of enteral feeding tube position, *Crit Care Med* 25:2055-2059, 1997.
2. Jaffe AR, et al: Validation of a blind transpyloric feeding tube placement technique in pediatric intensive care: rapid, simple, and highly successful, *Pediatr Crit Care* 1(2): 151-155, 2000.
3. Krafte-Jacobs B, et al: Rapid placement of transpyloric feeding tubes: a comparison of pH-assisted and standard insertion techniques in children, *Pediatrics* 98:242-248, 1996.
4. Powers J, et al: Bedside placement of small-bowel feeding tubes in the intensive care unit, *Crit Care Nurs* 23:16-24, 2003.
5. Chellis MJ, et al: Bedside transpyloric tube placement in the pediatric intensive care unit, *JPEN* 20:88-90, 1996.
6. Griffith DP, et al: Intravenous erythromycin facilitates bedside placement of postpyloric feeding tubes in critically ill adults: a double blind, randomized, placebo-controlled study, *Crit Care Med* 31:39-44, 2003.
7. Spalding HK, et al: Bedside placement of transpyloric feeding tubes in the pediatric intensive care unit using gastric insufflation, *Crit Care Med* 28:2041-2044, 2000.
8. Gharpure V, et al: Indicators of postpyloric feeding tube placement in children, *Crit Care Med* 28:2962-2966, 2000.

Additional Readings

Ellett ML, Beckstrand J: Predicting the distance for nasojejunal tube insertion in children, *J Soc Pediatr Nurs* 6:1231, 2001.

Lord LM, et al: Comparison of weighted vs. unweighted enteral feeding tubes for efficacy of transpyloric intubation, *JPEN* 17:271–273, 1993.

Metheny N, Titler M: Assessing placement of feeding tubes, *AJN* 101:36-45, 2001.

Zaloga GP: Bedside method for placing small bowel feeding tubes in critically ill patients, *Chest* 100:1643-1646, 1991.

AP

Enteral Nutrition: Initiation and Advancement

PURPOSE: Enteral nutrition is the optimal method for meeting the nutritional requirements of the child who has adequate gastrointestinal (GI) function but is unable to safely consume adequate oral nutrition

Dyana Burns Conway

PREREQUISITE KNOWLEDGE

- The GI tract should be used whenever possible unless contraindications exist.
- GI congenital anomalies, severe ischemic injury, necrotizing enterocolitis, hemodynamic instability with high vasopressor support, severe acute pancreatitis, GI obstruction or bleeding, and trauma or surgery to the bowel may lead the practitioner to limit enteral feedings.[1-3] If enteral feeding is initiated, the feeding is started at a low rate to provide trophic feeds and advanced slowly with assessment for feeding intolerance.
- Enteral nutrition can be the exclusive source of nutrition or can be administered in combination with oral or parenteral nutrition (PN). If fluid and caloric goals for enteral nutrition are not met within 72 hours, PN can be provided as an adjunct.
- Enteral feedings can be administered via the gastric (orogastric, nasogastric, or gastrostomic) route or via the transpyloric (nasoduodenal, nasojejunal, gastrojejunal, or jejunal) route (see Procedures 182 and 184).

- Considerations for the transpyloric route include delayed gastric emptying, GI dysmotility, poor gag reflex, gastroesophageal reflux disease, or ileus.
- The selection of formula is based on the child's age, nutritional requirements, digestive abilities, clinical status, and fluid limitations (see Procedure 180).
- Daily maintenance fluid requirements based on the child's age, size, and condition (see Table 180-1 in Procedure 180)
- Appropriate nutrient recommendations for the child's age, size, and condition. Several methods can be used to estimate energy needs. In calculation of suspected higher metabolic demands caused by such conditions as burns, cardiac disorders, failure to thrive, or trauma, estimation of the total energy expenditure (TEE) is recommended. The calculation for TEE is derived from resting energy expenditure (REE) plus the addition of factors for activity, injury, disease, and growth (see Figure 180-1 in Procedure 180).
- For the child who is critically ill, the use of the Recommended Dietary Allowance (RDA) may grossly overestimate caloric needs. Recent research has shown that energy needs may not be dependent on severity of illness but are tied to the phase of illness.[4,5] Caloric needs are reduced in the typical child in the pediatric intensive care unit who is mechanically ventilated, sedated, and paralyzed as a result of reduced activity.
- Overfeeding can cause many complications (hyperglycemia, fatty deposits in the liver, and increased carbon

dioxide production) that may hinder weaning mechanical ventilation and increase mortality.[3]

- Transpyloric feeding must be administered continuously. Gastric feedings may be administered continuously or with an intermittent schedule.
- Refeeding syndrome can occur with malnutrition. This syndrome is presumably caused by intracellular electrolyte shifts from glucose use and adenosine triphosphate production.[1,3] Correction of electrolyte disturbances and slow advancement of feeds are important to prevent further complications.

CHILD AND FAMILY ASSESSMENT

- Child's developmental level and ability to interact ➺➤*Rationale:* Influences preparation and interaction.
- Child's and family's understanding of the reasons for initiation and advancement of enteral nutrition ➺➤*Rationale:* Evaluates child's and family's understanding of the procedure and provides a gauge for ongoing education.
- Function of GI tract ➺➤*Rationale:* A functional GI tract is necessary for enteral feeding.
- Feeding and diet history ➺➤*Rationale:* Important considerations in determination of route and type of feeding.
- Historic growth data; birth weight, length, and head circumference are especially important for infants ➺➤*Rationale:* Comparison of growth parameters to normal values guides nutritional requirements (such as additional calories for catch-up growth, limiting of calories with obesity).
- Current anthropometric measurements, including admission weight, length or height, head circumference, body mass index for children >2yr of age, skin folds if available, and plots of these values on appropriate age and gender growth charts ➺➤*Rationale:* The measurement and evaluation of growth parameters are part of the foundation of the nutritional assessment. Admission measurements are necessary to determine effectiveness of enteral nutrition after initiation and advancement (see Procedure 181).
- History of conditions that impact GI malabsorption (e.g., cystic fibrosis, pancreatic insufficiency, short gut syndrome, intractable diarrhea, Crohn's disease, celiac disease, and hepatobiliary disorders), metabolic rate and fluid status (e.g., cardiac, hepatic, renal, or pulmonary disease), food allergy, and enteropathy (e.g., autoimmune or HIV associated)[4] ➺➤*Rationale:* These conditions influence the child's nutrition plan.
- History of developmental delay or mental retardation ➺➤*Rationale:* These children are at risk of development of obesity and osteopenia related to low REE and may need decreased caloric intake.

- Laboratory findings, including electrolytes (baseline sodium, potassium, calcium, phosphate, magnesium, blood urea nitrogen, creatinine, and glucose), liver function tests (LFT) (transaminases, alkaline phosphate, and bilirubin), serum proteins (total protein, albumin, prealbumin, and transferring), and hemoglobin (Hgb) and hematocrit (Hct) ➺➤*Rationale:* Baseline laboratory values provide data for selection of type and amount of formula and for the need for electrolyte supplementation. Depressed baseline protein levels indicate malnourishment. Hemoglobin and hematocrit values screen for anemia and iron status (see Table 185-1).
- Past and current medications ➺➤*Rationale:* Medications are evaluated to determine effect on nutrient intake and GI function. Assessment for potential drug and nutrient interactions (e.g., prednisone increases protein requirements).
- Cultural or religious dietary restrictions ➺➤*Rationale:* Individualized nutritional plans consider the child's cultural and religious preferences. Strict vegetarians may need soy-based formula.[4]

CHILD AND FAMILY EDUCATION

Individualized, developmentally appropriate education is provided to the family and to the child based on desire for knowledge, readiness to learn, and overall neurologic and psychosocial state.

- Explain the need for initiation of enteral nutrition and the process for advancement to meet full nutritional requirements to both the child and family ➺➤*Rationale:* Providing information decreases anxiety and fear and promotes understanding of treatment regimen and possible length of therapy.
- When indicated, discuss the need for long-term enteral nutritional support for the child ➺➤*Rationale:* Enteral tube feeding that is expected to exceed 4 to 6 weeks and long-term feeding necessitate gastrostomy/jejunostromy placement.
- Explain feeding route and schedule ➺➤*Rationale:* The explanation may increase compliance with prescribed feeding regimen.
- Encourage questions and answer questions as they arise ➺➤*Rationale:* Reinforcement of information is needed during periods of stress.

EQUIPMENT

- Properly placed feeding tube
- Enteral formula
- Feeding pump

| TABLE 185-1 | Suggested Monitoring for Enteral Nutrition Therapy |

Parameter	Baseline (before starting therapy)	Initiation	Follow-up
Electrolytes, including potassium, glucose, calcium, magnesium, phosphorus, sodium	Yes	Daily until stable (usually 3 days)	Weekly
Triglycerides	Yes	Weekly	Weekly
CBC with diff	Yes	Twice weekly	Weekly
Liver function tests (transaminases, bilirubin, alkaline phosphatase)	Yes	Weekly	Weekly
Serum proteins (total protein, albumin, prealbumin, transferrin)	Yes	Weekly one time	Every 2 weeks
Heme-test stools	Yes	Each stool	Daily
Urine dipstick (glucose, ketones, specific gravity, pH)	Yes	Daily	Weekly
Weight, length, head circumference	Yes	Daily (weight) Weekly (length/height, head circumference)	2-3 times/week Weekly/monthly
I & O	Yes	Daily	Daily

* Depending on age of child.
CBC with diff, Complete blood cell count; *I & O,* intake and output.
From American Society for Parenteral and Enteral Nutrition, Board of Directors: Guidelines for the use of parenteral and enteral nutrition in adult and pediatric patients, *JPEN* 26(suppl):1SA-138A, 2002.

Procedure for Enteral Nutrition: Initiation and Advancement

Steps	Rationale	Considerations
1. Determine maintenance fluid/caloric/protein requirements (see Table 180-1 and Figure 180-1). *(Level V*)*	Enteral feeding is based on the individual needs of the child. Determination of the child's fluid requirements and caloric/protein needs helps in development of an individualized nutritional plan of care.[1,3]	
2. Determine route of feeding (e.g., gastric or transpyloric). *(Level VI*)*	Transpyloric feeding is preferred in children at risk for aspiration and gastric feeding intolerance.[1]	Continuous enteral feeding is the preferred method of nutrient delivery in the child who is critically ill.[6,7]
3. Determine appropriate formula and begin with full strength. *(Level VI*)*	Children with normal GI tract function and no history of hemodynamic instability are started with full-strength formula to meet the fluid volume and caloric goals within 24 hours.[1,3]	Lower strength (e.g., half-strength) formula may be used for children with GI dysfunction. Trophic feeds may be initiated and advanced slowly. Once fluid goal is reached, the caloric strength is slowly increased to meet caloric goals.
4. Determine volume of feeding that meets caloric goal. Divide total volume by 24 (Box 185-1). *(Level II*)*	Determines the total fluid hourly goal per day.[1]	For most children, the total feeding volume equals the maintenance fluid requirement. In patients with fluid restriction, subtract the 24-hour volume of other infusions to determine total feeding volume.
5. Divide this volume by 4 for starting infusion rate. *(Level II*)*	Determines the initial infusion rate.[1]	Trophic feeds may be administered initially with concern for GI intolerance. Trophic feeds are administered at a lower infusion rate, typically 1 to 5 mL/h.

* Level II: Theory-based; no research data to support recommendations; recommendations from expert consensus group may exist
Level V: Clinical studies in more than one or two patient populations and situations to support recommendations
Level VI: Clinical studies in a variety of patient populations and situations to support recommendations

Procedure **for Enteral Nutrition: Initiation and Advancement**—*Continued*

Steps	Rationale	Considerations
6. Increase by same rate every 6 hours until goal is reached. *(Level II*)*	Increasing the rate every 6 hours achieves the fluid/caloric/protein needs of the patient in a 24-hour period.[1,3]	Advancement is child specific. The rate can be increased less frequently in children with GI dysfunction or hypoperfusion to the gut.
7. Maximize calories by increasing fluid limit, concentrating formula, or adding calorie modifiers. *(Level VI*)*	May be necessary to attain adequate growth and development [1,3,8,9]	As feeding is advanced, perform only one change (i.e., concentration, rate, or formula) at a time. For children with a fluid restriction, consider concentrating formula (e.g., 27 cal/oz) or adding caloric modifiers.

Procedure for Transitioning to Gastric Bolus Feeds

Steps	Rationale	Considerations
8. Multiply hourly infusion rate by 3 and infuse over 2 hours with a 1-hour rest. Monitor for 24 hours. *(Level II*)*	Compress feeds slowly and monitor for tolerance.	If feeding delivery is transpyloric (i.e., nasojejunal), the transpyloric tube must be pulled back to the gastric position before transitioning to bolus feeds. During transitions, observation for vomiting, diarrhea, abdominal discomfort, increased abdominal girth, and increased gastric residuals is especially important.[1]
9. Take the previous amount infused and compress to infuse over 1½ hours with 1½ hours rest. Monitor for 24 hours. *(Level II*)*	Rate of feeding compression is based on child's daily signs and symptoms of feeding tolerance.	Compression can be done every other day if child shows clinical signs of intolerance (e.g., mild abdominal distension, increased gastric residuals).
10. Compress further and infuse total amount over 1 hour with a 2-hour rest. Monitor for 24 hours. *(Level II*)*		
11. Last compression is to bolus feed. Amount is given over 30 minutes or with gravity every 3 hours. *(Level II*)*		

Procedure for Transitioning to Oral Feeds

Steps	Rationale	Considerations
12. Assess the following to determine readiness to transition from tube to oral feeds: Toleration of gastric bolus feeding. Resolution of the initial problem that precipitated the use of the tube. Quality of oral motor skills. Documentation of adequate or safe swallowing skills. *(Level VI*)*	Determines the children's readiness for safe transitioning to oral feeds.[3]	Consider bedside swallow examination with speech therapy or consider a modified barium swallow if child has had major neurologic sequelae from illness or is not at baseline status.

Procedure continues on following page

* Level II: Theory-based; no research data to support recommendations; recommendations from expert consensus group may exist
  Level VI: Clinical studies in a variety of patient populations and situations to support recommendations

AP This procedure should be performed only by physicians, advanced practice nurses, and other health care professionals (including critical care nurses) with additional knowledge, skills, and demonstrated competence per professional licensure or institutional standard.

Procedure	for Enteral Nutrition: Initiation and Advancement—*Continued*	
Steps	**Rationale**	**Considerations**
13. For the infant, offer the previous bolus amount orally with a bottle. Attempt to feed over a maximum of 30 minutes. The amount of formula not taken orally should be given as bolus feed via gastric tube. For the child who normally eats table food, begin with liquids from a cup and advance as tolerated. *(Level II*)*	For children with inconsistent oral intake, supplementation with enteral tube feeding is necessary to meet growth and developmental needs.[3]	Children recovering from critical illness are assessed for signs of clinical distress (e.g., tachypnea, diaphoresis, agitation) with initiation of oral feeds.
14. Once the infant or child is able to safely consume 100% of the nutritional requirements, the tube feeding can be discontinued. *(Level II*)*		The feeding tube may be removed earlier for the child or adolescent

* Level II: Theory-based; no research data to support recommendations; recommendations from expert consensus group may exist

Box 185-1	**Initiation and Advancement of Continuous Enteral Feeding for a 6-kg Infant**

Maintenance fluid requirement = 600 mL/d (100 mL/kg/d)
Daily energy requirement = 600 kcal/d (100 kcal/kg/d)
Daily protein requirement = 12 g/d (2 g/kg/d)

Day 1
600 mL/d ÷ 24 = 25 mL ÷ 4 = 6 mL/h (round number)
Full strength Enfamil with Iron at 6 mL/h via transpyloric tube; increase by 6 mL/h every 6 h to goal of 25 mL/h = 100 mL/kg/d

Day 2
Maintenance fluid volume increased to 120 mL/kg/d = 30 mL/h or 720 mL/d

Day 3
Increase caloric content of Enfamil to 24 cal/oz = 96 kcal/kg/d
(24 cal ÷ 30 cal/oz = 0.8 × 720 mL/d = 576 kcal/d or 96 kcal/kg/d)

Day 4
Add safflower oil 3 mL TID (8 cal/mL) = 100 kcal/kg/d
[8 cal/mL × 3 = 24 cal ÷ 6 (wt in kg) = additional 4 kcal/kg/d]

Increasing fluid/calories is dependent on the child's disease process and status. If child has fluid restriction, consider increasing caloric content (i.e., 27 cal/oz or with caloric modifiers).

TID, Three times per day.

Expected Outcomes	**Unexpected Outcomes**
• Maintain growth velocity appropriate for age and gender • Provide nutrients safely and without complications	• Failure to meet growth targets • Abdominal distention • Emesis • Diarrehea • Infection • Pulmonary aspiration • Drug or nutrient interactions
• Maintain stable fluid and electrolyte balance	• Dehydration • Hyperglycemia/hypoglycemia and electrolyte imbalance

Monitoring and Care of the Child

Activities and Interventions	Rationale	Reportable Conditions
1. Monitor for proper tube placement with radiographic confirmation before usage.	Prevents delivery of feeding into the esophagus or lungs.[1,3,8,10,11]	• Improper tube placement
2. Monitor feeding tolerance by noting presence or absence of vomiting, abdominal distension, and diarrhea. For gastric feedings, checking the residual formula volume is necessary to evaluate feeding tolerance. *(Level V*)*	Increased abdominal girth and large residuals indicate decreased gastric motility or emptying. Continuation of feeds with large residuals increases the risk for vomiting and pulmonary aspiration.[1,3,8,10,11]	• Abdominal girth increased more than 10% from baseline • For continuous feeds, residual greater than amount delivered in previous 2 hours • For intermittent or bolus feeds, residual greater than one half the volume delivered[3]
3. Monitor fluid status, including intake and output (urine output, emesis and stools).	Malabsorption and GI irritation can impact feeding tolerance.[1,3,8]	• Fluid imbalance • Vomiting • Oliguria • Diarrhea • Constipation
4. Monitor laboratory values (electrolytes, LFT, serum proteins, Hgb, Hct), including serum glucose levels.	Metabolic complications, such as electrolyte imbalances, dehydration, overhydration, hypoglycemia, and anemia, can occur with artificial modes of providing nutrition.[1,3,9] Infants are especially vulnerable to hypoglycemia or hyperglycemia.	• Electrolyte imbalance • Elevated LFT results • Decreased total protein, albumin, and prealbumin levels • Increased transferrin value • Decreased Hgb and Hct values • Glucose level of more than 120 mg/L or less than 60 mg/L (or as indicated)
5. Monitor for refeeding syndrome in children with a prolonged period without nutrition or in the malnourished child.	A prolonged period with nutrition and a malnourished state can lead to significant electrolyte disturbances.	• Hypophosphatemia • Hypomagnesemia • Hypokalemia • Respiratory distress

* Level V: Clinical studies in more than one or two patient populations and situations to support recommendations

Documentation

• GI assessment
• Fluid balance (weight, intake and output, emesis, stools)
• Laboratory values
• Date and time of initiation
• Type and strength of enteral nutrition, including modifiers
• Goal for total fluid volume, caloric intake, and protein needs
• Total mL/kg/d and kcal/kg/d delivered
• If bolus feeds, total volume delivered and frequency given
• If continuous feeds, initial rate of infusion and amount and frequency of advancement to achieve fluid goal
• Any signs of feeding intolerance
• Child and family education
• Unexpected outcomes and related treatment

References

1. Irving SY, et al: Nutrition for the critically ill child: enteral and parenteral support, *AACN Clin Issues* 11(4):541-558, 2000.
2. McClave SA, et al: Enteral tube feeding in the intensive care unit: factors impeding adequate delivery, *Crit Care Med* 27(7):1252-1256, 1999.
3. Nevin-Folino NL: *Pediatric manual of clinical dietetics,* ed 2, 2003, Pediatric Nutrition Practice Group, Chicago, American Dietetic Association.
4. Briassoulis G, et al: Energy expenditure in critically ill children, *Crit Care Med* 28:1166-1172, 2000.
5. White MS, et al: Energy expenditure in 100 ventilated, critically ill children: improving the accuracy of predictive equations, *Crit Care Med* 28:2307-2312, 2000.
6. Javid PJ, Jaksic T: The critically ill child. In Walker WA, et al, editors: *Nutrition in pediatrics,* ed 3, London, 2003, BC Decker.
7. Meert KL, et al: Gastric vs. small-bowel feeding in critically ill children receiving mechanical ventilation: a randomized controlled trial, *Chest* 126(3):872-878, 2004.
8. Adam S: Standardization of nutritional support: are protocols useful? *Intens Crit Care Nurs* 16:283-289, 2000.
9. Bettler J, Roberts KE: Nutrition assessment of the critically ill child, *AACN Clin Issues* 11(4):498-506, 2000.
10. Lynn-McHale Wiegand DJ, Carlson KK: *AACN procedure manual for critical care,* ed 5, Philadelphia, 2005, Elsevier.
11. Parrish CR: Enteral feeding: the art and the science, *Nutr Clin Pract* 18(1):76-85, 2003.
12. Grant MC, Martin S: Delivery of enteral nutrition, *AACN Clin Issues* 11(4):507-516, 2000.

Additional Readings

Burd RS, Lentz CW: The limitations of using gastric residual volumes to monitor enteral feedings: a mathematical model, *Nutr Clin Pract* 16(6):349-354, 2001.

Davies AR, et al: Randomized comparison of nasojejunal and nasogastric feeding in critically ill patients, *Crit Care Med* 30(3):586-590, 2002.

Hildebrandt LA, et al: Comparison of post-pyloric vs. gastric enteral formula administration, *Topics Clin Nutr* 17(3):44-51, 2002.

Neumann DA, DeLegge MH: Gastric versus small-bowel tube feeding in the intensive care unit: a prospective comparison of efficacy, *Crit Care Med* 30(7):1436-1438, 2002.

AP
Parenteral Nutrition: Initiation and Advancement

P U R P O S E : Parenteral nutrition (PN) is intended to safely provide nutritional support to children who are unable to receive adequate enteral nutrition

Sharon Y. Irving

PREREQUISITE KNOWLEDGE

- Child's baseline nutritional status and effects of disease process on metabolic needs
- Minimum fluid, caloric, protein, and electrolyte requirements for the child (see Table 180-1, Figure 180-1, and Table 183-1)
- Fluid requirements are often based on kilogram of body weight. Body surface area (m^2) is also frequently used to determine fluid needs (1500 mL/m^2/d). This method is particularly useful for obese children.
- The child's total body water is approximately 70% of body weight (between 75 and 85 mL/kg).
- Children who are unable to fully use the oral or enteral route for nutrition are prescribed PN as sole or adjunct therapy to meet nutritional requirements.
- PN consists of a complex hyperosmolar formulation of dextrose, amino acids, electrolytes, minerals, vitamins, and trace elements. The composition of these components makes it suitable to meet the child's nutritional needs.
- PN is indicated when the child's gastrointestinal (GI) function is inadequate to support nutritional needs or when enteral feeding is contraindicated in conditions such as GI obstruction, bleeding, or hemodynamic instability with high vasopressor support.[1,2]
- Relative contraindications for PN include inadequate intravenous (IV) access, short duration of therapy (usually less than 5 days), unstable fluid and electrolyte status, and imminent death from underlying disease state or patient condition.[3,4]
- Central access is usually preferred over peripheral access for long-term delivery of maximum fluid and nutrient requirements; however, peripheral PN has less complications associated with its administration.[5]
- Peripheral PN has a final dextrose concentration of 12.5% or less and is intended to supplement dietary intake.
- Centrally delivered PN therapy is intended to provide the child's total nutritional needs with dextrose concentrations 15% or greater.
- Pediatric formulations of amino acids for use in PN have profiles tailored to meet growth requirements of infants and children. TrophAmine contains tyrosine, cysteine, and glutamine (similar to amounts in breast milk, which is considered the standard).[6] Aminosyn and Novamine are recommended for children more than 6 months of age.[6]
- Lipid solutions (i.e., intralipids) provide fats and essential fatty acids. Lipid solutions may be infused separately or as an admixture (three-in-one solution with lipid emulsion mixed with amino acid–glucose solution and administered through a single line). When administered from a

separate bottle, intralipids are "piggy-backed" into the PN infusion distal to the PN in-line filter, close to the child's IV site. A separate infusion pump is used.

- Although solutions are available in 10% and 20% concentrations, 20% solution is most often the infusion of choice because of the increased caloric content (2 kcal/mL). The use of a filter with lipid solutions is not necessary unless the lipids are delivered in an admixture or combined PN intralipid solution. In this case, a 1.2-micron filter is appropriate.
- Cycling of PN may be preferred. Physiologically, cycled PN allows enzymes and hormones to regulate similar to regular eating and fasting patterns.[1,5,7] Cycled PN is typically infused over 10 to 16 hours per day. To decrease the delivery time, the cycled time is compressed by 2 to 4 hours daily until the goal is met. A common indication for cycled PN is to optimize normalcy for children on long-term therapy. Cycled PN may also be prescribed to boost the child's appetite.[1]
- Laboratory findings, including electrolytes (sodium, potassium, calcium, phosphate, magnesium, blood urea nitrogen, creatinine, and glucose), liver function tests (transaminases, alkaline phosphate, and bilirubin), serum proteins (total protein, albumin, prealbumin, and transferrin), and hemoglobin and hematocrit (Table 186-1)
- Institution-specific protocol policy regarding PN handling and administration
- Knowledge of operation of electronic infusion device suitable for PN and intralipid delivery

CHILD AND FAMILY ASSESSMENT

- Child's developmental level and ability to interact ➠*Rationale:* Influences preparation and interaction.

- Child's and family's understanding of the reasons for and risks and benefits of administering PN ➠*Rationale:* Evaluates child's and family's understanding of the procedure and provides a gauge for ongoing education.
- Family's desire and ability to be involved with child's care ➠*Rationale:* The family can provide support to the child.
- Child's underlying diagnosis and indication for therapy ➠*Rationale:* Provides direction for initiation and advancement of PN administration.
- Child's preillness nutritional status, including anthropometric measurements and biochemical and laboratory markers (i.e., albumin, prealbumin, electrolytes, liver function tests, triglyceride, and complete blood count) ➠*Rationale:* Identifies risk factors and challenges associated with meeting the child's nutritional needs.[3,7,8]
- Use and function of child's GI tract, including tolerance and ability for oral or tube feeding ➠*Rationale:* Adequate motor skills and a functional GI tract are needed to administer enteral feeding. PN may provide partial or full nutritional support.[2,5,9]
- Child's IV access ➠*Rationale:* Access (either central or peripheral) determines the concentration of nutrients that can be supplied.[2,7,10]

CHILD AND FAMILY EDUCATION

Individualized, developmentally appropriate education is provided to the family and to the child based on desire for knowledge, readiness to learn, and overall neurologic and psychosocial state.

- Explain the procedure for administering PN, including the purpose, steps, and rationale ➠*Rationale:* Providing information decreases fear and anxiety.

TABLE 186-1	Suggested Monitoring for PN Therapy		
Parameter	Baseline (before starting therapy)	Initiation	Follow-up
Blood chemistries	Yes	Daily until stable (usually 3 days)	Weekly
Triglycerides	Yes	4 hours after initiation, then daily for 3 days	Weekly
CBC w/diff	Yes	Twice weekly	Weekly
Liver function tests (transaminases, bilirubin, alkaline phosphate)	Yes	Weekly	Weekly
Albumin/prealbumin	Yes	Weekly once	Every 2 weeks
Glucose	Yes	Every hour for 4 hours until consistently <150, mg/dl	Daily
Urine metabolic indices (glucose, ketones, urea nitrogen)	Yes	Daily	Weekly
Weight, length/height, head circumference	Yes	Daily (weight) Weekly (length/height, head circumference)	Two to three times a week Weekly/monthly*
I & O	Yes	Daily	Daily

* Depending on age of child.
CBC with diff, Complete blood count with differential; *I & O,* intake and output.

From American Society for Parenteral and Enteral Nutrition, Board of Directors: Guidelines for the use of parenteral and enteral nutrition in adult and pediatric patients, *JPEN* 26(suppl):1SA-138SA, 2002.
Irving SY, Simone SD, Hicks RW, et al: Nutrition for the critically ill child: enteral and parenteral support, *AACN Clin Issues* 11:541-558, 2000.

- Discuss appropriate expected outcomes for the administration of PN ➤➤*Rationale:* The family and medical team can formulate similar goals and expectations.
- Provide developmentally appropriate information to the child and family regarding PN therapy ➤➤*Rationale:* If the child is able to understand the importance of therapy, external complications (e.g., child can help "protect" IV access, child will not play with the tubing or infusion device, etc) may be decreased. Appropriate education can minimize or avoid contradiction or omission of information.[3]
- Use written materials as appropriate; discuss provision of essential fluids, nutrients, and calories and body's reaction and use of these with the child and family ➤➤*Rationale:* A

family handbook or pamphlet gives a reference source for questions and a better understanding of PN therapy. The family and child should understand that all essential nutritional components are provided by PN therapy.
- Encourage and answer questions as they arise ➤➤*Rationale:* Reinforcement of information is needed during periods of stress.

EQUIPMENT

- Peripheral or central IV access
- Institution-specific PN order form

Procedure for Parenteral Nutrition: Initiation and Advancement

Steps	Rationale	Considerations
1. Discuss the child's nutritional needs with the multidisciplinary team. *(Level II*)*	A multidisciplinary approach with documented recommendations for PN therapy supports positive outcomes and minimizes cost and associated complications. An accurate plan also serves as an evaluation tool for the child's progress.[3,7,8]	Written recommendations are essential to plan and direct the necessary nutrition support and to monitor adequacy of the therapy. Must be evaluated and revised on a daily basis.
2. Identify appropriate route of administration. *(Level IV*)*	Central PN is the preferred route of delivery for complete nutritional support. Peripheral PN is useful for a short period (less than 14 days) and can assist in prevention of malnutrition and as adjunctive therapy with enteral feedings.	Children with fluid restriction and increased metabolic needs require central PN to meet nutritional and fluid requirements.[2,7,8]
3. Complete a comprehensive evaluation of the child's nutritional needs and a plan for PN advancement (Figure 186-1).		
4. Calculate the child's maintenance fluid requirements as a starting point for prescribing PN.	Specific fluid needs are dependent on child's age, weight, current fluid status, and degree of illness.[5,9,11]	
5. Calculate the child's resting energy expenditure (REE; see Figure 180-1)	The REE reflects energy at rest in a thermoneutral environment and is the basis for determining the caloric needs of the child. *(Level II*)*	In acute and critical illness, adjustments are made to the REE by the addition of a stress factor typically multiplied by 1.5 to 1.6.[11]

Procedure continues on following page

---

* Level II: Theory-based; no research data to support recommendations; recommendations from expert consensus group may exist
Level IV: Limited clinical studies to support recommendations

Procedure | **for Parenteral Nutrition: Initiation and Advancement**—*Continued*

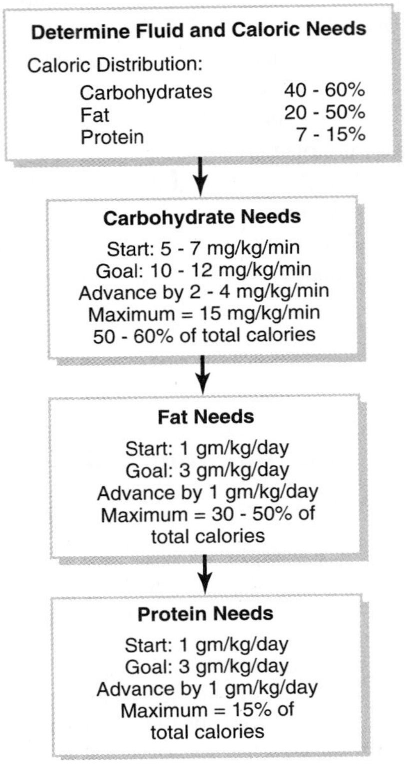

Steps	Rationale	Considerations

Determine Fluid and Caloric Needs

Caloric Distribution:

Carbohydrates	40 - 60%
Fat	20 - 50%
Protein	7 - 15%

Carbohydrate Needs

Start: 5 - 7 mg/kg/min
Goal: 10 - 12 mg/kg/min
Advance by 2 - 4 mg/kg/min
Maximum = 15 mg/kg/min
50 - 60% of total calories

Fat Needs

Start: 1 gm/kg/day
Goal: 3 gm/kg/day
Advance by 1 gm/kg/day
Maximum = 30 - 50% of
total calories

Protein Needs

Start: 1 gm/kg/day
Goal: 3 gm/kg/day
Advance by 1 gm/kg/day
Maximum = 15% of
total calories

FIGURE 186-1   Fluids and calories are based on patient needs and degree of injury or illness. Monitoring of electrolyte and metabolic laboratory values is necessary to determine degree of advancement for each parameter of parenteral nutrition. Advancement of protein and fat is based on normal renal and hepatic function in addition to clearance of triglycerides. *From Irving SY, et al: Nutrition for the critically ill child: enteral and parenteral support,* AACN Clin Issues *11(4):541-558, 2000.*

Steps	Rationale	Considerations
6. Determine grams of dextrose to be used to meet the child's caloric needs.	Dextrose is the major form of non-protein calories in PN. Approximately 40% to 60% of calories should come from carbohydrates in the form of dextrose.	IV dextrose provides 3.4 kcal/g. The glucose infusion rate (GIR; Table 186-2) is gradually increased to allow for appropriate insulin response, thus avoiding hyperglycemia.[2,5,8,9,12] A linear relationship exists between increased glucose energy intake, carbon dioxide (CO_2) production, and increased minute ventilation.[2,9,12]
7. Determine protein calories to be delivered as amino acid preparations. *(Level IV*)*	Between 7% and 15% of calories are given via amino acids.	Protein intake is usually maintained between 1 and 3 g/kg/d to promote a positive nitrogen balance. Protein provides 4 kcal/g (see Table 186-2).[5,8,9,12,13]
8. Determine electrolyte additive concentration for PN. *(Level V*)*	Electrolytes are essential in PN because they perform crucial physiologic functions.	Sodium and potassium are the major electrolytes added to PN. Calcium, magnesium, chloride, phosphorus, and acetate are other electrolytes added to PN formulas. Maintenance requirements are added unless deficits are identified (Table 186-3).[8,9,11]

* Level IV: Limited clinical studies to support recommendations
  Level V: Clinical studies in more than one or two patient populations and situations to support recommendations

Procedure for Parenteral Nutrition: Initiation and Advancement—*Continued*		
Steps	**Rationale**	**Considerations**
		Depending on individual require-ments, sodium and potassium are available in salt forms of chloride, acetate, and phosphate. Infants and young children have high calcium and phosphorus requirements for skeletal growth and may exceed compatibility limits of PN. TrophAmine (S. Braun Medical, Inc., Bethlehem PA) amino acid formulation allows for higher concentrations of these electrolytes.
9. Determine vitamins and mineral concentrations. *(Level IV*)*	Vitamins are necessary for cell function and metabolism. Vitamin deficiencies can rapidly develop and cause life-threatening compli-cations if vitamins are not included in PN.	Optimal requirements for vitamins are not yet determined; however, overdosing may lead to toxicity.[2,7,12] Standard multivitamin formulas are available in pediatric forms for children less than 11 years of age (see Table 186-3). Standard adult preparations are suitable for children 11 years of age and older.
10. Fat is provided via IV lipid emulsions and contributes to non-protein calories of PN. Use of 20% lipids is recommended. *(Level V*)*	Between 20% and 50% of daily calories are derived from fat. A 20% intralipid (IL) solution is used and provides 2 kcal/mL. A 20% IL solution is recommended because it is cleared more efficiently than 10% formulations.[6,8]	Minimum of 0.5 g/kg/d prevents essential fatty acid deficiency.[9,11] Increased rate of infusion can result in hyperlipidemia. Identify allergy to eggs and soy before prescribing. Traditionally, IL are egg-based formulations. Infants and small children have increased fat requirements for growth.[11]
11. Determine appropriate amounts of trace elements and minerals necessary for homeostasis and adequate growth. *(Level V*)*	Standard dosing is prescribed except with known deficiency or identified increased needs (Table 186-4).	In addition to promoting growth and development, trace elements and minerals assist in enzymatic processes and transport across cell membranes. Decreased copper and manganese are recommended with liver cholestasis.[10] Zinc deficiencies are rare; increased amounts are essential for tissue repair and wound healing.[1,4]
12. Determine the ratio of nonprotein calories (carbohydrates and fats) to protein calories in children with high protein needs. *(Level V*)*	To prevent negative nitrogen balance, PN must provide at least 80 to 100 nonprotein calories per gram of protein.[14]	Children with burns, intractable diarrhea, chest tubes with exces-sive drainage, and large blood losses have increased protein needs.

Procedure continues on p. 1361

* Level IV: Limited clinical studies to support recommendations
  Level V: Clinical studies in more than one or two patient populations and situations to support recommendations

TABLE 186-2	Parenteral Nutrition Initiation Calculations for a 3-year-old 15-kg Child	
Calculation	**Range**	**Example**
1. Determine child's fluid requirements	Determined by child's weight (see Table 180-1)	A 15-kg child's minimum fluid need = 1250 mL/d or 83.3 mL/kg/d or 52 mL/h
2. Determine patient's REE and TEE	REE for 3-year-old = 50 kcal/kg TEE = REE + [REE × (factors to account for growth, stress, etc)] Average TEE = REE + [REE × (0.5)]	REE = 750 kcal/d TEE = 750 + [750 × 0.5] = 1125 kcal/d Typically takes 3 days to reach caloric goal if electrolyte and fluid statuses remain stable
3. Calculate fat requirements (20% to 50% of total calories)	Start at 1 g/kg/d Use 20% IL solution = 2 kcal/mL 1 g of 20% IL solution = 5 mL	A 15-kg child = 15 g/d of IL IL hourly rate: 15 g × 5 mL = 75 mL/d or 3.1 m/L/h Calories from fat: = 75 mL/d × 2 kcal/mL = 150 kcal/d To determine remaining fluid volume for PN: Subtract IL volume from total daily fluid requirement Example: 1250 mL/d − 75 mL/d (IL) = 1175 mL/d (78 mL/kg/d or 50 mL/h) for PN
4. Calculate protein requirements (7% to 15% of total calories)	Start at 1 g/kg/d Amino acid solutions = 4 kcal/g Advance no more than 1 g/kg/d to goal	15 kg × 1 = 15 g/d Calories from protein: 15 × 4 kcal/g = 60 kcal/d To determine % amino acid solution: Divide grams of protein by the PN total fluid volume and multiply by 100 (for % protein) 15 g/d ÷ 1175 mL/d × 100 = 1.3% amino acid
5. Calculate carbohydrate requirements provided as dextrose. For central PN, start with 15% dextrose concentration (40% ÷ 60% of total calories). Gradually increase GIR over subsequent 2 to 3 days	IV dextrose yields 3.4 kcal/g GIR: [(% dextrose ÷ 100) × (mL/kg/d) × (1000) ÷ 1440 min/d]= mg/kg/min	Calories from dextrose: % dextrose ÷ mL/kg/d × 3.4 kcal [(15% ÷ 100) × (78 mL/kg/d) × (3.4 kcal/g)] = 39.8 kcal/kg/d or 597 kcal/d GIR = 8.1 mg/kg/min (15% ÷ 100) × (78 ml/kg/day) × (1000) ÷ 400
6. Calculate electrolyte requirements in accordance with child's needs and in parallel with minimum daily requirements	See Table 183-1	To determine electrolyte concentration per liter bag: mEq/kg/d ÷ (PN volume) mL/kg/d × 1000 mL = mEq/L Example: sodium = 3 mEq/kg/d (3 × 15 kg) ÷ 1175 × 1000 = 38 mEq/L
7. Determine need for addition or deletion of additives	Based on disease process, noted deficiencies, or necessary supplements	Examples: Standard heparin 500 U/L Delete copper and manganese with liver disease Add zinc for wound healing

REE, Resting energy requirements; *TEE*, total energy requirements; *GIR*, glucose infusion rate; *IL*, intralipid; *IV*, intravenous.

TABLE 186-3	Standard Vitamin Solution: Multivitamins for Infusion
Vitamin	**Dosage (per each 5 mL)***
A	700 µg
D	10 µg
E	7 mg
K	200 µg
Ascorbic acid (vitamin C)	80 mg
Thiamine (B-1)	1.2 mg
Riboflavin (B-2)	1.4 mg
Pyridoxine CL (B-2)	1 mg
Niacin	17 mg
Biotin	20 µg
Folic acid	140 µg
B-12	1 µg

*Infants greater than 3 kg receive 100% or 5 mL per PN solution.
Dosing reference: Manufacturer insert, DSM Pharmaceuticals, Inc, Greenville, NC.
Nevin-Folino NL: *Pediatric manual of clinical dietetics,* ed 2, 2003, Pediatric Nutrition Practice Group: Chicago, American Dietetic Association.

TABLE 186-4	Trace Element Requirements	
Trace Element	**Amount (kg/d)**	**Standard Dosage per Milliliter (neonatal injection)***
Zinc	100 to 300 µg	1.5 mg
Copper	20 µg	100 µg
Manganese	2 to 10 µg	77 µg
Chromium	0.14 to 0.2 µg	0.85 µg
Selenium	3 µg; maximum, 40 µg/d	
Iodide	1 µg	
Molybdenum	0.25 µg	

*Also pediatric 5 mL solution.
References: Manufacturer insert, American Regent Laboratories, Inc, Shirley, NY.
Nevin-Folino NL: *Pediatric manual of clinical dietetics,* ed 2, 2003, Pediatric Nutrition Practice Group: Chicago, American Dietetic Association.

Procedure for Cycling Parenteral Nutrition

Steps	Rationale	Considerations
13. Cycling is initiated by infusing PN volume over 20 hours. PN is "tapered up" to hourly rate during the first hour of infusion. Determine hourly rate and start at one fourth the rate and increase infusion every 15 minutes by same rate to hourly rate goal. For example, hourly rate is 20 mL/h. Start at 5 mL and increase by 5 mL every 15 minutes until at 20 mL/h.	Cycled PN optimizes normalcy for the child on long-term PN therapy. It may also boost the child's appetite. Cycling PN also decreases hepatic steatosis (fatty degeneration) and hyperinsulinemia. Graduated increase in starting cycled PN prevents hyperglycemia and helps achieve a steady state GIR.[5,8,9,12] *(Level V*)*	The child must have stable fluid and electrolyte status. Older children on a stable PN solution are candidates for cycled PN.[8] Steatosis is the result of excess caloric infusions, usually in the form of glucose.[6] Monitor blood glucose 1 to 2 hours into PN therapy when goal rate is achieved. As PN volume is compressed, the volume is decreased to one half to three fourths total maintenance fluid requirements. In addition, the amino acid and dextrose concentrations are decreased to limit protein to 2 to 3 g/kg/d and GIR to 10 mg/kg/min or less.
14. Infuse at goal rate for 18 hours. With previous example: 20 mL/h.	One to 2 hours are reserved as time to taper the PN infusion.	
15. During the last hour of infusion, PN is "tapered down" by decreasing rate by one fourth every 15 minutes until off. Using the previous example: decrease to 15 mL, then by 5 mL every 15 minutes until off.	Graduated decrease in stopping cycled PN prevents hypoglycemia in children with a high GIR. *(Level V*)*	Check glucose 1 hour after PN discontinued.
16. Increase time off PN by 2 to 4 hours daily. Goal is 10 to 12 h/d.	Weaning to the goal PN infusion rate and volume may take 3 days or more depending on the child's response.	As PN is cycled to fewer hours of infusion, the volume and concentration of PN is decreased. Monitor chemistries daily until at goal infusion.

* Level V: Clinical studies in more than one or two patient populations and situations to support recommendations

Procedure for Transitioning to Enteral or Oral Feeding

Steps	Rationale	Considerations
1. Determine tolerance of enteral or oral feeding.	Initiation of enteral feeding begins as soon as the GI tract is functional.	
2. *For enteral feeding:* Decrease PN/lipid volume milliliter per milliliter as enteral feeding is increased. If the child tolerates feeding advancement over 24 hours, discontinue PN.	Prevents hypoglycemia. Allows assessment of feeding tolerance before discontinuing PN therapy.	Monitor enteral feeding tolerance. Monitor blood glucose 1 hour after each decrease in PN therapy.

Procedure continues on following page

Procedure | for Transitioning to Enteral or Oral Feeding—*Continued*

Steps	Rationale	Considerations
3. *For oral feeds:* Decrease the PN hourly rate by one half for 2 hours, then decrease the rate by one half again for 2 hours, then discontinue PN	The PN therapy is not discontinued until the child can consume greater than half of nutritional requirements.[6]	Monitor oral intake and output. If less than half of daily fluid requirements are consumed during day, consider supplemental IV fluids over night. Reevaluate nutritional needs and route of administration. Monitor blood chemistries as indicated.

Expected Outcomes

- Maintenance of growth velocity appropriate for age and gender
- Balanced fluid status
- Chemistry/metabolic panel, complete blood cell count (CBC), and lipid levels within normal limits for the child
- Catheter site is free of infection

Unexpected Outcomes

- Failure to meet growth targets

- Fluid overload or dehydration
- Metabolic derangements

- Infection at catheter site or systemic infection

Monitoring and Care of the Child

Activities and Interventions	Rationale	Reportable Conditions
1. Weigh and measure child routinely; compare with baseline measurements. Document measurements on appropriate growth chart.	Evaluates response to enteral feeding. Growth measures reflect nutrition adequacy.	• Significant changes in growth velocity • Growth measures plotted at less than 5th percentile or more than 95th percentile
2. Triglyceride level 4 hours after intralipid infusion initiated. If level is 400 mg/dL or more, stop infusion and recheck every 4 hours until level is 200 mg/dL or less or what has been determined acceptable for the child	Hyperlipidemia usually occurs within 4 hours of initiating the infusion.[6] Intralipids are not continued if triglyceride level equals or exceeds 400 mg/dL.[3,12]	
3. Laboratory values: chemistry/metabolic panel every 12 hours for initial 24 to 48 hours of infusion.	Monitoring of laboratory values ensures adequate fluid, electrolyte, and nutrition needs are being met and the adjustments that are made to PN infusion are necessary.	• Abnormal values • Dehydration • Fluid overload
4. Complete blood count every 24 hours for first 48 hours, then twice each week.	Acute changes may be the first sign of infection.	• More than 10% variation from child's baseline values
5. Monitor child's ongoing tolerance of PN formulation. Make adjustments in the prescription as indicated.	Chemistry/metabolic values are compared with baseline values and followed daily until steady state of the PN formulation and normal laboratory values are attained (see Table 186-2).	• Electrolyte imbalance • Elevated liver function test (LFT) results • Decreased total protein, albumin, and prealbumin levels • Increased transferrin value • Decreased hemoglobin and hematocrit levels • Glucose level more than 120 mg/L or less than 60 mg/L (or as indicated)[15]
6. Monitor for complications related to PN therapy (see Table 183-2).	Complexity of PN therapy necessitates close observation to prevent deleterious effects.[2,7-9]	• Metabolic, infectious, or mechanical complications associated with initiation and advancement of PN

Documentation

- Date and time of initiation of PN
- Baseline and routinely measured laboratory values
- Assessment of catheter insertion site
- Growth parameters
- Vital signs and physical assessment findings
- Additional interventions necessary
- Child and family education
- Unexpected outcomes and related treatment

References

1. Donahue M: Parenteral nutrition. In McHale DJ, Carlson KK, editors: *AACN procedure manual for critical care,* ed 4, Philadelphia, 2001, Saunders.
2. Worthington P, Gilbert KA, Wagner BA: Parenteral nutrition for the acutely ill, *AACN Clin Issues* 11(4):559-579, 2000.
3. American Society for Parenteral and Enteral Nutrition, Board of Directors: Guidelines for the use of parenteral and enteral nutrition in adult and pediatric patients, *JPEN* 26(suppl):1SA-138SA, 2002.
4. University of South Carolina School of Medicine, Section 14: adult parenteral nutrition, from http://www.med.sc.edu:1060/nutrition/nm.htm. Retrieved October 10, 2006.
5. Irving SY, et al: Nutrition for the critically ill child: enteral and parenteral support, *AACN Clin Issues* 11(4):541-558, 2000.
6. Kleinman RE: Parenteral nutrition. In: *Pediatric nutrition handbook,* 2004, Chicago, American Academy of Pediatrics.
7. Worthington P, Reyen L: Administration and management of parenteral nutiriton. In Worthington PH, editor: *Practical aspects of nutritional support: an advanced practice guide,* Philadelphia, 2004, Saunders.
8. McGinnis C: Parenteral nutrition focus: nutrition assessment and formula composition, *J Infus Nurs* 25:54-64, 2002.
9. Teitelbaum DH, Coran AG: Perioperative nutritional support in pediatrics, *Nutrition* 14:130-142, 1998.
10. Nevin-Folino NL: *Pediatric manual of clinical dietetics,* ed 2, 2003, Pediatric Nutrition Practice Group, Chicago, American Dietetic Association.
11. Verger J, Schears G: Nutrition support. In Curley MAQ. Moloney-Harmon PA, editors: *Critical care nursing of infants and children,* ed 2, Philadelphia, 2001, Saunders.
12. Shulman RJ, Phillips S: Parenteral nutrition in infants and children, *J Pediatr Gastroenterol Nutr* 36:587-607, 2003.
13. Worthington P, Reyen L: Parenteral nutrition: indications and composition of formulas. In Worthington PH, editor: *Practical aspects of nutritional support: an advanced practice guide,* Philadelphia, 2004, Saunders.
14. Hart DWS, et al: Efficacy of a high-carbohydrate diet in catabolic illness, *Crit Care Clin* 29:1318-1324, 2001.
15. Syrinivasan V, et al: Association of timing, duration, and intensity of hyperglycemia with intensive care unit mortality in critically ill children, *Pediatr Crit Care Med* 5:329-336, 2004.

Additional Readings

Deckelbaum RJ: Intravenous lipid emulsions in pediatrics: time for a change? *J Pediatr Gastroenterol Nutr* 37:112-114, 2003.

Heine RG, Bines JE: New approaches to parenteral nutrition in infants and children, *J Pediatr Child Health.* 38:433-437, 2002.

Lipman TO: Grains or veins: is enteral nutrition really better than parenteral nutrition? a look at the evidence, *JPEN* 22:167-182, 1998.

Rogers EJ, Gilbertson HR, Heine RG, et al: Barriers to adequate nutrition in critically ill children, *Nutrition* 19:865-868, 2003.

Hypothermia/Hyperthermia Blanket and Use of BAIR Hugger® Warming Unit and Warming Cover

P U R P O S E : Hypothermia/hyperthermia units are used to increase or decrease body temperature or to maintain a desired temperature with an external source

Denise Ruffalo

PREREQUISITE KNOWLEDGE

- *Hypothermia* is any core temperature less than 35°C. Hypothermia is categorized as mild (32°C to 35°C), moderate (28°C to 32°C), and severe (<28°C). At body temperatures of less than 34°C, the hypothalamus functions minimally; and at temperatures of less than 29°C, it cannot regulate temperature at all.
- See Table 187-1 for the risk factors for hypothermia.
- Infants and children are among the high-risk groups for hypothermia, especially if they are unconscious, immobile, sedated, or malnourished.
- Infants and children are predisposed to thermal instability because of large body surface area, limited nutritional reserve, and impaired behavioral, neural, and endocrine response.
- When the temperature drops to a low enough level, shivering thermogenesis occurs. Shivering is triggered by a discrepancy between the temperature measured with peripheral temperature receptors and the temperature set point in the hypothalamus.[1] Shivering increases carbon dioxide production, metabolic rate, oxygen consumption, and myocardial demand. Neonates and infants less than 6 months of age cannot shiver to generate heat. The infant uses nonshivering thermogenesis, which breaks down

brown fat for the creation of heat. Nonshivering thermogenesis is a process that requires energy, so the infant's oxygen consumption increases when this occurs. Shivering may be treated with sedatives and neuromuscular blocking agents, which decrease the body's ability to shiver. Covering of the arms and legs during cooling decreases the temperature gradient during cooling; this decrease is associated with less frequent severe shivering.[1]
- See Table 187-2 for physiologic responses to hypothermia.[2]
- See Table 187-3 for complications of rewarming
- Hypothermia produces a decrease in the metabolic rate, which causes biochemical reactions to slow considerably. As a result, drug levels and drug effects are hard to determine. Intramuscular and subcutaneous injections may not be properly absorbed during hypothermia.
- Certain cardiac dysrhythmias are common in hypothermia. At less than 34°C, atrial fibrillation may occur; at less than 30°C, first-degree atrioventricular block may occur; and at less than 20°C, third-degree atrioventricular block may occur.
- Passive rewarming includes prevention of further exposure, removal of wet clothing, provision of a warm environment, and application of warm blankets.
- Active measures that may be implemented to rewarm are heated humidified air, warmed intravenous fluids, and

1365

TABLE 187-1	Risk Factors for Hypothermia

Cause	Mechanism
Exposure Trauma Drowning	Increased heat loss, especially conductive heat loss (wet clothes or immersion) or convective losses (wind)
CNS Depression Head injury Cerebral hemorrhage, tumor, infection	Direct central effect on thalamic temperature center
Drug-Induced Narcotics Barbiturates Phenothiazines Alcohol General anesthesia	CNS depression and vasodilation CNS depression Alpha-adrenergic block, lowered set point CNS depression CNS depression with vasodilation
Endocrine Abnormalities Hypoglycemia Hypothyroidism Hypopituitarism	Impaired thermogenesis, limited metabolic response Impaired hypothalamic response to cold
Spinal Cord Transection	Interrupted sensory afferent Inability to sense cold Impaired central reflex and behavioral responses
Skin Disorders Erythrodermas Burns Stevens-Johnson syndrome	Increased transdermal water and heat losses
Therapeutic Treatment of Reye's syndrome Cardiopulmonary bypass	CNS depression

CNS, Central nervous system.

gastric lavage with warmed solution. An external device such as a hypothermia/hyperthermia blanket, which circulates warmed water through coils in a pad or blanket, may be used to warm the child. In severe circumstances, cardiopulmonary bypass may be used to allow for direct perfusion of the central circulation with warmed blood.

- Continuous monitoring of the child's temperature is necessary during active rewarming therapy.
- The literature suggests that rewarming should not occur faster than 1°C every hour.[3] More recent literature suggests that rewarming should occur over a longer period of time (exact time has not been determined) to help improve neurocognitive outcome and decrease potential complications from rewarming.[4]
- In the state of *hyperthermia,* the child has a sustained elevation in body temperature (>37.8°C orally or 38.8°C rectally) because of internal or external forces.[5]
- Internal factors for hyperthermia are fever, malignant hyperthermia, and heat-related illnesses. External factors are environmental factors and accidental overheating.
- See Table 187-4 for physiologic responses to hyperthermia.
- Oxygen consumption rises 10% to 12% for every 1°C of temperature elevation.
- Methods of fever reduction are sponging with tepid water with or without the use of antipyretics and use of a hypother-

mia/hyperthermia blanket that circulates cooled water or air through coils in a pad or blanket placed under the child.

- Continuous monitoring of the child's temperature is necessary during active cooling therapy.
- Refer to manufacturer-specific guidelines regarding controls, alarms, safety features, and troubleshooting for the hypothermia/hyperthermia unit used. These instructions must be understood before the equipment is used.
- Child development as it relates to clinical assessment and active warming or cooling of the child

CHILD AND FAMILY ASSESSMENT

- Assess any existing cardiac abnormalities or inadequate heart function, including dysrhythmias ➤➤*Rationale:* Cooling may worsen preexisting cardiovascular dysfunction. Assessment of the child's response to therapy and potential side effects. Cardiac dysrhythmias are associated with the cooling and warming process. Bradycardia may occur as a result of sinus node depression from slowing of conduction through the atrioventricular node.
- Assess current medications administered ➤➤*Rationale:* Decreased cardiac output, dehydration, slowed hepatic metabolism, impaired glomerular filtration, and abnormal renal filtration can result in reduced drug clearance.[5]

TABLE 187-2	Physiologic Responses to Hypothermia
Central Nervous System	Decreased cerebral blood flow Progressive paralysis of central nervous system Reduced cerebral metabolic demand
Cardiovascular System	Decreased heart rate, contractility, and cardiac output Delayed depolarization in pacemaker tissue Electrocardiogram characteristics: increased PR, QRS, and QT intervals; J wave (J wave is deflection of QRS-ST junction); ST elevation; and T wave inversion Decreased transmembrane resting potential that results in atrial fibrillation or ventricular fibrillation
Pulmonary System	Hypoventilation Decreased cough reflex Increased airway secretions Paralysis of mucociliary mechanism
Gastrointestinal System	Hypomotility Decreased hepatic metabolism Decreased insulin release from pancreas Stress ulceration
Renal System	Impaired renal tubular transport that causes decreased sodium and water reabsorption Decreased antidiuretic hormone Fluid shift from vascular compartment to interstitial spaces
Acid-Base Balance	Decreased systemic carbon dioxide production Early respiratory alkalosis Eventual metabolic acidosis in severe hypothermia
Hematologic System	Shift of oxyhemoglobin dissociation curve to left, causing decreased oxygen delivery to tissues Increased blood viscosity Coagulopathy caused by inhibition of enzyme reactions of coagulation cascade and splenic sequestration of platelets
Immunologic System	Leukocyte sequestration in spleen Decreased neutrophil function Reduced collagen deposition

From Kelly EM: External warming/cooling devices. In Lynn-McHale DJ, Carlson KK, editors: *AACN procedure manual for critical care,* ed 4, Philadelphia, 2001, Saunders. Used with permission.

TABLE 187-3	Complications Of Rewarming
Complication	**Mechanism**
Acidosis	Rewarming causes peripheral vasodilation. Carbon dioxide production is increased associated with temperature increase and from return of accumulated acids in peripheral circulation to heart. Slow rewarming avoids sudden recirculating of these acids.
Rewarming shock	Hypothermia vasoconstriction masks hypovolemia. If child's circulation volume is insufficient during rewarming vasodilation, sudden decrease occurs in blood pressure, systemic vascular resistance, and preload.
Dysrhythmia	Rewarming places additional stress on already stressed myocardium.
Deep-ended hypothermia	As colder surface blood is returned to core, core temperatures may drop. Also referred to as "after fall" or "after drop."

- Assess baseline neurologic status ➤➤*Rationale:* Mental status and level of consciousness may change from either hyperthermia or hypothermia. Seizures may occur with hyperthermia. Muscle weakness, decreased coordination, lethargy, and poor judgment may occur with hypothermia.
- Assess baseline gastrointestinal function ➤➤*Rationale:* An ileus may occur with hypothermia because of decreased intestinal motility. Vomiting may occur with hyperthermia.
- Assess baseline skin integrity ➤➤*Rationale:* Application of a heating or cooling process may damage the child's skin and cause tissue damage. Disease processes that affect

peripheral circulation may put the child at increased risk. Hypothermia may cause immunosuppression; skin integrity is a child's first defense against infectious agents.
- Assess blood gases, electrolytes, and coagulation studies ➤➤*Rationale:* Alterations in temperature may change the acid-base balance, cause electrolyte imbalances (especially K+), and cause increased blood viscosity and coagulopathy. Hypoxemia may occur. Hypothermia causes a shift of the oxyhemoglobin dissociation curve to the left; therefore, less oxygen is released to the tissues. Hyperthermia causes a shift to the right, and oxygen is readily released.

TABLE 187-4	Physiologic Responses to Hyperthermia

System	Responses
Central nervous	Convulsions
	Increased cerebral metabolic rate, resulting in increased needs for oxygen and glucose
	Mental status changes
Cardiovascular	Increased metabolic rate
	Increased cardiovascular demand
	Increased heart rate
	Vasoconstriction or vasodilatation
Pulmonary	Increased carbon dioxide production
Musculoskeletal	Shivering
Skin	Diaphoresis, which may lead to electrolyte and fluid imbalances
Gastrointestinal	Vomiting
Hematologic/cellular	Increased inflammatory activity
	Destruction of body proteins and cells
	Elevated oxygen consumption
	Shift of oxyhemoglobin curve to right causing oxygen to be readily released

- Assess child's developmental level and ability to interact ➤➤*Rationale:* These factors influence preparation of the child and interaction.
- Assess child's and family's understanding of the reasons for and risks and benefits of the hypothermia/hyperthermia blanket ➤➤*Rationale:* Evaluates child's and family's understanding of the procedure and provides a gauge for ongoing education.

CHILD AND FAMILY EDUCATION

Individualized, developmentally appropriate education is provided to the family and to the child based on desire for knowledge, readiness to learn, and overall neurologic and psychosocial state.

- Provide information about the cooling or warming procedure to the child's family and in a developmentally appropriate manner to the child. Information should include reason for therapy, anticipated length of therapy, and temperature goal. ➤➤*Rationale:* Providing information decreases anxiety and fear.
- Encourage the child to verbalize any discomfort. Use age-appropriate pain scales per institution- or unit-specific protocol. See Procedure 173 for further information. ➤➤*Rationale:* Early detection of pain can optimize the child's comfort.
- Encourage questions and answer questions as they arise ➤➤*Rationale:* Reinforcement of information is needed during periods of stress.
- If the BAIR Hugger® (Augustine Medical, Inc., Eden Prairie, MN) is used, explain that the child's gown will be removed so that the BAIR Hugger® blanket is directly against the child's skin. Emphasize that the child's privacy will be maintained at all times. ➤➤*Rationale:* Child and family know what to expect, which decreases stress and anxiety and increases compliance.
- Encourage questions and answer questions as they arise ➤➤*Rationale:* Reinforcement of information is needed during periods of stress.

EQUIPMENT

- Sheet or light blanket
- Temperature probe and module to monitor child's temperature
- Cardiac monitor
- Hypothermia/hyperthermia unit with appropriately sized blanket
- Distilled water to refill water reservoir chamber as needed

BAIR Hugger® System

- Sheet and cotton blanket
- Temperature probe and module to monitor child's temperature
- Cardiac monitor
- BAIR Hugger® console with appropriately sized blanket

Procedure	for Hypothermia/Hyperthermia Blanket	
Steps	**Rationale**	**Considerations**
1. Ensure child and family understand procedure and all questions are answered.	Evaluates and reinforces understanding of previously taught information.	Developmental level, cognitive ability, and anxiety level determine approach to and effectiveness of teaching.
2. Collect equipment and supplies needed.	Facilitates completion of task in a timely manner.	Consider the child's size in selection of the appropriate blanket size.
3. Collect equipment needed for continuous monitoring of a core temperature.	Continuous monitoring of body temperature is necessary during warming and cooling therapy.	Some hypothermia/hyperthermia devices have a patient temperature probe integrated into the machine.

Procedure for Hypothermia/Hyperthermia Blanket—*Continued*		
Steps	**Rationale**	**Considerations**
4. Ensure the alarm system for the temperature monitoring system is functional and the alarm is sufficiently audible.	Promotes patient safety by avoiding inadvertent over-warming or cooling of the child.	
5. Insert power cord plug into a grounded AC receptacle.	Establishes a power source. A grounded power source promotes patient safety.	
6. Wash hands; put on clean gloves.	Standard precautions; reduces transmission of microorganisms.	
7. Apply the hypothermia/hyperthermia blanket flat on the bed and place a single dry sheet or blanket over the hypo/hyperthemia blanket.	Sheet or blanket protects the child's skin from moisture.	Avoid the use of heavy blankets or pads over the hypothermia/ hyperthermia blanket because this interferes with the heating or cooling process. Children may be at greater risk for skin breakdown because of the placement of the hypothermia/hyperthermia blanket beneath them. The hypothermia/ hyperthermia blanket may make pressure-reducing beds less effective.
8. Initially position the child with the back on the blanket.	The blanket warms or cools the child through conduction-transfer of temperature from one surface to another. Supine position ensures maximum body surface exposure to the heated or cooled blanket.	Any supports used to turn the child should be placed under the hypothermia/hyperthermia blanket.
9. Fill the water reservoir with distilled water to the designated level. *(Level I*)*	Insufficient water level causes damage to the internal components of the unit.	Do not use alcohol to fill the reservoir. Alcohol may accelerate blanket deterioration. Water level should be checked regularly during therapy and refilled as needed.
10. Attach the connection hoses to the blanket and machine. Close all clamps on the connection hoses and blanket before connecting.	Attachment of connections without clamping of hoses results in leaking of water.	
11. When all connections have been made, ensure that all connections are tight. Check for kinks in the tubing of the system. Release all clamps.	Failure to release clamps or correct kinks in the tubing prevents water flow to the blanket. Ensuring tight connections prevents spraying or leaking.	
12. Ensure appropriate privacy.	Decreases fear and respects child's right to privacy.	School-aged children may be especially modest. Ensuring privacy for this age group promotes feelings of security.
13. Place lubricated thermometer probe into the child's rectum and connect to the monitor or hypothermia/ hyperthermia unit temperature monitoring system.	Failure to monitor the child's temperature may result in skin damage or inappropriate temperature.	Rectal probes are contraindicated in children with neutropenia and should only be placed in these children with a prescribing practitioner's order. Attach probe securely to the child's leg to prevent dislodgement.

Procedure continues on following page

* Level I: Manufacturer's recommendations only

Procedure for Hypothermia/Hyperthermia Blanket—*Continued*

Steps	Rationale	Considerations
14. Turn on the machine.	Activates the machine.	

Procedure for Use of the Hypothermia/Hyperthermia Blanket in Manual Mode

Steps	Rationale	Considerations
1. Press the manual mode button.	Activates manual mode.	
2. Adjust the set point to the desired blanket temperature.	The machine monitors the water temperature and heats or cools the water circulating through the blanket to maintain the selected set point temperature.	The child's temperature must be monitored when manual mode is used. Manually adjust the blanket set point as needed to maintain the child's temperature at the desired level.

Procedure for Use of the Hypothermia/Hyperthermia Blanket in Automatic Mode

Steps	Rationale	Considerations
1. Press the automatic mode button.	The machine monitors and automatically adjusts the water temperature to maintain the child's temperature at the selected set point.	The temperature probe must be inserted and connected to the machine for this mode to be activated and to function properly.
2. Obtain the child's temperature as displayed on the hypothermia/hyperthermia blanket's display screen.	Baseline temperature is obtained before treatment is started.	Ensure the temperature probe is not dislodged.
3. Take the child's temperature with a thermometer and compare the two readings.	Ensures the hypothermia/hyperthermia blanket probe is functioning correctly.	
4. Adjust the set point to the desired temperature for the child.	Allows the machine to warm or cool the water as appropriate in response to the child's current and desired temperature.	
5. Discontinue cooling or warming treatment when the child's desired temperature is achieved and maintained.	Therapy is no longer required.	
6. When the hypothermia/hyperthermia treatment is discontinued, the child's temperature can still be monitored by pressing the monitor mode button.	Allows temperature monitoring with or without hypothermia/hyperthermia therapy.	
7. Discontinue continuous rectal temperature monitoring when therapy is no longer indicated.	Monitoring is no longer required.	

Procedure for BAIR Hugger Warming Unit and Warming Cover

Steps	Rationale	Considerations
1. Refer to steps 1 to 3 and 5 to 7 in the section Procedure for Hypothermia/Hyperthermia Blanket.	Initial steps are the same.	
2. Connect the hose of the warming unit to the blanket.	Supplies the blanket with warm or cool air to blow on the child.	Do not warm the child with the warming unit hose alone. Cases of thermal injury have been reported. *(Level I*)*
3. Ensure appropriate privacy.	Decreases fear and respects child's right to privacy.	School-aged children may be especially modest. Ensuring privacy for this age group promotes feelings of security.
4. Place lubricated thermometer probe into the child's rectum and connect to the monitor.	Supplies continuous temperature monitoring.	Rectal probes are contraindicated in children with neutropenia and should only be placed in these

---

* Level I: Manufacturer's recommendations only

Procedure	**for Hypothermia/Hyperthermia Blanket**—*Continued*	
Steps	**Rationale**	**Considerations**
		children with a prescribing practitioner's order. Attach probe securely to the child's leg to prevent dislodgement.
5. Remove the child's gown and blankets.	The blanket warms or cools with convection; warmed or cooled air is distributed around the child and directly on to the skin.	Respect the child's privacy with removal of gown.
6. Place the BAIR Hugger blanket directly on the child with the perforated side against the child's skin. (*Level I**)	The warmed or cooled air is delivered through these holes.	Do not leave children unattended during administration of therapy to prevent suffocation.
7. Press the on/off button and select the appropriate temperature setting.	Begins the air delivery.	
8. Place a cotton blanket over the BAIR Hugger blanket.	Prevents heat loss.	
9. Discontinue therapy when desired temperature is achieved and maintained.	Prevents overheating or overcooling.	
10. Monitor child's temperature.	Child's temperature is monitored with or without therapy.	
11. Discontinue continuous rectal temperature monitoring when therapy is no longer indicated.	Continuous monitoring is no longer required.	
12. Discard used supplies and equipment in appropriate receptacle; wash hands.	Standard precautions; reduces transmission of microorganisms.	

* Level I: Manufacturer's recommendations only

Expected Outcomes

- Desired temperature is achieved and maintained

- Child's skin remains intact
- Child is free from complications of hypothermia/hyperthermia

Unexpected Outcomes

- Inability to achieve desired temperature
- Overheating or overcooling of the child
- Breakdown in skin integrity
- Acid/base abnormality
- Cardiac/hemodynamic instability
- Shivering
- Neurologic changes from baseline

Monitoring and Care of the Child

Activities and Interventions	**Rationale**	**Reportable Conditions**
1. Complete physical assessment every hour.	Temperature changes can affect all body systems.	• Significant change in assessment
2. Continuously monitor core temperature.	Assesses child's response to intervention.	• Continued hypothermia or hyperthermia
3. Continuous cardiac monitoring.	Cardiac arrhythmias are a possible side effect of cooling or warming.	• Cardiac arrhythmia

Continued

Monitoring and Care of the Child—Cont'd

Activities and Interventions	Rationale	Reportable Conditions
4. Monitor blood pressure every 15 minutes for first hour of therapy and every hour thereafter, unless child's condition warrants more frequent monitoring.	Vasodilatation occurs with warming therapy. Vasoconstriction occurs with cooling therapy.	• Hypertension or hypotension
5. Assess skin integrity every hour; focus assessment on bony prominences.	Warming or cooling process may damage the child's skin.	• Skin injuries
6. Assess neurologic status.	Mental status and level of consciousness may change as result of hyperthermia or hypothermia.	• Change in mental status or level of consciousness
7. Monitor arterial or venous blood gases and electrolytes.	Alterations in temperature may change the acid-base balance and cause electrolyte imbalances.	• Abnormal blood gas or electrolyte values
8. Assess child's comfort and effectiveness of comfort strategies.	Ensures child tolerates therapy.	• Unrelieved pain
9. Assess shivering with palpation of the mandible for vibration and close inspection of facial, neck, and chest muscles for fasciculation.[3]	Shivering increases carbon dioxide production and increases metabolic rate, oxygen consumption, and myocardial demands. (Level V*)	• Shivering that persists
10. Monitor intake and output.	Insensible water loss can be increased during warming therapy.	• A positive or negative fluid balance

* Level V: Clinical studies in more than one or two patient populations and situations to support recommendations

Documentation

- Child and family education
- Child's temperature and route of temperature assessment
- Time of initiation and discontinuation of therapy and type of therapy used, including manual or automatic mode for hypo/hyperthermia blanket
- Temperature of warming/cooling blanket
- Child's response to therapy
- Vital signs and laboratory results
- Child's comfort level using a pain scale appropriate to the child's age and development level (see Procedure 173 and any specific interventions provided)
- Unexpected outcomes and related treatment

References

1. Cairns C, Andrews P: Management of hyperthermia in traumatic brain injury, *Curr Opin Crit Care* 8(2):106-110, 2002.
2. Kelly EM: External warming/cooling devices. In Lynn-McHale DJ, Carlson KK, editors: *AACN procedure manual for critical care,* ed 4, Philadelphia, 2001, Saunders.
3. Bernard SA, Buist M: Induced hypothermia in critical care medicine: a review, *Crit Care Med* 31970:2041-2051, 2003.
4. Grigore AM, et al: The rewarming rate and increased peak temperature alter neurocognitive outcome after cardiac surgery, *Anesthesia Analgesia* 94(1):4-10, 2002.
5. Pate MF: Thermal regulation. In Curley MAQ, Moloney-Harmon PA, editors: *Critical care nursing of infants and children,* ed 2, Philadelphia, 2001, Saunders.

Additional Readings

Casey G: Fever management in children, *Nurs Stand* 14(40): 36-42, 2000.
de Caen A: Management of profound hypothermia in children without the use of extracorporeal life support therapy, *Lancet* 360:1394-1395, 2002.
Kober A, et al: Effectiveness of resistive heating compared with passive warming in treating hypothermia associated with minor trauma: a randomized trial, *Mayo Clin Proceedings* 76(4): 369-375, 2001.
Lapointe L, Von Rueden KT: Coagulopathies in trauma patients, *AACN Clin Iss* 13(2):192-203, 2002.
O'Neill KA, et al: The effects of core and peripheral warming methods on temperature and physiologic variables in injured children, *Pediatr Emerg Care* 17(2):138-142, 2001.
Thoresen M, Whitelaw A: Cardiovascular changes during mild therapeutic hypothermia and rewarming in infants with hypoxic-ischemic encephalopathy, *Pediatrics* 106(1):92-99, 2000.

Obtaining an Accurate Temperature Measurement

P U R P O S E : Because the risk for alterations in body temperature is greater for infants and children who are critically ill, accurate evaluation of body temperature is essential. Alterations in temperature may indicate potentially life-threatening processes.

Annette M. Fleck

PREREQUISITE KNOWLEDGE

- Body temperature is the measurement of the presence or absence of heat. Normal body temperature results when heat production and heat loss are balanced. Heat production occurs in the body as a byproduct of all metabolic reactions. Body temperature is influenced by factors such as age, circadian rhythm, and hormones. Core body temperature varies by 1.1°C with circadian cycles throughout the day.[1]
- Receptor cells in the skin, sensitive to heat and cold, respond to changes in temperature. This response triggers nerve impulses transmitted through the cerebral cortex to the hypothalamus. The hypothalamus is the integrating center for regulation of body temperature. A heat-sensitive area of the hypothalamus protects the body by initiating physiologic responses. When heat reduction is necessary, the hypothalamus sends out impulses that dilate cutaneous blood vessels and stimulate sweat glands. The radiation of heat from the large volume of blood brought to the skin's surface, together with evaporation by perspiration, helps eliminate heat from the body. The hypothalamus can send impulses to increase heat production and reduce heat loss when body temperature drops below normal. The impulses inhibit secretion of sweat, increase the basal metabolic rate, and constrict superficial blood vessels to meet the body's thermoregulatory demands.
- Heat-producing processes of the body such as metabolism, disease processes, exercise, shivering, unconscious tensing of muscles, and increased thyroid activity can sometimes produce more heat than necessary. To offset excessive heat production and restore normothermia, the body uses these four processes: convection, radiation, conduction, and evaporation.
- Mechanisms of heat loss
  - *Convection* refers to heat transfer by air movement or liquid carrying heat away from an object. This transfer is dependent on air velocity, temperature, and exposed surface area. Convection losses increase with shivering and wind conditions.
  - *Radiation* is an energy transfer via electromagnetic waves to surrounding cooler surfaces without direct contact. The degree of heat loss by radiation is directly related to core and ambient temperature and the exposed body surface area. The large head size in proportion to body size of infants and children also predisposes them to hypothermia. Most losses emanate from the unprotected head, which accounts for the majority of heat loss in the operating room.
  - *Conduction* is the transfer of heat to surrounding objects through direct physical contact. Conduction heat loss increases five times if the child is wet and up to 30 times with cold water immersion.[2]
  - *Evaporation* occurs primarily through perspiration, which is removed from the skin as transdermal water loss by changing from a liquid into a vapor. These losses can also occur from the respiratory tract and open body cavities.

- For older children, shivering is a means of increasing heat production; however, it is not effective over the long term because of muscle fatigue. Shivering ceases at body temperatures below 33°C.
- Infants maintain body temperature through a chemical nonshivering thermogenesis. This process begins with the secretion of norepinephrine and results in the breakdown of brown fat to create heat. This process requires energy and increases the infant's oxygen consumption, which may not be effective in the critically ill infant. Cold stress can produce hypoxemia, lactic acidosis, and hypoglycemia; can stimulate pulmonary vasoconstriction; and may worsen any existing cardiovascular dysfunction, increase heart failure, and permit right to left intracardiac shunting. Cold stress may be prevented through the maintenance of a neutral thermal environment (NTE). NTE provides a set environmental temperature in which a neonate is able to maintain a normal core temperature with minimal oxygen and caloric expenditure. This narrow range of temperature tolerance in infants varies with gestational and postnatal age. The NTE range broadens with increased age and weight of the infant. A closed isolette is useful for infants who need maintenance of a controlled thermal environment. See Procedure 190 for further discussion of this topic.
- Children have higher metabolic rates than adults, and in turn increasing oxygen consumption and nutritional needs, which may further tax the child and lead to thermoregulatory issues. Children and infants also have larger surface area–to–volume ratios; thus, more heat is lost to the environment through evaporation, conduction, and convection than in adults. The mechanisms for temperature regulation are so efficient in health that a departure from normal body temperature has become a cardinal sign of illness. Critically ill infants and children are at risk for ineffective thermoregulation from environmental and maturational factors (see Table 188-1 for a review of these factors).[3]
- Critical care nurses play an essential role in identification of and protection from factors that put the child at risk for thermal instability. See Box 188-1 for a listing of these factors.
- Assessment of body temperature is an evaluation tool that provides information about the severity and nature of illness. In the intensive care setting, safety, speed, accuracy, infection control, and convenience are important considerations in the selection of a temperature measurement device and appropriateness to the individual child's condition. Various devices are used to measure core, regional, and skin temperature in critically ill infants and children, each with relative advantages and disadvantages unique to the child.
- The mode for measurement of temperatures should be kept as constant as possible. Modes typically used are: infrared scanners, dot matrix disposable, digital, electronic, and thermistor within catheters or probes. The glass mercury bulb thermometer has been used as the gold standard and is identified by the National Bureau of Standards for comparison with other instruments. Concerns regarding potential mercury exposure on breakage have prompted the American Association of Pediatrics recommendation to

Table 188-1	Factors Related to Ineffective Thermoregulation
Environmental	**Maturational**
Changing environmental temperature	Extremes of age
Insufficient heating or humidification	Large ratio of body surface to body mass
Physical contact with or proximity to cold or warm objects	Metabolic immaturity and decreased heat production
Wet or exposed body surfaces	Rapid metabolic rate
Excessive or insufficient clothing or coverings	Thin layer of subcutaneous fat

From Pate MF: Thermal regulation. In Curley M, Moloney-Harmon P, editors: *Critical care nursing of infants and children,* St Louis, 2001, Saunders.

Box 188-1	Factors That Predispose Infants and Children to Thermal Instability

- Relatively large body surface area
- Relatively limited nutritional reserve
- Impaired cardiac, renal, hepatic, or endocrine function
- Impaired behavioral, neural, and endocrine responses (from underlying physical and physiologic states)
- Impaired neuroendocrine response (from pharmacologic agents)
- Cardiopulmonary resuscitation, anesthesia, or extended radiographic procedures

From Pate MF: Thermal regulation. In Curley MAQ, Moloney-Harmon P, editors: *Critical care nursing of infants and children,* ed 2, St Louis, 2001, Saunders.

phase out mercury glass bulb thermometers and eliminate usage in the hospital setting.[3]

- Temperature monitoring sites can be categorized by tissue blood flow. The site and the device must be individually evaluated based on relative advantages and disadvantages unique to the child, safety, comfort, and availability. The rectal temperature remains the standard with which all others are compared.
  - High blood flow areas that represent core or internal temperatures are: pulmonary artery, lower esophageal, nasopharyngeal, and tympanic membrane. These sites detect core temperature changes rapidly.
  - Intermediate blood flow areas that are good reflections of core temperature during steady state conditions include: bladder, rectal, oral, and axillary route
  - Noninvasive cutaneous monitoring of low blood flow areas such as the toe, forehead, or temporal artery is the least reliable indicator of rapid core temperature[5,6]
- Consistent skin temperature site monitoring is imperative with use of a warming or cooling device. Normal thermoregulation maintains body temperature within a narrow range, 36.2°C to 37.2°C, with an average normal temperature of 37.0°C.[6] See Table 188-2 for a comparison of temperature measurements obtained at various sites.
- Extremes of life for human body temperature range between 24°C and 44°C.[7] Internationally, the Celsius scale is the standard unit of temperature measurement. The conversion of Celsius to Fahrenheit is: $C \times 9/5 + 32 = F$. Thermometers are often only calibrated down to 34.4°C. Accurate temperature

TABLE 188-2 Normal Variations in Body Temperature on Basis of Rectal Temperature of 37°C

Type of Temperature Measurement	Degrees Lower than Rectal Temperature
Oral	0.3°C -0.5° C
Esophageal	0.2°C
Pulmonary artery	0.2°C -0.3°C
Tympanic membrane	0.05°C -0.25°C
Bladder	0.1°C -0.2°C
Axillary	0.6°C -0.8°C

From Kelly EM: External warming/cooling devices. In Lynn-McHale DJ, Carlson K, editors: *AACN procedure manual for critical care,* ed 4, Philadelphia, 2001, Saunders.

measurement then necessitates the use of a thermometer capable of reading to a temperature of 15°C.[8]

- Relevant points that concern high blood flow methods are as follows:
  - The ideal spot for continuous core temperature is a pulmonary artery catheter; however, this is also the most invasive
  - An esophageal temperature probe is also reliable when positioned in the lower third of the esophagus, behind the right atrium, with radiographic verification. The temperature reading may be falsely lowered if an accompanying gastric tube is present with applied continuous suction. Therefore, the gastric tube is better placed on a low intermittent setting. An open chest for thoracic or cardiac procedure makes measurement with this method inaccurate.
  - Nasopharyngeal temperatures provide an estimate of hypothalamic temperature. Often used in the operating room, this probe must be positioned in the nasopharyngeal area posterior to the soft palate. This method is inaccurate with uncuffed endotracheal tubes and can cause trauma to the soft tissue of the nasopharynx. Trauma or bleeding to the nasopharynx or tympanic membrane may result in inaccurate temperature readings, and thus, this method may be inadvisable.
- Hypothermia is a temperature measurement below 36.4°C that may be caused by an increase in heat loss, a decrease in heat production, an alteration in thermoregulation, or other miscellaneous conditions. Hypothermia may be classified as mild (34°C to 36.4°C), moderate (27.5°C to 33.9°C), deep (17°C to 27.4°C), or profound (<16.9°C). If body temperature drops to 34.8°C, functioning of the hypothalamus is impaired. As the body temperature drops below 30°C, the hypothalamus stops functioning, metabolic processes slow, and shivering stops, thus accelerating the development of hypothermia.[8] Children's high body surface areas, low body fat mass, and greater degree of brown fat metabolism make them especially susceptible to accidental hypothermia. Neonates have further vulnerability to hypothermia because of their inability to produce heat by shivering.[2]
- Hyperthermia is a sustained elevation in body temperature of greater than 37.8°C orally or 38.8°C rectally. Hyperthermia may be caused by internal factors such as fever, malignant hyperthermia, or heat-related illnesses. External factors of hyperthermia include accidental overheating or extreme environmental exposure.
- Fever is a symptom that may have several causes, such as traumatic brain injury, congenital central nervous system (CNS) malformations, the presence of toxins that affect the brain's temperature control areas, infection, dehydration, endocrine disorders, hypothalamic lesions, drugs, or iatrogenic causes. Fever is the body's natural response to a viral or bacterial infection. A febrile state increases the heart rate and metabolic demand, which may be detrimental to critically ill children, especially those with an underlying disease involving the heart or lungs. Fever itself may cause convulsions in some children when the temperature rises quickly.
- Malignant hyperthermia is a rare hereditary condition of the skeletal muscles that occurs with exposure to triggering agents (most commonly anesthetic agents and succinylcholine) and causes a hypermetabolic crisis. The instability of the muscle cell membrane causes a sudden increase in myoplasmic calcium and skeletal muscle contractures. Initial signs include increased end-tidal carbon dioxide, tachypnea, and tachycardia followed by ventricular ectopy. Muscle rigidity may or may not occur. Fever, resulting from many biochemical derangements, is the hallmark sign. The muscle relaxant dantrolene is administered as treatment for malignant hyperthermia.
- See Table 188-3 for additional terms related to temperature.
- Not all sites and temperature measuring devices are created equal, and each child is unique. The most commonly used methods of body temperature measurement include oral, tympanic, axillary, and rectal sites, with use of infrared thermometers or electronic devices. For critically ill children, a combination of temperature measuring techniques is often indicated. Specific information about temperature monitoring devices is available from each manufacturer and must be understood by the nurse before the equipment is used.
- Placement of continuous skin temperature leads and placement of indwelling thermistors should be checked every time the child is repositioned.
- Child development as it relates to clinical assessment and obtaining an accurate temperature measurement

CHILD AND FAMILY ASSESSMENT

- The temperature mode selected should be appropriate to the individual's age and condition ➺***Rationale:*** Assists in anticipating, recognizing, and assessing child's individual response to temperature monitoring.
- Risk factors, medical history, and cause of the child's underlying condition ➺***Rationale:*** Assists in recognizing and responding to child's current state of health.
- Current medication therapy ➺***Rationale:*** Medications such as vasopressors and vasodilators may affect heat transfer, increase the potential for skin injury, and contribute to an adverse response. Anticoagulation therapy may increase potential for skin injury.

TABLE 188-3	Terms Associated with Temperature
Euthermia	Range of body temperature associated with health
Hypothermia	Temperature below 36.4°C
Induced hypothermia	Intentional cooling with surface (transfer of heat from skin to coolant circulating through coils of cooling device) or central (circulatory heat exchange in cardiopulmonary bypass machine) means
Fever	Response to pyrogen: Hypothalamus either resets its range higher, maintaining thermoregulation, or change occurs in sensitivity of hypothalamus neuron activity to warmth and coolness
Hyperthermia	Dysfunction of thermoregulation caused by injury to hypothalamus or when heat loss mechanisms are overwhelmed by high environmental heat
Malignant hyperthermia	Rare hereditary condition of skeletal muscles that occurs on exposure to triggering agents (most commonly anesthetic agents), causing hypermetabolic crisis
Heat stroke	Failure of heat-regulating mechanisms of body when temperature-humidity index is high
Poikilothermia	Loss of ability to thermoregulate from loss of hypothalamic function, as seen in management with high-dose pentobarbital and with child with brain death

Modified from Kelly EM: External warming/cooling devices. In Lynn-McHale DJ, Carlson K, editors: *AACN procedure manual for critical care*, ed 4, Philadelphia, 2001, Saunders.

- Laboratory values for coagulopathy and platelet dysfunction ➤➤*Rationale:* Bleeding tendencies may preclude invasive monitoring of temperature or obtaining a rectal temperature.
- Preexisting neutropenia ➤➤*Rationale:* Less invasive methods of temperature monitoring may be indicated in oncology patients and with other potential immunocompromised conditions.
- Child's developmental level and ability to interact ➤➤*Rationale:* These factors influence preparation of the child and interaction.
- Child's and family's understanding of the reasons for, and risks and benefits of the procedure ➤➤*Rationale:* Evaluates child's and family's understanding of the procedure and provides a gauge for ongoing education.

CHILD AND FAMILY EDUCATION

Individualized, developmentally appropriate education is provided to the family and to the child based on desire for knowledge, readiness to learn, and overall neurologic and psychosocial state.

- Explain the reason for monitoring temperature, the site selected, the device to be used, and the frequency of monitoring ➤➤*Rationale:* Child and family know what to expect.
- Determine child's and family's understanding of mode selected ➤➤*Rationale:* Providing information about site selected may facilitate cooperation with procedure.
- Explain normal body temperature ranges, indications for obtaining measurements, and what deviations from base-

line may be pertinent to the individual child ➤➤*Rationale:* Encourages child and family to ask questions and verbalize concerns regarding temperature monitoring, significance of readings, and associated interventions.
- Explain what interventions may be needed to assist with the child's body temperature regulation ➤➤*Rationale:* Prepares the child and family for further interventions.

EQUIPMENT

The ideal thermometer should be easy to use, accurately reflect core temperature, minimize spread of infection, provide rapid results, and cause no undue discomfort or embarrassment.[9] An understanding of the proper use and limitations of each monitoring device is important in prevention of errors. Equipment varies with site selection and temperature monitoring device to be used.

High blood flow core temperature reading

- Pulmonary artery catheter requires pulmonary artery catheter, temperature probe, cables, and modules adaptable to the monitor in use
- Distal esophageal temperature monitoring, with sensor immediately behind the left atrium, is primarily used in the operating room, as is nasopharyngeal method with cable and modules adaptable to monitor in use
- Tympanic membrane digital thermometer and disposable temp probe covers

Intermediate blood flow area temperature monitoring

- Bladder mode of temperature monitoring is usually performed via an indwelling urinary catheter and electronic collection device. Accuracy is dependent on urinary flow and volume.
- Rectal temperature may be obtained via electronic handheld device with disposable temperature probe cover or via a continuous rectal probe connected by a cable to the monitoring device. A water-soluble lubricating substance should be used to ease probe placement.
- Oral temperature monitoring may be obtained with a single-use chemical dot plastic strip thermometer or handheld electronic device with disposable probe covers.[10]
- An axillary temperature may be obtained via electronic handheld device with disposable probe cover or via a continuous monitoring probe placed over the axillary artery. Continuous monitoring requires probe wire, cable, module, and monitoring device.
- A temporal artery temperature may be obtained via electronic handheld device moved over the skin in the area of the temporal artery.

Low blood flow area temperature monitoring

- Peripherally placed skin temperature measurements are the most convenient but may be the least accurate. Noninvasive temperature-sensitive pacifiers and forehead strips have not been found to be consistent or reliable.

Procedure for Obtaining an Accurate Temperature Measurement

Steps	Rationale	Considerations
For All Routes		
1. Ensure the child and family understand the procedure and questions are answered.	Evaluates and reinforces under standing of previously taught information.	Developmental level, cognitive ability and anxiety level influence approach to and effectiveness of teaching.
2. Gather needed equipment and supplies	Facilitates completion of the procedure in a timely manner.	
3. Wash hands.	Standard precautions; reduces the transmission of microorganisms	
4. Explain the procedure to the child in developmentally appropriate language.	The child knows what to expect.	
5. Obtain measurement. Record value, mode, time, and date.	Establishes temperature measurement and completes the assessment.	Documenting mode allows comparison of subsequent measurements obtained.
6. Take the child's temperature with the same method at intervals delineated by prescribing practitioner's order or institution or unit-specific protocol. Recommendation is to monitor the temperature every hour until temperature stabilizes; then every 2 hours until normal; and then every 4 hours when stable unless otherwise indicated. *(Level II*)*	Vital signs should be taken as often as necessary considering the child's current condition and status. Temperature monitoring should not be delayed if a deleterious trend is suspected to be developing.	
7. To decrease the possibility of inaccuracy, electronic and infrared devices should be regularly scheduled for calibration and necessary battery changes per the manufacturer's specifications. *(Level I*)*	Question the accuracy of any temperature reading that does not correlate with the child's present state. The temperature should be double checked with an alternate device or site. Inaccurate temperature measurement can result in serious errors in diagnosis and treatment.	
For Oral Temperature Measurement Refer to previous steps 1-7.		
8. Wait at least 10 minutes after administration of oral medication, mouth care, or drinking of hot or cold fluids.	Prevents falsely influenced readings.	
9. Instruct the child to close lips and mouth and not to bite or talk with the thermometer in place.	Requires child's cooperation to keep mouth closed and not bite on the thermometer.	The oral mode of temperature monitoring may be ineffective in children with mouth breathing, oxygen therapy, respiratory distress, tachypnea, oral intubation, altered level of consciousness, or developmental level that prevents cooperation with the procedure. This mode is contraindicated if the child has oral injuries or has had oral surgery.
10. Insert oral temperature device under the tongue, slightly off midline in	Ensures accurate probe placement.	

Procedure continues on following page

---

* Level I: Manufacturer's recommendation
  Level II: Theory-based; no research data to support recommendations; recommendations from expert consensus group may exist

Procedure for Obtaining an Accurate Temperature Measurement—*Continued*

Steps	Rationale	Considerations
the sublingual pocket. Digital thermometer with or without disposable probe cover may be used.		
11. Hold in place for recommended time period for the device used. *(Level I*)*	Digital thermometer signals when reading completed.	The use of an electronic thermometer intended for multiple patients becomes problematic when children need protective isolation; therefore, single-use digital thermometers may be indicated. The single-use chemical dot thermometer made of flexible polystyrene strip may be considered. Disposable or single-use thermometers have negligible risk of cross contamination and spread of infection.
12. Keep one hand on the thermometer at all times while in place.	For safety and injury prevention, never leave the child alone during an oral temperature assessment.	
13. Remove thermometer when device indicates temperature measurement is complete. *(Level I*)*	Procedure is complete.	

For Tympanic Temperature Measurement
Refer to previous steps 1-7.

Steps	Rationale	Considerations
14. Place a new disposable cap over the tympanic probe.	Disposable caps or probe covers reduce risk of cross contamination.	The American Academy of Pediatrics advises against ear temperature measurements in infants less than 3 months of age.[11] *(Level II*)*
15. Switch on the tympanic ear thermometer.	Ensures readiness of device.	
16. Gently position probe into ear canal, aligning probe tip towards the child's opposite eye.	The ear is easily accessible and highly accepted by children.	The ear canal radiates energy in the form of electromagnetic waves. Infrared thermometers detect this thermal radiation. Narrow ear canals impede reading this energy, which causes inconsistent and falsely low readings.[12]
17. Pull the ear lobe down and back for children less than 3 years of age and up and back for the older child.	Use of ear tug straightens curvature of the ear canal.	Tympanic measurements can be affected by whether the child has been lying on that ear or has been exposed to extremes in temperature and are limited by cerumen, sizing of probe covers, and positioning of the thermometer. The presence of otitis media may result in local heat production.[13]
18. Press and hold activation button until a reading appears or an audible sound indicates completion. *(Level I*)*	The device obtains tympanic temperature.	For safety and injury prevention, never leave the child alone when obtaining temperature measurement.

* Level I: Manufacturer's recommendation
Level II: Theory-based; no research data to support recommendations; recommendations from expert consensus group may exist

Procedure	**for Obtaining an Accurate Temperature Measurement**—*Continued*	
Steps	**Rationale**	**Considerations**
19. Remove the thermometer and read the temperature.	Procedure is complete.	Tympanic membrane thermometer readings closely parallel core body temperatures because the hypothalamus and tympanic membrane both receive the blood supply from the internal carotid artery. Operator variability is common with the use of tympanic membrane thermometers when used in pediatric patients. *(Level IV*)*
20. Discard cap/probe cover.	Use of a new cap/probe cover for every reading helps prevent cross contamination.	
For Axillary Temperature Measurement Refer to previous steps 1-7.		
21. Place the tip of the thermometer under the armpit, ensuring contact between the skin of the arm and skin of the chest.	Ensures accurate probe placement; prevents ambient air from affecting reading.	
22. Hold the arm next to the side of the chest, keeping the thermometer under the arm for the recommended time period for the device used. The digital device will display a reading or signal an audible sound when reading is completed. *(Level I*)*	Keeping the arm in close proximity to the chest decreases the effect of environmental temperature on the measurement.	For safety and injury prevention, never leave the child alone when taking a temperature measurement. Keep one hand on the thermometer at all times while it is in place.
23. Remove the thermometer.	Procedure is complete.	
For Rectal Temperature Measurement Refer to previous steps 1-7.		Rectal temperatures are contraindicated with neutropenia, diarrhea, and recent rectal surgery. This method is preferred for children who are unable to cooperate and may bite the thermometer. The Academy of Pediatrics no longer recommends the rectal mode for routine monitoring of temperature in neonates because of increased risk of bowel perforation or vagal stimulation. For infants and toddlers, a rectal temperature remains the most accurate method of assessment.[11]
24. Put on clean gloves.	Standard precautions; reduces transmission of microorganisms.	
25. Ensure adequate privacy.	Limits negative emotional response; maintains modesty and respects child's right to privacy.	School-aged children may be especially modest. Ensuring privacy for this age group promotes feelings of security.
26. Positioning may be prone, supine, or side lying with the hips flexed; depending on child's present status and condition.	Ensures accurate probe placement.	Side lying with flexed hips may facilitate insertion.

Procedure continues on following page

Procedure   for Obtaining an Accurate Temperature Measurement—*Continued*

Steps	Rationale	Considerations
27. Expose only necessary area during the procedure.	Exposure of the buttocks may cause the infant to urinate. Placement of the probe may also initiate a defecation stimulus and a potential vagal stimulus in the neonate.	
28. Separate the buttocks with thumb and forefinger of one hand while gently inserting with the other hand a well-lubricated rectal thermometer inclined toward the child's umbilicus, through the anal sphincter into the rectum.	To prevent damage to the rectal mucosa, water-soluble nongreasy nonirritating lubricating jelly is recommended.	Depths of insertion: preterm, 2.5 cm; full term, 3 cm; to 4 cm on children with a maximum depth of rectal probe insertion of 5 cm. Do not place thermometer directly into fecal matter, which may falsely lower the reading.[12]
29. Steadily hold probe in place for recommended time period for the device used. An electronic device signals completion of reading by audible sound or display of reading. *(Level I*)*	Prevents injury, ensures probe remains in the rectum.	For safety and injury prevention, never leave the child unattended when taking a temperature measurement. Keep one hand on the thermometer at all times.
30. Remove rectal thermometer. Discard disposable probe if used.	Procedure is complete.	
For all methods:		
31. Obtain measured value from device readout.	Establishes temperature measurement.	
32. Dispose of used supplies and equipment in appropriate receptacle.	Standard precautions; reduces transmission of microorganisms.	
33. Remove gloves, if worn; wash hands.	Standard precautions; reduces transmission of microorganisms.	

* Level I: Manufacturer's recommendation

Expected Outcomes

- Baseline body temperature measurement is obtained

- Accurate body temperature measurements are obtained
- Body temperature measurements obtained result in appropriate therapy

- Child is free from injury related to body temperature measurement

Unexpected Outcomes

- Body temperature not within normal limits
- Inability to obtain body temperature
- Reading does not correlate with child's current signs and symptoms
- False-positive reading triggers initiation of unnecessary therapy
- False-negative reading delays treatment response
- Mercury exposure if glass bulb thermometer is broken
- Cross contamination of children with use of same thermometer results in infection
- Skin injury specific to individual route used
  - ❖ Oral mucosa injury: oral route
  - ❖ Skin tears: axillary route
  - ❖ Injury to the inner ear: tympanic route
  - ❖ Mucosal tear of rectum or colon: rectal route

Monitoring and Care of the Child

Activities and Interventions	Rationale	Reportable Conditions
1. Perform physical assessment of all body systems every 1 to 2 hours.	Alterations in temperature can affect all body systems.	• Significant changes in assessment
2. Monitor body temperature per institution-specific protocol.	Vital signs, including temperature, should be taken as often as necessary	• Hypothermia or hyperthermia

Monitoring and Care of the Child—Cont'd

Activities and Interventions	Rationale	Reportable Conditions
Recommendation for frequency is every hour until temperature stabilizes, then every 2 hours until normal, then every 4 hours when stable unless otherwise indicated.	with consideration of the child's current condition and status. Temperature monitoring should not be delayed if a deleterious trend is suspected to be developing.	
3. Confirm accuracy of temperature measurement obtained by comparing value with child's other signs and symptoms.	Falsely high or low temperature reading could trigger unnecessary therapy. Confirmation of accuracy may be aided by temperature taken via an alternate site or mode or selection of a continuous mode of monitoring.	• Variation in temperature from child's baseline
4. Ensure child's comfort; assess using developmentally and age-appropriate pain scale. Refer to Procedure 173 for further information.	Optimize child's comfort.	• Unrelieved discomfort
5. Initiate nursing measures for hypothermia/hyperthermia as indicated by child's condition.	Additional treatment may be necessary.	• Unrelieved temperature imbalance

Documentation

- Child's temperature, site used, and time and date of assessment
- Deviation from child's baseline temperature
- Comfort assessment
- Child and family education
- Unexpected outcomes and related treatment

References

1. Pate MF: Thermal regulation. In Curley MAQ, Moloney-Harmon PA, editors: *Critical care nursing of infants and children,* ed 2, Philadelphia, 2001, Saunders.
2. Lange Varga J: Warming procedures. In Henretig FM, King C, editors: *Textbook of pediatric emergency procedures,* Baltimore, 1997, Williams & Wilkins.
3. Jones H, Kleber C, Eckert G, et al: Comparison of rectal temperature measured by digital vs. mercury glass thermometer in infants under two months old, *Clin Pediatr* 42:357-359, 2003.
4. Sweeney MF, Madisen MS, Belan KG, et al: Noninvasive vital monitoring in children. In Furman B, Zimmerman JJ, editors: *Pediatric critical care,* St Louis, 1988, Mosby-Year Book, Inc.
5. Roy S, et al: Temporal artery temperature measurements in healthy infants, children, and adolescents, *Clin Pediatr* 42:433-437, 2003.
6. Coursan DB, et al: *Critical care medicine: perioperative management,* Philadelphia, 2002, Williams and Wilkins.
7. Aun CTS: Thermal disorders. In Oh TE, editor: *Intensive care manual,* ed 4, Oxford, 1997, Butterworth-Heinemann.
8. Petty KJ: Hypothermia. In Fauci AS, et al, editors: *Harrison's principles of internal medicine,* New York, 1998, McGraw-Hill.
9. Biehler J, Barnes B: Evaluation of vital signs. In Henretig FM, King C, editors: *Textbook of pediatric emergency procedures,* Baltimore, 1997, Williams & Wilkins.
10. Potter P, et al: Evaluation of chemical dot thermometer for measuring body temperature of orally intubated patients, *Am J Crit Care* 12(5):403-407, 2003.
11. Kiernan BS: Taking a temperature: which way is best? *JSPN* 6(4):192-195, 2001.
12. Jiropaet V, Jiropaet K: Comparison of tympanic membrane, abdominal, skin, axillary, and rectal temperature measurements in term and preterm neonates, *Nurs Health Sci* 2(1):1, 2000.
13. Craig JV, et al: Infrared ear thermometry compared with rectal thermometry in children: a systematic review, *Lancet* 360(9333):603, 2002.

Additional Readings

Charkoudian N: Skin blood flow in adults human thermoregulation: how it works, when it does not, and why, *Mayo Clin Proc* 78:603-612, 2003.

Dollberg S, et al: Continuous measurement of core body temperature in preterm infants, *Am J Perinatol* 17(5):257-264, 2000.

Fabri B, Fox M, Grayson A, et al: Should we rely on nasopharyngeal temperature during cardiopulmonary bypass? *Perfusion* 17:145-151, 2002.

Kahyaoglu O: Effects of crying on infrared tympanic temperature measurement in pediatrics, *Clin Pediatr* 36(8):487, 1997.

Kelly EM: External warming/cooling devices. In Lynn-McHale DJ, Carlson KK, editors: *AACN procedure manual for critical care,* ed 4, Philadelphia, 2001, Saunders.

Melnyk BM, Houlder LC: The accuracy and reliability of tympanic thermometry compared to rectal and axillary sites in young children, *Pediatr Nurs* 26(3):311, 2000.

Robinson JL, et al: Comparison of esophageal, rectal, axillary, bladder, tympanic, and pulmonary artery temperatures in children, *J Pediatr* 133(4):553-556, 1998.

Rush M: Temperature measurement: practice guidelines, *Paediatr Nurs* 15(9):9, 2003.

Holtzclaw BJ: Monitoring body temperature in critical and acute-care settings, *Safe Pract Patient Care* 1:2, 2004.

Warming Devices: Radiant

P U R P O S E : External radiant warming devices provide maintenance of normothermia and enhanced thermoregulation in infants and children with mild hypothermia

Annette M. Fleck

PREREQUISITE KNOWLEDGE

- Body temperature is the measurement of the presence or absence of heat. Normal body temperature results when heat production and heat loss are balanced. Heat production occurs in the body as a byproduct of all metabolic reactions. Body temperature is influenced by factors such as age, circadian rhythm, and hormones. Core body temperature varies by 1.1°C with circadian cycles throughout the day.[1]
- Mechanisms of temperature regulation in the body should be understood (See Procedure 188 for a discussion of these mechanisms.)
- Radiant warmers are typically used with infants but can also be used with young children less than 2 years of age and for warming a specific site (e.g., a surgical site) on an older child. Use of a hypothermia/hyperthermia blanket should be considered in children greater than 2 years of age for thermoregulatory therapy. An isolation incubator that provides warm ambient air and humidity is best suited to infants less than 36 weeks gestation, to very low–birth weight (VLBW) infants (weight less than 1500 g), and to extremely low–birth weight (ELBW) infants (weight less than 1000 g). See Procedure 190 for a discussion of thermoregulation and use of radiant warmer devices in this population.
- Mechanisms of heat loss and thermoregulation should be understood (See Procedure 188 for a discussion of these mechanisms.)
- Infants produce heat through nonshivering thermogenesis, which requires breakdown of brown fat. This is an energy-requiring process that increases the infant's oxygen consumption and glucose use; the critically ill infant may not have effective thermogenesis. Cold stress can produce hypoxemia, lactic acidosis, and hypoglycemia; can stimulate pulmonary vasoconstriction; and may worsen any existing cardiovascular dysfunction, increase heart failure, and permit right to left intracardiac shunting.
- For children, shivering is a means of increasing heat production; however, it is not effective over the long term because of muscle fatigue. Shivering ceases at body temperatures less than 33°C.
- The physiologic consequences of cold stress in infants should be understood and are outlined in Figure 189-1.
- Children have higher metabolic rates than do adults, which results in increased oxygen consumption and nutritional needs that may further tax the child, leading to thermoregulatory issues. Children and infants have large ratios of surface area to volume; thus, more heat is lost to the environment through heat loss mechanisms than in adults. The mechanisms for temperature regulation are so efficient in health that a departure from normal body temperature (increase or decrease) has become a cardinal sign of illness.
- Critically ill infants and children are at risk for ineffective thermoregulation from environmental and maturational factors. Critical care nurses play an essential role in identification and protection of neonatal/pediatric patients from specific risks related to ineffective thermoregulation. (See Table 188-1 in Procedure 188 for a discussion of these risks.)

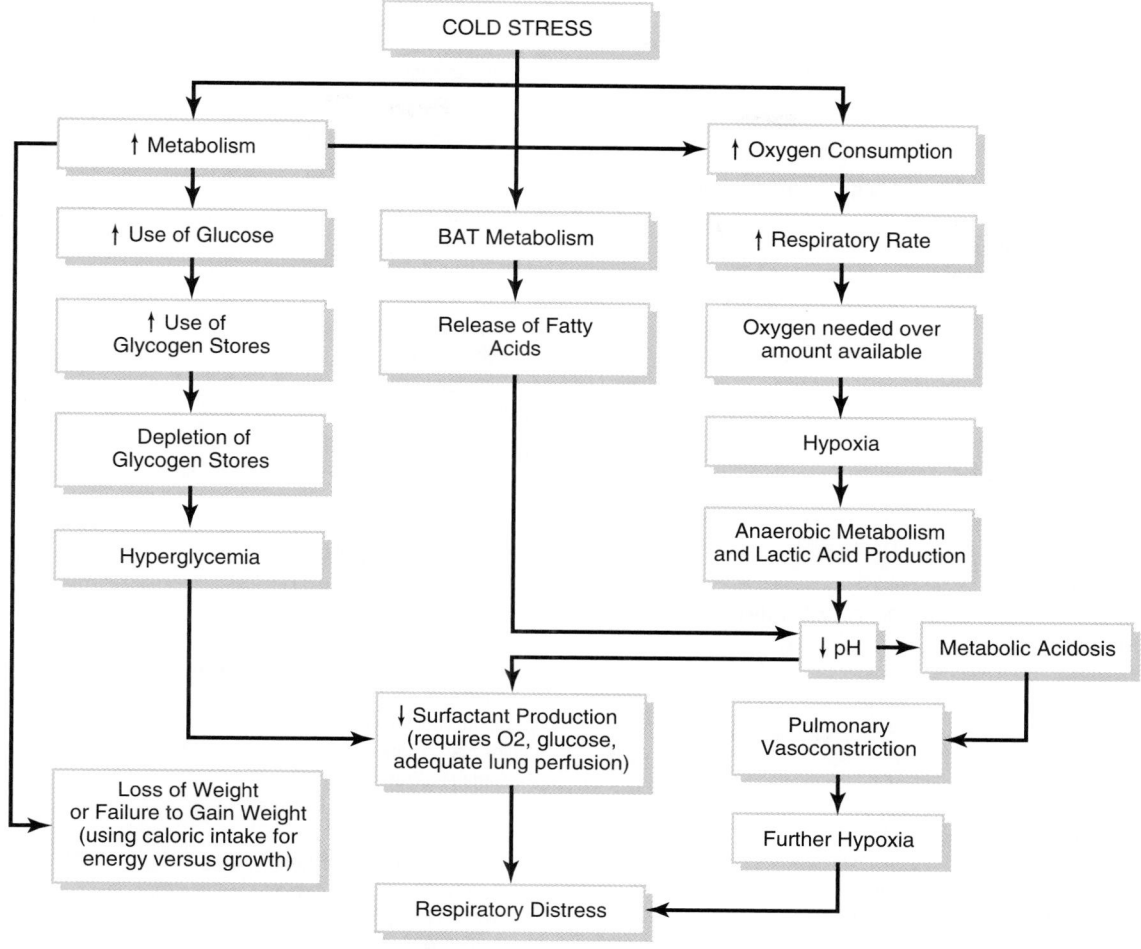

FIGURE 189-1 Physiologic Consequences of Cold Stress in Infants. *From Blackburn ST, Loper DL:* Maternal, fetal and neonatal physiology, *Philadelphia, 1992, Saunders.* (BAT=Brown adipose tissue.)

- Critically ill infants and young children under certain circumstances need support for maintenance of body temperature so that energy expended for metabolic heat production is minimized.
- The mechanism by which a radiant warmer provides warmth should be understood. These devices provide warmth via radiant energy from electrically heated elements. The element emits radiation within the infrared region of the electromagnetic spectrum, which allows for optimal absorption of energy by the skin.
- Radiant warmers are used to warm a newborn directly after birth, to regulate an infant's temperature during long-term care in a hospital, to keep a child warm during or after surgery, and to keep a child warm with minimal coverage because of a procedure or accessibility needs.
- The radiant warmer can be placed over the child to heat the face, hands, feet, legs, torso, or, more typically, the entire body of an infant. Radiant infrared heating can warm the blood by passing through the skin's dermal vasculature.
- These devices are usually regulated with servo control to keep the skin temperature constant, which is achieved via a skin temperature monitor from a thermistor in direct contact with the skin
- Consistent skin temperature monitoring is imperative with a warming device. The normal range of skin temperature is 36.2°C to 37.2°C, with an average normal temperature of 37.0°C.
- Warming lamps are not preferred because they have no feedback sensor to monitor the child's temperature. Thermal injuries have been reported with the use of heat lamps.
- Hypothermia is a temperature measurement below 36.4°C that may result from numerous causes. Hypothermia may be classified as mild (34°C to 36.4°C), moderate (27.5°C to 33.9°C), deep (17°C to 27.4°C), or profound (<16.9°C). If body temperature drops to 34.8°C, functioning of the hypothalamus is impaired. As the body temperature drops to less than 30°C, the hypothalamus stops functioning, metabolic processes slow, and shivering stops, thus accelerating the development of hypothermia.[2] Physiologic characteristics that occur with hypothermia depend on the cause and degree of hypothermia. Box 189-1 outlines the causes of hypothermia.

Box 189-1	**Causes of Hypothermia**

I. Excessive heat loss
   A. Environmental exposure
      1. Accidental
      2. Iatrogenic
   B. Increased cutaneous blood flow: burns, psoriasis, toxic epi-
      dermal necrolysis
II. Inadequate heat production
   A. Decreased metabolism
      1. Malnutrition
      2. Hypothyroidism
      3. Adrenal insufficiency
      4. Hepatic failure
      5. Hypoglycemia
      6. Diabetic ketoacidosis
   B. Altered thermoregulation
      1. Sepsis
      2. Uremia
      3. Hypothalamic dysfunction
      4. Spinal cord injury: T1 or above
      5. Episodic spontaneous hypothermia with hyperhidrosis
   C. Drug-induced
      1. Phenothiazines
      2. Barbiturates
      3. Ethanol
      4. Opiates
      5. Clonidine
      6. Lithium
      7. Benzodiazepines

From Petty KJ: Hypothermia. In Fauci AS, et al, editors: *Harrison's principles of internal medicine,* New York, 1998, McGraw-Hill.

Box 189-2	**Significant Findings of Hypothermia**

Cardiovascular
   Decreased heart rate
   Decreased cardiac output
   Decreased contractility
   Arrhythmias
   Decreased perfusion
   Pale cool skin
   Delayed capillary refill
Pulmonary
   Apnea or shallow breathing
   Hypoventilation
   Decreased cough reflex
Central nervous system
   Pupillary dilation with core temperature less than 35°C
   Decreased level of consciousness; lethargy
   Diminished reflexes
   Possible amnesia
   Decreased cerebral blood flow
   Potential for seizures
Renal
   Decreased renal perfusion
   Decreased tubular reabsorption that leads to electrolyte imbal-
   ances
   Acute tubular necrosis
Acid-base balance
   Early respiratory alkalosis
   Eventual metabolic acidosis
Gastrointestinal
   Decreased intestinal motility; ileus
   Decreased insulin release from the pancreas
   Decreased hepatic metabolism
   Stress ulceration
Hematologic
   Decreased oxygen delivery to tissue
   Increased blood viscosity
   Coagulopathy
   Splenic sequestration of platelets
Immunologic
   Leukocyte sequestration in the spleen
   Decreased neutrophils
   Decreased collagen deposition

- The effect of hypothermia on all body systems should be understood (see Box 189-2 for a listing of these findings).
- High body surface area, low body fat mass, and greater degree of brown fat metabolism make children especially susceptible to accidental hypothermia. Neonates have further vulnerability to hypothermia because of an inability to produce heat with shivering.[3] See Box 189-1 for a review of additional factors that predispose the infant and child to temperature instability.
- Metabolism of medications is dependent on organ function and thus is temperature sensitive as well. Hypothermia alters the pharmacologic dynamics of various drugs, especially muscle relaxants and anesthetics.[4]
- Radiant warmers may increase convective and evaporative heat loss and insensible water loss but may eliminate radiant heat loss. Insensible water loss (IWL) may be as high as twice the normal rate.[5] Adequate hydration is necessary for *all* infants and children who undergo radiant warmer therapy, and fluid requirements must be individualized.
- A disadvantage of having an infant lie in an open bed is lack of a barrier to infection.[6]
- Major advantages of the radiant warmer versus the incubator with an infant are provision of quick access and facilitation of procedures.

- Newer infrared patient warmers are now undergoing trials for use in the operating room, emergency room, intensive care unit, recovery room, and burns and plastic units. These designs are more compact and mobile and permit better patient access.
- Overly aggressive active external warming exposes the child to unnecessary risks of core temperature after-drop, metabolic acidosis, and shock.[3] After-drop occurs as warming relieves peripheral vasoconstriction; cooler peripheral blood enters the central circulation and can cause core temperature to drop even further.
- Rewarming shock occurs when hypothermic vasoconstriction masks hypovolemia. If the child's circulating blood volume is insufficient during rewarming vasodilatation, a sudden decrease in blood pressure, systemic vascular return, and preload occurs.[7]

- Children who are hypothermic with a stable condition may undergo safe warming with external active techniques, including radiant warmer devices.
- External rewarming of body temperature should not exceed 0.5°C to 2.0°C per hour.[2]

CHILD AND FAMILY ASSESSMENT

- Current medication therapy ➤*Rationale:* Medications such as vasopressors and vasodilators may affect heat transfer, increase the potential for skin injury, and contribute to an adverse response. Anticoagulation therapy may increase the potential for skin injury.
- Presence of coagulopathy and platelet dysfunction, which may affect mode of continuous temperature monitoring ➤*Rationale:* Invasive monitoring of temperature may aggravate existing bleeding tendencies.
- Baseline temperature via continuous monitoring ➤*Rationale:* Determines initial temperature and verifies indication for warming device; ongoing monitoring is allowed for prevention of rapid rewarming or overheating.
- Presence of acid-base imbalances ➤*Rationale:* Hypothermia may cause metabolic acidosis.
- Indications of dehydration; evaluation of intake and output and serum electrolytes ➤*Rationale:* Child may have increased insensible water loss from therapy. Fluid status should be known before therapy is initiated.
- Child's level of consciousness and neurologic function ➤*Rationale:* Determines baseline neurologic status.
- Presence or absence of bowel sounds and baseline abdominal and gastrointestinal function ➤*Rationale:* Determines baseline status. Children with hypothermia may develop an ileus from decreased intestinal motility.
- Baseline skin integrity ➤*Rationale:* Provides baseline data regarding skin integrity. Externally applied warming can cause burns or skin irritation.

CHILD AND FAMILY EDUCATION

Individualized, developmentally appropriate education is provided to the family and to the child based on desire for knowledge, readiness to learn, and overall neurologic and psychosocial state.

- Instruct the child and family how the radiant warmer device can be used to treat mild hypothermia ➤*Rationale:* Knowledge base concerning child's condition and procedure is increased.
- Explain the reason for temperature monitoring and how a deviation from normal body temperature range affects the child's condition ➤*Rationale:* The child and family are encouraged to ask questions and verbalize concerns regarding the child's condition, temperature ranges, and associated therapy.
- Determine the child's and family's understanding of therapy through open discussion ➤*Rationale:* Clarification and reinforcement of information may be needed in times of stress and anxiety.
- Discuss expectations for the duration of therapy and parameters for discontinuation of the device ➤*Rationale:* An explanation of what is expected and the length of therapy decreases child and family anxiety and enhances cooperation.

EQUIPMENT

- Cardiac monitor
- Continuous temperature monitoring device (in addition to skin thermistor of warming unit), including temperature probe, cable, and module
- Overhead radiant warmer (stand-alone resuscitation warmer unit or radiant warmer with built-in open care infant bed), skin thermistor, and power supply

Procedure   for Warming Devices: Radiant

Steps	Rationale	Considerations
1. Ensure child and family understand procedure and questions are answered.	Evaluates and reinforces understanding of previously taught information.	Developmental level, cognitive ability, and anxiety level determine approach to and effectiveness of teaching.
2. Wash hands.	Standard precautions; reduces transmission of microorganisms.	
3. Obtain baseline temperature.	Indicates current temperature.	
4. Place the child on a cardiac monitor.	Children with hypothermia are more susceptible to cardiac arrhythmias.	

Procedure continues on following page

Procedure for Warming Devices: Radiant—*Continued*

Steps	Rationale	Considerations
5. Adjust height of adjustable warming fixture (available on some models to suit varying bed heights). Consult manufacturer's instructions for the specific warmer unit.	Maintains optimal distance for operation of device and prevents thermal skin injury.	
6. Ensure adequate privacy.	Limits negative emotional response, maintains modesty, and respects child's right to privacy.	School-aged children may be especially modest. Ensuring privacy for this age group promotes feelings of security.
7. Determine area to be warmed. Expose skin surface area and apply skin thermistor probe with foiled back shield to area of trunk or abdomen that is not directly over a bony prominence and does not interfere with other necessary equipment. Insert the probe plug into the heater unit.	Transfer of energy necessitates direct exposure of skin. Placement of linens or drapes blocks this energy. Child's skin temperature should be monitored continuously and heat control mechanism adjusted accordingly during therapy.	If child is prone, attach probe to the skin over either flank, not between the scapulae.
8. Plug warming device into grounded outlet.	Establishes a power source. Grounded outlet promotes patient safety.	
9. Select desired skin temperature (typically 36°C to 36.5°C).	To achieve and maintain desired temperature.	
10. Turn on device and set warmer device in automatic (skin) servo control mode. Pre-warm the unit when possible to reduce conductive heat loss. *(Level II*)*	The warmer automatically increases or decreases heat delivered to the child in response to the feedback loop from the child's skin temperature sensor.	Non-servo control manual mode can be used but necessitates close observation to avoid wide temperature swings and the possibility of thermal injury to the child.
11. Read skin temperature from gauge on heater unit. If measurement registers at less than set point, verify that heater is functional.	High and low temperature alarm limits alert staff with audible alarm to further adjust skin temperature control.	Heat emitted to the child should never exceed 45°C because tissue damage could occur.[5]
12. Comparison of temperature obtained via axilla, rectum, or core measurement with skin thermistor probe temperature is an important safety factor.	Safety adjunct to prevent equipment malfunction. Ensures warmer temperature probe is functioning and correlates with the child's temperature obtained with another method.	If the child has decreased perfusion, the warmer may continue to generate heat regardless of child's actual core temperature, which may differ from skin temperature in the presence of cardiovascular compromise.
13. Check thermistor probe frequently to ascertain that it is in solid contact with skin and that it is free from foreign matter.	Covering the foil-shielded probe or poor skin contact of the probe and foil shield may cause overheating.	
14. Continuously reassess child and readings. Monitor for visual and audible alarms that indicate deviation from set parameters.	Prevents overheating or insufficient warmth.	External warming should only be applied to head and truncal areas to minimize peripheral vasodilatation.[3] The head must be kept covered if warmer is directed at the trunk because as much as 30% of body heat can be lost from the head.

* Level II: Theory-based; no research data to support recommendations; recommendations from expert consensus group may exist

Procedure for **Warming Devices: Radiant**—*Continued*

Steps	Rationale	Considerations
15. Record both the radiant warmer temperature setting and skin temperature hourly.	A clear increase or decrease trend in skin thermistor temperature may indicate development of sepsis or a neurologic problem.	
16. Visually inspect skin routinely for the duration of therapy.	Skin integrity and tissue perfusion (skin color, temperature, and capillary refill) must be routinely monitored as child rewarms to detect potential tissue injury.	Consider protective eye lubrication and use of eye patches if eye blinking is not observed or the lids are fixed open to prevent corneal scarring. Precautions should be considered, although studies have yet to document these potential complications to infrared energy.[5] *(Level II*)* The risk of tissue injury is increased when heat or pressure is combined with chemical irritants such as cleaning solutions or lotions. The thin delicate skin of the neonate or the edema of the child with gross fluid overload is susceptible to burns and pressure irritation.
17. Continue warming procedures until child's condition is normothermic and hemodynamic stability is achieved.	External warming is no longer needed once body temperature is corrected and child's condition is stabilized.	Radiant warmer therapy may be needed for several weeks in preterm infants because they are unable to produce their own heat.

* Level II: Theory-based; no research data to support recommendations; recommendations from expert consensus group may exist

Expected Outcomes	Unexpected Outcomes
• Rewarming is achieved at appropriate rate • Normothermia is maintained • Child is free from complications of external warming	• Overheating, which can cause hyperthermia and increased oxygen consumption and skin injury • Inability to achieve desired core body temperature with this device • Dehydration from exaggerated insensible water loss • Cardiac arrhythmia • Hemodynamic instability • Acid-base imbalances • Skin irritation and burns • Corneal irritation • Rewarming shock

Monitoring and Care of the Child

Activities and Interventions	Rationale	Reportable Conditions
1. Provide continuous cardiac monitoring.	Necessary for assessment of cardiac rhythm.	• Arrhythmias
2. Monitor vital signs during therapy.	Apnea, hypotension, and seizures have been associated with rapid rewarming.	• Vital sign measurements outside the child's normal values
3. Monitor all body systems every 1 to 2 hours and as indicated by child's status and condition.	Provides ongoing assessment of child's condition.	• Significant change in assessment results
4. Monitor skin and set temperatures displayed on unit. Additional temperature measurements from alternate sites should be obtained when systemic perfusion is compromised.	Monitors child's progress. Comparison of simultaneous temperature values permits added control and accuracy.	• Simultaneous temperature values that do not closely correlate • Hyperthermia or uncorrected hypothermia
5. Obtain daily weights; monitor fluid and electrolyte status to maintain adequate hydration.	Prevents dehydration or fluid overload. Insensible water loss may be as high as twice the normal rate.[5]	• Negative or positive fluid balance
6. Monitor serum glucose.	Radiant warmers may increase metabolic rates in infants, which may accentuate hypoglycemia. A transient hyperglycemic response is common in older infants and children with alterations in temperature.	• Hypo or hyperglycemia
7. Examine skin integrity and tissue perfusion hourly and provide eye protection as needed.	Detects skin injury and burns and prevents potential corneal irritation from excess exposure to infrared energy/light.	• Skin irritation, burns • Corneal irritation
8. Monitor arterial blood gases and electrolytes as indicated and per prescribing practitioner's order.	Detects acid-base and electrolyte imbalances.	• Abnormal blood gas or electrolyte values for child
9. Ensure child's comfort; assess pain using developmentally appropriate and institution-specific approved pain scale.	Optimizes comfort.	• Unrelieved pain or discomfort

Documentation

- Child and family education
- Initial and subsequent temperature measurements, including site, time, and date of measurements
- Vital signs, hemodynamic status, cardiac rhythm, and other pertinent physical assessment findings
- Radiant warmer set point and skin temperature
- Time and date that warming therapy was initiated and discontinued
- Child's symptoms and degree of comfort during therapy
- Skin integrity and tissue perfusion
- Unexpected outcomes and related treatment

References

1. Pate MF: Thermal regulation. In Curley MAQ, Moloney-Harmon PA, editors: *Critical care nursing of infants and children,* ed 2, Philadelphia, 2001, Saunders.
2. Petty KJ: Hypothermia. In Fauci AS, et al, editors: *Harrison's principles of internal medicine,* New York, 1998, McGraw-Hill.
3. Lange Varga J: Warming Procedures. In Henretig FM, King C, editors: *Textbook of pediatric emergency procedures,* Baltimore, 1997, Williams & Wilkins.
4. Sessler D: Complications and treatment of mild hypothermia, *Anesthesiology* 95:531-543, 2001.
5. Webster HF: Bioinstrumentation: Principles and techniques. In Hazinski MF, editor: *Nursing care of the critically ill child,* ed 2, St Louis, 1992, Mosby.
6. Greenspan J, et al: Thermal stability and transition studies with hybrid warming device for neonates, *J Perinatol* 21:167-173, 2001.
7. Kelly EM: External warming/cooling devices. In Lynn-McHale DJ, Carlson KK, editors: *AACN procedure manual for critical care,* ed 4, Philadelphia, 2001, Saunders.

Additional Readings

Buhre W, Rossaint R: Perioperative management and monitoring in anesthesia, *Lancet* 362:93-98, 2003.
Maayan-Metzer A, et al: Effect of radiant warmer on trans-epidermal water loss (TEWL) and skin hydration in preterm infants, *J Perinatol* 24(6):372-5, 2004.
Meyer M, et al: A clinical comparison of radiant warmer and incubator care for preterm infants from birth to 1800 grams, *Pediatrics* 108:2, 2001.
Morcom F: Chill out: therapeutic hypothermia improves survival, *Emerg Nurs* 11:4, 2003.

Neonatal Thermoregulation

PURPOSE: A neutral thermal environment is provided and/or maintained for the high-risk or preterm infant because of their limited neonatal thermoregulation. These infants often have an inability to stabilize and maintain body temperature without support; providing a neutral thermal environment allows conservation of limited resources for other necessary bodily functions.

Jacqueline M. McGrath

PREREQUISITE KNOWLEDGE

- Anatomy and physiology of the skin of the high-risk infant; infants have a thinner layer of subcutaneous fat[1,2]
- Principles of heat loss via the skin. Infants, especially preterm infants, have a larger surface-to-body mass ratio.[1-5]
- An understanding of thermogenesis and brown fat metabolism is needed to provide care based in a sound physiologic foundation for these infants.[3,6-9]
- Normal core body temperature for these infants should range from 36.5°C to 37°C; however, the normal range for a particular infant is noted to be when the infant's caloric expenditures and oxygen consumption are minimized. Normal axillary temperatures range from 36.5°C to 37.3°C.[1-4,10-12]
- Rectal temperature measurement, although reflective of core body temperature, is an invasive procedure and should only be done with extreme care. The thermometer can only be inserted 2 cm in a preterm infant and 3 cm in a full-term infant before it hits the curvature of the bowel. A thermometer can easily perforate the bowel and cause damage if inserted too far or too forcefully.[10]
- Axillary temperature measurements are most often used to reflect core body temperature in infants. They are less invasive and easily obtained.[1-4,10-12]
- The differences between and implications of core versus skin temperatures[1-3]

- Equipment such as double-walled incubators and overhead warmers are often used to support thermoregulation in infants. Care providers must understand how the equipment used to support the infant operates and how skin temperature is monitored. An ability to troubleshoot this equipment in support of the infant is also necessary.[4,13-16]
- An incubator is believed to be a more optimal environment for the high-risk infant than a radiant warmer unit because both conductive and convective losses are more easily stabilized for the infant. In addition, infants are often touched and disturbed less in an incubator, which could promote sleep and increase energy available for use in other processes.[14-17]
- All gases delivered to the infant must be considered a source of heat loss and should be warmed and humidified to decrease heat loss and prevent irritation to the infant's orifices.[1,3]
- Child development as it relates to clinical assessment and neonatal thermoregulation

CHILD AND FAMILY ASSESSMENT

- Gestational age and postconceptional age of the infant
  ➤Rationale: Permeability of the skin is greatest in extremely early born preterm infants (those less than 26 weeks gestation). The skin becomes less permeable with increasing postconceptional age (PCA) and thus less

susceptible to heat loss. Low–birth weight infants also have decreased stores of brown fat needed for thermogenesis.[1,3,5,6]

- Baseline core axillary temperature of the infant; axillary temperatures are considered core temperatures because of the deposits of brown fat found there ➤➤*Rationale:* Baseline and ongoing temperature monitoring is the basis for decision-making and intervention.
- Glucose levels ➤➤*Rationale:* Heat is a byproduct of energy production; glucose is needed for the production of heat through chemical thermogenesis.[3,6,10]
- Status of the respiratory system ➤➤*Rationale:* Oxygen consumption is increased during heat production. If the respiratory system is already compromised by prematurity or illness, heat production is also compromised.[3,6,10]
- Function or maturation of the gastrointestinal system ➤➤*Rationale:* A functional gut is needed for the administration of enteral or oral feedings. If the infant's condition is stable and mature enough to tolerate feedings, enteral or oral is the route of choice to provide nutrition to support glucose stores. An intravenous route for glucose administration is needed if the gut cannot tolerate feedings.[1,2,9]
- Any object that touches the infant's skin must be assessed for its contribution to heat loss in the infant; this includes the care provider's hands, stethoscope, and other medical equipment.[1-3,15,16,18]

CHILD AND FAMILY EDUCATION

Individualized, developmentally appropriate education is provided to the family based on desire for knowledge, readiness to learn, and overall psychosocial state.

- Provide information about the mechanics of heat loss in the high-risk infant through evaporation, convection, conduction, and radiation; assure the family that this is an expected area of intervention for all high-risk and preterm infants[1-3,14,17] ➤➤*Rationale:* Providing information decreases anxiety and fear related to the need for equipment to support the body temperature in these infants. In addition, this information contributes to the family's management of thermoregulation in the home environment.[18]

- Explain the need to regularly monitor body temperature and how the need for heat production can affect energy reserves and oxygen consumption in these infants ➤➤*Rationale:* Providing information on range of temperature, assessment of temperature changes, and the effects of temperature management on the body is helpful for understanding the need for interventions to better support the infant.
- Explain the need to consider the environment and all objects that touch the infant as potential avenues of heat loss ➤➤*Rationale:* All caregivers have the opportunity to affect temperature management and must be aware of the environment and their personal contributions to heat loss.[14,19]
- Explain the possible need for equipment such as radiant warmers and double-walled incubators to provide thermal support for infants[3,4,14] ➤➤*Rationale:* Providing information about the equipment used to support the high-risk or preterm infant can decrease anxiety and fear. In addition, this information can provide families with the ability to appropriately interact with and touch the infant in these environments.
- Encourage questions and answer questions as they arise ➤➤*Rationale:* Reinforcement of information is needed during periods of stress.

EQUIPMENT

- Head covering greater than ½ inch thick
- Warmed blankets
- Heat shields
- Plastic bubble wrap
- Warming pads
- Prewarmed radiant warmer
- Prewarmed double-walled incubator
- Humidification source for air in incubator
- Porthole sleeves for incubator
- Mechanism to warm and humidify gases delivered to the infant
- Thermometers (electric, ear, skin tapes, etc.)
- Temperature probes/covers for incubators and radiant warmers

Procedure for Neonatal Thermoregulation

Steps	Rationale	Considerations
In the Delivery Room		
1. If the temperature of the room can be adjusted, make the room warmer for the birth of the infant.[5,20] *(Level IV*)*	Heat loss during the delivery process is high and interventions to decrease all circumstances that could influence heat loss are necessary.	Decreases convective sources of heat loss for the infant; conserves energy for other processes.
2. Close doors and adjust vents in the room.	Decreases convective sources of heat loss for the infant; conserves energy for other processes.	
3. Before delivery of the high-risk or preterm infant, place a radiant warmer in the delivery room.[5,20] *(Level IV*)*	Decreases conductive sources of heat loss for the infant; conserves energy for other processes.	If the infant to be delivered is less than 28 weeks gestation, delivery into an incubator or combination incubator/radiant warmer bed should be considered as the environmental intervention of choice when available.[5,19,20] *(Level IV*)*
4. If the stabilization nursery is not next door to the delivery room, prewarm a transport incubator ready for use to transport the infant to the nursery.[5,19,20] *(Level IV*)*	Decreases convective and conductive sources of heat loss during transport to the nursery; conserves energy for other processes necessary for survival.	
5. Place the radiant warmer in the delivery room out of the way so that it is not in a walkway or near air drafts.	Decreases convective sources of heat loss for the infant; conserves energy for other processes necessary for survival.	
6. Turn on and prewarm the radiant warmer with manual settings to a temperature of 37°C.	Decreases convective and conductive sources of heat loss for the infant; conserves energy for other processes necessary for survival.	
7. Place all supplies that will be used for resuscitation or will touch the infant on the warmer. This step includes warming the hands and stethoscopes of care providers.[19-21] *(Level IV*)*	Decreases conductive sources of heat loss for the infant; conserves energy for other processes necessary for survival.	
8. Ensure head covering greater than ½ inch thick is available. *(Level II*)*	Increased numbers of heat receptors are found on the face and head; covering the head is especially important when evaporative losses after the birth process are great.	The trigeminal area of the neonate's face is most receptive to changes in temperature. Most stockinet capping used in the delivery room is not ½ inch thick and should not be considered adequate for temperature management in the ill or preterm infant.
9. Ensure blankets from a nearby blanket warmer are available.	Decreases conductive sources of heat loss for the infant; conserves energy for other processes necessary for survival.	
10. Ensure that the family understands the rationale for these interventions and the need for this equipment.	Evaluates and reinforces understanding of previously taught information.	Developmental level, cognitive ability, and anxiety level determine approach to and effectiveness of teaching.

* Level II: Theory-based; no research data to support recommendations; recommendations from expert consensus group may exist
  Level IV: Limited clinical studies to support recommendations

Procedure for Neonatal Thermoregulation—*Continued*

Steps	Rationale	Considerations
11. Once the infant is born, catch the infant in a warmed sterile towel or blanket.	Decreases conductive and radiant sources of heat loss for the infant; conserves energy for other processes necessary for survival.	
12. Stop momentarily for the mother and family to see and touch the infant, then proceed to the radiant warmer.	Allowing the parents to see the infant increases bonding and decreases anxiety and fear during a time when fears might be high given the high-risk nature of the birth.	
13. An occlusive polyethylene body bag may be used immediately after delivery during stabilization; place the torso and extremities in the bag and secure. Remove the wrapping after the neonate's condition has been stabilized in the delivery room or after admission to Neonatal Intensive Care Unit (NICU).[22] *(Level II*)*	Reduces the postnatal temperature decrease caused by excessive evaporative heat loss.	
14. Dry the infant quickly, remove the wet towels or blankets from the bed space, and wrap the infant in dry warmed blankets.[5,19,20] Cover the infant's head with a hat. *(Level IV*)*	Decreases evaporative, radiation, and conductive sources of heat loss for the infant; conserves energy for other processes necessary for survival.	
15. Allow the parents to touch the infant, warming their hands if possible.	Allowing the parents to touch and see the infant increases bonding and decreases anxiety and fear during a time when fears might be high given the high-risk nature of the birth. Warming the hands should decrease conductive sources of heat loss and stress for the infant.	
16. Provide oxygen support as needed.	Heat production requires energy and could increase metabolic needs for the infant, necessitating increased oxygen support if the infant's respiratory system is already stressed or immature.	Oxygen and all gases should be warmed and humidified, especially because the trigeminal area of the neonate's face is most receptive to changes in temperature. However, little or no research examines these particular issues in temperature management.
17. Transport the infant in a prewarmed double-walled transport incubator to the NICU.	Decreases convective and conductive sources of heat loss during transport to the nursery; conserves energy for other processes necessary for survival.	
18. On entry into the NICU, the infant is routinely weighed. Place a heating lamp over the scale to prewarm it. Also prewarm the covering on the scale on which the infant lays. Perform the weight measurement quickly and smoothly and place the infant in an incubator or radiant warmer.	Decreases convective and conductive sources of heat loss for the infant; conserves energy for other processes necessary for survival.	Extremely early born preterm infants (those less than 28 weeks) should be placed in an incubator or radiant warmer with a bed scale so that continued monitoring of weights does not compromise thermal regulation.[18,20,21,23] *(Level IV*)*

Procedure continues on following page

---

* Level II: Theory-based; no research data to support recommendations; recommendations from expert consensus group may exist
Level IV: Limited clinical studies to support recommendations

Procedure | for Neonatal Thermoregulation—*Continued*

Steps	Rationale	Considerations
Use of Double-Walled Incubator		
19. Once the decision to bring the infant to the NICU has been made, a double-walled incubator or radiant warmer should be prewarmed on air control (manual) to 37°C. On the infant's arrival to the NICU, the air control inside the incubator should be set on basis of the gestational age of the infant.[5,19,20] *(Level IV*)*	Decreasing all avenues of heat loss during the admission process allows the infant to conserve energy for other processes necessary for survival.	Incubators are the environment of choice for the high-risk or preterm infant. Thermal regulation is easier to stabilize in this environment, and the external environment is not as great a concern if an incubator is used.
20. Place the double-walled incubator or radiant warmer in a bed space that is free of drafts and away from doorways or air vents and outside windows if it is winter.	Decreases convective and conductive sources of heat loss for the infant; conserves energy for other processes necessary for survival.	
21. Secure the temperature probe on the abdomen according to the manufacturer's guidelines. Choose a site that is away from bony areas and a place where the infant is not to be positioned or lying on top of the probe. Switch the incubator to skin (servo) control set at 36.5°C.[2,24] *(Level IV*)*	Servo control regulates the environment of the incubator in response to the infant's skin temperature and conserves energy for other processes necessary for survival.[10,13,24,25] *(Level IV*)*	A set point of 36.5°C is most often recommended for support of the infant. Over warming can be just as stressful to a high-risk infant as an environment that is too cold. The temperature probe may need to be moved when the infant's position is changed.[13,24] A displaced or inaccurately placed probe can cause inaccurate temperature readings.[10,13,24,25] *(Level IV*)*
22. Obtain an axillary core temperature. Although standard practice in many NICUs is still to obtain the initial core temperature rectally, no rationale exists for this procedure and it is no longer recommended.	Core temperatures are a late sign of hypothermia in an infant and are not considered the best indication of temperature stability. Infants move in and out of hypothermic states on the basis of skin temperature alone, and assessment leading to appropriate intervention must be the guiding force for the practice for monitoring thermal regulation in the infant.	Rectal temperature should be done with caution; perforation of the bowel is possible. This method should not be used as the routine route for temperature monitoring. If this site is used, the probe should be inserted downward and backward at a 30-degree angle to a depth of 3 cm in a term infant and 2 cm in a preterm infant. The probe should be held in place for 3 or more minutes to ensure an accurate reading.
23. Place all supplies that will be used to care for the infant or will touch the infant in the incubator. Warm the hands and stethoscopes of care providers before use on the infant.[19,20,23] *(Level IV*)*	Decreases convective and conductive sources of heat loss for the infant; conserves energy for other processes necessary for survival.	A small number of diapers and other routine supplies can be stored at the foot of the incubator so they are always ready for caregiving. The stethoscope can also be left inside the incubator so that it is warm before it touches the infant's skin.

* Level IV: Limited clinical studies to support recommendations

Procedure for Neonatal Thermoregulation—*Continued*

Steps	Rationale	Considerations
24. Axillary temperature can be used for routine monitoring of core temperature. The probe must be held in place for 3 or more minutes for an accurate reading.[5,10,11,14] *(Level IV*)*	Axillary temperatures are noninvasive and approximate core temperatures.[1,3]	In a cold environment, core temperatures are not indicative of thermal stability in an infant. The infant uses all resources to maintain core temperature, and skin temperatures have been known to fluctuate widely even when core temperatures appear stable.
25. Add 70% humidity to double-walled incubators for infants less than 30 weeks gestation for the first 7 days of life (depending on the gestation of the infants and the permeability of the skin). After the first week, continue humidity at 50% to 60% until the infant reaches 30 to 32 weeks postconceptional age.[26] *(Level IV*)*	Generally, 40% humidity in the incubator may lower the environmental needs of the preterm infant by 1°C or more. Humidity also decreases insensible water loss through the skin and can make stabilization of electrolytes easier to achieve.	Aquaphor and other ointments have also been used as a barrier to decrease heat loss in the very low–birth weight infant. More research is needed in this area to better justify this practice.
26. If recommended by the manufacturer, use sleeves on portholes, especially if the infant is early born, is low birth weight, or has thermal instability.[19,20] *(Level IV*)*	Decreases convective sources of heat loss for the infant; conserves energy for other processes necessary for survival.	Newer incubators generally do not require sleeves on the portholes to maintain temperature stability within the incubator environment.
27. When incubators are covered with blankets or incubator covers and then uncovered, monitoring of temperature regulation may need to be more frequent.[27] *(Level IV*)*	Uncovering the incubator may result in increased heat loss for the infant.	As a result of developmental care in the NICU, incubators are often hooded with blankets or incubator covers for extended periods of time and until a thermal effect has been noted.

Use of Radiant Warmer

Steps	Rationale	Considerations
28. Secure the temperature probe on the abdomen according to the manufacturer's guidelines. Choose a site that is away from bony areas and brown fat deposits; the infant should not be positioned lying on top of the probe. Switch the radiant warmer to skin (servo) control set at 36.5°C.	Servo control regulates the environment under the radiant warmer in response to the infant's skin temperature and conserves energy for other processes necessary for survival.[10,13,24,25]	Servo control is optimal under a radiant warmer. Instances of over-warming an infant have occurred when the probe was not placed appropriately or the warmer was not switched to skin control to monitor the infant's temperature appropriately.[13,15,16,24,25] *(Level IV*)* The temperature probe may need to be moved when the infant's position is changed.[10,13,24,25] *(Level IV*)* A displaced probe can cause temperature fluctuations.[10,13,24,25]
29. All supplies that will be used to care for the infant or will touch the infant should be placed on the warmer; this step includes warming the hands and stethoscopes of care providers.	Decreases convective and conductive sources of heat loss for the infant; conserves energy for other processes necessary for survival.	A small number of diapers and other routine supplies can be stored at the foot of the warmer so they are always ready for caregiving. The stethoscope can also be left in the bed space so that it is warm before it touches the infant's skin.

Procedure continues on following page

* Level IV: Limited clinical studies to support recommendations

Procedure   for Neonatal Thermoregulation—*Continued*

Steps	Rationale	Considerations
30. Warming pads can be placed under infants in radiant warmers or incubators.	Decreases conductive sources of heat loss for the infant; conserves energy for other processes necessary for survival.	May cause burns if used without appropriate protective covers or if temperature is not monitored appropriately.
31. Saran wrap or plastic blankets and plastic shields can be placed over the infant in radiant warmers or incubators.	Decreases convective sources of heat loss for the infant; conserves energy for other processes necessary for survival.[1-3]	Ensure that if plastic shields are used the chance of decreasing the amount of radiant heat that reaches the infant is considered. Plexiglas has been found to be opaque to radiant waves.[1-3]
Bathing the Infant		
32. Bathing should be delayed until the infant's temperature is stabilized in the normal range for 2 to 4 hours; consider the metabolic effects of temperature stability such as glucose needs and oxygen requirements.[5,19-21,26] *(Level IV*)* Excessive vernix may be removed, but removal of all vernix is not necessary for hygienic purposes.[20,26]	Bathing decreases the infant's temperature.	Extremely early born preterm infants, those less then 28 weeks, should have stable conditions for at least 4 hours before the first bath; consider the metabolic needs of the infant and their decreased ability to meet those needs.[5,19,20] *(Level IV*)*
33. Temperature should be monitored closely before, during, and after the bath; warmed towels and bedding should be available, and the bath should be discontinued if the infant displays distress.	Assesses for significant change in temperature.	
Weaning to an Open Crib		
34. Weaning to an open crib should occur slowly. The incubator temperature should be decreased 1°C to 1.5°C daily until the incubator is at room temperature.[28,29] *(Level IV*)*	Once an infant has had 5 days of consistent weight gain, has not had apnea or bradycardia, is tolerating enteral feedings, is not on mechanical ventilation, and has a medically stable condition, weaning to an open crib may be considered.[28,29] *(Level IV*)*	
35. During weaning, the infant should be dressed with a hat and two blankets.[28,29] *(Level IV*)*	Hats and blankets decrease heat loss.	
36. Place the infant into an open crib. Axillary temperature should be monitored closely during this time.	Assesses infant's tolerance of weaning process.	If the weaning process fails, the infant should be returned to the incubator with servo control and the trial to wean should not begin again until the infant has medical stability and stable weight gain for at least 48 hours.

* Level IV: Limited clinical studies to support recommendations

Expected Outcomes

- Core temperature as measured with axillary temperature remains 36°C to 37°C

- Energy for other process such as growth is available because heat production by the infant is unnecessary

Unexpected Outcomes

- Infant temperature drops below 36°C and infant needs rewarming[1,3,7]
- Infant temperature rises above 37.5°C and intervention is needed to decrease to a normal range.
- Infant fails to gain weight appropriately[1,3,7,17]
- Infant needs increased oxygen and glucose support because energy has been used for heat production rather than growth and development[1-3,7,17]

Monitoring and Care of the Child

Activities and Interventions	Rationale	Reportable Conditions
1. Monitor core temperature every 2 to 4 hours as needed to maintain infant temperature between 36°C and 37°C.	Regular assessment of core temperature allows prompt intervention for abnormalities.[1,3]	• Infant core temperature less than 36°C • Air temperature greater than 37°C
2. Monitor glucose levels every hour until stable and then every 8 hours as needed and per prescribing practitioner's order or unit-specific protocol.	Glucose is needed for energy production and chemical thermogenesis in the infant; allows prompt intervention for low levels.[3,6,10]	• Glucose level less than 40 mg/dL • Low glucose level not responsive to interventions
3. Monitor probe placement every 4 to 8 hours.	Monitors for presence of a steady environment; core temperature may not always be reflective of an unstable environment. Probes may need to be moved with position changes for optimal readings. A displaced probe may cause temperature fluctuations.	• Infant core temperature less than 36°C • Air temperature greater than 37°C
4. Monitor oxygen consumption.	Oxygen is needed for energy and heat production; therefore, oxygen consumption may be increased.[3,6,10]	• Increasing oxygen needs above baseline for infant
5. Monitor caloric expenditures.	If energy is used for chemical thermogenesis, energy for growth and other bodily functions may not be available.[3,6,10]	• Weight loss • Consistent inability to gain weight
6. Monitor for other signs and symptoms of hypothermia and/or cold stress, such as peripheral vasoconstriction, increased production of ketone bodies, dissociation of albumin and bilirubin (increased bilirubin levels, not falling even in the presence of phototherapy).[1,3]	Signs and symptoms of hypothermia or adverse physiologic effects may be present even when the core temperature appears stable.	• Instability even with appropriate interventions

Documentation

- Core temperature
- Alarm set point on incubator or warmer
- Control mode: skin, air, or servo control
- Environmental temperature
- Air temperature and skin temperature readings of incubator
- Set point of incubator or warmer
- Oxygen requirements
- Glucose level
- Indicators of calorie expenditure such as weight gain or loss
- Feeding tolerance
- Interventions used to maintain temperature
- Family education
- Unexpected outcomes and related treatment

References

1. Armstrong V: Neonatal thermoregulation. *NANN guidelines for practice,* Petaluma, CA, 1997, National Association of Neonatal Nurses.
2. Blackburn ST: *Maternal, neonatal, and fetal physiology: a clinical perspective,* ed 2, Philadelphia, 2003, Saunders.
3. Bach V, et al: Body temperature regulation in the newborn infant: interaction with sleep and clinical implications, *Neurophysiol Clin* 2:379-402, 1996.
4. Dodman N: Newborn temperature control, *Neonatal Network* 4(3):19-23, 1987.
5. Smales ORC, Kime R: Thermoregulation in babies immediately after birth, *Arch Dis Childhood* 53:58-61, 1978.
6. Buczkowski-Bickermann MK: Thermoregulation in the neonate and the consequences of hypothermia, *CRNA: Clin Forum Nurs Anesthetists* 3(2):77-82, 1992.
7. Davis V: The structure and function of brown adipose tissue in the neonate, *J Obstet Gynecol Neonatal Nurs JOGNN* Nov/Dec:368-372, 1980.
8. Gluckman PD, et al: Transition from fetus to neonate—an endocrine perspective, *Acta Paediatr Suppl* 428:7-11, 1999.
9. Himms-Hagen J: Does thermoregulatory feeding occur in newborn infants? A novel view of the role of brown adipose tissue thermogenesis in control of food control, *Obesity Res* 3(4):361-369, 1995.
10. Bliss-Holtz J: Methods of newborn infant temperature monitoring: a research review, *Iss Comprehens Pediatr Nurs* 18:287-298, 1995.
11. Keeling EB: Thermoregulation and axillary temperature measurements in neonates: a review of the literature, *Maternal Child Nurs J* 20(3,4):124-140, 1992.
12. Stephen SB, Sexton PR: Neonatal axillary temperatures: increases in readings over time, *Neonatal Network* June:25-28, 1987.
13. Boyd H, Lenhart P: Temperature control: servo versus nonservo—which is best? *Neonatal Network* 15(2):75-76, 1996.
14. Choudhary SP, et al: Knowledge, attitude and practices about neonatal hypothermia among medical and paramedical staff, *Indian J Pediatr* 67(7):491-496, 2000.
15. LeBlanc MH: Thermoregulation: incubators, radiant warmers, artificial skins, and body hoods, *Clin Perinatol* 18(3),403-422, 1991.

16. LeBlanc MH, Donnelly MM: Thermoregulation: the design of incubators and radiant warmers. In Brans YW, Hay WW, editors: *Physiologic monitoring and instrument diagnosis in perinatal and neonatal medicine,* New York, 1995, Cambridge University Press.
17. Hackman PS: Recognizing and understanding the cold-stressed term infant, *Mother-Baby J* 5(4):10-25, 1995.
18. Thomas K: Infant weight and gestational age effects on thermoneutrality in the home environment, *J Obstet Gynecol Neonatal Nurs* 32(6):745-752, 2003.
19. Thomas KA: Preterm infant thermal responses to caregiving differ by incubator control mode, *J Perinatol* 23(8):640-645, 2003.
20. Longhead MK, Longhead JL, Reinhart MJ: Incidence and physiologic characteristics of hypothermia in the very low birth weight infant, *Pediatr Nurs* 23(1):11-15, 1997.
21. Penny-MacGillivray T: A newborn bath: when? *J Obstet Gynecol Neonatal Nurs* 25(6):481-487, 1996.
22. Vohra S, Frent G, Campbell V, et al: Effect of polyethylene occlusive skin wrapping on heat loss in very low birth weight infants at delivery: a randomized trial, *J Pediatr* 134:547–551, 1999.
23. Fardig JA: A comparison of skin-to-skin contact and radiant heat in promoting neonatal thermoregulation, *J Nurse-Midwifery* 25(1):19-28, 1980.
24. Blackburn ST, et al: Neonatal thermal care, part I: survey of temperature probe practices, *Neonatal Network* 20(3):15-18, 2001.
25. Blackburn ST, et al: Neonatal thermal care, part III: the effects of infant position and temperature probe placement, *Neonatal Network* 20(3):25-30, 2001.
26. Lund et al: *Neonatal skin care: evidence-based clinical practice guideline: Association of Women's Health, Obstetric and Neonatal Nurses (AWHONN),* Washington, 2001, National Association of Neonatal Nurses (NANN).
27. Nelson H, Thomas K, Stein M: Thermal effects of hooding incubators, *J Obstet Gynecol Neonatal Nurs* 21(5):377-381, 1992.
28. Medoff-Cooper B: Transition of the preterm infant to an open crib, *J Obstet Gynecol Neonatal Nurs* 23(4):329-335, 1994.
29. Meier PP: Transition of the preterm infant to an open crib: process of the project group, *J Obstet Gynecol Neonatal Nurs* 23(4):321-326, 1994.

Neonatal Positioning

P U R P O S E : Neonatal positioning is used to position the preterm and term neonate in a manner that promotes physiologic and behavioral development

Barbara McFadden

PREREQUISITE KNOWLEDGE

- Extremely low–birth weight infants are at higher risk for neuromotor problems than are other infants.
- Preterm infants, especially very low–birth weight (VLBW) infants, have an inability to change static posture, which may result in muscle imbalance (Figure 191-1).
- The benefits of prone positioning in regards to respiratory function, apnea, and sleep state in the preterm infant
- Despite the benefits of prone positioning, the preterm infant is at risk for postural abnormalities.
- Supine positioning is the recommended position for sleep in term, near-term, and preterm infants greater than 34 weeks corrected age in preparation for discharge.
- The risks associated with prone positioning for sleep
- The risks of soft bedding and stuffed animals in relation to sudden infant death syndrome (SIDS)
- The importance of incorporation of supine sleep positioning before discharge
- The importance of prone time in achievement of developmental milestones

CHILD AND FAMILY ASSESSMENT

- Family's previous experience with a preterm infant or child with neurodevelopmental abnormalities ➡*Rationale:* Assesses family's current knowledge related to prevention of neurodevelopmental abnormalities or developmental delays.
- History of SIDS or SIDS-related event in a sibling or family history of SIDS ➡*Rationale:* Identifies high risk

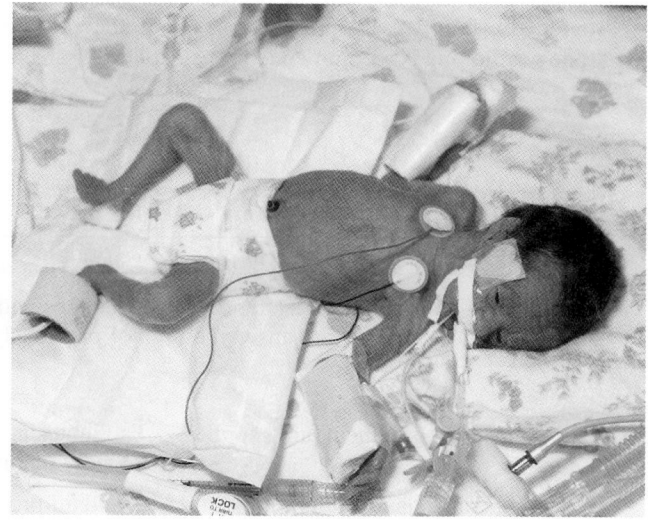

FIGURE 191-1 Hypotonic infant. *From Hunter JG: The neonatal intensive care unit. In Case-Smith J, editor:* Occupational therapy for children, *ed 4, St Louis, 2001, Mosby.*

infants; the families of high risk infants must be educated on the importance of supine positioning.
- Neonate's post conception age ➡*Rationale:* This information is necessary for identifying appropriate positioning interventions.
- Support mechanisms within the family ➡*Rationale:* Education must be provided to all possible caregivers.
- Family's understanding of the reasons for and risks and benefits of appropriate neonatal positioning ➡*Rationale:*

Evaluates family's understanding of the procedure and provides a gauge for ongoing education.

CHILD AND FAMILY EDUCATION

Individualized, developmentally appropriate education is provided to the family based on desire for knowledge, readiness to learn, and overall psychosocial state.

- Provide the family with information about the role of prone positioning in physiologic development of the VLBW infant; the prone position promotes development of the pulmonary, cardiovascular, sleep state, organizational, and gastrointestinal functions of preterm infants ➤*Rationale:* Providing information may increase the family's knowledge base, improve cooperation, and decrease anxiety.
- Explain that the VLBW infant is at increased risk for abnormal neuromotor development and positional deformities because prone positioning leads to static posture as a result of immature muscle development and the effects of gravity. ➤*Rationale:* Providing information may increase the family's knowledge base, improve cooperation, and decrease anxiety.
- Explain that variation of head position during sleeping prevents abnormal head molding (plagiocepahly) ➤*Rationale:* Providing information may increase the family's knowledge base, improve cooperation, facilitate the family's participation in the infant's care and decrease anxiety.
- Provide the family with information about the reason supine positioning is recommended for sleep. Prone sleep is believed to be associated with hypoxia and hypercarbia from rebreathing carbon dioxide trapped near the infant's face. Most SIDS deaths occur during the first 1 to 6 months of life. ➤*Rationale:* Providing information may increase the family's knowledge base, improve cooperation, and decrease anxiety.
- Explain the reason prone positioning during waking hours is necessary; prone to play allows the infant the time to strengthen the muscles of the neck, arms, and trunk and allows the acquisition of developmental milestones ➤*Rationale:* Providing information may increase the family's knowledge base, improve cooperation, and decrease anxiety.
- Demonstrate the use of facilitative tuck to aid in hand-to-mouth and flexed position of infant and explain that facilitative tuck allows for positive touch and normal flexion and also aids in calming the infant during noxious procedures ➤*Rationale:* Providing information may increase the family's knowledge base, improve cooperation, facilitate the family's participation in the infant's care and decrease anxiety.
- Encourage questions and answer questions as they arise ➤*Rationale:* Reinforcement of information is needed during periods of stress.

EQUIPMENT

- Appropriate positioning tools such as gel mattress, pillows, bunting, and snuggle-up
- Small blankets when these tools are not available

Procedure for **Neonatal Positioning**

Steps	Rationale	Considerations
1. Ensure child and family understand procedure and questions are answered.	Evaluates and reinforces understanding of previously taught information.	Developmental level, cognitive ability, and anxiety level determine approach to and effectiveness of teaching.
2. Gather needed equipment and supplies.	Facilitates completion of task in a timely manner.	
3. Wash and warm hands before all interventions.	Standard precautions; reduces transmission of microorganisms. Prevents cold stress of the infant.	
4. Use water or gel pillow under head. (*Level I**)	Reduces bilateral head flattening.	These supports may be expensive.
5. Change position of head for sleep. (*Level II**)	Reduces bilateral head flattening.	Infants often develop "favorite" position.
6. Supine: Head near midline; support under shoulder and humerus; rolls under legs and against lateral thighs.[1] (*Level II**)	Skull shaping; prevents shoulder retraction, allows hand-to-mouth contact, promotes flexion, and prevents hip abduction and external rotation.	Provide boundaries for the infant with blankets or preformed devices to assist in maintenance of position.

* Level I: Manufacturer's recommendations only
  Level II: Theory-based; no research data to support recommendations; recommendations from expert consensus group may exist

Procedure | **for Neonatal Positioning**—*Continued*

Steps	Rationale	Considerations
7. Side-lying: Ensure neutral head-trunk alignment. Place support roll behind head and trunk. Alternate sides routinely (Figure 191-2).[1] *(Level II*)*	Promotes hand-to-mouth and hand midline; prevents shoulder retraction.	If shoulder retraction persists, use swaddling to stabilize arm toward midline. Provide boundaries with blankets or preformed devices to assist in maintenance of position.

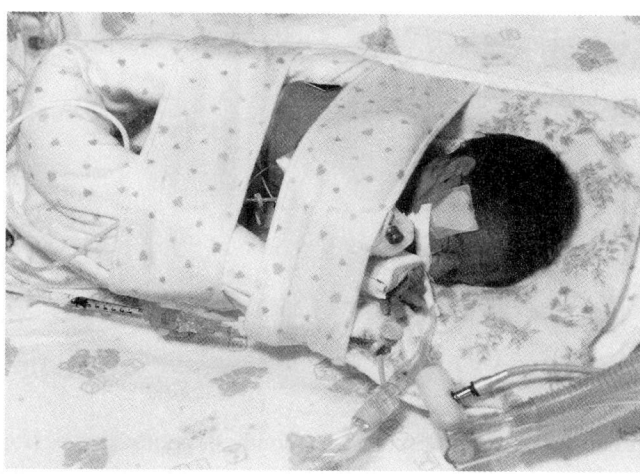

FIGURE 191-2 Side-lying position. *From Hunter JG: The neonatal intensive care unit. In Case-Smith J, editor: Occupational therapy for children, ed 4, St Louis, 2001, Mosby.*

Steps	Rationale	Considerations
8. Prone: Place a horizontal diaper roll under trunk and hips to maintain posterior pelvic tilt and hip flexion; lateral support to legs and feet (Figure 191-3).[1] *(Level II*)*	Prevents shoulder retraction; prevents foot eversion and excessive hip abduction.	Provide boundaries with blankets or preformed devices to assist in maintenance of position.

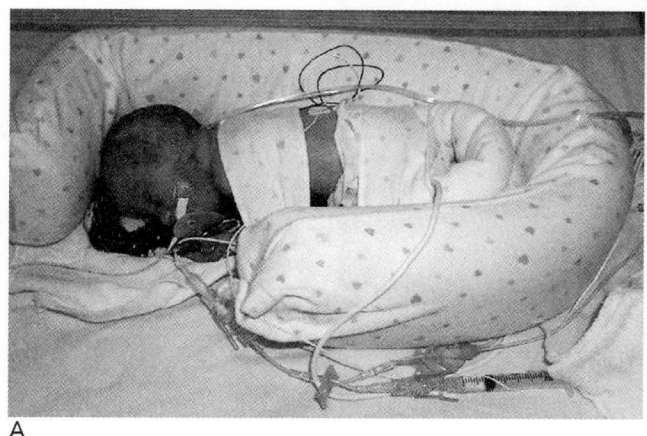 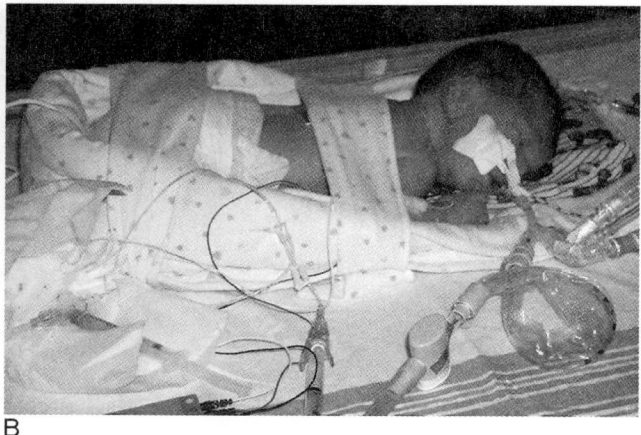

A   B

FIGURE 191-3 Prone position. *From Hunter JG: The neonatal intensive care unit. In Case-Smith J, editor: Occupational therapy for children, ed 4, St Louis, 2001, Mosby.*

Procedure continues on following page

* Level II: Theory-based; no research data to support recommendations; recommendations from expert consensus group may exist

Procedure for Neonatal Positioning—*Continued*

Steps	Rationale	Considerations

9. At 34 weeks after conception, infants should begin transition to supine position.[2] *(Level IV*)*	Promotes supine sleep position in preparation for discharge.	Hospitalized preterm infants are routinely placed in the prone position. Once conditions are stable and without clinical indications for prone positioning, infants should be transitioned to supine position for sleep.
		Possible exceptions:
		  Infants with respiratory distress, oxygen requirement, or tachypnea.
		  Infants with symptomatic apnea.
		  Infants with suspected airway obstruction.
		  Infants with symptomatic gastroesophageal reflux.
		  Infants with clinical conditions in which supine positioning is contraindicated (e.g., neural tube defects).

10. Use facilitative tuck during procedures to aid in calming infant and promote flexed position (see Figure 191-4).	Promotes hand-to-mouth, provides positive touch, counteracts noxious stimuli, and prevents long-term developmental sequelae from effects of noxious procedures.	Important for infants with increased length of stay, poor weight gain, or developmental delay.

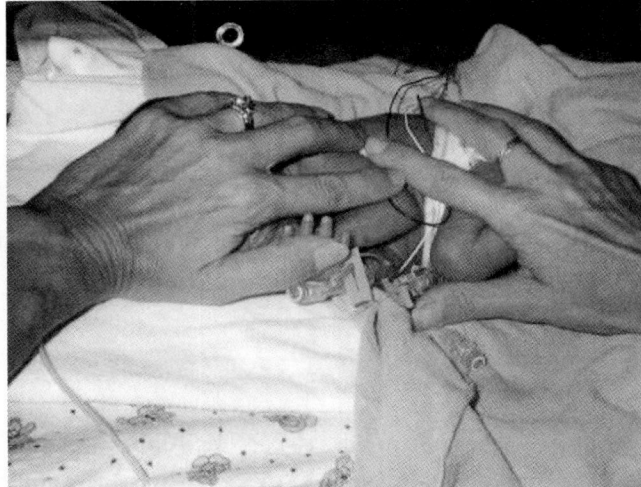

FIGURE 191-4   Facilitative tuck. *From Hunter JG: The neonatal intensive care unit. In Case-Smith J, editor: Occupational therapy for children, ed 4, St Louis, 2001, Mosby.*

Steps	Rationale	Considerations
11. Limit amount of soft bedding or procedural aids for sleeping. *(Level II*)*	These objects increase risk for SIDS.	Soft bedding or stuffed animals may cover the infant's face and increase hypoxia and hypercarbic effects.
12. Ensure that the parent and family understand the reason for transition to supine positioning.	Reinforces appropriate sleep position for home and potential consequences of prone positioning for sleep.	Especially important to stress with history of SIDS-related event in family.

* Level II: Theory-based; no research data to support recommendations; recommendations from expert consensus group may exist
Level IV: Limited clinical studies to support recommendations

Expected Outcomes

- Infant tolerates supine positioning for sleep

- Normal neurodevelopmental outcome
- Normal head shaping
- Infant is free from positional deformities
- Family understands need for supervised prone positioning for play
- Ability to self-calm
- Normal sleep patterns

Unexpected Outcomes

- Increased respiratory rate and work of breathing, apnea, desaturations
- Airway obstruction
- Increased gastroesophageal reflux
- Developmental delays
- Plagiocephaly
- Positional deformities
- Family is not able to describe or state reason for supervised prone positioning
- Extended periods of agitation
- Irregular sleep patterns

Monitoring and Care of the Infant

Activities and Interventions	Rationale	Reportable Conditions
1. Monitor for signs and symptoms of gastroesophageal reflux: apnea, bradycardia, desaturations, and emesis.	Indications of gastroesophageal reflux need further investigation and possible changes in positioning.	• Apnea • Bradycardia • Increased oxygen requirement, persistent with feedings
2. Monitor infant's ability to self calm and sleep patterns.	Periods of calm and adequate sleep result in improved weight gain and duration of REM sleep. Ability to self-calm promotes tolerance of procedures.	• Extended periods necessary to recover after procedures • Poor weight gain
3. Monitor infant for signs of respiratory distress.	Increase in respiratory distress may indicate underlying pathology or worsening condition.	• Increased respiratory rate • Increased work of breathing • Increased oxygen requirement • Apnea or cyanosis
4. Monitor infant's tolerance of supine positioning.	Infants used to prone sleep positioning may need short periods of supine positioning to increase tolerance to position.	• Increased wakefulness, crying, or poor weight gain
5. Monitor infant's comfort level with changes in position.	Early identification of discomfort facilitates prompt treatment.	• Infant's inability to tolerate a particular position

Documentation

- Family education
- Positions used and time in each position
- Infant's tolerance of positioning
- Amount of time in prone position for play and tolerance
- Changes in infant status
- Comfort assessment and any specific interventions provided
- Unexpected outcomes and related treatment

References

1. Sweeney JK, Gutierrez: Musculoskeletal implications of preterm infant positioning in the NICU, *J Perinatal Neonatal Nurs* 16(1):58-70, 2002.
2. American Academy of Pediatrics, Task Force on Infant Sleeping and Sudden Infant Death Syndrome: Changing concepts of sudden infant death syndrome: implications for sleeping environment and sleeping position (RE 9946), *Pediatrics* 105:650-656, 2000.

Additional Readings

Davis BE, et al: Effects of sleep position on infant motor development, *Pediatrics* 102(5):1135-1140, 1998.
Fox MD, Molesky MG: The effects of prone and supine positioning on arterial oxygen pressure, *Neonatal Network* 8(4):25-29, 1990.
Jones MW, McMurray JL: The other side of "back to sleep," *Neonatal Network* 22(4):49-52, 2003.
Monterosso L, et al: Neuromotor development and the physiologic effects of positioning in very low birth weight infants, *JOGNN* 31(2):138-146, 2002.

Phototherapy

P U R P O S E :   Phototherapy (the application of specific light waves to the skin of the infant to decrease bilirubin concentrations) is the treatment of choice for hyperbilirubinemia. The main demonstrated value of phototherapy is a reduction in the risk that total serum bilirubin level will reach a level at which an exchange transfusion is recommended.

Ann Schwoebel

PREREQUISITE KNOWLEDGE

- The causes of hyperbilirubinemia, factors that affect its severity, and identification of infants at risk for hyperbilirubinemia
- The goal of phototherapy and other hyperbilirubinemia treatment is avoidance of bilirubin concentrations that may result in kernicterus and prevention of elevated bilirubin levels associated with permanent sequelae.[1-3]
- The syndrome of bilirubin-induced neurologic dysfunction refers to a wide spectrum of disorders caused by severe hyperbilirubinemia. The three phases in acute bilirubin encephalopathy are early, intermediate, and advanced. In the beginning phase, the infant is lethargic and hypotonic and has a poor suck; fever, irritability, high-pitched cry, and hypertonia then develop. In the last phase, in which central nervous system damage is probably irreversible, the infant has a shrill cry, no feeding, apnea, fever, deep stupor to coma, sometimes seizure, and death. Kernicterus is the chronic form of bilirubin encephalopathy.
- No standardized method exists for delivery of phototherapy (PT).[1]
- PT units vary widely as do the types of lamps used in the unit: cool white/daylight, special blue, halogen, fiberoptic, and light-emitting diode (LED). Blue-green spectrum is most effective. At these wavelengths, light penetrates skin well and is absorbed maximally by bilirubin.[2]
- Thorough understanding of the type of PT unit used and the manufacturer's recommendations regarding usage

- The effectiveness of PT is related to the area of skin exposed and the radiant energy and the wavelength of the light.[3]
- PT changes bilirubin through structural photoisomerization into water-soluble lumirubin that is excreted in the urine.[3]
- A clear relationship exists between the dose of PT and the decline in the total serum bilirubin (TSB) levels. Factors that determine the dose are: spectrum of light emitted, irradiance of light source, design of PT unit; surface of infant exposed to the light; distance of infant from light source, and the cause of the jaundice.[4]
- The irradiance (dose) from the PT light is measured in units of microwatts per square centimeter per nanometer (μW/cm^2 per nm) with a radiometer. Standard PT units deliver 8 to 15 μW/cm^2 per nm, and intensive PT requires more than 30 μW/cm^2 per nm.[5]
- Fiberoptic pads are less effective than conventional PT but more effective than no treatment in near-term/term infants. Both treatments, however, are effective for the preterm infant because of the infant's smaller surface area and thinner skin, which allows light to penetrate deeper into the tissues.[6]
- Home PT should be used only in infants with bilirubin levels in the "optimal" PT range; it is not appropriate for an infant with higher bilirubin concentrations.[1]
- Halogen lamps cannot be brought close to the infant (to increase the irradiance) without the risk of a burn.
- Periodic checks of PT units are necessary to ensure that an adequate irradiance is delivered.

- No standard exists for discontinuation of PT. The TSB level for discontinuation of PT depends on the age at which PT is initiated and the cause of the hyperbilirubinemia.[1]
- Congenital porphyria or a family history of porphyria is an absolute contraindication to the use of PT.[7]

CHILD AND FAMILY ASSESSMENT

- Prenatal diagnosis of ABO/Rh(D) blood type serum screen for unusual isoimmune antibodies ➻***Rationale:*** Allows team caring for the infant to educate the family on the need for PT.
- Evaluation of the infant's laboratory test results that indicate the necessity for PT, such as total and direct bilirubin level, type and Coombs', complete blood count with differential and reticulocyte count, and G6PD if available ➻***Rationale:*** Allows team caring for the infant to determine the necessity for PT.
- Function of gastrointestinal tract ➻***Rationale:*** A functional gut is needed to decrease bilirubin levels.
- Evaluation of the adequacy of intake in breastfeeding infant ➻***Rationale:*** Identifies breastfed infants who are at risk for dehydration because of inadequate intake and, subsequently, elevated bilirubin levels.
- Desire of parents to be present with the infant during PT ➻***Rationale:*** Family may provide caretaking activities and comfort for the infant.
- Family history of siblings with jaundice or familial disorder associated with jaundice, such as G6PD deficiency ➻***Rationale:*** Allows the team caring for the infant to educate the family on the possibility of the need for PT and complications.
- Status of neurologic system (i.e., lethargy, hypotonia, poor suck followed by hypertonia, arching retrocollis, and opisthotonos) ➻***Rationale:*** These symptoms may be related to acute bilirubin encephalopathy and kernicterus.
- Family's understanding of the reasons for and risks and benefits of PT ➻***Rationale:*** Evaluates family's understanding of the procedure and provides a gauge for ongoing education.

CHILD AND FAMILY EDUCATION

Individualized, developmentally appropriate education is provided to the family based on desire for knowledge, readiness to learn, and overall psychosocial state.

- Provide information about PT, including an explanation of newborn jaundice and hyperbilirubinemia ➻***Rationale:*** Providing information can help to decrease family stress and fear.
- Explain the need to cover the infant's eyes ➻***Rationale:*** Providing information can help to decrease family stress and fear and promote compliance.
- Provide information about the potential complications of PT ➻***Rationale:*** Providing information can help to decrease family stress and aid in the family's decision-making abilities.
- Provide information on the institution-specific or unit-specific protocol regarding feeding and holding the infant undergoing PT ➻***Rationale:*** Providing information can help to decrease family stress and inform the family when they can feed and hold the baby.
- Provide information on the institution-specific or unit-specific protocol regarding supplementation of calories and fluids to improve enteroheptic circulation of bilirubin and help lower the bilirubin level ➻***Rationale:*** Supplemental fluid intake may be necessary to correct mild dehydration; milk-based formula is best because it inhibits the enterohepatic circulation.
- Encourage questions and answer questions as they arise ➻***Rationale:*** Reinforcement of information is needed during periods of stress.

EQUIPMENT

- Phototherapy unit
- Photometer
- Eye shield
- Incubator, crib, or radiant warmer
- Diaper (optional)

Procedure for Phototherapy

Steps	Rationale	Considerations
1. Ensure family understands the reason and procedure for PT and questions are answered.	Evaluates and reinforces understanding of previously taught information.	Developmental level, cognitive ability, and anxiety level determine approach to and effectiveness of teaching.
2. Select the appropriate PT unit for use on the basis of the need for either standard or intensive PT. *(Level IV*)*	Units vary in their output (i.e., PT dose). Daylight, cool white, blue, tungsten-halogen, and fiberoptic units deliver 8 to 15 $\mu W/cm^2$ per nm.[1,3]	Most of the devices deliver enough output for standard PT; but when bilirubin levels approach the range for intensive

Procedure continues on following page

* Level IV: Limited clinical studies to support recommendations

Procedure **for Phototherapy**—*Continued*

Steps	Rationale	Considerations
	Special-blue, fluorescent, and LED units deliver 30 $\mu W/cm^2$ per nm or more.[1,3]	PT (high TSB or near exchange level), special blue fluorescent tubes or LED units should be used.[3]
3. Before and during use, periodically check intensity (irradiance) of unit with photometer. *(Level I*)*	Confirms that an adequate irradiance is delivered.	Efficacy of PT depends on the dose of PT administered. Replace unit if intensity falls by 10% to 20% of the setting.
4. Wash hands. *(Level VI*)*	Standard precautions; reduces the transmission of microorganisms.	
5. Identify the infant with two patient identifiers.	Confirms correct patient as recommended by the Joint Commission for Accreditation of Healthcare Organizations (JCAHO); prevents unnecessary medical procedures.	Two patient identifiers should be used for patient identification per institution-specific protocol; most commonly name and birth date or name and medical record number are used.
6. Undress infant, except for diaper, for PT.[1,3] *(Level IV*)*	Increase in surface area exposed to PT leads to an increased rate of decline in TSB; diaper protects gonads against possible chromatic radiant damage.	Consider removal of diaper when bilirubin levels approach the exchange transfusion range.
7. Place infant in either a crib or incubator or under a radiant warmer depending on type of unit used and infant's gestational age and illness. *(Level II*)*	Lights used for PT produce heat, except for the LED units.	Open crib is the preferred method in term/near-term infants for intensive PT (the top of the incubator prevents the light from being brought sufficiently close to the infant).
8. Place protective eye shields on infant, if a fiberoptic blanket is not used.[1,3] *(Level IV*)*	Prevents possible retinal damage from exposure to the light.	Eye patches should be checked frequently to verify they do not occlude the nares or cause corneal abrasion.
9. Position PT unit over the infant. Light should be no further than 10 to 15 cm from the infant. *(Levels I and II*)*	Distance of the light source from the infant affects the irradiance.	Halogen PT lamps *cannot* be positioned closer to the infant than recommended by the manufacturer without the risk of burn.
10. Assess infant, including temperature, every 4 hours.	Avoids hyperthermia caused by the PT units and assesses skin color.	Assessment of skin color while infant is under special blue/blue fluorescent bulbs and LEDs is difficult.
11. Switch off PT unit and remove protective eye shield for 15 to 30 minutes every 3 to 4 hours. *(Level II*)*	Facilitates provision of direct infant care and drawing of blood specimens; allows parent interactions and a respite to the infant.	If bilirubin level is approaching the exchange transfusion zone, PT should be administered continuously until a decline in serum bilirubin level occurs.
12. When PT is discontinued, clean the unit with a hospital disinfectant.	Reduces the risk of health care associated infections.	

* Level I: Manufacturer's recommendations only
Level II: Theory-based; no research data to support recommendations; recommendations from expert consensus group may exist
Level IV: Limited clinical studies to support recommendations
Level VI: Clinical studies in a variety of patient populations and situations to support recommendations

Expected Outcomes

- Standard PT: In the first 24 hours, a decrease of 6% to 20% of the initial bilirubin level is seen
- Intensive PT: A decrease of 30% to 40% of the initial bilirubin level is seen by 24 hours; the most significant decline occurs in the first 4 to 6 hours
- Infant is free from complications of PT

- Overall decrease in TSB level over several hours to days

Unexpected Outcomes

- Bilirubin levels continue to rise, necessitating an exchange transfusion

- Increased insensible H_2O loss that results in dehydration
- Retinal damage
- Corneal abrasion
- Obstructed nasal breathing
- Hyperthermia
- Interruption of bonding process
- Skin breakdown from frequent stools
- Bronze baby syndrome seen in infants with cholestasis
- The TSB level does not decrease to desired level and further intervention is necessary

Monitoring and Care of the Infant

Activities and Interventions	Rationale	Reportable Conditions
1. Monitor intake and output.	Photoproducts responsible for decline in serum bilirubin are excreted in urine and bile; maintenance of an adequate intake and output should help improve the efficacy of PT.	- Decrease in urine or stool output - Decrease in the amount of oral intake or change in feeding pattern - Weight loss of more than 8% to 10%
2. Monitor infant's vital signs, skin color, and neurologic status.	Changes in vital signs or neurologic status may indicate bilirubin encephalopathy/kernicterus. The infant may appear cyanotic under blue lights.	- Lethargy, hypotonia, poor suck - Fever, high-pitched cry, irritability - Hypertonia, apnea, shrill cry
3. Monitor TSB levels.[1]	PT "bleaches" the skin; visual assessments of jaundice and transcutaneous bilirubin (TcB) measurements in infants undergoing PT are not reliable.	- Increasing TSB
4. Assess skin integrity with all interventions.	Allows prompt identification of skin excoriation from loose stools and urinary excretion of byproduct of bilirubin.	- Excessive skin breakdown from frequent/loose stools

Documentation

- Family education
- Vital signs/neurologic assessment
- Intake and output
- Type and number of PT units in use
- Irradiance measurement
- Assessment of jaundice
- Total time away from PT for direct care and parent bonding
- Unexpected outcomes and related treatment

References

1. American Academy of Pediatrics Subcommittee on Hyperbilirubinemia: Management of hyperbilirubinemia in the newborn infant 35 or more weeks of gestation, *Pediatrics* 114(1):297-316, 2004.
2. Ennever JF: Bluelight, green light, white light, more light treatment of neonatal jaundice, *Clin Perinatol* 17:4467-4481, 1990.
3. Maisels MJ, Watchko JF: Treatment of jaundice in low birthweight infants, *Arch Dis Childhood Fetal Neonatal Ed* 88(6):F459-F463, 2003.
4. Maisels MJ: Phototherapy-traditional and nontraditional, *J Perinatol* l 21(suppl 1):S93-S97, 2001.
5. Bhutani VK, et al: Diagnosis and management of hyperbilirubinemia in the term neonate: for a safer first week, *Pediatr Clin North Am* 51:843-861, 2004.
6. Mills JF, Tudehope D: Fiberoptic phototherapy for neonatal jaundice, *Cochrane Database Systematic Rev* 3:1-54, 2003. Text available at http://gateway.ut.ovid.com/gwl/ovidweb.cgi.
7. Paller AS, et al: Purpuric phototherapy-induced eruption in transfused neonates: relation to transient porphyrinemia, *Pediatrics* 100:360-364, 1997.

Additional Readings

Agency for Health Research and Quality: *Management of neonatal hyperbilirubinemia; summary, evidence report/technology assessment: number 65,* Rockville, MD, 2002, AHRQ Publication Number 03-E005. Text available at http://www.ahrq.gov/clinic/epcsums/neonatalsum.htm.

Association of Women's Health, Obstetric and Neonatal Nurses: Hyperbilirubinemia in the neonate: risk assessment, screening and management, presented in Washington, DC, 2002.

Bhutani VK, et al: *Guidelines for home management and phototherapy for neonatal hyperbilirubinemia; guidelines for pediatric home health care,* Chicago, 2002, American Academy of Pediatrics.

Johnson LH, Bhutani VK: System-based approach to management of neonatal jaundice and prevention of kernicterus, *J Pediatr* 140:396-403, 2002.

Joint Commission on Accreditation of Health Care Organizations: Kernicterus threatens healthy newborns, *Sentinel Event Alert* 18: 2001.

Joint Commission on Accreditation of Health Care Organizations: Revised guidance to help prevent kernicterus, *Sentinel Event Alert* 31: 2004.

Kang JH, Shankaran S: Double phototherapy with high irradiance compared with single phototherapy in neonates with hyperbilirubinemia, *Am J Perinatol* 12:178-180, 1995.

Maisels MJ: Neonatal hyperbilirubinemia. In Klaus M, Fanaroff, editors: *Care of the high-risk neonate,* ed 5, Philadelphia, 2001, Saunders.

Reiser D: *Hyperbilirubinemia: identification and management in healthy term and near term newborns,* Washington, DC, 2001, Association of Women's Health, Obstetric and Neonatal Nursing.

Sari SU, et al: Double versus single phototherapy in term newborns with significant hyperbilirubinemia, *J Tropical Pediatr* 46:36-39, 2000.

Schwoebel A, Sakraida S: Hyperbilirubinemia: new approaches to an old problem, *J Perinatol Neonatal Nurs* 11(3):78-97, 1997.

Seidman DS, et al: A new blue light-emitting phototherapy device: a prospective randomized controlled study, *J Pediatrics* 136:771-774, 2000.

Shinwell ES, et al: Effect of position changing on bilirubin levels during phototherapy, *J Perinatol* 22(3):226-229, 2002.

Stokowski L: Early recognition of neonatal jaundice and kernicterus, *Adv Neonatal Care* 2(2):101-114, 2002.

Skin-to-Skin Contact/Kangaroo Care

P U R P O S E : Skin-to-skin contact provides both emotional and physiologic benefits to infants and parents

Diane Hudson-Barr

PREREQUISITE KNOWLEDGE

- Principles of family-centered care
- Principles of developmental care
- Skin-to-skin contact (SSC), also known as kangaroo care, kangaroo mother care, or skin-to-skin care, was originally used in the late 1970s in Bogotá, Columbia. In an attempt to reduce the infection rate in an overcrowded nursery and decrease infant abandonment, mothers were encouraged to provide skin-to-skin care to their infants 24 hours a day. The mothers stayed at the hospital and held the infants until the infant's condition was stable enough for discharge home. With this intervention, the infant mortality rate related to infection decreased dramatically, along with decreases in apnea and bradycardia, improved rates of breastfeeding, and decreased infant abandonment.[1]
- SSC was introduced in the late 1980s to neonatal intensive care units (NICUs) in the United States. SSC has been used successfully with intubated infants, low–birth weight infants, in the immediate postpartum period, during phototherapy, and with adoptive parents.[1]
- Parents are encouraged to provide SSC for as long as the infant and the parent tolerate the procedure. The SSC time frame may be as short as 20 minutes or as long as 4 or more hours.
- Emotional benefits of SSC include promotion of parent-infant attachment.
- Physiologic benefits of SSC for the infant include improved oxygenation, stabilization of vital signs, increased weight gain, increased sleep, and increased duration of and milk production in breastfeeding.

- Long-term benefits of SSC include promotion of parent-infant interactions and infant development.
- Skill in safe infant transfer techniques is necessary to promote safe transition from infant incubator or bed to parent's chest.
- Recognition of infant physiologic and behavioral cues that indicate stress and nonstress conditions to promote effective infant monitoring during procedure.

CHILD AND FAMILY ASSESSMENT

- Family's understanding of the reasons for and risks and benefits of the procedure; successful SSC requires both participants to tolerate the procedure because the stress of the parent or infant is communicated to the other participant and decreases the benefits of SSC **➥Rationale:** Evaluates family's understanding of the procedure and provides a gauge for ongoing education.
- Parent interest in participation in SSC **➥Rationale:** Parents may feel ambivalent towards SSC; they may want to hold the infant and yet may be afraid that the infant will not tolerate the experience well. Review the benefits of SSC, including this unique aspect of parent-infant interaction, yet be supportive of decision that the parent makes.

CHILD AND FAMILY EDUCATION

Individualized, developmentally appropriate education is provided to the family based on desire for knowledge, readiness to learn, and overall neurologic and psychosocial state.

- Explain the procedure to the parents ➤➤*Rationale:* Providing information decreases anxiety and fear; parents understand how to participate in the process.
- Explain behavioral and physiologic cues that suggest the infant is tolerating or not tolerating the procedure ➤➤*Rationale:* Assists parent in learning the infant cues that indicate stress and nonstress responses.
- Encourage questions and answer questions as they arise ➤➤*Rationale:* Reinforcement of information is needed during periods of stress.

EQUIPMENT

- Infant diaper
- Infant hat (optional)
- Temperature probe (if currently used with infant)
- Blanket
- Gown or button-down shirt/blouse for parent
- Comfortable chair, rocker or recliner with arm supports and foot stool
- Pillows or blankets to assist in comfortable positioning
- Privacy screen
- Tape

Procedure for Skin-to-Skin Contact/Kangaroo Care

Steps	Rationale	Considerations
1. Ensure parent understands SSC teaching and questions are answered.	Evaluates and reinforces understanding of previously taught information.	Developmental level, cognitive ability, and anxiety level determine approach to and effectiveness of teaching.
2. Position rocker and privacy screen at infant's bedside.	Provides privacy; decreases parent's anxiety.	
3. Have parent wear button-down shirt/blouse or provide hospital gown that opens in the front.	Promotes privacy for parents and facilitates direct placement of infant on parent's chest.	Parent should remove bra or t-shirt so that infant is directly against the skin.
4. Wash hands; have parents wash hands. (*Level VI**)	Standard precautions; reduces transmission of microorganisms.	
5. Remove infant clothing except for diaper. Optional: place hat on infant's head.	Promotes direct contact between infant's skin and parent's skin.	Depending on unit-specific protocol, a hat may or may not be used with the infant.
6. Place infant in supine position.	Facilitates transfer.	
7. If infant is intubated or has several indwelling catheters, move the tubing to the front of the incubator.	Facilitates transfer.	
8. If desired, slide out mattress tray.	Facilitates transfer.	
9. Have parent stand as close to the incubator/bed as possible.	Facilitates transfer.	Especially with infants who are intubated, the infant transfer may be easier to complete with two nurses.
10. Have parent support the infant's back and buttocks by sliding hands under the infant. The nurse supports the infant's head and ventilator/catheter equipment.	Two-person transfer facilitates safer movement of the infant from the incubator/bed to the parent's chest.	
11. Moving at the same time, the nurse and parent turn the infant to the vertical position and move infant to the parent's chest. (*Level IV**)	Vertical positioning increases oxygen saturation.[2]	

* Level IV: Limited clinical studies to support recommendations
  Level VI: Clinical studies in a variety of patient populations and situations to support recommendations

Procedure for Skin-to-Skin Contact/Kangaroo Care—*Continued*

Steps	Rationale	Considerations
12. The parent slowly sits in the rocker/chair.	Facilitates safe transfer of infant to parent's chest.	Secure the ventilator/oxygen tubing and catheter tubing to the parent's shoulder.
13. Reposition the infant as needed so that the infant's head is turned to the side with the ear resting above the parent's heart. *(Level IV*)*	Positioning the infant in this manner facilitates regulation of infant vital signs in response to parent's heart rate and breathing pattern.[2,3]	
14. Close the parent's shirt/gown around the infant.	Promotes temperature stability in the infant.	
15. Use pillows and blankets to provide comfortable positioning for the parent; reposition foot stool as needed.	Comfortable positioning promotes extended time in SSC.	
16. Position privacy screen around parent and infant.	Decreases parental anxiety about exposure to staff and visitors in the nursery.	
17. If infant is warmed by servo, turn the bed to manual setting at the current temperature. *(Level I*)*	Use of current bed temperature prevents cooling or heating changes in response to changes in the infant's temperature.	Remember to return the incubator setting to servo once the baby has been returned to the incubator to resume servo function of the incubator.
18. Check infant's temperature within 15 minutes of transfer. If stable, temperature can be checked per unit-specific protocol or every 1 to 2 hours. *(Level IV*)*	Verifies infant is tolerating procedure.[2,4,5]	Do not leave the temperature probe positioned so that it is against both the infant and the parent's skin. Reposition the temperature probe to the lateral aspect of the costal margin.
19. Monitor infant's physiologic cues (heart rate, color, respiratory rate, oxygen saturation) and behavioral cues (comfort level, presence of agitation) frequently throughout SSC. *(Level V*)*	Detects early any indications the infant is not tolerating the procedure.[2,3,6-8]	The infant may need 5 or more minutes to settle down after transfer from incubator/bed to parent's chest.
20. To return the infant to the incubator/bed, wash hands; loosen tape securing ventilator/ oxygen/catheter tubing to parent's clothing.	Facilitates easy movement of infant back to incubator/bed.	
21. Parent slowly rises to a standing position while the nurse supports the infant's head and any tubing.	Prevents accidental dislodgement of tubes/catheters.	
22. Have the parent provide support to the infant's back and buttocks and slowly lower the infant to the mattress.	Decreases stress associated with movement from parent's chest to incubator/bed.	
23. The nurse positions the infant and equipment.	Facilitates developmentally appropriate positioning.	
24. Encourage the parent to remain at the bedside as the infant is repositioned.	Parent continues to be involved in infant's care.	

Procedure continues on following page

* Level I: Manufacturer's recommendations only
Level IV: Limited clinical studies to support recommendations
Level V: Clinical studies in more than one or two patient populations and situations to support recommendations

Procedure for Skin-to-Skin Contact/Kangaroo Care—*Continued*

Steps	Rationale	Considerations
25. Reposition temperature probe to appropriate location on the infant's skin, if needed.	Positions temperature probe to accurately read infant's skin temperature.	
26. Return incubator to servo setting if that is setting being used.	Facilitates neutral thermal environment for infant.	

Expected Outcomes

- Enhanced infant-parent attachment
- Infant remains hemodynamically stable (temperature, heart rate, respiratory rate)
- Improved infant oxygenation
- Decreased parental/infant distress, increased parental/infant relaxation
- Increased parental satisfaction
- Increased incidence and length of breastfeeding
- Increased milk supply

Unexpected Outcomes

- Poor infant-parent attachment
- Increased infant physiologic distress (bradycardia, apnea, desaturation)
- Decreased infant body temperature
- Deterioration in infant oxygenation
- Increased infant behavioral distress (facial grimacing, agitation, crying)
- Parent is tense, unable to relax during SSC
- Parent does not like SSC
- Decrease in duration or frequency of breastfeeding
- No improvement or decrease in milk supply

Monitoring and Care of the Infant

Activities and Interventions	Rationale	Reportable Conditions
1. Monitor infant's physiologic stability.	Changes in infant's vital signs may indicate infant is not tolerating SSC.	- Bradycardia - Decreased temperature - Apnea - Desaturations
2. Monitor infant's behavioral stability.	Changes in infant's behavior may indicate infant is not tolerating SSC.	- Agitation - Inconsolable crying

Documentation

- Parent education
- Length of time of SSC
- Parent feedback related to SSC
- Infant tolerance of SSC
- Unexpected outcomes and related treatment

References

1. Gale G: Kangaroo care, *Neonatal Network* 17(5):69-71, 1998.
2. Fohe K, et al: Skin-to-skin contact improves gas exchange in premature infants, *J Perinatol* 20(5):311-315, 2000.
3. Swinth JY, et al: Kangaroo (skin-to-skin) care with a preterm infant before, during, and after mechanical ventilation, *Neonatal Network* 22(6):33-38, 2003.
4. Eichel P: Kangaroo care: expanding our practice to critically ill neonates, *Newborn Infant Nurs Rev* 1(4):224-228, 2001.
5. Kirsten GF, et al: Kangaroo mother care in the nursery, *Pediatr Clin North Am* 48(2):443-451, 2001.
6. Feldman R, et al: Comparison of skin-to-skin (kangaroo) and traditional care: parenting outcomes and preterm infant development, *Pediatrics* 110(1):16-26, 2002.

7. Ludington-Hoe SM, Swinth JY: Kangaroo mother care during phototherapy: effect on the bilirubin profile, *Neonatal Network* 20(5):41-48, 2001.

8. Moran M, et al: Maternal kangaroo (skin-to-skin) care in the NICU beginning 4 hours postbirth, *MCN* 24(2):74-79, 1999.

Additional Readings

Anderson GC, et al: Mother-newborn contact in a randomized trial of kangaroo (skin-to-skin) care, *JOGNN* 32(4):604-611, 2003.

Bohnhorst B, et al: Skin-to-skin (kangaroo) care, respiratory control, and thermoregulation, *J Pediatr* 138(2):193-197, 2001.

Charpak N, et al: A randomized, controlled trial of kangaroo mother care: results of follow-up at 1 year of corrected age, *Pediatrics* 108(5):1072-1079, 2001.

Charpak N, et al: Kangaroo mother care: 25 years after. *Acta Paediatr* 94(5), 512-522, 2005.

Chow MJ, et al: A randomized control trial of early kangaroo care for preterm infants: effects on temperature, weight, behavior, and acuity, *Nurs Res* 10(2):129-142, 2002.

Engler AJ, et al: Kangaroo care: national survey of practice, knowledge, barriers, and perceptions, *MCN Am J Maternal Child Nurs* 27:146-161, 2002.

Furman L, et al: Correlates of lactation in mothers of very low birthweight infants, *Pediatrics* 109(4):e57, 2002.

Johnston CC, et al: Kangaroo care is effective in diminishing pain response in preterm neonates, *Arch Pediatr Adolesc Med* 157(11): 1084-1088, 2003.

Ludington-Hoe SM, Golant SK: *The best you can do to help your premature infant,* New York, 1993, Bantam Books.

Ludington-Hoe SM, et al: Skin-to-skin contact (Kangaroo Care) analgesia for preterm infant heelstick, *AACN Clinical Issues,* 16(3): 373-387, 2005.

Ludington-Hoe SM, Swinth JY: Developmental aspects of kangaroo care, *JOGNN* 25(8):691-703, 1996.

Nyqvist, KH: How can kangaroo mother and high technology be compatible? *J Hum Lact,* 20(1): 72-74, 2004.

Roberts KL, et al: A comparison of kangaroo mother care and conventional cuddling care, *Neonatal Network* 19(4):31-35, 2000.

Umbilical Vessel Catheter: Care and Management

P U R P O S E : Proper care and management of umbilical vessel catheters prevents potential complications such as accidental dislodgement, hemorrhage and infection; ensures proper placement and patency of the catheter; and facilitates accurate, direct measurement of arterial blood pressure

Karen Helton Rapoport and Colleen Salazar Young

PREREQUISITE KNOWLEDGE

- Anatomy of fetal and newborn circulatory system
- Proper placement of catheters
  - ❖ Umbilical arterial catheter (UAC) should be within the aorta either high-lying (T6-T9) or low-lying (L3-L4).
  - ❖ Umbilical venous catheter (UVC) should be within the inferior vena cava above the diaphragm (T9-T10).[1-4]
- Umbilical catheters are designed specifically for catheterization of the umbilical artery and umbilical vein. Double lumen catheters are available. UACs require infusion of heparin-containing fluid and may be attached to blood pressure transducers.[1]
- UACs are inserted to obtain arterial blood samples, directly measure arterial blood pressure or to facilitate the administration of fluids and medications.
- UVCs are inserted to facilitate the administration of fluids and medications or provide venous access for exchange transfusion.
- Complications of UAC: False aneurysm, lower limb ischemia, refractory hypoglycemia, hypertension, and intestinal necrosis
- Complications of UVC: Pericardial effusion, cardiac arrhythmias, hepatic necrosis, portal hypertension, perforation of the vessel/peritoneum, and perforation of the colon
- Contraindications for insertion of umbilical vessel catheter include: Abdominal wall defects, necrotizing enterocolitis

(NEC), peritonitis, infant age more than 7 days, vascular compromise below level of umbilicus, or omphalitis[3-5]
- Catheters must be secured, both with initial suturing and secondary securing methods, to ensure proper placement is maintained and to avoid complications such as hemorrhage from a displaced arterial catheter.[1,2,6]
- Pressure monitoring systems and waveform interpretation
- Principles of aseptic technique
- Child development as it relates to clinical assessment and umbilical vessel catheter

CHILD AND FAMILY ASSESSMENT

- Presence of abdominal wall defects, NEC, vascular compromise below level of umbilicus, omphalitis, or peritonitis ➙*Rationale:* These factors may preclude placing an umbilical vessel catheter.
- Patency of umbilical vessels ➙*Rationale:* If vessels are not patent, false tracking may occur, which prevents proper placement of the umbilical vessel catheter.
- History of hematologic issues within the family or of the newborn ➙*Rationale:* The likelihood of thrombus may be increased with certain hematologic disorders.
- Family's understanding of the reasons for and risks and benefits of the procedure ➙*Rationale:* Evaluates family's understanding of the procedure and provides a gauge for ongoing education.

CHILD AND FAMILY EDUCATION

Individualized, developmentally appropriate education is provided to the family based on desire for knowledge, readiness to learn, and overall psychosocial state.

- Provide information on what the catheters, monitor, and transducer look like; what they monitor/infuse; where the catheters go when they enter the skin. If possible show examples ➤*Rationale:* Providing information decreases anxiety and fear; examples enhance understanding.
- Depending on institution-specific protocol, the family may not be able to hold the newborn because of the difficulty of monitoring the catheters and ensuring their security while the infant is held; provide the family with information about complications if the catheter is displaced, such as hemorrhage, new catheter placement, and repeat x-rays ➤*Rationale:* Providing information increases understanding and may promote compliance with the protocol.
- Provide information on the reasons for catheter placement and the procedure ➤*Rationale:* Providing information decreases anxiety and fear.
- Explain that having the catheter in place provides a painless means for obtaining blood from the infant ➤*Rationale:* Providing information decreases anxiety and fear; knowledge that pain is reduced for the infant may provide comfort to the family.

- Encourage questions and answer questions as they arise ➤*Rationale:* Reinforcement of information is needed during periods of stress and is especially important if the procedure is emergent.

EQUIPMENT[1-7]

- Clean gloves
- Heparinized saline solution
- Hydrocolloid skin barrier (for placement under tape or adhesive to protect skin against epidermal stripping from tape or adhesive removal)
- One half–inch to 1-inch paper, cloth, or plastic tape for bridge to secure catheter or commercial umbilical catheter securing device (e.g., UMB-E Umbilical Catheter Anchor by Kendall-LTP [Chicopee, MA]) or transparent nonocclusive dressing for securing catheter
- Fluids to be infused
- Infusion pump
- Pressure transducer system for arterial or central venous pressure (CVP) monitoring
- Measuring tape
- Three-way stopcock
- One-mL and 3-mL syringes
- Padded hemostats

Procedure | for Umbilical Vessel Catheter: Care and Management

Steps	Rationale	Considerations
Securing the Catheter		
1. Gather needed equipment and supplies.	Facilitates completion of task in a timely manner.	
2. Wash hands.	Standard precautions; reduces transmission of microorganisms.	
3. Put on clean gloves.	Standard precautions.	
4. Verify catheter position before securing catheter. Place hydrocolloid barrier on skin, under adhesive tape.	Prevents tape removal and replacement if catheter position must be adjusted. Removal of tape can result in epidermal stripping, especially in preterm infants. Use of a pectin barrier (i.e., Neutraskin by Incutech Inc., Kernersville, NC) allows reapplication of tape as needed and minimizes trauma to skin.[1,4,6]	

Procedure continues on following page

Procedure	**for Umbilical Vessel Catheter: Care and Management**—*Continued*	
Steps	**Rationale**	**Considerations**
5. Methods of securing catheter. Bridge/goal post method: Apply two t-pieces of tape to abdomen parallel to each other on either side of catheter. Use two tape strips to enclose catheter and vertical t-pieces (Figure 194-1).	Secure taping helps to ensure that catheter is not dislodged, reducing the risk of complications such as hemorrhage or necrosis.[1,3-6,8]	Approved methods for securing catheters vary among institutions; be familiar with institution-specific protocol.

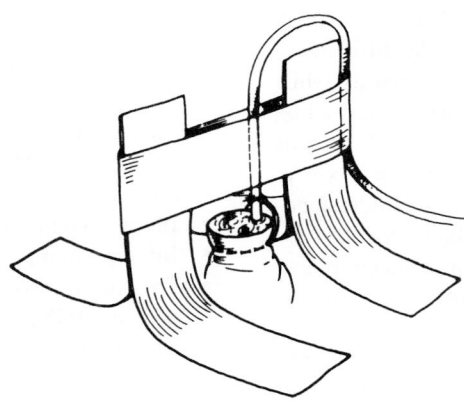

FIGURE 194-1   Bridge/t-piece method of securing UVC catheter. *From Klaus M, Fanaroff A:* Care of the high-risk neonate, *ed 5, Philadelphia, 2001, Saunders.*

  Apply two pieces of tape to enclose catheter; suture the line up one side of tape, across top, down opposite side; place final suture in cord.
  Use commercial umbilical securing device, such as UMB-E Umbilical Catheter Anchor (Figure 194-2).
  Alternative method for securing catheters may be the use of a transparent nonocclusive dressing. *(Level V*)*

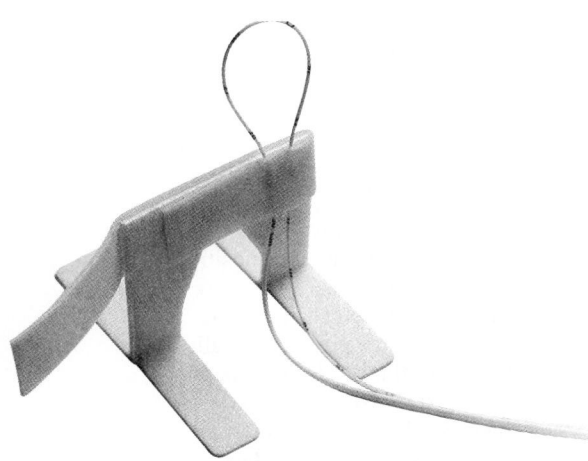

FIGURE 194-2   UMB-E commercial securing device for umbilical catheter. *Photo courtesy of Kendall-LTP, www.kendall-ltp.com, 2005.*

* Level V: Clinical studies in more than one or two patient populations and situations to support recommendations

Procedure for Umbilical Vessel Catheter: Care and Management—*Continued*

Steps	Rationale	Considerations
6. Dispose of used supplies and equipment in appropriate receptacles.	Standard precautions; reduces transmission of microorganisms.	
7. Wash hands.	Standard precautions.	
Blood Sampling from UAC		
8. Gather needed equipment and supplies.	Facilitates completion of task in a timely manner.	Commercially available set-ups for blood draws from UACs are intended to decrease the number of times the line is entered, decreasing the risk of infection.
9. Wash hands.	Standard precautions; reduces transmission of microorganisms.	
10. Identify infant with two patient identifiers per institution-specific protocol.	Ensures correct patient and procedure as recommended by the Joint Commission on Accreditation of Healthcare Organizations (JCAHO).	Patient identification process is institution-specific; refer to institution-specific protocol.
11. Put on clean gloves.	Standard precautions; reduces transmission of microorganisms.	
12. Ensure a heparinized flush solution in a 3-mL syringe (or per manufacturer's recommendations) is attached to luer-lock stopcock at all times. Turn stopcock off to syringe when fluid is infusing. Stop infusion before sampling blood.[1,3,6,9]	Proper use of a stopcock is essential to safe care of umbilical vessel catheters. A 3-mL syringe is needed both to clear the line and for accuracy of laboratory values.[8] Avoid use of larger syringes to prevent accidental fluid overload and avoid use of excessive negative pressure during withdrawal from catheter.	
13. Clean luer-lock stopcock connections with povidone-iodine, alcohol, or chlorhexidine before opening the line per institution-specific protocol.[1-3,5] *(Level IV*)*	Maintenance of sterility decreases likelihood of infection transmission to the infant.[1-3,5]	Maintain aseptic technique with all open connections.
14. To clear line: turn stopcock off to infant; remove heparinized syringe and replace with empty 3-mL syringe with use of aseptic technique. Once syringe is in place, turn stopcock off to intravenous (IV) fluid and slowly withdraw 1 to 4 mL of blood. *(Level IV*)*	Removal of 1 mL is generally adequate clearance of blood before specimen is obtained for blood gas, sodium, and potassium levels. If specimen is obtained for glucose level, 3 mL should be removed from a 3.5 Fr and 4 mL from a 5 Fr catheter.[9]	Labeling the syringe used to clear the line prevents confusion of waste with laboratory specimen. In calculation of volume of blood removed to clear line, consider dead space of catheter and tubing before stopcock.
15. Turn stopcock off to infant and remove syringe containing blood; place in location that maintains sterility. *(Level IV*)*	Maintenance of sterility decreases likelihood of infection transmission to the infant.[1-3,5]	Placing an open sterile 4×4 near the workspace can provide a location for the blood-containing syringe. Place it where the infant cannot disturb it.

Procedure continues on following page

* Level IV: Limited clinical studies to support recommendations

Procedure for Umbilical Vessel Catheter: Care and Management—*Continued*

Steps	Rationale	Considerations
16. Attach sterile syringe to stopcock port; turn stopcock off to IV fluid. Slowly withdraw volume of blood needed for ordered laboratory specimens. *(Level IV*)*	Quicker blood sampling and infusion via a high-lying umbilical arterial catheter may affect cerebral blood flow and therefore oxygenation.[8]	A separate heparinized syringe may be used for arterial blood gas sample, usually 0.2 to 0.4 mL.
17. Turn stopcock off to infant. Remove syringe and place in location that maintains sterility. Reattach the syringe containing the initial blood removed. Turn stopcock off to IV fluid. Gently draw back to aspirate any air into the syringe. Tap the syringe to remove any air bubbles to the base of the syringe; slowly infuse blood to infant. *(Level IV*)*	Maintenance of sterility decreases likelihood of infection transmission to the infant.[1-3,5] Slow blood sampling from high UACs may be useful, with withdrawal and reinfusion of samples over 40 seconds.[8] *(Level IV*)*	Concerns with reinfusion of sample used to clear line include possible contamination of the syringe, potential that discard volume contains clots, and exposure of the clinician to blood.[10,11] Assess ease of reinfusion; do not force.
18. Ensure no air bubbles or clots are infused and that all blood is reinfused to prevent unnecessary iatrogenic blood loss, with consideration of the neonate's small circulating blood volume. *(Level V*)*	Prevents complications of air embolism and thromboembolism.[1-3]	
19. Turn stopcock off to infant. Remove syringe and discard. With a new 3-mL flush-filled syringe, flush dead space of stopcock to remove any blood that may be present. Attach syringe to stopcock. Open stopcock to infant and syringe; aspirate gently for air. Gently tap syringe to raise any air bubbles toward plunger. Flush catheter with the minimum amount of flush necessary to clear catheter. *(Level IV*)*	Prevents complications of air embolism and thromboembolism.[1-3]	
20. Turn stopcock off to flush syringe. Resume fluid infusion. Place blood in appropriate laboratory tubes and label at the bedside.[2,3]	Maintains patency of UAC. Promotes patient safety; ensures accurate and efficient processing of specimen.	
21. Dispose of used supplies and equipment appropriately.	Standard precautions; reduces transmission of microorganisms.	
22. Remove gloves; wash hands.	Standard precautions.	
Umbilical Catheter Infusions		
23. Do not infuse vasoactive medications, including epinephrine, dopamine, and dobutamine, via UAC. *(Level V*)*	These drugs cause vasoconstriction and should not be administered via an UAC.[12]	
24. Blood products should be given preferably via an UVC. *(Level II*)*	Administration of blood product via UAC increases risk of clot formation.	

* Level II: Theory-based; no research data to support recommendations; recommendations from expert consensus group may exist
  Level IV: Limited clinical studies to support recommendations
  Level V: Clinical studies in more than one or two patient populations and situations to support recommendations

Procedure for Umbilical Vessel Catheter: Care and Management—*Continued*

Steps	Rationale	Considerations
25. Glucose-containing fluids may be given either via UVC or high-lying UAC.[13,14] *(Level IV*)*	Glucose administration via UAC has been linked to refractory hypoglycemia when malpositioned at the level of the celiac axis because hyperinsulinemia results from infusion of glucose into the pancreatic artery.[13] Recent publications have indicated that high-lying UACs are preferred to low-lying UACs because of lower risk of vascular complications with high lines.[15] Maximum glucose infusion rates may be determined by manufacturer's recommendations.	
26. Heparin infusion is recommended via UAC.[16] *(Level IV*)*	Heparin infusion can decrease the likelihood of catheter occlusion from fibrin clots, which prolongs patency and prevents thrombotic complications.[15,16]	
27. Administration of certain medications is not recommended via UAC, including phenytoin, phenobarbital, calcium gluconate, and indomethacin. *(Level V*)*	The UAC may be frequently entered for blood draws; therefore, continuous medications are better administered via UVC. Medications that are irritating or hyperosmolar can be damaging to the aorta.[12] Indomethacin can alter blood flow to the mesenteric arteries if administered via UAC.[12]	
28. Use infusion pumps to administer fluid and medications.	An infusion pump maintains an infusion pressure greater than aortic pressure.[1,3,13]	

Use of Double Lumen Catheter in Umbilical Vein

Steps	Rationale	Considerations
29. Draw blood samples from the larger lumen. The other lumen's infusion should be paused to prevent contamination of blood sample. Administer blood preferably via larger lumen. *(Level II*)*	Pausing of adjacent lumen's infusion during blood draw decreases likelihood of contaminated blood sample and altered laboratory results. Administration of blood via larger lumen decreases likelihood of red blood cell destruction on transfusion.[1,2]	
30. If both lumens are not used, the smaller lumen line should be heparin locked. Heparin flush should be administered a minimum of every 12 hours. If infusion of fluids via both lumens is needed, which may have questionable interaction, consult with prescribing practitioner/pharmacist. *(Level II*)*	Heparinized flush is used to ensure patency and avoid thrombus formation. Infusion of fluids through separate lumens does not indicate that these fluids stay separated once entering the vein or artery because both lumens open at the end of the catheter.[1,2]	

* Level II: Theory-based; no research data to support recommendations; recommendations from expert consensus group may exist
Level IV: Limited clinical studies to support recommendations
Level V: Clinical studies in more than one or two patient populations and situations to support recommendations

Expected Outcomes

- The UAC is correctly placed at T6-T9 or L3-L4

- The UVC is correctly placed at T9-T10 above the diaphragm

- Catheter shows brisk blood return and appropriate waveform (arterial or central venous pressure)
- Infant is free from catheter complications

- Fluids infuse without difficulty
- Infant's condition remains hemodynamically stable

Unexpected Outcomes

- Malposition of UAC that results in false aneurysm, lower limb ischemia, refractory hypoglycemia, hypertension, or intestinal necrosis
- Malposition of UVC that results in pericardial effusion, cardiac arrhythmias, hepatic necrosis, portal hypertension, perforation of the vessel/peritoneum, or perforation of the colon
- Inability to withdraw blood
- Dampened or absent waveform
- Hemorrhage, thrombosis, air embolism, infection, or knot in UAC
- Vasospasm and lower limb ischemia (UAC)
- Inability to administer fluids
- Hypotension/bradycardia as result of blood loss from inadvertent catheter disconnection

Monitoring and Care of the Child

Activities and Interventions	Rationale	Reportable Conditions
All Umbilical Catheters		
1. Ensure luer lock is used for all connections. Check security of connection every shift and with every entry into line.	Blood loss and infection can result from accidental disconnections.[1-3,9,13,17]	• Accidental blood loss
2. Keep catheter, stopcock, and syringes free of air and blood; never flush air or clots through line.	Flushing of air or clots can result in embolism to major organs.[3,9,13,17]	• Presence of clot or air in line that cannot be aspirated and cleared
3. Do not place stopcock and other connections under linen.	Prevents immediate detection of an accidental disconnection that could lead to severe blood loss from the infant.[5]	• Accidental blood loss
4. Monitor infant closely to prevent accidental self-dislodgement of catheter or disconnection. Use the least restrictive measure possible to ensure patient safety (e.g., positioning, blanket rolls). If immobilization of extremity is necessary, use soft restraints, following institution-specific protocol regarding ordering and monitoring of medical immobilization devices or restraints.	Refer to institution-specific guidelines for the safe use of medical immobilization devices or restraints in accordance with state regulations, accrediting agencies such as JCAHO, and community and national standards. Guidelines include how often medical immobilization devices or restraints are to be ordered and monitored.[3,5]	• Accidental blood loss • Catheter is dislodged • Medical immobilization or use of restraints is required
5. Do not use occlusive or nontransparent dressing over the umbilicus.	Nontransparent dressings obscure inspection of umbilicus and evaluation of the catheter insertion site.[3,5]	• Unable to assess catheter insertion site
6. Check catheter centimeter marking at umbilicus every shift and compare with initial placement measurement.	Movement of catheter can result in malposition of catheter and lead to unexpected outcomes. A catheter should never be advanced if dislodged.[2,3,9]	• Change in catheter position of more than 1 cm
7. Continually monitor insertion site for signs of bleeding, redness, or drainage.	Drainage from umbilicus or redness of umbilicus may indicate infection (omphalitis).[3,4]	• Redness or drainage from umbilicus • Bleeding • Persistent oozing

Monitoring and Care of the Child—Cont'd

Activities and Interventions	Rationale	Reportable Conditions
8. Check security of tape to catheter and abdomen every shift.	Movement in catheter can result in malposition of catheter.[1,3,9]	• Loose tape that results in catheter movement
9. Perform cleansing of luer-lock or stopcock connections with povidone-iodine, alcohol, or chlorhexadine before opening the line as per institution-specific protocol. Maintain aseptic technique with all open connections.	Minimizes risk of infection.[1-3,9]	• Signs and symptoms of sepsis
10. Keep rubber-tipped or padded hemostats at bedside for accidental disconnections or breaks in the line. If catheter is accidentally removed, use a 2×2 and apply pinching pressure to stump of umbilicus.	Blood loss and infection can result from accidental disconnections.[1,3,9,17] Padded hemostats may prevent further damage to the catheter.[1,3]	• Break in catheter • Inadvertent catheter removal
11. Intravenous tubing and add-on devices, which include transducer tubing, should be changed at no less than 72-hour intervals or per institution-specific protocol. *(Level VI*)*	Limits the number of entries into the system, thereby decreasing likelihood of introduction of infection.[15]	• Failure to change tubing or add-on devices at indicated interval
Umbilical Arterial Catheter		
12. Use minimum amount of flush necessary to clear line; 0.3 to 0.5 mL, administered slowly over at least 5 seconds.	Excessive use of flush can lead to volume overload and electrolyte disturbances. Rapid bolus can result in spikes in blood pressure, which can increase intracranial pressure.	• Electrolyte abnormalities/fluid overload • Indications of increased intracranial pressure

13. Continuously monitor waveform and pressure; set alarm limits appropriately.
   Perform zero referencing with transducer leveled to infant's phlebostatic axis on initial set-up and per manufacturer's recommendations.
   Electronic calibration of monitor should be performed per manufacturer's recommendation. *(Level I*)*
   See Procedure 137 for further discussion of arterial catheter waveform.
	Arterial pressure is represented by a waveform, which reflects systole, valve closure, and diastole.[11,16]
	Dampening of the waveform (loss of dicrotic notch) or sluggish blood return/flushing may indicate clot formation.
	Blood clot development can occur from vessel wall trauma or presence of the catheter.[1,3,9,13]
	Appropriately set alarms facilitate prompt identification of hypotension or hypertension or catheter disconnection.
	Errors in leveling can result in inaccurate pressure readings.[18]
	Zeroing and calibration ensures that the displayed pressure is accurate.[13,18]
		• Dampening or absence of waveform
		• Difficulty in obtaining blood from or flushing catheter
		• Hypotension or hypertension

14. Assess pedal or posttibial pulses with initial assessment and care.
   Keep toes exposed to identify early changes in perfusion
   Check perfusion to lower back and buttocks with care.
	UAC lines are associated with lower limb vasospasm, which can develop into ischemia and possible loss of limb.[3,9,14]	• Decreased perfusion or lower limb ischemia

---

* Level I: Manufacturer's recommendations only
  Level VI: Clinical studies in a variety of patient populations and situations to support recommendations

Continued

Monitoring and Care of the Child—Cont'd

Activities and Interventions	Rationale	Reportable Conditions
15. If "catheter toes" (bluish discoloration of toes on one leg) are noted, apply warm compress to contralateral limb.	Application of warmth to contralateral extremity may relieve vasospasm of lower limb. Do not apply warm compress to compromised limb.[3,13]	• Catheter toes that do not resolve within 15 minutes or that worsen despite warm compress

16. Refer to institution-specific protocol regarding appropriate use of infusion solutions, heparin, and medications.
 	
    Change fluid and tubing per institution-specific protocol.
    Correct position of UAC must be verified before use.[1-3,9,13,17]
	The UAC permits introduction of solutions and drugs directly into major arteries
	Drugs that cause vasoconstriction, are irritating, or are extremely hyperosmolar should not be administered per UAC.[12]
		• Solution infusing/ordered other than identified as acceptable per institution-specific protocol

17. Label line as arterial	Identification of correct line, especially when UVC/multiple lines are in place, can prevent accidental administration of drugs/solutions into the wrong vessel.[1,3]	• Administration of vasoactive or other contraindicated medications via UAC
Umbilical Venous Catheter 18. Refer to institution-specific protocol regarding appropriate use of infusion solutions, heparin, and medications.	The UVC permits introduction of solutions and drugs directly into major veins/organs.	• Solutions infusing/ordered other than identified as acceptable per institution-specific protocol
19. Correct position must be verified before use of UVC.	If catheter is in the liver, necrosis of liver tissue can result.[1-,3,9,13,17]	• Incorrect position of UVC
20. Label line as venous.	Identification of correct line, especially when UAC/multiple lines are in place, can prevent accidental administration of drugs/solutions into the wrong vessel.[1,3]	• Administration of contraindicated medications via UVC
21. Change fluid and tubing as identified by institution-specific protocol. Replace tubing used to administer blood or lipid emulsions within 24 hours of the start of infusion; intralipid hang time is no greater than 24 hours.[15]	Prolonged hang time increases microbial growth in lipid emulsion.	• Tubing used to administer blood or lipids not changed at indicated time interval

Documentation

- Family education
- Use of medical immobilization devices or restraints per institution-specific protocol
- Blood return, ease of flushing, waveform
- Catheter insertion depth in centimeters
- Rate, type and amount of fluid infused, including flushes
- Lower limb perfusion
- Condition of insertion site hourly
- Amount of blood withdrawn/removed and not returned to infant
- Unexpected outcomes and related treatment

References

1. Altimer L, et al: *Neonatal nursing policies, procedures, competencies, & clinical pathways,* 1999, National Association of Neonatal Nurses.
2. Gomella T: *Neonatology: management, procedures, on-call problems, diseases and drugs,* ed 5, New York, 2004, McGraw-Hill.
3. Perinatal Advisory Council Los Angeles Communities: *Neonatal guidelines of care,* 1998, PAC LAC.
4. Verklan M, Walden M, editors: *Core curriculum for neonatal intensive care nursing,* ed 3, Philadelphia, 2004, Saunders.
5. Merenstein G, Gardner S: *Handbook of neonatal intensive care,* ed 5, St Louis, 2002, Mosby-Year Book, Inc.
6. Kenner C, Lott J: *Comprehensive neonatal nursing: a physiologic perspective,* ed 3, Phildelphia, 2002, Saunders.
7. Jaimovich D, Vidyasagar D: *Handbook of pediatric and neonatal transport medicine,* ed 2, Philadelphia, 2002, Hanley and Belfus, Inc.
8. Schulz G, et al: Slow blood sampling from an umbilical artery catheter prevents a decrease in cerebral oxygenation in the preterm newborn, *Pediatrics* 111(1):e73-e76, 2003.
9. MacDonald M, Ramasethu J: *Atlas of procedures in neonatology,* ed 3, Philadelphia, 2002, JB Lippincott Company.
10. Dech ZF, Szaflarski NL: Nursing strategies to minimize blood loss associated with phlebotomy, *AACN Clin Iss* 7(2):277-287, 1996.
11. Frey AM: Drawing blood samples from vascular access devices: evidence-based practice, *J Infusion Nurs* 26(5):285-293, 2003.
12. Zenk K, et al: *Neonatal medications & nutrition: a comprehensive guide,* ed 3, Santa Rosa, CA, 2003, NICU INK.
13. Avery G, et al: *Neonatology: pathophysiology and management of the newborn,* ed 5, Philadelphia, 1999, JB Lippincott Company.
14. Barrington KJ: Umbilical artery catheters in the newborn: effects of position of the catheter tip (Cochrane Review), *The Cochrane Library* 3: 2004.
15. O'Grady N: Guidelines for prevention of intravascular catheter-related infections, *Morbidity Mortality Weekly Rep* 51(RR-10), 2002.
16. Barrington KJ: Umbilical artery catheters in the newborn: effects of heparin (Cochrane Review). *The Cochrane Library* 4: 2004.
17. Klaus M, Fanaroff A: *Care of the high-risk neonate,* ed 5, Philadelphia, 2001, Saunders.
18. Curley M, Moloney-Harmon P, editors: *Critical care nursing of infants and children,* ed 2, Philadelphia, 2001, Saunders.

AP

Umbilical Vessel Cannulation and Removal: Perform

P U R P O S E : To place an indwelling umbilical catheter into the umbilical vein or artery of a neonate for administration of medications, blood products, or fluids. An umbilical venous catheter may also be placed emergently for neonatal resuscitation after delivery.

Mildred Kenney-Lau and Carrie C. Steele

PREREQUISITE KNOWLEDGE

- Anatomy and physiology of the cardiovascular system, including circulation
- Anatomy of the umbilical cord stump
- Indications for umbilical catheter (UC) placement include:
  - ❖ Administration of intravenous fluids
  - ❖ Administration of parenteral nutrition
  - ❖ Administration of medications
  - ❖ Continuous monitoring of blood pressure (umbilical artery catheter [UAC])
  - ❖ Continuous monitoring of central venous pressure (umbilical venous catheter [UVC])
  - ❖ Frequent blood sampling
  - ❖ Exchange transfusion
  - ❖ Blood sampling for arterial blood gas monitoring
- Contraindications to UC placement
- Complications of UC placement
- Aseptic technique, including sterile field preparation and maintenance
- Institution-specific medical immobilization and physical restraint protocols; also see Procedure 200.

- Mastery of neonatal resuscitation principles and techniques
- Radiologic techniques for evaluation of proper placement of UC
- Skill in basic suturing technique
- Informed consent is required before placement of a UC, except in emergent situations

CHILD AND FAMILY ASSESSMENT

- Prenatal diagnosis of congenital malformations indicating need for placement of UC, such as congenital heart disease, pulmonary malformations, and confirmed low birth weight fetus ➪*Rationale:* Allows team caring for the neonate to prepare for the delivery and educate parents on the need for placement of indwelling umbilical lines.
- Prenatal diagnosis of congenital malformations contraindicating the placement of UC, such as abdominal wall defects or congenital diaphragmatic hernia ➪*Rationale:* Allows team caring for the neonate to prepare for the delivery.
- Neonate's clinical status indicating necessity for UC placement, such as hypoglycemia, respiratory distress, cardiovascular instability, or difficulty obtaining peripheral intravenous lines ➪*Rationale:* Allows team caring for the neonate to prepare for the procedure and educate parents on the need for placement of indwelling umbilical lines.

- Neonate's clinical status contraindicating placement of UC, such as lower extremity vascular compromise, necrotizing enterocolitis, omphalitis, or peritonitis ➤➤*Rationale:* Allows team caring for the neonate to prepare for alternative line placement.
- Neonate's gestational age, estimated birth weight, and umbilical vessels and cord anatomy ➤➤*Rationale:* The team caring for the neonate can prepare for the procedure.
- Family's understanding of the reasons for and risks and benefits of the procedure ➤➤*Rationale:* Evaluates the family's understanding of the procedure and provides a gauge for ongoing education.

CHILD AND FAMILY EDUCATION

Individualized, developmentally appropriate education is provided to the family prenatally or postnatally based on desire for knowledge, readiness to learn, and overall psychosocial state and the clinical status of the neonate.

- Provide information about the necessity of UC placement and the various uses of the catheter ➤➤*Rationale:* Providing information can help to decrease the family's anxiety and aid in their decision-making abilities and informed consent.
- Provide information about the potential complications of UC placement and continued usage ➤➤*Rationale:* Providing information can help to decrease the family's stress and aid in their decision-making abilities and informed consent.
- Provide information on institution-specific protocols regarding the holding of neonates with indwelling umbilical lines ➤➤*Rationale:* Providing information can help to decrease the family's anxiety and inform the family when they will be able to hold the baby.
- Provide information on institution-specific protocols regarding infant positioning with indwelling umbilical lines ➤➤*Rationale:* Providing information can help to decrease the family's anxiety.
- Provide information on institution-specific protocols regarding dressing or swaddling the neonate with indwelling umbilical lines ➤➤*Rationale:* Providing information decreases the family's stress and informs the family of when they will be able to dress or swaddle the baby.
- Encourage questions and answer questions as they arise ➤➤*Rationale:* Reinforcement of information is needed during periods of stress and is especially important if the procedure is emergent.

EQUIPMENT

- Sterile small scissors
- Sterile curved mosquito hemostat
- Sterile curved Kelly clamp
- Sterile prepackaged UV insertion tray
- Sterile tissue forceps
- Sterile eye straight forceps
- Sterile gauze (4×4 and 2×2)
- Sterile Mayo needle holder
- Sterile probe
- Sterile knife holder
- Sterile scalpel blade
- Sterile 4.0 silk suture with a curved needle
- Sterile syringes (1 mL, 3 mL, 5 mL, and 10 mL)
- Sterile three-way stopcock
- Sterile Luer stub adaptors
- Sterile umbilical catheters, 3.5F and 5.0F (single or double lumen)
- Sterile heparinized flush solution
- Sterile medicine cups
- Three sterile drapes or towels
- Umbilical tape
- Povidone-iodine solution
- Measuring tape
- Four soft restraints
- Sterile gloves and gowns
- Caps and masks
- Blood gas syringe and specimen tubes

Procedure for Insertion of Umbilical Vessel Catheters

Steps	Rationale	Considerations
1. Ensure family understands procedure and questions are answered.	Evaluates and reinforces understanding of previously taught information and facilitates informed consent.	Developmental level, cognitive ability, and anxiety level determine approach to and effectiveness of teaching. In an emergency situation, preprocedural teaching may be limited.
2. Obtain informed consent.	Ensures medical-legal compliance as suggested by the Joint Commission on Accreditation of Healthcare Organizations (JCAHO).	Refer to institution-specific protocols for obtaining and documenting informed consent. In emergency situations, follow institution-specific protocol for assumption of consent.

Procedure continues on following page

Procedure for Insertion of Umbilical Vessel Catheters—*Continued*

Steps	Rationale	Considerations
3. Gather needed equipment and supplies and place in a sterile fashion onto sterile working tray/field to create a sterile working field.	Facilitates completion of task in a timely manner; facilitates maintenance of sterile field.	
4. Wash hands.	Standard precautions; reduces transmission of microorganisms.	
5. Conduct final patient verification process (e.g., "Time out") per institution-specific protocol.	Confirms correct patient, procedure, and site as recommended by JCAHO; prevents unnecessary medical procedures.	Use active communication techniques.
6. Position infant supine under a radiant warmer and restrain all four extremities.	Helps to maintain the sterile field.	Monitor restraints per JCAHO recommendations and institution-specific protocol.
7. Measure the shoulder to umbilical (SU) length or use the birth weight (BW) to determine the length of catheter to be inserted for UAC or UVC.[1,2] (*Level V**)	Most commonly used methods to determine insertion depth/length of the catheter.	For resuscitation, the UVC is inserted to 2 to 4 cm.[3] Refer to the appropriate chart after obtaining either the SU length or BW to determine insertion depth.[1,2]
8. Put on cap and mask. Scrub and then dress for a sterile procedure.	Use of maximal sterile barrier precautions decreases catheter-related bloodstream infections (CRBSI).[4]	
9. Prepare tray for the procedure by sorting equipment and preparing catheters.	Facilitates completion of procedure without delays.	Catheter should have a stopcock attached to the end and be flushed with a sterile solution and left with a syringe with flush connected to the stopcock. Ensure that the stopcock is closed to the infant and atmosphere.
10. Cleanse umbilical cord, cord clamp, and abdomen with povidone-iodine solution.	Decreases risk of infection.	
11. Place the sterile drapes/towels around the umbilical cord so that it is exposed but the abdomen, chest and lower extremities are covered.	Creates a sterile working field.	
12. Tie umbilical tape around the base of the cord stump.	Minimizes blood loss.	Tie tight enough to minimize blood loss but not so tight that the catheter cannot pass easily.
13. With a scalpel, cut the umbilical cord 1 to 2 cm above the skin.	Improves visualization of vessels.	
14. Stabilize cord with the forceps or hemostat to visualize and identify vessels.	Identifies insertion site.	
15. Identify vessel to be cannulated.	Ensures proper vessel cannulation.	Three vessels should be identified (two arteries and one vein). The vein is the large thin-walled vessel.
16. Gently insert curved iris forceps into the lumen of the vessel and dilate. Repeat this procedure until the lumen is dilated.	Facilitates passage of catheter.	Remove any blood clots from the umbilical vein before dilation.

* Level V: Clinical studies in more than one or two patient populations and situations to support recommendations

Procedure for Insertion of Umbilical Vessel Catheters—*Continued*

Steps	Rationale	Considerations
17. Insert catheter into the dilated lumen of the vessel and gently advance the catheter to the desired insertion length.	Prevents perforation of vessel wall.	A double catheter technique for misdirected UVC can be attempted.[5]
18. Gently pull back on the syringe to obtain blood return.	Confirms location of catheter in a blood vessel.	
19. Flush catheter clear of all blood.	Helps to ensure patency of catheter.	
20. Secure catheter with suture material.	Prevents accidental dislodgement of catheter.	
21. Discard used supplies and equipment, including sharps, in appropriate receptacles.	Standard precautions; reduces transmission of microorganisms. Protects personnel health.	
22. Remove protective equipment and wash hands.	Standard precautions.	
23. Verify catheter tip position via an anterior/posterior chest radiograph, echocardiography, or ultrasound scan.[6-12] *(Level V*)*	Desired placement must be verified before infusion of fluids or medications to prevent complications related to incorrect UC placement.	*Chest radiography verification:* High umbilical artery catheter (UAC): Level of thoracic vertebrae 6 to 10. Low UAC: Level of lumbar vertebrae 3 to 4. Umbilical vein catheter (UVC): Level of thoracic vertebrae 8 to 9 or above the diaphragm. *Echocardiography or ultrasound scan verification:* High UAC: Thoracic aorta. Low UAC: Abdominal aorta. UVC: Inferior vena cava.

* Level V: Clinical studies in more than one or two patient populations and situations to support recommendations

Expected Outcomes	Unexpected Outcomes
• Appropriate placement of the UAC (for a high positioned line at the level of thoracic vertebrae 6 to 10 and for a low positioned line at the level of lumbar vertebrae 3 to 4) confirmed via an anterior/posterior chest radiograph	• Malpositioned catheter
• Appropriate placement of the UVC (at the level of thoracic vertebrae 8 to 9 or above the diaphragm) confirmed via an anterior/posterior chest radiograph	• Malpositioned catheter
• Placement of the UVC to 2 to 4 cm for use as access in resuscitation[3]	• Inability to advance catheter to desired location
• Infant is free from cardiovascular complications of UC placement	• Dysrhythmias, heart failure, cardiac tamponade, endocarditis, myocardial perforation, pericardial effusion[13-17]
• Infant is free from gastrointestinal complications of UC placement	• Hepatic necrosis, intestinal perforation or necrosis, necrotizing enterocolitis, omphalitis, peritoneal perforation[14,18,19]
• Infant is free from neurologic complications of UC placement	• Intraventricular hemorrhage, paraplegia, sciatic nerve palsy

Continued

Expected Outcomes

- Infant is free from renal complications of UC placement
- Infant is free from pulmonary complications of UC placement
- Infant is free from vascular complications of UC placement

- Infant is free from complications of UC placement

- Catheter remains in place until elective removal

Unexpected Outcomes

- Bladder injury, hematuria
- Pulmonary effusion, hemorrhage, infarction[20]

- Embolism: Air, Wharton-jelly, cotton-fiber, systemic, pulmonary
- Hemorrhage, thrombosis, vasospasm[14,15,19-22]
- Breaks in catheter
- Electrical hazards
- Infection
- Loss of extremity[13,19]
- Accidental dislodgement of catheter

Procedure for Removal of Umbilical Catheters

Steps	Rationale	Considerations
1. Ensure family understands procedure and questions are answered.	Evaluates and reinforces understanding of previously taught information.	Cognitive ability and anxiety level determine approach to and effectiveness of teaching.
2. Gather needed supplies and equipment and place on sterile working field.	Facilitates completion of procedure in a timely manner.	Sterile gloves, gauze, sterile barrier, and suture removal kit are needed for procedure.
3. Remove all tape or securing devices from catheter.	Allows for optimal access to catheter.	
4. Wash hands and put on sterile gloves.	Standard precautions; reduces transmission of microorganisms.	
5. Cut and remove all suture material.	Retained sutures may cause an infection.	
6. Remove catheter slowly; ensure that entire catheter is removed.	Minimizes blood loss. Retained catheter fragments may embolize.	Place pressure on cord with gauze to decrease blood loss if needed.
7. Discard used supplies and equipment in appropriate receptacles.	Standard precautions; reduces transmission of microorganisms.	
8. Remove gloves; wash hands.	Standard precautions.	

Expected Outcomes

- Entire UC is removed
- Minimal blood loss
- Removal of all sutures
- Infant is free from complications of UC removal

Unexpected Outcomes

- Retention of a piece of or the whole catheter
- Significant blood loss
- Retained sutures that cause infection
- Dysrhythmias
- Heart failure
- Cardiac tamponade
- Endocarditis
- Myocardial perforation
- Pericardial effusion

Monitoring and Care of the Infant

Activities and Interventions	Rationale	Reportable Conditions
1. Monitor insertion length of catheter.	Ensures proper placement of catheter.	• Catheter not sutured at documented insertion length
2. Monitor perfusion to lower extremities, genital, perianal, sacral, and buttock areas.	Perfusion to these areas may become compromised.	• Cyanosis or decreased perfusion
3. Monitor waveform of UAC.	Indicates correct positioning, absence of vasospasm.	• Dampening of waveform
4. Monitor heart rate and electro-cardiographic (EKG) tracing.	Malpositioned lines may cause arrhythmias.	• Arrhythmias
5. Monitor blood loss from blood draws and oozing from insertion site.	Excessive blood loss may indicate idiopathic anemia.	• Amount of blood loss and volume of blood drawn from line

Documentation

- Informed consent or emergency assumption of consent
- Patient and procedure verification process
- Date and time of catheter insertion; individual who placed catheter
- Vessels cannulated
- Catheter size and type (e.g., single or double lumen)
- Insertion length of catheter
- Catheter tip location on radiologic study
- Centimeter mark on catheter at suture
- Adjustments to catheter position performed after insertion
- Lower extremity perfusion
- Time, date, and reason for catheter removal
- Family education
- Unexpected outcomes and related treatment

References

1. Dunn PM: Localization of the umbilical catheter by postmortem measurement, *Arch Dis Childhood* 41:69-75, 1965.
2. Shukla H, Ferrara A: Rapid estimation of insertion length of umbilical catheters in newborns, *AJDC* 140:786-788, 1986.
3. Kattwinkel J, editor: *Textbook of neonatal resuscitation,* ed 4, Dallas, 2000, American Academy of Pediatrics and American Heart Association.
4. O'Grady NP, et al: Guidelines for the prevention of intravascular catheter related infections, *MMWR* 51(No.RR-10): 1-29, 2002.
5. Mandel D, et al: Double catheter technique for misdirected umbilical vein catheter, *J Pediatr* 139(4):591-592, 2001.
6. Ades A, et al: Echocardiographic evaluation of umbilical venous catheter placement, *J Perinatol* 23:24-28, 2003.
7. Baker DH, et al: Proper localization of umbilical arterial and venous catheters by lateral roentgenograms, *Pediatrics* 43(1):34-39, 1969.
8. Barrington KJ: Umbilical artery catheters in the newborn: effects of positioning of the catheter tip (Cochrane Review), 1998, retrieved January 8, 2004, from http://nichd.nih.gov/cochrane/Barring1/Barrington.htm.
9. Greenberg M, Movahed H, Peterson B, et al: Placement of umbilical venous catheters with use of bedside real-time ultrasonography, *J Pediatr* 126(4):633-635, 1995.
10. Paster SB, Middleton P: Roentgenographic evaluation of umbilical artery and vein catheters, *J Am Med Assoc* 231(7):742-746, 1975.
11. Raval N, et al: Umbilical venous catheters: to determine position and associated complications of malpositioned umbilical venous catheters, *Am J Perinatol* 12(3):201-204, 1995.
12. Schlesinger AE, et al: Neonates and umbilical venous catheters: normal appearance, anomalous positions, complications, and potential aid to diagnosis, *Am J Roentgenol* 180(4):1147-1160, 2003.
13. Kotnis R, et al: Retained umbilical arterial catheter presenting as an umbilical abscess, *Arch Dis Childhood* 83(1):74, 2000.
14. Loisel DB, et al: Intravenous access in newborn infants: impact of extended umbilical venous catheter use on requirement for peripheral venous lines, *J Perinatol* 16(6):461-466, 1996.
15. Lussky RC: Radiology casebook, *J Perinatol* 20:562-564, 2000.
16. Nowlen TT, et al: Pericardial effusion and tamponade in infants with central catheters, *Pediatrics* 110(1):137-142, 2002.
17. Symchych PS, Winchester P: Endocarditis following intracardiac placement of umbilical venous catheters in neonates, *J Pediatr* 90(2):287-289, 1977.

18. Moens E, et al: Hepatic abscesses associated with umbilical catheterization in two neonates, *Eur J Pediatr* 162(6): 406-409, 2003.

19. Mokrohisky ST, et al: Low positioning of umbilical-arterial catheters increases associated complications in newborn infants, *N Engl J Med* 299(11):561-564, 1978.

20. Fletcher MA, et al: Umbilical arterial catheter use: report of an audit conducted by the study group for complications of perinatal care, *Am J Perinatol* 11(2):94-99, 1994.

21. Baserga MC, et al: The use of topical nitroglycerin ointment to treat peripheral tissue ischemia secondary to arterial line complications in neonates, *J Perinatol* 22:416-419, 2002.

22. Egan EA, Eitzman DV: Umbilical vessel catheterization, *Am J Disabled Child* 121:213-218, 1971.

Additional Readings

Diamond LK, et al: Erythroblastosis fetalis; VII, treatment with exchange transfusion, *N Engl J Med* 244(2):39-49, 1951

Kitterman JA, et al: Catheterization of umbilical vessels in newborn infants, *Pediatr Clin N Am* 17(4):895-912, 1970.

Symansky MR, Fox HA: Umbilical vessel catheterization: indications, management, and evaluation of the technique, *J Pediatr* 80(5):820-826, 1972.

Todd NA: Procedural flowchart job aid for umbilical arterial line placement, *Neonatal Network* 12(8):63-64, 1993.

PROCEDURE **196**

Admission

PURPOSE: Safe admission of an infant, child, or adolescent to the hospital

Lucy R. Paskus

PREREQUISITE KNOWLEDGE

- Pediatric anatomy and physiology
- Pediatric pathophysiology
- Pediatric physical assessment skills
- Pediatric cognitive and psychosocial assessment skills
- Child developmental as it relates to hospitalization of the infant, child, and adolescent
- Elements of family-centered care
- Signs and symptoms of communicable diseases in children
- Indications for institution of isolation procedures
- Equipment needed to set up the room specific to the child's reason for admission

CHILD AND FAMILY ASSESSMENT

- General appearance of child ➤➤*Rationale:* The initial assessment of color, systemic perfusion, level of activity and responsiveness, position of comfort, and feeding behavior in infants provides information required to assess the need for emergent medical intervention.[1]
- The presence of a language or communication barrier with the child or family ➤➤*Rationale:* Identifies the need for an interpreter or an alternative form of communication, such as a communication board.
- Family structure ➤➤*Rationale:* Identifies individuals available to provide support to the child and individuals who can provide legal permission for the child's treatment.
- Individual who can provide legal permission for the child's treatment ➤➤*Rationale:* Except in emergency situa-

tions, consent for treatment is required. In most states, children less than 18 years of age are not allowed to provide consent for medical treatment. Exceptions such as the emancipated minor vary among jurisdictions.
- As appropriate, assess if the adolescent or young adult has an Advanced Directive ➤➤*Rationale:* The Patient Self-determination Act is a federal law that requires hospitals to ask patients if they have an Advanced Directive. Emancipated minors and those 18 years of age and older may have or may choose to implement an Advanced Directive. Regulations about Advanced Directives vary from state to state.[2]
- The reason for hospitalization and history of current illness ➤➤*Rationale:* Provides the basis for interventions.
- Child's and family's understanding of the reasons for and risks and benefits of hospitalization ➤➤*Rationale:* Evaluates child's and family's understanding of hospitalization and provides a gauge for ongoing education.
- Recent history of cold symptoms or exposure to a contagious disease ➤➤*Rationale:* Child may need isolation procedures/precautions and screening for infectious diseases.
- Residence in a long-term care facility or group-living situation ➤➤*Rationale:* Child may need isolation procedures/precautions and screening for drug-resistant organisms.
- Child's known allergies ➤➤*Rationale:* Promotes patient safety; the presence of allergies may require alterations in interventions, food allergy alerts, or latex alerts.
- Presence of pain, assessed with age-appropriate or developmentally appropriate tools (see Procedure 173 for further information) ➤➤*Rationale:* Facilitates immediate implementation of comfort measures and interventions.
- Complete nursing assessment, including physical, cultural, social, emotional, and spiritual elements ➤➤*Rationale:*

Identifies the child's and family's physical, social, cultural, emotional, and spiritual needs and strengths; contributes to the formulation of a comprehensive plan of care.

- Child's and family's previous experiences with hospitalization **→Rationale:** Previous experiences influence response to and ability to cope with current hospitalization.[3]
- The child's and family's ability to cope with the stress of illness and hospitalization **→Rationale:** Identifies the need for emotional or spiritual support.
- Child's developmental level and ability to interact **→Rationale:** Allows for the adaptation of interventions to fit the developmental level of the child and degree of interaction. Child Life services may be used to provide developmentally appropriate play and diversional activities for the child.
- Need for economic assistance **→Rationale:** Facilitates referral to Social Work to assist with identification of financial resources.
- Family's desire and ability to remain with the child during the hospitalization **→Rationale:** The presence of family provides comfort and support for the child; family presence is a tenet of family-centered care.[1,3-5] *(Level VI[*])*

CHILD AND FAMILY EDUCATION

Individualized, developmentally appropriate education is provided to the family and to the child based on desire for knowledge, readiness to learn, and overall neurologic and psychosocial state.

- If admission is elective, the child and family should be educated and prepared in advance of the admission **→Rationale:** Preparation reduces anxiety and fear, and absorption of information is improved in a less stressful situation before admission.
- Introduce members of health care team **→Rationale:** Child's and family's comfort level is increased by knowing who is providing care to the child.
- Orient the child and family to the room, unit, and facility **→Rationale:** Facilitates ability to independently use the equipment in the room (bed, call bell, television, etc) and to access restrooms, playroom, and cafeteria as appropriate; promotes patient safety.
- Review unit guidelines and visitation policy **→Rationale:** Understanding of regulations increases compliance.

- Explain the purpose of monitoring devices and the meaning behind the numbers/waveforms on the monitors **→Rationale:** Providing information decreases anxiety and fear.
- Explain the purpose of the various tubes and equipment **→Rationale:** Providing information decreases anxiety and fear.
- With traumatic injury or intensive care unit (ICU) admission, preparation for the family and siblings regarding the child's appearance may be necessary **→Rationale:** Advanced preparation assists the family and siblings in coping with the child's altered appearance.
- Share information regarding the child's condition **→Rationale:** Providing information decreases anxiety and fear.
- Prepare the child and family for any procedures to be undertaken **→Rationale:** Preparation reduces anxiety and fear.
- Encourage the family to be involved in care of the child and to comfort and reassure the child as able **→Rationale:** The family's involvement, a key element of family-centered care, provides comfort for the child.
- Encourage questions and answer questions as they arise **→Rationale:** Reinforcement of information is needed during periods of stress and is especially important if the admission is emergent.

EQUIPMENT

- Bed, crib, or radiant warmer appropriate for child's size and needs
- Cardiac and respiratory monitoring equipment as ordered/anticipated
- Blood pressure monitoring equipment
- Ventilator with circuit as needed
- Oxygen source and flow meters
- Bag-valve-mask system appropriately sized for the child
- Suction source and suction canister with tubing
- Yankauer and appropriately sized suction catheters
- Stethoscope
- Intravenous pump and tubing as needed
- Scale appropriate for weight or in-bed scale, zeroed
- Tape measure
- Stadiometer, length board, or arm-length measuring device
- Thermometer

---

* Level VI: Clinical studies in a variety of patient populations and situations to support recommendations

Procedure | for Admission

Steps	Rationale	Considerations
1. Before the child's arrival, set up the room based on the child's age and reason for admission.[6]	Ensures appropriate equipment is available to safely admit the child to the hospital.	To avoid moving the child after arrival, the need for a specialized room, isolation or positive pressure should be considered before admission.
2. Observe standard precautions; implement transmission-based precautions as applicable.[6] *(Level II*)*	Standard and transmission-based precautions are the primary strategies for successful nosocomial infection control.	Children with upper respiratory infection symptoms should be placed on appropriate isolation precautions per institution-specific protocol, pending further investigation and treatment.
3. Introduce self and explain role to child and family; discuss with the child and family the rationale for this acute care/ICU admission.	Identifying yourself and your role as the nurse initiates a professional relationship with the child and family, increasing their comfort level.	This step may need to be repeated several times because the child and family may be overwhelmed by the information they receive.
4. As the child arrives, conduct a focused assessment of airway, breathing, and circulation.[1,3,7] *(Level II*)*	Allows the identification of conditions that need emergent intervention.	In children, untreated respiratory distress may lead to respiratory arrest and subsequent cardiac arrest.[1,2,7]
5. Attach the child to appropriate monitoring devices per prescribing practitioner's order or unit-specific or institution-specific protocol; obtain initial vital signs, including pain assessment.[3,6] *(Level II*)*	Baseline vital signs provide a comparison point for future assessments and are used to identify the need for urgent/emergent interventions.	Assessment of peripheral perfusion provides a useful indication of cardiac output in children; hypotension is often a late sign of inadequate cardiac output.[1,3,7]
6. Measure length or height and weight; obtain occipitofrontal circumference (OFC) on children less than 2 years old. Plot this information on appropriate growth charts (see Procedure 181 for further information).[1,3,4,6] *(Level II*)*	An accurate weight is necessary for appropriate dosing of many pediatric medications. The child's height, weight, OFC, and body mass index (BMI) plotted on a growth chart may identify the need for further nutritional interventions.	In emergent situations, a weight-based resuscitation tape may be used to quickly estimate the child's weight.[8] If a child is unable to stand or lie flat, upper or lower arm length can be used to calculate length.[8,9]
7. Obtain an emergency drug sheet based on the child's weight; verify the accuracy of the child's name and weight on the sheet.[6] *(Level II*)*	All pediatric advanced life support medications are dosed based on the child's weight.[7] Calculation of doses before an emergency situation allows for prompt intervention.	Emergency drug doses calculated by the nurse should be independently verified by a second nurse or pharmacist.[6]
8. Place an identification band on the child that contains two patient identifiers; verify that the information is correct.[4,6] *(Level II*)*	The identification band is used throughout the child's hospitalization to verify identity. The Joint Commission on Accreditation of Healthcare Organizations (JCAHO) lists identification of patients with two patient identifiers as a National Patient Safety Goal to ensure the correct patient receives the correct treatment or therapy.	Two patient identifiers should be used for patient identification per institution-specific protocol; most commonly, name and birth date or name and medical record number are used. Other identifiers, such as a digital photograph or individual specific bar code, may be used to identify the child per institution-specific protocol. In extenuating circumstances, an identification band may be secured to the radiant warmer or crib rather than the child.

Procedure continues on following page

---

* Level II: Theory-based; no research data to support recommendations; recommendations from expert consensus group may exist

Procedure | for Admission—*Continued*

Steps	Rationale	Considerations
9. If the child has known allergies, identify those allergies per institution-specific protocol.	Clear identification of child's known allergies in a highly visible way promotes patient safety.	Institution-specific protocols may include the use of an arm band to identify the child's specific allergies.
10. The child should not eat or drink until approved by medical care team.[6]	The child may need sedation or a procedure that necessitates nothing by mouth (NPO) status.	Intravenous fluid may be necessary if a lengthy NPO time is anticipated, especially in infants at risk for hypoglycemia.[7]
11. Notify medical team of child's arrival.[6]	The medical care team is responsible for timely medical assessment and intervention.	When notifying medical care team, communicate the need for urgent/emergent medical intervention as appropriate.
12. Discuss immediate tests and interventions with the child and family.	Preparation and education may decrease anxiety of child and caregivers. Families consistently report information as a key factor in reducing stress and anxiety.[5,10]	In emergent situations, tests and interventions may be explained as they occur and even after they occur.
13. Assist the child and family with completion of an admission information sheet or database (including screens for domestic violence and evidence of child abuse/neglect).[6]	Collects basic biographic and historic information; assesses current needs of the child and family. If domestic violence or child abuse/neglect is suspected or documented, institution-specific guidelines for reporting can be quickly implemented.	Provide appropriate resources for language barriers, literacy concerns, or other obstacles to completing the form.[6]
14. Review with the child and family all medications the child receives.	The JCAHO recommends medication reconciliation as the child moves from the home to the hospital setting to promote patient safety.	
15. Review unit and hospital layout with the child and family, including unit and hospital rules and available services.	Provides the child and family an increased comfort level with their surroundings.	Provision of written resources (e.g., maps, visitation guidelines, cafeteria hours, etc.) may be helpful for the child and family.
16. Address needs identified by the child and family on admission information sheet.[6] *(Level II*)*	Meets the needs identified by the child and family.	Specific needs may necessitate referral to the chaplain, Child Life specialist, social worker, etc.
17. Implement prescribing practitioner's orders.[6] *(Level II*)*	Begins medical interventions.	Sharing the nursing assessment with the medical team may assist in directing interventions towards the needs identified by the child and family.
18. Develop an individualized plan of care for the child in conjunction with the child and family.[6] *(Level II*)*	Involving the child and family in development of the plan of care is a key element of family-centered care.	If the child or family is unable to participate at the initial development of the plan, encourage participation when there is the ability to do so.
19. Regularly solicit questions from the child and family.	The child and family may be hesitant to ask questions without prompting.	Continually solicit questions from the child and family because new questions may arise or clarification may be necessary.

* Level II: Theory-based; no research data to support recommendations; recommendations from expert consensus group may exist

Procedure for Admission—*Continued*

Steps	Rationale	Considerations
20. Begin discharge planning. *(Level II*)*	Initiation of discharge planning at the time of admission facilitates a smooth discharge process.	In addition to discharge home, discharge planning might also include death or transfer to hospice or rehabilitation setting or long-term care facility.

* Level II: Theory-based; no research data to support recommendations; recommendations from expert consensus group may exist

Expected Outcomes

- The child is safely admitted to the hospital

- The child's and family's psychosocial, developmental, and physical needs are met
- An individualized plan of care, based on the nursing assessment, is developed for the child with input from the child and family
- The child and family understand and agree with the plan of care for the child

Unexpected Outcomes

- The child has injury as a result of incomplete admission process, including failure to obtain or communicate information
- The child's and family's psychosocial, developmental, or physical needs are not met
- The plan of care is not developed with input from the child or family and is not individualized

- The child or family lack understanding as to the child's plan of care

Monitoring and Care of the Child

Activities and Interventions	Rationale	Reportable Conditions
1. Vitals signs and reassessment are repeated based on the child's condition, unit routines, and prescribing practitioner's orders.	Unit routines and prescribing practitioner's orders typically represent the maximum time frame for frequency of obtaining vital signs and assessments; nursing judgment may indicate the need for more frequent evaluation based on changes in the child's condition.	• Significant changes in vital signs • Hemodynamic instability • Respiratory distress • Other concerns as identified by the nurse, child, or family
2. Review the plan of care regularly to identify the need for modifications to meet the changing needs of the child and family over the course of the child's hospitalization.	The plan of care is a dynamic tool and may need frequent adjustment based on the changing needs of the child and family.	• Inability to meet the child's and family's needs despite adjustments to the plan of care

Documentation

- Vital signs and assessments
- Medications taken regularly
- Child and family education
- Medications administered in the hospital
- Plan of care
- Height or length, weight, and OFC (as applicable)
- Review of admissions forms
- Initiation of referrals
- Presence of emergency equipment at bedside (where applicable)
- Unexpected outcomes and related treatment
- Discharge planning

References

1. Hazinski MF: *Manual of pediatric critical care*, St Louis, 1999, Mosby.
2. Omnibus Budget Reconciliation Act of 1990 (OBRA-90): Patient Self-Determination Act, Pub L10-508; 4206-4751, 1990.
3. Smith JB, Martin SA: Caring practices: providing developmentally supportive care. In Curley M, Moloney-Harmon P, editors: *Critical care nursing of infants and children,* ed 2, Philadelphia, 2001, Saunders.
4. Wong DL, Hockenberry MJ, editors: *Wong's nursing care of infants and children,* St Louis, 2003, Mosby.
5. Miles MS: Support for parents during a child's hospitalization: a nurse's guide to helping parents cope, *Am J Nurs* 103(2):62-64, 2003.
6. Children's Hospital: Admission of the child to the hospital. In *Children's hospital nursing policy and procedure manual,* Denver, 2003, The Children's Hospital.
7. Hazinski MF, editor: *PALS provider manual*, Dallas, 2002, American Heart Association.
8. Jarzem PF, Gledhill RB: Predicting height from arm measurements, *J Pediatr Orthoped* 13(6):761-765, 1993.
9. Spender QW, et al: Assessment of linear growth of children with cerebral palsy: use of alternative measures to height or length, *Development Med Child Neurol* 31(2):206-214, 1989.
10. Curley MAQ, Meyer EC: Caring practices: the impact of the critical care experience on the family. In Curley M, Moloney-Harmon P, editors: *Critical care nursing of infants and children,* ed 2, Philadelphia, 2001, Saunders.

Additional Reading

Schrey C, Schrey M: A parents' perspective: our needs and our message . . . the experience and wisdom of two parents who have a child with a congenital cardiac defect, *Crit Care Nurs Clin North Am* 6(1):113-119, 1994.

Discharge

PURPOSE: The safe transition or discharge of the child from the critical or acute care unit, with the family able to care for the child after discharge by monitoring the child's progress, monitoring the effectiveness or side effects of medications, and recognizing adverse signs and symptoms to report immediately to the health care provider

Kathryn A. Beauchamp

PREREQUISITE KNOWLEDGE

- Discharge planning should begin early in the child's hospitalization.
- Members of the multidisciplinary health care team must work together with the family to formulate a plan that results in a smooth discharge process.
- Pediatric anatomy and physiology
- Pediatric growth and development
- Psychologic and sociocultural needs of the child and family
- Psychosocial principles that alleviate the stressors of hospitalized children and their families
- Indicators of changes in a child's status
- Potential long-term effects of hospitalization on the child
- Effects of hospitalization on family dynamics
- Outcomes of multidisciplinary team discharge planning meetings
- Community resources for child and family referrals
- Institution-specific or unit-specific policy on discharge criteria
- Effective teaching methodologies and the ability to assess learning
- Teaching parents to provide care for the child and providing positive reinforcement fosters parental self esteem and facilitates involvement in the discharge process[1] *(Level IV*)*
- Transfer of a child from a critical care unit to the general care unit is a stressful experience for the family; interven-

tions that can minimize the stress have been identified[2,3] *(Level IV*)*

CHILD AND FAMILY ASSESSMENT

- Child's and family's knowledge, learning style, and primary language **→Rationale:** Assessment before teaching facilitates the effectiveness and success of the teaching-learning process.
- Child's and family's knowledge about diagnosis, purpose of medications, assessment of the child, and care necessary in the home **→Rationale:** Assesses current knowledge level; identifies areas in which further teaching is necessary before discharge.
- Child's and family's knowledge of and ability to use and troubleshoot medical equipment that will be used in the home **→Rationale:** Assesses current knowledge level; identifies areas in which further teaching is necessary before discharge.
- Child's and family's knowledge of and ability to administer formula (including preparation) and medications **→Rationale:** Assesses current knowledge level; identifies areas in which further teaching is necessary before discharge, facilitates safe administration of formula and medications in the home.
- Community resources identified to facilitate child's transition to the home environment **→Rationale:** Identifies

---

* Level IV: Limited clinical studies to support recommendations

referrals completed and those that must be made to facilitate the transition to home care.

- Child's and family's knowledge of emergency response plan ➻*Rationale:* Assesses family's knowledge of information needed in the event of an emergency in the home setting; identifies areas in which further teaching is necessary before discharge.
- For the child whose condition is dependent on technology, assess the family's ability to appropriately intervene in an emergency situation (e.g., cardiopulmonary arrest, equipment failure) ➻*Rationale:* Ensures the family can identify and manage life-threatening situations in the home; identifies areas in which further teaching is needed before discharge.
- Child's needs related to transport to the home environment ➻*Rationale:* Ensures appropriate transportation home (e.g., ambulance) or safety equipment (car seat, car bed) is available at time of discharge.
- Child's participation in school as consistent with age and medical condition ➻*Rationale:* Assists child and family with a school support plan and school reentry.
- Shortly before discharge, assess the family's ability to independently care for the child in the home environment ➻*Rationale:* Assures that the family is ready to care for the child in the home environment at time of discharge.

CHILD AND FAMILY EDUCATION

Individualized, developmentally appropriate education is provided to the family and to the child based on desire for knowledge, readiness to learn, and overall neurologic and psychosocial state.

- Educate the family about the child's diagnosis, purpose of medications, assessment of the child, and care needed in the home after discharge; include return demonstration of skills as appropriate ➻*Rationale:* Provides the child and family with the tools needed to manage the child's care in the home; return demonstration allows evaluation of learning.
- For children who have needed intensive care, educate the family about potential negative emotional, behavioral, and academic outcomes, such as posttraumatic stress disorder, regression, difficulty sleeping, acting out, difficulty with school adjustment, and attention difficulties ➻*Rationale:* A study done in the Pediatric Intensive Care Unit (PICU) setting showed that children of mothers who were given education about possible negative outcomes of PICU admission and tools to manage those negative outcomes had improved outcomes compared with children of mothers who did not receive the education.[4] (*Level IV**)

---

* Level IV: Limited clinical studies to support recommendations

- Educate the family in the use and trouble shooting of medical equipment that will be used in the home; include return demonstration of skills as appropriate ➻*Rationale:* Provides the child and family with the tools needed to manage the child's care in the home; return demonstration allows evaluation of learning.
- Teach the family to administer formula (including preparation) and medications; include return demonstration of skills as appropriate ➻*Rationale:* Provides the child and family with the tools needed to manage the child's care in the home; return demonstration allows evaluation of learning.
- Educate the family about the emergency response plan developed specifically for the child ➻*Rationale:* Provides the child and family with the tools needed to safely manage the child's care in the home.
- For the child whose condition is dependent on technology, teach the family appropriate interventions in an emergency situation (e.g., cardiopulmonary arrest, equipment failure); include return demonstration of skills as appropriate ➻*Rationale:* Provides the family with the skills needed to manage an emergency situation in the home while awaiting additional resources identified in the emergency response plan; return demonstration allows evaluation of learning.
- Provide child and family with educational material (pamphlets, videotapes, audiovisual aids, audiotapes) appropriate to child's and family's needs ➻*Rationale:* Increased knowledge of diagnosis and treatment options reduces anxiety and allows child and family to participate in plan-of-care; these materials serve as a reference and reinforce previously taught information.
- Encourage questions and answer questions as they arise ➻*Rationale:* Reinforcement of information is needed during periods of stress.

EQUIPMENT

Dependent on needs of individual child:

- Monitoring: Cardiovascular, respiratory, blood pressure, oxygen saturation
- Respiratory support: Ventilator, continuous positive airway pressure (CPAP), Bilevel positive airway pressure (BiPAP), tracheostomy mask, supplemental oxygen
- Medications and intravenous fluids
- Nutritional supplements
- Child transportation safety equipment (e.g., car seat or car bed)
- Prescriptions
- Copy of follow-up appointments
- Copy of posthospital patient care plan, discharge instructions, or similar documents

Procedure for Discharge

Steps	Rationale	Considerations
1. Anticipate discharge status. *(Level II*)*	Child is evaluated and considered for discharge based on the reversal of the disease process or resolution of physiologic condition that prompted admission to the unit.[5]	Children with chronic management with illness that has been reversed or resolved and condition that is stable may be discharged to a designated patient care unit, rehabilitation unit, or home.[5]
2. If child is to be transferred from the intensive care unit (ICU) to the general care unit, ensure that family is provided information about the transfer before the event. If possible, take the family on a tour of the new unit. *(Level IV*)*	Transfer from the ICU is stressful for the family; ensuring information has been provided decreases stress.[2,3] *(Level IV*)*	Written information about the transfer has been shown to decrease the family's stress.[2] Provide positive information about the receiving unit. Framing the transfer as an indication of the child's improving status may ease the transition for the family.
3. Ensure family and child teaching is completed and family and child understand all teaching and can safely perform all activities/ interventions in teaching plan.	Teaching must be completed for safe discharge of the child to the home environment.	Teaching must be ongoing throughout the child's hospital stay to allow the family time to assimilate information and ensure the family is ready to assume care at discharge.
4. Coordinate collaborative discharge planning with multidisciplinary team.[6] *(Level II*)*	Team meetings provide consensus for complicated discharges.	Consider cultural and religious beliefs and complicated medical or psychosocial situations in discharge planning.
5. Coordinate discharge with Primary Care Provider (PCP).[6] *(Level II*)*	Child will continue to need monitoring of health status after hospitalization.	Address need for PCP if child had no prior health care provider.
6. Contact Case Management.[2] *(Level II*)*	Provides discharge support services (medical equipment, nursing services, insurance issues).	Rehabilitation referral is appropriate when child's level of acuity cannot be managed at home.
7. Obtain Social Services consult.	Provides resources to the child and family with new diagnosis, chronic illness, complicated family dynamics, and legal and ethical issues.	Consider consult if discharge plan necessitates a life style change for child or family.
8. Develop discharge plan in collaboration with child and family.[6] *(Level II*)*	Provides child and family with the information needed to administer care, monitor progress, and recognize adverse signs or symptoms to report.	Provide interpreter services where applicable.
9. Support increasing independence in care.	Child and family must demonstrate competence in providing care by discharge.	Return demonstration of routine and specialized care should be documented per institution-specific protocol.
10. Provide instruction on preparation of special formula or dietary supplements.	Prevents incorrect mixing of formula or dietary supplement.	Check that formula or dietary supplement is available to child and family from local supplier. Provide opportunity for return demonstration by family.

Procedure continues on following page

* Level II: Theory-based; no research data to support recommendations; recommendations from expert consensus group may exist
  Level IV: Limited clinical studies to support recommendations

Procedure | for Discharge—*Continued*

Steps	Rationale	Considerations
11. Provide prescriptions and letters of medical necessity for equipment as applicable.	Prevents disruption in medication administration and medical management.	Prescriptions for compounded medications should be given to family 48 hours before discharge. Check that local pharmacy can fill special prescriptions. Consult with Social Service if family has financial concerns.
12. As appropriate, provide letters to notify school of child's absence.	Prevents miscommunication with school administration.	Family may need a letter to the employer to access federal leave programs (e.g., Family Medical Leave Act).
13. Identify discharge date, time, and transportation home in advance.[6] (*Level II**)	Prevents miscommunication and provides for a timely discharge.	Consult with Case Management for special transportation needs and the use of car seats for appropriate age group.
14. Review plan for child to return to school or work and discuss restrictions to any activities (i.e., stairs, gym).	Prevents disruption in school/day care/preschool participation.	Document on School Nurse Referral form where applicable.
15. Complete Post Hospital Patient Care Plan or institution-specific document.	Provides child and family with written instructions for care, medication administration, and follow-up care.	Use interpreter services and translate instructions if necessary.
16. Complete Nursing Discharge Note or institution-specific document.	Provides documentation of child's hospitalization.	Refer to institution-specific protocol.
17. Ensure presence of a discharge order from the appropriate prescribing practitioner.	Ensures prescribing practitioner responsible for child's inpatient care has authorized the discharge.	Refer to institution-specific protocol.

* Level II: Theory-based; no research data to support recommendations; recommendations from expert consensus group may exist

Expected Outcomes	Unexpected Outcomes
• Child is discharged when discharge criteria have been met	• Child's condition becomes unstable, necessitating delay in discharge or readmission to hospital
• If child is transferred to the general care unit, family and child perceive that transfer process is implemented without complications	• Family feels unprepared for transfer • Family does not receive notification of transfer
• Child and family participate in formulating a discharge plan of care	• Family is unable to participate in formulating discharge plan of care
• Child and family show competence in providing care after hospitalization	• Child's level of acuity increases and family is unable to care for child at home • Family is unable to show competence in providing posthospitalization care
• Child and family are able to state when and whom to contact in case of questions or problems	• Child and family cannot state when or whom to contact in case of questions or problems

Monitoring and Care of the Child

Activities and Interventions	Rationale	Reportable Conditions
1. Continually monitor to ensure that discharge criteria have been met.	Child's condition can change unexpectedly.	• Change in child's condition from predischarge baseline • Signs and symptoms of infection • Increased oxygen requirement • Feeding intolerance
2. Medication administration is changed from intravenous to oral (as appropriate) in preparation for discharge.	Ensures child tolerates oral medications before discharge.	• Child has adverse reaction to change in medication route • Vomiting • Diarrhea
3. Monitor progress of discharge teaching.	Ensures teaching is completed before discharge.	• Family does not meet teaching goals
4. Monitor coordination of home care services.	Ensures services are available at time of discharge.	• Difficulty in obtaining home care services

Documentation

- Nursing discharge note
- Post Hospital Patient Care Plan or similar document
- Posthospital follow-up care
- Child and family teaching, including evaluation of learning and written documents provided to the family and child
- Medications and intravenous fluids
- Multidisciplinary referrals
- Treatments
- School/day care/ preschool referrals

References

1. Miles MS: Support for parents during a child's hospitalization, *Am J Nurs* 103(2):62-64, 2003.
2. Bouve IR, et al: Preparing parents for their child's transfer from the PICU to the pediatric floor, *Appli Nurs Res* 12:114-120, 1999.
3. Saarman L: Transfer out of critical care: freedom or fear? *Crit Care Nurs Q* 16:78-85, 1993.
4. Melnyk BM, et al: Creating opportunities for parent empowerment: program effects on the mental health/coping outcomes of critically ill young children and their mothers, *Pediatrics* 113(6):597-607, 2004.
5. American Academy of Pediatrics Committee on Hospital Care and Pediatric Section of the Society of Critical Care Medicine: Guidelines and levels of care for pediatric intensive care units, *Crit Care Med* 21:931-937, 1993.
6. National Association of Neonatal Nurses: *Discharge guidelines for the technology dependent infant,* Glenview, IL, 1999, National Association of Neonatal Nurses.

Additional Readings

Andrus S, et al: Teaching documentation tool: building a successful discharge, *Crit Care Nurs* 23:39-48, 2003.

Henderson A, Zernike W: A study of the impact of discharge information for surgical patients, *J Adv Nurs* 35:435-441, 2001.

Kinney MR, et al: *AACN's clinical reference for critical care nursing,* ed 4, St Louis, 1998, Mosby, Inc.

Krozek C, Scoggins A: *Patient and family education . . . amended to comply with 2001 JCAHO standards,* Glendale, CA, 2001, Cinahl Information Systems.

Intrahospital Transport

PURPOSE: The prevention of adverse effects during intrahospital transport with use of guidelines regarding organization, equipment, personnel, and assessment skills needed to promote safe, consistent, and comprehensive management of the child throughout the transport process

E. Marsha Elixson and Elizabeth Ristuccia-Semegran

PREREQUISITE KNOWLEDGE

- Intrahospital transport (IHT) of children is part of the critical care continuum.
- With the high acuity and complex diagnoses that necessitate IHT, efficacious completion of the process is vital to optimize the child's comfort and safety.
- American Heart Association Pediatric Advanced Life Support (PALS) or Advanced Pediatric Life Support (APLS) principles of assessment, monitoring, intervention, communication, and documentation should be used during IHT of the child.[1]
- Because IHT is associated with adverse physiologic changes and adverse events, transport of the child must be justified (benefits must outweigh risks).[2-5]
- Mastery of pediatric CPR is necessary; mastery of pediatric advanced life support is preferred.[1-6]
- Ability to monitor the child and recognize changes in status
- Communication systems available within the facility to contact health care providers as needed to manage physiologic changes or adverse events
- Ability to provide a comfortable and secure environment during transport
- Ability to use monitoring devices and equipment
- Potential risks and complications of IHT with consideration of the status of the individual child[3-5]:
  - ❖ Deterioration in physiologic status
  - ❖ Alterations in ventilation
  - ❖ Dislodgement of artificial airway
  - ❖ Loss of oxygen supply
  - ❖ Lack of needed equipment
  - ❖ Equipment malfunction
  - ❖ Loss or infiltration of vascular access
  - ❖ Removal of indwelling line or tube (e.g., indwelling urinary catheter, chest tube)
  - ❖ Omission of required medication dose
- Management of intravenous (IV) access devices
- Ability to identify and troubleshoot malfunctioning monitoring devices and equipment
- Pharmacology and appropriate pediatric dosing of medications used during IHT
- Oxygen concentration of 100% is generally used for transport. Children who should not receive this default concentration may include[4]:
  - ❖ Neonates
  - ❖ Children with congenital heart disease with single ventricle physiology
  - ❖ Children with congenital heart disease dependent on right-to-left shunt to maintain systemic blood flow
- Safety considerations with IHT
- Positive IHT outcomes in children are dependent on availability of expert knowledgeable staff and available correctly functioning state-of-the-art monitoring technology and equipment.[2-5]
- Institution-specific protocols or procedures regarding IHT of the child
- Child development as it relates to clinical assessment and IHT

TABLE 198-1	Acuity Levels/Levels of Care

Level I: Floor/ward patient	Clinically stable No cardiorespiratory monitoring requirements
Level II: Monitored patient	Clinically stable on monitoring May be receiving oxygen Sedation is not planned during transport
Level III: Monitored patient	Clinically stable but at risk for loss of protective airway reflexes Diagnosis puts child at risk for desaturation
Level IV: Patients post conscious sedation;transfer to or from catheterization laboratory, recovery room, postanesthesia care unit, emergency department	Clinically stable but sedated At risk for loss of protective airway reflexes At risk for hemodynamic compromise At risk for potential requirement of medication administration during IHT
Level V: All patients for intensive care unit, trauma, critical illness, post resuscitation, or clinical instability	At risk for hemodynamic compromise Unstable/artificial airway in place requires a respiratory therapist Receiving pharmacologic infusions At risk for additional medication requirements during IHT

Levels of Care are based on acuity, observation requirements, medical needs, and equipment necessities.
From Children's Healthcare of Atlanta: 3.24: Intrahospital transport of patients. *Children's Healthcare of Atlanta policy and procedure manual*, Atlanta, 2003, Children's Healthcare of Atlanta. Used with permission.

CHILD AND FAMILY ASSESSMENT

- Child's developmental level and ability to interact ➤➤*Rationale:* These factors influence preparation of the child for IHT and interaction with the child.
- Child's and family's understanding of the reasons for and risks and benefits of the IHT ➤➤*Rationale:* Evaluates child's and family's understanding of the procedure and provides a gauge for ongoing education.
- Impact of a planned IHT versus an emergency IHT ➤➤*Rationale:* Urgent situations create stress and decrease time to plan ahead or prepare.
- Child's and family's concerns related to the child's temporary separation from a known environment and care team ➤➤*Rationale:* Allows identification of family's concerns; facilitates reinforcement of information concerning availability of consistent comprehensive care.
- Child's hemodynamic parameters, level of consciousness, and activity ➤➤*Rationale:* Rapid status changes can occur in children during transport; the alert and agitated child with an artificial airway may need sedation during transport to ensure the airway remains in place.[1-5]
- Anticipated duration of transport ➤➤*Rationale:* Allows the transport team to ensure adequate volumes of continuous medication infusions (e.g., inotropes), IV fluids, oxygen, and medications that may need to be administered while the child is away from the unit.[2,4,5]
- Personnel needed for transport and potential or known need for medical interventions that necessitate a physician or other advanced care provider (e.g., nurse practitioner) ➤➤*Rationale:* Ensures availability of all individuals needed to safely transport child (Tables 198-1 and 198-2 for an example of an IHT classification system).

TABLE 198-2	Minimum Staff Minimum Staff Requirements for Patient Care Transport Based on Acuity Levels

Level II	RN PCT
Level III	RN PCT Consider RCT
Level IV	RN PCT Consider RCT Consider advanced care provider (NP, PA)
Level V	RN PCT, if needed for equipment transport RCT Advanced care provider or physician as condition warrants

RN, Registered nurse; *PCT,* patient care technician; *RCT,* respiratory care professional; *NP,* nurse practitioner; *PA,* physician assistant.
From Children's Healthcare of Atlanta: 3.24: Intrahospital transport of patients. *Children's Healthcare of Atlanta policy and procedure manual*, Atlanta, 2003, Children's Healthcare of Atlanta. Used with permission.

- Presence or need for artificial airway ➤➤*Rationale:* The child may decompensate during the transport; children at risk for decompensation of respiratory status should have a secured airway before transport.[2-4]
- Patency, security, and position of endotracheal tube (ETT), if present ➤➤*Rationale:* Airway must be patent and secure before transport, and position of tube tip must be noted; transport involves a risk of airway dislodgement.[1-5]
- Security of invasive lines and tubes ➤➤*Rationale:* All invasive lines and tubes must be secure before transport;

transport involves a risk of invasive line and tube dislodgement.[1-5]

- Volume of pharmacologic agents and IV fluids ➧**Rationale:** Continuous infusions must be continued throughout transport; adequate volume must be available for entire duration of transport to prevent potential changes in the child's hemodynamic status.
- Presence of equipment that increases difficulty of transport (e.g., traction or other equipment that cannot fit in elevator available en route) ➧**Rationale:** Transporters can plan for alternative routes or change of equipment, which prevents an increase in transport time.
- Required equipment or patient-specific devices that cannot function in a specific procedure area (e.g., metal in a magnetic resonance imaging area) ➧**Rationale:** Decreases risk to child by preventing transport that must be aborted.
- Child's risk for hypothermia ➧**Rationale:** Environmental temperature may vary greatly during transport, which puts the child at risk for hypothermia; cold stress may result in acidosis or hemodynamic instability.[3,4]
- Desire of family members to be present during the transport ➧**Rationale:** Family members may provide comfort and support to the child during IHT but should have the choice not to accompany the child.

CHILD AND FAMILY EDUCATION

Individualized, developmentally appropriate education is provided to the family and to the child based on desire for knowledge, readiness to learn, and overall neurologic and psychosocial state.

- Provide information that explains the need for and the mode of IHT ➧**Rationale:** Providing pertinent information helps to decrease the child's and family's anxiety levels.
- Provide information on the purpose of the test or procedure and the location of the child's transport. If the family will stay in a waiting area at the transport location, provide this information before transport. ➧**Rationale:** Providing pertinent information increases knowledge and decreases fear and anxiety related to the procedure.
- Explain how the transport will occur, who will accompany the child, the anticipated duration of the transport, and how the level of care will be maintained ➧**Rationale:** Providing pertinent information increases knowledge and decreases fear and anxiety related to the procedure.
- Use interpretation services if the child's or family's preferred language is not English ➧**Rationale:** Decreases barriers to communication
- Encourage questions and answer questions as they arise ➧**Rationale:** Reinforcement of information is needed

during periods of stress and is especially important if the IHT is emergent.

EQUIPMENT

- Appropriate staff according to level of acuity (see Table 198-2)
- Appropriate size and type of transport vehicle (e.g., stretcher, isolette)
- Chart or hard copy of medical record; identification/addressograph card
- X-ray films or hard copy of other diagnostic studies as indicated
- Emergency medication/code sheet, based on child's weight
- Emergency medications per PALS guidelines
- Cardiorespiratory monitor with visual/audible alarms
- Pulse oximeter
- Blood pressure monitoring device
- Invasive monitoring device specific to the individual child (e.g., arterial catheter or intracranial pressure monitoring)
- Back-up battery supply for monitors as indicated or available
- Stethoscope
- Pharmacologic infusions and pumps specific to the individual child
- Respiratory equipment:
  - ❖ Oxygen tank
  - ❖ Appropriately sized face mask
  - ❖ Appropriately sized endotracheal or tracheostomy tubes specific to the individual child
  - ❖ Laryngoscope with appropriate size and type of blades specific to the individual child
  - ❖ Self-inflating manual resuscitation bag
  - ❖ Flow-inflating manual resuscitation bag if indicated
  - ❖ Appropriately sized suction catheters
  - ❖ Portable suction
  - ❖ Portable ventilator as required or available
- Other equipment and supplies specific to the individual child
  - ❖ Sedation or neuromuscular blocking agents
  - ❖ Fluid for volume administration
  - ❖ Reversal agents
  - ❖ Tape
  - ❖ Medications scheduled for administration while the child is away from the unit
  - ❖ Equipment to obtain vascular access
  - ❖ Syringes
  - ❖ Clean gloves
  - ❖ Gowns
- Requisition, consent, other procedure-specific paperwork as indicated

Procedure for Intrahospital Transport

Steps	Rationale	Considerations
1. Ensure child and family understand transport requirement and procedure and questions are answered. *(Level II*)*	Evaluates and reinforces understanding of previously taught information.	Developmental level, cognitive ability, and anxiety level determine approach to and effectiveness of teaching.
2. Contact receiving location to identify anticipated time of arrival and special needs of the child (e.g., artificial airway, special precautions such as communicable disease isolation).[2,4,5] *(Level II*)*	Ensures receiving location is ready for the child; prevents delay in performing procedure on child's arrival to location.	
3. Collect all needed equipment and supplies.[2-5] *(Level V*)*	Ensures safe transport of the child.	Ensure equipment is functioning correctly. Plug in equipment until actual departure to ensure battery pack is charged before transport.
4. If transport staff has responsibilities for other children, ensure responsibility for care has been transferred to another staff member and complete report given.[2] *(Level II*)*	Promotes safety of all patients; facilitates continuity of care.	
5. Wash hands.	Standard precautions; reduces transmission of microorganism.	Put on appropriate protective garb if specific precautions or isolation are necessary.
6. Ensure patient identification armband or other institution-specific mechanism for patient identification is present. *(Level VI*)*	Promotes patient safety; allows receiving location to verify correct patient, procedure, and site as recommended by the Joint Commission for Accreditation of Healthcare Organizations (JCAHO). Prevents unnecessary medical procedures.	Mechanism for patient identification process and verification process is institution specific. Use active communication techniques.
7. Ensure transport equipment is secure and is not placed on the child.[2-5] *(Level V*)*	Promotes safety and stability of equipment during IHT. Ensuring equipment is not lying on the child prevents injury.	Equipment that is dropped or falls may result in equipment failure, inability to monitor the child, or displacement of invasive lines or tubes.
8. Determine adequate supplies, medications, intravenous fluids, oxygen required based on estimated length of transport.[1-5] *(Level III*)*	Prevents destabilization related to loss of oxygen, inability to provide continuous medication infusions, or inability to treat child's agitation.	Maintain consistent level of care.
9. Immediately before transport, notify receiving location that child is en route.[2,4,5] *(Level II*)*	Ensures receiving location is ready for child on arrival; minimizes time child is away from the unit.	
10. Position child for comfort/safe travel; ensure transport staff can see child and monitors.[2,4] *(Level II*)*	Facilitates rapid identification of changes in child's status.	Soft restraints are used as needed to maintain child's safety.[2,4]
11. Immediately before transport, assess child's physiologic status.[2,4] *(Level II*)*	Establishes baseline; ensures child can be safely transported.	

Procedure continues on following page

---

* Level II: Theory-based; no research data to support recommendations; recommendations from expert consensus group may exist
Level III: Laboratory data; no clinical data to support recommendations
Level V: Clinical studies in more than one or two patient populations and situations to support recommendations
Level VI: Clinical studies in a variety of patient populations and situations to support recommendations

Procedure for Intrahospital Transport—*Continued*

Steps	Rationale	Considerations
12. Immediately before transport, ensure that all monitors/equipment and alarms are functioning properly and adequate supplies of medications and oxygen are available.[2-5] *(Level II[*])*	Ensures deterioration of child's status can be identified and managed. Adequate supplies prevent deterioration.	Failure of equipment and inadequate supplies are two common reasons for complications related to transport.[2-5]
13. Ensure child's privacy is maintained during transport.	Promotes child's rights; complies with Health Insurance Portability and Accountability Act.	
14. Maintain standard precautions and any special precautions needed for communicable diseases throughout transport.[2,4] *(Level VI[*])*	Reduces transmission of micro-organisms; protects other patients and personnel.	Specific isolation or precaution needs must be communicated before actual transport begins.
15. Maintain airway patency and security throughout transport.[2-5] *(Level V[*])*	Promotes adequate ventilation.	
16. For children undergoing mechanical ventilation, ensure ventilator parameters (e.g., tidal volume, positive end expiratory pressure (PEEP), peak inspiratory pressure) are maintained during transport.[2,4,5] *(Level II[*])*	Prevents destabilization from inadequate/inappropriate ventilation.	If the child's current mode of ventilation cannot be reproduced for transport, alternate mode of ventilation should be trialed before transport.[4] *(Level II[*])*
17. On arrival to transport location and if monitoring and equipment are transferred to equipment available at transport location, assess child's physiologic status.[2,4] *(Level II[*])*	Assesses physiologic status of the child; ensures that equipment and monitoring are functioning correctly and that child's condition remains stable on new equipment.	
18. The IHT staff maintains responsibility for the child until completion of the transport or report is accepted at the receiving location.[2,4] *(Level II[*])*	The IHT staff is accountable for child throughout transport.	Responsibility ends after report has been accepted by receiving team.
19. On return to unit and after child is transferred to unit monitors and equipment; assess child's physiologic status and intactness of all invasive lines and tubes. Ensure that all alarms are activated.[2,4] *(Level II[*])*	Assesses physiologic status of the child; ensures that equipment and monitoring are functioning correctly and that child's condition remains stable on new equipment. Activation of alarms promotes patient safety.	
20. Dispose of used supplies and equipment in appropriate receptacles.	Standard precautions; reduces transmission of microorganisms.	
21. Remove protective items; wash hands.	Standard precautions.	
22. Ensure transport equipment is cleaned, restocked, checked, and returned to storage location per institution-specific or unit-specific protocols. *(Level II[*])*	Ensures functioning and availability of equipment for future transports.	

* Level II: Theory-based; no research data to support recommendations; recommendations from expert consensus group may exist
  Level V: Clinical studies in more than one or two patient populations and situations to support recommendations
  Level VI: Clinical studies in a variety of patient populations and situations to support recommendations

Expected Outcomes

- Child's condition remains hemodynamically stable throughout transport
- All invasive lines and tubes remain intact and functioning throughout transport

- All equipment functions correctly throughout transport
- Child is free from known adverse effects of IHT

Unexpected Outcomes

- Hemodynamic instability

- Inadvertent removal of ETT
- Inadvertent removal of intravascular catheter
- Inadvertent removal of drain or tube
- Equipment malfunction or failure
- Injury
- Cardiopulmonary arrest
- Death

Monitoring and Care of the Child

Activities and Interventions	Rationale	Reportable Conditions
1. Monitor child consistently and continuously during IHT.	Maintains level of care throughout transport; facilitates prompt identification of problems.	• Change in hemodynamic status • Deterioration in respiratory status
2. Continuously monitor child's tolerance of IHT.	Changes in child's condition may indicate complications arising during IHT. Agitation may increase likelihood of loss of invasive lines or tubes.	• Change in hemodynamic status • Change in respiratory status • Agitation or pain
3. Monitor all invasive lines and devices for functioning and intactness throughout transport.	Risk of dislodgement of invasive lines or devices is increased with transport and moving child in and out of bed.	• Inadvertent removal of invasive line or device • Invasive line or device does not function

Documentation

- Child and family education
- Child's physiologic status before, during, and at completion of IHT
- Child's response to and tolerance of IHT
- Mode of transport
- Equipment and monitoring used during transport
- If appropriate, ETT position before and at completion of transport
- Accompanying personnel
- Fluids infused; medications and treatments administered during IHT
- Interventions during IHT
- Indications for transport
- Unexpected outcomes and related treatment

References

1. Post-arrest stabilization and transport. In: Hazinski MF, editor: *Pediatric advanced life support provider manual*, Dallas, 2002, American Heart Association.
2. Australasian College for Emergency Medicine, Australian and New Zealand College of Anaesthetists and Joint Faculty of Intensive Care Medicine: Minimum standards for intrahospital transport of critically ill patients, *Emerg Med* 15:202-204, 2003.
3. Wallen E, et al: Intrahospital transport of critically ill pediatric patients, *Crit Care Med* 23:1588-1595, 1995.
4. Warren J, et al: Guidelines for the inter- and intrahospital transport of critically ill patients, *Crit Care Med* 32(1): 256-262, 2004.
5. Waydhas C: Equipment review: intrahospital transport of critically ill patients, *Crit Care* 3(5):83-89, 1999.
6. Venkataraman ST, Orr RA: Intrahospital transport of critically ill patients, *Crit Care Clin* 8(3):525-531, 1992.

Additional Readings

Guidelines Committee ACoCCM, Society of Critical Care Medicine and the Transfer Guidelines Task Force: Guidelines for the transfer of critically ill patients, *Crit Care Med* 21:931-937, 1993.

Pope BB: Providing safe passage for patients, *Nurs Manage* 34(9):41-46, 2003.

Outside Facility Transport

P U R P O S E : Maintenance of the critical care environment and delivery of the child in stable or improved condition from the referring to the receiving center

Susan Ingrid Maeder-Chieffo and Robyn Neely Funk

PREREQUISITE KNOWLEDGE

- "Neonatal-pediatric inter-facility transports should be performed rapidly and safely by qualified personnel who are employed by transport programs that have established prospectively developed operational guidelines, consultation services, and transfer agreements" *(American Academy of Pediatrics).*[1] Registered nurses employed as staff on a unit or ward of an institution should not perform transports unless hired by a transport team or accompanying a team as a pediatric expert.
- Emergency Medical Treatment and Labor Act (EMTALA), Consolidated Budget Reconciliation Act (COBRA), Omnibus Budget Reconciliation Act (OBRA), and Joint Commission for the Accreditation of Health Care Organizations (JCAHO) laws and regulations that govern interfacility transport[1-3]
- Transport of critically ill children from one facility to another is based on the receiving hospital's ability to deliver a higher level of care (e.g., services not available at the referring facility).[3]
- Levels of care offered by Basic Life Support (BLS), Advanced Life Support (ALS), Critical Care, and Specialty Transport Services
- Mastery of Advanced Cardiac Life Support (ACLS) protocols; certification as required by State regulations or institution-specific protocols
- Mastery of Pediatric Advanced Life Support (PALS) or Advanced Pediatric Life Support (APLS) and Neonatal Resuscitation Program (NRP) protocols; certification as

required by state regulations or institution-specific protocols and dependent on patient population
- Altitude physiology and gas laws (Boyle's, Dalton's, Henry's, and Charles')[1,4]
- Appropriate pediatric dosing of sedatives, analgesics, paralytics, and emergency medications
- Transport environment limitations and safety considerations
- Transport equipment must[1]:
  - Be portable, sturdy, lightweight, and securable
  - Be compatible with other equipment (i.e., regulators and hoses)
  - Have AC/DC compatible batteries able to last twice the estimated time of the transport
  - Meet federal, state, and Federal Aviation Association (FAA) regulations
  - Be able to withstand vibration, altitude, and temperature changes
  - Be able to fit through facility and transport vehicle doors
  - Be able to be lifted by two personnel
- State certification requirements for interfacility transport personnel and specialized skill requirements
- State requirements for transport vehicle and supplies
- Knowledge of modes of transport (ground, rotor, and fixed wing) and ability to troubleshoot equipment, location, and modes to secure supplies within each
- Competence and experience caring for infants and children in the inpatient setting[1,2]
- Ability to calculate volume of oxygen and medical air cylinder supplies that are necessary based on child's requirements and anticipated length of transport

- Knowledge of appropriate safety devices for child (i.e., car seat) and crew (i.e., nonflammable uniforms, appropriate weather gear in the event of vehicular breakdown, rubber-soled shoes, helmets, ear protection) in the transport environment[1,2,4]
- Risks of interfacility transport, including[1-3]:
  - ❖ Possibility of vehicle crash
  - ❖ Instability of child's condition as a result of change in environment
  - ❖ Possibility of death because of inability to perform needed procedures/surgery as a result of space limitations and resource limitations
- Understanding that the ambulance/rotor-wing/fixed-wing company's Medical Director is the physician responsible for the child's care and orders unless a prearranged legal agreement exists between said company and the receiving facility
- Registered nurses employed as staff on a unit or ward of an institution should be considered an adjunct to the child's care during a transport by a qualified and appropriately triaged transport team.
- Informed consent is required before transport of the child to another facility except in the case of true medical emergency.[1-3]

CHILD AND FAMILY ASSESSMENT

- Child's developmental level and ability to interact ➤➤*Rationale:* Influences preparation of the child and interaction.
- Parent's or legal guardian's language skills and preferred language ➤➤*Rationale:* Facilitates provision of a medical interpreter if the family does not speak English or verbal review of the consent forms in the event of illiteracy so the family can provide informed consent.
- Child's and family's understanding of the reasons for and risk and benefits of transfer to another facility ➤➤*Rationale:* Evaluates child's and family's understanding of the procedure and provides a gauge for ongoing education.
- Child's airway status and risk for respiratory decompensation ➤➤*Rationale:* Identifies need for artificial airway placement before transport, decreasing risk to the child.
- Desire of family members to accompany the team during the transport ➤➤*Rationale:* The presence of familiar family members is comforting, but the family should have the choice not to accompany the child; type of transport vehicle may limit ability to transport a family member with the child.
- Level of comfort and anxiety during the transport ➤➤*Rationale:* Patient may need antianxiety or pain medications during the transport. Family members may not be able to retain treatment information if they have high levels of stress.

CHILD AND FAMILY EDUCATION

Individualized, developmentally appropriate education is provided to the family and to the child based on desire for knowledge, readiness to learn, and overall neurologic and psychosocial state.

- Review the benefits of the services of the accepting facility with the family ➤➤*Rationale:* Providing information decreases anxiety and fear.
- Discuss the risks of transport with the family ➤➤*Rationale:* The family must be informed of risks before signing consent to provide informed consent.
- Provide family with directions and contact numbers for the accepting facility if they are unable or not permitted to travel with the child ➤➤*Rationale:* Providing information decreases anxiety and fear; facilitates communication while the family and child are separated.
- Obtain contact numbers of the family if they are not traveling with the child; mobile phone service may be most useful ➤➤*Rationale:* Certain treatments may not be covered by the transport consent such as surgery, blood products, or anesthesia. The mobile phone number can be used to update the family of changes in the child's condition during the transport or diversion to a nearer facility and to obtain unanticipated consent.
- In the event of an ambulance transport, if the family wishes to follow in their own vehicle, inform them not to follow the ambulance in the event emergency lights and sirens are being used ➤➤*Rationale:* Following emergency vehicles that are using lights and sirens is illegal and dangerous for the personnel and child on board.
- Encourage questions and answer questions as they arise ➤➤*Rationale:* Reinforcement of information is needed during periods of stress and is especially important given the usually emergent nature of the transport.

EQUIPMENT

- Equipment supplies and checks typically include items that the staff nurse does not normally consider: Oxygen tanks and regulator checks, back-up plans for all critical systems, vehicle checks, and appropriate licensures for states team may have to cross into or out of during the transport
- Appropriately triaged and licensed vehicles based on distance and child's acuity and EMTALA compliance issues
- Transport and ACLS supplies and equipment, as recommended by American Association of Pediatrics (AAP) transport division or Air and Surface Transport Nurses Association (ASTNA) publications, which also meet individual state requirements
- Ambulance stretcher, flight litter, or transport isolette (latter generally limited to infants less than 5 kg)[1]
- Transport monitor and charge cord appropriate for child's weight/size with audible and visual alarms and waveforms that also have capabilities specific for child's needs; ability to monitor heart rate (HR), respiratory rate (RR), blood pressure (BP), oxygen saturation, temperature, invasive lines, or end tidal CO_2
- Intravenous pumps and charge cords with high and low flow capabilities to meet child's needs, including mechanism to secure pumps to stretcher, pole, or isolette

- Transport ventilator, tubing, and humidification system appropriate for child's size and ventilation settings[1-3]
- Portable suction unit and charge cord
- Transport defibrillator/external pacemaker and pads appropriate for child's size
- Emergency medications, generally enough to cover a full code during the time it takes to divert to the nearest facility (not necessarily the receiving facility); medications must be stored in a temperature-controlled setting to avoid adulteration

- Intravenous (IV) fluids, electrolytes, and antibiotics as recommended by individual state requirements and AAP or ASTNA guidelines
- Mobile phone service and two-way radio that has been deemed operational in region of transport
- Medical command physician (MCP) or responsible physician available to respond to emergent phone calls or requests from team
- Approved transport protocols or written orders
- Weather-appropriate and vehicle-appropriate clothing for all caregivers[1,2,4]

Procedure for Outside Facility Transport

Steps	Rationale	Considerations
1. Obtain demographic data, child's specific location, and assessment of child from referring facility staff.[1,2] *(Level II*)*	Receiving facility's Admissions department requires demographics to admit the child before arrival. Specific location of child at referring facility is imperative for directions and timely transfer. Acuity level dictates mode of transport and personnel required.	Type of facility requesting transport should be known: teaching hospital or community medical center is appropriate location to request interfacility transport team. Physician's office or clinic should be referred to Emergency Medical Services instead of waiting for interfacility team to arrive.[1]
2. Ascertain whether parent or legal guardian is present. *(Level II*)*	Consent for transport must be obtained before assuming care of child unless it is a case of medical emergency and every effort has been made to contact parent or legal guardian.[1-3]	Ask parent to stay with the child. If family needs to go home first for items, negotiate time they must be available at the referring facility or obtain verbal consent for the transport.
3. Select appropriate transport vehicle.[1-3] *(Level II*)*	Promotes safety of transport team and child. **EMTALA compliance regulation:** Qualified personnel with equipment appropriate for the transport environment must perform patient transfers.	In selection of appropriate vehicle, consider distance, transport time, timely treatment, transport delays, critical care requirements, inaccessible area, and local ground resources. In the event of an air transport, the pilot decides whether a family member can accompany the team and child. If a family member does not accompany the child, obtain consent and mobile phone number (if available) before family leaves to travel to receiving facility.[4]
4. Contact accepting physician and review child's status and mode of transport.[1,2] *(Level II*)*	The physician is ultimately responsible for the medical transportation of the child.	Medical report and nursing report, when performed separately, often yield a more complete status of the child.
5. Evaluate oxygen and medical air levels in the transport vehicle's tanks.[1-3] *(Level II*)*	Support of airway and breathing is an essential component in transport care; adequate gas supplies must be available.	High flow ventilators or nebulizer systems, distance, and potential for vehicle breakdown all must be considered in calculation of gas supply required.

* Level II: Theory-based; no research data to support recommendations; recommendations from expert consensus group may exist

Procedure for Outside Facility Transport—*Continued*

Steps	Rationale	Considerations
6. Obtain directions to referring facility if ground transport and check for availability of maps covering area. *(Level II*)*	Timeliness of transport is dependent on accurate directions.	Have team member sit in front with emergency medical technician (EMT) driving if driver is unfamiliar with destination.
7. Pack special equipment or medications that may be required based on triage and report.[1-3] *(Level II*)*	Ensures transport team is prepared to care for the child; anticipates child's individual care needs.	Referring facilities may loan their equipment in emergent situation; however, they no longer have the equipment for their own use and the cost of sending the equipment back can be significant. The perception of competency in caring for a child may be in doubt if the team is unprepared.[1]
8. Notify supervisor or dispatch center of team departure and names of all personnel on board.[1,2,4] *(Level II*)*	Motor vehicle accident or catastrophic event may occur while team is en route; promotes team safety.	Supervisor or dispatch center should have emergency contact numbers of all personnel on transport.
9. Plug in any necessary equipment and turn on inverter. *(Level II*)*	Prevents equipment batteries from draining.	Consideration of back up for all critical systems and policies for intervention should be in place for power failure and or truck breakdown.[1,2]
10. Notify referring facility of departure time and estimated time of arrival (ETA); ask if parents are still available. *(Level II*)*	Facilitates planning of referring facility; parental consent must be obtained on team's arrival.	Lack of or inaccurate ETA can delay a transport if a team arrives and the child is not ready to leave. For example, waiting at the bedside for charts and x-rays to be copied.
11. Turn off inverter once transport vehicle engine is turned off and unload necessary equipment to take into child's room/unit.	Saves ambulance battery. Maintains adequate level of care and prevents unexpected emergency; team must maintain adequate level of care with necessary equipment and medications for unexpected emergency from equipped transport vehicle to patient floor and back to equipped transport vehicle.	Consideration of back up for all critical systems and policies for intervention should be in place for power failure and/or truck breakdown.[1,2] Child's level of care should never decrease.
12. Call receiving facility to notify them of arrival at the child's bedside. Request to speak with MCP if the child's assessment differs from triaged assessment to obtain orders that fall out of the transport protocol ordered for the child.[1,2] *(Level II*)*	Facilitates planning at receiving hospital; allows for all appropriate equipment to be set up at bedside. Keeps MCP updated regarding child's condition.	Depending on child's diagnosis, transport team may need to make a decision to "stay and play" (stabilize and resuscitate) or "swoop and scoop" (for children with continued decompensation without receiving facility intervention, such as cardiac surgery) at the referral center. In most cases, stabilization before transport is recommended.[1-3]
13. Obtain consent for transport and admission from the parent or legal guardian.[1-3] *(Level II*)*	Ensures medical-legal compliance.	Ascertain whether family member with child is the actual legal guardian. In emergent situation, the referring Attending Physician may sign consent.

Procedure continues on following page

Procedure for Outside Facility Transport—*Continued*

Steps	Rationale	Considerations
14. Verify referring facility has completed EMTALA transport consent with legal guardian.[1-3] *(Level II*)*	Ensures medical-legal compliance; must be completed by a representative of the organization that requests transport.	Legal guardian must be informed of all risks to provide informed consent (vehicular accident, death, inability to perform surgery on transport, etc).
15. Offer the family directions and telephone numbers of the receiving facility.[1,2] *(Level II*)*	Decreases family's anxiety; even if one parent accompanies the child in the transport vehicle, other family members usually drive or are driven to the receiving facility.	If parents are upset, consider suggesting that, for their own safety, they find a relative or friend to drive them to the receiving facility.
16. On arrival at referral hospital, complete a primary survey by assessing airway, breathing, and circulation (ABC).[1,2] *(Level II*)*	Reassesses child's status; identifies emerging problems and facilitates prompt intervention.	At minimum, ABC/primary survey should be stabilized before departing referring facility, which differs from prehospital EMS practice.
17. Complete a secondary survey (head to toe) and perform any necessary interventions for stabilization.[1,2] • Review chest x-ray (CXR) and recent laboratory work if applicable to determine effectiveness of ventilation and endotracheal tube (ETT) placement. • Assess sufficiency and patency of venous and arterial access. • Secure all lines and tubes. *(Level II*)*	Facilitates identification of problems that necessitate management/stabilization before transport.	Any hospital environment is considered a higher level of care than a transport setting; initial stabilization should be completed within the hospital setting. Radiology is not available in the transport setting.
18. Secure the child and necessary equipment to either the isolette or stretcher and transport to vehicle.[1-3] *(Level II*)*	Prevents child and equipment from becoming projectiles in event of accident and ensures child, family, and caregiver safety.	Pediatric-designed restraint systems should be used.[1-3]
19. Contact the receiving facility to alert them of departure; communicate with MD or RN accepting the child, depending on institution-specific protocol.[1-3] *(Level II*)*	Allows receiving facility to anticipate and plan for child's approximate arrival time.	Allows Operating Room to contact staff if off hours or emergent procedure is necessary. Isolation needs can be reviewed at this time.
20. Plug in any necessary equipment and turn on inverter. Observe equipment to evaluate whether charge light indicator is on. *(Level II*)*	Prevents equipment batteries from draining.	Consideration of back up for all critical systems and policies for intervention should be in place for power failure and/or truck breakdown.[1,2]
21. Continue to assess child frequently throughout transport. *(Level II*)*	Reassesses child's status; identifies emerging problems and facilitates prompt intervention.	Changes in assessment must be relayed to MCP.
22. Perform any necessary treatments child may need to ensure continued stabilization during the transport process.[1-3] *(Level II*)*	Maintains level of care.	MCP/protocols are required for orders.

* Level II: Theory-based; no research data to support recommendations; recommendations from expert consensus group may exist

Procedure for Outside Facility Transport—*Continued*

Steps	Rationale	Considerations
23. On arrival at receiving facility, deliver child to bed/nursing unit with all necessary equipment to manage ABC and maintain level of care.[1,2] *(Level II*)*	Team must maintain adequate level of care with necessary equipment and medications for unexpected emergency from equipped ambulance to patient floor.	Child's level of care should never decrease.[1-3]
24. Provide receiving team with report, including updates and changes in child's status.[1-3] *(Level II*)*	Promotes smooth transition of care.	For purposes of expediting transport, a detailed history may not always be possible; provide phone numbers and names of referring MD/RN.
25. Contact family if they did not accompany child and inform them of safe arrival. *(Level II*)*	Decreases family anxiety and concerns.	If unable to be completed in a timely manner, assign the responsibility to another individual.
26. Complete all documentation and paperwork.[1,2] *(Level II*)*	Provides new caregivers with documentation of care, interventions, and medications provided during transport.	On occasion, because of limited personnel on board, patient care takes precedence over documentation. Documentation must be completed once transport is completed.
27. Restock equipment and medications.[1-3] *(Level II*)*	Packs and equipment must be complete and ready for the next transport.	Equipment checks are part of the transport process.

* Level II: Theory-based; no research data to support recommendations; recommendations from expert consensus group may exist

Expected Outcomes

- Child is transferred from one facility to another via an appropriate level of care by individuals who have been trained to manage children in the transport environment
- Child arrives at the receiving facility in stable or improved condition

- Transport from one facility to another is carried out in a timely manner

- All systems and equipment function appropriately throughout the transport

Unexpected Outcomes

- Child is transported from one facility to another with a level of care that is lower than what they were receiving at the referring facility

- Child's condition deteriorates during the transport and the child arrives at the receiving facility in unstable condition
- Vehicular accident that results in injury to child, transport team members, or family
- Delay in transport because of lack of available transport team members
- Delay in transport because of road conditions
- Vehicular breakdown during transport
- Delay at referring facility because required documentation is not available
- Loss of power
- Inadequate medical gas supply
- Equipment malfunction
- Failure of backup systems or equipment

Monitoring and Care of the Child

Activities and Interventions	Rationale	Reportable Conditions
1. Maintain care and monitoring per institution-specific protocol and state guidelines; obtain vital signs at least every 15 minutes throughout transport.	Ensures safe transport of child and maintains established level of care. Facilitates identification of emerging problems.	• Contact MCP with any changes that require treatment or changes in accepting services: ❖ Pneumothorax ❖ Dislodged airway ❖ Changes in electrolytes/arterial blood gas (ABG)/glucose results from previous report ❖ Cardiovascular collapse ❖ Seizure activity or changes in level of consciousness ❖ Changes in vital signs: 10% or more deviation from baseline ❖ Any untoward events
2. Perform necessary stabilization interventions before departure.	Promotes patient safety because interventions are more difficult to perform in the transport environment. Ensures medical-legal compliance.	• Contact MCP to review stabilization interventions necessary (i.e., pneumothorax that requires needle decompression, cardiovascular collapse that requires CPR, emergency medication administration, and IV fluids)

Documentation

- Triaged assessment of child, location of child, and names of staff from referring facility
- Informed consent for transport and individual who provided consent
- Presence of appropriately completed EMTALA transport consent
- Members of transport team
- Transport team's primary and secondary survey of child at referring facility on arrival of team
- Interventions necessary for stabilization before departure from referring facility
- Method used to secure child for transport
- Vital signs and assessments performed throughout transport
- Time of departure from referring facility and arrival at receiving facility
- Individuals who assumed care of child on arrival at receiving unit
- Child and family education
- Contact numbers of family
- Unexpected outcomes and related treatment

References

1. MacDonald M, Ginzburg H, editors: *Guidelines for air and ground transport of neonatal and pediatric patients,* ed 2, Elk Grove Village, IL, 1999, American Academy of Pediatrics.
2. James S, editor: *Standards for critical care and specialty ground transport,* Lexington, KY, 2002, Air and Surface Transport Nurses Association.
3. Warren J, et al: Guidelines for the inter- and intrahospital transport of critically ill patients, *Crit Care Med* 32(1): 256-262, 2004.
4. Arndt K, editor: *Standards for critical care and specialty rotor-wing transport,* Chicago, 2003, Air and Surface Transport Nurses Association.

Additional Readings

Air and Surface Transport Nurses Association: available at www.ASTNA.org.
American Academy of Pediatrics: available at www.AAP.org.
Holleran R, editor: *Air and surface patient transport principles and practice,* ed 3, Cincinnati, 2003, Air and Surface Transport Nurses Association (ASTNA).
Shields R: Top 10 ways to prepare for a pediatric critical care transport, *J Emerg Nurs* 29:574-575, 2003.
Warren J: Guidelines for the inter- and intrahospital transport of critically ill patients, *Crit Care Med* 32(1):256-262, 2004.

Protective/Restraint Devices: Application and Monitoring

P U R P O S E : Protection of the child during acute medical-surgical care or rehabilitation if the child shows behavior that interferes with ongoing medical treatment and less restrictive interventions have been determined to be ineffective in managing the behavior

Paula M. Agosto and Patricia A. Hubbs

PREREQUISITE KNOWLEDGE

- *Restraint* is the involuntary restriction of a person's freedom of movement, physical activity, or normal access to one's body through the use of any manual method or mechanical device or equipment attached to or adjacent to the body that cannot be easily removed.[1]
- The child has the right to be free from restraint of any form that is not necessary for effective medical treatment or is used as a means of coercion, discipline, convenience, or retaliation by staff; restraint is a safety measure of the last resort.[1,2]
- Assessment skills to determine whether adequate clinical justification exists for the use of restraint for the child
- Knowledge of and skill in implementing less restrictive alternatives to restraints, such as[2]:
  - ❖ Diversion
  - ❖ Decreased sensory stimulation
  - ❖ Facilitation of normal sleep/wake cycle
  - ❖ Swaddling and bundling of infants
  - ❖ Reorientation
  - ❖ Family presence
  - ❖ Identification of cause of pain or agitation:
    - ○ Discomfort related to body position
    - ○ Child/ventilator dyssynchrony

- ○ Malfunctioning of medical devices, such as urinary catheter, intravenous catheter, endotracheal tube, or surgical drain
- ○ Hypoxia
- ○ Adverse reaction to medication
- In selection of protective device/restraint, the least invasive option that is effective should be used.[2]
- The Joint Commission for Accreditation of Healthcare Organizations (JCAHO) gives guidance around the use of protective/restraint devices in the *Comprehensive accreditation manual for hospitals: the official handbook*. With use of these guidelines, standard practices that limit mobility or temporarily immobilize the child, such as surgical positioning, intravenous arm board use, or protection of surgical and treatment sites in children, are considered protective devices rather than restraints.[1]
- Protective/restraint devices that are used with infants and children include soft wrist or ankle restraints, arm or foot boards for arterial or venous lines, mittens, bulky surgical dressings, and elbow immobilizers (e.g., Snuggle Wraps (the Able Co., James Island, SC); Heelbo L-Bow Arm Restraint System (Hollister, Inc., Libertyville, IL).
- Knowledge of proper and safe application and removal of restraint devices, including rapid removal in case of emergency

- Age-specific impact of restraint use
- Complications of the use of restraints, including circulatory compromise, alterations in skin integrity, increased agitation, hyperthermia, rhabdomyolysis, and death[1-3]
- Various terms, including medical immobilization, chemical restraint, behavioral restraint, and forensic restraint, are discussed in relation to restraint. This procedure deals specifically with protective/restraint devices implemented during medical care and postsurgical care. The purpose of a protective/restraint device is to support medical healing.[1]

CHILD AND FAMILY ASSESSMENT

- Child's developmental level and ability to interact **➤➤Rationale:** These factors influence preparation of the child, interaction, and less restrictive interventions that are appropriate to attempt.
- Child's and family's understanding of the reasons for and risks and benefits of a protective/restraint device **➤➤Rationale:** Evaluates child's and family's understanding of the procedure and provides a gauge for ongoing education.
- The use of protective/restraint device during acute medical-surgical care is based on the individual child's assessed needs **➤➤Rationale:** A protective device/restraint can only be used if the child has behavior that interferes with effective medical treatment and less restrictive interventions have been determined to be ineffective. The use of restraint may be warranted during the treatment of certain specific conditions or the use of certain clinical procedures for prevention of significant harm to the child.
- Invasive lines, tubes, or surgical repair present that could result in significant injury to the child if removed or disrupted **➤➤Rationale:** Assesses risk to the child and facilitates development of an individualized plan.
- Factors such as difficult airway, facial edema, cervical spine injury, hemodynamic instability, or presence of large bore catheters, such as those used for extracorporeal membrane oxygenation (ECMO) or continuous renal replacement therapy (CRRT), that could be anticipated to result in significant injury or death if medical devices were inadvertently removed **➤➤Rationale:** Identifies children at high risk and facilitates development of an individualized plan.

- Child's age, size, developmental level, and activity level **➤➤Rationale:** Facilitates selection of appropriate protective/restraint devices.
- Child's attempts or behaviors with high potential to dislodge or remove a medically necessary device **➤➤Rationale:** Identifies the child as needing a protective/restraint device.

CHILD AND FAMILY EDUCATION

Individualized, developmentally appropriate education is provided to the family and to the child based on desire for knowledge, readiness to learn, and overall neurologic and psychosocial state.

- Discuss the need for protective device/restraint when less restrictive alternatives have been ineffective **➤➤Rationale:** Protective device/restraint use during acute medical-surgical care may be considered as an intervention when other preventive measures have been ineffective in stopping behavior that could cause the child significant harm by interfering with medical treatment.
- Discuss the use of protective device/restraint with child and family when restraint during acute medical-surgical care is needed **➤➤Rationale:** Assures the family that the application or initiation of protective device/restraint during acute medical-surgical care is necessary to maintain child's safety, and the individual child's rights, dignity, and well being are respected.
- Discuss the plan to release the child from the restraint device as soon as safe and possible **➤➤Rationale:** Assures the family and child that the protective device/restraint will be used for the shortest time possible; when the child no longer shows behavior that interferes with acute medical-surgical care, the protective device/restraint will be removed.
- Encourage questions and answer questions as they arise **➤➤Rationale:** Reinforcement of information is needed during periods of stress.

EQUIPMENT

- Protective/restraint devices appropriate for the child's age, size, developmental level, and level of activity
- Institution-specific written restraint documentation record

Procedure for Protective/Restraint Devices: Application and Monitoring

Steps	Rationale	Considerations
1. Identify attempts to remove or observed behaviors with high potential to dislodge or remove a medically necessary device or prevent healing.	Identifies child who may need protective/restraint device.	
2. Attempt less restrictive alternatives.[1,2] *(Level II*)*	Child has the right to be free from restraint of any form that is not necessary for effective medical treatment.[1]	Less restrictive alternative may not be an option if child shows behavior that leads to imminent dislodgement or removal of a medically necessary device.
3. Ensure child and family understand the procedure and questions are answered.	Evaluates and reinforces understanding of previously taught information.	Developmental level, cognitive ability, and anxiety level determine approach to and effectiveness of teaching.
4. Gather needed equipment and supplies.	Facilitates completion of task in a timely manner.	
5. If restraints are used, obtain prescribing practitioner's order.[1,2] *(Level II*)*	Restraint is used only on the order of a licensed independent practitioner (LIP).	If LIP is not available to issue order, a registered nurse initiates restraint use on basis of appropriate assessment of the child and obtains an order from the LIP as soon as possible, preferably within 12 hours.[2]
6. Wash hands.	Standard precautions; reduces transmission of microorganisms.	
7. Select appropriate protective/ restraint device.	The least restrictive form of restraint should be used.[1,2] *(Level II*)*	
8. Apply protective device/restraint with appropriate technique; assess size and fit of restraint.	Appropriate size, fit, and application of restraint prevents entanglement, strangulation, and neurovascular injury.	Ensure restraint can be removed rapidly in case of emergency.
9. Assess the child at least every 2 hours or per institution-specific protocol and document appropriately; ensure the child's environment is clean and safe, modesty is maintained, and need for food, fluids, personal hygiene, and toileting is met.[1,2] *(Level II*)*	Monitoring determines the following: the child's physical and emotional well being; that the child's rights, dignity, and safety have been maintained; whether less restrictive methods are possible; when changes in the child's behavior or clinical condition warrant the removal of restraints.	Monitoring is accomplished by observation, interaction with the child, or related direct examination of the child by qualified staff. Documentation of monitoring is in accordance with institution-specific protocol.
10. Terminate use of restraint at the earliest possible time.	Child has the right to be free from restraint of any form that is not necessary for effective medical treatment.[1]	

* Level II: Theory-based; no research data to support recommendations; recommendations from expert consensus group may exist

Expected Outcomes

- Child remains safe; individual rights, dignity, and well-being are respected

- Safe and effective alternatives to restraint are successfully implemented as soon as possible
- Medically necessary devices remain intact and in place; medical healing occurs
- Child has an acceptable level of comfort

Unexpected Outcomes

- Injury or death related to:
  - ❖ Improper use or application of restraints
  - ❖ Accidental dislodgement of medically necessary devices
- Unnecessary restriction of freedom from continued use of device when no longer necessary
- Inadvertent dislodgement of medically necessary devices
- Unmanaged pain
- Unmanaged agitation or emotional distress

Monitoring and Care of the Child

Activities and Interventions	Rationale	Reportable Conditions
1. Assess the child at least every 2 hours for the following and document appropriately: a. Behaviors that indicate continued need for same level of restraint b. Pain c. Emotional distress d. Impaired circulation e. Altered skin integrity f. Range of motion g. Comfortable body position h. Nutrition and fluid needs i. Toileting and hygiene needs j. Readiness for removal of restraint	Monitoring determines the following: the child's physical and emotional well being; that the child's rights, dignity, and safety have been maintained; whether less restrictive methods are possible; when changes in the child's behavior or clinical condition warrant the removal of device/restraints. Adequate assessment usually necessitates temporary removal of the device.	• Unmanaged pain • Unmanaged agitation or emotional distress • Impaired circulation • Alterations in skin integrity • Alterations in range of motion • Inability to meet nutrition and fluid needs because of use of protective/restraint device
2. Monitor status of medical device, incision, or effectiveness of necessary medical treatment.	Protects device, incision; ability to provide medical treatment is reason for use of restraint.	• Device is inadvertently removed or moved out of position • Suture line is no longer intact • Inability to provide necessary medical treatment despite use of restraint
3. Assess continued requirement for restraint at least every 8 hours[2]; if restraint use is still necessary, ensure prescribing practitioner's order is renewed daily until device is no longer required.	Goal is removal of the restraint as soon as possible; frequent reassessment allows device to be discontinued as soon as possible.	• Twenty-four hours have elapsed since LIP order for restraint was provided

Documentation

- Child and family education
- Less restrictive interventions used before implementation of use of protective/restraint device
- Assessment of need for protective/restraint device
- Device used
- Time protective/restraint device use initiated
- Relevant orders for restraint use
- Results of initial monitoring and assessment
- Ongoing assessments
- Significant changes in the child's condition
- Removal of device
- Unexpected outcomes and related treatment

References

1. Joint Commission on Accreditation of Healthcare Organizations: *Comprehensive accreditation manual for hospitals: the official handbook,* Oakbrook Terrace, IL, 2006, Joint Commission Resources.
2. Maccioli GA, et al: American College of Critical Care Medicine, Society of Critical Care Medicine; clinical practice guidelines for the maintenance of patient physical safety in the intensive care unit: use of restraining therapies; American College of Critical Care Medicine Task Force 2001-2002, *Crit Care Med* 31(11):2665-2676, 2003.
3. Sorrentino A: Chemical restraints for the agitated, violent, or psychotic pediatric patient in the emergency department: controversies and recommendations, *Curr Opin Pediatr* 16(2):201-205, 2004.

Additional Readings

Dorfman DH, Kastner B: The use of restraint for pediatric psychiatric patients in emergency departments, *Pediatr Emerg Care* 20(3):151-156, 2004.

Joint Commission for Accreditation of Health Care Organizations: *Hospital standard FAQs,* retrieved March 4, 2006, from http://www.jcaho.org/accredited+organizations/hospitals/standards/hospital+faqs/provision+of+care/restraint+and+seclusion/restraint_seclusion.htm.

LeBel J, et al, National Association of State Mental Health Program Directors: *Publication 2000: best practices,* from http://www.nasmhpd.org/publications.cpm.

Staten P: Firmly grasp new restraint and seclusion standards, *Nurs Manage* 34(11):12-14, 2003.

Sudders M: Child and adolescent inpatient restraint reduction: a state initiative to promote strength-based care, *J Am Acad Child Adolesc Psychiatr* 43(1):37-45, 2004.

Providing a Safe Environment

P U R P O S E : Provides and maintains an environment that ensures infants and children are free from injury and adverse events during hospitalization

Lisa Thompson

PREREQUISITE KNOWLEDGE

- "Between 3% and 4% of hospitalized patients are harmed by care that is supposed to help them" (Lannon et al, 2003).[1]
- "Children are subject to unique vulnerabilities that may predispose them to higher rates of in-hospital safety events than the adult population. They are not able to directly question their care and may not have parents or guardians continuously at their bedside to oversee their care" (Miller et al, 2003).[2] Therefore, the responsibility of all health care providers is to ensure that children are provided with a safe environment.
- Normal vital sign parameters for infants and children
- Institution-specific protocol for patient identification
- Institution-specific implementation mechanisms for the Joint Commission on Accreditation of Healthcare Organizations (JCAHO) National Patient Safety Goals[3]
- Appropriate isolation techniques required for various communicable diseases
- Appropriate hand hygiene techniques
- Appropriate use of protective barriers
- Principles of aseptic technique
- Level of disinfection required after medical equipment is used
- Electrical hazards particular to the child undergoing acute or critical care and the acute or critical care environment
- Institution-specific mechanism for contacting the biomedicine department or other department responsible for maintenance of electrical safety of medical equipment and identification and referral of malfunctioning equipment
- Correct use of all equipment used in the care of the child

CHILD AND FAMILY ASSESSMENT

- Child's developmental level and cognitive functioning ➤➤*Rationale:* These factors influence preparation of the child and education and equipment and supplies needed to provide a safe environment as children explore and interact with their environment differently based on developmental level.
- Family's understanding of and reasons for described safety measures ➤➤*Rationale:* Influences compliance with safety measures; provides a gauge for ongoing education.
- Child's known allergies ➤➤*Rationale:* Facilitates screening the environment for substances, foods, and medications to which the child is known to be allergic; promotes patient safety.
- Desire of family members to be present during hospitalization ➤➤*Rationale:* Family may provide comfort and support to the child during hospitalization but should have the choice not to remain with the child. Monitoring requirements are increased when family members are not with the child.
- Accurate weight and length of child ➤➤*Rationale:* Medication dosing and fluid requirements in children are generally based on weight or body surface area; inaccurate weight or length measurement results in incorrect medication dosing or fluid calculations.

CHILD AND FAMILY EDUCATION

Individualized, developmentally appropriate education is provided to the family and to the child based on desire for knowledge, readiness to learn, and overall neurologic and psychosocial state.

- Educate the child and family that all electrical equipment brought into the hospital from home must be cleared with the biomedicine department. Instruct them that they should not manipulate any medical equipment at the child's bedside unless they have received education from the unit staff. ➤*Rationale:* Assures that all equipment at the bedside is in optimal functioning condition and is used appropriately and in compliance with electrical safety standards of the hospital.
- Educate the child and family in proper hand hygiene techniques and the use of protective barrier equipment if necessary ➤*Rationale:* Decreases transmission of microorganisms and unnecessary exposure for the already compromised condition of the child.
- Educate the child and family in the use of side rails ➤*Rationale:* Prevents injury from falls.
- Educate the child and family about medications, treatments, and procedures the child is to receive ➤*Rationale:* Teaching the family and child about treatments, proce-

dures, and medications facilitates active participation in the child's care and promotes patient safety; family is aware of planned interventions and may recognize an inappropriate treatment, procedure, or medication.
- Encourage questions and answer questions as they arise ➤*Rationale:* Reinforcement of information is needed during periods of stress.

EQUIPMENT

- Cardiorespiratory monitors with functioning alarms as prescribed or per unit-specific protocol
- Equipment for airway management at bedside: Suction, manual resuscitation bag, and mask
- Hospital bed, radiant warmer, or crib with functioning side rails
- Isolation equipment: Gloves, masks, protective eyewear, gowns, and hair covers as indicated
- Patient identification band or other institution-specific mechanism used for patient identification
- Allergy band or other institution-specific mechanism used to identify the child with allergies
- Institution-specific soap and dispenser
- Institution-specific alcohol-based hand disinfectant and dispenser

Procedure for Providing a Safe Environment

Steps	Rationale	Considerations
1. Ensure child and family understand teaching about maintenance of a safe environment and questions are answered.	Evaluates and reinforces understanding of previously taught information.	Developmental level, cognitive ability, and anxiety level determine approach to and effectiveness of teaching.
2. Ensure that child is wearing an institution-specific identification band or that institution-specific patient identification mechanism is present at all times.[3] *(Level II*)*	Ensures identification mechanism is present to prevent treatments, medications, and procedures to the wrong child.	Care must be taken when children have the same name to also check medical record numbers; refer to institution-specific or unit-specific name alert protocol.
3. Use two patient identifiers to identify the child before medication or treatment administration, and with laboratory specimens obtained, before blood administration. Conduct institution-specific final patient verification process before invasive procedures.[3] *(Level II*)*	Confirms correct child, procedure, and site, as recommended by the JCAHO.	Use active communication techniques. Two patient identifiers should be used for patient identification per institution-specific protocol; most commonly, name and birth date (outpatient setting) or name and medical record number (inpatient setting) are used.
4. For the child with known allergies, ensure allergy bracelet is present or institution-specific mechanism for allergy identification is in place; check bracelet before administration of medications and foods.	Prevents child from receiving a substance to which they are known to be allergic.	

Procedure continues on following page

* Level II: Theory-based; no research data to support recommendations; recommendations from expert consensus group may exist

Procedure for Providing a Safe Environment—*Continued*

Steps	Rationale	Considerations
5. If the child is monitored, ensure monitor alarms are turned on with alarm limits set based on child's age and condition. *(Level II*)*	Immediate interventions can be provided in the case of deterioration in child's condition.	Age-appropriate vital signs may not be appropriate for a specific child's condition.
6. Place child in the appropriately sized bed, warmer, isolette, or crib.	Prevents entrapment; promotes child's safety.	Crib mattress should fit crib. Beds and cribs used in the intensive care unit (ICU) should have side rails and head rails that come down fully and head boards that are easily removed to allow total access to the child in case of emergency.
7. Ensure side rails are up at all times.[4] *(Level II*)*	Prevents child falling from bed or crib.	Situations exists in which a side rail may interfere with the functioning of medical equipment (i.e., extracorporeal membrane oxygenation [ECMO], rigid oscillator tubing); other safety mechanisms should be initiated.
8. Ensure functioning suction device is present at every bedside.[4] *(Level II*)*	Prevents aspiration of gastric contents; protects airway.	Every bedside should have a Yankauer or tonsil tip suction for removal of oral secretions; a child with an artificial airway should have appropriately sized suction catheters at the bedside.
9. Ensure presence of an appropriately sized oxygen mask and manual resuscitation device at the bedside of any child receiving mechanical ventilation.[4] *(Level II*)*	In the event of ventilator malfunction or accidental extubation, bag-valve-mask ventilation can be provided.	Children with tracheostomies should have a spare tracheostomy tube of the same size and type and a second tube one size lower at the bedside at all times.
10. Ensure any child on prolonged bed rest has a pressure-relieving pad or mattress and is repositioned as medical condition permits, ideally every 2 hours.[4] *(Level III*)*	Prevents skin breakdown.	Children too unstable to turn should be placed on a pressure-relieving bed or mattress.
11. Ensure that all medical equipment in the child's environment has a tag that indicates date of most recent biomedical inspection and when next inspection is due.[3] *(Level II*)*	Regular assessment and inspection of equipment decreases likelihood of equipment malfunction.	
12. Identify any equipment that is not functioning appropriately and immediately return it to the biomedicine department.[3] *(Level II*)*	Prevents injury from malfunctioning equipment.	Use institution-specific reporting mechanism to report equipment malfunctions.
13. Ensure supplies and equipment are out of reach of child's crib or bed.[4] *(Level II*)*	Prevents harm to child from playing with medical equipment.	

* Level II: Theory-based; no research data to support recommendations; recommendations from expert consensus group may exist
  Level III: Laboratory data; no clinical data to support recommendations

Procedure for Providing a Safe Environment—*Continued*

Steps	Rationale	Considerations
14. Wash hands or use institution-specific alcohol-based hand disinfectant and encourage family to use correct hand hygiene techniques before and after all patient contact.[4] *(Level VI*)*	Reduces transmission of microorganisms.	
15. Ensure standard precautions are used for all children; institute isolation techniques as appropriate on basis of individual child's disease process.[3,4] *(Level VI*)*	Reduces the transmission of micro-organisms; protects all children on the unit and health care providers.	
16. Ensure food and beverages are kept out of patient care areas.	Prevents an environment conducive to bacterial growth.	
17. Ensure live plants and flowers are not kept at child's bedside.[4] *(Level II*)*	Prevents introduction of gram-negative rods and other pathogens into the environment.	
18. Ensure latex balloons and other latex products are not allowed in pediatric areas.[4] *(Level III*)*	Avoids the danger of aspiration of balloon pieces; protects the child with latex sensitivity or allergy from exposure.	
19. Institute protective/restraint devices as indicated to support medical healing and prevent the child from removing medically necessary devices such as endotracheal tubes or damaging a healing incision (see Procedure 200 for further information). *(Level II*)*	Prevents falls or dislodgement of medically necessary tubes or catheters, protects wounds and incision sites.	Protective/restraint devices must be able to be removed quickly by the health care provider in the event of an emergency.
20. Ensure that institution-specific and unit-specific systems designed to protect the child from being removed from the facility without permission are in place and functioning.[3] *(Level II*)*	Prevents the child from being removed from the facility by an unauthorized individual or before completion of the child's treatment.	

* Level II: Theory-based; no research data to support recommendations; recommendations from expert consensus group may exist
Level III: Laboratory data; no clinical data to support recommendations
Level VI: Clinical studies in a variety of patient populations and situations to support recommendations

Expected Outcomes

- The child receives treatments, medications, blood products, and procedures that are prescribed

- The child is free from injury from a fall, inadvertent removal of tube or catheter, or equipment malfunction

- The child is free from nosocomial infection
- Child is discharged to the family or legal guardians after treatment is completed

Unexpected Outcomes

- The child receives a medication, procedure, blood product, or treatment prescribed for another child
- The child has an adverse reaction to a blood product, medication, or therapy that was prescribed for another child
- Fall that results in injury to the child
- Inadvertent removal of tube or catheter
- Equipment malfunction that results in injury to the child
- Child develops a nosocomial infection
- Child is removed from the facility by an unauthorized individual before completion of treatment

Monitoring and Care of the Child

Activities and Interventions	Rationale	Reportable Conditions
1. Monitor identification band or institution-specific patient identification mechanism to ensure that it remains in place and does not compromise circulation.	Patient identification mechanism must be in place at all times to promote patient safety. As child's condition changes, child may become edematous and the identification band may compromise circulation.	• Missing patient identification mechanism • Cool distal extremity with diminished pulse and poor capillary refill
2. Assess skin under monitoring leads and pulse oximeter probe regularly to ensure that skin integrity is not impaired.	Prolonged placement of monitoring devices can irritate skin and eventually cause breakdown.	• Skin breakdown
3. Monitor function of bedside emergency equipment every shift.	In the event of an emergency, equipment is ready for use; prevents compromise of child's therapy as result of faulty equipment.	• Equipment malfunction • Expired inspection date (report to the biomedicine department)
4. Reassess alarm limits at least every shift or with any significant change in child's status to ensure they are appropriate for child's condition.	Ensures notification of significant changes in vital signs and monitored parameters.	
5. Reassess the need for protective/restraint devices every shift; if restraint is used in medical/surgical care, use must be reevaluated daily and an order written for use.[3] (Level II*)	Ensures that protective/restraint devices are used for the shortest time necessary.	• See Procedure 200 for further information.
6. If restraints are used in medical/surgical care, assess the child at least every 2 hours.[3] (Level II*)	Ensures the appropriate use of protective/restraint devices.	• See Procedure 200 for further information.

* Level II: Theory-based; no research data to support recommendations; recommendations from expert consensus group may exist

Documentation

- Monitoring systems in use are functional with alarms on and functional and appropriate limits set
- Hospital-issued identification band or institution-specific patient identification system is on child
- Side rails are elevated
- Isolation precautions implemented
- Functioning suction device at bedside
- Functioning and appropriately sized resuscitation mask and manual resuscitation bag at bedside
- Documentation of malfunctioning equipment per institution-specific protocol
- Child and family education
- Unexpected outcomes and related treatment

References

1. Lannon CM, et al, National Initiative for Children's Health Care Quality Project Advisory Committee: Principles of patient safety in pediatrics, *Pediatrics* 107(6):1473-1475, 2003.
2. Miller MR, et al: Patient safety events during pediatric hospitalizations, *Pediatrics* 111(6):1358-1365, 2003.
3. Joint Commission on Accreditation of Healthcare Organizations: *2006 Comprehensive accreditation manual for hospitals: the official handbook,* Oakbrook Terrace, IL, 2006, Joint Commission Resources.
4. Wilson D, Perry KA: Pediatric variations of nursing interventions. In Wong DL, et al, editors: *Wong's essentials of pediatric nursing,* ed 6, St Louis, 2001, Mosby.

Additional Reading
Stower S: Keeping the hospital environment safe for children, *Paediatr Nurs* 12(6):37-43, 2000.

Index

Page reference followed by b indicates box, f indicates figure or illustration, t indicates table, and n indicates footnote.

A

a wave, 482b
a-A ratio (arterial-to-alveolar oxygen ratio), 128t
  calculation of, 130b
A-aDO$_2$ (alveolar-arterial oxygen difference), 128t
  calculation of, 130b
Abdominal compartment syndrome, definition of, 725
Abdominal paracentesis
  assistance with, 667-672
    child/family assessment and education in, 667-668
    documentation of, 671b, 672
    equipment in, 668
    monitoring and care of child in, 671b
    outcomes in, 671b
    procedure in, 669b-670b
  performance of, 759-765
    child/family assessment and education in, 759-760
    documentation in, 765b
    equipment in, 760
    landmark identification in, 762b, 762f
    monitoring and care of child in, 764b-765b
    outcomes in, 764b
    procedure in, 761b-764b
    references on, 765
    Z tract method in, 762b-763b, 763f
Abdominal perfusion pressure, 725
ABO groups and Rh type compatibilities, 988, 988t
A/C. *See* Assist/control (A/C) ventilation.
Acidosis, respiratory and metabolic, 117f, 119t
Adenosine, in advanced life support, dosage(s) and remarks, 298t
Adjunctive medications, 96t
Admission, to hospital, 1431-1436
  child/family assessment and education in, 1431-1432
  documentation in, 1435b
  equipment in, 1432
  monitoring and care of child in, 1435b
  outcomes in, 1435b
  procedure in, 1433b-1435b
  references on, 1436
AEGM. *See* Atrial electrogram.

Aerosolized medication. *See* Metered dose inhaler; Nebulized medication.
Afterload, hemodynamic, definition of, 425
Airway(s)
  nasopharyngeal and oropharyngeal, 35-40, 36f
  sizing guidelines for, 37t
Airway pressure release ventilation (APRV), 188f
Alkalosis, respiratory and metabolic, 117f, 120t
All absorbent combined wound dressings, 935t
Allen test, modified, 1121, 1122f
Alveolar gas exchange, mechanisms of, 166, 167f
Alveolar gas trapping, 155
Alveolar ventilation, definition of, 166
Alveolar-arterial oxygen difference (A-aDO$_2$), 128t
  calculation of, 130b
Amiodarone, in advanced life support, dosage(s) and remarks, 298t
Analgesia
  epidural, 1243-1244
  levels of, 1293
  patient controlled, 1253b, 1269-1279
Anatomic dead space, definition of, 166
Anesthesia, general, 1293
Anesthesia, local
  in endotracheal intubation, 96t
  via epidural catheter, dosages, 1244
  via infusion, 1255-1259
  in wound suturing, 982t-983t
Anthropometric measurements, obtaining, 1322-1327
  child/family assessment and education in, 1324
  documentation in, 1327b
  equipment in, 1323f, 1324
  monitoring and care of child in, 1327b
  outcomes in, 1327b
  procedure(s) in, 1324b-1326b
    body mass index (BMI), 1326b
    head circumference measurement, 1326b
    linear growth measurement, 1325b-1326b
    percent ideal body weight (IBW), 1326b
    weight measurement, 1325b
  references on, 1327
Anti-tachycardia pacing, definition of, 355b
Anxiolysis, 1293

Apheresis, 767
  adverse effects of, 769
  assistance with, 767-777
    child/family assessment and education in, 769-770
    documentation in, 773b
    equipment in, 770
    monitoring and care of child in, 772b
    outcomes in, 771b
    procedure in, 771b
    references on, 773
  guidelines for therapeutic, 768t-769t
  prescribed medications and, 769
APRV. *See* Airway pressure release ventilation.
Arterial blood gas analysis, 115-120
  capillary blood gas values in, 118t
  child/family assessment and education in, 115-116
  determining acid-base disturbances in, 117f, 119t-120t
  documentation in, 120b
  flow chart of, 117f
  monitoring and care of child in, 120b
  normal arterial blood gases in, 117t
  oxygenation indicators in, 116t
  oxyhemoglobin dissociation curve in, 116f
  procedure for, 118b-119b
  references on, 120
Arterial blood gases, normal, 117t
Arterial blood oxygen saturation (SaO$_2$), 117t
  and venous oxygen saturation, 134-135
Arterial catheter, 1121-1122
  blood sampling from, 1034-1041
    child/family assessment and education in, 1034-1035
    closed blood conservation method of, 1039b-1040b
    documentation in, 1041b
    equipment in, 1035
    monitoring and care of child in, 1041b
    outcomes in, 1040b
    procedures in, 1035b-1040b
    references on, 1041
    stopcock method of, 1036b-1039b
  dressing change procedure for, 1028b
  insertion assist and management of, 1023-1033
    child/family assessment and education in, 1023-1024
    documentation in, 1032b